Mayo Clinic
Internal Medicine Review

EIGHTH EDITION

Mayo Clinic
Internal Medicine Review

EIGHTH EDITION

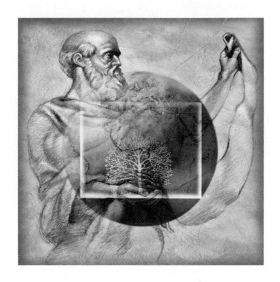

Editor-in-Chief
Amit K. Ghosh, MD

Associate Editors
Christopher M. Wittich, MD, PharmD
Deborah J. Rhodes, MD
Thomas J. Beckman, MD
Randall S. Edson, MD
Dennis K. McCallum, PharmD

MAYO CLINIC SCIENTIFIC PRESS
INFORMA HEALTHCARE

MAYO CLINIC

ISBN-13 9781420084788

The triple-shield Mayo logo and the words MAYO, MAYO CLINIC, and MAYO CLINIC SCIENTIFIC PRESS are marks of Mayo Foundation for Medical Education and Research.

For order inquiries, contact Informa Healthcare, Kentucky Distribution Center, 7625 Empire Drive, Florence, KY 41042 USA.

E-mail: orders@taylorandfrancis.com

www.informahealthcare.com

Catalog record is available from the Library of Congress

Care has been taken to confirm the accuracy of the information presented and to describe generally accepted practices. However, the authors, editors, and publisher are not responsible for errors or omissions or for any consequences from application of the information in this book and make no warranty, express or implied, with respect to the contents of the publication. This book should not be relied on apart from the advice of a qualified health care provider.

The authors, editors, and publisher have exerted efforts to ensure that drug selection and dosage set forth in this text are in accordance with current recommendations and practice at the time of publication. However, in view of ongoing research, changes in government regulations, and the constant flow of information relating to drug therapy and drug reactions, the reader is urged to check the package insert for each drug for any change in indications and dosage and for added warnings and precautions. This is particularly important when the recommended agent is a new or infrequently employed drug.

Some drugs and medical devices presented in this publication have Food and Drug Administration (FDA) clearance for limited use in restricted research settings. It is the responsibility of the health care providers to ascertain the FDA status of each drug or device planned for use in their clinical practice.

Printed in Canada

DEDICATED TO

All students of medicine, whatever their level of experience
and whatever their needs

FOREWORD

The eighth edition of *Mayo Clinic Internal Medicine Review* is a reflection of the continued commitment by the faculty of the Department of Internal Medicine to its mission to "serve the patient and advance the science." There are substantial differences from the previous edition as a result of extensive revisions. All chapters were updated, 12 new authors and 2 new associate editors were recruited, a new chapter on hospital medicine was added, and new tables, figures, and questions and answers were included. These changes and improvements are consistent with the theme eloquently articulated by William J. Mayo, MD, in 1928: "The glory of medicine is that it is constantly moving forward, that there is always more to learn."* My hope is that the reader will find the contents of this book informative, enjoyable, and, most of all, useful in our shared objective of understanding, preventing, diagnosing, and treating the diseases that still plague the human race.

Nicholas F. LaRusso, MD
Chair, Department of Internal Medicine
Mayo Clinic, Rochester, Minnesota

*Mayo WJ. The aims and ideals of the American Medical Association. Proceedings of the 66th Annual Meeting of the National Education Association of the United States, 1928. p. 158-63.

PREFACE

Medical advances have been occurring at breathtaking speed, with diagnostic and treatment options becoming available for conditions for which none previously existed. However, several aspects of health care remain the same. Patients continue to rely heavily on clinicians for help in understanding the burgeoning evidence in medical research and for providing optimal health care. Clinicians remain steadfast in their quest to meet the needs of their patients and to encourage innovation in meeting those needs. The focus on patient safety and quality of care remains a keystone of medical practice, and multidisciplinary care with a system-based approach is increasingly being adopted to manage chronic disorders. The associated demands and challenges mandate that physicians remain abreast of the latest developments in medicine. To assist physicians in this endeavor, the Department of Internal Medicine at Mayo Clinic provides continuing medical education updates and resources in a timely manner. This book, *Mayo Clinic Internal Medicine Review*, is designed to meet the needs of practicing clinicians and physicians-in-training by updating their knowledge of internal medicine and helping to prepare them for the internal medicine certification and maintenance of certification examinations administered by the American Board of Internal Medicine (ABIM).

The success of the earlier editions of this textbook is exemplified by the number of books published. The positive reaction to and the success enjoyed by the earlier editions prompted the Department of Internal Medicine to proceed with the publication of the eighth edition. Each chapter has been thoroughly updated, and a new chapter on hospital medicine has been added. The goal is to provide an update in internal medicine that is readable and easy to study.

This book is divided into chapters based on subspecialty topics and written by authors with expertise in the respective fields of medicine. Bulleted items highlight elements that are important concepts. The repetition of important points in the chapters reinforces the essential aspects of the topics and serves as an additional aid in review of the subjects. Multiple-choice questions appear at the end of each chapter; there are more than 350 multiple-choice questions in this edition. Correct answers and detailed explanations follow the questions.

I am grateful to all the individuals who contributed ideas and suggestions for improvement during the development of this book. I thank the esteemed authors of the previous editions for their input into this edition and for permitting the use of some of the materials from previous editions. I am indebted to all authors for their immense effort and contributions to this edition. I thank the staffs of the Section of Scientific Publications, Department of Medicine, and Division of Media Support Services at Mayo Clinic for their contributions to this edition. The support and cooperation of the publisher, Informa Healthcare, are also gratefully acknowledged.

I trust that the eighth edition of *Mayo Clinic Internal Medicine Review* will continue to update and advance the reader's knowledge of internal medicine.

Amit K. Ghosh, MD
Editor-in-Chief

PREFACE TO THE FIRST EDITION

For more than 2 decades, the staff of the Mayo Clinic and faculty of the Mayo Graduate School of Medicine have provided in-house didactic presentations for residents and fellows preparing for the internal medicine certifying examination administered by the American Board of Internal Medicine (ABIM). The extreme popularity of the Mayo "board reviews" among the residents and fellows and other physicians prompted the initiation of "Mayo Internal Medicine Board Review" courses in August 1992 to all physicians. Nearly 200 physicians in 1992 and twice that number in August 1993 attended the courses offered in Rochester, Minnesota. The popularity and the great demand for the course syllabus inspired us to write this book for candidates preparing for the ABIM examinations in internal medicine. This book, *Mayo Internal Medicine Board Review 1994-95*, will be used as the course syllabus for the "Mayo Internal Medicine Board Review" courses to be held in 1994 (July 24-30) and 1995 (July 23-29) in Rochester, Minnesota.

This is not a comprehensive textbook of medicine. It is rather analogous to a guide or a notebook containing selected topics deemed important for candidates preparing for the certifying or recertifying examinations offered by the ABIM in 1994 and 1995. The authors of this book assume that the candidates preparing for the board examinations will have studied at length a standard textbook of medicine before reading this review. The chapters are divided by subspecialty topics. As a means of underscoring the important clinical points for the boards, many paragraphs are followed by selected "pearls." Some of these pearls may seem repetitious, but this approach is intentional. We hope this format will aid readers in recapitulating the salient points of the topic under discussion. The questions at the end of each chapter are intended to familiarize the candidates with the format of the ABIM examination. Answers to these questions and their explanations are at the end of the book.

My coauthors and I are truly pleased to present this book and anticipate that it will be valuable to anyone preparing for the certifying and recertifying examinations in internal medicine of the ABIM. We look forward to hearing comments and suggestions from readers.

Udaya B. S. Prakash, MD
January 1994

PRODUCTION STAFF

Mayo Clinic Section of Scientific Publications

Randall J. Fritz, DVM	Editor
LeAnn M. Stee	Editor
Roberta J. Schwartz	Production editor
Traci J. H. Post	Scientific publications specialist
Alissa K. Baumgartner	Copy editor/proofreader
John P. Hedlund	Copy editor/proofreader

Mayo Clinic Section of Illustration and Design

Jonathan Goebel	Designer
James E. Rownd	Cover illustrator
Deborah A. Veerkamp	Production designer
Jonalle M. Sauer	Production designer

CONTRIBUTORS

Haitham S. Abu-Lebdeh, MD
Consultant, Division of General Internal Medicine, Mayo Clinic, Rochester, Minnesota; Assistant Professor of Medicine, College of Medicine, Mayo Clinic

Timothy R. Aksamit, MD
Consultant, Division of Pulmonary and Critical Care Medicine, Mayo Clinic, Rochester, Minnesota; Assistant Professor of Medicine, College of Medicine, Mayo Clinic

Robert C. Albright, Jr., DO
Consultant, Division of Nephrology and Hypertension, Mayo Clinic, Rochester, Minnesota; Assistant Professor of Medicine, College of Medicine, Mayo Clinic

Thomas J. Beckman, MD
Consultant, Division of General Internal Medicine, Mayo Clinic, Rochester, Minnesota; Associate Professor of Medicine, College of Medicine, Mayo Clinic

Margaret Beliveau Ficalora, MD
Consultant, Division of General Internal Medicine, Mayo Clinic, Rochester, Minnesota; Instructor in Medicine, College of Medicine, Mayo Clinic

Eduardo E. Benarroch, MD
Consultant, Department of Neurology, Mayo Clinic, Rochester, Minnesota; Professor of Neurology, College of Medicine, Mayo Clinic

Peter A. Brady, MB,ChB, MD
Consultant, Division of Cardiovascular Diseases, Mayo Clinic, Rochester, Minnesota; Assistant Professor of Medicine, College of Medicine, Mayo Clinic

Robert D. Brown, Jr., MD
Chair, Department of Neurology, Mayo Clinic, Rochester, Minnesota; Professor of Neurology, College of Medicine, Mayo Clinic

Sean M. Caples, DO
Senior Associate Consultant, Division of Pulmonary and Critical Care Medicine, Mayo Clinic, Rochester, Minnesota; Assistant Professor of Medicine, College of Medicine, Mayo Clinic

Brian A. Crum, MD
Consultant, Department of Neurology, Mayo Clinic, Rochester, Minnesota; Assistant Professor of Neurology, College of Medicine, Mayo Clinic

Lisa A. Drage, MD
Consultant, Department of Dermatology, Mayo Clinic, Rochester, Minnesota; Assistant Professor of Dermatology, College of Medicine, Mayo Clinic

Stephen B. Erickson, MD
Consultant, Division of Nephrology and Hypertension, Mayo Clinic, Rochester, Minnesota; Assistant Professor of Medicine, College of Medicine, Mayo Clinic

Lynn L. Estes, PharmD
Infectious Diseases Pharmacy Specialist, Mayo Clinic, Rochester, Minnesota; Assistant Professor of Pharmacy, College of Medicine, Mayo Clinic

Fernando C. Fervenza, MD, PhD
Consultant, Division of Nephrology and Hypertension, Mayo Clinic, Rochester, Minnesota; Associate Professor of Medicine, College of Medicine, Mayo Clinic

Amit K. Ghosh, MD
Consultant, Division of General Internal Medicine, Mayo Clinic, Rochester, Minnesota; Associate Professor of Medicine, College of Medicine, Mayo Clinic

William W. Ginsburg, MD
Consultant, Division of Rheumatology, Mayo Clinic, Jacksonville, Florida; Associate Professor of Medicine, College of Medicine, Mayo Clinic

C. Christopher Hook, MD
Consultant, Division of Hematology, Mayo Clinic, Rochester, Minnesota; Assistant Professor of Medicine, College of Medicine, Mayo Clinic

Barry L. Karon, MD
Consultant, Division of Cardiovascular Diseases, Mayo Clinic, Rochester, Minnesota; Assistant Professor of Medicine, College of Medicine, Mayo Clinic

Kyle W. Klarich, MD
Consultant, Division of Cardiovascular Diseases, Mayo Clinic, Rochester, Minnesota; Assistant Professor of Medicine, College of Medicine, Mayo Clinic

Scott C. Litin, MD
Consultant, Division of General Internal Medicine, Mayo Clinic, Rochester, Minnesota; Professor of Medicine, College of Medicine, Mayo Clinic

Conor G. Loftus, MD
Consultant, Division of Gastroenterology and Hepatology, Mayo Clinic, Rochester, Minnesota; Assistant Professor of Medicine, College of Medicine, Mayo Clinic

Karen F. Mauk, MD, MSc
Consultant, Division of General Internal Medicine, Mayo Clinic, Rochester, Minnesota; Assistant Professor of Medicine, College of Medicine, Mayo Clinic

Bryan McIver, MB,ChB, PhD
Consultant, Division of Endocrinology, Diabetes, Metabolism, Nutrition, Mayo Clinic, Rochester, Minnesota

Virginia V. Michels, MD
Emeritus Consultant, Department of Medical Genetics, Mayo Clinic, Rochester, Minnesota; Professor of Medical Genetics, College of Medicine, Mayo Clinic

Clement J. Michet, Jr., MD
Consultant, Division of Rheumatology, Mayo Clinic, Rochester, Minnesota; Associate Professor of Medicine, College of Medicine, Mayo Clinic

Martha P. Millman, MD, MPH
Consultant, Division of Preventive, Occupational and Aerospace Medicine, Mayo Clinic, Rochester, Minnesota; Instructor in Preventive Medicine, College of Medicine, Mayo Clinic

Kevin G. Moder, MD
Consultant, Division of Rheumatology, Mayo Clinic, Rochester, Minnesota; Associate Professor of Medicine, College of Medicine, Mayo Clinic

Timothy J. Moynihan, MD
Consultant, Division of Medical Oncology, Mayo Clinic, Rochester, Minnesota; Assistant Professor of Oncology, College of Medicine, Mayo Clinic

Paul S. Mueller, MD
Consultant, Division of General Internal Medicine, Mayo Clinic, Rochester, Minnesota; Associate Professor of Medicine, College of Medicine, Mayo Clinic

James S. Newman, MD
Consultant, Division of Hospital Internal Medicine, Mayo Clinic, Rochester, Minnesota; Assistant Professor of History of Medicine, College of Medicine, Mayo Clinic

Robert Orenstein, DO
Consultant, Division of Infectious Diseases, Mayo Clinic, Rochester, Minnesota; Assistant Professor of Medicine, College of Medicine, Mayo Clinic

John G. Park, MD
Consultant, Division of Pulmonary and Critical Care Medicine, Mayo Clinic, Rochester, Minnesota; Assistant Professor of Medicine, College of Medicine, Mayo Clinic

John J. Poterucha, MD
Consultant, Division of Gastroenterology and Hepatology, Mayo Clinic, Rochester, Minnesota; Associate Professor of Medicine, College of Medicine, Mayo Clinic

Abhiram Prasad, MD
Consultant, Division of Cardiovascular Diseases, Mayo Clinic, Rochester, Minnesota; Associate Professor of Medicine, College of Medicine, Mayo Clinic

Rajiv K. Pruthi, MBBS
Consultant, Division of Hematology, Mayo Clinic, Rochester, Minnesota; Assistant Professor of Medicine, College of Medicine, Mayo Clinic

Deborah J. Rhodes, MD
Consultant, Division of Preventive, Occupational and Aerospace Medicine, Mayo Clinic, Rochester, Minnesota; Assistant Professor of Medicine, College of Medicine, Mayo Clinic

Otis B. Rickman, DO
Consultant, Division of Pulmonary and Critical Care Medicine, Mayo Clinic, Rochester, Minnesota; Assistant Professor of Medicine, College of Medicine, Mayo Clinic

David J. Rosenman, MD
Consultant, Division of Hospital Internal Medicine, Mayo Clinic, Rochester, Minnesota; Assistant Professor of Medicine, College of Medicine, Mayo Clinic

Thomas R. Schwab, MD
Consultant, Division of Nephrology and Hypertension, Mayo Clinic, Rochester, Minnesota; Associate Professor of Medicine, College of Medicine, Mayo Clinic

Gary L. Schwartz, MD
Consultant, Division of Nephrology and Hypertension, Mayo Clinic, Rochester, Minnesota; Associate Professor of Medicine, College of Medicine, Mayo Clinic

Robert E. Sedlack, MD, MHPE
Consultant, Division of Gastroenterology and Hepatology, Mayo Clinic, Rochester, Minnesota; Assistant Professor of Medicine and of Medical Education, College of Medicine, Mayo Clinic

Lynne T. Shuster, MD
Consultant, Division of General Internal Medicine, Mayo Clinic, Rochester, Minnesota; Assistant Professor of Medicine, College of Medicine, Mayo Clinic

Peter C. Spittell, MD
Consultant, Division of Cardiovascular Diseases, Mayo Clinic, Rochester, Minnesota; Assistant Professor of Medicine, College of Medicine, Mayo Clinic

David P. Steensma, MD
Consultant, Division of Hematology, Mayo Clinic, Rochester, Minnesota; Associate Professor of Medicine and of Oncology, College of Medicine, Mayo Clinic

Bruce Sutor, MD
Consultant, Division of Assessment and Consultation, Mayo Clinic, Rochester, Minnesota; Assistant Professor of Psychiatry, College of Medicine, Mayo Clinic

Karen L. Swanson, DO
Consultant, Division of Pulmonary and Critical Care Medicine, Mayo Clinic, Rochester, Minnesota; Assistant Professor of Medicine, College of Medicine, Mayo Clinic

Zelalem Temesgen, MD
Consultant, Division of Infectious Diseases, Mayo Clinic, Rochester, Minnesota; Associate Professor of Medicine, College of Medicine, Mayo Clinic

Charles F. Thomas, Jr., MD
Consultant, Division of Pulmonary and Critical Care Medicine, Mayo Clinic, Rochester, Minnesota; Associate Professor of Medicine, College of Medicine, Mayo Clinic

Prathibha Varkey, MD, MPH
Consultant, Division of Preventive, Occupational and Aerospace Medicine, Mayo Clinic, Rochester, Minnesota; Associate Professor of Medical Education, of Medicine, and of Preventive Medicine, College of Medicine, Mayo Clinic

Thomas R. Viggiano, MD
Consultant, Division of Gastroenterology and Hepatology, Mayo Clinic, Rochester, Minnesota; Professor of Medicine, College of Medicine, Mayo Clinic

Abinash Virk, MD
Consultant, Division of Infectious Diseases, Mayo Clinic, Rochester, Minnesota; Assistant Professor of Medicine, College of Medicine, Mayo Clinic

Gerald W. Volcheck, MD
Consultant, Division of Allergic Diseases, Mayo Clinic, Rochester, Minnesota; Assistant Professor of Medicine, College of Medicine, Mayo Clinic

Amy W. Williams, MD
Consultant, Division of Nephrology and Hypertension, Mayo Clinic, Rochester, Minnesota; Assistant Professor of Medicine, College of Medicine, Mayo Clinic

John W. Wilson, MD
Consultant, Division of Infectious Diseases, Mayo Clinic, Rochester, Minnesota; Assistant Professor of Medicine, College of Medicine, Mayo Clinic

CONTRIBUTORS FOR PHARMACY REVIEW

Alma N. Adrover, PharmD, MS

Scott E. Apelgren, MS, BCPS, BCOP, BCNSP

Jeffrey J. Armon, PharmD

Sansana Donna Boontaveekul, PharmD, MS

Lisa K. Buss, PharmD

Sarah L. Clark, PharmD

Julie L. Cunningham, PharmD, BCPP

Magali P. Disdier, PharmD, PhD

Lynn L. Estes, PharmD

Anna C. Gunderson, PharmD

Heidi D. Gunderson, PharmD

Robert W. Hoel, RPh, PharmD

Todd M. Johnson, PharmD

Philip J. Kuper, PharmD, BCPS

Scott Luther Larson, PharmD, BCPS

Jennifer D. Lynch, PharmD

Kari L. B. Matzek, PharmD

Kevin W. Odell, PharmD

John G. O'Meara, PharmD

Narith N. Ou, PharmD

Lance J. Oyen, PharmD

Virginia H. Thompson, RPh

Roger A. Warndahl, RPh

Christopher M. Wittich, MD, PharmD

Robert C. Wolf, PharmD

TABLE OF CONTENTS

Mayo Clinic
Internal Medicine Review

EIGHTH EDITION

1

The Board Examination

Amit K. Ghosh, MD

Many physicians take the American Board of Internal Medicine (ABIM) certifying examination in internal medicine (IM) annually. The total number of candidates who took the ABIM certifying examination for the first time in 2005 was 7,051. Of these, 92% passed the examination. Currently, greater importance is being placed on achieving board certification. In a 2003 Gallup poll of 1,001 US adults aged 18 years or older, 98% wanted their physicians to be board-certified, and 79% thought that the recertification process was very important. Moreover, 54% would choose a new internist if their physicians' board certification had expired, and 75% said that they would choose a new specialist in a similar event. Many managed-care organizations now require board certification before employment.

This chapter is aimed primarily at candidates preparing for the ABIM's certifying or maintenance of certification examination in IM. However, candidates preparing for non-ABIM examinations also may benefit from the information, which covers various aspects of preparation for an examination, strategies to answer the questions effectively, and avoidance of pitfalls.

Aim of the Examination

The ABIM has stated that the certifying examination tests the breadth and depth of a candidate's knowledge in IM to ensure that the candidate has attained the necessary proficiency required for the practice of IM. According to the ABIM, the examination has 2 goals: the first is to ensure competence in the diagnosis and treatment of common disorders that have important consequences for patients, and the second is to ensure excellence in the broad domain of IM.

Examination Format

The examination for ABIM certification in IM is 1 day in duration and consists of 4 sections; there are 60 questions in each section, and each section is 2 hours in duration. These examinations are all computer-based and allow considerable flexibility to candidates to decide on the duration of the breaks between sessions. Details regarding the examination, training requirements, eligibility requirements,

application forms, and other related information can be obtained from the ABIM, 510 Walnut Street, Suite 1700, Philadelphia, PA 19106-3699; telephone numbers: 215-446-3500 or 800-441-2246; fax number: 215-446-3590; e-mail address: request@abim.org; Internet address: http://www.abim.org.

Almost all of the questions are clinical and based on correct diagnosis and management. Because there is no penalty for guessing the answers, candidates should *answer every question*. Most questions are based on the presentations of patients. Among these, 75% are in the setting of outpatient or emergency department situations, and the remaining 25% are in the inpatient setting, including the critical care unit and nursing home. The ability to answer these questions requires integration of information provided from several sources (such as history, physical examination, laboratory test results, and consultations), prioritization of alternatives, or use of clinical judgment. Candidates should know that a portion of questions are known as field questions, or pretest questions, and are included for experimental purposes only and to test the question quality. Although field questions are not scored, they cannot be identified during the examination. The overall ability to manage a patient in a cost-effective, evidence-based fashion is stressed. Questions that require simple recall of medical facts have essentially been eliminated. The examination is reviewed by practicing internists to ensure the questions are relevant to a general internal medicine practice.

* Candidates should answer every question; there is no penalty for guessing.
* Most questions are based on presentations of patients.
* Questions that require simple recall of medical facts are in the minority.

A list of normal laboratory values and illustrative materials (electrocardiograms, blood smears, Gram stains, urine sediments, chest radiographs, and photomicrographs) necessary to answer questions are provided. Candidates should interpret the abnormal values on the basis of the normal values provided and not on the basis of the normal values to which they are accustomed in their practice or training. Candidates for the certifying examination receive an e-mail communication from the ABIM highlighting several aspects of the computer-based testing and examination instructions several weeks before the examination. Although much of the information contained in this chapter is available on the ABIM Web site, candidates for ABIM examinations should read information that is sent to them because the ABIM may change various components of the format of the examination.

- A list of normal laboratory values and illustrative materials necessary to answer questions are provided.
- An e-mail with all examination information is sent by the ABIM several weeks before the examination and should be read by candidates.

Scoring

The passing scores reflect predetermined standards set by the ABIM. Passing scores are determined before the examination and therefore are not dependent on the performance of any group of candidates taking the examination.

- Passing scores are set before the examination.

The Content

The questions in the examination cover a broad area of IM. They are divided into primary and cross-content groups. The subspecialties in the primary content areas have included cardiovascular diseases, gastroenterology, pulmonary diseases, infectious diseases, rheumatology/orthopedics, endocrinology/metabolism, oncology, hematology, nephrology/urology, neurology, psychiatry, allergy/immunology, dermatology, obstetrics/gynecology, ophthalmology, otolaryngology, and miscellaneous. The specialties in the cross-content group have included adolescent medicine, critical care medicine, clinical epidemiology, ethics, geriatrics, nutrition, palliative/end-of-life care, occupational/environmental medicine, preventive medicine, women's health, patient safety, and substance abuse. Approximately 75% of the questions test knowledge in the following major specialties in IM: cardiology, endocrinology, gastroenterology, hematology, infectious diseases, nephrology, oncology, pulmonary diseases, and rheumatology. The remaining 25% of questions cover allergy/immunology, dermatology, gynecology, neurology, urology, ophthalmology, and psychiatry. Independent of primary content, about 50% of the questions encompass the cross-content topics. Table 1-1 shows the distribution of the contents for a recent ABIM certifying examination in IM.

- About 75% of the questions test knowledge in the major specialties.
- About 25% of the questions cover allergy/immunology, dermatology, gynecology, neurology, urology, ophthalmology, and psychiatry.
- About 50% of all questions encompass the cross-content topics: geriatrics, critical care medicine, adolescent medicine, clinical epidemiology, medical ethics, nutrition, occupational medicine, preventive medicine, substance abuse, patient safety, and women's health.

Table 1-1   Contents of the Certification Examination of the American Board of Internal Medicine

Area	% of Test
Primary content	
Cardiovascular disease	14
Gastroenterology	9
Pulmonary disease	10
Infectious disease	9
Rheumatology/orthopedics	8
Endocrinology/metabolism	8
Medical oncology	7
Hematology	6
Nephrology/urology	6
Allergy/immunology	3
Psychiatry	4
Neurology	4
Dermatology	4
Obstetrics/gynecology	3
Ophthalmology	2
Otorhinolaryngology	2
Miscellaneous	3
	100
Cross-content	
Critical care medicine	10
Geriatric medicine	10
Preventive medicine	6
Women's health	6
Medical ethics	3
Clinical epidemiology	3
Nutrition	3
Palliative/end-of-life care	3
Adolescent medicine	2
Occupational/environmental medicine	2
Substance abuse	2
Patient safety	2

From ABIM. Internal medicine: certification examination blueprint. [cited 2007 Mar 22.] Available from: https://www.abim.org/pdf/blueprint/im_cert.pdf. Used with permission.

Question Format

Each session contains 60 multiple-choice, single-best–answer questions. The question may include a case history, a brief statement, a radiograph, a graph, or a picture (such as a blood smear or Gram stain). Each question has 5 possible answers, and the candidates should identify the *single-best* answer. More than 1 answer may appear correct or partially correct for a question. Also, the traditionally correct answer may not be listed as an option. In that situation, the one answer that is better than the others should be selected. As noted above, most questions are based on interactions with patients.

The examples in this chapter, the questions at the end of each chapter in this book, and the examples included on the ABIM's Web site (https://www.abim.org/cert/im.shtm) should help candidates become familiar with the question format. Furthermore, the national in-training examination taken by most second-year residents in IM provides ample opportunity to become familiar with the question format.

* All questions are of the single-best–answer type.
* Various study guides should be used to become familiar with the question format.

Examples

Select the *best answer* for each of the following questions.

1. A 55-year-old woman presents with a history of having noticed a blood stain from her left breast on her nightgown. She has a past history of hyperprolactinemia, treated with bromocriptine. She has no family history of breast cancer. No masses are found on clinical examination. On manual expression there is a drop of bright red blood from a solitary duct at the 2-o'clock position of the left breast. Breast imaging with mammography and ultrasonography is negative for worrisome lesions. What is the most appropriate next step in her management?

   a. Advise reassessment in 6 months with mammography and ultrasonography.
   b. Reassure the patient, because the breast imaging was negative.
   c. Surgically excise the duct.
   d. Do an endocrine work-up in view of the history of hyperprolactinemia.
   e. Have the patient undergo MRI of the breast.

2. A 20-year-old male military recruit returns home from several weeks of summer training in boot camp. He comes to your office the following day with a 12-day history of fever (38°C), coryza, pharyngitis, and cough. Physical examination discloses a bullous lesion over the right tympanic membrane and scattered crackles in both lung fields. Blood cell count shows mild thrombocytopenia. A chest radiograph shows patchy alveolar-interstitial infiltrates in both lungs. Which of the following is the best treatment for this patient?

   a. Erythromycin
   b. Penicillin
   c. Trimethoprim
   d. Clindamycin
   e. Ceftazidime

3. A 56-year-old man presents with a 1-year history of abnormal results of liver function tests. He has a history of hypertension. He has no risk factors for viral hepatitis or a family history of liver disease. He drinks a glass of wine 2 or 3 times a week. On examination, his body mass index is 36, blood pressure 154/90 mm Hg, pulse 80 beats per minute. Results of the rest of the examination are normal. Laboratory study results include aspartate aminotransferase, 88 U/L; alanine aminotransferase, 90 U/L; bilirubin, 1.2 mg/dL; albumin, 4.0 g/dL; prothrombin time, normal. Total cholesterol was 260 mg/dL, and low-density lipoprotein cholesterol was 158 mg/dL. The patient wants to know more about the significance of the increased laboratory values. Which of the following statements about this patient's condition is true?

   a. The chance of cirrhosis developing is more than 40%.
   b. His estimated survival is lower than expected survival for the general population.
   c. Statins are absolutely contraindicated in this case.
   d. The patient is underreporting his alcohol intake.
   e. The patient needs to have a liver biopsy for diagnosis.

4. A 50-year-old woman is admitted for abdominal pain and vomiting. At operation, a ruptured appendix is removed. That evening, fever, hypotension, and oliguria develop. After a 2-L infusion of 0.9% saline, blood pressure was 80/60 mm Hg, and heart rate was 120 beats per minute. Laboratory study results were hemoglobin 9.0 g/dL and leukocytes 18×10^9/L. Findings on pulmonary catheterization include right atrial pressure 8 mm Hg, pulmonary artery pressure 28/10 mm Hg, wedge pressure 12 mm Hg, and cardiac output 9.0 L/min. Which of the following is the most appropriate intervention?

   a. Additional saline infusion
   b. Albumin infusion
   c. Red cell transfusion
   d. Dobutamine therapy
   e. Norepinephrine therapy

5. A 70-year-old man is seen in the clinic for evaluation before elective total hip replacement. His medical history is significant for hypertension and hyperlipidemia. He has no prior history of thromboembolism or coronary artery disease. The family history is positive for diabetes mellitus and hyperlipidemia. His medications include amlodipine 10 mg daily, aspirin 81 mg daily, and simvastatin 40 mg daily. You have been consulted for "clearance for surgery." What is the most appropriate recommendation for this patient?

   a. Enoxaparin 30 mg every 12 hours for 7 days postoperatively
   b. Enoxaparin 30 mg every 12 hours for 30 days postoperatively
   c. Aspirin and pneumatic compression boots during the immediate postoperative period, aspirin continued on dismissal indefinitely
   d. Enoxaparin 30 mg every 12 hours for 14 days postoperatively
   e. Warfarin therapy to keep the international normalized ratio at 2 to 3 for 14 days postoperatively

6. A 65-year-old man is referred to your practice for a 4-month history of swallowing difficulties. His wife reports that the patient starts coughing and choking immediately after he drinks any fluid and that he has lost 2.3 kg. He denies any hematemesis

or melena. He denies any history of food "sticking" in the suprasternal region. His past medical history includes a cerebrovascular accident with a right-sided hemiplegia 8 months ago, diabetes mellitus, gastroesophageal reflux, and hypertension. On physical examination, the patient is alert and cooperative and has right-sided hemiparesis. His hematocrit value is 42% and blood glucose 122 mg/dL. What is the next best step in the evaluation of his symptoms?

a. Upper endoscopy
b. Upper gastrointestinal barium study
c. Esophageal manometry
d. MRI of head
e. CT of neck

7. A 68-year-old woman was recently admitted to another hospital with severe back pain. At that time, MRI of the spine showed moderate bulging disks at L3-4 and L4-5 causing moderate compression of the L4 nerve root. Her other medical problems included hypertension and diet-controlled diabetes mellitus. Medications included hydrochlorothiazide 25 mg once daily. On physical examination, the blood pressure was 148/96 mm Hg, and the pulse rate was 78 beats per minute. On neurologic examination, there was an antalgic gait and the straight leg raising test was negative. Results of the remainder of the examination were normal. Laboratory values were hematocrit 30%, platelet count 110×10^9/L, blood urea nitrogen 60 mg/dL, creatinine 4.0 mg/dL, serum sodium 132 mEq/L, serum chloride 112 mEq/L, serum bicarbonate 15 mEq/L, serum calcium 12.5 mg/dL, and serum glucose 120 mg/dL. On urinalysis, there was trace proteinuria, no ketonuria or glucosuria, and no casts. Arterial pH was 7.32, and PCO_2 was 30 mm Hg. What is the most likely diagnosis?

a. Sarcoidosis
b. Primary hyperparathyroidism
c. Multiple myeloma
d. Aggressive hydrochlorothiazide therapy
e. Milk-alkali syndrome

8. A patient who is positive for human immunodeficiency virus and has low CD4 counts is receiving multidrug treatment. He complains of colicky flank pain, and many crystals are subsequently noted on urinalysis. Which of the following drugs is most likely causative?

a. Ribavirin
b. Trimethoprim-sulfamethoxazole
c. Indinavir
d. Acyclovir
e. Ganciclovir

9. A 34-year-old woman comes to your office with a 4-week history of hemoptysis, intermittent wheeze, and generalized weakness. On examination, her blood pressure is 186/112 mm Hg.

She appears cushingoid and has noted these changes taking place during the past 12 weeks. Auscultation discloses localized wheezing in the left mid lung area. The chest radiograph indicates partial atelectasis of the left upper lobe. The patient is referred to you for further evaluations. Which of the following is *least likely* to provide useful information for diagnosis and treatment?

a. Serum adrenocorticotropic hormone level
b. 24-Hour urine test for 5-hydroxyindoleacetic acid level
c. Bronchoscopy
d. CT of the chest
e. Serum potassium level

10. A 62-year-old woman presents with the onset of eye discomfort and diplopia. She has not noted any other new neurologic symptoms. Neurologic examination shows a normal mental status and neurovascular findings. Reflexes are slightly decreased in the lower extremities. Gait and coordination are normal. Cranial nerves show an inability to adduct, elevate, and depress the eye. Pupillary reaction is normal. Motor strength testing is negative. Sensation is normal, except there is decreased vibratory and joint position sensation in the feet. What abnormality would be expected?

a. Saccular aneurysm of the cavernous sinus on CT
b. Brainstem neoplasm on MRI
c. Left temporal sharp waves on electroencephalography
d. Increased fasting blood glucose level
e. Increased erythrocyte sedimentation rate

11. A 45-year-old woman presents with symptoms of fatigue, cold intolerance, and constipation. Hypothyroidism was diagnosed 7 years ago, and the patient remains euthyroid while receiving levothyroxine 0.125 mg daily. She is compliant with her medications and has not received any new prescription medications. Physical examination shows a pulse rate of 55 beats per minute. Blood pressure is 140/80 mm Hg. The deep tendon reflexes are delayed. Investigations show a hemoglobin level of 12.1 g/dL, thyroid-stimulating hormone 12.1 mIU/L, and free thyroxine 0.75 ng/dL. All of the following drugs could affect levothyroxine metabolism *except*:

a. Calcium carbonate
b. Sertraline
c. Oral iron
d. Sucralfate
e. Vitamin C

12. In a 34-year-old man with acute myelomonocytic leukemia, fever and progressive respiratory distress develop, and the chest radiograph shows diffuse alveolar infiltrates. The patient completed intensive chemotherapy 6 weeks earlier. The total leukocyte count has remained less than 0.5×10^9/L for more than 3 weeks. He is currently (for at least 10 days) receiving a

cephalosporin (ceftazidime). Which of the following is the most appropriate therapy for this patient?

a. Clindamycin
b. Blood transfusion to increase the number of circulating leukocytes
c. Antituberculous (triple-drug) therapy
d. Amphotericin intravenously
e. Pentamidine aerosol

The answers to the questions are as follows:

1. Answer c.

2. Answer a (*Mycoplasma* infection).

3. Answer b.

The patient has a history consistent with nonalcoholic steatohepatitis (NASH). A population-based study in the United States showed that patients with NASH had a slightly lower survival rate than expected for the general population (standard mortality ratio of 1.34). In patients with NASH, the progression to cirrhosis over a 7-year period is 8% to 26% (compared with 38%-50% in alcoholic hepatitis over a similar period) (Gastroenterology. 2005;129:113-21).

4. Answer a.

The patient has a history consistent with septic shock. The management of septic shock includes resuscitation with rapid infusion of large volumes of intravenous fluids to correct intravascular hypovolemia, supportive care, monitoring, and treatment of infection with antimicrobial therapy and surgical drainage (if necessary). Colloids have not been shown to be more beneficial than crystalloids in the management of shock. Vasopressors (norepinephrine or dopamine) are second-line agents and should be used in patients who remain hypotensive after adequate fluid resuscitation or in patients in whom pulmonary edema has developed.

5. Answer b.

Recent recommendations suggest anticoagulation for prophylaxis in venous thromboembolism (VTE) for 30 days after hip replacement. The choices of anticoagulants (duration 30 days) include enoxaparin 30 mg every 12 hours, dalteparin 5,000 international units every 12 hours, fondaparinux 2.5 mg daily, or warfarin with a target international normalized ratio between 2.0 and 3.0.

The recommended duration of prophylaxis for knee replacement is 2 weeks. The 2004 guidelines of the American College of Chest Physicians recommend that aspirin should not be used for prophylaxis against VTE in any patient group (Chest. 2004:126(3 Suppl);338S-400S).

6. Answer b (oropharyngeal dysphagia).

7. Answer c.

8. Answer c.

9. Answer b (bronchial carcinoid).

10. Answer d.

11. Answer e.

The following drugs decrease absorption of levothyroxine: calcium carbonate, iron, sucralfate, bile-acid binding resins, and aluminum hydroxide. Patients should be instructed to take levothyroxine at least 2 hours apart from these medications. Drugs that increase the metabolism of levothyroxine include sertraline, phenytoin, and phenobarbiturate.

12. Answer d (disseminated aspergillosis in a leukopenic patient).

Questions 1 through 3 are examples of questions that are aimed at evaluating knowledge and judgment about problems that are frequent in clinical practice and for which physician intervention makes a considerable difference. These questions judge the candidate's minimal level of clinical competence. These questions include descriptions of the work-up of a patient with bloody nipple discharge despite a negative physical examination and mammography, typical clinical features of *Mycoplasma* pneumonia, and recognition of slightly lower than normal survival in patients with nonalcoholic steatohepatitis. Therefore, the decision making is relatively easy and straightforward and requires knowledge of disease patterns and prognosis. Questions 4 through 12 are more difficult to answer because they are structured to reflect excellence in clinical competence rather than just minimal competence. In other words, they require more extensive knowledge (ie, knowledge beyond that required for minimal competence) in IM and its subspecialties. Although most of the questions on the examination are based on encounters with patients, some require recall of well-known medical facts.

Preparation for the Test

Training during medical school forms the foundation on which advanced clinical knowledge is accumulated during residency training. However, the serious preparation for the examination actually starts at the beginning of the residency training in IM. Most candidates will require a minimum of 6 to 8 months of intense preparation for the examination. Cramming just before the examination is counterproductive and is unlikely to be successful. Some of the methods of preparation for the board examination are described below. Additionally, each candidate may develop her or his own system.

- Preparation for the ABIM examination should start at the beginning of the residency training in IM.

Each candidate should use a standard textbook of IM. Any of those available should provide good basic knowledge in all areas of IM. Ideally, the candidate should use 1 good textbook and not jump from 1 to another, except for reading certain chapters that are outstanding in a particular textbook. The most effective way to use the textbook is with patient-centered reading; this should occur throughout the residency program. The candidate should read the descriptions of the symptoms and signs carefully because often they are part of the questions in the examination. Table 1-2 provides several examples of the common descriptions of symptoms and signs that could be part of the examination. Rather than reading chapters at random, candidates are encouraged to read the literature in a structured manner to assist in future recall of facts. This book and similar board review syllabi are excellent tools for brushing up on important board-relevant information several weeks to months

Table 1-2   Common Descriptions of Signs and Symptoms in Examination Questions

History (Symptoms)	Physical Findings (Signs)	Likely Diagnosis
Cardiology		
Shortness of breath or asymptomatic	Late peaking systolic murmur, intensity decreases with handgrip & increases with squatting	Hypertrophic obstructive cardiomyopathy
Asymptomatic, headache	Hypertension, diminished or absent lower extremity pulses, systolic murmur, bruit over chest wall	Coarctation of aorta
Neurology		
Gait impairment, falls, dysphagia, dysarthria	Inability to look up & side to side	Progressive supranuclear palsy
Diplopia, oscillating images, reading fatigue, loss of depth perception	Impaired adduction on lateral gaze, with nystagmus in the contralateral abducting eye	Internuclear ophthalmoplegia (consider multiple sclerosis, cerebrovascular disease)
Fluctuating memory, confusion, visual hallucinations	Mild parkinsonism, dementia	Lewy body dementia
Inappropriate behavior, dementia, poor social skills	Dementia	Frontotemporal dementia
Paroxysmal pain affecting the side of the face	Usually normal	Trigeminal neuralgia affecting 1 of the branches of cranial nerve V
Muscle stiffness, clumsiness, occasional emotional lability	Brisk reflexes, spasticity (upper motor neuron signs), atrophy, fasciculation (lower motor neuron signs)	Amyotrophic lateral sclerosis
Altered mental status, fever, headache	Flaccid paralysis, neck rigidity ±, altered mental status	West Nile virus encephalitis
Infectious disease		
Recurrent sinusitis, skin, or pulmonary infections due to *Staphylococcus aureus*	Sinus tenderness, abnormal lung sounds	Chronic granulomatous disorder
Recurrent *Neisseria* infections	Neck rigidity ±, altered mental status	Inherited deficiencies of complement (C5, 6, 7, 8, 9), factor D, or properdin
Recurrent episodes of bacterial pneumonia, sinusitis, diarrhea due to *Streptococcus pneumoniae*	Malnourished, abnormal lung sounds	Common variable immuno-deficiency
Gastroenterology		
Cirrhosis of liver, ingestion of raw oysters	Fever, hypotension, hemorrhagic bullae, signs of cirrhosis of liver	*Vibrio vulnificus*
Diarrhea	Pruritus, grouped vesicles over the elbow, knee, scalp, or back of neck	Dermatitis herpetiformis due to celiac sprue
Hepatitis C, photosensitivity	Skin fragility, erosions, blisters on dorsum of hand, hyperpigmentation	Porphyria cutanea tarda
Dermatology		
Facial rash, photosensitivity	Papules & pustules on bridge of nose, face, telangiectasia	Rosacea
Rash	Sharply demarcated erythematous papules, silvery white scales over scalp, extensor surfaces of extremities, & nails	Psoriasis
Cough with sore throat	Tender, erythematous pretibial nodules	Erythema nodosum
Ulcerative colitis	Irregular, undermined ulcer with violaceous border or scarring in lower extremities	Pyoderma gangrenosum
Flushing, diarrhea, rapid heart rate	Brown-red macules, urticaria on stroking skin	Systemic mastocytosis

before the examination. They, however, cannot take the place of comprehensive textbooks of internal medicine. This book is designed as a study guide rather than a comprehensive textbook of medicine. Therefore, it should not be used as the sole source of medical information for the examination.

* Candidates should thoroughly study a standard textbook of IM.
* This book is designed as a study guide and should not be used as the sole source of information for preparation for the examination.
* Candidates should pay considerable attention to the descriptions of signs and symptoms.

The Medical Knowledge Self-assessment Program (MKSAP) prepared by the American College of Physicians is extremely valuable for obtaining practice in answering multiple-choice questions. The questions and answers from the MKSAP are very useful to learn the type of questions asked and the depth of knowledge expected for various subjects.

Some candidates find it helpful to prepare for the examination in study groups. Formation of 2 to 5 candidates per group permits study of different textbooks and review articles in journals. The group should meet regularly as each candidate is assigned reading materials. Selected review articles on common and important topics in IM should be included in the study materials. Indiscriminate reading of articles from many journals should be avoided. In any case, most candidates who begin preparation 6 to 8 months before the examination will not find time for extensive study of journal materials. The newer information in the recent (within 6-9 months of the examination) medical journals is unlikely to be included in the examination. Notes and other materials the candidates have gathered during their residency training are also good sources of information. These clinical "pearls" gathered from mentors will be of help in remembering certain important points.

* Study groups may help cover large amounts of information.
* Indiscriminate reading of articles from many journals should be avoided.
* Information in the recent (within 6-9 months of the examination) medical journals is unlikely to be included in the examination.

Candidates should try to remember some of the uncommon manifestations of the most common diseases (such as polycythemia in common obstructive pulmonary disease) and common manifestations of uncommon diseases (such as pneumothorax in eosinophilic granuloma). The large majority of the questions on the examination involve conditions most commonly encountered in clinical practice. Several formulas and points should be memorized (such as the anion gap equation). The clinical training obtained and the regular study habits formed during residency training are the most important aspects of preparation for the examination.

In general, the examination rarely has questions about specific drug dosages or specific chemotherapy regimens used in oncology. Rather, questions are geared toward concepts regarding the treatment of patients. Questions regarding adverse effects of medications are common on the examination, especially when the adverse effect occurs frequently or is potentially serious. The candidate is also expected to recognize when a clinical condition is a drug-related event.

* Study as much as possible about board-eligible topics.
* Learn about the uncommon manifestations of common diseases and the common manifestations of uncommon diseases.

Day of the Examination

Adequate time is allowed to read and answer all the questions; therefore, there is no need to rush or become anxious. You should watch the time to ensure that you are at least halfway through the examination when half of the time has elapsed. Start by answering the first question and continue sequentially. Almost all of the questions follow a case presentation format. At times, subsequent questions will give you information that may help you answer a previous question. Do not be alarmed by lengthy questions; look for the question's salient points. When faced with a confusing question, do not become distracted by that question. Mark it so you can find it later, then go to the next question and come back to the unanswered ones at the end. Extremely lengthy stem statements or case presentations are apparently intended to test the candidate's ability to separate the essential from the unnecessary or unimportant information. You may want to highlight important information presented in the question in order to review this information after reading the entire question and the answer options.

* Look for the salient points in each question.
* If a question is confusing, mark it to find it and come back to the unanswered questions at the end.

Some candidates may fail the examination despite the possession of an immense amount of knowledge and the clinical competence necessary to pass the examination. Their failure to pass the examination may be caused by the lack of ability to understand or interpret the questions properly. The ability to understand the nuances of the question format is sometimes referred to as *boardsmanship*. Intelligent interpretation of the questions is very important for candidates who are not well versed in the format of multiple-choice questions. Tips on boardsmanship include the following:

* All questions whose answers are known should be answered first.
* Spend adequate time on questions for which you are certain of the answers to ensure that they are answered correctly. It is easy to become overconfident with such questions and thus you may fail to read the questions or the answer options carefully. Make sure you never make mistakes on easy questions.
* Read the final sentence (that appears just before the multiple answers) several times to understand how an answer should be selected. Recheck the question format before selecting the correct answer. Read each answer option completely. Occasionally a response may be only partially correct. At times, the traditionally correct answer is not listed. In these situations, select the best alternative listed. Watch for qualifiers such as *next*, *immediately*, or *initially*.

* Avoid answers that contain absolute or very restrictive words such as *always*, *never*, or *must*. Answer options that contain absolutes are likely incorrect.
* Try to think of the correct answer to the question before looking at the list of potential answers. Assume you have been given all the necessary information to answer the question. If the answer you had formulated is not among the list of answers provided, you may have interpreted the question incorrectly. When a patient's case is presented, think of the diagnosis before looking at the list of answers. It will be reassuring to realize (particularly if your diagnosis is supported by the answers) that you are on the right track.
* Abnormalities on, for example, the photographs, radiographs, and electrocardiograms will be obvious.
* If you do not know the answer to a question, very often you are able to rule out 1 or several answer options and improve your odds at guessing.
* Occasionally you can use information presented in 1 question to help you answer other difficult questions.

Candidates are well advised to use the basic fund of knowledge accumulated from clinical experience and reading to solve the questions. Approaching the questions as real-life encounters with patients is far better than trying to second-guess the examiners or trying to analyze whether the question is tricky. As indicated above, the questions are never tricky, and there is no reason for the ABIM to trick the candidates into choosing wrong answers.

It is better not to discuss the questions or answers (after the examination) with other candidates. Such discussions usually cause more consternation, although some candidates may derive a false sense of having performed well in the examination. In any case, the candidates are bound by their oath to the ABIM not to discuss or disseminate the questions. Do not study between examination sessions.

* Approach questions as real-life encounters with a patient.
* There are no trick questions.

Connections

Associations, causes, complications, and other relationships between a phenomenon or disease and clinical features are important to remember and recognize. For example, Table 1-3 lists some of the connections in infectious and occupational entities in pulmonary medicine. Each subspecialty has many similar connections, and candidates for the ABIM and other examinations may want to prepare lists like this for different areas.

Computer-based Testing

Candidates currently can take the computer-based test for the certification test examination. The computer-based test provides a more flexible, quiet, and professional environment for examination. The computer-based test is administered by Pearson VUE, a company with around 200 centers in the United States. Candidates are encouraged to schedule their examination date by calling Pearson VUE (800-601-

3549) as soon as possible. Candidates can now select to take their test on any 1 of the 8 available days in the month of August.

Candidates are encouraged to access the online tutorial at www.abim.org/cert/cbt.shtm. This tutorial allows the candidate to become familiar with answering questions, changing answers, making notes electronically, accessing the table of normal laboratory values, and marking questions for review.

Maintenance of Certification

The diplomate certificates issued to candidates who have passed the ABIM examination in IM since 1990 are valid for 10 years. The total number of candidates who took the ABIM maintenance of certification examination for the first time in 2005 was 4,242. Of these, 82% passed the examination.

Enhancements to Maintenance of Certification Program

In January 2006, the ABIM enhanced the maintenance of certification program to increase flexibility, incorporate programs developed by other organizations, and assess performance in clinical practice. The 3 general components (credentialing, self-evaluation, and secure examination) were retained, and all self-evaluation modules now have a points value.

Every candidate needs to complete a total of 100 points in self-evaluation modules. Unlike the previous system, renewal of more than 1 certificate does not necessitate taking additional self-evaluation modules (ie, the same number of points, 100, satisfies the requirement to sit for these examinations). Candidates have to complete at least 20 points in medical knowledge and at least 20 points in practice performance. The remaining 60 points may be obtained from completion of modules developed by ABIM and other organizations that meet the ABIM standards. Thus, one could combine an ABIM knowledge module (20 points) and an ABIM practice improvement module (20 points) with the American College of Physicians MKSAP (3 modules, 60 points), or one could combine an ABIM practice improvement module (20 points) with 3 ABIM knowledge modules (60 points) and the ABIM peer and patient feedback module (20 points). In 2007, the ABIM introduced annual updates of topics consisting of 25-question modules (10 points) and a structured phaseout of the 60-question medical knowledge modules (Table 1-4). All points are valid for 10 years.

The all-inclusive fee structure started in 2006 allows unlimited access to ABIM self-evaluation modules and 1 examination. Thus, continuous medical education credits can be earned without any additional fees for 10 years.

The self-evaluation modules evaluate performance in clinical skills, preventive services, practice performance, fund of medical knowledge, and feedback from patients and colleagues. Successfully completed self-evaluation modules are valid for 10 years. Candidates may apply to begin the maintenance of certification process any time after initial certification. The ABIM recommends that completion of the self-evaluation modules be spread out over time. It is anticipated that a candidate will complete 1 self-assessment module every 1 to 2 years. The ABIM encourages candidates to enroll within 4 years of certification in order to have adequate time to complete the program.

Table 1-3   Example of Connections Between Etiologic Factors and Diseases

Etiologic Factor	Agent, Disease
Cattle, swine, horses, wool, hide	Anthrax
Abattoir worker, veterinarian	Brucellosis
Travel to Southeast Asia, South America	Melioidosis
Squirrels, chipmunks, rabbits, rats	Plague
Rabbits, squirrels, infected flies, or ticks	Tularemia
Birds	Psittacosis, histoplasmosis
Rats, dogs, cats, cattle, swine	Leptospirosis
Goats, cattle, swine	Q fever
Soil, water-cooling tower	Legionellosis
Military camps	Mycoplasmosis
Chicken coops, starling roosts, caves	Histoplasmosis
Soil	Blastomycosis
Travel in southwestern United States	Coccidioidomycosis
Ohio and Mississippi river valleys	Histoplasmosis
Decaying wood	Histoplasmosis
Gardeners, florists, straw, plants	Sporotrichosis
Progressive, massive fibrosis	Silicosis, coal, hematite, kaolin, graphite, asbestosis
Autoimmune mechanism	Silicosis, asbestosis, berylliosis
Monday morning sickness	Byssinosis, bagassosis, metal fume fever
Metals and fumes producing asthma	Baker's asthma, meat wrapper's asthma, printer's asthma, nickel, platinum, toluene diisocyanate (TDI), cigarette cutter's asthma
Increased incidence of tuberculosis	Silicosis, hematite lung
Increased incidence of carcinoma	Asbestos, hematite, arsenic, nickel, uranium, chromate
Welding	Siderosis, pulmonary edema, bronchitis, emphysema
Centrilobar emphysema	Coal, hematite
Generalized emphysema	Cadmium, bauxite
Silo filler's lung	Nitrogen dioxide
Farmer's lung	*Thermoactinomyces, Micropolyspora*
Asbestos exposure	Mesothelioma, bronchogenic carcinoma, gastrointestinal cancer
Eggshell calcification	Silicosis, sarcoid
Sarcoid-like disease	Berylliosis
Diaphragmatic calcification	Asbestosis (also ankylosing spondylitis)
Nonfibrogenic pneumoconioses	Tin, emery, antimony, titanium, barium
Minimal pathology in lungs	Siderosis, baritosis, stannosis
Bullous emphysema	Bauxite lung

- Candidates who passed the ABIM certification examination in IM in 1990 and thereafter have certificates that are valid for 10 years.
- The maintenance of certification process is called continuous professional development and consists of a 3-step process.

Medical Knowledge and Clinical Skills Self-evaluation Modules

The medical knowledge module is an open-book examination containing 60 single-best–answer multiple-choice questions regarding recent clinical advances in IM. As mentioned previously, ABIM has introduced the 25-question annual update modules, and a phase-in schedule is in place to replace the existing modules by 2010. This module tests the candidate's knowledge of IM and clinical judgment. The questions are written by board members and ABIM diplomates. Candidates may choose a module in IM or a subspecialty (focused content). The module is available on paper (it is being phased out), CD-ROM, or the Internet. Candidates must achieve a predetermined passing score to establish credit for the module. The module may be repeated as often as necessary to achieve a passing score.

The clinical skills self-evaluation module consists of an open-book examination containing audio and visual information pertaining to

Table 1-4   Annual Update Medical Knowledge Modules, 3-Year Phase-In

Year	New Modules	Other ABIM Modules Available	To Be Discontinued
2007	2007 annual update	Recent advances, general A	General B
2008	2008 annual update	2007 annual update, recent advances	General A
2009	2009 annual update	2008 annual update, 2007 annual update	Recent advances
2010	2010 annual update	2009 annual update, 2008 annual update	2007 annual update

Abbreviation: ABIM, American Board of Internal Medicine.

physical examination and physical diagnosis and physician-patient communication skills. The module contains 60 single-best–answer multiple-choice questions. It is available on a CD-ROM with Web access. Candidates must achieve a predetermined passing score to establish credit for the module. The module may be repeated as often as necessary to achieve a passing score.

Performance-based Practice Improvement Module

This module is a computer-based instrument to help candidates assess the care they provide to patients and to help them develop a plan for improvement. Areas of the practice that have potential for quality improvement are identified. Completion of this module involves review of patient charts and comparing them with national guidelines. Data are submitted electronically to the ABIM to provide feedback. Candidates can implement the changes and measure their impact over a 2-week to 2-year period.

Patient- and Peer-Feedback Module

Confidential and anonymous feedback regarding the candidate's professionalism, physician-patient communication skills, and overall patient care skills is obtained from colleagues and patients of the candidate by an automated telephone survey. The candidate selects 10 colleagues and 25 patients, who are asked to complete a brief, anonymous telephone survey. The candidate receives a summary of the survey findings.

Secure Examination

A comprehensive, secure, computer-based examination is offered 2 times yearly, currently in May and November. The examination consists of 3 modules of 60 single-best–answer multiple-choice questions. Each module is 2 hours in duration, although the candidate might finish early and choose to take the next module immediately or after a brief break (recommended). Successful completion of the self-evaluation modules is not required before taking this examination. Questions are based on well-established information and assess clinical judgment more than pure recall of medical information. The examination contains clinically relevant questions. To pass the final examination, the candidate must achieve a predetermined passing score. The examination may be repeated as often as it takes to achieve a passing score. The blueprint of the number of questions for the maintenance of certification examination is described at http://www.abim.org/moc/im.shtm.

Details of the maintenance of certification program can be obtained from the ABIM, 510 Walnut Street, Suite 1700, Philadelphia, PA 19106-3699; telephone number: 800-441-2246; fax number: 215-446-3590; Internet address: http://www.abim.org.

2

Allergy

Gerald W. Volcheck, MD

Allergy Testing

Standard allergy testing relies on identifying the IgE antibody specific for the allergen in question. Two classic methods of doing this are the immediate wheal-and-flare skin prick tests (a small amount of antigen is introduced into the skin and evaluated at 15 minutes for the presence of an immediate wheal-and-flare reaction) and in vitro testing.

Allergy testing that does not have a clear scientific basis includes cytotoxic testing, provocation-neutralization testing or treatment, and "yeast allergy" testing.

Patch Tests and Prick (Cutaneous) Tests

Many seem confused about the concept of patch testing of skin as opposed to immediate wheal-and-flare skin testing. Patch testing is used only to investigate contact dermatitis, a type IV hypersensitivity reaction. Patch tests require about 96 hours for complete evaluation (similar to tuberculin skin reactivity, which requires 72 hours). Most substances that cause contact dermatitis are small organic molecules that can penetrate various barriers inherent in the skin surface. The mechanisms of hypersensitivity postulated to explain these reactions usually involve the formation of haptens of endogenous dermal proteins.

Inhalant allergens, in comparison, generally are sizable intact proteins in which each molecule can be multivalent with respect to IgE binding. These molecules penetrate the skin poorly and are seldom involved in cutaneous type IV hypersensitivity reactions. They cause respiratory symptoms, such as allergic rhinitis and asthma, and are identified by skin prick testing. Their sources include dust mites, cats, dogs, cockroaches, molds, and tree, grass, and weed pollens.

* Patch testing is used to investigate contact dermatitis.
* Skin prick (immediate) testing is used to investigate respiratory allergy to airborne allergens.

Prick, scratch, and intradermal testing involve introducing allergen to the skin layers below the external keratin layer. The deeper techniques are more sensitive but less specific. With the deeper, intradermal tests, allergen is introduced closer to responding cells and at higher doses. Allergen skin tests performed by the prick technique

adequately identify patients who have important clinical sensitivities without identifying a large number of those who have minimal levels of IgE antibody and no clinical sensitivity. Intradermal testing is used in selected cases, including evaluating allergy to stinging insect venoms and to penicillin. Drugs with antihistamine properties, such as H_1 receptor antagonists, and many anticholinergic and tricyclic antidepressant drugs can suppress immediate allergy skin test responses. The H_2 receptor antagonists have a small suppressive effect. Corticosteroids can suppress the delayed-type hypersensitivity response but not the immediate response.

* Intradermal skin tests are more sensitive but less specific than prick skin tests.
* Intradermal skin testing is used to investigate allergy to insect venoms and penicillin.

In Vitro Allergy Testing

In vitro allergy testing initially involves chemically coupling allergen protein molecules to a solid-phase substance. The test is then conducted by incubating serum (from the patient) that may contain IgE antibody specific for the allergen that has been immobilized to the membrane for a standard time. The solid phase is then washed free of nonbinding materials from the serum and incubated in a second solution containing a reagent (eg, radiolabeled anti-IgE antibody). The various wells are counted, and the radioactivity is correlated directly with the preparation of a standard curve in which known amounts of allergen-specific IgE antibody were incubated with a set of standard preparations of a solid phase. In vitro allergy testing uses the principles of radioimmunoassay or chromogen activation.

It is important to understand that this test only identifies the presence of allergen-specific IgE antibody in the same way that the allergen skin test does. Generally, in vitro allergy testing is not as sensitive as any form of skin testing and has some limitations because of the potential for chemical modification of the allergen protein while it is being coupled to the solid phase by means of covalent reaction. Generally, it is more expensive than allergen skin tests and has no advantage in routine clinical work. In vitro allergy testing may be useful clinically for patients who have been taking antihistamines and are unable to discontinue their use or for patients who have primary cutaneous diseases that make allergen skin testing impractical or inaccurate (eg, severe atopic eczema with most of the skin involved in a flare).

* Skin testing is more sensitive and less expensive than in vitro allergy testing.

Asthma

Pathology

The pathologic features of asthma have been studied chiefly in fatal cases; some bronchoscopic data are available for mild and moderate asthma. The histologic hallmarks of asthma are listed in Table 2-1.

* The histologic hallmarks of asthma include mucous gland hypertrophy, mucus hypersecretion, epithelial desquamation, widening of the basement membrane, and infiltration by eosinophils.

Pathophysiology

Bronchial hyperresponsiveness is common to all forms of asthma. It is measured by assessing pulmonary function before and after exposure to methacholine, histamine, cold air, or exercise. Prolonged aerosol corticosteroid therapy reduces bronchial hyperresponsiveness. Prolonged therapy with certain other anti-inflammatory drugs (eg, cromolyn sodium, nedocromil) also reduces bronchial hyperresponsiveness. Note that although both cromolyn and nedocromil were originally touted as "antiallergic" (they inhibit mast cell activation), they affect most cells involved in inflammation; also, the effects on these cells occur at lower doses than those that inhibit mast cell activation.

* Bronchial hyperresponsiveness generally is present in all forms of asthma.
* Prolonged aerosol corticosteroid therapy reduces bronchial hyperresponsiveness.

Persons who have allergic asthma generate mast cell and basophil

Table 2-1   Histologic Hallmarks of Asthma

Mucous gland hypertrophy
Mucus hypersecretion
Alteration of tinctorial & viscoelastic properties of mucus
Widening of basement membrane zone of bronchial epithelial
  membrane
Increased number of intraepithelial leukocytes & mast cells
Round cell infiltration of bronchial submucosa
Intense eosinophilic infiltration of submucosa
Widespread damage to bronchial epithelium
        Large areas of complete desquamation of epithelium into
            airway lumen
        Mucous plugs filled with eosinophils & their products

mediators that have important roles in the development of endobronchial inflammation and smooth muscle changes that occur after acute exposure to allergen. Mast cells and basophils are prominent during the immediate-phase reaction.

* In the immediate-phase reaction, mast cells and basophils are important.

In the so-called late-phase reaction to allergen exposure, the bronchi display histologic features of chronic inflammation and eosinophils become prominent in the reaction.

* In the late-phase reaction, eosinophils become prominent.

Patients who have chronic asthma and negative results on allergy skin tests seem to have an inflammatory infiltrate in the bronchi and histologic findings dominated by eosinophils when asthma is active. Patients with sudden asphyxic asthma may have a neutrophilic rather than an eosinophilic infiltration of the airway.

Various hypotheses explain the development of nonallergic asthma. One proposal is that the initial inflammation represents an autoimmune reaction arising from a viral or other microbial infection in the lung and, for reasons unknown, inflammation becomes chronic and characterized by a lymphocyte cytokine profile in which interleukin (IL)-5 is prominent. The intense eosinophilic inflammation is thought to come from the IL-5 influence of T cells in the chronic inflammatory infiltrate.

* IL-5 stimulates eosinophils.

The 2 types of helper T cells are TH1 and TH2. In general, TH1 cells produce interferon-γ and IL-2, and TH2 cells produce IL-4 and IL-5. IL-4 stimulates IgE synthesis. Hence, many clinical scientists believe that atopic asthma is caused by a preferential activation of TH2 lymphocytes.

* IL-4 stimulates IgE synthesis.
* TH2 lymphocytes produce IL-4 and IL-5.

Important characteristics of cytokines are summarized in Table 2-2. IL-1, IL-6, and tumor necrosis factor are produced by antigen-presenting cells and start the acute inflammatory reaction against an invader; IL-4 and IL-13 stimulate IgE synthesis; IL-2 and interferon-γ stimulate a cell-mediated response; and IL-10 is the primary anti-inflammatory cytokine.

Genetics of Asthma

The genetics of asthma is complex and confounded by environmental factors. No "asthma gene" has been discovered.

The gene encoding the β subunit of the high-affinity IgE receptor is located on chromosome 11q13 and is linked to total IgE, atopy, and bronchial hyperreactivity. Polymorphic variants of the β_2-adrenergic receptor are linked to bronchial hyperreactivity. The gene for IL-4 is located on chromosome 5q31 and is linked to total IgE.

Table 2-2   Characteristics of Cytokines

Cytokine	Major Actions	Primary Sources
IL-1	Lymphocyte activation	Macrophages
	Fibroblast activation	Endothelial cells
	Fever	Lymphocytes
IL-2	T- & B-cell activation	T cells (TH1)
IL-3	Mast cell proliferation	T cells
	Neutrophil, macrophage maturation	Mast cells
IL-4	IgE synthesis	T cells (TH2)
IL-5	Eosinophil proliferation & differentiation	T cells (TH2)
IL-6	IgG synthesis	Fibroblasts
	Lymphocyte activation	T cells
IL-8	Neutrophil chemotaxis	Fibroblasts
		Endothelial cells
		Monocytes
IL-10	Inhibits IFN-γ & IL-1 production	T cells
		Macrophages
IL-13	Promotes IgE synthesis	T cells
IFN-α	Antiviral activity	Leukocytes
IFN-γ	Activates macrophages	T cells (TH1)
	Stimulates MHC expression	
	Inhibits TH2 activity	
TNF-γ	Antitumor cell activity	Lymphocytes
		Macrophages
TNF-β	Antitumor cell activity	T cells
GM-CSF	Stimulates mast cells, granulocytes, macrophages	Lymphocytes
		Mast cells
		Macrophages

Abbreviations: GM-CSF, granulocyte-macrophage colony-stimulating factor; IFN, interferon; IL, interleukin; MHC, major histocompatibility complex; TH, helper T cell; TNF, tumor necrosis factor.

Occupational Asthma

Every patient interviewed about a history of allergy or asthma must be asked to provide a detailed occupational history. A large fraction of occupational asthma escapes diagnosis because physicians obtain an inadequate occupational history. An enormous range of possible industrial circumstances may lead to exposure and resultant disease. The most widely recognized types of occupational asthma are listed in Table 2-3.

* Inquiry into a possible occupational cause of asthma is important for all patients with asthma.

As new industrial processes and products evolve, occupational asthma may become more common. An example of this is latex-induced asthma among medical workers, associated with the widespread use of latex gloves. The incidence of occupational asthma is estimated to be 6% to 15% of all cases of adult-onset asthma.

* Allergy to latex is an important cause of occupational asthma.

Gastroesophageal Reflux and Asthma

The role of gastroesophageal reflux in asthma is not known. Two mechanistic hypotheses involve 1) reflex bronchospasm from acid in the distal esophagus and 2) recurrent aspiration of gastric contents. Although a well-documented reflex in dogs links acid in the distal esophagus to vagally mediated bronchospasm, this reflex has not been demonstrated consistently in humans. The other hypothesis is that gastric contents reach the tracheobronchial tree by ascending to the hypopharynx.

Asthma-Provoking Drugs

It is important to recognize the potentially severe adverse response that patients with asthma may show to β-blocking drugs (β_1- and β_2-blockers), including β_1-selective β-blocking agents. Patients with asthma who have glaucoma treated with ophthalmic preparations of timolol or betaxolol (betaxolol is less likely to cause problems) may experience bronchospasm.

* β-Blocking drugs, including eyedrops, can cause severe adverse responses.

Table 2-3   Industrial Agents That Can Cause Asthma

Metals
  Salts of platinum, nickel, chrome
Wood dusts
  Mahogany
  Oak
  Redwood
  Western red cedar (plicatic acid)
Vegetable dusts
  Castor bean
  Cotton
  Cottonseed
  Flour
  Grain (mite, weevil antigens)
  Green coffee
  Gums
Industrial chemicals & plastics
  Ethylenediamine
  Phthalic & trimellitic anhydrides
  Polyvinyl chloride
  Toluene diisocyanate
Pharmaceutical agents
  Phenylglycine acid chloride
  Penicillins
  Spiramycin
Food industry agents
  Egg protein
  Polyvinyl chloride
Biologic enzymes
  Bacillus subtilis (laundry detergent workers)
  Pancreatic enzymes
Animal emanations
  Canine or feline saliva
  Horse dander (racing workers)
  Rodent urine (laboratory animal workers)

* So-called β_1-selective β-blocking agents such as atenolol may also provoke asthma.

Persons taking angiotensin-converting enzyme inhibitor drugs may develop a chronic cough that can mimic asthma. This cough may not be accompanied by additional bronchospasm.

* Angiotensin-converting enzyme inhibitors can cause coughing.

Aspirin ingestion can cause acute, severe, and fatal asthma in a small subset of patients with asthma. The cause of the reaction is unknown but probably involves the generation of leukotrienes. Most of the affected patients have nasal polyposis and hyperplastic pansinus mucosal disease and are steroid-dependent for control of asthma. However, not all asthma patients with this reaction to aspirin fit the profile. Many nonsteroidal anti-inflammatory

drugs can trigger the reaction; the likelihood correlates with a drug's potency for inhibiting cyclooxygenase enzyme. Structural aspects of the drug seem unrelated to its tendency to provoke the reaction. Only nonacetylated salicylates such as choline salicylate (a weak cyclooxygenase inhibitor) seem not to provoke the reaction. Leukotriene-modifying drugs may be particularly helpful in aspirin-sensitive asthma.

* Aspirin and other nonsteroidal anti-inflammatory drugs can cause acute, severe asthma.
* Asthma, nasal polyposis, and aspirin sensitivity form the "aspirin allergy triad."
* Leukotriene modifiers may be helpful in aspirin-sensitive asthma.

Traditionally, asthma patients have been warned not to take antihistamines because the anticholinergic activity of some antihistamines was thought to cause drying of lower respiratory tract secretions, further worsening the asthma. However, antihistamines do not worsen asthma, and, in fact, some studies have shown a beneficial effect. Thus, occasionally an antihistamine is specifically prescribed for asthma because it may have some beneficial effect on asthmatic inflammation.

* Antihistamines are not contraindicated in asthma.

Cigarette Smoking and Asthma
A combination of asthma and cigarette smoking leads to accelerated chronic obstructive pulmonary disease. Because of accelerated decline in irreversible obstruction, all asthma patients who smoke should be told to stop smoking.
   Environmental tobacco smoke is an important asthma trigger. In particular, children with asthma who are exposed to environmental smoke have more respiratory infections and asthma attacks.

Medical History
A medical history for asthma includes careful inquiry about symptoms, provoking factors, alleviating factors, and severity. Patients with marked respiratory allergy have symptoms when exposed to aeroallergens and often have seasonal variation of symptoms. If allergy skin test results are negative, one can be reasonably certain that the patient does not have allergic asthma.

* In allergic asthma, symptoms either are sporadic and consistently related to exposure or are seasonal.

Respiratory infections (particularly viral), cold dry air, exercise, and respiratory irritants can trigger allergic and nonallergic asthma.

* Patients with allergic asthma are likely to respond to many nonimmunologic triggers.
* Cold dry air and exercise can trigger asthma.

Assessment of Severity
Asthma is *mild intermittent* if 1) the symptoms are intermittent (≤ 2 times weekly), 2) continuous treatment is not needed, and 3) the

flow-volume curve during formal pulmonary function testing is normal between episodes of symptoms. Even for patients who meet these criteria, inflammation (albeit patchy) is present in the airways and corticosteroid inhaled on a regular basis diminishes bronchial hyperresponsiveness.

* Corticosteroid inhaled regularly diminishes bronchial hyperresponsiveness.

Asthma is *mild persistent* or *moderate* when 1) the symptoms occur with some regularity (>2 times weekly) or daily, 2) there is some nocturnal occurrence of symptoms, or 3) asthma exacerbations are troublesome. For many of these patients, the flow-volume curve is rarely normal and complete pulmonary function testing may show evidence of hyperinflation, as indicated by increased residual volume or an increase above expected levels for the diffusing capacity of the lung for carbon dioxide. Patients with mild, moderate, or severe persistent asthma should receive treatment daily with anti-inflammatory medications, usually inhaled corticosteroids.

Asthma is *severe* when symptoms are present almost continuously and the usual medications must be given in doses at the upper end of the dose range to control the disease. Most patients with severe asthma require either large doses of inhaled corticosteroid or oral prednisone daily for adequate control. Most of them have been hospitalized more than once for asthma. The severity of asthma can change over time, and 1 of the first signs that asthma is not well controlled is the emergence of nocturnal symptoms.

* Nocturnal symptoms suggest that asthma is worsening.

Methacholine Bronchial Challenge
If a patient has a history suggestive of episodic asthma but has normal results on pulmonary function tests on the day of the examination, the patient is a reasonable candidate for a methacholine bronchial challenge. The methacholine bronchial challenge is also useful in evaluating patients for cough in whom baseline pulmonary function appears normal. Positive results indicate that bronchial hyperresponsiveness is present (Table 2-4). Some consider isocapneic hyperventilation with subfreezing dry air (by either exercising or breathing a carbon dioxide–air mixture) or exercise testing as alternatives to a methacholine challenge.

Do not perform a methacholine challenge in patients who have severe airway obstruction or a clear diagnosis of asthma. Usually, a 20% decrease in forced expiratory volume in 1 second (FEV_1) is considered a positive result.

* Patients with suspected asthma and normal results on pulmonary function tests are candidates for methacholine testing.

Differential Diagnosis
The differential diagnosis of wheezing is given in Table 2-5.

Medications for Asthma
Medications for asthma are listed in Table 2-6. They can be divided into bronchodilator compounds and anti-inflammatory compounds.

Bronchodilator Compounds
Currently, the only anticholinergic drug available in the United States for treating asthma is ipratropium bromide, although it is approved only for treating chronic obstructive pulmonary disease. Several short-acting β-adrenergic compounds are available, but albuterol, levalbuterol, and pirbuterol are probably prescribed most. More side effects occur when these medications are given orally rather than by inhalation. Nebulized β-agonists are rarely used long-term in adult asthma, although they may be lifesaving in acute attacks. For home use, the metered-dose inhaler or dry powdered inhalation is the preferred delivery system. Salmeterol and formoterol are 2 long-acting inhaled β-agonists. Both should be used in combination with inhaled corticosteroids. Theophylline is effective for asthma, but it has a narrow therapeutic index, and interactions with other drugs (cimetidine, erythromycin, and quinolone antibiotics) can increase the serum level of theophylline.

* Theophylline has a narrow therapeutic index.
* β-Agonists are best delivered by the inhaler route.

Table 2-4   Medical Conditions Associated With Positive Findings on Methacholine Challenge

Current asthma
Past history of asthma
Chronic obstructive pulmonary disease
Smoking
Recent respiratory infection
Chronic cough
Allergic rhinitis

Table 2-5   Differential Diagnosis of Wheezing

Pulmonary embolism
Cardiac failure
Foreign body
Central airway tumors
Aspiration
Carcinoid syndrome
Chondromalacia/polychondritis
Löffler syndrome
Bronchiectasis
Tropical eosinophilia
Hyperventilation syndrome
Laryngeal edema
Vascular ring affecting trachea
Factitious (including psychophysiologic vocal cord adduction)
α_1-Antiprotease deficiency
Immotile cilia syndrome
Bronchopulmonary dysplasia
Bronchiolitis (including bronchiolitis obliterans), croup
Cystic fibrosis

Table 2-6   Medications for Asthma

Bronchodilator compounds
    Anticholinergic drugs (ipratropium bromide)
    β_2-Agonist drugs
        Short-acting (albuterol, pirbuterol)
        Long-acting (salmeterol, formoterol)
    Methylxanthines (theophylline)
"Antiallergic" compounds
    Cromolyn
    Nedocromil
Glucocorticoids
    Systemic
        Prednisone
        Methylprednisolone
    Topical
        Triamcinolone acetonide
        Beclomethasone
        Flunisolide, budesonide, fluticasone, mometasone
Antileukotrienes
    Leukotriene receptor antagonists (zafirlukast, montelukast)
    Lipoxygenase inhibitors (zileuton)

Anti-inflammatory Compounds

Cromolyn and nedocromil are inhaled anti-inflammatory medications that are appropriate for treatment of mild or moderate asthma. The 5-lipoxygenase inhibitor zileuton and the leukotriene receptor antagonists zafirlukast and montelukast are approved for treatment of mild persistent asthma. These agents work by decreasing the inflammatory effects of leukotrienes. Zileuton can cause increased liver function test results. Cases of Churg-Strauss vasculitis have also been linked to zafirlukast, although a clear cause-and-effect relationship has not been established.

Corticosteroid Therapy

Many experts recommend inhaled glucocorticoids for mild persistent asthma because of the potential long-term benefits of reduced bronchial hyperresponsiveness and reduced airway remodeling (fibrosis). Long-term use of β-agonist bronchodilators may adversely affect asthma; this also argues for earlier use of inhaled glucocorticoids. Asthma mortality has been linked to the heavy use of β-agonist inhalers. This association may simply reflect that patients with more severe asthma (who are more likely to die of an asthma attack) use more β-agonist inhalers. However, prolonged and heavy use of inhaled β-agonists may have a direct, deleterious effect on asthma, although this has not been proved. Certainly, asthma patients with regularly recurring symptoms should receive inhaled corticosteroids (or cromolyn or nedocromil) as part of the treatment.

* Prescribe inhaled glucocorticoids for mild, moderate, and severe persistent asthma.
* Long-term use of β-agonist bronchodilators may worsen asthma.

The inflammatory infiltrate in the bronchial submucosa of asthma patients likely depends on cytokine secretory patterns. Corticosteroids may interfere at several levels in the cytokine cascade.

Bronchoalveolar lavage and biopsy studies show that corticosteroids inhibit IL-4, IL-5, and granulocyte-macrophage colony-stimulating factor in asthma.

Monocytes or platelets may be important in the asthmatic process. Corticosteroids modify activation pathways for monocytes and platelets. Furthermore, corticosteroids have vasoconstrictive properties, which reduce vascular congestive changes in the mucosa, and they tend to decrease mucous gland secretion.

* Corticosteroids reduce airway inflammation by modulating cytokines.
* Corticosteroids can inhibit the inflammatory properties of monocytes and platelets.
* Corticosteroids have vasoconstrictive properties.
* Corticosteroids decrease mucous gland secretion.

The most common adverse effects of inhaled corticosteroids are dysphonia and thrush. These unwanted effects occur in about 10% of patients and can be reduced by using a spacer device and rinsing the mouth after administration. Usually, oral thrush can be treated successfully with oral antifungal agents. Dysphonia, when persistent, may be treated by decreasing or discontinuing the use of inhaled corticosteroids.

Detailed study of the systemic effects of inhaled corticosteroids shows that these agents are much safer than oral corticosteroids. Nevertheless, there is evidence that high-dose inhaled corticosteroids can affect the hypothalamic-pituitary-adrenal axis and bone metabolism. Also, high-dose inhaled corticosteroids may increase the risk of future development of glaucoma, cataracts, and osteoporosis. Inhaled corticosteroids can decrease growth velocity in children and adolescents. The effect of inhaled corticosteroids on adult height is not known, but it appears to be minimal.

Poor inhaler technique and poor compliance can result in poor control of asthma. Therefore, all patients using a metered-dose inhaler or dry powder inhaler should be taught the proper technique for using these devices. Most patients using metered-dose inhaled corticosteroids should use a spacer device with the inhaler.

* The most common cause of poor results is poor inhaler technique.
* Patients should use a spacer device with metered-dose inhaled corticosteroids.

Anti-IgE Treatment With Omalizumab

Omalizumab is the first recombinant humanized anti-IgE monoclonal antibody approved for use in asthma. It blocks IgE binding to mast cells and is indicated for refractory moderate to severe persistent allergic asthma. It is approved for use in patients 12 years or older with positive skin or in vitro allergy testing. Dosing is based on the patient's IgE level and body weight. The dosage is typically 150 to 375 mg subcutaneously every 2 to 4 weeks.

* Omalizumab is approved for use in refractory moderate to severe persistent asthma.

Goals of Asthma Management

The goals of asthma management are listed in Table 2-7.

Management of Chronic Asthma

Baseline spirometry is recommended for all patients with asthma, and home peak flow monitoring is recommended for those with moderate or severe asthma (Figure 2-1).

* Spirometry is recommended for all asthma patients.
* Home peak flow monitoring is recommended for patients with moderate or severe asthma.

Environmental triggers should be discussed with all asthma patients, and allergy testing should be offered to those with suspected allergic asthma or with asthma that is not well controlled. Although allergy immunotherapy is effective, it is recommended only for patients with allergic asthma who have had a complete evaluation by an allergist.

Management of Acute Asthma

Inhaled β-agonists, measurements of lung function at presentation and during therapy, and systemic corticosteroids (for most patients) are the cornerstones of managing acute asthma (Figure 2-2). Generally, nebulized albuterol, administered repeatedly if necessary, is the first line of treatment. Delivery of β-agonist by metered-dose inhaler can be substituted in less severe asthma attacks. Inhaled β-agonist delivered by continuous nebulization may be appropriate for more severe disease.

* Inhaled β-agonist can be delivered by intermittent nebulization, continuous nebulization, or metered-dose inhaler.

It is important to measure lung function (usually peak expiratory flow rate but also FEV_1 whenever possible) at presentation and after administration of bronchodilators. These measurements provide invaluable information that allows the physician to assess the severity of the asthma attack and the response (if any) to treatment.

Patients who do not have a prompt and full response to inhaled β-agonists should receive a course of systemic corticosteroids. Patients with the most severe and poorly responsive disease (FEV_1 <50%, oxygen saturation <90%, and moderate to severe symptoms) should be treated on a hospital ward or in an intensive care unit.

Table 2-7   Goals of Asthma Management

No asthma symptoms
No asthma attacks
Normal activity level
Normal lung function
Use of safest & least amount of medication necessary
Establishment of therapeutic relationship between patient & provider

* Measure pulmonary function at presentation and after giving bronchodilators.
* Most patients with acute asthma need a course of systemic corticosteroids.

Allergic Bronchopulmonary Aspergillosis

Allergic bronchopulmonary aspergillosis is an obstructive lung disease caused by an allergic reaction to *Aspergillus* in the lower airway. The typical patient presents with severe steroid-dependent asthma. Most patients with this condition have coexisting asthma or cystic fibrosis.

* Allergic bronchopulmonary aspergillosis develops in patients with asthma or cystic fibrosis.

The diagnostic features of allergic bronchopulmonary aspergillosis are summarized in Table 2-8. Fungi other than *Aspergillus fumigatus* can cause an allergic bronchopulmonary mycosis similar to allergic bronchopulmonary aspergillosis.

Chest radiography can show transient or permanent infiltrates and central bronchiectasis, usually affecting the upper lobes (Figure 2-3). Advanced cases show extensive pulmonary fibrosis.

Allergic bronchopulmonary aspergillosis is treated with systemic corticosteroids. Total serum IgE may be helpful in following the course of the disease. Antifungal therapy has not been effective.

Chronic Rhinitis

Medical History

Vasomotor rhinitis is defined as nasal symptoms occurring in response to nonspecific, nonallergic irritants. Common triggers of vasomotor rhinitis are strong odors, respiratory irritants such as dust or smoke, changes in temperature, changes in body position, and ingestants such as spicy food or alcohol. This is considered a *nonallergic* rhinitis.

* *Vasomotor rhinitis* is defined as nasal symptoms in response to nonspecific stimuli.

Historical factors favoring a diagnosis of *allergic* rhinitis include a history of nasal symptoms that have a recurrent seasonal pattern (eg, every August and September) or symptoms provoked by being near specific sources of allergens, such as animals. Factors favoring *vasomotor* rhinitis include symptoms provoked by strong odors and changes in humidity and temperature.

* Allergic rhinitis has a recurrent seasonal pattern and may be provoked by being near animals.
* Triggers of vasomotor rhinitis include strong odors and changes in humidity and temperature.

Factors common to allergic rhinitis and vasomotor rhinitis (thus, without differential diagnostic value) include perennial symptoms, intolerance of cigarette smoke, and history of "dust" sensitivity. Factors that suggest fixed nasal obstruction (which should prompt

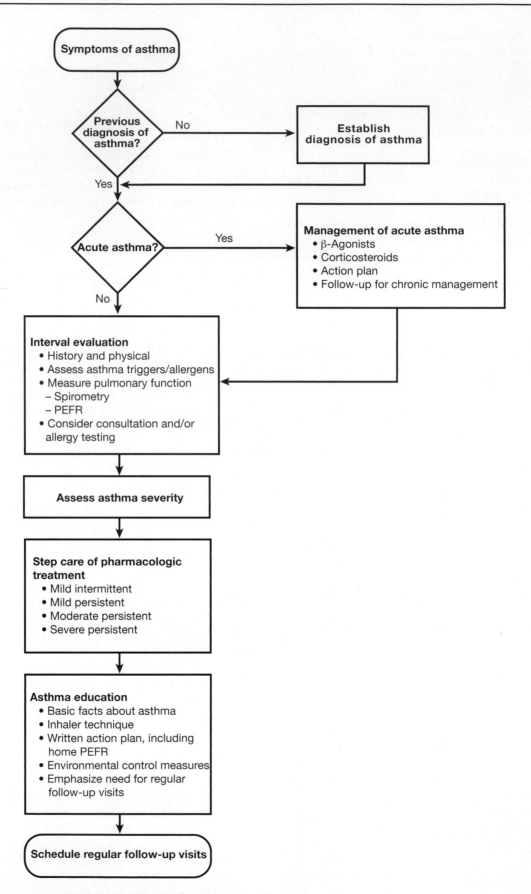

Figure 2-1. Diagnosis and Management of Asthma. PEFR indicates peak expiratory flow rate.

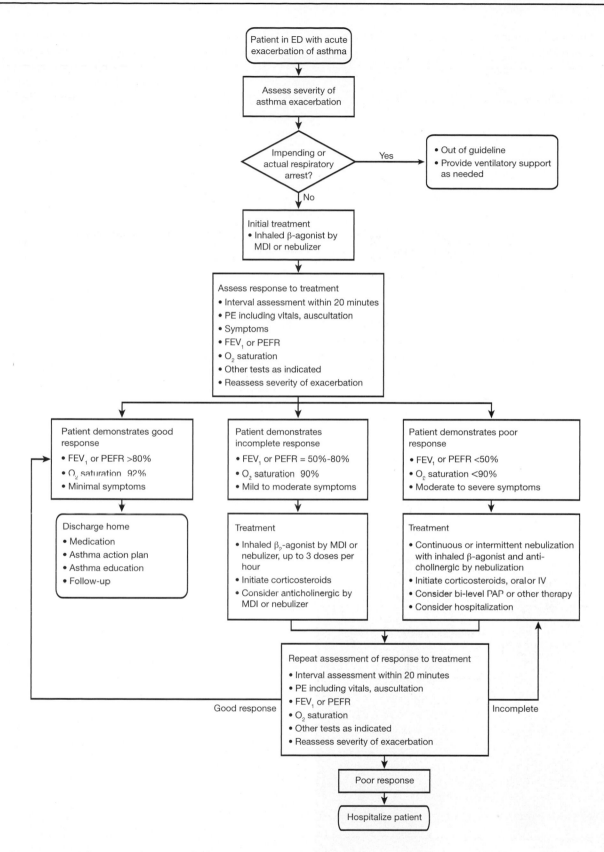

Figure 2-2. Management of Acute Asthma in Adults. ED indicates emergency department; FEV$_1$, forced expiratory volume in 1 second; IV, intravenous; MDI, metered-dose inhaler; PAP, positive airway pressure; PE, physical examination; PEFR, peak expiratory flow rate. (From ICSI Health Care Guideline: Emergency and Inpatient Management of Asthma. 2nd ed. Institute for Clinical Systems Improvement; Bloomington, Minnesota, March 2006. Used with permission.)

Table 2-8   Diagnostic Features of Allergic Bronchopulmonary Aspergillosis

Clinical asthma
Bronchiectasis (usually proximal)
Increased total serum IgE
IgE antibody to *Aspergillus* (by skin test or in vitro assay)
Precipitins or IgG antibody to *Aspergillus*
Radiographic infiltrates (often upper lobes)
Peripheral blood eosinophilia

physicians to consider other diagnoses) include unilateral nasal obstruction, unilateral facial pain, unilateral nasal purulence, nasal voice but no nasal symptoms, disturbances of olfaction without any nasal symptoms, and unilateral nasal bleeding (Table 2-9).

• Perennial symptoms, intolerance of cigarette smoke, and history of "dust" sensitivity are common to allergic and vasomotor rhinitis.
• House dust mite sensitivity is a common cause of perennial allergic rhinitis.

Allergy Skin Tests in Allergic Rhinitis

The interpretation of allergy skin test results must be tailored to the unique features of each patient.

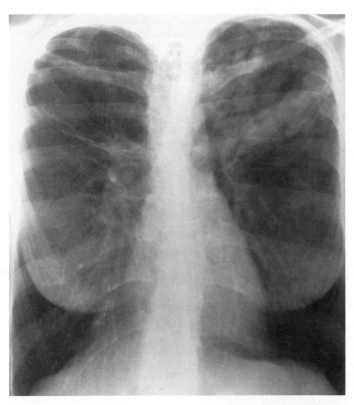

Figure 2-3. Allergic Bronchopulmonary Aspergillosis. Chest radiograph shows cylindrical infiltrates involving the upper lobes.

1. For patients with perennial symptoms and negative results on allergy skin tests, the diagnosis is vasomotor rhinitis.
2. For patients with seasonal symptoms and appropriately positive allergy skin tests, the diagnosis is seasonal allergic rhinitis.
3. For patients with perennial symptoms, allergy skin tests positive for house dust mite suggest house dust mite allergic rhinitis. In this case, dust mite allergen avoidance should be recommended. Patients should encase their bedding with allergy-proof encasements, remove carpeting from the bedroom, and keep the relative humidity in the house at 40% to 50% or less.

Corticosteroid Therapy for Rhinitis

The need for systemic corticosteroid treatment for rhinitis is limited. Occasionally, patients with severe symptoms of hay fever may benefit greatly from a short course of prednisone (10 mg 4 times daily by mouth for 5 days). This may induce sufficient improvement so that topical corticosteroids can penetrate the nose and satisfactory levels of antihistamine can be established in the blood. Severe nasal polyposis may warrant a longer course of oral corticosteroids. Sometimes, recurrence of nasal polyps can be prevented by continued use of topical corticosteroids. Polypectomy may be required if nasal polyps do not respond to treatment with systemic and intranasal corticosteroids.

• Treatment of nasal polyposis can include oral prednisone, followed by topical corticosteroids.

In contrast to systemic corticosteroid therapy, topical corticosteroid agents for the nose are easy to use and have few adverse systemic effects. Intranasal corticosteroids may decrease growth velocity in children.

• Intranasal corticosteroids may decrease growth velocity in children.

Long-term treatment with decongestant nasal sprays may have "addictive" potential (a vicious cycle of rebound congestion called *rhinitis medicamentosa* caused by topical vasoconstrictors). In contrast, inhaled corticosteroid does not induce dependence.

• Unlike decongestant nasal sprays, intranasal corticosteroid does not induce tachyphylaxis and rebound congestion.

Table 2-9   Differential Diagnosis of Chronic Rhinitis

Allergic rhinitis
Vasomotor rhinitis
Rhinitis medicamentosa
Sinusitis
Nasal polyposis
Nasal septal deviation
Foreign body
Tumor

A substantial number of patients with vasomotor rhinitis also have a good response to intranasal (topical aerosol) corticosteroid therapy, especially if they have the nasal eosinophilia or nasal polyposis form of vasomotor rhinitis.

* Many patients with vasomotor rhinitis have a good response to topical aerosol corticosteroid therapy.

If a patient with hay fever does not receive adequate relief with topical corticosteroid plus antihistamine therapy, it may indicate the need for systemic corticosteroid treatment and the initiation of immunotherapy. Unilateral symptoms suggest anatomical causes, including polyps, septal deviation, and tumor.

* If pharmacologic management fails, allergy immunotherapy should be considered for patients with allergic rhinitis.

An unusual side effect of intranasal corticosteroids is nasal septal perforation. Dry powder spray cannisters deliver a powerful jet of particulates, and a few patients have misdirected the jet to the nasal septum.

* Rarely, topical corticosteroid nasal sprays cause perforation of the nasal septum.

Antihistamines and Decongestants
Antihistamines antagonize the interaction of histamine with its receptors. Histamine may be more causative than other mast cell mediators of nasal itch and sneezing. These are symptoms most often responsive to antihistamine therapy.

Pseudoephedrine is the most common agent in nonprescription drugs for treating cold symptoms and rhinitis and usually is the active agent in widely used proprietary prescription agents. Phenylpropanolamine has been removed from the market because of its association with hemorrhagic stroke in women. Several prescription and nonprescription combination agents combine an antihistamine and decongestant. Decongestant preparations are often the only therapeutic option for patients with vasomotor rhinitis unresponsive to topical glucocorticoids.

* Pseudoephedrine is the most common decongestant in nonprescription preparations.

Men who are middle-aged or older may have urinary retention caused by antihistamines (principally the older drugs that have anticholinergic effects) and decongestants. Although there has been concern for years that decongestants may exacerbate hypertension because they are α-adrenergic agonists, no clinically significant hypertensive response has been seen in patients with hypertension that is controlled medically.

* Antihistamines and decongestants may cause urinary retention in men.
* The elderly are more sensitive to the anticholinergic effects of antihistamines.

Immunotherapy for Allergic Rhinitis
Until topical nasal glucocorticoid sprays were introduced, allergen immunotherapy was considered first-line therapy for allergic rhinitis when the relevant allergen was seasonal pollen of grass, trees, or weeds. Immunotherapy became second-line therapy after topical corticosteroids were introduced because immunotherapy 1) requires more time commitment during the build-up phase and 2) carries a small risk of anaphylaxis to the immunotherapy injection itself. However, immunotherapy for allergic rhinitis can be appropriate first-line therapy in selected patients and is highly effective.

Immunotherapy is usually reserved for patients who do not receive satisfactory relief from intranasal corticosteroids or who cannot tolerate antihistamines. Controlled trials have shown a benefit for pollen, dust mite, and cat allergies and a variable benefit for mold allergy. Immunotherapy is not used for food allergy or nonallergic rhinitis. The practice is less uniform with respect to mold allergens, with endorsement divided in the subspecialty. Immunotherapy has been shown to decrease the incidence of the development of asthma in children with allergic rhinitis and to decrease the onset of new allergen sensitivities in those treated for a single allergen.

* Immunotherapy usually is reserved for patients who do not receive relief from intranasal glucocorticoids or who cannot tolerate antihistamines.
* Controlled trials have shown that immunotherapy is effective for allergic rhinitis.
* Anaphylaxis is a risk of immunotherapy.
* Immunotherapy for allergic rhinitis can be first-line therapy in selected patients.

Environmental Modification

House Dust Mites
House dust mites are so small that they cannot maintain their own internal water unless the ambient humidity is high. They eat all kinds of organic matter but seem to favor mold and epidermal scales shed by humans. They occur in all human habitations, although the population size varies with local conditions. The only geographic areas free of house dust mites are at high elevations with extreme dryness.

* House dust mites require high humidity to survive.
* They are found in nearly all human habitations.

Areas in the home harboring the most substantial mite populations are bedding and fabric-upholstered furniture (heavily used) and any area where carpeting is on concrete (when concrete is in contact with the ground). Although carpeting is often cited as an important mite-related problem, carpet on wooden floors in a dry, well-ventilated house usually harbors only a small number of dust mites. Aerosol dispersion of allergen from this source is not great compared with that from bedding and furniture. To prevent egress of allergen when the mattress and pillows are compressed by occupancy of the bed, encase the bedding (and sometimes, when practical, furniture cushions) in dust-proof encasements. To some degree, this also prevents infusion of water vapor into the bedding matrix. These 2 factors combine to markedly decrease the amount of airborne allergen. In contrast, recently marketed acaricides that kill mites or denature their protein allergens have not proved useful in the home. Measures for controlling dust mites are listed in Table 2-10.

* Dust mites are an important source of respiratory allergen.
* The most substantial mite populations are in bedding and fabric-upholstered furniture.
* Impermeable encasements prevent egress of allergen.
* Chemical sprays (acaricides) capable of either killing mites or denaturing the protein allergens are not substantially helpful when applied in the home.

Pollen

Air conditioning, which enables the warm-season home to remain tightly closed, is the principal defense against pollinosis. Most masks purchased at local pharmacies cannot exclude pollen particles and are not worth the expense. Some masks can protect the wearer from allergen exposure. These include industrial-quality respirators designed specifically to pass rigorous testing by the Occupational Safety and Health Administration (OSHA) and the National Institute for Occupational Safety and Health (NIOSH) and be certified as capable of excluding a wide spectrum of particulates, including pollen and mold. These masks allow persons to mow the lawn and do yard work, which would be intolerable otherwise because of exposure to pollen allergen.

* Only industrial-quality masks are capable of excluding pollen particles.

Animal Dander

No measure for controlling animal dander can compare with getting the animal completely out of the house. No air filtration scheme that is feasible for average homeowners to install can eliminate allergen from an actively elaborating animal. If complete removal is not tenable, some partial measure must be considered.

If the house is heated or cooled by a forced-air system with ductwork, confining the pet to a single room in the house is only partially effective in reducing overall exposure, because air from every room is collected through the air-return ductwork and redistributed through a central plenum. If air-return ducts are sealed in the room where the animal is kept and air can escape from the room only by infiltration, exposure may be reduced. The room selected for this measure should be as far as possible from the bedroom of the person with the allergy. Naturally, the person should avoid close contact with the animal and should consider using a mask if handling the animal or entering the room where the animal is kept is necessary. Most animal danders have little or no relation to animal hair, so shedding status is irrelevant. Bathing cats about once every other week may reduce the allergen load in the environment.

* Complete avoidance is the only entirely effective way to manage allergy to household pets.

Sinusitis

Sinusitis is closely associated with edematous obstruction of the sinus ostia (the osteomeatal complex). Poor drainage of the sinus cavities predisposes to infection, particularly by microorganisms that thrive in low oxygen environments (eg, anaerobes). In adults, *Streptococcus pneumoniae, Haemophilus influenzae,* anaerobes, and viruses are common pathogens. In addition, *Branhamella catarrhalis* is an important pathogen in children.

Important clinical features of acute sinusitis are purulent nasal discharge, tooth pain, cough, and poor response to decongestants. Findings on paranasal sinus transillumination may be abnormal.

* Purulent nasal discharge, tooth pain, and abnormal findings on transillumination are important clinical features of sinusitis.

Physicians should be aware of the complications of sinusitis, which can be life-threatening (Table 2-11). Mucormycosis can cause recurrent or persistent sinusitis refractory to antibiotics. Allergic fungal sinusitis is characterized by persistent sinusitis, eosinophilia, increased total IgE, antifungal (usually *Aspergillus*) IgE antibodies, and fungal colonization of the sinuses. Wegener granulomatosis, ciliary dyskinesia, and hypogammaglobulinemia are medical conditions that can cause refractory sinusitis (Table 2-12).

Untreated sinusitis may lead to osteomyelitis, orbital and periorbital cellulitis, meningitis, and brain abscess. Cavernous sinus thrombosis, an especially serious complication, can lead to retrobulbar pain, extraocular muscle paralysis, and blindness.

Persistent, refractory, and complicated sinusitis should be evaluated by a specialist. Sinus computed tomography (CT) is the preferred imaging study for these patients (Figure 2-4).

Table 2-10 Dust Mite Control

Encase bedding & pillows in airtight encasements
Remove carpeting in bedroom
Remove upholstered furniture from bedroom
Remove all carpeting laid on concrete
Discontinue use of humidifier
Wash bedding in hot water
Run dehumidifier

Table 2-11 Complications of Sinusitis

Osteomyelitis
Meningitis
Subdural abscess
Extradural abscess
Orbital infection
Cellulitis
Cavernous sinus thrombosis

Table 2-12 Causes of Persistent or Recurrent Sinusitis

Nasal polyposis
Mucormycosis
Allergic fungal sinusitis
Ciliary dyskinesia
Wegener granulomatosis
Hypogammaglobulinemia
Tumor

Amoxicillin (500 mg 3 times daily) or trimethoprim-sulf-amethoxazole (1 double-strength capsule twice daily) for 10 to 14 days is the treatment of choice for uncomplicated maxillary sinusitis.

The sensitivity of plain radiography of the sinuses is not as good as that of CT (using the coronal sectioning technique). Good-quality coronal CT scans show greater detail about sinus mucosal surfaces, but CT usually is not necessary in acute uncomplicated sinusitis. CT is indicated, though, for patients being considered for a sinus operation and for those in whom standard treatment of sinusitis fails. However, patients with extensive dental restorations that contain metal may generate too much artifact for CT to be useful. For these patients, magnetic resonance imaging techniques are indicated.

* Sinus imaging is indicated for recurrent sinusitis.
* Sinus CT is preferred to sinus radiography for complicated sinusitis.

Urticaria and Angioedema

The distinction between acute and chronic urticaria is arbitrary and based on the duration of the urticaria. If it has been present for 6 weeks or longer, it is called *chronic urticaria*.

Secondary Urticaria

Most patients simply have urticaria as a skin disease (*chronic idiopathic urticaria*). A large number of these patients have an antibody that interacts with their own IgE or IgE receptor that produces the urticaria. Occasionally urticaria is the presenting sign of more serious internal disease. It can be a sign of lupus erythematosus and other connective tissue diseases, particularly the "overlap" syndromes that are more difficult to categorize. Thyroid disease, malignancy (mainly of the gastrointestinal tract), and lymphoproliferative diseases may be associated with urticaria, as may be occult infection, particularly of the stool, gallbladder, and dentition. Immune-complex disease has been associated with urticaria, usually with urticarial vasculitis, and hepatitis B virus has been identified as an antigen in cases of urticaria and immune-complex disease.

* Urticaria can be associated with lupus erythematosus and other connective tissue diseases, thyroid disease, malignancy, infection, and immune-complex disease.

A common cause of acute urticaria and angioedema (other than the idiopathic variety) is drug or food allergy. However, drug or food allergy usually does not cause chronic urticaria.

* Chronic urticaria and angioedema are often idiopathic.
* A common secondary cause of acute urticaria and angioedema is drug or food allergy.

Relation Between Urticaria and Angioedema

In common idiopathic urticaria, which lasts 2 to 18 hours, the lesions itch intensely because histamine is 1 of the causes of wheal formation.

* Typical urticarial lesions last 2-18 hours and are pruritic.

The pathophysiologic mechanism is similar for urticaria and angioedema. The critical factor is the type of tissue in which the capillary leak and mediator release occur. Urticaria occurs when the capillary events are in the tightly welded tissue wall of the skin—the epidermis. Angioedema occurs when the capillary events affect vessels in the loose connective tissue of the deeper layers—the dermis. Virtually all patients with the common idiopathic type of urticaria also have angioedema from time to time. When urticaria is caused by allergic reactions, angioedema may also occur. The only exception is hereditary angioneurotic edema (HANE), which is not related to mast cell mediator release but is a complement disorder. Patients with this form of angioedema rarely have urticaria.

C1 Esterase Inhibitor Deficiency

HANE is characterized by recurrent episodes of angioedema. If HANE is strongly suspected, the diagnosis can be proved by the appropriate measurement of complement factors (decreased levels

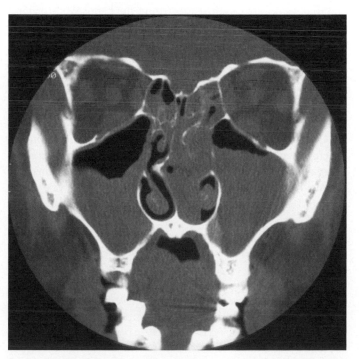

Figure 2-4. Sinusitis. Sinus computed tomogram shows opacification of the osteomeatal complex on the left, subtotal opacification of the right maxillary sinus, and an air-fluid level in the left maxillary antrum.

of C1 esterase inhibitor [quantitative and functional] and C4 [also C2, during an episode of swelling]).

* Levels of C1 esterase inhibitor and C4 are decreased in HANE.

The duration of individual swellings varies. Many patients with HANE have had at least 1 hospitalization for what appeared to be intestinal obstruction. If they avoid laparotomy on these occasions, the obstruction usually resolves in 3 to 5 days. Cramps and diarrhea may occur.

Lesions in HANE do not itch. The response to epinephrine is a useful differential point: HANE lesions do not respond well to epinephrine, but common angioedema usually resolves in 15 minutes or less. Laryngeal edema almost never occurs in the common idiopathic type of disease (although it may occur in allergic reactions, most often in insect-sting anaphylaxis cases); however, it is relatively common in HANE (earlier articles cited a 30% mortality rate in HANE, with all deaths due to laryngeal edema). HANE episodes may be related to local tissue trauma in a high percentage of cases, with dental work often regarded as the classic precipitating factor.

* Most patients with HANE have been hospitalized for "intestinal obstruction."
* HANE lesions do not respond well to epinephrine.
* In HANE, laryngeal edema is relatively common.
* Dental work is the classic precipitating factor for HANE.

The common idiopathic form of urticaria and angioedema is usually unrelated to antecedent trauma except in special cases of delayed-pressure urticaria, in which hives and angioedema occur after minor trauma or pressure to soft tissues (eg, to the hands while playing golf). The response to pressure distinguishes this special form of physical urticaria from HANE.

It is reasonable to perform C4 and C1 esterase inhibitor assays (functional and quantitative) for all patients with unexplained recurrent angioedema, especially if urticaria is not present.

The 3 major types of HANE-like disorders are the following:

1. Classic HANE is a genetic dysregulation of gene function for C1 inhibitor that is inherited in an autosomal dominant pattern. Therapy with androgens (testosterone, stanozolol, and danazol) reverses the dysregulation and allows expression of the otherwise normal gene, resulting in half-normal plasma levels of C1, which are sufficient to eliminate the clinical manifestations of the disease.

* Classic HANE is a genetic dysregulation (autosomal dominant).
* Testosterone, stanozolol, and danazol reverse the dysregulation.

2. In some cases of HANE, the gene for the C1 inhibitor mutates, rendering the molecule functionally ineffective but quantifiable in the blood. Thus, plasma levels of the C1 inhibitor molecule may be within the reference range in these patients. This is the basis for requesting immunochemical and functional measures of serum C1 inhibitor (with immunochemical measures only, the diagnosis is missed in cases of normal levels of an inactive molecule). Both classic HANE (low levels of C1 esterase inhibitor) and classic HANE

with the mutated gene for C1 inhibitor (nonfunctional C1 esterase inhibitor) are inherited forms of the disease. However, the proband may start the mutational line in both forms of HANE, so the family history is not positive in all cases.

* HANE with normal levels of C1 esterase inhibitor that is nonfunctional (by esterase assay) indicates a gene mutation.

3. C1 esterase inhibitor deficiency may be an acquired disorder with malignancy or lymphoproliferative disease. Plasma levels for C1q, C4, and C1 esterase inhibitor are low in acquired C1 esterase inhibitor deficiency. The hypothesis for the pathogenesis of this form of angioedema is that the tumor has or releases determinants that fix complement, and with constant consumption of complement components, a point is reached at which the biosynthesis of C1 inhibitor cannot keep up with the consumption rate, and the relative deficiency of C1 inhibitor allows episodes of swelling.

* C1 esterase inhibitor deficiency can be an acquired disorder in malignancy or lymphoproliferative disease.
* C1q levels are low in acquired C1 esterase inhibitor deficiency.

Physical Urticaria

Heat, light, cold, vibration, and trauma or pressure have been reported to cause hives in susceptible persons. Obtaining the history is the only way to suspect the diagnosis, which can be confirmed by applying each of the stimuli to the patient's skin in the laboratory. Heat can be applied by placing coins (soaked in hot water for a few minutes) on the patient's forearm. Cold can be applied with coins kept in a freezer or with ice cubes. For vibration, a laboratory vortex mixer or any common vibrator can be used. A pair of sandbags connected by a strap can be draped over the patient to create enough pressure to cause symptoms in those with delayed pressure urticaria. Unlike most cases of common idiopathic urticaria, in which the lesions affect essentially all skin surfaces, many cases of physical urticaria seem to involve only certain areas of skin. Thus, challenges will be positive only in the areas usually involved and negative in other areas. Directing challenges to the appropriate area depends on the history.

* For physical urticaria, the history is the only way to suspect the diagnosis, which can be confirmed by applying stimuli to the patient's skin.

Food Allergy in Chronic Urticaria

Food allergy almost never causes chronic urticaria. However, urticaria (or angioedema or anaphylaxis) can be an acute manifestation of true food allergy.

* Food allergy almost never causes chronic urticaria.
* Food allergy may cause acute urticaria, angioedema, or anaphylaxis.

Histopathology of Chronic Urticaria

Chronic urticaria is characterized by mononuclear cell perivascular cuffing around dermal capillaries, particularly involving the capillary loops that interdigitate with the rete pegs of the epidermis.

Urticarial vasculitis shows the usual histologic features of leukocytoclastic vasculitis.

* The characteristic histopathologic feature of chronic urticaria is a mononuclear cell perivascular cuff around capillaries.

Management of Urticaria

The history is of utmost importance for discovering the 2% to 4% of cases of chronic urticaria actually due to allergic causes. A complete physical examination is needed, with particular attention paid to the skin (including some test for dermatographism) to evaluate for the vasculitic nature of the lesions and to the liver, lymph nodes, and mucous membranes. Laboratory testing need not be exhaustive: chest radiography, a complete blood cell count with differential count (to discover eosinophilia), liver enzymes, erythrocyte sedimentation rate, serum protein electrophoresis, total hemolytic complement, antinuclear antibody, urinalysis, and stool examination for parasites. Allergy skin testing is indicated only if the patient has strong allergic tendencies and some element in the history suggests an allergic cause. However, patients with idiopathic urticaria often have fixed ideas about an allergy causing their problem, and skin testing often helps to dissuade them of this idea.

* The history is of utmost importance in diagnosing allergic urticaria.
* Laboratory testing may include chest radiography, eosinophil count, liver enzymes, erythrocyte sedimentation rate, serum protein electrophoresis, total hemolytic complement, and stool examination for parasites.

Management of urticaria and angioedema consists of blocking histamine, beginning usually with nonsedating H_1 antagonists. The addition of leukotriene antagonists may be helpful. The role of H_2 antagonists is unclear; they may help a small percentage of patients. Tricyclic antidepressants, such as doxepin, have potent antihistamine effects and are useful. Systemic corticosteroids can be administered for acute urticaria and angioedema or for very severe chronic idiopathic urticaria and angioedema.

* Urticaria and angioedema: management is usually with H_1 antagonists.
* Urticaria and angioedema: systemic corticosteroids are used for severe cases.

Anaphylaxis

Anaphylaxis is a generalized reaction characterized by flushing, hypotension, and tachycardia. Urticaria and angioedema may occur in many cases, and in patients with moderate to severe asthma or rhinitis as a preexisting condition, the asthma and rhinitis can be made worse. This definition of *anaphylaxis* is based on clinical manifestations. A cellular and molecular definition of *anaphylaxis* is a generalized allergic reaction characterized by activated basophils and mast cells releasing many mediators (preformed and newly synthesized). The dominant mediators of acute anaphylaxis are histamine and prostaglandin D_2. The serum levels of tryptase may be increased for

a few hours after clinical anaphylaxis. Physiologically, the hypotension of anaphylaxis is caused by peripheral vasodilatation and not by impaired cardiac contractility. Anaphylaxis is characterized by a hyperdynamic state. For these reasons, anaphylaxis can be fatal in patients with preexisting fixed vascular obstructive disease in whom a decrease in perfusion pressure leads to a critical reduction in flow (stroke) or in patients in whom laryngeal edema develops and completely occludes the airway.

* The clinical hallmarks of anaphylaxis are flushing, hypotension, and tachycardia.
* Urticaria and angioedema may be present.
* Histamine and prostaglandin D_2 are the dominant mediators of acute anaphylaxis.
* Peripheral vasodilatation causes hypotension of anaphylaxis.

Latex allergy is an important cause of intraoperative anaphylaxis. Patients with intraoperative anaphylaxis should be evaluated for possible latex allergy, usually by a skin test or in vitro assay. When persons with known latex allergy undergo invasive procedures, a latex-free environment is necessary. Patients with spina bifida or those with dermatitis, rhinitis, or asthma caused by latex allergy are at increased risk of anaphylaxis to latex.

* Latex allergy is an important cause of intraoperative anaphylaxis.

Food Allergy

Clinical History

The clinical syndrome of food allergy should prompt patients to provide a history containing some or all the following: For very sensitive persons, some tingling, itching, and a metallic taste in the mouth occur while the food is still in the mouth. Within 15 minutes after the food is swallowed, some epigastric distress may occur. There may be nausea and rarely vomiting. Abdominal cramping is felt chiefly in the periumbilical area (small-bowel phase), and lower abdominal cramping and watery diarrhea may occur. Urticaria or angioedema may occur in any distribution, or there may be only itching of the palms and soles. With increasing clinical sensitivity to the offending allergen, anaphylactic symptoms may emerge, including tachycardia, hypotension, generalized flushing, and alterations of consciousness.

In extremely sensitive persons, generalized flushing, hypotension, and tachycardia may occur before the other symptoms. Most patients with a food allergy can identify the offending foods. The diagnosis should be confirmed by skin testing or in vitro measurement of allergen-specific IgE antibody.

* Allergic reactions to food usually include pruritus, urticaria, or angioedema.

Common Causes of Food Allergy

Items considered to be the most common allergens are listed in Table 2-13.

Food-Related Anaphylaxis

Food-induced anaphylaxis is the same process involved in acute urticaria or angioedema to food allergens, except the severity of the reaction is greater in anaphylaxis. Relatively few foods are involved in food-induced anaphylaxis; the main ones are peanuts, shellfish, and nuts. Patients with latex allergy can develop food allergy to banana, avocado, kiwifruit, and other fruits.

* Anaphylaxis to food can be life-threatening.
* There is cross-sensitivity between latex and banana, avocado, and kiwifruit.

Allergy Skin Testing in Food Allergy

Patients presenting with food-related symptoms may have food allergy, food intolerance, irritable bowel syndrome, nonspecific dyspepsia, or 1 of many nonallergic conditions. A careful and detailed history on the nature of the "reaction," the reproducibility of the association of food and symptoms, and the timing of symptoms in relation to the ingestion of food can help the clinician form a clinical impression.

In many cases, allergy skin tests to foods can be helpful. If the allergy skin tests are negative (and the clinical suspicion for food allergy is low), the patient can be reassured that food allergy is not the cause of the symptoms. If the allergy skin tests are positive (and the clinical suspicion for food allergy is high), the patient should be counseled about the management of the food allergy. For highly sensitive persons, this includes strict and rigorous avoidance of the offending foods. These patients should also be given an epinephrine kit for self-administration in case of emergency. Although some food allergies may be outgrown, peanut, tree nut, fish, and shellfish allergies are typically lifelong.

If the diagnosis of food allergy is uncertain or if the symptoms are mild and nonspecific, sometimes oral food challenges are helpful. An open challenge is usually performed first. If negative, the diagnosis of food allergy is excluded. If positive, a blinded placebo-controlled challenge can be performed if there is suspicion about the positive result.

* Positive results on skin tests and double-blind food challenges can confirm the diagnosis of food allergy.
* If results of food skin tests are negative, food allergy is unlikely.
* Patients with anaphylaxis to food should strictly avoid the offending food and carry an epinephrine kit.

Stinging Insect Allergy

In patients clinically sensitive to Hymenoptera, reactions to a sting can be either large local reactions or systemic, anaphylactic reactions. With a large local sting reaction, swelling at the sting site may be dramatic, but there are no symptoms distant from that site. Stings of the head, neck, and dorsum of the hands are particularly prone to large local reactions.

Anaphylaxis caused by allergy to stinging insects is similar to all other forms of anaphylaxis. Thus, the onset of anaphylaxis may be very rapid, often within 1 or 2 minutes. Pruritus of the palms and soles is the most common initial manifestation and frequently is followed by generalized flushing, urticaria, angioedema, or hypotension (or a combination of these). The reason for attaching importance to whether a stinging insect reaction is a large local or a generalized one is that allergy skin testing and allergen immunotherapy are recommended only for generalized reactions. Patients who experience a large local reaction are not at increased risk of future anaphylaxis.

* Two varieties of reaction to sting: large local and anaphylactic.

Bee and Vespid Allergy

Yellow jackets, wasps, and hornets are vespids, and their venoms cross-react to a substantial degree. The venom of honeybees (family Apidae) does *not* cross-react with that of vespids. Unless the patient actually captures the insect delivering the sting, uncertainty will likely attend many cases of insect-stinging anaphylaxis. Thus, usually it is appropriate to conduct skin testing to honeybee and to each of the vespids. To interpret skin tests accurately, it is helpful to know which insect caused the sting producing the generalized reaction. Often, the circumstances of the sting can help determine the type of insect responsible. Multiple stings received while mowing the grass or doing other landscape jobs that may disturb yellow-jacket burrows in the ground are likely causes of yellow-jacket stings. A single sting received while near picnic tables or refuse containers at picnic areas is likely from a yellow jacket or possibly a hornet. Stings received while working around the house exterior (painting, cleaning eaves and gutters, or attic work) are most likely from wasps.

* Yellow jackets, wasps, and hornets are vespids, and their venoms cross-react.
* The venom of bees does not cross-react with that of vespids.
* It is helpful to know which insect caused the sting.

Allergy Testing

Patients who have had a generalized reaction warrant allergen skin testing. Patients who have had a large local reaction to 1 of the Hymenoptera stings do *not* warrant allergen skin testing because they are not at increased risk of future anaphylaxis.

* A generalized reaction warrants allergen skin testing.
* A large local reaction does not warrant allergen skin testing.

In many cases, skin testing should be delayed for at least 1 month after a sting-induced general reaction because tests conducted closer to the time of the sting have a substantial risk of being falsely negative. Positive results on skin testing that correlate with the clinical history are sufficient evidence for considering Hymenoptera venom immunotherapy.

Table 2-13 Common Causes of Food Allergy

Eggs	Shellfish
Milk	Soybean
Nuts	Wheat
Peanuts	

- Skin testing should be delayed for at least 1 month after a sting-induced general reaction.
- Patients with clinical anaphylaxis and positive results on venom skin tests may benefit from venom immunotherapy.

Venom Immunotherapy

The decision to undertake venom immunotherapy can be reached only after a discussion between the patient and the physician. General indications for venom immunotherapy are listed in Table 2-14. Patients must understand that once initiated, the immunotherapy injection schedule must be maintained and that there is a small risk of immunotherapy-induced anaphylaxis. It is important that patients understand that despite receiving allergy immunotherapy, they must carry epinephrine when outdoors because of the 2% to 10% possibility that immunotherapy will not provide suitable protection. Most, but not all, patients can safely discontinue venom immunotherapy after 5 years of treatment.

- There is a small risk that venom immunotherapy will induce anaphylaxis.
- There is a 2%-10% chance that venom immunotherapy will not provide adequate protection.

Avoidance

The warnings that every patient with stinging insect hypersensitivity should receive are listed in Table 2-15. The circumstances of each patient may require additional entries to this list. Also, patients need to know how to use self-injectable epinephrine in its several forms. Many patients wear an anaphylaxis identification bracelet.

- All patients with stinging-insect sensitivity should carry an epinephrine kit.

Drug Allergy

Drug Allergy Not Involving IgE or Immediate-Type Reactions

Patients with drug allergy not involving IgE or immediate-type reactions have negative results on skin prick and intradermal testing.

Stevens-Johnson Syndrome

Stevens-Johnson syndrome is a bullous skin and mucosal reaction; very large blisters appear over much of the skin surface, in the mouth, and along the gastrointestinal tract. Because of the propensity of the blisters to break down and become infected, the reaction often is life-threatening. Treatment consists of stopping use of the drug that

Table 2-14 Indications for Venom Immunotherapy

History of mild, moderate, or severe anaphylaxis to a sting
Positive results on skin tests to venom implicated historically in the anaphylactic reaction
Urticaria distant from the site of the sting (adults only)

Table 2-15 Dos and Don'ts for Patients With Hypersensitivity to Insect Stings

Avoid looking or smelling like a flower
  Avoid flowered prints for clothes
    Avoid cosmetics & fragrances, especially ones derived from flowering plants
Never drink from a soft-drink can outdoors during the warm months—a yellow jacket can land *on* or *in* the can while you are not watching, go inside the can, & sting the inside of your mouth (1 of the most dangerous places for a sensitive patient to be stung) when you take a drink
Avoid doing outdoor maintenance & yard work
Never reach into a mailbox without first looking inside it
Never go barefoot
Always look at the underside of picnic table benches & park benches before sitting down
Never attempt to eject a stinging insect yourself from the interior of a moving automobile; pull over, get out, & let someone else remove the insect

causes the reaction, giving corticosteroids systemically, and providing supportive care. The patients are often treated in burn units. Penicillin, sulfonamides, barbiturates, diphenylhydantoin, warfarin, and phenothiazines are well-known causes. A drug-induced Stevens-Johnson reaction is an absolute contraindication to administering a causative drug to the patient.

- Stevens-Johnson syndrome is life-threatening and is an absolute contraindication for rechallenge with the drug.

Toxic Epidermal Necrolysis

Clinically, toxic epidermal necrolysis is almost indistinguishable from Stevens-Johnson syndrome. Histologically, the cleavage plane for the blisters is deeper than in Stevens-Johnson syndrome. The cleavage plane is at the basement membrane of the epidermis, so even the basal cell layer is lost. This makes toxic epidermal necrolysis even more devastating than Stevens-Johnson syndrome because healing occurs with much scarring. Often, healing cannot be accomplished without skin grafting, so the mortality rate is even higher than for Stevens-Johnson syndrome. Patients with toxic epidermal necrolysis should always be cared for in a burn unit because of full-thickness damage over 80% to 90% of the skin. The very high mortality rate is similar to that for burn patients with damage of this extent.

- Toxic epidermal necrolysis is a life-threatening exfoliative dermatitis.

Morbilliform Skin Reaction

Morbilliform skin reaction is the most common dermatologic manifestation of a drug reaction. It is an immune-mediated drug rash without IgE involvement, manifested by a macular-papular exanthem. The rash can be accompanied by pruritus but has no other systemic symptoms. It typically occurs more than 5 days after use of a medication was begun. It is not associated with anaphylaxis or other serious sequelae.

- Morbilliform skin reaction is the most common dermatologic manifestation of a drug reaction and is not associated with anaphylaxis.

Ampicillin-Mononucleosis Rash

Ampicillin-mononucleosis rash is a unique drug rash that occurs when ampicillin is given to an acutely ill, febrile patient who has mononucleosis. The rash is papular, nonpruritic, rose-colored, and usually on the abdomen and has a granular feel when the fingers brush lightly over the surface of the involved skin. It is not known why the rash is specific for ampicillin and mononucleosis. This rash does not predispose to allergy to penicillin.

- Ampicillin-mononucleosis rash is papular, nonpruritic, rose-colored, and on the abdomen.
- This rash does not predispose to penicillin allergy.

Fixed Drug Eruptions

Fixed drug eruptions are red to red-brown macules that appear on a certain area of the patient's skin; any part of the body can be affected. The macules do not itch or have other signs of inflammation, although fever is associated with their appearance in a few patients. The unique aspect of this allergic phenomenon is that if a patient is given the same drug in the future, the rash develops in exactly the same skin areas. Resolution of the macules often includes postinflammatory hyperpigmentation. Except for cosmetic problems due to skin discolorations, the phenomenon does not seem serious. Antibiotics and sulfonamides are the most frequently recognized causes.

- In fixed drug eruptions, the same area of skin is always affected.

Erythema Nodosum

Erythema nodosum is a characteristic rash of red nodules about the size of a quarter, usually nonpruritic and appearing only over the anterior aspects of the lower legs. Histopathologically, the nodules are plaques of infiltrating mononuclear cells. Erythema nodosum is associated with several connective tissue diseases, viral infections, and drug allergy.

- Erythema nodosum rash is usually nonpruritic, appearing only over the anterior aspect of the lower legs.
- It is associated with several connective tissue diseases, viral infections, and drug allergy.

Contact Dermatitis

Contact dermatitis can occur with various drugs. Commonly, it is a form of drug allergy that is an occupational disease in medical or health care workers. In some patients receiving topical drugs, allergy develops to the drug or to various elements in its pharmaceutical formulation (eg, fillers, stabilizers, antibacterials, and emulsifiers).

Contact dermatitis is a manifestation of type IV hypersensitivity and clinically appears as an area of reddening on the skin that progresses to a granular weeping eczematous eruption of the skin, with some dermal thickening and a plaque-like quality of the surrounding skin. Histopathologically, the affected area is infiltrated by mononuclear cells. When patients are receiving treatment for a dermatitis, and contact hypersensitivity develops to corticosteroids or other drugs used in treatment, a particularly difficult diagnostic problem arises unless the physician is alert to this possibility. When contact hypersensitivity to a drug occurs, it does not increase the probability of acute type I hypersensitivity and is not associated with serious exfoliative syndromes. However, patients can develop exquisite cutaneous sensitivity of this type so that almost no avoidance technique in the workplace completely eliminates dermatitis; even protective gloves are only partly helpful. Thus, it can be occupationally disabling.

- Contact dermatitis is a form of drug allergy.
- It is a manifestation of type IV hypersensitivity.

Drug Allergy Involving IgE or Immediate-Type Reactions

Penicillin Allergy

Penicillin can cause anaphylaxis in sensitive persons. It is an IgE-mediated process that can be evaluated with skin testing to the major and minor determinants of penicillin. Patients with positive results on skin testing and a clinical history of penicillin allergy can be desensitized to penicillin, but the procedure may be hazardous.

- Penicillin can cause anaphylaxis.
- It is an IgE-mediated process diagnosed with penicillin skin testing to the major and minor determinants.
- Patients can be desensitized, but the procedure may be hazardous.

Penicillin skin tests can be helpful in determining whether it is safe to administer penicillin to a patient with suspected penicillin allergy. About 85% of patients who give a history of penicillin allergy have negative skin tests to the major and minor determinants of penicillin. These patients generally are not at increased risk of anaphylaxis, and most can receive penicillin safely. If penicillin skin tests are positive, there is a 40% to 60% chance that an allergic reaction will develop if the patient is challenged with penicillin. Most of these patients should avoid penicillin and related drugs. However, if there is a strong indication for penicillin treatment, desensitization can be considered. The desensitization procedure involves the administration of progressively increasing doses of penicillin. Desensitization can be accomplished by the oral or intravenous route and is usually performed in a hospital setting.

Ampicillin, amoxicillin, nafcillin, and other β-lactam antibiotics cross-react strongly with penicillin. Early studies suggested that up to 20% to 30% of patients with penicillin allergy were also allergic to cephalosporins. More recent studies have suggested that the cross-sensitivity of penicillin with cephalosporins is much less, about 5%. Most studies have suggested that aztreonam does not cross-react with penicillin.

- About 5% of patients with penicillin allergy are also allergic to cephalosporins.
- Aztreonam does not cross-react with penicillin.

Radiographic Contrast Media Reactions

Radiographic contrast media can cause reactions that have the clinical appearance of anaphylaxis. Estimates of the frequency of these reactions are 2% to 6% of procedures involving intravenous contrast media. The incidence of intra-arterial contrast-induced reactions is lower. The anaphylactoid reactions do *not* involve IgE antibody (thus, the reason for the term *anaphylactoid*). Radiocontrast media appear to induce mediator release on the basis of some other property intrinsic to the contrast agent. The tonicity or ionic strength of the media seems particularly related to anaphylactoid reactions. With the availability of low ionic strength media, the incidence of reactions has been lower.

- The frequency of contrast media reactions is 2%-6% of procedures.
- The reaction does not involve IgE antibody.
- Nonionic or low osmolar contrast media cause fewer anaphylactoid reactions than standard contrast media.

The frequency of radiocontrast media reactions can be decreased with the use of low ionic strength media in patients with a history of asthma or atopy. Patients with a history of reaction to radiocontrast media who subsequently need radiographic contrast media procedures can be pretreated with a protocol of 50 mg oral prednisone every 6 hours for 3 doses, with the last dose 1 hour before the procedure. At the last dose, 50 mg of diphenhydramine or an equivalent H_1 antagonist is recommended. Some studies show that the addition of oral ephedrine can be beneficial. However, most studies show that the addition of an H_2 antagonist is unnecessary.

- Patients with a history of systemic reactions to radiocontrast media should be pretreated with systemic corticosteroids and an H_1 antagonist and should be offered nonionic contrast agents.

Other Allergic Conditions

Mastocytosis

Systemic mastocytosis is a disorder of abnormal proliferation of mast cells. The skin, bone marrow, liver, spleen, lymph nodes, and gastrointestinal tract can be affected. The clinical manifestations vary but can include flushing, pruritus, urticaria, unexplained syncope, fatigue, and dyspepsia. Bone marrow biopsies with stains for mast cells (toluidine blue, Giemsa, or chloral acetate esterase) and immunochemical stains for tryptase are the most direct diagnostic studies. Fluorescence in situ hybridization and polymerase chain reaction may detect a clonal disorder of systemic mastocytosis, Fip1-like-platelet-derived growth factor receptor α-1. Serum levels of tryptase and urinary concentrations of histamine and histamine metabolites may be increased.

Treatment initially consists of antihistamines. Cromolyn sodium given orally can be beneficial, especially in patients with gastrointestinal tract symptoms. Corticosteroids should be considered in severe cases, and interferon is a promising investigational treatment.

Eosinophilia

Eosinophilia is idiopathic, secondary (reactive), or primary. Idiopathic hypereosinophilic syndrome is a well-defined entity. Secondary causes include the following: infectious (tissue-invasive parasitosis); drugs; toxins; inflammation; atopy and allergies (asthma); malignancy (lymphoma, Hodgkin lymphoma, cutaneous T-cell lymphoma, and metastatic cancer); collagen vascular disease (eosinophilic vasculitis); pulmonary (hypereosinophilic pneumonitis and Löffler syndrome); and eosinophilic myalgia syndrome. The primary clonal and monoclonal disorders include acute leukemia (myeloid and lymphoid); chronic myeloid leukemia; myelodysplastic syndrome and chronic myelomonocytic leukemia; classic and atypical myeloproliferative disorders (systemic mastocytosis); and unclassified (chronic eosinophilic leukemia). The clinical diagnostic approach is to exclude secondary eosinophilic disorders; to evaluate bone marrow aspirates and biopsy specimens with genetic and molecular studies; and to perform tests to assess eosinophilia-mediated tissue injury (chest radiography, pulmonary function tests, echocardiography, and serum trypsin levels). The differential diagnosis of eosinophilia is given in Table 2-16.

The clinical manifestations include weight loss, muscle weakness, and cutaneous induration. The laboratory hallmark is peripheral and tissue eosinophilia. Follow-up studies show that many affected patients continue to have marked disability months and years after the acute illness. Although corticosteroids are used in the treatment

Table 2-16 Common Causes of Eosinophilia

Atopic
    Allergic rhinitis
    Allergic bronchopulmonary aspergillosis
    Asthma
    Atopic dermatitis
    Drug hypersensitivity
Pulmonary
    Eosinophilic pneumonia
    Löffler syndrome
Proliferative/neoplastic
    Idiopathic hypereosinophilic syndrome
    Eosinophilic leukemia
Vasculitis/connective tissue
    Churg-Strauss vasculitis
    Eosinophilic fasciitis
Eosinophilic gastroenteritis
Infectious
    Visceral larva migrans
    Helminth
Toxic
    Eosinophilia-myalgia syndrome
    Toxic oil syndrome

of this disorder, there is no evidence that corticosteroid therapy alters long-term disability or mortality.

Hypereosinophilia syndrome is an idiopathic eosinophilic disorder characterized by an absolute eosinophil count of more than 1,500/mcL (1.5×10^9/L); chronic course of 6 months or longer; organ involvement as manifested by eosinophilia-mediated tissue injury (cardiomyopathy, dermatitis, pneumonitis, sinusitis, gastrointestinal tract inflammation, left or right ventricular apical thrombus, and stroke); and no other causes of eosinophilia. The syndrome typically affects persons in the third through sixth decades of life; women are affected more often than men. Symptoms include fatigue, cough, shortness of breath, or rash. Cardiac involvement in hypereosinophilia syndrome is especially significant: endomyocardial fibrosis, mural thrombi, and mitral and tricuspid incompetence can occur. The clinical syndrome is 1 of a restrictive cardiomyopathy with congestive heart failure. Echocardiography and endomyocardial biopsy are important diagnostic tests.

Hypereosinophilia syndrome is treated with prednisone, 1 mg/kg per day, alone or in combination with hydroxyurea. Second-line therapy is recombinant interferon-alfa.

Common Variable Immunodeficiency

Common variable immunodeficiency can affect persons of all ages, both males and females. It is not a hereditary disorder. Patients have recurrent infections and hypogammaglobulinemia (low IgG levels). Recurrent pyogenic infections include chronic otitis media, chronic or recurrent sinusitis, pneumonia, and bronchiectasis.

Patients with common variable immunodeficiency often have autoimmune or gastrointestinal tract disturbances. About one-half of patients have chronic diarrhea and malabsorption. There may be steatorrhea, protein-losing enteropathy, ulcerative colitis, or Crohn disease. Other gastrointestinal tract problems associated with the disease are atrophic gastritis, pernicious anemia, giardiasis, and chronic active hepatitis. Pathologic changes in the gastrointestinal tract mucosa include loss of villi, nodular lymphoid hyperplasia, and diffuse lymphoid infiltration.

Autoimmune anemia, thrombocytopenia, or neutropenia is present in 10% to 50% of the patients. Inflammatory arthritis and lymphoid interstitial pneumonia are other associated conditions. Also, patients have an increased risk of a malignancy developing, particularly a lymphoid malignancy such as non-Hodgkin lymphoma.

The diagnosis of common variable immunodeficiency should be considered in patients with recurrent pyogenic infections and hypogammaglobulinemia. Associated gastrointestinal tract or autoimmune disease and the exclusion of hereditary primary immunodeficiencies support the diagnosis. Treatment is with intravenous gamma globulin.

Terminal Complement Component Deficiencies

Patients with deficiency of the terminal complement component C5, C6, C7, or C8 have an increased susceptibility to meningococcal infections. The terminal complement components form the membrane attack complex that causes cell lysis; hence, deficiency of 1 of these components results in defective microbial killing. The terminal component C9 participates in membrane pore formation but is not essential for complement-mediated cell lysis. Thus, patients with the rare C9 deficiency have a limited increased susceptibility to infections.

Terminal complement component deficiency should be suspected in patients with recurrent meningococcal disease, a family history of meningococcal disease, or systemic meningococcal infection or in those infected with an unusual serotype of meningococcus. Diagnosis is confirmed with assay of total hemolytic complement and measurement of individual complement components.

Allergy Pharmacy Review
Sansana Donna Boontaveekul, MS, PharmD

Drug (Trade Name)	Toxic/Adverse Effects	Drug Interactions	Comments

Bronchodilators
  Albuterol (Proventil HFA, Ventolin HFA, Vospire ER)
  Epinephrine (Primatene Mist)
	Palpitations, tachycardia, hypertension, arrhythmia, tremor, nervousness, headache, insomnia, GERD or pharyngitis	β-Blockers may inhibit bronchodilator effect in patients with asthma
		Tricyclic antidepressants & sympathomimetics may cause hypertension
			Bronchodilators must be used cautiously for those with DM, cardiovascular disorders, hyperthyroidism, or seizure
			β-Blockers may precipitate asthma in asthmatics

Formeterol (Foradil)	Palpitations, headache, tremor, nervousness	MAO inhibitors may cause tachycardia or agitation	
Ipratropium (Atrovent)	Ipratropium may cause blurred vision & dry mouth		
Ipratropium & albuterol (Combivent)			
Isoetharine (Bronkosol) Isoproterenol (Isuprel)	Isoetharine may cause hypertension, tachycardia, & palpitations	Isoproterenol or epinephrine may sensitize myocardium to effects of general anesthetics	

Levalbuterol (Xopenex)
  Metaproterenol (Alupent)
  Pirbuterol (Maxair autoinhaler)
  Salmeterol (Serevent)
  Terbutaline (Brethine)
  Tiotropium (Spiriva)			

Leukotriene receptor antagonists	Rarely may cause systemic eosinophilia with vasculitis consistent with Churg-Strauss syndrome		
Montelukast (Singulair) Zafirlukast (Accolate)		Zafirlukast & zileuton can increase warfarin effects	
Zileuton (Zyflo)		Zileuton can double theophylline concentrations	

Anti-inflammatory inhalant products
  Beclomethasone (Qvar)
  Budesonide (Pulmicort)
  Cromolyn (Intal)
  Flunisolide (Aerobid)
  Fluticasone (Flovent HFA)
  Fluticasone & salmeterol (Advair Diskus)
  Mometasone (Asmanex)
  Nedocromil (Tilade)
  Triamcinolone (Azmacort)
			Corticosteroids, cromolyn, & nedocromil are not effective for relieving acute bronchospasm
			When stopping use of systemic corticosteroids, inhaled corticosteroids do not provide systemic effects needed to prevent symptoms of adrenal insufficiency

First-generation antihistamines[a,b]
  Brompheniramine maleate (Dimetapp elixir)
  Chlorpheniramine maleate (Chlor-Trimeton)
  Clemastine fumarate (Tavist)
  Cyprohepatidine (Periactin)
  Dexchlorpheniramine maleate
	CNS depression (most frequent, sedation)
	Some patients, especially children, may have paradoxical excitement (restlessness, insomnia, tremors, nervousness, palpitation)
	Sensitivity reaction & photosensitivity
		Alcohol may potentiate CNS effects & should be avoided while taking antihistamines
		Additive CNS suppressant effects may occur in patients taking other CNS suppressants (sedatives, tranquilizers)
			Histamine H_1 receptor antagonists block H_1 receptor sites, preventing action of histamine on cells; they do not chemically inactivate or prevent histamine release

Allergy Pharmacy Review (continued)

Drug (Trade Name)	Toxic/Adverse Effects	Drug Interactions	Comments
First-generation antihistamines[a,b] (continued)			
Diphenhydramine HCl (Benadryl) Hydroxyzine HCl (Atarax) Hydroxyzine pamoate (Vistaril) Promethazine HCl (Phenergan)	Cardiovascular effects are uncommon & usually limited to overdosage Promethazine may lower seizure threshold Adverse anticholinergic effects: dryness of mouth, nose, throat; dysuria; urinary retention; blurred vision; thickening of bronchial secretions		Antihistamines exert various degrees of antihistaminic, anticholinergic, & antimuscarinic activities & are useful as sedatives, antiemetics, anti–motion sickness, antitussive, & anti-parkinsonism agents Unlabeled use: increased appetite, weight gain (cyproheptadine) Caution for patients with angle-closure glaucoma, prostatic hypertrophy, stenosing peptic ulcer, pyloroduodenal obstruction, bladder neck obstruction
Second-generation antihistamines[a,c]			
Cetirizine HCl (Zyrtec)	Nausea, dyspepsia, dry mouth, headache, drowsiness	No clinically important drug interactions have been reported in patients taking cetirizine concomitantly with azithromycin, erythromycin, or ketoconazole	Cetirizine is a carboxylic acid metabolite of hydroxyzine The increase in polarity of cetirizine may decrease its distribution in CNS; thus, reduced potential for CNS adverse effects compared with first-generation antihistamines; incidence of certain adverse CNS effects (somnolence) is higher in patients taking cetirizine than in those taking other second-generation antihistamines
Desloratadine (Clarinex)		Although AUC of desloratadine increases with concomitant use of erythromycin or ketoconazole, no clinically important changes measured by ECG, laboratory evaluations, vital signs, adverse events	Desloratadine, fexofenadine, & loratadine are selective for peripheral H_1 receptors & less sedating than first-generation antihistamines Desloratadine is a major metabolite of loratadine Dosage adjustment is recommended in patients with renal or hepatic impairment (or both) (cetirizine, desloratadine, loratadine, & fexofenadine—renal impairment only)

Allergy Pharmacy Review (continued)

Drug (Trade Name)	Toxic/Adverse Effects	Drug Interactions	Comments
Second-generation antihistamines[a,c] (continued)			
Fexofenadine HCl (Allegra)		Fexofenadine is active metabolite of terfenadine, but does not have cardiotoxic & drug interaction potentials of terfenadine; no clinically important adverse effects or changes in QT_c interval reported with concomitant use of erythromycin or ketoconazole despite increases in AUC & peak plasma concentration of fexofenadine	
Loratadine (Claritin, Claritin Reditabs, Tavist ND, Alavert)		Although AUC of loratadine increases with concomitant use of erythromycin or ketoconazole, no clinically important changes are indicated by ECG, laboratory evaluation, vital signs, adverse effects	
Nasal solution products	Bitter/bad taste, nasal burning/ stinging/irritation, pharyngitis, sneezing	No clinically important drug interactions known	
Azelastine HCl (Astelin)	Somnolence & headache can occur		Histamine H_1 receptor antagonist
Cromolyn sodium (Nasalcrom)			Mast cell stabilizer; begin therapy before & continue at regular intervals during allergenic exposure
Corticosteroid nasal spray products	Mild nasopharyngeal irritation, occasional sneezing attacks, nasal stuffiness, epistaxis, rhinorrhea, headache	No clinically important drug interactions known	Should be used at regular intervals; shake well before each use; if used at excessive doses, systemic corticosteroid effects may appear; the pump must be primed with first use
Beclomethasone dipropionate (Beconase AQ), 42 mcg			
Budesonide (Rhinocort Aqua), 32 mcg			
Flunisolide (Nasarel), 25 mcg			
Fluticasone propionate (Flonase), 50 mcg			
Mometasone furoate (Nasonex), 50 mcg			
Triamcinolone acetonide (Nasacort AQ), 55 mcg			
Histamine H_1 receptor antagonist ophthalmic products[d]			
Emedastine difumarate (Emadine) 0.05% ophthalmic solution	Transient eye burning/stinging, blurred vision, dry eyes, foreign body sensation, headache, bitter taste	Benzalkonium (preservative) may be absorbed by soft contact lens; wait at least 10 min after applying drug before inserting contact lenses	
Epinastine (Elestat) 0.05% ophthalmic solution			
Levocabastine (Livostin) 0.05% ophthalmic suspension			Levocabastine: shake well before use

Allergy Pharmacy Review (continued)

Drug (Trade Name)	Toxic/Adverse Effects	Drug Interactions	Comments
Mast cell stabilizer ophthalmic products[d]			
Cromolyn sodium (Crolom) 4% ophthalmic solution	Same as above	Same as above	
Lodoxamide tromethamine (Alomide) 0.1% ophthalmic solution			
Pemirolast potassium (Alamast) 0.1% ophthalmic solution	Preservative in pemirolast is lauralkonium Cl; wait at least 10 min after applying drug before inserting contact lenses		
Nedocromil sodium (Alocril) 2% ophthalmic solution	Same as above	Same as above	
Histamine H$_1$ receptor antagonists and mast cell stabilizer ophthalmic products[d]			
Azelastine HCl (Optivar) 0.5 mg/mL ophthalmic solution			
Ketotifen fumarate (Zaditor) 0.025% ophthalmic solution			
Olopatadine HCl (Patanol) 0.1% ophthalmic solution			
Monoclonal Antibody			
Omalizumab (Xolair)	Anaphylactic reactions within 2 h of initial dose (<0.1%), malignant neoplasm (0.2%), headache, injection site reaction, upper respiratory tract infection, sinusitis, pharyngitis, viral infection	No formal drug interaction studies have been performed	IgG monoclonal antibody that inhibits IgE binding to high-affinity IgE receptors on mast cells & basophils; for subcutaneous use only; dose is based on pretreatment IgE serum levels & body weight

Abbreviations: AUC, area under curve; CNS, central nervous system; DM, diabetes mellitus; ECG, electrocardiography; GERD, gastroesophageal reflux disease; MAO, monoamine oxidase.

[a] Histamine H$_1$ receptor antagonists.

[b] Oral or parenteral products.

[c] Available in oral products only.

[d] To prevent contamination of products, care should be taken not to touch eyelids or surrounding areas with dropper tip of bottle.

Questions

Multiple Choice (choose the best answer)

1. A 19-year-old male basketball player presents with breathing difficulty during his basketball games. He reports that his respiratory symptoms start within a minute of playing basketball—primarily in games and not during practice—and that the feeling is that he "can't breath in deeply." He also notes a change in his voice at the time. After he is on the bench, his symptoms subside. He does not have breathing difficulties at other times. Pretreatment with an albuterol metered-dose inhaler has not helped him. Which of the following would be present on testing?

   a. Flattening of the inspiratory loop with normal expiratory loop on spirometry when symptomatic
   b. Flattening of the inspiratory loop with normal expiratory loop on spirometry when asymptomatic
   c. Flattening of the inspiratory loop and expiratory loop on spirometry when symptomatic
   d. Normal inspiratory loop and expiratory loop on spirometry when symptomatic
   e. Normal inspiratory loop and concavity of the expiratory loop on spirometry when symptomatic

2. A 31-year-old woman presents in her fifth month of pregnancy with increasing asthma symptoms. Her asthma had been well controlled throughout pregnancy but worsened over the past 4 days with the onset of an upper respiratory tract infection. She is having daily symptoms and nighttime awakenings due to dyspnea. She is using her albuterol inhaler every 3 hours and has been compliant with her usual inhaler regimen of budesonide, 2 puffs daily. She denies fever or purulent mucus. On examination she has scattered expiratory wheezes throughout all lung fields, a respiratory rate of 18 breaths per minute, oxygen saturation of 97%, and a forced expiratory volume in 1 second (FEV_1) that is 64% of the predicted value, which improves to 72% of the predicted value after use of albuterol. At this point, what should be done to improve her current exacerbation?

   a. Begin use of prednisone, 40 mg daily for 5 days.
   b. Begin use of montelukast (Singulair), 10 mg daily.
   c. Increase budesonide dosage to 2 puffs twice daily.
   d. Begin use of amoxycillin, 500 mg 3 times daily for 10 days.
   e. Discontinue use of budesonide inhaler.

3. A 59-year-old man with a history of moderate persistent asthma and nasal polyposis is being evaluated for degenerative arthritis. He reports that several years ago the administration of aspirin resulted in a significant flare of his asthma and increased nasal congestion. He has avoided taking analgesic medications since then. Which of the following analgesic medications would be most likely to provoke an asthma exacerbation?

   a. Acetaminophen
   b. Ibuprofen
   c. Celecoxib
   d. Rofecoxib
   e. Tramadol

4. A 78-year-old man reports a 5-month history of recurrent swelling of the orbits, lips, and tongue. The swelling occurs every 2 to 3 weeks and lasts for 3 days. There is no associated pruritus or hives. He denies the use of any blood pressure medications. He also reports fatigue and a 4.5-kg weight loss. He cannot relate the swelling episodes to food ingestion, over-the-counter medication ingestion, or environmental changes. What is the most likely underlying cause of the angioedema?

   a. Hereditary C1 esterase inhibitor deficiency
   b. Hematologic malignancy
   c. Superior vena cava syndrome
   d. Mastocytosis
   e. Allergy to food preservative

5. A 43-year-old woman reports a history of pruritic hives and wheezing after her second dose of intravenous penicillin approximately 10 years ago. She has avoided penicillin since then and has not had any further drug reactions. She is being treated for endocarditis, and penicillin in high doses is considered the drug of choice. What recommendation can be given for penicillin use?

   a. Penicillin cannot be given; use an alternate medication.
   b. Skin test to the major determinant of penicillin; if results are negative, penicillin can be given.
   c. Skin test to the major and minor determinants of penicillin; if results are negative, penicillin can be given.
   d. Patch test to penicillin; if results are negative, penicillin can be given.
   e. Avoid penicillin, but other β-lactam antibiotics may be used.

6. A 44-year-old woman presents for evaluation of nasal symptoms with a 10-month duration. She describes unilateral nasal congestion and rhinorrhea that is unchanged during the different seasons. Over-the-counter antihistamine-decongestant preparations have not been helpful. She lives in an older house with a dog and a cat. Her physical examination reveals decreased air flow through the right nare. What is the next step in management?

   a. Skin prick testing to dust mite, cat, dog, and regional trees, grasses, weeds, and molds
   b. Intradermal skin testing to dust mite, cat, dog, and regional trees, grasses, weeds, and molds
   c. Rhinoscopy
   d. A trial of an intranasal corticosteroid
   e. Plain film sinus radiography

7. A 62-year-old man presents with a 3-year history of recurrent sinopulmonary infections documented by sinus CT scan and chest radiography. Before the past 3 years, he does not recall having recurrent infections, allergic rhinitis, or asthma. Sputum cultures have shown growth of *Streptococcus pneumoniae* and *Haemophilus influenzae*. Currently, he reports having a chronic productive cough. Which of the following laboratory tests is most likely to yield abnormal results from this patient?

    a. White blood cell count
    b. IgG level
    c. Neutrophil adhesion assay
    d. Total complement level
    e. IgE level

Answers

1. Answer a.
The vignette describes a typical presentation of vocal cord dysfunction characterized by abrupt onset of symptoms in an anxiety-provoking situation. The classic spirometry finding in vocal cord dysfunction is flattening of the inspiratory loop when symptomatic (due to the variable extrathoracic obstruction) with a normal expiratory loop. When the patient is asymptomatic, normal spirometry results make diagnosis difficult.

2. Answer a.
This pregnant asthmatic is having a significant flare of her asthma, and aggressive treatment is warranted because of her decreased FEV_1, increased use of albuterol, and wheezing. In this situation, systemic corticosteroids are required. The main risk to the mother and child is hypoxia. Systemic corticosterids, inhaled corticosteroids, long- and short-acting inhaled β-agonists, and leukotriene receptor blockers are acceptable for use in the treatment of the pregnant asthmatic. For ongoing management, adding montelukast or increasing her budesonide dosage may be helpful, but these options are not the most effective in treating her acute exacerbation.

3. Answer b.
This patient has Samter Triad, a combination of nasal polyps, asthma, and aspirin sensitivity. In these patients, ingestion of aspirin results in significant asthma and rhinitis exacerbations through the inhibition of the cyclooxygenase-1 (COX-1) enzyme. Of the medications listed, ibuprofen is also primarily a COX-1 inhibitor as are the other commonly used anti-inflammatory agents, including naproxen, oxaprozin, nabumetone, and etodolac. Celecoxib and rofecoxib are COX-2 inhibitors and do not exacerbate asthma and rhinitis.

4. Answer b.
In an adult with intermittent angioedema, angiotensin-converting enzyme inhibitors are the most common cause, but this patient was not taking any blood pressure medications. There were no clear food or medication sensitivities in the history. The recurrent angioedema, coupled with fatigue and weight loss, is suggestive of an acquired C1 esterase inhibitor deficiency. Unlike hereditary angioedema, which typically presents within the first 3 decades, acquired C1 esterase inhibitor deficiency typically has an onset after the fifth decade. Hematologic malignancies are the underlying diseases most commonly associated with acquired C1 esterase inhibitor deficiency. Other malignancies have also been associated with C1 esterase inhibitor deficiency, although less commonly.

5. Answer c.
The clinical history is consistent with an IgE-mediated reaction to penicillin. Over time, the majority of patients lose their sensitivity to penicillin. Penicillin allergy can be assessed by skin testing to the major and minor determinants of penicillin. These are allergenic metabolites of penicillin. If the testing is negative, the patient can receive penicilllin, with the risk of a serious reaction being the same as for someone in the general population who has never had a reaction. Skin testing to only the major determinant will miss approximately 25% of patients who are penicillin allergic. If the skin testing is positive, the patient is at high risk of an IgE-mediated reaction and penicillin could be given only under a desensitization protocol.

6. Answer c.
Whenever nasal and sinus symptoms are unilateral, further anatomical evaluation is required to assess for tumor. This can be accomplished with rhinoscopy or CT scan of the sinuses. Plain film radiography is not sensitive for this evaluation. Allergic rhinitis should cause bilateral nasal symptoms. Skin prick testing is the test of choice for evaluation of airborne allergens (cat, dog, dust mite, molds, trees, grasses, and weeds). Intradermal skin testing is associated with a high false-positive rate for evaluation of airborne allergens, but it is helpful for evaluation of venom and drug allergy.

7. Answer b.
Recurrent sinopulmonary infections with common respiratory microorganisms are the primary manifestations of common variable immunodeficiency disease (CVID). The main laboratory abnormality in CVID is a depressed level of IgG. The hypogammaglobulinemia predisposes to recurrent sinus and pulmonary infections. Other manifestations include autoimmune processes and infectious diarrhea. The treatment of CVID is gamma globulin given intravenously or subcutaneously. The neutrophil adhesion assay is decreased in chronic granulomatous disease, which is characterized by recurrent skin and pulmonary abscesses. Deficiencies of the late complement system (C5, C6, C7, C8, and C9) typically manifest as recurrent infections with meningococci and gonococci.

3

Cardiology

Kyle W. Klarich, MD
Peter A. Brady, MB,ChB, MD
Abhiram Prasad, MD
Barry L. Karon, MD

Part I

Kyle W. Klarich, MD

Physical Examination

Even given all the recent technologic advances in medical testing and imaging, it is imperative that physicians be able to accurately assess patients at the bedside so that the clinician can order the appropriate and cost-effective test efficiently. This chapter outlines the salient features of a thorough physical examination.

Jugular Venous Pressure

Jugular venous pressure indicates the pressure of the right atrium (Figure 3-1). Changes in amplitude of waves may indicate structural disease and rhythm changes. The jugular venous pressure is normally 6 to 8 cm H_2O (1 mm Hg is equal to 1.36 cm H_2O) and is best evaluated with the patient supine at an angle of 45° or more. The right atrium lies about 5±1 cm below the sternal angle, and thus the estimated jugular venous pressure is equal to the height of the jugular venous pressure above the sternal angle + 5 cm. The normal waves profile contains an *a* deflection, which reflects atrial contraction; *c* deflection, closure of tricuspid valve; followed by the *x* descent, downward motion of right ventricle; and *v* deflection, atrial filling deflection while the tricuspid valve is closed followed by the *y* descent, representing ventricular filling as the tricuspid valve opens.

* Normal jugular venous pressure is 6-8 cm H_2O.
* Normal waves are *a*, atrial contraction; *c*, closure of tricuspid valve; and *v*, atrial filling.
* *x* descent, downward motion of right ventricle.
* *y* descent, early right ventricular filling phase.

The examiner should distinguish jugular venous pressure from carotid pulsations: jugular venous pressure varies with respiration, is nonpalpable with gentle pressure, and can be eliminated by obstructing pressure at the diastolic end. When the pressure is increased, consideration should be given to not only biventricular failure but also constrictive pericarditis, pericardial tamponade, cor pulmonale (especially pulmonary embolus), and superior vena cava syndrome.

Abnormalities of the waves indicate various conditions, as follows:

1. Increased jugular venous pressure, increased pressure indicating possible fluid overload. Common in congestive heart failure
2. Large *a* wave: tricuspid stenosis, right ventricular hypertrophy, pulmonary hypertension (ie, increased right ventricular end-diastolic pressure)
3. Cannon *a* wave: atria contracting intermittently against a closed atrioventricular valve (atrioventricular dissociation)
4. Rapid *x* + *y* descent: constrictive pericarditis
5. Kussmaul sign: venous filling with inspiration, pericardial tamponade, or constriction. Paradoxical increase in venous pressure with inspiration occurs in pericardial tamponade, constriction, and right ventricular failure
6. Large, fused *cv* wave: tricuspid regurgitation

* Increased jugular venous pressure increases the likelihood of congestive heart failure 4-fold.

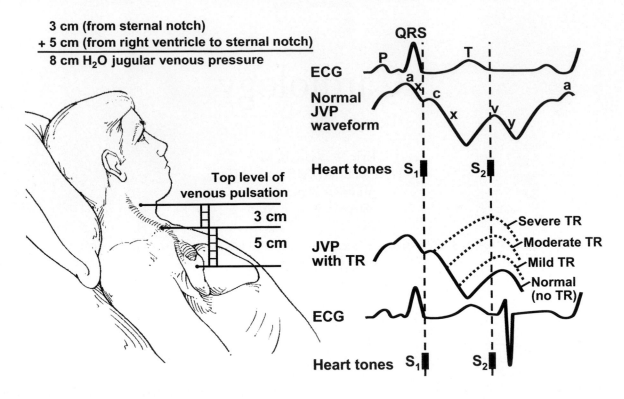

Figure 3-1. Evaluation of Jugular Venous Pressure (JVP). ECG indicates electrocardiogram; TR, tricuspid regurgitation.

• Increased jugular venous pressure can be associated with pulmonary embolus, superior vena cava syndrome, tamponade, and constriction.
• Abnormalities of waves:
    large *a* wave: tricuspid stenosis, right ventricular hypertrophy, pulmonary hypertension
    cannon *a* wave: atria contracting against a closed atrioventricular valve (atrioventricular dissociation)
    rapid *x* + *y* descent: constrictive pericarditis

Arterial Pulse

Palpation of the radial pulse is useful for rate; the brachial or carotid pulse is checked for contour. Tardus is the timing and rate of rise of upstroke, and parvus is the volume. In hypertension, a radial-femoral delay (checking radial and femoral pulses simultaneously) may indicate accompanying aortic coarctation.

Abnormalities of the arterial pulse and their indicated conditions are as follows (Figure 3-2):
1. Parvus and tardus: aortic stenosis
2. Parvus only: low output, cardiomyopathy
3. Bounding: aortic regurgitation or atrioventricular fistulas
4. Bifid (2 systolic peaks): hypertrophic obstructive cardiomyopathy (from midsystolic obstruction)
5. Bisferiens (2 systolic peaks, occurs when a large volume is ejected rapidly, and a distinct systolic dip): aortic regurgitation
6. Dicrotic (a systolic peak followed by diastolic pulse wave): left

ventricular failure with hypotension, low output, and increased peripheral resistance
7. Pulsus paradoxus (exaggerated inspiratory decrease [>10 mm Hg] in pulse pressure): suggestive of tamponade
8. Pulsus alternans (alternating strong and weak pulse): severe depression of left ventricular function

Apical Impulse

This is normally a discrete area of localized contraction. It is usually maximal at the fifth intercostal space, midclavicular line.

Abnormalities of the apical impulse and their indicated conditions are as follows:
1. Apex displaced (laterally or downward or both), impulse poor and diffuse: cardiomyopathy
2. Sustained, but not necessarily displaced: left ventricular hypertrophy, aortic stenosis, often with large *a* wave
3. Trifid (or multifid): hypertrophic cardiomyopathy
4. Hyperdynamic, descended, and diffuse with rapid filling wave: mitral regurgitation, aortic regurgitation
5. Tapping quality, localized, nondisplaced; normal, or can occur in mitral stenosis

• Abnormalities of apical impulse:
    Apex displaced, impulse poor and diffuse: cardiomyopathy
    Trifid: hypertrophic cardiomyopathy
    Tapping quality, localized: normal or mitral stenosis

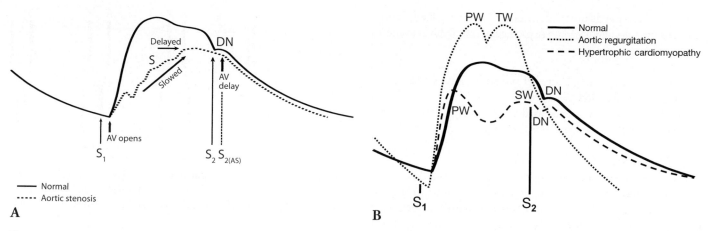

A

B

Figure 3-2. Variations in Arterial Pulse. A, Solid line indicates normal contour. Dotted line indicates typical contour of calcific aortic stenosis (AS; slowed and delayed). S_2 is delayed in aortic stenosis as ejection time prolongs. AN indicates anacrotic notch; AV, aortic valve; DN, dicrotic notch. B, Solid line indicates normal contour. Dotted line indicates aortic regurgitation (bisferiens pulse, rapid upstroke, percussion wave [PW], tidal wave [TW], rapid runoff). Dashed line indicates hypertrophic cardiomyopathy (bifid pulse, also known as "spike and dome," rapid PW, then often a secondary wave [SW]).

Additional Cardiac Palpation

A palpable aortic valve component (A_2) at the right upper sternum suggests a dilated aorta (eg, aneurysm, dissection, severe aortic regurgitation, poststenotic dilatation in aortic stenosis, hypertension).

Severe tricuspid regurgitation may result in a pulsatile liver palpable in the right epigastrium. One should look for accompanying hepatojugular reflux, that is, distention of the external jugular vein 3 to 4 beats after compression of the liver. In patients with severe emphysema, the apical impulse rotates medially and also may be appreciated in the epigastrium and could be confused with a pulsatile liver.

Right ventricular hypertrophy results in sustained lift, best appreciated in the fourth intercostal space 2 to 3 cm left parasternally. Diastolic overload (eg, atrial septal defect, anomalous pulmonary venous return) results in a vigorous outward and upward motion but may not be sustained. In significant pulmonary hypertension, the pulmonary valve component (P_2) may be palpable (this may be physiologic in slender people with small anteroposterior diameter).

- Pressure overload of the right ventricle usually results in sustained, lateralized impulses.
- Volume overload (eg, regurgitant lesions, atrial septal defect) usually is appreciated as dynamic and forceful but not sustained impulses.
- Palpable A_2 or P_2 components are considered pathologic in adults with average body habitus.

Thrills

Thrills indicate turbulent flow (such as aortic stenosis, ventricular septal defect).

Heart Sounds

The art of cardiac auscultation is best understood by keeping in mind the relationship of the cardiac cycle (Figure 3-3).

First Heart Sound

The first heart sound (S_1) consists of audible mitral valve closure followed shortly by tricuspid valve closure. Shortly after, the normally silent aortic and pulmonary valve openings occur after a period known as the isovolumic contraction time. A loud S_1 occurs with, for example, mitral stenosis and short PR intervals because the mitral valve is wide open when the left ventricle begins to contract and then slaps shut (assumes some preserved pliability of the mitral valve leaflets). S_1 also is augmented in hypercontractile states (eg, fever, exercise, thyrotoxicosis, pheochromocytomas, anxiety, anemia). The intensity of S_1 is *decreased* if the mitral valve is heavily calcified and immobile (severe mitral stenosis) and with a long PR interval (occurs

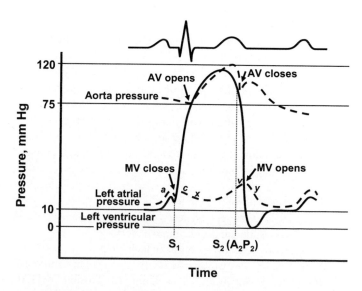

Figure 3-3. The Normal Cardiac Cycle. AV indicates aortic valve, MV, mitral valve.

classically with acute rheumatic fever), poor left ventricular function, and rapid diastolic filling leading to premature mitral valve closure, as in aortic regurgitation.

* Loud S_1 occurs with a short PR interval, mitral stenosis, and hypercontractile states.
* The intensity of S_1 is decreased with heavily calcified mitral valve, long PR interval, and aortic regurgitation.

Second Heart Sound

The second heart sound (S_2) consists of aortic valve closure followed by pulmonary valve closure. Intensity of both is increased by hypertension (ie, loud or tympanic A_2 with systemic hypertension and a loud P_2 with pulmonary hypertension, P_2 is then audible at apex). Intensity is decreased with heavily calcified valves (severe aortic stenosis). Normally, the split between A_2 and P_2 widens on inspiration and narrows on expiration as a result of the relative increase in blood return to the right side of the heart during inspiration and greater capacitance of the lungs, such that A_2 moves slightly closer to S_1 and P_2 moves farther away (Figure 3-4). The sequence is reversed during expiration. This is normal physiologic splitting of S_2. This is best heard in the left second intercostal space with the patient seated.

* The intensity of S_2 is increased by hypertension.
* The intensity of S_2 is decreased with heavily calcified valves.
* Physiologic splitting of S_2 occurs in inspiration as a result of increased blood return to the right side of the heart.

The interplay of multiple factors can affect the timing of the closure of semilunar values: electrical activation, duration of ventricular ejection, gradient across semilunar valves, and elastic recoil properties of the great vessels.

Common conditions leading to abnormalities of splitting of the S_2 and their indicated conditions are as follows:

1. Physiologic splitting: normal splitting due to respiratory variation of blood flow; on inspiration, A moves to the "left" closer to S_1, and P moves to the "right" away from S_1
2. Fixed split: atrial septal defect, widest split occurs with a combination of atrial septal defect and pulmonary stenosis
3. Paradoxic split (caused by delay in aortic closure so it closes after pulmonary valve): left bundle branch block
4. Persistent splitting: occurs during right bundle branch block. A_2 and P_2 are separated because of delayed electromechanical activation of the right ventricle; this effect is accentuated further by inspiration

* Abnormalities of splitting of S_2:
  Fixed split: atrial septal defect
  Paradoxic split: left bundle branch block
  Persistently split: right bundle branch block
* Mnemonic for normal valve sequence: S_1-S_2 (right ventricular-left ventricular sequence): "Many Things Are Possible" (MTAP; S_1 = mitral opens before tricuspid; S_2 = aortic closes before pulmonic).

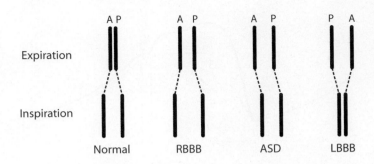

Figure 3-4. Effects of Respiration and Conduction on the Second Heart Sound. The A indicates aortic closure; ASD, atrial septal defect; LBBB, left bundle branch block; P, pulmonary closure; RBBB, right bundle branch block.

Third Heart Sound

The third heart sound (S_3) occurs in early diastole, coinciding with maximal early diastolic left ventricular filling. Its origin is debated, but it may be caused by tensing of the chordae as the blood distends the left ventricle during diastole. It is a low-pitched sound best heard with the bell of the stethoscope. It is normally heard in young people (younger than 30 years—a normal variant due to excellent ventricular distensibility) and pathologically in heart failure. In adults, it is associated with volume load on the left ventricle, such as aortic regurgitation, mitral regurgitation, and cardiomyopathy.

* S_3 is a normal variant in children and very fit young adults.
* S_3 in adults is associated with volume load on the left ventricle (aortic regurgitation, mitral regurgitation, cardiomyopathy).

Fourth Heart Sound

Like S_3, the fourth heart sound (S_4) is a low-pitched sound best heard with the bell of the stethoscope, loudest at the apex. This occurs with the atrial "kick" as blood is forced into the left ventricle by atrial contraction when the left ventricle is stiff and noncompliant. Examples, such as in aortic stenosis, systemic hypertension, hypertrophic cardiomyopathy, and ischemia, often present with the generation of S_4. It cannot occur with loss of atrial contraction (ie, atrial fibrillation).

* S_4 occurs in aortic stenosis, systemic hypertension, hypertrophic cardiomyopathy, and ischemia.
* S_4 cannot occur with loss of atrial contraction (ie, atrial fibrillation).

Opening Snap

Opening snap is an early diastolic sound caused by opening of the pathologic rheumatic mitral valve. It is virtually always caused by mitral stenosis, and the interval from the S_2 to the opening snap helps determine the severity. With severe mitral stenosis, the left atrial pressure is very high and thus the valve opens earlier, and the interval is less than 60 m/s.

* Opening snap is virtually always caused by mitral stenosis.

Murmurs

The specific murmurs are discussed with the individual valvular lesions described later in this chapter, but some broad guidelines follow here.

A systolic ejection murmur begins after S_1 and ends before S_2. It may have a diamond-shaped quality with crescendo and decrescendo components, but, in general, the more severe the obstruction (the narrower the orifice), the louder the murmur and the later the peak of the murmur. It may be preceded by an ejection click, if the pliability of the valve is preserved. Echocardiography may be required if there is a diastolic murmur or a systolic murmur of grade 3 or higher or if there are other signs or symptoms of cardiac disease (Figure 3-5).

- For systolic ejection murmur, in general, the more severe the obstruction, the louder the murmur and the later the peak.

A holosystolic murmur occurs when blood goes from a high-pressure to a low-pressure system (eg, mitral regurgitation, ventricular septal defect). It engulfs S_1 and S_2.

- A holosystolic murmur occurs with mitral regurgitation and ventricular septal defect.

Maneuvers That Alter Cardiac Murmurs

Inspiration increases venous return and thus increases right-sided sounds (S_3 and S_4) and murmurs, tricuspid and pulmonary stenosis, and tricuspid and pulmonary regurgitation. *Valsalva maneuver* increases intrathoracic pressure, inhibiting venous return and thus decreasing preload. Most cardiac murmurs and sounds diminish in intensity during Valsalva maneuver because of decreased ventricular filling and decreased cardiac output (except hypertrophic obstructive cardiomyopathy, which increases because of dynamic left ventricular outflow obstruction accentuated by decreased preload). *Handgrip* increases cardiac output and systemic arterial pressure, decreasing the gradient producing the murmur across the aortic valve. A *change in posture* from supine to upright causes a decrease in venous return; therefore, stroke volume decreases, and this decrease causes a reflex increase in heart rate and peripheral resistance. *Squatting* and the

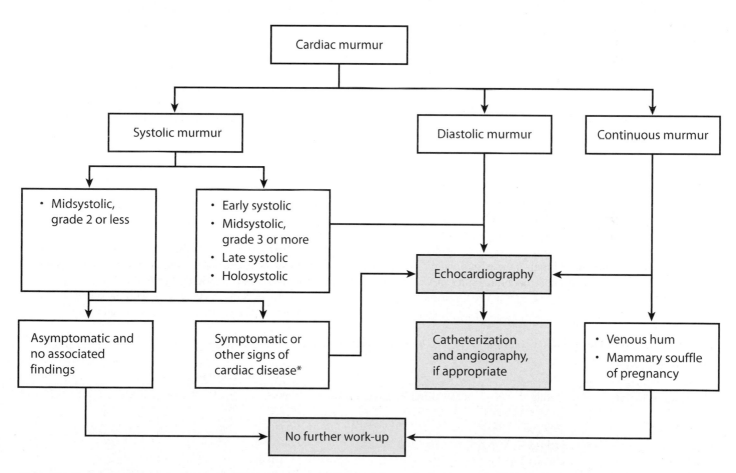

Figure 3-5. Recommendations for Evaluating Heart Murmurs. *If electrocardiography or chest radiography has been performed and the results are abnormal, echocardiography is recommended. (From Bonow RO, Carabello BA, Chatterjee K, de Leon AC Jr, Faxon DP, Freed MD, et al. ACC/AHA 2006 guidelines for the management of patients with valvular heart disease: a report of the American College of Cardiology/American Heart Association Task Force on Practice Guidelines [Writing Committee to Revise the 1998 Guidelines for the Management of Patients With Valvular Heart Disease]. Circulation. 2006;114:e84-e231. Used with permission.)

Valsalva maneuver have opposite hemodynamic effects. Squatting increases peripheral resistance and increases venous return. *Amyl nitrite* pharmacologically decreases afterload. It is supplied in a vial that can be crushed; the amyl nitrite is inhaled by the patient and works transiently. It increases the murmur, producing gradient between the left ventricle and the aorta. It increases the murmurs of hypertrophic obstructive cardiomyopathy and aortic stenosis. The effects of maneuvers are shown in Table 3-1.

- Bedside maneuvers that alter cardiac murmurs:
    Inspiration
    Valsalva maneuver
    Handgrip
    Change in posture
    Squatting
    Inhalation of amyl nitrite
- The maneuver used to distinguish aortic stenosis and hypertrophic cardiomopathy is the Valsalva maneuver.

Valvular Heart Disease

Aortic Stenosis

The pathophysiologic effect of aortic stenosis on the heart is that of a pressure load, leading to pressure hypertrophy of the left ventricle. Although cases of supravalvular and subvalvular aortic stenosis are appreciated, these are beyond the scope of this review. The vast majority of cases of aortic stenosis are due to valvular stenosis.

Types

The *congenital bicuspid* type of aortic stenosis occurs in 2% of the population. It may be associated with obstruction in infancy through early adulthood. It is the most common cause of aortic stenosis in adults younger than 55 years. Frequently, when a patient is young and the valve is still pliable, the auscultation is different from that of degenerative aortic valve disease. An ejection click often precedes the systolic murmur. The earlier the click (ie, the closer to S_1), the more severe the stenosis. A_2 is delayed with progressive stenosis, and when severe, there may be paradoxic splitting of the second sound. Bicuspid aortic valve may be associated with coarctation of the aorta (10% of

patients). If bicuspid aortic valve is suspected, the diagnosis usually can be made successfully with 2-dimensional and Doppler echocardiography without the need for cardiac catheterization in young people. If the diagnosis is confirmed, the aorta should be imaged with ultrasonography or computed tomography to rule out coarctation.

- Congenital bicuspid valvular aortic stenosis occurs in 2% of the population.
- It is the most common cause of aortic stenosis in adults younger than 55 years.
- An ejection click often precedes the systolic murmur.
- The earlier the click (closer to first heart sound), the more severe the stenosis.
- A_2 is delayed with progressive stenosis; when severe, there may be paradoxic splitting of the second sound.

Degenerative aortic valve disease is the most common cause of aortic stenosis in adults older than 55 years. The valve is tricuspid and calcified. When calcification is extensive, A_2 becomes inaudible.

- Degenerative aortic valve disease is the most common cause of aortic stenosis in adults older than 55 years.
- When calcification is extensive, A_2 becomes inaudible.

The *rheumatic* type of aortic valve disease is less common. It is associated with thickening and fusion of the aortic cusps at the commissures. It always occurs with a rheumatic mitral valve, although considerable mitral stenosis or regurgitation may not always be evident. It usually occurs in adulthood (age 40-60 years), usually 15±5 years after acute rheumatic fever.

- The rheumatic type of aortic valve disease is a less common cause of valvular aortic stenosis.
- It usually occurs at 40-60 years of age.

Symptoms

The classic symptoms of the valvular type of aortic stenosis (regardless of type) include exertional dyspnea, syncope, angina, and sudden cardiac death. The onset of symptoms is an ominous sign. The

Table 3-1   Effects of Physical Maneuvers and Other Factors on Valvular Diseases

Maneuver or Factor	Result	Effect on Murmur			
		Mitral Regurgitation	MVP	Aortic Stenosis	HOCM
Amyl nitrite	↓ afterload	↓	↑/0	↑	↑
Valsalva	↓ preload	↓	↑	↓	↑
Handgrip	↑ afterload	↑	↓/0	↓	↓
Post-PVC	↑ contractility ↓ afterload	=	↓	↑	↑[a]

Abbreviations: HOCM, hypertrophic obstructive cardiomyopathy; MVP, mitral valve prolapse; PVC, premature ventricular complex.
[a] Although the murmur increases, the peripheral pulse decreases because of the increase in outflow obstruction.

presence of angina does not necessarily indicate coexisting coronary disease; rather, it is related to increased left ventricular filling pressure causing subendocardial ischemia.

- Symptoms of aortic stenosis: exertional dyspnea, syncope, angina, and sudden cardiac death.
- Angina does not necessarily indicate coexisting coronary disease.

Physical Examination

The pulse is parvus and tardus in hemodynamically significant aortic stenosis. The left ventricular impulse is localized, lateralized, and sustained. Arterial thrills may be palpable at the carotid artery, suprasternal notch, second intercostal space, or left and right sternal borders. A fourth heart sound may be present, both palpable and audible. A$_2$ is diminished and delayed and may even become absent with decreasing pliability of the aortic cusps. The ejection systolic murmur becomes louder and peaks later with increasing severity, radiating to the carotid arteries and the apex.

- The pulse is parvus (small) and tardus (delayed) in hemodynamically significant aortic stenosis.
- The ejection systolic murmur becomes louder with increasing severity.
- A$_2$ is diminished, delayed, or absent with progressive aortic stenosis.

Diagnosis

Electrocardiography in aortic stenosis may show left ventricular hypertrophy (not a sensitive index; echocardiography is better), but the results often are normal in young patients. Left bundle branch block is common, and in later stages of the condition conduction abnormalities may develop (eg, complete heart block) if the calcium impinges on the conducting system. On chest radiography, the heart size is normal, until left ventricular remodeling occurs in the late stages, even when the stenosis is severe. The aortic root may show poststenotic dilatation. In degenerative aortic valve disease, calcium in the valve leaflets may be seen, especially on a penetrated lateral view.

- Electrocardiography is often normal in young patients with aortic stenosis.
- Left bundle branch block is common on electrocardiography.
- The aortic root may show poststenotic dilatation on chest radiography.

Differential diagnoses include 1) hypertrophic cardiomyopathy (note different carotid upstroke and change in murmur with Valsalva maneuver) and 2) mitral regurgitation (murmur may radiate anteriorly and upward along the aorta, particularly if there is rupture of chordae of the posterior mitral valve leaflet; however, there is no radiation to the carotid arteries).

Aortic stenosis can be diagnosed with bedside physical examination. The most important physical finding is the parvus and tardus pulse. However, the degree of aortic stenosis can be difficult to determine, particularly in older patients. Doppler echocardiography is useful for assessing gradients and correlates well with cardiac

catheterization. Severe aortic stenosis is present when the mean Doppler gradient is more than 40 mm Hg, the valve area is less than 1.0 cm^2, and the valve index is 0.6 cm^2/ m^2. Progression to symptoms can be insidious. Progression is about 0.12 cm^2 per year. With onset of symptoms, survival is 1 to 3 years (Figure 3-6).

- Aortic stenosis can be diagnosed with bedside physical examination.
- The most important physical finding is the parvus and tardus pulse.
- Two-dimensional and Doppler echocardiography is useful for diagnosis.
- Severe aortic stenosis: gradient is >40 mm Hg, valve area is <1.0 cm^2, and valve index is 0.6 cm^2/m^2.

Treatment

All patients with aortic stenosis should receive antibiotic prophylaxis for bacterial endocarditis. They should be educated about symptoms that may develop and should promptly report any evidence of symptoms: dyspnea, chest pain, angina, syncope, or congestive heart failure (Table 3-2). Aortic valve replacement is the only effective treatment for patients with severe obstruction.

- Aortic valve replacement is the only effective treatment of aortic stenosis.

Aortic Regurgitation

The pathophysiology of aortic regurgitation is that of volume and pressure overload on the left ventricle, leading to hypertrophy and dilatation. The cause can be related to either the aortic root or aortic valve and the condition can be acute or chronic (Table 3-3).

Valvular

Causes of valvular aortic regurgitation include 1) congenital bicuspid valve, 2) rheumatic fever, 3) endocarditis, 4) degenerative aortic valve disease, 5) seronegative arthritis, 6) ankylosing spondylitis, and 7) rheumatoid arthritis.

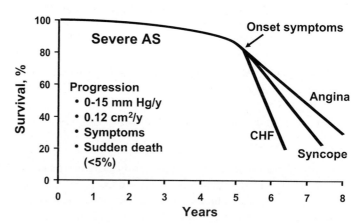

Figure 3-6. Natural History of Aortic Stenosis (AS). CHF indicates congestive heart failure. (Modified from Ross J Jr, Braunwald E. Aortic stenosis. Circulation. 1968;37 Suppl 5:61-7. Used with permission.)

Table 3-2   Quantitation of the Severity of Aortic Stenosis and Treatment Guidelines

Severity	AVA, cm^2	AVA Index, cm^2/m^2	Gradient, mm Hg	Follow-up or Treatment
Normal	3.0-4.0		<10	
Mild	>1.5	>0.8	<30	Echo every 5 y or if symptoms
Moderate	1.0-1.5	0.5-0.8	30-40	Monitor for symptoms
				Echo every 1-2 y
Severe	<1.0	<0.6	>40	Symptoms: operate
				No symptoms: echo every 6-12 mo

Abbreviations: AVA, aortic valve area; echo, echocardiography.
Data from Bonow RO, Carabello BA, Chatterjee K, de Leon AC Jr, Faxon DP, Freed MD, et al. ACC/AHA 2006 guidelines for the management of patients with valvular heart disease: a report of the American College of Cardiology/American Heart Association Task Force on Practice Guidelines (Writing Committee to Revise the 1998 Guidelines for the Management of Patients With Valvular Heart Disease). Circulation. 2006;114:e84-e231.

Aortic Root Dilatation

Various conditions have been associated with aortic root dilatation. Marfan syndrome can be associated with progressive dilatation of the aortic root and sinuses (so-called cystic medial necrosis). Prophylactic β-adrenergic blocker therapy is effective for slowing the rate of aortic dilatation and reducing the development of aortic complications in some patients with Marfan syndrome. When the aortic root reaches 5 to 5.5 cm or more in diameter, it should be replaced. Syphilis is an uncommon cause of aortic regurgitation and usually causes aortic root dilatation above the sinuses (syphilis spares the sinuses). It should be remembered that syphilis is associated with calcium in the aortic root on chest radiography. Age is also a related factor. With advancing age, the aorta dilates; hypertension also tends to accelerate this process. Acute aortic regurgitation may be associated with an aortic dissection.

* Marfan syndrome can be associated with aortic root dilatation.
* Hypertension is a common cause of (usually mild) aortic regurgitation.
* Syphilis is an uncommon cause of aortic regurgitation.

Symptoms

The symptoms of acute aortic regurgitation are extreme: pulmonary edema, shock, and, often, chest pain (in the setting of aortic dissection). The symptoms of chronic aortic regurgitation include fatigue, dyspnea, palpitations, and exertional angina.

Physical Examination

With severe aortic regurgitation, several physical signs have been

Table 3-3   Aortic Regurgitation: Symptoms and Findings on Examination

	Acute	Chronic
Symptoms	Pulmonary edema Shock Arrhythmia Chest pain Dissection, RCA infarct	Dyspnea Fatigue Exercise intolerance Night sweats Palpitations
Examination	Faint, short murmur	Peripheral pulses Quincke and Duroziez signs, pistol-shot pulse Enlarged, diffuse, hyperdynamic LV Murmur LSB—valve etiology RSB—root etiology
Chest radiography	Wide mediastinum Pulmonary edema	Enlarged heart Enlarged aorta
Electrocardiography	Low voltage (if pericardial effusion) ST elevation II, III, F (if aortic dissection into RCA)	LVH

Abbreviations: LSB, left sternal border; LV, left ventricle; LVH, left ventricular hypertrophy; RCA, right coronary artery; RSB, right sternal border.

reported. A bounding, rapidly collapsing Corrigan pulse resulting from wide pulse pressure is found. A bisferiens pulse may be present. Other findings are de Musset head nodding, Duroziez sign (systolic and diastolic ["to-and-fro"] murmur of gentle compression with stethoscope) over the femoral artery, and Quincke sign (pulsatile capillary nail bed). Müller sign (systolic pulsations of the uvula) is often noted. The left ventricular impulse is diffuse and hyperdynamic, and the apex beat is often displaced downward. A diastolic decrescendo murmur is heard at either the left or the right sternal border, and the S$_2$ may be paradoxically split because of increased left ventricular volume.

The duration of the murmur is related to the rate of pressure equilibration between the aorta and the left ventricle. Mild aortic regurgitation with physiologic diastolic pressures results in a holodiastolic murmur. The shorter the murmur, the faster the pressure equilibration, the more severe the aortic regurgitation, or the higher the left ventricular end-diastolic pressure. The loudness of the murmur does not correlate with the severity of aortic regurgitation, particularly in acute aortic regurgitation (such as with dissection). A systolic flow murmur is common, because of the increased ejection volume. It does not necessarily indicate coexistent structural aortic stenosis.

- Findings indicative of aortic regurgitation: bounding, rapidly collapsing Corrigan pulse, diastolic decrescendo murmur, and an S_2 that may be paradoxically split.
- The duration, but not the loudness, of the murmur, is related to the severity of the aortic regurgitation (shorter is more severe).

Diagnosis

Although the diagnosis of aortic regurgitation can be made at bedside clinical examination, it can be missed if a patient with acute aortic regurgitation presents with little or no murmur. Electrocardiography often shows left ventricular hypertrophy. Echocardiography is best suited to gather the important functional and hemodynamic data needed to make management decisions in patients with aortic regurgitation.

Because aortic regurgitation has a long, silent, well-compensated natural history, key factors should be routinely followed with echocardiography: left ventricular size, aortic root size and morphology, valve morphology, and left ventricular function (ejection fraction).

Chest radiography shows an enlarged cardiac shadow and prominence of the left ventricular enlargement in a leftward and inferior pattern. The aorta also may be enlarged, especially in Marfan syndrome.

Table 3-4 outlines the natural history of severe aortic regurgitation.

- In aortic regurgitation, electrocardiography may show left ventricular hypertrophy.
- Echocardiography is useful to confirm the diagnosis and guide therapy.

Treatment

Acute severe aortic regurgitation is a surgical emergency. As a bridge to operation, nitroprusside to reduce peripheral resistance and encourage forward flow or inotropic agents may be considered to augment cardiac output. An intra-aortic balloon pump is contraindicated because it will worsen regurgitation.

Chronic aortic regurgitation is a combined volume and pressure overload on the left ventricle. The left ventricle compensates by dilating and increasing compliance. Hence, patients with aortic regurgitation may remain asymptomatic for decades. The development of symptoms, however, usually reflects left ventricular dysfunction, and survival is limited unless surgical intervention is prompt. Medical management, such as an angiotensin-converting enzyme inhibitor or nifedipine, has been shown to slow ventricular dilatation in patients with severe aortic regurgitation and may help to delay operation. However, compensation cannot be maintained indefinitely and eventually left ventricular filling pressure increases, coronary flow reserve diminishes, and left ventricular dysfunction develops insidiously. Angina in the absence of epicardial coronary stenosis may be present. Asymptomatic dysfunction may develop in a subset of patients. In an attempt to operate before left ventricular dysfunction develops, several factors have been suggested: a systolic dimension more than 55 mm, a diastolic dimension more than 75 mm, or an ejection fraction less than 50%. Asymptomatic patients with dilated left ventricles need to be followed carefully; if there is evidence of resting left ventricular systolic dysfunction, progressive diastolic dysfunction, or rapidly progressive left ventricular dilatation, operation should be performed.

Table 3-4   Natural History of Severe Aortic Regurgitation

Status of Patient	% of Patients/y
Asymptomatic with normal LV systolic function	
Progression to symptoms or LV dysfunction	<6
Progression to asymptomatic LV dysfunction	<3.5
Sudden death	<0.2
Asymptomatic with LV dysfunction	
Progression to cardiac symptoms	>25
Symptomatic	
Mortality rate	>10

Abbreviation: LV, left ventricular.
From Bonow RO, Carabello BA, Chatterjee K, de Leon AC Jr, Faxon DP, Freed MD, et al. ACC/AHA 2006 guidelines for the management of patients with valvular heart disease: a report of the American College of Cardiology/American Heart Association Task Force on Practice Guidelines (Writing Committee to Revise the 1998 Guidelines for the Management of Patients With Valvular Heart Disease). Circulation. 2006;114:e84-e231. Used with permission.

The possibility for valve preservation (repair vs replacement) may favor earlier operation before left ventricular dilatation has occurred.

- Acute aortic regurgitation is a surgical emergency.
- Patients with aortic regurgitation can be asymptomatic for several years.
- If symptoms develop, survival is limited unless surgical intervention is prompt.
- If ejection fraction decreases below normal, operation is needed.

Mitral Stenosis

Mitral stenosis is obstructive to the flow of blood from the left atrium to the left ventricle, preventing proper diastolic filling and leading to pulmonary congestion. Mitral stenosis is almost always due to rheumatic heart disease causing leaflet thickening with fusion of the commissures and later calcification.

Symptoms

Symptoms of mitral stenosis do not usually develop for decades after rheumatic fever. The murmur of mitral stenosis is apparent on physical examination about 10 years after rheumatic fever. Then, in another 10 years, symptoms develop, usually dyspnea and later orthopnea with paroxysmal nocturnal dyspnea, which can be insidious. Atrial fibrillation often causes considerable deterioration of clinical status. Hemoptysis and pulmonary hypertension with signs of right-sided failure (ie, ascites and peripheral edema) are late manifestations. Systemic emboli also may result from atrial fibrillation (about 20% without anticoagulation).

- Mitral stenosis is almost always due to rheumatic heart disease.
- Symptoms do not develop for decades after mitral stenosis is found on physical examination.

- Symptoms: dyspnea, orthopnea with paroxysmal nocturnal dyspnea.
- Atrial fibrillation causes considerable deterioration of clinical status.

Physical Examination

The S_1 in mitral stenosis is loud. The shorter the interval from S_1 (A_2) to the opening snap, the more severe the mitral stenosis. An opening snap occurs only with a pliable valve, and it disappears when the valve calcifies. The stenosis is mild if this interval is more than 90 milliseconds, moderate if it is 80 milliseconds, and severe if it is less than 60 milliseconds. The diastolic murmur is a low-pitched, holodiastolic rumble, heard best at the apex with the bell of the stethoscope. The murmur may have presystolic accentuation if sinus rhythm is present. Right ventricular lift and increased P_2 are associated with pulmonary hypertension.

- Physical examination in mitral stenosis:
  Loud S_1
  The shorter the interval from A_2 to the opening snap, the more severe the stenosis
  Diastolic murmur is a low-pitched holodiastolic rumble
  The longer the murmur, the more severe the stenosis

Diagnosis

Electrocardiography shows P mitrale and later right ventricular hypertrophy. Chest radiography (Figure 3-7) shows straightening of the left heart border with a large left atrial shadow and dilated upper lobe pulmonary veins. With pulmonary hypertension, the central pulmonary arteries become prominent. In severe stenosis, Kerley B lines may be present, indicating a pulmonary wedge pressure of more than 20 mm Hg.

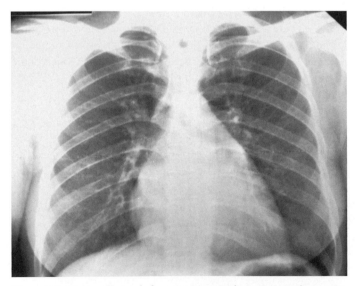

Figure 3-7. Chest radiograph from a patient with severe mitral stenosis, showing a typical straight left heart border, prominent pulmonary artery, large left atrium, right ventricular contour, and pulmonary venous hypertension.

- In mitral stenosis, electrocardiography shows P mitrale and later right ventricular hypertrophy.
- Chest radiography shows straightening of the left heart border, a large left atrial shadow, and dilated upper lobe pulmonary veins.
- In severe stenosis, Kerley B lines may be present.

Two-dimensional and Doppler echocardiography is the test of choice to diagnose mitral stenosis and determine its severity. Information is gained about valve gradient and valve area (Table 3-5), and pulmonary artery pressures can be noninvasively assessed. Cardiac catheterization is usually unnecessary unless the coronary arteries need to be studied or the echocardiographic findings do not concur with the clinical situation. Severe stenosis usually correlates with a mean gradient of 12 mm Hg or more.

- Two-dimensional and Doppler echocardiography is used to diagnose mitral stenosis and determine its severity.
- For diagnosis of mitral stenosis, cardiac catheterization is usually unnecessary.
- Severe stenosis correlates with a mean gradient ≥12 mm Hg.

Treatment

Rheumatic fever is the cause of mitral stenosis, and prophylaxis for rheumatic fever is warranted.

Because mitral stenosis represents obstruction to diastolic filling, anything that shortens diastolic filling time will worsen the severity and symptoms of the disease (eg, tachycardia, atrial fibrillation, exercise). Therefore, β-adrenergic blockers and calcium channel blockers are reasonable choices to help with better left ventricular filling. Salt restriction and diuretic therapy are useful for early symptoms.

The left ventricle is unaffected, protected from volume or pressure overload. It is small, vigorous, and possibly underfilled late in mitral stenosis. Intervention is not needed until there are symptoms of exertional dyspnea, pulmonary edema, or moderate pulmonary hypertension. Marked volume overload of the left atrium leads to increased stroke risk and intervention. Because atrial fibrillation is frequent and intermittent in the early stages, intermittent screening with Holter electrocardiography may be warranted, and anticoagulation should be considered early. With a pliable valve that is noncalcified and has no regurgitation, a mitral valve balloon valvuloplasty can be performed percutaneously, and this may preclude the need for valve replacement for at least 10 years.

Table 3-5   Severity of Mitral Stenosis, by Valve Area, Gradient, and Pulmonary Pressure

Severity	Valve Area, cm²	Mean Gradient, mm Hg	Systolic PAP, mm Hg
Mild	1.5-2	<6	Normal
Moderate	1-1.5	6-11	≤50
Severe	<1	≥12	>50

Abbreviation: PAP, pulmonary artery pressure.

- Intervention for mitral stenosis is indicated with exertional dyspnea, pulmonary edema, or moderate pulmonary hypertension (>50 mm Hg).
- Atrial fibrillation is a common consequence of left atrial volume overload.
- Anticoagulation should be considered for stroke prophylaxis.
- Percutaneous balloon valvuloplasty is the procedure of choice if the valve leaflets are pliable.

Mitral Regurgitation

Etiology

The mitral valve is a complex structure, and regurgitation can result from 3 general anatomical abnormalities: leaflet, tensor apparatus (chordal and papillary muscles), and alteration of myocardium. Common causes of mitral regurgitation include mitral valve prolapse syndrome and myxomatous degeneration, infective endocarditis, collagen vascular disease, ischemia, and rheumatic heart disease (Table 3-6). In the case of ischemic mitral regurgitation, the posterior medial papillary muscle with its single blood supply (compared with anterolateral, which has dual blood supply) is more susceptible.

- Most common causes of mitral regurgitation are mitral valve prolapse and myxomatous degeneration, ischemia, and infective endocarditis.

Symptoms

Chronic mitral regurgitation is a volume overload on the left ventricle with reduced afterload. Given time, the left ventricle can compensate by increasing stroke volume. Therefore, a long asymptomatic phase is possible. The most common symptoms of mitral regurgitation include fatigue, dyspnea (due to increased left atrial pressure), and pulmonary edema. Symptoms often worsen with atrial fibrillation.

Physical Examination

The findings of mitral regurgitation include a diffuse and hyperdynamic left ventricular impulse, which may be visible, and a palpable rapid filling wave. The S_1 is usually obliterated, and there is a holosystolic murmur. The S_2 is widely split (early A_2), and there is an S_3. A low-pitched early diastolic rumble indicates severe regurgitation; it represents a volume murmur and usually not coexisting mitral stenosis.

In acute mitral regurgitation, the murmur may be short because of increased left atrial pressure. In severe mitral regurgitation, the carotid upstroke may appear parvus, because of the low forward stroke volume, but not tardus. The left atrium may be palpable with systole, and the left ventricle, with diastole; there may be both S_3 and S_4. If the cause is ruptured chordae, an anterior leaflet murmur radiates to the axilla and back, and a posterior leaflet murmur radiates to the base and carotid arteries. Consider acute mitral regurgitation with a normal-sized heart, pulmonary edema, and acute onset of symptoms.

- Physical examination in mitral regurgitation:
  S_1 is usually obliterated
  Holosystolic murmur is present

S_2 is widely split (early A_2)
Low-pitched early diastolic rumble indicates severe regurgitation

Diagnosis

Chest radiography may first show a dilated left atrium and then, as mitral regurgitation increases, dilatation of the left ventricle.

Pathophysiology

Mitral regurgitation is a volume overload with marked decrease in afterload which "offloads" the left ventricle. Filling volume must increase to maintain adequate forward output. This results in a hyperdynamic ventricle, and thus many patients with considerable mitral regurgitation remain asymptomatic for many years. However, as with chronic aortic regurgitation, there may be development of asymptomatic left ventricular dysfunction. A low or low-normal ejection fraction therefore suggests substantial ventricular dysfunction.

- Many patients with mitral regurgitation remain asymptomatic for many years.
- A low or low-normal ejection fraction suggests substantial ventricular dysfunction.

There is no universally accepted medical treatment for mitral regurgitation. Symptoms indicate that intervention (mitral repair or replacement) is warranted. Most patients experience a decrease in ejection fraction after mitral valve repair or replacement.

Table 3-6   Types of Mitral Regurgitation

| Anatomical Type | Clinical Presentation | |
	Chronic	Acute or Subacute
Leaflets	Rheumatic Prolapse Annular calcification Connective tissue disease Congenital cleft Drug-related	Infective endocarditis
Tensor apparatus (chordal and papillary muscles)	Prolapse	Rupture of chordae Myocardial infarction Papillary muscle rupture
Myocardium	Regional ischemia or infarctions Dilated cardiomyopathy Hypertrophic cardiomyopathy	

Modified from McGoon MD, Schaff HV, Enriquez-Sarano M, Fuster V, Callahan MJ. Mitral regurgitation. In: Giuliani ER, Gersh BJ, McGoon MD, Hayes DL, Schaff HV, editors. Mayo Clinic practice of cardiology. 3rd ed. St Louis: Mosby; 1996. p. 1450-69. Used with permission of Mayo Foundation.

Treatment

Asymptomatic patients with a normal or hyperdynamic ejection fraction can continue to undergo regular observation. Operation should be considered for symptomatic patients (note that ventricular function considerably influences the postoperative outcome), and, because afterload is increased when the mitral valve is replaced, left ventricular function may actually deteriorate. In mildly symptomatic patients, operation may be considered, particularly if serial examinations show progressive cardiac enlargement. Earlier operation may be indicated in patients who are suitable for mitral valve repair rather than replacement, especially when the ejection fraction is less than 60% or the left ventricular end-diastolic dimension is more than 45 mm.

* In symptomatic patients with severe mitral regurgitation, operation should be considered.
* In asymptomatic patients with an ejection fraction <60% or left ventricular end-systolic dimension >45 mm, operation may be considered, especially if mitral valve repair is possible and surgical risk is relatively low.

Mitral Valve Prolapse

Pathophysiology and Natural History

Mitral valve prolapse is the most common valvular heart disease and is the most common cause of mitral regurgitation in the United States. Mitral valve prolapse refers to a systolic billowing of 1 or both mitral leaflets into the left atrium with or without mitral regurgitation. Estimates of prevalence in the general population range from 2% to 6%.

In patients with mitral valve prolapse, as with other causes of mitral regurgitation, the degree of left atrial and left ventricular dilatation depends on the severity of mitral regurgitation. In Marfan syndrome, the supporting apparatus is often involved with dilatation of the mitral anulus in addition to elongated chordae and redundant leaflets.

Other valves also may be involved with the same myxomatous degeneration, leading to tricuspid valve prolapse (occurring in approximately 40% of patients with mitral valve prolapse), pulmonic valve prolapse (~10%), and aortic valve prolapse (2%). Mitral valve prolapse is associated with secundum atrial septal defect and supraventricular arrhythmias (Curr Probl Cardiol. 1982;7:1-48).

The mitral valve prolapse syndrome is associated with a benign course in most patients. Patients with diagnostic auscultatory findings of click-murmur, thickened mitral leaflets on echocardiography, and left ventricular and atrial enlargement are at high risk for future complications, including atrial fibrillation, systemic embolism, and pulmonary hypertension. There is also a lifelong risk of ruptured mitral valve chordae, which may lead to acute decompensation. Infective endocarditis is a serious complication of mitral valve prolapse, although the overall incidence is low. There is also a small risk of sudden cardiac death (Figure 3-8).

Physical Examination

Mitral valve prolapse is most commonly diagnosed with cardiac auscultation in asymptomatic patients or found incidentally on echocardiography performed for another reason. Yet, primary evaluation of the patient with mitral valve prolapse is a careful physical examination. The classic auscultatory finding is the midsystolic click, a high-pitched sound of short duration. There may be multiple clicks. Clicks result from sudden tensing of the mitral valve apparatus as the leaflets prolapse into the left atrium during systole. The midsystolic click(s) is frequently followed by a mid-late systolic murmur that is high-pitched, musical, or honking and often loudest at the cardiac apex. The character and intensity of the clicks and the murmur vary under loading conditions of the left ventricle. Dynamic auscultation is helpful for establishing the diagnosis of mitral valve prolapse syndrome. Changes in left ventricular end-diastolic volume result in changes in the timing of the midsystolic click(s) and murmur. When end-diastolic volume is decreased (such as with standing), the critical volume is achieved earlier in systole and the click-murmur complex occurs earlier after S_1. By contrast, any maneuver that augments the volume of blood in the ventricle (eg, squatting), reduces myocardial contractility, or increases left ventricular afterload lengthens the time from onset of systole to initiation of mitral valve prolapse, and the systolic click or murmur moves toward S_2 (Figure 3-9) (Curr Probl Cardiol. 1976;1:1-60; J Am Coll Cardiol. 1998;32:1486-588).

Diagnosis

Results of electrocardiography most often are normal, although 24-hour ambulatory electrocardiographic recordings or event monitors may be useful for documenting arrhythmias. Chest radiography may show skeletal abnormalities such as pectus excavatum.

Echocardiography is the most useful noninvasive test for defining mitral valve prolapse. The definition includes more than 2 mm of posterior displacement of 1 or both leaflets into the left atrium. All patients with mitral valve prolapse should have an initial echocardiogram to determine the diagnosis, stratify risk, and define possible

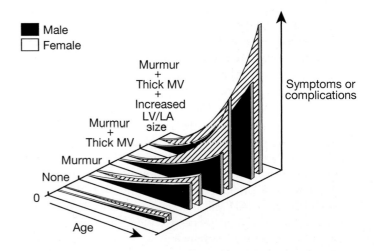

Figure 3-8. Risk Factors for Complications in Mitral Valve Prolapse. LA indicates left atrial; LV, left ventricular; MV, mitral valve. (From Boudoulas H, Kolibash AJ Jr, Wooley CF. Mitral valve prolapse: a heterogeneous disorder. Primary Cardiol. 1991;17:29-43.)

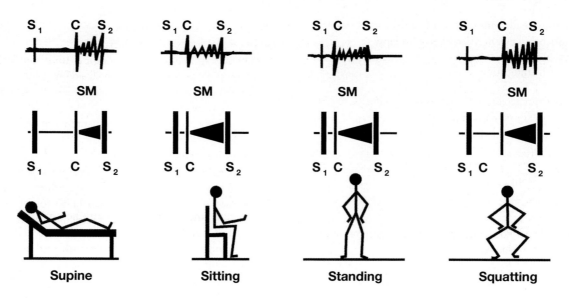

Figure 3-9. Auscultation Findings in Mitral Valve Prolapse. C indicates click; SM, systolic murmur; ◀, murmur.

associated lesions (eg, atrial septal defect). Serial echocardiograms are not usually necessary in asymptomatic patients with mitral valve prolapse unless there are clinical indications of worsening status.

Treatment

Reassurance is a major part of the management of patients with mitral valve prolapse because most are asymptomatic and lack a high-risk profile. A normal lifestyle and regular exercise are encouraged. Patients should be educated about when to seek medical advice (worsening symptoms).

Common symptoms include palpitations, atypical chest pain that rarely resembles classic angina pectoris, dyspnea, and fatigue. Patients should be advised in cessation of the use of caffeine, alcohol, and cigarettes. Patients with recurrent palpitations often respond to therapy with β-adrenergic blockers or calcium channel blockers. Orthostatic symptoms due to postural hypotension and tachycardia are best treated with volume expansion, preferably by liberalizing fluid and salt intake. Transient cerebral ischemic episodes occur with increased incidence in patients with mitral valve prolapse, and some patients need long-term anticoagulation (Table 3-7).

Asymptomatic patients with mitral valve prolapse and no serious mitral regurgitation can be evaluated clinically every 3 to 5 years. Serial echocardiography is necessary only in patients who have high-risk features on the initial echocardiogram.

Surgery may be required for mitral valve prolapse. The thickened, redundant mitral valve often can be repaired rather than replaced, a procedure associated with a low operative mortality rate and excellent short- and long-term results, particularly in patients who have a flail mitral leaflet due to rupture of chordae tendineae or their marked elongation. Recommendations for surgery in patients with mitral valve prolapse and mitral regurgitation are the same as those for patients with other forms of severe mitral regurgitation.

Tricuspid Stenosis

The cause of tricuspid stenosis is almost always rheumatic, and it is never an isolated lesion. Carcinoid syndrome may cause tricuspid valve retraction and a relative stenosis (usually causes worse tricuspid regurgitation), and in rare cases atrial tumors may be the cause.

- The cause of tricuspid stenosis is almost always rheumatic.

Tricuspid Regurgitation

Mild tricuspid regurgitation is relatively common, occurring in up to 85% to 90% of patients. Significant tricuspid regurgitation is usually caused by dilatation of the right ventricle. When there is pulmonary hypertension, tricuspid regurgitation is common, but not mandatory. Tricuspid regurgitation often accompanies mitral valve disease, but it may be related to 1) biventricular infarction, 2) primary pulmonary hypertension, 3) congenital heart disease (such as Ebstein anomaly), or 4) carcinoid syndrome—more commonly associated with tricuspid regurgitation than tricuspid stenosis.

- Tricuspid regurgitation is usually caused by dilatation of the right ventricle.
- It often accompanies mitral valve disease.

Tricuspid Valve Prolapse

This may occur as an isolated entity or in association with other connective tissue abnormalities. The tricuspid valve may prolapse or become flail as a result of trauma or endocarditis (commonly fungal or staphylococcal in drug addicts).

Physical Examination

Findings on physical examination include jugular venous distention with a prominent *v* wave, a prominent right ventricular impulse, a

Table 3-7   Recommendations for Use of Aspirin and Oral
Anticoagulants in Mitral Valve Prolapse

Indication	Class
1. Aspirin therapy for cerebral transient ischemic attacks	I
2. Warfarin therapy for patients aged ≥65 years, in atrial fibrillation with hypertension, mitral regurgitation murmur, or history of heart failure	I
3. Aspirin therapy for patients aged <65 years, in atrial fibrillation with no history of mitral regurgitation, hypertension, or heart failure	I
4. Warfarin therapy after stroke	I
5. Warfarin therapy for transient ischemic attacks despite aspirin therapy	IIa
6. Aspirin therapy after stroke in patients with contraindications to anticoagulants	IIa
7. Aspirin therapy for patients in sinus rhythm with echocardiographic evidence of high-risk mitral valve prolapse	IIb

Data from Bonow RO, Carabello BA, Chatterjee K, de Leon AC Jr, Faxon DP, Freed MD, et al. ACC/AHA 2006 guidelines for the management of patients with valvular heart disease: a report of the American College of Cardiology/American Heart Association Task Force on Practice Guidelines (Writing Committee to Revise the 1998 Guidelinees for the Management of Patients With Valvular Heart Disease). Circulation. 2006;114:e84-e231.

pansystolic murmur at the left sternal edge, possibly a right-sided S_3, and peripheral edema, ascites, and hepatomegaly.

Surgical Therapy

Tricuspid annuloplasty may be helpful if regurgitation is a result of right ventricular dilatation. However, if there is considerable pulmonary hypertension, tricuspid valve replacement is usually required with either a biologic or a mechanical valve. Biologic prostheses in the tricuspid position do not degenerate as quickly as prostheses in the left side of the heart. In patients with endocarditis, the tricuspid valve can be removed completely, and patients may tolerate this well for several years.

Congenital Heart Disease

Atrial Septal Defect

There are multiple types of atrial septal defects (Table 3-8).

Secundum Atrial Septal Defect

Patients with secundum atrial septal defect often survive to adulthood and may be asymptomatic. The condition is often detected on routine examination with the finding of a systolic flow murmur and "fixed" split S_2. If the defect has gone undetected, atrial fibrillation frequently develops in their 50s along with onset of symptoms, usually dyspnea with subsequent tricuspid regurgitation and right-sided heart failure. Stroke may occur as a result of paradoxical embolism.

- Patients with secundum atrial septal defect often survive to adulthood and may be asymptomatic.
- The condition is found on routine examination with the finding of a systolic flow murmur and "fixed" split S_2.
- Atrial fibrillation often develops in patients in their 50s with onset of symptoms.
- Stroke may occur as a result of paradoxical embolism.

Physical Examination

Findings include a normal or slightly prominent jugular venous pressure, a right ventricular heave or lift, an ejection systolic murmur in the pulmonary artery due to increased flow (usually less than grade 3/6), a fixed splitting of the S_2, and a tricuspid diastolic flow rumble if the shunt is large.

- Physical findings of secundum atrial septal defect:
  Ejection systolic murmur in the pulmonary artery (never more than grade 3/6)
  Fixed splitting of S_2
  Tricuspid diastolic flow rumble with large shunts

Diagnosis

Electrocardiography characteristically shows right bundle branch block and right axis deviation. Chest radiography shows pulmonary plethora, a prominent pulmonary artery, and right ventricular enlargement (Figure 3-10). Young patients (younger than 40 years) with secundum atrial septal defect and sinus rhythm do not have left atrial enlargement. If the chest radiograph shows left atrial enlargement, consider another lesion, particularly primum atrial septal defect with mitral regurgitation.

- If the chest radiograph shows left atrial enlargement, consider primum atrial septal defect with mitral regurgitation.

Table 3-8   Types of Atrial Septal Defects

Type	%	Location	Associated Findings	ECG Findings
Ostium secundum	75	Fossa ovalis	None	Incomp RBBB, R axis
Sinus venosus	10	Vena cava	Anomalous PV	Incomp RBBB, ectopic P wave, R axis
Ostium primum	10-15	Lower septum	Cleft MV, Down syndrome	Incomp RBBB, L axis (LAHB)

Abbreviations: ECG, electrocardiography; Incomp, incomplete; L axis, left axis deviation; LAHB, left anterior hemiblock; MV, mitral valve; P wave, atrial depolarization wave on ECG; PV, pulmonary veins; R axis, right axis deviation; RBBB, right bundle branch block.

Two-dimensional and color Doppler echocardiography usually can show the defect and right ventricular enlargement with volume overload. If visualization is poor, transesophageal echocardiography can be performed. Cardiac catheterization is usually unnecessary, unless coexisting coronary artery disease is suspected.

Sinus Venosus Atrial Septal Defect

An uncommon condition, this occurs in the superior portion of the atrial septum. It is often associated with anomalous pulmonary veins, usually the right upper. If echocardiography shows right ventricular volume overload and no secundum defect (because surface echocardiography can miss the sinus venosus area), consider sinus venosus atrial septal defect or anomalous pulmonary veins.

Primum Atrial Septal Defect (Partial Atrioventricular Canal)

This is a defect in the lower portion of the septum due to partial atrioventricular canal defect. The mitral valve is usually congenitally cleft and produces various degrees of regurgitation.

Diagnosis

On electrocardiography, findings are different from those of secundum type; left axis deviation and right bundle branch block are evident. More than 75% of patients have first-degree atrioventricular block. The chest radiographic findings are the same as those for secundum atrial septal defect, although there may be left atrial enlargement because of mitral regurgitation. Atrioventricular canal defects are the most common cardiac anomaly associated with Down syndrome.

* Electrocardiography shows left axis deviation with right bundle branch block and, commonly, first-degree atrioventricular block.
* Atrioventricular canal defects are the most common cardiac anomaly of Down syndrome.

Treatment of Atrial Septal Defects

Infective endocarditis is rare in patients with atrial septal defect, and antibiotic prophylaxis for endocarditis is not recommended (unless there is associated complex congenital heart disease). Patients with atrial septal defect have variable symptoms depending on the size of the shunt. Intervention should be considered once there is evidence of hemodynamic compromise: left-to-right shunting of more than 30% or evidence of right-sided chamber enlargement.

Surgical treatment has been successful for more than 30 years with very low complication rates. Recently, percutaneous closure with an occluder device was approved for use.

Ventricular Septal Defect

Ventricular septal defect occurs in different parts of the ventricular septum, most commonly classified as either in the membranous septum or in the muscular septum. Small restrictive defects produce a loud murmur, and patients are often asymptomatic. The size of the hole determines the degree of left-to-right shunting. Small defects may have a long holosystolic murmur, often with a thrill at the left sternal edge, usually around the fourth interspace. Large defects may produce a mitral diastolic flow rumble at the apex, especially when the shunt is more than 2.5:1.

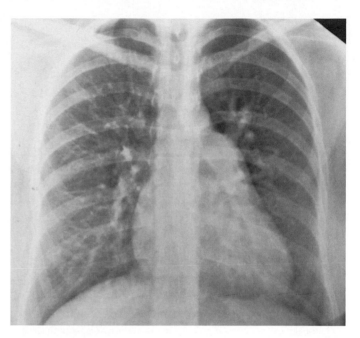

Figure 3-10. Chest radiograph from a patient with a large left-to-right shunt due to a secundum atrial septal defect. Note cardiac enlargement with right ventricular contour, prominent pulmonary artery, and pulmonary plethora.

Typical clinical scenario: In adults, ventricular septal defect generally presents as a loud murmur in an asymptomatic patient. Large defects cause considerable symptoms early in life and are, in the United States, usually closed when discovered. In adults, a large ventricular septal defect generally has progressed to Eisenmenger syndrome (pulmonary hypertension) and cannot be closed (see Eisenmenger Syndrome below). It is critical to recommend prophylaxis for subacute bacterial endocarditis. Sometimes patients present with symptoms of this infection.

* Ventricular septal defects are most common in the membranous septum or the muscular septum.
* Small, restrictive defects produce a loud murmur.
* The size of the hole determines the degree of left-to-right shunting.

Patent Ductus Arteriosus

This condition is associated with maternal rubella. It produces essentially an arteriovenous fistula. A small ductus is compatible with a normal lifespan. The ductus may calcify in adult life. A continuous "machinery" murmur envelops the S_2 around the second interspace beneath the left clavicle. A large patent ductus arteriosus may produce ventricular failure. Surgical ligation is curative; subsequently, patients do not need prophylaxis for endocarditis.

All significant shunt lesions, when large, may produce increased pulmonary pressures and subsequently pulmonary vascular disease and pulmonary hypertension.

Typical clinical scenario: A patient in an ambulatory clinic is an asymptomatic adult with a loud continuous "machinery" murmur.

It is crucial to recommend prophylaxis for subacute bacterial endocarditis.

- Patent ductus arteriosus is associated with maternal rubella.
- A small ductus is compatible with a normal lifespan.
- A continuous "machinery" murmur is present.
- Surgical ligation is curative; subsequently, prophylaxis for endocarditis is not needed.
- All of the above-described shunt lesions, when large, may produce increased pulmonary pressures and subsequently pulmonary vascular disease.

Eisenmenger Syndrome

Eisenmenger syndrome develops in the first few years of life when a large shunt (usually a ventricular septal defect or patent ductus arteriosus, less often atrial septal defect) produces pulmonary hypertension and irreversible pulmonary vascular disease. This condition causes the shunt to reverse so that blood flows from the right to the left, and subsequent cyanosis occurs. The condition is then inoperable. Death commonly occurs in the third or fourth decade of life as a result of exercise-induced syncope, arrhythmia, hemoptysis, and stroke. The cyanosis produces marked erythrocytosis, often with hemoglobin values in the teens or 20s. There is no need for phlebotomy in patients with a hemoglobin value less than 20 g/dL or a hematocrit value less than 65%. Also, repeated phlebotomies frequently lead to iron deficiency, and iron-deficient erythrocytes are more rigid than ordinary ones, and the risk of stroke is thereby increased. Phlebotomy may be necessary in symptomatic patients with a hemoglobin value more than 20 g/dL. Fluid should be replaced concomitantly in patients with Eisenmenger syndrome because hypotension and syncope may be fatal as a result of exacerbation of right-to-left shunting and hypoxia.

Typical clinical scenario: Patients have a long medical history because of the huge right-to-left shunts. A patient presents with syncope and erythrocytosis. Phlebotomy should not be used unless the patient has neurologic symptoms and a hemoglobin value more than 20 g/dL.

- Eisenmenger syndrome develops in the first few years of life.
- The syndrome produces pulmonary hypertension and irreversible pulmonary vascular disease.
- Death is common in the third or fourth decade of life.
- Associated conditions: exercise-induced syncope, arrhythmia, hemoptysis, and stroke.
- Cyanosis produces marked erythrocytosis.

Pulmonary Stenosis

This may occur as an isolated lesion or in association with a ventricular septal defect. Valvular pulmonary stenosis often causes few or no symptoms. The valve is frequently pliable, and it may be bicuspid. Thickened dysplastic valves, often stenotic, occur in association with the Noonan syndrome.

- Thickened dysplastic valves, often stenotic, occur with the Noonan syndrome.

Physical Examination

Findings include a prominent *a* wave in the jugular venous pulse; right ventricular heave; ejection systolic click—the earlier the click, the more severe the stenosis (the click indicates that the valve is pliable and noncalcified); ejection systolic murmur—the longer the murmur and the later peaking, the more severe the stenosis; and soft and late P_2 (with severe stenosis P_2 becomes inaudible). The pulmonary opening click is the only right-sided sound that gets softer with inspiration as the pulmonary valve partially opens with the inspiratory increase in venous return. Later in life, the valve may become so thick, calcified, and immobile that the ejection click disappears.

- Findings of pulmonary stenosis:
  Prominent *a* wave in the jugular venous pulse
  Ejection systolic click
  The pulmonary opening click is the only right-sided sound that gets softer with inspiration

Diagnosis

Electrocardiography shows right ventricular hypertrophy. On chest radiography, poststenotic pulmonary dilatation, especially of the left pulmonary artery (Figure 3-11), is the hallmark.

The diagnosis can be reliably made with 2-dimensional echocardiography, and Doppler reliably predicts the gradient and estimates right ventricular pressure. In asymptomatic patients, treatment is indicated when the right ventricular systolic pressure approaches two-thirds or more that of the systemic blood pressure. The treatment of choice for a pliable noncalcified valve is percutaneous balloon valvuloplasty, which has essentially replaced surgical valvotomy.

Typical clinical scenario: A young patient presents with dyspnea on exertion or exertional syncope. On examination, there is a murmur that is late-peaking and louder with inspiration. A systolic click is also heard, but it is softer with inspiration. A prominent *a* wave is seen on jugular venous profile. On echocardiography, the condition is diagnosed with a gradient more than 50 mm Hg across the pulmonary valve. If the valve is still pliable (usually to middle age), balloon valvuloplasty is the procedure of choice.

- The diagnosis of pulmonary stenosis is made with 2-dimensional and Doppler echocardiography.
- The treatment for a pliable valve is percutaneous balloon valvuloplasty when the right ventricular systolic pressure is two-thirds or more that of the systemic pressure.

Coarctation of the Aorta

This is usually either a discrete or a long segment of narrowing adjacent to the left subclavian artery. It is more common in males and frequently is associated with a bicuspid aortic valve. Most cases of coarctation are diagnosed in childhood; only about 20% are diagnosed in adulthood. This is the most common cardiac anomaly associated with Turner syndrome. Other associations include aneurysms of the circle of Willis and aortic dissection or rupture. There is an increased incidence of aortic dissection or rupture in Turner syndrome, even in the absence of coarctation. As a result of the coarctation, systemic collateral vessels develop from

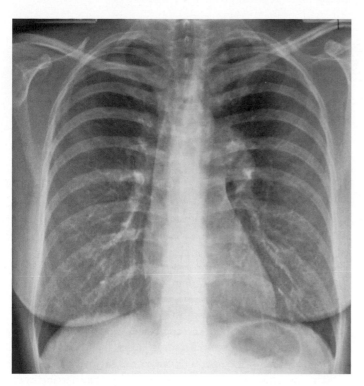

Figure 3-11. Typical chest radiograph from a patient with valvular pulmonary stenosis, showing normal cardiac size and marked prominence of main and left pulmonary arteries, representing poststenotic dilatation. This does not occur with infundibular pulmonary stenosis. Lung fields appear mildly oligemic.

the subclavian and axillary arteries through the internal mammary, scapular, and intercostal arteries.

* Coarctation of the aorta is more common in males.
* The condition is frequently associated with a bicuspid aortic valve.
* Only 20% of cases are diagnosed in adulthood.
* It is the most common cardiac anomaly associated with Turner syndrome.
* The incidence of aortic dissection or rupture is increased in Turner syndrome, even in the absence of coarctation.

There are 5 major complications of coarctation of the aorta: 1) cardiac failure, 2) aortic valve disease, 3) aortic rupture or dissection, 4) endarteritis, and 5) rupture of an aneurysm of the circle of Willis—this is exacerbated by the presence of hypertension, which occurs in the upper limbs. Systemic hypertension may be the presenting feature in adults. Some patients complain of pain and fatigue in the legs on exercise, reminiscent of claudication.

Symptoms
Typical clinical scenario: Coarctation should be considered in patients with hypertension who are younger than 50 years. There may be coexistent claudication of the lower extremities. Examination shows differentiated blood pressure: upper extremity hypertension and lower extremity hypotension. On simultaneous palpation of the radial and femoral pulses, there is a delay, smaller in the femoral arteries. Patients may present with symptoms of aortic rupture, dissection, congestive heart failure, or associated conditions of Turner syndrome, circle of Willis aneurysm, or bicuspid valve.

Physical Examination
Findings include an easily palpable brachial pulse; the femoral pulse is weak and delayed. There are differences in systolic pressure between the upper and the lower extremities. Exercise may exaggerate the systemic hypertension. An ejection click is present when there is an associated bicuspid valve. A_2 may be loud as a result of hypertension. An S_4 may be present with associated left ventricular hypertrophy and hypertension. Murmurs may originate from 1) the coarctation, which can produce a systolic murmur over the left sternal edge and over the spine in the midthoracic region, and it sometimes extends into diastole in the form of a continuous murmur; 2) arterial collateral vessels, which are spread widely over the thorax; and 3) the bicuspid aortic valve, which may generate a systolic murmur.

* Physical findings of coarctation of the aorta: easily palpable brachial pulse, weak and delayed femoral pulse, differences in systolic pressure between the upper and the lower extremities.
* Coarctation can produce a systolic murmur over the left sternal edge and over the spine in the midthoracic region.
* Arterial collateral vessels are spread widely over the thorax.

Diagnosis
Results of electrocardiography may be normal. The more severe the coarctation stenosis and hypertension, the more likely the finding of left ventricular hypertrophy with or without repolarization changes. Chest radiography may show rib notching from the dilated and pulsatile intercostal arteries and a "3" configuration of the aortic knob, which represents the coarctation site with proximal and distal dilatation.

* Chest radiographic findings in coarctation of the aorta are rib notching and a "3" configuration of the aortic knob.

The condition may be shown on echocardiography and Doppler, although imaging may be difficult in this area, and additional visualization may be necessary with digital subtraction angiography, magnetic resonance imaging, computed tomography, or angiography.

Treatment
Balloon angioplasty has been performed in some patients, although it has been associated with aneurysm formation and re-coarctation. Surgical treatment has been an accepted approach since 1945. Even after coarctation repair, there is a considerable rate of hypertension. As many as 75% of patients are hypertensive at 30-year follow-up. Surgically treated patients still often die prematurely of coronary artery disease, heart failure, stroke, or ruptured or dissected aorta. Age at operation is important. The 20-year survival rate is 91% in patients who have operation when they are younger than 14 years and 79% in patients who have operation when they are older than 14 years.

* Surgical repair is the accepted treatment of coarctation of the aorta.

- Even after successful operation, there is a high rate of cardiovascular complications.
- Surgically treated patients often die prematurely of coronary artery disease, heart failure, stroke, or ruptured or dissected aorta.

Ebstein Anomaly

This is a congenital lesion of the right side of the heart that has a variable clinical spectrum. It involves an inferior displacement of the tricuspid valve ring into the right ventricular cavity, causing a sail-like elongated anterior cusp or tricuspid valve on echocardiography. The degree of displacement is variable, as is the degree of abnormality of the tricuspid valve. The inferior displacement of the tricuspid valve results in "atrialization" of the right ventricle. Maternal lithium ingestion during pregnancy has been associated with this anomaly.

- Ebstein anomaly is thought to be associated with maternal lithium ingestion during pregnancy.
- The anomaly involves inferior displacement of the tricuspid valve ring into the right ventricular cavity, causing a sail-like tricuspid valve on echocardiography.

Symptoms

Ebstein anomaly has a protracted natural history.

Typical clinical scenario: Although findings are highly variable, most patients present with cyanosis and dyspnea with or without atrial arrhythmias. The cyanosis is due to right-to-left shunting at the atrial level.

Physical Examination

The extremities are usually cool, often with peripheral cyanosis (a reflection of low cardiac output). A prominent a wave and, if tricuspid regurgitation is present, a v wave are present in the jugular venous pressure (although this is variable because the large right atrium may accommodate a large tricuspid regurgitant volume). A right ventricular lift is noted. The S_1 has a loud tricuspid (T_1) component. A holosystolic murmur increases on inspiration at the left sternal edge from tricuspid regurgitation. One or more systolic clicks are noted (often may be multiple). Common associated conditions are secundum atrial septal defect, preexcitation syndrome, and bundle of Kent (atrioventricular accessory pathway in 13% of patients in a Mayo Clinic series). Patients with secundum atrial septal defects are often very cyanotic because of the increased right-to-left shunting, and they may present with neurologic events due to paradoxical embolism.

- Findings of Ebstein anomaly include cool extremities, often with peripheral cyanosis.
- A holosystolic murmur increases on inspiration.
- One or more systolic clicks are noted.
- Associated conditions: secundum atrial septal defect, preexcitation syndrome, and bundle of Kent.
- Patients with secundum atrial septal defects are often very cyanotic.

Diagnosis

Chest radiography shows a narrow pedicle with an enlarged globular silhouette and right atrial enlargement. The lung fields are normal or oligemic. On electrocardiography, a tall P wave (Himalayan P waves) and right bundle branch block are found.

Two-dimensional and Doppler echocardiography delineates the anatomy precisely, and cardiac catheterization is unnecessary. Electrophysiologic study may be necessary to delineate the bypass tract, if present.

Treatment

The long asymptomatic phase supports a policy of postponing surgical intervention until the patient has significant symptoms. Patients may require anticoagulation if an atrial septal defect is present and paradoxical emboli have occurred. In addition, there is high frequency of accessory atrioventricular pathways leading to tachycardia.

Pregnancy and Cardiac Disease

Physiologic Changes of Pregnancy

Plasma volume starts to increase in the first trimester and continues to increase through the third trimester to almost 50% more than normal. An increase in red cell mass also begins early and peaks in the second trimester, but not to the same degree as the plasma volume; thus, there is a relative anemia. The cardiac output increases by 30% to 50%, and peripheral resistance decreases. Heart rate also increases throughout pregnancy. Increased venous pressure in the lower extremities leads to pedal edema in 80% of healthy pregnant women.

- Physiologic changes of pregnancy include markedly increased plasma volume and a moderate increase in red cell mass, which cause a relative anemia.
- Peripheral resistance decreases.
- Cardiac output increases.

Because of these changes, the physical examination may suggest cardiac abnormalities to the unwary. Normal results of physical examination in a healthy pregnant woman include increased jugular venous pressure, bounding carotid pulses, and an ejection systolic murmur in the pulmonary area (should not be more than grade 3/6). The S_2 is loud, and there is often an S_3 or diastolic filling sound. An S_4 occasionally may be heard.

- Ejection systolic murmur in the pulmonary area (not more than grade 3/6) is a normal finding in pregnancy.
- An S_3 or S_4 is common.

Although an S_3 or diastolic filling sound is common, a long rumble should raise the possibility of mitral stenosis. Because of the decrease in peripheral resistance and increased output changes, stenotic lesions are less well tolerated than regurgitant ones; for example, a patient with aortic stenosis has exaggeration of the aortic valve gradient, whereas a patient with mitral regurgitation experiences "afterload reduction" with peripheral vasodilatation and so tolerates pregnancy better. Functional class of the patient is a consideration in terms of whether pregnancy is possible. Patients who are in New York Heart Association functional class III or IV have a maternal mortality rate approaching 7%.

- An S_3 or diastolic filling sound is common in pregnancy, but a long rumble should raise the possibility of mitral stenosis.
- For patients in functional class III or IV, the maternal mortality rate approaches 7%.

Pregnancy is *absolutely contraindicated* in patients with the following conditions: 1) Marfan syndrome with a dilated aortic root—there is an increased risk of dissection and rupture because hormonal changes soften the connective tissue (there is unpredictable risk of dissection and rupture in Marfan syndrome and pregnancy even when the aortic root has normal size), 2) Eisenmenger syndrome (maternal mortality rate is 50%), 3) primary pulmonary hypertension, 4) symptomatic severe aortic stenosis, 5) symptomatic severe mitral stenosis, and 6) symptomatic dilated cardiomyopathy.

Although not absolute contraindications, the following conditions are also of concern in pregnancy: 1) atrial septal defect (deep venous thrombosis may lead to paradoxical embolus) and 2) coarctation (increased risk of dissection and rupture).

Patients at risk during pregnancy should minimize activity (decreases cardiac output), reduce sodium in the diet, and minimize anemia with iron and vitamin supplements.

If symptoms deteriorate and congestive heart failure supervenes, bed rest may need to be instituted. Arrhythmias such as atrial fibrillation need to be treated promptly in these situations. If necessary, cardioversion can be performed with apparently low risk to the fetus. Fetal cardiac monitoring should be performed at the same time. Occasionally patients need operative intervention. Operation during the first trimester is associated with a markedly increased rate of fetal loss. Percutaneous aortic, mitral, and pulmonary balloon valvuloplasty have been performed during pregnancy and may obviate cardiopulmonary bypass. Careful lead shielding of the fetus is needed during these procedures.

Drugs
Many cardiac drugs cross the placenta into the fetus but yet can be used safely when necessary and are not absolutely contraindicated in pregnancy. These include digoxin, quinidine, procainamide, β-adrenergic blockers, and verapamil. The β-adrenergic blockers can be associated with growth retardation of the fetus, neonatal bradycardia, and hypoglycemia. They may need to be used, however, in large doses in patients with hypertrophic cardiomyopathy, and fetal growth must be monitored.

Drugs that should be avoided are angiotensin-converting enzyme inhibitors (ie, captopril), which cause fetal renal dysgenesis; phenytoin, which causes hydantoin syndrome and teratogenicity; and warfarin, which causes teratogenicity and abortion (should be especially avoided in the first and third trimesters). One noncardiac drug to avoid is tetracycline, which stains fetal teeth.

- Drugs to avoid in pregnancy: angiotensin-converting enzyme inhibitors (ie, captopril), phenytoin, warfarin, and tetracycline.

Delivery
Delivery is a time of rapid hemodynamic swings. With each uterine contraction, about 500 mL of blood is released into the circulation.

Cardiac output goes up with advancing labor. Oxygen consumption increases 3-fold. High-risk patients need careful monitoring with Swan-Ganz catheterization to maintain preload at an optimal level, maternal and fetal electrocardiographic monitoring, careful analgesia and anesthesia to avoid hypotension, delivery in the left lateral position so the fetus is not lying on the inferior vena cava (this position maintains venous return), and a short second stage of labor (delivery may need to be facilitated if labor progresses slowly).

Vaginal delivery is safer for most women because the average blood loss is less than 500 mL; with cesarean section it is 800 mL. Usually, cesarean section is performed only for obstetric indications. The new guidelines of the American Heart Association state that there is no need for antibiotic prophylaxis in an uncomplicated vaginal delivery.

- With each uterine contraction, 500 mL of blood is released into the circulation.
- There is no need for antibiotic prophylaxis in uncomplicated vaginal delivery.

Prosthetic Valves and Pregnancy
Most women of childbearing age who need a valve replacement will receive a biologic valve, and if they are in sinus rhythm they will usually not be receiving anticoagulants. Women with mechanical valves will be taking warfarin, and this poses a problem with teratogenicity (first trimester) and increased risk of spontaneous abortion. Anticoagulation in pregnancy is complex and controversial. In general, pregnancy should be diagnosed as soon as possible, therapy should be switched to unfractionated subcutaneous heparin (low-molecular-weight heparin has not yet been approved for this indication), and the activated partial thromboplastin time should be monitored. Many physicians now advocate that the patient be returned to warfarin therapy until delivery. Heparin also is associated with significant maternal complications (valve thrombosis and fetal loss). High-risk pregnancy teams adept at management are essential.

- In pregnant patients with mechanical valves, therapy should be switched from warfarin to unfractionated subcutaneous heparin, at least for the first trimester.
- Warfarin is associated with embryopathy.
- Heparin is associated with increased fetal loss.
- Warfarin is contraindicated in the first and third trimesters.

Hypertension and Pregnancy
High blood pressure during pregnancy is defined as an increment in systolic blood pressure of 30 mm Hg, an increment in diastolic blood pressure of 15 mm Hg or more, or an absolute diastolic blood pressure of 90 mm Hg or more. Hypertension during pregnancy may be 1) chronic hypertension (blood pressure ≥140/80 mm Hg before pregnant state), 2) transient hypertension (develops during pregnancy), 3) preeclampsia (starts ≥20 weeks of pregnancy), or 4) a combination of these.

For the medical management of hypertension, methyldopa is most extensively studied and is safe. β-Adrenergic blockers are safe and efficacious but may lead to growth retardation and fetal bradycardia.

Angiotensin-converting enzyme inhibitors are contraindicated because they cause fetal renal failure. Hydralazine is used when additional drug treatment is needed, but it may be associated with fetal thrombocytopenia. Calcium channel blockers are not extensively studied. Diuretics are effective because the hypertension of pregnancy is "salt-sensitive." Although there is not total agreement, the Working Group on Hypertension in Pregnancy allows continuation of the use of diuretics if they had been prescribed before gestation.

Pericardial Disease

The pericardium has an inner layer, the visceral pericardium, and an outer layer, the parietal pericardium. The space between the 2 layers contains 15 to 25 mL of clear fluid. The pericardium has 3 main functions: prevent cardiac distention, limit cardiac displacement because of its attachment to neighboring structures, and protect the heart from nearby inflammation.

Acute or Subacute Inflammatory Pericarditis

Symptoms
The chest pain of pericarditis is often aggravated by movement of the trunk, by inspiration, and by coughing. The pain is often relieved by sitting up. Low-grade fever and malaise are other findings.

Diagnosis
Pericardial friction rub may be variable. Chest radiography is usually normal. It may show globular enlargement if pericardial effusion is marked (at least 250 mL). Occasionally, pulmonary infiltrate or small pleural effusion is noted. Left pleural effusion predominates, and the cause is unknown. Electrocardiography shows acute concave ST elevation in all ventricular leads. The PR segment is also depressed in the early stages. Echocardiography allows easy diagnosis of pericardial effusion and determination of whether the pericardial effusion is hemodynamically significant.

* Chest pain is the presenting symptom of pericarditis.
* Electrocardiography shows concave ST elevation and a depressed PR segment.

Causes
The causes of pericarditis include viral pericarditis, idiopathic pericarditis, autoimmune and collagen diseases (eg, systemic lupus erythematosus, rheumatoid arthritis, scleroderma), and postmyocardial infarction. The postcardiotomy syndrome follows open heart procedures. It presents with pyrexia, increased sedimentation rate, and pleural or pericardial chest pain. It occurs weeks to months after open heart operation. Its incidence decreases with age, and it usually responds to anti-inflammatory agents. Pericarditis also is associated with radiation and neoplasm, namely, Hodgkin disease, leukemia, and lymphoma. Breast, thyroid, and lung tumors can metastasize to the pericardium and cause pericarditis or pericardial effusion. Melanoma also metastasizes to the heart. Uremia and tuberculosis also can cause pericarditis. If no cause can be documented, idiopathic viral pericarditis is the most likely diagnosis, and treatment

with nonsteroidal anti-inflammatory agents or high-dose aspirin usually resolves the condition.

* Causes of pericarditis: autoimmune and collagen diseases; postmyocardial infarction; radiation; neoplasm; breast, thyroid, and lung tumors; uremia; tuberculosis.

Pericardial Effusion
The response of the pericardium to inflammation is to exude fluid, fibrin, and blood cells, causing a pericardial effusion. The condition is not seen on chest radiography until the amount of effusion is 250 mL. If fluid accumulates slowly, the pericardial sac distends slowly with no cardiac compression. If fluid accumulates rapidly, such as with bleeding, tamponade can occur with relatively small amounts of fluid. Tamponade restricts the blood entering the ventricles and causes a decrease in ventricular volume. The increased intrapericardial pressure increases the ventricular end-diastolic pressure and mean atrial pressure, and the increased atrial pressure increases the venous pressure. The decreased ventricular volume and filling diminish cardiac output. Any of the previously listed causes of pericarditis can cause tamponade, but other acute causes of hemopericardium should be considered, such as ruptured myocardium after infarction, aortic dissection, ruptured aortic aneurysm, and sequelae of cardiac operation.

* Pericardial effusion is not seen on chest radiography until the amount is 250 mL.
* Tamponade can occur with small amounts of fluid.
* Tamponade restricts the blood entering the ventricles and decreases ventricular volume.

Clinical Features
Tamponade produces a continuum of features, depending on its severity. The blood pressure is low, the heart is small and quiet, tachycardia may be present, jugular venous pressure is increased, and pulsus paradoxus develops (increased flow of blood into the right heart during inspiration, decreased flow into the left heart). An increase in inspiratory distention of the neck veins (Kussmaul sign) may occur, as with constrictive pericarditis.

Treatment
Emergency pericardiocentesis is performed with echocardiography-directed guidance.

Constrictive Pericarditis
Diastolic filling of both ventricles is prevented by the pericardium. The smaller the ventricular volume, the higher the end-diastolic pressure. The most common causes are recurrent viral pericarditis, irradiation, previous open heart operation, tuberculosis, and neoplastic disease.

Symptoms
Dominantly right-sided failure, peripheral edema, ascites, and often dyspnea and fatigue are present.

* Symptoms of constrictive pericarditis: peripheral edema, ascites, dyspnea, and fatigue.

Physical Examination

The jugular venous pressure is increased (the patient should be observed when he or she is sitting or standing), and inspiratory distention of neck veins (Kussmaul sign) is present. The jugular venous pressure may show rapid descents, and pericardial knock is present in fewer than 50% of cases (sound is probably due to sudden cessation of ventricular filling). Ascites and peripheral edema are usually present. Chest radiography may show pericardial calcification, but no specific changes are found on electrocardiography.

* Signs of constrictive pericarditis: increased jugular venous pressure, inspiratory distention of neck veins, rapid descents of jugular venous pressure, and pericardial knock (fewer than 50% of cases).
* Chest radiography may show pericardial calcification.
* No specific changes are found on electrocardiography.

Diagnosis

Echocardiography and Doppler may be helpful, particularly Doppler, which shows hemodynamic effects of respiratory changes in mitral and tricuspid inflow velocities. Other methods such as computed tomography and magnetic resonance imaging help to delineate the thickness of the pericardium. The major confounding diagnosis is restrictive cardiomyopathy, and the distinction can be very difficult. Diastolic expansion of both ventricles is affected equally; therefore, diastolic pressure is increased and equal in all 4 chambers. Ventricular pressure curve shows characteristic "√" (square root sign) from rapid ventricular filling and equalization of pressures (also may be seen in restrictive cardiomyopathy). The a and v waves are usually equal, and x and y descents are rapid. If pulmonary artery systolic pressure is more than 50 mm Hg, myocardial disease is likely. If the end-diastolic pulmonary artery pressure is more than 30% of systolic pressure, myocardial disease is likely. Both of these findings are nonspecific, however.

Treatment

The treatment of choice for constrictive pericarditis is thoracotomy to remove the pericardium.

* Constrictive pericarditis is diagnosed from respiratory changes in mitral and tricuspid inflow velocities.
* The major confounding diagnosis is restrictive cardiomyopathy.
* Diastolic pressure is increased and equal in all 4 chambers.

The Heart and Systemic Disease

Many systemic diseases may have manifestations in the heart. This section describes those that are most likely to be included on the examination.

Hyperthyroidism

Effects

The cardiovascular manifestations of hyperthyroidism include an increase in heart rate, stroke volume, and cardiac output. Peripheral vascular resistance is decreased, and thus there is a widened pulse pressure. All of these lead to an increase in myocardial oxygen consumption and therefore may precipitate angina. Other potential symptoms include palpitations, tachycardia, presyncope or syncope, and shortness of breath on exertion.

* The effects of hyperthyroidism lead to increased myocardial work and oxygen consumption and therefore may precipitate angina and arrhythmias.

Symptoms

Typical clinical scenario: An elderly woman (hyperthyroidism is 4-8 times as common in women as in men) presents with weight loss, weakness, and tachycardia and may or may not have angina or atrial fibrillation (15%). Examination shows tremor of fingers and tongue; goiter may or may not be present.

Physical Examination

Common physical findings are tachycardia and a bounding pulse with a wide pulse present with forceful apical pulse and a systolic ejection murmur due to increased flows. Cardiac arrhythmias are common, particularly supraventricular tachycardia and atrial fibrillation. Atrial fibrillation occurs in 10% to 20% of patients with hyperthyroidism. Therefore, thyrotoxicosis should always be suspected in patients with atrial fibrillation and the thyroid function should be checked.

* Findings of hyperthyroidism: tachycardia, bounding pulse, forceful apical impulse, widened pulse pressure, and systolic ejection murmur.
* Cardiac arrhythmias are common, especially atrial fibrillation.
* Thyrotoxicosis should be suspected in patients with atrial fibrillation.

Treatment

Treatment of underlying hyperthyroidism usually leads to reversal of cardiac symptoms. If atrial fibrillation is present, the risk of embolization is high and anticoagulation should be instituted. Cardioversion should not be attempted until a euthyroid state is achieved.

Hypothyroidism

Effects

Hypothyroidism leads to cardiac enlargement and decreased function due to infiltration of the myocardium with mucoproteins. This disorder decreases the metabolic rate and circulatory demand and causes bradycardia, decreased myocardial contractility and stroke volume, and an increase in peripheral resistance. In one-third of patients, a pericardial effusion is present. The cardiomyopathy of hypothyroidism is reversible if detected early. The hypothyroid state can increase cholesterol levels and accelerate atherosclerosis.

Symptoms

Typical clinical scenario: An elderly patient presents with depression, lethargy, and slowed mentation. Examination shows hair loss on the scalp and eyebrows and macroglossia. Sinus bradycardia usually is present. Chest radiography shows increased cardiac size.

Electrocardiography shows low voltage of QRS with prolonged intervals of QRS, PR, and QT.

* Hypothyroidism may lead to a reversible dilated cardiomyopathy.

Physical Examination

There may be cardiac enlargement due to the myocardial disease or to a commonly found pericardial effusion. The volume of pulses is decreased because of a decrease in myocardial contractility.

* Physical findings in hypothyroidism: cardiac enlargement, reduced myocardial contractility, and pericardial effusion (this occurs in a third of patients).
* Heart failure is less common, but it is reversible if found early.
* Atherosclerosis is accelerated.

Treatment

Treating the underlying cause and hypothyroidism likely leads to reversal of cardiac involvement.

Diabetes Mellitus

Effects

This condition frequently is associated with premature development of atherosclerosis. It is 2 times more prevalent in diabetic men and 3 times more prevalent in diabetic women than in a nondiabetic population. Patients with diabetes have an increased prevalence of hypertension and hyperlipidemia. Angina and myocardial infarction may often manifest as either atypical symptoms or silent ischemia. In fact, congestive heart failure may be the first manifestation of coronary artery disease among the diabetic population. There is also some evidence that cardiomyopathy unassociated with epicardial coronary atherosclerosis exists. This is speculated to be caused by small-vessel disease.

Treatment

The BARI (Bypass and Angioplasty Revascularization Investigation) trial found that coronary artery bypass grafting reduced the death rate more than percutaneous transluminal coronary angioplasty in patients with diabetes mellitus and multivessel coronary artery disease. However, stents and glycoprotein IIb/IIIa inhibitors were not routinely used in that trial. Patients with diabetes seem to have a higher complication rate than nondiabetics regardless of the interventional strategy chosen. If percutaneous intervention is chosen, glycoprotein IIb/IIIa inhibition and stent placement have better long-term control.

Preventive strategy is important. Trials have shown that aggressive management of traditional risk factors for coronary artery disease lowers mortality. Diabetic-specific risk factors for coronary artery disease include glycemic control and urinary protein excretion.

Randomized control trials have found that the use of antihypertensives for aggressive lowering of blood pressure (systolic pressure ≤120 mm Hg, diastolic pressure ≤80 mm Hg) reduces mortality. Statins and fibrates are effective for primary and secondary prevention of coronary artery disease in patients with both diabetes and hyperlipidemia. Aspirin also is effective for primary and secondary prevention. Angiotensin-converting enzyme inhibitors as a class reduce cardio-vascular events and mortality in patients with diabetes who are older than 55 years and have additional risk factors (HOPE trial).

* Fatal myocardial infarction is more common in diabetics than in nondiabetics.
* Lipid lowering and glycemic control are important in the prevention of coronary artery disease.
* The prevalence of hypertension is increased in diabetes, but aggressive control lowers mortality.
* The incidence of silent myocardial ischemia is high.
* Angiotensin inhibition should be considered for primary and secondary prevention in diabetics with known vascular disease or with 1 or more traditional risk factors.
* Aspirin is beneficial for primary and secondary prevention in diabetes.

Amyloidosis

Effects

Amyloidosis is the result of multiple diseases leading to the extracellular deposition of insoluble proteins in organs. It is estimated that there are 1,275 to 3,200 new cases annually in the United States. Amyloidosis is classified by the precursor plasma proteins that form the extracellular fibril deposits. The primary systemic type, AL, is due to monoclonal immunoglobulin free light chains, the hereditary (familial) type is due to mutant transthyretin deposition, the wild-type transthyretin type (wild type TTR, or senile type) is due to normal wild-type transthyretin deposition, and the secondary type (AA type) is related to amyloid A protein, usually the result of multiple myeloma. Amyloidosis, especially the AL type, frequently involves the heart and can cause arrhythmias, heart failure with left ventricular diastolic dysfunction, and sudden cardiac death. Organs involved typically are the liver, kidney, heart, gastrointestinal tract, and nervous tissue. In primary amyloidosis, nearly 90% of patients have clinical manifestations of cardiac dysfunction.

The heart is enlarged, most often a result of thickened ventricular myocardium from the protein infiltration. Abnormalities of diastolic function, conduction, and ultimately systolic dysfunction can occur. Amyloid deposition in the cardiac valves leads to atrioventricular valvular regurgitation, which is usually not severe.

Secondary amyloidosis occurs in association with chronic diseases such as rheumatoid arthritis, tuberculosis, chronic infection, neoplasia (especially multiple myeloma), and chronic renal failure. Cardiac involvement occurs in secondary amyloidosis, but it is usually not a prominent feature. In senile amyloidosis the heart is the organ most commonly involved. The prevalence of this disorder increases after age 60 years. Familial amyloidosis is autosomal dominant.

Clinical Features

The following can occur in cardiac amyloid involvement: congestive heart failure, arrhythmias, sudden death, angina, chest pain, pericardial effusion (usually not hemodynamically significant), and murmurs. The natural history of the disease is usually intractable because of ventricular cardiac failure. Diastolic abnormalities are early common manifestations and are classic for restrictive cardiomyopathy. The restrictive classification indicates a poor prognosis.

Symptoms

Typical clinical scenario: The diagnosis of amyloidosis should be given particular consideration when a patient (usually 40-70 years) presents with dyspnea and progressive edema of the lower extremity. Ancillary conditions such as vocal hoarseness, carpal tunnel syndrome, or peripheral neuropathy may be present and point to the systemic nature of the disease. The patient often has received treatment with digoxin and a diuretic but has had little improvement. The key finding is a low-voltage QRS complex with or without other conduction abnormalities (such as increased PR interval or bundle branch block) coupled with echocardiographic findings of thick walls and usually preserved ventricular function.

Diagnosis

The diagnosis of cardiac involvement is made on the basis of electrocardiography, which shows a classic low-voltage QRS complex, which is nonspecific. In addition, echocardiography is particularly useful. Classically, echocardiography shows an increase in left ventricular wall thickness, in contradistinction to the small (or normal) voltage on electrocardiography (Figure 3-12). Tissue characteristics on echocardiography are often described as granular. The atria generally are dilated. The cardiac valves may show some thickening and regurgitation. There may be a small pericardial effusion. Diastolic function generally is abnormal; in the early stages of the disease it shows a prolongation of the relaxation, and in the later stages it shows restrictive filling (consistent with high left ventricular filling pressures).

- In primary amyloidosis, 90% of patients have cardiac dysfunction.
- Echocardiographic features: thickened ventricular walls, granular myocardial appearance, dilated atria.
- Abnormal diastolic function: consistent with delay and relaxation in the early stages and with restrictive (increased ventricular filling pressure) patterns in the later stages.
- Hallmark: normal to reduced voltage on electrocardiography, in the face of "thick" walls on echocardiography.

Treatment

Treatment of the underlying cause may lead to a better prognosis. However, once cardiac amyloidosis is diagnosed, the prognosis generally is poor. Referral to a tertiary center with expertise in amyloidosis is warranted because experimental protocols have evolved into worthy treatments, such as stem cell transplant in primary amyloidosis.

Hemochromatosis

Effects

Hemochromatosis is an iron-storage disease. There is a primary or a secondary form related to exogenous iron (usually from repeated blood transfusions) deposits within the cardiac cells. Cardiac hemochromatosis generally does not occur alone and is accompanied by involvement of other organ systems, primarily the tetrad of diabetes, liver disease, brown skin pigmentation, and congestive heart failure. The condition may present with cardiomegaly, congestive heart

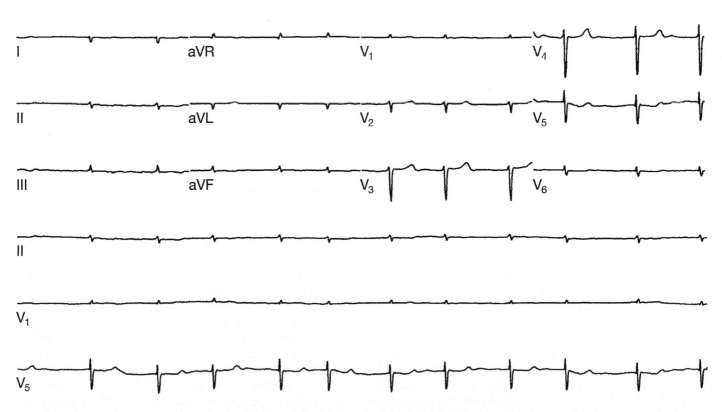

Figure 3-12. Electrocardiography in Cardiac Amyloidosis. Classic finding is low-voltage complexes.

failure, and arrhythmias. This disease has features of poor systolic and diastolic function. Once clinical cardiac symptoms appear, the prognosis is very poor unless treatment is initiated with a combination of phlebotomy and iron chelation.

Symptoms

Typical clinical scenario: Patients are middle-aged and present with symptoms and signs of heart failure. Clues to hemochromatosis are a well-tanned patient with diabetes or, at minimum, increased blood glucose value, arthralgias, and loss of libido. The diagnosis is made on the basis of increased transferrin saturation and increased serum ferritin value.

* Hemochromatosis is related to iron deposits within cardiac cells.
* Cardiac involvement in hemochromatosis does not occur alone; other organs are involved.
* The key to diagnosis is the tetrad of diabetes, liver disease, skin hyperpigmentation, and congestive heart failure.

Carcinoid Heart Disease

Effects

Carcinoid tumor is a malignant tumor. The primary site, usually gastrointestinal (terminal ileum), can produce a classic syndrome (in about 4% of patients) when metastatic to the liver or lungs. Malignant carcinoid tumors produce serotonin-like substances that cause cutaneous flushing, wheezing, and diarrhea, which is the carcinoid syndrome. These circulating substances are also toxic to valvular tissues. They are metabolized in the liver and lungs. Cardiac involvement occurs in approximately 50% of patients after hepatic or pulmonary metastasis. Therefore, toxic effects generally affect right-sided cardiac valves unless there is a shunt (generally a patent foramen ovale) that allows right-to-left movement of blood substances. Carcinoid lesions are fibrous plaques that form on valvular endocardium. The valve leaflets become thickened, relatively immobile, and retracted. The result is regurgitation with an element of stenosis of both the tricuspid and the pulmonary valves.

Symptoms

Typical clinical scenario: A 50- to 70-year-old patient presents with weight loss, fatigue, watery diarrhea (>10 stools daily), dyspnea on exertion, and audible wheezes. The patient has a red complexion and notes feeling hot flashes intermittently.

Physical Examination

Examination typically reveals a prominent v wave in an increased jugular venous pressure profile, a pulsatile liver that may be enlarged, ascites, and usually considerable peripheral edema.

Diagnosis

Electrocardiography typically shows right ventricular hypertrophy and right bundle branch block. Diagnosis is made by identification of a thickened tricuspid valve and pulmonary valve (left-sided valves only if a shunt is present) and the finding of liver metastasis on computed tomography, confirmed by a 24-hour urine study for 5-hydroxy-indoleacetic acid. Acquired tricuspid and pulmonary stenosis with or without regurgitation is rare and should always raise the possibility of carcinoid heart disease.

* Carcinoid tumors produce serotonin-like substances that cause flushing, wheezing, and diarrhea.
* Changes occur in the tricuspid and pulmonary valves. Dominant lesions are tricuspid regurgitation, pulmonary regurgitation, and stenosis.
* Acquired tricuspid and pulmonary stenosis with or without regurgitation is rare and should always raise the possibility of carcinoid heart disease.

Treatment

Treatment of underlying carcinoid tumor is important for relief of symptoms. If there is evidence of right heart failure (eg, intractable edema, ascites, dyspnea), then intervention may be warranted. Surgical therapies include tricuspid valve replacement and pulmonary valve resection.

Hypereosinophilic Syndrome

Effects

This syndrome affects young patients, generally male, who have a persistent eosinophil concentration of more than 1.5×10^9/L. The causes are several, including idiopathic hypereosinophilia, Löffler endocarditis, reactive or allergic eosinophilia, leukemic or neoplastic eosinophilia, or Churg-Strauss syndrome. All of these may have cardiac manifestations.

Clinical Features

Patients present with weight loss, fatigue, dyspnea, syncope, and systemic embolization. Cardiac manifestations include arrhythmias, myocarditis, conduction abnormalities, and thrombosis. Eosinophilic deposition occurs in the heart, where a clot forms in the apices of the ventricles and in the inflow portions under the mitral and tricuspid valves. This ultimately leads to matting down of the atrioventricular valve and causes considerable regurgitation. The clot ultimately scars, leading to endomyocardial fibrosis and restrictive cardiomyopathy.

* Hypereosinophilic syndrome may be present in patients with a persistent eosinophil value >1.5×10^9/L.
* Hypereosinophilic syndrome presents with restrictive cardiomyopathy, atrioventricular valve regurgitation, and systemic embolization.
* Unexpected thromboembolism in the presence of normal left ventricular function should raise suspicion of this syndrome.
* Churg-Strauss syndrome should be considered if pulmonary involvement is present.
* Typical clinical scenario: A young patient has fatigue, weight loss, and dyspnea of relatively recent onset (months) and presents to the emergency department because of new right-sided weakness. Echocardiography shows a normal to small left ventricle, mitral valve abnormalities, and apical ventricular thrombus. The diagnosis is confirmed on the basis of a complete blood count with differential count.

Systemic Lupus Erythematosus

Systemic lupus erythematosus may involve any of the cardiac structures. Special features of involvement include the antiphospholipid syndrome, Libman-Sacks endocarditis, and congenital heart block in the offspring of mothers with lupus.

Offspring of mothers with anti-La and anti-Ro antibodies are at risk for development of neonatal lupus, characterized by myocarditis and inflammation and fibrosis of the conduction system, which may lead to congenital heart block.

Cardiac involvement in patients with systemic lupus erythematosus may include pericarditis, which is characterized by a positive antinuclear antibody in the pericardial fluid, myocarditis (more common in patients with anti-Ro antibody), a valvulopathy, coronary arteritis, and Libman-Sacks endocarditis.

Libman-Sacks endocarditis is a noninfective vegetation that may be present in up to 50% of patients with systemic lupus erythematosus. It does not generally embolize or interfere with valvular function.

- The offspring of mothers with anti-La and anti-Ro antibodies are at risk for congenital heart block.
- Approximately a third of patients with systemic lupus erythematosus may have clinical evidence of cardiac involvement, including pericarditis, endocarditis, myocarditis, and coronary arteritis.
- Typical clinical scenario: A mother with a history of multiple spontaneous abortions carries a baby to term, and the baby is born with complete heart block.

Scleroderma

Scleroderma affects the skin with sclerotic changes, the esophagus with dysphagia, and small vessels with manifestations such as Raynaud phenomenon. Cardiac involvement is manifested by intramural coronary involvement and immune-mediated endothelial injury, which is often associated with the Raynaud phenomenon clinically. Cardiac involvement is the third most common cause of mortality in patients with scleroderma. Conduction defects occur in up to 20% of patients, and a pericardial effusion is found in a third of patients, but it is often asymptomatic. Indirect cardiac involvement due to pulmonary hypertension and cor pulmonale is frequent.

- Cardiac involvement is the third most common cause of mortality in patients with scleroderma.
- Coronary vasculitis is associated with clinical Raynaud phenomenon.
- Conduction defects may occur in up to 20% of patients.

Rheumatoid Arthritis

Rheumatoid arthritis may be associated with involvement of nearly all cardiac components, including pericardium, myocardium, valves, coronary arteries, and aorta. Rheumatoid arthritis may cause both granulomatous and nongranulomatous inflammation of valve leaflets, which rarely leads to severe valvular incompetence. Pericarditis of rheumatoid arthritis usually is associated with a low glucose level and complement depletion in the pericardial fluid. Rheumatoid nodules may be deposited in the conduction system, leading to degrees of heart block. Aortitis and pulmonary hypertension due to pulmonary vasculitis are very rare complications of rheumatoid arthritis.

- Pericardial fluid accumulation in patients with rheumatoid pericarditis will be low in glucose and complement and is associated with nodular rheumatoid arthritis.
- Granulomatous involvement in the conduction system may lead to heart block.
- Nongranulomatous and granulomatous involvement of valvular tissue may lead to incompetence of cardiac valve structures.

Ankylosing Spondylitis

Aortic dilatation and aortic regurgitation may be present in approximately 10% of patients. Aortic valve cusps become distorted and retracted, leading to considerable aortic regurgitation. The conduction system may become involved as a result of both fibrosis and inflammation.

Marfan Syndrome

Marfan syndrome is an autosomal dominant condition associated with degenerative elastic tissues, leading to arachnodactyly, tall stature, pectus excavatum, kyphoscoliosis, and lenticular dislocation.

Common cardiac manifestations include mitral valve prolapse, aortic regurgitation due to aortic dilatation, and increased risk of aortic dissection. Long-term β-adrenergic blockade has been shown to decrease the rate of aortic dilatation and potential for dissection. Dissection occurs rarely in an aorta less than 55 mm in diameter. When dissection occurs, it tends to start in the ascending aorta and extend along the entire aorta.

Friedreich Ataxia

This is an autosomal recessive neurologic disorder that involves the heart in up to 90% of cases. It usually manifests as a symmetric hypertrophy and less commonly as a dilated cardiomyopathy.

Osteogenesis Imperfecta

Brittle bones, blue sclera, and deafness are the hallmarks of this condition, which leads to a lack of collagen-supporting matrix. Ultimately, there is a degeneration of elastic tissues, including aortic root dilatation, aortic regurgitation, annular dilatation, and chordal stretch leading to marked atrioventricular regurgitation.

Lyme Disease

Lyme disease is a spirochete infection by *Borrelia burgdorferi* organisms. Up to 10% of cases have clinical cardiac involvement. Cardiac manifestations include atrioventricular block and Lyme carditis. The diagnosis is generally made by biopsy of the right ventricular myocardium or gallium scanning.

Acquired Immunodeficiency Syndrome (AIDS)

Clinically apparent cardiac involvement may occur in up to 10% of patients with AIDS. Cardiac involvement has been reported as a myocarditis in up to 50% of patients at autopsy. This may be associated with ventricular arrhythmias, dilated cardiomyopathy, pericarditis, or infectious or malignant invasion of the cardiac structures.

Cardiac Trauma

Contusion, in the acute stage, may lead to arrhythmia, increased cardiac enzyme values, transient regional wall motion abnormalities, and pericardial effusion or tamponade. It also has been reported to cause disruption of the aorta or valves (tricuspid valve most often) or right ventricular rupture.

Commotio cordis is sudden cardiac death due to trauma, characteristically mild trauma to the chest wall, which is generally a non-penetrating blow such as that delivered by a baseball or softball. This can occur in the absence of underlying cardiac disease and leads to instantaneous cardiac arrest. Research indicates that the trauma must be delivered during the vulnerable phase of the cardiac cycle, which is described as 15 to 30 milliseconds before and after the T wave.

Typical clinical scenario: An 11-year-old boy playing baseball is pitched a ball errantly and takes a blow to the chest. He falls to the ground pulseless.

Prosthetic Valve

Bioprostheses

These are made of animal or human tissue, which may be unmounted or mounted in a frame. Different types include 1) homograft (human tissue), either aortic or pulmonary; 2) heterograft (porcine valve), for example, Hancock or Carpentier-Edwards; and 3) pericardial (bovine valve), for example, Ionescu-Shiley. Tissue valves have the advantage that they are not as thrombogenic as mechanical valves; thus, most patients in sinus rhythm do not require anticoagulation in the long term, although they will need it for the first 3 to 6 months after valve replacement. There is a risk of systemic embolism, however, with biologic prostheses in patients with atrial fibrillation, particularly with a mitral prosthesis. The disadvantage is that tissue valves degenerate and calcify, and thus patients need reoperation. Approximately 50% of patients need valve replacement at 10 to 15 years. In young patients (20 years or younger), these valves may calcify very rapidly. Tissue valves last a little longer in the tricuspid position than in positions on the left side of the heart. Aortic valves have a slightly better durability than mitral valves. Prosthesis failure can be detected by clinical evaluation and 2-dimensional and Doppler echocardiography.

- Tissue valves are not as thrombogenic as mechanical valves.
- Most patients with tissue valves who are in sinus rhythm do not require anticoagulation.
- Tissue valves degenerate and calcify.
- About 50% of patients need valve replacement 10 to 15 years after original valve placement.

Mechanical Valves

An example of a *ball valve* is the Starr-Edwards. It has excellent longevity and is a so-called high-profile valve. Newer valves such as the *bileaflet* St. Jude or *tilting disc valve* (ie, Björk-Shiley) have a lower profile. All mechanical valves have a risk of thromboembolism and necessitate long-term anticoagulation. Hemolysis may occur with mechanical prostheses, especially if there is a perivalvular leak. Anticoagulation complications include hemorrhage, especially when the international normalized ratio is too high, and thrombosis, when the ratio is subtherapeutic. The rate of minor hemorrhages is 2% to 4% per year, and that of major hemorrhages is 1% to 2% per year. Risk of complications from mechanical prostheses, including endocarditis, is approximately 1% per year. All patients with a valvular prosthesis require antibiotic prophylaxis for endocarditis.

- All mechanical valves have a risk of thromboembolism.
- Hemolysis may occur with mechanical prostheses, especially in association with perivalvular leak.
- Anticoagulation can be associated with hemorrhage and thrombosis.
- All patients with a valvular prosthesis require antibiotic prophylaxis for endocarditis.

Tumors of the Heart

Most cardiac tumors are metastatic. The most common primary cardiac tumor is myxoma.

Cardiac Myxoma

Most cardiac myxomas are sporadic, but there have been some reports of familial occurrence. A syndrome of cardiac myxomas with lentiginosis (spotty pigmentation) and recurrent myxomas has been recognized. About 75% to 85% are in the left atrium, 18% are in the right atrium, and the rest are in the ventricles. Most of the atrial tumors arise from the atrial septum, usually adjacent to the fossa ovalis. About 95% are single. Most myxomas have a short stalk, are gelatinous and friable, and tend to embolize. They occasionally calcify, so they may be visible on a chest radiograph.

The main clinical features are obstruction to blood flow, embolization, and systemic effects. Left atrial tumors prolapse into the mitral valve orifice and produce mitral stenosis. They mimic mitral valvular stenosis, with symptoms of dyspnea, orthopnea, cough, pulmonary edema, and hemoptysis. Classically, symptoms occur with a change in body position. Physical findings suggest mitral stenosis. Pulmonary hypertension also may occur. An early diastolic sound, the tumor "plop," may be heard. This has a lower frequency than an opening snap.

- Most cardiac tumors are metastatic.
- The most common primary cardiac tumor is myxoma.
- About 75%-85% of cardiac myxomas are in the left atrium and 18% are in the right atrium; the rest are in the ventricles.
- Clinical features are obstruction to blood flow, embolization, and systemic effects.
- Symptoms occur with a change in body position.
- An early diastolic sound, the tumor "plop," may be heard.

Embolization

Systemic emboli may occur in 30% to 60% of patients with left-sided myxoma, frequently to the brain and lower extremities. Histologic examination of embolized material is important. Coronary embolization is rare, but it should be considered in a young patient with no known previous cardiac disease. Systemic effects are fatigue, fever, weight loss, and arthralgia. Systemic effects may be associated with an increased sedimentation rate, leukocytosis, hypergammaglobulinemia, and anemia. Increased immunoglobulins are usually of IgG class.

Echocardiography is the preferred approach to diagnosis. Transesophageal echocardiography helps delineate the precise site of origin and accurately assesses tumor size and degree of mobility. Operation is indicated when the diagnosis is made.

* Systemic emboli occur in 30% to 60% of cases of left-sided myxoma, frequently to the brain and lower extremities.
* Coronary embolization is rare.
* Systemic effects: fatigue, fever, weight loss, and arthralgia.
* Systemic effects may be associated with an increased sedimentation rate, leukocytosis, hypergammaglobulinemia, and anemia.
* Increased immunoglobulins are usually of IgG class.
* Echocardiography is the preferred approach to diagnosis.
* Operation is indicated.

Primary Cardiac Neoplasm

Rhabdomyoma is most common in women and children. It can produce obstruction of cardiac valves, simulating other abnormalities, and can cause cardiac arrhythmias. Other tumors, such as Kaposi sarcoma associated with acquired immunodeficiency syndrome (AIDS), do not usually cause cardiac symptoms.

Secondary tumors most often originate from bone, breast, lymphoma, leukemia, and thyroid. More than half of patients with malignant melanoma have metastases to the heart.

* Rhabdomyoma is most common in women and children.
* More than half of patients with malignant melanoma have metastases to the heart.

Imaging in Cardiology

An important part of cardiology is the appropriate choice of an imaging method to aid in the diagnosis, quantification, and prognosis of various diseases. The most commonly ordered test is assessment of left ventricular function. Various techniques are available, as outlined in Table 3-9. It is important for the clinician to have a focused question and subsequently choose the most appropriate technique to answer the clinical question.

Contrast Angiography

This imaging method was the first to visualize the cardiac chambers and directly assess left ventricular size and function with x-rays by injecting radiopaque material (iodine dye) into the cardiac chamber. Intracardiac access usually is required, and thus it is an invasive procedure, although new techniques (eg, intravenous digital subtraction angiography) may allow a more noninvasive approach. With use of a 30° right ventricular oblique and an orthogonal (60°) left anterior oblique view (sometimes with a 20°-30° cranial tilt to avoid foreshortening of the left ventricle), biplane views are obtained over several cycles to assess left ventricular volumes and regional wall motion abnormalities. Several algorithms have been developed to extrapolate the information of these 2 views to the entire heart. This requires certain

assumptions about the ventricular shape (regularity) and contraction pattern (concentric), which may not hold true in ischemia with resting wall motion abnormalities and previous myocardial infarction. Other concerns include the need for ionizing radiation, possible allergies to iodine, and impairment of renal function. These usually are managed with appropriate preparation (eg, hydration, corticosteroids, antihistamine, acetylcysteine) and by minimizing the amount of contrast agent used. Because coronary angiography, that is, the selective visualization of the coronary arteries, is the reference technique to assess the location (not necessarily the hemodynamic significance) of coronary artery stenosis, assessment of left ventricular function by contrast ventriculography should be performed only during accompanying coronary angiography. If the dye load needs to be minimized (renal failure), an alternative technique should be considered to save approximately 20 to 50 mL of contrast agent.

Echocardiography

Echocardiography uses a high-frequency (2-10 MHz) ultrasonic beam produced by a piezoelectric crystal from a transducer to generate images and acquire and process the various acoustic echoes. Currently, 3 methods are readily available: M-mode, 2-dimensional, and Doppler-color Doppler. A single cursor (beam) traverses the object of interest and traces its motion through time and gives excellent temporal-spatial resolution for timing of motion of structures in the cardiac cycle. M-mode echocardiography provides only limited information about the structures and has largely been replaced by 2-dimensional echocardiography.

Two-Dimensional Echocardiography

Two-dimensional imaging provides a beat-to-beat tomogram of the heart. Outlining the endocardial and epicardial borders allows determination of left ventricular volumes in end-diastole and end-systole and subsequently stroke volume, ejection fraction, cardiac output, and muscle mass. The algorithms used are similar to those used in contrast ventriculography, requiring certain assumptions about ventricular shape and contraction. The technique is, however, completely noninvasive and thus lends itself to serial image acquisition. Its easy availability has made it the most widely used imaging technology in cardiology today. With assessment of endocardial motion and wall thickening from various transducer positions, regional wall motion abnormalities also can be assessed. The morphologic features of valves (eg, pliability, degree of calcification, morphologic abnormalities, flail segments) and intracardial and pericardial structures also can be analyzed. With exercise or pharmacologic (usually dobutamine) stress, regional wall motion can be assessed both at rest and at stress for the diagnosis of coronary artery disease. Regional wall motion analysis requires a highly skilled interpreter, particularly in the presence of preexisting regional wall motion abnormalities.

Doppler-Color Doppler Echocardiography

Doppler-color Doppler echocardiography allows direct measurements of blood velocities across valves and along conduits (eg, left ventricular outflow tract, vessels), which permit calculation of stroke volume, cardiac output, valve gradients, and severity of regurgitant lesions and semiquantitation of intracardiac and extracardiac shunts.

Table 3-9   Cardiac Imaging Methods

| Method | Variable Assessed | | | | Cost Effectiveness[a] |
	LVEF	RV Function	LV Mass	RWMA	
Contrast angiography	Yes	No	No	Yes	++++[b]
Two-dimensional echocardiography	Yes	Yes	Yes	Yes	++
First-pass RNA	Yes	Yes, quantitative[c]	No	No	+
Blood pool RNA	Yes	No	No	Yes	+
Magnetic resonance imaging	Yes	Yes, quantitative[c]	Yes	Yes	+++/+
Electron beam computed tomography	Yes	Yes, quantitative[c]	Yes	Yes	+++

Abbreviations: LV, left ventricular; LVEF, left ventricular ejection fraction; RNA, radionuclide angiography; RV, right ventricular; RWMA, regional wall motion abnormalities.

[a] +, Least expensive; ++++, most expensive.

[b] If performed without coronary angiography.

[c] Quantitative, absolute measurements of global ventricular volumes possible to facilitate measure of RV ejection fraction.

The crucial element for optimal echocardiographic image acquisition is the availability of appropriate acoustic "windows" to allow proper directing of the ultrasound beam to the structure of interest. Obese patients, very cachectic patients, and patients with extensive lung disease (eg, smokers, chronic obstructive pulmonary disease, restrictive lung disease) may pose insurmountable problems for transthoracic echocardiography in a small percentage of cases. Transesophageal echocardiography may overcome this problem, but it is an invasive approach. Echocardiography also requires the most operator experience and is more dependent on the operator for both image acquisition and interpretation. Neither technique can currently visualize the coronary arteries in the way that angiography does.

Contrast Echocardiography
Contrast echocardiography is a new technology, enhancing the echocardiographic signal with injection of an enhancing agent. Some of these agents are now smaller than red blood cells and cross the pulmonary vascular bed. Applications in the clinical arena include better visualization of the endocardium that is not conducive to sonographic access (caused by obesity, emphysema, chest deformities). Work is also progressing to use echocardiographic contrast agents as "flow" agents to assess myocardial perfusion, an additional, independent factor complementing regional wall motion analysis and cardiac function. Standardization of testing algorithms is in progress.

Radionuclide Imaging
Radionuclide imaging principally uses 2 techniques: labeling erythrocytes with an isotope to assess endocardial motion or using perfusion tracers (thallium, sestamibi) to assess differences between resting and stress blood flow.

Radionuclide Angiography
Erythrocytes are labeled with technetium, which can be imaged by a gamma camera, which usually is placed in the anteroposterior, left anterior oblique, and lateral positions. Sufficient photon cap-

ture is ensured by acquiring images over multiple cardiac cycles. This procedure requires electrocardiographic gating, which opens the aperture of the camera for fractions during the cardiac cycle. Patients with atrial fibrillation and markedly variable RR intervals are not suited for this approach. Quantification of left ventricular function is based on the number of photons in the ventricle at end-diastole and end-systole. This count-based method obviates any geometric assumptions and thus provides a very accurate assessment of left ventricular function, especially in patients with poor function. Because radionuclide angiography is dependent on the number of photons available at end-diastole and end-systole, there is a very good signal with little noise in large, poorly contractile ventricles, allowing excellent discrimination between low ejection fractions, particularly during serial assessment. In contrast, echocardiography relies on the endocardial inward motion, which is poor in severely dysfunctional ventricles, introducing a higher signal-to-noise ratio that makes discrimination between low ejection fractions difficult.

First-Pass Radionuclide Angiography
Recently, techniques have been developed to follow the passage of a radioisotope bolus through the right and left cardiac system, allowing assessment of left ventricular function. Subsequently, the tracer distributes according to coronary blood flow, and perfusion images are obtained. This technique, based on dye-dilution and videodensitometric principles, allows easy, economical assessment of both right and left ventricular function. Drawbacks are difficulties in administering the bolus (poor intravenous access), which lead to early diffusion of the bolus with poor discrimination of the dextro-phase and levo-phase. Similar to radionuclide angiography, first-pass radionuclide angiography is extremely sensitive to arrhythmias, particularly when they occur during the calculation phase of the first-pass acquisition.

Myocardial Perfusion Imaging
The 2 most commonly applied isotopes are thallium and sestamibi, which distribute to the myocardium according to blood flow. They

are avidly taken up by the myocytes. These isotopes can subsequently be imaged at rest and after exercise (Figure 3-13). Images are acquired by a planar technique in which the camera is positioned similar to that in radionuclide angiography in 3 positions. More accurate is a single-photon emission computed tomography approach in which a camera rotates around the patient and takes images at certain narrow-angle intervals to compose a complete 3-dimensional image of the entire heart without superpositrons. The views are then commonly displayed as short-axis tomograms spanning the entire heart (Figure 3-13, upper left at stress; upper right at rest). The images are then compared with each other. During stress (exercise or pharmacologic), there is usually reduced uptake in the affected myocardium. Subsequently, at rest, there is redistribution of the isotope (thallium) where a preferential washout of the previously normal myocardium and a preferential uptake of the previously hypoperfused myocardium take place. With sestamibi, the isotope is taken up essentially irreversibly into the myocardium, and a repeat resting injection is mandatory to reflect the resting flow conditions. The extent and the severity of the perfusion defect provide additional important information in regard to the prognosis of the disease which goes beyond the mere diagnosis of the presence or absence of coronary artery disease. It is also helpful to assess residual ischemia in patients with previous myocardial infarction and to assess therapeutic efficacy in patients treated medically or by intervention. The result of the

imaging studies should always be viewed in conjunction with the data available from the exercise or stress electrocardiogram.

Gated Sestamibi Imaging

Improved imaging techniques and shortened image acquisition time due to dual- or triple-camera configurations have made gated imaging available, a technique similar to radionuclide angiography. Unlike multiple-gated acquisition scanning, in which the isotope remains in the left ventricular cavity (a "lumenogram"), with gated single-photon emission computed tomography the motion of myocardium is imaged throughout the cardiac cycle. This allows regional wall motion analysis similar to that of echocardiography. Because of technical circumstances, poststress images are acquired with a considerable time delay and thus reflect mostly resting contractility.

Magnetic Resonance Imaging

Magnetic resonance imaging (MRI) is a noninvasive, 3-dimensional imaging technique that allows noninvasive assessment of left ventricular size, function, and muscle mass. The technique is extremely precise. Recent technical advances have considerably shortened the acquisition time. Clinical applications are emerging aside from study of left ventricular function and anatomical structure. It has the potential to differentiate plaque composition and thus may be able to identify vulnerable plaques. Additional work indicates its usefulness for

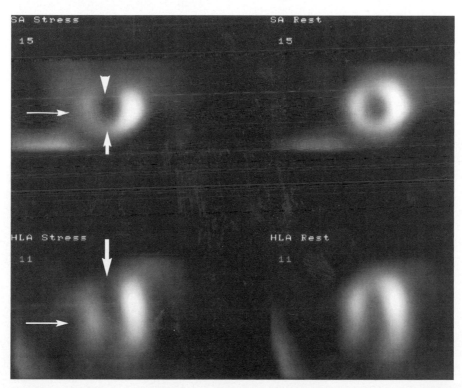

Figure 3-13. Myocardial Perfusion Image for a Patient With Exertional Angina (Class III) of Recent Onset. Low-level exercise with 1-mm ST-segment depression at 2 minutes into exercise. The left column depicts the stress images with a representative short-axis tomogram (upper left panel) and the horizontal long axis (lower left panel). In the right column are the rest images, with corresponding short-axis tomogram in the right upper panel and the corresponding horizontal long-axis tomogram in the right lower panel. Note the severely reduced uptake in the apical (thick arrow), septal (thin arrows), anterior (arrowhead), and inferior (short arrow) segments. At rest there is nearly complete normalization in all segments. Subsequent angiography indicated complete occlusion of the right coronary artery and 80% stenosis in the proximal left anterior descending coronary artery. The circumflex coronary artery did not show a critical lesion.

assessing myocardial perfusion and, although MRI for this purpose is not yet widely available, it will undoubtedly add to our diagnostic armamentarium in the near future.

Electron Beam Computed Tomography

Electron beam computed tomography (EBCT) uses a scanner without any movable parts in which an electron beam is deflected, via magnetic fields, rapidly on several rings around the patient, allowing high-fidelity, high-resolution, 3-dimensional images of the entire heart in rapid succession. Like all complex imaging techniques it is dependent on electrocardiographic gating; however, it requires only 1 beat to complete a cycle. Because the entire heart is encompassed in the scan, no geometric assumptions need to be made. It is ideally suited for serial studies in left ventricular remodeling because of its high precision and accuracy. Drawbacks are the requirements for a contrast agent to be administered into a peripheral vein and for ionizing radiation.

EBCT has raised considerable interest for the early detection of coronary atherosclerosis because it opens the possibility for early, effective, and targeted intervention (primary prevention). It is currently the most widely used technique in this field because of its ease of application (rapid acquisition time, no contrast agent) and standardized imaging and analysis algorithms. It detects coronary calcium, an essential component of coronary plaque. Databases are being generated to assess the degree of calcification in relation to age, sex, and ethnic background. This information has been correlated with future risk for cardiac events, surpassing any currently available algorithm containing the conventional risk factor array (eg, lipid profile, smoking history, family history, hypertension, and diabetes). Interest in the early detection of atherosclerosis has resulted in other scanning technology. It is not yet clear whether these other scanners are equivalent in their predictive accuracy.

Positron Emission Tomography

Positron emission tomography depends on the detection of a simultaneous pair of photons radiating into exact opposite directions. This principle, not unlike radionuclide angiography, allows high-spatial and temporal resolution imaging. Positron emission tomography currently is the reference standard for the assessment of myocardial viability. However, the complexity of the technology and the cost currently limit its use to tertiary academic centers.

Part II

Peter A. Brady, MB,ChB, MD

Mechanism of Arrhythmias: Reentry

Reentry is the most common mechanism responsible for cardiac arrhythmias. Reentrant rhythms may be micro-reentrant or macro-reentrant. For reentry to occur, 3 conditions must be met (Figures 3-14 and 3-15): 1) 2 or more anatomically or functionally distinct pathways (connected proximally and distally to form a closed circuit) must be present (eg, slow and fast pathways in patients with supraventricular tachycardia due to atrioventricular [AV] nodal reentry), 2) unidirectional block must occur in 1 pathway, and 3) slowed conduction must occur in the second pathway to an extent that conduction in the first pathway has recovered by the time the impulse reaches its distal connection. Examples of micro-reentrant circuits include the sinus node, AV node, or injured myocardium bordering a myocardial infarction (myocardial scar). Macro-reentrant circuits include reentry within the atrium (as in atrial flutter), AV conduction system, ventricle, or an accessory pathway (as in Wolff-Parkinson-White syndrome).

* Reentry is the most common mechanism for cardiac arrhythmias. Other less common mechanisms of arrhythmias are those due to triggered activity and increased automaticity.
* Automaticity is enhanced by increased sympathetic tone, hypoxia, acid-base and electrolyte disturbances, and atrial or ventricular stretch.

Investigations Commonly Used in the Evaluation and Management of Patients With Suspected Rhythm Disorders

Electrocardiography

Electrocardiography (ECG) remains a valuable tool in the evaluation of heart rhythm disorders. In many cases, ECG performed during symptoms of tachycardia is diagnostic of the tachycardia mechanism and is all that is needed to plan management. In other cases, ECG may provide clues to the probable diagnosis of symptoms. Whenever possible, a current ECG should be compared with previous recordings.

Ambulatory ECG Monitoring and Transtelephonic Event Recording

Ambulatory (Holter) monitoring is useful for the evaluation of both symptomatic and asymptomatic rhythm disturbances and their relationship to daily activity (eg, exercise). Symptoms, if present, must, however, occur frequently enough to be recorded during the 24- or 48-hour recording period. A diary in which patients record their activity and specific symptoms and precise duration of both allows correlation with heart rhythm recordings.

Ambulatory monitoring is also useful for assessing the impact of treatment on arrhythmias (eg, determining the adequacy of ventricular rate control during drug therapy for atrial fibrillation because control at rest may not reflect response during exercise or daily activity).

* Ambulatory monitoring allows correlation of (frequent) symptoms with heart rhythm and helps assess response to treatment and pacemaker function.

Transtelephonic event recording is similar to ambulatory recording but is more useful for documenting heart rate and rhythm when

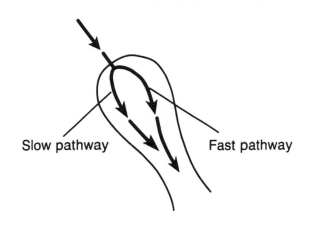

Figure 3-14. Reentry Within the Atrioventricular (AV) Node. The 2 limbs of reentrant circuit are shown. Recent evidence suggests that a portion of the reentrant pathway is separate from the AV node.

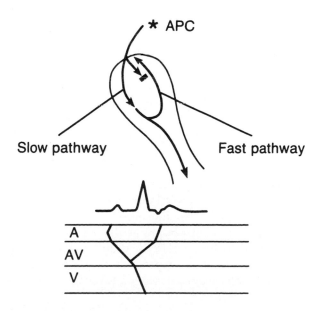

Figure 3-15. Atrioventricular (AV) Nodal Reentrant Tachycardia. An atrial premature complex (APC) blocks in fast pathway but conducts over slow pathway to ventricle. Impulse then returns to atria over recovered fast pathway and can reenter slow pathway and initiate tachycardia. The A indicates atrium; V, ventricle.

symptoms are less frequent (<1 episode per 24-48 hours). Typically, patients either wear the recording device continuously for several days or weeks or briefly attach it to themselves during symptoms. The ECG is permanently stored in memory when the device is activated during symptoms by the patient. In most cases, continuous loop recorders record the ECG obtained 30 seconds to 4 minutes before the activation button is depressed. This feature is useful in patients whose symptoms are brief or of sudden onset. When convenient, the ECG then can be transmitted over the telephone for evaluation. In most cases, depending on the specific population of patients in which the device is used, about 20% of transmissions document abnormal heart rhythm. However, even when completely normal, transmissions can be helpful for patient management when a normal rhythm is identified. Implantable loop event recorders also may be used when symptoms are more infrequent or are of such sudden onset that activation is not possible. These devices, which are implanted subcutaneously in the pectoral region, can be programmed to provide information regarding rhythm disturbances over several months.

- Transtelephonic event recording documents heart rate during symptoms that occur infrequently.
- About 20% of transmissions document abnormal heart rhythm.
- Transtelephonic event recording is often helpful for patient management even if a normal rhythm is identified.

Implantable Loop Recorder

For patients with infrequent and sudden-onset symptoms, activation of a loop recorder may be difficult. In such cases, an implantable loop recorder should be considered. An implantable loop recorder is inserted subcutaneously in the anterior part of the chest and can be programmed to record both patient-activated and automatically activated events. Event data can be retrieved noninvasively (much like a pacemaker), allowing correlation with symptoms and rhythm.

Exercise Testing

Treadmill exercise testing is useful when symptoms occur during exercise because it allows evaluation of cardiac rhythm in a controlled setting with ECG monitoring. Exercise testing is also useful to determine whether the beneficial effect of a drug at rest is reversed with exercise. For example, patients with atrial fibrillation may have adequate control of heart rate at rest but poor control with moderate exercise. Similarly, patients with ventricular tachycardia or complex ventricular ectopy may have adequate suppression of the arrhythmia at rest in response to medical therapy only to have ventricular tachycardia with exercise. Not infrequently, proarrhythmic effects of antiarrhythmic drugs may be provoked by exercise testing. This is particularly the case for class IC drugs (eg, flecainide and propafenone) because of use-dependence (ie, the pharmacologic effect of a drug is affected by heart rate) and their long unbinding times from the sodium channel.

- Exercise testing allows evaluation of cardiac rhythm disturbance during exercise.
- Exercise testing is useful for assessing whether the effect of a drug is reversed with exercise.

Premature ventricular complexes (PVCs) occur during exercise testing in 10% of patients without and 60% of those with coronary artery disease. The response of PVCs *during* exercise does not predict the severity of coronary artery disease. Elimination of PVCs with exercise is not an indication that coronary artery disease is less severe. Recent data suggest that appearance of frequent PVCs (defined as 7 or more per minute, ventricular bigeminy or trigeminy, ventricular couplets or triplets, ventricular tachycardia or flutter, torsades de pointes, or ventricular fibrillation) during the recovery phase of treadmill exercise testing may be a better predictor of outcome than PVCs occurring during exercise.

- PVCs occur during exercise in 10% of patients without and in 60% of those with coronary artery disease.
- The response of PVCs during exercise does not predict the severity of coronary artery disease.
- Elimination of PVCs with exercise does not indicate less severe coronary artery disease.

Exercise testing is useful for assessing sinus node function, for diagnosing chronotropic incompetence in a patient who complains of dyspnea on exertion or fatigue, and for assessing AV block. Exercise testing is most useful for assessing second-degree AV block in which the site of block is unknown (ie, within the AV node vs. His-Purkinje system). This distinction is important because AV block occurring within the AV node (Wenckebach [Mobitz I]) is usually benign and does not require pacing. Characteristically, block within the AV node improves with exercise because increased catecholamines enhance AV node conduction. In contrast, AV block due to failure of conduction in the His-Purkinje system (Mobitz II) has a worse prognosis and a high incidence of progression to complete heart block and thus is an indication for permanent pacing. In contrast to block within the AV node, Mobitz II block typically worsens during exercise because enhanced AV node conduction increases the frequency of activation of the diseased His-Purkinje system, thus putting greater strain on the already diseased conducting system.

- Exercise testing is useful for assessing sinus node function.
- Mobitz I block usually improves with exercise.
- Mobitz II block usually worsens with exercise.
- Mobitz II block frequently progresses to complete AV block and therefore requires permanent pacing.

Electrophysiologic Testing

Electrophysiologic study involves the placement of electrode catheters in the heart to record and to stimulate heart rhythm. In most cases, pacing and recording electrodes (catheters) are positioned in the high right atrium, across the tricuspid valve in the region of the AV node and His bundle, and in the right ventricular apex (Figure 3-16). In select patients, additional catheters are placed (most commonly within the coronary sinus) to record from the left atrium and ventricle. Electrophysiologic testing is indicated in patients with cardiogenic syncope of undetermined origin, for determining the mechanism of supraventricular tachycardia, for assessing symptomatic patients with Wolff-Parkinson-White syndrome, and for evaluating patients

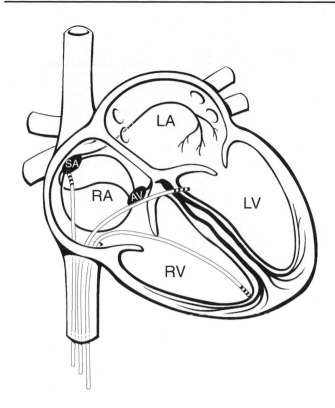

Figure 3-16. Locations of Intracardiac Catheters for Pacing and During Cardiac Electrophysiologic Study. AV indicates atrioventricular node; LA, left atrium; LV, left ventricle; RA, right atrium; RV, right ventricle; SA, sinoatrial node.

with sustained ventricular tachycardia and survivors of out-of-hospital cardiac arrest. As part of the evaluation of patients with syncope, electrophysiologic study (including measurement of sinus and AV nodal function and ventricular stimulation to exclude ventricular arrhythmias), when normal, also can be used in combination with tilt-table testing. Complications resulting from electrophysiologic study are infrequent, occurring in less than 0.5% to 1.0% of cases. Most common complications include vascular injury and hematoma at the puncture site.

- Electrophysiologic testing is invasive.
- Indications for electrophysiologic study include a history of syncope suggestive of cardiogenic syncope or to determine the mechanism of a clinically documented or suspected heart rhythm disorder.
- Complications are uncommon and usually minor.

Therapy for Heart Rhythm Disorders

Several therapeutic options are available for heart rhythm disorders. These include drug therapy, radiofrequency ablation, and device therapy (pacing for bradyarrhythmias and implantable cardioverter-defibrillators for tachyarrhythmias).

Antiarrhythmic Drugs
Therapeutic range, half-life, and routes of metabolism of antiarrhythmic drugs are listed in Table 3-10. The relative effectiveness

of these drugs for treating PVCs, ventricular tachycardia, paroxysmal tachycardia that uses the AV node as part of the reentrant circuit, and atrial fibrillation is given in Table 3-11. The predominant target of the antiarrhythmic drugs is shown in Figure 3-17.

Half-life is an important concept in the use of antiarrhythmic drugs. It is the time required for 50% of the drug within the body to be eliminated. It takes 5 half-lives for a drug to reach steady state or to be eliminated completely. If a drug has a half-life of 90 minutes (eg, lidocaine), a steady state will be reached in 6 hours; therefore, a loading dose is given to achieve a therapeutic level more promptly.

- Half-life is an important concept in the use of antiarrhythmic drugs.
- Half-life is the time required for 50% of the drug within the body to be eliminated.
- It takes 5 half-lives for a drug to reach steady state or to be eliminated completely.

Proarrhythmic effect (Table 3-12), a common and important problem of all antiarrhythmic drugs, occurs when the drug creates an adverse rhythm disturbance (Figure 3-18), including sinus node suppression and sinus bradycardia, AV block, or increased frequency of or new-onset atrial or ventricular arrhythmias. All antiarrhythmic agents should be considered proarrhythmic. The effect was first described in association with quinidine and causes quinidine syncope, which occurs in an estimated 3% of patients who take this drug. In such patients, a rapid polymorphic ventricular tachycardia, termed *torsades de pointes*, develops. The frequency of proarrhythmia is higher in patients with decreased ventricular function and a history of sustained ventricular tachycardia or ventricular fibrillation. Unfortunately, it is these patients who most often require antiarrhythmic drugs. Also, proarrhythmia can occur in structurally normal hearts.

- Proarrhythmic effect occurs when a drug creates a rhythm disturbance.
- All antiarrhythmic drugs can cause arrhythmias (ie, have proarrhythmic potential).
- Quinidine syncope due to polymorphic ventricular tachycardia (torsades de pointes) is an example of a proarrhythmic effect.

The results of recent pharmacologic trials for the prevention of sudden cardiac death are summarized in Table 3-13.

Class I Antiarrhythmic Drugs
The Cardiac Arrhythmia Suppression Trial (CAST) evaluated the use of flecainide, encainide, and moricizine to suppress asymptomatic or mildly symptomatic ventricular ectopy after myocardial infarction. The hypothesis tested was that patients in whom spontaneous ventricular ectopy could be suppressed would have improved outcome. In fact, patients who received class I agents showed a decrease in survival rates despite the adequate suppression of ventricular ectopy when compared with placebo. At the time, this was a totally unexpected and alarming finding. Similar results have been reported with class IA drugs (eg, quinidine, procainamide, and disopyramide) and the class IB drug mexiletine.

Table 3-10 Properties of Antiarrhythmic Drugs

Drug	Therapeutic Range, mcg/mL	Half-life, h	Route of Metabolism	
			Hepatic, %	Renal, %
Class IA				
Quinidine	2-5	6-8	80	20
Procainamide	4-10	3-6	50	50
Disopyramide	2-5	4-8	50	50
Class IB				
Lidocaine	1.5-5	1-4	100	...
Mexiletine	1-2	8-16	100	...
Phenytoin	10-20	24	~100	...
Class IC				
Flecainide	0.2-1	12-27	75	25
Propafenone	Not helpful[a]	2-10	100	...
Class III				
Amiodarone	1-2.5	25-110 days	80	...
Sotalol	~2.5	7-18	...	100
Ibutilide	Not established	2-12	...	80
Dofetilide	1-3.5	10	...	80

[a] Therapeutic effects for propafenone are generally associated with a QRS width increase of 10% above baseline.
Modified from MKSAP IX: Part C, Book 1, 1992. American College of Physicians. Used with permission.

Table 3-11 Relative Effectiveness of Antiarrhythmic Drugs

Drug	Effectiveness[a]			
	PVCs	VT	PSVT	AF
Quinidine	2+	2+	2+	2+
Procainamide	2+	2+	2+	2+
Disopyramide	2+	2+	2+	2+
Lidocaine	2+	2+	0	0
Mexiletine	2+	2+	0	0
Ibutilide[b]	-	-	-	2+
Flecainide	4+	2+	3+	2+
Propafenone	4+	2+	3+	2+
Dofetilide[c]	2+	2+	-	2+
Amiodarone	4+	3+	3+	3+
Sotalol	3+	2-3+	3+	2+

Abbreviations: AF, atrial fibrillation (prevention of paroxysmal AF); PSVT, paroxysmal tachycardia that uses atrioventricular node as part of reentrant circuit; PVCs, premature ventricular complexes; VT, ventricular tachycardia.
[a] Effectiveness: 0, not effective; 1+, least effective; 4+, most effective.
[b] Only intravenous form available; approved for acute cardioversion.
[c] An option to maintain sinus rhythm in patients with atrial fibrillation and underlying heart disease.

- CAST reported decreased survival rate with drug therapy in patients with asymptomatic ventricular ectopy after infarction.

Amiodarone

Results from 2 randomized trials of amiodarone after myocardial infarction (European Myocardial Infarction Amiodarone Trial [EMIAT] and Canadian Amiodarone Myocardial Infarction Arrhythmia Trial [CAMIAT]) suggested that amiodarone may decrease arrhythmia-related death. However, overall mortality was not improved. Results from amiodarone trials among patients with congestive heart failure are also mixed. The Survival Trial of Antiarrhythmic Therapy in patients with Congestive Heart Failure arrhythmia (STAT-CHF) study showed that overall mortality was not significantly different between patients treated with amiodarone and those receiving placebo. In contrast, the Gruppo de Estudio de la Sobrevida en la Insuficiencia Cardiaca en Argentina (GESICA) study (randomized trial of low-dose amiodarone in severe congestive heart failure) showed that low-dose amiodarone therapy reduced total mortality in comparison with placebo therapy in patients with congestive heart failure. The differences in outcome may be explained by differences in patient population. In the STAT-CHF study, approximately 70% of the study population had coronary artery disease, compared with 30% in the GESICA study. Currently, the routine use of amiodarone after myocardial infarction or in unselected patients with congestive heart failure is not recommended. However,

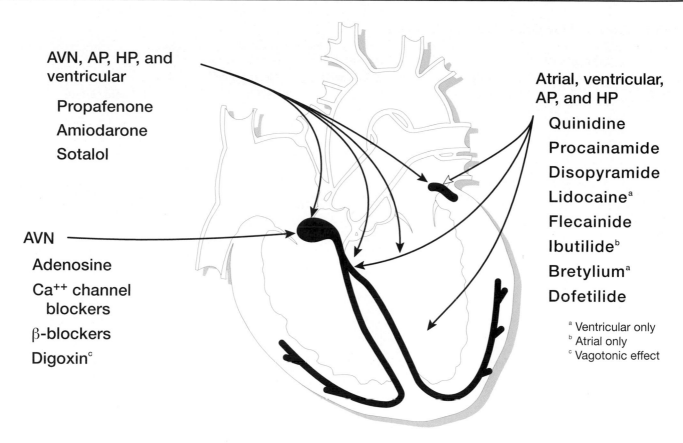

AVN, AP, HP, and ventricular

Propafenone

Amiodarone

Sotalol

AVN

Adenosine

Ca++ channel blockers

β-blockers

Digoxin[c]

Atrial, ventricular, AP, and HP

Quinidine

Procainamide

Disopyramide

Lidocaine[a]

Flecainide

Ibutilide[b]

Bretylium[a]

Dofetilide

[a] Ventricular only
[b] Atrial only
[c] Vagotonic effect

Figure 3-17. The Predominant Targets of Frequently Used Antiarrhythmic Agents. AP indicates accessory pathway; AVN, atrioventricular node; HP, His-Purkinje system.

if patients have frequent and complex PVCs associated with documented symptoms in the setting of compromised left ventricular dysfunction, it is not unreasonable to consider a trial of amiodarone therapy.

• The routine use of amiodarone after myocardial infarction or in unselected patients with congestive heart failure for PVC suppression or primary prevention of sudden cardiac death is not recommended.

Adenosine

Adenosine slows conduction in the AV node and is eliminated by uptake in endothelial cells and erythrocytes. Its half-life is 10 seconds. Adenosine is indicated in supraventricular reentrant tachycardia that uses the AV node as part of the reentrant circuit (ie, AV nodal reentry or reentry using an accessory pathway). The drug does not terminate atrial fibrillation, flutter, or tachycardia, and it slows the ventricular rate for only a few seconds because of its short half-life. Both adenosine and verapamil have equal efficacy at the highest recommended doses (adenosine, 12 mg; verapamil, 10 mg). Because of the short half-life of adenosine, approximately 10% of patients have recurrent supraventricular tachycardia after its administration, whereas recurrent supraventricular tachycardia is rare after termination by verapamil. In patients who present with wide QRS tachycardia (ventricular tachycardia) or atrial fibrillation and associated Wolff-Parkinson-White syndrome, hemodynamic collapse is common

when they are given verapamil. This hemodynamic collapse is not associated with adenosine. The cost of adenosine is approximately twice that of verapamil.

• Adenosine slows conduction in the AV node.
• Adenosine can terminate supraventricular reentrant tachycardia that relies on conduction through the AV node.
• Adenosine does not terminate atrial fibrillation, flutter, or atrial tachycardia (exceptions exist, so adenosine should not be used to "diagnose" atrial tachycardia by exclusion).
• The efficacy of 12 mg of adenosine is equal to that of 10 mg of verapamil.
• The cost of adenosine is twice that of verapamil.

Electrophysiology Study

Because of the widespread availability and use of implantable cardioverter-defibrillators, electrophysiologic testing is less commonly used. Most commonly, an electrophysiologic study is performed to attempt induction of a suspected heart rhythm disorder in patients who present with syncope.

Among patients presenting with ventricular tachycardia due to coronary disease, the chance of inducing clinical tachycardia in the laboratory is 95% but decreases to 75% in patients with dilated cardiomyopathy or valvular heart disease. Among patients who present with out-of-hospital cardiac arrest or ventricular fibrillation, the

Table 3-12 Toxicity and Side Effects of Antiarrhythmic Drugs

Drug	Frequency of Side Effects, %	Organ Toxicity	% Proarrhythmia During Treatment for VT	Risk of Congestive Heart Failure[a]		Side Effects
				EF >30%	EF ≤30%	
Quinidine	30	Moderate	3	0	0	Nausea, abdominal pain, diarrhea, thrombocytopenia, hypotension, ↓ warfarin clearance
Procainamide	30	High	2	0	1+	Lupus-like syndrome, rash, fever, headache, nausea, hallucinations, diarrhea
Disopyramide	30	Low	2	1+	4+	Dry mouth, urinary hesitancy, blurred vision, constipation, urinary retention
Lidocaine	40	Moderate	2	0	0	L-H, seizure, tremor, confusion, memory loss, nausea
Mexiletine	40	Low	2	0	0	L-H, tremor, ataxia, confusion, memory loss, altered liver function
Ibutilide[b]	25	Low	4	0	0	Nausea, headache
Flecainide	30	Low	5	1+	3+	L-H, visual disturbance, headache, nausea
Propafenone	30	Low	5	0-1+	2+	L-H, headache, nausea, constipation, metallic taste, ↓ warfarin clearance
Dofetilide	20	Low	4	0	0	Headache, chest pain, dizziness
Amiodarone	65	High	4	0	1+	Corneal deposits, photosensitivity, sleep disturbance, nausea, anorexia, tremor, ataxia, neuropathy, pulmonary fibrosis, thyroid disorders, hepatotoxicity, ↓ warfarin clearance
Sotalol	30	Low	5	1+	3+	L-H, fatigue, dyspnea, nausea

Abbreviations: EF, ejection fraction; L-H, light-headedness; VT, sustained ventricular tachycardia.

[a] Congestive heart failure risk: 0, no risk; 4+, high risk.

[b] Intravenous therapy for acute cardioversion in patients with atrial fibrillation.

Modified from MKSAP IX: Part C, Book 1, 1992. American College of Physicians. Used with permission.

chance of life-threatening ventricular arrhythmia being induced at testing decreases to 70%.

Transcatheter Radiofrequency Ablation

Transcatheter ablation therapy using a radiofrequency energy source to heat tissue has revolutionized the treatment of almost all heart rhythm disorders. With currently available technology, supraventricular tachycardias such as AV nodal reentrant tachycardia or tachycardia due to an accessory pathway (such as Wolff-Parkinson-White syndrome) are completely curable with radiofrequency ablation in more than 95% of cases. Ectopic atrial tachycardias are curable in more than 90% of cases. Table 3-14 lists heart rhythm disorders amenable to catheter ablation therapy. In addition, considerable progress has been made in recent years in the treatment of atrial fibrillation (especially paroxysmal atrial fibrillation) and ventricular tachycardia due to reentry around a scar after myocardial infarction.

The technique of radiofrequency ablation is similar to that described for electrophysiologic testing and, in most cases, is performed during the same procedure if an abnormal rhythm is found or has been documented clinically. When an area of tissue critical for initiating or sustaining the abnormal rhythm has been identified (mapped), a specially designed electrode catheter capable of delivering radiofrequency energy is maneuvered in proximity and radiofrequency energy is delivered. This procedure prevents further conduction of electrical impulses and prevents the abnormal rhythm from occurring.

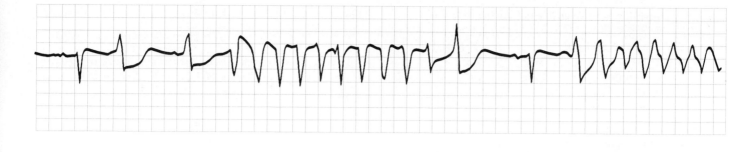
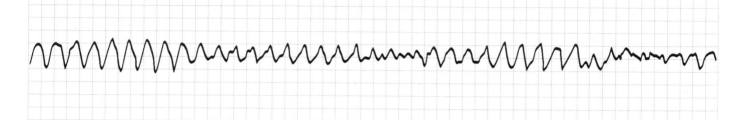
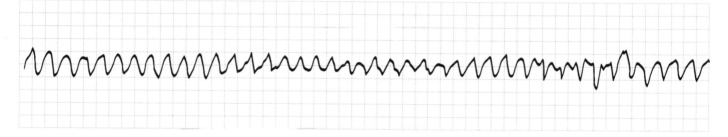

Figure 3-18. Proarrhythmic Response to Quinidine. Quinidine resulted in prolongation of QT interval, and late-coupled premature ventricular complex initiated polymorphic ventricular tachycardia, termed *torsades de pointes*.

Table 3-13 Results of Trials on Pharmacologic Prevention of Primary Sudden Cardiac Death

Trial	Patients	No.	Drug	Follow-up, mo	Total Mortality, % Placebo	Drug	Significance
Julian et al., 1982	MI <2 wk	1,456	*d*-, *l*-Sotalol	12	8.9	7.3	No
CAST, 1989	MI, EF <55%, >6 PVCs/h	1,455	Flecainide Encainide	10	3.0	7.7	Yes
CAST II, 1992	MI, EF ≤40%, >6 PVCs/h	1,155	Moricizine	18	12.4	15.0	No
SWORT, 1996	MI, EF ≤40%	3,121	*d*-Sotalol	5	3.1	5.0	Yes
Diamond-MI, 1997	MI	1,510	Dofetilide	≥12	32.0	31.0	No
GESICA, 1994	CHF	516	Amiodarone	24	41.4	33.5	Yes
STAT-CHF, 1995	CHF, EF <40%	674	Amiodarone	45	29.2 (2 y)	30.6 (2 y)	No
CAMIAT, 1997	MI, ≥10 PVCs/h or ± NSVT	1,202	Amiodarone	22	11.4	9.4	No
EMIAT, 1997	MI, EF ≤40%	1,486	Amiodarone	21	13.7	13.9	No

Abbreviations: CHF, congestive heart failure; EF, ejection fraction; MI, myocardial infarction; NSVT, nonsustained ventricular tachycardia; PVCs, premature ventricular complexes.

Table 3-14 Heart Rhythms Amenable to Catheter Ablation

Rhythm	Curable	Treatable
SVT	AVNRT AVRT (bypass tract) EAT AFL (without fibrillation)	AF
Ventricular	RV outflow tract tachycardia Idiopathic LV tachycardia	VT due to coronary disease and scar after MI

Abbreviations: AF, atrial fibrillation; AFL, atrial flutter; AVNRT, atrioventricular node reentry tachycardia; AVRT, atrioventricular reentry tachycardia; EAT, ectopic atrial tachycardia; LV, left ventricular; MI, myocardial infarction; RV, right ventricular; SVT, supraventricular tachycardia; VT, ventricular tachycardia.

* Supraventricular tachycardia due to AV nodal reentrant tachycardia, accessory pathway in Wolff-Parkinson-White syndrome, automatic atrial focus, atrial flutter, and some cases of atrial fibrillation and ventricular tachycardia can be cured with radiofrequency ablation.
* Ablation is performed with radiofrequency energy passed through a catheter.

About 1% to 2% of patients experience complications, including vascular injury at the site of catheter insertion, cardiac perforation, and infection. In addition, if the site of the critical area, such as an accessory pathway, is close to the normal conduction system, or if AV nodal reentrant tachycardia is ablated, there is a 5% risk of creating complete heart block that requires permanent pacing. When compared with previous surgical approaches for the treatment of similar tachycardias, the technique has reduced the hospital stay from 7 days to 1 to 2 days and the time to return to work or school from 6 to 8 weeks to 3 to 5 days. The cost is approximately 40% of the surgical cost.

* Catheter ablation is successful in 95% of cases of accessory pathway or reentrant tachycardia in the AV node.
* The complication rate is 1%-2%.
* Catheter ablation reduces hospital stay to 1-2 days.
* The cost is 40% of the surgical cost.

Catheter ablation also may be used to achieve complete heart block in some cases of supraventricular tachycardias (usually atrial fibrillation or atrial flutter) that are refractory to medications and associated with rapid ventricular rates. With either direct-current ablation or radiofrequency ablation, complete heart block can be achieved in more than 95% of patients. In such cases, permanent pacing is required. In select patients, this approach results in substantial improvement in symptoms (because of regularization of the heart rate) and in exercise capacity with use of rate-responsive pacing.

However, a disadvantage is that patients are pacemaker-dependent and require long-term follow-up.

* Catheter ablation achieves complete heart block in supraventricular tachycardias that are refractory to medication and associated with rapid ventricular rate.
* Catheter ablation results in heart block in >95% of patients; permanent pacing then is required.
* Symptoms improve substantially.

Current therapeutic interventions available to patients with symptoms due to tachycardia are summarized in Table 3-15.

Device Therapy
Device therapy is used for abnormal heart rhythms due to bradycardias (permanent cardiac pacemaker implantation) and tachycardias (implantable cardioverter-defibrillators [ICDs]).

Permanent Cardiac Pacemaker Implantation
An internationally recognized 4-letter system is used to classify different types of implantable pacemakers and ICDs (Table 3-16). The initial letter is used to denote the chamber paced, the second letter the chamber sensed, and the third letter the programmed mode of response of the pacemaker (eg, inhibited, triggered, or both). Recently, a fourth letter was added to denote whether rate-responsiveness is possible. In a pacemaker with rate-responsiveness, the programmed rate automatically increases in response to sensor-detected activity. Usually, the sensor is located within the pulse-generator or is part of the implanted lead system. Common pacing modes include VVI (ventricular paced, ventricular sensed, inhibited in response to a ventricular event), VVIR (same as previous entry but also has rate responsiveness), DDD (atrial and ventricular pacing and sensing with triggered and inhibited response to a sensed atrial or ventricular event), and DDDR (same as previous entry but also has rate responsiveness). The precise choice of pacemaker used depends in large part on clinical circumstances.

Table 3-15 Summary of Tachyarrhythmia Therapy

Supraventricular Tachycardia	Drug	Ablation	ICD
AVNRT	+	++	-
AVRT	+	++	-
EAT	+	+	-
IAST	++	o	-
Typical A flutter	+	++	-
AFib	++	+	o

Symbols: +, effective; ++, preferred; o, investigational; -, no indication.
Abbreviations: A, atrial; AFib, atrial fibrillation; AVNRT, atrioventricular nodal reciprocating tachycardia; AVRT, atrioventricular reciprocating tachycardia; EAT, ectopic atrial tachycardia; IAST, inappropriate sinus tachycardia; ICD, implantable cardioverter-defibrillator.

Table 3-16 Code of Permanent Pacing

Chamber(s) Paced	Chamber(s) Sensed	Mode(s) of Response	Programmable Capabilities
V = Ventricle A = Atrium D = Dual (atrium and ventricle)	V = Ventricle A = Atrium D = Dual (atrium and ventricle) O = None	T = Triggered I = Inhibited D = Dual (triggered and inhibited) O = None	R = Rate modulated

Physiologic pacing (with a DDD pacemaker) attempts to maintain heart rate with normal AV synchrony and to increase heart rate in response to physical activity. In patients with normal sinus node activity, DDD pacemakers can "track" atrial activation. This tracking has the advantage that as sinus node activity increases (eg, in response to exercise or some other stress), the pacemaker rate increases accordingly so that the ventricle is paced at the appropriate rate but with normal AV conduction delay (PR interval). In patients with chronic atrial fibrillation, rate-modulated pacing (the *R* in VVIR) is used to increase heart rate in response to physical demand. In such cases, a sensor that responds to body motion, respiratory rate, blood temperature, or some other variable is used to drive the pacemaker so that the rate at which pacing occurs is appropriate to metabolic demands. Patients fitted with this type of pacemaker have increased exercise endurance during treadmill testing. Patients with both sinus node dysfunction and AV conduction system disease benefit most from DDDR pacing.

* Physiologic pacing maintains heart rate with normal AV synchrony and increases the rate during physical activity.
* Rate-modulated pacing increases exercise endurance during treadmill testing.

Complications of Permanent Pacing

Complications of device therapy (pacing and ICD) may be classified as early (usually within 30 days of implant) or late. Early complications are most commonly related to vascular injury, hematoma, pneumothorax, dislodgment of the lead, and extracardiac stimulation (eg, diaphragmatic stimulation). In most cases, repositioning of the lead or reprogramming of the device remediates the problem. Late complications include lead fracture or insulation defect, infection, pacemaker syndrome, and pacemaker-mediated tachycardia.

Pacemaker syndrome may develop during dominant ventricular pacing in a minority of patients with intact retrograde conduction between the ventricle and the atrium (Figure 3-19). When the ventricle is paced, the impulse conducts retrogradely to the atrium and simultaneous atrial and ventricular contraction results. Because the atria are contracting against closed tricuspid and mitral valves, the atrial contribution to ventricular filling is prevented and the atria are distended. The increased atrial pressure distends the neck veins, leading to a sensation of "fullness in the neck" and symptoms due to decreased forward cardiac output such as light-headedness and fatigue.

Symptoms and signs due to pacemaker syndrome can be eliminated with dual-chamber pacing.

* In pacemaker syndrome, atria contract against closed tricuspid and mitral valves, resulting in backward blood flow and decreased forward blood flow (cardiac output).
* Symptoms are typically "fullness in the neck," light-headedness, and fatigue.
* Dual-chamber pacing eliminates symptoms.

Pacemaker-mediated tachycardia is a well-recognized complication of dual-chamber pacemakers (DDD pacing) and occurs when retrograde conduction between the ventricle and atrium is intact. In this type of tachycardia, the pacemaker generator acts as 1 limb of the reentrant circuit. Typically, a spontaneous PVC occurs which conducts retrogradely to the atrium. This early retrograde atrial activity is sensed by the pacemaker, which awaits the normal AV delay and then paces the ventricle. The "early" ventricular activity generated by the pacemaker then conducts retrogradely to the atrium, and

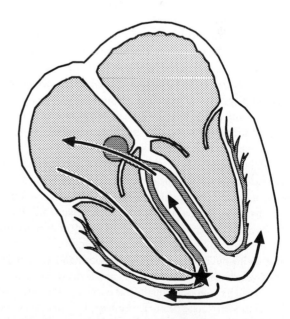

Figure 3-19. Pacemaker Syndrome. Retrograde atrial activation during ventricular pacing (star) results in simultaneous atrial and ventricular contractions.

the reentrant circuit is completed. Typically, the tachycardia rate is close to the upper rate limit of the device. Most pacemaker devices possess algorithms that recognize and attempt to abort pacemaker-mediated tachycardia. Alternatively, the device can be programmed to reduce or eliminate it.

- Pacemaker-mediated tachycardia occurs with DDD pacing when there is intact retrograde conduction between the ventricle and atrium.
- The abnormality is corrected by programming changes of the pacemaker generator.

Indications for Permanent Pacemaker Implantation

Guidelines for permanent pacemaker implantation are well established. Indications for specific conduction system diseases are listed in Table 3-17. Indications are generally grouped according to the following classification: class I indication—conditions for which there is general agreement that permanent pacemakers should be implanted; class II—conditions for which permanent pacemakers are frequently used but opinions differ about the necessity of implantation; and class III—conditions for which there is general agreement that pacemakers are not necessary. Clinical symptoms such as syncope, presyncope, or exercise intolerance that can be correlated with and attributed to a bradycardia disorder usually constitute a class I indication for permanent pacemaker implantation. If symptoms cannot be correlated with bradycardia, it is less certain that permanent pacemaker implantation is indicated.

Implantable Cardioverter-Defibrillators

ICDs continuously monitor heart rhythm and can detect and treat abnormal ventricular arrhythmia with overdrive pacing (antitachycardia pacing), low-energy cardioversion, or up to 30- to 40-J shocks. In most cases, an ICD can be implanted in the pectoral region in a fashion similar to that of permanent pacemakers. Moreover, with improvements in ICD technology, earlier problems with limited battery life, larger pulse generators, and frequent inappropriate shocks (often due to atrial fibrillation with rapid ventricular response being confused with a rapid ventricular tachycardia) are rapidly being resolved.

ICDs improve mortality outcomes among patients who survive a sudden cardiac death episode when compared with historical controls. Historically, such patients had a 70% survival rate at 1 year without treatment or with empiric antiarrhythmic drug therapy. Use of the ICD has improved the overall 1-year survival rate to 90%; recurrent sudden cardiac death occurs in 2% of patients at 1 year and in 4% of patients at 4 years. In terms of secondary prevention, the Antiarrhythmic Versus Implantable Defibrillator (AVID) trial reported that an ICD is superior for reducing overall mortality in comparison with empiric amiodarone therapy in patients with a history of out-of-hospital cardiac arrest or symptomatic sustained ventricular tachycardia (secondary sudden cardiac death prevention).

Several trials have reported on the role of the ICD among patients at high risk of sudden cardiac death (ie, primary prevention). One of the first was the Multicenter Automatic Defibrillator Implantation Trial (MADIT), which found that patients with prior myocardial infarction, ejection fraction less than 35%, and nonsustained ventricular

Table 3-17 Indications for Pacemaker Implantation

Sinus node dysfunction
    Class I
        Documented symptomatic bradycardia
    Class II
        HR <40 bpm, symptoms present but not clearly correlated
          with bradycardia
    Class III
        Asymptomatic bradycardia (<40 bpm)
AV block
    Class I
        Symptomatic 2° or 3° AV block, permanent or intermittent
        Congenital 3° AV block with wide QRS
        Advanced AV block 14 days after cardiac surgery
    Class II
        Asymptomatic type II 2° or 3° AV block with ventricular
          rate >40 bpm
    Class III
        Asymptomatic 1° and type I 2° AV block
Myocardial infarction
    Class I
        Recurrent type II 2° AV block and 3° AV block with wide
          QRS
        Transient advanced AV block in presence of BBB
    Class II
        Persistent advanced AV block with narrow QRS
        Acquired BBB in absence of AV block
    Class III
        Transient AV block in absence of BBB

Abbreviations: AV, atrioventricular; BBB, bundle branch block; bpm, beats per minute; HR, heart rate.

tachycardia with electrophysiologically inducible sustained monomorphic ventricular tachycardia not suppressible with procainamide had improved survival with ICD when compared with the best medical (including antiarrhythmic) therapy. Similar observations were confirmed in the Multicenter Unsustained Tachycardia Trial (MUSTT). MADIT II addressed prophylactic implantation of an ICD in a group of patients with prior myocardial infarction and reduced ejection fraction (<30%), without additional risk stratification, and found improved survival with ICD therapy compared with best medical therapy. The Sudden Cardiac Death in Heart Failure Trial (SCD-HeFT) enrolled patients with mild to moderate congestive heart failure (New York Heart Association [NYHA] class II and III) and depressed left ventricular ejection fraction (≤35%) with both ischemic and nonischemic cardiomyopathy but with no prior history of ventricular arrhythmia. ICD therapy was associated with a significant reduction in risk of death compared with medical therapy.

Current Indications for ICD Implantation

The following are indications for ICD implantation:

1. Documented episode of cardiac arrest due to ventricular fibrillation, not due to a transient or reversible cause

2. Documented sustained ventricular tachyarrhythmia, either spontaneous or induced by an electrophysiology study, not associated with an acute myocardial infarction and not due to a transient or reversible cause

3. Documented familial or inherited conditions with a high risk of life-threatening ventricular tachycardia, such as long QT syndrome or hypertrophic cardiomyopathy

4. Coronary artery disease with a documented prior myocardial infarction, a measured left ventricular ejection fraction less than 35%, and inducible, sustained ventricular tachycardia or ventricular fibrillation at electrophysiologic study. The myocardial infarction must have occurred more than 4 weeks before defibrillator insertion. The electrophysiologic test must be performed more than 4 weeks after the qualifying myocardial infarction

5. Documented prior myocardial infarction and a measured left ventricular ejection fraction less than 30%

6. Ischemic dilated cardiomyopathy, documented prior myocardial infarction, NYHA class II and III heart failure, and measured left ventricular ejection fraction less than 35%

7. Nonischemic dilated cardiomyopathy for more than 9 months, NYHA class II and III heart failure, and measured left ventricular ejection fraction less than 35%

   Patients must not have:

   a. Cardiogenic shock or symptomatic hypotension while in a stable baseline rhythm

   b. Had a coronary artery bypass graft or percutaneous transluminal coronary angioplasty within the past 3 months

   c. Had an acute myocardial infarction within the past 40 days

   d. Clinical symptoms or findings that would make them a candidate for coronary revascularization

   e. Irreversible brain damage from preexisting cerebral disease

   f. Any disease, other than cardiac disease (eg, cancer, uremia, liver failure), associated with a likelihood of survival less than 1 year

- ICD is indicated for *any* symptomatic ventricular arrhythmia that does not have a reversible cause.
- For primary prevention of sudden cardiac death, the ejection fraction is used for risk stratification in most cases.
- An ICD is indicated for an ejection fraction <30% in patients with ischemic cardiomyopathy (prior myocardial infarction). If the ejection fraction is <35%, then an additional qualifier (congestive heart failure class II or III) is required.
- Ejection fraction >35% is not an indication for ICD implantation.

Cardiac Resynchronization Therapy (CRT)

Several recently published clinical trials have shown benefit, in terms of symptom response and mortality, from placement of a lead via the coronary sinus to allow "synchronized" pacing of both the right and left ventricles.

Current indications for CRT, which in most cases combines pacing therapy (CRT) with a defibrillator (CRT-D), include sinus rhythm with an ejection fraction less than 35%, QRS width more than 120 milliseconds, and moderate to severe symptoms due to heart failure (NYHA class III or IV). Beyond these current guidelines, indications for CRT and CRT-D continue to evolve.

Part III
Peter A. Brady, MB,ChB, MD

Specific Arrhythmia Problems

Sinus Node Dysfunction

Sinus node dysfunction, also called sick sinus syndrome, includes sinus bradycardia, sinus pauses, tachycardia-bradycardia syndrome (Figure 3-20), sinus arrest, and chronotropic incompetence. The diagnosis is made from the medical history and results of electrocardiographic (ECG) and Holter monitoring, which are the most useful diagnostic tests. Electrophysiologic testing generally is not helpful for evaluating patients with a history consistent with sinus node disease because it has low sensitivity. In some cases, prolonged monitoring with an event recorder may be required to correlate symptoms with bradycardia. If a patient is able to exercise, a treadmill test is useful for determining whether the sinus node rate can increase appropriately to meet metabolic need.

- Sinus node dysfunction includes sinus bradycardia, sinus pauses, tachycardia-bradycardia syndrome, sinus arrest, and chronotropic incompetence.
- The diagnosis is made from the history and the results of ECG and Holter monitoring.
- Electrophysiologic testing is reserved for patients in whom the arrhythmia mechanism cannot be determined by ECG or Holter monitoring.

Asymptomatic patients with sinus node dysfunction do not require specific therapy. Symptomatic patients usually receive a pacemaker. Often, patients with tachycardia-bradycardia have atrial fibrillation that at times presents with rapid ventricular rates and at other times with inappropriate, symptomatic bradycardia. Pacemakers are used to prevent the bradycardia, and drugs may be used to slow conduction through the atrioventricular (AV) node and to prevent episodes of rapid ventricular rate.

- Asymptomatic patients with sinus node dysfunction do not require specific therapy.
- Symptomatic patients with sinus node dysfunction receive a pacemaker.

Conduction System Disorders

First-degree AV block results in a prolonged PR interval. If the QRS is narrow, the conduction delay is most likely within the AV node. In patients with associated bundle branch block, the conduction delay may be distal to the AV node in the His-Purkinje system or bundle branches. Two subtypes of second-degree AV block are described: Mobitz I (Wenckebach) manifests as gradual prolongation of the PR interval before a nonconducted P wave. Classically, the PR interval after the nonconducted P wave is shorter than the PR interval before the nonconducted P wave (Figures 3-21 and 3-22). Also, the RR interval that encompasses the nonconducted P wave is shorter than 2 RR intervals between conducted beats. Wenckebach conduction is frequently observed after an inferior myocardial infarction, which can result in ischemia of the AV node. Generally, this does not require pacing (temporary or permanent) unless hemodynamic problems are associated with the slow heart rate.

- First-degree AV block results in a prolonged PR interval.
- Second-degree AV block of Mobitz I type results in gradual prolongation of the PR interval before a nonconducted P wave.
- Wenckebach conduction may accompany inferior myocardial infarction.
- Wenckebach conduction does not require pacing unless hemodynamic problems are associated with the slow heart rate.

Mobitz II second-degree AV block usually is caused by conduction block within the His-Purkinje system and frequently is associated with bundle branch block (Figure 3-23). This conduction abnormality is shown on the ECG as a sudden failure of a P wave to conduct to the ventricle, with no change in the PR interval either before or after the nonconducted P wave. This problem may herald complete heart block, and therefore strong consideration should be given to permanent pacing. Complete heart block is diagnosed when there is no relation between the atrial rhythm and the ventricular rhythm and *the atrial rhythm is faster than the ventricular escape rhythm* (Figure 3-24). The ventricular escape rhythm is either a junctional escape focus, with a conduction pattern similar to that seen during normal

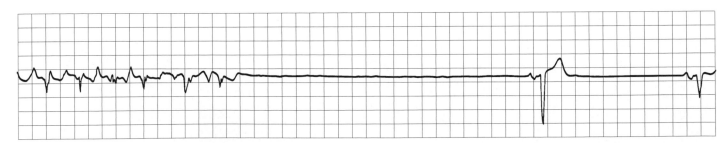

Figure 3-20. Tachycardia-bradycardia with episode of atrial fibrillation terminating spontaneously, followed by a 4.5-second pause until the sinus node recovers. (From MKSAP IX: Part C, Book 1, 1992. American College of Physicians. Used with permission.)

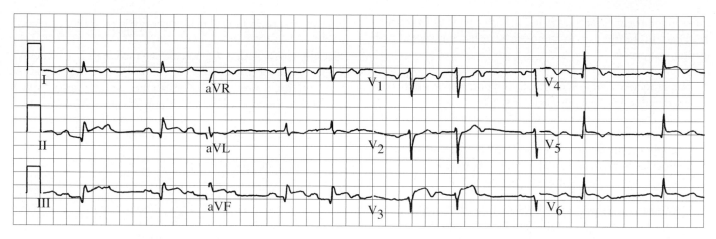

Figure 3-21. 3:2 Mobitz I (or Wenckebach) second-degree atrioventricular block in a patient with acute inferior myocardial infarction.

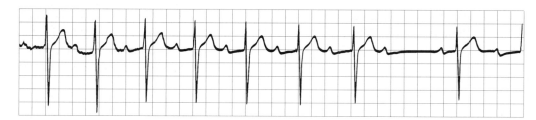

Figure 3-22. Mobitz I second-degree atrioventricular block; note gradual PR prolongation. The PR interval after a nonconducted P wave is shorter than the PR interval preceding the nonconducted P wave.

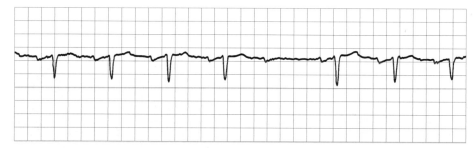

Figure 3-23. Mobitz II second-degree atrioventricular block with no change in the PR interval before or after a nonconducted P wave.

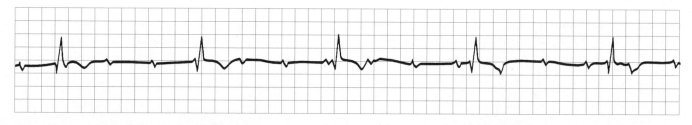

Figure 3-24. Complete heart block with an atrial rate at 70 beats per minute and a ventricular escape rhythm at 30 beats per minute.

rhythm, or a ventricular escape focus, with a wide QRS conduction pattern. In most cases, complete heart block is treated with permanent pacing.

- Second-degree AV block of Mobitz II type usually is due to conduction disease in the His-Purkinje system.
- It often heralds complete heart block; permanent pacing should be considered.
- Complete heart block: no relation between atrial rhythm and ventricular rhythm, and atrial rhythm is faster than ventricular escape rhythm. Treatment is with pacing.

Bifascicular block refers to left bundle branch block, right bundle branch block with left anterior fascicular block (marked left axis deviation), or right bundle branch block with left posterior fascicular block (right axis deviation). Bifascicular block usually is associated with underlying structural heart disease and has a 1% chance of progressing to complete heart block in asymptomatic persons. Patients presenting with syncope and bifascicular block may have intermittent complete heart block caused by conduction system disease or ventricular tachycardia caused by the underlying myocardial disease. Permanent pacing can be used to treat syncope due to complete heart block.

- Bifascicular block usually is associated with structural heart disease.
- Bifascicular block progresses to complete heart block in 1% of asymptomatic persons.

- Permanent pacing is used to treat syncope in complete heart block.

High-degree AV block is diagnosed when there is a 2:1 or higher AV conduction block (Figure 3-25). It can be due to a Wenckebach or Mobitz II mechanism. A Wenckebach mechanism is more likely if the QRS conduction (duration) is normal, and a Mobitz II-type mechanism is more likely if the QRS complex demonstrates additional conduction disease, such as bundle branch block.

Carotid Sinus Syndrome

Carotid sinus massage is performed to identify carotid sinus hypersensitivity (Figure 3-26). Approximately 40% of patients older than 65 years have a hyperactive carotid sinus reflex (3-second pause or a decrease in systolic blood pressure of 50 mm Hg), although most of these patients do not have spontaneous syncope. In patients without evidence of carotid bruit on carotid auscultation or a history of cerebrovascular disease, carotid sinus massage should be performed over the carotid bifurcation at the angle of the jaw for 5 seconds while monitoring heart rate and blood pressure. Approximately 35% of patients with a hyperactive carotid sinus reflex have a pure cardioinhibitory component manifested only by a pause in ventricular activity exceeding 3 seconds. Fifteen percent of patients have a pure vasodepressor component, with a normal heart rate maintained but a decrease in systolic blood pressure of more than 50 mm Hg. Sixty percent of patients have a combined response of both cardioinhibitory and vasodepressor components. In such patients, permanent pacing

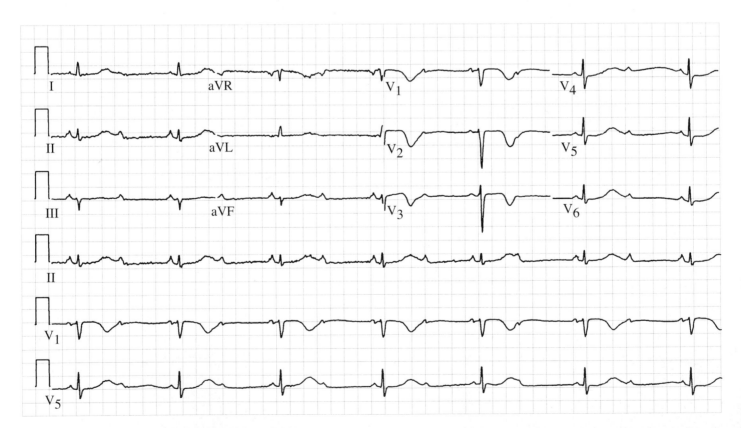

Figure 3-25. High-grade 2:1 atrioventricular conduction block.

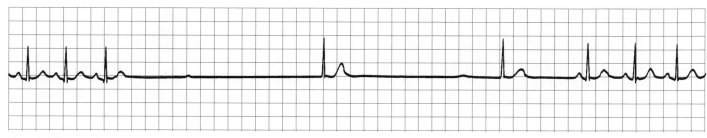

Figure 3-26. Carotid sinus massage resulting in sinus pause with junctional escape beats before sinus rhythm returns.

may prevent the cardioinhibitory response, but the vasodepressor response continues to produce symptoms.

- Carotid sinus massage is used to identify carotid sinus hypersensitivity.
- About 40% of patients >65 years have a hyperactive carotid sinus reflex (3-second pause or decrease in systolic blood pressure of 50 mm Hg).

Rarely, neck abnormalities, such as lymph node enlargement, prior neck surgery, or a regional tumor, can cause a carotid sinus syndrome. Often, surgical techniques to treat this condition are unsuccessful, and the primary form of therapy is AV sequential pacing for the cardioinhibitory component and elastic stockings for the vasodepressor component. Occasionally, the condition responds to anticholinergic medications.

Summary of Indications for Pacemakers

Symptomatic bradycardia is a class I indication for pacemaker implantation. Commonly, this is due to AV block (second-degree Mobitz II, high-grade, or third-degree), sinus node dysfunction, and carotid sinus hypersensitivity. Correlation of symptoms and bradycardia is important but may not be possible in some cases (class II indication). In asymptomatic patients, pacing should be considered in complete heart block (particularly with escape <40 beats per minute or pauses >3 seconds), Mobitz II block (especially associated with bifascicular or trifascicular block), and postoperative AV block.

- Pacing is indicated for symptomatic bradycardias due to second- or third-degree heart block, sinus node dysfunction, and carotid sinus hypersensitivity.
- Asymptomatic patients with complete heart block, Mobitz II AV block, or postoperative AV block should also be considered for pacing.

Atrial Flutter

Atrial flutter is identified by the characteristic sawtooth pattern of atrial activity at a rate of 240 to 320 beats per minute. Patients with normal conduction systems maintain 2:1 AV conduction; thus, the ventricular rate is often close to 150 beats per mintue. Higher degrees of AV block (3:1 or higher) in the absence of drugs that slow AV nodal conduction (digoxin, β-adrenergic blocker, calcium antagonist) suggest the presence of intrinsic AV conduction disease (Figure 3-27). In patients with 2:1 AV conduction and a heart rate of 150 beats per minute, 1 of the flutter waves is often buried in the QRS complex. Carotid sinus massage (or use of adenosine to transiently block AV conduction) may be helpful for revealing the flutter waves and establishing the diagnosis.

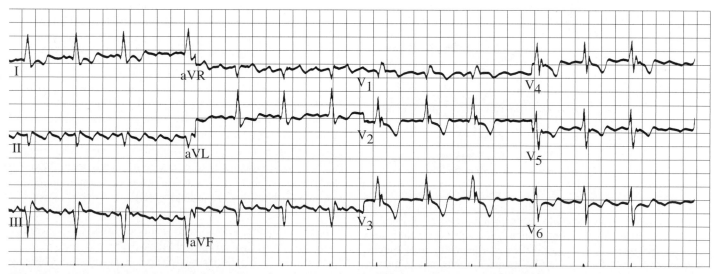

Figure 3-27. Atrial flutter with 3:1 conduction in a patient with atrioventricular conduction disease.

* Atrial flutter is atrial activity at 240-320 beats per minute.
* The ventricular rate is close to 150 beats per minute.

Pharmacologic therapy for atrial flutter is used to slow AV node conduction and to control the ventricular rate or to control the flutter itself. The same medications used to treat atrial fibrillation (discussed below) are used to treat atrial flutter. Success rates for the control of atrial flutter are 30% to 50%.

Nonpharmacologic therapy for typical atrial flutter has been well established. Unlike atrial fibrillation, which is composed of multiple reentrant wavelets that travel through the atria, typical atrial flutter consists of a single reentrant circuit that follows the tricuspid valve anulus (Figure 3-28). This fixed reentrant pathway results in a surface ECG with very stable flutter waves (Figure 3-27) and provides a target for ablation. Radiofrequency catheter ablation of this single circuit has a success rate higher than 90%. Ablation is performed within the atrium between the tricuspid anulus and the inferior vena cava to interrupt the atrial flutter circuit. Other options include ablation of the AV node and permanent pacemaker implantation (which is also useful in atrial fibrillation). In this case, the atria continue to fibrillate but symptoms are often much improved due to slower ventricular rate and regularity. Atrial flutter is associated with an identical risk of thromboembolism as atrial fibrillation and should be treated similarly with regard to anticoagulation.

* Typical atrial flutter ablation has a success rate >90%.
* Atrial flutter is associated with a similar risk of thromboembolism

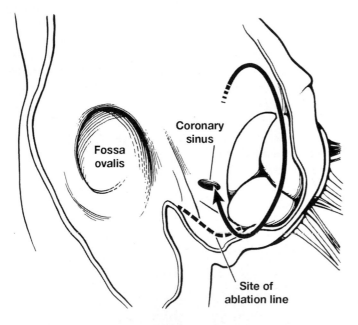

Figure 3-28. View of the Right Atrium. Tricuspid valve is on the right. The atrial flutter circuit is confined to the path depicted by the circular arrow adjacent to the valve. An ablation lesion along the dashed line ("Site of ablation line") interrupts the circuit, eliminating atrial flutter. In contrast to atrial flutter, atrial fibrillation has wandering wavefronts throughout the atria which will not respond to the flutter ablation line.

as atrial fibrillation and should be treated similarly to atrial fibrillation with regard to anticoagulation.

Atrial Fibrillation

Atrial fibrillation is the most common arrhythmia encountered in clinical practice. Its frequency increases with age. Atrial fibrillation is characterized by continuous and irregular activity of the ECG baseline caused by swarming electrical currents in the atria. According to population-based studies, its prevalence is 5% among persons 65 or older. Common associated conditions include hypertension, cardiomyopathy, valvular heart disease (particularly mitral stenosis), sick sinus syndrome, Wolff-Parkinson-White syndrome (especially in young patients), alcohol use ("holiday heart"), and thyrotoxicosis. The presence of these conditions should be sought in the history and physical examination. Atrial fibrillation is frequently initiated by discrete triggers, most often from muscle sleeves present in the proximal portions of the pulmonary veins. Atrial fibrillation should be distinguished from atrial flutter (uniform flutter waves) and multifocal atrial tachycardia (isoelectric interval between premature atrial contractions that have 3 or more different morphologic forms).

* Conditions commonly associated with atrial fibrillation include hypertension, cardiomyopathy, valvular heart disease, sick sinus syndrome, Wolff-Parkinson-White syndrome, thyrotoxicosis, and alcohol use.
* Atrial fibrillation should be distinguished from atrial flutter (uniform flutter waves) and multifocal atrial tachycardia (isoelectric interval between premature atrial contractions that have 3 or more different morphologic forms).

Therapy for Atrial Fibrillation

The therapeutic approach in patients with atrial fibrillation is determined by the severity of symptoms and comorbid conditions but can broadly be divided into rate control (using pharmacologic agents or ablation to slow conduction through the AV node) and stroke prophylaxis (for ongoing atrial fibrillation) in patients at risk of stroke. Assessment of stroke risk in atrial fibrillation is most easily evaluated using the CHADS2 scoring system (*c*ongestive heart failure, *h*ypertension, *a*ge >75 years, *d*iabetes, and previous *s*troke). Rhythm control is most often used in patients who experience symptoms due to atrial fibrillation and involves both pharmacologic and nonpharmacologic (usually catheter ablation) approaches to restore and maintain normal sinus rhythm. The choice of the approach depends for the most part on the presence and severity of symptoms, age, and comorbid conditions. In the absence of symptoms, a rate control strategy has been shown to have outcomes similar, in terms of mortality, to those of a rhythm control strategy. Initial management of atrial fibrillation usually involves rate control with use of AV nodal blocking agents and anticoagulation before deciding on long-term strategy, which needs to be individualized.

* It is important to know which agents are useful for rate control and which for rhythm control (Table 3-18).
* Treatment of atrial fibrillation is based on the presence or absence of symptoms.

- Adequate rate control (with anticoagulation therapy if risk of stroke is increased) is associated with outcomes similar to those of a rhythm control strategy.
- Initial management of atrial fibrillation usually involves rate control with use of AV nodal blocking agents and anticoagulation before deciding on long-term strategy, which needs to be individualized.

Rate Control and Anticoagulation

The 3 main categories of drugs used to blunt the AV node response in atrial fibrillation are digitalis glycosides, β-adrenergic blocking agents, and calcium channel blockers. These are summarized in Table 3-18. None of these agents have been shown to be effective for the prevention of recurrent atrial fibrillation.

Digoxin acts indirectly by increasing vagal tone and at therapeutic concentration has no direct effect in slowing AV node conduction. Because of its mechanism of action, digoxin is less effective than β-blockers or calcium channel blockers, particularly with exercise, when an increase in sympathetic tone results in more rapid AV node conduction. Thus, the optimal role for digoxin in atrial fibrillation is therapy for patients with left ventricular dysfunction (because of the drug's positive inotropy) or adjunctive therapy for patients receiving β-blockers or calcium channel blockers. Digoxin alone is no better than placebo for terminating atrial fibrillation.

- Digoxin alone is no better than placebo for terminating atrial fibrillation.
- Digoxin is less effective than β-blockers or calcium channel blockers in controlling ventricular rate and is best used as an adjunctive agent for its inotropic effect in patients with impaired ventricular function.

β-Blockers such as propranolol, metoprolol, and atenolol are effective in slowing AV node conduction and may be particularly useful when atrial fibrillation complicates hyperthyroidism or myocardial infarction (in which case they reduce the risk of death from myocardial infarction). β-Blockers also decrease the risk of postoperative myocardial infarction, making them well suited for postoperative atrial fibrillation. Carvedilol decreases mortality of patients with chronic heart failure and may be a good choice in that setting. Esmolol, because of its intravenous formulation and short half-life, is particularly useful for acute management of atrial fibrillation.

- β-Blockers are effective for slowing ventricular rate in atrial fibrillation, but they do not terminate atrial fibrillation (although they may prevent it postoperatively).
- β-Blockers are particularly useful postoperatively and in hyperthyroidism, acute myocardial infarction, and chronic heart failure.

Calcium channel blockers are broadly divided into 2 groups: dihydropyridines (eg, nifedipine, amlodipine, felodipine) and nondihydropyridines (diltiazem, verapamil). Dihydropyridine agents have little or no effect on AV node conduction and no role in the management of atrial fibrillation. Verapamil and diltiazem are both available as

Table 3-18 Pharmacologic Therapy for Atrial Fibrillation

Agents	Comments
Control of ventricular rate	
β-Blockers (eg, atenolol, metoprolol, propranolol, carvedilol)	Ideal postoperatively & in hyperthyroidism, acute MI, & chronic CHF (especially carvedilol)
Calcium channel blockers (eg, verapamil, diltiazem)	Nifedipine, amlodipine, & felodipine are not useful for slowing AV conduction
Digoxin	Less effective than β-blockers & calcium channel blockers, especially with exercise Useful in heart failure
Maintenance of sinus rhythm	
Class IA: quinidine, disopyramide, procainamide	Enhance AV conduction—rate must be controlled before use Monitor QTc
Class IC: propafenone, flecainide	Slow AV conduction Often first choice for patients with normal heart Monitor QRS duration
Class III: sotalol, amiodarone	Amiodarone is agent of choice for ventricular dysfunction & after MI

Abbreviations: AV, atrioventricular; CHF, congestive heart failure; MI, myocardial infarction.

intravenous and oral preparations and are well suited for acute and chronic rate control. Also, both agents have negative inotropic effects and should be used cautiously in congestive heart failure.

- Diltiazem and verapamil are both effective for rate control in atrial fibrillation; nifedipine, amlodipine, and felodipine are not and have no role in the management of atrial fibrillation.

Adenosine is very effective at slowing AV node conduction; however, because of its short half-life, it has no role in the treatment of atrial fibrillation. It can be useful diagnostically by slowing ventricular rate transiently, permitting visualization of atrial activity if the diagnosis is in question.

Nonpharmacologic AV Node Rate Control

If rate control using pharmacologic agents fails (whether due to persistent symptoms or intolerance of medications), catheter ablation of the AV junction may be considered. The advantages of this approach are that it is more than 95% effective for controlling symptoms due to atrial fibrillation and for preventing tachycardia-induced cardiomyopathy (a reversible form of ventricular dysfunction that can occur with long-standing poorly controlled ventricular rates of more than 110 beats per minute) and it can be performed with minimal risk. A disadvantage of this approach is that it creates dependence on ventricular pacing and is effectively irreversible. For patients in whom this approach is adopted, a single-lead ventricular pacemaker (programmed to VVIR mode) is implanted if atrial fibrillation is permanent (chronic), and a dual-chamber pacemaker is used for paroxysmal atrial fibrillation. The dual-chamber pacemaker has a mode-switching function. This device permits the tracking of P waves during sinus rhythm and reverts to VVIR (or DDIR) pacing when atrial fibrillation recurs. With ablation of the AV node, the risk of thromboembolism is unchanged because the fibrillation itself persists in the atria and risk factors remain; thus, appropriate stroke prophylaxis must be prescribed.

Rhythm Control

Pharmacologic Rhythm Control

Rhythm control (maintenance of sinus rhythm) can control symptoms effectively. However, maintaining sinus rhythm has not been shown to decrease the likelihood of thromboembolism, nor has it been shown to prolong survival. In fact, some drugs used to prevent recurrences may cause new arrhythmias (proarrhythmias).

Class IA agents (eg, quinidine, procainamide, and disopyramide) can be associated with torsades de pointes, particularly at the time of reversion of atrial fibrillation to normal sinus rhythm, and treatment should be initiated in a monitored setting. Class IA agents also enhance AV node conduction; thus, before these agents are used, rate control agents should be administered. Class IB agents (eg, lidocaine, mexiletine, tocainide) have no marked effect in treating atrial fibrillation and should not be used for that purpose. For patients with a normal heart, class IC agents (eg, propafenone, flecainide) are often a good first choice and often can be given safely in an outpatient setting (with ECG and treadmill testing at 3 days to exclude proarrhythmia). Amiodarone is safe for patients who have had myocardial infarction and those with systolic dysfunction and is preferable in these situations.

Nonpharmacologic Rhythm Control

With the recognition that atrial fibrillation frequently arises from rapid firing from within the pulmonary and other thoracic veins (even in patients with the usual risk factors for atrial fibrillation), catheter ablative approaches aimed at electrical isolation of these veins (the so-called pulmonary vein isolation procedure) have been developed and are being more frequently used with excellent success (in excess of 70% of patients are cured and the risk of complications is low). The major advantage of this procedure is that it is effective compared with drug therapy in atrial fibrillation and does not render the patient dependent on a permanent pacemaker, as is the case after ablation of the AV node.

Stroke Prevention

Acute Stroke Risk

Electrical cardioversion from atrial fibrillation is commonly used to control atrial fibrillation. According to current guidelines, patients with atrial fibrillation lasting more than 2 days should receive anticoagulation before cardioversion. Several weeks of warfarin therapy before cardioversion significantly decreases the incidence of cardioversion-associated thromboembolism to 0% to 1.6% (compared with up to 7% in the absence of anticoagulation). Anticoagulation should be continued for a minimum of 4 weeks after cardioversion because of the increased risk of thromboembolism in the weeks after cardioversion or indefinitely in select patients with risk factors for stroke. Although few data are available about cardioversion in the absence of anticoagulation for atrial fibrillation of recent onset (<48 hours), current guidelines do not mandate anticoagulation in this setting. Anticoagulation guidelines for atrial flutter are identical to those for atrial fibrillation. An alternative approach for patients who have had atrial fibrillation for more than 2 days is transesophageal echocardiography with cardioversion (if no thrombus is found) followed by anticoagulation for 3 to 4 weeks.

- Patients who have had atrial fibrillation for more than 2 days must receive anticoagulation for 3 weeks before cardioversion and for 4 weeks afterward.
- An alternative approach for patients who have had atrial fibrillation for more than 2 days is transesophageal echocardiography with cardioversion (if no thrombus is found) followed by anticoagulation for 3-4 weeks.

Chronic Stroke Prevention

Patients with atrial fibrillation due to rheumatic valvular disease have a markedly increased risk of stroke and should receive warfarin therapy. Most patients encountered in clinical practice have nonrheumatic atrial fibrillation. Warfarin decreases the incidence of thromboembolism close to 80% in this population. Risk of thromboembolism is determined by clinical and echocardiographic risk factors (Table 3-19). The risk factors are advanced age, previous transient ischemic attack or stroke, history of hypertension, diabetes mellitus, and congestive heart failure. Echocardiographic risk factors include depressed left ventricular function and left atrial enlargement. These are well validated using the CHADS2 scoring system. In this approach, 1 point is given for the presence of each of the conditions except prior stroke, for which 2 points are given (hence, CHADS2). A score of 2 or more indicates benefit from warfarin therapy regardless of the presence or absence of symptoms. The type of atrial fibrillation is not included in this scoring system. Patients who are younger than 60 years and have no clinical heart disease or hypertension are at extremely low risk and require no treatment, although some physicians recommend aspirin. For patients in whom warfarin therapy is indicated, an international normalized ratio (INR) should be maintained in the range of 2.0 to 3.0 (although 2.0-2.5 may be preferable for those older than 75 years). INR values are preferable to prothrombin times for management because prothrombin time assays vary among laboratories.

Table 3-19 Risk Factors for Thromboembolism in Nonrheumatic
          Atrial Fibrillation

Clinical Risk Factors	Echocardiographic Risk Factors
Congestive heart failure	Left ventricular dysfunction
Hypertension	Left atrial enlargement
Age >75 years	
Diabetes mellitus	
Prior stroke	
Other high-risk clinical settings	
Prosthetic heart valves	
Thyrotoxicosis	

- Clinical risk factors for stroke in nonrheumatic atrial fibrillation include congestive heart failure, hypertension, age >75 years, diabetes mellitus, and previous transient ischemic attack or stroke.
- Echocardiographic risk factors are depressed ventricular function and left atrial enlargement.
- Patients <60 years with structurally normal hearts and no hypertension are at low risk for thromboembolism and require no specific therapy.
- Warfarin should be used to maintain an INR of 2.0-3.0 (although 2.0-2.5 is preferable in the elderly).
- Studies have shown no difference between paroxysmal and chronic atrial fibrillation in stroke rate risk.

Supraventricular Tachycardia

Paroxysmal supraventricular tachycardia (PSVT) refers to cardiac arrhythmias of supraventricular origin using a reentrant mechanism with an abrupt onset and termination, a regular rate, and a narrow QRS complex, unless there is a rate-related or preexisting bundle branch block (Figure 3-29). Episodes usually respond to vagal maneuvers; if these fail, intravenously administered adenosine or verapamil terminates the arrhythmia in 90% of patients.

- PSVT is an arrhythmia with an abrupt onset and termination.
- Acutely, PSVT usually responds to vagal maneuvers; if not, adenosine or verapamil terminates the arrhythmia in 90% of patients.

PSVT generally is not a life-threatening arrhythmia and only occasionally is associated with near syncope or syncope. The rhythm is more serious when it is associated with severe heart disease and cardiac decompensation results, with the sudden increase in heart rate. This can occur in patients with congenital heart disease, cardiomyopathy, or ischemic heart disease.

- PSVT generally is not a life-threatening arrhythmia; it often occurs in an otherwise normal heart.
- PSVT is more serious when associated with heart disease.

Although pharmacologic agents that block the AV node or have antiarrhythmic properties can be used to manage patients with PSVT, most forms can be "cured" permanently with catheter ablation, which

has success rates of more than 90%. For patients with PSVT and hypertension, for example, in whom catheter ablation is not feasible or preferred, β-blockers or calcium channel blockers may be useful in hope of treating both conditions.

- PSVT responds to long-term treatment with most antiarrhythmic drugs.
- PSVT usually can be "cured" permanently with catheter ablation.

Multifocal atrial tachycardia is an automatic atrial rhythm diagnosed when 3 or more distinct atrial foci (P waves of different morphology) are present and the rate exceeds 100 beats per minute (Figure 3-30). The rhythm occurs primarily in patients with decompensated lung disease and associated hypoxia, increased catecholamines (exogenous and endogenous), atrial stretch, and local tissue acid-base and electrolyte disturbances. This rhythm is made worse by digoxin, which shortens atrial refractoriness, but it does respond to improved oxygenation and slow channel blockade with verapamil or diltiazem.

- Digoxin worsens multifocal atrial tachycardia.
- Multifocal atrial tachycardia is best treated with calcium channel blockers and correction of the underlying medical illnesses.

Differentiating Supraventricular Tachycardia With Aberrancy From Ventricular Tachycardia

Wide QRS tachycardia may be due to supraventricular tachycardia with aberrancy or to ventricular tachycardia. Useful findings to identify ventricular tachycardia are listed in Table 3-20.

Approximately 85% of wide QRS tachycardias are ventricular in origin and are often well tolerated. The absence of hemodynamic compromise during tachycardia is not a clue that the tachycardia is supraventricular in origin. In patients with a wide QRS tachycardia and a history of ischemic heart disease (eg, angina, myocardial infarction, Q wave on ECG), the tachycardia is ventricular in origin in 90% to 95%. Therefore, most wide QRS complex tachycardias are ventricular tachycardia (Figure 3-31).

- About 85% of wide QRS tachycardias are ventricular in origin.
- In patients with wide QRS tachycardia and ischemic heart disease, tachycardia is ventricular in origin in 90%-95%.

Intravenous administration of verapamil should be avoided in patients with a wide QRS tachycardia unless the tachycardia is supraventricular

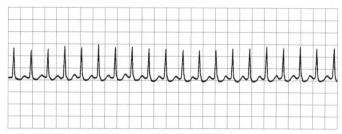

Figure 3-29. Paroxysmal Supraventricular Tachycardia.

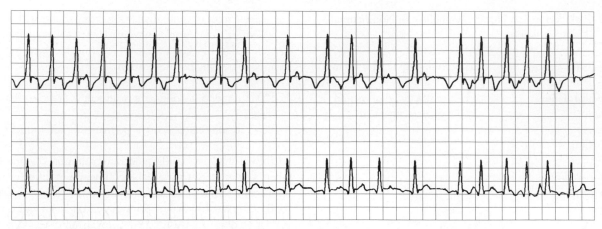

Figure 3-30. Simultaneous recordings from a patient with multifocal atrial tachycardia showing 3 or more P waves of different morphology. (Lower tracing, from MKSAP IX: Part C, Book 1, 1992. American College of Physicians. Used with permission.)

in origin. Most patients with a wide QRS tachycardia have ventricular tachycardia, and verapamil causes hemodynamic deterioration that requires cardioversion in more than half of the patients. The use of verapamil results in peripheral vasodilatation, further increase in catecholamines, and decreased cardiac contractility—all of which contribute to adverse hemodynamics.

* Intravenously administered verapamil should be avoided for wide QRS tachycardia.
* Verapamil causes hemodynamic deterioration requiring cardioversion in ventricular tachycardia.

Wolff-Parkinson-White Syndrome

This abnormality is defined as 1) symptomatic tachycardia, 2) short PR interval (<0.12 second), 3) a delta wave, and 4) prolonged QRS interval (>0.12 second).

In Wolff-Parkinson-White syndrome, a portion of the ventricular activation is due to conduction over the accessory pathway, with the remaining activation being due to conduction via the normal His-Purkinje conduction system. Not all patients with preexcitation have a short PR interval. Normal PR conduction may occur if the accessory pathway is far removed from the AV node. In patients

with a far left lateral accessory pathway, the heart is activated through the AV node before atrial activation reaches the accessory pathway. Thus, the PR interval may be normal before the onset of the delta wave.

Ventricular activation is abnormal in patients with Wolff-Parkinson-White syndrome. Infarction, ventricular hypertrophy, and ST-T wave changes should not be interpreted after the diagnosis is established, because these changes are usually due to the abnormal pattern of ventricular activation.

* In Wolff-Parkinson-White syndrome, the PR interval may be normal before the onset of the delta wave.
* Ventricular activation is abnormal in Wolff-Parkinson-White syndrome.

Preexcitation occurs in about 2 of 1,000 patients; tachycardia subsequently develops in 70%. The most serious rhythm disturbance is the onset of atrial fibrillation with rapid ventricular conduction over the accessory pathway resulting in ventricular fibrillation (Figure 3-32). Patients who are asymptomatic have a negligible chance of sudden death; for patients who are symptomatic, the incidence of sudden death is 0.0025 per patient-year.

* Preexcitation occurs in 2/1,000 patients; tachycardia develops in 70%.
* Asymptomatic patients have a negligible chance of sudden death.
* For symptomatic patients, the incidence of sudden death is 0.0025 per patient-year.

In most cases during tachycardia, conduction from the atria to the ventricles occurs over the normal conduction system and therefore results in a normal QRS complex (unless there is rate-related bundle branch block) and returns to the ventricle via the accessory pathway. This is often termed *orthodromic AV reentry* (Figure 3-33). Up to 5% of patients may have reentrant tachycardia that goes in the reverse direction (*antidromic AV reentry*), in which ventricular activation over the accessory pathway activates the ventricle from an ectopic location;

Table 3-20 Findings That Identify Ventricular Tachycardia

Evidence of AV dissociation with P waves "marching through" the QRS complexes

A QRS width >0.14 s if the tachycardia has a right bundle branch block pattern & >0.16 s if the tachycardia has a left bundle branch block pattern

Northwest axis (axis between −90° & −180°)

A different QRS morphology in patients with a preexisting bundle branch block

A history of structural heart disease

Abbreviation: AV, atrioventricular.

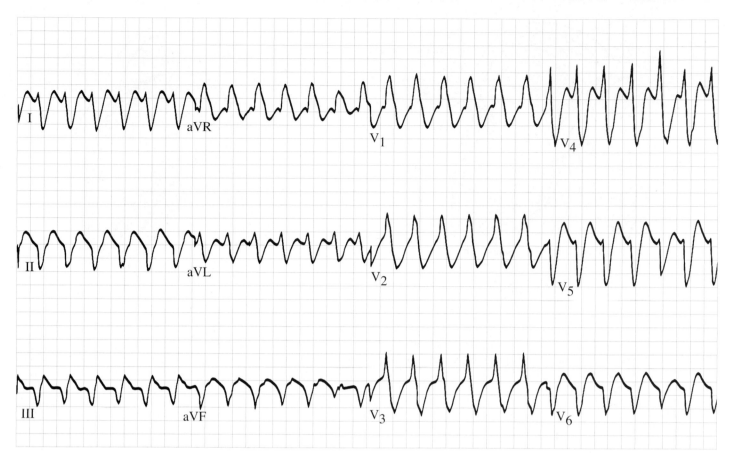

Figure 3-31. Ventricular tachycardia with a wide QRS complex, northwest axis, and fusion complexes in a patient with normal blood pressure.

the result is a wide QRS complex tachycardia that is often confused with ventricular tachycardia (Figure 3-34).

Electrophysiologic testing with catheter ablation of the accessory pathway is indicated in patients with *symptomatic* Wolff-Parkinson-White syndrome to identify pathway location and to determine whether it is an integral part of the reentrant circuit and not an innocent bystander (ie, the arrhythmia is AV node reentry).

Patients who have Wolff-Parkinson-White syndrome can safely take drugs that block the AV node. However, digoxin should be avoided. Also, AV nodal blocking drugs can be safely prescribed for attempted termination of PSVT when the QRS complex is narrow (ie, <100 milliseconds or so).

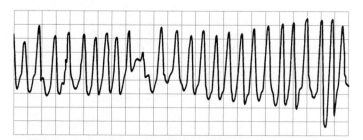

Figure 3-32. Atrial fibrillation in a patient with Wolff-Parkinson-White syndrome shows a wide QRS complex and irregular RR intervals.

Atrial Fibrillation in Wolff-Parkinson-White Syndrome

Wolff-Parkinson-White syndrome frequently has an association with atrial fibrillation, which is thought to be related to the presence of the accessory pathway because catheter ablation of the accessory pathway results, in most cases, in resolution of atrial fibrillation. Because the accessory pathway does not slow conduction in the same manner as the AV node, the ventricular response to atrial fibrillation can be very rapid and may precipitate ventricular fibrillation. During "preexcited" atrial fibrillation, wide, irregular, and rapid ventricular complexes are seen because activation down the accessory pathway does not use the normal His-Purkinje system (Figure 3-35). The use of agents such as adenosine, calcium channel blockers, β-blockers, or digoxin can result in an even more rapid ventricular response due to blocking of conduction down the AV node (which can limit concealed conduction into the pathway). Therefore, the agent of first choice is procainamide, which slows accessory pathway and intra-atrial conduction. Should a patient with Wolff-Parkinson-White syndrome and atrial fibrillation become hypotensive, cardioversion should be performed.

- Atrial fibrillation in Wolff-Parkinson-White syndrome should not be treated with digoxin, adenosine, β-blockers, or calcium channel blockers.
- In atrial fibrillation in Wolff-Parkinson-White syndrome, procainamide can be given to slow the ventricular rate (by slowing atrial and accessory pathway conduction) and to restore sinus rhythm.

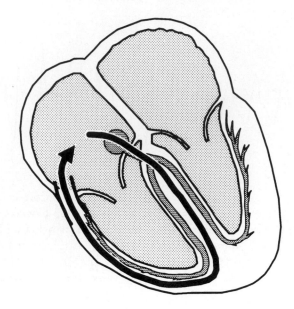

Figure 3-33. Typical mechanism of supraventricular tachycardia in patients with Wolff-Parkinson-White syndrome (orthodromic atrioventricular reentry): the result is a narrow QRS complex because ventricular activation is over the normal conduction system.

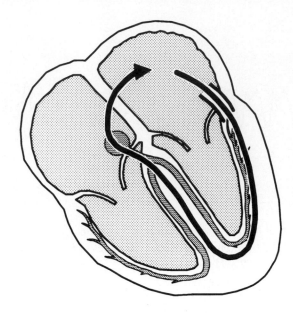

Figure 3-34. Unusual mechanism of supraventricular tachycardia in patients with Wolff-Parkinson-White syndrome; the result is a wide QRS complex because ventricular activation is over an accessory pathway. This arrhythmia is difficult to distinguish from ventricular tachycardia.

- If the heart rate is rapid and there is hemodynamic compromise, cardioversion should be performed.

PSVT in patients with an accessory pathway often terminates with vagal maneuvers or intravenously administered adenosine or verapamil. Additional episodes can be prevented with a β-blocker, a calcium antagonist, and class IA (quinidine, procainamide, disopyramide), class IC (propafenone, flecainide), and class III (amiodarone, sotalol) antiarrhythmic drugs. Radiofrequency ablation is used to ablate the accessory pathway and to cure the tachycardia, thus eliminating the need for medical therapy.

- Additional PSVT is prevented with a β-blocker, a calcium antagonist, and class IA, IC, and III antiarrhythmic drugs.
- Radiofrequency ablation is used to cure tachycardia and should be strongly considered for symptomatic patients.

Tachycardia-Mediated Cardiomyopathy

Persistent atrial fibrillation with a rapid ventricular rate may lead to progressive ventricular dysfunction (termed tachycardia-induced cardiomyopathy). This condition is reversible in most cases because control of the ventricular rate improves ventricular function. One issue in patients who present with tachycardia and congestive heart failure, or who are found to have left ventricular dysfunction during evaluation, is determining whether the heart failure is causing the tachycardia or the tachycardia has caused the heart failure. In a patient with heart failure who has a rhythm with an abnormal P-wave axis, tachycardia-mediated cardiomyopathy should be suspected.

Ventricular Ectopy and Nonsustained Ventricular Tachycardia

Management of frequent ventricular ectopy and nonsustained ven-

tricular tachycardia is predicated on the underlying cardiac lesion. For patients with structurally normal hearts, the long-term prognosis is excellent and no specific therapy is warranted in the absence of symptoms. If symptoms are present, management includes reassurance, β-blockers or calcium channel blockers for disturbing symptoms,

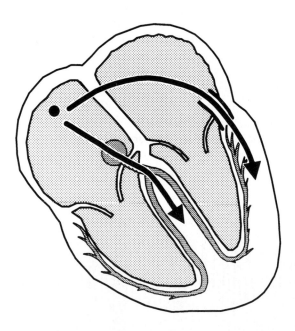

Figure 3-35. Conduction of sinus impulses in Wolff-Parkinson-White syndrome. The ventricles are activated over the normal atrioventricular node–His-Purkinje system and accessory pathway; the result is a fusion complex (QRS and delta wave).

and, in rare cases of frequent monomorphic symptomatic ventricular ectopy, catheter ablation.

In patients with previous myocardial infarction, depressed ventricular function (ejection fraction ≤35%), and nonsustained ventricular tachycardia, electrophysiologic study can stratify risk, even in the absence of symptoms. If, in this population, tachycardia is inducible, the mortality rate is decreased with implantation of a defibrillator. In patients with nonischemic (dilated) cardiomyopathy with ejection fraction less than 35%, recent evidence suggests potential mortality benefit with use of an implantable cardioverter-defibrillator. Use of amiodarone is not associated with mortality benefit in this population, as had previously been suggested.

* Patients with a structurally normal heart and complex ectopy or nonsustained ventricular tachycardia have an excellent prognosis; management includes reassurance or, if bothersome symptoms persist, calcium channel blockers or β-blockers.
* Patients with depressed ventricular function and nonsustained ventricular tachycardia are at increased risk for sudden cardiac death; in patients with previous myocardial infarction, risk can be stratified with electrophysiologic study.

Ventricular Tachycardia and Fibrillation

Patients who present with ventricular tachycardia or fibrillation or who survive sudden cardiac death (out-of-hospital cardiac arrest who were successfully resuscitated) have lethal ventricular arrhythmias and a substantial risk of recurrence. Survivors of sudden cardiac death have a risk of death approaching 30% in the first year after hospital dismissal. Current guidelines support the use of implantable cardioverter-defibrillators in this population. Antiarrhythmic drug therapy has not been shown to have benefit. Use of an implantable cardioverter-defibrillator reduces the recurrence rate of sudden death to 2% at 1 year and to 4% at 4 years; the overall mortality rate is 10% at 1 year and 20% at 4 years.

* Patients with ventricular tachycardia or fibrillation who survive sudden cardiac death have a substantial risk of recurrence.
* Survivors of sudden cardiac death have a risk of death of 30% at 1 year after hospital dismissal.
* Implantable cardioverter-defibrillator therapy improves outcome.

Torsades de Pointes

This is a form of ventricular tachycardia with a characteristic polymorphic morphology described as a "twisting of the points" (torsades de pointes) (Figure 3-18) and occurs in the setting of QT interval prolongation. Typically, polymorphic ventricular tachycardia is initiated by a late-coupled premature ventricular contraction. Common causes include medications (quinidine, procainamide, disopyramide, sotalol, tricyclic antidepressants), electrolyte disturbance (hypokalemia), or bradycardia (especially after myocardial infarction). After the tachycardia has been converted to sinus rhythm (electrically or spontaneously), treatment should be aimed at shortening the QT interval until the offending drug can be metabolized or the electrolyte disturbance or bradycardia corrected. Treatment options include temporary overdrive pacing, isoproterenol infusion, or

magnesium. Patients with a prolonged QT interval in the absence of medications, electrolytes, or bradycardia have a congenital form of this problem and are usually treated with a β-blocker.

* Torsades de pointes is a form of ventricular tachycardia involving a prolonged QT interval.
* Torsades de pointes usually is due to a medication, an electrolyte disturbance, or bradycardia.
* Treatment includes temporary overdrive pacing, isoproterenol, or magnesium.

Ventricular Arrhythmias During Acute Myocardial Infarction

Prevention of myocardial ischemia and the use of β-blockers are essential during and after acute myocardial infarction to decrease the frequency of life-threatening ventricular arrhythmias. Asymptomatic complex ventricular ectopy, including nonsustained ventricular tachycardia, should not be treated empirically in the acute phase of myocardial infarction because the risk of proarrhythmia outweighs the potential benefit of therapy for reducing the incidence of sudden cardiac death after hospital dismissal.

The routine use of lidocaine or amiodarone in suppressing ventricular arrhythmias in the acute phase of myocardial infarction is not recommended.

Ventricular tachycardia and fibrillation occurring within 24 hours after myocardial infarction are independent risk factors for in-hospital mortality at the time of the acute myocardial infarction but are not risk factors for subsequent total mortality or mortality due to an arrhythmic event after hospital dismissal and do not require antiarrhythmic therapy.

Ventricular tachycardia and fibrillation occurring 24 hours or longer after an acute myocardial infarction in the absence of reinfarction are independent risk factors for increased total mortality and death due to an arrhythmic event after hospital dismissal. Patients should be assessed with electrophysiologic testing, and the treatment option is usually an implantable cardioverter-defibrillator.

Episodes of refractory ventricular tachycardia and fibrillation during acute myocardial infarction should be treated with intravenously administered lidocaine, procainamide, bretylium, or amiodarone, and patients should have adequate oxygenation and normal electrolyte values. Recent data suggest that amiodarone may be a reasonable choice if lidocaine fails to control the arrhythmia. If these drugs are ineffective, alternative therapies to prevent recurrences of tachycardia include overdrive pacing if the tachycardia follows a bradycardia event, intra-aortic balloon pump, and coronary revascularization.

* Refractory ventricular tachycardia and fibrillation during acute myocardial infarction should be treated with intravenously administered lidocaine, procainamide, bretylium, or amiodarone.
* Alternative therapies are overdrive pacing and coronary revascularization.

Role of Pacing in Acute Myocardial Infarction

Among patients with an acute inferior myocardial infarction, 5% to 10% have Mobitz I second-degree or third-degree block in the absence of bundle branch block, and the site commonly is in the

AV node. This usually is transient, tends not to recur, and requires pacing only if there are symptoms as a result of bradycardia.

Bundle branch block occurs in 10% to 20% of patients with an acute myocardial infarction; in half of these patients, it is detected at the initial presentation, often representing preexisting conduction system disease. The appearance of a new bundle branch block is an indication for prophylactic temporary pacing.

Death of patients with myocardial infarction and bundle branch block usually is due to advanced heart failure and ventricular arrhythmias rather than to the development of complete heart block. Patients in whom transient complete heart block develops in association with a bundle branch block are at risk for recurrent complete heart block and should undergo permanent pacing. A new bundle branch block that never progresses to complete heart block is not an indication for permanent pacing.

- Death of patients with myocardial infarction and bundle branch block usually is due to advanced heart failure.
- New bundle branch block that never progresses to complete heart block is not an indication for permanent pacing.
- Second-degree (Mobitz II) block with bilateral bundle branch block and third-degree AV block warrants pacing.

Syncope

Syncope is defined as a transient loss of consciousness with spontaneous recovery. It is a frequent clinical syndrome that requires medical evaluation. Causes of syncope can be categorized as cardiovascular, noncardiovascular, and unexplained (Table 3-21). It is estimated that 30% of cases of syncope have a cardiogenic cause (bradycardia or tachycardia), 35% have a vasovagal cause, and 10% to 25% are related to a miscellaneous disorder such as orthostatic or situational syncope or seizures or are drug-related episodes. In 10% to 25% of cases, the cause is—and often remains—unknown.

The most important aspect of evaluation for syncope is the clinical history and physical examination, which provide key information in 40% to 75% of the patients for whom a diagnosis is eventually established. The factors associated with increased cardiogenic causes for syncope are listed in Table 3-22. In patients with increased risk of cardiogenic syncope, electrophysiologic testing should be considered. If an arrhythmogenic cause (bradycardia or tachycardia) for syncope has been established by noninvasive tests such as ECG, Holter monitoring, or transtelephonic monitoring, electrophysiologic testing is not indicated unless other arrhythmias are suspected. In patients at low risk for cardiogenic syncope, a noninvasive approach should be considered.

Table 3-21 Major Causes of Syncope

Cardiovascular	Noncardiovascular
Cardiogenic syncope	Neurologic
Structural heart disease	Metabolic
Coronary artery disease	Psychiatric
Rhythm disturbances	
Reflex syncope	
Vasovagal	
Carotid sinus hypersensitivity	
Situational	
Micturition	
Deglutition	
Defecation	
Glossopharyngeal neuralgia	
Postprandial	
Tussive	
Valsalva maneuver	
Oculovagal	
Sneeze	
Instrumentation	
Diving	
After exercise	
Orthostatic hypotension	

From Shen W-K, Gersh BJ. Syncope: mechanisms, approach, and management. In: Low PA, editor. Clinical autonomic disorders: evaluation and management. Boston: Little, Brown and Company; 1993. p. 605-40. Used with permission of Mayo Foundation for Medical Education and Research.

Table 3-22 Risk Stratification in Patients With Unexplained Syncope[a]

High-risk Factors	Low-risk Factors
Coronary artery disease, previous myocardial infarction	Isolated syncope without underlying cardiovascular disease
Structural heart disease	Younger age
Left ventricular dysfunction	Symptoms consistent with a vasovagal cause
Congestive heart failure	Normal ECG
Older age	
Abrupt onset	
Serious injuries	
Abnormal ECG (presence of Q wave, bundle branch block, or atrial fibrillation)	

Abbreviation: ECG, electrocardiogram.

[a] In patients who present with a prodrome (eg, nausea, diaphoresis), a neurocardiogenic mechanism is likely. Patients who experience rapid recovery (less than 5-10 minutes) rarely have a neurologic cause for syncope and are most unlikely to have syncope due to seizure or "brain hypoperfusion" because recovery in such circumstances takes hours. Thus, for cases in which recovery from syncope is rapid and no residual neurologic signs or symptoms are present, detailed (and expensive) neurologic evaluation should be avoided.

Modified from Shen W-K, Gersh BJ. Syncope: mechanisms, approach, and management. In: Low PA, editor. Clinical autonomic disorders: evaluation and management. Boston: Little, Brown and Company; 1993. p. 605-40. Used with permission of Mayo Foundation for Medical Education and Research.

Tilt-table testing is effective in eliciting a vasovagal response. For diagnostic purposes, tilt-table testing is indicated for patients with recurrent syncope without evidence of structural cardiac disease or for those with structural heart disease but after other causes of syncope have been excluded by appropriate testing. Tilt-table testing generally is not indicated for patients with a single episode of syncope without injury or in a high-risk setting with clear-cut vasovagal clinical features. Recommendations for evaluation of patients with syncope are outlined in Figure 3-36.

After the diagnosis of syncope has been established, the treatment usually is straightforward. Pacemaker therapy is appropriate for sinus node dysfunction and AV conduction disease. Various treatment options for tachyarrhythmias are discussed above. In patients with recurrent neurocardiogenic syncope (vasovagal syncope), education about the mechanism and triggering factors is important because in most cases recurrent episodes of syncope can be averted if appropriate action, such as sitting or lying down, is taken. Other therapeutic options include maintenance of increased intravascular volume and maneuvers to prevent venous pooling. One effective therapy is midodrine, which helps to promote an increase in venous return. Serotonin reuptake blockers may be effective in a subgroup of patients. Pacemaker therapy has a limited role in preventing syncope, even in patients with a predominant cardioinhibitory subtype of vasovagal syncope (ie, 1 that manifests with bradycardia), because vasodilatation is also a large component of these episodes. Indeed, although bradycardia is often a large component of vasovagal syncope, onset of symptoms is often only blunted, and unaffected, with pacing. However, the placebo effect of pacing was shown with the first and second vasovagal pacing studies (J Am Coll Cardiol. 1999;33:16-20 and JAMA. 2003;289:2224-9). The first trial randomized patients to a permanent pacemaker or no pacemaker; improvement was significant in patients who had pacing. However, in the second trial, all patients underwent pacemaker implantation but were randomized to pacemaker switched off (only sensing) or pacemaker switched on. There were no differences between groups in this study, a suggestion that any benefit of pacing in neurally mediated syncope was due to placebo effect.

Although β-blockers are frequently used, current evidence suggests they have limited or no benefit in the management of neurally mediated syncope. Indeed, the Prevention of Syncope Trial (POST) (Circulation. 2006;113:1164-70), which randomized 208 patients to metoprolol or placebo, found no differences in freedom from recurrent syncope between groups, even in patients with "adrenergically mediated" symptoms.

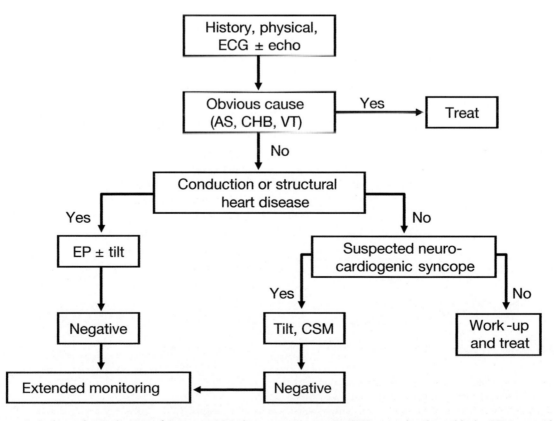

Figure 3-36. Diagnostic Pathway for Evaluation of Syncope. AS indicates aortic stenosis; CHB, complete heart block; CSM, carotid sinus massage; ECG, electrocardiogram; echo, echocardiography; EP, electrophysiologic study; tilt, tilt-table testing; VT, ventricular tachycardia.

Part IV

Abhiram Prasad, MD

Ischemic heart disease, principally myocardial infarction, accounts for approximately 1 of 3 deaths in the United States, or nearly 800,000 deaths annually. The substantial decrease in the death rate from acute myocardial infarction that has occurred since 1970 (Figure 3-37) is attributed to efforts in primary prevention and new interventions in the treatment of myocardial infarction. The variable presentation of patients with coronary heart disease includes patients who are asymptomatic (with or without silent ischemia), patients who have stable or unstable angina or myocardial infarction, and patients with sudden death.

- About one-third of the deaths annually in the United States are due to myocardial infarction.
- The substantial decrease in death from acute myocardial infarction since 1970 is due to primary prevention and new treatments of myocardial infarction.

Prevention of Coronary Heart Disease

The Framingham risk score is the most commonly used model to calculate the 10-year risk for development of coronary heart disease. The score is derived from the patient's age, sex, low-density lipoprotein (LDL) level, high-density lipoprotein cholesterol level, blood pressure, and the presence of diabetes and smoking (Circulation. 1998;97:1837-47). Risk factors for coronary artery disease for which intervention has been proved to reduce cardiac events include tobacco abuse, serum LDL cholesterol level, serum high-density lipoprotein level, and hypertension (Table 3-23).

Factors that clearly increase the risk of coronary artery disease and that intervention likely decreases include diabetes mellitus, physical inactivity, obesity, metabolic syndrome, and serum triglyceride levels. Factors for which intervention may improve subsequent risk include psychosocial factors (eg, anxiety and depression). Further information on primary prevention is available in the guidelines on stable angina of the American College of Cardiology and the American Heart Association (J Am Coll Cardiol. 2003;41:159-68).

- Smoking more than doubles the incidence of coronary heart disease and increases mortality by 50%.
- The relative risk of smokers who have quit smoking decreases rapidly, approaching the levels of nonsmokers within 2-3 years.
- Plasma levels of total cholesterol and LDL cholesterol are important risk factors for coronary heart disease. This relationship is strongest at high levels of cholesterol.
- A 1% decrease in total serum cholesterol yields a 2%-3% decrease in the risk of coronary heart disease.
- Lowering increased plasma levels of LDL cholesterol slows progression and promotes regression of coronary atherosclerosis.
- Lowering increased plasma levels of LDL cholesterol prevents coronary events, presumably because of stabilization of lipid-laden plaques.

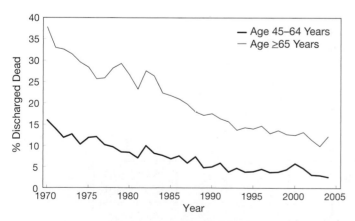

Figure 3-37. Case-Fatality Rate for Acute Myocardial Infarction in the United States, 1970-2004. (From National Heart, Lung, and Blood Institute. Morbidity and mortality: 2007 chart book on cardiovascular, lung, and blood diseases. Bethesda, MD: National Institutes of Health; 2007.)

Table 3-23 Risk Factors for Coronary Artery Disease

Modifiable Factor	Nonmodifiable Factor	Novel Factor
Increased LDL cholesterol level	Age	Inflammatory markers (eg, C-reactive protein)
Low HDL cholesterol level	Male sex	Small, dense LDL
Cigarette smoking	Family history of premature CAD[a]	Lipoprotein (a)
Hypertension		Homocysteine
Diabetes		Fibrinogen
Sedentary lifestyle		
Obesity		
Metabolic syndrome		
Stress and depression		
Socioeconomic factors		

Abbreviations: CAD, coronary artery disease; HDL, high-density lipoprotein; LDL, low-density lipoprotein.
[a] Age at onset <55 years in men and <65 years for primary relatives.

- The estimated decreased risk of myocardial infarction is 2%-3% for each 1-mm Hg decrease in diastolic blood pressure.
- The estimated decrease in the risk of myocardial infarction with the maintenance of an active compared with a sedentary lifestyle is 35%-55%.
- The adjusted mortality rates for coronary heart disease are 2-3 times higher in men with diabetes mellitus and 3-7 times higher in women with diabetes mellitus.
- Estrogen replacement therapy is not indicated in women with cardiovascular disease, and it may be harmful.
- Although heavy alcohol use increases the risk of cardiovascular disease, moderate consumption decreases the risk of heart disease.
- Metabolic syndrome is present in 20% of the US population, its prevalence is increasing, and it is associated with a 2-fold to 3-fold increase in mortality from cardiovascular disease.

Secondary prevention refers to efforts to prevent recurrent ischemic events in patients with known coronary artery disease. The role of antiplatelet agents, β-adrenergic blockers, and angiotensin-converting enzyme inhibitors is discussed below. Smoking cessation and optimum treatment of hypertension and diabetes mellitus are vital. Aggressive treatment of cholesterol levels is of value. The statin drugs reduce events after myocardial infarction to a greater degree than would be expected from their effect on atherosclerosis progression alone. This result may be related to stabilization of lipid-rich plaques, which are prone to rupture. In patients who have had a myocardial infarction and have increased levels of cholesterol (>220 mg/dL), treatment with a statin drug decreases overall mortality by 30% and disease mortality from coronary events by 42%. In patients who have had a myocardial infarction and have average levels of cholesterol (cholesterol, <240 mg/dL; LDL, >125 mg/dL), treatment with a statin drug reduces the chance of fatal heart disease or recurrent myocardial infarction by 24%.

Current guidelines for instituting cholesterol-lowering therapy were recommended by the National Cholesterol Education Program Expert Panel on Detection, Evaluation, and Treatment of High Blood Cholesterol in Adults (Adult Treatment Panel III). (J Am Coll Cardiol. 2004;44:720-32.)

- Therapeutic lifestyle changes, including a low-fat, low-cholesterol diet, weight management, and physical activity, are essential for cholesterol lowering.
- Viscous (soluble) fiber (10-25 g/day) and plant stanols or sterols (2 g/day) should be considered as therapeutic options.
- The following are indications for cholesterol-lowering therapy:
  1. Known coronary artery disease (or diabetes mellitus, peripheral vascular disease, multiple risk factors that confer a 10-year risk for coronary heart disease >20% calculated using a modified Framingham risk score): LDL >100 mg/dL. Goal LDL <100 mg/dL (optimal < 70 mg/dL)
  2. Two or more risk factors for coronary artery disease: LDL >130 mg/dL
  3. 0 or 1 risk factor for coronary artery disease: LDL >160 mg/dL
- Secondary therapeutic targets include treatment of metabolic syndrome, increased triglyceride levels, and low high-density lipopotein level.

Newer risk factors have been proposed for the diagnosis and management of patients with coronary heart disease. Abnormal levels of lipoprotein (a); homocysteine; small, dense LDL particle (phenotype B); and fibrinogen may be markers for coronary artery disease in patients who may not have the conventional risk factors. In patients with known coronary artery disease, inflammatory or infectious markers have been associated with adverse outcomes. These include inflammatory markers such as C-reactive protein, tumor necrosis factor-α, interleukin-1 and -6, and infectious agents such as *Chlamydia*, cytomegalovirus, and *Helicobacter*. New data suggest that increased levels of C-reactive protein are associated with a 2-fold to 3-fold increase in the rate of myocardial infarction. There is the suggestion that some drugs (ie, statins) may be beneficial in patients with inflammatory markers, although the data are preliminary.

Mechanism of Atherosclerosis

The response-to-injury hypothesis is the most prevalent explanation of atherosclerosis (N Engl J Med. 1992;326:242-50). According to this hypothesis, chronic minimal injury to the arterial endothelium is caused mainly by a disturbance in the pattern of blood flow (stage I injury), potentiated by high cholesterol levels, inflammation, infections, and tobacco smoke. Stage I injury leads to the accumulation of lipids, which are modified by oxidation and glycation. The modified LDL induces an inflammatory response in the vessel wall that results in the accumulation of macrophages and other leukocytes. Scavenger receptors on the macrophages mediate the uptake of the modified LDL into the cells to form macrophage foam cells. The release of toxic products by macrophages produces stage II injury, which is characterized by the adhesion of platelets. Macrophages and platelets with endothelial-release growth factors cause migration and proliferation of smooth muscle cells, which form a fibrointimal lesion or lipid lesion. Disruption of a lipid lesion that has a thin capsule causes stage III damage, with thrombus formation. The thrombus may organize and contribute to the growth of the atherosclerotic lesion or become totally occluded, culminating in unstable angina or myocardial infarction (Figure 3-38). Lipid-laden coronary artery lesions with less severe angiographic stenosis are more prone to rapid progression because of atherosclerotic plaque disruption. In up to two-thirds of cases of unstable angina or myocardial infarction, the culprit lesion is at a site with less than 50% stenosis.

- The most prevalent explanation for atherosclerosis is the response-to-injury hypothesis.
- Stage II injury is characterized by the adhesion of platelets.
- Stage III damage is disruption of a lipid lesion leading to thrombus formation.
- Lipid-laden coronary artery lesions with less severe angiographic stenosis are more prone to rapid progression because of atherosclerotic plaque disruption.
- In up to two-thirds of cases of unstable angina or myocardial infarction, the culprit lesion is at a site with <50% stenosis.

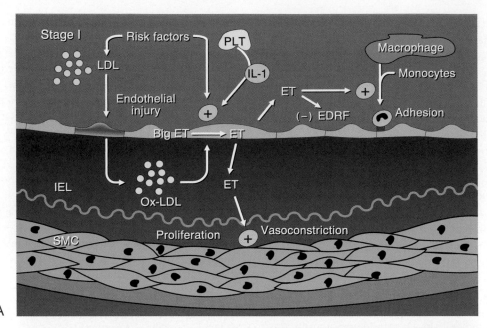

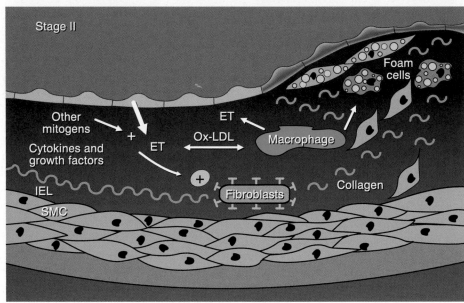

Figure 3-38. Stages of Vascular Injury. A, Stage I. B, Stage II. Interaction of endothelin (ET) and the atherosclerotic plaque. EDRF indicates endothelium-derived relaxing factor; IEL, internal elastic lamina; IL-1, interleukin 1; LDL, low-density lipoprotein particles; Ox-LDL, oxidized LDL particles; PLT, platelet; SMC, smooth muscle cell. "+" indicates stimulation. (From Lerman A. The endothelium. In Murphy JG, editor. Mayo Clinic cardiology review. 2nd ed. Philadelphia: Lippincott Williams & Wilkins; 2000. p. 99-112. Used with permission of Mayo Foundation for Medical Education and Research.)

Chronic Stable Angina

Pathophysiology

In chronic stable angina, myocardial ischemia is caused by a mismatch between myocardial oxygen demand and myocardial oxygen supply. Less important factors are perfusion pressure (aortic-to-right atrial gradient), autoregulation (maintenance of coronary blood flow through a physiologic range of perfusion pressures), autonomic tone, and compressive effect (high left ventricular end-diastolic pressure decreases subendocardial flow). Normally, coronary blood flow can increase up to 5 times to meet effort-related increases in myocardial oxygen demands. Ischemia occurs when flow reserve is inadequate, usually the result of fixed coronary artery disease. Restriction of resting blood flow to levels sufficient to cause ischemia at rest does not occur unless vessel stenosis is more than 95%. However, a decrease in overall flow reserve begins to occur with about 60% stenosis, at which point symptoms of exercise-induced ischemia may begin.

The 4 factors that determine myocardial oxygen consumption (demand) are heart rate, afterload, contractility, and wall tension [wall tension = (left ventricular radius) × (left ventricular pressure)]. With a dilated, poorly contractile left ventricle, the contribution of wall tension to myocardial oxygen consumption outweighs the other factors. The temporal sequence of events includes metabolic ischemia → diastolic dysfunction → perfusion abnormalities → regional wall motion abnormalities → electrocardiographic (ECG) changes → pain.

- In chronic stable angina, myocardial ischemia is caused by increased myocardial oxygen demand.
- Normally, coronary blood flow can increase up to 5 times to meet myocardial oxygen demand.
- Resting blood flow does not cause ischemia unless stenosis is >95%.
- The 4 factors of myocardial oxygen consumption: heart rate, afterload, contractility, and wall tension.
- The temporal sequence of events: ischemia → diastolic dysfunction → perfusion abnormalities → regional wall motion abnormalities → ECG changes → pain.

Clinical Presentation

Symptomatic Chronic Coronary Artery Disease
Typical angina is defined by the presence of all 3 of the following: characteristic retrosternal pain, the pain occurs with stress, and the pain is relieved by rest or nitroglycerin. Atypical angina is defined by the presence of 2 of these features. Noncardiac chest pain is defined by the presence of 1 or none of these features. Many patients have symptoms of angina pectoris during physical activity. The pain is described variously as pressure, burning, stabbing, ache, hurt, or shortness of breath. It can be substernal or epigastric and radiate to the neck, jaw, shoulder, elbow, or wrist. In chronic stable angina, the pain lasts 2 to 30 minutes and is usually relieved by rest. It generally is precipitated by any activity that increases myocardial oxygen consumption. Physical signs that occur with the pain include the onset of a fourth heart sound and mitral regurgitant murmur due to papillary muscle dysfunction. ST-segment depression may be found on the ECG, indicating subendocardial ischemia. The double product [(heart rate) × (systolic blood pressure)] is useful for defining myocardial oxygen demand. Nocturnal angina can be caused by unstable angina and also by increased wall tension with left ventricular dysfunction.

- Typical angina is defined by the presence of all 3 of the following: characteristic retrosternal pain, the pain occurs with stress, and the pain is relieved by rest or nitroglycerin. Atypical angina is defined by the presence of 2 of these features. Noncardiac chest pain is defined by the presence of 1 or none of these features.
- Physical signs occurring with the pain are a fourth heart sound and mitral regurgitant murmur due to papillary muscle dysfunction.
- The double product [(heart rate) × (systolic blood pressure)] is useful for defining myocardial oxygen demand.

Silent Ischemia
Silent ischemia is common in patients with symptomatic stable coronary artery disease or unstable angina or after myocardial infarction.

It is diagnosed by the presence of ST-segment depression in the absence of symptoms. The treatment is similar to that for chronic stable angina: risk factor modification, aspirin, and β-adrenergic blockers are effective. Whether percutaneous transluminal coronary angioplasty or coronary artery bypass grafting should be performed for silent ischemia alone is debated unless there are other markers of exceptionally high risk. The prognosis for this condition is the same as that for symptomatic ischemia.

- Silent ischemia is common in patients with symptomatic stable coronary artery disease or unstable angina or after myocardial infarction.
- Silent ischemia is diagnosed by the presence of ST-segment depression in the absence of symptoms.
- Treatment is similar to that for chronic stable angina.
- β-Adrenergic blockers are effective therapeutic agents in silent ischemia.
- Whether coronary angioplasty or bypass grafting should be performed for silent ischemia is debated.
- The prognosis for silent ischemia is the same as that for symptomatic ischemia.

Noninvasive Testing
Ancillary tests for coronary artery disease include measurement of left ventricular function, stress testing, and coronary angiography. Left ventricular function is the most important predictor of prognosis and should be measured in all patients with 2-dimensional echocardiography, radionuclide angiography, or left ventricular angiography. Exercise testing is performed with the treadmill or bicycle exertion test in conjunction with ECG monitoring, thallium or technetium-sestamibi scanning (perfusion of the myocardium), radionuclide angiography (left ventricular function), or echocardiography (left ventricular function) to assess for ischemia (J Am Coll Cardiol. 2002;40:1531-40). During a standard treadmill test (ie, exercise with stepped increases in workload every 2-3 minutes), heart rate, blood pressure, and the onset of subjective symptoms are monitored. The cardiac rhythm and the 12-lead ECG are monitored continuously. The ECG is positive for ischemia if there is a flat or downsloping ST-segment depression of 1 mm or more. The ECG response is uninterpretable when there is more than 1 mm of resting ST-segment depression, left bundle branch block, left ventricular hypertrophy, paced rhythm, digoxin therapy, or preexcitation (Wolff-Parkinson-White syndrome). For interpreting the results of any test, Bayes theorem is important. According to this theorem, the predictive value of a test depends on the prevalence of the disease in the population studied.

- The most important predictor of prognosis is left ventricular function.
- The ECG is positive for ischemia if there is a flat ST-segment depression of ≥1 mm.
- Complete left bundle branch block, resting ST-segment depression >1 mm, left ventricular hypertrophy, paced rhythm, digoxin therapy, or preexcitation render the exercise ECG uninterpretable.
- Bayes theorem: the predictive value of a test depends on the prevalence of the disease in the population studied.

ECG treadmill exertion testing has a sensitivity of about 70% and specificity of about 75%. Thus, a young patient with atypical chest pain and no risk factors (patient A in Figure 3-39) has a low pretest probability (5%) of coronary artery disease. If the test results are negative, the probability decreases to 3%. However, if the results are positive, the probability is less than 15%. In comparison, an older man (patient B in Figure 3-39) with typical chest pain and multiple risk factors has a high pretest probability (90%) of coronary artery disease, and even with negative test results the probability is higher than 70%. Thus, stress tests should not be used for the *diagnosis* of coronary artery disease in patients at high or low risk. Pretest probability of disease can be estimated with the following clinical criteria: age (men >40 years and women >60 years), male sex, and symptom status (in decreasing order of risk: typical angina, atypical angina, noncardiac chest pain, asymptomatic).

Several different types of cardiac imaging methods add to the sensitivity and specificity of ECG treadmill exertion testing. In thallium imaging, thallium Tl 201 injected at peak exercise labels areas of perfusion; "cold spots" are nonperfused regions. Scanning is repeated 3 to 24 hours later. Persistent cold spots indicate previous infarction, and reperfused areas indicate ischemia. Single-photon emission computed tomography thallium scanning (use of multiple tomographic planes) is more accurate than planar thallium scanning. In patients with left bundle branch block and severe left ventricular hypertrophy, thallium and sestamibi scanning give false-positive results during exercise stress.

Sestamibi scanning uses an isotope with a half-life different from that of thallium. Also, because this isotope has higher photon energy than thallium, it is routinely used in women and obese patients to avoid artifact. However, the results are interpreted in the same way as those of thallium scanning, with cold spots indicating lack of perfusion.

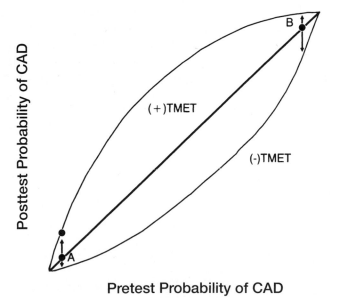

Figure 3-39. The effect of Bayes theorem on the ability of treadmill exertion testing (TMET) to diagnose coronary artery disease (CAD). Representative patients A and B are described in the text.

In radionuclide angiography (multiple gated acquisition scanning), erythrocytes are labeled with technetium Tc 99m and the left ventricular cavity is imaged during the cardiac cycle to measure (at rest and at peak exercise) left ventricular volume, ejection fraction, and regional wall motion abnormalities. The test result is positive if the ejection fraction decreases or new regional wall motion abnormalities appear. Because multiple cycles are gated, the test cannot be used with irregular rhythms.

In exercise echocardiography, 2-dimensional echocardiography is performed at rest and at peak exercise. Digital acquisition allows side-by-side comparisons of images from the same view. The test is positive for ischemia if global systolic function decreases or new regional wall motion abnormalities appear.

- The sensitivity and specificity of ECG treadmill exertion testing are about 70% and 75%, respectively.
- The treadmill exertion test should not be used to make the diagnosis of coronary artery disease.
- Thallium or sestamibi scanning gives false-positive results during exercise in patients with left bundle branch block and severe left ventricular hypertrophy.
- Multiple gated acquisition scanning is positive if the ejection fraction decreases or new regional wall motion abnormalities appear.
- Two-dimensional echocardiography is positive for ischemia if global systolic function decreases or new regional wall motion abnormalities appear.

All these imaging methods are more expensive than the ECG treadmill exertion test. Because Bayes theorem applies, imaging methods should not be used instead of ECG treadmill testing to diagnose coronary artery disease except in cases of an uninterpretable ECG or false-positive ECG results or for localizing specific regions of ischemia (for future revascularization procedures).

Pharmacologic stress tests that provoke ischemia have been developed for patients who cannot exercise. These tests include the use of dipyridamole thallium, which redistributes flow away from ischemic myocardium. Adenosine thallium works in the same way as dipyridamole. In dobutamine echocardiography, the myocardial oxygen demand is increased. Pacing echocardiography increases heart rate.

Treadmill exertion testing identifies high-risk patients. A patient is at high risk if the following results are obtained: a positive ECG in stage I of the Bruce protocol or at a heart rate less than 120 beats per minute, ST-segment depression more than 2 mm, ST-segment depression more than 6 minutes in duration after stopping, decreased blood pressure, multiple perfusion or wall motion defects (>25% of segments with exercise), and an increase in left ventricular end-systolic volume with exercise. In patients with poor prognostic factors, it is reasonable to proceed with coronary angiography to define the anatomy of the coronary arteries and the need for intervention. However, in patients who achieve a good workload without marked ST-segment depression and have appropriate blood pressure and heart rate responses, medical management may be indicated because of the excellent prognosis. The treadmill exertion test should not be performed on patients with high-risk unstable angina, patients who have had an acute myocardial infarction in the previous 2 days, or patients with symptomatic severe aortic stenosis, uncontrolled heart failure, uncontrolled arrhythmia, or severe aortic stenosis.

Noninvasive coronary angiography is being developed using computed tomography and magnetic resonance imaging. Rapid progress has been made, but the diagnostic accuracy is not good enough for these techniques to be considered an alternative to invasive coronary angiography. Computed tomography requires the use of contrast media and produces suboptimal images in patients with anything more than mild coronary calcification. Noninvasive imaging may have a role in symptomatic patients who have a low to moderate pretest probability of coronary heart disease because of its high negative predictive value. It is not recommended for screening asymptomatic patients or patients with established coronary heart disease. A valuable role for noninvasive angiography is for imaging coronary anomalies. The clinical utility of coronary calcium scores derived by computed tomography remains to be established.

- The major usefulness of stress testing is to identify high-risk patients, not to diagnose coronary artery disease.
- The treadmill exertion test should not be performed on patients with high-risk unstable angina, patients who have had an acute myocardial infarction in the previous 2 days, or patients with symptomatic severe aortic stenosis, uncontrolled heart failure, uncontrolled arrhythmia, or severe aortic stenosis.

Coronary Angiography

Although coronary angiography has many limitations, it is the standard method for defining the severity and extent of coronary artery disease. Subjective visual estimation of the percentage of stenosis may grossly underestimate the severity of the disease, especially if it is diffuse, because angiography outlines only the vessel lumen. The risk of serious complications of coronary angiography is approximately 0.2%. These complications include myocardial infarction (0.1%), stroke (0.1%), and death (0.1%). The risk is greater for older patients or for those with severe left ventricular dysfunction, left main coronary artery disease, or other coexistent diseases. Other complications include vascular complications (0.5%) and renal failure.

- Coronary angiography is the standard method for defining the severity of coronary artery disease.
- Visual estimation of the percentage of stenosis may grossly underestimate disease severity.
- The risk of serious complications in coronary angiography is approximately 0.2%.

Medical Therapy

Medical treatment for chronic stable angina should be given in a stepwise manner according to symptoms. Sublingual nitroglycerin should be given as needed. A first-line drug should be increased to the optimal dosage before a second or third drug is added. β-Adrenergic blockers are the most effective drugs for patients with coronary artery disease and should be the first-line drug of choice. They relieve angina mainly by decreasing heart rate, reducing contractility, and decreasing afterload (blood pressure). They are the

most effective drugs for reducing the double product (heart rate × blood pressure) with exercise. Also, these drugs may improve survival for some patients with known coronary artery disease, particularly those who have had a myocardial infarction and those with depressed left ventricular systolic function. β-Adrenergic blockers should not be prescribed if the patient has marked bronchospastic disease, severely symptomatic congestive heart failure, or bradycardia. However, they can and should be given to patients with left ventricular systolic dysfunction in the absence of overt heart failure. They should be given at a dosage that keeps the resting heart rate less than 70 beats per minute.

Long-acting nitrates should be added sequentially if symptoms continue. Nitrates relieve angina mainly by producing venodilatation, which decreases wall tension. Nitrate tolerance can occur with continuous exposure (use a nitrate-free interval with dosing 3 times daily). Isosorbide dinitrate, at least 20 to 30 mg 3 times daily, needs to be given.

Calcium channel blockers are effective for relieving angina by decreasing afterload, heart rate, and contractility; they may be used as a third-line drug. However, short-acting calcium channel blockers, specifically the dihydropyridines, may increase mortality of patients with ischemic heart disease. This detrimental effect probably does not occur with the longer-acting calcium channel blockers in patients with normal systolic function, but the use of these agents should be avoided if the patient has left ventricular systolic dysfunction. If a calcium channel blocker is required for patients with left ventricular systolic dysfunction, amlodipine should be given.

Ranolazine (Ranexa) is a new antianginal agent that is indicated for second-line therapy, as an adjunct to 1 of the above-discussed drugs. Experience with its use is limited. The mode of action is not known, but it is postulated to modulate myocardial metabolism.

Treatable underlying factors that contribute to ischemia (eg, anemia, thyroid abnormalities, and hypoxia) should always be sought. For patients with left ventricular dysfunction and nocturnal angina, diuretics and angiotensin-converting enzyme inhibitors may be helpful for decreasing wall tension. They may be beneficial for preventing future cardiovascular events in high-risk patients with known coronary artery disease regardless of the level of systolic function.

- The initial therapy for chronic stable angina is β-adrenergic blockade with sublingual nitroglycerin as needed.
- Long-acting nitrates should be added sequentially if symptoms continue.
- Nitrates relieve angina by producing venodilatation, which decreases wall tension.
- β-Adrenergic blockers relieve angina by decreasing heart rate, reducing contractility, and decreasing afterload (blood pressure).
- β-Adrenergic blockers are the most effective drugs for reducing the double product.
- Nitrate tolerance can occur with continuous exposure.
- β-Adrenergic blockers should not be prescribed if the patient has marked bronchospastic disease, severely symptomatic congestive heart failure, or bradycardia.
- β-Adrenergic blockers should be given at a dosage to keep the resting heart rate <70 beats per minute.

- Treatable underlying factors contributing to ischemia should be sought.
- Diuretics and angiotensin-converting enzyme inhibitors may be helpful for patients with left ventricular dysfunction and nocturnal angina.
- Short-acting calcium channel blockers should be avoided if the patient has coronary artery disease.
- For patients with left ventricular dysfunction, all calcium channel blockers except amlodipine should be avoided.

Antiplatelet agents may be helpful in patients with chronic stable angina pectoris. A low dose of aspirin probably does not prevent progression of atherosclerosis, but it may prevent acute myocardial infarction in patients with known coronary artery disease. In 2 large primary prevention trials, aspirin produced a 33% decrease in the risk for first, nonfatal myocardial infarction in men. The data are conflicting about the potential for a sex difference in the antithrombotic effects of aspirin; however, there is clear benefit for both men and women when aspirin is used in a secondary prevention strategy. The role of aspirin in primary prevention of stroke or overall cardiovascular mortality is uncertain.

- A low dose of aspirin probably does not prevent progression of atherosclerosis, but it may prevent acute myocardial infarction in patients with known coronary artery disease.
- The role of aspirin in primary prevention of stroke or overall cardiovascular mortality is uncertain.

Percutaneous Coronary Intervention
Percutaneous coronary intervention (PCI), a treatment for coronary artery disease, is performed at the time of coronary angiography. During percutaneous transluminal coronary angioplasty (PTCA), which is PCI with only a balloon, a small balloon is placed across a coronary stenosis and inflated to increase the area of the lumen at the site of stenosis. The mechanism of PTCA is a combination of "splitting" the atheroma and stretching the vessel. In experienced laboratories, the current success rate for PCI is more than 95%. Potential complications include myocardial infarction (<5%), vascular complications (1%), emergency coronary artery bypass grafting (0.2%), and mortality (<0.5%). The risks of the procedure are increased during emergency procedures, in elderly patients, and in patients with severely reduced ejection fraction, acute coronary syndromes, or severe diffuse coronary artery disease. Overall, more than 500,000 catheter-based therapies are performed annually in North America. The major problem with PTCA is restenosis, which occurs in 30% to 40% of patients within 6 months. Treatment with antiplatelet agents before PTCA may decrease the rate of acute closure but does not prevent restenosis. Glycoprotein IIb/IIIa inhibitors may decrease acute complications in high-risk patients but do not prevent restenosis. Other catheter-based therapies such as atherectomy, rotoblator, and laser have been used but they (and other therapies) have a high restenosis rate, similar to that of PTCA.

Placement of an intracoronary stent at the time of PCI is the only procedure that has been shown to decrease restenosis. Stents are used in approximately 90% of PCIs. The restenosis rate after successful bare-metal stent implantation is 20% to 30%. Stents also are effective for treating the acute complications of PTCA such as acute dissection and have decreased the need for emergency bypass operation. However, for patients who have restenosis within a stent, the rate of recurrent restenosis is high (>60%) if another procedure is performed. Drug-eluting stents that are coated with and elute drugs such as sirolimus (Rapamycin) and paclitaxel (Taxol) have been shown to significantly decrease the rate of restenosis (5%-10%). Drug-eluting stents are the predominant type of stents used in current practice. They seem to be associated with a slightly higher risk of stent thrombosis than bare-metal stents in the United States. Dual antiplatelet therapy is initiated at the time of stent deployment, and its duration varies according to the type of stent (Table 3-24). A loading dose of 300 mg (if a glycoprotein IIb/IIIa inhibitor is used) to 600 mg of clopidogrel is administered at the time of the PCI.

It is important to emphasize that for the treatment of chronic stable angina, PCI clearly relieves symptoms but does not reduce the risk of subsequent myocardial infarction or death.

- PTCA is a combination of splitting the atheroma and stretching the vessel.
- Currently, the initial success rate is >95%.
- Restenosis is a major problem of PTCA.
- Stents, particulary drug-eluting stents, can decrease the rate of restenosis.
- Antiplatelet agents reduce the risk of stent thrombosis but do not prevent restenosis.
- The duration of dual antiplatelet therapy typically ranges from 1-12 months depending on the type of stent deployed.

Surgical Treatment
The surgical treatment for severely symptomatic patients with chronic stable angina is coronary artery bypass grafting (CABG) with either saphenous vein or internal mammary artery grafts. CABG provides excellent relief from symptoms (partial relief in >90% of patients and complete relief in >70%). In-hospital mortality after CABG varies widely from less than 1% to 30%. Mortality increases

Table 3-24 Antiplatelet Therapy Used With Drug-Eluting Stents

Therapy	Duration
Aspirin	Indefinitely
Clopidogrel (Plavlix)	
Bare-metal stent implantation	At least 1 month
	Minimum of 2 weeks if patient is at ↑ risk of bleeding
Cypher stent	3 months
Taxus stent	6 months
Cypher or Taxus, in patients who are not at high risk of bleeding	Ideally up to 12 months

with age, poor ventricular function, female sex, left main coronary artery disease, unstable angina, diabetes mellitus, redo CABG, and emergency procedures. Complications of CABG include sternal wound infection (especially in patients with diabetes mellitus), severe left ventricular dysfunction (from perioperative myocardial infarction or inadequate cardioprotection), and late constrictive pericarditis. The procedure is not without latent problems. Closure rates of saphenous vein grafts are 20% at 1 year and 50% at 5 years. The patency rate is higher for internal mammary arteries, possibly up to 90% patency at 5 years. A minithoracotomy with a left internal mammary artery–left anterior descending artery anastomosis may shorten hospitalization, but long-term follow-up is needed.

* CABG provides excellent relief from symptoms.
* CABG gives partial relief in >90% of patients and complete relief in >70%.
* In-hospital mortality after CABG varies widely from <1%-30%.
* Mortality increases with age, poor ventricular function, female sex, left main coronary artery disease, unstable angina, diabetes mellitus, redo CABG, and emergency procedures.
* Closure rates of saphenous vein grafts are 20% at 1 year and 50% at 5 years.

Several randomized trials have compared CABG with medical therapy, and the intermediate-term follow-up results are as follows:

* CABG does not prevent myocardial infarction.
* CABG does not uniformly improve left ventricular function.
* CABG does not decrease ventricular arrhythmias.
* CABG improves survival only for patients with 1) left main coronary artery disease, 2) 3-vessel disease and moderately depressed left ventricular function, 3) 3-vessel disease and severe symptoms of ischemia at a low workload, and 4) multivessel disease with involvement of the proximal left anterior descending artery. For all other subsets of patients, CABG should not be performed to improve survival.
* The indications for CABG instead of medical therapy are 1) relieving symptoms in patients who have limiting symptoms unresponsive to medical management and 2) prolonging the life of the subsets of patients listed above.
* These recommendations were based on the randomized trials of CABG versus medical therapy, which all had a small number of patients and limited use of internal mammary artery grafts. In larger meta-analyses, there was a survival benefit for CABG versus medical therapy for all patients with 3-vessel disease.

Medical Versus Catheter-Based Versus Surgical Therapy

The decision about which therapy to use for a patient with chronic stable angina is individualized and must be based on the patient's age, lifestyle, and personal preference. However, randomized trials have compared the medical, catheter-based, and surgical therapies, and the results help in guiding decisions about which therapy to use for a selected subset of patients. The following summarizes the results of these trials.

1. Medical therapy versus PCI:

* PCI is associated with a similar or higher incidence of myocardial infarction and emergency CABG.
* The Clinical Outcomes Utilizing Revascularization and Aggressive Drug Evaluation (COURAGE) trial confirmed that, among patients with stable coronary artery disease, those who receive optimal medical therapy and those who receive PCI with bare-metal stents in addition to optimal medical therapy have equivalent outcomes with regard to death and myocardial infarction. High-risk patients with severe symptoms, markedly positive stress test, ejection fraction <30%, refractory heart failure, and PCI in the prior 6 months were excluded from the trial.
* PCI does not decrease the future risk of myocardial infarction.
* PCI does not improve resting left ventricular function.
* PCI does not increase survival.

2. PCI versus surgical therapy (multivessel disease—excluding left main coronary artery disease and totally occluded vessels):

* The rates of procedure-related mortality are similar (1%).
* There are more procedure-related Q-wave infarctions with CABG than with PCI (4.6% vs 2.1%), but events are well tolerated.
* The duration of initial hospitalization is longer with CABG than with PCI.
* The overall rates of death or myocardial infarction are similar at 5-year follow-up (85%-90% free of death and 80% free of myocardial infarction).
* Patients who have CABG have less angina, require less antianginal medication, and are less likely to need a repeat revascularization procedure than those who have PCI (8% vs 54% at 5-year follow-up). These data are derived from trials using PTCA and bare-metal stents. Repeat revascularization rates are likely to be much lower with drug-eluting stents.
* For patients with diabetes mellitus, 5-year survival is higher with CABG than with PCI (80% vs 65%). Increased survival is associated with a patent left internal mammary artery–left anterior descending artery graft.

Postcardiotomy Syndrome

Postcardiotomy syndrome occurs 2 weeks to 2 years postoperatively and consists of fever, pericarditis, and increased erythrocyte sedimentation rate. Rarely, it can present as pericardial tamponade. It probably is an autoimmune process (associated with antimyocardial antibodies); treatment is with aspirin and nonsteroidal anti-inflammatory drugs. Rarely, constrictive pericarditis may be a late complication. The diagnosis should be suspected in patients presenting months to years after cardiac surgery with congestive heart failure with predominantly right-sided signs of fluid overload, increased jugular venous pressure, but normal left ventricular ejection fraction.

Coronary Artery Spasm

The vasomotor tone of coronary arteries is important in the pathogenesis of coronary artery disease. Coronary artery vasoconstriction is a response to arterial injury. The endothelium affects vascular tone by releasing relaxing factors, for example, prostacyclin and nitric oxide, which prevent vasoconstriction and platelet deposition. With dysfunctional endothelium, these factors are absent and the coronary arteries may be more prone to spasm. Most clinical episodes of coronary artery spasm are superimposed on atherosclerotic plaques. However, patients may have primary coronary artery spasm and angiographically normal coronary arteries.

- Endothelium affects vascular tone by releasing relaxing factors (eg, prostacyclin and nitric oxide).
- With dysfunctional endothelium, coronary arteries may be more prone to spasm.
- Most episodes of spasm are superimposed on atherosclerotic plaques.
- Patients may have primary coronary artery spasm and angiographically normal coronary arteries.

The typical presentation of coronary artery spasm consists of recurrent episodes of rest pain in association with ST-segment elevation, which reverses with administration of nitrates. Coronary angiography with ergonovine or methylergonovine challenge has been used to diagnose coronary artery spasm, but the sensitivity and specificity are not known. The use of acetylcholine to provoke spasm may be helpful because it directly examines the status of the endothelium. ST-segment elevation on the resting 12-lead ECG during an episode of rest pain is the standard criterion for diagnosing coronary artery spasm. Coronary artery spasm is treated with long-acting nitrates or calcium channel blockers (or both).

- The typical presentation of coronary artery spasm is recurrent episodes of rest pain and ST-segment elevation that is reversed with nitrates.

Acute Coronary Syndromes

The term *acute coronary syndrome* refers to any constellation of clinical symptoms that are compatible with acute myocardial ischemia (Figure 3-40). Acute coronary syndromes encompass acute myocardial infarction (ST-segment elevation and non–ST-segment elevation) and unstable angina. Patients with these syndromes have to be differentiated from those with noncardiac chest pain on the basis of the clinical assessment (Table 3-25).

The resting ECG is essential in the evaluation of a patient presenting with an acute coronary syndrome. Patients without ST-segment elevation and myocardial ischemia may have unstable angina or they may have development of non–Q-wave myocardial infarction. Unstable angina and non–ST-segment elevation myocardial infarction have a similar pathogenesis. Patients with ST-segment elevation most likely have complete occlusion of an epicardial coronary artery that causes transmural injury. If untreated, a Q-wave myocardial infarction eventually develops. In a small proportion of patients with non–ST-segment elevation myocardial infarction, Q-wave myocardial infarction develops. In patients who have ST-segment elevation and receive thrombolytic therapy, non–Q-wave

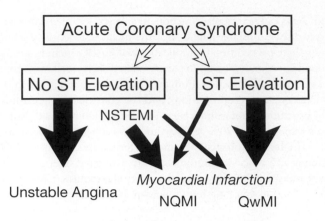

Figure 3-40. Nomenclature of Acute Coronary Syndromes. Patients with ischemic discomfort may present with or without ST-segment elevation on the electrocardiogram. In the majority of patients with ST-segment elevation (large arrows) a Q-wave anterior myocardial infarction (QwMI) ultimately develops, whereas in a small proportion (small arrow) a non–Q-wave anterior myocardial infarction (NQMI) develops. Patients who present without ST-segment elevation are experiencing either unstable angina or non–ST-segment elevation myocardial infarction (NSTEMI). The distinction between these 2 diagnoses is ultimately made on the basis of the presence or absence of a cardiac marker detected in the blood. In most patients with NSTEMI, a Q wave does not develop on the 12-lead electrocardiogram, and they are subsequently referred to as having sustained a non–Q-wave myocardial infarction (NQMI). In only a small proportion of patients with NSTEMI does a Q wave develop, and Q-wave myocardial infarction is later diagnosed. Not shown is Prinzmetal angina, which presents with transient chest pain and ST-segment elevation but rarely with myocardial infarction. The spectrum of clinical conditions that range from unstable angina to NQMI and QwMI is referred to as *acute coronary syndromes*. (From the Committee on the Management of Patients With Unstable Angina. ACC/AHA guidelines for the management of patients with unstable angina and non–ST-segment elevation myocardial infarction. A report of the American College of Cardiology/American Heart Association Task Force on Practice Guidelines. J Am Coll Cardiol. 2000;36:970-1062. Used with permission.)

myocardial infarction may develop. Acute coronary syndromes should be considered a continuous spectrum of diseases in patients who present with myocardial ischemia.

Early risk stratification is essential (Table 3-26). Patients presenting with a suspected acute coronary syndrome should be evaluated immediately in the emergency department, and those who have ST-segment elevation should be treated immediately (see below, ST-Segment Elevation Myocardial Infarction). For patients who do not have ST-segment elevation, chest pain units have been developed in emergency departments that allow dismissal of low-risk patients, observation of intermediate-risk patients, and admission of high-risk patients (Figure 3-41).

- *Acute coronary syndrome* refers to clinical symptoms compatible with acute myocardial ischemia.
- Early risk stratification is essential.

Table 3-25 Clinical Features Increasing the Likelihood of an Acute
Coronary Syndrome

History	Examination	Investigation Findings
Typical angina chest pain	Pulmonary edema	Pathologic Q waves
Age >70 y	Hypotension	Abnormal ST segments
Male sex	Extracardiac vascular disease	T-wave inversion ≥0.02 mV
Diabetes mellitus		Increased cardiac biomarkers

Table 3-26 High-Risk Features in Patients With Non–ST-
Segment Elevation Acute Coronary Syndrome

Age >75 y
Accelerating ischemic symptoms over 48 h
Ongoing rest pain for >20 min
Recurrent ischemic pain during observation
Hypotension
Reduced ejection fraction (<40%)
Pulmonary edema
Severe arrhythmia
ST-segment depression >0.05 mV
Increased cardiac biomarkers

Unstable Angina and Non–ST-Segment Elevation Myocardial Infarction

These conditions are characterized by an imbalance between myocardial oxygen supply and demand. They may be caused by an increased myocardial oxygen demand in the presence of a fixed myocardial oxygen supply. They also may be caused by a decrease in myocardial oxygen supply, which usually results from narrowing of the coronary artery due to a nonocclusive thrombus that developed on a disrupted atherosclerotic plaque. Superimposed spasm also may cause this syndrome.

All patients with the tentative diagnosis of an acute coronary syndrome should have continuous ECG monitoring and treatment to improve the myocardial oxygen demand-supply mismatch (J Am Coll Cardiol. 2002;40:1366-74). Sedation should be used to decrease anxiety and catecholaminergic stimulation of the heart. β-Adrenergic blocker is the treatment of choice for decreasing myocardial oxygen demand. Antiplatelet agents, such as aspirin, should be given immediately because they are effective for decreasing the incidence of progression to myocardial infarction. Heparin also decreases the incidence of progression to myocardial infarction and should be given to all patients who do not have contraindications to this treatment. Continuous intravenous administration of unfractionated heparin or subcutaneous injections of low-molecular-weight heparin can be given. Glycoprotein IIb/IIIa inhibitors should be prescribed for patients who are at high risk (eg, ongoing chest pain, transient ST-segment depression with angina at rest, increase in troponin levels), particularly if PCI is likely.

Unstable angina and non–ST-segment elevation myocardial infarction are differentiated on the basis of cardiac enzymes. Previously, creatine kinase-MB was the principal serum marker used in the evaluation of acute coronary syndromes. However, cardiac-specific troponin T and cardiac-specific troponin I are now the preferred biomarkers. An increase in the level of these markers in patients with an acute coronary syndrome indicates myocardial necrosis and identifies patients who are at high risk for future events.

There are 2 accepted therapeutic pathways for patients who present with unstable angina or non–ST-segment elevation myocardial infarction (Figure 3-42). The first is a conservative approach in which medical management is used to stabilize the patient's condi-

tion. Coronary angiography is indicated if 1) additional ischemic episodes occur despite optimal medical therapy, 2) there is left ventricular dysfunction or heart failure, and 3) serious arrhythmias occur. The second accepted therapeutic pathway is an early invasive approach in which all high-risk patients have coronary angiography within 48 hours and high-grade coronary lesions are treated. If the conservative pathway is taken, patients should undergo stress testing before dismissal, and patients with positive results of stress testing should also have coronary angiography. The early invasive strategy is preferred in high-risk patients.

- Unstable angina differs from non–ST-segment elevation myocardial infarction in that cardiac-specific biomarker values are increased in the latter.
- An early invasive strategy is preferred in high-risk patients with a non–ST-elevation acute coronary syndrome.

ST-Segment Elevation Myocardial Infarction

The underlying pathogenesis of ST-segment elevation myocardial infarction is usually rupture of an intracoronary plaque. This leads to platelet adhesion, aggregation, thrombus formation, and sudden, complete occlusion of an epicardial coronary artery. Without collateral circulation, 90% of the myocardium that is supplied by the occluded coronary artery is infarcted within 3 hours. If untreated, transmural myocardial infarction develops. Patients with ST-segment elevation myocardial infarction require urgent diagnosis and therapy to preserve the myocardium. It is for this group of patients that aggressive reperfusion therapy has improved survival.

- ST-segment elevation myocardial infarction usually implies acute occlusion of an epicardial coronary artery.
- If untreated, a transmural myocardial infarction will develop within 3 hours.

Myocardial infarction accounts for a large percentage of morbidity and mortality in the United States. More than 800,000 patients are admitted annually to a hospital with a primary diagnosis of an acute coronary syndrome. ST-segment elevation accounts for one-fifth

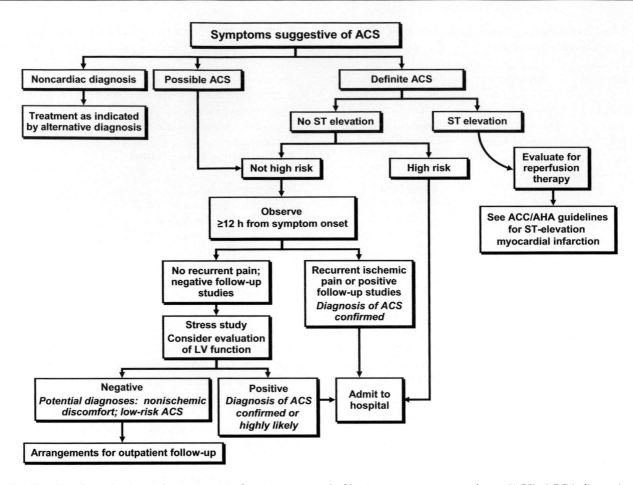

Figure 3-41. Algorithm for evaluation and management of patients suspected of having acute coronary syndrome (ACS). ACC indicates American College of Cardiology; AHA, American Heart Association; ECG, electrocardiography; LV, left ventricular. (Modified from Anderson JL, Adams CD, Antman EM, Bridges CR, Califf RM, Casey DE Jr, et al. ACC/AHA 2007 guidelines for the management of patients with unstable angina/non–ST-elevation myocardial infarction: a report of the American College of Cardiology/American Heart Association Task Force on Practice Guidelines [Writing Committee to Revise the 2002 Guidelines for the Management of Patients With Unstable Angina/Non–ST-Elevation Myocardial Infarction]. J Am Coll Cardiol. 2007;50:e1-157. Used with permission.)

of these patients. More than 50% of patients who have a myocardial infarction die before reaching the hospital. With the advent of coronary care units 4 decades ago, mortality from myocardial infarction decreased, primarily because of treatment of ventricular arrhythmias. β-Adrenergic blockade has further decreased in-hospital and posthospital mortality by 30% to 40%. In the 1980s, reperfusion therapy became the standard of care and has been shown to further improve survival. Currently, the overall in-hospital mortality for a patient with ST-segment elevation myocardial infarction is 5% to 10%.

Stunned myocardium occurs when a coronary artery is completely occluded and then opened, and transient akinesis of the myocardium occurs. If reperfusion occurs early enough, systolic contraction of the affected myocardium may be decreased after the event, but the myocardium is viable. Systolic contraction returns hours to days later. Currently, no clinical test differentiates stunned myocardium from infarcted, dead myocardium. *Infarct remodeling* occurs mainly after a large anteroapical myocardial infarction. An area of infarction may undergo thinning, dilatation, and dyskinesis. This

remodeling is associated with a high incidence of congestive heart failure and posthospital mortality. Angiotensin-converting enzyme inhibitors may help prevent infarct remodeling.

- Stunned myocardium: a coronary artery is completely occluded and then opened, and transient akinesis of the myocardium occurs.
- Infarct remodeling: occurs after a large anteroapical myocardial infarction.
- Angiotensin-converting enzyme inhibitors may help prevent infarct remodeling.

Presentation and Diagnosis

The usual presentation of ST-segment elevation myocardial infarction is angina-like pain that lasts longer than 20 minutes and is associated with typical ECG changes and increased levels of creatine kinase-MB fraction or troponin (Figure 3-43). However, more than 25% to 30% of myocardial infarctions are silent and present later as new ECG abnormalities or regional wall motion abnormalities.

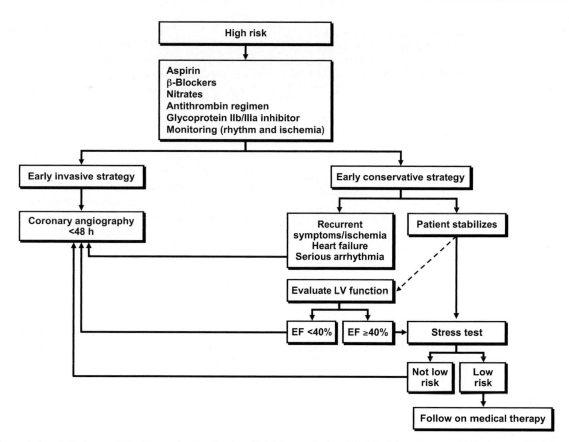

Figure 3 42. Acute Ischemia Pathway. EF indicates ejection fraction; LV, left ventricular. (Modified from Braunwald E, Antman EM, Beasley JW, Califf RM, Cheitlin MD, Hochman JS, et al. ACC/AHA 2002 guideline update for the management of patients with unstable angina and non–ST-segment elevation myocardial infarction: a report of the American College of Cardiology/American Heart Association Task Force on Practice Guidelines [Committee on the management of patients with unstable angina]. 2002 [cited 2006 March 1]. Available from: http://www.acc.org/clinical/guidelines/unstable/unstable.pdf.)

Silent myocardial infarctions occur especially in patients with diabetes mellitus and in the elderly. The increased incidence of myocardial infarction in the early morning is perhaps related to increased platelet aggregation. The pain of myocardial infarction mimics that of other diseases, for example, gastrointestinal tract or pericardial disease or musculoskeletal pain.

* More than 25%-30% of myocardial infarctions are silent.
* Silent myocardial infarctions occur especially in patients with diabetes mellitus and in the elderly.
* The increased incidence of myocardial infarction in the early morning is perhaps related to increased platelet aggregation.
* The pain of myocardial infarction mimics that of other diseases.

Basic and Drug Treatments

Bed rest and sedation are essential and beneficial in the acute stage of myocardial infarction for decreasing myocardial oxygen demand. Analgesics, particularly morphine, are beneficial for recurrent pain. Currently, prolonged bed rest is not recommended, and the effort to shorten hospitalization is increasing. Many physicians recommend a gradual increase in activity level over 3 to 6 days for an uncomplicated myocardial infarction. During the acute 3- to 4-day period, ECG monitoring is recommended for both tachyarrhythmias and bradyarrhythmias. Oxygen can be given at the initial presentation but has little benefit after 2 or 3 hours unless hypoxia (oxygen saturation < 90%) is present. However, modest hypoxemia is not uncommon, even with uncomplicated myocardial infarction, and is due to ventilation-perfusion lung mismatch.

* Prolonged bed rest is not recommended for myocardial infarction.
* Oxygen has little benefit beyond 3 hours after the initial presentation unless hypoxia is present.

Heparin is important for treating acute myocardial infarction. It prevents recurrent infarction (especially after thrombolytic therapy, when it should be administered for at least 24 hours), deep vein thrombosis, and intracardiac thrombus formation. Historically, intracardiac thrombus formation occurred in up to 40% of patients with anterior myocardial infarction in whom patency of the occluded vessel is not restored, and almost 50% of these patients had a systemic embolic event. Intravenous unfractionated heparin therapy is indicated for higher-risk patients (large or anterior myocardial infarction,

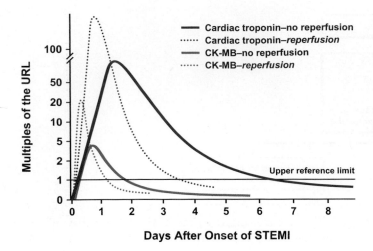

Figure 3-43. Cardiac Biomarkers in ST-segment Elevation Myocardial Infarction (STEMI). Typical cardiac biomarkers that are used to evaluate patients with STEMI include the MB isoenzyme of creatine kinase (CK-MB) and cardiac-specific troponins. The horizontal line depicts the upper reference limit (URL) for the cardiac biomarker in the clinical chemistry laboratory. The URL is that value representing the 99th percentile of a reference control group without STEMI. The kinetics of release of CK-MB and cardiac troponin in patients who do not undergo reperfusion are shown in the solid blue and red curves as multiples of the URL. Note that when patients with STEMI undergo reperfusion, as depicted in the dotted blue and dotted red curves, the cardiac biomarkers are detected sooner, increase to a higher peak value, but decline more rapidly, resulting in a smaller area under the curve and limitation of infarct size. (From Antman EM, Anbe DT, Armstrong PW, Bates ER, Green LA, Hand M, et al. ACC/AHA guidelines for the management of patients with ST-elevation myocardial infarction: a report of the American College of Cardiology/American Heart Association Task Force on Practice Guidelines [Committee to Revise the 1999 Guidelines for the management of patients with acute myocardial infarction]. J Am Coll Cardiol. 2004;44:E1-E211.)

atrial fibrillation, previous embolus, reperfusion therapy not given or unsuccessful). Low-molecular-weight heparin given subcutaneously may be more effective. Thromboembolism is uncommon in patients in whom reperfusion therapy is successful. Aspirin 325 mg should be administered immediately on admission to all patients. It decreases recurrent infarction by 50% in patients not receiving thrombolytic therapy. It also reduces mortality when given in addition to thrombolytic therapy. Clopidogrel (75 mg daily) is an alternative in patients with aspirin allergy or intolerance. Clopidogrel is also indicated in patients treated with thrombolytics starting on day 1 and its use is continued for 4 weeks.

- Heparin is important for treating acute myocardial infarction. It should be administered for at least 24 hours after thrombolytic therapy.
- Heparin prevents recurrent infarction, deep vein thrombosis, and intracardiac thrombus formation.
- Intracardiac thrombus formation occurs in up to 40% of patients

with anterior myocardial infarction in whom patency of the occluded vessel is not restored.

- Aspirin decreases recurrent infarction by 50% in patients not receiving thrombolytic therapy.
- Clopidogrel is an alternative in patients with aspirin allergy or intolerance.

Nitroglycerin is useful for subsets of patients with myocardial infarction—for those with pulmonary edema (by decreasing wall tension), severely increased blood pressure, and persistent myocardial ischemia. To prevent acute decreases in blood pressure in the early stages of myocardial infarction, intravenous nitroglycerin should be given instead of long-acting oral nitrates. The dosage of intravenous nitroglycerin is a 15-mcg bolus and an initial infusion of 10 mcg/min. This infusion should be increased every 5 to 10 minutes, up to a maximum of 150 to 200 mcg/min, until blood pressure decreases 10% to 15%. Mean blood pressure should be kept higher than 80 mm Hg. Nitrate intolerance develops with infusions that last longer than 24 hours. Intravenous nitroglycerin should not be given to patients with low blood pressure (systolic <90 mm Hg), patients with right ventricular infarction, and patients who have received a phosphodiesterase inhibitor for erectile dysfunction within the previous 24 hours (48 hours for tadalafil).

- Nitroglycerin is useful for patients with myocardial infarction who have pulmonary edema, uncontrolled hypertension, and persistent myocardial ischemia.
- Nitrate intolerance occurs with infusions that last longer than 24 hours.
- Intravenous nitroglycerin should not be given to patients with low blood pressure or right ventricular infarction or to patients who have received a phosphodiesterase inhibitor for erectile dysfunction within the previous 24 hours (48 hours for tadalafil).

β-Adrenergic blockers are useful during acute myocardial infarction and after myocardial infarction. If given early, they decrease in-hospital mortality. If given after myocardial infarction has been completed, β-adrenergic blockers can reduce posthospital reinfarction and mortality. In an acute setting, the typical dosage of metoprolol is 5 mg given intravenously 3 times, 5 minutes apart, followed by 100 mg given orally twice daily. β-Adrenergic blockers decrease pain and the incidence of ventricular fibrillation. The beneficial effects are probably multifactorial but include decreased myocardial oxygen demand, increased threshold for ventricular fibrillation, decreased platelet aggregability, and decreased sympathetic effects on the myocardium. β-Adrenergic blockers are most beneficial for patients with a large infarction, that is, those at higher risk for complications. Acute intravenous β-adrenergic blockers are also beneficial for patients receiving thrombolytic therapy. β-Adrenergic blockers are especially useful for patients with hyperdynamic circulation and continued postinfarction myocardial ischemia and should be given to patients presenting with less than 12 hours of pain who do not have contraindications, especially those with anterior myocardial infarction. Contraindications to β-adrenergic blockers are bradycardia (heart rate <60 beats per minute), second- or third-degree atrioventricular block, hypotension (systolic blood pressure <100 mm Hg), acute heart failure, cardiogenic shock, and cocaine-induced myocardial infarction.

* If given early, intravenous β-adrenergic blockers decrease in-hospital mortality.
* If given early, intravenous β-adrenergic blockers decrease the incidence of ventricular fibrillation.
* Contraindications to β-adrenergic blockers are bradycardia, second- and third-degree atrioventricular block, hypotension, acute heart failure, cardiogenic shock, and cocaine-induced myocardial infarction.

Calcium channel blockers have been used to treat myocardial infarction, but their routine use has no proven benefit. Routine use of verapamil and nifedipine has no benefit and may increase mortality. However, calcium channel blockers that block the atrioventricular node (eg, diltiazem) may be used to control ventricular rate in atrial fibrillation, especially if β-adrenergic blockers are contraindicated.

* Routine use of calcium channel blockers for myocardial infarction has no proven benefit.
* Routine use of verapamil and nifedipine to treat myocardial infarction may increase mortality.

In most patients, magnesium does not seem to have a therapeutic role after myocardial infarction. Although initial studies suggested that it may decrease infarct size, subsequent studies have not borne out this effect. Magnesium should be given only if a patient has documented hypomagnesemia (from diuretics) or for the treatment of torsades de pointes.

Angiotensin-converting enzyme inhibitors have been studied extensively in patients with ST-segment elevation myocardial infarction. These inhibitors seem to prevent the infarct remodeling, especially after a large anteroapical myocardial infarction. Although these drugs should not be given acutely via the intravenous route, data support the initiation of oral therapy within the first 24 hours after a myocardial infarction as long as blood pressure is stable and for chronic use. They are definitely indicated in patients with anterior infarction, pulmonary congestion, or left ventricular ejection fraction less than 40%, but it is reasonable to treat all patients after ST-segment elevation myocardial infarction in the absence of hypotension or contraindications. Angiotensin receptor blockers are recommended as an alternative in patients who are intolerant to angiotensin-converting enzyme inhibitors. However, data supporting their use are available only for patients with heart failure or ejection fraction less than 40%. Long-term aldosterone blockade (spironolactone or eplerenone) is indicated for patients without renal dysfunction (creatinine, ≤2.0 mg/dL for women and ≤2.5 mg/dL for men) or hyperkalemia (potassium, ≤5.0 mEq/L) who are receiving therapeutic doses of angiotensin-converting enzyme inhibitors and have symptomatic heart failure or diabetes mellitus with an ejection fraction of 40%.

Other medications are being studied for treating ST-segment elevation myocardial infarction. Although glycoprotein IIb/IIIa inhibitors are given routinely to high-risk patients with non–ST-segment elevation myocardial infarction, they are not indicated in patients treated with thrombolytics. There appears to be a modest benefit when abciximab is administerd during primary PCI. Several direct thrombin inhibitors have been studied in patients with acute ST-segment elevation myocardial infarction, but they are not yet approved for the treatment of acute coronary syndromes. Bivalirudin is approved for use for unstable angina during PCI and is also an acceptable alternative to unfractionated heparin for patients who have heparin-induced thrombocytopenia and require anticoagulation.

Reperfusion Therapy

Early reperfusion therapy has had a tremendous effect on the treatment of acute myocardial infarction. Overall, mortality is decreased 27%±3% when reperfusion is given early. For more than 50,000 patients in the Third International Study in Infarct Survival (ISIS-3) and Gruppo Italiano per lo Studio della Sopravvivenza nell'Infarcto Miocardico (GISSI-2) studies, the 35-day in-hospital mortality was only 10% with thrombolytic therapy. Time is of the essence when giving reperfusion therapy. The sooner the reperfusion, the better the extent of myocardial salvage and the better the effect on mortality. Without collaterals, 90% of the myocardium at risk is infarcted within 3 hours after occlusion. Very early reperfusion has a major effect on direct myocardial salvage. In a study in which thrombolysis was given less than 90 minutes after the onset of pain, mortality was 1%. In most US studies, the average time from pain onset to artery opening is 3.7 hours. The delay is in patient presentation (22%), transport (21%), in-hospital institution of the drug (35%), and reperfusion drug time (19%). Reperfusion at 2 to 6 hours salvages the peri-infarction zone, depending on the degree of collateral circulation. Thus, there is a lesser effect on myocardial salvage but an important effect on survival. The "open artery concept" describes a benefit in improvement in posthospital mortality in the presence of an open artery after thrombolytic therapy that is not reflected in improved ventricular function. The reason for this is unclear, but it may be related to improved electrical stability or prevention of ventricular remodeling.

* Overall, mortality is decreased 27%±3% when reperfusion is given early.
* For more than 50,000 patients, the 35-day in-hospital mortality was 10% with thrombolytic therapy.
* The sooner the reperfusion, the better the extent of myocardial salvage.
* Without collaterals, 90% of the myocardium at risk is infarcted within 3 hours after occlusion.

Reperfusion therapy with either fibrinolytics or primary PCI is indicated for patients presenting within 12 hours of onset of symptoms and either 1 mm of ST-segment elevation in 2 adjacent leads or new or presumably new left bundle branch block (J Am Coll Cardiol. 2004;44:671-719). ECG changes of a true posterior myocardial infarction also qualify for reperfusion therapy. Intravenous thrombolysis is not as effective (65%-70%) for restoring normal coronary blood flow (thrombolysis in myocardial infarction [TIMI] grade 3) as PCI (90%). However, this disadvantage is counterbalanced by faster administration of intravenous thrombolysis and wider availability of the fibrinolytics. Fewer than 10% of all hospitals have the capability of performing emergency PCI, and these centers must be able to provide rapid treatment, with door-to-balloon time of less than 90 minutes. Thus, the preferred strategy depends on 1) time since the onset of symptoms, 2) time required for transportation to a skilled PCI catheterization laboratory, 3) risk of ST-segment elevation myocardial infarction (Table 3-27), and 4) presence of contraindications to fibrinolytics (Table 3-28). At most medical centers that do not have the resources for primary PCI, intravenous thrombolysis is the treatment of choice for patients with acute myocardial infarction. Emergency PCI may be used for patients with 1) immediate access to a high-volume catheterization laboratory, 2) a contraindication for intravenous thrombolysis, 3) high-risk ST-segment elevation myocardial infarction (cardiogenic shock or pulmonary edema), or 4) continued ischemia after thrombolytic therapy (rescue PCI). Routine PCI after successful thrombolytic therapy is not indicated in the absence of ongoing symptoms or ischemia.

Thrombolytic therapy seems to be less beneficial for patients older than 75 years. Reperfusion therapy is not indicated for patients who have other ECG abnormalities (ST-segment depression) or for those who present late (>12 hours) and are asymptomatic with no hemodynamic compromise or serious arrhythmia.

Major complications of intravenous thrombolysis include major bleeding (5%-6% of patients), intracranial bleeding (0.5%), major allergic reaction (0.1%-1.7%), and hypotension (2%-10%). A higher incidence of myocardial rupture may occur in patients who are given thrombolytic therapy late (>12 hours after pain onset).

Table 3-27 Thrombolysis in Myocardial Infarction (TIMI) Risk Score for ST-Segment Elevation Myocardial Infarction[a]

Variable	Points	Risk Score	Odds of Death by 30-Day Mortality[b]	
Historical		0	0.8	
Age		1	1.6	
≥75 y	3	2	2.2	Low risk
65-74 y	2	3	4.4	
DM or HTN or		4	7.3	
angina	1	5	12	
Examination		6	16	
SBP <100 mm Hg	3	7	23	
HR >100 bpm	2	8	27	
Killip II-IV	2	>8	36	
Weight <67 kg				
(150 lb)	1			
Presentation				
Anterior STE or				
LBBB	1			
Time to Rx >4 h	1			
Risk score = total points (0-14)				

Abbreviations: DM, diabetes mellitus; HR, heart rate; HTN, hypertension; LBBB, left bundle branch block; Rx, therapy; SBP, systolic blood pressure; STE, ST-segment elevation.

[a] Entry criteria: chest pain >30 min, ST ↑, symptom onset <6 h, fibrinolytic-eligible.

[b] Referenced to average mortality (95% confidence interval).

From Morrow DA, Antman EM, Charlesworth A, Cairns R, Murphy SA, de Lemos JA, et al. TIMI risk score for ST-elevation myocardial infarction: a convenient, bedside, clinical score for risk assessment at presentation: an intravenous nPA for treatment of infarcting myocardium early II trial substudy. Circulation. 2000;102:2031-7. Used with permission.

Table 3-28 Contraindications and Cautions for Fibrinolysis Use in ST-Segment Elevation Myocardial Infarction

Absolute contraindications
Any prior ICH
Known structural cerebral vascular lesion
Known malignant intracranial neoplasm
Ischemic stroke within 3 months *except* acute ischemic stroke within 3 h
Suspected aortic dissection
Active bleeding or bleeding diathesis (excluding menses)
Significant closed head or facial trauma within 3 mo
Relative contraindications
History of chronic severe, poorly controlled hypertension
Severe uncontrolled hypertension on presentation (SBP >180 mm Hg or DBP >110 mm Hg)[a]
History of prior ischemic stroke >3 mo, dementia, or known intracranial pathology not covered in contraindications
Traumatic or prolonged (>10 min) CPR or major surgery (less than 3 weeks)
Recent (within 2 to 4 weeks) internal bleeding
Noncompressible vascular punctures
For streptokinase/anistreplase: prior exposure (more than 5 days ago) or prior allergic reaction to these agents
Pregnancy
Active peptic ulcer
Current use of anticoagulants: the higher the INR, the higher the risk of bleeding

Abbreviations: CPR, cardiopulmonary resuscitation; DBP, diastolic blood pressure; ICH, intracranial hemorrhage; INR, international normalized ratio; SBP, systolic blood pressure.

[a] Could be an absolute contraindication in low-risk patients with ST-segment elevation myocardial infarction.

From Antman EM, Anbe DT, Armstrong PW, Bates ER, Green LA, Hand M, et al. ACC/AHA guidelines for the management of patients with ST-elevation myocardial infarction: executive summary: a report of the ACC/AHA Task Force on Practice Guidelines (Committee to Revise the 1999 Guidelines on the Management of Patients With Acute Myocardial Infarction). J Am Coll Cardiol. 2004;44:671-719. Used with permission.

- Major complications of intravenous thrombolysis are major bleeding (5%-6% of patients), intracranial bleeding (0.5%), major allergic reaction (0.1%-1.7%), and hypotension (2%-10%).
- A higher incidence of myocardial rupture may occur in patients given thrombolytic therapy late (>12 hours after pain onset).

Several agents are available for intravenous thrombolysis. Streptokinase, a nonselective thrombolytic agent, combines with circulating plasminogen to split circulating and thrombus-bound plasminogen into plasmin, which splits fibrin. It lyses circulating fibrinogen and thus has systemic effects. The dosage is a 250,000-unit bolus and 1.5×10^6 units in 1 hour. Tissue plasminogen activator binds preferentially to preformed fibrin and lyses it without activating plasminogen in the general circulation. Thus, it has less effect on circulating fibrinogen and is "fibrin-specific." It has the fastest onset of action. The dosage is 100 mg over 90 minutes. Newer thrombolytic agents such as reteplase and tenecteplase offer better selectivity for active thrombus, but they seem to be equivalent in efficacy to tissue plasminogen activator in clinical trials. However, the greatest advantage is that they can be administered as a bolus, which reduces drug errors and speeds delivery.

The large European trials did not demonstrate any benefit of 1 thrombolytic therapy over the others. In the Global Utilization of Strategies To Open Occluded arteries (GUSTO) trial, the mortality rate was slightly lower when an accelerated dose of tissue plasminogen activator was given with intravenous heparin than with streptokinase. Compared with streptokinase, tissue plasminogen activator is more expensive and has a slightly increased risk of cerebral hemorrhage, especially in the elderly. It is reasonable to give tissue plasminogen activator preferentially to younger patients who present very early with a large myocardial infarction. However, in current practice, streptokinase is rarely used in the United States, and tenecteplase and reteplase are the most commonly used fibrinolytics.

After intravenous thrombolysis, a high-grade residual lesion is usually present. Reocclusion or ischemia occurs in 15% to 20% of patients and reinfarction occurs in 2% to 3%. Heparin should be given in conjunction with intravenous thrombolysis with the tissue-specific plasminogen activators to prevent reinfarction. A bolus of 60 U/kg (maximum, 4,000 units) followed by an initial infusion of 12 U/kg per hour (maximum, 1,000 U/h) adjusted to maintain activated partial thromboplastin time at 1.5 to 2.0 times control (approximately 50 to 70 seconds) is the recommended dose. The indications for coronary angiography or PCI after intravenous thrombolysis are spontaneous or inducible ischemia, cardiogenic shock, pulmonary edema, ejection fraction less than 40%, and serious arrhythmias. No benefit results from routine intervention in all patients.

- After intravenous thrombolysis, reocclusion or ischemia occurs in 15%-20% of patients and reinfarction occurs in 2%-3%.
- Heparin should be given in conjunction with intravenous thrombolysis with the tissue-specific plasminogen activators to prevent reinfarction.
- Streptokinase is the least expensive thrombolytic therapy.

Acute Mechanical Complications of Myocardial Infarction
Cardiogenic shock after myocardial infarction has a high rate of mortality, but with newer interventions the mortality rate has decreased from 90% to 50%. However, it is important to determine the cause of cardiogenic shock. Although most cases are due to extensive left ventricular dysfunction, there are other causes, for example, right ventricular infarction and mechanical complications of myocardial infarction. Pulmonary artery catheterization and 2-dimensional echocardiography may help in determining the cause (Table 3-29).

- The mortality from cardiogenic shock after contemporary therapy for myocardial infarction is 50%.
- Most cases of cardiogenic shock are due to extensive left ventricular dysfunction.
- Pulmonary artery catheterization and 2-dimensional echocardiography may help determine other causes of cardiogenic shock.

Right ventricular infarction occurs in up to 40% of patients with inferior myocardial infarction and is diagnosed from increased jugular venous pressure in the presence of clear lung fields. It can present anywhere from hours to several days after the onset of infarction. ST-segment elevation in a V_4R lead is diagnostic of a large right ventricular infarction and portends a high mortality rate. In extreme circumstances, right ventricular infarction can cause

Table 3-29 Diagnosis of Cause of Cardiogenic Shock

Cause	Pulmonary Artery Catheterization			Catheterization Findings	Two-Dimensional Echocardiography
	RA	PAWP	CO		
Left ventricular dysfunction	↑	↑↑	↓↓		Poor left ventricle
Right ventricular infarction	↑↑	↓	↓↓		Dilated right ventricle
Tamponade	↑↑	↑↑	↓↓	End-equalization	Pericardial tamponade
Papillary muscle rupture	↑	↑↑	↓↓	Large V	Severe mitral regurgitation
Ventricular septal defect	↑	↑↑	↑	Step-up	Defect seen
Pulmonary emboli	↑↑	=	↓	PADP > PAWP	Dilated right ventricle

Abbreviations: CO, cardiac output; PADP, pulmonary artery diastolic pressure; PAWP, pulmonary artery wedge pressure; RA, right atrial pressure.

cardiogenic shock because the right ventricle is not able to effectively pump enough blood to fill the left ventricle. Treatment includes large amounts of fluids given intravenously and infusion of dobutamine. If right ventricular infarction is recognized early, reperfusion therapy is indicated.

- Right ventricular infarction occurs in up to 40% of patients with inferior myocardial infarction and presents with increased jugular venous pressure with clear lung fields.

Myocardial free wall rupture may occur and cause abrupt decompensation. Free wall rupture occurs in 85% of all ruptures. It occurs suddenly, usually 2 to 14 days after transmural myocardial infarction, most commonly in elderly hypertensive women, and usually presents as electromechanical dissociation or death. If rupture is contained in the pericardium, tamponade may occur. If the diagnosis can be made by emergency echocardiography, surgery should be performed. If the rupture is sealed off, a pseudoaneurysm may occur; surgical treatment is required because of the high incidence of further rupture.

- Free wall rupture occurs in 85% of all ruptures.
- It occurs suddenly, usually 2-14 days after transmural myocardial infarction.

Papillary muscle rupture occurs in 5% of all ruptures and usually 2 to 10 days after myocardial infarction. It is associated with inferior myocardial infarction because of the single blood supply to the posteromedial papillary muscle. Rupture of papillary muscle is heralded by the sudden onset of dyspnea and hypotension. Although a murmur may be present, it may not be audible because of equalization of left atrial and left ventricular pressures. The diagnosis is made with echocardiography or pulmonary artery catheterization, which demonstrates a large V wave on pulmonary artery wedge pressure. The treatment is intra-aortic balloon pump and an emergency operation.

- Papillary muscle rupture occurs in 5% of all ruptures.
- It usually occurs 2-10 days after myocardial infarction.
- It is associated with inferior myocardial infarction.
- It is heralded by sudden dyspnea and hypotension.
- It is diagnosed with echocardiography or pulmonary artery catheterization.

Ventricular septal defects occur in 10% of all ruptures, usually 1 to 20 days after myocardial infarction, and are equally frequent in inferior and anterior myocardial infarctions. Ventricular septal defects associated with inferior myocardial infarctions have a poorer prognosis because of the serpiginous nature of the rupture and associated ventricular infarction. They are indicated by the sudden onset of dyspnea and hypotension. A loud murmur and systolic thrill are always present. The diagnosis is made with echocardiography or pulmonary artery catheterization, which demonstrates a step-up in oxygen saturation from the right atrium to the pulmonary artery. Treatment is intra-aortic balloon pump and an emergency operation.

- Ventricular septal defects occur in 10% of all ruptures.

- They are equally frequent in inferior and anterior myocardial infarctions.
- They are indicated by the sudden onset of dyspnea and hypotension.
- A ventricular septal defect almost always has a thrill and loud murmur.

Pre–Hospital-Dismissal Evaluation

For proper evaluation of a patient with myocardial infarction before dismissal from the hospital, the predictors of mortality must be determined. These include status of the left ventricle, ventricular arrhythmias, and presence of continued myocardial ischemia.

After myocardial infarction, most patients should have rehabilitation treadmill exertion testing to detect continued ischemia, particularly patients who did not have thrombolytic therapy. A submaximal treadmill test can be performed before dismissal, within 4 to 6 days after myocardial infarction. Alternatively, a symptom-limited treadmill test can be performed safely 10 to 21 days after myocardial infarction. If a submaximal treadmill test is performed before dismissal, a late symptom-limited treadmill test should be performed at follow-up evaluation 3 to 6 weeks after myocardial infarction. High-risk patients identified by treadmill exertion testing have an ST-segment depression greater than 1 mm, a decrease in blood pressure, or an inability to achieve 4 metabolic equivalents on the exercise test. Imaging exercise tests may identify additional high-risk patients by demonstrating multiple areas of ischemia. Pharmacologic stress tests (dobutamine echocardiography, dipyridamole thallium scanning, or adenosine thallium scanning) may be useful for patients unable to exercise. The role of stress testing for patients after thrombolytic therapy is less clear because most of them do well without intervention. However, stress testing is of value in providing an exercise prescription to patients.

- After myocardial infarction, most patients should undergo rehabilitation treadmill testing.
- It is a low-risk test for properly selected patients.

To prevent infarct remodeling and expansion, angiotensin-converting enzyme inhibitors should be given to all patients who have large anterior myocardial infarctions. In patients with an ejection fraction less than 40%, this therapy prevents future congestive heart failure and improves mortality. Data suggest that angiotensin-converting enzyme inhibitors may be beneficial for preventing recurrent myocardial infarction and cerebrovascular accidents in all high-risk patients who have coronary artery disease.

Coronary angiography is indicated after myocardial infarction if the results of a rehabilitation treadmill exertion test are highly positive or postinfarction angina occurs. Patients with these findings usually have substantial regions of myocardium at risk, and the coronary anatomy should be defined to determine whether they should undergo either catheter-based therapy or CABG. Coronary angiography is indicated in patients who have had hemodynamic instability. Patients who have had heart failure during hospitalization are at high risk and should be considered for coronary angiography. Because CABG improves mortality for patients with 3-vessel disease and depressed systolic function, it has been suggested that coronary angiography be performed in all patients who have a depressed ejection fraction to look for severe 3-vessel or left main coronary artery disease.

* Coronary angiography is indicated if the results of a rehabilitation treadmill exertion test are positive or postinfarction angina occurs.

No randomized trials have examined the benefit of PTCA or bypass grafting after myocardial infarction. However, in high-risk patients (ie, those with continued ischemia or positive results on a treadmill exertion test), it is reasonable to proceed with intervention. PCI can be undertaken if there is a single-vessel high-grade lesion amenable to the procedure. CABG should be performed if there is left main coronary artery or proximal 3-vessel disease or 2- or 3-vessel disease that supplies a large portion of the myocardium, especially when associated with moderate depression in left ventricular function.

Aggressive modification of risk factors is essential in the treatment of patients who have had a myocardial infarction. An exercise program, weight loss, and diet are mandatory for all patients after myocardial infarction. Many physicians determine the cholesterol level on admission to the hospital. The goal of treatment is to decrease LDL cholesterol to less than 100 (optimal <70) mg/dL. If LDL cholesterol is more than 100 mg/dL, the trend is to start treatment with a statin drug before dismissal, even before instituting diet and weight loss.

The following apply to patients who survive acute myocardial infarction:

* Aspirin decreases recurrent myocardial infarction by 31% and late mortality by 15%, more so in cases of non–ST-segment elevation myocardial infarction.
* Warfarin may cause a similar decrease in mortality and reinfarction, but it is not used routinely in the United States.
* Statin drugs reduce recurrent events and mortality in patients with increased cholesterol levels (total cholesterol >200 mg/dL).
* Statin drugs reduce recurrent events in patients with average cholesterol levels (LDL >125 mg/dL).
* β-Adrenergic blockers improve survival after myocardial infarction.
* β-Adrenergic blockers are most effective in high-risk patients (ie, decreased left ventricular function and ventricular arrhythmias) and may not be required for low-risk patients.
* β-Adrenergic blockers are also effective after thrombolytic therapy.
* Because antiarrhythmic agents are associated with increased mortality, they should not be used to suppress ventricular ectopy.
* Angiotensin-converting enzyme inhibitors decrease mortality after anterior myocardial infarction and depressed left ventricular function, presumably by inhibiting infarct remodeling.
* A rehabilitation program is essential for the patient's well-being and cardiovascular fitness.
* An automatic implantable cardioverter-defibrillator should be considered if the ejection fraction is <30% 1 month after a myocardial infarction in patients with an expected survival of at least 1 year.

Part V

Barry L. Karon, MD

Heart Failure

Heart failure is a clinical syndrome characterized by the inability of the heart to maintain adequate cardiac output to meet the metabolic demands of the body while still maintaining normal or near normal ventricular filling pressures. Heart failure may be present at rest, but often it is present only during exertion as a result of the dynamic nature of cardiac demands. For correct treatment of heart failure, the mechanism, underlying cause, and any reversible precipitating factors must be identified. Typical manifestations of heart failure are dyspnea and fatigue that limit activity tolerance and fluid retention leading to pulmonary or peripheral edema. These abnormalities do not necessarily dominate the clinical picture at the same time. Dyspnea may be due to impaired output or increased filling pressures or both. Heart failure, the symptomatic expression of cardiac disease, usually arises some time after cardiac disease has become established. The American College of Cardiology and and the American Heart Association stages of heart failure (Figure 3-44) emphasize that symptoms follow an asymptomatic phase of cardiac dysfunction. It is often clinically challenging to determine whether symptoms are cardiac due to structural disease or whether they are coincidental noncardiac symptoms coexisting with asymptomatic structural disease.

Heart failure may result from abnormalities of the pericardium, myocardium, endocardium, cardiac valves, or vascular or renal systems. Most commonly, however, it is due to impaired left ventricular myocardial function. In approximately half of cases, the left ventricle is enlarged and there is abnormal contractile function with demonstrable reduction in ejection fraction. This is referred to as dilated cardiomyopathy. In the other half of cases, the heart failure is occurring in the setting of normal ejection fraction; this is referred to as heart failure with preserved ejection fraction. Although isolated right ventricular failure can occur, the majority of cases of heart failure involve either the left ventricle alone or the left ventricle with associated right ventricular dysfunction. High ventricular filling pressures can cause dyspnea and edema.

* Heart failure is the inability of the heart to maintain adequate cardiac output to meet the metabolic demands of the body while still maintaining normal filling pressures.
* Heart failure may manifest at rest or only with exertion.
* Cardinal symptoms of heart failure are fatigue (related to impaired output) and fluid retention (resulting in pulmonary or peripheral edema). Dyspnea may be due to impaired output or increased filling pressures or both.
* The most common cause of heart failure is left ventricular myocardial dysfunction.
* High ventricular filling pressures cause dyspnea and edema.
* Myocardial dysfunction with preserved ejection fraction is as important as dilated cardiomyopathy in causing heart failure.

Ventricular diastolic function is a complex process. Three of its major components are relaxation, passive filling, and atrial contraction. Relaxation is an active, energy-requiring process during which calcium is removed from the actin-myosin filaments, causing contracted muscle to return to its original length. Relaxation properties are dynamic and are normally transiently enhanced during physical exertion. In disease states (eg, hypertension, ischemia), relaxation rates may not be able to augment or may even worsen. After active relaxation, filling of the ventricle continues along the pressure gradient from the left atrium to the left ventricle (passive filling). The amount of filling during this phase is determined by left atrial pressure and left ventricular compliance; compliance is the increase in ventricular volume per unit of driving pressure. Thus, abnormally low compliance impairs filling and produces high end-diastolic pressure. Ventricular filling is also affected by the duration of diastolic filling. The contribution from atrial contraction further increases ventricular volume by as much as 15% to 20% in normal subjects and 45% to 50% in those with abnormal ventricular relaxation and passive filling (Table 3-30).

* Three major components of ventricular diastolic function are relaxation, passive filling, and atrial contraction.
* Relaxation is impaired in myopathic ventricles and can worsen transiently in the setting of ischemia or hypertension.
* Impaired ventricular compliance means higher pressures are needed to produce volume changes.
* Atrial contraction takes on greater importance in patients with reduced ventricular relaxation or compliance.

Managing Heart Failure

Patients may present with asymptomatic ventricular dysfunction (usually dilated ventricles with reduced ejection fraction). These patients do not have heart failure, and they can usually be managed as outpatients; their treatment is discussed later in this chapter. Patients with heart failure (ie, symptoms and signs) may present either as outpatients or to acute care facilities, often depending on the severity of their symptoms. This heterogeneous group is said to have acute decompensated heart failure and includes both patients presenting for the first time with heart failure and patients presenting with a decompensation of known heart failure. Hospitalization is advisable when hypotension, worsening renal function, altered mentation, dyspnea at rest, significant arrhythmias (eg, new atrial fibrillation), or other complications such as disturbed electrolytes or lack of outpatient care options are present (Table 3-31). Patients without these factors who have exclusively exertional symptoms, are not severely congested, and have adequate perfusion (warm extremities, adequate blood pressure) may receive treatment as outpatients.

Managing patients with heart failure requires a disciplined thought process. The stages of heart failure development and management are outlined in Figure 3-44.

At risk for heart failure   Heart failure

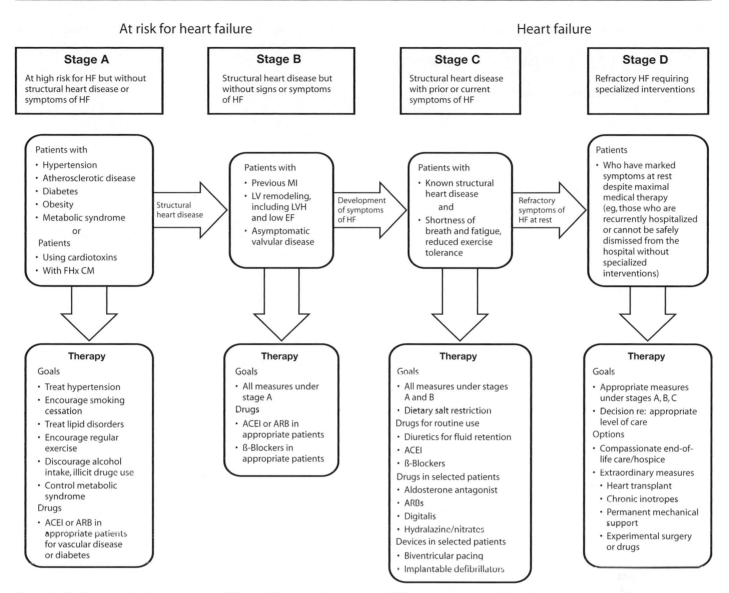

Figure 3-44. Stages in the Development of Heart Failure and Recommended Therapy by Stage. ACEI indicates angiotensin-converting enzyme inhibitors; ARB, angiotensin receptor blocker; EF, ejection fraction; FHx CM, family history of cardiomyopathy; HF, heart failure; LV, left ventricular; LVH, left ventricular hypertrophy; MI, myocardial infarction. (From Hunt SA, Abraham WT, Chin MH, Feldman AM, Francis GS, Ganiats TG, et al. ACC/AHA guideline update for the diagnosis and management of chronic heart failure in the adult: summary article. A report of the American College of Cardiology/American Heart Association Task Force on Practice Guidelines [Writing Committee to Update the 2001 Guidelines for the Evaluation and Management of Heart Failure]. J Am Coll Cardiol. 2005;46:1116-43. Used with permission.)

Diagnosis of Heart Failure

Heart failure is a clinical diagnosis made on the basis of symptoms, physical findings, and chest radiography. The symptoms typically include some combination of dyspnea, fatigue, and fluid retention. The dyspnea may be with exertion or with recumbency. Physical findings include evidence of low output or volume overload or both. These include narrow pulse pressure, poor peripheral perfusion, jugular venous distention, hepatojugular reflux, peripheral edema, ascites, and dull lung bases suggestive of pleural effusions. Lung crackles usually represent atelectatic compression rather than fluid in the alveoli, the latter being more common in acute heart failure. Edema usually affects the lower extremities but can also affect the abdomen. Cardiac findings include abnormalities of the cardiac apex (enlarged, displaced, sustained) and gallop rhythms. The liver may be enlarged, pulsatile, and tender if there is right heart failure. Clinical signs indicating high- and low-output heart failure could aid in patient management (Table 3-32).

Both the symptoms and signs of heart failure described above are nonspecific and can occur in other conditions. Use of the modified Framingham criteria for the clinical diagnosis of congestive heart failure retains an important place in clinical cardiology (Table 3-33).

By this scheme, the simultaneous presence of 2 major or 1 major and 2 minor criteria satisfies the clinical diagnosis of congestive heart failure. It is important to recognize that exertional dyspnea does not

Table 3-30 Abnormal Diastolic Function in Myocardial Disease

Phase	Influencing Factors	Treatment
Relaxation	Age, ischemia, hypertrophy	Treat ischemia, hypertension
Passive filling	Myocardial compliance, heart rate	Slow heart rate
Atrial contraction	Atrial contraction, atrioventricular synchrony	Maintain sinus rhythm, optimize atrioventricular delay

Table 3-31 Conditions That Prompt Hospitalization in Heart Failure

Hypotension
Worsening renal function
Altered mentation
Dyspnea at rest
Significant arrhythmias
Disturbed electrolytes
Lack of outpatient care

Table 3-32 Management of High-Output and Low-Output Heart Failure

Perfusion at Rest	Congestion at Rest	
	No	Yes
Normal	**Warm & dry** PCWP normal CI normal (compensated)	**Warm & wet** PCWP increased CI normal ↓ Hospitalize ± Nesiritide or vasodilators[a] Diuretics
Low	**Cold & dry** PCWP low or normal CI decreased ↓ Hospitalize Inotropic drugs[b]	**Cold & wet** PCWP increased CI decreased ↓ Hospitalize Nesiritide or vasodilators[a] Diuretics

Abbreviations: CI, cardiac index; PCWP, pulmonary capillary wedge pressure.
[a] Vasodilators: nitroglycerin or nitroprusside.
[b] Inotropic drugs: milrinone or dobutamine.

have the same weight as paroxysmal nocturnal dyspnea or orthopnea, and edema does not have the same weight as increased venous pressure. Patients with low-output heart failure may not have findings of volume overload (congestion) and thus may not satisfy Framingham criteria.

Natriuretic peptides are substances produced by the heart in increased amounts when there is increased intracardiac pressure or chamber dilatation. Accordingly, measurement of B-type natriuretic peptide or N-terminal pro-brain natriuretic peptide complements the clinical diagnosis of heart failure. In general, the degree of increase reflects the degree of myocardial dysfunction. Increased levels of these peptides do not distinguish systolic from diastolic, left from right, or acute from chronic cardiac dysfunction. Interpreting these levels has caveats (Table 3-34). In addition, there is substantial variability of levels in stable patients, up to 100%.

The utility of the natriuretic peptides for diagnosing heart failure has been best shown in patients without prior known cardiac disease. It can be difficult to interpret intermediately increased levels in patients with a prior history of ventricular dysfunction or heart failure who are receiving medical treatment. The negative predictive value of normal natriuretic peptide levels (in the absence of constriction, morbid obesity, or mitral stenosis) is more powerful than their positive predictive value.

- Heart failure is a clinical diagnosis based primarily on symptoms and physical findings.
- Use of the modified Framingham criteria can assist in diagnosing heart failure but will not be as helpful in patients with low-output heart failure without associated congestion.

- Natriuretic peptide levels are increased in patients with heart failure, although there are circumstances in which values may be higher or lower than expected. They are most useful in patients without a prior diagnosis of heart failure and in patients not receiving treatment for heart failure.

Management Phases in Acute Heart Failure

At the time of initial patient presentation, several things are done fairly simultaneously. The diagnosis of heart failure is made and common alternative diagnoses of pulmonary embolic or chronic obstructive pulmonary disease exacerbation are considered. The patient is then stratified clinically to guide initial treatment (usually parenteral) and improve symptoms (Figure 3-45).

After clinical improvement begins, the treatment is refined to optimize hemodynamics, minimize symptoms, and eventually transition to oral medications. The mechanism of heart failure and precipitating factors are defined, patient and family education are provided, and dismissal is planned (including heart failure follow-up).

Mechanisms of Heart Failure

The mechanism and causes of heart failure must be defined to select proper therapy. A simple categorical framework is given in Table 3-35.

Clinically, the most common cause of heart failure is left ventricular myocardial dysfunction. Because the treatment and prognosis are different for other causes of heart failure, accurate diagnosis is essential and is initially based on physical examination and noninvasive testing, such as echocardiography or radionuclide angiography.

Table 3-33 Framingham Criteria for Clinical Diagnosis of Congestive Heart Failure[a]

Major Criteria	Minor Criteria
PND	Peripheral edema
Orthopnea	Night cough
Increased JVP	DOE
Rales	Hepatomegaly
Third heart sound	Pleural effusion
Chest radiography	Heart rate >120 beats per minute
Cardiomegaly	Weight loss ≥4.5 kg in 5 days with diuretic
Pulmonary edema	

Abbreviations: DOE, dyspnea on exertion; JVP, jugular venous pressure; PND, paroxysmal nocturnal dyspnea.
[a] Validated congestive heart failure if 2 major or 1 major and 2 minor criteria are present concurrently.
Modified from Ho KKL, Anderson KM, Kannel WB, Grossman W, Levy D. Survival after the onset of congestive heart failure in Framingham heart study subjects. Circulation. 1993;88:107-15. Used with permission.

Precipitating Factors

The new appearance of or worsening of previous heart failure symptoms may merely represent natural disease progression. Often, however, 1 or more precipitating factors are responsible for symptomatic deterioration (Table 3-36). If these factors are not identified and corrected, symptoms of heart failure frequently return after initial therapy. The most common precipitants are dietary indiscretion (eg, sodium, fluid, alcohol), medication noncompliance (eg, cost, regimen complexity, patient understanding), and suboptimally controlled hypertension. The evaluation of each patient with heart failure follows these steps: 1) a medical history (include sodium and fluid intake, medication use and compliance, and sleep history from bedroom partners), 2) chest radiography to look for pneumonitis, 3) electrocardiography and measurement of cardiac biomarkers to document the rhythm and identify ischemia or myocardial injury, and 4) culture specimens of blood, urine, and sputum as appropriate from the history. Other tests should include determination of complete blood count and thyroid-stimulating hormone and creatinine levels.

* For different causes and mechanisms of heart failure, treatment and prognosis are different.
* For every patient with heart failure, precipitating factors must be sought and treated.
* Noncompliance, ischemia, rhythm changes, and uncontrolled hypertension are the most common precipitants of heart failure decompensation.

Cardiomyopathies

The classification of cardiomyopathies has proved troublesome and complex. The most recent proposed categorization divided them into primary and secondary cardiomyopathies, and the primary disorders

Table 3-34 Pitfalls in the Interpretation of Natriuretic Peptide Value

NP Higher Than Expected	NP Lower Than Expected
Women	Obesity
Elderly	Acute heart failure
Renal failure	Heart failure due to mitral stenosis
	Constriction

Abbreviation: NP, natriuretic peptide.

are further subdivided as genetic, acquired, or mixed. Although this proposal takes into account our progressive understanding of this heterogeneous group of disorders, the previous phenotypic classification of dilated, hypertrophic, and restrictive diseases still provides utility in day-to-day understanding and management of these disorders. The different anatomical and pathophysiologic processes for each cardiomyopathy are listed in Table 3-37.

Dilated Cardiomyopathy

Pathology and Etiology

The major abnormality in dilated cardiomyopathy is a remodeled left ventricle characterized by dilatation with a reduced ejection fraction. Left ventricular end-diastolic pressure typically is increased. The increased filling pressures and low cardiac output produce symptoms of shortness of breath and fatigue. The right ventricle may be normal, hypertrophied, or dilated.

An idiopathic dilated cardiomyopathy indicates left ventricular dysfunction without any known cause. Many of the cases are genetic; at least 1 affected family member can be identified in up to 30% of cases. Other causes of left ventricular dysfunction include severe coronary artery disease ("hibernating myocardium"), previous infarction, uncontrolled hypertension, ethanol abuse, hyperthyroidism or hypothyroidism, postpartum cardiomyopathy, toxins and drugs (including doxorubicin and trastuzumab), tachycardia-induced cardiomyopathy, infiltrative cardiomyopathy (ie, hemochromatosis, sarcoidosis), acquired immunodeficiency syndrome (AIDS), and pheochromocytoma.

* In dilated cardiomyopathy, the major abnormality is enlarged left ventricle with reduced ejection fraction.
* The most common cause of dilated cardiomyopathy in the United States is coronary artery disease.
* Other causes of left ventricular dysfunction: uncontrolled hypertension, ethanol abuse, thyroid disease, postpartum cardiomyopathy, toxins and drugs, and tachycardia-induced cardiomyopathy.
* Right ventricular contractile function may be normal or impaired in dilated cardiomyopathy.

Clinical Presentation

The presentation of dilated cardiomyopathy is highly variable. The patient may be asymptomatic and the diagnosis prompted

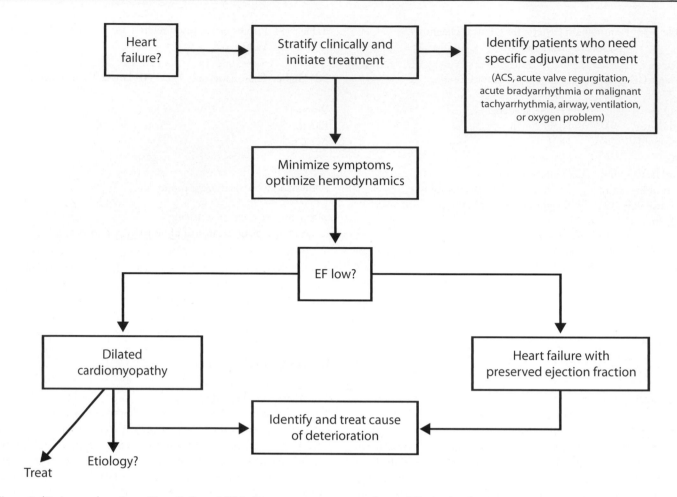

Figure 3-45. Approach to Acute Heart Failure. ACS indicates acute coronary syndrome; EF, ejection fraction.

by examination, chest radiography, electrocardiography (ECG), or imaging. Patients may have symptoms of mild to severe heart failure (New York Heart Association [NYHA] functional class II-IV). Atrial and ventricular arrhythmias are common in dilated cardiomyopathy. The following may be found on physical examination: jugular venous pressure is increased and a right ventricular lift is present (if there is right heart involvement), low-volume upstroke of the carotid artery, displaced and sustained left ventricular impulse (possibly with a rapid filling wave), audible third or fourth heart sounds, and an apical systolic murmur of mitral regurgitation. Pulmonary examination often has normal results but may reveal crackles or evidence of pleural effusion.

- Presentation of dilated cardiomyopathy is highly variable.
- Carotid volume is low, third heart sound is often present, and the apex is displaced and sustained.
- Jugular venous distention and a right ventricular lift signify right heart involvement.

ECG frequently shows left ventricular hypertrophy, intraventricular conduction delay, or bundle branch block. Rhythm abnormalities may include premature atrial contractions, atrial fibrillation, premature

ventricular contractions, or short bursts of ventricular tachycardia. The chest radiograph often shows left ventricular enlargement and pulmonary venous congestion. The diagnosis is made on the basis of left ventricular enlargement and reduced ejection fraction, which can be measured with echocardiography, radionuclide angiography, left ventriculography, cine computed tomography, or magnetic resonance imaging.

- ECG may show left ventricular hypertrophy, intraventricular conduction delay, or bundle branch block.
- Atrial and ventricular rhythm disturbances are common.
- The chest radiograph often shows left ventricular enlargement and pulmonary venous congestion.
- The diagnosis requires demonstration of left ventricular enlargement and reduced ejection fraction by any cardiac imaging method.

Evaluation
After impaired left ventricular contractile function is diagnosed, treatable secondary causes of left ventricular dysfunction should be excluded. Sensitive thyroid-stimulating hormone level should be determined to exclude hyperthyroidism or hypothyroidism.

Table 3-35 Causes of Heart Failure and Treatment

Cause	Treatment
Myocardial	
Dilated cardiomyopathy (including ischemic)	Angiotensin-converting enzyme inhibitors, angiotensin receptor blockers, β-adrenergic blockers (eg, carvedilol, metoprolol succinate, bisoprolol), diuretics, aldosterone antagonists, nitrates, digoxin, nitrates & hydralazine in combination, transplant, coronary revascularization, left ventricular aneurysmectomy (surgical ventricular remodeling), cardiac resynchronization therapy, cardiac defibrillator
Hypertrophic cardiomyopathy	β-Adrenergic blockers, verapamil, disopyramide, surgical myectomy, septal alcohol ablation, dual-chamber pacing
Restrictive cardiomyopathy	Diuretics, heart transplant, treatment of underlying systemic disease
Pericardial	
Tamponade	Pericardiocentesis
Constrictive pericarditis	Pericardiectomy
Valvular	Valve repair or replacement
Hypertension	Antihypertensive treatment
Pulmonary hypertension	Prostacyclin infusion, calcium channel blockers, heart-lung transplant, endothelin antagonists, phosphodiesterase type 5 inhibitor
High output	
Hyperthyroidism, Paget disease, arteriovenous fistula	Correction of underlying cause

Transferrin levels should be measured to screen for hemochromatosis. The serum angiotensin-converting enzyme level should be measured if sarcoidosis is a possibility. The metanephrine level should be measured if there is a history of severe labile hypertension or unusual spells. A history of ethanol or drug abuse must be sought.

In severe coronary artery disease, reversible left ventricular dysfunction can be caused by hibernating myocardium. However, with revascularization, left ventricular function may improve gradually. Identifying affected patients is difficult. Currently, the reference standard is positron emission tomography, which can show metabolic activity. Viability protocols used in stress echocardiography and radionuclide perfusion imaging are more widely available than positron emission tomography and are also useful for identifying hibernating myocardium.

Tachycardia-induced cardiomyopathy can occur in patients with prolonged periods of tachycardia (usually atrial fibrillation, flutter, or incessant atrial tachycardia). This is an important cause to establish because systolic dysfunction can be completely reversed after the tachycardia is treated.

* After depressed left ventricular function is diagnosed, treatable causes of reversible left ventricular dysfunction should be sought.
* Blood tests should be performed for thyroid dysfunction, sarcoidosis, and hemochromatosis, which are reversible causes of cardiomyopathy.
* Hibernating myocardium is a reversible cause of left ventricular dysfunction. Viability protocols by positron emission tomography, echocardiography, or nuclear scintigraphy can be used to make this diagnosis.
* Tachycardia-induced cardiomyopathy is reversible.

Some patients have left ventricular dysfunction caused by acute myocarditis. The natural history of these patients is unknown. Many patients have development of permanent left ventricular dysfunction, whereas others experience improvement with time. Thus, it is necessary to remeasure left ventricular function 3 to 6 months after making the diagnosis and initiating treatment. Although endomyocardial biopsy may help diagnose myocarditis, immunosuppressive therapy has not been shown to improve outcome and should be reserved for

Table 3-36 Precipitating Factors in Heart Failure

Diet (excessive sodium or fluid intake, alcohol)
Noncompliance with medication or inadequate dosing
Sodium-retaining medications (NSAIDs)
Infection (bacterial or viral)
Myocardial ischemia or infarction
Arrhythmia (atrial fibrillation, bradycardia)
Breathing disorders of sleep
Worsening renal function
Anemia
Metabolic (hyperthyroidism, hypothyroidism)
Pulmonary embolus

Abbreviation: NSAIDs, nonsteroidal anti-inflammatory drugs.

Table 3-37 Anatomical and Pathophysiologic Processes for Each Cardiomyopathy

Type	Left Ventricular Cavity Size	Left Ventricular Wall Thickness	Systolic Function	Diastolic Function	Other
Dilated cardiomyopathy	↑	N/↑	↓	↓	
Hypertrophic cardiomyopathy	↓/N	↑	↑	↓	Left ventricular outflow obstruction
Restrictive cardiomyopathy	N/↑	N	N	↓	

Abbreviation and symbols: ↓, decreased; N, normal; ↑, increased.

patients with giant cell myocarditis, concomitant skeletal myositis, or clinical deterioration despite standard pharmacologic therapy.

Pathophysiology

For understanding the treatment of heart failure associated with dilated cardiomyopathy, the hemodynamic, pathophysiologic, and biologic aspects of heart failure must be appreciated.

Preload can be thought of as the ventricular end-diastolic volume. The relationship of stroke volume to preload is shown on the Starling curve in Figure 3-46. *Afterload* is the tension, force, or stress acting on the fibers of the ventricular wall after the onset of shortening. Left ventricular afterload is increased by aortic stenosis and systemic hypertension but is decreased by mitral regurgitation. Importantly,

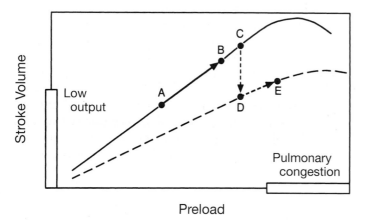

Figure 3-46. Starling Curve. Solid line is patient with normal contractility, and dotted line is one with depressed systolic function. Normally, stroke volume depends on preload of the heart. Increasing preload increases stroke volume (A to B). Myocardial dysfunction causes a shift of the curve downward and to the right (C to D), causing a severe decrease in stroke volume, which leads to symptoms of fatigue and lethargy. The compensatory response to decrease in stroke volume is an increase in preload (D to E). Because the diastolic pressure-volume relationship is curvilinear, increased left ventricular volume produces increased left ventricular end-diastolic pressure, causing symptoms of pulmonary congestion. Note flat portion of the curve at its upper end; here, there is little increase in stroke volume for increase in preload.

afterload is increased by ventricular enlargement and therefore the compensatory preload adjustment to contractile dysfunction (ie, cardiac enlargement) has a putative effect on stroke volume through its effects on afterload.

Figure 3-47 illustrates the neurohormonal hemodynamic response to decreased myocardial contractility. Decreased cardiac output activates baroreceptors and the sympathetic nervous system. Sympathetic nervous system stimulation causes an increased heart rate and contractility. α-Stimulation of the arterioles causes an increase in afterload. The renin-angiotensin system is activated by sympathetic stimulation, decreased renal blood flow, and decreased renal sodium. This system in turn activates aldosterone, causing increased renal retention of sodium and, thus, more pulmonary congestion. A low rate of renal blood flow results in renal retention of sodium. An increased level of angiotensin II causes vasoconstriction and an increase in afterload. In congestive heart failure, the compensatory mechanisms that increase preload eventually cause a malcompensatory increase in afterload, in turn causing further decrease in stroke volume.

Importantly, in the subacute and chronic stages of heart failure, neurohormonal (adrenergic, angiotensin II) and other signaling pathways lead to altered myocyte gene expression, impaired myocyte function, and progressive myocyte loss. Increased collagen production leads to progressive cardiac fibrosis. These structural changes are in addition to the hemodynamic effects of the same neurohormonal activation. This progressive myocardial dysfunction and remodeling are the natural history of untreated myocardial dysfunction.

- Within physiologic limits, an increase in preload causes an increase in stroke volume.
- An increase in afterload (which can result from hypertension, aortic valve stenosis, or increased left ventricular mass) decreases stroke volume.
- Either an increase in afterload or a decrease in myocardial contractility can shift the Starling curve downward and to the right.
- Initial compensatory neurohormonal mechanisms lead to long-term malcompensatory increase in afterload, with a further decrease in stroke volume.
- Neurohormonal activation modifies myocyte function with ultimate myocyte death and also increases myocardial fibrosis. This is known as remodeling.

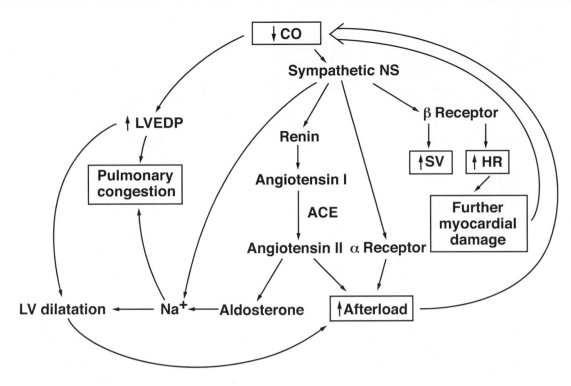

Figure 3-47. Neurohormonal Response to Decreased Myocardial Contractility. ACE indicates angiotensin-converting enzyme; CO, cardiac output; HR, heart rate; LV, left ventricular; LVEDP, left ventricular end-diastolic pressure; NS, nervous system; SV, stroke volume.

Treatment

In the treatment of dilated cardiomyopathy, it is important to identify and remove precipitating factors. Treatment of congestive heart failure in patients with dilated cardiomyopathy should be based on the pathophysiologic mechanisms described above (Figure 3-48).

Nonpharmacologic treatment is crucial to patient management. It includes sodium and fluid restriction, avoidance of alcohol, daily patient monitoring of weight (with a definition of, and plan for responding to, excessive gain), and regular aerobic exercise. Ongoing patient and family education and regular outpatient follow-up (often with nurse specialists) reduce heart failure exacerbations, emergency department visits, and hospitalizations.

The mainstays of pharmacologic therapy are angiotensin-converting enzyme (ACE) inhibitors, β-adrenergic blockers, and diuretics. By blocking conversion of angiotensin I to angiotensin II, ACE inhibitors decrease afterload by inhibition of angiotensin II and decrease sodium retention by inhibition of aldosterone. ACE inhibitors also directly affect myocyte gene expression, growth, and remodeling in a positive manner through the suppression of angiotensin and also by increasing bradykinin and vascular nitric oxide (Figure 3-49).

Overall, ACE inhibitors provide symptomatic improvement in patients with NYHA functional class II-IV failure and improve mortality in patients with moderate and severe heart failure. In asymptomatic patients, ACE inhibitors prevent onset of heart failure and reduce the need for hospitalization.

- ACE inhibitors decrease afterload, decrease sodium retention, and directly reduce adverse biologic effects on myocytes.

- ACE inhibitor use decreases mortality in patients with moderate and severe heart failure.
- ACE inhibitors provide symptomatic improvement in patients with NYHA class II-IV heart failure symptoms.
- In asymptomatic patients, ACE inhibitors reduce the incidence of heart failure and reduce the need for hospitalization.

ACE inhibitors are given initially in small doses because of possible hypotensive effects. Dosage should be titrated up as tolerated on the basis of symptoms and blood pressure, potassium, and creatinine measurements. Even if a patient is clinically compensated on a low or intermediate ACE inhibitor dose, upward dose adjustment as tolerated is beneficial. For optimal ACE inhibitor doses to be achieved, the diuretic dose may need to be reduced. Common side effects of ACE inhibitors include hypotension, hyperkalemia, azotemia, cough, angioedema (mild or severe), and dysgeusia. The benefits and potential side effects of ACE inhibitors are thought to be a class effect.

- ACE inhibitor doses are initially low but should be titrated upward; concomitant diuretic dose may need reduction.
- ACE inhibitor side effects: hypotension, hyperkalemia, azotemia, cough, angioedema, and dysgeusia.

Angiotensin II receptor blockers provide hemodynamic benefits similar to those of ACE inhibitors in patients with dilated cardiomyopathy. They cause less cough and angioedema than ACE inhibitors and should be tried in patients who cannot tolerate ACE inhibitors because of these bradykinin-mediated side effects. Because

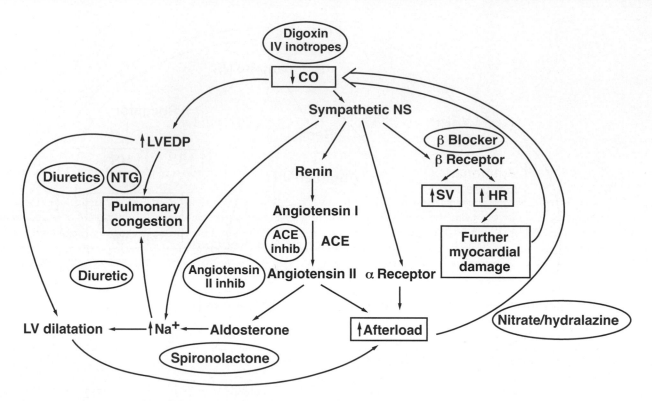

Figure 3-48. Effect of Drugs Used to Treat Heart Failure in Patients With Dilated Cardiomyopathy. inhib indicates inhibitor; IV, intravenous; NTG, nitroglycerin. Other abbreviations as in Figure 3-47.

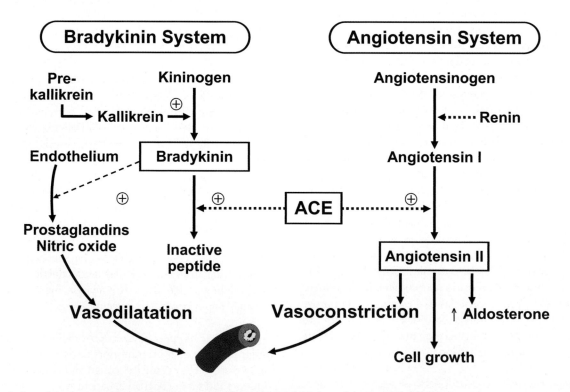

Figure 3-49. Action of Angiotensin-Converting Enzyme (ACE) on the Bradykinin and Angiotensin Systems.

they provide less reverse remodeling than ACE inhibitors, they remain second-line treatment, to be reserved for patients who cannot tolerate ACE inhibitors.

β-Adrenergic blockers (β-blockers) are effective adjuncts to ACE inhibitor therapy in patients with dilated cardiomyopathy; they improve symptoms, reverse remodeling of ventricles with improvement in ejection fraction, and decrease hospitalizations and mortality. Although acutely they may have unwanted hemodynamic effects (negatively inotropic, attenuation of heart rate response that may be maintaining cardiac output in the setting of reduced stroke volume), they provide long-term (may take up to 6 months) benefit by modifying the unfavorable biologic effects of enhanced adrenergic tone. These drugs are most useful for patients with asymptomatic left ventricular dysfunction and NYHA class II or III symptoms. They can be given cautiously to patients with class IV symptoms who have mild volume overload but should not be given to patients with more significant volume overload or cardiogenic shock. Initial dosing should be low, clinical follow-up should be close, and upward titration of the β-blocker dose should be slow and cautious. Well-studied β-blockers with established benefit for patients with heart failure include metoprolol succinate, carvedilol, and bisoprolol (although only metoprolol succinate and carvedilol currently have the approval of the US Food and Drug Administration for the treatment of heart failure). The benefits of β-blocking agents are not necessarily class effects.

* β-Blockers have been shown to be effective as adjunctive therapy to ACE inhibitors in patients with dilated cardiomyopathy.
* β-Blockers have a long-term beneficial effect on ventricular function and slow or reverse pathologic remodeling in dilated cardiomyopathy.
* β-Blockers need to be given carefully to avoid left ventricular decompensation.
* β-Blocker therapy is contraindicated in severely decompensated heart failure, especially when there is significant volume overload.

Diuretics are part of the routine management of patients with heart failure and either symptoms of pulmonary congestion or physical or radiographic evidence of fluid overload. Diuretic doses should be minimized because regular diuretic use causes neurohormonal activation and electrolyte imbalances. Mild fluid overload is initially treated with thiazide diuretics if renal function is normal. Loop diuretics are needed if there is significant fluid overload, renal dysfunction, or fluid overload resistant to thiazides. Occasionally, a combination of thiazides and loop diuretics is needed for severe fluid retention. The addition of spironolactone can help in patients with hypokalemia and may provide additional benefit by blocking aldosterone-mediated effects, as described below.

* Diuretics should be used for patients with heart failure and volume overload.
* Diuretic dose should be minimized so the renin-angiotensin-aldosterone system is not unnecessarily stimulated and to minimize unwanted metabolic side effects.

Drugs that directly affect contractility include digoxin and phosphodiesterase inhibitors (milrinone and amrinone). Digoxin provides symptomatic relief when the ejection fraction is less than 40%, but it does not improve survival. Because digoxin trials included few patients receiving β-blockers, it is not clear whether its benefit is maintained in the setting of contemporary therapy. Because digoxin is excreted by the kidneys, its dosage needs to be decreased with increased levels of creatinine and in older patients. The typical dosage is 0.25 mg/day but should be decreased to 0.125 mg/day if creatinine clearance is less than 70 mL/min. In patients with chronic renal failure, the digoxin dose is adjusted on the basis of trough digoxin levels and is ideally around 1 ng/dL. Because of drug-drug interactions, digoxin dosage should be decreased with concomitant administration of amiodarone, verapamil, and quinidine. Although short-term parenteral inotropic agents (milrinone and amrinone) may improve symptoms, long-term use increases mortality, and therefore these drugs should be used transiently and only in severe cases of congestive heart failure.

* Digoxin and phosphodiesterase inhibitors (milrinone and amrinone) directly affect contractility.
* Digoxin dosage needs to be decreased in azotemic and older patients and should be guided by trough digoxin levels.
* Digoxin dosage should be decreased with concomitant administration of amiodarone, verapamil, and quinidine.

Aldosterone antagonists may have added benefits mediated through inhibition of fibrosis and combating mechanical and electrical remodeling. A large study of spironolactone showed significant survival benefit in patients with NYHA class III and IV heart failure. There was little use of β-blocker therapy in these patients. In another study using selective aldosterone inhibitor, eplerenone was given to patients who had had infarction, left ventricular dysfunction, and either heart failure or diabetes; they had survival benefit at 30 days and 1 year. Both studies excluded patients with baseline renal failure and hyperkalemia; use of potassium supplements and potassium-sparing diuretics was discontinued. Nevertheless, there was still significant risk of hyperkalemia. Thus, these drugs need to be given carefully with cautious follow-up of laboratory values, avoidance of nonsteroidal anti-inflammatory drugs, and prompt attention to illnesses predisposing patients to dehydration.

* Aldosterone antagonists can be used in highly symptomatic patients already receiving baseline therapy or in patients with either heart failure or diabetes early after infarction.
* Patients with hyperkalemia or renal dysfunction should not receive these drugs.
* Patients treated with aldosterone antagonists need very careful laboratory follow-up.

Angiotensin receptor blockers can be used in combination with ACE inhibitor and β-blocker therapy in an effort to more completely block the renin-angiotensin-aldosterone pathway. This approach has been shown to reduce the combined end point of death and hospitalization for heart failure. Electrolyte disturbances and hypotension are more common with this approach, and it is not considered standard therapy. Routine use of combined therapy with ACE inhibitors, angiotensin receptor blockers, and aldosterone antagonists should be avoided.

Nitrates reduce preload and afterload through venodilatation. They also are anti-ischemic agents, may improve endothelial function, and combat ventricular remodeling. They should be given with a nitrate-free interval to prevent nitrate tolerance. Hydralazine may potentiate nitrate therapy by reducing nitrate tolerance when they are used in combination.

The combination of high-dose nitrates and hydralazine provides symptomatic improvement and improved mortality in patients with heart failure. However, the rate of intolerance to the necessary doses of medications is high, and their demonstrated mortality benefit is less than that achieved with ACE inhibitors. They are used in patients unable to tolerate ACE inhibitors or angiotensin receptor blockers. They have also been shown to benefit African-American patients when given as adjuvant therapy to ACE inhibitors and β-blockers.

- Diuretics and nitrates reduce pulmonary congestion.
- Nitrates reduce preload and afterload.
- Nitrate tolerance is best avoided by providing a nitrate-free interval.
- The combination of nitrates and hydralazine improves symptoms and mortality.

A 48-hour infusion of dobutamine may give symptomatic relief, but the effect is often temporary and mortality may be increased. Milrinone also may be used in this fashion and is preferred over dobutamine in patients who are chronically receiving β-blockers. Those therapies are reserved for severely symptomatic patients who are unresponsive to other therapies; they may receive continuous outpatient infusions.

Amlodipine and felodipine are safe in patients with dilated cardiomyopathy but do not provide any survival benefit. First-generation calcium channel blockers (verapamil, diltiazem, nifedipine), however, are relatively contraindicated because of their negative inotropic effects.

Anticoagulation with warfarin is recommended for patients in atrial fibrillation and those with intracardiac thrombus or a history of systemic or pulmonary thromboembolism. In 2 prospective studies, prophylactic warfarin use was not shown to decrease the composite end point of death, nonfatal stroke, or infarction when given to patients with dilated cardiomyopathy. Retrospective studies have suggested that aspirin may diminish the benefits of ACE inhibitors by blocking prostaglandin-induced vasodilatation. In addition, these studies showed an increased incidence of hospitalizations for heart failure in patients with dilated cardiomyopathy receiving aspirin. Accordingly, most advise aspirin use in small doses only in patients with coronary artery disease. Alternatively, clopidogrel may be given.

- Anticoagulation with warfarin is recommended in patients with atrial fibrillation, intracardiac thrombus, or a history of thromboembolism.
- Aspirin therapy should be reserved for patients with coronary artery disease.

Recapitulation of Drug Therapy for Dilated Cardiomyopathy

- ACE inhibitors and β-blockers improve symptoms and decrease mortality in patients with symptomatic dilated cardiomyopathy.
- ACE inhibitors and β-blockers prevent deterioration and subsequent hospitalizations in patients with asymptomatic dilated cardiomyopathy.
- Angiotensin receptor blockers can be used in patients intolerant of ACE inhibitors. There use in addition to ACE inhibitor and β-blocker therapy is less well established.
- Aldosterone antagonists have shown survival benefit in certain subgroups of patients with dilated cardiomyopathy but should not be used when hyperkalemia or renal failure is present.
- The combination of high-dose nitrates and hydralazine improves symptoms and survival (although the survival benefit is less than with ACE inhibitors), but intolerance to the high doses limits their usefulness.
- Nitrates should be used with a nitrate-free interval to prevent nitrate tolerance.
- Digoxin is useful for symptomatic treatment of patients with dilated cardiomyopathy but provides no survival benefit, and its role in patients receiving β-blockers is undefined.
- Phosphodiesterase inhibitors and prolonged infusion of dobutamine directly increase contractility and may improve symptoms transiently, but probably increase mortality.

Device Therapy

Implanted defibrillators improve survival as primary prevention in patients with ischemic and nonischemic dilated cardiomyopathies who have ejection fractions less than 30%. They should be offered to patients whose 1-year survival is not otherwise threatened. Patients should be thoroughly counseled about the role of these devices relative to survival and heart failure symptoms.

Patients with ventricular asynchrony may benefit from biventricular pacing, also known as cardiac resynchronization therapy. Current implantation criteria are sinus rhythm, QRS duration more than 120 milliseconds, NYHA class III-IV, ejection fraction less than 35%, and optimal medical management. Cardiac resynchronization therapy results in improvement in approximately 70% of patients.

- Patients receiving optimal medical management who have persistent qualifying degrees of left ventricular dysfunction should be considered for cardiac defibrillator or cardiac resynchronization therapy if they meet other selection criteria.

Cardiac Replacement Therapy

Heart transplantation is the procedure of choice for patients with severe dilated cardiomyopathy and severe symptoms. With successful transplantation, the 1-year survival is 90%. The major contraindication for transplantation in an otherwise healthy patient is a high pulmonary arteriolar resistance. Long-term complications after heart transplantation include rejection, infection, hypertension, hyperlipidemia, malignancy, and accelerated coronary vasculopathy.

In the United States, donor availability is the major limiting factor; in selected patients, left ventricular assist devices are used either as a bridge to transplantation or as final ("destination") therapy.

- The procedure of choice for patients with severely symptomatic dilated cardiomyopathy despite optimal medical management is heart transplantation. With successful transplantation, 1-year survival is 90%.
- Ventricular assist devices are an option for selected patients either as a bridge to transplantation or as destination therapy.

Heart Failure With Preserved Ejection Fraction

Approximately half of patients with a new diagnosis of heart failure have a normal ejection fraction. In addition, roughly half of US hospital admissions for acute decompensated heart failure are in patients with an ejection fraction of more than 40%. Although many, if not all, of these patients have contractile abnormalities that could be identified by more sophisticated evaluation techniques, the ejection fraction is the most widely available measure of systolic function and remains the standard in daily practice. This is a heterogeneous group and includes patients with hypertrophic and restrictive cardiomyopathies, infiltrative cardiac disorders, and constrictive pericarditis; all of these are further discussed below.

The remaining patients have some other form of diastolic dysfunction. Some patients have fairly normal diastolic filling properties at rest, but exertional hypertension or ischemia or both cause their diastolic filling properties to deteriorate (or at least the relaxation does not augment) with resultant increase in filling pressure. Others have abnormal baseline diastolic compliance with superimposed volume overload, which increases the diastolic filling pressures. Others have exhuberant heart rate responses to exercise with inadequate diastolic filling periods, and others rely on the atrial contribution to ventricular filling and suffer when atrial fibrillation develops. Some have low output due to severe regurgitant valve disease (including severe tricuspid regurgitation) or bradycardia. Severe occult renal insufficiency is also a common finding in this condition. Thus, it is highly desirable to try to understand the mechanism of diastolic dysfunction in any given patient in an effort to tailor the most effective treatment, which might include some combination of hypertension or ischemia treatment, diuretic treatment, ventricular rate slowing or support (pacemaker), restoration of sinus rhythm, valvular intervention, or renal replacement therapy.

- Heart failure with preserved ejection fraction represents a heterogeneous group of problems.
- There is not a standard therapy for heart failure with preserved ejection fraction; ideally, a tailored approach is applied.

Hypertrophic Cardiomyopathy

Etiology

Hypertrophic cardiomyopathy is a genetically and phenotypically heterogeneous family of disorders characterized by defects involving myocyte proteins with hypertrophy as a compensatory response. There may or may not be obstruction in the left ventricular outflow tract or mid-ventricular cavity. The diagnosis currently is based on the echocardiographic finding of increased myocardial wall thickness in the absence of an underlying cause such as hypertension, aortic stenosis, chronic renal failure, or infiltrative disease. Because hypertrophic cardiomyopathy is a hereditary disease, all patients should have their first-degree relatives screened, and genetic counseling is advised for potential parents.

- Hypertrophic cardiomyopathy is a heterogeneous family of genetic disorders of myocyte proteins with compensatory myocardial hypertrophy.
- Dynamic left ventricular outflow tract or mid-cavity obstruction occurs in some, but not all, patients.
- Diagnosis is based on the echocardiographic finding of increased myocardial wall thickness in the absence of a cause.
- Family screening and genetic counseling are advised.

Symptoms

Hypertrophic cardiomyopathy has several different manifestations. There appears to be a bimodal distribution of age at presentation. Young males (usually in the teens or early 20s) have a high propensity for syncope and sudden death. Older patients (in their 50s and 60s) present with symptoms of shortness of breath and angina and may have a better prognosis than young patients. The classic presentation of the younger group is a young athlete undergoing a physical examination to participate in sports who is found to have a heart murmur or left ventricular hypertrophy on ECG. The classic presentation of the older group is an older woman in whom pulmonary edema develops after noncardiac surgery and whose condition worsens with diuresis, afterload reduction, and inotropic support (all of which worsen dynamic left ventricular outflow tract obstruction). The classic symptom triad is syncope, angina, and dyspnea (symptoms similar to those of valvular aortic stenosis). Some hypertensive patients have a small hyperdynamic left ventricle with hypertrophy and dynamic left ventricular outflow tract obstruction—hypertensive hypertrophic cardiomyopathy. Although the pathophysiology is the same as in hypertrophic cardiomyopathy, these patients are not at increased risk for sudden death and ventricular fibrillation.

There is a 1.5% per year frequency of evolution from hypertrophic to dilated cardiomyopathy. This may reflect either the natural history or a superimposed secondary process such as ischemia. The treatment of a "burnt-out hypertroph" is then the same as that for other dilated cardiomyopathies.

- The classic presentation of hypertrophic cardiomyopathy is the triad of angina, syncope, and dyspnea.
- There is a bimodal distribution of presentation: young males with high incidence of sudden death and older patients with dyspnea and angina.
- The prognosis for older patients may be better than that for younger patients.
- Patients with hypertension may have hypertrophy and dynamic left ventricular outflow tract obstruction similar to those of patients with hypertrophic cardiomyopathy.

Pathophysiology

Signs and symptoms of hypertrophic cardiomyopathy are caused by 4 major abnormalities: diastolic dysfunction, left ventricular outflow tract obstruction, mitral regurgitation, and ventricular arrhythmias.

Diastolic dysfunction is caused by many mechanisms. Marked abnormality in calcium metabolism causes abnormal ventricular relaxation. High afterload due to left ventricular tract obstruction also delays ventricular relaxation. Severe hypertrophy and increased muscle mass produce decreased compliance so that there is increased pressure per unit volume entering the left ventricle during diastole. These combine to cause increased left ventricular diastolic pressure, which leads to angina and dyspnea.

In many patients, dynamic left ventricular tract obstruction is caused by the hypertrophied septum encroaching into the left ventricular outflow tract. This subsequently "sucks in" the anterior leaflet of the mitral valve (systolic anterior motion), creating left ventricular outflow tract obstruction. Because of this pathophysiologic process, dynamic outflow tract obstruction increases dramatically with decreased preload, decreased afterload, or increased contractility.

Systolic anterior motion of the mitral valve distorts the mitral valve apparatus during systole and may cause significant mitral regurgitation. Thus, the degree of mitral regurgitation is also dynamically influenced by the degree of left ventricular outflow tract obstruction. Patients with severe mitral regurgitation usually have severe symptoms of dyspnea.

Because of cellular disarray in patients with hypertrophic cardiomyopathy, the electrical conduction system is dispersed, leading to a high propensity for ventricular arrhythmias. The frequent occurrence of ventricular arrhythmias may cause sudden death or syncope.

* A major pathophysiologic abnormality in patients with hypertrophic cardiomyopathy is diastolic dysfunction.
* Left ventricular outflow tract obstruction and mitral regurgitation are caused by distortion of the mitral valve apparatus (systolic anterior motion), and they are dynamically influenced by preload, afterload, and contractility.
* The propensity for ventricular arrhythmias causing syncope and sudden death is high.

Examination

Hypertrophic cardiomyopathy is suspected on the basis of abnormal carotid artery upstroke and left ventricular impulse. The carotid artery upstroke is rapid compared with that of patients with aortic stenosis. If left ventricular outflow tract obstruction is extensive, the carotid artery upstroke has a bifid quality. The left ventricular impulse is sustained, indicating considerable left ventricular hypertrophy. It frequently has a palpable *a* wave. Patients with excessive left ventricular outflow tract obstruction may have a triple apical impulse. The first heart sound is normal, and the second heart sound is paradoxically split. A loud systolic ejection murmur indicates left ventricular outflow tract obstruction. The murmur changes in intensity with changes in loading conditions (Table 3-38). A holosystolic murmur of mitral regurgitation may be present; it increases in intensity with increases in the dynamic left ventricular outflow tract obstruction. Maneuvers affect the mitral regurgitant murmur of hypertrophic

obstructive cardiomyopathy differently than other mitral regurgitant murmurs. When mitral regurgitation is not due to hypertrophic obstructive cardiomyopathy, it increases with increasing afterload and varies little with changes in contractility and preload. When mitral regurgitation is due to hypertrophic cardiomyopathy, however, increased afterload decreases the dynamic left ventricular outflow obstruction and thus the amount of secondary mitral regurgitation.

In patients with hypertrophic obstructive cardiomyopathy, the intensity of the ejection murmur increases, whereas the arterial pulse volume decreases on the beat following a premature ventricular contraction. This is called the Brockenbrough sign, and it is due to post-ectopic increased contractility and decreased afterload, resulting in more dynamic obstruction. In contradistinction, in patients with fixed left ventricular outflow tract obstruction (eg, aortic stenosis), both the murmur intensity and the pulse volume increase with the beat following a premature contraction.

* The diagnosis of hypertrophic cardiomyopathy is suspected by palpating a sustained left ventricular impulse and rapid upstroke of the carotid artery.
* The outflow murmur intensity and carotid upstroke change with changes in loading conditions of the heart.
* In hypertrophic obstructive cardiomyopathy, the secondary mitral regurgitation murmur changes in the same direction as that of the left ventricular outflow obstruction murmur under different loading conditions. This differs from the auscultatory findings when mitral regurgitation is due to other conditions.

Table 3-38 Dynamic Left Ventricular Outflow Tract Obstruction

Increased obstruction
Decreased afterload
Amyl nitrite
Vasodilators
Increased contractility
Postpremature ventricular contraction beat
Digoxin
Dopamine
Decreased preload
Squat-to-stand
Nitrates
Diuretics
Valsalva maneuver (strain phase)
Decreased obstruction
Increased afterload
Handgrip
Stand-to-squat
Decreased contractility
β-Adrenergic blockers
Verapamil
Disopyramide
Increased preload
Fluids

Diagnostic Testing

Patients with hypertrophic cardiomyopathy usually have an abnormal ECG, which shows considerable left ventricular hypertrophy (Figure 3-50). Because ECG abnormalities may precede echocardiographically detected phenotypic expression, surveillance echocardiography is appropriate in patients with suspicious ECG results. Apical hypertrophic cardiomyopathy is a variant of hypertrophic cardiomyopathy in which the hypertrophy is localized at the apex of the left ventricle. Although patients with apical hypertrophic cardiomyopathy do not have outflow tract obstruction (no murmur or secondary mitral regurgitation), they do have diastolic dysfunction and a predisposition to ventricular arrhythmias. The ECG in these patients typically has large, diffuse, symmetric T-wave inversions across the precordium (Figure 3-51).

Hypertrophic cardiomyopathy is diagnosed with echocardiography, which shows severe hypertrophy of the myocardium (left ventricular wall thickness >16 mm in diastole) without any known cause. Formerly, asymmetric septal hypertrophy was required for the diagnosis, but it is now recognized that hypertrophy can be in any part of the myocardium. Doppler echocardiography can be used to diagnose left ventricular outflow tract obstruction, measure its severity, and detect mitral regurgitation. Cardiac catheterization is no longer necessary for diagnosing dynamic left ventricular outflow tract obstruction because all diagnostic data can be obtained with 2-dimensional and Doppler echocardiography.

Sudden death is a problem in patients with hypertrophic cardiomyopathy. Because of a strong association between ventricular arrhythmias and sudden death, 48- to 72-hour Holter monitoring is recommended for all patients with hypertrophic cardiomyopathy.

Predictors of sudden death include a personal or family history of sudden death, left ventricular hypertrophy, ventricular tachycardia at electrophysiologic study, young male, history of syncope, and non-sustained ventricular tachycardia. Genetic markers may identify patients with a strong propensity for sudden death. In some patients, carefully supervised stress testing also is indicated to search for ventricular tachycardia, to objectify symptom threshold, and to evaluate the variables contributing to symptoms.

* ECG usually shows evidence of left ventricular hypertrophy in cases of hypertrophic cardiomyopathy.
* Apical hypertrophy is suspected in the presence of large, symmetric, inverted T waves in precordial leads on ECG.
* The diagnosis of hypertrophic cardiomyopathy is made with echocardiography, which shows hypertrophy in the absence of any known cause.
* Predictors of sudden death: personal or family history of sudden death, young male, history of syncope, nonsustained ventricular tachycardia, massive left ventricular hypertrophy, and sustained ventricular tachycardia at electrophysiologic study.
* 48- to 72-Hour Holter monitoring is recommended for all patients with hypertrophic cardiomyopathy.

Treatment

Symptomatic Patients

For symptomatic patients with hypertrophic cardiomyopathy, initial treatment is with drugs that decrease contractility in an attempt to decrease left ventricular outflow tract obstruction (Figure 3-52). The

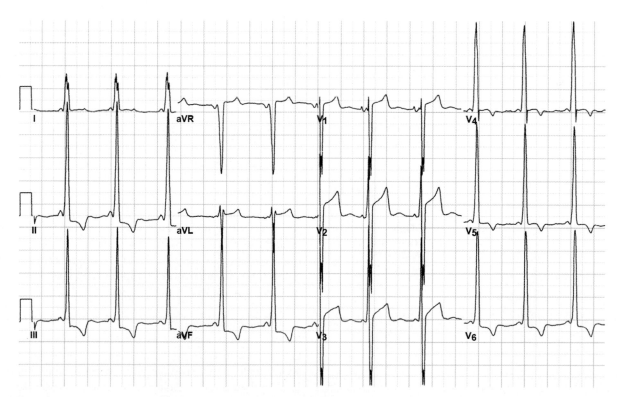

Figure 3-50. Electrocardiogram in hypertrophic cardiomyopathy, showing marked left ventricular hypertrophy.

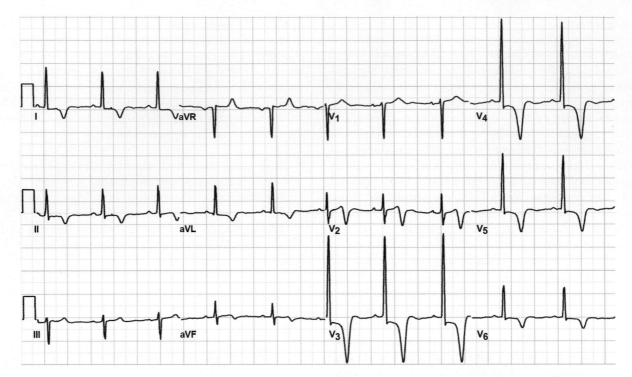

Figure 3-51. Electrocardiogram in apical hypertrophic cardiomyopathy with deep, symmetric T-wave inversions in precordial leads.

most effective medication is a high dose of β-blockers (>240 mg equivalent of propranolol/day). Although verapamil may be used if β-adrenergic blockade fails, it may cause sudden hemodynamic deterioration in patients with high resting left ventricular outflow tract gradients because of its vasodilating properties. Disopyramide may improve symptoms by decreasing left ventricular outflow tract obstruction, but anticholinergic side effects limit its use. All drugs

that reduce afterload or preload and those that increase contractility must be avoided in patients with hypertrophic cardiomyopathy. Cautious diuretic use for volume-overloaded states is permitted.

Septal reduction therapy (either surgical myectomy or alcohol septal ablation) is reserved for patients who are severely symptomatic despite optimal medical therapy and produces dramatic symptomatic relief. Mortality associated with surgical myectomy is less than 5% overall in experienced centers and less than 1% in patients younger than 40 years. Its complications are rare but include complete heart block, aortic regurgitation, and ventricular septal defect. Myectomy is a highly operator-dependent procedure and should be performed only at medical centers that specialize in this procedure. Alcohol septal ablation complications include complete heart block and ventricular arrhythmias. The long-term outcome of this procedure is unknown.

Dual-chamber pacing is an alternative to septal reduction therapy for occasional patients with hypertrophic cardiomyopathy and severe left ventricular outflow tract obstruction. Dual-chamber pacing can produce a reduction in gradient and symptomatic improvement in some patients, but this approach is not recommended for all patients with symptomatic hypertrophic obstructive cardiomyopathy.

Asymptomatic Patients
Whether to treat asymptomatic patients with nonsustained ventricular tachycardia is controversial (Figure 3-53). No antiarrhythmic agent is uniformly effective, and any may make the arrhythmia worse. In selected patients with multiple risk factors for sudden death, empiric amiodarone or an automatic implantable cardiac defibrillator

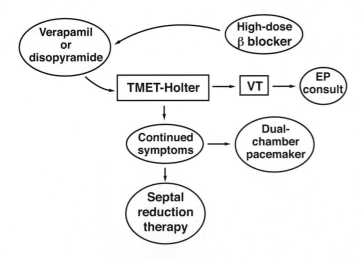

Figure 3-52. Treatment of Symptomatic Patients with Hypertrophic Cardiomyopathy. EP indicates electrophysiologic; TMET, treadmill exercise test; VT, ventricular tachycardia.

might be chosen. In patients who have already had an out-of-hospital arrest, the treatment of choice is an automatic implantable cardiac defibrillator.

- β-Blockade is the treatment of choice for patients with symptomatic hypertrophic cardiomyopathy.
- Verapamil may cause sudden hemodynamic deterioration in patients with high resting left ventricular outflow tract obstruction because of its vasodilating properties.
- Septal reduction therapy is reserved for severely symptomatic patients unresponsive to medical therapy.
- Dual-chamber pacing is an accepted treatment strategy in rare situations.
- No antiarrhythmic agent is uniformly effective, and any may worsen the arrhythmia.
- Automatic implantable cardiac defibrillator is the treatment of choice for patients with out-of-hospital arrest.

Restrictive Cardiomyopathy

Definition
The primary abnormality in restrictive cardiomyopathy is diastolic dysfunction, usually including abnormal relaxation, high compliance, and ineffectual atrial contribution to filling. Diastolic dysfunction causes abnormal left ventricular filling such that a greater-than-usual increase in filling pressure is required to fill the ventricle. This is reflected back to the pulmonary and systemic circulations, causing symptoms of shortness of breath and edema. In addition, the ventricle cannot fill adequately to meet its preload requirements, thus resulting in low cardiac output (Starling mechanism), fatigue, and lethargy. Normal or near-normal ejection fraction is present in most patients with restrictive cardiomyopathy.

- In restrictive cardiomyopathy, the primary abnormality is diastolic dysfunction.
- Diastolic dysfunction means a greater pressure per unit volume is required to fill the ventricle, causing dyspnea and edema.
- The left ventricle cannot fill to meet its preload requirements, causing low output, fatigue, and lethargy.

The cause of primary restrictive cardiomyopathy is unknown. There are 2 major categories: idiopathic restrictive cardiomyopathy and endomyocardial fibrosis. In idiopathic restrictive cardiomyopathy, there is progressive fibrosis of the myocardium. Familial cases, often with peripheral myopathy as well, have been reported. Endomyocardial fibrosis is probably an end stage of eosinophilic syndromes in which there is intracavitary thrombus filling of the left ventricle. This restricts filling and causes increased diastolic pressures. This fibrosis also may involve the mitral valve, causing severe mitral regurgitation. There may be 2 different forms of endomyocardial fibrosis: active inflammatory eosinophilic myocarditis in temperate zones and chronic endomyocardial fibrosis in tropical zones.

Diseases that cause infiltration of the myocardium (such as amyloidosis) have a presentation and pathophysiology similar to those of primary restrictive cardiomyopathy. Signs and symptoms similar

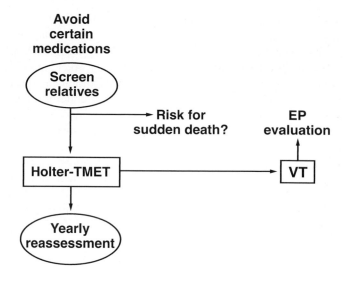

Figure 3-53. Treatment of Asymptomatic Patients With Hypertrophic Cardiomyopathy. Abbreviations as in Figure 3-52.

to those of restrictive cardiomyopathy also may develop after radiation therapy and anthracycline chemotherapy. Although other infiltrative diseases (eg, sarcoidosis, hemochromatosis) initially may mimic restrictive cardiomyopathy, they usually have progressed to a dilated cardiomyopathy by the time they cause cardiac symptoms.

- Restrictive cardiomyopathy may be idiopathic or due to infiltrative diseases (eg, amyloidosis).
- Endomyocardial fibrosis is probably an end stage of eosinophilic syndromes.
- Secondary fibrosis may involve the mitral valve, causing severe mitral regurgitation.

Signs and Symptoms
Patients with restrictive cardiomyopathy usually present with edema, dyspnea, ascites, and low output symptoms. Atrial arrhythmias due to passive atrial enlargement are frequently present, and the patient may present with atrial fibrillation. Jugular venous pressure is almost always increased, with rapid x and y descents. The precordium is quiet, and heart sounds are soft. There may be an apical systolic murmur of mitral regurgitation and a left sternal border murmur of tricuspid regurgitation. A third heart sound may be present. Dullness at the bases of the lungs is consistent with bilateral pleural effusions. ECG is usually low or normal voltage with atrial arrhythmias. Chest radiography shows pleural effusions with normal cardiac silhouette or atrial enlargement.

- Restrictive cardiomyopathy: biventricular failure, dyspnea, edema, and low output symptoms.
- Atrial arrhythmias are frequently present.
- Jugular venous pressure is increased, with rapid x and y descents.

Diagnosis
Restrictive cardiomyopathy is diagnosed with echocardiography. Typical findings are normal left ventricular cavity size and function

and marked enlargement of both atria. If there is right heart failure, the inferior vena cava is enlarged. Echocardiography is usually non-specific about the cause except in 2 instances. First, in amyloid heart disease, echocardiography demonstrates thickened myocardium with a scintillating appearance as well as pericardial effusion and thickened regurgitant valves. Second, in endomyocardial fibrosis, there is an apical thrombus (without underlying apical akinesis) or thickening of the endocardium under the mitral valve, which often tethers the valve, causing mitral regurgitation. Cardiac catheterization shows elevation and end-equalization of all end-diastolic pressures. A typical "square-root sign" or "dip-and-plateau" pattern consistent with early rapid filling is present. Endomyocardial biopsy usually is not helpful unless there is a systemic disease that has caused infiltration of the myocardium (ie, amyloidosis).

- Restrictive cardiomyopathy is diagnosed with echocardiography.
- Typical findings are normal left ventricular cavity size and function and marked enlargement of both atria.
- In amyloid heart disease, thickened myocardium has scintillating appearance, pericardial effusion, and valvular regurgitation.
- In endomyocardial fibrosis, there is thrombus in left ventricular apex (without apical akinesis) or posterior mitral leaflet tethering causing mitral regurgitation.

Treatment

There is no medical treatment for idiopathic restrictive cardiomyopathy. Diuretics decrease filling pressures and give symptomatic relief, but this may be at the expense of further decreasing cardiac output. Digoxin usually is not helpful because systolic contractility is maintained. Heart transplant is the only proven therapy for patients with severe restrictive cardiomyopathy. Corticosteroids and cytotoxic drugs are appropriate during the early stages of eosinophilic endocarditis. Endomyocardial fibrosis can be surgically resected and the mitral valve can be replaced, although mortality is significant.

- There is no medical treatment for idiopathic restrictive cardiomyopathy.
- Diuretics decrease filling pressures.
- Digoxin usually is not helpful.
- Heart transplant is the only proven therapy for severe restrictive cardiomyopathy.
- Medical therapy is used for early stages of eosinophilic endocarditis, and operation is used for endomyocardial fibrosis in selected cases.

It is important to differentiate restrictive cardiomyopathy from constrictive pericarditis. Both have similar presentations and findings on clinical examination and diagnostic studies. However, in constrictive pericarditis, pericardiectomy produces symptomatic improvement and, frequently, survival. Therefore, exploratory thoracotomy may be indicated in patients with normal left ventricular systolic function, large atria, and severe increase of diastolic filling pressures if doubt remains after anatomical (cine computed tomography or magnetic resonance imaging) and other tests (echocardiography, cardiac catheterization).

- It is important to differentiate restrictive cardiomyopathy from constrictive pericarditis.
- In constrictive pericarditis, pericardiectomy produces symptomatic improvement and may prolong survival.

Cardiology Pharmacy Review
Narith N. Ou, PharmD, Jeffrey J. Armon, PharmD

Drugs Commonly Used for Cardiac Resuscitation

Drug	Primary Use	Toxic/Adverse Effects	Comments: Precautions (P) and Contraindications (C)
Adenosine	Narrow complex PSVT	Chest pain, ischemia, bronchoconstriction, increased ICP, VF (infants)	Wide complex tachycardia (P) Drug/poison-induced arrest (C)
Amiodarone	Pulseless VT/VF, stable VT of unknown origin, AF	AV block, hypotension, proarrhythmias	Dose-related hypotension (P) Renal failure (P) Concomitant use of QT-prolonging drugs (eg, procainamide) (P)
Atropine	Sinus bradycardia, type IIa AVB, asystole	Tachyarrhythmias, ischemia	Hypothermic bradycardia (C) Avoid in advanced infranodal (type II) AVB or new 3rd-degree AVB with wide QRS (C)
β-Adrenergic blockers (atenolol, metoprolol, esmolol)	Myocardial infarction, supraventricular tachycardia	Bronchospasm, hypotension, bradycardia, exacerbation of heart failure	Bradycardia (<60 bpm) or 2nd- or 3rd-degree heart block (C) Poison/drug-induced arrest (C) Concomitant calcium channel blocker (P) Severe reactive airway disease (P) Wolff-Parkinson-White syndrome (P)
Calcium channel antagonists (diltiazem, verapamil)	Supraventricular tachycardia	AV block, hypotension, bradycardia, exacerbation of heart failure	Wolff-Parkinson-White syndrome (C) Ventricular arrhythmia (P) Concomitant use of β-blocker (P) Evolving MI (P)
Catecholamines (dobutamine, dopamine, epinephrine, norepinephrine)	Bradycardia, hypotension (except dobutamine), asystole (epinephrine)	Hypertension, tachycardia, ischemia, arrhythmia, hypotension (dobutamine)	Peripheral administration may cause severe extravasation (P) Use only after volume resuscitation (P) SBP <100 mm Hg and signs of shock (dobutamine) (P)
Digoxin	Supraventricular tachycardia	Proarrhythmia	Hypokalemia, hypercalcemia, or hypomagnesemia (C) Concomitant defibrillation (P) Wolff-Parkinson-White syndrome (P) AV block (P)
Lidocaine	Ventricular tachyarrhythmias	Proarrhythmia, seizures, exacerbation of heart failure	Prophylaxis after MI (C) Liver dysfunction or CHF (P) Evolving myocardial ischemia = more proarrhythmic (P)

Cardiology Pharmacy Review (continued)

Drugs Commonly Used for Cardiac Resuscitation (continued)

Drug	Primary Use	Toxic/Adverse Effects	Comments: Precautions (P) and Contraindications (C)
Procainamide	Ventricular & supraventricular tachyarrhythmias	Proarrhythmias (torsades de pointes), hypotension, exacerbation of heart failure	Low magnesium or potassium (P) Evolving myocardial ischemia = more proarrhythmic (P) Hypotension: slow infusion important (P) Polymorphic VT (C)
Vasopressin	Pulseless VT/VF, vasodilatory shock	Bradycardia, ?ischemia	Coronary artery disease (P)

Abbreviations: AF, atrial fibrillation; AV, atrioventricular; AVB, atrioventricular block; bpm, beats/minute; CHF, congestive heart failure; ICP, intracranial pressure; MI, myocardial infarction; PSVT, paroxysmal supraventricular tachycardia; SBP, systolic blood pressure; VF, ventricular fibrillation; VT, ventricular tachycardia.

Cardiology Pharmacy Review (continued)

Drugs Commonly Used in Cardiology

Drug	Toxic/Adverse Effects
Aldosterone antagonists (spironolactone, eplerenone)	Serious hyperkalemia if renally impaired, gynecomastia (less with eplerenone)
Angiotensin-converting enzyme inhibitors	Angioedema, renal failure, hypotension, hyperkalemia, hepatitis, neutropenia, cough, rashes, taste disturbance
Angiotensin II receptor antagonists	Rarely angioedema (<10% cross-reaction if h/o angiotensin-converting enzyme inhibitor angioedema), hepatitis, headache, dizziness, fatigue
β-Adrenergic blockers	Bronchospasm, hypotension, bradycardia, decompensated heart failure, CNS effects (lipophilic agents > nonlipophilic: depression, psychosis, dizziness, weakness, fatigue, vivid dreams, insomnia), GI effects, reduced peripheral vascular perfusion, impotence, hypo-/hyperglycemia
Calcium channel antagonists	Hypotension, bradycardia (verapamil, diltiazem), worsening of heart failure symptoms (verapamil, diltiazem), dizziness, flushing, peripheral edema, constipation, postural hypotension, taste disturbances
Centrally acting agents (clonidine, methyldopa)	Withdrawal hypertension, hypotension, hepatitis (methyldopa), bradycardia (clonidine), frequent CNS effects (depression, sedation), GI effects, sexual dysfunction, xerostomia (clonidine)
Clopidogren (Plavix)	Idiopathic thrombocytopenic purpura (rare), GI effects (loading dose)
Digoxin	Cardiovascular effects (heart block, ectopic arrhythmias, ventricular extra beats, ventricular tachycardia, paroxysmal supraventricular tachycardia), GI effects (anorexia, nausea, vomiting, diarrhea), CNS effects (drowsiness, dizziness, confusion, vision abnormalities, photophobia)
Direct thrombin inhibitors (lepirudin, argatroban, bivalirudin)	Bleeding (no available antidote for reversal), allergic reaction to reexposure & antibody formation (lepirudin)
Fondaparinux (Arixtra)	Bleeding risk in elderly, renal impairment
Hydralazine	Hypotension, hepatitis, neuropathy, flushing, GI effects, LLS
LMWH: (enoxaparin [Lovenox], dalteparin [Fragmin])	Bleeding, heparin-induced thrombocytopenia
Loop diuretics	Dehydration, hypokalemia, hyponatremia, pancreatitis, jaundice, deafness (high dose), thrombocytopenia, serious skin disorders, dizziness, postural hypotension, gout
Nesiritide (Natrecor)	Dose related hypotension, headache, renal impairment, increased mortality
Organic nitrates	Syncope, TIAs, headache, flushing, palpitations, peripheral edema
Potassium-sparing diuretics	Hyperkalemia, dehydration, GI effects (nausea, vomiting, diarrhea), CNS effects (headache, weakness), rashes, gynecomastia in men and breast enlargement/soreness in women (spironolactone)
Ranolazine (Ranexa)	Prolonged QT interval
Thiazide diuretics	Dehydration, rarely thrombocytopenia, cholestatic jaundice, pancreatitis, hepatic encephalopathy (in patients with cirrhosis), dizziness, gout, hyperglycemia, orthostasis, hypokalemia, hypermagnesemia, hypercalcemia, GI effects
Warfarin	Abnormal bleeding, rarely necrosis or gangrene of skin and other tissues, purple toe syndrome (cholesterol microembolization), osteoporosis

Abbreviations: CNS, central nervous system; GI, gastrointestinal tract; h/o, history of; LLS, lupuslike syndrome; LMWH, low-molecular-weight heparin; TIA, transient ischemic attack.

Cardiology Pharmacy Review (continued)

Selected Important Cardiac Drug Interactions

Drug	Drug	Net Effect and Suggested Actions
Amiodarone	Cyclosporine	Amiodarone increases serum cyclosporine Monitor cyclosporine levels
	Digoxin	Amiodarone increases serum digoxin levels Reduce digoxin dose by 25%-50% (monitor digoxin levels)
	Dofetilide	Amiodarone must be withdrawn for at least 3 mo or amiodarone level <0.3 mg/mL before initiating dofetilide therapy
	Fosphenytoin or phenytoin	Phenytoin level can increase × 2-3, amiodarone levels may decrease by >30% Monitor amiodarone effectiveness & phenytoin levels
	Procainamide	Amiodarone increases procainamide level; 20% reduction of procainamide dose is suggested Monitor procainamide levels; combination is rarely used
	Quinidine	Amiodarone increases quinidine levels; 50% reduction of quinidine dose is suggested Monitor quinidine levels; rarely used together
	Simvastatin	Amiodarone increases risk of myopathy or rhabdomyolysis with simvastatin. If >20 mg per day of simvastatin required, different agent is recommended
	Warfarin	Amiodarone increases warfarin effect Decrease warfarin dose by 25%-50%; monitor INR
Digoxin	Amiodarone	Amiodarone increases serum digoxin levels Reduce dose of digoxin by 25%-50% (monitor digoxin levels)
	Propafenone	Propafenone increases digoxin levels Empirically reduce digoxin dose; monitor levels & signs of increased digoxin
	Quinidine	Quinidine may increase digoxin levels Monitor ECG & digoxin levels
	Verapamil	Verapamil increases serum digoxin levels Reduction of digoxin dose may be required; monitor digoxin levels & signs of elevated digoxin
Dofetilide	Amiodarone	Torsades de pointes risk Amiodarone must be withdrawn for at least 3 mo or amiodarone level <0.3 mg/mL before initiating dofetilide therapy
	Cimetidine	Cimetidine is contraindicated because increased serum level of dofetilide = torsades de pointes effect
	Class I & III antiarrhythmic agents	Torsades de pointes risk Washout period of at least 3 half-lives of other antiarrhythmics before starting dofetilide
	Hydrochlorothiazide	Hydrochlorothiazide is contraindicated because increased serum level of dofetilide and decreased potassium = risk of torsades de pointes
	Ketoconazole	Ketoconazole is contraindicated because increased serum level of dofetilide = torsades de pointes effect
	Megestrol	Megestrol is contraindicated because increased serum level of dofetilide = torsades de pointes effect
	Prochlorperazine	Prochlorperazine is contraindicated because increased serum level of dofetilide = torsades de pointes effect
	Trimethoprim	Trimethoprim is contraindicated because increased serum level of dofetilide = torsades de pointes risk

Cardiology Pharmacy Review (continued)

Selected Important Cardiac Drug Interactions (continued)

Drug	Drug	Net effect and suggested actions
Dofetilide (continued)	Trimethoprim-sulfamethoxazole	Trimethoprim-sulfamethoxazole is contraindicated because increased serum level of dofetilide = torsades de pointes risk
	Verapamil	Verapamil is contraindicated because increased serum level of dofetilide = torsades de pointes risk
	Ziprasidone	Ziprasidone is contraindicated because increased serum level of dofetilide = torsades de pointes risk
Propafenone	Digoxin	Propafenone increases digoxin levels
		Empirically reduce digoxin dose; monitor levels & signs of increased digoxin
	Metoprolol	Propafenone increases metoprolol level 1.5-5 times
		Monitor cardiac function (especially blood pressure)
	Warfarin	Propafenone increases warfarin effect by 25%
		Monitor INR when adding/withdrawing propafenone
Ranolazine (Ranexa)	CYP3A inhibitors: azole antifungals, clarithromycin, diltiazem, erythromycin, protease inhibitors, verapamil, grapefruit	CYP3A inhibitors increase level of ranolazine & increase the risk of torsades de pointes
	QTc-prolonging drugs (class I & III antiarrhythmic agents)	QTc-prolonging drugs increase the risk of torsades de pointes
	Simvastatin	Ranolazine increases simvastatin level
		Reduce dose of simvastatin
Warfarin	Amiodarone	Amiodarone increases warfarin effect
		Decrease warfarin dose by 25%-50% & monitor INR
	Cholestyramine	Cholestyramine decreases effectiveness of warfarin
		Use colestipol as alternative
	Cyclooxygenase-2 inhibitors: celecoxib (Celebrex), rofecoxib (Vioxx)	These inhibitors increase INR (monitor INR closely)
	Propafenone	Propafenone increases warfarin effect by 25%
		Monitor INR when adding/withdrawing propafenone
	Glycoprotein IIb/IIIa inhibitors: abciximab (ReoPro), eptifibatide (Integrilin), tirofiban (Aggrastat)	These inhibitors increase hemorrhagic risk (use with caution)
	Thrombolytics	Thrombolytics increase hemorrhagic risk (use with caution)

Abbreviations: CYP, cytochrome P450; ECG, electrocardiogram; INR, international normalized ratio.

Questions

Multiple Choice (choose the best answer)

1. Under normal physiologic circumstances, the:

    a. Aortic valve closes before the pulmonary valve.
    b. Pulmonary valve closes before the aortic valve.
    c. Mitral valve opens before the tricuspid valve.
    d. Mitral valve and aortic valve are both open during isovolumic relaxation.
    e. Mitral valve and aortic valve are both open during isovolumic contraction.

2. Splitting of the semilunar valves (aortic valve and pulmonary valve):

    a. Occurs normally in expiration
    b. In left bundle branch block, occurs during inspiration
    c. In right bundle branch block, occurs during inspiration and expiration
    d. Occurs only in severe aortic stenosis
    e. Occurs in patients with mitral valve prolapse

3. The classic carotid finding in severe aortic regurgitation is:

    a. Pulsus alternans
    b. Bisferiens pulse
    c. Parvus and tardus
    d. Bifid carotid pulse
    e. Dicrotic pulse

4. Increased jugular venous pressure may be due to all of the following *except*:

    a. Increased intrathoracic pressure
    b. Increased pericardial pressure
    c. Tumor impinging on the drainage of the superior vena cava
    d. Increased intra-abdominal pressure
    e. Inspiration

5. A 55-year-old asymptomatic salesman with a history of chronic mitral regurgitation has an echocardiographic evaluation after his physical examination suggested a progressing murmur and left ventricular enlargement. The echocardiogram shows a normal ejection fraction of 65%, mild dilatation of left ventricular end-diastolic dimension, normal left ventricular end-systolic chamber size, and severe mitral regurgitation. Choose the correct statement about management in this patient:

    a. The risk of postoperative congestive heart failure increases if the preoperative ejection fraction decreases to less than 60%.
    b. Surgical correction is mandatory at this time.
    c. It is safe to wait for symptoms of congestive heart failure before intervening in this type of heart disease.
    d. Use of afterload reduction may improve the prognosis.
    e. β-Adrenergic blocker therapy will improve the prognosis.

6. A 35-year-old woman presents with mild exertional shortness of breath. She had rheumatic fever when she was a child. On examination, her blood pressure is 138/70 mm Hg and her pulse is 78 beats per minute and regular. The lungs are clear to auscultation. On cardiac examination, the first heart sound is loud and the second heart sound is physiologically split with a loud pulmonary component. The apical impulse is tapping, nondisplaced, and discrete. There is a high-pitched early diastolic snapping sound heard clearly at the apex and followed by a long, low-pitched, diastolic rumbling murmur, heard best with a bell in the left lateral decubitus position. There is a sternal lift. Jugular venous pressure is 10 cm H_2O. On the basis of the associated findings, you think the patient may have severe mitral stenosis. What other auscultatory finding would help confirm your clinical impression of severe mitral stenosis?

    a. A short interval from aortic closure (second heart sound) to mitral valve opening
    b. A grade 3/6 high-pitched, blowing diastolic murmur along the sternal border
    c. A grade 2/6 systolic ejection murmur best heard at the second rib interspace along the right sternal border
    d. Increased voltage of the QRS complex on electrocardiography
    e. Absence of opening snap

7. The patient described in question 6 is not interested in any further medical work-up or therapy. Three years later, however, she returns to your practice with considerable shortness of breath. She noted relatively sudden onset of dyspnea with minimal activity during the past week. She has had a prominent cough, that is productive of red-tinged sputum. She cannot lie flat and has been sleeping in a recliner. She can walk for only 20 feet before needing to rest. She denies chest pain or syncope. She wonders whether she has asthma or allergies because her chest is so "tight." What is the likely cause for her change in clinical status?

    a. Ruptured papillary muscle
    b. Ruptured mitral valve chordae
    c. Myocardial infarction
    d. New onset of atrial fibrillation
    e. Pulmonary embolism

8. A 33-year-old woman is admitted from the emergency department with fatigue, nausea, vomiting, and diarrhea. Diarrhea developed approximately a year ago; she has watery stools, about 2 dozen per day. Approximately 6 months ago, she started having trouble with weight loss and has lost about 60 pounds. She also started having flushes. Her husband noted

they came on when she exerted herself. In addition, the patient has become fatigued, has 2-pillow orthopnea, and can walk less than a block before stopping to rest.

Examination:

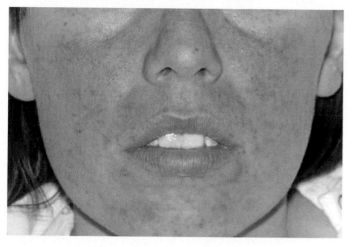

Question 8

Neck: jugular venous pressure to angle of the jaw, with large *v* wave
Chest: subtle lift of sternum
Auscultation: grade 3/6 holosystolic murmur and 1-2/6 diastolic rumble at left lower sternal border; grade 3/6 systolic ejection murmur, mid to late peaking at left upper sternal border. The systolic murmurs seemed to get louder with inspiration.
Abdomen: tender and firm
A CT scan obtained in the emergency department showed a complex pelvic mass. Echocardiogram showed thick, retracted tricuspid and pulmonary valve leaflets, with significant immobility and regurgitation.

The most likely diagnosis is:

a. Pulmonary embolism with right heart failure
b. Carcinoid syndrome
c. Aortic stenosis
d. Atrial septal defect
e. Eosinophilic heart disease

9. For the patient described in question 8, the next most appropriate test is:

a. CT of the chest to rule out pulmonary embolism
b. Transesophageal echocardiography with bubble study to assess intra-atrial septal integrity
c. Urine 5-hydroxyindoleacetic acid (5-HIAA) test
d. Hemodynamic cardiac catheterization
e. Complete blood count with differential analysis

10. A 56-year-old man presents with syncope. He has noted a 2-year history of chronic cough that is not productive of much sputum. He denies fever and chills. He has dyspnea on exertion at 2 blocks. His primary care provider has treated him twice with antibiotics without relief.
Examination:
   Pulse 80 beats per minute, blood pressure 120/65 mm Hg
   Lungs: crackles at bases
   Heart: Third heart sound present, no murmurs

Electrocardiogram

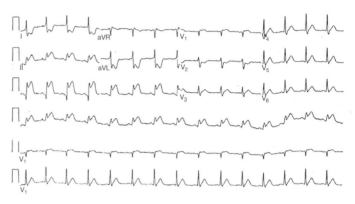

Question 10

Chest radiograph

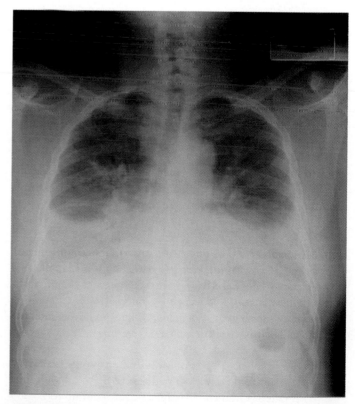

Question 10

The serum glucose level, complete blood count, ferritin level, and results of protein electrophoresis and urine electrophoresis were normal. Rhythm during your evaluation deteriorates to complete heart block. This patient likely has:

a. Hemochromatosis
b. Eosinophilic heart disease
c. Sarcoid disease
d. Cardiac amyloidosis
e. Hypothyroidism

11. For the patient described in question 10, the test and result that will make the diagnosis are:

a. Biopsy of myocardium with finding of noncaseating granulomatous disease
b. Subcutaneous fat aspirate: positive on Congo red stain
c. Complete blood count with differential: an increased eosinophil count
d. Determination of serum ferritin and iron levels: increased levels
e. Determination of sensitive thyroid-stimulating hormone level: increased

12. A 22-year-old male college student is referred to you because he was found to have hypertension during the dormitory blood drive and was not allowed to donate blood. He has no significant past medical history.

Examination:
  Blood pressure 160/86 mm Hg in the right arm, pulse 66 beats per minute and regular
  Carotid pulsations: brisk and equal; no bruits are noted
  Jugular venus pressure: normal
  Lungs: clear
  Heart: a normal first heart sound, an early systolic click heard best along the right upper sternal boarder, normal second heart sound, a soft grade 1-2/6 systolic ejection (crescendo-decrescendo) murmur along the left sternal border

All of the following tests might be helpful *except*:

a. Holter monitoring
b. Simultaneous palpation of the brachial-femoral pulse
c. Auscultation during a squat-to-stand maneuver
d. Valsalva maneuver
e. Passive leg lift and handgrip

13. All of the following statements about shunts, the atrial septum, and atrial septal defect (ASD) are true *except*:

a. A midsystolic ejection murmur and a diastolic rumble may be heard at the left lower sternal border.
b. A patent foramen ovale may be found in up to 25% of healthy adults.

c. The most common presenting symptoms of ASD in adults are fatigue and palpitations, whereas auscultation of a murmur on examination leads to discovery of ASD in most children.
d. Secundum ASD and patent foramen ovale require subacute bacterial endocarditis prophylaxis.
e. Anomalous pulmonary veins are associated with sinus venosus atrial septal defect.

14. A 19-year-old, asymptomatic, 6-foot 9-inch college basketball player is referred for evaluation after a murmur was found on a preparticipation physical examination. He has no prior history of cardiac disease; his only medical problem has been the need for corrective glasses. He has a family history of a paternal uncle dying unexpectedly in his 40s. He is a tall, fit-appearing man with pectus excavatum. Blood pressure is 120/72 mm Hg, and a grade 2/6 holodiastolic murmur is heard along the left sternal border to the apex. There is a third heart sound.

What do you most immediately need to do to determine his physical fitness to play sports?

a. Echocardiography to rule out a dilated aorta
b. Exercise stress test to rule out coronary artery disease
c. 24-Hour Holter monitoring to rule out sustained ventricular tachycardia
d. Genetic testing to rule out hypertrophic obstructive cardiomyopathy
e. No testing; you can reassure the patient that he can go back to competitive sports.

15. A 59-year-old man is admitted to the hospital after out-of-hospital cardiac arrest. He is successfully resuscitated and at the hospital is found to have acute ST elevation across chest leads V_1 through V_4, a suggestion of anterior wall myocardial infarction, and increased cardiac enzyme values. Revascularization with a stent placed at the left anterior descending artery is successful; perfusion is reportedly excellent. On day 3, clinical examination shows normal venous pressure and heart sounds and clear lung fields. No peripheral edema is present. His 12-lead electrocardiogram shows changes consistent with anterior wall myocardial infarction. On telemetry, however, several ventricular premature contractions, both singly and in couplets, give a bigeminal pattern. Bedside echocardiography shows an ejection fraction of 55% with mild anterior wall motion abnormalities consistent with the previous infarction. Predismissal exercise treadmill test shows appropriate workload without evidence of ischemia. At this time you advise:

a. Prophylactic cardioverter-defibrillator implantation
b. Diagnostic electrophysiologic study and implantable cardioverter-defibrillator if inducible ventricular tachycardia
c. Amiodarone loading dose and maintenance dose of 200 mg daily for at least 3 months

d. Assessment and treatment of modifiable cardiac risk factors

e. Holter monitoring at 1 month after dismissal and electro-physiologic study if results are positive

16. A 17-year-old boy comes for evaluation of a syncopal spell that occurred while he was waiting in the dentist's office. Although the spell was sudden, he remembers feeling hot and clammy and having a sensation of tunnel vision and of "not being there" shortly before losing consciousness. Afterward, he came around quickly and was fully oriented, although he felt somewhat fatigued. On examination in the office, there were no abnormal physical findings. No orthostatic symptoms or signs were apparent. Peripheral pulse and neurologic evaluation were normal. Your next step is:

a. Order a tilt-table test.

b. Give a β-adrenergic blocker to prevent further episodes of syncope.

c. Perform awake and sleep electroencephalography to rule out epilepsy.

d. Reassure the patient.

e. Advise an increased salt intake in the diet.

17. You are asked to see an 86-year-old man admitted after a syncopal spell. He described talking to his son on the telephone and next remembers stretching out his arm to break a fall. He sustained an injury to his right eye from the fall and was fully oriented immediately afterward. Clinical examination was unremarkable except for a grade 2/6 ejection-type murmur over the aortic area with a clearly audible split of the second heart that altered with respiration and a left carotid bruit. His 12-lead electrocardiogram is shown and is unchanged from 2 years previously. His ejection fraction is 65% by echocardiography. His aortic valve area is 1.85 cm².

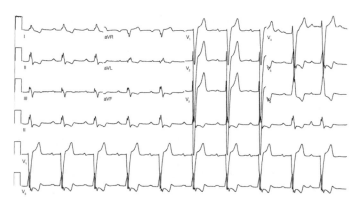

Question 17

Your next step is:

a. Order a neurologic evaluation and vascular studies of the carotid arteries.

b. Have a surgical evaluation for possible aortic valve replacement.

c. Order a treadmill exercise test to rule out ischemia.

d. Recommend permanent pacemaker implantation.

e. Order a tilt-table test.

18. A 27-year-old man has an episode of syncope while playing basketball. His health is otherwise excellent, and he tells you that he "feels a fraud" for bothering you. However, you learn that his brother died suddenly at age 25 years, and you obtain an echocardiogram which reveals a moderate degree of hypertrophy of the ventricular septum (maximum thickness, 2 cm). You also perform Holter monitoring, results of which are entirely normal, and a treadmill exercise test, during which the patient achieves 105% of functional aerobic capacity without symptoms. Your next step is:

a. Obtain genetic testing to further diagnose and stratify risk.

b. Advise implantation of a cardioverter-defibrillator.

c. Implant a permanent pacemaker to improve hemodynamics.

d. Order a tilt-table test to rule out a neurocardiogenic cause.

e. Reassure the patient but advise him to take up another sport.

19. An 85-year-old man who underwent permanent pacemaker implantation 6 months ago comes to your office complaining of frequent light-headedness and fatigue. He also describes a full sensation in the neck and the feeling of "heart pounding." On examination, his rhythm is regular. Intermittent pulsation is noted in his jugular veins, but jugular venous pressure is not increased. His chest radiograph is shown in the figure.

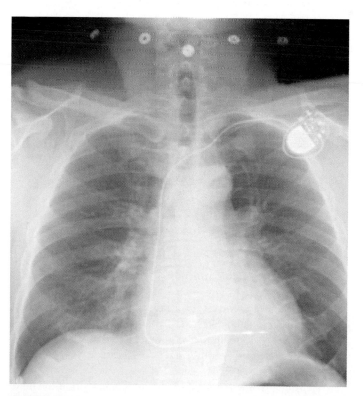

Question 19

What would you do next?

a. Start diuretic therapy.
b. Increase the rate of the pacemaker to avoid intrinsic (and possibly competing conduction).
c. Discuss placement of an atrial lead to promote atrioventricular synchrony.
d. Perform Holter monitoring; if results are negative, use an event recorder to assess for arrhythmias.
e. Perform a dobutamine stress test

20. A 65-year-old man who had his first myocardial infarction 10 years ago comes for evaluation. His most recent echocardiogram shows an ejection fraction of 25%. He denies syncope or palpitations. There is no history suggestive of angina or congestive heart failure. He is receiving maximal medical therapy. The 12-lead electrocardiogram is normal. You recommend:

a. Cardiac catheterization and possible revascularization
b. Exercise perfusion study to assess for ischemia
c. Implantation of a cardioverter-defibrillator
d. Prolonged Holter monitoring to assess for malignant arrhythmias
e. Reassure the patient and arrange for outpatient follow-up in 6 months.

21. A 68-year-old man presents with an ST-elevation myocardial infarction with changes noted in leads II, III and aVF. Thrombolytic therapy is administered immediately, along with aspirin, heparin, and morphine. Two hours later he is asymptomatic, but you observe the rhythm shown.

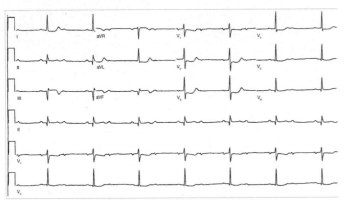

Question 21

At this time you recommend:

a. Urgent transthoracic echocardiography to rule out new ventricular septal defect
b. Urgent placement of a temporary pacemaker lead
c. Atropine intravenously, stat
d. Observation
e. Urgent coronary angiography in anticipation of the need for rescue revascularization

22. An 80-year-old woman presents to the emergency department with palpitations, dizziness, and shortness of breath. In the past, similar episodes have terminated spontaneously or with a Valsalva maneuver. Apart from increased cholesterol level and hypertension, which are both under good control, her health is otherwise excellent. When seen, she is mildly distressed but fully conscious and alert. You note that an electrocardiogram obtained in the past, when she was asymptomatic, was entirely normal.

Which of the following is most likely?

a. Sinus tachycardia
b. Supraventricular tachycardia due to atrioventricular node reentry
c. Atrial fibrillation
d. Ventricular tachycardia
e. Pacemaker-mediated tachycardia

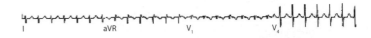

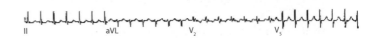

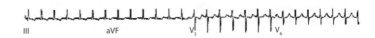

Question 22

23. Reasons for regularization of the rhythm in a patient being treated for atrial fibrillation include:

a. β-Adrenergic-blocker therapy
b. Radiofrequency ablation of the slow pathway to the atrioventricular node
c. Verapamil overdose
d. Digitalis toxicity
e. Overdose of flecainide

24. Atrial fibrillation in a 40-year-old patient is being treated with an antiarrhythmic drug. He becomes suddenly diaphoretic and syncopal, and the electrocardiogram shown here is obtained.

Which of the following is the most likely drug that was being administered to the patient?

a. Flecainide
b. Propafenone
c. Sotalol
d. Lidocaine
e. Mexiletine

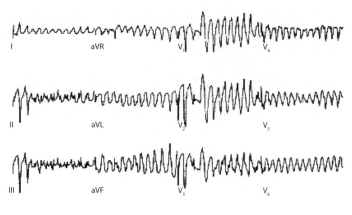

Question 24

25. A patient with first-degree atrioventricular block and PR interval of 270 milliseconds at a heart rate of 80 beats per minute may experience:

   a. Tachypalpitation
   b. Sudden cardiac death
   c. Pacemaker syndrome
   d. No symptoms
   e. Atrioventricular node reentrant tachycardia

26. You are asked to see a 65-year-old man because of an irregular rhythm. He is otherwise asymptomatic. You obtain a 12-lead electrocardiogram and observe the following:

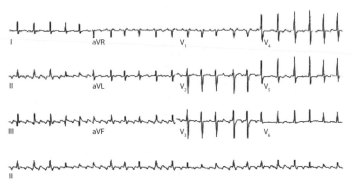

Question 26

What do you advise next?

   a. Schedule direct-current cardioversion within the next day or so.
   b. Start therapy with an antiarrhythmic agent such as flecainide.
   c. Assess stroke risk and consider anticoagulation if high.
   d. Obtain a transesophageal echocardiogram to rule out thrombus.
   e. Discuss possible benefit of ablation therapy.

27. An otherwise healthy 23-year-old woman complains of palpitations. There is no other cardiac history, and an echocardiogram obtained to rule out mitral valve prolapse 1 year ago was entirely normal. During exercise, you observe the 12-lead electrocardiogram shown here.

   Which of the following statements is true?

   a. The patient's palpitations are unrelated to the abnormality on the electrocardiogram.
   b. The rhythm is supraventricular tachycardia with aberrant conduction.
   c. This finding likely represents a structural abnormality in the patient's conduction system.
   d. Adenosine or verapamil might terminate this rhythm.
   e. A cardioverter-defibrillator should be implanted.

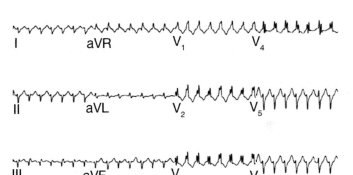

Question 27

28. A 36-year-old woman arrives in the emergency department complaining of palpitations and presyncope. Her 12-lead electrocardiogram is shown. On the basis of prior electrocardiograms, Wolff-Parkinson-White syndrome has been diagnosed. She is hypotensive (blood pressure, 70/40 mm Hg), and her heart rate is 180 beats per minute.

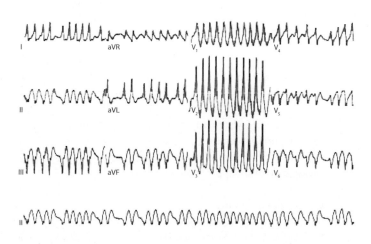

Question 28

Which of the following treatment options would be contraindicated?

a. Atrioventricular nodal blocking agents
b. Immediate cardioversion with direct-current shock
c. Antiarrhythmic therapy with procainamide or amiodarone
d. Radiofrequency ablation of the accessory pathway for recurrent tachycardia despite initial therapy
e. Amiodarone for recurrent arrhythmia

29. A 62-year-old man is referred by an orthopedic surgeon for a preoperative evaluation for elective left hip arthroplasty. He has a history of coronary artery disease with stable angina for many years. He uses nitroglycerin about twice a month. His exercise capacity is severely limited because of the pain in his hip. Current medications include aspirin 81 mg daily, atenolol 50 mg daily, and simvastatin 40 mg. His pulse rate is 72 beats per minute, blood pressure is 132/84 mm Hg, and results of cardiac examination are normal. What is the most appropriate next step in the patient's cardiac evaluation before his planned surgery?

a. Initiate β-adrenergic blocker therapy and proceed with operation.
b. Initiate nitrate therapy and proceed with operation.
c. Perform dobutamine echocardiography.
d. Perform treadmill exercise testing.
e. Perform coronary angiography.

30. A 69-year-old woman presents to a small community hospital with a 1-week history of intermittent chest pressure at rest. The pain became persistent on the day of admission and was associated with diaphoresis. She has a prior history of chronic stable angina treated with aspirin 81 mg daily and metoprolol 50 mg twice daily. Her past medical history is significant for diet-controlled diabetes mellitus and hypertension. She is not a smoker. Additional medications include hydrochlorothiazide 25 mg once daily. On physical examination, her pulse is regular at 66 beats per minute, blood pressure is 148/92 mm Hg, jugular venous pressure is normal, and all peripheral pulses are normal. On auscultation, the fourth heart sound is present but there is no murmur. There is no peripheral edema. The lungs are clear to auscultation. Electrocardiography shows a 1- to 2-mm ST-segment depression in the inferior leads and V_5-V_6. The troponin T value is increased at 0.1 ng/mL. The patient becomes asymptomatic after treatment with intravenous heparin and nitroglycerin with complete resolution of the electrocardiographic abnormalities. The following morning, recurrent, transient chest pressure and ST-segment depression develop. In addition to arranging transfer to a hospital with facilities for coronary angiography, which of the following is the most appropriate next step in her management?

a. Addition of amlodipine 5 mg daily
b. Exercise echocardiography
c. Administration of reteplase 10 units delivered intravenously over 2 minutes

d. Initiating an infusion of the glycoprotein IIb/IIIa inhibitor eptifibatide
e. Adenosine perfusion study

31. A 47-year-old man presents for a general medical examination. He is asymptomatic and runs 1 mile 3 times a week. His elder brother recently had coronary artery bypass grafting at the age of 49 years. The patient is a smoker. The physical examination is normal, and the blood pressure is 124/80 mm Hg. His body mass index is 26. In addition to recommendations regarding smoking cessation, which of the following set of investigations is most appropriate?

a. Lipid profile and CT for a coronary calcium score
b. Lipid profile and fasting plasma glucose and serum lipoprotein (a) tests
c. High-sensitivity C-reactive protein test and lipid profile
d. Exercise sestamibi stress test and C-reactive protein test
e. Lipid profile and fasting plasma glucose and plasma homocysteine tests

32. A 70-year-old woman presents with a 2-hour history of central chest pain radiating to her left arm. She is nauseated and diaphoretic. Her past medical history is remarkable for hypertension and a stroke 6 months ago from which she has made a good neurologic recovery. On physical examination, her pulse is 100 beats per minute, blood pressure is 122/78 mm Hg, jugular venous pressure is increased, and heart sounds are normal. There are no murmurs, and the lungs are clear to auscultation. Her medications include aspirin 325 mg daily and lisinopril 20 mg daily. The patient's electrocardiogram is shown below. In addition to the administration of oxygen, analgesic, and intravenous β-adrenergic blockers, what is the most appropriate next step in the management of this patient?

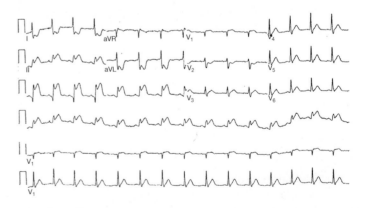

Question 32

a. Administer indomethacin.
b. Initiate an infusion of abciximab.
c. Administer a tenectaplase bolus.
d. Administer clopidogrel 300 mg.
e. Perform emergency coronary angiography.

33. A 59-year-old postmenopausal woman presents to the emergency department with severe retrosternal chest pain of 6 hours in duration that developed soon after she received the news of her son's death in a car accident. Her past medical history is unremarkable, and she has been in good health otherwise. The chest discomfort is not relieved by sublingual nitroglycerin. Her heart rate is 96 beats per minute, and her blood pressure is 168/88 mm Hg. Jugular venous pressure, carotid pulse, and peripheral pulses are normal. Cardiac auscultation is normal. Lungs are clear to auscultation. Cardiac troponin T is 0.06 (normal, ≤0.03). The 12-lead electrocardiogram shows 1-mm ST-segment elevation in precordial leads V_2-V_5. She is taken for emergency coronary angiography, which shows normal coronary arteries. Left ventriculography illustrates severe hypokinesis of the apical and midsegments of the heart with normal function at the base. Which of the following is the most likely diagnosis?

a. Apical ballooning syndrome (takotsubo cardiomyopathy)
b. Acute coronary syndrome
c. Myocarditis
d. Pericarditis
e. Dilated cardiomyopathy

34. A 55-year-old man returns for a clinic visit after an anterior myocardial infarction 2 months ago. Treatement with primary percutaneous coronary intervention was successful. Angiography had shown mild disease in the remainder of the coronary circulation. He has made an uncomplicated recovery, has completed cardiac rehabilitation, and is back at work as a salesman. Current medications are aspirin 81 mg daily, metoprolol 50 mg twice daily, clopidogrel 75 mg daily, simvastatin 40 mg daily, and lisinopril 30 mg daily. On examination, pulse rate is 64 beats per minute, blood pressure is 126/78 mm Hg, there are no murmurs or gallops noted on heart examination, and the lungs are clear. Resting echocardiography shows hypokinesis of the anterior wall, and left ventricular ejection fraction is 34%. Complete blood count and serum chemistry values are all within normal limits. With regard to his long-term outcome, what is the most important next step in his management?

a. Implantation of a cardioverter-defibrillator
b. An exercise stress test
c. Repeat coronary angiography
d. Continuation of long-term cardiovascular rehabilitation program
e. Isosorbide mononitrate 30 mg daily

35. A 66-year-old woman presents with progressive angina. Her past medical history is significant for hyperlipidemia, hypertension, and diabetes. On physical examination, her heart rate is 72 beats per minute and blood pressure is 144/88 mm Hg. The heart sounds are normal, and an additional fourth heart sound is present. The lungs are clear to auscultation, and the peripheral pulses are normal. Current daily medications include aspirin 325 mg, atenolol 25 mg, lisinopril 10 mg, atorvastatin 20 mg daily, insulin, and metformin. Laboratory tests show a normal complete blood count. The creatinine value is 1.6 mg/dL. A stress test is markedly positive for ischemia. The cardiologist has recommended proceeding with coronary angiography. In addition to taking steps to minimize the risk of contrast nephropathy, which of the following is the most important before angiography?

a. Start therapy with clopidogrel 75 mg daily.
b. Increase the dose of the atenolol to 50 mg daily.
c. Administer isosorbide mononitrate slow release 60 mg daily.
d. Decrease the dose of aspirin to 81 mg daily.
e. Discontinue the use of metformin.

36. A 42-year-old man is admitted to the hospital with worsening exertional and recumbent dyspnea. He has a prior diagnosis of primary restrictive cardiomyopathy. His blood pressure is 100/70 mm Hg. His heart rate is 80 beats per minute and regular. He has jugular venous distention and prominent x and y descents. Bibasilar crackles are present posteriorly. A third heart sound is present. He has moderate bilateral pitting edema of the lower extremities. Electrocardiography shows normal sinus rhythm with nonspecific repolarization changes. Chest radiography shows small bilateral pleural effusions. Echocardiography shows normal ventricular dimensions and a normal ejection fraction. Which of the following medications is expected to improve his symptoms?

a. Amiodarone
b. Carvedilol
c. Digoxin
d. Furosemide
e. Losartan

37. A 78-year-old man presents to the office with concerns about an abrupt decrease in exercise tolerance manifested as dyspnea accompanied by increasing abdominal girth and lower extremity edema. He has a history of ischemic dilated cardiomyopathy and previously was stable with New York Heart Association class III symptoms. He has no history of ventricular or supraventricular arrhythmias. His treatment includes digoxin 0.125 mg, metoprolol succinate 100 mg, enalapril 10 mg twice daily, and furosemide 40 mg daily. He has a biventricular pacemaker. His heart rate is 80 beats per minute. His blood pressure is 100/70 mm Hg. His jugular venous pressure is increased, and he has 3+ bilateral lower extremity pitting edema. His precordium is quiet with distant heart sounds. He has reduced air flow at the lung bases. Laboratory results include potassium 4.4 mmol/L, sodium 137 mmol/L, serum creatinine 1.4 mg/dL, and trough digoxin level 1.0 ng/mL. His chest radiography shows cardiomegaly, mild pulmonary venous congestion, and his cardiac resynchronization device. The rhythm strip from his electrocardiogram is shown here.

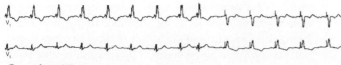

Question 37

His ejection fraction is unchanged at 35%. A nuclear perfusion study shows no ischemic regions. Which of the following steps is most appropriate?

a. Send the patient for coronary angiography.
b. Attempt to restore sinus rhythm.
c. Refer the patient to a cardiologist for explantation of a malfunctioning cardiac resynchronization device.
d. Double his digoxin dose to 0.25 mg daily.
e. Double his metoprolol succinate dose to 200 mg daily.

38. A 69-year-old man presents to the hospital with new orthopnea and edema. He is found to have a nonischemic dilated cardiomyopathy, ejection fraction 20%. Treatment includes furosemide intravenously and lisinopril and carvedilol. On the third hospital day, the patient notes persistent dyspnea. His medications include furosemide 40 mg per day, carvedilol 6.25 mg twice a day, and lisinopril 10 mg per day. His blood pressure is 95/60 mm Hg, and his pulse is 70 beats per minute. He has jugular venous distention, clear lungs, a displaced cardiac apex with a third heart sound but no cardiac murmurs, and mild lower extremity pitting edema. Which of the following medication changes is most appropriate at this time?

a. Increase the furosemide to 40 mg twice daily.
b. Double the carvedilol to 12.5 mg twice daily.
c. Increase the lisinopril to 20 mg daily.
d. Add spironolactone 25 mg twice daily.
e. Discontinue lisinopril and substitute valsartan.

39. A 60-year-old man presents to the office because of increasing exertional dyspnea, orthopnea, weight gain, and new lower extremity edema. On his own, he increased his furosemide dose and his symptoms have improved but have not totally disappeared. He has diabetes mellitus and coronary artery disease with prior silent myocardial infarctions. Angiography done 7 years earlier showed moderate diffuse coronary artery disease. His medications include metoprolol succinate, lisinopril, digoxin, furosemide, insulin, aspirin, and pravastatin. He indicates compliance with these medications. His examination shows a blood pressure of 120/70 mm Hg, heart rate 80 beats per minute and regular, mild jugular venous distention, trace edema, mild scattered end-expiratory wheezes, and a displaced and sustained cardiac impulse along with a right ventricular lift. Echocardiography shows an ejection fraction of 25%, and both left and right ventricular function have deteriorated compared with echocardiography done 3 years earlier. His creatinine level is 1.3 mg/dL, potassium 4.7 mmol/L, and hemoglobin A1C 13%. What is the next thing that you would do?

a. Add metformin 1 g twice daily in addition to his insulin.
b. Refer the patient to the pulmonary clinic.
c. Refer the patient for coronary angiography.
d. Refer the patient for transesophageal echocardiography.
e. Obtain cardiac MRI with gadolinium for delayed enhancement imaging.

40. A 30-year-old woman is transferred to your coronary care unit after presenting at her local hospital with pulmonary edema. One month earlier, she had a healthy child after an uneventful pregnancy. She is treated with diuretics, and echocardiography shows a global cardiomyopathy, ejection fraction 11%. She is supported with a balloon pump initially as well as intravenous inotropes. Coronary angiography is normal. The patient slowly improves and is weaned from the inotropes and the balloon pump. She is given metoprolol succinate 25 mg twice daily, captopril 6.25 mg 3 times daily, digoxin 0.25 mg daily, and furosemide 40 mg once daily. She is slowly ambulatory within her room and in the halls in the coronary care unit. Her heart rate is 105 beats per minute and regular. Her blood pressure is 90/60 mm Hg. Her jugular venous pressure is normal. Her lungs are clear. She has a left ventricular lift and a grade 2/6 mitral regurgitant murmur at the apex. A summation gallop is present. She has no hepatosplenomegaly, ascites, or edema. What is the most appropriate management at this time?

a. Dismiss from the hospital with follow-up within 2 weeks.
b. Increase the metoprolol succinate dose to 50 mg twice daily.
c. Increase the captopril dose to 12.5 mg 3 times daily.
d. Increase the doses of both metoprolol and captopril.
e. Insert a cardioverter-defibrillator for primary prevention.

41. Patients with dilated cardiomyopathy should be advised to avoid which of the following medications?

a. Allopurinol
b. Ferrous gluconate
c. Acetaminophen
d. Propoxyphene
e. Ibuprofen

42. Patients with heart failure should be advised of all of the following, *except*:

a. They should weigh themselves daily and report unexpected weight gain to care providers.
b. Follow a sodium-restricted diet as recommended by their care provider.
c. Be certain to take in at least eight 8-ounce glasses of water in addition to dietary intake to optimize kidney function.
d. They should self-assess their status (eg, breathing, ability to be active) daily and report any unexpected decline.
e. Check with health care providers before beginning treatment with any herbal remedies.

Answers

1. Answer a.

The mechanism of normal physiologic splitting of the second heart sound occurs as a result of the mechanics and hemodynamic changes of respiration. During the respiratory cycle, there is cyclic gradation of intrathoracic pressure (decreased intrathoracic pressure during inspiration and increased during expiration). This gradation of pressure affects the volume of blood returning to the right side of the heart and the gradient of pressure pushing blood from the lungs to the left side of the heart. Thus, there is relatively more blood on the right side during inspiration and relatively less on the left, and these volumes lead to delayed emptying to the right side of the heart. During isovolumic relaxation (and also contraction), the cardiac valves (mitral, tricuspid, aortic, and pulmonary) are all closed, because no volume is changing.

2. Answer c.

The physiologic splitting of the second heart sound occurs during inspiration and is due to the increased volume arriving in the right-sided chambers and prolonged ejection through the pulmonary valve. It is best heard during inspiration, in the left second intercostal space with the patient in the seated position. With left bundle branch block and severe aortic stenosis there is a delay in the ejection of blood through the left ventricle outflow tract, delaying atrioventricular closure so that the splitting is paradoxic and occurs during expiration. In right bundle branch block, the splitting occurs during inspiration, may be wider and even still split during expiration, and still moves in the normal fashion, longer in the inspiration phase of respiration. This abnormality is often referred to as persistent splitting, in contrast to fixed splitting, which is heard with an atrial septal defect.

3. Answer b.

The carotid upstroke can be described by its contour. Aortic regurgitation is usually referred to as a bisferiens pulse with a rapid upstroke, percussion wave, and a tidal wave. It feels like a shudder, with rapid runoff. Hypertrophic cardiomyopathy has a bifid pulse, also known as spike and dome, with rapid percussion wave and then often a secondary wave. The differential diagnosis of bisferiens pulse includes high-output states, such as anemia and hyperthyroidism. A difficult-to-palpate pulse with slow upstroke, often parvus and tardus, is classic for severe aortic stenosis. Pulsus alternans is a relatively strong pulse followed by a relatively weak pulse; it indicates a very weak ventricular performance and occurs in end-stage heart failure due to dilated cardiomyopathy.

4. Answer e.

Increased jugular venous pressure is classically due to congestive heart failure (either right or left ventricular failure). However, other causes should be considered: superior vena cava obstruction; pericardial disease (pericardial tamponade–Kussmaul pulsations, constrictive pericarditis causes rapid *y* descents); obstruction to right atrial emptying (tricuspid stenosis or tumor of right atrium); increased

intrathoracic pressure; pleural effusions; chronic obstructive pulmonary disease; and increased intra-abdominal pressure (eg, pregnancy, tense ascites, and straining). Inspiration is associated with a decrease in intrathoracic pressure and consequently a decrease in the jugular venous pressure. The phenomenon of Kussmaul sign is an inspiratory increase in the jugular venous pressure, signifying an increase in intracardiac pressure with inspiratory filling of the right ventricle. Kussmaul sign is often caused by pericardial disease, classically tamponade.

5. Answer a.

In the setting of severe mitral regurgitation, the optimal timing of surgical intervention has changed in recent years. It depends on the likelihood of surgical repair versus replacement and the hemodynamic consequences of the regurgitation on the left ventricle. The current goal is to intervene, even for asymptomatic patients, before irreversible left ventricular dysfunction leading to postoperative heart failure. If congestive heart failure, ventricular dysfunction, or symptoms are present, then surgery should be performed. If the left ventricular ejection fraction has decreased to less than 60% or the left ventricular end-systolic dimension is more than 45 mm, then surgical consultation should be sought, because the rates of development of postoperative left ventricular dysfunction and congestive heart failure are higher if surgery is delayed. Although the use of afterload reduction (ie, angiotensin-converting enzyme inhibitors) may reduce the regurgitant fraction, it has not yet been shown to improve long-term outcomes. (Heart. 2002;87:79-85; Heart. 2003;89:100-5; Circulation. 1998;98:1949-84.)

6. Answer a.

This patient presents with a typical history and findings of mitral stenosis. The presence of a pronounced first heart sound implies that the mitral valve leaflets are still pliable and are closing with force. In some patients with mitral stenosis, calcified leaflets that are not pliable or mobile have a very soft first heart sound. The increased jugular venous pressure, sternal lift, and increased pulmonary component of the second heart sound suggest considerable pressure overload on the left atrium in the setting of severe mitral stenosis and are associated with pulmonary hypertension. These physical findings are all consistent with *severe* mitral stenosis. The tapping, localized apical impulse is typical of the normal ventricular size and function in mitral stenosis (because the left ventricle is isolated from the valvular problem) and pressure builds in the left atrium, the pulmonary circuit, and the right cardiac chambers.

As the mitral stenosis worsens, the pressure increases, leading to earlier opening of the mitral valve and a shortening of the interval from aortic closure to mitral valve opening also known as aortic closure to opening snap (A_2-OS). Often, because the mitral valve is thickened and has lost some pliability, patients may present with a component of mitral regurgitation. Without considerable pressure overload of the left atrium (in the setting of early, mild mitral stenosis), this systolic murmur is generally holosystolic and begins with the first heart sound. As the mitral stenosis worsens (in the setting of moderate-severe stenosis), the pressure in the left atrium increases and mitral regurgitation murmur is shortened.

The blowing diastolic murmur and the systolic ejection murmur are both suggestive of aortic valve disease, which could coexist with the mitral valve involvement in rheumatic heart disease. However, they do not indicate the severity of the mitral valve disease.

The left ventricle is not affected in pure mitral stenosis. Therefore, left ventricular hypertrophy is not found on electrocardiography. Rather, the left atrium is pressure overloaded and enlarges; thus, left atrial enlargement is common on electrocardiography, as are, potentially, right ventricular and atrial enlargement.

7.   Answer d.

Mitral stenosis has a prolonged natural history: onset of rheumatic fever as a child, murmur and opening snap during the second decade, early exertional symptoms during the third decade, and atrial fibrillation leading to acute clinical decline in the fourth decade. Patients generally are not very aware of their decline in exercise tolerance during the first few stages of the disease until their rhythm changes abruptly to atrial fibrillation due to the enlarged left atrium. Loss of the atrial "kick" with resultant shortening of diastole leads to heart failure. Severe mitral stenosis in association with atrial fibrillation is associated with increasing pulmonary hypertension and frothy blood-tinged sputum. Although myocardial infarction and pulmonary embolism are in the differential diagnosis, they are less likely. Rupture of the papillary muscle most often is a rare complication of myocardial infarction and would be unlikely in a young woman. Rupture of a chordal attachment to the mitral valve is generally a complication of long-standing mitral valve prolapse due to myxomatous degeneration of the chordae tendineae and is not typically associated with rheumatic valvular disease.

8.   Answer b.

9.   Answer c.

The patient described in questions 8 and 9 gives a clinical history consistent with carcinoid syndrome. In addition to rheumatic fever and use of ergot alkaloids, carcinoid is one of the few diseases that can cause tricuspid stenosis. However, because of the stiff retracted tricuspid leaflets, carcinoid causes a combination of torrential tricuspid regurgitation and relative tricuspid stenosis.

The substances produced by the tumor (bradykinin, histamine, prostaglandins, and serotonin) are thought to lead to the valvular manifestations, which result in severe dysfunction of the right side of the heart due to tricuspid and pulmonary valve thickening and stenosis or regurgitation. These substances are metabolized in the lungs. Therefore, left-sided involvement is rare; it can occur when there is a shunt (patent foramen ovale), pulmonary metastasis, or overwhelming carcinoid syndrome.

Once suspected, the diagnosis is confirmed by measuring the 5-HIAA level in the urine. The left side of the heart is usually unaffected in the absence of intrapulmonary or intracardiac shunts. The tricuspid valve stenosis may lead to a prominent *a* wave in the jugular venous pressure, except when atrial fibrillation causes loss of atrial contraction. The tricuspid valve regurgitation is likely to cause a

predominant *v* wave. (Circulation. 1993;87:1188-96; Am J Cardiol. 1997;80:251-6.)

10.   Answer c.

11.   Answer a.

The patient described in questions 10 and 11 has sarcoidosis with cardiac involvement. Classic clinical findings of sarcoidosis are a chronic cough that is nonproductive and perihilar infiltrates. The diagnosis can be suggested by atypical regional wall motion abnormalities that do not respect the usual distribution of the coronary arteries. MRI may assist in the diagnosis. Cardiac sarcoidosis can be diagnosed from the pathognomonic finding of noncaseating granulomas on myocardial biopsy.

Other organs involved with sarcoidosis include lungs, eyes, skin, bones, and central nervous system. The heart is involved in 30% of autopsy cases. The most common cardiac manifestation is syncope due to conduction abnormalities and arrhythmias. Patients with late-stage disease may also present with heart failure due to a dilated or restrictive cardiomyopathy.

For the other possible tests included in the question: subcutaneous fat aspirate with positive Congo red staining is suggestive of amyloidosis; complete blood count with differential and increased eosinophil count is consistent with hypereosinophilic syndrome; and increased serum ferritin and iron levels suggest hemochromatosis. (N Engl J Med. 1997;336:1224-34; Mayo Clin Proc. 1985;60:549-54.)

12.   Answer a.

One of the most important maneuvers that should be performed in a younger patient with hypertension is simultaneous palpation of the brachial-femoral pulse. In this patient, the early systolic click and the systolic murmur might suggest the presence of a bicuspid aortic valve (typically heard at the right upper sternal border) or click of mitral valve prolapse. Mitral valve prolapse is associated with a mid-late systolic click, followed by a murmur. The squat-to-stand maneuver will help to rule out the possibility that this murmur and click are due to mitral valve prolapse syndrome. As the left ventricular volume increases with a squat, the click and murmur move later into systole. Bicuspid aortic valve is associated with the fixed early systolic click (tensing of the relatively less pliable bicuspid leaflets) and systolic ejection murmur characteristic of bicuspid aortic valve. In addition, the squat-to-stand maneuver will accentuate the murmur of hypertrophic cardiomyopathy, in the standing position, with dynamic left ventricular outflow obstruction due to decreased volume of the left ventricle. The Valsalva maneuver is also useful in patients with systolic murmurs, in which it will accentuate dynamic outflow tract murmurs (hypertrophic obstructive cardiomyopathy); the squat-to-stand maneuver will have the same effect on hypertrophic obstructive cardiomyopathy. Passive leg lift decreases the dynamic outflow murmur, as does the handgrip. Bicuspid valve is associated with coarctation, and coarctation is a cause of hypertension.

Coarctation is frequently associated with a bicuspid aortic valve. The symptoms of coarctation include headache, leg fatigue, and intermittent claudication. Unfortunately, patients may come to medical attention only after the development of congestive heart failure, endocarditis, or dissection of the aorta. Therefore, it is important to check for the radial-femoral delay in all patients with hypertension and pursue further testing if this finding is suspected or if bicuspid aortic valve is found.

Persistent hypertension is common in adults after repair of the aorta. Up to 30% of patients may have this finding. Patients need to be followed serially for hypertension, development of aortic aneurysms, and recoarctation. (J Am Coll Cardiol. 2003;41:2259-65; Lancet. 2001;358:89.)

13. Answer d.

Several clinical findings in ASD provide clues to the condition: right ventricular lift or sternal lift, palpable pulmonary artery pulse consistent with pulmonary artery volume and pressure overload, fixed split of the second heart sound and accentuation of the tricuspid valve closure leading to splitting of the first heart sound, midsystolic pulmonary ejection murmur due to increased volume of flow through the right ventricular outflow tract, and, if a large shunt is present, a mid to late diastolic rumble.

Chest radiography may also be helpful, classically (with large shunts) showing enlargement of the right atriuim (bulge of the right heart border), right ventricle (filled-in posterior sternal clear space), enlarged pulmonary artery, and increased pulmonary vascular markings.

Common anatomical types of ASD are ostium secundum, ostium primum, and sinus venosus. Subacute bacterial endocarditis prophylaxis is not necessary for secundum ASD or patent foramen ovale when this is an isolated finding. Sinus venosus defect is commonly accompanied by anomalous pulmonary venous return. Ostium primum ASD is commonly associated with a cleft Mitral valve and other complex congenital heart disease. (Circulation. 1968;37:476-88; Circulation. 1977;56:1047-53.)

14. Answer a.

The findings in this patient suggest Marfan syndrome, and the most immediate threat to his longevity and to his athletic participation is an enlarged aortic root. Aortic regurgitation in this patient's age group is commonly due to bicuspid aortic valve; however, a more concerning cause is due to aortic root dilatation, especially in a patient who has a family history of what could be sudden death due to dissection of the aorta. It is also important to quantify the aortic regurgitation that is suggested by the auscultation. However, it should not be severe given the lack of large pulse pressure (severe >100 mm Hg with a diastolic blood pressure <60 mm Hg). (N Engl J Med. 1992;326:905-9; Lancet. 1998;352:1722-3; J Am Coll Cardiol. 2004;43:665-9.)

15. Answer d.

Ventricular fibrillation (the most likely rhythm causing cardiac arrest in this patient) occurring in the setting of acute myocardial infarction is not currently an indication for implantation of a cardioverter-defibrillator. Given the relatively well-preserved left ventricular function, the patient will likely do well and would not benefit from placement of the device. There is no role for electrophysiologic study, amiodarone, or Holter monitoring in this patient at this time.

The option most likely to prevent further cardiac events is aggressive modification of risk factors and treatment of significant residual ischemia, if found.

16. Answer d.

There is no need for tilt-table testing unless the diagnosis is in doubt. Electroencephalography adds nothing, and increased salt and volume replacement are unnecessary unless symptoms are recurrent. Use of β-blocker therapy in most patients with neurocardiogenic syncope is not associated with a decrease in symptoms and is not routinely recommended, even in patients with recurrent episodes.

17. Answer d.

The clinical scenario is consistent with cardiogenic syncope. The electrocardiogram shows evidence of conduction system disease, and therefore the most likely mechanism of his syncope is high-grade atrioventricular block. A tilt-table test and treadmill exercise test are unlikely to be helpful. Importantly, extensive neurologic and vascular work-up is expensive and virtually never conclusive unless recovery is prolonged or focal neurologic signs are present. Patients with this type of presentation will most likely undergo implantation of a permanent pacemaker. The patient's aortic valve area is close to normal.

18. Answer b.

This patient most likely has a familial hypertrophic cardiomyopathy. Although results of the Holter and treadmill exercise tests are reassuring, the importance of the family history cannot be overstated. Genetic testing at this time is not clinically useful. The only way to prevent sudden cardiac death is implantation of a cardioverter-defibrillator.

19. Answer c.

The symptoms described are suggestive of pacemaker syndrome. Although this syndrome can occur with any variation of pacing device, whether single chamber or dual chamber, it is most common with single-chamber ventricular pacing, as in this case. Given the nature of his symptoms, upgrade to dual-chamber pacing is warranted.

20. Answer c.

The patient has markedly impaired left ventricular function in the setting of ischemic heart disease and he is at risk of sudden cardiac death and should be offered therapy with an implantable cardioverter-defibrillator. Because there is no history of angina or congestive heart failure, cardiac catheterization or exercise testing is not needed. In this setting, indication for a cardioverter-defibrillator is not predicated on the presence of ventricular arrhythmias, and therefore prolonged monitoring is unnecessary.

21. Answer d.

The patient has an acute coronary syndrome with ST-elevation myocardial infarction, most likely due to right coronary occlusion. Development of both Wenckebach, second-, and third-degree atrioventricular block is not uncommon in this setting. Because the patient is hemodynamically stable and without symptoms, a period of observation is reasonable because the majority of patients recover normal conduction and permanent pacing is not warranted.

22. Answer b.

For analysis of regular narrow complex tachycardias, the most common diagnoses to consider are atrioventricular node reentrant tachycardia, atrioventricular reentrant tachycardia using a retrograde conducting bypass tract, and atrial tachycardia. If the resting electrocardiogram is normal, the most likely is atrioventricular node reentrant tachycardia. If no P waves are visible, then the likelihood of this diagnosis is very high. The presence of a "concealed" accessory pathway can be determined only with electrophysiologic study. However, P waves are usually visible at least 90 milliseconds beyond the QRS (ie, more than 2 small squares on the electrocardiogram). An atrial tachycardia might be expected in about 10% of cases. There is no evidence of pacing to suggest pacemaker syndrome.

23. Answer d.

When the heart rhythm suddenly becomes regular in a patient with atrial fibrillation, the following possibilities must be considered: 1) conversion to sinus rhythm that will be apparent with easily discernible sinus P waves before each QRS, 2) organization of the rhythm to atrial flutter with either regular 1:1 atrioventricular conduction or regular 2:1 atrioventricular conduction, and 3) the development of complete heart block with a regular junctional escape rhythm. β-Adrenergic blockers and calcium channel blockers typically do not cause complete heart block, particularly at lower doses. In an overdose-type situation, complete heart block can result and unfortunately can also be associated with suppression of an escape junctional rhythm giving rise to asystole. Digitalis toxicity often presents with the development of complete heart block during atrial fibrillation and a relatively fast (>60 beats per minute) junctional escape rhythm giving the appearance on auscultation or pulse measurements of possible conversion to sinus rhythm. Flecainide typically enhances atrioventricular node conduction and may result in more rapid conduction, particularly of more relatively organized rhythms, and should not be used without an additional atrioventricular node-blocking agent.

24. Answer c.

The rhythm shown on the electrocardiogram is polymorphic ventricular tachycardia. When this is due to QT prolongation, it is often termed *torsades de pointes* (twisting of the points). Class III drugs such as sotalol and dofetilide increase the QT interval by blocking potassium channels, thereby prolonging repolarization. In contrast, sodium channel blocking drugs such as flecainide and propafenone prolong the QRS interval. In addition, sodium channel blockers have the property of use dependence, which means that they exert the greatest effect at *faster* heart rates, whereas class III agents such as sotalol have reverse use dependence, in which the maximum effect is at *slower* heart rates. Thus, a treadmill exercise test is useful in patients who are loaded with class I drugs, whereas measurement of the QT interval in patients loaded with class III agents such as sotalol is best done at *slower* heart rates.

25. Answer c.

Usually the term *pacemaker syndrome* is reserved for patients who have a pacemaker programmed to a ventricular pacing mode. If the patient has sinus rhythm, there may be dyssynchrony between the atrium and the ventricular paced beats, giving rise to the atrium contracting against a closed mitral and tricuspid valve. This produces large *a* waves and associated symptoms of headaches, nausea, near syncope, and fatigue and is referred to as the pacemaker syndrome. Although not a common finding, patients with a long PR interval even without a pacemaker may have contraction of the atrium simultaneous with a ventricle and have all the classic features of the pacemaker syndrome. First-degree atrioventricular block is not associated with sudden cardiac death and may be symptomatic, as noted above.

26. Answer c.

The electrocardiogram shows a narrow complex irregular tachycardia. No isoelectric segments are visible between each QRS complex. This is characteristic of atrial flutter. Because the patient is asymptomatic, attempts at restoration of sinus rhythm (at least initially) are unwarranted, and the most important first step is to assess stroke risk and consider anticoagulation therapy if high. Risk factors for stroke include *c*ongestive heart failure, *h*ypertension, *a*ge older than 75 years, *d*iabetes mellitus, and previous *s*troke or transient ischemic attack (CHADS score). Thus, direct-current cardioversion, antiarrhythmic drug, or ablative therapy for atrial fibrillation is usually reserved for patients with symptoms thought to be due to atrial fibrillation. Transthoracic echocardiography is more useful and less invasive than transesophageal echocardiography.

27. Answer d.

The differential diagnosis of a wide complex tachycardia in the setting of a structurally normal heart is 1) supraventricular tachycardia with aberrancy, 2) pre-excited tachycardia (impulses go from atrium to ventricle via the accessory pathway and return via the atrioventricular node), and 3) ventricular tachycardia. In each of these rhythms adenosine or verapamil may terminate the tachycardia. (Note: Verapamil should not be used in a patient who is known to have coronary artery disease and myocardial infarction because a wide complex tachycardia is most likely ventricular tachycardia and use of verapamil may lead to hemodynamic compromise.) The 2 main types of ventricular tachycardia in patients with structurally normal heart are right ventricular outflow tract ventricular tachycardia and idiopathic left ventricular tachycardia (the rhythm in the tracing). It is important to recognize these rhythms because they are amenable to catheter ablation with success rate of more than 95%. An implantable cardioverter-defibrillator is not indicated in a patient with normal heart and minimal or no symptoms.

28. Answer a.

Although it is often emphasized that atrioventricular nodal blocking agents should be avoided in patients with Wolff-Parkinson-White syndrome, it is important to note that a regular tachycardia, either orthodromic or antidromic, can be treated safely with atrioventricular nodal blocking agents because the atrioventricular node is an important limb for this reentrant arrhythmia. However, atrioventricular nodal blocking agents *are* contraindicated in patients with Wolff-Parkinson-White syndrome when the rhythm is *irregular*, such as in this case with atrial fibrillation, because blocking the atrioventricular node allows more rapid conduction directly to the ventricular myocardium through the accessory pathway and may precipitate ventricular fibrillation. Radiofrequency ablation should be offered to prevent risk of sudden death. Amiodarone may be used but is not first-line therapy.

29. Answer c.

This patient has not had prior coronary revascularization or a recent coronary evaluation. The first step is to determine his risk for perioperative cardiovascular adverse events on the basis of clinical predictors. The American College of Cardiology and American Heart Association guidelines on preoperative cardiovascular evaluation provide 3 categories: major, intermediate, and minor clinical predictors. A history of mild angina is an intermediate clinical predictor. The next consideration is the patient's exercise capacity, which in this case is poor (<4 metabolic equivalent tasks [METs]). The final consideration is the type of noncardiac surgical procedure. A hip replacement is not a high-risk surgical procedure. High-risk surgery includes emergency procedures, aortic and other major vascular surgery, peripheral vascular surgery, and surgical procedures associated with large fluid shifts or blood loss. The guidelines recommend the presence of 2 of the following: intermediate-risk clinical predictors, low exercise capacity, or high-risk surgery should lead to preoperative stress testing for myocardial ischemia before the noncardiac surgery. A stress test is indicated in the patient described here because he has an intermediate-risk clinical profile and a poor exercise capacity. The painful hip precludes exercise, thus dobutamine echocardiography is the most appropriate answer. The guidelines do not recommend proceeding directly to coronary angiography unless the patient has evidence of an unstable coronary syndrome. Low risk patients may proceed directly to noncardiac surgery after the initiation of β-adrenergic blocker therapy.

30. Answer d.

The patient presents with a non–ST-segment elevation myocardial infarction. She has a high-risk profile in view of her age, electrocardiographic changes, and increased biomarker levels. An initial conservative medical management strategy is reasonable in this patient because she presented to a small community hospital. However, recurrence of chest pain the following day is a clear indication for transferring her to a facility with a cardiac catheterization laboratory. Several studies have found that glycoprotein IIb/IIIa inhibitors are effective in the management of non–ST-segment elevation acute coronary syndromes, particularly in high-risk patients who require percutaneous coronary intervention. Initiation of a glycoprotein IIb/IIIa inhibitor such as eptifibatide is effective for reducing recurrent ischemia and recurrent myocardial infarction before coronary intervention and improves outcome after percutaneous coronary intervention. Amlodipine is an effective antianginal agent, but it is unlikely to be helpful in a patient with such unstable myocardial ischemia. Stress testing is absolutely contraindicated in patients with an acute coronary

syndrome. Similarly, thrombolytics such as reteplase are not indicated in non–ST-segment elevation acute coronary syndromes.

31. Answer b.

The patient is a relatively young man who is asymptomatic and appears to be otherwise healthy with a good exercise capacity. He has a family history of premature coronary artery disease and is a smoker. Management in this patient should center on modification of risk factors. It is important to focus attention on conventional risk factors such as hyperlipidemia and diabetes mellitus. Therefore, measurement of a full lipid profile, including total cholesterol, triglycerides, high-density lipoprotein cholesterol, and low-density lipoprotein cholesterol is important. Measurement of fasting plasma glucose to screen for diabetes is also indicated. His blood pressure seems to be normal. Several novel biomarkers have been introduced lately, but their clinical utility remains to be established. Of these, serum lipoprotein (a) has been associated with an increased risk of coronary artery disease. It is reasonable to measure this in patients with premature coronary artery disease. Although there is no specific treatment for an increased level of lipoprotein (a), current recommendations are to aggressively manage the conventional lipids, such as low- and high-density cholesterol. The link between high-sensitivity C-reactive protein levels and coronary artery disease has been established, but the clinical utility is not clear. Current recommendations suggest that it is reasonable to measure C-reactive protein levels in patients at intermediate risk for coronary artery disease. Increased homocysteine levels have been associated with coronary artery disease. However, 2 recent, large randomized trials found no benefit of vitamin B and folic acid supplementation in patients with hyperhomocysteinemia. Therefore, there is no indication for measuring the plasma homocysteine level.

32. Answer e.

The patient presents with acute chest pain, and the electrocardiogram is diagnostic of an ST-segment–elevation inferior myocardial infarction. There are extensive electrocardiographic changes consistent with a large territory at risk. The electrocardiogram is not consistent with pericarditis, and therefore indomethacin is not indicated. Similarly, glycoprotein IIb/IIIa inhibitors such as abciximab have been shown to result in worse outcomes in patients with ST-segment–elevation myocardial infarction. Such patients require reperfusion therapy with either a thrombolytic or primary percutaneous coronary intervention. However, this patient's history of a stroke 6 months previously is an absolute contraindication to thrombolytic therapy. Other absolute contraindications include a hemorrhagic stroke at any time in the past, known intracranial neoplasm, active internal bleeding or active peptic ulcer disease, suspected aortic dissection, and blood pressure more than 180/110 mm Hg despite therapy. Therefore, the most suitable treatment for this patient is emergency coronary angiography and revascularization.

33. Answer a.

The patient presents with symptoms consistent with an acute coronary syndrome with ST-segment elevation on electrocardiography. Therefore, it was reasonable to perform emergency angiography, which showed normal coronary arteries. The differential diagnosis in such patients includes coronary spasm, coronary embolism, and myocarditis. However, the patient had a very characteristic regional wall motion abnormality on left ventriculography which involved the mid and apical segments of the left ventricle with sparing of the basal segments. This entity was recently recognized as the apical ballooning syndrome (takotsubo cardiomyopathy). Apical ballooning syndrome occurs predominantly in postmenopausal women and frequently is preceded by mental or physical stress. The patient had received bad news immediately before the onset of her symptoms, a situation that is not unusual for the syndrome. In some patients, apical ballooning syndrome develops after a physical stress such as surgery. Acute coronary syndrome was ruled out by coronary angiography. Myocarditis is a differential diagnosis, although it typically produces global hypokinesis. Pericarditis is not associated with such extensive regional wall motion abnormalities. Dilated cardiomyopathy does not present with acute symptoms.

34. Answer a.

The patient had a large anterior myocardial infarction. He is currently receiving appropriate medical treatment, and echocardiography shows a reduced ejection fraction. Several clinical trials have confirmed the utility of an implantable cardioverter-defibrillator (ICD) in patients with coronary artery disease and reduced ejection fraction. The second Multicenter Automated Defibrillator Implantation Trial (MADIT II) found that patients with ejection fractions 35% or less benefited from ICD placement if they had had a myocardial infarction in the past. The patient fulfills these criteria and hence is a candidate for an ICD. Stress testing is not indicated for patients who have undergone primary percutaneous coronary intervention because their coronary anatomy has already been established. Repeat coronary angiography is also not indicated in patients who have undergone primary percutaneous coronary intervention unless there are other lesions that require revascularization. This patient had mild coronary artery disease in the remaining coronary circulation. Although cardiac rehabilitation for acute myocardial infarction is beneficial after hospital dismissal, there is no evidence that continuing hospital-based cardiac rehabilitation provides long-term benefit. The addition of isosorbide mononitrate in the absence of angina or myocardial ischemia is not indicated in patients with coronary artery disease.

35. Answer e.

This patient with diabetes mellitus has evidence of chronic renal failure. She requires coronary angiography, which places her at risk for contrast nephropathy. It would be reasonable to take prophylactic measures such as intravenous hydration and administration of *N*-acetylcysteine. In the presence of abnormal renal function, it is important to discontinue use of the metformin before coronary angiography. There is an increased risk of lactic acidosis among diabetic patients with renal impairment in whom contrast nephropathy develops while they are receiving metformin. Therefore, it is best practice to discontinue use of metformin before elective procedures and resume its use 48 hours after the administration of a radiologic contrast agent provided the patient has an uncomplicated recovery.

36. Answer d.

The patient's physical findings are consistent with right-sided heart failure, and his symptoms suggest biventricular heart failure. There are no examination or imaging features of dilated ventricle or reduced ejection fraction. The presentation is consistent with his prior diagnosis of restrictive cardiomyopathy. In the absence of dysrhythmia, hypertension, or impaired systolic function, there is no documented role for amiodarone, β-adrenergic blockade, digoxin, or an angiotensin-type II–receptor blocker. The only effective treatment for symptomatic improvement is diuretic therapy.

37. Answer b.

An abrupt change in status should always raise the question of a rhythm change. The rhythm strip shows atrial flutter. The patient was previously in sinus rhythm, and this might be the cause of his clinical change. He would require appropriate attention to anticoagulation and thrombus issues as one attempts to restore sinus rhythm. The absence of angina and the stable ventricular function without inducible ischemia on a perfusion study make ischemia less likely and coronary angiography less attractive. The pacemaker is having trouble with the rhythm change. It is clearly capturing the rhythm at the terminal portion of the rhythm strip, but the earlier portion reveals fusion between native QRS complex and pacing spikes. One might refer the patient to a pacemaker specialist for review of the electrocardiogram and device interrogation, but sending the patient for a device extraction for malfunction would not be correct. Doubling the digoxin dose would be expected to double his trough digoxin level, and it is currently at the upper limits of the desired level. Some situations might call for an increase in β-adrenergic blocker dose, but given his blood pressure and age it would be excessive to increase his metoprolol by such a large amount.

38. Answer a.

The patient is receiving an appropriate regimen for a dilated cardiomyopathy, including an angiotensin-converting enzyme inhibitor and a β-adrenergic blocker with proven benefit in this subset of patients. He remains volume overloaded despite low-dose furosemide. In the acute management of decompensated heart failure, volume and hemodynamic management is paramount. His hemodynamics are well controlled, and thus a higher dose of diuretic is appropriate. He has been receiving carvedilol and lisinopril for only a short time, and doubling doses when blood pressure and heart rate are already optimal is ill-advised. Aldosterone antagonists are appropriately added in patients who remain symptomatic after chronic therapy with an angiotensin-converting enzyme inhibitor and β-adrenergic blocker or in patients who are hypokalemic and require ongoing significant doses of diuretic. There is no proven value to substituting an angiotensin receptor blocker in place of an angiotensin-converting enzyme inhibitor unless the patient has cough or angioedema thought to be due to the angiotensin-converting enzyme inhibitor.

39. Answer c.

The patient has known coronary artery disease and poorly controlled diabetes with new deterioration in cardiac function. Progression of coronary artery disease is the most likely possibility, and this potentially would be treated with methods other than medication. The absence of angina is less helpful in diabetics or patients with a history of prior silent infarctions. One would not add metformin to the regimen of a patient with heart failure and impaired cardiac function because of the risk of lactic acidosis if acute heart failure occurs. Although he has dyspnea and some scattered wheezes, the orthopnea, weight gain, edema, and jugular venous distention all strongly suggest that this is cardiac rather than pulmonary disease, and an evaluation of the lungs would be deferred if all other cardiac avenues were unrevealing. There are no cardiac structural or functional issues that are unresolved that would require alternative cardiac imaging such as transesophageal echocardiography or MRI.

40. Answer a.

The patient is ambulatory and euvolemic and is receiving appropriate drugs. One hopes that her ventricle will reverse remodel, but this process will take place over time. Careful follow-up as an outpatient is important with medication doses titrated up no more often than every 2 weeks unless hypertension develops. The mild tachycardia is compensatory for her poor ventricular function. Increasing the metoprolol or captopril dose would either render her profoundly hypotensive or take away her compensatory tachycardia. Unlike acute coronary syndromes in which aggressive increases in medications to decrease myocardial oxygen demand are imperative, patients with cardiomyopathy need a more gentle and slow upward increase

in medications. An implantable cardioverter-defibrillator may be indicated if the patient continues to have sufficiently severe ventricular dysfunction after chronic optimal medical therapy. It is too early to implant now for primary prevention. Had the patient presented with out-of-hospital cardiac arrest, implantation for secondary prevention would have been appropriate.

41. Answer e.

Nonsteroidal anti-inflammatory agents should be avoided by patients with dilated cardiomyopathy. They are fluid-retaining and potentially nephrotoxic. Allopurinol, ferrous gluconate, acetaminophen, and propoxyphene can all be administered safely to patients with dilated cardiomyopathy.

42. Answer c.

Patients with heart failure should follow fluid restriction. This guideline varies from case to case, but generally the total should be 2 to 2.5 L daily (this includes dietary intake). Patients with heart failure should take an active role in their self-management, which includes assessing how they feel on a daily basis and following their weight. A sodium-restricted diet is a cornerstone of therapy for most patients with heart failure. Some over-the-counter medications contribute to fluid retention or interact with cardiac medications, and patients should always check with health care providers before beginning herbal therapies.

4

Critical Care Medicine

Otis B. Rickman, DO

Critical care medicine encompasses multidisciplinary aspects of the management of severely ill patients. All areas of medicine may have relevance for critically ill patients, but this review focuses on aspects of cardiopulmonary monitoring and life support, technologic interventions, and disease states typically managed in the intensive care unit (ICU).

Cardiopulmonary Resuscitation and Rapid Response Teams

Sudden cardiac arrest is the leading cause of death in the United States. Most persons with sudden cardiac arrest have ventricular fibrillation at some point in their arrest. Resuscitation is most effective if defibrillation is provided within 5 minutes after collapse. Effective cardiopulmonary resuscitation (CPR) is important both before and after shock delivery and can triple a patient's chance of survival.

The *2005 American Heart Association Guidelines for Cardiopulmonary Resuscitation and Emergency Cardiovascular Care* simplified the basic life support sequences, particularly for lay rescuers, and minimized the differences in the steps and techniques of CPR for infant, child, and adult victims. A universal compression-ventilation ratio (30:2) is recommended for all solo rescuers of infants (excluding newborns), children, and adults. Health care providers should deliver rescue breaths without chest compressions at a rate of 10 to 12 breaths per minute for adult patients with a pulse. They should also deliver cycles of compressions and ventilations when an advanced airway is not yet in place. After the airway is secured, there is no need to cycle between breathing and compressions: they should occur simultaneously at 12 breaths per minute and 100 compressions per minute without pauses for breaths. The guidelines should be consulted for more detail about the role of CPR, the coordination of CPR with defibrillation, the role of CPR in advanced life support, and basic and advanced life support for newborns, infants, and children.

Rapid response teams, also known as medical emergency teams, have emerged as a method to "expand the walls" of the ICU and attempt to identify critically ill patients before full cardiac arrest. These teams are generally made up of a physician, a critical care nurse, and a respiratory therapist. The key element for proper function of this system is that specific calling criteria have been developed, general ward staff have been educated to recognize these criteria, and the team can be activated by anyone. After implementing these teams, institutions have demonstrated a trend toward reduced mortality and have reduced unplanned ICU admissions.

- Sudden cardiac death is a leading cause of death in the United States.
- Effective CPR is important both before and after shock delivery and can triple a patient's chance of survival.
- The *2005 American Heart Association Guidelines for Cardiopulmonary Resuscitation and Emergency Cardiovascular Care* should be reviewed.
- Rapid response teams have demonstrated a trend toward reduced mortality and unplanned ICU admissions.

Airway Management

Expertise in management of the airway in critically ill patients, which pose unique challenges, is a required skill for anyone practicing in the ICU. Elective airway management in the operating room (OR) is associated with low rates of complication. However, emergent airway management in the ICU is associated with higher complication rates (about 25%) due to patient comorbidities, limited evaluation and planning time, and limited reserve of patients (respiratory failure and shock). With these limitations, many of the tools, equipment, and drugs that are available in the OR are not practical to use in the ICU. Components of successful management include assessment; preparation of the environment, patient, and equipment and drugs; and, most importantly, having a backup plan available to implement immediately if needed.

Endotracheal intubation allows maximal control of the airway, enables the delivery of specific inspired oxygen concentrations and positive pressure ventilation, and provides protection from aspiration. Indications for intubation include airway protection in cases of obstruction or loss of normal gag and cough reflexes, central nervous system injury or sedation with loss of normal control of ventilation, and any cause of respiratory failure requiring positive pressure–assisted ventilation. Orotracheal intubation is usually achieved through direct visualization with a laryngoscope. In experienced hands, this procedure should be relatively quick and safe.

Complications of intubation include vomiting and aspiration, hypoxemia during the procedure, and inadvertent intubation of the esophagus.

An airway assessment of difficulty in performing mask ventilation or difficult intubation should be attempted on all patients (Table 4-1). Since a full airway evaluation is possible in only a minority of ICU patients, alternative schemes such as the LEMON (*l*ook, *M*allampati, *o*bstruction, and *n*eck mobility) have been devised to help stratify risk. The Mallampati classification schema is widely used and consists of classes I (easy) to IV (difficult intubation).

1. Class I—entire tonsil is clearly visible
2. Class II—upper half of tonsil fossa is visible
3. Class III—soft and hard palate are clearly visible
4. Class IV—only hard palate is visible

Before intubation, the equipment, the environment, and the patient should be prepared. Being prepared for unforseen problems is of utmost importance. Table 4-2 lists elements required for proper preparation.

Successful intubation is often dependent on adequate pharmacotherapy (Table 4-3). The typical sequence followed in the OR is premedication, induction, and paralysis. Owing to unique challenges in the ICU, this is not always practical or advisable. Many induction agents used in the OR cause vasodilation and hypotension, a condition to which ICU patients are already predisposed. The majority of ICU patients should be considered to have a full stomach and would be candidates for rapid-sequence intubation; however, the risks of obliterating spontaneous ventilation should be carefully weighed against the probability of "cannot intubate or ventilate." It should also be noted that the most widely used short-acting paralytic, succinylcholine, often cannot be used owing to comorbidities (burns, upper motor neuron lesions, myopathy, crush injury, renal failure, and prolonged immobility) seen in the ICU population. In general, spontaneous breathing should be maintained in patients who are predicted to be difficult to intubate.

- Managing the airway in critically ill patients poses unique challenges.
- Successful management is predicated on proper preparation and planning.
- A backup method to direct laryngoscopy should be readily available.
- Use muscle relaxants with extreme caution.

Venous Access and Monitoring

Central Venous Catheterization

The first choices for access in patients requiring intravenous therapy are the peripheral veins. The most common locations for central access are the internal jugular, subclavian, and femoral veins. Indications for central venous access are lack of adequate peripheral veins, need for hypertonic or phlebitic medications or solutions, need for long-term access, measurement of central pressures, and access for procedures (hemodialysis, cardiac pacing).

Relative contraindications include inexperience of the practitioner, coagulopathy, inability to identify landmarks, infection or burn at the entry site, and thrombosis of the proposed central venous site. Central venous catheters are usually placed over a guidewire (modified Seldinger technique).

Complications of central venous catheterization include bloodstream infections, cardiac arrhythmias, pneumothorax, air embolism, catheter or guidewire embolism, catheter knotting, bleeding, and other potential complications of needle or catheter misplacement.

Table 4-1   Predictors of Difficult Mask Ventilation and Intubation

Difficult Mask Ventilation	Difficult Intubation
Age >55 y	Short thick neck
Body mass index >26 kg/m^2	Limited neck flexion or extension
Edentulous	Thyromental distance <3 finger breadths
Male	Long upper incisors
Mallampati class IV	Presence of overbite
Beard	Inability to jut mandibular incisors anterior to upper incisors
History of snoring	Inability to open mouth >3 cm
	Mallampati class >II
	High arched palate

Table 4-2   Elements and Equipment Required for Successful Endotracheal Intubation

Adequate personnel
Proper patient positioning
100% oxygen
Well-fitting bag valve mask
Suctioning equipment
Nasal & oral airways
Working laryngoscope
Various types & sizes of laryngoscope blades
Endotracheal tubes with intact cuffs
Tube stylet
10-mL syringe
Head rest
Working intravenous line
Induction drugs
Vasoconstrictor drugs
End-tidal carbon dioxide detector
Method to secure tube

Table 4-3   Commonly Used Drugs for Airway Management in the Intensive Care Unit

Midazolam
Fentanyl
Etomidate
Propofol
Succinylcholine
Nondepolarizing agents

- Pulmonary artery catheterization provides useful clinical information.
- Misinterpretation or artifacts may limit usefulness of data and may cause harm.
- Unique patterns are seen in the various shock states.

Pulmonary Artery Catheterization

Although common use (or overuse) of pulmonary artery catheterization has been criticized, data from pulmonary artery catheterization (Table 4-4) may aid in the diagnosis and treatment of many disorders encountered in ICUs. The usefulness of these measurements may be limited by the understanding of the physician interpreting the values. Table 4-5 shows hemodynamic patterns in the 4 shock states.

Indications for pulmonary artery catheterization include shock states, pulmonary edema, oliguric renal failure, indeterminate pulmonary hypertension, and myocardial and valvular disorders. Intravascular volume may be assessed more accurately, and the effects of therapeutic interventions (volume, vasodilator therapy, or inotropics) may be evaluated. Mixed venous oxygen saturation may also be measured (see detailed discussion later in this chapter). This may be particularly useful in assessing the effects of positive end-expiratory pressure (PEEP) on oxygen delivery (ie, improving arterial saturation but potentially decreasing cardiac output).

Complications of pulmonary artery catheterization include arrhythmias, right bundle branch block, complete heart block in patients with preexisting left bundle branch block, vascular or right ventricular perforation, thrombosis and embolism, catheter knotting, infection, and pulmonary infarction or rupture due to persistent wedging or overdistention of the balloon.

Systemic Oxygen Transport

In addition to providing numerous measured and calculated values, pulmonary artery catheters can facilitate measurement of systemic oxygen transport (Table 4-6). Under normal circumstances, oxygen demand by the tissues is met by the supply. Oxygen delivery is defined by cardiac output (CO) multiplied by arterial oxygen content (CaO_2):

$$O_2 \text{ delivery} = CO \times CaO_2$$

Although cardiac output may decrease, oxygen consumption per unit time ($\dot{V}O_2$) of the tissues may be maintained by increased oxygen extraction. The content of oxygen in the blood is the total amount of oxygen bound to hemoglobin (Hgb) plus the amount dissolved.

$$O_2 \text{ content: } CxO_2 = \underset{\text{(Bound)}}{(1.34 \times Hgb \times SxO_2)} + \underset{\text{(Dissolved)}}{(0.003 \times PxO_2)}$$

where x is arterial, venous, or capillary.

Under steady state conditions, the amount of oxygen used by the tissues equals the amount taken up by the lungs. The oxygen uptake ($\dot{V}O_2$) can be defined by the amount of oxygen leaving the lungs in pulmonary venous blood minus the amount of oxygen coming into the lungs in the pulmonary arteries. This should be familiar as the Fick equation:

$$\dot{V}O_2 = CO(CaO_2 - C\bar{v}O_2)$$

A shunt is defined by perfusion (Q) in the absence of ventilation ($\dot{V}$) (ie, $\dot{V}/Q$–0). With a pure shunt, PaO_2 does not increase even

Table 4-4   Hemodynamic Data Obtained With Pulmonary Artery Catheterization

Variable	Normal Values
Right atrial pressure (RAP)	2-8 mm Hg
Pulmonary arterial pressure (PAP)	16-24/5-12 mm Hg
Pulmonary capillary wedge pressure (PCWP)	5-12 mm Hg
Cardiac output (CO)	4-6 L/min
Cardiac index (CI = CO/body surface area)	2.5-3 L/min/m^2
Stroke volume (SV = CO/heart rate)	50-100 mL/beat
Stroke volume index (SVI = SV/body surface area)	35-50 mL/m^2

Systemic vascular resistance
    [SVR = (blood pressure – RAP)/CO]
	10-15 mm Hg/L/min
	    (×80 to convert to 800-1,200 dyne·s·cm^{-5})

Pulmonary vascular resistance
    [PVR = (PAP – PCWP)/CO]
	1.5-2.5 mm Hg/L/min
	    (100-200 dyne·s·cm^{-5})

Table 4-5   Hemodynamic Patterns in Various Shock States

Shock State	RAP	PCWP	SVR	CO
Hypovolemic	↓	↓	↑	↓
Distributive	↓→	↓→	↓	↑
Cardiogenic	↑	↑	↑	↓
Tamponade	Equalization of pressures			

Abbreviations: CO, cardiac output; PCWP, pulmonary capillary wedge pressure; RAP, right atrial pressure; SVR, systemic vascular resistance.

Table 4-6   Oxygen Transport Variables

Variable	Reference Values
Mixed venous oxygen saturation ($S\bar{v}O_2$), %	70-75
Oxygen delivery (DO_2), mL/min	950-1150
Oxygen uptake ($\dot{V}O_2$), mL/min	250
Oxygen extraction ratio (O_2ER), %	20-30

though the fraction of inspired oxygen (FIO_2) is increased to 100%. The normal shunt fraction is less than 3% to 5% of the total cardiac output. The shunt fraction is measured with the person breathing 100% oxygen and is expressed as follows:

$$\frac{Qs}{Qt} = \frac{CC'O_2 - CaO_2}{CC'O_2 - C\bar{V}O_2} = \frac{P(A\text{-}a)O_2 \times 0.003}{P(A\text{-}a)O_2 \times 0.003 + (Ca - C\bar{V})O_2}$$

where Qs is the portion of cardiac output shunted, Qt is the total cardiac output, $CC'O_2$ is capillary oxygen content, CaO_2 is arterial oxygen content, and $C\bar{V}O_2$ is venous oxygen content.

* Under normal conditions, oxygen demand is met by supply.
* When oxygen delivery is decreased, oxygen consumption can be maintained by increased extraction.
* The Fick equation can be used to calculate cardiac output.
* The normal shunt fraction is <5%; pure shunts do not improve with 100% oxygen.

Mixed Venous Oxygen Saturation
Many applications of the Fick equation are important in managing critically ill patients. One application involves continuous monitoring of mixed venous oxygen saturation ($S\bar{v}O_2$) by a specialized type of pulmonary artery catheter. Expressing oxygen content in terms of saturation and rearranging the Fick equation to solve for $S\bar{v}O_2$ yields the following:

$$S\bar{v}O_2 = SaO_2 - \frac{\dot{V}O_2}{CO \times Hgb \times 1.34}$$

where SaO_2 is arterial saturation, CO is cardiac output, and Hgb is hemoglobin concentration.

Note that decreased mixed venous oxygen saturation may be due to decreased arterial saturation, increased oxygen consumption, decreased cardiac output, or decreased hemoglobin. Certain disease states, particularly early sepsis, may be characterized by normal or increased mixed venous oxygen saturation because cardiac output initially increases along with impaired oxygen uptake by the tissues. Later in sepsis, due to decreased cardiac output, which causes decreased delivery of oxygen, the mixed venous oxygen saturation typically decreases.

* Decreased mixed venous oxygen saturation may result from decreased arterial saturation, increased oxygen consumption, decreased cardiac output, or decreased hemoglobin.
* In early sepsis, mixed venous oxygen saturation is normal or increased.

Pulmonary Artery Catheter Controversies
In case-control studies among patients who had a similar severity of illness, the use of a pulmonary artery catheter was associated with higher mortality than no use of a catheter. However, the validity of these findings is uncertain, and catheter use is still common clinical practice. Recent prospective trials of pulmonary artery catheterization in high-risk surgical patients and medical patients with acute respiratory distress syndrome (ARDS) randomly assigned to a conservative or liberal fluid management strategy showed no difference in outcome (ie, no clear evidence of benefit or harm) between catheterization and control groups.

Use of the pulmonary capillary wedge pressure (PCWP) as an indicator of left ventricular end-diastolic pressure assumes a continuous hydrostatic column extending from the pulmonary capillary to the left atrium. Although digital displays of PCWP are usually available, the pressure wave should be examined for potential artifacts and for the degree of respiratory variation. Because varying intrathoracic pressure may be sensed by the pulmonary artery catheter, the end-expiration PCWP should be recorded. Even with these measures, PCWP may be influenced by airway pressure and, thus, may not accurately reflect ventricular filling pressure, especially with high levels of PEEP.

* PCWP is an indicator of left ventricular end-diastolic pressure.
* PCWP may be influenced by airway pressure, especially with high levels of PEEP.

Catheter-Related Infections
Catheter-related infections are usually attributed to the migration of bacteria from the skin along the catheter tract. Catheter-related infection is usually defined by more than 15 colony-forming units per milliliter on semiquantitative culture of the catheter tip. Catheter-related bacteremia is defined by similar bacterial growth and blood cultures that are positive for the same organism as on the catheter tip. Risk factors include infected catheter site or cutaneous breakdown, multiple manipulations, the number of catheter lumens, and the duration of use of the same site (particularly after 3 or 4 days).

Treatment should include catheter removal and replacement at another site if necessary.

- Catheter-related infections usually are attributed to migration of bacteria from the skin along the catheter tract.
- Risk factors include infected catheter site or cutaneous breakdown, multiple manipulations, number of catheter lumens, and duration of use of same site.
- Catheters at an infected site should be removed.

Respiratory Failure

Effective functioning of the respiratory system requires normal central nervous system control, neuromuscular transmission and bellows function, and gas exchange at the alveolar-capillary level. Respiratory failure may result from disease at any of these levels. The 2 broad categories of respiratory failure are hypoxemic and hypercapnic.

Hypoxemic Respiratory Failure

Effective gas exchange requires adequate alveolar ventilation for the elimination of carbon dioxide, oxygen uptake across the alveolar-capillary membrane, and the delivery of oxygen to tissues. *Hypoxemia* may result from the following:

1. Decrease in the inspired partial pressure of oxygen (eg, at high altitude, including air travel or interruption of oxygen supply)
2. Hypoventilation
3. Ventilation-perfusion ($\dot{V}/Q$) mismatch
4. Shunt
5. Diffusion barrier

Estimation of the alveolar-arterial (A-a) gradient for oxygen is essential in analyzing the cause of hypoxemia (Table 4-7).

Alveolar Air Equation and the A-a Gradient

Alveolar gas consists of inspired gases saturated with water vapor. The alveolus also contains carbon dioxide delivered from the blood. The sum of the partial pressures of all gases present equals the ambient barometric pressure. The *alveolar air equation* defines this relationship as follows:

Table 4-7   Causes of Hypoxemia With Normal or Increased Alveolar-Arterial (A-a) Gradient

Normal A-a Gradient	Increased A-a Gradient
Low P_{IO_2} & low PB	$\dot{V}/Q$ mismatch
Low F_{IO_2}	Diffusion
Hypoventilation	Shunt

Abbreviations: F_{IO_2}, fraction of inspired oxygen; PB, barometric pressure; P_{IO_2}, partial pressure of inspired oxygen; $\dot{Q}$, perfusion; $\dot{V}$, ventilation.

$$P_{AO_2} = F_{IO_2}(PB - 47) - \frac{P_{aCO_2}}{R}$$

where P_{AO_2} is alveolar partial pressure, PB is barometric pressure (about 760 mm Hg at sea level), P_{H_2O} is water vapor pressure (47 mm Hg), and R is the respiratory quotient ($\dot{V}_{CO_2}/\dot{V}_{O_2}$, which is normally about 0.8). The simplified equation is

$$P_{AO_2} = F_{IO_2}(PB - 47) - \frac{P_{aCO_2}}{0.8}$$

Breathing room air ($F_{IO_2} = 0.21$) at sea level yields

$$P_{AO_2} = 150 - \frac{40}{0.8}$$

Normal P_{AO_2} is approximately 100 mm Hg.

The A-a oxygen difference is defined by P_{AO_2} minus P_{aO_2}, which is normally less than 10 to 20 mm Hg when breathing room air. The A-a gradient normally increases to approximately 50 to 100 mm Hg as the F_{IO_2} increases from 0.21 to 1.0, and it also increases slightly with age. Hypoxemia due to hypoventilation is characterized by increased P_{aCO_2} and decreased P_{aO_2} but a relatively normal A-a gradient. In hypoxemia due to ventilation-perfusion mismatch, an increased A-a gradient is present.

- Hypoxemia due to hypoventilation is characterized by an increased P_{aCO_2}, decreased P_{aO_2}, and a normal A-a gradient.
- Normal P_{AO_2} is approximately 100 mm Hg.

Hypercapnic Respiratory Failure

Hypercarbic or hypercapnic respiratory failure is caused by inadequate alveolar ventilation that is generally the result of airway obstruction, increased dead space or failure of respiratory bellows (chest wall, diaphragm, or neural control) (Table 4-8).

The partial pressure of carbon dioxide (P_{aCO_2}) in the blood is directly proportional to the amount of carbon dioxide produced ($\dot{V}_{O_2}$) and inversely proportional to alveolar ventilation ($\dot{V}_A$):

$$P_{aCO_2} = k \frac{\dot{V}_{CO_2}}{\dot{V}_A}$$

Alveolar ventilation is equal to total ventilation ($\dot{V}_E$) minus dead space ventilation ($\dot{V}_D$). Thus, physiologic dead space is defined by the portion of a breath that does not participate in gas exchange. Dead space volume (V_D) may be anatomical (conducting airways) or alveolar (areas of ventilation that receive no perfusion):

$$\dot{V}_A = \dot{V}_E - (V_D \times f)$$

where f = breaths per minute.

Table 4-8   Causes of Hypoventilation and Hypercapnic Respiratory Failure

Central nervous system	Muscular dysfunction
Drugs	Muscular dystrophies
Hyperthyroidism	Guillain-Barré syndrome
Ondine curse	Myasthenia gravis
Brainstem injury	Amyotrophic lateral sclerosis
Metabolic alkalosis	Malnutrition
Chest wall disorders	Acidosis
Kyphoscoliosis	Hypoxemia
Rib fractures	Anemia
Pain	Low cardiac output
Flail chest	Steroids
Diaphragm disorders	Aminoglycosides
Rupture, myopathy	Calcium channel blockers
Spinal cord & peripheral	Post-paralytic condition
nervous system	Detraining, atrophy,
Lesion at C3 to C5	overuse fatigue
Neuropathy	Increased workload
Trauma	

Dead space ventilation can be calculated using the following formula (Bohr equation):

$$\frac{V_D}{V_T} + \frac{PaCO_2 - PECO_2}{PaCO_2}$$

where PCO_2 is the partial pressure of expired carbon dioxide, and V_T is tidal volume. Normally V_D/V_T is less than 0.25 to 0.30.

The dead space-to-tidal volume ratio is calculated by measuring the partial pressure of carbon dioxide in an arterial blood gas sample ($PaCO_2$) and an expired gas sample ($PECO_2$).

- Physiologic dead space is defined by the portion of breath not participating in gas exchange.
- Increased dead space leads to decreased elimination of carbon dioxide at any given level of total minute ventilation.

Mechanical Ventilation

Mechanical ventilation may be valuable in various conditions of respiratory failure, including loss of respiratory control, neuromuscular or respiratory pump failure, and disorders of gas exchange. Many specific variables that have been suggested as criteria (or general guidelines) for ventilator support are listed in Table 4-9.

Physiologic Definitions and Relationships
To understand mechanical ventilation, including its targets, patient-ventilator interactions, and ventilator alarms, one must have a basic understanding of lung mechanics.

Lung Volumes
Total lung capacity (TLC) is the total volume of gas in the chest at the

Table 4-9   Criteria for Ventilator Support

Respiratory rate >30/min
Minute ventilation >10 L/min
Maximal inspiratory pressure <–20 cm H_2O
Vital capacity <10 mL/kg
PaO_2 <60 mm Hg with FIO_2 >0.60
PaO_2/FIO_2 <100-150
$P(A-a)O_2$ >300 mm Hg with FIO_2=1.0
V_D/V_T >0.60
$PaCO_2$ >50 mm Hg

Abbreviations: A-a, alveolar-arterial; FIO_2, fraction of inspired oxygen; V_D, dead space volume; V_T, tidal volume.

end of a maximal inspiration. *Vital capacity* (VC) is the volume of a maximal breath (expired or inspired). *Tidal volume* (V_T) is the volume of a normal breath. *Functional residual capacity* (FRC) is the lung volume at the end of a normal expiration. It reflects the relaxation point of the respiratory system or the point at which outward recoil of the chest wall is balanced by inward recoil of the lungs.

Compliance
Compliance (C) of the lungs or respiratory system is defined by the change in volume (ΔV) for a given change in pressure (ΔP):

$$C_{STATIC} = \frac{\Delta V}{\Delta P}$$

where ΔV is measured in milliliters and ΔP in centimeters of water. Normal compliance is approximately 200 mL/cm H_2O. Emphysema causes the loss of recoil and, thus, increased compliance. Most other disease states, particularly interstitial diseases, fibrosis, pulmonary edema, and ARDS, cause decreased compliance (ie, "stiff" lungs, or increased transpulmonary pressure for a given volume change).

- Normal compliance is approximately 200 mL/cm H_2O.
- Emphysema causes the loss of recoil and increased compliance.
- Interstitial diseases, fibrosis, pulmonary edema, and ARDS cause decreased compliance.

Resistance
Resistance (R) to airflow is defined by the change in pressure (ΔP) for a given change in flow ($\Delta \dot{V}$):

$$R = \frac{\Delta P}{\Delta \dot{V}}$$

where ΔP is measured in centimeters of water and $\Delta \dot{V}$ in liters per second. Common causes of increased airway resistance include biting of endotracheal tube, bronchospasm, and airway secretions.

- Common causes of increased airway resistance are biting of endotracheal tube, bronchospasm, and airway secretions.

The total pressure required to inflate the respiratory system (spontaneously or with a mechanical ventilator) is the pressure required to overcome elastic recoil (due primarily to lungs and chest wall) plus the pressure to overcome flow resistance (due primarily to airways and endotracheal tube):

$$P \text{ inflation} = \frac{\Delta V}{C_{STATIC}} + R \times \Delta \dot{V}$$

(Elastic Load)   (Resistive Load)

Modes of Mechanical Ventilation
Modes of mechanical ventilation refers to the pattern of cycling of the machine breath and its relation to the spontaneous breaths of the patient (eg, assist/control mode, intermittent mandatory ventilation, and pressure support ventilation). Table 4-10 shows the basic settings of a ventilator.

Volume Preset Assist/Control Mode
The *volume preset assist/control mode* is defined by a machine-assisted breath for every inspiratory effort by the patient. If no spontaneous breaths occur during a preset time interval, a controlled breath of predetermined tidal volume is delivered by the ventilator. The backup rate determines the minimum minute ventilation the patient will receive. The advantage of assist/control mode ventilation is that it allows maximal rest for the patient and maximal control of ventilation. The disadvantage is that hyperventilation or air trapping (or both) can occur in patients making rapid inspiratory efforts.

Pressure Support Ventilation
Pressure support ventilation may be used to assist spontaneously breath

Table 4-10   Basic Ventilator Settings

Mode
  Volume targeted
    Complete mechanical ventilation
    Assist/control
  Pressure targeted
    Pressure support
    Pressure control
    Pressure control inverse ratio
  Mixed
    Synchronized intermittent mandatory ventilation
Tidal volume
  Standard: 10mL/kg ideal body weight
  In adult respiratory distress syndrome: 6 mL/kg ideal body weight
Rate—titrated to desired minute ventilation for P_{CO_2}
Positive end-expiratory pressure & fraction of inspired oxygen
  (F_{IO_2})—titrated to F_{IO_2} <60%
Inspiratory flow rate
  Set to meet patient demand
  Allow adequate time for exhalation

ing patients, with or without intermittent mandatory ventilation (IMV) breaths. In this technique, for each inspiratory effort by the patient, the ventilator delivers a high rate of flow of inspired gas, up to a preset pressure limit. This pressure support occurs only during the spontaneous inspiratory effort, so that the rate and pattern of respiration are determined by the patient.

Volume Preset Intermittent Mandatory Ventilation
Volume preset intermittent mandatory ventilation allows a preset number of machine-assisted breaths of a given tidal volume. Between machine breaths, patients may breathe spontaneously. The IMV mode was developed as a mode for weaning patients from the ventilator so that the number of mechanical breaths could be decreased gradually, allowing for increasing spontaneous ventilation. However, recent trials have shown that this mode of weaning is inferior to weaning with T-piece trials or pressure support ventilation.

* Assist/control mode ventilation allows maximal rest for the patient and maximal control of ventilation, but it may result in hyperventilation in patients with high intrinsic breathing rates.
* IMV is inferior to other weaning techniques (T-piece trials or pressure support ventilation).
* Pressure support ventilation may improve patient ventilator synchrony.

Table 4-11 summarizes basic modes of ventilation.

PEEP
PEEP is intended to increase functional residual capacity, recruit partially collapsed alveoli, improve lung compliance, and improve ventilation-perfusion matching. An adverse effect of PEEP is an excessive increase in intrathoracic pressure with decreased cardiac output. Overdistention of lung units may also worsen gas exchange because of ventilator-induced lung injury. At levels of PEEP greater than 10 to 15 cm H_2O, barotrauma is of particular concern. The optimal, or best, PEEP may be defined as the lowest level of PEEP needed to achieve satisfactory oxygen delivery at a nontoxic F_{IO_2} (<60%).

* PEEP recruits partially collapsed alveoli, improves lung compliance, and decreases atelectotrauma (recruitment and derecruitment of alveoli).
* PEEP may decrease cardiac output due to an increase in intrathoracic pressure.
* The optimal, or best, PEEP is the lowest level of PEEP needed to achieve satisfactory oxygenation at a nontoxic F_{IO_2} (<60%).

Approach to the Alarming Ventilator
The approach to an alarming ventilator begins with disconnecting the patient from the ventilator and hand bagging the patient to relieve pressure in breath stacking or tension pneumothorax. Increasing sedation may be appropriate if evaluation shows no change in peak or plateau pressures and there was evidence of dyssynchrony with the ventilator. Mucous plugging, biting the tube, or bronchospasm causes an increase in airway resistance, resulting in an increase in peak pressure without a change in plateau pressure.

Table 4-11 Summary of Modes of Ventilation[a]

Ventilation	Rate	Volume	Trigger	Effect of Spontaneous Breath
CMV	Physician	Physician	Time	Nothing
PS	Patient	Compliance	Patient	Pressure supported
AC	Both	Physician	Time & patient	Volume supported
SIMV	Both	Physician	Time & patient	Pressure or volume supported

Abbreviations: AC, assist/control; CMV, complete mechanical ventilation; PS, pressure support; SIMV, synchronized intermittent mandatory ventilation.
[a] Table indicates whether patient or physician determines rate, time, and volume delivered and what happens when spontaneous breath occurs.

Both peak and plateau pressures increase when there is a change in compliance such as worsening edema, mainstem intubation, breath stacking (intrinsic PEEP), or tension pneumothorax.

Complications and Prophylaxis

Complications of mechanical ventilation may be related to airway access, physiologic responses to positive pressure, and complications related to other organ systems. Examples are given in Table 4-12. Other complications, such as pulmonary embolism or malnutrition, may also reflect the underlying disease state. Management of these complications requires ongoing surveillance and recognition. In patients receiving mechanical ventilation, pneumonia may be difficult to diagnose because pulmonary infiltrates are frequently present, tracheal secretions may be colonized by bacteria, and signs such as fever and leukocytosis are frequently blunted. In this setting, quantitative cultures of secretions obtained from bronchoalveolar lavage or protected-specimen brush may aid in the diagnosis of ventilator-associated pneumonia. Prophylaxis is commonly given to reduce stress-related gastritis and ulceration. H$_2$-blockers may increase colonization of the respiratory tract by gram-negative bacteria. Sucralfate or frequent use of antacids is an alternative. The hemodynamic complications of increased intrathoracic pressure may be overcome with the administration of fluid; however, there is often a coexisting condition of capillary leak and pulmonary edema that may worsen.

* Pneumonia may be difficult to diagnose in patients receiving mechanical ventilation.

Table 4-12 Complications of Mechanical Ventilation

Airway injury, bleeding, infection
Ventilator malfunction—leaks, power loss, incorrect settings, or alarm failures
Barotrauma; pneumothorax; interstitial, subcutaneous, or mediastinal air
Decreased right ventricular filling, increased right ventricular afterload, decreased cardiac output, hypotension
Gastrointestinal tract bleeding, stress gastritis, ulceration
Decreased urine output
Alteration in intracranial pressure

* Prophylaxis is commonly given to reduce stress-related gastritis and ulceration.
* H$_2$-blockers may increase colonization of the respiratory tract by gram-negative bacteria; sucralfate or frequent use of antacids is an alternative.

Intrinsic Positive End-Expiratory Pressure

An important and occasionally subtle complication of positive pressure ventilation is called *intrinsic PEEP*, *auto PEEP*, *breath stacking*, or *dynamic hyperinflation*. In this phenomenon, inadequate time during the expiratory phase of the respiratory cycle results in a mechanically assisted breath being delivered before passive expiration of the lungs is complete. Thus, a new machine breath is delivered before the previous breath is completely exhaled. This may worsen hyperinflation, increase intrathoracic pressure, reduce venous return, and worsen the associated complications (eg, barotrauma), especially in patients with airway obstruction. Intrinsic PEEP may occur in spontaneously breathing patients with obstructive airway disease, but the effect is most important in mechanically ventilated patients. Treatment typically involves optimizing bronchodilator therapy and altering the ventilator cycle to allow maximal expiratory time.

Oxygen Toxicity

Pulmonary oxygen toxicity appears to be the result of direct exposure to high tensions of inspired oxygen or alveolar oxygen. For adults, oxygen toxicity is not believed to be a major clinical concern if the FIO$_2$ is less than 0.40 to 0.50. Higher levels of inspired oxygen may be associated with acute tracheobronchitis (most likely an irritant effect). After several days of exposure, a syndrome of diffuse alveolar damage and lung injury may develop. The pathologic features may resemble those of ARDS.

* Pulmonary oxygen toxicity is the result of direct exposure to high tensions of inspired oxygen or alveolar oxygen.
* The syndrome of diffuse alveolar damage and lung injury may develop.

Tracheostomy

For patients who require prolonged mechanical ventilation or airway support, the timing of tracheostomy is controversial. The use of high-volume, low-pressure endotracheal tube cuffs has decreased the frequency of tracheal injury and stenosis caused by prolonged intubation. Tracheostomy has the advantages of decreased laryngeal injury, increased patient comfort, ease of suctioning, and, in certain patients, allowance for oral ingestion and speech. Complications may include tracheal injury and stenosis, bleeding, tracheoesophageal fistula, and possibly increased bronchial or pulmonary infections. Tracheostomy is commonly considered for patients who have needed or are expected to need intubation and mechanical ventilation for more than 2 to 4 weeks.

- High-volume, low-pressure endotracheal tube cuffs have decreased the frequency of tracheal injury and stenosis.
- Tracheostomy is considered for patients who have needed or are expected to need intubation and mechanical ventilation for more than 2 to 4 weeks.

Weaning

Patients are candidates for weaning from mechanical ventilation when they are hemodynamically stable and have adequately recovered from respiratory failure. It is important to identify these patients in order to decrease costs, ICU lengths of stay, and infectious and other complications of mechanical ventilation. The most effective way to wean patients is with a nursing or respiratory therapist protocol. General criteria are listed in Table 4-13. The rapid shallow breathing index (RSBI) is a sensitive and specific marker of weaning failure:

$$RSBI = \text{Respiratory frequency/Tidal volume} = f/V_T$$

If $f/V_T > 105$, there is a 95% chance of spontaneous breathing trial failure; if $f/V_T \leq 105$, there is an 80% chance of success.

If the patient seems ready for weaning, a spontaneous breathing trial should be instituted. This is typically done with a T-tube system. A daily interruption of sedation and institution of a 2-hour T piece trial leads to extubation 1.5 days earlier and decreases by half the rate of mechanical ventilation for more than 21 days. A weaning protocol is presented in Figure 4-1.

Acute Respiratory Distress Syndrome

Diffuse lung injury with acute hypoxic respiratory failure may result from various injuries. Acute lung injury is a frequent primary cause

Table 4-13 General Weaning Criteria

Inspiratory pressure >–20 cm
Tidal volume >5 mL/kg
Vital capacity >10 mL/kg
Resting minute ventilation <10 L/min
Able to double resting minute ventilation
Satisfactory gas exchange (PaO_2 >60 mm Hg on FIO_2 <40%)
Not unstable, no ischemia
Adequate mental status

Abbreviation: FIO_2, fraction of inspired oxygen.

of critical illness and may occur as a complication or a coexisting feature of multisystem disease. *ARDS* is commonly defined as diffuse acute lung injury with the following major features: diffuse pulmonary infiltrates, severe hypoxemia due to shunting and ventilation-perfusion mismatch, and normal or low pulmonary capillary wedge pressure (ie, noncardiogenic pulmonary edema) (Table 4-14). Mortality from all causes averages about 50%. For nearly 30 years after this syndrome was described, no single therapy was shown to alter outcome, although gradual improvement in overall mortality was attributed to multidisciplinary ICU management. Recently in prospective, controlled trials, a strategy of mechanical ventilation with reduced tidal volumes was associated with improved survival (discussed below).

- Diffuse lung injury with hypoxic respiratory failure may result from various injuries.
- Among patients with ARDS, mortality from all causes averages approximately 50%.

Etiology, Pathophysiology, and Prognosis

ARDS was described initially as a posttraumatic or shock-induced injury, but it occurs with various states (Table 4-15). The relative risks of developing ARDS have been estimated from studies of predisposed groups. The greatest frequency is among patients with sepsis (approximately 40%), gastric aspiration (30%), multiple transfusions (25%), pulmonary contusion (20%), disseminated intravascular coagulation (20%), pneumonia requiring ICU management (12%), and trauma with long-bone or pelvic fractures (5%).

The pathophysiologic mechanism of ARDS depends on damage to the alveolar-capillary unit. The earliest histologic changes are endothelial swelling, followed by edema and inflammation. Mononuclear inflammation, loss of alveolar type I cells, and protein deposition in the form of hyaline membranes may occur within 2 or 3 days. Fibrosis may develop after days or weeks of the process. Damage to type II alveolar cells leads to loss of surfactant. The surfactant that is produced may be inactivated by proteins present in the airways. Alveolar filling and collapse cause intrapulmonary shunting and ventilation-perfusion mismatch with hypoxemia.

Death from ARDS is not usually caused by isolated hypoxemic respiratory failure. The most frequent causes of death are complications of infection, sepsis syndrome, and failure of other organ systems. In addition to the clinical risk factors listed above, specific factors associated with death include less than 10% band forms on a peripheral blood smear, persistent acidemia, bicarbonate less than 20 mEq/L, or blood urea nitrogen greater than 65 mg/dL. Therefore, the systemic effects associated with ARDS may be important to the outcome.

- Death from ARDS is not usually caused by isolated hypoxemic respiratory failure.
- Infection, sepsis syndrome, and failure of other organ systems are the usual causes of death.
- Factors associated with death: <10% band forms on a peripheral blood smear, persistent acidemia, bicarbonate <20 mEq/L, or blood urea nitrogen >65 mg/dL.

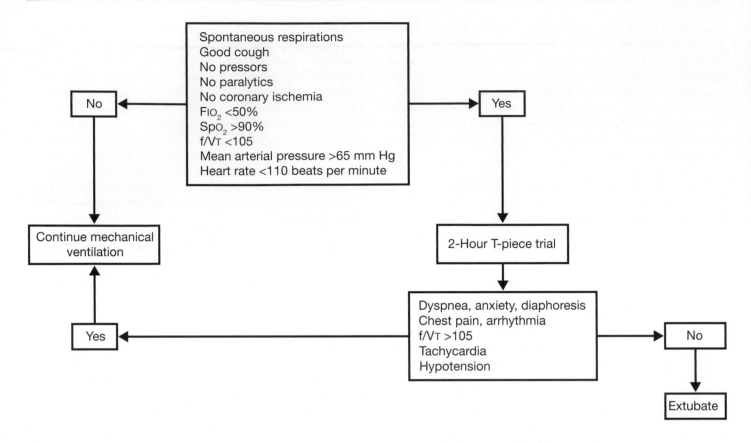

Figure 4-1. Ventilatory Weaning Protocol. FIO_2 indicates fraction of inspired oxygen; f/Vt, respiratory frequency divided by tidal volume (rapid shallow breathing index); SpO_2, arterial oxygen saturation.

Therapy for ARDS

The traditional therapy for ARDS involves optimization of physiologic variables and supportive management of associated complications. Measures include optimization of gas exchange and hemodynamics, nutrition, ambulation, and control of infections. Hypoxemia typically is corrected with positive pressure ventilation with supplemental oxygen and PEEP. PEEP provides potential benefits of increased lung volume and lung compliance and improvement in ventilation-perfusion relationships. Maintaining PEEP at a level adequate to prevent repetitive opening and closing (atelectotrauma) of gravitationally dependent lung units (ie, at a level greater than the *closing volume*) may be helpful in limiting tissue sheer forces that can potentiate capillary injury and worsen the degree of diffuse alveolar damage. Beyond the optimal level of PEEP, an increase in intrathoracic pressure may be associated with decreased venous return, increased pulmonary vascular resistance, decreased left ventricular filling, and a corresponding decrease in cardiac output.

Limiting the degree of alveolar distention during peak inflation may limit the potential for alveolar disruption and subsequent barotrauma, often referred to as *ventilator-associated lung injury*. This is achieved by delivering tidal volumes of limited size, either by a volume preset or a pressure-targeted mode of ventilation. In the management of ARDS, *protective ventilatory strategy* refers to the use of

PEEP levels chosen to prevent alveolar closure and tidal volumes chosen to prevent alveolar overdistention. A landmark randomized study found improved survival among ARDS patients receiving a tidal volume of 6 mL/kg ideal body weight compared with a control group receiving a tidal volume of 12 mL/kg ideal body weight. This is the only specific therapy for ARDS that has been shown to improve survival. In many patients supported according to these ventilator guidelines, the achieved level of alveolar ventilation results in an increase in arterial PCO_2. This phenomenon, *permissive hypercapnia*, does not appear to be harmful. Indeed, recent evidence indicates that mild hypercapnia and respiratory acidosis may decrease the degree of ventilator-induced lung injury.

- Hypoxemia typically is corrected with positive pressure ventilation with supplemental oxygen and PEEP.
- A protective ventilatory strategy in ARDS is designed to limit ventilator-induced lung injury.
- A tidal volume of 6 mL/kg ideal body weight is the only intervention shown to improve survival among ARDS patients.

Because increased capillary permeability allows greater intravascular fluid leak at any given hydrostatic pressure, intravascular volume is usually limited to that necessary for systemic perfusion.

Table 4-14 Criteria for Diagnosis of Acute Respiratory Distress Syndrome

Appropriate setting
  Pulmonary injury, shock, trauma
  Acute event
    Clinical respiratory distress, tachypnea
Diffuse pulmonary infiltrates on chest radiography
  Interstitial or alveolar pattern (or both)
Hypoxemia
  PaO_2/FIO_2 ratio <150
Exclude
  Chronic pulmonary disease accounting for the clinical features
  Left ventricular failure (most series require pulmonary artery wedge pressure <18 mm Hg)

Abbreviation: FIO_2, fraction of inspired oxygen.

Table 4-15 Disorders Associated With Acute Respiratory Distress Syndrome

Disorder	Cause
Shock	Any cause
Sepsis	Lung infections, other bacteremic or endotoxic states
Trauma	Head injury, lung contusion, fat embolism
Aspiration	Gastric, near-drowning, tube feedings
Hematologic	Transfusions, leukoagglutinin, intravascular coagulation, thrombotic thrombocytopenic purpura
Metabolic	Pancreatitis, uremia
Drugs	Narcotics, barbiturates, aspirin
Toxic	Inhaled—O_2, smoke
	Chemicals—paraquat
	Irritant gases—NO_2, Cl_2, SO_2, NH_3
Miscellaneous	Radiation, air embolism, altitude

However, associated shock states may demand volume expansion or increased inotropic support. Crystalloids can provide adequate filling pressures in patients with shock states, but large volumes may be required. Specific applications for colloids in ARDS include blood products (eg, for coagulopathies or anemia). Supplemental nutrition typically is provided throughout the course of critical illness. Many patients with ARDS have associated multiorgan injury and may have ileus or gastrointestinal tract dysfunction that precludes enteral feeding. Enteral feeding is recommended if tolerated. The consequences of malnutrition may include impairment of respiratory muscle function, depressed ventilatory drive, and limitation of host defenses. Mobilization, ambulation, and ventilator weaning are carried out as early as practical.

- Crystalloids can provide adequate filling pressures in patients with shock states.
- Many patients with ARDS have associated multiorgan injury.

Potential therapeutic and prophylactic agents have been directed against steps in the arachidonate pathways. Corticosteroids decrease cell membrane disruption and have other anti-inflammatory properties. Specifically, no differences in mortality have been observed in prospective, randomized studies of ARDS patients receiving methylprednisolone or placebo and a recent randomized controlled trial conducted by the ARDS Clinical Network found that mortality was increased if corticosteroid therapy was started after 2 weeks.

- Corticosteroids decrease cell membrane disruption and have other anti-inflammatory properties.
- Corticosteroids may decrease the time to resolution of fibroproliferative (late-phase) ARDS but should not be started after 2 weeks.

Pulmonary vasodilators, of which nitric oxide has been studied most widely, have been used as adjuncts to traditional therapy. Inhaled nitric oxide, delivered by a mechanical ventilator, naturally distributes to relatively well-ventilated regions of each lung. Nitric oxide acts as a dilator of the alveolar capillary and is rapidly inactivated in the bloodstream, thereby potentially improving perfusion to ventilated areas without systemic vasodilation.

Several studies of inhaled nitric oxide have shown dramatic short-term improvement in oxygenation and pulmonary artery pressures in patients with ARDS. However, outcome studies have not shown improved survival. Other vasodilating agents, including prostacyclin and prostaglandin E_1 have also been tried.

- Pulmonary vasodilators improve oxygenation with no documented effect on survival.

Prone positioning has been tried in an attempt to open flooded dependent alveoli and to improve ventilation-perfusion matching and oxygenation. Three randomized controlled trials of prone positioning in ARDS have been conducted: all showed improvements in oxygenation, none showed an improvement in mortality, and there was a high rate of complications, such as dislodgment of the endotracheal tube and central venous catheters, and obstruction of the endotracheal tube. Numerous other systemic and inhaled drugs and alternative ventilatory strategies have been tried; they have failed to improve survival among ARDS patients (Table 4-16).

- Prone positioning improves oxygenation with no effect on survival.

Prognosis

The prognosis for recovery of lung function in patients who survive ARDS is good. Studies of survivors have shown nearly normal lung volumes and airflow 12 months after the illness, with mild impairment in gas exchange—decreased diffusing capacity, desaturation with exercise, or widened A-a gradient. However, these patients are still severely impaired owing to neurologic complications such as

Table 4-16 Therapies That Have Not Improved Survival in Acute Respiratory Distress Syndrome

Drugs
  Corticosteroids
  N-acetylcysteine
  Dietary supplements
  Immunonutrition
  Prostaglandin E₁
  Lisofylline
  Ketoconazole
Other adjuncts
  Prone position
  Partial liquid ventilation
  High-frequency oscillation
  High positive end-expiratory pressure
  Ventilator modes other than volume control
Aerosol therapies
  Surfactant C & B
  Prostacyclin
  Nitric oxide

critical illness polyneuropathy and posttraumatic stress disorder. Therefore, the incentive is strong to continue aggressive measures in patients with otherwise reversible organ dysfunction who have a clear understanding of long-term outcomes.

- The prognosis for the recovery of lung function in patients surviving ARDS is good.
- Mild decreases in lung volumes, oxygenation, and diffusing capacity are typically observed after 6 to 12 months.
- Survivors are severely impaired owing to neurologic complications.

Shock

Shock is defined by evidence of end-organ hypoperfusion usually (but not necessarily) associated with hypotension. The most common classification is the Weil-Shubin classification: cardiogenic (decreased cardiac output), hypovolemic (decreased blood volume), obstructive, and distributive (variable cardiac output, decreased systemic vascular resistance). All forms of shock are usually characterized by end-organ hypoperfusion manifested as altered mental status, tachycardia, tachypnea, decreased urine output, and lactic acidosis. Hypotension is usually (but not always) present. The clinical history often helps determine the diagnosis (eg, blood loss, trauma, myocardial infarction, or systemic infection). Unlike other forms of shock, distributive shock is often characterized by relatively warm extremities and normal or increased cardiac output.

- Shock is defined by evidence of end-organ hypoperfusion, usually associated with hypotension.
- Common classification: cardiogenic, hypovolemic, obstructive, and distributive.

- Shock is usually characterized by hypotension, tachycardia, tachypnea, altered mental status, decreased urine output, and lactic acidosis.
- Distributive shock is often characterized by relatively warm extremities and normal or increased cardiac output.

After a rapid initial assessment, treatment of shock is directed at the presumed source, for example, volume (blood loss, hypovolemia), vasodilator or inotropic therapy (cardiogenic), or fluids, antibiotics, and drainage of any infected space (sepsis). Treatment of all forms of shock is usually aimed at stabilizing physiologic abnormalities and treating the underlying cause. Many times vasopressor agents are used; different agents are chosen for different states (Table 4-17).

Cardiogenic Shock
Cardiogenic shock typically manifests as low cardiac output, high systemic vascular resistance, and high filling pressures. This topic is covered in detail in Chapter 3 ("Cardiology").

Hypovolemic Shock
Causes of hypovolemic shock are listed in Table 4-18. Findings on physical examination and basic laboratory testing are diminished skin turgor, dry skin and mucosa, hypotension, low urine sodium levels and high urine osmolarity, oliguria, and a high serum urea nitrogen–creatinine ratio (>20:1). The hemodynamic pattern is one of decreased cardiac output and filling pressures and increased systemic vascular resistance. As in other forms of shock, physiologic abnormalities need to be corrected immediately and underlying processes (bleeding, dehydration, etc.) need to be treated. The American College of Surgeons defines blood loss in classes I through IV. Class III is defined as loss of more than 30% of the body's blood, with normal compensatory increases in heart rate and systemic vascular resistance unable to maintain normal perfusion. This marks the onset of hemodynamic collapse, end-organ hypoperfusion, and shock. Some clarification is needed for the traditional evaluation of the bleeding patient. Tachycardia is absent in most patients with moderate to severe blood loss. Orthostatic vital signs are of limited value in the ICU; to be effective they should be measured with the patient lying down and then standing. Even if measured correctly, for patients older than 65, the sensitivity is only 14% to 40%. Frequent checks (every 2-4 hours) of hemoglobin and the hematocrit are unnecessary. Changes in the hematocrit show poor correlation with blood volume in acute bleeding and are usually the result of infusion of crystalloid. Therefore, changes in the hematocrit most likely represent ongoing resuscitation and may not reflect active bleeding. Finally, the traditional practice of placing patients in the Trendelenburg position to increase blood pressure may increase blood pressure, but it does not increase cardiac output, which is the ultimate goal.

Obstructive Shock
Obstructive shock is associated with a physical impairment to adequate forward circulatory flow, involving mechanisms different from those of primary myocardial or valvular dysfunction. Several hemodynamic patterns may be observed, depending on the cause: a frank

Table 4-17 Vasoactive Agents, Common Dosages, and Hemodynamic Effects[a]

Agent	Dose	Cardiac		Vascular		
		HR	C	VC	VD	DA
Dopamine	1-4 mcg/kg/min	↑	↑	—	↑	↑↑↑↑
	4-20 mcg/kg/min	↑↑	↑↑↑	↑↑↑	—	↑↑
Norepinephrine	2-20 mcg/min	↑	↑↑	↑↑↑↑	—	—
Epinephrine	1-20 mcg/min	↑↑↑↑	↑↑↑↑	↑↑↑↑	↑↑↑	—
Vasopressin	0.03-0.04 U/h	—	—	↑↑↑	—	—
Phenylephrine	20-200 mcg/min	—	—	↑↑↑	—	—
Isoproterenol	1-5 mcg/min	↑↑↑↑	↑↑↑↑	—	↑↑↑↑	—
Dobutamine	2.5-15 mcg/kg/min	↑↑	↑↑↑↑	—	↑↑	—
Amrinone	0.75 mg/kg bolus; 5-15 mcg/kg/min	↑	↑↑↑	—	↑↑	—

Abbreviations: C, contractility; DA, dopaminergic; HR, heart rate; U, units; VC, vasoconstriction; VD, vasodilation.
[a] Number of arrows indicates relative strength of effect; dash indicates no clinically apparent effect.

decrease in filling pressures (as in mediastinal compressions of great veins); trends toward equalization of pressures (as in cardiac tamponade); or markedly increased right ventricular filling pressures with low pulmonary capillary wedge pressure (as in pulmonary embolism). Cardiac output is usually decreased with increased systemic vascular resistance. Common causes are tension pneumothorax, cardiac tamponade, and massive pulmonary embolus.

* Obstructive shock is associated with physical impairment of cardiac output not associated with primary myocardial or valvular dysfunction.

Distributive Shock

Of the many forms of distributive shock (Table 4-19), sepsis is probably the best known. Distributive shock manifests typically as a warm, vasodilated shock. The hemodynamic pattern is low filling pressures, high cardiac output, and low systemic vascular resistance. As in other forms of shock, treatment is supportive and is aimed at the underlying cause.

Table 4-18 Etiology of Hypovolemic Shock

Source	Cause
Trauma, postoperative	Bleeding
Gastrointestinal tract loss	Bleeding, vomiting, diarrhea
Renal loss	Diuretics, diabetes mellitus, diabetes insipidus
Skin	Burns, exudative skin lesions
Respiratory	Bronchorrhea
Third spacing	Pancreatitis, crush injuries
Disabled, bed-bound patients	Lack of access to water

Sepsis

Sepsis is an exaggerated inflammatory response to a noxious stimulus and is characterized by a severe catabolic reaction (up to 1% lean body mass per day), widespread endothelial dysfunction, and release of inflammatory agents. To achieve a common terminology, *systemic inflammatory response syndrome* (SIRS) was introduced for findings of fever or hypothermia, tachycardia, hyperventilation, and leukocytosis or leukopenia regardless of cause. *Sepsis* is defined as SIRS with a known or presumed source of infection, and *severe sepsis* is defined as sepsis associated with organ system dysfunction and systemic effects, including hypotension, decreased urine output, or metabolic acidosis. *Septic shock* refers to persistent signs of organ hypoperfusion despite adequate fluid resuscitation.

The mortality of patients with sepsis and multiorgan failure may be greater than 70% to 90%. Adverse risk factors include age older than 65 years, continued systemic signs of sepsis, persistent deficit in oxygen delivery, and preexisting renal or liver failure. Physiologic scoring systems (eg, Acute Physiology and Chronic Health Evaluation [APACHE]) may predict outcome more accurately for subgroups of patients.

* Mortality of patients with sepsis and multiorgan failure may be >70%-90%.

Table 4-19 Causes of Distributive Shock

Sepsis
Adrenal crisis/hemorrhage
Neurogenic
Anaphylactic
Hepatic failure
Pancreatitis
Thiamine deficiency

Multisystem organ failure, or *multiple organ dysfunction syndrome* (MODS), is usually defined as acute dysfunction of 2 or more organ systems lasting more than 2 days. Sepsis is the most common cause. The pathogenesis is attributed to the hemodynamic and immunologic effects of endotoxin, cytokines (tumor necrosis factor α), interleukins (ILs) (IL-1, IL-2, IL-6, IL-8), platelet-activating factor, arachidonic acid metabolites, polymorphonuclear leukocyte–derived toxic products, and myocardial depressant factors. Corticosteroids have no known benefit and may cause adverse effects in patients with sepsis syndrome, with or without ARDS. An exception is the use of relatively low doses of hydrocortisone or methylprednisolone in patients with documented adrenal insufficiency and severe sepsis, for which benefit has been reported.

Treatment

The Surviving Sepsis Campaign is a group of organizations and professional societies that have created guidelines for the treatment of sepsis (Table 4-20).

Antibiotics

The main recommendations are to collect samples for blood cultures before antibiotics are given; start other cultures and perform imaging studies as indicated; give appropriate antibiotics within 1 hour; and select specific antibiotics after 72 hours as appropriate and continue their use for 10 days. The source of the infection must be sought and drained if needed.

Early Goal-Directed Resuscitation

Early goal-directed resuscitation (EGDR) is an attempt to stabilize filling pressures, normalize physiologic abnormalities, and maintain cardiac output and systemic oxygen delivery to prevent the cascade of events leading to septic shock and multisystem organ failure. Previous ICU-based studies of goal-directed therapy did not show improved outcomes, presumably because the inflammatory cascade was well advanced and not reversible. A key component of the sepsis guidelines is the concept of EGDR, started immediately on recognition of sepsis. In these guidelines, resuscitation should begin as soon as severe sepsis or sepsis-induced tissue hypoperfusion is recognized. In a single-center study, this strategy decreased hospital mortality from 46% to 30% (absolute risk reduction, 16%). Goals of therapy within the first 6 hours (Figure 4-2) are as follows:

1. Mean arterial pressure ≥65 and ≤90 mm Hg
2. Urine output >0.5 mL/kg/h
3. Central venous oxygen saturation ($ScvO_2$) ≥70% or mixed venous oxygen saturation (SvO_2) ≥65%

If the goals are not achieved with fluid resuscitation during the first 6 hours, do 1 or both of the following:

1. Administer transfusion of packed red blood cells to increase the hematocrit to at least 30%
2. Administer dobutamine (maximal rate, 20 mcg/kg/min) to reach the goal

Typically a fluid challenge is performed in patients with suspected hypovolemia by giving 500 to 1,000 mL of crystalloid solution over 30 minutes, with additional doses based on response and tolerance. The input is typically greater than output owing to venodilation

Table 4-20 Summary of Surviving Sepsis Campaign Guidelines and Grade of Recommendation

Guideline	Grade
Deep vein thrombosis prophylaxis	A
Stress ulcer prophylaxis	A
Weaning protocol with spontaneous breathing trials	A
Early goal-directed resuscitation for severe sepsis	B
Do not use dopamine for renal protection	B
Activated protein C in patients with high risk of death	B
Avoid high tidal volumes & plateau pressures	B
Sedation protocols with daily awakening	B
Corticosteroids for 7 days in septic shock patients receiving vasopressors	C
Do not use bicarbonate if pH ≥7.15 in lactic acidemia	C
Cultures before beginning antibiotic therapy	D
Measure serum lactate to assess organ perfusion	D
Vasopressin if refractory to other pressors	D
Early empirical broad-spectrum antibiotic therapy	D, E
Vasopressors to keep mean arterial pressure 60-80 mm Hg (central & arterial access)	E
Provide rapid source control as appropriate	E
Maintain blood glucose <150 mg/dL	E
Reassessment of antimicrobials in 48-72 hours	E
Nutrition protocol, preferably enteral	E
Consider limitation of support when appropriate	E

and capillary leak. Most patients require continuing aggressive fluid resuscitation during the first 24 hours of management. Vasopressor therapy should be initiated if an appropriate fluid challenge fails to restore adequate blood pressure and organ perfusion or it should be used transiently in the face of life-threatening hypotension, even when fluid challenge is in progress. Norepinephrine and dopamine are first-line agents for correcting hypotension in septic shock. Norepinephrine is more potent than dopamine and may be more effective at reversing hypotension in septic shock patients. Dopamine may be particularly useful in patients with compromised systolic function but causes more tachycardia and may be more arrhythmogenic. Another agent, vasopressin, is being used more frequently in resistant shock and to help in weaning from catecholamines.

Activated Protein C

In a controlled prospective trial of recombinant human activated protein C (drotrecogin alfa) administered intravenously over 96 hours, the mortality among patients with severe sepsis had a 19% relative reduction (6% absolute decrease). Most of the benefit was in the sickest groups of patients. It is now recommended only for those with 2 or more dysfunctional organ systems (especially disseminated intravascular coagulation) or an APACHE II score of 25 or more. Activated protein C has anti-inflammatory and profibrinolytic properties that may contribute to this benefit. The main adverse effect of recombinant human activated protein C is bleeding.

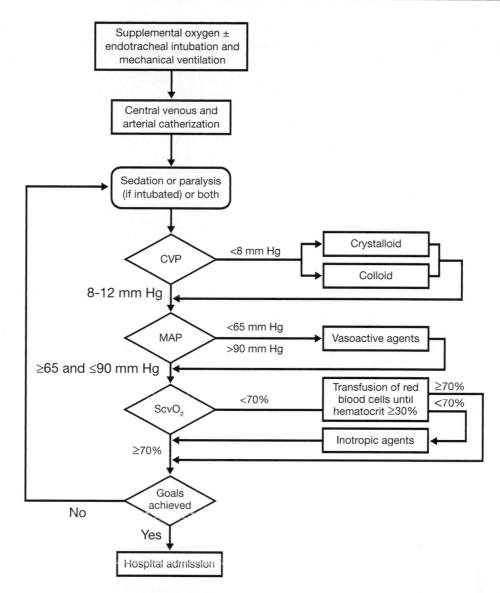

Figure 4-2. Protocol for Early Goal-Directed Therapy. CVP indicates central venous pressure; MAP, mean arterial pressure; ScvO$_2$, central venous oxygen saturation. (From Rivers E, Nguyen B, Havstad S, Ressler J, Muzzin A, Knoblich B, et al, for the Early Goal-Directed Therapy Collaborative Group. Early goal-directed therapy in the treatment of severe sepsis and septic shock. N Engl J Med. 2001;345:1368-77. Used with permission.)

Corticosteroids

High-dose corticosteroids are of no benefit in sepsis and have shown harm in the past. Recent randomized controlled trials have shown a mortality benefit from administration of low-dose hydrocortisone, 100 mg intravenously every 6 hours, and fludrocortisone, 50 mcg by mouth daily for 7 days, in patients who have sepsis and relative adrenal insufficiency. *Relative adrenal insufficiency* is defined as an increase in the serum cortisol level of less than 9 mg/dL in relation to baseline after intravenous administration of cosyntropin, 250 mcg, measured at 0, 30, and 60 minutes. The number needed to treat (NNT) to save 1 life is 7. This test should not be used in patients who have received etomidate for intubation since it is a selective inhibitor of β-hydroxylase and could therefore blunt the cortisol response to corticotropin.

- Sepsis syndrome typically is defined by a known or presumed source of infection associated with SIRS.
- Treatment is directed at the presumed source.
- Septic shock commonly is associated with multiorgan injury.
- Multisystem organ failure: acute dysfunction of ≥2 organ systems for >2 days.
- High-dose corticosteroid treatment is of no known benefit.

Miscellaneous

Glucose Control

There has been much interest in intensive insulin therapy for strict control of blood glucose. In 2 large randomized studies conducted in Belgium in surgical ICUs and medical ICUs, morbidity was prevented and, in the surgical population, mortality was improved. These studies have been widely criticized on internal and external validity. However, it is generally agreed that allowing blood glucose levels to increase to 200 mg/dL is unacceptable. The American Association of Clinical Endocrinologists recommends maintaining strict normoglycemia (<110 mg/dL) to see the benefits of tight control. This strict control, though, is associated with frequent episodes of hypoglycemia.

- Tight glucose control may be beneficial, but it is associated with hypoglycemia.
- Numerous subsequent validation studies are underway.

Stress Ulcer Prophylaxis

Definite risk factors for stress ulcer formation are mechanical ventilation for more than 48 hours and coagulopathy. H_2 blockers and sucralfate have both been shown to be effective prophylactic agents in this patient population. Owing to issues with medication binding and difficulty of administration, sucralfate is not the preferred agent. Proton pump inhibitors have not been studied as extensively and have not proved to be superior. Studies of head injury and burn patients have had conflicting results; however, it is reasonable to use prophylaxis in this population as well.

Management of Anemia and Transfusion

A restrictive transfusion strategy has been shown to be superior to a liberal strategy in ICU patients: Do not transfuse unless hemoglobin is less than 7 mg/dL for ICU patients in stable condition; if there is active ischemia, the threshold is less than 10 mg/dL. With use of this strategy, hospital mortality rates were significantly lower (22.3% vs 28.1%, P=.05).

Nutrition

Nutritional support improves body weight and mid arm muscle mass, but the effect of nutritional support on other outcomes such as survival and ICU length of stay is unclear. In general it is accepted that nutritional support should be given to patients who have preexisting malnutrition and to those who are expected to have inadequate intake for more than 5 days. The enteral route is preferred since there is no difference in outcomes between enteral and parenteral routes and enteral feeding is associated with fewer complications. Patients receiving enteral nutritional support should be maintained in a semirecumbent position, be given feedings slowly, and have gastric residual volumes checked. Reasonable goals for most ICU patients are 25 kcal/kg per day and 2 g of protein per day. There is no evidence that immunonutrition works. Previously it was believed that small-bowel feedings were superior to gastric feedings and were associated with fewer adverse events such as aspiration, but it is now known that there is no difference. Practically, it is much easier to feed into the stomach.

Disease-Severity Scoring Systems

The use of a severity-of-illness scoring system is increasingly prevalent in the ICU. These systems may define quantitative overall risks for populations of patients. An accurate quantifiable description of the pretreatment status of critically ill patients can allow improved precision in the evaluation and implementation of new therapies (ie, clinical research). Furthermore, these systems can be of great use in quality improvement efforts. In most systems, however, the role in individual case management is unclear. The types of clinical scoring systems have ranged from simple counts of failing organs to highly sophisticated methods that incorporate clinical and physiologic parameters (acute and chronic) into proprietary logistic regression prediction equations derived from large databases.

The Glasgow Coma Scale (GCS) was developed in the early 1970s as a triage tool for evaluation of patients with head injury. This scoring system assigns a weighted point score for 3 behavioral responses: eye opening (1-4 points), best verbal response (1-5 points), and best motor response (1-6 points). Thus, GCS scores range from 3 to 15 points and are categorized into 3 levels of dysfunction: severe dysfunction (3-8 points), moderate dysfunction (9-12 points), and mild dysfunction (≥13 points). The GCS system has been shown to correlate with mortality and the level of ultimate brain function in patients with traumatic brain injury. Because of its efficacy and simplicity, the GCS has been used within other scoring systems.

Several multisystem scoring systems have been developed for use in critically ill patients. Although a detailed review of these systems is beyond the scope of this text, they include the APACHE system, Simplified Acute Physiology Score (SAPS), Mortality Probability Model (MPM), Project IMPACT, and Therapeutic Intervention Scoring System (TISS).

- Severity scoring systems attempt to quantify overall risk for populations of patients.
- Severity scoring systems can be of great use in clinical research and quality assurance functions.
- The best role for most scoring systems in the care of individual patients is undefined.

Critical Care Medicine Pharmacy Review
Philip J. Kuper, PharmD, BCPS, Lance J. Oyen, PharmD

Review of Drugs Commonly Used in the ICU That Potentially Can Cause Delirium

Analgesics
  Opiates
  NSAIDs

Anesthetics & sedatives
  Benzodiazepines
  Bupivacaine
  Ketamine
  Lidocaine
  Propofol

Anticonvulsants
  Barbiturates
  Carbamazepine
  Phenytoin

Antifungals & antivirals
  Acyclovir
  Amphotericin
  Ketoconazole

Antihypertensives
  Captopril
  Clonidine
  Diltiazem
  Enalapril
  Hydralazine
  Methyldopa
  Nifedipine
  Nitroprusside
  Verapamil

Antimicrobials
  Aminoglycosides
  Cephalosporins
  Carbapenems
  Macrolides
  Metronidazole
  Monobactams
  Penicillins
  Quinolones
  Tetracyclines
  Trimethoprim-sulfamethoxazole
  (Cotrimoxazole)

Miscellaneous cardiac drugs
  Antiarrhythmics
  Atropine
  β-Blockers
  Digoxin

Miscellaneous
  Antihistamines
  Corticosteroids
  Theophylline
  Tricyclic antidepressants
  H_2-blockers

Abbreviations: ICU, intensive care unit; NSAIDs, nonsteroidal anti-inflammatory drugs.
Data from McGuire BE, Basten CJ, Ryan CJ, Gallagher J. Intensive care unit syndrome: a dangerous misnomer. Arch Intern Med. 2000;160:906-9, and Fish DN. Treatment of delirium in the critically ill patient. Clin Pharm. 1991;10:456-66.

Critical Care Medicine Pharmacy Review (continued)

Review of Drugs Commonly Used in the ICU for Agitation With Ventilation

Drug	Comments	
	Pros	**Cons**

Benzodiazepines
  Midazolam
  Lorazepam
  Diazepam
	Useful for anxiety-related agitation, inexpensive, minimal hemodynamic effects	Risk of oversedation & accumulation, especially prolonged use; depress respiratory drive; potential withdrawal reaction with long-term use

Anesthetic Propofol	Predictable, short-term sedative/hypnotic effects, no accumulation	Hypotension risk, depresses respiratory drive, high expense, deaths associated with acidosis
Neuroleptic Haloperidol	Specific for delirium, no effect on respiratory drive	Cardiac toxicity & hypotension risks, lowers seizure threshold
Sedative Dexmedetomidine	Pain and anxiolytic properties, does not depress ventilation	Short-term use only (until further research completed), potential withdrawal reaction

Opiates/analgesics
  Fentanyl
  Hydromorphone
  Methadone
  Morphine
	Useful for pain-induced agitation (accurate history for pain important)	May contribute to delirium & confusion, may contribute to hypotension due to histamine release

Abbreviation: ICU, intensive care unit.

Critical Care Medicine Pharmacy Review (continued)

Clinically Important Toxic Overdoses and Management

Drug Overdose	Clinical Syndrome	Basic Treatment
Acetaminophen (paracetamol)	0.5-24 h: Nausea, vomiting 24-72 h: Nausea, vomiting, RUQ pain, increased LFTs & PT 72-96 h: Liver necrosis, coagulation defects, jaundice, renal failure, hepatic encephalopathy 4 d to 2 wk: Resolution of liver dysfunction	Elimination: Gastric lavage (if <1 h after ingestion), activated charcoal (if <4 h after ingestion) (both longer if sustained-release product) Treatment: *N*-acetylcysteine for toxic ingestion based on Rumack-Matthew nomogram
Amphetamines	Hypertension, tachycardia, arrhythmias, myocardial infarction, vasospasm, seizures, paranoid psychosis, diaphoresis, tachypnea	Elimination: Activated charcoal for oral ingestion Agitation/seizures: Benzodiazepines Hypertension: Control agitation, α-antagonists (phentolamine), vasodilators (nitroglycerin, nitroprusside, nifedipine) Hyperthermia: Control agitation, external cooling
Iron	0.5-6 h: Nausea, vomiting, GI discomfort, GI bleeding, drowsiness, hypoglycemia, & hypotension 6-24 h: Latency/quiescence (may not occur in severe ingestions) 24-48 h: Shock, coma, seizures, coagulopathy, acidosis, cardiac failure 2-7 d: Hepatotoxicity & coagulopathy, metabolic acidosis, renal insufficiency 1-8 wk: GI disorders, achlorhydria	Elimination: Gastric lavage &/or whole bowel irrigation with polyethylene glycol–electrolyte solution, especially with tablets (radiopaque) present on KUB Shock: IV fluids & blood (if hemorrhage present); vasopressors if needed Antidote: Deferoxamine to chelate iron, when iron levels >500 mcg/dL or severe ingestion suspected (will change urine to "vin rosé" color)
Salicylate	Respiratory alkalosis (initially), metabolic acidosis (after substantial absorption), pulmonary edema, platelet dysfunction, nausea, vomiting, hearing loss, agitation, delirium	Elimination: Activated charcoal, hemodialysis (for severe poisoning), alkalinization of urine Agitation/delirium: Alkalize blood (acidemia enhances transfer into tissue, especially brain) with IV bicarbonate
Tricyclic antidepressants	Wide-complex tachyarrhythmias, hypotension, seizures	Tachyarrhythmias: Alkalizing blood (pH 7.5-7.55) with IV bicarbonate reduces binding to sodium channel Seizures: Benzodiazepines Hypotension: Fluid resuscitation, vasopressors

Abbreviations: GI, gastrointestinal tract; IV, intravenous; KUB, radiograph of kidneys, ureters, bladder; LFT, liver function test; PT, prothrombin time; RUQ, right upper quadrant.

Critical Care Medicine Pharmacy Review (continued)

Overview of Drotrecogin Alfa[a] (Activated Protein C)

Indication

Known or suspected infection that is being treated

and

Patient meets ≥3 SIRS criteria:

1. Core temperature >38°C or <36°C
2. HR >90 beats per minute unless a medical condition causes tachycardia or patient is receiving treatment to prevent tachycardia (eg, β-blocker)
3. RR >20 breaths per minute, $PaCO_2$ <32 mm Hg, or the use of a mechanical ventilator
4. WBC >12,000/mL

and

APACHE II score ≥25

or

At least 1 organ or system dysfunction:

1. Cardiovascular dysfunction (shock, hypotension, or the need for vasopressor support despite adequate fluid resuscitation)
2. Respiratory dysfunction (PaO_2/FiO_2 ratio <250)
3. Renal dysfunction (oliguria despite adequate fluid resuscitation)
4. Thrombocytopenia (platelet count <80,000/mcL or 50% decrease from the highest value in the past 3 d)
5. Metabolic dysfunction with elevated lactic acid concentrations

Contraindications

Clinical situations in which bleeding could be associated with increased risk of death:

1. Active internal bleeding
2. Recent (within 3 mo) hemorrhagic stroke
3. Recent (within 2 mo) intracranial or intraspinal surgery or severe head trauma
4. Trauma with an increased risk of life-threatening bleeding
5. Presence of an epidural catheter
6. Intracranial neoplasm or mass lesion or evidence of cerebral herniation
7. Known hypersensitivity to drotrecogin alfa or any of its metabolites

Warnings

Patients with single-organ dysfunction & recent surgery (within 30 d) had higher mortality, but sample was too small for statistical significance; these patients may not be at high risk of death irrespective of APACHE II score—therefore, the drug may not be indicated; carefully consider the risks & benefits

Precautions

The following conditions are likely to increase the risk of bleeding; therefore, the risks & benefits should be considered:

1. Concurrent therapeutic dosing of heparin; platelet count <30,000/mcL; INR >3.0
2. Recent (within 6 wk) GI bleeding
3. Recent (within 3 d) administration of thrombolytic therapy
4. Recent (within 7 d) administration of oral anticoagulants or glycoprotein IIb/IIIa inhibitors
5. Recent (within 7 d) administration of aspirin (>650 mg daily) or other platelet inhibitors
6. Recent (within 3 mo) ischemic stroke
7. Intracranial arteriovenous malformation
8. Known bleeding diathesis
9. Chronic severe hepatic disease
10. Any other condition in which bleeding constitutes a serious hazard

Adverse reactions

Serious bleeding occurred in 3.5% of patients in the drotrecogin alfa group compared with 2% in the placebo group

Dose

24 mcg/kg/h continuous infusion for 96 h

Abbreviations: APACHE, Acute Physiology and Chronic Health Evaluation; FiO_2, fraction of inspired oxygen; GI, gastrointestinal tract; HR, heart rate; INR, international normalized ratio; RR, respiration rate; SIRS, systemic inflammatory response syndrome; WBC, white blood cell count.

[a] Xigris; Eli Lilly and Co., Indianapolis, Indiana.

Questions

Multiple Choice (choose the best answer)

1. A 55-year-old nonsmoking woman with no past medical history and no use of medications was in her usual state of health until 1 day before admission, when epigastric pain began and gradually increased. In the local emergency department her lipase was 460 U/L. A diagnosis of pancreatitis was given. She received nothing by mouth and began receiving fluids intravenously. During the next 24 hours she became more dyspneic and was transported to your hospital for further evaluation. Immediate intubation was needed because of respiratory distress. Chest radiography showed diffuse, bilateral alveolar infiltrates. Arterial blood gas analysis showed pH 7.40, PCO_2 40 mm Hg, bicarbonate 24 mEq/L, and PaO_2 56 mm Hg. A pulmonary artery catheter was placed and showed the following: cardiac output 5.3 L/min, right atrial pressure 10 mm Hg, pulmonary artery pressure 45/12 mm Hg, and pulmonary capillary occlusion pressure 12 mm Hg. What is the most likely cause?

   a. Cardiogenic pulmonary edema
   b. Acute respiratory distress syndrome (ARDS)
   c. Acute eosinophilic pneumonia
   d. Chronic obstructive pulmonary disease (COPD) exacerbation
   e. Pulmonary embolus

2. A 63-year-old man with ARDS is transferred from another hospital. Examination findings include the following: height 60 inches (150 cm), weight 70 kg, temperature 37°C, pulse 120 beats per minute, blood pressure 123/64 mm Hg, arterial oxygen saturation (SpO_2) 88% on fraction of inspired oxygen (FIO_2) 1.0%, diffuse crackles, and jugular venous pressure 8 mm Hg. Mechanical ventilation is started in assist/control mode at 18 breaths per minute, positive end-expiratory pressure (PEEP) 10 cm H_2O, and FIO_2 1.0%. Which starting tidal volume is the most appropriate?

   a. 200 mL
   b. 270 mL
   c. 450 mL
   d. 700 mL
   e. 840 mL

3. A 50-year-old man who never smoked is admitted to the intensive care unit with respiratory distress. During the next several hours, respiratory failure ensues. He is presumed to have ARDS. The mechanical ventilator is set on assist/control mode with tidal volume 480 mL, rate 18 breaths per minute, PEEP 10 cm H_2O, and FIO_2 80%. After 4 hours the plateau pressure is 32 cm H_2O. How should the ventilator be adjusted?

   a. Increase FIO_2.
   b. Decrease tidal volume.
   c. Decrease rate to 12 breaths per minute.
   d. Increase tidal volume to 450 mL.
   e. Increase PEEP to 15 cm H_2O.

4. A 55-year-old man presents to the emergency department with altered mental status. Vital signs are as follows: temperature 39°C, pulse 130 beats per minute, blood pressure 85/30 mm Hg, respiratory rate 20 breaths per minute, and SpO_2 98% on room air. Physical examination findings include delirium; no murmurs, gallops, or rubs; clear lungs; mild epigastric tenderness; and intense erythema and warmth on the skin of his left thigh. The extremities are warm and without mottling. What is the most likely cause of the hypotension?

   a. Cardiogenic shock
   b. Adrenal crisis
   c. Sepsis
   d. Massive pulmonary embolus
   e. Severe acute pancreatitis

5. A 45-year-old woman with rheumatoid arthritis presents with hematemesis. Vital signs are as follows: temperature 37°C, respiration 17 breaths per minute, pulse 121 beats per minute, and blood pressure 98/65 mm Hg. What is the most appropriate next step for this patient?

   a. Consult a gastroenterologist.
   b. Order a complete blood cell count, blood chemistry panel, chest radiography, and lactate concentration.
   c. Insert a large-bore peripheral intravenous catheter.
   d. Insert a right internal jugular triple-lumen catheter.
   e. Administer an intravenous proton pump inhibitor.

6. Which of the following treatment strategies for sepsis has been shown to decrease mortality in randomized controlled trials?

   a. High-dose methylprednisolone
   b. Dopamine titrated to achieve a mean arterial pressure of 65 mm Hg
   c. Early appropriate antibiotics
   d. Supranormal oxygen delivery in the intensive care unit with a pulmonary artery catheter
   e. Goal-directed therapy started in the emergency department before admission to the intensive care unit

7. You are called emergently to the bedside of a 74-year-old woman who has received mechanical ventilation for the past 4 days for ARDS. The nurse tells you that the ventilator suddenly alarmed; the SpO_2 decreased over the next 2 minutes, from 95% to 80%, despite the administration of 100% oxygen. You determine that the peak and plateau pressures have both increased above baseline. On physical examination the trachea is midline and the breath sounds are decreased on the right. The patient was disconnected from the ventilator and bag-mask ventilated, but the SpO_2 remained 80% and the blood pressure decreased to 70/60 mm Hg. What should be done next?

   a. Increase sedation.
   b. Perform therapeutic bronchoscopy.
   c. Perform needle thoracostomy.
   d. Pull back the endotracheal tube.
   e. Resume use of ventilator and increase PEEP.

Answers

1.   Answer b.

This patient has hypoxemic respiratory failure. The chest radiographic findings of bilateral, diffuse alveolar infiltrates make both COPD exacerbation and pulmonary embolus extremely unlikely. The PaO_2/FiO_2 ratio is 56; less than 200 is consistent with ARDS and less than 300 is consistent with acute lung injury (ALI). Cardiogenic pulmonary edema could cause this degree of hypoxemia and account for the radiographic findings; however, the lack of symptoms and the normal cardiac output and pulmonary artery occlusion (wedge) pressure make this extremely unlikely. ARDS is the most likely explanation. The definition for ARDS from the American-European Consensus Conference on ARDS is acute-onset, bilateral alveolar infiltrates on chest radiography, pulmonary artery wedge pressure less than 18 mm Hg, or no clinical evidence of left atrial hypertension, and PaO_2/FiO_2 less than 300 for ALI and PaO_2/FiO_2 less than 200 for ARDS. There are many precipitating causes of ARDS: systemic inflammatory response syndrome (SIRS), trauma, shock from any cause, multiple transfusions (>10 units in 24 hours), disseminated intravascular coagulation, thrombotic thrombocytopenic purpura, and drugs such as narcotics, barbiturates, and aspirin. This patient had pancreatitis, a well-known risk factor for ALI and ARDS. Acute eosinophilic pneumonia is rare and would be unusual with acute pancreatitis.

2.   Answer b.

The most important factor in preventing ventilator-induced lung injury and improving survival among patients with ARDS is selecting an appropriate tidal volume based on ideal body weight (IBW). A low tidal volume mechanical ventilation strategy is now the standard of care for ARDS. The ARDS Clinical Network found a significant reduction in mortality (from 40% to 31%) in the group treated with lower tidal volumes. The tidal volume was set at 6 mL/kg IBW and was subsequently decreased stepwise by 1 mL/kg IBW as necessary to maintain a plateau pressure of no more than 30 cm H_2O. The minimal tidal volume was 4 mL/kg IBW. To answer this question correctly, the formula for IBW must be known: for males, 50 kg + [2.3 kg × (height in inches – 60)]; for females, 45.5 kg + [2.3 kg × (height in inches – 60)]. In this case, the IBW is 50 kg, so 200 mL is incorrect (4 mL/kg IBW) because it is too low to start with and will result in dyssynchrony, increased sedation, and respiratory acidosis. The correct answer is 270 mL (6 mL/kg IBW). The other tidal volumes are incorrect and would result in more ventilator-induced lung injury and worse patient outcomes: 450 mL (10 mL/kg IBW), 700 mL (10 mL/kg actual body weight), and 840 mL (12 mL/kg actual body weight).

3.   Answer b.

In the ARDS Clinical Network study, the tidal volume was initially set at 6 mL/kg IBW and was subsequently reduced stepwise by 1 mL/kg IBW if necessary to maintain a plateau pressure of no more than 30 cm H_2O. The minimal tidal volume was 4 mL/kg IBW. Increasing FiO_2 would not affect the elevated plateau pressure; elevated plateau pressures were associated with increased mortality in the ARDS Clinical Network trial. Decreasing the rate to 12 breaths per minute would lower the minute ventilation, worsening the respiratory acidosis. If changed at all, the rate should be increased. Increasing the tidal volume would cause more lung injury, and increasing PEEP would increase the plateau pressures further.

4.   Answer c.

Elevated temperature, hypotension, and altered mental status are associated with SIRS, which occurs in sepsis and in severe acute pancreatitis. However, the lesion on the skin is consistent with cellulitis, making sepsis more likely than pancreatitis. Cardiogenic shock and massive pulmonary embolus would be unlikely to cause SIRS. Physical examination findings in cardiogenic shock, hemorrhagic shock, and obstructive shock secondary to massive pulmonary embolus typically include cold, mottled extremities since the systemic vascular resistance increases to preserve oxygen delivery to vital organs. Adrenal crisis can cause distributive shock, as in this case; however, it is extremely rare and sepsis would be a much more common cause in this scenario.

5.   Answer c.

Dr. Osler said it best: "Patients don't die from their disease; they die from the physiologic consequences of their disease." Treat the patient before completing the history and physical examination, ordering tests, or requesting consultations. A simultaneous assessment of diagnosis and treatment is necessary for a critically ill, hemodynamically unstable patient. This approach contrasts with the traditional, linear approach: history, physical examination, investigation, diagnosis, and treatment. All these steps need to be done; however, they can be done after the patient's condition has begun to stabilize. This patient is hypovolemic from blood loss. The quickest, least invasive way to begin fluid administration is through a peripheral intravenous catheter. A triple-lumen catheter is required only if pressors are needed. There is a misconception that more fluid can be given through a triple-lumen central venous catheter than through a peripheral intravenous catheter.

6.   Answer e.

High-dose methylprednisolone has been shown to increase mortality and to increase rates of secondary infection. No vasoactive agents have ever been shown to improve mortality. Early appropriate antibiotics are clearly indicated and, along with source control, are cornerstones in the management of sepsis. In retrospective studies, antibiotics have been shown to improve survival, but randomized trials have not been conducted since it would be unethical to do so. Maximizing oxygen delivery in the intensive care unit with a pulmonary artery catheter is associated with a worsened mortality. However, in a study of septic shock patients randomly assigned to standard or early goal-directed therapy before admission to the intensive care units, a 500-mL bolus of crystalloid was given every 30 minutes to achieve a central venous pressure of 8 to 12 mm Hg. If the mean arterial pressure was less than 65 mm Hg after the bolus, vasopressors were given to maintain it at more than 65 mm Hg. The average amount of fluid given in the first 6 hours was 5 L. This significantly reduced hospital mortality from 46% to 30%. Interestingly, there was no difference in the 3-day period of the total amount of fluid given (ie, patients receiving the standard therapy received the same amount of fluid later and had a worse outcome).

7.   Answer c.
This question deals with how to approach an alarming ventilator. The first action is to disconnect the patient from the ventilator and begin hand-bag ventilation. This action relieves pressure in breath stacking or tension pneumothorax. Increasing sedation may be appropriate if the evaluation shows no change in peak or plateau pressures and if there was evidence of dyssynchrony with the ventilator. Mucous plugging, biting the tube, or bronchospasm would increase the airway resistance, resulting in an increase in peak pressure without a change in plateau pressure. Therefore, answer *b* is incorrect. Increases in both pressures are seen when there is a change in compliance, such as worsening edema, mainstem intubation, breath stacking, or tension pneumothorax. Pulling the endotracheal tube back is unlikely to help in this case since the majority of mainstem intubations are on the right; in this case, the breath sounds are absent on the right and mainstem intubation is not typically associated with hypotension. The lifesaving measure performed in this case was needle thoracostomy followed by chest tube placement.

5

Dermatology

Lisa A. Drage, MD

General Dermatology

Skin Cancer

Nonmelanoma skin cancers (basal cell, squamous cell) are the most common malignancies in the United States. More than 1 million skin cancers will be diagnosed in the United States this year. The cure rate for nonmelanoma skin cancer is more than 90% with early detection and appropriate treatment. The incidence of nonmelanoma skin cancer is increasing because of a combination of increased exposure to ultraviolet light, changes in clothing style, increased longevity, and atmospheric ozone depletion.

Both basal cell and squamous cell carcinomas commonly occur on sun-exposed skin areas. The ratio of basal cell carcinoma to squamous cell carcinoma is 4:1 in immunocompetent people. Basal cell carcinomas are usually slow-growing and locally invasive. They may invade vital structures and can cause considerable disfigurement. Basal cell carcinomas rarely metastasize to regional lymph nodes. In contrast, squamous cell carcinomas can metastasize to regional lymph nodes, and approximately 2% of all cutaneous squamous cell carcinomas lead to death.

- Skin cancer is the most common cancer in the United States, accounting for almost half of all cancers.
- Basal cell carcinoma constitutes approximately 80% of all skin cancers.
- Basal cell carcinoma and squamous cell carcinoma occur on sun-exposed skin.
- Cure rate is >90% with early detection and treatment.

Malignant Melanoma

In 2007, an estimated 59,940 Americans received a diagnosis of cutaneous melanoma and 8,110 died of the disease. The estimated lifetime risk of invasive melanoma is about 1% for Americans born in the 1990s.

The strongest risk factors for melanoma are a family history of melanoma, multiple benign or atypical nevi, and a previous melanoma. Additional risk factors include fair skin, blond or red hair, sun sensitivity, freckling, intermittent sun exposure, blistering sunburns, immunosuppression, human immunodeficiency virus (HIV), and tanning bed use. Inherited mutations in *CDKN2A* and *CDK4* genes, which have been documented in some families with melanoma, are associated with a 60% to 90% lifetime risk of melanoma. The familial atypical mole-melanoma syndrome is transmitted by an autosomal dominant gene. Patients with either familial or nonfamilial atypical nevi have an increased risk for development of malignant melanoma. Other risk factors that have been identified include a personal or family history of melanoma or nonmelanoma skin cancer, a large number of benign pigmented nevi, giant pigmented congenital nevus, and immunosuppression.

The key to improved survival with malignant melanoma is early detection and diagnosis. A full skin examination is recommended for persons at risk, including an evaluation for *a*ssymetry, *b*order irregularity, *c*olor variation, and a *d*iameter more than 6 mm or increasing in size (an ABCD evaluation). Changing or symptomatic moles or moles that stand out from other moles should be biopsied. Pathologic staging of the primary melanoma guides prognosis and further surgical decisions.

Increase in thickness of a melanoma (Table 5-1) and microscopic ulceration are both inversely correlated with survival. However, detection of intranodal deposits of melanocytes indicative of metastasis is now the most powerful staging and prognostic tool.

- The key to improved survival with malignant melanoma is early diagnosis.

Table 5-1   Survival in Malignant Melanoma, by Tumor Thickness[a]

Tumor, mm	5-Year Survival, %
<1.0	95.3
1.01-2.00	89.0
2.01-4.00	78.7
>4.00	67.4

[a] No nodal or distant metastasis.

* Increased tumor thickness is associated with decreased survival.
* Micrometastasis to the first draining lymph node is the most powerful staging and prognostic tool.

Stages I and II malignant melanomas consist of the cutaneous lesion without lymph node involvement. Stage III consists of the primary skin lesion plus microscopic or macroscopic lymph node involvement, and stage IV represents distant metastasis. Surgical management is recommended for treatment of the primary melanoma and consists of excision with tumor-free margins of 1 to 3 cm. Sentinel lymph node biopsy, whereby the first draining lymph node(s) is identified (with dye injection and lymphoscintigraphy) and sampled, improves prognostic accuracy in intermediate and thick melanomas and identifies candidates for systemic adjuvant treatment. Adjuvant high-dose interferon alfa-2b increases relapse-free survival rates and may improve overall survival rates in select patients. No form of adjuvant therapy has been shown to improve overall survival in patients with advanced (distant metastasis) disease. Ongoing therapeutic studies focus on vaccine immunotherapy and targeted chemotherapy.

* Surgical management of primary melanoma consists of excision with tumor-free margins of 1-3 cm.
* Node status, determined by sentinel lymph node biopsy, is the most powerful predictor of recurrence and survival.

Prevention of Melanoma and Nonmelanoma Skin Cancer

Dermatologists encourage regular use of sunscreens with a sun protection factor (SPF) of at least 30 and sun-protective clothing. Sun exposure during the first 18 years of life accounts for up to 80% of cumulative lifetime sun exposure. Persons with light skin types and outdoor workers need to be particularly vigilant with sun protection.

Cutaneous T-Cell Lymphoma

Cutaneous T-cell lymphoma is a non-Hodgkin lymphoma characterized by expansion of malignant T cells within the skin. The most common clinical presentations include mycosis fungoides and Sézary syndrome. Mycosis fungoides generally presents with discrete or coalescing patches, plaques, or nodules on the skin. Mycosis fungoides may progress to involve lymph nodes and viscera. Once extracutaneous involvement is recognized, the median duration of survival has been estimated at 2.5 years. The course of patients with patch- or plaque-stage cutaneous lesions, without extracutaneous disease, is less predictable, but the median duration of survival is approximately 12 years. Sézary syndrome, the more aggressive leukemic form of cutaneous T-cell lymphoma, is characterized by generalized erythroderma, keratoderma of the palms and soles, and a Sézary cell count of more than 1,000/mm³ in the peripheral blood. Most patients have severe pruritus.

* Mycosis fungoides and Sézary syndrome are forms of cutaneous T-cell lymphoma.
* Mycosis fungoides may progress to involve lymph nodes and viscera.
* The median survival for patients with mycosis fungoides is

12 years, but it decreases to 2.5 years with extracutaneous involvement.

Both mycosis fungoides and Sézary syndrome are characterized by the presence of Sézary cells (enlarged atypical lymphocytes with convoluted nuclei) involving the epidermis (epidermotrophism) and dermis. Immunohistochemical stains of cutaneous lesions demonstrate that these malignant T cells usually express CD3 and CD4 antigens (T-helper cell markers), and molecular genetic studies show clonal rearrangement of the T-cell receptor gene in lymphocyte populations from skin biopsy, lymph node, and peripheral blood specimens of patients with cutaneous T-cell lymphoma.

* Mycosis fungoides and Sézary syndrome are T-cell lymphomas characterized by the presence of Sézary cells in skin and peripheral blood.

Treatment of cutaneous T-cell lymphoma includes topical nitrogen mustard, psoralen with ultraviolet A (PUVA), radiotherapy (electron beam, orthovoltage), and systemic chemotherapy. Interferon, retinoids, and other agents also have been used. Most recently, extracorporeal photopheresis (ingestion of 8-methoxypsoralen, after which the patient's leukocytes are exposed to ultraviolet A and then reinfused) has been used in the treatment of cutaneous T-cell lymphoma.

Psoriasis

Psoriasis occurs in 1% to 3% of the US population. Onset is most common in the third decade of life, and about a third of patients have a family history of psoriasis. Psoriasis commonly presents with discrete papules and plaques covered with a silvery scale. Patterns of psoriasis include psoriasis vulgaris that presents with plaques involving the elbows, knees, and scalp. Guttate psoriasis is an acute form that often follows streptococcal throat infection and presents with small papules (5-10 mm in diameter) of psoriasis on the trunk and limbs. Other, less common forms of psoriasis include pustular psoriasis, which may be localized to the hands and feet or may be generalized. Approximately 50% of patients with psoriasis have nail abnormalities, most commonly onycholysis, pitting, and oil spots. Lesions of psoriasis may occur at previous sites of trauma (koebnerization). Medications such as lithium, β-adrenergic blockers, and antimalarials and discontinuation of the use of systemic corticosteroids can precipitate or exacerbate psoriasis. Psoriatic arthritis occurs in 5% to 8% of patients with skin psoriasis.

* The onset of psoriasis most often occurs in the third decade of life.
* One-third of patients have a family history of psoriasis.
* Psoriasis typically presents with red plaques with silver scale on elbows, knees, and scalp.
* About 50% of patients have nail abnormalities.
* Psoriasis occurs at sites of trauma (koebnerization).

The treatment of psoriasis includes topical corticosteroids, topical tar preparations, and phototherapy. Newer forms of treatment of localized psoriasis include a topical synthetic vitamin D analogue, calcipotriene, and a topical retinoid, tazarotene.

Systemic agents used in the treatment of resistant psoriasis include methotrexate, acitretin, and cyclosporine.

Targeted Therapy in Psoriasis
Research into the pathogenesis of psoriasis has shown that the disease is T-cell–mediated. This knowledge has led to the development of several targeted therapies. Alefacept is a fusion protein that interferes with lymphocyte activation by binding to T cells expressing CD2. Infliximab and etanercept (anti–tumor necrosis factor-α agents) have been effective in the treatment of psoriasis.

Phototherapy

Ultraviolet Light
Natural sunlight contains ultraviolet B (UVB, 280-320 nm), ultraviolet A (320-400 nm), and visible light. UVB radiation causes sunburn reaction. UVB has been used most commonly in combination with tar for treating inflammatory dermatoses, as in the Goeckerman therapy of psoriasis. UVB also may benefit atopic dermatitis, lichen planus, and certain other inflammatory dermatoses.

Narrow-Band UVB
The wavelength of UVB with therapeutic effect for psoriasis has been identified in the 311-nm range. Light units producing this wavelength have been developed (narrow-band UVB) and have been shown to be more effective than traditional UVB for the treatment of psoriasis.

Psoralen and Ultraviolet A (PUVA)
PUVA consists of ingestion of psoralen followed by exposure of the skin to ultraviolet A. PUVA has been used most commonly for therapy of generalized psoriasis, but it is also effective in the treatment of lichen planus, mycosis fungoides, urticaria pigmentosa, and vitiligo. PUVA therapy is associated with minimal systemic side effects but is associated with an increased risk of cutaneous squamous cell carcinoma and melanoma in patients who have received long-term therapy.

* Ultraviolet light is commonly used for therapy of generalized psoriasis.
* PUVA is a form of phototherapy consisting of oral psoralen followed by UVA light exposure.
* PUVA is associated with an increased risk of cutaneous squamous cell carcinoma and melanoma with long-term use.

Atopic Dermatitis
Atopy is manifested by the following: atopic dermatitis, asthma, and allergic rhinitis or conjunctivitis. Atopic dermatitis often presents in the neonatal period with scaling and erythema of the scalp and face, later spreading to the trunk. The distribution is often extensor in the older infant, and by the age of approximately 3 years distribution is the more classic flexural. In adolescence, facial involvement (perioral, eyelid, and forehead) is common. Generalized flares of eczema can occur at any age.

Disturbances in cell-mediated immunity lead to an increased incidence of bacterial and viral infections. Secondary infection with *Staphylococcus aureus* presents as a weeping, crusting dermatitis (impetiginization). Eczema herpeticum is a secondary infection with the herpes simplex virus, which may be generalized. Infections with the human papillomavirus and molluscum contagiosum are also more common and the lesions are more numerous in patients with atopic dermatitis.

* Eczema herpeticum, a generalized herpes simplex virus infection, may occur in patients with atopic dermatitis.

For many years, emollients and topical corticosteroids have been the mainstay of treatment in atopic dermatitis.

Allergic Contact Dermatitis
Allergic contact dermatitis is a form of localized or generalized dermatitis that results from exposure to an antigen. This is a type 4 hypersensitivity reaction (delayed, cell-mediated). Recognition of antigens by T lymphocytes requires participation of Langerhans cells, which are the "antigen-presenting" cells of the epidermis. One must consider the anatomical location of the cutaneous lesions and environmental exposure to allergens, including occupational, household, and recreational contactants, to define the cause of the contact dermatitis.

* Allergic contact dermatitis is a type 4 hypersensitivity reaction (delayed, cell-mediated).
* Langerhans cells are the "antigen-presenting" cells of the epidermis.

Patch testing is performed by applying substances to the patient's back; each substance is placed under a small aluminum disk covered with adhesive tape. These are left on the patient's back for 48 hours, and the results are interpreted at 48 and 96 hours. Positive reactions occur most often to the following antigens: nickel sulfate, potassium dichromate, thimerosal, paraphenylenediamine, ethylenediamine, neomycin sulfate, benzocaine, thiuram, formaldehyde, and fragrance.

Nickel sulfate allergies are mainly associated with inexpensive jewelry. Paraphenylenediamine is present in hair dyes and other cosmetics; para-aminobenzoic acid in sunscreens is immunologically related to paraphenylenediamine. Potassium dichromate sensitivity is one of the most common types of occupational allergic contact dermatitis and occurs in construction workers exposed to cement, leathers, and certain paints. Formaldehyde is a common preservative in cosmetics and shampoos. Neomycin sulfate and benzocaine are components of many topical antimicrobial and analgesic preparations. Thimerosal is a commonly used preservative in contact lens solutions and in some intramuscular injections. Thiuram is a rubber accelerator and fungicide and therefore may correlate with occupational dermatitis related to wearing shoes containing rubber or rubber gloves. Allergic contact dermatitis to thiuram and other rubber accelerators is associated with rubber glove use in health care workers.

- Nickel sulfate allergies are associated with inexpensive jewelry.
- Potassium dichromate sensitivity occurs in construction workers exposed to cement, leathers, and certain paints.
- Formaldehyde is a common preservative in cosmetics and shampoos.
- Allergic contact dermatitis to thiuram and other rubber accelerators is associated with rubber glove use in health care workers.

Acne Vulgaris

Acne vulgaris is one of the most common problems addressed in clinical dermatology. Acne occurs physiologically at puberty with varying degrees of severity but may persist into the second and third decades of life. The pathogenesis of acne is multifactorial; inheritance, increase in sebaceous gland activity, hormonal influences, disturbances of keratinization, and bacterial infection have all been implicated. The primary lesions of acne are noninflammatory and include microcomedones, closed comedones (whiteheads), and open comedones (blackheads). The secondary or inflammatory lesions include papules and pustules, nodules, and cysts. Treatment options for acne are given in Table 5-2.

Systemic Retinoid Use in Acne Vulgaris

Isotretinoin (13-*cis*-retinoic acid) is a synthetic vitamin A derivative used primarily for the treatment of severe nodulocystic acne vulgaris. The mechanism of action of 13-*cis*-retinoic acid in acne is probably multifactorial, including improvement in keratinization, decrease in sebum production, and decrease in inflammation. A 20-week course at a dosage of approximately 1 mg/kg per day is the standard regimen.

- Isotretinoin is used for the treatment of severe acne vulgaris.

The greatest risk associated with use of systemic retinoids is teratogenicity. Before isotretinoin is prescribed, female patients must be counseled on this side effect and use reliable contraception during therapy and for at least 1 month after use of the drug is discontinued.

- The greatest risk with the use of systemic retinoids is teratogenicity.

The systemic retinoids are associated with various side effects, including xerosis (dry skin), dermatitis, cheilitis, sticky skin, peeling skin, epistaxis, conjunctivitis, hair loss, and nail dystrophy. Symptoms of arthralgias and myalgias also may occur. Hyperlipidemia, including both hypertriglyceridemia and hypercholesterolemia, develops in most patients. Other *potential* laboratory abnormalities include increased liver enzyme values and leukopenia. Skeletal hyperostosis may occur, particularly in association with long-term use. Concerns regarding depression and suicidal ideation are being studied.

- Side effects of systemic retinoids include xerosis, dermatitis, cheilitis, sticky skin, peeling skin, epistaxis, conjunctivitis, hair loss, and nail dystrophy. Concerns regarding depression and suicidal ideation are being studied.

Autoimmune Bullous Diseases

Bullous pemphigoid (Figure 5-1) is the most common autoimmune bullous disease. The disease predominantly occurs in elderly patients and usually presents with large, tense bullae on an erythematous base with a predilection for flexural areas. Lesions often are generalized but may be localized.

- Bullous pemphigoid is the most common autoimmune bullous disease.
- It occurs predominantly in elderly patients.
- It presents as large, tense bullae with a predilection for flexural areas.

Immunofluorescence testing is important for the diagnosis of bullous pemphigoid. Direct immunofluorescence testing of perilesional skin shows deposition of C3 in a linear pattern at the basement membrane zone in almost all cases and of IgG in more than 90%. Indirect immunofluorescence testing of serum shows IgG anti–basement-membrane zone antibodies in approximately 70% of cases.

- Immunofluorescence testing is important for the diagnosis of bullous pemphigoid.
- Almost all cases have deposition of C3 and IgG in a linear pattern at the basement membrane zone.

Table 5-2   Treatment of Acne Vulgaris

Type of Acne	Treatment
Comedonal	Topical tretinoin, benzoyl peroxide
Papular or pustular	Same as above, plus topical or systemic antibiotics
Cystic	Systemic antibiotics; if severe, isotretinoin

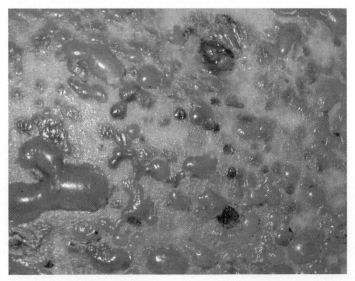

Figure 5-1. Bullous Pemphigoid.

Treatment of bullous pemphigoid includes systemic corticosteroids, dapsone, azathioprine, cyclophosphamide, and mycophenolate mofetil. In general, bullous pemphigoid requires less immunosuppressive therapy than does pemphigus and, in contrast to pemphigus, the titer of circulating antibodies does not correlate with disease activity.

Epidermolysis bullosa acquisita is another subepidermal bullous disease. It is characterized clinically by blisters or erosions induced by trauma, which predominantly occur on distal locations. A small subset of patients have generalized lesions, which clinically may be difficult to distinguish from bullous pemphigoid.

* Epidermolysis bullosa acquisita is characterized by blisters or erosions induced by trauma.
* It occurs predominantly on distal sites.

On direct immunofluorescence testing, epidermolysis bullosa acquisita has a pattern similar to that in bullous pemphigoid, namely, deposition of IgG and C3 in a linear pattern at the basement membrane zone. In contrast to bullous pemphigoid, C3 may be absent or IgG may be the dominant immunoreactant. Indirect immunofluorescence testing of serum demonstrates IgG anti–basement-membrane zone antibodies in 25% to 50% of patients. Epidermolysis bullosa acquisita tends to be resistant to immunosuppressive therapy.

* On direct immunofluorescence, epidermolysis bullosa acquisita shows deposition of IgG and C3 in a linear pattern at the basement membrane zone.
* Epidermolysis bullosa acquisita tends to be resistant to immunosuppressive therapy.

Cicatricial pemphigoid is characterized by mucosal lesions, with limited or no cutaneous lesions. The disease predominantly affects oral and ocular mucous membranes, and less frequently the genital, pharyngeal, or upper respiratory mucosa. This disease is also known as benign mucous membrane pemphigoid, which is a misnomer because untreated ocular involvement may lead to blindness. Patients may present with oral erosions or diffuse gingivitis.

* Cicatricial pemphigoid affects oral and ocular mucous membranes, and less frequently genital, pharyngeal, or upper respiratory mucosa.

Treatment of cicatricial pemphigoid is similar to that of bullous pemphigoid, with systemic corticosteroids, dapsone, azathioprine, cyclophosphamide, and mycophenolate. Cyclophosphamide has been used particularly in patients with ocular involvement.

Herpes gestationis, also referred to as pemphigoid gestationis, consists of intensely pruritic urticarial papules, plaques, or blisters usually occurring in the latter half of pregnancy. The lesions are histologically characterized by a subepidermal bulla with eosinophils.

* Herpes gestationis consists of intensely pruritic urticarial papules, plaques, or blisters.

Direct immunofluorescence testing is particularly useful because the other dermatoses of pregnancy (such as pruritic urticarial papules and plaques of pregnancy) are negative by immunofluorescence testing. The serum from approximately half of patients with herpes gestationis contains the HG factor, which is a complement-fixing IgG anti–basement-membrane zone antibody. The circulating antibody crosses the placenta, and the baby born to a mother with herpes gestationis may have a transient blistering eruption develop during the neonatal period.

* In herpes gestationis, direct immunofluorescence is useful because the other dermatoses of pregnancy are negative with such testing.

Linear IgA bullous dermatosis is characterized by vesicles or blisters on an erythematous base in a generalized distribution with a high rate of mucosal involvement. Drug-induced disease has occurred with vancomycin. This disease is characterized by the direct immunofluorescence finding of IgA deposition in a linear pattern at the basement membrane zone, with or without C3 or IgG deposition.

* In linear IgA bullous dermatosis, direct immunofluorescence shows IgA deposition in a linear pattern at the basement membrane zone.

Dermatitis herpetiformis (Figure 5-2) is characterized by extremely pruritic, grouped vesicles occurring predominantly over the elbows, knees, buttocks, back of the neck and scalp, and lower part of the back, usually beginning in the third or fourth decade of life. Virtually all patients have some degree of gluten-sensitive enteropathy (celiac sprue), although it is usually low-grade and subclinical. This association is important in terms of management of dermatitis herpetiformis. Dermatitis herpetiformis also is associated with thyroid disease.

* In dermatitis herpetiformis, virtually all patients have some degree of gluten-sensitive enteropathy (celiac sprue).

The hallmark of the diagnosis of dermatitis herpetiformis is the direct immunofluorescence finding of IgA deposits in a stippled, granular, or clumped pattern along the basement membrane zone. Skin biopsy specimens should be obtained from an area 0.5 to 1 cm from an active lesion. IgA deposits tend to persist in the skin over time. A small percentage of patients who strictly adhere to a gluten-free diet may show diminution in IgA deposits after many years, but IgA deposits in the skin are unaffected by pharmacologic therapy. Testing for endomysial antibodies and tissue transglutaminase is useful for both diagnosis and management of dermatitis herpetiformis, although these antibodies correlate with the degree of gluten-sensitive enteropathy rather than the skin lesions per se.

* In dermatitis herpetiformis, direct immunofluorescence shows IgA deposits in a stippled, granular, or clumped pattern.
* Testing for endomysial antibodies and tissue transglutaminase is useful for diagnosis and management.

The mainstay of treatment of dermatitis herpetiformis consists of dapsone and a gluten-free diet. Patients who strictly adhere to a gluten-free diet may have a decreased need for dapsone. Patients

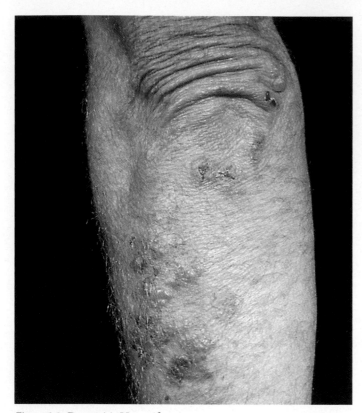

Figure 5-2. Dermatitis Herpetiformis.

must adhere to the diet for at least 8 months before it is effective. The titer of IgA anti-endomysial antibodies decreases during strict adherence to a gluten-free diet. Patients with gluten-sensitive enteropathy have an increased risk for small bowel lymphoma. Only adherence to a gluten-free diet will affect this risk. Systemic corticosteroids are not helpful for the treatment of dermatitis herpetiformis.

* Treatment of dermatitis herpetiformis consists of dapsone and a gluten-free diet.

Bullous eruption of systemic lupus erythematosus shares clinical and histologic features with dermatitis herpetiformis. The blisters were therefore originally thought to represent the coexistence of dermatitis herpetiformis and lupus erythematosus, but they are now established as a distinct subset of lupus.
    Direct immunofluorescence testing shows deposition of IgG, IgM, IgA, or C3 in a linear or granular pattern at the basement membrane zone, similar to the classic lupus band.

* In bullous eruption of systemic lupus erythematosus, direct immunofluorescence shows deposition of IgG, IgM, IgA, or C3 in a linear or granular pattern at the basement membrane zone.

The clinical variants of *pemphigus* include pemphigus vulgaris and pemphigus foliaceus (with the subsets pemphigus erythematosus and fogo selvagem, the latter being an endemic form of pemphigus

that occurs in South America). There is also a drug-induced variant of pemphigus, particularly associated with D-penicillamine, captopril, or other thiol-containing medications.
    More than 50% of patients with pemphigus vulgaris present with oral lesions, and more than 90% have oral mucosal involvement at some point in the course of the disease. Pemphigus vulgaris is characterized by coalescing blisters and erosions, often with generalized involvement. In contrast, pemphigus foliaceus (Figure 5-3), considered to represent the superficial variant of pemphigus, may present with superficial scaling-crusting lesions of the head and neck area (in a seborrheic dermatitis-like pattern) or generalized distribution.

* Pemphigus vulgaris is characterized by coalescing blisters and erosions.
* Pemphigus foliaceus may present with superficial scaling-crusting lesions of the head and neck.

All types of pemphigus are characterized by the deposition of IgG and C3 at the intercellular space (epidermal cell surface) on direct immunofluorescence testing (intercellular substance [ICS] antibody). On indirect immunofluorescence testing, IgG anti-ICS antibodies are found in approximately 90% of cases. The titer of IgG anti-ICS antibodies is useful in both diagnosis and management of pemphigus.

* All types of pemphigus are characterized by the direct immunofluorescence finding of IgG and C3 deposition at the epidermal cell surface.
* The titer of IgG anti-ICS antibodies is useful in diagnosis and management.

Pemphigus antibodies are pathogenic in that they have been shown to induce acantholysis in vitro and in animal models.

* Pemphigus antibodies induce acantholysis.

High-dose corticosteroids generally are required to control pemphigus. Various steroid-sparing immunosuppressive agents have been

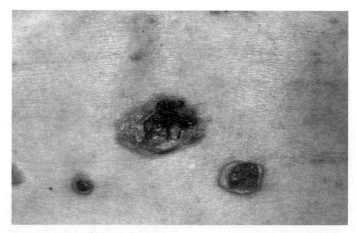

Figure 5-3. Pemphigus Foliaceus.

used, including azathioprine, mycophenolate mofetil, cyclophosphamide, gold, and dapsone.

* High-dose corticosteroids generally are required to control pemphigus, followed by institution of a steroid-sparing agent.

Erythema Multiforme

Erythema multiforme (Figure 5-4) is an acute, usually self-limited eruption of maculopapular, urticarial, occasionally bullous lesions characterized by iris or target morphology. A subset of patients with erythema multiforme may have recurrent lesions. When erythema multiforme presents with extensive cutaneous and mucosal lesions, it is referred to as Stevens-Johnson syndrome. Various etiologic factors have been implicated in erythema multiforme. The most commonly cited precipitating factor is viral infection, particularly herpes simplex virus. This is responsible for a considerable percentage of recurrent erythema multiforme. Other infectious agents that have been noted to cause erythema multiforme include *Mycoplasma pneumoniae* and *Yersinia enterocolitica*. Drugs have been reported to induce erythema multiforme, particularly sulfonamides, barbiturates, and anticonvulsants. Erythema multiforme also may be associated with underlying connective tissue disease or malignancy. A small subset of patients with erythema multiforme have disease limited to the oral mucosa. Erythema multiforme tends to involve the lips, buccal mucosa, and tongue, in contrast to pemphigus vulgaris, which typically involves the pharynx, buccal mucosa, and tongue, and pemphigoid, which most often involves gingivae. Neither pemphigus nor pemphigoid involves the lips.

* The most commonly cited precipitating factor for erythema multiforme is viral infection, particularly herpes simplex.
* Other infectious agents: *Mycoplasma pneumoniae* and *Yersinia enterocolitica*.
* Drugs also induce erythema multiforme: sulfonamides, barbiturates, anticonvulsants.

Erythema Nodosum

Erythema nodosum (Figure 5-5) typically presents as tender, erythematous, subcutaneous nodules localized to the pretibial areas. The nodules may be acute and self-limited or chronic, lasting for months to years. The most common cause is streptococcal pharyngitis. Other infectious agents that have been implicated in the development of erythema nodosum include *Yersinia enterocolitica*, *Coccidioides*, and *Histoplasmosis*. Drug-induced erythema nodosum most often is associated with oral contraceptives and sulfonamides. Other associations with erythema nodosum include sarcoidosis, inflammatory bowel disease, and Behçet syndrome.

* The most common cause of erythema nodosum is streptococcal pharyngitis.
* Drug-induced erythema nodosum most often is associated with oral contraceptives and sulfonamides.
* Other associations: sarcoidosis, inflammatory bowel disease, Behçet syndrome.

Drug Reactions

The morphologic spectrum of reactions that may be induced by medications is broad, and hundreds of drugs may produce a given cutaneous reaction. Types of cutaneous lesions induced by drugs include maculopapular eruptions, acne folliculitis, necrotizing vasculitis, vesiculobullous lesions, erythema multiforme, erythema nodosum, fixed drug eruptions, lichenoid reactions, photosensitivity reactions, pigmentary changes, and hair loss.

Approximately 2% of hospitalized patients have cutaneous drug reactions, and penicillin, sulfonamides, and blood products are responsible for approximately two-thirds of such reactions. The most common types of clinical presentations (in descending order of frequency)

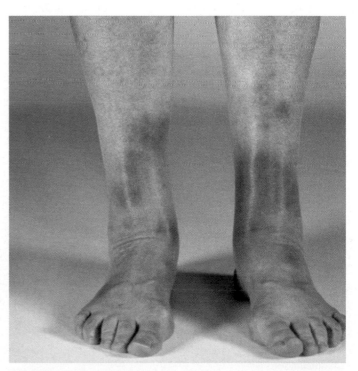

Figure 5-5. Erythema Nodosum.

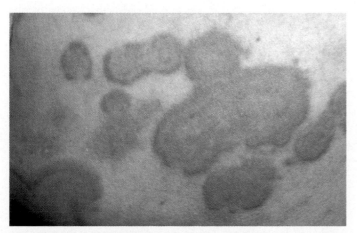

Figure 5-4. Erythema Multiforme.

are exanthematous or morbilliform eruptions, urticaria or angioedema, fixed drug eruptions, and erythema multiforme. Stevens-Johnson syndrome, exfoliative erythroderma, and photosensitive eruptions are less common. Table 5-3 outlines the types of cutaneous reactions to drugs.

- About 2% of hospitalized patients have cutaneous drug reactions.
- Penicillin, sulfonamides, and blood products are responsible for about two-thirds of drug reactions.
- Urticarial drug reactions are most often related to aspirin, penicillin, and blood products.
- Photoallergic reactions are most often associated with sulfonamides, thiazides, griseofulvin, or phenothiazines.
- Phototoxic reactions may be induced by tetracyclines.

Exanthematous or morbilliform eruptions are the most common type of cutaneous drug reaction. This type of eruption usually begins within a week of onset of therapy, but it may occur more than 2 weeks after initiation of the therapy or up to 2 weeks after use of the drug has been discontinued. Ampicillin, penicillin, and cephalosporins are commonly associated with morbilliform eruptions. A fixed drug eruption is one or several lesions that recur at the same anatomical location on rechallenge with the medication. The genital and facial areas are common sites of involvement. Phenolphthalein, barbiturates, salicylates, and oral contraceptives have been implicated in the cause of fixed drug eruptions.

- Exanthematous or morbilliform eruptions are the most common cutaneous drug reaction.
- A fixed drug eruption is one or several lesions that recur at the same location on rechallenge.
- Phenolphthalein, barbiturates, salicylates, and oral contraceptives are implicated in fixed drug eruptions.

Lichenoid drug eruptions are morphologically similar to lichen planus (with violaceous papules of the skin) and most often have been associated with gold and antimalarial drugs, although various medications may induce this type of reaction.

Table 5-3   Cutaneous Reactions to Drugs

Type of Skin Reaction	Cause
Urticarial	Aspirin, penicillin, blood products
Photoallergic	Sulfonamides, thiazides, griseofulvin, phenothiazines
Phototoxic	Tetracyclines
Slate-gray discoloration	Chlorpromazine
Slate-blue discoloration	Amiodarone
Yellow or blue-gray pigmentation	Antimalarials

Cutaneous Signs of Underlying Malignancy

Cutaneous metastasis occurs in 1% to 5% of patients with metastatic neoplasms. The types of malignancy metastatic to the skin are lung, breast, kidney, gastrointestinal, melanoma, and ovary. Lesions usually present on the scalp, face, or trunk.

- Cutaneous metastasis occurs in 1%-5% of patients with metastatic neoplasms.
- Lesions usually present on the scalp, face, or trunk.

Paget disease of the nipple is an erythematous, scaly, or weeping eczematous eruption of the areola. Virtually all patients with Paget disease have an underlying ductal carcinoma of the breast. In contrast, *extramammary Paget disease*, a morphologically similar eruption that usually occurs in the anogenital region, is associated with underlying carcinoma in only about 50% of cases. Extramammary Paget disease may be associated with underlying cutaneous adnexal carcinoma or with underlying visceral carcinoma (particularly of the genitourinary or distal gastrointestinal tracts).

- Patients with Paget disease have underlying ductal carcinoma of the breast.
- Extramammary Paget disease may be associated with underlying carcinoma in only 50% of cases.

Acanthosis nigricans (Figure 5-6) consists of velvety brown plaques of the intertriginous regions, particularly the axillae and groin. It has been associated with adenocarcinoma of the gastrointestinal tract, particularly the stomach. It also occurs with insulin-resistant diabetes. Acanthosis nigricans also may be associated with obesity or certain medications (such as prednisone and nicotinic acid). There is an autosomal dominant variant of acanthosis nigricans.

- Acanthosis nigricans is associated with adenocarcinoma of the gastrointestinal tract, particularly the stomach.
- It also may be associated with obesity, certain medications, and insulin-resistant diabetes.

Pyoderma gangrenosum (Figure 5-7) consists of ulcers with irregular, undermined, inflammatory, violaceous borders that heal with cribriform scarring. The lesions are most commonly associated with inflammatory bowel disease or rheumatoid arthritis. Pyoderma gangrenosum may be associated with malignancy of the hematopoietic system, particularly leukemia.

- Pyoderma gangrenosum is most commonly associated with inflammatory bowel disease or rheumatoid arthritis.
- It may be associated with leukemia.

The skin lesions of *glucagonoma syndrome* (*necrolytic migratory erythema*) (Figure 5-8) consist of erosions, crusting, and peeling involving the perineum and perioral areas, but they may be generalized. The syndrome also includes stomatitis, glossitis (beefy tongue), anemia, diarrhea, and weight loss. It is associated with an islet cell (α) tumor of the pancreas.

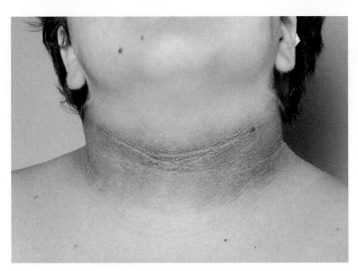

Figure 5-6. Acanthosis Nigricans.

* Glucagonoma syndrome consists of erosions, crusting, and peeling involving the perineum and perioral areas.
* It is associated with an islet cell tumor of the pancreas.

Gardner syndrome is a hereditary (autosomal dominant) form of colon polyposis. Clinical features include adenomatous polyps of the colon, osteomas of the skull and face, scoliosis, soft tissue tumors (including dermoids, lipomas, and fibromas), and sebaceous (epidermal inclusion) cysts of the face and scalp. There is a high incidence of colon carcinoma. In approximately 60% of patients, adenocarcinoma of the colon develops by age 40 years. Malignancies of other sites have been associated with this syndrome, including adrenal, ovarian, and thyroid.

* Gardner syndrome is a hereditary (autosomal dominant) form of colon polyposis.
* Clinical features are soft tissue tumors and sebaceous cysts of the face.
* There is a high incidence of colon cancer.

Acquired ichthyosis most often has been associated with Hodgkin disease, but it has been reported with other types of lymphoma, multiple myeloma, and various carcinomas.

* Acquired ichthyosis is associated with Hodgkin disease.

Hirsutism may reflect androgen excess due to an adrenal or ovarian tumor.
   Hypertrichosis is an increase in hair unrelated to androgen excess, such as hypertrichosis lanuginosa acquisita (growth of soft downy hair). It has been associated with carcinoid tumor, adenocarcinoma of the breast, lymphoma, gastrointestinal malignancy, and other types of neoplasms.
   Sweet syndrome (*acute febrile neutrophilic dermatosis*) has skin lesions that consist of erythematous plaques and nodules, most commonly located on the proximal aspects of the extremities and face. The association is with leukemia, particularly acute myelocytic or acute myelomonocytic leukemia, although many other diseases also have been associated.

* Sweet syndrome is associated with leukemia (acute myelocytic or acute myelomonocytic).

Generalized pruritus is the presentation for many cutaneous and systemic disorders. Pruritus may be the presenting symptom in lymphoma.

* Pruritus may be the presenting symptom in lymphoma.

In *dermatomyositis*, the pathognomonic skin lesions are Gottron papules (Figure 5-9) involving the skin over the joints of the fingers, elbows, and knees. Poikilodermatous lesions or erythematous maculopapular eruptions may diffusely involve the face, particularly the periorbital area (heliotrope rash [Figure 5-10]), and the trunk and extremities. The cutaneous lesions are photosensitive and pruritic. The disease is characterized by proximal myositis. Although creatine kinase and aldolase levels usually are increased in patients with myositis, it is important to verify the diagnosis by obtaining an

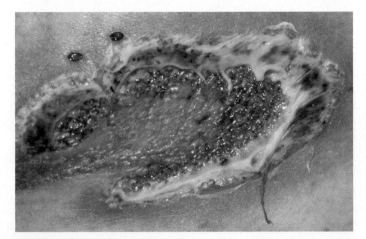

Figure 5-7. Pyoderma Gangrenosum.

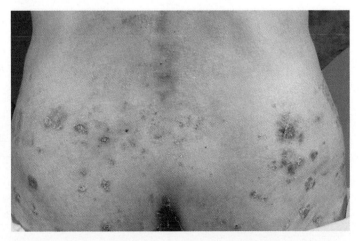

Figure 5-8. Glucagonoma Syndrome (Necrolytic Migratory Erythema).

electromyogram and a muscle biopsy specimen. Dermatomyositis is associated with an increased incidence of underlying malignancy.

- Dermatomyositis may involve the periorbital area (heliotrope rash) or the dorsal aspect of the hands (Gottron papules).
- The lesions are photosensitive and pruritic.
- Dermatomyositis is characterized by proximal myositis.
- Dermatomyositis is associated with an increased risk of internal malignancy.

Cutaneous amyloidosis may present clinically as macroglossia (Figure 5-11), waxy papules on the eyelids or nasolabial folds, pinch purpura, and postproctoscopic purpura (Figure 5-12). Multiple myeloma may be associated with amyloid.

- Amyloidosis may be associated with multiple myeloma.

Tylosis is a rare disorder characterized by palmar-plantar keratoderma associated with esophageal carcinoma. It has autosomal dominant inheritance.

- Tylosis is associated with esophageal carcinoma.

The *autoimmune bullous diseases* are a heterogeneous group of disorders characterized by antibody deposition at the basement membrane zone or epidermis. An association with malignancy has been found in several of these disorders.

- Pemphigus is associated with thymoma with or without myasthenia gravis.
- Paraneoplastic pemphigus presents with clinical and histologic features of pemphigus and erythema multiforme and is associated with lymphoma and leukemia.
- Small bowel lymphoma rarely develops in patients with dermatitis herpetiformis.
- Epidermolysis bullosa acquisita is associated with amyloidosis and multiple myeloma.

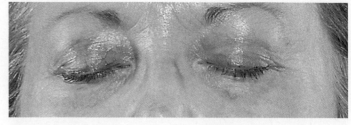

Figure 5-10. Dermatomyositis: Heliotrope Discoloration.

- Bullous pemphigoid has not been associated with an increased risk of underlying malignancy.

Dermatology: An Internist's Perspective

Pulmonary

The skin is involved in 15% to 35% of patients with *sarcoidosis*. Lesions may present as 1) lupus pernio (erythematous swelling of the nose), 2) translucent papules around the eyes and nasolabial folds, 3) annular lesions with central atrophy, 4) nodules on the trunk and extremities, and 5) scar sarcoid.

- The skin is involved in 15%-35% of patients with sarcoidosis.
- Lesions may present as lupus pernio (erythematous swelling of the nose).

Acute sarcoidosis may present with a combination of erythema nodosum, bilateral hilar lymphadenopathy, fever, and arthralgias (Löfgren syndrome). *Erythema nodosum* (Figure 5-5) is a reactive condition that may be associated with acute sarcoidosis. Erythema nodosum typically presents as tender, erythematous, subcutaneous nodules localized to pretibial areas.

- Erythema nodosum may be associated with acute sarcoidosis (Löfgren syndrome).

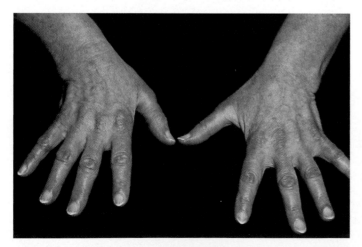

Figure 5-9. Dermatomyositis: Gottron Papules.

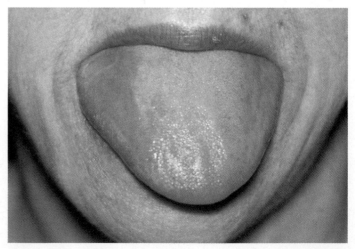

Figure 5-11. Amyloidosis: Macroglossia.

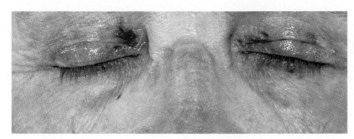

Figure 5-12. Amyloidosis: Postproctoscopic Purpura.

In antineutrophil cytoplasmic autoantibody (ANCA)-associated granulomatous vasculitis, cutaneous involvement occurs in more than 50% of patients and is manifested by cutaneous infarction, ulceration, hemorrhagic bullae, purpuric papules, or urticaria. A skin biopsy may show hypersensitivity vasculitis or granulomatous vasculitis.

* In antineutrophil cytoplasmic autoantibody (ANCA)-associated granulomatous vasculitis, cutaneous involvement occurs in >50% of patients.
* Manifestations are ulceration, hemorrhagic bullae, purpuric papules, and urticaria.

Churg-Strauss granulomatosis (*allergic granulomatosis*) is characterized by a combination of adult-onset asthma, peripheral eosinophilia, and pulmonary involvement with recurrent pneumonia or transient infiltrates. Skin lesions have been reported in up to 60% of patients and consist of palpable purpura, cutaneous infarcts, and subcutaneous nodules.

* Skin lesions of Churg-Strauss granulomatosis occur in up to 60% of patients.
* Skin lesions include palpable purpura, cutaneous infarcts, and subcutaneous nodules.

In *relapsing polychondritis*, there is episodic destructive inflammation of cartilage of the ears, nose, and upper airways. There may be associated arthritis and ocular involvement. In the acute stage, the ears may be red, swollen, and tender. Later, they become soft and flabby. Nasal chondritis may lead to saddle-nose deformities. Relapsing polychondritis is mediated by antibodies to type II collagen.

* Relapsing polychondritis is characterized by episodic destructive inflammation of cartilage of ears, nose, and upper airways.
* Nasal chondritis may lead to saddle-nose deformities.

Cardiovascular
Pseudoxanthoma elasticum may be transmitted by autosomal dominant or autosomal recessive inheritance. Yellow xanthoma-like papules are seen on the neck (plucked-chicken skin), axillae, groin, and abdomen. Angioid streaks may be seen in the fundus. Skin biopsy shows degeneration of elastic fibers. Systemic associations include stroke, myocardial infarction, peripheral vascular disease, and gastrointestinal hemorrhage.

* Pseudoxanthoma elasticum is associated with stroke, myocardial infarction, peripheral vascular disease, and gastrointestinal hemorrhage.

Ehlers-Danlos syndrome includes 10 subgroups that vary in severity and systemic associations. Cutaneous findings are skin hyperextensibility with hypermobile joints and fish-mouth scars. Angina, peripheral vascular disease, and gastrointestinal bleeding may be associated.

* Ehlers-Danlos syndrome is associated with angina, peripheral vascular disease, and gastrointestinal bleeding.

Erythema marginatum is one of the diagnostic criteria for acute rheumatic fever. This uncommon eruption occurs on the trunk and is characterized by erythematous plaques with rapidly mobile serpiginous borders.

* Erythema marginatum is one of the diagnostic criteria for acute rheumatic fever.

Gastrointestinal
Osler-Weber-Rendu syndrome (*hereditary hemorrhagic telangiectasia*), with autosomal dominant inheritance, is manifested by cutaneous and mucosal telangiectasias. Frequent nosebleeds and gastrointestinal bleeds may be a presenting feature. Pulmonary arteriovenous malformations and central nervous system angiomas are also features of this syndrome.

* Osler-Weber-Rendu syndrome has autosomal dominant inheritance.
* Features are cutaneous and mucosal telangiectasia, nosebleeds, gastrointestinal bleeds, pulmonary arteriovenous malformations, and central nervous system angiomas.

Acrodermatitis enteropathica is an inherited (autosomal recessive) or acquired disease characterized by zinc deficiency (failure of absorption or failure to supplement). The clinical features include angular cheilitis, a seborrheic dermatitis-like eruption, erosions, blisters, and pustules, with skin lesions particularly involving the face, hands, feet, and perineum. Alopecia and diarrhea are other features of this syndrome.

* Acrodermatitis enteropathica is an inherited (autosomal recessive) or acquired disease.
* The disease is characterized by zinc deficiency (failure of absorption or failure to supplement).

Peutz-Jeghers syndrome is an inherited (autosomal dominant) syndrome of intestinal polyposis. Patients have hamartomas, mostly involving the small bowel, and a slightly increased risk for carcinoma. Cutaneous lesions include macular pigmentation (freckles) of the lips, periungual skin, fingers, and toes and pigmentation of the oral mucosa.

* Peutz-Jeghers syndrome is an inherited (autosomal dominant) syndrome of intestinal polyposis.
* Patients have an increased risk for carcinoma.

Dermatitis herpetiformis (Figure 5-2) is an immune-mediated bullous disease that presents with intensely itchy vesicles on extensor surfaces (elbows, knees, buttocks, scapulae). Gluten-sensitive enteropathy occurs in almost all patients, although it may be subclinical. Gluten-sensitive enteropathy is associated with an increased risk of small B-cell lymphoma.

- Dermatitis herpetiformis is an immune-mediated bullous disease.
- Gluten-sensitive enteropathy occurs in almost all patients.
- Gluten-sensitive enteropathy is associated with an increased risk of small B-cell lymphoma.

Extensive *aphthous ulceration* may be associated with Crohn disease or gluten-sensitive enteropathy.

- Aphthous ulceration may be associated with Crohn disease or gluten-sensitive enteropathy.

Pyoderma gangrenosum (Figure 5-7) presents with ulceration, predominantly on the lower extremities, with inflammatory undermined borders. The lesions heal with cribriform scarring. The occurrence of the disease at sites of trauma is classic (pathergy). Systemic disease associations include inflammatory bowel disease (ulcerative colitis more commonly than Crohn disease), rheumatoid arthritis, and paraproteinemia.

- Pyoderma gangrenosum occurs at sites of trauma.
- Associated diseases are inflammatory bowel disease (ulcerative colitis more than Crohn disease), rheumatoid arthritis, and paraproteinemia.

Cutaneous Crohn disease may present as skin nodules with granulomatous histologic findings. Other manifestations include pyostomatitis vegetans (granulomatous inflammation of the gingivae), granulomatous cheilitis, oral aphthous ulceration, perianal skin tags, perianal fistulas, and peristomal pyoderma gangrenosum.

- A manifestation of Crohn disease is pyostomatitis vegetans (granulomatous inflammation of gingivae).

Bowel bypass syndrome presents with a flu-like illness with fever, malaise, arthralgias, myalgias, and inflammatory papules and pustules on the extremities and upper trunk. The disease is recurrent and episodic and occurs in up to 20% of patients after jejunoileal bypass. The condition responds to antibiotics or to reversal of the bypass procedure.

- Bowel bypass syndrome presents with a flu-like illness and inflammatory papules and pustules.
- It occurs in up to 20% of patients after jejunoileal bypass.

Gardner syndrome and *glucagonoma syndrome* are described earlier in this chapter.

Nephrology
Partial lipodystrophy is associated with C3 deficiency and the nephrotic syndrome.

Uremic pruritus is associated with end-stage renal disease and responds to UVB therapy.

Neurocutaneous
Fabry disease is an X-linked recessive disorder due to deficiency of the enzyme α-galactosidase A. The skin changes consist of numerous vascular tumors (angiokeratomas) that develop during childhood and adolescence. Corneal opacities are present in 90% of patients. Systemic manifestations include paresthesias and pain due to involved peripheral nerves, renal insufficiency, and vascular insufficiency of the coronary and central nervous system.

- Fabry disease is a recessive disorder due to deficiency of α-galactosidase A.
- Systemic manifestations are paresthesias, renal insufficiency, and vascular insufficiency.

The clinical features of *ataxia-telangiectasia* include cutaneous and ocular telangiectasia, cerebellar ataxia, choreoathetosis, IgA deficiency, and recurrent pulmonary infections.

Tuberous sclerosis may be inherited in an autosomal dominant pattern (25%) or may occur sporadically (new mutation). Predominant cutaneous lesions include hypopigmented macules, adenoma sebaceum, subungual or periungual fibromas, and shagreen patch (connective tissue nevus) (Figure 5-13). This syndrome is associated with epilepsy (80%) and mental retardation (60%). Rhabdomyomas may occur in the heart in childhood. Angiomyolipomas occur in the kidneys in up to 80% of adults with this syndrome.

- Tuberous sclerosis may be inherited in an autosomal dominant pattern or be sporadic.
- It is associated with epilepsy (80%) and mental retardation (60%).
- Angiomyolipomas occur in the kidneys in up to 80% of affected adults.

Neurofibromatosis (von Recklinghausen disease) (Figure 5-14) occurs in 1 in 3,000 births. Inheritance is autosomal dominant, and approximately 50% of cases are new mutations. The major signs of the disease are café au lait spots, axillary freckling (Crowe sign), neurofibromas, and Lisch nodules of the iris.

- Neurofibromatosis is autosomal dominant.
- Major signs: café au lait spots, axillary freckling, neurofibromas.

The associated central nervous system tumors include acoustic neuromas, optic gliomas, and meningiomas. Other associated tumors include pheochromocytoma, neuroblastoma, and Wilms tumor. Café au lait spots and neurofibromas frequently occur in the absence of neurofibromatosis. The diagnostic criteria for neurofibromatosis include 2 or more of the following:

1. Six or more café au lait macules more than 0.5 cm in greatest diameter in prepubertal patients, or more than 1.5 cm in diameter in adults
2. Two or more neurofibromas of any type, or 1 plexiform neurofibroma
3. Freckling of skin in axillary or inguinal regions

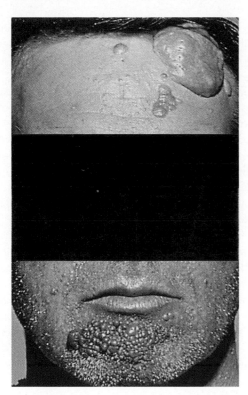

Figure 5-13. Tuberous Sclerosis: Adenoma Sebaceum and Forehead Plaque.

4. Optic gliomas
5. Lisch nodules
6. An osseous lesion such as sphenoid dysplasia or thinning of long bone cortex with or without pseudarthrosis
7. A first-degree relative with neurofibromatosis that meets the above diagnostic criteria

Sturge-Weber-Dimitri syndrome is characterized by capillary angioma (port-wine stain) in the distribution of the upper or middle branch of the trigeminal nerve. There may be associated meningeal angioma in the same distribution. Intracranial tramline calcification, mental retardation, epilepsy, contralateral hemiparesis, and visual impairment may be associated.

* Sturge-Weber-Dimitri syndrome is characterized by capillary angioma in the distribution of the upper or middle branch of the trigeminal nerve.
* Associated features are intracranial calcification, mental retardation, epilepsy, contralateral hemiparesis, and visual impairment.

Rheumatology

Psoriatic arthritis occurs in 5% to 8% of patients with cutaneous psoriasis. Several different patterns of arthritis occur. An asymmetric oligoarthritis occurs in 70% of patients. This group includes patients with "sausage digits" and monoarthritis. The second most common presentation is asymmetric arthritis clinically similar to rheumatoid arthritis, which occurs in 15% of patients with psoriatic arthritis. Distal interphalangeal involvement, arthritis mutilans, and a spinal

form of arthritis similar to ankylosing spondylitis each occurs in 5% of patients with psoriatic arthritis.

* Psoriatic arthritis occurs in 5%-8% of patients with psoriasis.
* Asymmetric oligoarthritis is most common.
* 5% of patients have ankylosing spondylitis.

Reiter syndrome consists of the triad of urethritis, conjunctivitis, and arthritis. The disease usually affects young men. Two-thirds of patients have skin lesions, namely, circinate balanitis, consisting of erythematous plaques of the penis, and keratoderma blennorrhagicum, a pustular psoriasiform eruption of the palms and soles. Most patients are positive for HLA-B27.

* Reiter syndrome triad: urethritis, conjunctivitis, arthritis.
* Skin signs are circinate balanitis and keratoderma blennorrhagicum.
* Most patients are positive for HLA-B27.

Erythema migrans is an annular, sometimes urticarial, erythematous plaque presenting as a manifestation of Lyme disease. The plaque develops subsequent to and surrounding the site of a tick bite. Lesions are single in 75% of patients and multiple in 25%. Other acute features of Lyme disease include fever, headaches, myalgias, arthralgias, and lymphadenopathy. The deer tick *Ixodes scapularis* contains a spirochete, *Borrelia burgdorferi*, that is responsible for the syndrome. Arthritis is a late complication of Lyme disease. Weeks or months after the initial illness, meningoencephalitis, peripheral neuropathy, myocarditis, atrioventricular node block, or destructive erosive arthritis may develop.

* Erythema migrans presents as a manifestation of Lyme disease.
* The lesion develops subsequent to and surrounding the site of a tick bite.
* Lesions are single in 75% of patients and multiple in 25%.

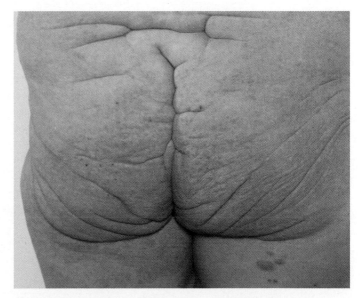

Figure 5-14. Neurofibromatosis: Plexiform Neurofibroma.

In *rheumatoid arthritis*, nodules may occur over the extensor surfaces of joints, most commonly on the dorsal aspects of the hands and elbows. Rheumatoid vasculitis with ulceration may occur in the setting of rheumatoid arthritis with a high circulating rheumatoid factor.

During the late stages of *gout*, tophi (urate deposits with surrounding inflammation) occur in the subcutaneous tissues. Improved methods of treatment account for the decrease in the incidence of tophaceous gout in recent years.

* Gouty tophi may occur in subcutaneous tissues.

In *lupus erythematosus* (LE), cutaneous abnormalities occur in approximately 80% of patients. LE can be classified into acute cutaneous LE (malar rash, generalized maculopapular eruption, or bullous LE), subacute cutaneous LE, and chronic cutaneous LE (localized discoid LE, generalized discoid LE, and lupus panniculitis).

* In LE, cutaneous abnormalities occur in 80% of patients.

Skin lesions are present in up to 85% of patients with acute systemic LE. A butterfly rash with erythema involving the nose and cheeks is characteristic. Erythematous papules and plaques also may occur on the dorsal aspect of the hands, and the skin overlying the interphalangeal and metacarpal phalangeal joints is spared. Maculopapular erythema also may occur on sun-exposed areas.

Subacute cutaneous LE (Figure 5-15) usually presents with generalized annular or polycyclic plaques. The lesions may appear papulosquamous or vesiculobullous. Subacute cutaneous LE is characterized by the presence of anti-Ro (anti-SSA) antibodies in serum and photosensitivity. These antibodies cross the placenta, and children born to mothers with subacute cutaneous LE may develop congenital heart block or a transient photodistributed skin eruption during the neonatal period.

* Subacute cutaneous LE presents with annular or polycyclic plaques.
* Subacute cutaneous LE is characterized by the presence of anti-Ro (anti-SSA) antibodies and photosensitivity.

Discoid LE (Figure 5-16) is characterized by erythematous papules and plaques with follicular hyperkeratosis and scaling. Localized discoid LE is usually not associated with progression to systemic LE. Generalized discoid LE or disseminated discoid LE refers to lesions involving the head and neck area and also the trunk and extremities. Discoid LE most commonly affects the face, scalp, and ears. Although most patients with discoid LE lack manifestations of systemic LE, approximately 25% of patients with systemic LE have had cutaneous lesions of discoid LE at some point during the course of their illness. Circulating antinuclear antibodies are demonstrable in most patients with systemic LE and subacute cutaneous LE, but they are present in only a small percentage of patients with discoid LE.

* Discoid LE is characterized by erythematous papules and plaques with follicular hyperkeratosis and scaling.

* Discoid LE most commonly affects the face, scalp, and ears.
* 25% of patients with systemic LE have had cutaneous manifestations of discoid LE.

The term *scleroderma* encompasses a wide spectrum of diseases ranging from generalized multisystem disease to localized cutaneous disease. The systemic end of the spectrum is represented by diffuse scleroderma and the CREST (*c*alcinosis cutis, *R*aynaud phenomenon, *e*sophageal involvement, *s*clerodactyly, and *t*elangiectasia) syndrome. The middle area of the spectrum is represented by eosinophilic fasciitis and linear scleroderma, which may have systemic involvement. Localized scleroderma (also known as morphea) may be a single plaque or may be multiple plaques in a generalized distribution.

Systemic scleroderma consists of diffuse sclerosis associated with smoothness and hardening of the skin, with masklike face and microstomia. Sclerodactyly, periungual telangiectasia, telangiectatic mats, hyperpigmentation, and cutaneous calcification may be observed. Esophageal, pulmonary, renal, and cardiac involvement may be associated with systemic scleroderma. The CREST syndrome (Figure 5-17) is associated with circulating anticentromere antibodies.

* Systemic scleroderma may include sclerodactyly, periungual telangiectasia, telangiectatic mats, hyperpigmentation, and cutaneous calcification.

Eosinophilic fasciitis manifests as tightly bound thickening of the skin and underlying soft tissues of the extremities. Other features include arthralgias, hypergammaglobulinemia, and peripheral blood eosinophilia.

* Eosinophilic fasciitis manifests as tightly bound thickening of the skin and underlying soft tissue of the extremities.

Morphea manifests as discrete sclerotic plaques with a white, shiny center and erythematous or violaceous periphery. Localized or linear scleroderma may have various presentations depending on extent, location, and depth of sclerosis. Most lesions are characterized by

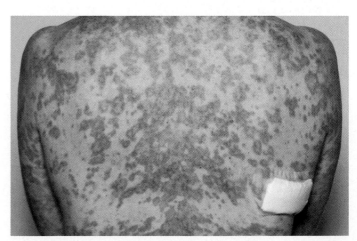

Figure 5-15. Subacute Cutaneous Lupus Erythematosus.

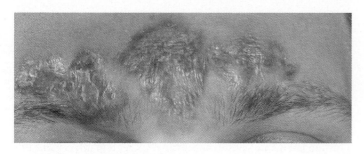

Figure 5-16. Discoid Lupus Erythematosus.

sclerosis and atrophy associated with depression or "delling" of the soft tissue; underlying bone may be affected in linear scleroderma.

* Morphea manifests as discrete sclerotic plaques with a white, shiny center.
* Underlying bone may be affected in linear scleroderma.

Hematologic

Graft-versus-host disease (GVHD) most commonly occurs after bone marrow transplantation and represents the constellation of skin lesions, diarrhea, and liver enzyme abnormalities. GVHD occurs in 60% to 80% of patients who undergo allogeneic bone marrow transplant.

* GVHD commonly occurs after bone marrow transplant.
* GVHD includes skin lesions, diarrhea, and liver enzyme abnormalities.

GVHD generally occurs in 2 phases. Acute GVHD begins 7 to 21 days after transplant, and chronic GVHD begins within months to 1 year after transplant. One or both phases may occur in the same patient. Acute GVHD results from attack of donor immunocompetent T lymphocytes and null lymphocytes against host histocompatibility antigens. Chronic GVHD results from immunocompetent lymphocytes that develop in the recipient.

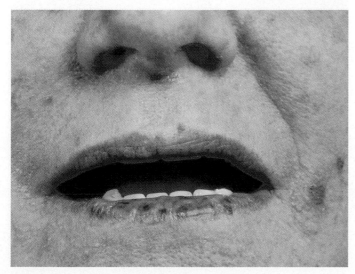

Figure 5-17. Scleroderma: CREST Syndrome.

The cutaneous abnormalities of acute GVHD include pruritus, numbness or pain of the palms and soles, an erythematous maculopapular eruption of the trunk, palms, and soles, and blisters that, when extensive, resemble toxic epidermal necrolysis. Acute GVHD also includes intestinal abnormalities resulting in diarrhea and liver function changes.

* Cutaneous abnormalities of GVHD are pruritus, numbness or pain of palms and soles, and erythematous maculopapular eruption of trunk, palms, and soles.

Chronic GVHD mainly affects skin and liver. Early chronic GVHD is characterized by a lichenoid reaction consisting of cutaneous and oral lesions that resemble lichen planus, with coalescing violaceous papules on the skin and white reticulated patches on the buccal mucosa. Late chronic GVHD is characterized by cutaneous sclerosis, poikilodermatous-reticulated lesions, and scarring alopecia. The cutaneous infiltrate is composed predominantly of suppressor/cytotoxic T cells.

* Chronic GVHD is a lichenoid reaction consisting of cutaneous and oral lesions.

Mastocytosis (mast cell disease) can be divided into 4 groups, depending on the age at onset and the presence or absence of systemic involvement: 1) urticaria pigmentosa arising in infancy or adolescence without substantial systemic involvement, 2) urticaria pigmentosa in adults without substantial systemic involvement, 3) systemic mast cell disease, and 4) mast cell leukemia.

The cutaneous lesions may be brown to red macules, papules, nodules, or plaques that urticate on stroking. Less commonly, the lesions may be bullous, erythrodermic, or telangiectatic. The systemic manifestations are due to histamine release and consist of flushing, tachycardia, and diarrhea.

* Cutaneous lesions of mastocytosis are brown to red macules, papules, nodules, or plaques that urticate on stroking.
* Systemic manifestations are due to histamine release.

Necrobiotic xanthogranuloma—indurated plaques with associated atrophy and telangiectasia with or without ulceration—may occur on the trunk or periorbital areas. Serum electrophoresis shows an IgG κ paraproteinemia or multiple myeloma.

Endocrine

Diabetes Mellitus

Several dermatologic disorders have been described in diabetes.

Necrobiosis lipoidica diabeticorum (Figure 5-18) classically occurs on the shins and presents as yellow-brown atrophic telangiectatic plaques that occasionally ulcerate. Two-thirds of patients with this skin disorder have diabetes.

* Necrobiosis lipoidica diabeticorum occurs on the shins.
* Two-thirds of patients have diabetes.

Granuloma annulare (Figure 5-19) is an asymptomatic eruption consisting of small, firm, flesh-colored or red papules in an annular configuration (less commonly nodular or generalized). The association with diabetes is disputed.

* Granuloma annulare consists of small, firm, flesh-colored or red papules in an annular configuration.

Rarely, patients with poorly controlled diabetes present with spontaneously occurring *subepidermal blisters* (bullosa diabeticorum) on the dorsal aspects of the hands and feet.

The *stiff-hand syndrome* has been reported in juvenile-onset insulin-dependent diabetes. Patients have limited joint mobility and tight waxy skin on the hands. There is an increased risk of subsequent renal and retinal microvascular disease.

* Stiff-hand syndrome is associated with an increased risk of subsequent renal and retinal microvascular disease.

In *scleredema*, there is an insidious onset of thickening and stiffness of the skin on the upper back and posterior neck. The condition is more common in middle-aged men with diabetes. The diabetes is often long-standing and poorly controlled.

* Scleredema is more common in middle-aged men with diabetes.
* Diabetes is often long-standing and poorly controlled.

Thyroid
Pretibial myxedema and thyroid acropachy are cutaneous associations of Graves disease.

Metabolic
The *porphyrias* are a group of inherited or acquired abnormalities of heme synthesis. Each type is associated with deficient activity of a particular enzyme. The porphyrias are usually divided into 3 types: erythropoietic, hepatic, and mixed.

Erythropoietic porphyria is a hereditary form (autosomal recessive) characterized by marked photosensitivity, blisters, scarring alopecia, hirsutism, red-stained teeth, hemolytic anemia, and splenomegaly. The skin lesions are severely mutilating. Onset is in infancy or early childhood.

* Erythropoietic porphyria is autosomal recessive.
* Skin lesions are severely mutilating.

Erythropoietic protoporphyria is an autosomal dominant syndrome that usually begins during childhood. It is characterized by variable degrees of photosensitivity and a marked itching, burning, or stinging sensation that occurs within minutes after sun exposure. It is associated with deficiency of ferrochelatase.

* Erythropoietic protoporphyria is autosomal dominant.
* It is associated with deficiency of ferrochelatase.

Porphyria cutanea tarda (Figure 5-20), one of the hepatic porphyrias, is an acquired or hereditary (autosomal dominant) disease associated with a defect in uroporphyrinogen decarboxylase. The disease may be precipitated by exposure to toxins (such as chlorinated phenols or hexachlorobenzene), alcohol, estrogens, iron overload, underlying hemochromatosis, and infection with hepatitis C. Porphyria cutanea tarda usually presents in the third or fourth decade of life.

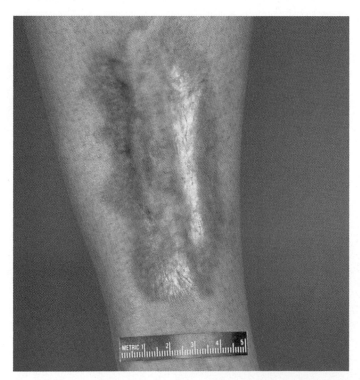

Figure 5-18. Necrobiosis Lipoidica Diabeticorum.

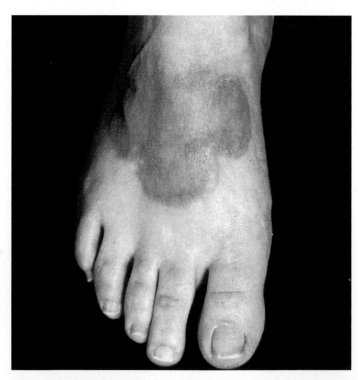

Figure 5-19. Granuloma Annulare.

Clinical manifestations include photosensitivity, skin fragility, erosions and blisters (particularly on dorsal surfaces of the hands), hyperpigmentation, milia, hypertrichosis, and facial suffusion. Sclerodermoid skin changes develop in some patients. The diagnosis is confirmed by the finding of increased porphyrin levels in the urine. Treatment includes phlebotomy or low-dose chloroquine.

* Porphyria cutanea tarda is acquired or inherited (autosomal dominant).
* It is associated with a defect in uroporphyrinogen decarboxylase.
* It may be precipitated by exposure to toxins, infection with hepatitis C, or underlying hemochromatosis.

Acute intermittent porphyria lacks skin lesions and is characterized by acute attacks of abdominal pain or neurologic symptoms.

* Acute intermittent porphyria lacks skin lesions.
* It involves acute attacks of abdominal pain or neurologic symptoms.

Variegate porphyria (mixed porphyria) also follows autosomal dominant inheritance. Variegate porphyria is characterized by cutaneous abnormalities that are similar to those of porphyria cutanea tarda and by acute abdominal episodes, as in acute intermittent porphyria. Variegate porphyria tends to be precipitated by drugs such as barbiturates and sulfonamides.

* Variegate porphyria is autosomal dominant.
* It tends to be precipitated by drugs such as barbiturates and sulfonamides.

Nail Clues to Systemic Disease

Onycholysis consists of distal and lateral separation of the nail plate from the nail bed. Onycholysis may be due to psoriasis, lichen planus, infection (such as *Candida* or *Pseudomonas*), a reaction to nail cosmetics, or a drug reaction. Drugs that have been noted to induce onycholysis include tetracycline and chlorpromazine. Association with thyroid disease (hyperthyroidism more than hypothyroidism) has also been observed.

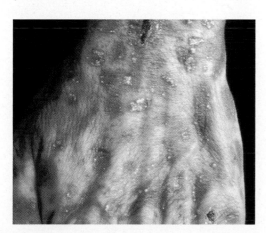

Figure 5-20. Porphyria Cutanea Tarda.

* Onycholysis may be due to psoriasis, lichen planus, infection (*Candida* or *Pseudomonas*), nail cosmetics, or a drug reaction.

Pitting is a common feature of psoriatic nails. Graphlike pits have been associated with alopecia areata.

Terry nails consist of whitening of the proximal or entire nail as a result of changes in the nail bed. This abnormality is associated with cirrhosis.

* Terry nails are associated with cirrhosis.

Muehrcke lines consist of white parallel bands associated with hypoalbuminemia.

* Muehrcke lines are associated with hypoalbuminemia.

Half-and-half nails (*Lindsay nails*) are nails in which the proximal half is white and the distal half is red. This abnormality may be associated with renal failure.

* Half-and-half nails may be associated with renal failure.

Yellow nails are associated with chronic edema, pulmonary disease, pleural effusion, chronic bronchitis, bronchiectasis, and lung carcinoma.

Beau lines are transverse grooves in the nail associated with high fever, chemotherapy, systemic disease, and drugs.

Koilonychia (*spoon nails*) is associated with iron deficiency anemia, but it also may be idiopathic, familial, or related to trauma.

* Koilonychia is associated with iron deficiency anemia.

Blue-colored lunula is associated with hepatolenticular degeneration (Wilson disease) and argyria.

Mees lines are white bands associated with arsenic.

* Mees lines are associated with arsenic.

Cutaneous Manifestations of HIV Infection

Primary infection with human immunodeficiency virus (HIV) results in a flu-like illness and an exanthem in 30% to 60% of patients. The exanthem may be morbilliform or pityriasis rosea-like. Oral ulceration and erosions and erosive esophagitis also may occur at this stage. The acute exanthem and enanthem are self-limited and often go undiagnosed.

In the early stage of the disease, cutaneous manifestations include genital warts, genital herpes, psoriasis, mild seborrheic dermatitis, and pruritic papular eruption. With symptomatic HIV infection (CD4 count of 200-400/mcL), both infections and inflammatory dermatoses occur more frequently. These include psoriasis, oral hairy leukoplakia, candidiasis, herpes zoster, drug reactions, herpes simplex, tinea pedis, and onychomycosis. In patients with a family history of atopy, atopic dermatitis may be a manifestation at this stage.

As the CD4 count decreases to less than 200/mcL, patients may present with a disseminated fungal infection, recurrent or severe herpes zoster, persistent herpes simplex, bacillary angiomatosis, and molluscum contagiosum. *Bacillary angiomatosis* consists of 1 or more vascular papules or nodules caused by the gram-negative bacteria *Bartonella quintana* and *Bartonella henselae*. Eosinophilic folliculitis, a pruritic eruption primarily involving the head, neck, trunk, and proximal extremities, is characteristic of symptomatic HIV infection.

With advanced HIV infection (CD4 counts of <50/mcL), overwhelming infection is characteristic. Infectious agents include cytomegalovirus, *Cryptococcus*, *Acanthamoeba*, and extensive molluscum contagiosum.

Oral hairy leukoplakia is caused by Epstein-Barr virus infection of the oral mucosa and usually occurs in patients with advanced HIV infection.

Molluscum contagiosum, a common viral infection of otherwise healthy children, occurs in 10% to 20% of patients with HIV infection.

- Molluscum contagiosum occurs in 10%-20% of patients with HIV infection.

Epidemic Kaposi sarcoma usually presents as oval papules or plaques oriented along skin lines of the trunk, extremities, face, and mucosa. This presentation is in contrast to that of classic Kaposi sarcoma in elderly patients, which occurs predominantly on the distal lower extremities. Human herpesvirus 8 (HHV-8) has been identified in tissue from patients with both epidemic and classic Kaposi sarcoma.

- Epidemic Kaposi sarcoma presents as oval papules or plaques along skin lines of the trunk, extremities, face, and mucosa.
- It is most commonly associated with HIV infection.

Dermatology Pharmacy Review
Roger A. Warndahl, RPh

Drug	Toxic/Adverse Effects[a]	Drug Interactions[b]
Systemic antibacterials		
Cephalosporins	Nausea, vomiting, diarrhea Anaphylaxis Hemolytic anemia Nephrotoxicity Neutropenia, thrombocytopenia Pseudomembranous colitis Rash, erythema multiforme	
Clindamycin	Nausea, vomiting, diarrhea, abdominal pain Granulocytopenia, neutropenia Hypotension Pseudomembranous colitis Rash, Stevens-Johnson syndrome	
Fluoroquinolones (ciprofloxacin, gatifloxacin, levofloxacin, lomefloxacin, moxifloxacin, norfloxacin, ofloxacin, sparfloxacin, trovafloxacin)	Nausea, vomiting, diarrhea, abdominal pain Increased liver enzymes Increased serum creatinine Nephrotoxicity Phototoxicity Pseudomembranous colitis QT interval prolongation Rash, erythema multiforme, toxic epidermal necrolysis	Cardiac arrythmias: amiodarone, bepridil, bretylium, disopyramide, erythromycin, phenothiazine, procainamide, quinidine, sotalol, tricyclic antidepressants Increased cardiovascular side effects: cisapride Increased levels or effects: astemizole, terfenadine, probenecid Increased toxicity: cyclosporine Increased levels of theophylline or caffeine
Macrolides (azithromycin, clarithromycin, dirithromycin, erythromycin)	Abdominal pain, nausea, diarrhea Oral candidiasis Increased liver enzymes Pseudomembranous colitis Anaphylaxis Stevens-Johnson syndrome	Cardiotoxicity: astemizole, terfenadine, cisapride, pimozide, quinolones (gatifloxacin, sparfloxacin, moxifloxacin) Increased levels or effects: warfarin, carbamazepine, digoxin, ergot alkaloids, vinblastine, cyclosporine, tacrolimus, methylprednisolone Severe myopathy, rhabdomyolysis: HMG-CoA reductase inhibitors (atorvastatin, lovastatin, simvastatin, cerivastatin)
Penicillins	Nausea, vomiting, mild diarrhea Anaphylaxis Acute interstitial nephritis Hemolytic anemia Pseudomembranous colitis	Decreased penicillin effects: tetracyclines (demeclocycline, doxycycline, minocycline, oxytetracycline, tetracycline)
Sulfonamides	Nausea, vomiting, diarrhea Hematologic reactions Hepatitis Nephrotoxicity Rash, photosensitivity, Stevens-Johnson syndrome	Increased effect: warfarin Increased nephrotoxicity & decreased effect: cyclosporine Bone marrow suppression: methotrexate Enhanced hypoglycemia: glipizide, glyburide
Tetracyclines (doxycycline, minocycline, tetracycline)	Photosensitivity Nausea, diarrhea Acute renal failure Exfoliative dermatitis Discoloration of teeth (young children)	Decreased effects: penicillin Increased levels: digoxin Risk of pseudotumor cerebri: isotretinoin Renal toxicity: methoxyflurane

Dermatology Pharmacy Review (continued)

Drug	Toxic/Adverse Effects[a]	Drug Interactions[b]
Systemic immunomodulators and antiproliferatives		
Azathioprine	Nausea, vomiting, diarrhea Hepatoxicity Malignancies Rash Thrombocytopenia, leukopenia, anemia Veno-occlusive disease	Increased effects: allopurinol Possible myelosuppression: ACE inhibitors Increased hepatoxicity: methotrexate Decreased anticoagulant effectiveness: warfarin

Corticosteroids	Increased appetite, fluid retention
	Insomnia
	Hirsutism, hyperpigmentation
	Glucose intolerance
	Cataracts
	Osteoporosis
		Antagonized effects: neostigmine,
		  pyridostigmine
		Decreased steroid effects: rifampin,
		  phenytoin
		Increased steroid effects: macrolides,
		  ketoconazole, fluconazole, itraconazole
		Should not be given with live vaccines

Cyclophosphamide	Alopecia
	Sterility
	Nausea, vomiting, stomatitis
	Hemorrhagic cystitis
	Malignancies
	Thrombocytopenia, anemia, leukopenia
	Stevens-Johnson syndrome, toxic
	  epidermal necrolysis
		Cardiac toxicity potentiated:
		  anthracyclines
		Decreased effects of digoxin
		Increased effects: phenytoin, barbiturates,
		  allopurinol, thiazides

Cyclosporine	Nausea, diarrhea, gum hyperplasia
	Hypertension
	Psoriasis
	Hirsutism, hypertrichosis
	Increased triglycerides
	Nephropathy
	Headache
	Tremor
		Increased risk of rhabdomyolysis:
		  atorvastatin, cerivastatin, lovastatin,
		  pravastatin, simvastatin
		Increased toxicity: digoxin, prednisone,
		  protease inhibitors, calcium channel
		  blockers
		Decreased cyclosporine concentrations:
		  phenytoin, orlistat, rifampin,
		  sulfonamides, grapefruit juice,
		  azathioprine, macrolides, azole antifungals
		Increased renal failure: foscarnet
		Increased nephrotoxicity: sulfonamides,
		  NSAIDs, aminoglycosides

Dapsone	Nausea, vomiting
	Hemolytic anemia, methemoglobinemia,
	  leukopenia, agranulocytosis
	Skin rash, exfoliative dermatitis
	Hepatitis
	Peripheral neuropathy
	Psychosis
		Increased levels of both drugs:
		  trimethoprim
		Increased hematologic reactions:
		  pyrimethamine
		Decreased dapsone effects: rifampin

Gold compounds (auranofin, aurothioglucose, gold sodium thiomalate)	Rash Stomatitis Conjunctivitis Proteinuria, hematuria Alopecia Eosinophilia, leukopenia, thrombocytopenia Hepatotoxicity	Increased levels: immunosuppressants

Dermatology Pharmacy Review (continued)

Drug	Toxic/Adverse Effects[a]	Drug Interactions[b]
Systemic immunomodulators and antiproliferatives (continued)		
Interferons	Flu-like symptoms Hypertension Psychiatric disturbances Rash Hypocalcemia, hyperglycemia Aplastic anemia Acute renal failure	
Methotrexate	Nausea, vomiting Vasculitis Stomatitis Leukopenia, thrombocytopenia Renal failure Rash, photosensitivity Hepatotoxicity	Increased methotrexate toxicity: penicillins, salicylates, nonsteroidal anti-inflammatory drugs, probenecid, cyclosporine Increased bone marrow suppression: sulfonamides, trimethoprim Decreased levels: phenytoin
Psoralen (methoxsalen, trioxsalen)	Nausea Pruritus, erythema Painful blistering Depression	Other photosensitizing agents
Retinoids (isotretinoin, acitretin)	Teratogenicity Hematologic changes Arthralgias Acute pancreatitis Hirsutism, alopecia Photoallergic reactions Rash, vasculitis Lipid abnormalities Visual disturbances Psychiatric disorders Osteoporosis Hepatotoxicity Hearing impairment	Increased risk of pseudotumor cerebri: tetracyclines Hepatotoxicity: methotrexate Additive toxic effects: vitamin A Progestin-only birth control may have decreased efficacy
Thalidomide	Teratogenicity Stevens-Johnson syndrome Somnolence, headache Permanent nerve damage Acute renal failure Neutropenia Thrombotic events	Increased sedation: barbiturates, chlorpromazine, reserpine, alcohol
Tumor necrosis factor inhibitors		
Etanercept	Infections, sepsis New or worsening heart failure Blood dyscrasias Neurologic effects Hematologic effects Malignancies	Increased malignancies: cyclophosphamide Decreased neutrophil count: sulfasalazine Increased risk of severe infections & neutropenia: anakinra Should not be given with live vaccines
Adalimumab	Infections Malignancies Hematologic effects Congestive heart failure	Increased risk of severe infections & neutropenia: anakinra Should not be given with live vaccines

Dermatology Pharmacy Review (continued)

Drug	Toxic/Adverse Effects[a]	Drug Interactions[b]
Tumor necrosis factor inhibitors (continued)		
Infliximab	Infections, sepsis Heart failure Hepatotoxicity Hematologic effects Hypersensitivity reactions Malignancies Hepatitis B reactivation Arthralgias, myalgias	Increased risk of severe infections & neutropenia: anakinra Increased risk of hepatosplenic T-cell lymphomas: azathioprine, mercaptopurine Should not be given with live vaccines
Topical antibacterials		
Azelaic acid	Pruritus, burning, peeling Depigmentation	
Bacitracin	Allergic dermatitis	
Benzoyl peroxide	Excessive drying Dermatitis	Skin irritation: tretinoin
Clindamycin	Dryness, peeling of skin	Antagonism: erythromycin
Erythromycin	Skin irritation	Antagonism: clindamycin Cumulative irritant effect with topical acne therapies
Metronidazole	Skin irritation	
Mupirocin	Skin irritation Contact dermatitis Headache	
Neomycin	Contact dermatitis (>10% of users)	
Sodium sulfacetamide	Skin irritation Stevens-Johnson syndrome, toxic epidermal necrolysis	
Tetracycline	Skin irritation Temporary follicular staining	
Topical immunomodulators & antiproliferatives		
Anthralin	Skin irritation Contact allergic reactions Stains skin, hair Should not be applied to eyes, mucous membranes, or intertriginous skin areas	Before use, 1 week should be allowed after use of topical steroids, because of rebound phenomenon of psoriasis
Calcipotriene	Skin irritation Hypercalcemia Worsening of psoriasis Skin atrophy, hyperpigmentation	
Coal tar	Skin irritation Contact dermatitis Folliculitis Phototoxicity Psoriasis Staining of skin	
Corticosteroids	Systemic absorption Local irritation Skin atrophy Skin infection	

Dermatology Pharmacy Review (continued)

Drug	Toxic/Adverse Effects[a]	Drug Interactions[b]
Topical immunomodulators & antiproliferatives (continued)		
Mechlorethamine	Contact sensitivity Hyperpigmentation Irritant dermatitis Telangiectases	
Retinoids (adapalene, tretinoin, alitretinoin, tazarotene, bexarotene)	Skin irritation Photosensitivity	Considerable skin irritation: topical sulfur, resorcinol, benzoyl peroxide, salicylic acid Increased phototoxicity: thiazides, tetracyclines, fluoroquinolones, phenothiazides, sulfonamides
Tacrolimus, pimecrolimus	Carcinogenesis Increased risk of viral infections Phototoxicity Skin burning, pruritus	
Topical keratolytics		
Masoprocol	Local irritation Allergic contact dermatitis	Should not be used with other skin care products or makeup
Resorcinol	Mild irritant Hyperpigmentation Methemoglobinemia Green discoloration of urine	Considerable skin irritation: retinoids
Salicylic acid	Local irritation	Increased irritation of skin: other medications
Sulfur	Skin irritation	Increased irritation of skin: other topical medications

Abbreviations: ACE, angiotensin-converting enzyme; HMG-CoA, 3-hydroxy-3-methylglutaryl coenzyme A; NSAIDs, nonsteroidal anti-inflammatory drugs.

[a] Toxic/adverse effects: focus is on dermatologic, very common, or life-threatening effects.

[b] Drug interactions: focus is on other dermatology drugs and very common or life-threatening interactions.

Questions

Multiple Choice (choose the best answer)

1. A 19-year-old man presents with fever, malaise, headache, and skin signs that develop rapidly during the 2 hours the patient is evaluated in the emergency department. He is a healthy college student who is not receiving any medications. Physical examination shows fever, tachycardia, and normal results of neurologic examination. Laboratory examination shows an increased leukocyte count. Results of cultures and further studies are pending. The skin signs, shown in the figure, are characteristic and are scattered over the lower extremities, upper extremities, and trunk. The most likely diagnosis is:

    a. Meningococcemia
    b. Primary rash of human immunodeficiency virus
    c. Rocky Mountain spotted fever
    d. Streptococcal toxic shock syndrome
    e. Scalded skin syndrome

2. Your patient presents with recurrent episodes of the skin findings shown in the figure. The most likely infectious association is:

    a. Herpes simplex virus
    b. *Pseudomonas*
    c. Dermatophyte
    d. *Borrelia burgdorferi*
    e. *Mycobacterium marinum*

3. On the basis of the skin findings shown in the figure, the most likely diagnosis is:

    a. Necrobiosis lipoidica
    b. Erythema multiforme
    c. Sarcoidosis
    d. Kaposi sarcoma
    e. Bacillary angiomatosis

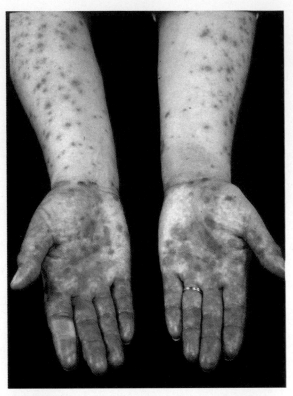

Question 2

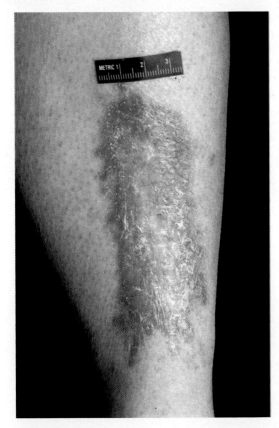

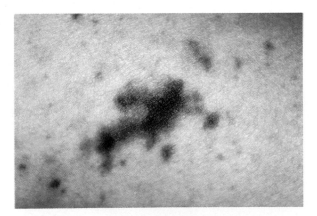

Question 1

Question 3

4. A patient you are seeing for a general medical evaluation presents with the signs shown in the figures. The most likely diagnosis is:

a. Neurofibromatosis
b. Tuberous sclerosis
c. Acanthosis nigricans
d. Muir-Torre syndrome
e. Cowden disease

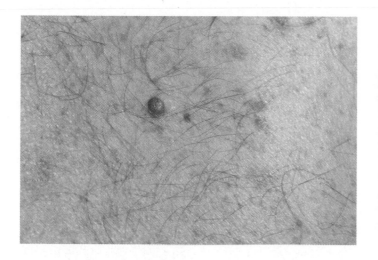

Question 4

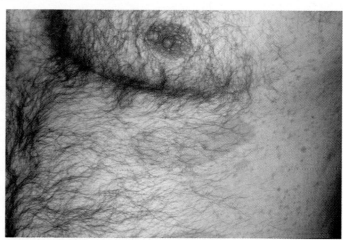

Question 4

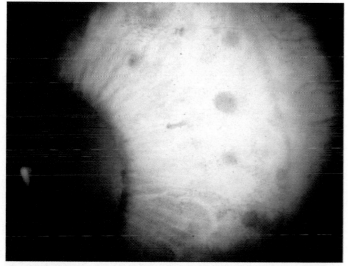

Question 4

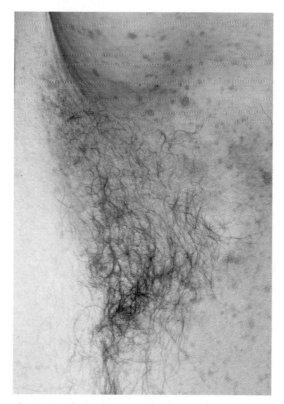

Question 4

5. A patient has had recurrent bouts of the skin findings shown in the figure. He is asymptomatic when the skin findings develop, which on examination present as nonblanching bright-red papules. The most likely diagnosis is:

    a. Leukocytoclastic vasculitis
    b. Porphyria cutanea tarda
    c. Erythema nodosum
    d. Contact dermatitis
    e. Stasis dermatitis

6. A 28-year-old man presents with a new itchy rash. He has no previous history of skin problems and is not receiving any medications. He has not used any new products on the skin or been in a wooded area. He has red papules and excoriations on the wrist, groin, underarms, and between the fingers. The best laboratory test is:

    a. Scabies preparation
    b. Tissue transglutaminase test
    c. Patch test
    d. Lyme disease test
    e. Chest radiography

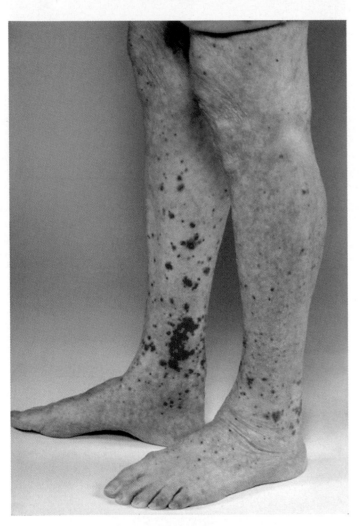

Question 5

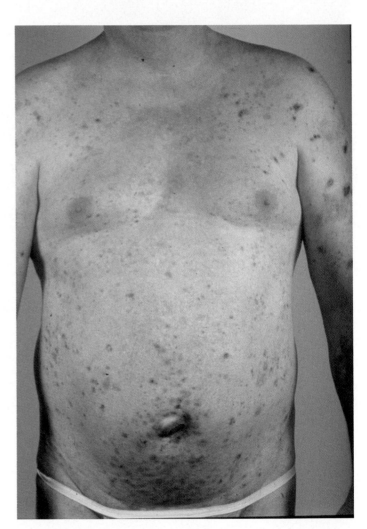

Question 6

7. A 34-year-old man presents with recurrent episodes of blisters on the backs of his hands. His skin burns easily and breaks easily, and he has difficulty in his construction job because of the involvement of his hands. The physical findings in the figure are areas of healing skin and scores. He has some healing erosions on the face but no mucosal involvement or involvement of other sites. The most likely diagnosis is:

a. Porphyria cutanea tarda
b. Pemphigus vulgaris
c. Bullous pemphigoid
d. Bullous lupus erythematosus
e. Dermatomyositis

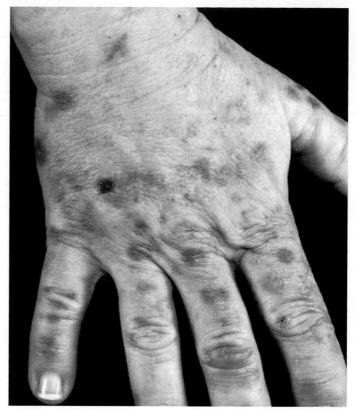

Question 7

Answers

1.   Answer a.
Meningococcemia and meningococcal meningitis are caused by *Neisseria meningitidis*, an encapsulated gram-negative diplococcus. The majority of cases occur in patients younger than 5 years, but up to 33% of cases occur in adults. People in crowded situations, such as college students living in dormitories, are at moderately increased risk for this diesease, which has a mortality rate of 10% to 20%. A seasonal disease, occurring in winter and spring, it is known for its rapid progression of signs and symptoms. The skin signs may be an early clue to diagnosis and classically appear as petechiae on the trunk and extremities which evolve into purpura with gun-metal–gray centers and geographic borders.

2.   Answer a.
Erythema multiforme presents with target lesions, often located on palms and soles, but generalized eruptions also occur. Although drugs such as sulfonamides, barbiturates, and anticonvulsants are commonly associated with development of erythema multiforme, recurrent lesions are most often linked to a herpes simplex infection. Although the skin signs of active herpes simplex may be apparent, the herpes simplex outbreak may be subclinical. Discontinuation of use of any culprit drugs and a trial of acyclovir or other appropriate antiviral is appropriate in cases of recurrent erythema multiforme.

3.   Answer a.
Necrobiosis lipoidica is a skin sign of internal disease. It presents with red (or violet) plaques on the anterior surface of the lower aspect of the legs. Over time, the area expands and the central area turns yellow-brown. This central area atrophies, and telangiectasia or ulcers may develop. Necrobiosis lipoidica is more frequent in patients with diabetes mellitus. Once the association is confirmed, the condition is termed *necrobiosis lipoidica diabeticorum*. Other skin signs of diabetes mellitus include *Candida* infections of the mouth and

genitalia, diabetic bullae, diabetic dermopathy (brown shin spots), scleredema, foot ulcers, acanthosis nigricans, granuloma annulare, insulin lipodystrophy, and eruptive xanthoma.

4. Answer a.

Neurofibromatosis is one of the most common mutations in humans and has multiple skin manifestations. These include café au lait macules (light tan macules), intertriginous freckling (Crowe sign), and neurofibromas. Lisch nodules of the iris are also prominent. Associated tumors include acoustic neuromas, optic gliomas, meningiomas, pheochromocytoma, neuroblastoma, and Wilms tumor.

Tuberous sclerosis presents with adenoma sebaceum (facial angiofibromas), periungual fibroma, shagreen patch (connective tissue nevus), and ash leaf spots (white oval macules). It is associated with rhabdomyomas and angiomyolipomas of the kidneys.

Acanthosis nigricans presents with velvety brown plaques in intertriginous areas (neck, axilla, and groin). Although usually a marker of obesity and insulin resistance syndromes, acanthosis nigricans can be a skin sign of internal malignancy. It is associated with adenocarcinoma of the gastrointestinal tract, especially gastric carcinoma.

Muir-Torre syndrome is also a skin sign of internal malignancy and presents with sebaceous gland tumors (sebaceous adenoma, sebaceous epithelioma, and sebaceous carcinoma) in association with colorectal carcinoma. Genitourinary, breast, and other cancers may also occur.

Cowden disease (multiple hamartoma syndrome) presents with central facial papules (trichilemmomas), oral papules, and hand keratosis. It can be associated with breast and thyroid cancer.

5. Answer a.

The patient with leukocytoclastic vasculitis (also known as hypersensitivity vasculitis or small vessel vasculitis) presents with palpable purpura in dependent areas. Leukocytoclastic vasculitis affects the small vessels, specifically the postcapillary venules. Commonly occurring in crops or waves, it usually occurs on the skin of the lower extremities, but it may also affect the kidneys, muscles, joints, gastrointestinal system, and peripheral nerves. Often a cause is not identified, but associations include infections, drugs, connective tissue diseases, dysproteinemia, and malignancy.

6. Answer a.

Scabies is caused by infestation of the epidermis with the mite *Sarcoptes scabiei* var *hominis*. It causes epidemics in school-age children and patients in nursing homes. Pruritus is the major complaint, prominent at night, and there is often a history of itching or rash in family members and close personal contacts. The rash is due to sensitivity to the mite protein. Clinical features include inflammatory, excoriated papules in the web spaces of the hands and feet, axillae, groin, wrists, and submammary sites. Facial involvement is uncommon, except in children. The pathognomonic finding is a burrow commonly located on the hands. Identification of mites, eggs, or fecal material on a scabies preparation is diagnostic. In immunocompromised patients, scabies may appear as a generalized scaling eruption (Norwegian scabies or crusted scabies) and cause epidemics in hospitals.

7. Answer a.

Porphyria cutanea tarda is usually an acquired disease associated with a defect in uroporphyrinogen decarboxylase. The disease is precipitated by exposure to liver toxins, commonly alcohol and estrogens, but also viral hepatitis and hexachlorobenzene. It may be precipitated by underlying hemochromatosis or iron overload. Clinical findings include photosensitivity, blisters, milia, skin fragility, scarring, and facial hirsutism. In contrast to acute intermittent porphyria, there are no neurologic symptoms. Diagnosis is established with a 24-hour urine porphyrin study. Treatment is phlebotomy and management or discontinuation of the precipitating factors.

6

Endocrinology

Bryan McIver, MB,ChB, PhD

Basic Principles of Endocrinology

Numerous chemical messages control various functions at the level of cells, organs, and organ systems. Such messages may be *autocrine* (the chemical message directly affects the cell producing it), *paracrine* (the message has local effects), or *endocrine* (the message has distant sites of action). Typically, endocrine effects are caused by hormones that are produced by specialized organs, although several important endocrine functions are performed by nonglandular tissues, most prominently the liver (eg, insulinlike growth factor 1 [IGF-1] production and thyroid hormone activation) and the kidney (eg, renin production and vitamin D activation).

Hormones act at the cell surface or within the cell or in both places. For example, steroid hormones and thyroid hormones exert effects on most cells in the body through nuclear receptors that regulate gene transcription and protein synthesis. In contrast, glycoprotein hormones such as corticotropin (ACTH) act through specific cell surface receptors that produce their effects through second messenger systems. Typically, hormones in the latter group exert their effects rapidly, whereas hormones that act through nuclear hormone receptors produce slower responses. Because of this lag in response, the serum concentrations of these hormones measured at any given time may not truly reflect the amount of "signal" that nuclear receptors have been exposed to over the preceding hours.

Most hormone actions are determined by the interaction of multiple hormones secreted by different tissues. In the classic example of a negative-feedback loop, the thyroid gland produces thyroxine (T_4), which is regarded as the regulated "end product" or active hormone. The secretion of T_4 is stimulated by thyrotropin (TSH), which is produced by the pituitary gland. TSH is a trophic hormone that is required both for secretion of thyroid hormone and for maintenance of the gland itself. It is secreted in response to decreasing levels of T_4 and triiodothyronine (T_3), and its secretion is suppressed by increasing levels of T_4 and T_3. This negative-feedback control maintains a constant concentration of thyroid hormone. The process is more complex, however, because T_4 itself is a prohormone, which is converted to the active form (T_3) in the liver, kidneys, and several end organs in which it exerts its physiologic effects. The conversion of T_4 into T_3 requires the activity of microsomally located deiodinases, which may either activate (into T_3) or inactivate (into reverse T_3) the prohormone. At least some aspects of this deiodination reaction appear to be regulated, although details of the additional control mechanism remain unclear. Even the apparently straightforward negative-feedback control of thyroid hormone concentrations encompasses a complexity and subtlety that may have significant physiologic impact.

Because the structure of hormone systems maintains homeostasis in response to changes in the internal and external environments, it is important to recognize that in certain situations endocrine abnormalities may be a consequence, rather than a cause, of systemic illness. For example, with extreme weight loss, such as anorexia nervosa, secretion of the trophic hormones that regulate gonadal function is decreased or absent. This is not a result of a primary endocrine disease but rather represents a physiologic response to the depletion of the body's energy reserves (fat) necessary for successful reproduction. Treatment should be directed at the underlying cause. A precisely analogous situation affects TSH production in starvation or other severe illness, resulting in the euthyroid sick syndrome, which is easily mistaken for thyrotoxicosis because of the low circulating concentration of TSH.

One important principle to consider in the evaluation of patients with suspected endocrine disease is the need to clearly document endocrine dysfunction before proceeding with imaging studies. Imaging studies performed in isolation may be misleading because of the propensity of modern, detailed imaging studies to detect incidental abnormalities of endocrine glands that have no functional significance and often reflect normal variation or aging. Specifically, endocrine glands seem to exhibit a remarkable propensity to develop benign hyperplastic or neoplastic nodules, the finding of which may confuse the evaluation of a putative endocrine disorder.

- Hormones typically act either through nuclear receptors that regulate gene transcription mechanisms or through membrane-bound receptors that alter the concentration of intracellular second messenger systems.

- Hormone systems are finely regulated by the interaction between trophic hormones and end hormones (negative and positive feedback).
- Endocrine dysfunction may be a consequence of systemic disease.

Hypothalamic-Pituitary Disorders

The pituitary and hypothalamus control several peripheral hormone systems. The hypothalamus contains centers vital to the regulation of sleep/wake cycles, appetite, metabolic rate, and thirst. It responds to many neural and endocrine inputs, and integrates these signals directly to control pituitary function through the secretion of releasing factors into a portal system running down the pituitary stalk. The pituitary can be divided, anatomically and physiologically, into anterior and posterior parts. The anterior component responds to those portal signals; the posterior pituitary secretions are manufactured in the cell bodies of the hypothalamus and released under direct neurologic control from the nerve endings in the pituitary itself.

The anterior pituitary secretes a number of trophic hormones that act on endocrine glands elsewhere in the body. Disease (particularly adenomas) of this region may result in syndromes of hormone excess or deficiency. The posterior pituitary is not a gland in the classic sense but instead represents the terminus of axons of neurons in the supraoptic and paraventricular nuclei of the hypothalamus. It functions as a storehouse and is the site of release for vasopressin and oxytocin. The main consequence of posterior pituitary disease is disordered water homeostasis.

In addition to their effects on systemic hormone systems, pituitary and hypothalamic lesions can cause local compressive effects on the visual pathway or the cavernous sinus (with consequent lesions of cranial nerves II, III, IV, and VI) and on hypothalamic centers, leading to disordered appetite and sleep/wake cycles.

Hypopituitarism

Etiology

Anterior pituitary diseases can cause hypopituitarism, with deficiency of 1, several, or all of the anterior pituitary hormones. Causes of hypopituitarism include primary pituitary disease, hypothalamic disease, interruption of the pituitary stalk, and extrasellar disorders. The most common causes are pituitary tumors, pituitary surgery or trauma, and radiotherapy. Hypopituitarism can also be functional, resulting from suppression of hypothalamic regulation of the anterior pituitary gland. Common causes include suppression of the hypothalamic-pituitary-adrenal axis following the use of exogenous corticosteroids; suppression of gonadotropin-releasing hormone (GnRH) related to significant weight loss, exercise, or systemic illness; and suppression of TSH in response to systemic illness (the euthyroid sick syndrome). Treatment in these cases should be directed at the underlying cause.

An extrasellar lesion, such as a craniopharyngioma (most commonly) or Rathke cleft cyst, may impinge on and impair the function of the hypothalamic-pituitary unit.

- Hypopituitarism may be functional. Treatment should be aimed at the underlying cause.

- Anterior pituitary hormone deficiency can be total, multiple, or selective.
- The most common causes of hypopituitarism are pituitary tumors, pituitary surgery, and radiotherapy.
- Exogenous corticosteroid use or significant weight loss can lead to functional suppression of hypothalamic regulation of the anterior pituitary gland.
- The commonest extrasellar cause of hypopituitarism is a craniopharyngioma.

Clinical Presentation in Adults

Adults with hypopituitarism can present with the features of deficiency of 1 or more anterior pituitary hormones. The clinical presentation depends on the age at onset, the hormone(s) affected, and the extent, speed of onset, and duration of the deficiency (Table 6-1). Hypopituitarism typically occurs as a chronic process of insidious onset. With the exception of prolactin, the manifestations of hypopituitarism are not related directly to anterior pituitary hormone deficiency but to secondary deficiency of end hormones.

Gonadotropin Deficiency

In women, gonadotropin deficiency causes oligomenorrhea or amenorrhea, loss of libido, vaginal dryness and dyspareunia, and loss of secondary sex characteristics (estrogen deficiency). In men, gonadotropin deficiency leads to loss of libido, erectile dysfunction, infertility, loss of secondary sex characteristics, atrophy of the testes, and, under some circumstances, gynecomastia (testosterone deficiency).

ACTH Deficiency

In ACTH deficiency, the consequent hypocortisolism causes malaise, anorexia, weight loss, gastrointestinal tract disturbance, and hyponatremia. Because ACTH helps maintain skin pigmentation, patients often have a pale complexion ("alabaster skin") and are unable to develop or maintain a tan. Patients do not have features of mineralocorticoid deficiency because aldosterone secretion is unaffected, although adrenal crisis is still possible in affected individuals, particularly with severe physical stress.

Patients with hypopituitarism may also present with acute symptoms and signs of cortisol deficiency. This occurs most commonly following withdrawal of prolonged high-dose glucocorticoid therapy that has caused suppression of the hypothalamic-pituitary-adrenal axis. Patients with acute destruction of the pituitary by trauma, pituitary surgery, or hemorrhage (pituitary apoplexy) can also present in this fashion. In the case of pituitary apoplexy, a "thunderclap headache" is a typical accompaniment to the abrupt onset of systemic illness. Medical or surgical illness or thyroid hormone replacement therapy in a patient with unrecognized ACTH deficiency also exacerbates the symptoms of cortisol deficiency and may precipitate an adrenal crisis.

TSH Deficiency

TSH deficiency leads to secondary hypothyroidism and an atrophic thyroid gland. Low concentrations of thyroid hormone may cause the full spectrum of hypothyroid symptoms (detailed in the "Disorders of the Thyroid Gland" section), which overlap with the symptoms of steroid deficiency (which may coexist with central hypothyroidism). Treatment of steroid deficiency should precede treatment with thyroid hormone to avoid a potentially life-threatening adrenal crisis. The clinical challenge is to recognize that this rare condition could be represented by a low TSH in the presence of a symptom complex that does not clearly indicate thyrotoxicosis.

Prolactin Deficiency
The only clinical consequence of prolactin deficiency is the inability to initiate and sustain postpartum lactation, which may be the first manifestation of Sheehan syndrome (typically triggered by postpartum hemorrhage).

Growth Hormone Deficiency
In adults, growth hormone (GH) deficiency is often asymptomatic. However, some patients may complain of fatigue, decreased exercise tolerance, abdominal obesity, and loss of muscle mass. The use of human GH supplementation in patients with putative isolated GH deficiency is currently a growth industry, which is not supported by the evidence. Despite this, a small number of patients with true GH

Table 6-1   Hypothalamic-Pituitary Hormones: Functions and Clinical Syndromes

Feature	GH	PRL	LH/FSH	ACTH/LPH/END	TSH	ADH
Anterior pituitary cell type	Somatotroph	Lactotroph	Gonadotroph	Corticotroph	Thyrotroph	Supraoptic & paraventricular nuclei
Regulation (*the dominant regulators are italicized*)	*GHRH* (+) GHRIH (−)	*DA* (−) TRH, VIP (+)	*GnRH* (+) DA, opioids (−)	*CRH* (+) AVP (+)	*TRH* (+) GHRIH, DA (−)	Plasma osmolality (osmoreceptors) & blood volume (volume & baroreceptors)
Secretion	Episodic Sleep-related surge	Episodic Sleep-related surge	Phasic throughout life Episodic Cyclic in women of reproductive age	Episodic Diurnal Stress-responsive	Episodic Minimal diurnal change	Exquisitely sensitive to changes in plasma osmolality
Physiologic functions	IGF-1–mediated growth Intermediary metabolism	Lactogenesis Others (?)	Initiation & maintenance of sexual/reproductive functions	ACTH: initiation & maintenance of cortisol production by adrenal cortex LPH/END: pigmentary effects	Initiation & maintenance of T_4/T_3 secretion by thyroid	Maintenance of plasma osmolality Maintenance of blood volume & pressure
Deficiency in adult	Syndrome of GH deficiency?	Loss of postpartum lactation	Hypogonadotropism	Secondary cortisol deficiency	Secondary hypothyroidism	Central diabetes insipidus
Deficiency in child	Shortness of stature Hypoglycemia	Not recognized	Hypogonadotropism in adolescent	Secondary cortisol deficiency	Secondary hypothyroidism	Central diabetes insipidus
Hypersecretion in adult	Acromegaly	Hyperprolactinemic syndrome	No distinct syndrome	Cushing disease	TSH-induced hyperthyroidism	SIADH
Hypersecretion in child	Gigantism	Hyperprolactinemic syndrome in adolescent	Precocious puberty	Cushing disease	TSH-induced hyperthyroidism	SIADH

Abbreviations: ACTH, corticotropin; ADH, vasopressin; AVP, arginine vasopressin; CRH, corticotropin-releasing hormone; DA, dopamine; END, β-endorphin; FSH, follicle-stimulating hormone; GH, growth hormone; GHRH, GH-releasing hormone; GHRIH, GH-releasing inhibiting hormone or somatostatin; GnRH, gonadotropin-releasing hormone; IGF-1, insulinlike growth factor 1; LH, luteinizing hormone; LPH, β-lipotropin; PRL, prolactin; SIADH, syndrome of inappropriate ADH secretion; TRH, thyrotropin-releasing hormone; TSH, thyrotropin; VIP, vasoactive intestinal polypeptide.

deficiency do exist and may benefit significantly from replacement therapy.

* Gonadotropin deficiency manifests as hypogonadism and infertility.
* ACTH deficiency causes glucocorticoid deficiency without mineralocorticoid deficiency.
* Patients with acute hypopituitarism present with rapidly progressive features of steroid deficiency accompanied by headache in the presence of pituitary apoplexy.
* TSH deficiency leads to secondary hypothyroidism.
* Prolactin deficiency manifests as a failure of lactation in the postpartum period.
* In adults, GH deficiency leads to an ill-defined syndrome of weakness, altered body fat distribution, and malaise.
* In a typical clinical scenario for hypopituitarism, the patient has an insidious onset of numerous signs and symptoms caused by several end-hormone deficiencies. The broad spectrum and overlapping nature of the symptoms can make diagnosis more challenging.

Diagnosis

It is essential to document both the degree and the extent of endocrine dysfunction and to determine the cause of hypopituitarism. Functional causes of hypopituitarism are common and should be considered before searching for an organic cause.

Endocrine Evaluation

Gonadotropin Axis—Deficiencies in the gonadotropin axis are manifested as a low serum concentration of testosterone or estradiol, with low or inappropriately normal levels of luteinizing hormone (LH) and follicle-stimulating hormone (FSH). The menstrual cycle is a sensitive indicator of hypothalamic-pituitary-gonadal function in women, and a woman with a normal menstrual cycle can be assumed to have normal gonadotropin secretion. No biochemical testing is necessary under those conditions. Hyperprolactinemia is a common cause of central hypogonadism.

ACTH-Adrenocortical Axis—A normal plasma level of ACTH and cortisol does not necessarily confirm that the pituitary can secrete sufficient ACTH during conditions of stress. Morning and afternoon cortisol measurements may help to establish a normal diurnal rhythm (higher in the morning, lower in the afternoon), providing evidence of an intact hypothalamic regulatory system, but adrenal insufficiency may still be present. An ACTH stimulation test (cosyntropin test) may provide additional information, although again, recent onset of hypopituitarism may leave the adrenal response to exogenous ACTH entirely intact. With chronic ACTH deficiency, the adrenal cortex is atrophic and typically a cortisol secretory response to exogenous ACTH is absent. The cosyntropin test cannot distinguish between ACTH deficiency (chronic secondary adrenal insufficiency) and primary adrenal insufficiency. Therefore, in the presence of low cortisol levels, it is important to measure ACTH levels: a low or inappropriately normal ACTH level is consistent with pituitary dysfunction, whereas an increased ACTH level is consistent with primary adrenal disease. Assessment of renin and aldosterone may also be useful in the assessment of primary adrenal insufficiency, in which

aldosterone production capacity is also lost. Other provocative tests include the use of insulin-induced hypoglycemia or metyrapone to stimulate ACTH secretion, although these are used rarely. Because the most common cause of adrenal insufficiency is prior exposure to exogenous steroids, a careful drug history (including topical lotions and steroids that are inhaled or injected) and a synthetic steroid screen (serum) are crucially important to establish a diagnosis of adrenal failure.

TSH-Thyroid Axis—Low serum levels of free thyroxine (FT$_4$) and an inappropriately normal or low serum level of TSH support the diagnosis of central hypothyroidism. Consideration should be given to the effects of systemic illness and adrenal insufficiency, both of which can alter TSH secretion, giving the impression of secondary hypothyroidism.

GH—Random determinations of GH concentrations are not useful in the evaluation of GH deficiency. Low serum concentrations of IGF-1 suggest the diagnosis. Provocative testing with insulin-induced hypoglycemia is the standard way to stimulate GH secretion. However, this is contraindicated for the elderly and for patients with ischemic heart disease. The stimulation test with arginine plus growth hormone–releasing hormone (GHRH) has a diagnostic accuracy similar to that of insulin-induced hypoglycemia and has become the test of choice for diagnosing GH deficiency in adults.

Prolactin—Deficiency is suggested by low serum concentrations. Note that interruption of the pituitary stalk often increases prolactin concentrations through the release of lactotrophs from tonic inhibition by dopamine ("stalk effect").

Structural Evaluation

Structural evaluation requires imaging of the hypothalamic-pituitary region, preferably with magnetic resonance imaging (MRI). If a space-occupying lesion in the region of the sella is detected, the visual fields should be assessed. Modern high-resolution MRI scanning may detect small nonfunctioning lesions of the pituitary (incidentalomas) in 5% to 10% of patients. Many of these lesions are of no medical significance, but clinical and biochemical correlation is essential.

Therapy in Adults

Therapy includes correction, if possible, of the cause (functional or structural) and administration of the deficient hormone(s) of the target gland(s) or, in selected cases, of the pituitary hormones.

ACTH Deficiency

Glucocorticoid replacement is essential and should be initiated before introducing other replacement hormones. Hydrocortisone should be given twice daily. An average daily dose is 10 to 20 mg in the early morning and 5 to 10 mg in the early or mid afternoon. Alternatively, a longer-acting corticosteroid such as prednisone 5 mg once daily is sufficient. Patients should double or triple the steroid dose during times of acute illness and should receive steroid parenterally when unable to take it orally. For patients with combined deficiency of ACTH and TSH, glucocorticoid replacement should be initiated before thyroid hormone replacement therapy to avoid precipitation of an acute adrenal crisis.

TSH Deficiency

The drug of choice is levothyroxine sodium. Levels of serum FT4 (rather than TSH) must be monitored to ensure the adequacy of replacement therapy.

Gonadotropin Deficiency

If fertility is not desired, conjugated estrogens in combination with progesterone (on a cyclical or continuous basis) are prescribed for women with an intact uterus. Induced menopause should be considered for women at the appropriate age. In men, testosterone can be delivered intramuscularly or transdermally, using patches or gel. For the restoration of fertility, gonadotropin therapy is indicated.

GH Deficiency

GH therapy may be considered for symptomatic patients with documented hypothalamic-pituitary disease and evidence of an impaired response to provocative testing. The goal of therapy is to restore serum levels of IGF-1 to normal while avoiding side effects. In the short term, GH therapy may enhance the sense of well-being and increase muscle strength, exercise tolerance, and bone mineral density. The long-term effects of this therapy remain unknown.

- Instruct patients about glucocorticoid dose modification during acute illness.
- For the combined deficiency of ACTH and TSH, initiate glucocorticoid therapy before thyroid hormone replacement therapy.
- Use FT4 to monitor the adequacy of therapy in secondary hypothyroidism.

Pituitary Tumors

Pituitary tumors can be sporadic or part of multiple endocrine neoplasia type 1 (MEN-1). They may be present in patients who have the clinical features of a mass effect or endocrine dysfunction, or they may be discovered incidentally when the head is imaged for other reasons. Tumors smaller than 1 cm are *microadenomas* and those 1 cm or larger are *macroadenomas*. Evaluation of a pituitary tumor should address 4 questions:

1. Is the tumor causing a mass effect? Superior extension of the tumor may compromise the optic pathways, leading to impaired visual acuity and visual field defects. Rarely, it produces a hypothalamic syndrome, with disturbed thirst, satiety, sleep, and temperature regulation. Lateral extension of the tumor may compress cranial nerves III, IV, and VI, leading to diplopia and strabismus. Extension of the tumor inferiorly may lead rarely to cerebrospinal fluid (CSF) rhinorrhea. Ophthalmologic evaluation, including assessment of visual acuity, visual fields, and optic discs, is important, particularly if there is suprasellar extension of the tumor. Headaches may accompany enlarging pituitary tumors, particularly in the presence of suprasellar extension.

2. Is hypopituitarism present? Hypopituitarism may be caused by compressive destruction of the pituitary gland or interruption of the pituitary stalk by tumor growth. Stalk compression can cause increased production of prolactin, with secondary hypogonadism. Rarely, patients with pituitary tumors present acutely with pituitary apoplexy, which may be the first clinical expression of the underlying tumor. Endocrine evaluation is essential (see "Hypopituitarism" section).

3. Is there evidence of hormone excess? Approximately 30% to 40% of pituitary tumors are nonfunctioning. The remainder are hyperfunctioning: prolactinomas (40%-50%); GH tumors causing acromegaly (10%-15%); ACTH tumors resulting in Cushing disease (10%-15%); and TSH tumors resulting in hyperthyroidism (<5%). A small percentage of tumors secrete more than 1 hormone, most commonly both prolactin and GH. Although the clinical history and examination findings are useful, formal biochemical evaluation is recommended in every case.

4. What is the nature of the tumor? Although the majority of intrasellar masses reflect pituitary adenomas, alternative possibilities exist, including Rathke cleft cyst, craniopharyngioma, inflammatory masses, and metastatic disease. Evaluation should be guided by the clinical setting, but on occasion a pituitary biopsy may be necessary to establish the diagnosis accurately.

- Ophthalmologic evaluation is important, particularly with suprasellar extension of a tumor.
- Endocrine evaluation should determine hormonal excess or deficiency.

Treatment

Treatment includes surgical excision, irradiation, or medical therapy. The first-line treatment for functioning pituitary tumors is surgical excision, except in the case of prolactinomas, for which dopamine agonist therapy is usually effective. Large tumors that compress or threaten the optic chiasm should also be considered for resection, even in the absence of a hormonal effect, although again, macroprolactinomas may resolve rapidly with dopamine agonist therapy, which should be the first-line therapy for these tumor types. Drug therapy is available for some functional tumors (see below). Simple observation is an option if the tumor is small, does not have a local mass effect, and is nonfunctional.

- Treatment of a pituitary tumor includes surgical excision, irradiation, or medical therapy.
- Observation is an option when the tumor is small and nonfunctioning or, in the case of a microprolactinoma, when it is not associated with clinical features that affect quality of life.

Surgery

Transsphenoidal surgery is the operation of choice for most pituitary tumors (except prolactinoma). Rarely, craniotomy may be necessary for tumors with significant suprasellar extension. Both operations require considerable neurosurgical expertise. The morbidity (bleeding, infection, transient diabetes insipidus, CSF rhinorrhea, and anterior pituitary dysfunction) associated with transsphenoidal surgery is less than 1% for microadenomas and about 5% for macroadenomas; mortality is less than 1%. Persistence or recurrence rate of the tumor is less than 20% to 30% for microadenomas but may be as high as 50% to 70% for macroadenomas.

Radiotherapy

Radiotherapy is reserved for pituitary macroadenomas after surgical or medical therapy fails or as primary therapy for patients who are poor surgical candidates or who refuse operation. Radiotherapy may be delivered by conventional external beam radiation or stereotactic gamma knife radiosurgery. The latter delivers a single dose of highly focused radiation and is reserved for the treatment of small-volume pituitary adenomas or smaller macroadenomas that may involve the cavernous sinus. Both forms of radiotherapy have a long latent period (from a few months to years) before the onset of action, and postradiation hypopituitarism may occur (30%-40% of patients receiving conventional therapy).

Drug Therapy

Dopamine agonists (bromocriptine or cabergoline) are used for the management of prolactinomas. The somatostatin analogue octreotide may be useful in the management of GH- or TSH-producing tumors. GH-receptor antagonist therapy is also available for the treatment of acromegaly that has failed to respond to conventional therapy.

Follow-up

Sequential MRI scanning is used to monitor tumor size. Assessment of endocrine function is essential to assess the development of hypopituitarism, especially in patients who have undergone surgical treatment or radiotherapy. Measurement of hormone concentrations in the serum is the mainstay of hormone monitoring, although this is not an accurate means to monitor steroid hormone replacement. Monitoring of the trophic hormones (eg, TSH) should be avoided in the management of hypopituitarism.

Prolactinoma

Pituitary tumors associated with hyperprolactinemia may be prolactinomas or nonfunctioning tumors that produce a "stalk effect." In the latter situation, the impingement of the tumor on the pituitary stalk interferes with the tonic inhibition of pituitary lactotrophs by dopamine (secreted by the hypothalamus), leading to excess secretion of prolactin by normal lactotrophs. Minor increases in the concentration of prolactin may occur through several physiologic mechanisms (eg, drugs, stress, direct nipple stimulation, or pregnancy) and may not reflect the effect of a pituitary lesion.

- Pituitary tumors associated with hyperprolactinemia are prolactinomas or any tumor or mass lesion with a suprasellar extension and stalk effect.

Clinical Features

Women typically present with galactorrhea and oligomenorrhea or amenorrhea. In men, the recognition of hyperprolactinemia is often delayed because symptoms of hypogonadism, including decreased libido and impotence, may be attributed to other factors. For this reason, men are more likely to present late, with a macroprolactinoma. Galactorrhea is unusual in men because of the absence of estrogen priming of the breast. Gynecomastia in men may occur in hyperprolactinemia, because of secondary hypogonadism, but does not reflect a direct action of prolactin on the breast.

- Clinical features of prolactinoma in women: ovulatory or menstrual dysfunction and galactorrhea.

- Clinical features of prolactinoma in men: decreased libido and impotence. Galactorrhea is rare.

Diagnosis

Differential Diagnosis

Pituitary tumors are not the only cause of hyperprolactinemia. Physiologic causes of hyperprolactinemia include pregnancy, the postpartum state, and stressful conditions such as surgery or seizure. Stalk disruption may occur with infiltrative disorders, including lymphoma and hypophysitis, which lead to disinhibition of prolactin secretion by normal lactotrophs.

Drugs are a common cause of hyperprolactinemia. Neuroleptic agents, antidepressants, cimetidine, verapamil, opiates, and marijuana are all associated with hyperprolactinemia. The mechanism of action is interference with the synthesis, secretion, or action of dopamine. In primary hypothyroidism, hyperprolactinemia is often encountered because of the stimulatory effect of thyrotropin-releasing hormone (TRH) on the synthesis and secretion of prolactin. Chest wall lesions such as herpes zoster, thoracotomy, tumors, or trauma increase prolactin concentrations, possibly through stimulation of thoracic nerve terminals that eventually signal the hypothalamus. Hyperprolactinemia may also be seen in renal failure and cirrhosis because of slowed metabolism of the hormone. Organic hypothalamic disorders that cause hyperprolactinemia include surgery or irradiation, sarcoidosis or Langerhans cell histiocytosis, and neoplastic disorders such as craniopharyngioma and metastatic disease.

- Physiologic hyperprolactinemia occurs in pregnancy and in the postpartum period.
- Pathologic hyperprolactinemia occurs with prolactinomas or conditions that interrupt the pituitary stalk.
- Functional disorders leading to hyperprolactinemia include neuroleptics, primary hypothyroidism, chest wall lesions, and chronic renal or liver failure.

A diagnostic approach to hyperprolactinemia is outlined in the following steps:

1. Rule out pregnancy, which is the commonest cause of amenorrhea and galactorrhea in women of reproductive age.
2. Measure the TSH concentration to rule out primary hypothyroidism.
3. Review medications and drug use history.
4. Image the hypothalamus and pituitary with MRI if other causes of hyperprolactinemia have been ruled out.
5. If a tumor is present, evaluate other pituitary function and visual fields if necessary.

The main diagnostic dilemma is to differentiate a macroprolactinoma from a nonfunctioning tumor that causes a stalk effect. This distinction has therapeutic implications because medical therapy is the first-line treatment for a prolactinoma, whereas nonfunctioning tumors with suprasellar extension should be surgically resected. A serum concentration of prolactin greater than 200 ng/mL supports the diagnosis of prolactinoma; a concentration less than 75 ng/mL is more consistent with a stalk effect, particularly in the presence of a macroadenoma. If the value is between 75 and 200 ng/mL, a trial of dopamine agonist therapy is reasonable. Regression of the tumor mass and a decrease in prolactin concentrations with this therapy support the diagnosis of prolactinoma.

If evaluation fails to identify the cause of hyperprolactinemia, follow-up is appropriate because some patients may harbor a microadenoma or other hypothalamic-pituitary space-occupying lesion that is below the limit of radiographic detection, and follow-up examinations may show evidence of a mass at a later date. The serum level of prolactin should be checked every 6 to 12 months, and MRI should be repeated in 1 year, or earlier if deemed necessary by the development of new symptoms.

Therapy

Treatment is indicated for the management of infertility, hypogonadism, or galactorrhea. Medical treatment with a dopamine agonist is usually the first choice. Transsphenoidal surgery is usually reserved for patients who are intolerant or resistant to dopamine agonist therapy or who require urgent decompression of the sella for visual field defects that have not responded to a trial of dopamine agonist.

Dopamine Agonists

Dopamine agonists (bromocriptine or cabergoline) are very effective in the treatment of hyperprolactinemia caused by prolactinoma. In most cases, these agents also lead to rapid shrinkage of the tumor. Consequently, these drugs are indicated as first-line therapy even for large prolactinomas causing a visual field defect. Frequent assessment of the visual fields and tumor size is indicated in these cases. Neither tumor size nor the degree of prolactin elevation predicts tumor response. Side effects of these drugs may include nausea, fatigue, nasal stuffiness, nightmares, and postural hypotension. Long term therapy with a dopamine agonist may cause tumor fibrosis and shrinkage. After 3 to 5 years of dopamine agonist therapy, withdrawal of the therapy and monitoring of prolactin levels should be considered in patients with prolactinomas because the disorder may resolve spontaneously. Intervening pregnancy may also accelerate the resolution of a microprolactinoma.

Restoration of gonadal function and fertility is a major goal of drug therapy for a prolactinoma. In pregnancy, the risk of growth for microprolactinomas is less than 5% and for macroprolactinomas, 20% to 40%. Patients should be observed closely with clinical and visual field evaluations, especially if they have a macroprolactinoma. If tumor growth is suspected, the head should be examined with MRI. Although treatment with dopamine agonists usually is discontinued during pregnancy, it is reasonable to continue maintenance therapy if the patient has a macroprolactinoma. An increase in tumor size may be an indication for surgical excision.

* The treatment of choice for prolactinomas is medical therapy with a dopamine agonist.
* During pregnancy, the risk of growth for microprolactinomas is <5% and for macroprolactinomas, 20%-40%.
* If marked tumor growth complicates pregnancy, consider surgical excision.

Surgical Treatment of Prolactinomas

For microadenomas, the surgical cure rate is 60% to 80%, and for macroadenomas, 0% to 30%.

GH Tumors: Acromegaly

GH-producing pituitary tumors account for more than 99% of acromegaly cases. Rarely, acromegaly may be caused by ectopic GH-producing tumors or hypothalamic or extra-hypothalamic GHRH-producing tumors. It is preferable to diagnose acromegaly early because the disease is associated with substantial morbidity and premature mortality.

Clinical Features

The clinical features of acromegaly are due to excess IGF-1 and the mass effects of the pituitary tumor. In adults, characteristic features are prominent supraorbital ridges, macroglossia, prognathism, and an increase in hand and foot size. Patients may complain of excessive sweating, increased skin oiliness, headache, and symptoms of carpal tunnel syndrome. The prevalence of colon polyps is increased 3-fold among patients with acromegaly, who also are at increased risk of colon cancer. Currently, it seems prudent to perform colonoscopy on all patients when acromegaly is diagnosed. Cardiovascular disease is the most common cause of premature death. Many patients have hypertension and glucose intolerance. Sleep apnea is a common feature that may resolve or improve with successful treatment of acromegaly.

* Acromegaly is associated with an increased risk of premalignant colon polyps and colon cancer.
* Other common features include hypertension, glucose intolerance, and sleep apnea.

Diagnosis

Biochemical Diagnosis

Measuring the serum concentration of IGF-1 is the best screening test for acromegaly (physiologic increases can occur in pregnancy and adolescence and with sleep apnea). If the IGF-1 serum level is mildly to moderately increased, it is appropriate to proceed with an oral glucose tolerance test to document nonsuppressible GH secretion. Following ingestion of a glucose load, GH levels do not suppress to less than 1 ng/mL in active acromegaly. A random serum level of GH is not helpful because of the pulsatile secretion of GH.

Radiologic Diagnosis

After the diagnosis has been confirmed biochemically, the sella should be examined with MRI. If a pituitary tumor is not delineated (a rare event) or diffuse pituitary hypertrophy is noted, measure the serum level of GHRH to exclude a GHRH-producing tumor and search for evidence of an ectopic GH-producing tumor.

* The serum concentration of IGF-1 is increased in all patients with active acromegaly.
* Failure of GH to suppress to <1 ng/mL with an oral glucose tolerance test is diagnostic of acromegaly.
* A random serum level of GH is not helpful.

Therapy

Surgical excision of the GH-secreting tumor is the treatment of choice. Excision may be curative (40%-80% of cases depending on the size of the tumor and the degree of lateral extension) and facilitates adjunctive therapy. For persistent disease, treatment with octreotide or gamma knife radiosurgery (plus interim octreotide) is used to control GH secretion.

Radiotherapy has a cure rate of 70% after 10 years; hypopituitarism can occur in up to 50% of patients at 10 years, but other morbidity is rare. The major disadvantage of radiotherapy is the long latent period (months to years) before disease activity is controlled. During this wait for the full effects of radiotherapy, pharmacologic therapy is needed.

Octreotide is an effective therapeutic option. Treatment should be initiated with short-acting octreotide administered subcutaneously 3 times daily to assess tolerance. This can be switched quickly to the long-acting depot form of octreotide administered monthly. Octreotide can normalize GH and IGF-1 levels in 80% of patients and produce shrinkage of the tumor in 30% to 50%. Side effects include nausea, flatulence, orthostatic hypotension, headache, cholelithiasis (10% of patients), and impairment of glucose tolerance. Pegvisomant (a GH-receptor antagonist) is indicated for patients who do not respond to, or cannot tolerate, octreotide therapy. The goal of therapy is to achieve and sustain a normal level of IGF-1, and the definition of *cure* should include restoration of GH suppressibility to a glucose load.

- Surgical excision is the treatment of choice.
- For persistent disease after excision, pharmacologic therapy or radiotherapy should be considered.
- Pharmacologic therapy is required while awaiting the full effects of adjunctive radiotherapy.

ACTH-Producing Tumors

ACTH-producing tumors are discussed below in the "Cushing Syndrome" section.

Gonadotropin-Producing Tumors

Gonadotropin-producing tumors constitute the largest fraction of "nonfunctioning" pituitary tumors, as indicated by positive immunohistochemical staining of resected tumor specimens. Although more than 80% of these tumors are able to synthesize gonadotropins or their subunits (or both), increased serum levels of FSH, LH, or their subunits are found in less than 35% of patients. Clinically, the tumors are macroadenomas at presentation. The patients may be any age, but the tumors usually occur in middle-aged or elderly persons and predominantly in males. Mass effects dominate the clinical features, and some degree of hypopituitarism is usually present together with hyperprolactinemia caused by a stalk effect. Currently, no effective medical therapy is available. Surgical excision is required.

TSH-Producing Tumors

Primary TSH tumors are rare, and patients may present with diffuse goiter and mild hyperthyroidism. Laboratory evaluation demonstrates an increased or inappropriately normal TSH level with an increased concentration of FT_4. The α-glycoprotein subunit levels are high, and there is no TSH response to stimulation with TRH. Often such tumors cosecrete GH. Treatment options include excision, pharmacologic therapy with octreotide, and ancillary measures for the management of thyrotoxicosis, targeting the thyroid gland.

Pituitary Incidentaloma

With advances in the resolution of imaging methods, pituitary incidentaloma is increasingly recognized. Autopsy studies suggest that approximately 10% of persons harbor small pituitary tumors, and modern MRI scanning can identify anomalies in 5% to 10% of adults. Evaluation should determine whether the tumor affects pituitary endocrine function (hypopituitarism and hyperfunction) or causes a mass effect (or both). Screening tests should include the measurement of prolactin, FT_4, testosterone (in men), and cortisol. Active intervention is dictated by the finding of a functioning pituitary tumor that can cause morbidity or mortality or an incidentaloma larger than 1 cm in diameter. Otherwise, the patient should be observed and the imaging study repeated in 6 to 12 months and at less frequent intervals thereafter.

Miscellaneous Pituitary Disorders

Craniopharyngioma

Craniopharyngioma is a slow-growing encapsulated benign squamous cell tumor that originates from remnants of the Rathke pouch. It is the most common tumor in the pituitary region in childhood but can occur at any age. Two-thirds of the tumors are suprasellar, and one-third originate in or extend into the sella. Most are cystic, and some have solid and cystic areas. Calcification is often present within the tumor. Mass effects and the consequences of hypopituitarism dominate the clinical presentation.

Surgical excision is possible only for small craniopharyngiomas. Treatment is often complicated by panhypopituitarism and diabetes insipidus. Larger craniopharyngiomas may be decompressed, and radiotherapy should be considered for persistent or recurrent disease.

Pituitary Apoplexy

Pituitary apoplexy is a clinical syndrome produced by sudden hemorrhage or infarction of the pituitary gland. Apoplexy usually occurs in a gland with a preexisting cyst or adenoma, but it has been described in normal pituitary glands. The onset of symptoms may be acute or subacute. The majority of patients present with headache, visual field defects, ophthalmoplegia, and, often, altered mental status. The immediate threat to the patient's life is from cortisol deficiency. Therapy includes hormonal support and neurosurgical decompression.

Lymphocytic Hypophysitis

Lymphocytic hypophysitis is presumed to be autoimmune in origin. Classically, it occurs in women during the postpartum period. The clinical presentation may be due to a mass effect (a sellar mass) but more commonly to deficiency of 1 or more anterior pituitary hormones (ACTH deficiency is the most common). Corticosteroid therapy is often used in an attempt to shrink the sellar mass, but its effects are often disappointing. In many cases, the diagnosis is made only postoperatively because the process may be radiologically indistinguishable from a pituitary adenoma. Hormonal replacement therapy is given as needed.

Diabetes Insipidus

Etiology
Central diabetes insipidus may result from decreased production of vasopressin (ADH) because of granulomatous infiltration of the posterior pituitary and the pituitary stalk (eg, sarcoidosis, tuberculosis, or Langerhans cell histiocytosis), closed head trauma or neurosurgery, or primary neoplasms such as craniopharyngioma or metastatic neoplasms primarily from the breast or lung. However, idiopathic hypothalamic diabetes insipidus is the most common cause of the syndrome and may be an autoimmune disorder. Nephrogenic diabetes insipidus may be caused by chronic renal disease, electrolyte abnormalities (hypercalcemia or hypokalemia), and drugs such as lithium and demeclocycline, which antagonize the effects of ADH on the renal tubules.

* Diabetes insipidus may result from decreased production of ADH or lack of renal responsiveness to the hormone.

Clinical Features
Patients typically present with polyuria and polydipsia, often with a preference for ice-cold water. Nocturia is usually present, and enuresis may be the presenting complaint of children. The absence of nocturia, intermittent symptoms, and a 24-hour urine output greater than 18 L suggest psychogenic polydipsia. It is important to remember that because patients with diabetes insipidus rely solely on their thirst mechanism to regulate water balance, lack of access to water or loss of the sensation of thirst will lead to extreme hyperosmolar dehydration.

Cortisol and, to a lesser extent, thyroid hormones are necessary for the excretion of a water load. In patients with central diabetes insipidus, the development of hypopituitarism may mask the symptoms of diabetes insipidus, which become apparent only after adequate cortisol replacement therapy.

* Diabetes insipidus is characterized by polyuria and polydipsia.
* The absence of nocturia suggests psychogenic polydipsia.
* When thirst sensation is impaired or access to water is restricted, hyperosmolar dehydration may ensue.
* Cortisol is necessary for the kidney to excrete a water load.

Diagnosis

Endocrine Diagnosis
The diagnosis of diabetes insipidus is often complicated by the disorder being partial. Also, prolonged periods of polyuria, regardless of the primary cause, may decrease the maximal urine-concentrating ability of the kidney, creating a nephrogenic component to the condition.

In a patient with polyuria and dilute urine, a random plasma osmolality greater than 295 mOsm/kg or sodium greater than 145 mg/dL suggests the diagnosis of diabetes insipidus. Plasma osmolality less than

280 mOsm/kg implies psychogenic polydipsia. If plasma osmolality is between 280 and 295 mOsm/kg, a water deprivation test is indicated. A random plasma osmolality greater than 295 mOsm/kg (or at the end of a water deprivation test) and urine osmolality less than 300 mOsm/kg at the end of a water deprivation test exclude primary polydipsia and confirm diabetes insipidus. To differentiate between central and nephrogenic diabetes insipidus, 1 mcg desmopressin (DDAVP) is injected subcutaneously immediately following the water deprivation test, and urine osmolality is measured at 30, 60, and 120 minutes. A postinjection urine osmolality more than 150% of the preinjection osmolality is consistent with central diabetes insipidus.

A partial response to water deprivation, with urine osmolality greater than 300 mOsm/kg, can occur in partial central or nephrogenic diabetes insipidus as well as in primary polydipsia. In these circumstances, it is also necessary to collect plasma for ADH levels at the end of the water deprivation test.

* A random plasma osmolality >295 mOsm/kg suggests diabetes insipidus.
* A random plasma osmolality <280 mOsm/kg, in an untreated patient, suggests psychogenic polydipsia.
* Central diabetes insipidus can be distinguished from nephrogenic diabetes insipidus by the response to exogenous desmopressin.
* The absence of response to water deprivation (urine osmolality <300 mOsm/kg) is diagnostic of diabetes insipidus.

Etiologic Diagnosis
Imaging of the hypothalamus and neurohypophysis as well as the sella is essential. Systemic diseases involving the hypothalamus or pituitary stalk must be considered.

Therapy
The underlying cause should be treated. However, in central diabetes insipidus, treatment seldom restores ADH secretion. There is no need for intervention in patients with mild diabetes insipidus (urine output, 2-5 L daily) who have free access to water. For greater degrees of central diabetes insipidus, which interfere with the patient's sleep, desmopressin is the drug of choice. It is administered by nasal spray (5-10 mcg once or twice daily) or orally (0.1-0.8 mg daily in divided doses). For patients who are unconscious or allergic to nasal desmopressin, the drug can be given parenterally (1-2 mcg subcutaneously or intravenously 1 or 2 times daily). Thiazides may be useful in treating nephrogenic diabetes insipidus. Psychiatric assessment is needed for patients with psychogenic polydipsia.

Syndrome of Inappropriate Secretion of ADH

Etiology
The syndrome of inappropriate secretion of ADH (SIADH) occurs when excessive ADH is secreted in the absence of a hyperosmolar stimulus or a hypovolemic or hypotensive (or both) stimulus. SIADH may be a consequence of the following:

1. Central nervous system or hypothalamic disorders (including trauma) or inflammatory, degenerative, vascular, or neoplastic disorders

2. The use of drugs that enhance ADH secretion or action (eg, chlorpropamide, carbamazepine, vincristine, vinblastine, cyclophosphamide, phenothiazines, monoamine oxidase inhibitors, and tricyclic antidepressants)
3. Neurogenic influences such as pain or nausea
4. Benign and malignant pulmonary disorders (eg, pneumonia, lung abscess, empyema, mesothelioma, and small cell lung carcinoma)

Pathophysiology

SIADH leads to hyponatremia, with low serum osmolality and inappropriately concentrated urine. The expansion of the extracellular fluid volume leads to natriuresis (from an increase in glomerular filtration rate, atrial natriuretic hormones, and suppression of the renin-angiotensin-aldosterone axis). Natriuresis exacerbates plasma hypo-osmolality, thus explaining the absence of edema despite an expanded extracellular fluid volume.

* Physiologic or appropriate ADH hypersecretion occurs in response to plasma hyperosmolality or hypovolemia or hypotension.
* SIADH is characterized by hypervolemia, hyponatremia, and hypo-osmolality of body fluids and inappropriately concentrated urine. Edema is absent.

Clinical Features

The clinical features depend on the degree and rapidity of the development of hyponatremia. Patients with SIADH may be asymptomatic if the hyponatremia develops gradually over weeks and months. Symptoms include lethargy, malaise, nausea and vomiting, and confusion. Severe or rapidly developing hyponatremia can lead to alterations in mental status or seizures.

* Clinical features depend on the degree and rapidity of the development of hyponatremia.

Diagnosis

The diagnosis of SIADH is one of exclusion. Pseudo-hyponatremia due to hyperlipidemia (normal plasma osmolality) and hyperosmolar states due to water loss, as in hyperglycemia (increased plasma osmolality), must be excluded. Diseases in which increased secretion of ADH is appropriate (eg, congestive heart failure, ascites, nephrosis, hypovolemia, hypothyroidism, and hypocortisolism) must also be excluded.

The main diagnostic challenge is to differentiate SIADH from subclinical hypovolemia. In subclinical hypovolemia, the urinary concentration of sodium is less than 20 mEq/L (in the absence of diuretic use) and the serum levels of creatinine and uric acid are increased, as are plasma renin activity and the plasma level of aldosterone. An accurate diagnosis is essential since water deprivation, the main treatment of SIADH, is inappropriate in dehydrational hyponatremia.

* The main diagnostic challenge is to differentiate SIADH from subclinical hypovolemia. Determine plasma renin activity and the concentrations of urinary sodium, serum creatinine and uric acid, and plasma aldosterone.

Therapy

Therapy for SIADH includes treating the underlying disorder. Water intake is restricted to 800 to 1,000 mL daily. If necessary, an ADH antagonist (demeclocycline, 900-1,200 mg daily) can be given. If acute neurologic sequelae are present, hypertonic saline is administered intravenously (200-300 mL of 5% saline over 3-4 hours) to achieve a gradual increase in serum sodium (do not exceed 0.5 mEq per hour or 12 mEq in 24 hours). Rapid correction of hyponatremia can lead to central pontine myelinolysis.

* Identify and treat the underlying disorder.
* Therapy for hyponatremia consists of water restriction and, if needed, demeclocycline.
* In the presence of acute neurologic sequelae, administer hypertonic saline to increase serum sodium by 0.5 mEq per hour.
* Rapid correction of hyponatremia can lead to potentially fatal central pontine myelinolysis.

Disorders of the Thyroid Gland

Laboratory Assessment of Thyroid Function

Several thyroid tests to determine thyroid function and structure are being used increasingly in healthy adult screening studies. However, abnormal test results can be obtained in euthyroid patients with nonthyroidal illness. Consequently, the history and physical examination are as important as laboratory investigation in the evaluation of thyroid disease.

Total T_4

Serum total T_4 concentration is a measurement of T_4 bound to thyroid hormone–binding proteins such as thyroxine-binding globulin (TBG). Therefore, conditions that affect TBG concentration affect total T_4 measurements. Androgens, anabolic steroids, glucocorticoids, chronic liver disease, niacin, and familial TBG deficiency decrease total TBG. Estrogens, pregnancy, acute hepatitis, and familial TBG excess increase TBG and total T_4 concentrations.

Total T_3

Serum total T_3 concentration is decreased in hypothyroidism, in nonthyroidal illness and caloric deprivation, and by drugs such as propranolol, amiodarone, and glucocorticoids. Serum T_3 levels are increased in thyrotoxicosis and peripheral hormone resistance. Serum T_3 concentrations should be measured to establish or exclude the diagnosis of T_3 thyrotoxicosis in a patient with a suppressed TSH level and a normal serum concentration of FT_4.

FT_4

The serum concentration of FT_4 is decreased in hypothyroidism and nonthyroidal illness and increased in hyperthyroidism, nonthyroidal illness, and peripheral hormone resistance.

Thyroid Hormone–Binding Proteins

Thyroid hormone–binding proteins can be measured directly by radioimmunoassay or, more commonly, with the T_3 resin uptake test, which provides an indirect measurement of unoccupied T_4 binding sites on binding proteins. The normal range is 30% to 40%. A decrease in T_4 binding sites, and thus an increase in T_3 resin uptake, occurs in hyperthyroidism, in low TBG states, and in the presence of binding inhibitors, as in nonthyroidal illness or with the use of certain drugs (see above). An increase in T_4 binding sites, and thus a decrease in T_3 resin uptake, occurs in hypothyroidism and high TBG states.

Serum TSH
Current fourth-generation TSH assays measure TSH concentrations as low as 0.01 mIU/L, allowing clinicians to differentiate low-normal values from suppressed values. TSH is increased in primary hypothyroidism, during recovery from nonthyroidal illness, and with peripheral resistance to thyroid hormones. TSH is suppressed in hyperthyroidism of any cause (except that due to TSH-producing tumors), in nonthyroidal illness, and by drugs such as somatostatin, dopamine, and glucocorticoids. Measurement of TSH is the best single test of thyroid function. However, TSH levels are unreliable in cases of pituitary disease because values can be "inappropriately" normal relative to thyroid hormone concentrations. Thus, TSH levels may be normal or increased with TSH-producing tumors and normal or decreased in central hypothyroidism.

Thyroid Scanning
Thyroid scanning may be performed with technetium pertechnetate or radioactive iodine. Thyroid scanning is reserved for the documentation of toxic thyroid nodules, ectopic thyroid tissue in struma ovarii, and metastatic disease in the postoperative evaluation and follow-up of patients with differentiated thyroid cancer.

Radioactive Iodine I 131 Uptake
The normal range for 24-hour radioactive iodine I 131 uptake (RAIU) depends on the dietary iodine intake in a given population. In the US population, the normal range is 10% to 25%. A 24-hour RAIU study is indicated during the evaluation of hyperthyroidism to distinguish low-uptake states from high-uptake states and to aid in dose calculations when radioactive iodine is used to treat Graves disease.

Serum Thyroglobulin
Thyroglobulin is used mainly as a tumor marker in follow-up evaluations of patients with differentiated thyroid carcinoma. It also may be useful in the differential diagnosis of suppressed TSH with low RAIU (lymphocytic thyroiditis or exogenous hyperthyroidism). Serum thyroglobulin levels are usually elevated in lymphocytic thyroiditis and low in exogenous hyperthyroidism.

TSH Receptor–Stimulating Immunoglobulins
Measurement of TSH receptor–stimulating immunoglobulins (TSIs), sometimes called TSH-receptor antibodies (TRAbs), which are immune markers of Graves disease, is important in the differential diagnosis of hyperthyroidism in pregnant women who cannot undergo RAIU. TSI levels may help to predict the occurrence of neonatal thyrotoxicosis in infants born to women with active Graves disease or a history of it. TSI measurement is also helpful in the diagnosis of euthyroid Graves ophthalmopathy.

Antithyroglobulin and Antimicrosomal (Antiperoxidase) Antibodies
Antithyroglobulin and antimicrosomal antibodies are used as markers of autoimmune thyroid disease. However, the absence of these antibodies does not exclude autoimmune thyroid disease. Conversely, the presence of these antibodies is not diagnostic of autoimmune thyroid disease; they can be found in otherwise healthy persons. High titers occur in more than 90% of patients with Hashimoto thyroiditis, and modestly increased titers are found in primary atrophic hypothyroidism and Graves disease. Antithyroglobulin antibodies, when present, make measurement of thyroglobulin unreliable for follow-up of thyroid malignancies.

Thyroid Ultrasonography
Ultrasonography is used for the assessment of thyroid nodules and goiter and for follow-up of patients with thyroid cancer. Altered blood flow can be documented in patients with Graves disease.

Hyperthyroidism

Etiology
Primary thyroid disorders that cause hyperthyroidism can be divided into those characterized by increased production and release of T_4 (high RAIU) and those characterized by unregulated release of T_4 due to gland destruction (suppressed RAIU) (Table 6-2).

The most common cause of hyperthyroidism in iodine-sufficient areas is Graves disease. Other frequent causes include toxic nodular goiter, lymphocytic and subacute thyroiditis, and exogenous hyperthyroidism.

Clinical Features
Typical symptoms include heat intolerance, palpitations, increased sweating, diarrhea, weight loss, menstrual irregularities, insomnia, nervousness, irritability, and emotional lability. In severe, prolonged hyperthyroidism, proximal muscle weakness may be present. Ocular manifestations include findings due to sympathetic overactivity from

Table 6-2   Causes of Increased and Suppressed 24-Hour Radioactive Iodine Uptake (RAIU)

High RAIU	Low RAIU
Graves disease	Lymphocytic thyroiditis (postpartum thyroiditis)
Autonomous nodular goiter	Subacute thyroiditis
HCG-dependent hyperthyroidism of trophoblastic disease	Exogenous hyperthyroidism
TSH-secreting pituitary adenoma	Recent iodine load (eg, contrast dye)
Metastatic follicular thyroid carcinoma	Struma ovarii (if RAIU is measured over thyroid only)
Selective pituitary resistance to thyroid hormones	

Abbreviations: HCG, human chorionic gonadotropin; TSH, thyrotropin.

hyperthyroidism of any cause (retraction of the upper lid, stare, and lid lag) or findings unique to Graves disease (puffiness of the lids, conjunctival injection and chemosis, proptosis, and extraocular muscle weakness). Patients with Graves ophthalmopathy may complain of a gritty sensation in the eyes, excessive lacrimation, photophobia, and diplopia. Most patients with hyperthyroidism have a small, firm goiter, but its presence and characteristics vary according to the cause.

Atypical presentations of hyperthyroidism, particularly in the elderly, include apathy, weight loss, supraventricular tachycardia, atrial fibrillation, and congestive heart failure. Young adult males may develop gynecomastia.

- The clinical features of hyperthyroidism reflect the effects of excess thyroid hormone. However, some features, such as Graves ophthalmopathy, may be specific to the underlying cause.
- The presence of goiter and its characteristics vary according to the cause.
- Atypical presentations of hyperthyroidism in the elderly include weight loss, apathy, atrial fibrillation, and congestive heart failure.

Diagnosis of Hyperthyroidism

The biochemical diagnosis of hyperthyroidism rests on the demonstration of suppressed TSH and an increased serum level of FT_4. Normal FT_4 values should prompt the measurement of serum T_3 concentrations to determine the presence of T_3 toxicosis. An increased or inappropriately normal TSH level in the presence of an increased FT_4 level indicates hyperthyroidism due to pituitary TSH-secreting tumors or selective pituitary resistance to thyroid hormones. A low level of serum TSH by itself is not diagnostic of hyperthyroidism and can be encountered in nonthyroidal illness, glucocorticoid therapy, dopamine therapy, and secondary hypothyroidism.

Specific Causes

Graves Disease

Graves disease is characterized by the triad of hyperthyroidism, ophthalmopathy, and dermopathy, which may occur singly or in combination. Management of hyperthyroidism does not influence the clinical course of eye or skin manifestations. The hyperthyroidism is caused by autoantibodies with TSH-like activity (ie, TSIs). Although Graves disease occurs most often in young women, it can occur at any age and in either sex. The disease tends to relapse and remit spontaneously. Usually, the thyroid is diffusely enlarged and smooth, with a firm consistency.

- Hyperthyroidism, ophthalmopathy, and dermopathy characterize Graves disease.
- Hyperthyroidism is caused by the production of TSI.

Painless Lymphocytic Thyroiditis (Postpartum Thyroiditis or Silent Thyroiditis)

Painless lymphocytic thyroiditis is usually a self-limiting disease that occurs most commonly in the postpartum period (although it may occur in males) and tends to recur with subsequent pregnancies in two-thirds of women with the disease. Patients with a history of lymphocytic thyroiditis also have an increased incidence of chronic autoimmune thyroiditis. The classic presentation is a triphasic pattern of thyroid function: an initial hyperthyroid phase (suppressed TSH, low RAIU, and increased levels of FT_4) is followed by a hypothyroid phase and subsequent recovery of normal thyroid function. However, patients may present at any stage of the disorder or may have thyroid recovery without having a hypothyroid phase.

β-Blockers may be prescribed in the hyperthyroid phase for symptomatic tachycardia or tremor. There is no indication for antithyroid medications or radioactive iodine therapy because the hyperthyroidism is due to the release of preformed thyroid hormone into the circulation and not to increased production of thyroid hormone. Temporary thyroid hormone replacement therapy may be necessary for symptomatic patients during the hypothyroid phase. In some cases, the hypothyroidism may be permanent.

- Painless lymphocytic thyroiditis may occur in both sexes, but it is more common in women in the postpartum period.
- Patients typically present with transient hyperthyroidism, followed by transient hypothyroidism before thyroid recovery.
- Treatment is symptomatic: β-blockers for hyperthyroid symptoms and temporary thyroid hormone replacement therapy for hypothyroidism.
- Two-thirds of women with postpartum thyroiditis have recurrence of disease with subsequent pregnancies.

Subacute Painful Thyroiditis (de Quervain Thyroiditis)

Subacute painful thyroiditis is characterized by a painful, tender goiter. Patients often complain of fever, malaise, myalgia, and a history of upper respiratory tract infection. Odynophagia may be a prominent symptom. Transient hyperthyroidism (low RAIU) is often present at diagnosis and may be followed by transient hypothyroidism. The erythrocyte sedimentation rate is invariably increased.

The differential diagnosis includes hemorrhage into a thyroid nodule. With hemorrhage, the onset of pain is similarly abrupt, but the features of a systemic illness are absent and a tender nodule can often be palpated. In this case, thyroid function is unaffected, and the erythrocyte sedimentation rate is normal. Treatment options for painful thyroiditis include nonsteroidal anti-inflammatory drugs (NSAIDs) for mild or moderate disease and corticosteroid therapy for severe disease. The response to corticosteroid therapy is dramatic, typically with relief of symptoms within 24 hours.

- Subacute thyroiditis is characterized by a tender thyroid gland.
- The erythrocyte sedimentation rate is markedly increased.
- Symptomatic therapy includes NSAIDs or corticosteroid therapy.

Multinodular Goiter

Toxic multinodular goiter occurs in patients with a long-standing nodular goiter in which autonomous nodules develop. The hyperthyroidism is usually mild, and cardiovascular manifestations may dominate the clinical features. The goiter is large, nodular, and asymmetrical. The thyroid may be difficult to palpate in some patients because of substernal extension or a short neck.

- Toxic multinodular goiter occurs in patients with nodular goiter.
- Hyperthyroidism may be characterized by organ-specific manifestations, particularly cardiovascular ones.
- A goiter may be difficult to palpate because of a short neck or substernal extension.

Toxic Thyroid Adenoma

A hyperfunctioning autonomous follicular adenoma ("toxic thyroid adenoma"), found most often in middle-aged women, may lead to hyperthyroidism. The solitary nodule is usually larger than 3 cm, is easy to palpate, and has a firm consistency. A radioisotope scan demonstrates intense uptake in the nodule, with suppressed uptake in the rest of the gland.

- A radioisotope scan demonstrates intense uptake in the nodule, with suppressed uptake in the rest of the gland.
- Most solitary hyperfunctioning nodules are >3 cm.

Exogenous Hyperthyroidism

Exogenous hyperthyroidism can result from the use of T_4 or T_3 (or both). Factitial thyrotoxicosis should be suspected in thyrotoxic patients who do not have a palpable goiter and do not have suppressed RAIU. Low serum levels of thyroglobulin help to differentiate this disorder from painless lymphocytic thyroiditis.

- The absence of goiter and the absence of suppressed RAIU in a thyrotoxic patient should prompt consideration of factitial thyrotoxicosis.

Therapy

Thionamides

Methimazole and propylthiouracil are used to treat the hyperthyroidism of Graves disease. They act by blocking thyroid hormone synthesis and may have immunomodulating properties that decrease the production of TSI. At very high doses, propylthiouracil decreases the peripheral conversion of T_4 to T_3. The effect of thionamides is temporary, and hyperthyroidism often recurs after discontinuation of treatment. Therefore, these drugs are used in Graves disease to control hyperthyroidism with the hope of spontaneous remission of the disease during therapy. Treatment is given for 12 to 18 months and then discontinued. The safety of long-term antithyroid drug therapy is not well documented. In more than 50% of patients, the disease relapses within the first 3 to 6 months. Adverse effects are uncommon (<5%) but potentially serious and include agranulocytosis and hepatitis. Agranulocytosis can develop abruptly within a few hours; commonly, it initially manifests with an extreme sore throat. Thionamides can cross the placenta and, in high doses, block thyroid hormone synthesis in the fetal thyroid. For pregnant women, the lowest dose that controls symptoms is used.

- Thionamides block thyroid hormone synthesis and may decrease production of TSI.
- Agranulocytosis can develop abruptly.
- Thionamides can cross the placenta and affect the fetal thyroid.

Radioactive Iodine

Radioactive iodine therapy is effective in ablating the thyroid gland and is commonly used to treat the hyperthyroidism of Graves disease or toxic multinodular goiter. This therapy has not been associated with long-term risks, but pregnancy and breastfeeding are contraindications. Most physicians avoid administering radioactive iodine to very young patients. The goal of therapy is to render the patient hypothyroid. The maximal effect from radioactive iodine is apparent within 2 to 3 months. Treatment of toxic multinodular goiter requires higher doses of radioactive iodine and often more than 1 course of treatment. Painful thyroiditis may develop within a week after treatment, as can transient worsening of hyperthyroidism. Radiation-induced enlargement of the gland may worsen obstructive symptoms, particularly in patients with a substernal goiter. Currently, it is debated whether radioactive iodine therapy may worsen Graves ophthalmopathy. It has been suggested that this risk is decreased if corticosteroid treatment is given before radioactive iodine therapy to patients with symptomatic ophthalmopathy.

- Pregnancy and breastfeeding are contraindications to treatment with radioactive iodine.
- Radioactive iodine therapy may be given in Graves disease or toxic multinodular goiter.
- The dose of radioactive iodine is intended to make the patient hypothyroid.
- Radiation-induced enlargement of the gland may worsen obstructive symptoms, particularly in patients with a substernal goiter.

Surgery

Subtotal or near-total thyroidectomy is rarely performed to treat Graves disease but is indicated in certain situations, including a large obstructive gland and pregnancy. Thyrotoxic patients with thyroid nodules that look suspicious on fine-needle aspiration should be referred for surgery. To prevent a thyroid storm as well as excessive bleeding from the overactive friable gland, the patient should be rendered euthyroid with antithyroid drug therapy and then given stable iodine for 7 to 10 days preoperatively. Damage to the recurrent laryngeal nerves or parathyroid glands is not common (<1% to 2%) with experienced surgeons.

- Subtotal thyroidectomy is indicated for thyrotoxic patients with large goiters or suspicious-looking nodules and for patients with Graves disease who are young or pregnant.

Supportive Therapy

β-Blockers are used to control the adrenergic manifestations of hyperthyroidism. Propranolol (a nonselective β-blocker) is prescribed most commonly. These drugs are administered to patients with severe symptomatic hyperthyroidism while awaiting the effects of more definitive therapy.

Thyroid Storm

Thyroid storm is a state of severe hyperthyroidism in untreated or inadequately treated hyperthyroid patients who are undergoing surgical treatment or who have acute intercurrent illness. It is characterized by delirium, fever, tachycardia, hypotension, vomiting, diarrhea, and, eventually, coma. Treatment should be initiated immediately. Together with other supportive therapy, propylthiouracil is given to block thyroid hormone synthesis, sodium iodide is given to inhibit the release of thyroid hormones, and propranolol is given to control the adrenergic manifestations.

Thyrotoxicosis in Pregnancy

Antithyroid drug therapy is the first-line treatment of thyrotoxicosis during pregnancy. Surgical excision may be an option after the first trimester. Radioactive iodine is contraindicated because of its ablative effects on the fetal thyroid. Because antithyroid drugs cross the placenta, the lowest dose necessary to control the disease should be given.

Hypothyroidism

Hypothyroidism can be primary (intrinsic thyroid disease) or secondary (hypothalamic-pituitary disease). Primary hypothyroidism accounts for more than 90% of all cases. The commonest causes of primary hypothyroidism in iodine-replete areas of the world are Hashimoto thyroiditis (goitrous hypothyroidism) and Ord disease (atrophic hypothyroidism), both caused by autoimmune thyroid disease. Hashimoto thyroiditis, which tends to cluster in families, is a common disease, particularly in middle-aged and elderly women.

Other common causes include hypothyroidism occurring after radioactive iodine treatment of hyperthyroidism, surgical thyroidectomy, and radiotherapy for neck malignancies. Hypothyroidism may be transient during the course of subacute or painless thyroiditis.

* The commonest cause of hypothyroidism is autoimmune thyroid disease (Hashimoto thyroiditis or Ord disease).

Clinical Features

The clinical presentation of hypothyroidism depends on the degree and duration of the deficiency. In current practice, many patients are asymptomatic, having received a diagnosis through routine screening. Early symptoms include leg cramps, ankle swelling, dry skin, and dry hair. Patients often complain of fatigue, achiness, and mental slowing. Cold intolerance and a mild degree of weight gain are frequently present. The thyroid gland is typically firm or rubbery, with a bosselated texture.

Uncommon manifestations include psychosis, deafness, and cerebellar ataxia. Some patients experience central hypoventilation and apnea because of respiratory depression. Macrocytic anemia, pernicious anemia (associated autoimmune disease), or microcytic anemia (iron deficiency due to menorrhagia) may be present. Patients with dramatic increases in TSH may experience galactorrhea (TRH stimulates prolactin secretion). Hyponatremia due to SIADH may be present. Associated laboratory findings include hyperlipidemia and increased aspartate aminotransferase, lactate dehydrogenase, or creatine kinase.

Autoimmune thyroiditis may be a manifestation of polyglandular autoimmunity (Addison disease, type 1 diabetes mellitus, hypoparathyroidism, or pernicious anemia). It also is associated with vitiligo and other autoimmune and connective tissue diseases.

Diagnosis

The TSH concentration is increased in primary hypothyroidism and low or inappropriately normal in secondary hypothyroidism. A low FT_4 or FTI confirms the diagnosis of hypothyroidism, provided nonthyroidal illness has been excluded. Serum measurements of T_3 are not usually helpful in the diagnosis and may be normal in hypothyroid patients, as a result of up-regulation in the conversion of T_4 to T_3.

Hashimoto thyroiditis is usually associated with a bosselated (micronodular), firm goiter and a high titer of antimicrosomal antibodies. In contrast, Ord disease demonstrates an atrophic, often impalpable gland, although antibodies are typically detectable in this condition also. Hypothyroidism occurring after radioactive iodine therapy, thyroid surgery, or radiotherapy to the neck or occurring transiently during the course of subacute or silent thyroiditis is usually evident from a careful clinical evaluation. The diagnosis of central hypothyroidism should prompt imaging of the head and testing of pituitary function.

* Low FT_4 or FTI and increased TSH levels are diagnostic of primary hypothyroidism if nonthyroidal illness has been excluded.
* Low FT_4 or FTI and inappropriately normal or low TSH levels indicate central hypothyroidism. MRI of the head and pituitary function tests should be performed.

Therapy

Thyroid hormone replacement therapy is initiated with synthetic T_4. The usual daily replacement dose of T_4 is 1.6 mcg T_4/kg body weight. In patients with ischemic heart disease, treatment usually is initiated at a lower dose (eg, 25 mcg), with dose increments every few weeks. Care should be taken, particularly in Ord disease, in which autonomous function of the gland remnant may result in thyrotoxicosis if T_4 therapy is initiated at full replacement doses. The goals of therapy are to normalize TSH in primary hypothyroidism and to normalize FT_4 in central hypothyroidism.

Failure to normalize TSH concentrations may be indicative of poor compliance, malabsorption due to concomitant use of medications (eg, cholestyramine, sucralfate, calcium supplements, or ferrous sulfate within 4 hours of T_4), or gastrointestinal tract disease. Other reasons include progressive thyroid disease, pregnancy, and increased hormone clearance (with use of estrogen, phenytoin, or rifampin). A suppressed TSH level in a patient treated for primary hypothyroidism may indicate reduced T_4 requirements of aging, decreased clearance, or (rarely) reactivation of the thyroid remnant with development of Graves disease. It is important to assess TSH annually or as indicated by the patient's symptoms to ensure compliance and to determine whether dose adjustment is needed.

* Monitor TSH in primary hypothyroidism.
* Monitor FT_4 in central hypothyroidism.
* Avoid medications that may interfere with intestinal absorption for at least 4 hours after ingestion.

Miscellaneous Circumstances

Thyroxine Replacement Therapy in Pregnancy

Women who are receiving T_4 replacement therapy should be counseled about the importance of ensuring adequate replacement before conception. Most patients with primary hypothyroidism who are receiving an adequate dosage before pregnancy require an increased dose as the pregnancy progresses (an average dose increase of 25%-50%). TSH levels should be assessed periodically during pregnancy, and the T_4 dose should be adjusted as necessary to maintain a normal TSH.

Thyroxine Replacement Therapy in Patients With Angina
Hypothyroid patients with progressive, symptomatic ischemic heart disease should be evaluated by a cardiologist. Hypothyroidism does not contraindicate intervention, although there is an increased risk of hyponatremia and other perioperative complications. Replacement therapy typically is initiated with 25 mcg daily, and the dose is increased gradually to the replacement dosage.

Subclinical Hypothyroidism
In subclinical hypothyroidism, serum TSH levels are increased in clinically euthyroid patients with normal FT_4 concentrations. It is a relatively common disorder and affects 5% to 15% of elderly persons. Patients are usually asymptomatic or have minimal nonspecific symptoms that may be unrelated to hypothyroidism. A trial of replacement therapy is indicated for symptomatic patients and for patients at risk of progressive disease. The risk of progression to overt hypothyroidism increases with age, the presence of thyroid antibodies, and TSH levels greater than 10 mIU/L.

Myxedema Coma
Myxedema coma occurs in patients who have severe, untreated hypothyroidism, and although it may be spontaneous, it usually is precipitated by acute illness (eg, infection, surgery, or myocardial infarction), exposure to cold, or the use of sedatives or opiates. The mortality rate (20%-50%) is high. The onset is insidious, with progressive stupor culminating in coma. Seizures, hypothermia, hypotension, hypoventilation, hyponatremia, and hypoglycemia may be present.

Treatment should be initiated promptly with intravenous T_4. This is usually given as a single daily dose (50-100 mcg). Aggressive treatment of associated conditions such as hypothermia should be initiated. The use of glucocorticoids in myxedema coma is controversial. The optimal approach is to administer corticosteroids if there is clinical and laboratory evidence of hypocortisolism. An effort should be made to conserve body heat; external warming is likely to cause cutaneous vasodilatation, with increased hypotension. Often, the prognosis is determined by the coexisting conditions.

Thyroid Nodules
Thyroid nodules are extremely common and increase in frequency with age. Nodules may be detected during a routine medical examination, noticed by the patient, or detected during neck ultrasonography performed for other reasons. With the discovery of a nodule, the primary concern is whether the underlying process is benign or malignant. In addition to considering primary thyroid malignancies, consider metastatic disease (renal cell carcinoma is the most common malignancy metastatic to the thyroid). Patients with benign adenomas and cysts may present with thyroid nodules, and patients with a multinodular goiter may present with a dominant nodule. Occasionally, the goiter of Hashimoto thyroiditis may simulate a solitary thyroid nodule.

At least 95% of palpable thyroid nodules are benign, but the likelihood of malignancy increases with solitary nodules, older age, male gender, and a history of irradiation to the head and neck (especially during childhood). The initial step in the evaluation of a thyroid nodule is measurement of TSH to determine whether autonomy is present. Thyroid malignancy is substantially less likely if the TSH level is suppressed. If the TSH level is suppressed, a thyroid scan and an RAIU study should be performed. A thyroid scan is not helpful in the evaluation of a thyroid nodule unless the TSH is suppressed and a hyperfunctioning nodule is suspected.

Following TSH measurement, ultrasound-guided fine-needle aspiration should be performed in a palpable nodule. Fine-needle aspiration has high sensitivity and specificity for excluding malignancy if performed and interpreted by experienced personnel. If the aspirate has benign characteristics, annual follow-up with palpation and measurement of TSH is adequate, provided no change is noted in the size and characteristics of the nodule. A nondiagnostic aspirate requires repetition (under ultrasonographic guidance if needed). If the aspirate is interpreted as suspicious or compatible with malignancy, surgical intervention is required.

- Of palpable thyroid nodules, ≥95% are benign.
- TSH measurement is the first test in the evaluation of thyroid nodules.
- Fine-needle aspiration has high sensitivity and specificity for excluding malignancy if performed and interpreted by experienced personnel.
- A thyroid scan is not helpful in the evaluation of a thyroid nodule unless the TSH is suppressed and a hyperfunctioning nodule is suspected.

Thyroid Cancer

Differentiated Thyroid Cancer
Papillary thyroid carcinoma is the most common type of thyroid cancer (80%-90% of cases). Its incidence peaks in early adulthood and again in late adulthood. Dissemination is generally via the lymphatics to lymph nodes; other sites of metastases include the lungs and bone. Typically, manifestation is as a thyroid nodule, as cervical lymphadenopathy, or as an incidental finding in an excised gland.

Follicular carcinoma (10%-15% of cases) spreads preferentially by the hematogenous route. The usual manifestation is as a thyroid mass or metastatic deposits to the lungs, bones, or brain. Rarely, especially if the tumor burden is large, follicular carcinoma can cause thyrotoxicosis.

Patients with undifferentiated *anaplastic carcinoma* usually present with a rapidly progressive thyroid mass with pain and compressive local neck symptoms. It has an extremely poor prognosis, and patients have a median survival of less than 3 months after diagnosis.

Conversely, among patients with differentiated cancer, the 20-year cause-specific mortality rate varies from less than 5% to 15%, with papillary cancer having the best prognosis. Factors associated with a poorer prognosis include age older than 45 at diagnosis, incomplete resection, extensive local invasion, large size of primary tumor, and the presence of distant metastases (metastases to the cervical lymph nodes do not affect prognosis).

Surgical excision is the therapy of choice for differentiated thyroid cancer. For anaplastic cancer, excision is sometimes undertaken to palliate compression of the trachea and to prevent or delay asphyxiation. The extent of surgical excision in differentiated thyroid cancer is a subject of debate, but near-total thyroidectomy is usually performed. The affected lymph nodes are selectively excised.

Patients at low risk of recurrent disease are treated with a dose of T_4 to maintain TSH between 0.1 and 0.4 mIU/L. Those at higher risk undergo radioactive iodine imaging at 4 to 8 weeks postoperatively, after thyroid hormone withdrawal. If necessary, a sufficient dose of radioactive iodine is administered to ablate the thyroid remnant. Suppressive therapy is initiated, with the target TSH level being less than 0.1 mIU/L.

Reevaluation in 3 to 6 months and annually thereafter is required. Chest radiography, determination of serum levels of TSH and thyroglobulin, and neck ultrasonography are performed at each visit. Whole body iodine scanning is also in widespread use in the routine follow-up of patients with thyroid cancer. Most differentiated thyroid malignancies synthesize and secrete thyroglobulin, which can be used as a marker of recurrent or persistent disease. If a patient has little or no thyroid tissue and is receiving suppressive T_4 therapy, the serum thyroglobulin level should be less than 5 ng/mL; a higher (or increasing) level implies persistent or recurrent disease.

- Papillary cancer spreads via the lymphatics to the lymph nodes and has the best prognosis. Manifestation is as a thyroid mass or cervical lymphadenopathy or as an incidental finding.
- Follicular carcinoma spreads preferentially by the hematogenous route. Manifestation is as a thyroid mass or distant metastatic deposits.
- Patients with anaplastic carcinoma present with rapidly progressive local symptoms.
- Surgical excision is the definitive therapy for differentiated thyroid cancer.
- Follow-up evaluation requires determination of TSH and thyroglobulin levels, neck ultrasonography, and chest radiography. Radioactive iodine imaging is performed if there is evidence of recurrent or persistent disease.
- Recurrences are treated, depending on location, with excision or radioactive iodine.

Miscellaneous Thyroid Disorders

Sick Euthyroid Syndrome
Patients who require hospitalization for a systemic illness, psychiatric disorder, or trauma frequently have abnormal thyroid function test results without identifiable intrinsic thyroid disease. The abnormalities resolve with recovery from the associated illness. Specific therapy is not required. During the acute illness, the TSH level may be normal or low (approximately 0.01 mcU/L) because of the central effects of the illness. TSH levels may be increased during recovery.

The main challenge in sick hospitalized patients is to distinguish between nonthyroidal illness and intrinsic thyroid or pituitary disease. Helpful features in the differential diagnosis include the presence of goiter, extrathyroidal manifestations of Graves disease, hypothalamic-pituitary mass effects, or hypopituitarism. A high serum level of T_3 suggests hyperthyroidism, whereas a TSH level greater than 20 mIU/L supports the diagnosis of primary hypothyroidism.

Amiodarone and the Thyroid
Amiodarone is a class III antiarrhythmic agent. Iodine comprises 40% of the drug by weight. This drug can affect thyroid function in several ways, including causing drug-induced thyroiditis. In persons with impaired thyroid autoregulation (underlying autoimmune thyroid disease or nodular goiter), iodide excess can lead to hyperthyroidism or hypothyroidism. When using amiodarone, it is important to monitor thyroid function, particularly in the elderly (consider the high prevalence of Hashimoto thyroiditis and nodular goiter and the difficulty with detecting thyroid dysfunction in this age group).

Lithium and the Thyroid
Lithium decreases the synthesis and secretion of thyroid hormones. Its use has been associated with the development of goiter and hypothyroidism, especially in patients who have underlying autoimmune thyroid disease.

Disorders of Calcium and Bone Metabolism

Hypercalcemia
Clinically, the causes of hypercalcemia are best categorized as either parathyroid-dependent or parathyroid-independent.

Parathyroid-Dependent Hypercalcemia

Primary Hyperparathyroidism
Etiology—Primary hyperparathyroidism is the most common cause of hypercalcemia in ambulatory patients. It is more common in women. A single parathyroid adenoma is the cause in 80% of patients, multiple adenomas are the cause in 5% of patients, and hyperplasia of all 4 glands is the cause in 15%. Rarely, patients with parathyroid carcinoma present with a neck mass and hypercalcemia. In 6% to 10% of patients with hyperparathyroidism, the adenoma may be found in the thyroid, thymus, or mediastinum. The disease may be sporadic or familial. Familial hyperparathyroidism may be a manifestation of MEN-1 or MEN-2A. Parathyroid hyperplasia is usually present in familial hyperparathyroidism.

- Primary hyperparathyroidism is a common disorder that may be sporadic or familial.
- Parathyroid adenoma is the usual cause.
- Hyperplasia is common in the familial forms of hyperparathyroidism. It may be an isolated feature or occur in association with MEN-1 or MEN-2A.

Clinical Features—Most patients with primary hyperparathyroidism are asymptomatic, and the hyperparathyroidism is identified by routine laboratory testing. Symptomatic hypercalcemia may be manifested as polyuria and polydipsia. Hypercalciuria can cause nephrolithiasis. Nephrocalcinosis and band keratopathy may occur in severe disease. Nonspecific symptoms of fatigue, weakness, myopathy, and depression may be present. Skeletal manifestations include osteopenia or osteoporosis and, in severe disease, bone pain and pathologic fractures.

* Primary hyperparathyroidism is commonly asymptomatic.
* When the disease is symptomatic, symptoms may involve the kidneys, skeleton, and nervous and cardiovascular systems.

Laboratory Features—Hypercalcemia is usually mild and often has existed for several years before diagnosis. In most cases, serum phosphate concentrations are normal, but with prolonged hyperparathyroidism, they may decrease. The serum level of parathyroid hormone (PTH) is usually increased or inappropriately normal for the degree of hypercalcemia. Urinary calcium excretion is often increased or at the upper limits of normal. Its measurement is important not only to assess the risk of nephrolithiasis but also to exclude disorders characterized by low rates of calcium excretion (familial hypocalciuric hypercalcemia and thiazide use).

Radiographic Features—Primary hyperparathyroidism is associated with loss of cortical bone. Characteristic radiographic skeletal changes include subperiosteal bone resorption (visible on the radial borders of the phalanges), a "salt-and-pepper" appearance of the skull, and osteitis fibrosa cystica (fibrous replacement of the resorbed bone, with bone pain, tenderness, deformity, or fracture). Brown tumors are collections of osteoclasts intermixed with poorly mineralized woven bone. Renal stones or nephrocalcinosis may be visible on abdominal radiographs.

* The principal laboratory findings are hypercalcemia and increased PTH or inappropriately normal PTH for the degree of hypercalcemia.
* Urinary calcium measurement is important in the differential diagnosis and helps guide management.
* Characteristic skeletal findings in severe disease are subperiosteal bone resorption and cortical bone loss. A "salt-and-pepper" appearance of the skull and osteitis fibrosa cystica may be present.

Therapy—Surgical parathyroidectomy is the treatment of choice for primary hyperparathyroidism. Preoperative imaging (sestamibi subtraction scanning or ultrasonography) often identifies a solitary parathyroid adenoma, allowing a minimal access surgery. Intraoperative measurement of PTH confirms a surgical cure or may guide the surgeon to a more extensive exploration when necessary. In patients with parathyroid hyperplasia, subtotal parathyroidectomy is performed, leaving about 50 mg of parathyroid tissue intact. Later, it may be necessary to remove this tissue if hypercalcemia persists or recurs. Reversible, mild, asymptomatic hypocalcemia is common in the early postoperative period. However, in patients with severe preexisting parathyroid-induced bone disease, correction of hyperparathyroidism may lead to marked and prolonged hypocalcemia.

Conservative therapy may be indicated for mild uncomplicated disease, especially in the elderly. Indications for excision include serum calcium level greater than 1 unit above the upper limit of normal, nephrolithiasis or pronounced hypercalciuria, osteopenia or osteoporosis, and symptomatic hypercalcemia. Imaging studies to localize the parathyroid neoplasm usually are reserved for patients with persistent or recurrent hyperparathyroidism. However, with the advent of minimally invasive parathyroid surgery, preoperative localization with sestamibi scanning is increasingly being used.

* Parathyroidectomy is the treatment of choice.
* Indications for parathyroidectomy include serum calcium >1 unit above the upper limit of normal, nephrolithiasis, marked hypercalciuria, osteopenia, osteoporosis, and symptomatic hypercalcemia.

Familial Hypocalciuric Hypercalcemia

Familial hypocalciuric hypercalcemia, an autosomal dominant disorder, results from an altered set point of the calcium-sensing receptor in the parathyroid glands and renal tubules. Characteristically, it is an uncomplicated, asymptomatic, mild hypercalcemia in a patient with a normal or slightly increased level of PTH, low urinary calcium, and a positive family history. The diagnosis is strongly supported by a calcium to creatinine clearance ratio less than 0.01. Parathyroid surgery is not indicated because the complications of hyperparathyroidism do not develop.

* Familial hypocalciuric hypercalcemia is not associated with symptoms and does not require treatment.

Thiazide-Induced Hypercalcemia

Mild hypercalcemia may occur in patients taking thiazide diuretics. The hypercalcemia is multifactorial (dehydration, decreased renal calcium clearance, and possibly increased PTH secretion). PTH levels are inappropriately normal or mildly increased. The hypercalcemia usually resolves within a few weeks after the discontinuation of drug therapy. Thiazide-induced hypercalcemia is more likely to occur in patients with underlying mild primary hyperparathyroidism.

Lithium

Lithium raises the threshold of inhibition of PTH secretion by serum calcium. PTH levels are inappropriately normal or mildly increased. The hypercalcemia resolves after discontinuation of lithium.

Parathyroid-Independent Hypercalcemia

Hypercalcemia of Malignancy

Hypercalcemia of malignancy often develops acutely and may be severe and life-threatening. It is the most common cause of hypercalcemia in hospitalized patients and may be due to the destructive effects of skeletal metastases or the paraneoplastic effect of a malignancy. Patients in the latter group have few or no skeletal metastases, and the hypercalcemia resolves after treatment of the malignancy. Most of these tumors secrete parathyroid hormone–related peptide (PTHrp), which mediates this humoral hypercalcemia of malignancy. Serum PTH is suppressed in all cases of hypercalcemia due to malignancy.

Vitamin D Intoxication

Hypercalcemia, hypercalciuria, renal insufficiency, and soft tissue calcification follow prolonged ingestion of toxic doses of vitamin D or its metabolites. Because vitamin D is stored in fat, the condition may persist for months after treatment has been discontinued. Hypercalcemia also occurs in vitamin A intoxication.

Sarcoidosis, Other Granulomatous Disorders, and Some Lymphomas

The hypercalcemia and hypercalciuria in these disorders are due to the presence of vitamin D–dependent granulomas and some lymphomas that express high concentrations of the 1α-hydroxylase enzyme and thus can autonomously generate 1,25-dihydroxyvitamin D from circulating 25-hydroxyvitamin D. The serum levels of 25-hydroxyvitamin D are normal, and those of 1,25-dihydroxyvitamin D are increased. The hypercalcemia is responsive to glucocorticoid therapy.

Miscellaneous Causes

Hyperthyroidism enhances bone turnover and may lead to net bone loss. Hypercalcemia and, more frequently, hypercalciuria may be present. The hypercalcemia resolves with the treatment of thyrotoxicosis. In an addisonian crisis, hypercalcemia is often present and may be symptomatic. It is related to dehydration and increased albumin concentration and is reversible with glucocorticoid therapy. Immobilization may result in hypercalcemia in patients with rapid bone turnover, as in Paget disease of bone.

* Hypercalcemia of malignancy may be due to skeletal metastases, the secretion of a humoral factor such as PTHrp, or to the production of 1,25-dihydroxyvitamin D (typically by lymphomas).

Management of Hypercalcemia

When feasible, treatment of the primary cause may be the most important intervention. Glucocorticoids are the drugs of choice for the hypercalcemia of granulomatous disorders. Humoral hypercalcemia of malignancy may be treated by complete resection of the tumor.

In severe hypercalcemia or hypercalcemia in which the primary cause is not immediately treatable, calcium concentrations should be decreased. Aggressive rehydration with volume expansion promotes calciuresis (saline diuresis) and has a transient hypocalcemic effect. Loop (but not thiazide) diuretics help promote renal calcium excretion but should only be given after volume expansion. Pamidronate (a bisphosphonate) given as a single intravenous dose of 30 to 90 mg inhibits bone resorption and mobilization of calcium from bone and has a marked and prolonged effect on calcium concentrations. Calcitonin is used rarely because of its modest effects and the rapid onset of tachyphylaxis. Dialysis is reserved for patients with renal failure.

* Volume expansion and calciuresis (saline diuresis) form the cornerstone of therapy. Loop diuretics are useful adjuncts after rehydration.
* Pamidronate decreases calcium concentrations by inhibiting bone resorption and has a marked and prolonged effect on calcium concentrations.
* Dialysis is reserved for patients with renal failure.

Hypoparathyroidism

Etiology

Hypoparathyroidism may be due to decreased PTH production by the parathyroid glands or to resistance of the target tissue to the actions of PTH. The parathyroid glands may be damaged during thyroidectomy or neck dissection, or they may be excised completely for the treatment of primary hyperparathyroidism due to parathyroid hyperplasia. Hypoparathyroidism may be transient or permanent, and it may appear within hours after the operation. Hypocalcemia after neck surgery often is manifested by symptoms of neuromuscular excitability, for example, Chvostek and Tinel signs.

Hypoparathyroidism also may result from an autoimmune or infiltrative process (hemochromatosis or Wilson disease) or from defective formation of the branchial arches associated with thymic aplasia (DiGeorge syndrome). Hypomagnesemia (from use of diuretics, malabsorption, or malnutrition) impairs the secretion and action of PTH.

Pseudohypoparathyroidism is characterized by end-organ resistance to the actions of PTH because of a receptor or postreceptor defect. Patients often have a characteristic appearance: short stature, round face, short metacarpals and metatarsals, calcification of the basal ganglia, and mild mental retardation. A defect in the Gs subunit of the receptor is commonly identified. Pseudopseudohypoparathyroidism is a variant of the disorder, and the patients have the same characteristic physical features but not the biochemical abnormalities.

* Hypoparathyroidism may result from surgical damage to the parathyroids or from an autoimmune, infiltrative, or congenital process.
* Hypomagnesemia is a cause of functional hypoparathyroidism.

Clinical Features

Hypoparathyroidism leads to decreased mobilization of calcium from bone, decreased renal distal tubular calcium reabsorption, decreased proximal renal tubular phosphate excretion, and decreased renal production of 1,25-dihydroxyvitamin D. This leads to hypocalcemia and hyperphosphatemia. In hypoparathyroidism, PTH is low or inappropriately normal in the presence of hypocalcemia. In contrast, PTH is increased in pseudohypoparathyroidism.

Symptoms reflect the degree as well as the rate of development of hypocalcemia and include paresthesias, carpopedal spasm, laryngeal stridor, and convulsions. Apathy and depression may occur. Calcification of the basal ganglia and benign intracranial hypertension also occur. Gastrointestinal tract manifestations include abdominal pain, nausea, vomiting, and malabsorption. A prolonged QT interval may be present. Hypoparathyroidism is also associated with the development of cataracts and alopecia. Mucocutaneous candidiasis may be a manifestation of DiGeorge syndrome.

* Symptoms of hypocalcemia reflect its degree and the rate of its development.
* Hypoparathyroidism is characterized by hypocalcemia and hyperphosphatemia in the presence of normal renal function.

- PTH is low in hypoparathyroidism and increased in pseudohypoparathyroidism.

Diagnosis

Differential Diagnosis

Hypoparathyroidism with resultant hypocalcemia must be differentiated from other causes of hypocalcemia. Hypocalcemia may result from decreased secretion of PTH, PTH resistance, decreased production of vitamin D, vitamin D resistance, and disorders associated with decreased mobilization of calcium from bone or increased calcium deposition in tissues. Vitamin D deficiency may be caused by malnutrition, malabsorption, or liver or kidney disease. In vitamin D deficiency, hypocalcemia triggers secondary hyperparathyroidism with renal phosphate wasting. In acute or chronic renal failure, the pathogenesis of hypocalcemia is multifactorial, resulting from hyperphosphatemia and decreased production of 1,25-dihydroxyvitamin D.

Hypocalcemia may occur in osteoblastic metastases (eg, prostate cancer) and in the hungry bone syndrome seen after parathyroidectomy for hyperparathyroidism with severe bone disease. Hypocalcemia and soft tissue calcification may occur in acute pancreatitis. Hypocalcemia is also associated with the use of loop diuretics.

Diagnostic Approach

When evaluating hypocalcemia, it is important to correct the total calcium value for the prevailing albumin levels or to determine the level of ionized calcium. The next step is to measure the serum level of PTH. In a hypocalcemic patient, a low serum level of PTH is diagnostic of hypoparathyroidism. A high serum level of PTH suggests vitamin D deficiency or pseudohypoparathyroidism. Low plasma levels of 25-hydroxyvitamin D occur from poor nutrition, malabsorption, or liver disease. Low plasma levels of 1,25-dihydroxyvitamin D occur in renal failure. The measurement of serum concentrations of creatinine and magnesium will identify renal failure and magnesium deficiency states.

Therapy

For acute, severe hypocalcemia, urgent treatment with intravenous calcium is indicated to prevent tetany, laryngeal stridor, or convulsions. Calcium gluconate, 10 to 20 mL of a 10% solution (90 mg elemental calcium per 10 mL), is infused over 5 to 10 minutes. The serum calcium level is maintained between 7.0 and 8.5 mg/dL by a subsequent infusion of calcium (10-15 mg/kg infused over 4-6 hours). Continuous electrocardiographic monitoring is essential; extravasation of calcium gluconate can cause severe tissue necrosis, so that central administration may be recommended.

For chronic hypocalcemia, treatment is oral calcium supplements (2.0-3.0 g daily). Ergocalciferol is given as 50,000 to 100,000 international units daily. It has a slow onset and offset of action. A suitable fast-acting alternative is calcitriol (1,25-dihydroxyvitamin D). Thiazide diuretics may be given to decrease the risk of marked hypercalciuria, and oral phosphate binders may be given to control hyperphosphatemia.

It is critical to monitor therapy closely because patients are at risk of hypercalciuria, nephrolithiasis, and nephrocalcinosis. Therapeutic doses are adjusted to keep the serum level of calcium just below the lower limits of normal, around 8.5 mg/dL, and the urinary level of calcium at less than 300 mg in 24 hours.

- Severe, acute hypocalcemia requires treatment with intravenous calcium.
- Chronic hypocalcemia requires treatment with oral calcium and vitamin D.

Osteoporosis

Osteoporosis is the most common skeletal disorder encountered in clinical practice. It is characterized by decreased bone mass, with thinning of the cortices and loss of trabeculae, leading to increased bone fragility and risk of fracture. Bone density (and bone loss) can be quantified with dual energy x-ray absorptiometry. Osteopenia is defined as a bone mass 1.0 to 2.5 standard deviations below the mean peak bone mass of a sex- and height-matched control population. Osteoporosis is defined as a bone mass value more than 2.5 standard deviations below the peak bone mass of a sex- and height-matched control population.

Etiology

The most common types of osteoporosis are postmenopausal osteoporosis, characterized by high turnover of bone, and senile osteoporosis, which occurs in older men and women. Osteoporosis may be secondary to hypogonadism, hyperparathyroidism, hyperthyroidism, or hypercortisolism. It is associated with malnutrition (eg, calcium deficiency, protein malnutrition, vitamin C deficiency, and alcoholism), malabsorption, neoplastic disorders (eg, multiple myeloma, leukemia, lymphoma, and systemic mastocytosis), and abnormalities of bone collagen (eg, osteogenesis imperfecta). Drugs such as corticosteroids, heparin, methotrexate, and GnRH analogues all increase bone loss. Immobilization also promotes bone loss.

- Osteoporosis may be primary or secondary.
- Osteoporosis may be secondary to endocrine, nutritional, intestinal, neoplastic, or genetic disorders. It also may be induced by drugs or immobilization.

Clinical Features

Fractures can occur with minor trauma and be axial or appendicular. Osteoporotic fractures heal normally. Vertebral fractures lead to loss of height and spinal deformity (kyphoscoliosis and dowager hump). Other osteoporotic fractures include those of the hip and distal radius (Colles fracture).

The serum levels of calcium, phosphate, and alkaline phosphatase are normal in osteoporosis. The serum level of alkaline phosphatase may be increased slightly during fracture healing.

Lateral spine radiographs show a loss of horizontal trabeculae and an apparent prominence of the vertical trabeculae, biconcave vertebrae, and a decrease in vertebral height. Bone mineral density can be assessed by dual energy x-ray absorptiometry of the lumbar vertebrae (although vessel wall calcification and vertebral deformity with advancing age can make this measurement unreliable) or the hip. A decrease of 1 standard deviation from peak bone density of a control population leads to a doubling of the fracture risk.

• Osteoporosis is characterized by the occurrence of fracture with minimal trauma and normal serum levels of calcium, phosphate, and alkaline phosphatase.

Diagnosis

The diagnosis of osteoporosis is based on the finding of low bone mass with or without fractures and the exclusion of other causes of osteopenia, such as osteomalacia, multiple myeloma, and metastatic disease. Bone densitometry should be used as a screening study for patients at risk of osteoporosis (eg, postmenopausal women not taking preventive measures). Whether routine screening for baseline values should be performed for asymptomatic postmenopausal women who receive estrogen replacement therapy is debated. Bone densitometry is indicated for patients who have radiologic evidence of previous vertebral fracture. It also is helpful in determining the need for surgery in hyperparathyroidism.

During the evaluation of a patient who has a fracture, it is important to remember that osteomalacia may coexist with osteoporosis. Myeloma or metastatic disease should be excluded as a cause of pathologic fracture. Secondary causes of osteoporosis should be actively excluded during history taking and the physical examination as well as by appropriate laboratory and radiographic investigations. The evaluation should include serum levels of calcium (and, if necessary, PTH), 25-hydroxyvitamin D, and TSH. If indicated, the patient should undergo screening for Cushing syndrome with a 1-mg overnight dexamethasone suppression test or 24-hour urinary free cortisol measurement. Measurement of testosterone is indicated for males.

• The diagnosis of osteoporosis requires the exclusion of other causes of low bone mineral density. Osteomalacia, malignancy, and other secondary causes of osteoporosis should be actively excluded by the judicious use of history taking, physical examination, and laboratory evaluation.

Prevention and Treatment of Osteoporosis

To a certain extent, bone loss can be prevented by timely estrogen replacement in women at and beyond menopause and by the provision of adequate calcium and vitamin D intake in all adults (in premenopausal women and men younger than 65 years, 1,000 mg daily of elemental calcium; in postmenopausal women and men older than 65 years, 1,500 mg daily). Other measures to ensure attainment (and maintenance) of adequate bone mass include regular weight-bearing exercise and avoidance of alcohol and tobacco abuse.

Estrogen replacement is effective for the prevention and treatment of osteoporosis in women who do not have contraindications to it. It decreases bone resorption and has been shown in epidemiologic and retrospective studies to decrease the incidence of osteoporotic fractures. Estrogen can be given orally or transdermally. Women receiving estrogen replacement therapy require a breast examination and mammography annually. To decrease the risk of endometrial hyperplasia, progesterone is also administered in a cyclical or continuous fashion if the patient has an intact uterus. Because of the increase in breast cancer risk and the adverse effect on vascular disease (at least among high-risk women), estrogen therapy has fallen out of style in recent years.

Alendronate and risedronate are oral bisphosphonates with potent antiresorptive effects; they prevent bone loss and increase bone density. They have been shown to reduce fracture risk and to be effective in preventing steroid-induced bone loss. Bisphosphonates are now regarded as first-line therapy in the treatment of osteoporosis. Side effects include dyspeptic symptoms and esophagitis, particularly if the medication is taken incorrectly. Oral bisphosphonates should be taken in the morning with a glass of water and on an empty stomach (any food or other drink may interfere with intestinal absorption), and the patient should not lie down for 30 to 60 minutes after the dose. These medications are available as a once-weekly or once-monthly dose, which increases tolerability and may improve compliance. Preliminary studies have shown that combination therapy with estrogen and alendronate may increase bone density more effectively than single-agent therapy. No decrease in fracture risk has been demonstrated.

Calcitonin is a weak antiresorptive agent and is administered by nasal spray. The advent of alternative medications with greater efficacy means that calcitonin is rarely indicated. The exception is for the management of painful vertebral fractures.

• Bisphosphonate drugs are the therapy of choice for the prevention and treatment of osteoporosis.
• Replacement of calcium and vitamin D remains central in prevention and treatment of osteoporosis.
• Nasal calcitonin is a weak antiresorptive agent.

Recombinant PTH is also now available for treatment of osteoporosis after clinical trials demonstrated the ability of this agent to increase bone formation and bone mass when given by daily subcutaneous injection. This treatment is indicated for patients who have not shown improvement with bisphosphonate therapy or who are unable to tolerate those drugs orally or intravenously. Prior radiotherapy is a contraindication to PTH therapy because of the risk of sarcoma.

Osteomalacia

In adults, osteomalacia is characterized by defective mineralization of newly formed bone matrix, with the accumulation of unmineralized osteoid. Normal mineralization of bone requires adequate calcium and phosphate concentrations in the extracellular fluid, functional osteoblasts, and optimal conditions for the mineralization of mature osteoid. Osteomalacia results when any or a combination of these prerequisites is not met.

Vitamin D deficiency is the most common cause of osteomalacia and results from poor intake (chronic alcoholism and institutionalized patients), malabsorption (celiac disease), and decreased exposure to the sun. Other causes include decreased liver production of 25-hydroxyvitamin D due to liver disease or increased metabolism to inactive compounds (phenytoin or rifampin). Renal disease and vitamin D–dependent rickets type I lead to decreased production of 1,25-dihydroxyvitamin D.

Phosphate deficiency may result from malnutrition or increased renal losses. This is seen in hereditary X-linked hypophosphatemia, acquired tubular phosphate leak due to production of a phosphaturic substance from an occult mesenchymal tumor (oncogenic osteomalacia), and a generalized tubular defect (Fanconi syndrome) that may be hereditary or acquired.

- Osteomalacia is characterized by defective mineralization and accumulation of unmineralized osteoid.
- The common causes of vitamin D deficiency are malnutrition, malabsorption, and liver disease.

Clinical Features

In addition to fractures or pseudofractures, typical symptoms of osteomalacia include diffuse bone pain and tenderness, muscle weakness, and a waddling gait. The serum level of alkaline phosphatase is usually increased in osteomalacia except in cases due to hypophosphatasia. In vitamin D deficiency, secondary hyperparathyroidism is usually present and the level of 25-hydroxyvitamin D is decreased. The serum level of calcium is low or normal.

Radiography may not be helpful, although radiographic features of secondary hyperparathyroidism may be apparent. In later stages, there may be radiographic evidence of pseudofractures (Looser zones). These are narrow lines of radiolucency that are perpendicular to the cortical bone surface and are typically bilateral and symmetrical. They are found most commonly in the pubic rami, the medial aspect of the femur near the femoral head, the scapulae, and the metatarsals.

Therapy

Effective therapy is based on identifying and treating the underlying disorder as well as providing adequate calcium and phosphate at the areas of mineralization. This usually is achieved with calcium, vitamin D, and, when indicated, phosphate supplementation. Calcium supplementation should provide 1,000 to 2,000 mg of elemental calcium daily, whereas the degree of vitamin D supplementation varies according to the underlying diagnosis. In nutritional deficiency, 2,000 to 4,000 international units daily of vitamin D_2 is given until healing occurs, and then 400 international units daily is given for maintenance. Higher doses (25,000-50,000 international units daily) are used to treat vitamin D deficiency caused by malabsorption.

The goals of therapy are to achieve bone healing and to normalize the serum concentrations of calcium, phosphate, and alkaline phosphatase. Complications of treatment include hypercalciuria, hypercalcemia, and renal impairment. Hypercalciuria is the first sign of overdosage.

- Diffuse bone pain, tenderness, and muscle weakness are typical symptoms of osteomalacia.
- Serum alkaline phosphatase is increased in all cases of osteomalacia except for cases due to hypophosphatasia.
- Vitamin D deficiency is characterized by a low or normal serum level of calcium and secondary hyperparathyroidism.
- Treatment is directed at the underlying cause and at providing adequate mineral and vitamin D supplementation.

- Complications of treatment include hypercalciuria, hypercalcemia, and renal impairment.

Paget Disease

Paget disease affects 3% of the population older than 45 years. It is a monostotic or polyostotic bone disorder characterized by the presence of abnormal osteoclasts, which lead to an increased rate of bone resorption and, subsequently, disorganized bone remodeling. This results in decreased tensile strength, skeletal pain, and bone deformities. Commonly affected sites include the sacrum, spine, femur, tibia, skull, and pelvis. Its pathogenesis is not fully understood.

Clinical Features

Most patients present with increased serum levels of alkaline phosphatase or a radiographic abnormality. The 2 main clinical features are pain and deformity. The pain may be related to pagetoid involvement, fracture, degenerative changes in adjoining joints, or, rarely, the development of osteosarcoma. Deformity may affect the long bones, skull, or spine. The serum level of alkaline phosphatase is the most useful marker of disease activity and its response to therapy.

Neurologic complications are caused by nerve entrapment or hydrocephalus due to the development of platybasia. High-output cardiac failure is rare but can occur when more than 20% of the skeleton is affected, because of the increased vascularity of affected bone. Hypercalciuria and hypercalcemia can occur in an immobilized patient.

Diagnosis

Paget disease should be suspected if serum alkaline phosphatase concentrations are increased and serum calcium, phosphate, and 25-hydroxyvitamin D levels are normal. A bone scan is the most sensitive test for identifying pagetic bone lesions. Typical radiographic findings demonstrate the characteristic bone expansion, deformity, trabecular expansion, sclerosis, and pseudofractures.

Therapy

Many patients require only monitoring of alkaline phosphatase levels. Indications for active therapy include the presence of pain, disease involving weight-bearing bones, disease in proximity to joints, neurologic complications, or marked increase in alkaline phosphatase level (>1,000 U/L). Medical therapy consists of bisphosphonates administered intravenously or orally. Alkaline phosphatase levels are used to monitor therapy. Orthopedic surgery may be needed to treat deformity, fracture, or degenerative joint disease. Pretreatment with an antiresorptive agent reduces bleeding and postoperative hypercalcemia. Neurosurgical intervention may be required for nerve entrapment syndromes.

- Typical findings in Paget disease include normal serum levels of calcium, phosphate, and 25-hydroxyvitamin D and increased serum levels of alkaline phosphatase.
- Pseudofractures are characteristic radiographic findings.
- Indications for active therapy include the presence of pain, disease involving weight-bearing bones, disease in proximity to joints, neurologic complications, or a marked increase in the alkaline phosphatase level (>1,000 U/L).

Disorders of the Adrenal Glands

Adrenal Failure

Etiology

Primary Adrenal Failure

Primary adrenal failure is manifested clinically by glucocorticoid and mineralocorticoid deficiency. It may result from autoimmune adrenalitis (Addison disease), the most common cause in the United States; destruction of the adrenals by a granulomatous process such as tuberculosis; bilateral adrenal hemorrhage related to sepsis, anticoagulation therapy or a lupus anticoagulant; congenital adrenal enzyme deficiency; or the use of drugs, such as aminoglutethimide or ketoconazole, that inhibit steroidogenesis. Adrenal metastases are common in metastatic malignancies such as lung cancer, but clinically pronounced adrenocortical failure is uncommon.

Secondary Adrenal Failure

Secondary adrenal failure is due to ACTH deficiency. Mineralocorticoid deficiency is not present. ACTH deficiency may occur alone (exogenous steroid use or lymphocytic hypophysitis) or, more often, in association with other features of hypopituitarism. Functional ACTH deficiency is the most common cause of secondary adrenal failure and is a consequence of the suppression of the hypothalamic-pituitary-adrenal axis by the prolonged use of pharmacologic doses of glucocorticoids.

* In the United States, the most common cause of primary adrenocortical failure is autoimmune adrenalitis (Addison disease).
* Primary adrenal failure: deficiencies of cortisol, adrenal sex steroids, and aldosterone.
* Secondary adrenal failure: deficiencies of cortisol and adrenal sex steroids. Aldosterone secretion is intact.

Clinical Features

Patients with adrenal failure usually have an insidious presentation, with fatigue, muscle weakness, anorexia, weight loss, nausea, vomiting, and diarrhea. Hyponatremia, lymphocytosis, and eosinophilia may be present. Aldosterone deficiency leads to hypovolemia, orthostatic hypotension, hyperkalemia, and hyperchloremic acidosis. In females, the loss of adrenal androgens leads to decreased pubic hair. Because ACTH levels are increased (lack of negative feedback by cortisol), patients with primary adrenal failure become hyperpigmented, particularly on the elbows, knees, and buccal mucosa and on surgical scars. In contrast, patients with secondary adrenal failure are pale (low ACTH levels). Because aldosterone secretion is unaffected, hyperkalemia does not occur.

Acute Adrenocortical Failure or Adrenal Crisis

Adrenal crisis usually occurs in patients with unrecognized adrenal failure who develop an intercurrent illness such as pneumonia. They experience dehydration and hypotension out of proportion to the severity of the illness. Abdominal pain in combination with nausea and vomiting may mimic an acute abdomen. Unexplained fever, hyponatremia, hyperkalemia, azotemia, hypercalcemia, and eosinophilia may all be present. Adrenal crisis may occur with inadequate cortisol replacement or it may be the first manifestation of bilateral adrenal hemorrhage.

* Addison disease develops insidiously with both glucocorticoid and mineralocorticoid deficiency.
* Adrenal crisis may develop during intercurrent illness in a patient with unrecognized adrenal failure, with inadequate cortisol replacement, or after bilateral adrenal hemorrhage.

Diagnosis

Endocrine Diagnosis

The diagnosis of adrenal failure is confirmed with the cosyntropin test, which assesses the cortisol response to synthetic ACTH (1 mcg or 250 mcg). An appropriate response to cosyntropin is an increase in plasma cortisol by more than 7 mcg/dL from the baseline value (this may not be achieved in healthy patients with a high basal level of cortisol) or to an absolute value greater than 18 mcg/dL.

A high ACTH level suggests primary adrenal insufficiency, whereas a low or "inappropriately normal" level indicates secondary failure. A normal response to cosyntropin rules out Addison disease but does not completely exclude ACTH deficiency (although the 1-mcg test is more sensitive in this regard) that is partial or of recent onset. If the diagnosis is still suspected, an insulin-hypoglycemia or metyrapone test may be performed; these test the ACTH response to hypoglycemia (insulin) or to inhibition of adrenal steroidogenesis (metyrapone).

* An abnormal cosyntropin test establishes the diagnosis of adrenal failure but cannot differentiate primary from secondary adrenal failure.
* A normal cortisol response excludes primary adrenal failure but does not completely exclude secondary adrenal failure that is partial or of recent onset.

Therapy

Primary adrenal failure requires glucocorticoid and mineralocorticoid replacement, whereas secondary adrenal failure requires only glucocorticoid replacement. Patients should be educated about the need to increase their steroid dosage during acute illness and the use of injectable glucocorticoid when oral replacement therapy is not possible. Patients should always wear a medical identification bracelet or necklace. Usually glucocorticoid replacement is with hydrocortisone or prednisone. The adequacy of therapy can be assessed only by the patient's sense of well-being and the absence of manifestations of glucocorticoid excess. Mineralocorticoid replacement is provided by fludrocortisone. Dose adjustment is guided by the presence of orthostatic hypotension, edema, hyperkalemia or hypokalemia, and, if needed, plasma renin activity.

In mild or moderate acute illness, the glucocorticoid dosage is doubled or tripled for the duration of the illness. Dexamethasone (4 mg intramuscularly) is given when the patient cannot take oral medications (nausea or vomiting). Intravenous hydrocortisone is given in stress doses before and during recovery from surgery. The management of an adrenal crisis requires intravenous rehydration, electrolyte replacement, and hydrocortisone (usually 100 mg every 6 hours). The cortisol and serum ACTH levels should be checked, but management should not be delayed while awaiting results. A search should be undertaken for a precipitating illness.

- Primary adrenal failure requires both glucocorticoid and mineralocorticoid replacement, whereas secondary failure requires only glucocorticoid replacement.
- Patient education is a critical component of effective management.
- Glucocorticoid replacement needs to be modified in acute illness.

Cushing Syndrome

Etiology

The most common cause of Cushing syndrome is the prolonged use of supraphysiologic doses of glucocorticoids. Endogenous Cushing syndrome is caused by overproduction of cortisol by the adrenal cortex (Cushing disease in 60% of cases, adrenal tumors in 25%, and ectopic ACTH-producing tumors in 15%). This may be the result of adrenal autonomy (ACTH-independent) or unregulated, excessive secretion of ACTH (ACTH-dependent). ACTH-independent disorders include autonomous adrenal adenomas, adrenal carcinoma (which also usually produces adrenal androgens), and, rarely, macronodular or micronodular adrenal hyperplasia. ACTH-dependent Cushing syndrome may be caused by a small pituitary corticotroph adenoma (Cushing disease) or ectopic secretion of ACTH. Ectopic ACTH-secreting tumors can be aggressive and malignant (eg, squamous cell carcinoma of the lung) or indolent (eg, pheochromocytoma, medullary carcinoma of the thyroid, or bronchial carcinoid). Very rarely, corticotropin-releasing hormone (CRH)-producing tumors, such as a bronchial carcinoid, cause pituitary hyperplasia and excess ACTH secretion.

- Exogenous glucocorticoid therapy is the most common cause of Cushing syndrome.
- Endogenous Cushing syndrome comprises ACTH-independent and ACTH-dependent disorders.
- The most common causes of endogenous Cushing syndrome are Cushing disease (60% of cases), adrenal tumors (25%), and ectopic ACTH-producing tumors (15%).

Clinical Features

Many of the clinical features of Cushing syndrome are nonspecific and include weight gain, diabetes mellitus, hypertension, and changes in mood and affect. Symptoms and signs that appear to be more specific for the disorder include central obesity, supraclavicular fat pads, thin skin, easy bruising, wide (>1 cm) purple striae, and proximal muscle weakness. In severe and rapidly progressive disease (usually ectopic ACTH production by a malignant tumor), the main features are weight loss, weakness, secondary diabetes, and mineralocorticoid excess (hypertension, edema, and hypokalemia). Often, there is not sufficient time for the development of the classic features of cortisol excess.

Adrenal androgen excess may produce acne, hirsutism, and menstrual irregularities. However, in adrenal carcinoma, the overproduction of androgens may be more extreme and lead to virilization. When ACTH is produced in marked quantities, as in the syndrome of ectopic ACTH, hyperpigmentation may occur.

- The clinical picture of cortisol excess varies according to the rapidity of onset and the underlying disorder.
- Central obesity, supraclavicular fat pads, thin skin, easy bruising, wide purple striae, and proximal muscle weakness are the more specific features of the disease.

Diagnosis

Confirmation of Cushing Syndrome

The diagnosis of Cushing syndrome involves a 2-step approach: biochemical confirmation of the disorder and determination of the underlying cause. The best screening test for Cushing syndrome is measurement of 24-hour urinary free cortisol excretion. An increase in urinary free cortisol suggests but does not confirm the diagnosis of Cushing syndrome (levels increased more than 3-fold the upper limit of normal in a 24-hour collection are considered diagnostic if the clinical suspicion for the disorder is high). The differential diagnosis includes pseudo-Cushing states (eg, depression, alcohol use, and acute illness). If the clinical suspicion of Cushing syndrome is high, a normal urinary free cortisol excretion does not rule out the disorder (of the 24-hour urinary cortisol collections from 10% of patients with established Cushing syndrome, 1 in 4 is normal). In this situation, it is best to repeat the test in 1 month. The 1-mg dexamethasone suppression test is best reserved for screening for subclinical Cushing syndrome in a patient with an adrenal incidentaloma (see below). The 2-day low-dose dexamethasone suppression test (0.5 mg every 6 hours for 2 days) has limited usefulness in the diagnosis of Cushing syndrome (except for cases in which the clinical suspicion for the disorder is low). False-positive results may be obtained in patients with pseudo-Cushing states or those taking estrogen-containing medications that increase cortisol-binding globulin. False-negative results may also occur, particularly in the case of ACTH-producing pituitary adenomas, some of which show unusual suppressibility to dexamethasone. Therefore, the 2-day low-dose dexamethasone suppression test has been replaced by the dexamethasone-CRH test.

- The best screening test for Cushing syndrome is measurement of the 24-hour urinary free cortisol level. A level increased more than 3-fold in 24 hours is considered diagnostic, particularly if the clinical features of the disorder are prominent.
- The 24-hour urinary free cortisol level may be intermittently normal in some patients with Cushing syndrome. If clinical suspicion is high but the 24-hour urinary free cortisol level is normal, the test should be repeated.
- The 24-hour urinary free cortisol level may be increased in pseudo-Cushing states, including psychiatric disorders and acute illness. In these conditions, false-positive results may be obtained on a low-dose dexamethasone suppression test.

- The 2-day low-dose dexamethasone suppression test has limited usefulness in the diagnosis of Cushing syndrome and has been largely replaced by the dexamethasone-CRH test.

Cause of Cushing Syndrome

After the diagnosis of Cushing syndrome has been confirmed biochemically, the next step is to determine whether the disease is ACTH-dependent or ACTH-independent. A suppressed ACTH (<5 pg/mL) implies adrenal autonomy, and computed tomography (CT) of the abdomen should be performed. A normal (10-80 pg/mL) or modestly increased (<200 pg/mL) concentration is observed in an ACTH-dependent process. Extreme increases in ACTH (>200 pg/mL) suggest—but do not confirm—ectopic ACTH secretion.

The differentiation of pituitary-dependent disease from ectopic ACTH production can be one of the most difficult evaluations in endocrinology. Most causes of ACTH-dependent disease are due to pituitary disease; thus, if the clinical features are consistent with pituitary disease (eg, middle-aged woman, slow onset, progression of disease), magnetic resonance imaging (MRI) of the pituitary gland should be considered. A pituitary lesion larger than 4 mm is suggestive of an ACTH-producing pituitary tumor, and the patient may proceed directly to transsphenoidal exploration. The absence of a pituitary lesion on MRI does not rule out Cushing disease because 50% of the tumors are not visible on MRI. If no abnormality is found on imaging of the sella, sampling of the inferior petrosal sinuses (together with CRH provocative testing) should be performed. Documentation of a central-to-peripheral ACTH concentration gradient confirms that the source of excess ACTH is from a pituitary tumor. The 2-day high-dose dexamethasone suppression test was used to distinguish between pituitary-dependent disease and ectopic ACTH secretion. However, this test is considered obsolete when traditional criteria are used for interpretation because one-third of bronchial carcinoid tumors respond like pituitary adenomas. Also, the clinical presentation of bronchial carcinoids may be indistinguishable from that of pituitary-dependent disease.

- After biochemical confirmation of Cushing syndrome, the next step is to measure ACTH levels.
- If the ACTH level is <5 pg/mL, proceed to CT of the adrenal glands.
- If the ACTH level is >10 pg/mL, distinguish between a pituitary-dependent tumor and ectopic ACTH production.
- Clinically, bronchial carcinoid tumors may be indistinguishable from pituitary disease.
- Inferior petrosal sinus sampling should be performed to distinguish between pituitary disease and ectopic disease.
- The 2-day high-dose dexamethasone suppression test is considered obsolete in the differential diagnosis of ACTH-dependent Cushing syndrome.

Therapy

Removal of the source of ACTH secretion is the treatment of choice in ACTH-dependent Cushing syndrome. However, this is not always possible; transsphenoidal surgery has about a 30% failure rate, and an ectopic source of ACTH may not be resectable or even detectable. In these cases, bilateral adrenalectomy is the treatment of choice.

In ACTH-independent Cushing syndrome, resection of the adrenal adenoma or carcinoma is indicated. In adrenal carcinoma, complete resection may not be possible and adjuvant treatment with inhibitors of steroidogenesis, such as ketoconazole, may be indicated.

In all cases, surgical excision of the causative tumor is followed by a period of cortisol deficiency because of suppression of the hypothalamic-pituitary-adrenal axis. This may take 1 year to recover, and glucocorticoid replacement is required during this time. Lifelong replacement of glucocorticoid and mineralocorticoid is necessary after bilateral adrenalectomy.

- A period of suppression of the normal axis occurs after removal of the causative tumor and may last up to 1 year.

Primary Aldosteronism

Etiology

Primary aldosteronism results from autonomous (renin-independent) aldosterone production by the zona glomerulosa. It may be due to an aldosteronoma, idiopathic bilateral hyperplasia, adrenocortical carcinoma, or, rarely, familial glucocorticoid-remediable aldosteronism.

Clinical Features

Most patients present with hypertension and hypokalemia. The hypertension can be of variable severity. The hypokalemia is often mild and may be absent (30% of patients are normokalemic). However, it may be exacerbated by diuretic therapy. Most patients are asymptomatic, but a few experience myopathic symptoms and paresthesias due to hypokalemia and alkalosis. Edema is usually absent.

Diagnosis

The diagnosis of primary aldosteronism requires documentation of autonomous aldosterone secretion and, subsequently, definition of the underlying cause. Although hypokalemia is often present in primary aldosteronism, it is a nonspecific finding and may not occur in patients treated with angiotensin-converting enzyme inhibitors or potassium-sparing diuretics such as spironolactone. A urinary potassium concentration greater than 30 mEq/L in a patient with hypokalemia suggests renal wasting of potassium and increases suspicion for mineralocorticoid excess.

The measurement of the ratio of plasma aldosterone (PA in ng/dL) to plasma renin activity (PRA in ng/mL per hour) is used to screen for primary aldosteronism. It is important to measure PA after correction of hypokalemia because the latter decreases aldosterone secretion. Increased PA and suppressed PRA, with a PA:PRA ratio greater than 20, is suggestive of primary aldosteronism. The diagnosis is confirmed by the demonstration of a nonsuppressed 24-hour urinary aldosterone in the salt-replete state (instruct patients to add salt to their food during the collection).

Hypertension caused by excess of a mineralocorticoid other than aldosterone is seen in deoxycorticosterone-producing tumors, congenital adrenal hyperplasia due to 11- or 17-hydroxylase deficiency, Cushing syndrome, and genetic or acquired (use of licorice or chewing tobacco) deficiency of 11β-hydroxysteroid dehydrogenase. This enzyme is present in the distal renal tubule and catalyzes the inactivation of cortisol. Inactivation of this enzyme potentiates the mineralocorticoid effect of cortisol.

- It is estimated that 30% of patients with primary aldosteronism have normokalemia.
- If hypokalemia occurs with the use of diuretics, suspect primary aldosteronism.
- Urinary potassium concentration >30 mEq/L in a patient with hypokalemia suggests renal wasting of potassium and increases suspicion for primary aldosteronism.
- A PA:PRA ratio >20 suggests primary aldosteronism.

The major challenge is to distinguish between an aldosterone-secreting adenoma and bilateral adrenal hyperplasia. This is important because an aldosterone-secreting adenoma can be treated surgically. However, bilateral hyperplasia can be treated only medically. CT of the adrenals may be misleading if the functional tumor is small and not visualized. Furthermore, a visible adrenal mass may be an incidental finding or the mass may be a hyperplastic nodule superimposed on a background of bilateral adrenal hyperplasia. Selective adrenal venous sampling is the most useful localizing procedure; a unilateral aldosterone gradient helps direct surgical excision.

- An adrenal mass seen on CT may not be an aldosteronoma.
- The most reliable localizing test is selective adrenal venous sampling.

Therapy
Unilateral adrenalectomy is indicated for aldosteronoma unless the patient is a poor surgical risk. Surgical resection corrects the hypokalemia (100%) and normalizes or markedly improves the hypertension in about 70% of patients. Persistent postoperative hypertension should be treated with standard antihypertensive therapy.

Medical treatment is indicated for the management of bilateral adrenal hyperplasia and for patients with aldosteronoma who are not candidates for surgery. Spironolactone, an aldosterone antagonist, restores potassium concentrations and normalizes blood pressure in most patients. Adverse effects include gastrointestinal tract upset, menstrual irregularity, and, in men, gynecomastia, decreased libido, and impotence. Women of childbearing age who take spironolactone should use effective contraception because the drug may cause feminization of the male fetus through its androgen-blocking effects.

Pheochromocytoma

Etiology
Pheochromocytomas arise in chromaffin cells of neural crest origin in the adrenal medulla or, less frequently, along the sympathetic chain and rarely in sympathetic tissue in the walls of the urinary bladder. Of these tumors, 10% are malignant, 10% are extra-adrenal, and 10% are familial. Familial pheochromocytomas are more likely to be intra-adrenal, bilateral, and malignant. Pheochromocytomas can secrete catecholamines continuously or episodically.

Clinical Features
Pheochromocytomas may present as an incidental finding on abdominal imaging performed for other reasons. More commonly, they are suspected because of the presence of hypertension that is paroxysmal, refractory to treatment, or associated with paroxysmal symptoms of headache, palpitations, sweating, anxiety, and pallor. Some patients present with hypermetabolism that is manifested as heat intolerance, sweating, and weight loss. The tumor may be part of MEN-2A or MEN-2B, von Hippel-Lindau disease, or neurofibromatosis. In most patients, the paroxysmal symptoms are stereotyped and vary only in severity or frequency.

- Pheochromocytomas can be asymptomatic and discovered incidentally.
- Common symptoms include headache, palpitations, and sweating. The symptoms may be paroxysmal.
- Some patients may have a family history of pheochromocytoma. The tumor may be a manifestation of MEN-2A or MEN-2B.

Diagnosis
The diagnosis of pheochromocytoma requires documentation of increased urinary excretion of free catecholamines and metanephrines. Catecholamine-containing drugs, α-methyldopa, labetalol, and monoamine oxidase inhibitors cause falsely elevated concentrations. Severe stress, intercurrent illness, acute myocardial ischemia, drug and food interaction with monoamine oxidase inhibitors, abrupt withdrawal of clonidine, or excessive use of sympathomimetic amines also causes increased excretion of urinary catecholamines. Normal values in a hypertensive or otherwise symptomatic patient are sufficient to exclude the diagnosis. In patients with paroxysmal symptoms, the diagnostic yield is increased by collecting urine during or shortly after a paroxysm.

For screening purposes, 24-hour urinary metanephrines are preferred over plasma metanephrine levels because the latter is a less specific test. Plasma catecholamines have limited usefulness in the diagnosis of pheochromocytoma.

- Normal urinary catecholamine values in a hypertensive patient exclude the diagnosis. In patients with paroxysmal symptoms, the diagnostic yield is increased substantially by initiating collection during or shortly after a paroxysm.
- Increased values in hypertensive patients establish the diagnosis only if other disorders associated with hypertension and catecholamine excess are excluded (eg, severe stress, intercurrent illness, acute myocardial ischemia, certain medications, or abrupt withdrawal of clonidine).

CT or MRI of the abdomen (and, if indicated, the pelvis, thorax, and neck) is used to localize a pheochromocytoma. On MRI, pheochromocytomas have a high-intensity signal on T2-weighted images. 123I-metaiodobenzylguanidine (123I-MIBG) is taken up by pheochromocytomas and is used as an adjunct to CT or MRI if metastatic disease is suspected.

- Radiographic localization of the pheochromocytoma is attempted only if the biochemical diagnosis is firm.
- Pheochromocytomas appear as a high-intensity signal on T2-weighted MRI.
- ^{123}I-MIBG is used as an adjunct to CT or MRI if metastatic disease is suspected.

Therapy

Complete excision of a pheochromocytoma is curative. Medical treatment is used preoperatively to diminish perioperative morbidity and mortality. Ongoing treatment is required if resection is incomplete and if recurrent or metastatic disease is present. α-Adrenergic blockade should be instituted with phenoxybenzamine, starting with 10 mg twice daily. β-Adrenergic blockers may be necessary to control reflex tachycardia after maximal α-blockade has been achieved. If cure is achieved, urinary catecholamine concentrations return to normal within 2 weeks. Long-term follow-up is important to assess for persistent or recurrent disease.

- Surgical excision of the tumor is curative.
- α-Adrenergic blockade should be initiated when the diagnosis is made.
- β-Blockade may be necessary to control reflex tachycardia after effective α-blockade.

Adrenal Incidentaloma

Etiology

Small (1-6 cm) adrenal masses are found in about 10% of autopsies and increasingly are being detected on abdominal CT performed for other reasons. Although most of them are nonfunctioning adenomas, a few are functioning adenomas or carcinomas of the adrenal gland. Metastatic disease to the adrenals may also present in this way.

Evaluation

Evaluation should address the following 2 questions:
1. Is the lesion benign or malignant?
2. Is the lesion hyperfunctioning?

The size of the adrenal mass can help to distinguish between a benign tumor and a malignant tumor. Most adenomas are smaller than 4 cm in diameter. The incidence of carcinoma exceeds 35% in masses larger than 6 cm. Needle biopsy cannot distinguish between a benign and a malignant adrenal neoplasm and should not be attempted if pheochromocytoma is suspected. Needle biopsy is useful to confirm a suspicion of disease metastatic to the adrenals.

For all patients, screen for pheochromocytoma (24-hour urinary metanephrines) and subclinical Cushing syndrome (1-mg overnight dexamethasone suppression test). It is important to determine the functional status of the adrenal mass before surgical management. An unsuspected pheochromocytoma may provoke a hypertensive crisis. Similarly, removal of the cortisol-producing tumor may be followed by an adrenal crisis. Such patients need perioperative and postoperative cortisol replacement until the ACTH-adrenal axis recovers, and this may take up to 1 year. Also, screen for primary aldosteronism (PA:PRA ratio) if the patient has hypertension. An

androgen-producing or a feminizing adrenal tumor needs to be considered only when clinical findings suggest overproduction of sex steroids.

Therapy

A functioning tumor should be excised. Patients with nonfunctioning tumors smaller than 4 cm should have CT repeated in 3 months to assess for growth. If the size is stable after 3 months, additional scans are performed 1 year after the diagnosis. An adrenal mass larger than 4 cm in diameter or a mass that is increasing in size on serial observation should be excised.

- Laboratory investigation of an adrenal incidentaloma should include measurement of 24-hour urinary catecholamines, a 1-mg overnight dexamethasone suppression test, and, if the patient is hypertensive, determination of the PA:PRA ratio.
- Pheochromocytoma or subclinical cortisol production should be excluded before surgical excision.
- Needle biopsy of an adrenal incidentaloma is not indicated unless metastatic disease is suspected (first, rule out pheochromocytoma).
- Excision is indicated for a functioning tumor, a mass >4 cm, and a mass that is increasing in size on serial observation.

The Testis

Male Hypogonadism

Etiology

Decreased testosterone production may be a result of testicular failure (hypergonadotropic hypogonadism or primary hypogonadism) or LH deficiency due to a hypothalamic or pituitary disorder (hypogonadotropic hypogonadism or secondary hypogonadism). Hypergonadotropic hypogonadism may result from Klinefelter syndrome, testicular trauma, radiotherapy or chemotherapy, autoimmune or infectious (mumps) disorders, or orchitis and degenerative disorders such as dystrophia myotonica. Hypogonadotropic hypogonadism may be due to a functional hypothalamic disorder (eg, constitutional delay in puberty, use of neuroleptic drugs, nutritional disorders, severe systemic illness, moderate to severe sleep apnea, major depression, hyperprolactinemia, or thyroid or adrenal disorders). Organic disorders of the hypothalamus and pituitary can also lead to hypogonadism (eg, a pituitary tumor).

Androgen resistance may be genetic or acquired. Genetic androgen resistance includes testicular feminization and 5α-reductase deficiency. Acquired androgen resistance may occur with the use of the androgen receptor blockers spironolactone or flutamide.

- Decreased testosterone production may result from primary testicular failure or from a central hypothalamic or pituitary disorder.
- Central hypogonadotropism may result from functional or organic hypothalamic disorders or from organic diseases of the anterior pituitary gland.

Clinical Features

Adult males with hypogonadism present with decreased libido and potency, decreased ejaculate volume, infertility, decreased stamina, decreased sexual hair growth, and gynecomastia. Hot flashes may occur if testosterone deficiency is rapid in onset. In men with chronic and severe testosterone deficiency, physical findings may include pallor, a female pattern of fat distribution, testicular atrophy, and gynecomastia.

Adolescents with hypogonadism present with delayed puberty and growth. Sexual infantilism is associated with the absence of a pubertal growth spurt, eunuchoid habitus (ratio of arm span to height is >1), high-pitched voice, poor muscle development, and a female pattern of fat distribution. The testes usually are small and soft. Small, firm testes in a hypogonadal male suggest Klinefelter syndrome, and the presence of midline defects or anosmia in an adolescent with sexual infantilism suggests Kallmann syndrome.

Diagnosis

The diagnosis is confirmed by documenting low serum levels of testosterone. Measurement of LH and FSH helps to differentiate primary from secondary hypogonadism. Gonadotropin concentrations are increased in primary testicular failure, but they are decreased or inappropriately normal in secondary hypogonadism. Additional tests that may be indicated include karyotyping to confirm Klinefelter syndrome. Secondary hypogonadism requires exclusion of Kallmann syndrome, measurement of the serum concentration of prolactin, pituitary function testing, and MRI of the head to exclude organic hypothalamic-pituitary disease.

* Serum levels of LH and FSH help to differentiate primary from secondary hypogonadism.
* Hypogonadotropic hypogonadism mandates assessment of pituitary function and MRI of the head. Evaluate for the presence of midline defects or anosmia in adults (Kallmann syndrome).

Therapy

Androgen Therapy

In adults, androgen therapy is aimed at the restoration and maintenance of secondary sex characteristics. Testosterone replacement cannot stimulate spermatogenesis. In secondary hypogonadism, gonadotropins can be used to induce spermatogenesis and to restore fertility.

Androgens can be replaced by 17-hydroxyl esters of testosterone (eg, testosterone enanthate) administered intramuscularly every 2 weeks. However, this mode of delivery produces a supraphysiologic level of testosterone shortly after the injection, and the level gradually decreases to a low level before the next injection. A more physiologic mode of delivery is transdermal testosterone by means of a patch or gel applied to the skin. Also, 17α-alkylated derivatives of testosterone can be administered orally; however, they are associated with substantial hepatotoxicity and should not be used.

Testosterone replacement therapy is contraindicated in the presence of prostate cancer (the prostate-specific antigen [PSA] level should be checked before treatment is initiated) or psychosis, and it may worsen the symptoms of prostatism. Side effects include acne, edema, erythrocytosis, and exacerbation of obstructive sleep apnea. Patients receiving testosterone replacement therapy should have a prostate examination and a PSA test annually.

* In adults, androgen therapy restores and maintains secondary sex characteristics.
* An annual prostate examination and serum PSA level are recommended for patients receiving testosterone replacement therapy.

Selected Disorders of Male Hypogonadism

Klinefelter Syndrome

Klinefelter syndrome is common (1:400-1:500) and arises because of the presence of 1 or more extra X chromosomes. The classic karyotype is 47,XXY. The disorder is characterized by hyalinization of the seminiferous tubules and dysfunction of the Leydig cells, which is manifested at puberty. The testes are small and firm, gynecomastia is present, FSH levels are increased, and testosterone levels are decreased. If more than 1 X chromosome is present, the incidence of mental retardation and somatic abnormalities is increased. In mosaicism, the clinical manifestations are less severe and if an XY line is present, fertility may be possible.

Patients with Klinefelter syndrome have a slightly increased incidence of diabetes mellitus, chronic obstructive pulmonary disease, autoimmune disorders, varicose veins, malignancy of the breast, lymphoma, and germ cell neoplasm. Therapy includes testosterone replacement. Breast reduction surgery is indicated if the patient's gynecomastia is a source of emotional distress.

* Klinefelter syndrome is due to 1 or more extra X chromosomes; the classic karyotype is 47,XXY.
* Characteristic findings include small, firm testes, gynecomastia, increased FSH levels, and various degrees of testosterone deficiency.

Kallmann Syndrome

This syndrome is characterized by secondary hypogonadism and anosmia. It is a congenital disorder, often familial, that is due to defective migration of GnRH-producing neurons during embryogenesis. Patients present with delayed puberty. Anosmia is present in 80% of patients. Other midline defects such as a cleft lip or palate, color blindness, cryptorchidism, and skeletal abnormalities may occur. Laboratory evaluation shows isolated hypogonadotropic hypogonadism. On MRI, the olfactory bulbs may be abnormal or absent, but the hypothalamic-pituitary region is normal. Therapy for Kallmann syndrome consists of testosterone replacement to allow for the development of secondary sex characteristics. The administration of gonadotropin is required for fertility.

* Kallmann syndrome is characterized by hypogonadotropic hypogonadism and anosmia.

Gynecomastia

Etiology

Gynecomastia, the most common disorder of the male breast, is caused by some degree of estradiol excess that can be 1) a relative estrogen excess due to decreased testosterone production or the use of an androgen receptor blocker (spironolactone, cimetidine, or flutamide) or 2) an absolute increase in estradiol production because of adrenal cancer, a Leydig cell tumor, or a human chorionic gonadotropin (HCG)-producing tumor. Androgen-secreting tumors or exogenous androgen use can produce gynecomastia through the peripheral conversion of testosterone to estrogen.

In young, healthy, pubertal males, gynecomastia is physiologic and tends to be transient. The use of anabolic steroids or Klinefelter syndrome may account for a small number of cases. All other causes are rare in this age group. In adults, the 2 common causes are drugs and alcohol-related liver disease. Ectopic HCG-producing tumors, feminizing adrenal and testicular tumors, and pituitary tumors are rare causes of gynecomastia. In about 10% of cases, the cause of gynecomastia is indeterminate.

- The basic mechanism underlying the development of gynecomastia is an increase in the estrogen to androgen ratio.
- In adults, the 2 most common causes of gynecomastia are drugs and alcoholic liver disease.
- In about 10% of cases, the cause of gynecomastia is indeterminate.

Clinical Features
Patients usually present with breast enlargement or tenderness (or both) that may be unilateral or bilateral. Rarely, a patient may complain of galactorrhea. Gynecomastia is firm, with a fine nodularity, and spreads radially with a well-defined outer border.

Diagnosis
The differential diagnosis includes pseudogynecomastia (bilateral fatty enlargement) and malignancy (if unilateral gynecomastia). A history of alcohol consumption and medications should be part of the initial evaluation. Endocrine tests should include measurement of testosterone, estradiol, LH and FSH, β-HCG, TSH, and prolactin levels. If indicated, karyotyping should be performed.

An increase in β-HCG implies the presence of an HCG-secreting tumor. A high level of estradiol should prompt evaluation for feminizing adrenal or testicular tumors. If LH, FSH, and sex steroid concentrations are normal, an underlying endocrine disorder is unlikely.

- If the gynecomastia is bilateral, consider pseudogynecomastia. If unilateral, consider malignancy.
- Evaluation includes measurement of testosterone, LH, FSH, β-HCG, TSH, estradiol, and prolactin levels.

The Ovary

Amenorrhea
Primary amenorrhea is present when menarche has not occurred by age 16 years in a young female who has normal secondary sex characteristics or by age 14 in the absence of secondary sex characteristics. Secondary amenorrhea is present when a woman with previously established menstrual function does not menstruate for a period longer than 3 of her previous cycle intervals or for 6 months.

Etiology
Amenorrhea may be physiologic, as in pregnancy or after menopause. Pathologic amenorrhea may result from a hypothalamic disorder that leads to the loss of cyclical GnRH production, a pituitary disorder resulting in hypogonadotropic hypogonadism, an ovarian disorder, or a uterine disorder or genital tract disorder that prevents the egress of shed endometrium. The common causes of primary amenorrhea are gonadal dysgenesis (45% of cases), constitutional delay of puberty (20%), and müllerian agenesis (15%). The common causes of secondary amenorrhea are hypothalamic dysfunction (40% of cases), polycystic ovarian syndrome (30%), pituitary disease (20%), and ovarian failure (10%).

- Amenorrhea can result from impaired function of any component of the hypothalamic-pituitary-gonadal axis or from an anatomical abnormality of the genital tract.
- The common causes of amenorrhea are physiologic, for example, pregnancy.

Primary Amenorrhea
Developmental anomalies in patients who present with primary amenorrhea include imperforate hymen, isolated absence of the uterus, and vaginal atresia. However, ovarian disorders account for most of the causes of primary amenorrhea. Functional suppression of the hypothalamic GnRH cell population by a nutritional or psychiatric disorder, prolonged heavy exercise, systemic illness, hyperprolactinemia, or thyroid or adrenal disorders also cause amenorrhea. Organic hypothalamic-pituitary disease is an uncommon cause of primary amenorrhea; in young adults, craniopharyngioma is more common than prolactinoma.

- Outflow tract disorders are uncommon causes of primary amenorrhea.
- Ovarian disorders are the most common cause of primary amenorrhea.
- Hypothalamic-pituitary disease may be functional or organic.

Secondary Amenorrhea
Patients who have polycystic ovary syndrome, autoimmune oophoritis, abdominal radiotherapy, chemotherapy with cyclophosphamide or vincristine, or ovarian tumors that secrete excessive androgen can present with secondary amenorrhea.

Functional hypogonadotropism may be triggered by situational stress, weight loss, or systemic illness (eg, hyperthyroidism). In organic hypothalamic-pituitary disorders, secondary hypogonadism occurs alone or in association with other pituitary function abnormalities. The incidence of postpartum pituitary necrosis (Sheehan syndrome), previously a common cause, has decreased with improved obstetric care.

Acquired outflow tract abnormalities are rare causes of secondary amenorrhea. Such disorders may be the result of postpartum endometritis or destruction of the basal layer of the endometrium by overzealous dilatation and curettage, with subsequent obliteration of the endometrial cavity (Asherman syndrome).

- Functional or organic hypothalamic-pituitary disorders are the common causes of secondary amenorrhea.
- Ovarian causes of secondary amenorrhea include polycystic ovary syndrome and autoimmune oophoritis.

- Acquired outflow tract abnormalities are uncommon causes of secondary amenorrhea.
- Patients with hyperthyroidism may present with amenorrhea.

Clinical Features

In addition to amenorrhea, patients may experience symptoms of estrogen deficiency. These include vaginal dryness, hot flashes, and loss of secondary sex characteristics. Other findings are those related to the etiologic disorder, such as galactorrhea, hirsutism, shortness of stature, or features of Turner syndrome.

Diagnosis

Secondary Amenorrhea

The first step in the work-up of amenorrhea is to exclude pregnancy (measure HCG level) regardless of the patient's history of sexual activity or contraceptive use. The serum levels of prolactin and TSH should be measured to exclude hyperprolactinemia and thyroid dysfunction, respectively. Serum levels of estradiol, LH, and particularly FSH help to differentiate ovarian from hypothalamic-pituitary disorders. An increase in FSH in a patient with low estradiol levels confirms primary ovarian failure. If ovarian failure has no readily apparent cause, autoimmune oophoritis should be considered and appropriate tests to exclude other autoimmune endocrine disorders are indicated. A low estradiol level and inappropriately low levels of FSH and LH indicate a hypothalamic-pituitary disorder, and pituitary function testing and appropriate imaging should be performed. Hirsutism and acne suggest hyperandrogenism and should be investigated by measuring the serum concentration of testosterone and dehydroepiandrosterone sulfate (DHEAS).

- The evaluation of secondary amenorrhea should include measurement of HCG, prolactin, TSH, estradiol, FSH, LH, and, if indicated, testosterone and DHEAS.
- Low estradiol and increased FSH levels indicate primary ovarian failure.
- Low estradiol and inappropriately low FSH and LH levels indicate a hypothalamic-pituitary disorder: rule out functional and organic disease.

Primary Amenorrhea

If the appearance is that of an adult female and there is no evidence of pregnancy (check a pregnancy test in all cases), consider outflow tract obstruction or androgen insensitivity (eg, testicular feminization). A pelvic assessment is an important part of the evaluation. Normal findings on pelvic examination should prompt an evaluation similar to that for secondary amenorrhea. The absence of a uterus should prompt measurement of testosterone; a normal female testosterone concentration supports the diagnosis of müllerian agenesis, whereas a high serum level of testosterone suggests androgen insensitivity.

If sexual infantilism is present, gonadotropins should be measured. An increase in FSH suggests primary gonadal failure and dictates karyotyping. Normal or low FSH levels suggest hypogonadotropic hypogonadism or delayed puberty.

- Adult female sex characteristics and a negative pregnancy test should lead to a consideration of genital tract anomalies or androgen insensitivity.
- The presence of sexual infantilism suggests a disorder of the hypothalamic-pituitary-gonadal axis or delayed puberty.

Therapy

Management is directed at the underlying disorder and restoration of normal gonadal function. However, if successful treatment of the underlying disorder is not possible, estrogen replacement therapy and, when feasible, restoration of fertility are indicated.

Estrogen Replacement Therapy

Estrogen replacement therapy is undertaken to help control hot flashes, prevent atrophic vaginitis, promote secondary sex characteristics, and prevent osteoporosis. Estrogen therapy is contraindicated if the patient has an estrogen-dependent neoplasm, cholestatic liver disease, or a history of venous thrombosis. Progesterone replacement therapy is indicated only for women with an intact uterus. Estrogen and progesterone replacement therapy can be administered sequentially or in combination. Sequential therapy usually results in predictable cyclic withdrawal bleeding. The goal of combination therapy is to induce endometrial atrophy and amenorrhea and may be preferred by patients who find cyclic withdrawal bleeding inconvenient.

Estrogen replacement therapy increases the risk of endometrial cancer (although this is prevented by progesterone), and it is associated with an increase in the risk of breast cancer.

Ovulation Induction

Hypogonadal women who desire fertility can be given clomiphene citrate, exogenous gonadotropin, or GnRH therapy. The treatment of choice for hyperprolactinemia is bromocriptine or cabergoline.

Selected Disorders Associated With Amenorrhea

Turner 45/XO Gonadal Dysgenesis

Turner syndrome is the most common cause of primary amenorrhea and affects 1 in 3,000 newborn females. It is characterized by a missing X chromosome, which leads to the development of streak gonads, primary ovarian failure, and sexual infantilism. Physical abnormalities associated with Turner syndrome include a webbed neck, low-set ears, micrognathia, a shield-like chest, short metacarpals and metatarsals, an increased carrying angle at the elbows, renal developmental abnormalities, and cardiovascular anomalies (including coarctation and aortic stenosis). Mosaics tend to have less severe manifestations of the syndrome, and the degree of ovarian dysgenesis varies depending on the ratio of XO to XX germ cells.

Anorexia Nervosa

This syndrome occurs most often in females younger than 25 years, although cases in males are increasingly reported. It is characterized by a distorted perception of weight and body image that leads to poor nutrition. Patients deny the nature of the problem, arguably because they do not perceive it. Amenorrhea occurs in most females with anorexia nervosa and often precedes the weight loss. Other features of the disorder include bradycardia, hypotension, constipation, growth of lanugo hair, and, in severe cases, dependent edema. Endocrine findings include secondary hypogonadism, low IGF-1 levels, increased reverse T_3 levels, and increased serum cortisol concentrations that are suppressed in response to exogenous dexamethasone.

Androgens in Healthy Females

Circulating androgens in adult females originate from the ovaries and adrenal cortex. Testosterone is synthesized by the ovaries and adrenals and from conversion of androstenedione in the peripheral tissues. Dehydroepiandrosterone (DHEA) is produced mainly by the adrenals and, to a lesser extent, the ovaries. DHEAS is derived almost exclusively from the adrenal cortex. Ovarian androgens are synthesized by thecal cells in an LH-dependent fashion. Adrenal androgens are synthesized in the zona fasciculata and zona reticularis in an ACTH-dependent manner. These androgens are metabolized to testosterone or dihydrotestosterone at their target tissues. In females, androgens mediate increased hair growth and maintain libido and muscle mass.

- Testosterone originates from the ovaries and adrenals, but DHEAS is produced almost exclusively by the adrenal cortex.
- Ovarian androgen production is LH-dependent. Adrenal androgen production is ACTH-dependent.

Hirsutism and Virilization

Hirsutism refers to excessive androgen-induced hair growth in the androgen-sensitive areas of the female body. *Virilization* refers to the masculinization of secondary sex characteristics and the sex organs and is the result of pronounced androgen stimulation. Although virilization always is associated with hirsutism, hirsutism frequently occurs without virilization.

Etiology

Androgen excess may result from increased production of androgens by the ovaries or adrenal cortex (or both). Ovarian (LH-dependent) disorders include polycystic ovarian syndrome. Adrenocortical (ACTH-dependent) disorders include congenital adrenal hyperplasia and ACTH-dependent Cushing disease. Hirsutism also can occur because of increased sensitivity of the hair follicles to androgen. Hirsutism and virilization may be the consequence of exposure to exogenous androgens, anabolic steroids, or some progestational agents derived from testosterone.

Clinical Features

The clinical features depend on the severity of the hyperandrogenism. Manifestations include acne, hirsutism of androgen-sensitive areas (including the upper lip, chin, chest, and lower abdomen), menstrual abnormalities, and masculinization (temporal hair recession, deepening voice, increased muscle mass, and clitorimegaly).

Diagnosis

A benign cause is suggested by onset at puberty with an indolent, slowly progressive course. In contrast, rapid onset with a severe, progressive course suggests a malignant disorder.

A positive family history is often elicited in facial hirsutism, polycystic ovarian syndrome, and late-onset congenital adrenal hyperplasia. Generally, a young woman who has mild hirsutism of pubertal onset and normal menstrual function and who does not have any major disorder does not need to undergo detailed endocrine testing. Hirsutism of pubertal onset associated with menstrual irregularity but no virilization may be due to polycystic ovaries or late-onset congenital adrenal hyperplasia.

Diagnostic testing should include measurement of serum levels of testosterone, DHEAS, and prolactin as well as screening for Cushing syndrome (overnight 1-mg dexamethasone suppression test or 24-hour urinary free cortisol). If a neoplastic disorder is suspected (serum testosterone >200 ng/dL or plasma DHEAS >7 ng/dL), pelvic ultrasonography and abdominal CT are indicated. In selected patients, determination of the serum level of 17-hydroxyprogesterone, with or without ACTH stimulation, may be necessary to confirm congenital adrenal hyperplasia.

- The most important diagnostic clues are the time of onset, tempo of progression, and severity of hyperandrogenic state.
- DHEAS >7 ng/dL suggests an adrenal tumor.
- Serum testosterone >200 ng/dL suggests an ovarian neoplasm. Serum testosterone <200 ng/dL suggests polycystic ovarian syndrome (see "Polycystic Ovarian Syndrome" section).

Selected Hyperandrogenic States

Idiopathic Hirsutism

Idiopathic hirsutism is usually due to a modest increase in ovarian androgen production, with increased peripheral androgen production and increased sensitivity of hair follicles to androgens. The hyperandrogenicity is usually mild and LH-dependent. Onset occurs at puberty and progresses slowly. Menstrual cycles are regular and findings on pelvic examination are unremarkable. The serum levels of testosterone and DHEAS are normal.

Polycystic Ovarian Syndrome

Polycystic ovarian syndrome is the most common cause of hyperandrogenism. The diagnosis is made when the following criteria are present: 1) oligomenorrhea or amenorrhea, 2) clinical or biochemical hyperandrogenism, and 3) exclusion of other causes of hyperandrogenism (eg, Cushing syndrome or congenital adrenal hyperplasia). The onset of the disorder is at puberty, and progression is slow. Most patients experience some degree of infertility. The serum levels of testosterone are usually at the upper limits of normal or modestly increased (usually <200 ng/dL). DHEAS levels are normal or mildly increased in 25% of patients. Serum levels of estradiol are normal. Gonadotropin secretion is abnormal, and approximately 60% of patients have an increased LH:FSH ratio. In most patients, the ovaries have a characteristic appearance on ultrasonography, with multiple peripherally located cysts. This radiologic finding, however, is not specific for polycystic ovarian syndrome; it is seen also in women with other causes of hyperandrogenism and in nonhirsute women with normal menses.

Polycystic ovarian syndrome is also considered a metabolic disorder: most patients are obese and have insulin resistance. Patients are at increased risk of glucose intolerance or type 2 diabetes mellitus. Treatment with metformin may be considered for patients with established glucose intolerance. This agent and insulin-sensitizing agents are increasingly being used for treatment of hirsutism in women with polycystic ovarian syndrome who have normal glucose levels. Studies have shown that these agents may restore ovulation; thus, the patient should be counseled about contraception.

* Hirsutism, menstrual abnormality, infertility, and anovulation characterize polycystic ovarian syndrome.
* Serum concentrations of testosterone are normal or modestly increased but usually <200 ng/dL.
* Ultrasonographic findings of polycystic-appearing ovaries are not sufficient to make the diagnosis.
* Patients are usually obese, have insulin resistance, and are at increased risk of glucose intolerance or type 2 diabetes mellitus.

Late-Onset Congenital Adrenal Hyperplasia

Congenital adrenal hyperplasia (CAH) is due to an inherited (autosomal recessive) deficiency of 1 of the steroidogenic enzymes necessary for the synthesis of corticosteroid hormones by the adrenal gland. Patients may present in a classic fashion in the neonatal or postnatal period. This usually occurs with severe enzyme deficiency. However, patients with mild enzyme deficiency can present after puberty. The most common cause is 21-hydroxylase deficiency (90%), but deficiency of 11β-hydroxylase or 3β-hydroxysteroid dehydrogenase also leads to CAH. Such blocks in the steroidogenic pathway result in the accumulation of precursor molecules proximal to the site of block. These precursors are shunted into pathways that lead to the synthesis of androgens. The process is ACTH-dependent and, thus, can be suppressed by dexamethasone. In 21-hydroxylase deficiency, the concentration of 17-hydroxyprogesterone is usually increased (>300 ng/dL), and if it is normal, an ACTH stimulation test is indicated. A concentration of 17-hydroxyprogesterone greater than 1,200 ng/dL 30 minutes after stimulation is diagnostic.

Virilizing Tumors of the Ovary and Adrenal Gland

Virilizing tumors of the ovary and adrenal gland can occur at any age; they produce severe hyperandrogenism, with a rapid onset and progression. Adrenal tumors characteristically are associated with high levels of DHEAS, whereas ovarian tumors produce high levels of testosterone. Diagnosis requires appropriate imaging. Rarely, selective venous sampling is required to localize the source of androgen excess.

Therapy of Hirsutism

Oral contraceptives are used in the management of idiopathic hirsutism and polycystic ovarian syndrome. They suppress LH production, which in turn decreases ovarian testosterone production. It is important to avoid agents with androgenic progestins. Spironolactone is an androgen receptor blocker. Because it causes menstrual dysfunction, it often is combined with an oral contraceptive agent (some form of contraception is required because spironolactone may cause abnormal development of genitalia in a male fetus). A patient who receives medical therapy should be counseled

that an effect may not be seen for 6 months. Also, because treatment is not effective against established hair, some form of mechanical hair removal is desirable early during therapy.

* In hirsutism, medical therapy is used to decrease androgen production or to inhibit the effect of androgens on hair follicles.

Hyperlipidemias

Disorders of lipoprotein metabolism predispose to premature ischemic heart disease and vascular disease. In some patients, an extreme increase in triglyceride concentrations can lead to acute pancreatitis.

Etiology

Increases in total cholesterol and triglyceride concentrations may be caused by a coexisting disorder (eg, poorly controlled diabetes mellitus, hypothyroidism) or the use of drugs (eg, corticosteroids). In the absence of precipitating factors, an increase in lipoprotein concentration is termed *primary hyperlipidemia*. It is the result of genetic defects (eg, absence of the low-density lipoprotein [LDL] receptor) or acquired defects (due to an interaction of aging, weight gain, poor diet, sedentary lifestyle, and genetic predisposition).

* Hyperlipidemias: genetic or acquired disorders that can result from increased production or reduced clearance (or both).

Some of the primary hyperlipidemias are outlined in Table 6-3, and the causes of secondary hyperlipidemia are outlined in Table 6-4.

Clinical Features

Most patients with hyperlipidemia have no physical findings attributable directly to increased concentrations of lipoprotein. Some patients have a corneal arcus (arcus senilis), but the significance of this finding decreases with increasing age. Patients with an extreme increase in LDL cholesterol (LDL-C) may exhibit tendon xanthomas or thickening of the Achilles tendon. Other patients with an increase in intermediate-density lipoprotein (IDL) may have palmar tuboeruptive xanthomas. In hyperchylomicronemia, eruptive xanthomas may develop on the buttocks.

Increased LDL-C, increased IDL, increased Lp(a) lipoprotein, and decreased high-density lipoprotein cholesterol (HDL-C) all confer an increased risk of atherosclerotic vascular disease. Increased HDL-C is associated with decreased atherogenic risk. Hypertriglyceridemia may be atherogenic by inducing alterations in other lipoproteins (eg, it may decrease HDL-C and increase small-density LDL-C, very low-density lipoprotein [VLDL] remnants, and IDL); in addition, it may have an unidentified direct atherogenic action. Pancreatitis may develop with increases in triglyceride-rich lipoproteins (>1,000 mg/dL).

* Clinical presentations: ischemic vascular disease, pancreatitis, or xanthomas.

Diagnosis

The Adult Treatment Panel of the National Cholesterol Education Program has recommended that all adults older than 20 be evaluated for hypercholesterolemia to identify those at risk of coronary artery disease. Lipid screening tests should not be performed during an acute illness or hospitalization, which may transiently lower LDL-C. Plasma triglyceride concentrations vary considerably after meals and should be measured in the fasting state. Provided plasma triglyceride concentrations are less than 400 mg/dL, LDL-C concentrations can be reliably estimated by use of the Friedewald equation:

$$LDL\text{-}C = \text{total cholesterol} - HDL\text{-}C - \frac{\text{triglycerides}}{5}$$

Lp(a) lipoprotein is an independent risk factor for vascular disease. It should be measured in patients with a strong family history of premature ischemic heart disease who do not have conventional risk factors and in patients with established coronary artery disease who have progressive disease despite control of conventional risk factors.

- Lipid screening tests should not be conducted during an acute illness or hospitalization.

Nonmodifiable risk factors for cardiovascular disease include age older than 45 for men and 55 for women. A family history of pre-

Table 6-3 Features of Primary Hyperlipidemias

Feature	Familial Hypercholesterolemia	Familial Combined Hyperlipidemia	Familial Dysbetalipoproteinemia	Familial Hypertriglyceridemia	Severe Hypertriglyceridemia	
					Early Onset	Adult Onset
Pathophysiology	Defective LDL receptor or defective apo B-100; impaired catabolism of LDL	Overproduction of hepatic VLDL–apo B-100 but not of VLDL-Tg	Defective or absent apo E; excess of CM remnants and VLDL in fasting state	Overproduction of hepatic VLDL–Tg but not of apo B-100	Lipoprotein lipase deficiency Apo C-II deficiency; defect in CM & VLDL catabolism	Overproduction of hepatic VLDL–Tg Delayed catabolism of CMs & VLDL
Mode of inheritance	Autosomal codominant	Autosomal dominant	Autosomal recessive	Autosomal dominant	Autosomal recessive	Autosomal recessive
Estimated population frequency	1:500	1:50	1:5,000	1:50	<1:10,000	Rare
Risk of CAD	+++	++	+	+ In families in which HDL-C is deficient	–	+
Physical findings	Arcus senilis Tendinous xanthomas	Arcus senilis	Arcus senilis Tuberoeruptive & palmar xanthomas	None	Lipemia retinalis Eruptive xanthomas	Milky plasma Lipemia retinalis Eruptive xanthomas Pancreatitis
Associated findings		Obesity Glucose intolerance Hyperuricemia HDL-C deficiency	Obesity Glucose intolerance Hyperuricemia	Obesity Glucose intolerance Hyperuricemia HDL-C deficiency	HDL-C deficiency Recurrent abdominal pain Pancreatitis Hepatosplenomegaly	Obesity Glucose intolerance Hyperuricemia HDL-C deficiency Pancreatitis
Treatment	Diet Niacin & resin Statin & resin Probucol & resin	Diet Drugs singly or in combination with niacin, statin, gemfibrozil, resin	Diet Niacin Gemfibrozil Statin	Diet Niacin Gemfibrozil Abstain from alcohol, estrogen	Diet Fish oil	Diet Control diabetes when present Avoid alcohol, estrogen Gemfibrozil Fish oil

Abbreviations: apo, apolipoprotein; CAD, coronary artery disease; CM, chylomicron; HDL-C, high-density lipoprotein cholesterol; LDL, low-density lipoprotein; Tg, triglyceride; VLDL, very low-density lipoprotein; +++, very high; ++, high; +, moderate; –, no increased risk.

Table 6-4   Causes of Secondary Hyperlipidemia

Increased LDL-C	Increased Triglycerides	Decreased HDL-C
Hypothyroidism	Obesity	Hypertriglyceridemia
Dysglobulinemia	Diabetes mellitus	Obesity
Nephrotic syndrome	Hypothyroidism	Diabetes mellitus
Obstructive liver disease	Sedentary life	Cigarette smoking
Progestins	Alcohol	Sedentary life
Anabolic steroids, glucocorticoid therapy	Renal insufficieny	β-Blockers
Anorexia nervosa	Estrogens	Progestins
Acute intermittent porphyria	β-Blockers	Anabolic steroids
	Thiazides, steroids	
	Dysglobulinemias	
	Systemic lupus erythematosus	

Abbreviations: HDL-C, high-density lipoprotein cholesterol; LDL-C, low-density lipoprotein cholesterol.

mature coronary artery disease (a parent or sibling with myocardial infarction or sudden death before age 55) confers increased risk. Modifiable risk factors include smoking, hypertension, diabetes mellitus, and an HDL-C less than 35 mg/dL. An HDL-C greater than 60 mg/dL confers protection against cardiovascular disease.

- Assessment of other coronary risk factors is important for evaluating the overall atherogenic risk and planning effective management.

Therapy

The National Cholesterol Education Program Guidelines are used to guide therapy (Table 6-5). The target LDL-C level depends on the presence of ischemic heart disease (secondary prevention) or risk factors for ischemic heart disease (primary prevention). High-risk patients have 2 or more risk factors.

Treatment requires dietary and lifestyle modification and correction of secondary causes when feasible (eg, treatment of hypothyroidism or diabetes mellitus) in conjunction with the appropriate use of lipid-lowering agents.

Diet Therapy

Dietary therapy is used to achieve and maintain a normal body weight. A typical healthy diet can be provided by following the American Heart Association step I diet, which provides for 30% or fewer calories from fat and 10% or fewer calories from saturated fat. Alcohol restriction often decreases triglyceride concentrations.

Behavior Modification

Weight reduction enhances the cholesterol-lowering effect of an appropriate diet, decreases triglycerides, increases HDL-C, decreases blood pressure, and improves glucose tolerance. Smoking cessation and regular exercise also increase HDL-C.

Drug Therapy

After drug therapy for hyperlipidemia has been instituted, it is likely to be lifelong. Therefore, drug therapy should be embarked upon only after vigorous efforts at dietary and lifestyle modification. Both the physician and the patient should be made aware of the potential risks associated with lipid-lowering agents. The teratogenic potential of most of these drugs should also be borne in mind when prescribing them for women of childbearing age. Patients should be monitored for potential side effects as well as for the efficacy of the medication in reaching the predetermined goals. Lipid concentrations should be checked approximately 3 months after therapy has been instituted. If the lipid goals are not achieved, the dose may need to be increased. However, combination therapy may need to be considered for some patients. Because of the increased risk of myositis or hepatitis (or both), combination therapy should be reserved for secondary prevention in established cardiovascular disease.

Treatment of Increased LDL-C

In most instances, a statin is the drug of choice for the treatment of increased concentration of LDL-C. In estrogen-deficient women, estrogen replacement therapy is effective in decreasing LDL-C and increasing HDL-C, and it is appropriate in women up to the age of menopause. However, oral estrogens should not be given to patients with hypertriglyceridemia; for these patients, a transdermal estrogen patch may be considered. Recent studies of long-term estrogen use do not provide evidence of benefit in cardiovascular outcomes, and the risk of myocardial infarction may actually be increased by estrogen, at least among women at high risk. Patients who do not reach their therapeutic goals will benefit from the addition of a resin (colesevelam or cholestyramine) to the statin. Niacin can also be used for the treatment of increased LDL-C. However, many patients are unable to tolerate this medication long-term because of its side effects, most notably facial flushing and worsening of glucose tolerance.

Treatment of Hypertriglyceridemia

Extreme hypertriglyceridemia (>1,000 mg/dL) requires timely treatment to reduce the risk of pancreatitis. This includes cessation of

Table 6-5   Overview of Therapy for Hyperlipidemia[a]

Clinical Risk Assessment	Initiate Diet Therapy	Initiate Drug Therapy	Goal of Therapy
No CAD; <2 risk factors	>160 mg/dL	>190 mg/dL	<130 mg/dL
No CAD; ≥2 risk factors	>130 mg/dL	>160 mg/dL	<100 mg/dL
CAD; step II AHA diet	Any level	Any level	<70-80 mg/dL

Abbreviations: AHA, American Heart Association; CAD, coronary artery disease.
[a] Values refer to low-density lipoprotein cholesterol levels.

oral estrogen or alcohol use, improved control of diabetes, and restriction of caloric intake. In severe cases, insulin treatment may prove useful. Fibrates such as gemfibrozil or fenofibrate are the drugs of choice. Many patients with hypertriglyceridemia have glucose intolerance or diabetes. These disorders are a relative contraindication to niacin, which increases insulin resistance and may worsen glycemic control. Fish oil capsules (1 g) at a dosage of 8 to 10 capsules daily may be effective for hypertriglyceridemia.

Treatment of Low HDL-C
In the absence of heart disease, lifestyle modification is the intervention of choice in conjunction with an attempt to discontinue drugs that can lower HDL-C (eg, androgens). In the presence of ischemic heart disease, lowering LDL-C to less than 100 mg/dL is indicated. Drugs that can increase HDL-C include niacin, statins, and, to a lesser extent, fibrates. In postmenopausal women, estrogen replacement therapy can increase HDL-C concentrations.

Treatment of Increased Lp(a) Lipoprotein
There is no proven treatment for increased concentrations of Lp(a) lipoprotein, although niacin may produce some modest decrease. Some authorities advocate intervention to lower LDL-C to less than 100 mg/dL in patients with increased Lp(a) lipoprotein. Estrogen replacement therapy may be effective in postmenopausal women.

Diabetes Mellitus

Etiology and Classification
Diabetes mellitus is a metabolic disorder characterized by increased fasting and postprandial concentrations of glucose. It is the most common metabolic disorder and affects about 10% of the US population. The classification of this disorder into 2 broad categories is somewhat artificial and the reader should recognize that a degree of overlap exists. Type 1 diabetes mellitus (T1D) is characterized by immune destruction of the insulin-producing beta cells in the islets of Langerhans. It represents 10% to 20% of the diabetic population and usually appears at a younger age. Most patients eventually lose all endogenous insulin secretion and are prone to the development of ketoacidosis.

A complex interaction between genes and the environment leads to the development of T1D. This is illustrated by the 50% concordance for the disease seen in monozygotic twins. This disease is associated frequently with certain histocompatibility antigen (HLA)

types, with polymorphisms of the insulin gene and other variants in immune response genes having weak contributions to the pathogenesis of this disorder. Antibodies to islets or some constituent of the islets are frequently present, at least in the early stages of the disease (islet-cell antibodies and glutamic acid decarboxylase [GAD] antibodies) and may help to differentiate T1D from type 2 diabetes mellitus (T2D). Often, a "honeymoon" period occurs, during which insulin requirements decrease dramatically after restoration of euglycemia. The duration of this phase is highly variable.

- T1D is characterized by immune destruction of the islets, which leads to insulin deficiency.
- Concordance is seen in 50% of monozygotic twins.

The pathogenesis of T2D is more complex. It is characterized by abnormalities of insulin secretion and insulin action in target tissues such as the liver, muscle, and adipose tissue. The ability of glucose to stimulate its own uptake and to suppress its own release is also defective. Impaired suppression of glucagon secretion after the ingestion of a meal also contributes to postprandial hyperglycemia in these patients. Although T2D usually appears in older, obese patients, it increasingly has been described in obese, sedentary children and adolescents. T2D is more common among certain ethnic groups. Monozygotic twins exhibit almost 100% concordance if 1 of the twins is affected. The overall genetic contribution to the pathogenesis of T2D is greater than in T1D. However, individual genes have a weaker contribution than in T1D (eg, HLA polymorphisms in T1D). Environmental factors such as obesity also have a definite role in the development of the disease.

- T2D is characterized by defective insulin secretion and action.
- Environmental factors such as obesity have an important role in the development of T2D.
- T2D can occur at any age.

Maturity-onset diabetes of the young (MODY) describes a group of single-gene disorders in patients who present with diabetes at a young age. MODY is usually inherited as an autosomal dominant trait. Various mutations are responsible for this disorder, and the clinical expression is variable.

Clinical Features
The onset of T1D is usually dramatic, with weight loss, polyuria, and polydipsia. Often, the presentation is precipitated by an infection

or other severe physical stress because patients lack the reserve of endogenous insulin secretion to overcome the effects of counter-regulatory hormones (eg, glucagon, cortisol, growth hormone, and epinephrine) on glucose metabolism. Severe dehydration and ketoacidosis may be present. In very young children, nocturnal enuresis may signal the onset of disease.

T2D usually has a more insidious onset. Often, the disease is diagnosed during routine laboratory testing by the presence of glycosuria or fasting hyperglycemia. Patients may complain of blurring of vision, myopia, episodes of recurrent skin infections, or monilial vaginitis (females) or balanitis (males). Occasionally, patients may present with evidence of chronic diabetic complications (eg, neuropathy, nephropathy, retinopathy, or vascular disease) but without symptoms related to glucose intolerance. Symptoms such as polyuria, polydipsia, and polyphagia may only develop in situations of increased insulin resistance such as pregnancy, infection, or steroid use. Also, patients occasionally present with hyperosmolar nonketotic coma.

- T1D has a rapid onset related to abrupt, severe insulin deficiency, with polyuria, polydipsia, weight loss despite polyphagia, severe dehydration, and ketoacidosis.
- T2D has an insidious onset, and patients may present with complications. Under certain conditions, polyuria, polydipsia, and polyphagia may develop.

Diagnosis
The normal fasting plasma glucose concentration is less than 105 mg/dL. In adults (but not pregnant women), fasting values of 126 mg/dL or greater on 2 or more occasions confirm the diagnosis of diabetes mellitus. Fasting values between 110 mg/dL and 125 mg/dL encompass the class of impaired fasting glucose. These thresholds were recommended by the American Diabetes Association because epidemiologic data demonstrated a progressive increase in microvascular complications with progressive impairment in fasting glucose concentrations greater than 105 mg/dL.

- In adults (but not pregnant women), fasting plasma glucose values ≥126 mg/dL on 2 or more occasions confirm the diagnosis of diabetes mellitus.

Oral Glucose Tolerance Test
Currently, the main utility of glucose tolerance testing is during pregnancy, when it is used to screen for gestational diabetes mellitus. Epidemiologic data have demonstrated that impaired glucose tolerance is a marker for increased cardiovascular morbidity (in some cohorts) and mortality. However, the clinical application of glucose tolerance testing in this situation is unknown.

Therapy for T1D
Insulin replacement is the appropriate therapy for T1D, and oral agents have no role in its management. The optimal regimen allows the patient to maintain a healthy, active lifestyle, with optimal glycemic control and minimal hypoglycemia. This can be achieved with intensive insulin therapy but requires considerable commitment from the patient to self-monitor plasma glucose concentrations and to

adjust the insulin dosage accordingly. The Diabetes Control and Complications Trial demonstrated conclusively that intensive therapy with tight glycemic control prevents or markedly decreases the risks of chronic microvascular complications of diabetes.

Nutrition
Intake should allow for maintenance of a reasonable weight and for growth in children and adolescents. Protein should account for 10% to 20% of the total calories; total fat, less than 30% (saturated fat, <10%); and complex carbohydrates, the rest.

Exercise
The glycemic response to exercise varies depending on the duration and type of exercise, the fitness of the person, and the relationship of exercise to meals and insulin injections. Blood glucose levels should be monitored before and after exercise to determine the response to exercise and to prevent hypoglycemia. Patients should always carry appropriate identification and have access to glucose or glucagon (or both).

Insulin Therapy
Intensive insulin therapy allows the use of insulin in a fashion that mimics insulin secretion by the healthy pancreas. Short-acting insulin (regular or lispro) is injected at mealtimes to facilitate disposal of the meal, and a once-daily long-acting insulin (glargine insulin) is taken to replace basal insulin secretion.

An insulin pump provides a continuous subcutaneous infusion of insulin in a programmed fashion. It also is used to provide meal-stimulated insulin secretion, and it allows the patient to change the infusion rate of "basal" insulin (during exercise or at night).

The insulin dosage required for a typical patient with T1D who is within 20% of ideal body weight and does not have intercurrent illness is approximately 0.5 to 1.0 U/kg daily. The insulin requirements may increase markedly during intercurrent illness.

The glycemic goals are individualized according to the presence of intercurrent disease (ischemic heart disease or cerebrovascular disease), diabetic complications, and the ability to perceive hypoglycemia. If a female who has T1D is considering pregnancy or is pregnant, tighter control is important to decrease the risk of birth defects or macrosomia.

- Intensive insulin therapy attempts to simulate normal insulin secretion, with a combination of short-acting and long-acting insulin.
- An insulin pump allows the patient to adjust basal insulin levels as needed.

Glycemic Goals of Optimal Therapy
Blood glucose targets are as follows: fasting, 70 to 130 mg/dL; bedtime, 100 to 140 mg/dL. Hemoglobin A_{1c} should be less than 6.5%. Higher target levels are required for patients at risk of hypoglycemia because of their inability to recognize hypoglycemic symptoms.

Monitoring
On most days, the blood glucose concentration should be self-monitored 4 times daily—before meals and at bedtime. If the patient

has unexplained morning hypoglycemia or hyperglycemia, blood glucose should be measured at 2 AM to 4 AM. Hemoglobin A_{1c} should be measured every 2 to 3 months.

- Hemoglobin A_{1c} should be monitored every 2-3 months; the goal is <6.5%.
- The patient should self-monitor blood glucose at least 4 times daily. The goal is 70-130 mg/dL fasting and 100-140 mg/dL at bedtime.

Therapy for T2D

Most patients with T2D are obese and lead sedentary lifestyles. Often, they have multiple cardiovascular risk factors such as hypertension and dyslipidemia. Therapy should include appropriate modification of these risk factors, appropriate exercise and nutrition, and achievement of appropriate glycemic control with a near-normal hemoglobin A_{1c}.

Calorie restriction while consuming a healthy, balanced diet is appropriate to promote weight reduction. Exercise improves insulin action, facilitates weight loss, reduces cardiovascular risks (increases HDL-C and decreases VLDL-triglycerides), and increases a patient's sense of well-being. If the patient has preexisting coronary or peripheral vascular disease, exercise recommendations should be modified appropriately.

- The treatment goals for T2D include appropriate lifestyle modification, modification of cardiovascular risk factors, and optimal glycemic control.
- Calorie restriction is appropriate to promote weight reduction.
- A prudent exercise program facilitates weight reduction and improves insulin action, cardiovascular fitness, and the sense of well-being.

Drug Therapy for T2D

Sulfonylureas are insulin secretagogues. These agents bind to the sulfonylurea receptor on beta cells, causing closure of potassium channels, with the subsequent influx of calcium and exocytosis of insulin. The efficacy of these medications depends on the presence of endogenous insulin secretion. Primary failure occurs in the absence of endogenous insulin secretion. Secondary failure occurs with progression of disease, when sulfonylureas are no longer effective in achieving glycemic control.

Repaglinide and *nateglinide* have an extremely short half-life and act in a fashion similar to sulfonylureas. These agents are taken before each meal (the dose is skipped if the meal is missed).

Metformin is a biguanide, a class of drugs that improves the liver action of insulin. Lactic acidosis is extremely rare if the specific exclusion criteria for the use of metformin are followed: 1) renal impairment—plasma creatinine value of 1.5 mg/dL or greater for men and 1.4 mg/dL or greater for women, 2) cardiac or respiratory insufficiency that is likely to cause central hypoxia or reduced peripheral perfusion, 3) history of lactic acidosis, 4) severe infection that could lead to reduced tissue perfusion, 5) liver disease, 6) alcohol abuse with binge drinking, and 7) use of intravenous radiographic contrast agents. For hospitalized patients, it is prudent to withhold metformin therapy.

Thiazolidinediones chiefly improve peripheral insulin action. Troglitazone, the first member of the class to be used clinically, was withdrawn because of its association with severe hepatotoxicity. The newer members of the group, rosiglitazone and pioglitazone, do not contain a vitamin E moiety, which is thought to account for the hepatotoxicity associated with troglitazone. Nevertheless, it is recommended that liver function be monitored closely during treatment with these drugs. Thiazolidinediones can cause marked fluid retention and should not be prescribed if the patient has congestive heart failure.

Exenatide (Byetta) is the first of a new class of drugs (the incretin mimetics) that alter gastrointestinal hormone action, slowing the absorption of carbohydrates in the meal and altering insulin response to eating. The incretin mimetics promote improved glycemic control, including postprandial glycemia. In addition, they promote satiety and may assist in weight loss efforts.

Although all these newer agents seem to be effective in improving hemoglobin A_{1c}, their effect on clinical outcomes (vascular disease, microvascular complications) remains unknown. Until appropriate outcomes-based trials are completed, it seems appropriate to reserve these agents for patients whose therapy with more traditional drugs has failed.

- Sulfonylureas are insulin secretagogues. Their efficacy depends on the presence of some degree of endogenous insulin secretion.
- Metformin improves the action of insulin in the liver. Its use should be avoided in certain circumstances because of the risk of lactic acidosis.
- Thiazolidinediones improve peripheral insulin action but are associated with fluid retention.
- Repaglinide and nateglinide are short-acting agents that increase insulin secretion; they are taken before meals.

Insulin is reserved for patients with T2D in whom diet and oral agents (monotherapy and combination therapy) have not provided adequate glycemic control. It is the preferred therapy when patients are pregnant, are undergoing surgical treatment, or are severely ill. Patients with T2D often have some degree of meal-stimulated endogenous insulin secretion, which allows treatment with simpler insulin regimens than for T1D. Once-daily injections of intermediate-acting insulin in combination with an oral agent or twice-daily injections of intermediate-acting insulin are commonly used to manage T2D. Insulin therapy is associated with some degree of weight gain in most patients. For this reason, insulin sometimes is given in combination with metformin to help limit weight gain. In patients who have a more severe insulin deficiency, an intensive insulin program or a split-mix program may be used (eg, NR-0-NR-0).

- Simple insulin regimens are useful for patients with T2D who have experienced secondary treatment failure (eg, intermediate insulin once or twice daily; supplement once-daily dosing with an oral agent if necessary).
- Prescribe an intensive insulin program or split-mix program (eg, NR-0-NR-0) for patients with severe insulin deficiency.

Combination Therapy

Combination therapy is frequently prescribed for patients with T2D if maximal therapy with a single agent fails to achieve adequate glycemic control. This takes advantage of the different mechanisms of action of oral agents. A commonly used regimen is the combination of a sulfonylurea with metformin.

- Combination therapy with metformin and a sulfonylurea significantly improves control when therapy with 1 agent fails.

Hypoglycemia in Diabetes

Hypoglycemia occurs when there is a mismatch between glucose availability and glucose requirements. This may be due to unplanned exercise, inappropriate dosing of insulin, or inadequate caloric intake. Patients with T1D are prone to hypoglycemia unawareness, which develops after repeated neuroglycopenia. This may require appropriate adjustment of glycemic goals because the prevention of hypoglycemia has been shown to reverse or ameliorate hypoglycemia unawareness. Many episodes of severe hypoglycemia occur at night and may not be apparent if glucose is checked at bedtime and at breakfast. Occasionally, patients report symptoms such as nightmares, morning headache, or night sweats. It is important to emphasize the need for periodic self-monitoring of blood glucose between 1 AM and 3 AM. Preventive strategies for nocturnal hypoglycemia include increasing the bedtime snack or modifying the insulin regimen.

Patients with long-standing T1D also develop defective counterregulation because they are unable to secrete glucagon and become dependent on the autonomic nervous system to respond to hypoglycemia. The use of β-blockers in these situations can abolish all acute responses to hypoglycemia.

Insulin clearance is delayed by renal impairment and by circulating insulin antibodies. Alcohol may interfere with gluconeogenesis and with the perception of hypoglycemic symptoms. Hypoglycemia may be a manifestation of cortisol deficiency (patients with T1D are at increased risk of other autoimmune endocrinopathies).

- Patients with T1D are especially prone to hypoglycemia.
- Episodes of severe hypoglycemia may occur during the night—check the blood glucose level between 1 AM and 3 AM.
- Hypoglycemia may be precipitated by exercise, decreased caloric intake, renal insufficiency, and cortisol deficiency.

Acute Complications of Diabetes Mellitus

Diabetic Ketoacidosis

Diabetic ketoacidosis occurs in patients with T1D and may be the initial presentation of diabetes. It is characterized by polyuria, polydipsia, dehydration, anorexia, nausea and vomiting, abdominal pain, tachypnea, mental obtundation, and coma. The physical findings include clinical evidence of dehydration, decreased mentation, deep and rapid Kussmaul respiration, and a characteristic breath odor (acetone). Often, diabetic ketoacidosis is precipitated by a failure to take insulin or to increase insulin and consume extra fluids during acute illness, infection, or other intercurrent illness such as myocardial infarction, pancreatitis, stroke, or trauma.

The diagnosis is based on the demonstration of moderate or severe hyperglycemia, ketonemia, and metabolic acidosis. Associated biochemical abnormalities include hyponatremia, azotemia, and hyperamylasemia. Serum levels of potassium, phosphate, and magnesium (despite large body losses) may be normal. However, concentrations of these ions often decrease precipitously as the acidosis is corrected.

- Diabetic ketoacidosis occurs with severe insulin deficiency and is often precipitated by intercurrent illness.
- It may be the initial manifestation of T1D.
- Diagnosis requires the presence of pronounced hyperglycemia, ketonemia, and metabolic acidosis.
- Serum levels of potassium may be normal despite large body losses.
- A thorough search for precipitating factors should be undertaken in all cases.

Treatment

Treatment of diabetic ketoacidosis requires correction of the metabolic state and electrolyte depletion. These goals are achieved by the administration of insulin, the replacement of fluid and electrolytes, and treatment of precipitating factors.

Insulin—Insulin infusion is preferred over subcutaneous or intramuscular injection. A continuous low dose (2-4 units per hour) is recommended and should continue until the acidosis has resolved. It is important not to terminate the insulin treatment early, based purely on resolution of hyperglycemia, since recurrent acidosis may occur. This insulin infusion allows suppression of lipolysis and ketogenesis and stimulates glucose uptake.

Fluids—Fluids are given intravenously to restore volume and to correct electrolyte and fluid losses. The average fluid deficit in adults is 5 to 8 L. Approximately 4 L should be replaced in the first few hours. As plasma glucose values approach 250 mg/dL, change to 0.45% saline in 5% dextrose in water. This allows maintenance of intravenous insulin while keeping the plasma glucose at about 200 mg/dL during the first 12 hours, permitting correction of ketosis and avoiding a rapid decrease in osmolarity with its risk of cerebral edema.

Electrolytes—The potassium deficit is about 300 to 500 mEq. Regardless of the initial serum level of potassium, the total body stores of potassium are low. With correction of the acidosis, the serum level of potassium decreases. Potassium should be added to the intravenous fluids as soon as renal perfusion and urine flow are assured. Add 40 mEq of potassium, as potassium chloride, to each liter of intravenous fluid. Phosphate repletion is indicated by phosphate levels less than 1 mg/dL. Give phosphate in a dose of 0.08 mM/kg intravenously over 6 hours. (Neutral potassium phosphate: 1 ampule contains 3 mM phosphate and 15 mEq of potassium.) Monitor the serum level of phosphate carefully because of the risk of hypocalcemia, seizures, and death.

Prognosis

The mortality rate of diabetic ketoacidosis is 5% to 15% and, in most patients, is due to an associated precipitating illness such as myocardial infarction, stroke, or sepsis. After successful therapy, the goal is to avoid recurrence by educating the patient.

- Prognosis: 5%-15% mortality, usually from associated illness.
- After successful therapy, the goal is to avoid recurrence.

Hyperglycemic Hyperosmolar Nonketotic Coma

Hyperglycemic hyperosmolar nonketotic coma is characterized by hyperglycemia, hyperosmolar dehydration, and the absence of ketoacidosis. It usually occurs in poorly treated T2D when there is sufficient insulin to inhibit excess lipolysis and ketogenesis but not enough to suppress hepatic glucose production or to stimulate peripheral glucose uptake. High concentrations of urinary glucose provoke an osmotic diuresis, with marked dehydration and subsequently decreased renal function. It often is precipitated by acute illness such as myocardial infarction, pancreatitis, infection, or surgery.

Diagnosis

Hyperglycemic hyperosmolar nonketotic coma should be suspected in any patient with diabetes who presents with an altered level of consciousness and severe dehydration. Laboratory abnormalities include marked hyperglycemia (often >600 mg/dL), absence of ketones, and increased plasma osmolarity (>320 mOsm/L). A search for an underlying disorder is an integral part of the evaluation.

- Hyperglycemic hyperosmolar nonketotic coma is characterized by hyperglycemia and dehydration without ketoacidosis.
- The disorder should be suspected in any patient with diabetes who has altered sensorium and severe dehydration.
- Laboratory evaluation demonstrates marked hyperglycemia (>600 mg/dL), no significant ketosis, and plasma hyperosmolarity (>320 mOsm/L).
- Always search for a precipitating disorder.

Therapy

The objectives of treatment are to restore volume and osmolarity and to control the hyperglycemia. Fluid resuscitation with normal saline should be followed by 0.45% saline to correct the hyperosmolarity. Insulin is administered intravenously, but it is important to decrease the plasma glucose level gradually to a level between 200 and 300 mg/dL to avoid cerebral edema. At this stage, the infusion of insulin can be discontinued, and it should be given subcutaneously. Electrolyte replacement as outlined above for diabetic ketoacidosis is also important. Repeated neurologic evaluation is essential because focal deficits or seizures may become apparent during therapy. Complications include vascular events such as myocardial infarction or stroke, cerebral edema, and hypokalemia. The mortality rate is 50%.

- Treatment: fluid and electrolyte replacement and management of hyperglycemia.
- Hyperglycemic hyperosmolar nonketotic coma has a mortality rate of 50%.

Chronic Complications of Diabetes Mellitus

Microvascular Disease in Diabetes

Chronic hyperglycemia and other metabolic abnormalities associated with diabetes lead to damage of the microcirculation. This is manifested clinically as diabetic retinopathy, nephropathy, and neuropathy. Some degree of diabetic retinopathy occurs in 50% to 70% of patients with T1D within 10 years after diagnosis and reaches a prevalence of 95% by 15 to 20 years; it is rare in those who have had T1D for less than 5 years. Diabetic retinopathy is present in 15% to 20% of patients at the time of diagnosis of T2D and reaches 50% by 15 years. Background diabetic retinopathy is characterized by microaneurysms, hard exudates, hemorrhages, and macular edema. Proliferative retinopathy occurs when areas of the retina are ischemic; this provides a stimulus to the growth of new vessels. These vessels are fragile and prone to hemorrhage, which can lead to loss of vision. Panretinal photocoagulation is used to treat proliferative retinopathy. The destruction of ischemic areas of the retina decreases the stimulus for neovascularization and progression of proliferative retinopathy. The treatment of hypertension, hyperglycemia, glaucoma, and dyslipidemia is also important in these circumstances. Patients should have an annual dilated ophthalmic examination by an experienced ophthalmologist to identify those at risk.

Infections and Diabetes

Cutaneous skin infections are often a presenting feature of poorly controlled T2D. Typical infections include candidiasis as well as furuncles and carbuncles (caused by *Staphylococcus aureus* infection). Malignant external otitis due to infection with *Pseudomonas* is peculiar to diabetes and is life-threatening.

Ischemic Heart Disease in Diabetes

Ischemic cardiovascular disease appears earlier and is more extensive in persons with diabetes than in the general population. Coronary artery disease accounts for about 70% of deaths among those with diabetes, and patients may present with sudden cardiac death. Epidemiologic studies have shown that persons with T2D have the same risk of myocardial infarction as patients who have already had a myocardial infarction. For this reason, treatment of dyslipidemia is considered to be secondary prevention in diabetes. Patients with ischemic heart disease may present in an atypical manner; patients with angina may present with epigastric distress, heartburn, and neck or jaw pain; myocardial infarction may be silent (in 15% of patients) and patients may present with sudden onset of left ventricular failure. The role of screening for vascular disease in asymptomatic patients with diabetes remains uncertain.

Hyperlipidemia in Diabetes

In poorly controlled T2D, the concentrations of triglyceride-rich lipoproteins are increased because of an overproduction of VLDL together with decreased lipoprotein lipase activity. HDL-C levels are low, and levels do improve but usually do not normalize with control of glucose and triglyceride levels. Compositional changes in LDL (small, dense LDL) that increase the atherogenicity of these particles are more likely to occur in patients with T2D.

Diabetes and Pregnancy

Both fasting and postprandial glucose concentrations decrease in normal pregnancy. Because of an increase in the concentration of circulating hormones such as human placental lactogen, estrogen, progesterone, and cortisol (which increase insulin resistance), insulin secretion also increases. Glucose is a major metabolic substrate for the fetus and traverses the placenta by facilitated diffusion.

Pregnancy is a diabetogenic state and may worsen glucose control in women with established diabetes. Inadequate glycemic control early in pregnancy increases the risk of congenital malformations, whereas poor control in late pregnancy increases the risk of macrosomia, neonatal hypoglycemia, hypocalcemia, polycythemia, hyperbilirubinemia, and respiratory distress. Pregnancy may exacerbate diabetic retinopathy, and nephropathy may lead to pregnancy-induced hypertension and toxemia.

Gestational diabetes complicates 2% to 3% of all pregnancies. All pregnant women older than 25 years should be evaluated at 24 to 28 weeks with a 50-g oral glucose tolerance test. Plasma glucose levels higher than 140 mg/dL 1 hour after ingestion of the glucose drink require formal testing with a 100-g glucose drink. Gestational diabetes is diagnosed if glucose values exceed 105 mg/dL (fasting), 190 mg/dL (1 hour), 165 mg/dL (2 hours), and 145 mg/dL (3 hours).

- Early detection and optimal management of diabetes during pregnancy can prevent congenital malformations and decrease neonatal morbidity and mortality.
- Gestational diabetes complicates 2%-3% of all pregnancies.
- Screen all pregnant women older than 25 years at 24-28 weeks.

Treatment

Tight glycemic control is essential in pregnancy and before conception to decrease the risk of fetal malformations. The goals of therapy are to ensure tight control of diabetes (while avoiding hypoglycemia and fasting ketonemia) and adequate nutrition and optimal weight gain. Home monitoring for blood glucose and urine ketones is important. Because postprandial glucose concentrations are closely associated with malformations and macrosomia, they are often used to guide therapy. The blood glucose concentration should be between 60 and 90 mg/dL while fasting and 70 to 140 mg/dL 1 hour after a meal.

Women with gestational diabetes who become euglycemic in the postpartum state should be followed up periodically. They are at high risk of T2D (60% develop the disease within 15 years after the diagnosis of gestational diabetes) and should be encouraged to exercise, consume an appropriate diet, and make an effort to lose weight.

- Periodic follow-up of patients with gestational diabetes is necessary because 60% develop T2D within 15 years.

Hypoglycemia in Nondiabetic Patients

Etiology

Hypoglycemic disorders may be classified into *insulin-mediated* (insulin levels not appropriately suppressed) and *noninsulin-mediated* (insulin levels suppressed). Causes of insulin-mediated hypoglycemia include insulinoma, use of sulfonylurea or exogenous insulin, and autoimmune hypoglycemia mediated by insulin antibodies that bind insulin and prevent its degradation. Noninsulin-mediated hypoglycemia may be related to alcohol use, cortisol insufficiency, or GH deficiency in

children. Renal failure, liver failure, and sepsis are the common causes of noninsulin-mediated hypoglycemia in hospitalized patients. Mesenchymal or epithelial tumors may cause hypoglycemia through production of an insulinlike growth factor (IGF) such as IGF-2.

- Insulin-mediated causes of hypoglycemia include insulinoma, exogenous insulin use, sulfonylurea use, and autoimmune hypoglycemia.
- Noninsulin-mediated causes of hypoglycemia include alcohol use, cortisol deficiency, childhood GH deficiency, renal failure, liver failure, sepsis, and tumors secreting IGF-2.

Clinical Features

Hypoglycemia may result in hyperadrenergic and neuroglycopenic symptoms. Hyperadrenergic symptoms include palpitations, sweating, tremor, and nervousness. Neuroglycopenic symptoms include confusion, inappropriate affect, blurred vision, diplopia, seizures, and loss of consciousness. Often, confusion or inappropriate affect are recognized by the patient's family or work colleagues. Symptoms are relieved promptly after oral nutrient intake. Patients with fasting hypoglycemia often learn to reduce symptoms by increasing the frequency of their meals; they may gain weight.

- Hypoglycemia may cause symptoms related to activation of the sympathoadrenal system and neuroglycopenia.

Diagnosis

The first essential step in the evaluation of a patient with a history suggestive of hypoglycemia is to document a low level of plasma glucose (<50 mg/dL) in the presence of symptoms and the prompt resolution of symptoms when the plasma glucose level is increased to the normal range (the Whipple triad). This can be achieved during a spontaneous episode or after provocation of symptoms by fasting. Capillary blood glucose monitoring devices are inaccurate and unreliable when used to record low blood glucose levels and should not be used to confirm hypoglycemia or the Whipple triad.

After hypoglycemia has been confirmed, the next step is to establish its mechanism (insulin-mediated or noninsulin-mediated). This is achieved by simultaneously measuring the beta-cell polypeptides, insulin, and C peptide during a hypoglycemic episode (spontaneous or provoked). In insulin-mediated hypoglycemia, insulin levels do not suppress appropriately (insulin = 6 mU/mL). In patients with hyperinsulinemia, C peptide is measured to determine whether the source of insulin is endogenous or exogenous. Endogenous insulin is secreted from the pancreas with equimolar concentrations of C peptide, whereas exogenous insulin does not contain C peptide. Thus, C peptide is not suppressed (C peptide = 200 pmol/L) in endogenous hyperinsulinemia and is undetectable in exogenous hyperinsulinemia. It is essential to measure plasma sulfonylurea levels when the person is hypoglycemic because beta-cell polypeptide levels in a patient taking sulfonylureas are indistinguishable from those associated with insulinoma. The use of sulfonylureas is not always surreptitious: it may also be the result of pharmacy error or the patient mixing up his or her medications with those belonging to a family member.

- It is essential to document the Whipple triad in all patients with suspected hypoglycemic disorder: low plasma glucose at the time of symptoms and prompt resolution of symptoms following normalization of plasma glucose level.
- Capillary blood glucose monitors should not be used to confirm hypoglycemia or the Whipple triad because they are inaccurate.
- Plasma insulin levels should be measured to determine the mechanism of hypoglycemia: insulin is not appropriately suppressed in insulin-mediated causes of hypoglycemia.
- C-peptide levels distinguish between exogenous and endogenous insulin: if the patient is injecting insulin, C-peptide levels are undetectable.
- Endogenous hyperinsulinemic hypoglycemia caused by insulinoma is indistinguishable from sulfonylurea use: plasma sulfonylurea levels should be measured in all cases of insulin-mediated hypoglycemia (while the patient is hypoglycemic).

Insulinoma

The diagnosis of insulinoma is confirmed with the demonstration of endogenous hyperinsulinemic hypoglycemia in the absence of detectable sulfonylurea in the blood. Diagnostic criteria for insulinoma include plasma concentration of insulin 6 mU/mL or greater (radioimmunoassay) and C peptide of 200 pmol/L or greater when the plasma glucose level is less than 50 mg/dL. The next step in the evaluation is an attempt at preoperative localization of the insulinoma with ultrasonography and spiral CT of the pancreas. This is not always successful because ultrasonography and CT have a detection rate for insulinoma of only 60%. The key to successful removal of an insulinoma in patients with both positive and negative preoperative localization studies is surgical exploration of the pancreas by an experienced surgeon in combination with intraoperative ultrasonography. Almost all insulinomas can be identified and excised in this manner. Patients with insulinoma who refuse surgical excision or who have persistent or recurrent malignant insulinoma may be treated with diazoxide, which inhibits insulin secretion.

- Diagnostic criteria for insulinoma are plasma insulin ≥6 mU/mL and C peptide ≥200 pmol/L when plasma glucose is <50 mg/dL and plasma sulfonylurea is undetectable.
- Preoperative abdominal ultrasonography and spiral CT of the pancreas localize approximately 60% of insulinomas.
- Intraoperative ultrasonography of the pancreas is a useful localization tool.

Postprandial Hypoglycemia

Postprandial hypoglycemia is defined as symptomatic hypoglycemia occurring 1 to 5 hours after a meal. It can occur in patients who have had gastrectomy or who have rapid gastric emptying of unknown cause. The mechanism is believed to be due to the rapid entry of glucose into the small bowel, causing a rapid increase in the plasma level of glucose and dramatic secretion of insulin. A similar syndrome may affect patients after bariatric surgery and seems to be the result of beta-cell hyperplasia. So-called reactive hypoglycemia is most likely not a true clinical entity. This disorder has been diagnosed in many patients

on the basis of the results of an oral glucose tolerance test. However, this test is not reliable: normal subjects may demonstrate low plasma levels of glucose after an oral glucose load and remain asymptomatic, symptomatic patients often do not have associated low plasma levels of glucose, and patients who have "hypoglycemia" after oral glucose frequently have normal glucose levels after a mixed meal test.

- The oral glucose tolerance test is not useful in the evaluation and diagnosis of postprandial hypoglycemia.

Therapy

Treatment is directed at the hypoglycemia and underlying cause. For patients unable to eat or drink, 1 mg of glucagon can be administered subcutaneously or intramuscularly to stimulate endogenous glucose production. Alternatively, in the appropriate setting, 25 to 50 mL of 50% dextrose may be given intravenously and repeated in 15 minutes if necessary, although this may be associated with superficial phlebitis and pain.

- Glucagon injected subcutaneously or intramuscularly may be used to treat hypoglycemia if the oral route is not available.

Multiple Endocrine Neoplasia

MEN-1

MEN-1 is a syndrome characterized by neoplasms of the parathyroid, endocrine pancreas, and anterior pituitary. It is familial and inherited as an autosomal dominant trait with high penetrance. The gene for MEN-1 belongs to the family of tumor suppressor genes and is located on chromosome 11.

Primary Hyperparathyroidism

Primary hyperparathyroidism is the most common manifestation of MEN-1, exhibiting almost 100% penetrance by middle age. Parathyroid hyperplasia is usually the underlying cause. The differential diagnosis includes familial hyperparathyroidism (positive family history with no other features of MEN-1) and familial hypocalciuric hypercalcemia. Treatment requires removal of most parathyroid tissue. Half of 1 gland may be left in situ or transplanted to the forearm to facilitate reexploration if hypercalcemia recurs.

Islet Cell Neoplasia

Islet cell neoplasia is the second most common neoplasm in MEN-1. Tumors may secrete pancreatic polypeptide (75%-85% of tumors), gastrin (60%), insulin (25%-35%), vasoactive intestinal peptide (VIP) (3%-5%), glucagon (5%-10%), and somatostatin (1%-5%). Islet cell tumors may also secrete other peptide hormones, including ACTH, CRH, and GHRH. One-third of these tumors are malignant and many are metastatic by the time of diagnosis. Malignant islet cell tumors are the leading cause of death in patients with MEN-1. Diagnosis depends on the clinical recognition and appropriate investigation of the characteristic syndromes.

Pituitary Tumors

More than 10% to 50% of patients with MEN-1 have pituitary tumors. The most common tumor is a prolactinoma. Acromegaly in MEN-1 may be due to a pituitary tumor that secretes GH or to ectopic secretion of GHRH. Similarly, Cushing syndrome in MEN-1 may be caused by an ACTH-secreting pituitary tumor or ectopic secretion of ACTH or CRH.

Other Manifestations of MEN-1

Other manifestations of MEN-1 include carcinoid tumors (secretion of serotonin, calcitonin, or CRH), thyroid or adrenal adenomas, and subcutaneous or visceral lipomas.

Screening for MEN-1

Family screening is best undertaken with the use of genetic screening if the causative mutation can be identified in the proband. Alternatively, measurement of serum calcium and PTH will identify hyperparathyroidism, the most likely initial presenting feature of MEN-1. Laboratory evaluation or imaging studies (or both) for pancreatic or pituitary tumors may be indicated in the presence of relevant symptoms. Currently, there is only scanty evidence that aggressive screening decreases the morbidity and mortality of MEN-1.

MEN-2

MEN-2 is subdivided into MEN-2A (medullary carcinoma of the thyroid [MTC], pheochromocytoma, and primary hyperparathyroidism) and MEN-2B (MTC, pheochromocytoma, mucosal neuromas, and marfanoid habitus). These 2 familial syndromes are inherited in an autosomal dominant pattern with a high degree of penetrance.

MEN-2A

MTC is the most common manifestation (>90% of cases) and is preceded by C-cell hyperplasia. Pheochromocytomas occur in about 50% of patients, and one-half are bilateral. These tumors have an increased incidence of malignancy (20%-40%). Hyperparathyroidism develops in 15% to 20% of patients.

MEN-2B

MEN-2B, unlike MEN-2A, is characterized by the absence of hyperparathyroidism and the presence of mucosal neuromas. The MTC of MEN-2B develops earlier in life and is more aggressive. Hypercalcemia may indicate bone metastases. Mucosal neuromas are the most distinctive feature of MEN-2B and may occur on the tongue, eyelids, or lips and along the gastrointestinal tract. Intestinal neuromas may cause intermittent obstruction or diarrhea.

Genetics of MEN-2

MEN-2 is caused by mutations in the RET proto-oncogene, which is present in 95% to 98% of affected persons. Screening for RET mutations allows early identification of patients at risk of MTC. This should be undertaken as early as possible in childhood. The presence of an RET mutation in a family member of a proband with MEN-2 is an indication for thyroidectomy.

Endocrinology Pharmacy Review
Lisa K. Buss, PharmD

Drug	Toxic/Adverse Effects	Drug Interactions
Hypoglycemic agents		
Insulin	Hypoglycemia, localized reaction at injection site	See following table
Sulfonylureas Glipizide Glyburide Glimepiride	Hypoglycemia, GI effects (nausea, diarrhea), dermatologic effects (pruritus, erythema, urticaria, photosensitivity)	See following table
Biguanides Metformin	GI effects (diarrhea, nausea, vomiting, abdominal cramping, flatulence), metallic/abnormal taste, lactic acidosis, decreased vitamin B_{12} levels	Cimetidine, ethanol, iodinated contrast media, cationic drugs (amiloride, digoxin, morphine, quinine, procainamide, quinidine, ranitidine, vancomycin, trimethoprim)
α-Glucosidase inhibitors Acarbose Miglitol	Flatulence, abdominal bloating & pain, diarrhea	Digoxin, sulfonylurea, digestive enzymes, intestinal absorbents
Thiazolidinediones Pioglitazone Rosiglitazone	Myalgias, respiratory effects (URI, pharyngitis, sinusitis), headache, edema	Oral contraceptives, rosiglitazone-gemfibrozil, rifampin
Repaglinide	Hypoglycemia, GI effects (nausea, diarrhea), musculoskeletal effects (arthralgia, back pain), respiratory effects (URI, sinusitis), headache	Gemfibrozil, itraconazole, ketoconazole
Nateglinide	Respiratory effects (URI, flulike symptoms), dizziness	None reported
Pramlintide	Nausea, vomiting, abdominal pain, anorexia, headache, hypoglycemia	Avoid with medications that alter GI motility (eg, anticholinergics), administer oral medications 1 h before or 2 h after pramlintide
Incretin mimetics		
Exenatide	Hypoglycemia, nausea, vomiting, diarrhea	Use with caution if medication requires rapid GI absorption; administer medications requiring a threshold concentration for efficacy (oral contraceptive, antibiotics) 1 h before exenatide
Dipeptidyl peptidase-4 inhibitor		
Sitagliptin	Headache, upper respiratory tract infection, nasopharyngitis	None reported
Osteoporosis		
Calcium	Constipation	Decreased calcium absorption with iron, fiber laxatives, fluoride, quinolones, phenytoin, tetracyclines
Vitamin D	None unless dose exceeds physiologic requirements	Decreased vitamin D absorption with mineral oil & cholestyramine
Calcitonin—salmon	Nasal symptoms (irritation, redness, sores), taste disorders, rhinitis	
Bisphosphonates Alendronate Ibandronate Risedronate	Nausea, diarrhea, abdominal pain, esophagitis, constipation	Antacids, calcium, salicylates (increased risk of GI effects); do not take other medications ≤30 min after alendronate or risedronate (≤60 min after ibandronate)
Raloxifene	Hot flashes, GI effects (nausea, dyspepsia), musculoskeletal effects (arthralgia, myalgia), weight gain, depression, insomnia	Cholestyramine, warfarin, estrogen

Endocrinology Pharmacy Review (continued)

Drug	Toxic/Adverse Effects	Drug Interactions
Osteoporosis (continued)		
Teriparatide	Arthralgia, asthenia, leg cramps, constipation, diarrhea, dizziness, syncope, increased cough, rhinitis, nausea, hyperuricemia, hypercalcemia	None identified
Thyroid agents		
Thyroid replacement	Unusual if dose is appropriate	Antacids, iron, colestipol, antidiabetic agents, cholestyramine, oral anticoagulants
Levothyroxine	If overdosed, weight loss, increased	
Liothyronine	appetite, palpitations, tachycardia, &	
Liotrix	increased pulse rate & blood pressure	
Thyroid, desiccated	may result	
Antithyroid agents	Dermatologic effects (pruritus, rash,	Warfarin
Methimazole	arthralgia), GI effects (nausea,	
Propylthiouracil	vomiting), loss of taste, headache	
Male reproductive drugs		
Androgenic agents	Females: amenorrhea or oligomenorrhea, virilism	Anticoagulants, tricyclic antidepressants
Fluoxymesterone		
Methyltestosterone	Males: gynecomastia, changes in libido,	
Testosterone	headache, depression, sleep apnea, acne, hirsutism, male pattern baldness	
Erectile dysfunction agents		
Sildenafil	Headache, flushing, dyspepsia, dizziness, priapism	Nitrates, α_1-adrenergic blockers, erythromycin, antifungals, protease inhibitors
Tadalafil		
Vardenafil		
Papaverine	Priapism, penile fibrosis, pain at injection site	
Phentolamine		
Alprostadil	Penile pain, penile fibrosis, priaprism, warmth/burning in urethra	None identified
Contraception	Thrombosis, hypertension, increased risk of cervical cancer	Antibiotics, anticoagulants, anticonvulsants, antifungals, corticosteroids, tricyclic antidepressants
Estrogens	Estrogen-related: nausea, bloating,	
Ethinyl estradiol	migraine headache, breast tenderness,	
Mestranol	edema, cervical discharge, melasma	
Progestins	Progestin-related: increased appetite,	
Ethynodiol diacetate	weight gain, fatigue, acne, hair loss,	
Desogestrel	hirsutism, depression, breast regression,	
Gestodene	hypomenorrhea	
Levonorgestrel		
Norethindrone		
Norethindrone acetate		
Norgestimate		
Norgestrel		
Norelgestromin		
Etonogestrel		
Drospirenone		

Endocrinology Pharmacy Review (continued)

Drug	Toxic/Adverse Effects	Drug Interactions
Hormone replacement therapy	Breast tenderness, breast enlargement, increased risk of ovarian cancer, possible increased risk of breast cancer	No significant interactions have been reported
Estrogens	Estrogen-related: breakthrough bleeding,	
Conjugated estrogens	spotting, thromboembolism, increased	
Esterified estrogens	risk of endometrial cancer if estrogen	
Estradiol	therapy is unopposed, increased risk	
Estropipate	of gallbladder disease	
Progestins	Progestin-related: menstrual periods	
Medroxyprogesterone	may resume, breast tumors,	
Micronized progesterone	abdominal cramping	
Antihyperlipidemic agents		
Bile acid sequestrants		
Cholestyramine	GI effects (bloating, constipation, flatulence)	Administer ≥4 h before or 2 h after other drugs
Colestipol	Same as above	Same as above
Colesevelam	Dyspepsia, constipation	
HMG-CoA reductase inhibitors		
Lovastatin	Headache, myalgia, increased liver enzymes, diarrhea, rhabdomyolysis	CYP3A4 inhibitors[a], fibrates
Pravastatin	Same as lovastatin	Cholestyramine, colestipol, fibrates, cyclosporine
Simvastatin	Same as lovastatin	Same as lovastatin
Atorvastatin	Same as lovastatin	Same as lovastatin
Fluvastatin	Same as lovastatin	Potent CYP2C9 inhibitor, warfarin
Rosuvastatin	Same as lovastatin	Cyclosporine, niacin, warfarin, gemfibrozil
Fibric acid derivatives		
Gemfibrozil	Dyspepsia, diarrhea, myopathy, hepatotoxicity, cholelithiasis	Warfarin, statins, sulfonylureas
Fenofibrate		
Nicotinic acid	GI distress, skin flushing, tingling &	Statins, colestipol, cholestyramine
Immediate-release	warmth, headache, hypotension,	
Extended-release	hyperglycemia, hyperuricemia, hepatotoxicity (>2 g/d, increased risk with extended-release form)	
Selective cholesterol absorption inhibitor		
Ezetimibe	Diarrhea, arthralgia, abdominal pain, headache, fatigue	Cyclosporine, fibric acid derivatives

Abbreviations: GI, gastrointestinal tract; URI, upper respiratory tract infection.

[a] CYP3A4 inhibitors include azole antifungals, macrolide antibiotics, diltiazem, verapamil, cyclosporine, nefazodone, fluvoxamine, ritonavir, nelfinavir, indinavir, & grapefruit juice.

Endocrinology Pharmacy Review (continued)

Drugs That Affect Hypoglycemic Effect of Insulin

Decrease Effect	Increase Effect
Acetazolamide	ACE inhibitors
AIDS antivirals	Alcohol
Albuterol	Anabolic steroids
Asparaginase	Antidiabetic agents
Calcitonin	β-Blockers
Contraceptives, oral	Calcium
Corticosteroids	Chloroquine
Cyclophosphamide	Clonidine
Danazol	Disopyramide
Diazoxide	Fluoxetine
Diltiazem	Guanethidine
Diuretics	Lithium carbonate
Dobutamine	MAO inhibitors
Epinephrine	Mebendazole
Estrogens	Pentamidine
Isoniazid	Propoxyphene
Lithium	Pyridoxine
Morphine	Salicylates
Niacin	Sulfonamides
Nicotine	Tetracyclines
Phenothiazine	
Phenytoin	
Terbutaline	
Thiazide diuretics	
Thyroid hormones	

Abbreviations: ACE, angiotensin-converting enzyme; AIDS, acquired immunodeficiency syndrome; MAO, monoamine oxidase.

Drugs That Affect Hypoglycemic Effect of Oral Hypoglycemic Agents

Decrease Effect	Increase Effect
β-Blockers	Androgens
Calcium channel blockers	Anticoagulants
Cholestyramine	Azole antifungals
Contraceptives, oral	Gemfibrozil
Corticosteroids	H$_2$ antagonists
Diazoxide estrogens	Magnesium salts
Hydantoins	MAO inhibitors
Isoniazid	Methyldopa
Niacin	Probenecid
Phenothiazine	Salicylates
Rifampin	Sulfonamides
Sympathomimetics	Tricyclic antidepressants
Thiazide diuretics	Urinary acidifiers
Thyroid agents	

Abbreviation: MAO, monoamine oxidase.

Questions

Multiple Choice (choose the best answer)

Pituitary and Adrenal Medulla

1. A 28-year-old woman, whose method of contraception is condoms, complains of secondary amenorrhea for the past 6 months. She does not "feel pregnant" and an over-the-counter pregnancy test was negative after 3 months. She has noticed a small amount of white discharge from both nipples, although not enough to dampen her undergarments. There are no other symptoms of pituitary insufficiency and no neurologic symptoms. She takes no prescription medication but used marijuana occasionally during college. On examination, there is evidence of an upper, outer quadrantanopia, most prominent on the right. The pulse is 78 beats per minute and the blood pressure is 102/64 mm Hg. There is expressible white discharge from both breasts. CT scan of the head reveals a 1.5-cm pituitary mass, which distorts the optic chiasm. Laboratory data include the following: morning cortisol 22 mcg/dL (reference range, 10-24 mcg/dL), sodium 140 mEq/L, potassium 3.8 mEq/L, free thyroxine 0.6 ng/dL (reference range, 0.8-1.8 ng/dL), hemoglobin 12.9 g/dL, and creatinine 1.1 mg/dL. What should you do next?

   a. Measure serum prolactin level.
   b. Refer her to a neurosurgeon for transsphenoidal surgery.
   c. Measure serum thyrotropin (TSH) level.
   d. Measure serum insulinlike growth factor 1 (IGF-1) level.
   e. Check visual fields.

2. A 62-year-old man complains of a 5-year history of progressive erectile failure and recent loss of libido. He acknowledges worsening fatigue and lethargy, morning headaches, and about 6.8 kg of weight gain over the past year, but he denies other neurologic symptoms. He has become less physically active in recent years because of his occupation as a business manager. His current medications include atorvastatin 20 mg daily, aspirin 81 mg daily, and atenolol 50 mg daily, prescribed for high blood pressure 10 years ago. A permanent pacemaker was inserted for heart block 6 years ago. On physical examination, he is overweight with abdominal adiposity. His pulse is 68 beats per minute and the blood pressure is 144/86 mm Hg. There is assymetric (right > left) gynecomastia, with mild breast tenderness bilaterally. Testicular examination reveals normal-sized testes (20 mL), which are soft. Male secondary sexual characteristics are normal. His visual fields are normal to confrontation. A CT scan reveals no evidence for a pituitary macroadenoma. Laboratory data include the following: total testosterone 127 ng/dL, TSH 0.8 mIU/L, free thyroxine 0.9 ng/dL, morning cortisol 18 mcg/dL, prolactin 35 ng/mL, sodium 138 mEq/L, potassium 4.2 mEq/L, and creatinine 1.2 mg/dL. What would you do next?

   a. Refer to a neurosurgeon for transsphenoidal surgery.
   b. Prescribe bromocriptine or other dopamine-agonist therapy.

   c. Prescribe testosterone supplementation through a percutaneous route.
   d. Check serum luteinizing hormone (LH) and follicle-stimulating hormone (FSH) concentrations.
   e. Perform an MRI to obtain adequate imaging of the pituitary gland.

3. A 48-year-old man complains of headaches for 3 to 4 months and erectile dysfunction for 6 to 8 months, with recent loss of libido. A CT scan conducted at the local emergency department, where he was evaluated for the headaches, reveals a possible pituitary mass. He is referred to you. At presentation, you note that he has large hands, a prominent jaw, and rather acromegalic facial features. Neither ring nor shoe size has changed recently, but his wife complains that he snores loudly. On examination, he exhibits large spade-like hands, prominent jaw, and a large tongue, but there is no gap between the front teeth. He has an enlarged thyroid, which does not feel nodular. Laboratory data include the following: growth hormone 4 ng/mL (reference range, 0-5 ng/mL), TSH 1.2 mIU/L, glucose 189 mg/dL, and hemoglobin A_{1c} 9.2%. What would you do next?

   a. Perform a glucose tolerance test to assess growth hormone suppression.
   b. Request pituitary MRI.
   c. Measure testosterone level.
   d. Check free thyroxine level.
   e. Request a lateral skull radiograph.

4. A 38-year-old woman complains of 2 months of excessive thirst, polyuria, and nocturia up to 6 times each night. She keeps a 2-L bottle of water beside her bed and drinks 8 oz (237 mL) every time she awakens at night. During the day, she estimates that she drinks up to 5 L of water and other fluids. These symptoms began a few weeks after a motor vehicle accident, in which she was involved in a head-on collision with another vehicle. She was wearing a seatbelt, her air bag deployed, and she does not believe that she struck her head on the steering wheel as a result. She was never unconscious. Emergency department evaluation demonstrated no neurologic abnormalities, and a head CT scan was negative. She had considerable chest and abdominal bruising from the seatbelt. She had some hematuria, but an abdominal CT scan was negative. She was advised to drink "plenty of fluids" but did not require hospital admission. She had a minor whiplash injury and wore a support collar for a few weeks. She denies any additional symptoms of pituitary or hypothalamic disease and has had no subsequent hematuria. Examination reveals an apparently healthy, well-hydrated woman, with no neurologic or endocrine findings. Laboratory data include the following: sodium 135 mEq/L, potassium 3.4 mEq/L, creatinine 0.8 mg/dL, TSH 2.0 mIU/L, glucose 88 mg/dL, and calcium 9.6 mg/dL. What would you do next?

a. Refer the patient for MRI of the head to assess the pituitary and hypothalamus.

b. Perform a water deprivation test.

c. Measure plasma vasopressin (ADH) concentration.

d. Measure urine osmolalities before and after desmopressin administration.

e. Advise fluid restriction to no more than 3 L daily to avoid renal "washout."

5. A 28-year-old woman is referred by a cardiologist for a possible pheochromocytoma. She has been anxious since the birth of her daughter 3 years ago, immediately before which her boyfriend left home abruptly. During the last few weeks of her pregnancy, she was hypertensive without evidence of preeclampsia. The pregnancy was terminated early with cesarean section because of pregnancy-related hypertension. In the postpartum period, she developed worsening anxiety attacks, which now occur 2 or 3 times daily, with the symptoms dominated by heart racing and palpitations, shortness of breath, fear, and nausea. In addition, she notes sweating with these spells, and she has been told that she looks pale and unwell at the time. She was prescribed a selective serotonin reuptake inhibitor (SSRI), which she took for only a few weeks because it did not seem to help. When she visited a cardiologist because of the palpitations, she had hypertension, with a blood pressure of 152/96 mm Hg on repeated testing. On examination, the pulse is 88 beats per minute, there are no cardiac murmurs, the lungs are clear, and she appears anxious but otherwise well. During a spell, she hyperventilates, appears pale and anxious, and has dilated pupils. Rebreathing into a paper bag settles the symptoms within a few minutes. At the time of the spell, her pulse was 120 beats per minute and the blood pressure was 160/100 mm Hg. Laboratory data include the following: sodium 139 mEq/L, potassium 3.9 mEq/L, glucose 88 mg/dL, and 24-hour urinary metanephrines 3.6 mg in 24 hours (reference range, <1.3 mg in 24 hours) (at least 1 spell occurred during the collection). Chest radiographs and cardiograms were negative, and Holter monitoring revealed episodes of sinus tachycardia associated with her symptoms. What would you do next?

a. Check a 24-hour urine collection for fractionated catecholamines, and check plasma metanephrine levels.

b. Request a CT scan of the adrenal glands.

c. Reassure the patient that this is not a pheochromocytoma.

d. Undertake a metaiodobenzylguanidine (MIBG) scan.

e. Measure 24-hour urinary dopamine levels.

6. A 22-year-old female college student is referred for evaluation of secondary amenorrhea over the past 3 to 4 years. She underwent menarche at age 12 and has had erratic and intermittently heavy periods since then. She has noticed increasing acne over the past 2 years, with some annoying hair growth in the mustache area, inner thigh, and central chest. She takes no medication and denies drug use. She has gained 6.8 to 9.0 kg since starting college 3 years before. She has been sexually active over the past 2 years with 1 boyfriend, and he uses condoms for contraception. On examination, she is overweight with a body mass index (BMI) of 26.8 kg/m^2. The examination findings are otherwise normal, including normal secondary sexual characteristics and modest hirsutism in the areas the patient is aware of. There is no clitoromegaly. Laboratory study results include the following: TSH 2.2 mIU/L, free thyroxine 1.2 ng/dL, estradiol 75 pg/mL, FSH 1.0 IU/L, prolactin 12 ng/mL, and pregnancy test negative. What would you do next?

a. Request MRI of the head to exclude a pituitary tumor.

b. Prescribe medroxyprogesterone, 10 mg daily for 10 days.

c. Check LH, testosterone, dehydroepiandrosterone (DHEA), and DHEA-sulfate levels.

d. Request ultrasonography of the ovaries.

e. Start estrogen replacement therapy for hypothalamic amenorrhea.

7. A 48-year-old man has noticed vision changes over the past 18 months, and his optometrist diagnosed bitemporal hemianopia. MRI demonstrated a 3.5-cm pituitary mass consistent with a pituitary adenoma, with invasion of the right cavernous sinus and distortion of the optic chiasm. The patient complains of fatigue, malaise, anorexia, and weight loss of 4.5 kg over the past 6 to 8 months. He acknowledges loss of libido and erectile dysfunction during the same period. On examination, he is pale and sallow but with no abnormal pigmentation. Secondary sexual characteristics are normal, and testicular volumes are also normal, although the testicular texture is soft. The thyroid is palpable and of normal size, and he is clinically euthyroid. There is a clinically evident bitemporal hemianopia. There are no features of acromegaly or Cushing syndrome. Laboratory data include the following: prolactin 360 ng/mL, morning cortisol 2.1 mcg/dL, free thyroxine 0.6 ng/dL, TSH 2.5 mIU/L, total testosterone 130 ng/dL, and LH 0.7 IU/L. What would be your initial management?

a. Refer for urgent surgical decompression of the pituitary tumor.

b. Start bromocriptine therapy.

c. Recommend gamma knife irradiation.

d. Start octreotide therapy.

e. Begin steroid replacement therapy.

Thyroid and Parathyroid

8. A 28-year-old woman complains of a 3-week history of palpitations and shakiness. She attributes her insomnia to her baby, born 5 weeks previously. On examination there is increased sweating, a fine tremor of outstretched hands, and a small nontender goiter. Laboratory investigations show TSH <0.002 mIU/L and free thyroxine 2.1 ng/dL (reference range, 0.8-1.8). She is breastfeeding. Which of the following investigations is indicated to help establish the diagnosis?

a. TSH receptor antibodies
b. Radioactive iodine uptake
c. Erythrocyte sedimentation rate (ESR)
d. Thyroglobulin
e. Epstein-Barr virus testing

9. A 48-year-old woman undergoes a carotid Doppler study to investigate a carotid bruit detected on physical examination. No significant carotid stenosis is discovered, but the study reveals a 1.4-cm nodule in the right lobe of the thyroid gland. She is otherwise asymptomatic and denies dysphagia, dysphonia, and dyspnea. There is no prior history of thyroid disease and a negative family history. There is no history of radiation exposure. Examination is unremarkable. No thyroid nodule is palpable. Laboratory investigations reveal a TSH of 1.2 mIU/L. What is the next step in management?

a. Perform a thyroid isotope scan.
b. Perform fine-needle aspiration (FNA) of the thyroid nodule under ultrasonographic guidance.
c. Begin levothyroxine therapy at a dose that suppresses TSH and repeat the neck examination in 6 months.
d. Advise surgical removal of the nodule.
e. Arrange a follow-up visit in 6 months to 1 year.

10. A 74-year-old woman is referred because of concerns regarding her coordination and sense of balance. Over the past year, her hearing has deteriorated and she has had several episodes of disorientation. On examination there is decreased hearing, an apathetic appearance, and some degree of delay in her tendon reflexes. Relevant laboratory results include the following: hemoglobin 9 g/dL (normochromic, normocytic), aspartate aminotransferase (AST) 60 U/L, alanine aminotransferase (ALT) 75 U/L, and creatine kinase 900 U/L. What is the next step in management?

a. Measure TSH level.
b. Perform electromyography.
c. Perform vestibular function testing.
d. Perform MRI of the head.
e. Prescribe L-dopa.

11. A 55-year-old woman with a 20-year history of type 1 diabetes mellitus is referred for management of osteoporosis, diagnosed after a wrist fracture. Bone mineral density revealed T scores of –3.6 at the femoral neck and –3.2 at the lumbar spine. Her history is remarkable for significant dyspepsia, incompletely controlled on proton pump inhibitors. Levels of serum calcium, parathyroid hormone (PTH), 25-hydroxyvitamin D (25-OH-D), and bone-specific alkaline phosphatase are normal. Which of the following would be the ideal first-line treatment in this case?

a. Parenteral bisphosphonate
b. Oral bisphosphonate
c. Recombinant PTH
d. Calcitonin
e. Vitamin D and calcium supplementation alone

12. A 44-year-old man is referred for evaluation of proximal muscle weakness and bone pain. There is no history of bowel surgery, no history of fracture, and no symptoms suggestive of malabsorption. Examination is remarkable only for quadriceps weakness and tenderness and a waddling gait. He is not taking any medications. Laboratory investigation results (and reference ranges) include the following: serum calcium 9.1 mg/dL (8.9-10.1 mg/dL), alkaline phosphatase 252 U/L (<115 U/L), PTH 11.2 pmol/L (1.0-5.2 pmol/L), 25-OH-D 30 ng/mL (8-38 ng/mL), and 1,25-dihydroxyvitamin D (1,25-[OH]$_2$-D) <22 pg/mL (22-67 pg/mL). The bone mineral density T score was –2.6 in the femoral neck. What is the next step in management?

a. Measure serum phosphate level.
b. Perform a parathyroidectomy.
c. Perform a bowel biopsy.
d. Perform a muscle biopsy.
e. Perform a positron emission tomographic (PET) scan.

13. A 64-year-old woman is referred for evaluation of hypercalcemia detected on routine testing 2 days ago. She is asymptomatic, but her serum calcium level is elevated (13.4 mg/dL). A chest radiograph shows mediastinal lymphadenopathy. Which test result does *not* support a diagnosis of granuloma-associated hypercalcemia?

a. Normal serum phosphate concentrations
b. PTH 4.8 pmol/L (reference range, 1.0-5.2 pmol/L)
c. Undetectable PTH-related peptide (PTHrP)
d. 25-OH-D 30 ng/mL
e. 1,25-(OH)$_2$-D >70 pg/mL

14. You are asked to evaluate a 25-year-old woman with hypercalcemia, fatigue, and weakness, which have been ongoing for the previous 3 months. Laboratory data (and reference ranges) include the following: serum calcium 10.2 mg/dL (8.9-10.1 mg/dL), PTH 5.2 pmol/L (1.0-5.2 pmol/L), and urinary calcium excretion 40 mg in 24 hours (20-275 mg in 24 hours). She is not known to be taking any medications, and there is no history of nephrolithiasis or fracture. Which of the following is indicated?

a. Parathyroidectomy
b. Measurement of 25-OH-D
c. Parathyroid imaging
d. Calculation of fractional calcium excretion and thiazide screen
e. Measurement of PTHrP

Adrenal Cortex and Gonads

15. A 32-year-old woman has a 2-year history of muscle weakness, weight gain, oligomenorrhea, hirsutism, easy bruising, and facial fullness. She denies other symptoms, and her periods

are normal while she takes an oral contraceptive. She is taking no other medications. On examination, the pulse rate is 88 beats per minute and regular; blood pressure is 145/95 mm Hg. She exhibits truncal obesity, plethoric facies, and mild hirsutism on the chin and neck area. There are no abdominal striae. The 24-hour urinary cortisol level is 200 mcg/dL (by high-performance liquid chromatography). What would you do next?

a. Perform a 1-mg overnight dexamethasone suppression test.
b. Measure the serum level of corticotropin (ACTH).
c. Measure morning and evening cortisol levels to assess the diurnal rhythm.
d. Request CT of the adrenal glands.
e. Request MRI of the pituitary gland.

16. A 33-year-old man sees you for the first time to discuss the possibility of having children. His puberty was delayed, and, after a detailed endocrine evaluation, he began testosterone therapy at age 14 years. He has continued to receive testosterone, and he now receives it percutaneously. He is getting married soon and hopes that he and his wife will be able to have a family "naturally." He is in good general health, with no symptoms of pituitary insufficiency and with normal erectile function. On examination he appears well. The pulse rate is 72 beats per minute, blood pressure is 110/70 mm Hg, and he has normal beard growth, normal musculature, and normal secondary sexual characteristics but soft, pea-sized testes (<1 mL bilaterally). Total testosterone is 546 ng/dL. What would you do next?

a. Request MRI of the head.
b. Measure the serum levels of LH, cortisol, and thyroid hormone.
c. Advise him to adopt or to use donor sperm, since there is no chance of recovery of testicular function.
d. Perform testicular ultrasonography.
e. Offer a trial of gonadotropin treatment, while warning him that the chance of successful restoration of fertility is low, even after prolonged gonadotropin therapy.

17. A 43-year-old man has a history of hypertension, first diagnosed at the age of 26. He also has a past medical history that includes type 2 diabetes mellitus. The hypertension is controlled with a hydrochlorothiazide diuretic and an angiotensin-converting enzyme inhibitor. On examination, the blood pressure is 144/92 mm Hg. There are no signs of Cushing syndrome. Laboratory studies show the following: sodium 140 mEq/L, potassium 3.1 mEq/L, creatinine 1.0 mg/dL, and morning cortisol 20 mcg/dL. What is the next step in management?

a. Perform CT of the abdomen to identify an adrenal mass.
b. Measure plasma renin and aldosterone levels.
c. Measure 24-hour urinary metanephrine levels.
d. Request MRI of the abdomen.
e. Perform overnight dexamethasone suppression testing.

18. A 32-year-old woman complains of a 2-year history of progressive fatigue and muscle aching. Previous assessment revealed a TSH level of 7.2 mIU/L, and she began levothyroxine therapy. Her symptoms worsened, and fibromyalgia was diagnosed. Over the past 6 months she has lost 4.5 kg, and she complains of anorexia. She has also begun to experience abdominal pain, bloating, and mild nausea, but evaluation of her gastrointestinal tract was negative and irritable bowel syndrome was diagnosed. She was prescribed an antidepressant, which she began taking 3 months ago, but she has not found it useful. She has heard that T_3 therapy or natural thyroid hormone is better than synthetic thyroid hormone. Her current medication consists of levothyroxine, 0.1 mg daily. On examination, she appears sallow and unwell, with a pulse rate of 100 beats per minute and blood pressure of 90/60 mm Hg. The thyroid gland is slightly enlarged, firm, and nontender with no nodules. No pigmentation of the buccal mucosa or skin is noted. Laboratory testing shows the following: hemoglobin 10.3 g/dL, leukocytes 9.4×10^9/L, sodium 136 mEq/L, potassium 5.1 mEq/L, TSH 5.1 mIU/L, and morning cortisol 7 mcg/dL. What would you do next?

a. Measure the serum level of ACTH.
b. Measure the serum levels of free thyroxine and triiodothyronine (T_3).
c. Request CT of the adrenal glands.
d. Perform a cosyntropin stimulation test.
e. Perform an insulin hypoglycemia test.

19. A 29-year-old woman is evaluated for hirsutism, which began in her teenage years and has worsened over the past decade. She now plucks the most prominent hairs weekly and shaves monthly. In addition, she notes hair growth increasing on her inner thighs and lower abdomen, and recently she has developed some dark hair on her central chest in addition to the periareolar hair that has been present for several years. She underwent menarche at age 11, but her periods have always been erratic, occurring at 40- to 60-day intervals. She has no current plans for pregnancy but would like to maintain that option for the future. Her past medical history includes hypothyroidism, for which she takes levothyroxine, 0.1 mg daily. Her only other medication is a daily multivitamin, although in the past she took an oral contraceptive to control her periods. She quit taking it 6 months ago because of weight gain and fluid retention. On examination, she is overweight with a body mass index (BMI) of 31 kg/m². She has normal secondary sexual characteristics, and there is moderate hirsutism affecting the upper lip, chin, anterior chest, and inner thigh. There are no signs of virilization. Laboratory evaluation shows the following results: total testosterone 45 ng/dL, dehydroepiandrosterone sulfate (DHEAS) 2.37 mcg/mL, glucose 96 mg/dL, and TSH 3.1 mIU/L. How would you treat this patient?

a. Prescribe medroxyprogesterone (10 mg for 10 days every 3 months) to induce withdrawal bleeding and spironolactone (100 mg daily) to treat hirsutism.

b. Prescribe medroxyprogesterone (10 mg for 10 days every 3 months) to induce withdrawal bleeding and metformin (1,000 mg daily) to treat hirsutism.

c. Prescribe spironolactone (100 mg daily) and a combined oral contraceptive agent.

d. Prescribe medroxyprogesterone (10 mg for 10 days every 3 months) to induce withdrawal bleeding and pioglitazone (Actos) to treat hirsutism.

e. Advise the patient to continue plucking and shaving hairs and to avoid medical therapy at this stage because the hirsutism is only moderate.

20. A 26-year-old man complains of a 2-year history of decreased libido and inability to maintain an erection. Five years ago, he noticed bilateral, nontender breast enlargement. He shaves daily, but his beard growth has always been sparse. There is no change in muscle strength or in axillary or pubic hair growth. His growth and pubertal development were normal. He takes no medication and denies illegal drug use. On examination, his secondary sexual characteristics are normal and the testes are small and firm, with no masses. He has bilateral, nontender gynecomastia. Laboratory results are as follows: total testosterone 100 ng/dL, FSH 36 IU/L, TSH 1.5 mIU/L, free thyroxine 1.0 ng/dL, and prolactin 16 ng/mL. What would you do next?

a. Request MRI of the head.

b. Request chromosome analysis.

c. Request semen analysis.

d. Measure the serum level of LH.

e. Measure the serum level of estradiol.

21. A 51-year-old man is referred for further evaluation of long-standing hypertension, which has been resistant to therapy. He also has received diagnoses and therapy for the following: hyperlipidemia, glucose intolerance, and gastroesophageal reflux disease. Current medications include aspirin, 81 mg daily; amlodipine, 5 mg daily; metoprolol, 100 mg twice daily; hydrochlorothiazide, 50 mg daily; atorvastatin, 10 mg daily; and omeprazole, 20 mg daily. On examination, his pulse rate is 68 beats per minute, the blood pressure is 150/98 mm Hg, the heart and lungs are normal, and there is no pulmonary or peripheral edema. Laboratory results are as follows: sodium 140 mEq/L, potassium 3.9 mEq/L, creatinine 1.0 mg/dL, fasting glucose 124 mg/dL, and 24-hour urinary metanephrines 0.7 mg. What would you do next?

a. Measure plasma levels of renin and aldosterone.

b. Discontinue use of antihypertensive medication for 2 weeks and measure plasma levels of renin and aldosterone.

c. Salt-load the patient and measure 24-hour urinary sodium excretion.

d. Measure 24-hour urinary potassium excretion.

e. Measure 24-hour urinary norepinephrine and epinephrine.

Diabetes and Hypoglycemia

22. A 48-year-old man is referred to you for further management of his diabetes, which he has had for the past 5 years. Initially treated with diet alone, he subsequently required additional therapy with glyburide and metformin. He is active but slightly overweight, with a BMI of 26 kg/m². He checks his blood glucose approximately 4 times a day, with readings between 100 and 180 mg/dL, and his hemoglobin A_{1c} is 8.4% (reference range, 4.0%-6.1%). One sibling has type 1 diabetes mellitus, his mother has rheumatoid arthritis, and his father has hypothyroidism. Further management could include all of the following *except*:

a. Discontinue use of glyburide; start insulin therapy.

b. Discontinue use of metformin; start insulin therapy.

c. Discontinue use of glyburide and metformin; start insulin therapy.

d. Add a thiazolidinedione.

e. Review lifestyle and diet, and attempt to modify them for 3 months before making changes.

23. You are asked to see an 18-year-old male who had a fasting glucose of 143 mg/dL during a physical fitness evaluation. He has a BMI of 22 kg/m². His hemoglobin A_{1c} is 6.7% (reference range, 4.0%-6.1%). There is no history of malaise or weight loss. Diabetes was diagnosed in his mother at an early age (24 years), and she has been using insulin since then. Urine ketones are negative as are islet cell and glutamic acid decarboxylase (GAD-65) antibodies. What should be the next step in management?

a. Refer to a dietitian for advice about caloric intake.

b. Request CT scan of the abdomen.

c. Start treatment with insulin.

d. Start treatment with metformin.

e. Observe; also screen for diabetes in other family members.

24. You have been observing a 74-year-old man with type 2 diabetes mellitus diagnosed 18 months previously, when he had a fasting glucose of 143 mg/dL. At diagnosis, his hemoglobin A_{1c} was 6.8% (reference range, 4.0%-6.1%). Dietary therapy and lifestyle modification were instituted, and the patient quit smoking. He returns seeking advice for lower extremity weakness that has developed progressively over the past 3 months in association with a weight loss of 4.6 to 6.8 kg. For the past week he has required assistance with stairs and getting out of bed. He has not experienced peripheral sensory symptoms, but thigh discomfort keeps him awake at night. Examination reveals intact reflexes at the ankle, but absent patellar reflexes, with 3/5 power in the hip flexors. Currently, his fasting glucose is 165 mg/dL and his hemoglobin A_{1c} is 7%. Which is the next step in management?

a. Electromyography

b. Blood culture

c. MRI of the thoracolumbar spine
d. Chest radiograph
e. Chest CT scan

25. A 28-year-old woman has a 6-month history of weekly episodes of light-headedness, sweating, tremor, slurred speech, and blurred vision. These symptoms occur at various times during the day but mostly before meals. They are relieved within a few minutes of drinking orange juice or eating a candy bar. There is no other notable past medical history, and she takes no medications. She has a family history of type 2 diabetes mellitus. Investigations during a spell showed the following: plasma glucose 38 mg/dL, insulin 10 mcIU/mL (reference range, 5-25 mcIU/mL), and C peptide 4.2 ng/mL (reference range, 1.5-3.5 ng/mL). Plasma glucose concentration after ingestion of orange juice was 82 mg/dL. Which of the following would be the next step in management?

a. Refer for abdominal surgery for insulinoma.
b. Request a CT scan of the abdomen.
c. Endoscopic ultrasonography because the patient may have multiple endocrine neoplasia type 1 (MEN-1).
d. Screen for the presence of sulfonylureas at the time of hypoglycemia.
e. Begin a 72-hour fast.

26. An 80-year-old woman is hospitalized after a fall at home, which resulted in a painful L2 compression fracture. Four hours after admission she has an acute confusional episode. Capillary blood glucose is 40 mg/dL and plasma glucose confirms this (43 mg/dL). Her mental state returns to normal after injection of 50 mL 10% dextrose, and subsequent plasma glucose is 95 mg/dL. Relevant laboratory data (and reference ranges) obtained with the first plasma glucose include the following: creatinine 1.6 mg/dL (0.9-1.2 mg/dL), cortisol 18 mcg/dL (10-22 mcg/dL in morning), insulin <1.4 mcIU/mL, and C peptide undetectable. Which of the following would be the next step in management?

a. Perform a cosyntropin stimulation test.
b. Get a detailed drug history.
c. Perform a 72-hour fast.

d. Administer 10% dextrose infusion for 36 hours to ensure clearance of all oral hypoglycemic agents.
e. Perform abdominal CT to localize the insulinoma.

27. A 40-year-old woman with primary biliary cirrhosis (PBC) is referred for an evaluation of her lipid status. A brother who is 10 years older has recently begun taking a lipid-lowering agent, but there is no family history of premature ischemic heart disease. The patient has been in stable health for the past 6 months with only pruritus, thought to be related to her PBC. On examination she no cutaneous features of hyperlipidemia, but she has mild scleral icterus and hepatosplenomegaly. Notable laboratory results (and reference ranges) include cholesterol 388 mg/dL, triglycerides 166 mg/dL, high-density lipoprotein cholesterol (HDL-C) 22 mg/dL, calculated low-density lipoprotein cholesterol (LDL-C) 333 mg/dL, TSH 9.5 mIU/L, creatinine 1.3 mg/dL, total bilirubin 15.5 mg/dL (<1.2 mg/dL), AST 75 U/L (<31 U/L), and alkaline phosphatase 700 U/L (<98 U/L). What treatment is indicated in this situation?

a. No therapy
b. Lipoprotein apheresis
c. A resin such as cholestyramine or colesevelam
d. Thyroid hormone replacement
e. Niacin

28. A 52-year-old man who has had diabetes for 10 years has been treated with diet, glyburide, and metformin. He has a known history of hyperlipidemia and is taking aspirin (325 mg) and simvastatin (20 mg) daily. At his annual examination, he has the following laboratory results: fasting glucose 170 mg/dL, hemoglobin A_{1c} 7.5% (reference range, 4.0%-6.1%), TSH 3.5 mIU/L, creatinine 1.3 mg/dL, cholesterol 240 mg/dL, triglycerides 280 mg/dL, HDL-C 25 mg/dL, and calculated LDL-C 159 mg/dL. Which treatment is most likely to achieve a beneficial decrease in cholesterol?

a. Add a resin such as cholestyramine or colesevelam.
b. Add gemfibrozil.
c. Change to 10 mg atorvastatin.
d. Begin thyroid hormone replacement therapy.
e. Add niacin.

Answers

1. Answer a.
The combination of secondary amenorrhea and breast secretion suggests hyperprolactinemia, although it is essential to exclude pregnancy in any woman of childbearing age in whom secondary amenorrhea develops. Causes of hyperprolactinemia include a secreting pituitary tumor, a pituitary or hypothalamic tumor causing a so-called stalk compression effect, prescription medications, marijuana and other illegal drugs, pregnancy, breastfeeding, and nipple stimulation. The presence of a pituitary mass in this patient suggests the diagnosis of a macroprolactinoma. Her low free thyroxine level raises the possibility of early hypopituitarism. Further assessment should include a more detailed biochemical evaluation of pituitary function and visual fields measurement to assess for a possible mass effect of the tumor on the optic chiasm. However, the first step in management is to confirm the presence and degree of hyperprolactinemia by measurement of the serum prolactin level since a significant elevation would strongly support the diagnosis of prolactinoma, which can be treated medically even in the presence of visual field dysfunction.

2. Answer d.
He has clear evidence of acquired hypogonadism, with symptoms, signs, and biochemical support for low testosterone concentrations. The initial evaluation of hypogonadism should be to distinguish primary (gonadal) from secondary (central) causes since this indicates the appropriate approach to further evaluation and therapy. The prolactin concentration is not high enough to strongly suggest a pituitary prolactinoma and may reflect the stress of drawing a blood sample or of concurrent illness. MRI cannot be performed in a patient with a pacemaker in situ. Although testosterone replacement would correct the low testosterone, this is not an appropriate treatment for this man with probable central hypogonadism, which may reflect his untreated sleep apnea.

3. Answer b.
He has symptoms and signs strongly suggestive of acromegaly. The normal level of growth hormone does not exclude the diagnosis, because growth hormone is secreted in a pulsatile fashion. Although a glucose tolerance test is one of the best available tests for the detection of growth hormone excess, it is not reliable (or easily interpreted) in patients with uncontrolled diabetes. Serum IGF-1 provides a better confirmatory test in these patients. Pituitary MRI is necessary, however, given the CT findings, since a large compressive tumor requires surgical debulking, independent of any hormonal effect. Assessment of pituitary function should certainly include measurement of free thyroxine in addition to TSH, but this is not a primary issue in this patient. Lateral skull radiographs can demonstrate erosion of the sella in response to pituitary tumor growth, but this is neither sensitive nor specific for acromegaly and has been replaced by the more accurate technologies of CT and MRI.

4. Answer b.
The symptoms are in keeping with diabetes insipidus (DI), which could be central or nephrogenic, but they could also be a consequence of primary (psychogenic) polydipsia. The fact that she is well hydrated and has normal levels of creatinine and electrolytes does not distinguish these diagnoses because the thirst mechanism and her free access to fluids protects her from dehydration even with complete DI. Nevertheless, her low-normal sodium, potassium, and creatinine suggest overhydration. Establishing the diagnosis is crucial, and this requires assessment of urinary concentrating capacity in response to fluid deprivation. Measurement of responsiveness to desmopressin can distinguish central from nephrogenic DI. Fluid restriction is appropriate only for primary polydipsia. MRI of the pituitary and hypothalamus is useful only if central DI is confirmed. Measurement of plasma vasopressin is possible, but it is not useful in this evaluation since the level would be low in primary polydipsia and in central DI.

5. Answer a.
The combination of spells, palpitations, hypertension, and pallor suggests catecholamine excess and is consistent with either severe anxiety and panic attacks or episodic release of catecholamines from a pheochromocytoma or paraganglioma. The elevated metanephrines level is also consistent with either diagnosis, although most pheochromocytomas would cause at least a 3-fold elevation of metanephrines above the upper limit of the reference range. Nevertheless, measuring levels of urinary fractionated catecholamines and plasma metanephrines is more sensitive and specific for assessing catecholamine excess in the evaluation of pheochromocytoma and is the appropriate next step in the evaluation of this patient. CT of the adrenals should be performed only after the diagnosis is clear since incidental adrenal tumors are common and may be misleading. Similarly, an MIBG scan is only useful to localize the source of excess catecholamines and has significant false-positive and false-negative rates.

6. Answer c.
The history is characteristic of polycystic ovarian syndrome, and the laboratory evaluation excludes central hypogonadism. Significant pituitary disease is effectively excluded by the normal prolactin and thyroid function, and assessment by MRI is not necessary. Although the ovaries are typically "cystic" in polycystic ovarian syndrome, MRI is not a useful test beecause it is neither sensitive nor specific for this diagnosis. A progesterone challenge can be useful to evaluate estrogen status, but again the results neither confirm nor refute the diagnosis. For this young woman, with no immediate desire for pregnancy, the therapeutic use of an oral contraceptive to suppress endogenous ovarian androgens makes sense. First, though, the diagnosis should be confirmed by measuring adrenal and ovarian androgens.

7. Answer e.
The patient has symptoms and signs of adrenal insufficiency, with biochemical confirmation. Consequently, he needs immediate introduction of steroid therapy before any other treatment is initiated. Although this is a large tumor with significant compression of the chiasm, his visual changes are relatively long-standing. Therefore, immediate surgical decompression may not be necessary

or worthwhile, particularly if medical therapy (bromocriptine) is available. The tumor is surgically incurable because of the invasion of the cavernous sinus. The increased concentration of prolactin is unlikely to be the result of a "stalk effect." Useful and significant shrinkage of the tumor may be achieved by dopamine agonist therapy, perhaps avoiding the need for neurosurgery. Gamma knife irradiation may be useful in the management of surgically incurable pituitary tumors, but its utility is limited close to the optic chiasm, so it would not be recommended for this tumor. The role of octreotide therapy in this context is unclear.

8. Answer a.

The differential diagnosis includes Graves disease and postpartum thyroiditis. Radioactive iodine uptake is elevated in the former and suppressed in the latter. However, this investigation is contraindicated in this setting because radioactive iodine is excreted in breast milk. The ESR may be elevated in thyroiditis but is nonspecific. Thyroglobulin is elevated in thyroiditis and in Graves disease. TSH receptor antibodies are likely to be present in Graves disease and absent in postpartum thyroiditis (>98% specificity; 90% sensitivity).

9. Answer b.

This is a thyroid incidentaloma which, given its size (>1.0 cm), should be investigated by ultrasonographically guided FNA. A history of radiation exposure to the head and neck would be a criterion for FNA even if the incidentaloma were <1.0 cm. Levothyroxine suppression therapy is not recommended; it may have adverse side effects and will not clearly distinguish benign from malignant thyroid nodules.

10. Answer a.

This patient's vertigo and deafness are uncommon manifestations of hypothyroidism. The anemia and altered liver function test results may reflect the same problem. All patients with unexplained neurologic symptoms should undergo screening for hypothyroidism.

11. Answer a.

Vitamin D and calcium supplementation alone or calcitonin administration is inadequate therapy in this situation. The patient's reflux symptoms preclude the use of an oral bisphosphonate. Parenteral bisphosphonate therapy is a reasonable option, although data are incomplete for appropriate dosage, monitoring, and frequency of administration. PTH therapy should also be considered, although typically this approach is reserved for patients for whom bisphosphonate therapy has failed.

12. Answer a.

This presentation suggests hypophosphatemia, the result of renal phosphate wasting. The new onset of the condition in a middle-aged man strongly suggests tumor-induced osteomalacia, caused by a mesenchymal tumor secreting phosphatonin, which causes renal phosphate wasting. If the diagnosis is confirmed, detection of the tumor may require multiple imaging methods. The discrepancy between 25-OH-D and 1,25-$(OH)_2$-D levels is often encountered because of the interference of phosphatonin with 1-α-hydroxylase activity.

13. Answer b.

Asymptomatic hypercalcemia in an otherwise asymptomatic patient is most often caused by primary hyperparathyroidism. If the parathyroid glands are normal, secretion of PTH is suppressed by hypercalcemia. Granulomas and some lymphomas express 1-α-hydroxylase and activate vitamin D to produce excess 1,25-$(OH)_2$-D, the mediator of the hypercalcemia. 25-(OH)-D levels are typically normal.

14. Answer d.

This patient has a mild elevation in serum calcium with an inappropriately normal PTH (ie, nonsuppressed). This would be compatible with primary hyperparathyroidism. However, if this were the case, one would expect a higher 24-hour urinary calcium excretion. Hypercalcemic hypocalciuria is a familial disorder in which the PTH receptor has a marginally elevated set point. A family history of mild asymptomatic hypercalcemia with a low fractional calcium excretion is diagnostic. A similar biochemical picture is seen with thiazide use; in fact, this patient had hypokalemia and was using diuretics for weight loss. Hypocalcemia would accompany PTH elevation due to 25-OH-D deficiency.

15. Answer b.

This patient has symptoms and signs strongly suggesting Cushing syndrome. The elevated urinary cortisol is high enough to provide a presumptive diagnosis of Cushing syndrome. Before proceeding to imaging, the most important step is to distinguish ACTH-dependent from ACTH-independent Cushing syndrome. Adrenal and pituitary imaging should be performed only when peripheral or central hypercortisolism is confirmed. Beware of plasma cortisol measurements during use of oral contraceptives, which can alter steroid-binding proteins, increasing the measured cortisol concentration.

16. Answer e.

The diagnosis is almost certainly isolated hypogonadotropic hypogonadism, and there is nothing to suggest other pituitary dysfunction. Nevertheless, at some point MRI might be worthwhile since pituitary imaging 20 years ago was far less sensitive than currently available technology. However, the main question at present is whether restoration of endogenous testicular function is possible. Although testicular fibrosis may limit functional recovery, case reports do exist of successful restoration of fertility in this situation. It is reasonable to consider pulsatile gonadotropin therapy, followed by sperm collection and storage. The alternatives of donor sperm or adoption should also be discussed during counseling.

17. Answer b.

The patient has diabetes and hypertension, but there are no other supporting features to suggest Cushing syndrome, and his plasma cortisol level is normal. However, the patient has both hypertension and hypokalemia, making Conn syndrome a possibility. Although the hydrochlorothiazide may explain the low potassium, measurement of renin and aldosterone is appropriate. Screening for pheochromocytoma by measuring urinary metanephrines may also be appropriate since sustained, young-onset hypertension is a feature of this condition. MRI is useful in the further evaluation of some adrenal masses, but abdominal CT scans are typically insufficient to identify an adenoma in Conn syndrome. However, biochemical confirmation should always precede anatomical imaging.

18. Answer d.

The patient's symptoms strongly suggest adrenal insufficiency, most likely due to Addison disease. Although ACTH concentration may be elevated, the cosyntropin test is a more sensitive and specific test for primary adrenal failure. Given the high level of clinical suspicion, the patient should begin receiving steroid replacement therapy immediately after the cosyntropin test is completed and before the results are available. Thyroid hormone concentrations are often abnormal in adrenal insufficiency, and increased thyroid hormone dosages (and particularly the use of T_3) can precipitate an adrenal crisis. A recheck of thyroid status is appropriate some weeks after starting steroid replacement therapy. CT scan of the adrenal glands is not a useful test in this condition. The insulin hypoglycemia test is unsafe in the context of adrenal failure and should not be used in this evaluation.

19. Answer c.

The patient's symptoms, signs, and biochemical profile all point to polycystic ovary syndrome. Her degree of hirsutism is troublesome and warrants antiandrogenic therapy with spironolactone. It must be emphasized that she should not become pregnant during treatment with this drug, which can influence fetal development. Consequently, she should receive an oral contraceptive rather than progesterone withdrawal therapy for her menstrual irregularity. Fluid retention and weight gain can be minimized by careful selection of a low-dose estrogen preparation, and further androgenization can be avoided with careful selection of a nonandrogenizing progestin. Weight loss through diet and exercise should be strongly recommended and supported, and insulin sensitization can be useful adjunctive treatment in some patients.

20. Answer b.

This man has a history of incomplete pubertal development and progressive hypogonadism. Biochemically, this has been shown to be primary gonadal failure, because of the high FSH level. Consequently, MRI of the head and measurement of estradiol would not be useful. His semen analysis will show azoospermia or severe oligospermia since he has hypogonadism with testicular atrophy. Consequently, this test is not necessary at this stage. The possible causes of his hypogonadism include Klinefelter syndrome, testicular irradiation or injury, chemotherapy, infectious (mumps) or autoimmune orchitis, or a degenerative condition such as dystrophia myotonica. Treatment should include testosterone replacement therapy and genetic counseling, if appropriate.

21. Answer a.

This patient has poorly controlled hypertension despite taking 3 antihypertensive agents. Exclusion of secondary causes, including hyperaldosteronism, is essential. The best test for hyperaldosteronism is measurement of plasma renin activity and aldosterone concentration. An aldosterone to renin ratio >20 strongly suggests hyper-

aldosteronism. Aldosterone antagonists and angiotensin-converting enzyme inhibitors can influence the test, and their use should be stopped before the renin and aldosterone are measured; however, the use of other antihypertensives can be continued. Although most patients with this condition are hypokalemic as a consequence of increased renal potassium wasting, measurement of urinary potassium losses is not an accurate diagnostic test and not all patients are hypokalemic. Primary hyperaldosteronism can be confirmed by measurement of 24-hour urinary sodium excretion during liberal salt intake. Measurement of urinary metanephrine levels is usually a sufficiently sensitive test to rule out pheochromocytoma.

22. Answer d.

This patient most likely has slow-onset autoimmune diabetes, suggested by his relatively young age at onset, his modest BMI, and his family history of both type 1 diabetes mellitus and the connective tissue and autoimmune diseases. Control is suboptimal at present with the use of 2 antidiabetic medications. Insulin therapy will probably be required. The addition of an insulin sensitizer is unlikely to help his control further since there is no evidence of significant insulin resistance. Combined use of sulfonylurea and insulin (as would result from answer *b*) has doubtful benefit over insulin alone.

23. Answer e.

The absence of autoantibodies does not exclude type 1 diabetes mellitus, but it makes the diagnosis less likely. His hemoglobin A_{1c} value is elevated, implying that hyperglycemia has been present for some time. His family history is a possible clue to maturity-onset diabetes of the young (MODY), and his family members should be evaluated for diabetes. Making the correct (genetic) diagnosis would help determine the correct treatment since these patients respond to insulin secretagogues but not to sensitizers.

24. Answer a.

Diabetes may cause lower extremity weakness as a result of diabetes-associated polyradiculopathy or femoral amyotrophy. In these cases, clinical findings are compatible with a lower motor neuron lesion with muscle weakness and hyporeflexia. Sensory changes are absent in amyotrophy, although myalgia is common. Weight loss is also a commonly associated finding. Because of the possibility of a paraneoplastic process, in this ex-smoker, chest imaging may also be indicated, but the diagnostic study for his current symptoms would be electromyography.

25. Answer d.

The elevated C peptide value with hypoglycemia indicates that endogenous insulin is the mediator of the hypoglycemia. A 72-hour fast is not indicated since inappropriate insulin secretion has been documented. Before embarking on surgery or localization studies for a pancreatic tumor, surreptitious sulfonylurea use should be considered and excluded.

26. Answer b.

Hypoglycemia in a hospitalized 80-year-old is unlikely to be caused by endogenous hyperinsulinemia, which is excluded by the insulin and C peptide measurements. Exogenous insulin use is also excluded on the basis of these results, which also rule out oral hypoglycemic agents. Therefore, a 72-hour fast, CT, and dextrose infusion are not indicated. A cortisol level of 19 mcg/dL excludes Addison disease. In this case, propoxyphene used as an analgesic was the cause of hypoglycemia, which, although the mechanism is poorly understood, sometimes occurs when the drug is used in patients with renal impairment.

27. Answer d.
Pharmacologic treatment of her lipids raises safety concerns with hepatic dysfunction. Lipoprotein apheresis would be the only safe intervention if treatment was felt to be necessary. Her thyroid status may not merit thyroid hormone replacement therapy in its own right, but her PBC increases the probability of progressive thyroid failure. However, in the context of dyslipidemia, correction of hypothyroidism should always be the first therapeutic step.

28. Answer b.
Niacin is poorly tolerated and may worsen glycemic control in this setting. His thyroid status is normal, so the addition of thyroxine is not recommended. In this situation, doubling the statin dose may achieve a further 10% to 20% reduction in cholesterol, but the 10-mg dose of atorvastatin has an efficacy comparable to that of 20 mg of simvastatin. Although addition of a fibrate may not achieve the targets, an improvement in both triglycerides and HDL-C could be expected, and a future increase in the statin dose is probably necessary to decrease his LDL-C to the target range.

7

Gastroenterology and Hepatology

Robert E. Sedlack, MD, MHPE
Conor G. Loftus, MD
Thomas R. Viggiano, MD
John J. Poterucha, MD

Part I

Robert E. Sedlack, MD, MHPE
Conor G. Loftus, MD
Thomas R. Viggiano, MD

Esophagus

Esophageal Function

The upper esophageal sphincter (or cricopharyngeal muscle) and the muscle of the proximal one-third of the esophagus are striated muscle under voluntary control. A transition from skeletal to smooth muscle occurs in the midesophagus. In the distal one-third of the esophagus, the muscle is smooth muscle that is under involuntary control. The lower esophageal sphincter is a zone of circular muscle located in the distal 2 to 3 cm of the esophagus. To transport food from the mouth, the esophagus must work against a pressure gradient, with negative pressure in the chest and positive pressure in the abdomen. The lower esophagus has a sphincter for unidirectional flow that prevents reflux of gastric contents. Normal esophageal motility both transports food and prevents reflux.

- The esophagus transports food against a pressure gradient and prevents reflux of gastric contents.

Normal Motility

After a person swallows, the upper esophageal sphincter relaxes within 0.5 second. A primary peristaltic wave then passes through the body of the esophagus at a rate of 1 to 5 cm/s, generating an intraluminal pressure of 40 to 100 mm Hg. Within 2 seconds after the swallow, the lower esophageal sphincter relaxes and stays relaxed until the wave of peristalsis passes through it. Next, the lower esophageal sphincter contracts again and maintains its resting tone. Two major symptom complexes result if the esophagus is unable to perform its 2 major functions: dysphagia (transport dysfunction) and reflux (lower esophageal sphincter dysfunction).

- Dysphagia: transport dysfunction.
- Reflux: lower esophageal sphincter dysfunction.

Dysphagia

Dysphagia is the defective transport of food and is usually described as "sticking." *Odynophagia* is pain on swallowing. The 3 causes of dysphagia must be distinguished: mechanical (obstructed lumen), functional (motility disorder), and oropharyngeal (faulty transfer of a food bolus to the esophagus). Answers to 3 questions frequently suggest the diagnosis (Figure 7-1): 1) What type of food produces the dysphagia? 2) What is the course of the dysphagia? 3) Is there heartburn? Dysphagia with an intermittent course is caused by a ring, a web, or a motility disorder.

- Mechanical dysphagia must be distinguished from functional dysphagia.
- Intermittent dysphagia is caused by a ring, a web, or a motility disorder.

Mechanical Cause

Mechanical obstruction occurs if the lumen diameter is less than 12 mm. The course is progressive, dysphagia with solids is greater than with liquids, and there is associated weight loss.

- Mechanical obstruction: progressive course, weight loss, and dysphagia with solids is greater than with liquids.

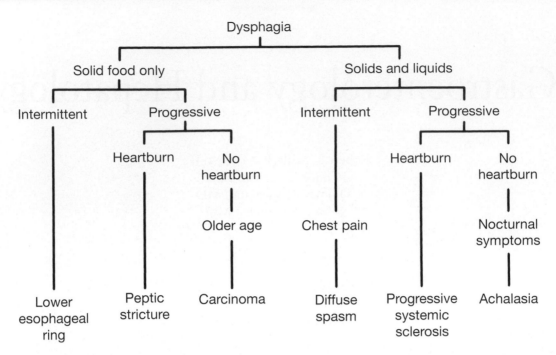

Figure 7-1. Diagnostic Scheme for Dysphagia. Obtaining answers to 3 questions (see text) often yields the most likely diagnosis. (From MKSAP VI: part 1:44, 1982. American College of Physicians. Used with permission.)

Peptic stricture results from prolonged reflux and is usually a short (<2-3 cm long) narrowing in the distal esophagus.

- Peptic stricture results from prolonged reflux, usually in the distal esophagus.

Alkali is more injurious to the esophagus than acid and can produce a lye stricture (in postgastrectomy patients, alkaline reflux can produce severe esophagitis). Do not induce vomiting after the ingestion of lye. Stricture tends to occur at the 3 physiologic narrowings where the initial passage of the corrosive may have been delayed. Bougienage or temporary stenting of the esophagus after 3 or 4 weeks may prevent occurrence of stricture. There is an increased incidence of squamous cell cancer in patients with lye stricture.

- Postgastrectomy alkaline reflux can produce severe esophagitis.
- Do not induce vomiting after the ingestion of lye.
- Lye stricture is associated with an increased incidence of squamous cell cancer.

Leiomyoma is the most common benign tumor. It is usually asymptomatic. Radiographically, a leiomyoma appears as a smooth filling defect with normal mucosa. It arises from the esophagus at a 90° angle, and its border is distinct from the esophageal wall. Perform endoscopy even if classic changes are seen on barium swallow.

The conditions that predispose to esophageal squamous cell carcinoma include achalasia, lye stricture, Plummer-Vinson syndrome, human papillomavirus, tylosis, smoking, and alcohol. In the United States, 20% of malignant tumors are squamous cell carcinoma and 80% are adenocarcinoma. Progressive dysphagia with weight loss is typical. The diagnosis is established by endoscopy with biopsy and cytology. The 5-year survival rate is only 7% to 15%; 28% of patients have lung metastases, and 25% have liver metastases. The prognosis is poor in the United States because of late detection of the tumor. In China, the prognosis is excellent because of screening programs and early detection.

Squamous cell carcinoma is more radiosensitive than adenocarcinoma. Surgery is difficult for proximal lesions. Surgery and preoperative irradiation are used for lesions in the distal one-third of the esophagus. Palliation strategies include laser endoscopy, bougienage, and stent placement. Chemotherapy has not traditionally been beneficial. Squamous cell carcinoma can produce ectopic parathyroid hormone; therefore, hypercalcemia does not mean that the tumor is unresectable.

- Conditions that predispose to esophageal squamous cell cancer: achalasia, lye stricture, Plummer-Vinson syndrome, human papillomavirus, tylosis, smoking, and alcohol.
- Esophageal malignancies are usually unresectable; palliative treatment includes laser endoscopy, bougienage, and stent placement.
- The 5-year survival of US patients is only 7%-15%.

A *lower esophageal ring* (Schatzki ring) is a mucosal membrane that marks the junction of the esophageal mucosa and gastric mucosa. Muscular rings are rare. Patients present with intermittent dysphagia with solids or with a sudden obstruction from a food bolus ("steak house syndrome"). On radiographs, a lower esophageal ring is a thin annulus at the esophagogastric mucosal junction. Treatment is dilatation.

- Esophageal ring: intermittent dysphagia and food bolus impaction.
- Treatment is dilatation.

An *esophageal web* is a membrane of squamous mucosa that occurs anywhere in the esophagus. Patients present with intermittent dysphagia. *Plummer-Vinson syndrome* is a cervical esophageal web and iron deficiency anemia. It is associated with a 15% chance of oropharyngeal or esophageal squamous cell cancer.

- Esophageal web: intermittent dysphagia.
- Plummer-Vinson syndrome: cervical esophageal web and iron deficiency anemia, with a 15% chance of oropharyngeal or esophageal squamous cell cancer.

Functional Cause

Functional obstruction (motility disorders) is characterized by dysphagia with solids and liquids and an intermittent course; weight loss may or may not occur. The 3 important motor abnormalities of the esophagus are achalasia, diffuse esophageal spasm, and scleroderma.

- Functional obstruction: intermittent dysphagia with solids and liquids, with or without weight loss.

Achalasia results from esophageal denervation, specifically the degeneration of Auerbach ganglion cells. Chest radiography shows an air-fluid level. Barium swallow fluoroscopy shows a dilated esophagus with a beak-like tapering. The motility pattern is characterized by incomplete relaxation of the lower esophageal sphincter, hypertensive lower esophageal sphincter (usually without reflux), and aperistalsis in the esophageal body (most important feature). Patients with achalasia should be examined endoscopically because cancer of the esophagogastric junction may have the radiographic appearance and motility pattern of achalasia (*pseudoachalasia*). A clue would be an older patient with dysphagia and heartburn. Treatment is with surgical methods (myotomy), with injection of botulinum toxin into the lower esophageal sphincter, or more commonly with pneumatic dilatation (rather than bougienage). Pneumatic dilatation is as effective as Heller myotomy. Botulinum toxin blocks the release of acetylcholine from presynaptic cholinergic neurons and decreases lower esophageal pressure for 3 to 12 months. Botulinum toxin provides short-term relief of symptoms, is safe, and has few side effects. Currently, it is given to elderly patients and to patients who have a high surgical risk.

In Brazil, the parasite *Trypanosoma cruzi* (which causes Chagas disease) produces a neurotoxin that destroys the myenteric plexus. Esophageal dilatation identical to that of achalasia, megacolon, and megaureter occurs in Chagas disease.

- Achalasia: chest radiography shows air-fluid level.
- Dilated esophagus with beak-like tapering on barium swallow fluoroscopy.
- Most important motility pattern in achalasia: aperistalsis in the esophageal body.
- Endoscopically examine patients who have achalasia.
- Treat achalasia with surgery, botulinum toxin injection, or pneumatic dilatation.

- Chagas disease has esophageal dysfunction identical to that of achalasia.

Patients with *diffuse esophageal spasm* usually present with chest pain but may have intermittent dysphagia, which is aggravated by stress and hot or cold liquids. Barium swallow fluoroscopy demonstrates a corkscrew esophagus. Motility studies demonstrate simultaneous contractions of high amplitude in the body of the esophagus. If the patient is asymptomatic during the test, motility may be normal. The lower esophageal sphincter is hypertensive or has defective relaxation in one-third of patients. Medical treatment (nitrates, anticholinergic agents, and nifedipine) has unpredictable results. Surgical treatment is long myotomy.

- Diffuse esophageal spasm usually causes chest pain.
- It is aggravated by stress and hot or cold liquids.
- Barium swallow fluoroscopy shows a corkscrew esophagus.
- Medical treatment has unpredictable results.

Esophageal involvement with *scleroderma* is associated with Raynaud phenomenon. Barium swallow fluoroscopy shows a common esophagogastric tube. Aperistalsis in the body of the esophagus and incompetence of the lower esophageal sphincter, which causes severe reflux, is demonstrated with motility studies.

- Scleroderma: Raynaud phenomenon, aperistalsis, and reflux.

Oropharyngeal Dysphagia

Oropharyngeal dysphagia is the result of faulty transfer of a food bolus from the oropharynx to the esophagus caused by structural abnormalities or disorders of either neural regulation or skeletal muscle (Table 7-1). Patients with oropharyngeal dysphagia present with high esophageal dysphagia associated with coughing, choking, or nasal regurgitation. After the presence of oropharyngeal dysphagia is recognized, other associated symptoms may lead to the diagnosis of the underlying illness (eg, a young person with oropharyngeal dysphagia, central scotoma, and neurologic symptoms has multiple sclerosis).

- Oropharyngeal dysphagia is the result of faulty transfer of a food bolus from the oropharynx to the esophagus caused by structural or neuromuscular disorders.
- Patients present with cervical esophageal dysphagia associated with coughing, choking, or nasal regurgitation.

Gastroesophageal Reflux Disease

Reflux

The lower esophageal sphincter is the major barrier to reflux. This sphincter is a 2- to 4-cm–long specialized segment of circular smooth muscle in the terminal esophagus. The pressure of this sphincter varies markedly during the day, but the normal resting pressure is 15 to 30 mm Hg. Swallowing causes the pressure to decrease promptly (within 1-2 seconds after the onset of swallowing) and the sphincter to remain relaxed until the peristaltic wave passes over it. The sphincter then contracts to maintain the increased resting

Table 7-1   Causes of Oropharyngeal Dysphagia

Muscular Disorders	Neurologic Disorders	Structural Causes
Amyloidosis	Amyotrophic lateral sclerosis	Cervical osteophytes
Dermatomyositis	Cerebrovascular accident	Cricopharyngeal dysfunction
Hyperthyroidism	Diphtheria	Goiter
Hypothyroidism	Huntington disease	Lymphadenopathy
Myasthenia gravis	Multiple sclerosis	Zenker diverticulum
Myotonia dystrophica	Parkinson disease	
Oculopharyngeal myopathy	Polio	
Stiff-man syndrome	Tabes dorsalis	
	Tetanus	

pressure that prevents reflux. The pressure of the lower esophageal sphincter decreases markedly for 2 hours after a meal. Transient relaxations of the lower esophageal sphincter cause some gastroesophageal reflux to occur in everyone during the day but do not cause symptoms or esophagitis. Patients with clinically symptomatic reflux or inflammation have more frequent transient relaxations of the lower esophageal sphincter of unknown cause and have more frequent and longer episodes of reflux.

- Lower esophageal sphincter pressure decreases for 2 hours after a meal.
- Patients with clinically symptomatic reflux show relatively frequent, transient relaxations of the lower esophageal sphincter.

The degree of tissue damage is the real concern in gastroesophageal reflux disease (GERD). Factors that determine whether reflux esophagitis occurs include the frequency of transient relaxations of the lower esophageal sphincter, the volume of gastric contents, the rate of gastric emptying (if delayed, reflux may develop), the potency of the refluxate (acid, pepsin, and bile), the efficiency of esophageal clearance (motility and salivary bicarbonate), and the resistance of esophageal tissue to injury and the ability to repair it.

The evaluation of esophagitis is designed to answer 4 important questions (Table 7-2): 1) Does the patient have reflux and, if so, how severe? 2) Does the patient have esophagitis and, if so, to what extent? 3) Are the patient's symptoms due to reflux? 4) What is the mechanism of reflux?

For most patients, the medical history is sufficiently typical to warrant a trial of therapy without expensive tests being conducted. However, testing should be performed if patients have an atypical medical history, refractory symptoms, long-standing reflux, dysphagia, iron deficiency anemia, weight loss, or possible complications of esophagitis. Test elderly patients who have onset of reflux.

Atypical symptoms of GERD include noncardiac chest pain, asthma, chronic cough, and hoarseness. Reflux is the most common cause of noncardiac chest pain. Asthmatic patients with coexisting reflux should receive treatment for reflux because it may improve control of respiratory symptoms. Reflux should be considered in asthmatic patients who have postprandial or nocturnal wheezing.

Complications of reflux include ulceration, bleeding, stricture, aspiration, Barrett esophagus, and adenocarcinoma of the esophagus.

- For most patients, the medical history is sufficiently typical to warrant a trial of therapy without tests.
- Testing should be performed if patients have an atypical medical history, refractory symptoms, long-standing reflux, dysphagia, iron deficiency anemia, weight loss, or possible complications of esophagitis. Test elderly patients who have onset of reflux.
- Atypical symptoms of GERD: noncardiac chest pain, asthma, chronic cough, and hoarseness.
- Complications of gastroesophageal reflux: ulceration, bleeding, stricture, aspiration, Barrett esophagus, and adenocarcinoma of the esophagus.

Barrett Esophagus

Barrett esophagus is a complication of chronic gastroesophageal reflux in which the normal esophageal squamous mucosa is replaced by columnar epithelium. Patients with Barrett esophagus are at increased risk of adenocarcinoma developing in this columnar epithelium. Patients with Barrett esophagus should have aggressive antireflux treatment. Although the matter is controversial, most experts recommend a screening endoscopy in high-risk patients (older than 50 years, Caucasian, and male) with chronic reflux for more than 5 to 7 years. If the mucosal characteristics are seen endoscopically, biopsies are needed to confirm the diagnosis as well as to look for

Table 7-2   Evaluation of Esophagitis

Question	Tests for Reflux
Is reflux present?	pH probe, isotope scan[a]
Is esophagitis present?	Biopsy, endoscopy[a]
Are symptoms due to reflux?	Acid perfusion (Bernstein test)
What is the mechanism of reflux?	Motility

[a] The first test in this pair is more sensitive than the second.

dysplasia. There is some debate on surveillance frequency after the diagnosis is made, but in general, after dysplasia has been excluded on 2 endoscopies 1 year apart, the screening interval can be increased to every 3 years. If low-grade dysplasia is identified at any time, the screening frequency should be increased to every year. If high-grade dysplasia is identified (and confirmed by 2 pathologists), the patient should be referred for an esophagectomy. Photodynamic therapy, or another mucosal ablation technique, could also be considered for patients who are not surgical candidates.

- Barrett esophagus predisposes to adenocarcinoma.
- Esophagogastroduodenoscopy should be performed to screen for Barrett esophagus in high-risk patients (older than 50 years, Caucasian, and male) with chronic reflux for more than 5-7 years.

Tests for Reflux
During barium swallow fluoroscopy, reflux of barium occurs in 60% of patients with esophagitis but also in 25% of control subjects. It is a qualitative test and does not distinguish between normal and abnormal reflux. Upper gastrointestinal radiography is used primarily as a screening test to exclude other diagnoses (eg, ulcer) and to identify complications of reflux (eg, strictures, ulcers, and cancer or mass). Radiography may not detect Barrett esophagus.

- Reflux of barium occurs in 60% of patients with esophagitis but also in 25% of control subjects.

Esophagoscopy is the definitive test if gross inflammation is present. However, 40% of patients may have symptomatic reflux with no gross inflammation. This is the preferred first test for long-standing cases of reflux to rule out Barrett esophagus. It is also the first test for patients with reflux without dysphagia.

- Esophagoscopy is the test preferred first for long-standing cases of reflux to rule out Barrett esophagus.
- Esophagoscopy is the first test for patients with reflux without dysphagia.

Esophageal biopsy findings in patients with reflux but without gross esophagitis include elongation of the basal cell layer and papillae. Esophagoscopy and distal esophageal biopsies are about 60% sensitive for detecting reflux. Eosinophilia in the biopsy specimen is 100% sensitive for the diagnosis of esophagitis. If Barrett esophagus is found, biopsy specimens should be obtained from along the length of Barrett epithelium as surveillance for dysplasia (premalignant changes) or malignancy.

- Biopsy may detect esophagitis when gross inflammation is not present.
- With Barrett esophagus, it is important to obtain biopsy specimens from along the length of the mucosa as surveillance for dysplasia (premalignant changes) or malignancy.

Monitoring of the pH in the distal esophagus of patients during a 24-hour period of normal routine allows a more physiologic evaluation of reflux during daily activities. This test is valuable for patients with atypical symptoms, reflux symptoms refractory to therapy, a non-diagnostic evaluation, or pulmonary symptoms.

- With 24-hour pH monitoring, a more physiologic evaluation of reflux during daily activities is possible.
- This test is valuable for patients with atypical symptoms.

Esophageal impedance testing can be used to detect the presence of nonacidic reflux in patients who are receiving proton pump inhibitor therapy or who have achlorhydria or bile reflux.

The acid perfusion test (Bernstein test) involves administering a saline perfusion for 10 minutes, which should not cause symptoms, and then infusing 0.1 N hydrochloric acid to determine whether the pain is reproduced. If heartburn and chest pain occur with acid instillation, treat for reflux.

- If heartburn and chest pain are reproduced with acid instillation, treat for reflux.

Esophageal manometry is reserved for patients with suspected esophageal motility disorders or for preoperative evaluation of surgical candidates.

- Esophageal manometry is reserved for suspected esophageal motility disorders.

Treatment of Reflux
The treatment of GERD is divided into 3 phases:

Phase 1 therapy includes lifestyle modifications. The patient should elevate the head of the bed 6 inches, modify the diet so it contains less fat and more protein, eat 3 meals a day, not eat for 3 hours before reclining, lose weight if overweight, and avoid specific foods (fatty foods, chocolate, alcohol, citrus juices, tomato products, coffee, and carminatives). The patient should stop smoking and avoid alcohol. Avoid drugs that decrease pressure in the lower esophageal sphincter: anticholinergic agents, sedatives, tranquilizers, theophylline, progesterone or progesterone-containing birth control pills, nitrates, β-adrenergic agonists, and calcium channel blockers. Therapy is with antacids or alginic acid 30 minutes after meals and at bedtime.

Phase 2 therapy includes drugs that decrease gastric acid output. All histamine (H_2) receptor antagonists are equally effective, and a twice-daily dose is preferable for treating gastroesophageal reflux. Proton pump inhibitors (eg, omeprazole) are the most effective agents to relieve symptoms and to promote mucosal healing. It is best to treat gross esophagitis for 6 weeks. Long-term use of these agents is safe. Drugs that increase lower esophageal sphincter pressure and esophageal clearance (eg, metoclopramide and bethanechol) have a limited role in treating reflux and often cause side effects.

Phase 3 therapy includes antireflux surgery, which is reserved for younger patients who want to avoid lifelong medical treatment and for patients who have reflux that is refractory to medical therapy or who develop complications. Nissen fundoplication is the preferred operation; fundoplication increases lower esophageal sphincter pressure. Although a new endoscopic suturing procedure has been developed, its long-term results are not available.

- Phase 1 therapy: modify lifestyle, avoid drugs that decrease pressure in the lower esophageal sphincter, and use antacids as the first line of treatment.
- Phase 2 therapy: H_2-blockers or omeprazole.
- Phase 3 therapy: antireflux surgery is reserved for younger patients who want to avoid lifelong medical treatment and for patients who have reflux that is refractory to medical therapy or who develop complications.

Noncardiac Chest Pain

Chest pain is a frightening symptom, and patients are often referred to internists and gastroenterologists when the findings of a cardiac evaluation are negative for cardiac disease. Internists must understand the limitations of the diagnostic studies used to evaluate noncardiac chest pain. First, important cardiac disease must be ruled out. GERD is the most common cause of noncardiac chest pain, but esophageal pain may be due to a motor disorder (eg, spasm) or esophageal inflammation (eg, infection or injury). Esophageal spasm can closely mimic angina. Esophagogastroduodenoscopy is used to rule out mucosal disease (eg, inflammation, neoplasms, and chemical injury). An esophageal motility study is performed to look for motor disorders (eg, esophageal spasm and "nutcracker esophagus"), and 24-hour pH monitoring can be used to document the presence of reflux and its correlation with episodes of chest pain. Therapy for noncardiac chest pain includes avoidance of precipitants. Antacids, H_2 receptor antagonists, and proton pump inhibitors may be beneficial for patients with reflux. Sublingual nitroglycerin or calcium channel blockers are sometimes helpful in motor disorders, but their efficacy is unproven. If appropriate, reassurance that cardiac disease is not present may be all that is necessary.

- For all chest pain, first rule out important cardiac disease.
- GERD is the commonest cause of noncardiac chest pain.
- Esophageal spasm can closely mimic angina.
- Esophagogastroduodenoscopy is used to detect mucosal disease.
- Motility studies are used to detect motility disorders.
- Use of 24-hour pH monitoring documents episodic reflux and correlation with symptoms.
- Sublingual nitroglycerin or calcium channel blockers are sometimes helpful.

Infections of the Esophagus

Patients with immunodeficiency disorders (acquired immunodeficiency syndrome [AIDS]), diabetes mellitus, malignancies (especially lymphoma and leukemia), or esophageal motility disorders are susceptible to opportunistic infections of the esophagus. Patients with these infections present with odynophagia. The most important infections to recognize are those caused by *Candida*, herpesvirus, or cytomegalovirus. In Candidal infection, barium radiography shows small nodules in the upper one-third of the esophagus, and endoscopy shows cottage cheese–like plaques. Diagnosis is made by demonstrating pseudohyphae on potassium hydroxide preparations. Treatment is with nystatin or clotrimazole for colonization and

ketoconazole or fluconazole for esophagitis. Rarely, amphotericin B is used. In herpesviral infection, barium radiography and endoscopy show small discrete ulcers without plaques. Diagnosis is based on finding intranuclear inclusions (Cowdry type A bodies) in biopsy specimens from an edge of the ulcer. Treatment is with acyclovir. In cytomegaloviral infection, radiography and endoscopy show severe inflammation with large ulcers. Intranuclear inclusions may be seen in biopsy specimens from the ulcer base, but viral cultures are unreliable. Treatment is with ganciclovir or foscarnet (if resistant to ganciclovir).

- Immunosuppressed patients with opportunistic infections present with odynophagia.

Other Esophageal Problems

Medication-Induced Esophagitis

Patients with medication-induced esophagitis present with odynophagia (or, less frequently, dysphagia). Pill esophagitis is more likely to occur if there is abnormal motility, stricture, or compression (left atrial enlargement). It is more common in the elderly and is recognized as inflammation in the midesophagus, with sparing of the distal esophagus. Medications commonly associated with esophagitis include tetracycline, doxycycline, quinidine, potassium supplements, bisphosphonates (alendronate and risedronate), ferrous sulfate, and ascorbic acid. The use of these medications in patients with known esophageal strictures or symptoms of dysphagia should be avoided if possible.

- Midesophageal inflammation is associated with abnormal motility, stricture, or compression and is more common in the elderly.
- Medicines responsible for esophagitis: tetracycline, doxycycline, quinidine, potassium supplements, bisphosphonates (alendronate and risedronate), ferrous sulfate, and ascorbic acid.

Mallory-Weiss Syndrome

Mallory-Weiss syndrome is mucosal laceration at the gastric side of the esophagogastric junction. It accounts for about 10% of the cases of upper gastrointestinal tract bleeding: 75% of the patients have a history of retching or vomiting before bleeding and 72% have diaphragmatic hernias. In 90% of the patients, the bleeding stops spontaneously. Vasopressin, endoscopic injection, or electrocautery may control bleeding. Surgical treatment for persistent bleeding is rarely necessary. Angiography with intra-arterial infusion of vasopressin is successful in 70% of patients with continued bleeding.

- Mallory-Weiss syndrome: mucosal laceration at the esophagogastric junction.
- Accounts for about 10% of cases of upper gastrointestinal tract bleeding. Bleeding stops spontaneously in 90%.
- Among patients with Mallory-Weiss syndrome, 75% have a history of retching and vomiting before bleeding.

Esophageal Perforation

Esophageal perforation commonly occurs after dilatation in an area of stricture. Spontaneous perforation of the esophagus (Boerhaave syndrome) follows violent retching, often after an alcoholic binge. It also occurs after heavy lifting, defecation, seizures, and forceful labor (childbirth). The most common site of perforation is the left posterior part of the distal esophagus. If pleural fluid is present, it may have an increased concentration of amylase. Zenker diverticulum, cervical osteophytes (difficult intubations), and endoscopy (intubation) are causes of perforation of the cervical esophagus.

- Esophageal perforation commonly occurs after dilatation.
- Boerhaave syndrome follows violent retching, often after an alcoholic binge.

Stomach and Duodenum

Peptic ulcers are defects in the gastric or duodenal mucosa that result from an imbalance between the digestive activity of acid and pepsin in the gastric juice and the host's protective mechanisms to resist mucosal injury. Peptic ulcers are categorized as being associated with 3 possible etiologic factors: 1) *Helicobacter pylori*; 2) nonsteroidal anti-inflammatory drugs (NSAIDs), including aspirin; or 3) miscellaneous causes. Miscellaneous causes include ulcers due to hypersecretion from gastrinomas (Zollinger-Ellison syndrome), idiopathic hypersecretion, and duodenogastric reflux of gastric mucosal barrier–breaking agents such as bile salts or lysolecithin. Recent reports estimate that less than 5% of ulcers have a miscellaneous cause. Thus, at least 95% of peptic ulcers are due to either *H pylori* or NSAIDs.

Helicobacter pylori

The Organism

H pylori is a gram-negative, spiral-shaped microaerophilic bacillus that contains 4 to 6 unipolar, sheathed flagella. This fastidious organism resides beneath and within the mucous layer of the gastric mucosa and produces several enzymes, such as urease and mucolytic proteases, that are important for its survival and pathogenic effect. After it has been ingested, the organism moves into and through the mucous layer of the stomach. It has been postulated that several virulent factors are needed for successful colonization of the gastric mucosa, including the organism's motility, adhesins, proteases, phospholipases, cytokines, cytotoxins, and urease. Urease is thought to protect the organism from the acidic environment. After colonization, the organism multiplies in the gastric mucous layer. Defense mechanisms may help control the infection, but unless treated, the organism remains in the gastric mucous layer for life.

H pylori causes persistent gastric infection and chronic inflammation. Ingestion of *H pylori* can cause acute gastritis symptoms (nausea, vomiting, and dyspepsia), but within weeks to months after infection, a chronic superficial gastritis develops, and after years to decades, chronic atrophic gastritis or gastric malignancy may develop.

Epidemiology

In the United States, *H pylori* has an age-related prevalence, occurring in 10% of the general population younger than 30 and in 60% of those older than 60. *H pylori* is present in 40% to 50% of the general population overall; it is more prevalent among blacks and Hispanics, poorer socioeconomic groups, and institutionalized persons. In developing countries such as India and Saudi Arabia, 50% of the population is infected by age 10 and 70% by age 20, and 85% to 95% of the population overall is infected. Evidence of person-to-person transmission includes clustering within families, higher than expected prevalence among institutionalized persons, transmission by endoscopy and biopsy, and a higher prevalence of infection among gastroenterologists. The fecal-oral route of transmission has been postulated, and indeed, *H pylori* has been isolated from human feces.

Associated Diseases

Active Chronic Gastritis

H pylori infection (type B gastritis) is found universally in patients with active chronic gastritis that is not associated with autoimmunologic mechanisms (type A gastritis—pernicious anemia) or chemical injury (alcohol, NSAIDs, and bile salts). *H pylori*–induced active chronic gastritis is the most common type of chronic gastritis, and in some patients, it may progress to chronic atrophic gastritis. An important concept is that *H pylori*–induced gastritis is the basic disease, and the development of duodenal or gastric ulcers or malignancy is a complication of the gastritis.

Duodenal Ulcer

H pylori is found in 60% to 95% of patients with duodenal ulcers. The most important link between *H pylori*–induced gastritis and the development of duodenal ulcers is the presence of gastric metaplasia in the duodenal bulb. Some data suggest that the metaplastic cells must be infected by *H pylori* to permit the development of duodenitis or duodenal ulcer. Among *H pylori*–positive patients with duodenal ulcer who do not receive treatment, most have ulcer relapse within 1 year. However, if the infection is eradicated, the rate of relapse approaches zero. *H pylori* infection causes an increase in basal and meal-stimulated gastrin release. Asymptomatic carriers of the bacillus may have a protective mechanism that prevents the hypersecretion of gastric acid. Enhanced gastric acid secretion occurs only in ulcer patients.

Gastric Ulcer

H pylori is found in about 80% of patients with gastric ulcer. Eradication of the bacteria decreases the relapse rate of gastric ulcers.

Gastric Tumors

Studies from the United States and Great Britain have established a strong association between *H pylori* infection (diagnosed through serum samples) and the emergence of noncardia gastric adenocarcinoma. It has been postulated that *H pylori* gastritis progresses to atrophic gastritis, and, in the presence of other risk factors, gastric adenocarcinoma eventually develops. This appears to be a rare occurrence. A cause-and-effect relationship has not been established, and further studies are needed to determine the exact role of *H pylori* in the development of gastric adenocarcinoma.

H pylori has also been associated with MALT lymphoma of the stomach. Of 450 patients with *H pylori*–positive gastritis, 125 (28%) had mucosal lymphoid follicles and 8 (1.8%) had B lymphocytes infiltrating the epithelium, consistent with the development of early lymphoma. Simple eradication of the *H pylori* infection can induce regression or even complete remission in a significant percentage of these early lymphomas.

Nonulcer Dyspepsia

Nonulcer dyspepsia is common, affecting about 20% of the US population. Among persons with functional dyspepsia, approximately 50% are infected with *H pylori*, which is similar to the prevalence of *H pylori* in asymptomatic persons. There is no convincing evidence that treatment of *H pylori*–positive patients with nonulcer dyspepsia results in marked clinical improvement.

Diagnostic Tests for H pylori *Infection*

Various diagnostic tests are available for determining whether *H pylori* infection is present. The choice of which test to use is determined by the clinical setting and the cost.

Serology

H pylori produces not only a local immune response but also a systemic immune response. Current detection methods exist for antibodies of the IgG, IgA, and IgM classes. Serologic testing is the most cost-effective, noninvasive way to diagnose primary *H pylori* infection, but serologic results remain positive over time, which limits the usefulness of this test in follow-up evaluation. The sensitivity is 95%, the specificity is 90% to 95%, and the cost is $40 to $100.

Breath Test

A radiolabeled dose of urea is given orally to the patient. If *H pylori* is present, the urease splits the urea and radiolabeled carbon dioxide is exhaled. The advantage of this test is that it is quick, easy to perform, and does not require endoscopy. The sensitivity is 95% to 98%, the specificity is 95% to 98%, and the cost is $100 to $200.

Biopsy Urease Tests

A biopsy specimen is impregnated into agar that contains urea and a pH indicator. As the urea is split by *H pylori*–produced urease, the pH of the medium changes the color of the agar from yellow to red. This test depends on bacterial urease: the more organisms present, the more rapidly the test becomes positive. The sensitivity is 95%, the specificity is 98%, and the cost is $20 (plus the cost of endoscopy to obtain tissue).

Stool Antigen Test

The *H pylori* stool antigen test is simple and noninvasive and can be used to assess the success of eradication efforts. The sensitivity is 94%, and the specificity is 92%.

Histologic Examination

An advantage of histologic examination is being able to evaluate the underlying inflammatory reaction. *H pylori* can be demonstrated with the following stains: Gram, hematoxylin-eosin, Giemsa, and Warthin-Starry silver. The sensitivity is 98%, the specificity is 98%, and the cost is $250.

Culture

Culturing *H pylori* is tedious and expensive and should be reserved for special circumstances (eg, if an antibiotic-resistant organism is suspected or if virulence testing is being done). The sensitivity is 90% to 95%, the specificity is 100%, and the cost is $150.

Currently, because many symptomatic patients undergo endoscopy, histologic examination and biopsy urease tests are used most commonly in the initial evaluation. Newer, inexpensive serologic tests that can be performed in minutes are being investigated.

Treatment

With an *H pylori*–positive duodenal or gastric ulcer, the treatment goal is to heal the ulcer and eradicate (not suppress) the bacteria. Combination therapy with antisecretory agents and antimicrobial therapy for *H pylori* is most effective. There has been extensive research to determine the simplest and most efficacious agents for combination therapy, and specific recommendations for treatment regimens are constantly changing. The following general principles should guide treatment:

1. All patients with gastric or duodenal ulcer who are infected with *H pylori* should receive combination therapy.
2. Patients with a well-documented ulcer who are infected with *H pylori* but whose disease is in remission with maintenance antisecretory therapy should receive combination therapy; then maintenance antisecretory therapy will not be necessary.
3. Maintenance antisecretory therapy is unnecessary except for patients with recurrent *H pylori*–negative ulcers and for some patients with a previous history of bleeding from an ulcer.
4. Currently, treatment is not recommended for nonulcer dyspepsia and asymptomatic *H pylori*–infected patients.

NSAID-Induced Ulcers

NSAIDs inhibit gastroduodenal prostaglandin synthesis, which results in decreased secretion of mucus and bicarbonate and reduced mucosal blood flow. NSAID-induced ulcers occur more commonly in the stomach than in the duodenum. They are located typically in the prepyloric area or antrum of the stomach.

The risk of peptic ulcer disease with NSAIDs is dose dependent. It is important for physicians to understand that the anti-inflammatory properties of NSAIDs predispose patients to ulceration (prostaglandin inhibition) and that there are different dose-response relationships for the analgesic and anti-inflammatory properties of NSAIDs. The maximal analgesic effect plateaus well below the effective anti-inflammatory dose. Low doses of aspirin or NSAIDs give pain relief but have little anti-inflammatory activity. The newer NSAIDs have been marketed with more convenient (less frequent) dosing intervals and in dosages that have marked anti-inflammatory activity. Thus, the use of newer NSAIDs may subject the patient to an increased risk of ulcer without providing increased analgesia. Selective cyclooxygenase (COX)-2 inhibitors have been shown to decrease the rate of ulcer formation as well as ulcer complications such as bleeding, perforation, and pain. However, data suggest that even low-dose aspirin may reduce or eliminate any protective benefit of COX-2 drugs. In many instances, the use of NSAIDs can be discontinued and simple analgesic therapy with acetaminophen substituted. For patients who require NSAIDs, an attempt should be made to use the lowest possible dose. It also is important for physicians to know that the risk of peptic ulcer disease with NSAID use is maximal in the first month of treatment (ulcers may occur shortly after treatment is begun) and that elderly patients and patients with a previous history of peptic ulcer disease are at highest risk.

The first step in the treatment of an NSAID-induced ulcer is to discontinue use of the drug. H₂-receptor antagonists and sucralfate are ineffective in preventing gastric ulcers and in decreasing the frequency of NSAID-induced mucosal erosions. Prostaglandin replacement with the synthetic prostaglandin misoprostol decreases the incidence of NSAID-induced gastric ulcers. However, diarrhea develops in many patients, thus limiting the usefulness of misoprostol. Proton pump inhibitors are effective in healing and preventing ulcers and have few side effects.

Duodenal Ulcer

H pylori infection and associated antral gastritis occur in approximately 95% of patients with duodenal ulcer. However, an ulcer develops in only 10% to 20% of all patients who are infected with H pylori; therefore, other risk factors must be involved. Other risk factors that contribute to duodenal ulceration include use of NSAIDs, acid hypersecretion, cigarette smoking, cirrhosis, chronic pulmonary disease, and chronic renal disease. The use of NSAIDs is the second most common cause of duodenal ulcer. There is no evidence that diet, alcohol, corticosteroids, caffeine, or stress increases the risk of duodenal ulceration.

* H pylori or NSAIDs, including aspirin, cause 95% of duodenal ulcers.
* Risk factors for duodenal ulcers: H pylori, NSAIDs, acid hypersecretion, cigarette smoking, cirrhosis, chronic pulmonary disease, and chronic renal disease.

Gastric Ulcer

H pylori infection and associated antral gastritis are present in 80% of patients with gastric ulcer. Most gastric ulcers occur in areas of gastritis on the lesser curvature of the stomach near the junction of the body and antrum. Because acid secretion is normal or low in patients with gastric ulcer, gastric ulceration is believed to occur when the gastric mucosal barrier of mucus and bicarbonate is damaged. The risk factors other than H pylori infection that contribute to gastric ulceration include NSAIDs, bile reflux, and cigarette smoking. Bile reflux may occur from previous gastroduodenal surgery or from abnormal antral motility or pyloric sphincter function. Alcohol can cause gastritis, but there is no evidence that alcohol predisposes to gastric ulceration.

* Risk factors for gastric ulcers: H pylori, NSAIDs, bile reflux, and cigarette smoking.

Zollinger-Ellison Syndrome

Zollinger-Ellison syndrome is characterized by the triad of peptic ulceration, acid hypersecretion, and diarrhea caused by a gastrin-producing tumor. The tumor usually is located in the pancreas, but it can occur in the wall of the duodenum. Two-thirds of gastrinomas are malignant and can metastasize to regional lymph nodes and the liver. One-fourth of gastrinomas are related to a multiple endocrine neoplasia type 1 (MEN-1) syndrome and are associated with pituitary adenoma and hyperparathyroidism.

The most common clinical presentation is duodenal bulb ulceration, although multiple postbulbar ulcers or the coexistence of a duodenal ulcer with diarrhea or a duodenal ulcer with hypercalcemia increases the likelihood of Zollinger-Ellison syndrome. A duodenal ulcer that is not related to H pylori infection or to NSAID use should also increase the likelihood of Zollinger-Ellison syndrome. Gastrinoma also should be considered in patients with recurrent ulcers, intractable ulcers, a family history of ulcer disease or MEN-1 syndrome, or evidence of gastric acid hypersecretion (enlarged rugal folds, dilated duodenum, and increased acid output).

The serum level of gastrin should be determined if Zollinger-Ellison syndrome is suspected. Serum levels of gastrin greater than 1,000 pg/mL in patients who produce gastric acid are essentially diagnostic of gastrinoma. Increased serum levels of gastrin may also be present in atrophic gastritis, pernicious anemia, postvagotomy states, proton pump inhibitor therapy, and renal failure because gastric acid output is low in these conditions. Basal and stimulated gastric acid secretory studies should be performed in all patients who have increased levels of gastrin. The basal acid output is more than 10 mEq per hour. When the laboratory results are equivocal, a secretin test should be performed. An intravenous bolus of secretin produces a paradoxical increase in the serum level of gastrin in patients with gastrinoma.

The test of choice to localize a gastrinoma is an octreotide scan. Almost all gastrinomas have somatostatin receptors, and radiolabeled octreotide, a somatostatin analogue, produces a positive scan in approximately 80% of cases. Endoscopic ultrasonography has been reported to localize approximately 70% of gastrinomas. Computed tomography (CT) of the abdomen localizes 50% of gastrinomas, and selective arteriography localizes 33%. In combination, these studies localize 80% to 85% of gastrinomas. If a tumor cannot be localized, surgical exploration is indicated in patients who do not have evidence of metastases or MEN-1.

Approximately 20% to 25% of gastrinomas can be completely removed surgically. If the tumor cannot be removed, a parietal cell vagotomy may help control acid secretion. Patients who are not candidates for surgery or who have an unresectable tumor can be managed medically with acid suppression and chemotherapy. High-dose, long-term treatment with proton pump inhibitors is safe and effective. Chemotherapy with streptozocin and 5-fluorouracil is effective in 50% of patients with metastatic disease.

* Zollinger-Ellison syndrome: peptic ulceration, acid hypersecretion, and diarrhea caused by a gastrin-secreting tumor.
* Rule out Zollinger-Ellison syndrome in patients with duodenal ulcers not related to H pylori or NSAID use or with duodenal ulcers with diarrhea, multiple postbulbar ulcers, or hypercalcemia.
* Do not explore surgically if metastatic disease or MEN-1 is present.

Stress Ulcers

Stress ulceration is caused by gastric mucosal ischemia due to an underlying illness. *H pylori* is not an important pathogenic factor. The underlying conditions for stress ulcers are trauma, sepsis, and serious illness. Most of the hemorrhages occur 3 to 7 days after the traumatic event. Burns, especially those involving more than 35% of the body, may cause ulcers. Central nervous system trauma produces Cushing ulcer, which occurs in 50% to 75% of patients with head injury. This ulcer tends to be deep and perforate more often than other ulcers.

* Underlying conditions for stress ulcers: trauma, sepsis, and serious illness.
* Hemorrhaging occurs 3-7 days after the traumatic event.
* Burns involving >35% of the body may produce ulcers.
* Stress ulcers occur in 50%-75% of patients with head injury (Cushing ulcers).

Prophylaxis against bleeding is to maintain intragastric pH greater than 4.0. Antacids clearly decrease the incidence of bleeding compared with placebo. H₂ receptor antagonists are as effective as antacids and sometimes easier to use. Sucralfate is as effective as antacids and H₂-blockers, according to some studies. Also, sucralfate may decrease nosocomial pneumonia in ventilator-dependent patients because gastric pH is not decreased (decreased bacterial overgrowth). Prostaglandins may have a role in prophylaxis. Enteral feedings can maintain intragastric pH greater than 3.5. If antacids cannot be used, give H₂-blockers or sucralfate; combination treatment may be helpful.

* Prophylaxis: maintain intragastric pH >4.0.
* Antacids, H₂ receptor antagonists, and sucralfate decrease the incidence of bleeding.
* Sucralfate may decrease nosocomial pneumonia in ventilator-dependent patients.

The medical therapy for acute gastric mucosal ulcers that are bleeding is to correct the underlying predisposing condition. Generally, upper gastrointestinal tract bleeding stops spontaneously about 85% of the time. Angiographic therapeutic techniques include intra-arterial vasopressin and transcatheter embolization. Endoscopic techniques include epinephrine injection and cautery (BiCap/heater probe) or laser photocoagulation. Surgical therapy for acute gastric mucosal ulcers that are bleeding must be considered when the blood requirement is more than 4 to 6 units per 24 to 48 hours. The mortality rate with all forms of surgical therapy is 30% to 40%.

Nonerosive Nonspecific Chronic Gastritis

Chronic gastritis is divided into type A and type B. *Type A gastritis*, or *autoimmune gastritis*, involves the body and fundus of the stomach. A subset of patients develops atrophic gastritis (inflammation of the gland zone with variable gland loss). Pernicious anemia with hypochlorhydria or achlorhydria and megaloblastic anemia may result. Antiparietal cell antibodies are found in 90% of patients. Intrinsic factor antibodies are detected less commonly. Other autoimmune diseases, such as Addison disease and Hashimoto thyroiditis, are often present. The serum levels of gastrin are increased, which may give rise to gastric carcinoid tumors. Gastric polyps occur, and intestinal metaplasia may be a precursor to gastric adenocarcinoma.

* Type A gastritis is associated with three A's: *a*utoimmune, *a*trophic gastritis, and pernicious *a*nemia.
* The serum levels of gastrin are increased.
* Type A gastritis is associated with gastric carcinoids, polyps, and adenocarcinoma.

Type B gastritis involves the antrum and is associated with *H pylori* infection. Serum levels of gastrin are normal or increased. Gastric ulcers and duodenal ulcers occur commonly, and the incidence of gastric adenocarcinoma is increased.

* Type B gastritis is associated with *H pylori* infection.
* The serum levels of gastrin are normal or increased.
* Type B gastritis is associated with gastric and duodenal ulcers and with adenocarcinoma.

Gastric Cancer

In the 1940s, gastric cancer was the most common malignant disease in the United States. Since then, the decrease in incidence has been dramatic. Japan has the highest mortality rate from gastric cancer. Migration studies show a decrease in incidence among persons who move from high-risk areas to low-risk areas and a suggestion of increased risk among persons who move from low-risk areas to high-risk areas. Environmental factors include diet: there is an increased association with increased consumption of starch, pickled vegetables, salted fish and meat, smoked foods, nitrate and nitrite, and salt. The population at risk is persons older than 50. The male to female ratio is as high as 2:1. Also, gastric cancer is more common in lower socioeconomic groups. There is a 2-fold to 3-fold greater incidence among relatives.

* The incidence of gastric cancer has decreased dramatically in the United States since the 1940s.
* The incidence decreases among persons who move from high-risk areas.
* Increased association with increased consumption of starch, pickled vegetables, salted fish and meat, smoked foods, nitrate and nitrite, and salt.
* A 2-fold to 3-fold greater incidence among relatives.

Possible Precancerous Lesions or Situations

H pylori infection, chronic atrophic gastritis, and intestinal metaplasia frequently occur in patients with gastric cancer; however, all 3 conditions are found frequently in older persons without gastric carcinoma. Chronic benign gastric ulcer rarely progresses to cancer. Previous autopsy studies showed that the prevalence of pernicious anemia was 10%. An endoscopic screening study of 123 patients with pernicious anemia showed a prevalence of gastric neoplastic lesions of 8.1%. The risk is minimally increased after gastrectomy, but surveillance endoscopy is not necessary.

- *H pylori*–positive chronic atrophic gastritis is found frequently in patients with gastric cancer.
- Chronic benign gastric ulcer rarely progresses to cancer.
- Pernicious anemia: prevalence of 10%.
- Postgastrectomy: minimal increased risk, but endoscopy screening is not necessary.

Clinical Aspects

Gastric cancer is often asymptomatic, but abdominal discomfort and weight loss are the common presenting complaints. Physical examination is often unrevealing, but up to 30% of patients have an epigastric mass. Endoscopy, with multiple (7 or 8) biopsies, and CT of the abdomen (to identify extragastric extension) are indicated.

- Abdominal discomfort and weight loss are common presenting complaints.
- Up to 30% of patients have an epigastric mass.
- Perform endoscopy, with multiple (7 or 8) biopsies.

Treatment and Prognosis

For local disease, resection often requires total gastrectomy for tumor-free margins. The omentum and spleen (splenic hilar nodes) are often removed in curative resection.

For disseminated disease, surgical treatment is necessary only for palliation. Response to chemotherapy is generally poor. The only consistent factor is extent of disease. Five-year survival is 90% if the tumor is confined to the mucosa and submucosa, 50% if the tumor is through the serosa, and 10% if the tumor involves lymph nodes.

Gastric Polyps

Gastric polyps are rare; a 0.5% prevalence has been reported in an autopsy series. The 3 types of polyps are hyperplastic, fundic gland, and adenomatous. Hyperplastic and fundic gland polyps are more common and are not premalignant. No therapy is needed. Adenomatous polyps are premalignant, especially if larger than 2 cm. They occur most often in achlorhydric stomachs (ie, in patients with pernicious anemia) and are usually localized to the antrum. If pedunculated, the polyp can be removed endoscopically.

- Hyperplastic polyps are more common and not premalignant.
- Adenomatous polyps are premalignant, especially if >2 cm.

Gastroduodenal Dysmotility Syndromes

Symptoms of abnormal gastric motility may include nausea, vomiting, bloating, early satiety, dyspepsia, heartburn, anorexia, weight loss, and food avoidance. The specific cause of abnormal gastric motor function is unknown but is believed to be related to autonomic neuropathy. Diabetes mellitus is probably the most common medical cause of symptomatic gastric motor dysfunction. Causes of gastroparesis are listed in Table 7-3.

- Nausea, vomiting, bloating, early satiety, dyspepsia, heartburn, anorexia, weight loss, and food avoidance may suggest abnormal gastric motility.

- Abnormal gastric motor function is believed to be related to autonomic neuropathy.
- Diabetes mellitus: the most common medical cause of symptomatic gastric motor dysfunction.

Treatment

Currently, several prokinetic drugs are available in the United States. These drugs augment motility, thus enhancing the movement of luminal contents. Metoclopramide is a dopamine antagonist and a cholinergic agonist that increases the rate and amplitude of antral contractions. It crosses the blood-brain barrier and frequently causes such side effects as drowsiness, athetosis, and the release of prolactin. Domperidone is a selective dopamine antagonist that works only on peripheral receptors in the gut. It has no cholinergic effects and fewer side effects than metoclopramide. Bethanechol is a systemic cholinergic agonist with side effects. It may be useful in low dosage in combination with other agents. Erythromycin stimulates both cholinergic and motilin receptors.

- Metoclopramide is a dopamine antagonist and a cholinergic agonist.
- Domperidone is a selective dopamine antagonist.
- Erythromycin stimulates both cholinergic and motilin receptors.

Small Intestine

Diarrhea

Patients use the term *diarrhea* to refer to any increase in the frequency, fluidity, or volume of the stool or to any change in its consistency. Normally, stools are generally solid and brown, but these features vary with diet. The frequency of stools varies among persons, from 1 to 3 daily to 2 or 3 stools weekly. Blood, pus (leukocytes), and oil are not present in normal stools (Table 7-4).

Diarrhea is defined as an increase in stool weight or volume. Because a stool is 65% to 80% water, stool weight is proportional to stool water. Because dietary fiber content influences the water content of the stool, stool weight can vary according to the diet of a culture. In the United States, normal daily stool weight is less than 200 g per day and normal stool volume is less than 200 mL per day (compared with <400 g per day and 400 mL per day in rural Africa).

Table 7-3 Conditions Causing Gastroparesis

Acute Conditions	Chronic Conditions
Anticholinergic drug use	Amyloidosis
Hyperglycemia	Diabetes mellitus
Hypokalemia	Gastric dysrhythmias
Morphine use	Pseudo-obstruction
Pancreatitis	Scleroderma
Surgical procedure	Vagotomy
Trauma	

Table 7-4   Normal Stool Composition

Feature	Value
Weight, g	<200
Water, %	65-80
Fat, g	<7
Nitrogen, g	<2.5
Electrolytes, mEq/L	
Sodium	40
Potassium	90
Chloride	15
Bicarbonate	30

Normal daily intestinal fluid balance is important to understand. Each day, 9 to 10 L of isotonic fluid is presented to the proximal small intestine (2 L from diet; 8 L from endogenous secretions). The small bowel absorbs most of the fluid (7-9 L), and the colon absorbs all the 1 to 2 L presented to it each day (except for <200 mL) and forms a soft, solid stool. There is considerable reserve because the maximal absorptive capacity is 12 L per day for the small bowel and 4 to 6 L per day for the colon.

Mechanisms of Diarrhea

Osmotic diarrhea occurs when water-soluble molecules are poorly absorbed, remain in the intestinal lumen, and retain water in the intestine. Osmotic diarrhea follows ingestion of an osmotically active substance and stops with fasting. Stool volume is less than 1 L per day, and the stool has an osmolar gap—stool osmolality is greater than the sum of the electrolyte concentrations.

$$\text{Stool osmolar gap} = 290 - 2 \text{ (stool sodium + potassium)}$$

A normal stool osmolar gap is less than 50. Often, stool pH is less than 6.0 in carbohydrate malabsorption (most commonly lactase deficiency) owing to colonic fermentation of the undigested sugars. Clinical causes of osmotic diarrhea that produce an osmolar gap greater than 50 include carbohydrate malabsorption, lactase deficiency, sorbitol-sweetened foods, saline cathartics, and magnesium-based antacids.

- In osmotic diarrhea, stool volume is <1 L per day.
- Diarrhea stops with fasting.
- Stool has an osmolar gap.
- Causes of osmotic diarrhea: lactase deficiency, sorbitol foods, and antacids.

In secretory diarrhea, fluid and electrolyte transport is abnormal, (ie, the intestine secretes rather than absorbs fluid). Stool volume is greater than 1 L per day, and its composition is similar to that of extracellular fluid, so there is no osmolar gap. The diarrhea persists despite fasting, and hypokalemia is often present. Causes of secretory diarrhea include bacterial toxins, neuroendocrine tumors, surreptitious ingestion of laxative, bile acid diarrhea, and fatty acid diarrhea.

- In secretory diarrhea, stool volume is >1 L per day.
- There is no osmolar gap.
- Diarrhea persists despite fasting.
- Causes of secretory diarrhea: bacterial toxins, neuroendocrine tumors, surreptitious ingestion of laxative, bile acid diarrhea, and fatty acid diarrhea.

Many disease processes have more than 1 mechanism for causing diarrhea (*mixed mechanisms*). For example, generalized malabsorption (such as in celiac disease) has osmotic components (from carbohydrate malabsorption) and secretory components (unabsorbed fatty acids cause secretion in the colon).

In exudative diarrhea, membrane permeability is abnormal and serum proteins, blood, or mucus is exuded into the bowel from sites of inflammation, ulceration, or infiltration. The volume of feces is small and the stools may be bloody. Examples include invasive bacterial pathogens (eg, *Shigella* and *Salmonella*) and inflammatory bowel disease.

- Exudative diarrhea: abnormal membrane permeability.
- Volume of feces is small.
- Causes: invasive bacterial pathogens (*Shigella* and *Salmonella*) and inflammatory bowel disease.

In motility disorders, both *rapid transit* (inadequate time for chyme to contact the absorbing surface) and *delayed transit* (bacterial overgrowth) can cause diarrhea. Rapid transit occurs after gastrectomy or intestinal resection and with hyperthyroidism or carcinoid syndrome. Delayed transit occurs with structural defects (strictures, blind loops, and small-bowel diverticula) or with underlying illnesses that cause visceral neuropathy (diabetes) or myopathy (scleroderma), that is, pseudo-obstruction.

- Rapid transit: diarrhea results from malabsorption.
- Delayed transit: diarrhea results from bacterial overgrowth.

Clinical Approach

It is useful to differentiate small-bowel ("right-sided") diarrhea from colonic ("left-sided") diarrhea (Table 7-5). *Right-sided diarrhea* is characterized by large-volume stools, and the increase in the number of stools is modest. Symptoms attributed to inflammation of the rectosigmoid are absent, and proctoscopic examination findings are normal. *Left-sided diarrhea* is characterized by frequent, small-volume stools with obvious evidence of inflammation, and proctosigmoidoscopic examination usually confirms inflammation. Left-sided diarrhea usually suggests an exudative mechanism, whereas the mechanism for right-sided diarrhea is nonspecific.

Acute Diarrhea

Acute diarrhea is abrupt in onset and usually resolves in several days (3-10 days). It is self-limited, and the cause (possibly viral) usually is not found. No evaluation is necessary unless the stools are bloody and fever or infection is suspected (eg, from travel history or a common

Table 7-5   Right-Sided and Left-Sided Diarrhea: Contrasts in Clinical Presentation

Feature	Right-Sided (Small-Bowel) Diarrhea	Left-Sided (Colonic) Diarrhea
Reservoir capacity	Intact	Decreased
Stool volume	Large	Small
Increase in number of stools	Modest	Large
Urgency	Absent	Present
Tenesmus	Absent	Present
Mucus	Absent	Present
Blood	Absent	Present

source outbreak). If these conditions exist, do not treat with antimotility agents. Begin the evaluation with stool studies for bacterial pathogens, ova, and parasites and proctosigmoidoscopy. Recognize the common situations that predispose to specific infections (see "Infectious Diarrheas" subsection).

- For acute diarrhea, no evaluation is necessary unless the stools are bloody and fever or infection is suspected.
- Do not administer antimotility agents if the stools are bloody and fever or infection is suspected.

Chronic Diarrhea

Chronic diarrhea is an initial episode lasting longer than 4 weeks or diarrhea that recurs after the initial episode. The most common cause of chronic diarrhea is irritable bowel syndrome, but lactase deficiency should always be considered. Several features are used to differentiate organic diarrhea from functional diarrhea (Table 7-6).

- The most common cause of chronic diarrhea is irritable bowel syndrome.

- Always consider lactase deficiency in suspected irritable bowel syndrome.
- Differentiate organic diarrhea from functional diarrhea.

Chronic Watery Diarrhea

The evaluation of chronic watery diarrhea usually requires distinguishing between secretory diarrhea and osmotic diarrhea (Table 7-7). This can be done by collecting stools and measuring volume, osmolality, and electrolyte content and observing the patient's response to fasting.

- Evaluation of chronic watery diarrhea requires distinguishing between secretory diarrhea and osmotic diarrhea.

Physiology of Nutrient Absorption

The sites of nutrient, vitamin, and mineral absorption are the following: The duodenum absorbs iron, calcium, magnesium, folate, water-soluble vitamins, and monosaccharides. The jejunum absorbs fatty acids, amino acids, monosaccharides, and water-soluble vitamins. The ileum absorbs monosaccharides, fatty acids, amino acids, fat-soluble vitamins (A, D, E, and K), vitamin B_{12}, and conjugated bile salts. The distal small bowel can adapt to absorb nutrients. The proximal small bowel cannot adapt to absorb vitamin B_{12} or bile salts.

- The distal small bowel can adapt to absorb nutrients.
- The proximal small bowel cannot adapt to absorb vitamin B_{12} or bile salts.

Fat absorption is the most complex process. Dietary fat consists mostly of long-chain triglycerides that must be digested by pancreatic lipase, which cleaves 2 of the 3 long-chain fatty acids from the glycerol backbone. The resultant free fatty acids and monoglycerides are solubilized by micelles for absorption. The fatty acids and monoglycerides are reesterified by intestinal epithelial cells into chylomicrons that are absorbed into the circulation via lymphatic vessels. Conversely, medium-chain triglycerides are absorbed directly into the portal vein and do not require micellar solubilization.

Table 7-6   Features Differentiating Organic Diarrhea From Functional Diarrhea

Feature	Organic Diarrhea	Functional Diarrhea
Weight loss	Often present	Absent
Duration of illness	Variable (weeks to years)	Usually long (>6 mo)
Quantity of stool	Variable but usually large (>200 g in 24 h)	Usually small (<200 g in 24 h)
Blood in stool	May be present	Absent (unless from hemorrhoids)
Timing of diarrhea	No special pattern	Usually in the morning or after meals
Nocturnal symptoms	May be present	Absent
Fever, arthritis, skin lesions	May be present	Absent
Emotional stress	No relation to symptoms	Usually precedes or coincides with symptoms
Cramping abdominal pain	Often present	May be present

From Matseshe JW, Phillips SF. Chronic diarrhea: a practical approach. Med Clin North Am. 1978;62:141-54. Used with permission.

Table 7-7   Features Differentiating Osmotic Diarrhea From Secretory Diarrhea

Feature	Osmotic Diarrhea	Secretory Diarrhea
Daily stool volume, L	<1	>1
Effect of 48-hour fasting	Diarrhea stops	Diarrhea continues
Fecal fluid analysis		
Osmolality, mOsm	400	290
([Na] + [K]) × 2,[a] mEq/L	120	280
Solute gap[b]	>125	<50

Abbreviations: K, potassium; Na, sodium.

[a] Multiplied by 2 to account for anions.

[b] Calculated by subtracting ([Na] + [K]) × 2 from osmolality.

From Krejs GJ, Hendler RS, Fordtran JS. Diagnostic and pathophysiologic studies in patients with chronic diarrhea. In Field M, Fordtran JS, Schultz SG, eds. Secretory diarrhea. Bethesda, MD: American Physiological Society; 1980, pp 141-51. Used with permission.

Mechanisms of fat malabsorption are summarized in Table 7-8. Malabsorption should be suspected if the medical history suggests steatorrhea or if there is diarrhea with weight loss (especially if intake is adequate), chronic diarrhea of indeterminate nature, or nutritional deficiency. The causes of symptoms in malabsorption are summarized in Table 7-9.

Various features suggest specific conditions, as follows:

1. Diarrhea with iron deficiency anemia (evaluation for blood loss is negative)—proximal small-bowel malabsorption (eg, sprue)
2. Diarrhea with metabolic bone disease—decreased calcium and protein; thus, proximal small-bowel malabsorption
3. Hypoproteinemia with normal fat absorption—protein-losing enteropathy (with eosinophilia, eosinophilic gastroenteritis; with lymphopenia, intestinal lymphangiectasia)
4. Oil droplets (neutral fat) or muscle fibers (undigested protein) present in stool—pancreatic insufficiency (maldigestion)
5. Normal (usually) serum levels of calcium, magnesium, and iron—pancreatic insufficiency (serum levels of albumin may also be normal)
6. Howell-Jolly bodies (if there is no history of splenectomy) or dermatitis herpetiformis—celiac sprue (characteristic findings on small-bowel biopsy are not specific for sprue, but the response to a gluten-free diet is)
7. Fever, arthralgias, and neurologic symptoms—Whipple disease

Helpful hints in the medical history, physical examination, or laboratory results may suggest the possibility of diarrhea or malabsorption (Table 7-10). For example, the medical history may include previous surgery (resulting in short-bowel syndrome, dumping syndrome, blind loop syndrome, postvagotomy diarrhea, or ileal resection), irradiation, or systemic disease. Other hints in the history might include any of the following:

1. Age—youth suggests lactase deficiency, inflammatory bowel disease, or sprue
2. Travel—parasites or toxicogenic agents (exposure to contaminated food or water)
3. Drugs—laxatives, antacids, antibiotics, colchicine, or lactulose
4. Family history—celiac sprue, inflammatory bowel disease, polyposis coli, or lactase deficiency

• Hints in the medical history may suggest diarrhea or malabsorption: previous surgery (short-bowel syndrome, dumping syndrome, blind loop syndrome, postvagotomy diarrhea, and ileal resection), irradiation, or systemic disease.

Diseases Causing Diarrhea

Osmotic Diarrhea

Lactose is normally split by the brush border enzyme lactase into glucose and galactose, which are absorbed in the small bowel. In

Table 7-8   Mechanisms of Fat Malabsorption

Alteration	Mechanism	Disease State
Defective digestion	Inadequate lipase	Pancreatic insufficiency
Impaired micelle formation	Duodenal bile salt concentration	Common duct obstruction or cholestasis
Impaired absorption	Small-bowel disease	Sprue and Whipple disease
Impaired chylomicron formation	Impaired β-globulin synthesis	Abetalipoproteinemia
Impaired lymphatic circulation	Lymphatic obstruction	Intestinal lymphangiectasia & lymphoma

Table 7-9 Causes of Symptoms in Malabsorption

Extragastrointestinal Symptom	Cause
Muscle wasting, edema	Decreased protein absorption
Paresthesias, tetany	Decreased vitamin D & calcium absorption
Bone pain	Decreased calcium absorption
Muscle cramps	Weakness, excess potassium loss
Easy bruisability, petechiae	Decreased vitamin K absorption
Hyperkeratosis, night blindness	Decreased vitamin A absorption
Pallor	Decreased vitamin B_{12}, folate, or iron absorption
Glossitis, stomatitis, cheilosis	Decreased vitamin B_{12} or iron absorption
Acrodermatitis	Zinc deficiency

lactase deficiency, lactose is not split in the small intestine but enters the colon, where it is fermented in the lumen by bacteria, forming lactic acid and liberating hydrogen. The result is diarrhea of low pH and increased intestinal motility. Several other disaccharidase deficiencies can also result in malabsorption of specific carbohydrates; however, the most common disaccharidase deficiency involves lactase. "Acquired" lactase deficiency (possibly genetic) is common in blacks, Eskimos, and people from Asia and the Middle East. Diarrhea, abdominal cramps, and flatulence occur after ingestion of dairy products. There is improvement with dietary changes. The pH of the stool is less than 6.0. In the lactose tolerance test, blood glucose levels increase less than 20 mg/100 mL after ingestion of lactose. Results of the hydrogen breath test may be abnormal. Jejunal biopsy results are normal (disaccharidase levels are decreased). Transient lactose intolerance can occur in any clinical setting in which the intestinal mucosa is damaged, including simple viral gastroenteritis. In patients on a weight-reduction diet who drink soda or chew sugarless gum, osmotic diarrhea may develop from excessive ingestion of fructose or other artificial sweeteners.

* Lactase deficiency: lactose is not split in the small intestine.
* Diarrhea is characterized by stool with low pH and increased intestinal motility.
* The most common disaccharidase deficiency is lactase deficiency.
* Diarrhea, abdominal cramps, and flatulence occur after ingestion of dairy products.
* Results of the hydrogen breath test may be abnormal.
* In patients on a weight-reduction diet who drink diet soda or chew sugarless gum, osmotic diarrhea may develop from artificial sweeteners.

Secretory Diarrhea

VIPoma

The syndrome of watery diarrhea, hypokalemia, and achlorhydria (*WDHA*), also called *Verner-Morrison syndrome* or *pancreatic cholera*, is a massive diarrhea (5 L daily) with dehydration and hypokalemia. The patient may have numerous endocrine tumors (with hypercalcemia or hyperglycemia). This diarrhea is associated with a non–beta islet cell tumor of the pancreas. Vasoactive intestinal peptide is the most common mediator; other mediators are prostaglandin, secretin, and calcitonin. It is diagnosed with pancreatic scan or angiography and measurement of hormone levels. Treatment is with somatostatin or surgery.

* Pancreatic cholera: massive diarrhea, dehydration, and hypokalemia.
* Patients may have multiple endocrine tumors.
* Diarrhea is associated with a non–beta islet cell tumor of the pancreas.

Carcinoid Syndrome

Carcinoid tumors arise from enterochromaffin cells of neural crest origin. About 90% of the tumors are in the terminal ileum. There

Table 7-10 Associated Signs and Symptoms of Systemic Illnesses Causing Diarrhea

Sign or Symptom	Diagnosis To Be Considered
Arthritis	Ulcerative colitis, Crohn disease, Whipple disease, *Yersinia* infection
Marked weight loss	Malabsorption, inflammatory bowel disease, cancer, thyrotoxicosis
Eosinophilia	Eosinophilic gastroenteritis, parasitic disease
Lymphadenopathy	Lymphoma, Whipple disease
Neuropathy	Diabetic diarrhea, amyloidosis
Postural hypotension	Diabetic diarrhea, Addison disease, idiopathic orthostatic hypotension, autonomic dysfunction
Flushing	Malignant carcinoid syndrome
Proteinuria	Amyloidosis
Peptic ulcers	Zollinger-Ellison syndrome
Hyperpigmentation	Whipple disease, celiac disease, Addison disease, pancreatic cholera, eosinophilic gastroenteritis

Modified from Fine KD. Diarrhea. In Feldman M, Scharschmidt BF, Sleisenger MH, editors. Sleisenger & Fordtran's gastrointestinal and liver disease: pathophysiology, diagnosis, management. 6th ed., Vol. 1. Philadelphia: WB Saunders Company; 1998. p. 128-52 . Used with permission.

is episodic facial flushing (lasting up to 10 minutes), watery diarrhea, wheezing, right-sided valvular disease (endocardial fibrosis), and hepatomegaly. If the gut is normal, look for bronchial tumors or gonadal tumors. Dietary tryptophan is converted into serotonin (which causes diarrhea, abdominal cramps [intestinal hypermotility], nausea, and vomiting), histamine (responsible for flushing), and other chemicals (bradykinin and corticotropin). Intestinal tumors are usually asymptomatic because of the high hepatic first-pass clearance of these mediators. Carcinoid syndrome arises when these mediators are released into the systemic bloodstream; this suggests that liver metastases or bronchial tumors are present. The diagnosis of carcinoid syndrome is made by finding increased urinary levels of 5-hydroxyindoleacetic acid (5-HIAA) and by liver biopsy. This syndrome is not associated with hypertension, as in pheochromocytoma. Treatment is with octreotide.

Laxative Abuse

Of the population older than 60 years, 15% to 30% take laxatives regularly. This is laxative abuse. With the surreptitious ingestion of laxatives, patients complain of diarrhea but do not admit taking laxatives. In referral centers, this is the commonest cause of watery diarrhea. Proctoscopy shows melanosis coli. Barium enema demonstrates "cathartic colon," that is, the colon is dilated, hypomotile, and lacking haustra. Laxatives that cause melanosis coli include anthracene derivatives (senna, cascara, and aloe). Stool phenolphthalein is the diagnostic test. Underlying emotional problems should be addressed.

- Proctoscopy demonstrates melanosis coli.
- Barium enema shows "cathartic colon" (ie, dilated, hypomotile, and lacking haustra).
- Address underlying emotional problems.

Bile Acid Malabsorption

Bile acid malabsorption is caused by ileal resection or disease. Diarrhea due to bile acid malabsorption may produce 2 clinical syndromes, each requiring a different treatment. In a *limited resection* (<100 cm), malabsorbed bile acids enter the colon and stimulate secretion. Liver synthesis can compensate, so bile acid concentration in the upper small bowel is sufficient to achieve the critical micelle concentration and allow for normal fat absorption. There is no steatorrhea. The fecal fat test result is less than 20 g in 24 hours. The treatment is cholestyramine, which binds excess bile acids.

In an *extensive resection* (>100 cm), bile acid malabsorption is severe and enterohepatic circulation is interrupted. This limits synthesis, and the liver cannot compensate. Bile acid concentration is decreased in the upper small bowel, micelles cannot be formed, and fat malabsorption results. The malabsorbed fatty acids themselves stimulate secretion in the colon. Fat-soluble vitamins (A, D, E, and K) may be malabsorbed. Additionally, excess fatty acids bind intestinal calcium; this allows an increase in oxylate absorption, which increases the risk of oxylate renal stones. The treatment of this bile acid malabsorption is a low-fat diet (<50 g daily) rich in medium-chain triglycerides. Cholestyramine would further decrease bile acid concentration and increase steatorrhea.

- Limited resection: treat with cholestyramine.
- Extensive resection: treat with a low-fat diet rich in medium-chain triglycerides.

Bacterial Overgrowth

The proximal small intestine is usually sterile, and its major defense mechanisms are gastric acid, normal peristalsis (the most important defense), and intestinal IgA. When defenses are altered, bacterial overgrowth results. The mechanism of steatorrhea is deconjugation of bile acids by bacteria that normally do not occur in the proximal intestine. Deconjugation of bile acids changes the ionization coefficient, and the deconjugated bile acids can be passively absorbed in the proximal small bowel. (Normally, conjugated bile acids are actively absorbed distally in the ileum.) As a result, the critical micellar concentration is not reached, and mild steatorrhea results from the intraluminal deficiency of bile acids.

- Normal peristalsis is the most important defense in the proximal small bowel.
- Deconjugated bile acids can be absorbed passively.
- Mild steatorrhea results from the intraluminal deficiency of bile acids.

Clinical features of bacterial overgrowth are steatorrhea (10-20 g daily), vitamin B_{12} malabsorption (macrocytic anemia), positive jejunal cultures (>10^5 organisms), increased serum folate levels from bacterial production, and abnormal bile acid breath test results. In the bile acid breath test, ^{14}C-labeled bile acids release $^{14}CO_2$ when deconjugated by bacteria in the gut. This test has low sensitivity (false-negative rate, 20%-30%).

Associated conditions include postoperative conditions (blind loops, enteroenterostomy, or gastrojejunocolic fistula), structural conditions (diverticula, strictures, or fistulas), motility disorders (diabetes mellitus, scleroderma, or pseudo-obstruction), achlorhydria (atrophic gastritis or gastric resections; achlorhydria is corrected with antibiotics), and impaired immunity. Two examples of impaired immunity are hypogammaglobulinemic sprue (in small-bowel biopsy specimens, no plasma cells are seen in the lamina propria and the villi are flat) and nodular lymphoid hyperplasia associated with IgA deficiency, which predisposes to *Giardia lamblia* infection.

- Diarrhea, vitamin B_{12} deficiency, postoperative or structural conditions, motility disorders, achlorhydria, and impaired immunity suggest bacterial overgrowth.

Infectious Diarrheas

The toxicogenic and invasive causes of bacterial diarrhea and the associated features are outlined in Tables 7-11 and 7-12.

Noninvasive Bacterial Diarrhea (Toxicogenic)

Toxicogenic bacterial diarrhea, characterized by watery stools without fecal leukocytes, is caused by several organisms, including the following:

Staphylococcus aureus—The diarrhea is of rapid onset and lasts for 24 hours. There is no fever, vomiting, or cramps. The toxin is ingested with egg products, cream, and mayonnaise. Treatment is supportive.

Clostridium perfringens ("church picnic diarrhea")—The toxin is ingested with precooked foods, usually beef and turkey. Heat-stable spores produce toxins. Although the bacteria are killed and the toxin is destroyed, the spores survive. When food is rewarmed, the spores germinate, producing toxin. The diarrhea is worse than the vomiting and is later in onset. It lasts 24 hours. Treatment is supportive.

Escherichia coli (traveler's diarrhea)—The toxin is ingested with water and salads. It is a plasmid-mediated enterotoxin. Treatment is rehydration with correction of electrolytes and ciprofloxacin, norfloxacin, or trimethoprim-sulfamethoxazole. *E coli* may be important in nursery epidemic diarrhea.

Vibrio cholerae—The toxin is ingested with water. It is the only toxicogenic bacterial diarrhea in which antibiotics clearly shorten the duration of the disease. Treatment is with tetracycline.

Bacillus cereus—The source of the toxin is fried rice in Asian restaurants. One type has rapid onset and resembles *S aureus* infection; the other type has a slower onset and resembles *C perfringens* infection. The diagnosis is made by isolating the organism from contaminated food and by the medical history. Treatment is supportive.

Other toxicogenic bacteria—*Clostridium botulinum* produces a neurotoxin that is ingested in improperly home-processed vegetables, fruits, and meats. It interferes with the release of acetylcholine from peripheral nerve endings. *Clostridiuim difficile*—See "Antibiotic Colitis" subsection.

- Toxicogenic bacterial diarrhea: watery, no fecal leukocytes.
- *S aureus*: rapid onset.
- *C perfringens*: "church picnic diarrhea" from precooked foods; delayed onset of diarrhea is the predominant symptom.
- *E coli*: traveler's diarrhea.
- *V cholerae*: the only toxicogenic diarrhea in which antibiotics shorten the duration of the disease. Tetracycline is the treatment of choice.
- *B cereus*: source of toxin is fried rice in Asian restaurants.

Invasive Bacterial Diarrhea

Invasive bacterial diarrhea is characterized by fever, bloody stools, and fecal leukocytes. It is caused by several organisms, including the following:

Shigella—*Shigella* infection is often acquired outside the United States. Bloody diarrhea is characteristic, and fever and bacteremia occur. Diagnosis is based on positive stool and blood cultures. Treatment is with ampicillin. Resistant strains are emerging for which chloramphenicol is an alternative. (Plasmids are responsible for antibiotic deactivation resistance.)

Salmonella (non-*typhi*)—In the United States, *Salmonella typhimurium* is the most common agent. The toxin is ingested with poultry. Fever is present. The absence of bloody diarrhea is the main characteristic that distinguishes it from *Shigella* infection. Diagnosis is based on positive stool culture. Treatment is supportive. Severe symptoms should be treated with ciprofloxacin.

Table 7-11 Toxicogenic Causes of Bacterial Diarrhea

Organism	Onset, h	Mediated by Cyclic AMP	Fever	Intestinal Secretion
Staphylococcus aureus	1-6	+	−	+
Clostridium perfringens	8-12	−	±	+
Escherichia coli	12	+	+	+
Vibrio cholerae	12	+	Due to dehydration	++++
Bacillus cereus	1-6	+	−	+

Abbreviation: AMP, adenosine monophosphate.

Table 7-12 Invasive Causes of Bacterial Diarrhea

Organism	Fever	Bloody Diarrhea	Bacteremia	Antibiotic Effectiveness
Shigella	+	+	+	+
Salmonella	+	−	−	−
Vibrio parahaemolyticus	+	+	−	+(?)
Escherichia coli	+	+	−	
Staphylococcus aureus (enterocolitis)	+	+	±	+
Yersinia enterocolitica	+	+	+	+
Campylobacter jejuni	+	+	±	+
Vibrio vulnificus	+	+	+	+

Treating mild symptoms with other antibiotics may result in a prolonged carrier state.

Vibrio parahaemolyticus—The toxin is ingested with undercooked shellfish. This infection is increasing in frequency in the United States (it is common in Japan). Fever and bloody diarrhea are the chief characteristics. Diagnosis is based on positive stool culture. Antibiotics are of questionable value in treating this infection, but erythromycin may be most effective.

E coli—In the United States, enteroinvasive *E coli* is a rare cause of diarrhea. Enteroinvasive *E coli* involves the colon and causes fever, bloody diarrhea, and profound toxicity (similar to *Shigella* infection). Enterohemorrhagic *E coli* (serotype O157:H7) produces a cytotoxin that damages vascular endothelial cells. *E coli* O157:H7 can cause sporadic or epidemic illness from contaminated meat and raw milk. Enterohemorrhagic *E coli* infection should be suspected when bloody diarrhea occurs after eating hamburger and when bloody diarrhea is complicated by hemolytic uremic syndrome or thrombotic thrombocytopenic purpura. Antibiotic treatment has not been effective and is not recommended because it may increase the risk of development of hemolytic uremic syndrome or thrombotic thrombocytopenic purpura from the rapid release of toxin during bacterial death.

S aureus (enterocolitis)—Diagnosis is based on positive stool culture or Gram stain, which shows a predominance of gram-positive cocci and a paucity of other organisms.

- Invasive bacterial diarrhea: fever, bloody stools, and fecal leukocytes.
- *Shigella*: bloody diarrhea.
- *S typhimurium*: no bloody diarrhea. Treat with antibiotics only if blood cultures are positive.
- *V parahaemolyticus*: undercooked shellfish, bloody diarrhea.
- *E coli*: bloody stools, abdominal pain with fever. Occurs after eating hamburgers; may cause hemolytic uremic syndrome and thrombotic thrombocytopenic purpura.

Other Pathogens That Cause Invasive Bacterial Diarrhea
Yersinia enterocolitica—The spectrum of disease includes acute enteritis and chronic enteritis. Acute enteritis is similar to shigellosis and usually lasts 1 to 3 weeks. It is characterized by fever, diarrhea, leukocytosis, and fecal leukocytes. Chronic enteritis occurs especially in children, with diarrhea, failure to thrive, hypoalbuminemia, and hypokalemia. Other features are acute abdominal pain (mesenteric adenitis), right lower quadrant pain, tenderness, nausea, and vomiting. It mimics appendicitis or Crohn disease. This gram-negative rod is hardy and can survive in cold temperatures. It grows on special medium (cold enriched). It is an invasive pathogen, with fecal-oral transmission in water and milk.

Extraintestinal manifestations are nonsuppurative arthritis and ankylosing spondylitis (in HLA-B27). Skin manifestations are erythema nodosum and erythema multiforme. Thyroid manifestations are Graves disease and Hashimoto disease. Multiple liver abscesses and granulomata are present.

Treatment is with aminoglycosides or trimethoprim-sulfamethoxazole. The bacteria are variably sensitive to tetracycline and chloramphenicol. β-Lactamases are frequently produced, making penicillin resistance common.

- *Y enterocolitica* infection: acute abdominal pain (differential diagnosis includes appendicitis and Crohn disease).
- Fecal-oral transmission in water and milk.
- Manifestations include nonsuppurative arthritis and ankylosing spondylitis (in HLA-B27).

Campylobacter jejuni—*C jejuni* are comma-shaped, motile, microaerophilic gram-negative bacilli. Transmission is linked to infected water, unpasteurized milk, poultry, sick dogs, and infected children. The incubation period is 2 to 4 days before invasion of the small bowel. Infection results in the presence of blood and leukocytes in the stool. It may mimic granulomatous or idiopathic ulcerative colitis. It also may mimic small-bowel secretory diarrhea, with explosive, frequent watery diarrhea due to many species that produce a cholera-type toxin. The diarrhea usually lasts 3 to 5 days but may recur. Antibiotic treatment is with erythromycin when severe, but treatment often is not needed. Postdiarrheal illnesses are hemolytic uremic syndrome and postinfectious arthritis.

- *C jejuni*: transmission is linked to infected water, unpasteurized milk, poultry, sick dogs, and infected children.
- It may mimic granulomatous or idiopathic ulcerative colitis.
- Diarrhea usually lasts 3-5 days but may recur.

Vibrio vulnificus (noncholera)—The organisms are extremely invasive and produce necrotizing vasculitis, gangrene, and shock. They are routinely isolated from seawater, zooplankton, and shellfish along the Gulf of Mexico and both coasts of the United States, especially in the summer. The 2 clinical syndromes are 1) wound infection, cellulitis, fasciitis, or myositis after exposure to seawater or cleaning shellfish and 2) septicemia after the ingestion of raw shellfish (oysters). Patients at high risk of septicemia include those with liver disease, congestive heart failure, diabetes mellitus, renal failure, an immunosuppressive state, or hemochromatosis. Treatment is with tetracycline.

- *V vulnificus* is extremely invasive, producing necrotizing vasculitis, gangrene, and shock.
- Wound infection, cellulitis, fasciitis, or myositis occurs after exposure to seawater or cleaning shellfish.
- Septicemia occurs after the ingestion of raw shellfish (oysters).

Aeromonas hydrophila—Previously, the pathogenicity of *A hydrophila* was questioned. Although the infection is often mistaken for that of *E coli*, *A hydrophila* is now recognized as an increasingly frequent cause of diarrhea after a person has been swimming in freshwater or salt water. The organism produces several toxins. Treatment is with trimethoprim-sulfamethoxazole and tetracycline.

Malabsorption Due to Diseases of the Small Intestine

Celiac Sprue
Celiac sprue is a gluten-sensitive enteropathy characterized in children as growth retardation and in adults as an iron deficiency that is unresponsive to iron taken orally. Osteomalacia can be present without steatorrhea if the proximal small bowel is involved. Splenic

atrophy and an abnormal blood smear with Howell-Jolly bodies may be clues to the diagnosis in 10% to 15% of patients. The skin manifestation is dermatitis herpetiformis. The measurement of circulating antigliadin, endomysial, or tissue transglutaminase antibodies is useful for noninvasive screening. If the results are positive, a small-bowel biopsy should be performed. False-negative results can occur in the IgA-based tests because roughly 5% of patients with sprue also have IgA deficiency. IgG-based testing or confirmation of normal total IgA levels should be performed with all sprue screening. If the result of the antibody testing is negative, another diagnosis should be considered. Small-bowel biopsy findings are not diagnostic, but response to a gluten-free diet is diagnostic. If the patient has no response to the diet, the diet should be reviewed for inadvertent gluten ingestion. If symptoms recur after 10 to 15 years of successful dietary management, small-bowel lymphoma should be considered (especially if there is also abdominal pain).

* Celiac sprue: iron deficiency that is unresponsive to iron taken orally; osteomalacia may be present with or without steatorrhea.
* Splenic atrophy and abnormal blood smear with Howell-Jolly bodies may be clues to the diagnosis in 10%-15% of patients.
* Lymphoma is a late complication.

Tropical Sprue
In tropical sprue, diarrhea occurs 2 to 3 months after travel to the tropics. After 6 months, megaloblastic anemia develops because of folate deficiency and possible coexisting vitamin B_{12} deficiency. The pathogenesis is presumed to be due to a type of bacterial overgrowth in the small bowel; however, the specific organism is somewhat controversial. Small-bowel biopsy specimens show blunted villi similar to those in celiac sprue. Treatment is with tetracycline (250 mg 4 times daily) and folate with or without vitamin B_{12}.

* Tropical sprue: diarrhea and megaloblastic anemia after travel to the tropics.
* Cause: controversial.
* Treatment: tetracycline (250 mg 4 times daily) and folate with or without vitamin B_{12}.

Whipple Disease
Whipple disease is a systemic infectious disease involving the central nervous system (CNS), heart, kidneys, and small bowel. It is caused by gram-positive bacilli. Small-bowel biopsy specimens show periodic acid-Schiff (PAS)–positive granules in the macrophages. Whipple disease should be suspected in patients who have recurrent arthritis, pigmentation, adenopathy, or CNS symptoms (dementia, myoclonus, ophthalmoplegia, visual disturbances, coma, or seizures). Treatment is with trimethoprim-sulfamethoxazole or tetracycline for 1 year.

* Suspect Whipple disease in patients who have recurrent arthritis, pigmentation, adenopathy, or CNS symptoms.
* Small-bowel biopsy specimens show PAS-positive granules in the macrophages.
* Treatment: trimethoprim-sulfamethoxazole or tetracycline for 1 year.

Eosinophilic Gastroenteritis
Patients with eosinophilic gastroenteritis have a history of allergies (eg, asthma) and food intolerances and episodic symptoms of nausea, vomiting, abdominal pain, and diarrhea. Laboratory findings include peripheral eosinophilia, iron deficiency anemia, and steatorrhea or protein-losing enteropathy. Small-bowel radiographs show coarse folds and filling defects, and biopsy specimens show infiltration of the mucosa by eosinophils and, occasionally, absence of villi. Parasitic infection should be ruled out. Treatment with corticosteroids produces a rapid response.

* Mucosal eosinophilic gastroenteritis: allergies, food intolerances, eosinophilia, and episodic intestinal symptoms.
* Rule out parasitic infection.
* Corticosteroids produce a rapid response.

Systemic Mastocytosis
Systemic mastocytosis is a proliferation of mast cells in the skin (urticaria pigmentosa), bones, lymph nodes, and parenchymal organs. Histamine is released, and 50% of patients have gastrointestinal tract symptoms (ie, diarrhea and peptic ulcer). "Bath pruritus" (itching after a hot bath) is a clue to the diagnosis.

* Systemic mastocytosis causes urticaria pigmentosa.
* Gastrointestinal tract symptoms occur in 50% of patients.
* "Bath pruritus" is a clue to the diagnosis.

Intestinal Lymphangiectasia
Intestinal lymphangiectasia is a disorder caused by lymphatic obstruction. Hypoplastic lymphatics cause lymph to leak into the intestine. The clinical features are edema (often unilateral leg edema), chylous peritoneal or pleural effusions, and steatorrhea or protein-losing enteropathy. Laboratory findings include lymphocytopenia (average, 0.6×10^9/L) due to enteric loss. All serum proteins are decreased, including immunoglobulins. Small-bowel radiographs show edematous folds, and small-bowel biopsy specimens show dilated lacteals and lymphatics in the lamina propria that may contain lipid-laden macrophages. The same biopsy findings are seen in obstruction of mesenteric nodes (lymphoma, Whipple disease, and Crohn disease) and obstruction of venous inflow to the heart (constrictive pericarditis and severe right heart failure). Diagnosis is based on abnormal small-bowel biopsy findings and documented enteric protein loss by increased α_1-antitrypsin levels in the stool. Treatment is with a low-fat diet and medium-chain triglycerides (they enter the portal blood rather than the lymphatics). Occasionally, surgical excision of the involved segment is useful if the lesion is localized.

* Intestinal lymphangiectasia: unilateral lymphedema of the leg and chylous peritoneal or pleural effusions.
* Lymphocytopenia is universal.
* Decreased serum proteins.
* Small-bowel biopsy specimens show dilated lacteals and lymphatics.
* Treatment: low-fat diet and medium-chain triglycerides.

Amyloidosis

Systemic amyloidosis is characterized by a diffuse deposition of an amorphous eosinophilic extracellular protein polysaccharide complex in the tissue. The main sites of amyloid deposition are the walls of blood vessels and the mucous membranes and muscle layers of the intestine. Any portion of the gut may be involved. Amyloid damages tissues by infiltration (muscle and nerve infiltration causes motility disorders and malabsorption) and ischemia (obliteration of vessels causes ulceration and bleeding). Intestinal dysmotility can produce diarrhea, constipation, pseudo-obstruction, megacolon, and fecal incontinence. Clinical findings in amyloidosis include macroglossia, hepatomegaly, cardiomegaly, proteinuria, and peripheral neuropathy. Pinch (posttraumatic) purpura or periorbital purpura after proctoscopic examination may occur. Small-bowel radiography shows symmetrical, sharply demarcated thickening of the plicae circulares. Fat aspirate confirms the diagnosis in 80% of patients and rectal biopsy stained with Congo red in 70%.

Miscellaneous Small-Bowel Disorders

Meckel Diverticulum

Meckel diverticulum, the persistence of the vitelline duct, is the most frequent developmental abnormality of the gut. It usually occurs within 100 cm of the ileocecal valve on the antimesenteric border of the ileum. It contains all layers of the intestinal wall and so is a true diverticulum. The mucosa is usually ileal but may be gastric (pancreatic or intestinal). Complications include obstruction due to intussusception and volvulus around the band that fixes the diverticulum to the bowel wall. Benign (leiomyomas) and malignant (carcinoids or leiomyosarcoma) tumors have been found in diverticula. Diverticulitis is uncommon. Incarceration in an indirect inguinal hernia (Littre hernia) and perforation that causes peritonitis may occur. Hemorrhage is the common complication and results from ulceration of the ileal mucosa adjacent to the gastric mucosa. This accounts for 50% of the cases of lower gastrointestinal tract bleeding in children and young adults. Radiography usually is not helpful in making the diagnosis. A nuclear scan (parietal cells concentrate technetium) may show the diverticulum, but false-positive and false-negative results can occur.

- Meckel diverticulum is the most frequent developmental abnormality of the gut.
- It accounts for 50% of the cases of lower gastrointestinal tract bleeding in children and young adults.

Aortoenteric Fistula

A history of gastrointestinal tract bleeding in a patient who has had a previous aortic graft demands immediate evaluation to rule out an aortoenteric fistula. If the patient presents with massive bleeding, do not attempt endoscopy or arteriography. Emergency surgery is indicated.

Management of a smaller bleeding episode is more controversial, and urgent CT or extended upper endoscopy has been suggested as a possible alternative to surgical exploration. If the presence of a graft fistula is confirmed (by air in the vessel wall on CT or erosion of a graft into the intestinal lumen on endoscopy), emergent surgery is indicated.

- If a patient presents with massive bleeding, do not attempt endoscopy or arteriography. Emergency surgery is indicated.

Chronic Intestinal Pseudo-Obstruction

Pseudo-obstruction is a syndrome characterized by the clinical findings of mechanical bowel obstruction but without occlusion of the lumen. The 2 types are primary and secondary.

The primary type, also called *idiopathic pseudo-obstruction*, is a visceral myopathy or neuropathy. It is associated with recurrent attacks of nausea, vomiting, cramping abdominal pain, distention, and constipation, which are of variable intensity and duration. If the cause is familial, the patient has a positive family history and the condition is present when the patient is young. Esophageal motility is abnormal (achalasia) in most patients. Occasionally, urinary tract motility is abnormal, and diarrhea or steatorrhea results from bacterial overgrowth. Upper gastrointestinal tract and small-bowel radiographs show dilatation of the bowel and slow transit (not mechanical obstruction).

- Idiopathic pseudo-obstruction is due to a familial cause or to a sporadic visceral myopathy or neuropathy.
- Recurrent attacks have variable frequency and duration.
- Abnormal esophageal motility occurs in most patients.
- Steatorrhea is caused by bacterial overgrowth.

Secondary pseudo-obstruction is due to underlying systemic disease or precipitating causes. These causes include the following (the most important causes are in italics):

1. Diseases involving the intestinal smooth muscle: *amyloidosis*, scleroderma, systemic lupus erythematosus, myotonic dystrophy, and muscular dystrophy
2. Neurologic diseases: *Parkinson disease*, Hirschsprung disease, Chagas disease, and familial autonomic dysfunction
3. Endocrine disorders: *myxedema* and hypoparathyroidism
4. Drugs: *antiparkinsonian medications* (*L-dopa*), phenothiazines, tricyclic antidepressants, ganglionic blockers, clonidine, and narcotics

Approach to the Patient With Chronic Intestinal Pseudo-Obstruction

If a patient has chronic intestinal psudo-obstruction, first rule out a mechanical cause for the obstruction. Second, look for an underlying precipitating cause such as metabolic abnormalities, medications, or an underlying associated disease. If a familial idiopathic cause is suspected, assess esophageal motility. Suspect scleroderma if intestinal radiography shows large-mouth diverticula of the small intestine. Suspect amyloidosis if the skin shows palpable purpura and if proteinuria and neuropathy are present.

- Secondary pseudo-obstruction is due to an underlying systemic disease or precipitating cause.
- Patients with scleroderma present with large-mouth diverticula of the intestine.
- Patients with amyloidosis present with palpable purpura, proteinuria, and neuropathy.

Inflammatory Bowel Disease

Idiopathic inflammatory bowel disease refers to 2 disorders of unknown cause: chronic ulcerative colitis and Crohn disease. Other possible causes of inflammation, especially infection, should be excluded before making the diagnosis of idiopathic inflammatory bowel disease.

Ulcerative colitis is a mucosal inflammation involving only the colon. *Crohn disease* is a transmural inflammation that can involve the gastrointestinal tract anywhere from the esophagus through the anus. The rectum is involved in about 95% of patients with ulcerative colitis and in only 50% of patients with Crohn disease. Ulcerative colitis is a continuous inflammatory process that extends from the anal verge to the more proximal colon (depending on the extent of the inflammation). Crohn disease is a segmental inflammation in which inflamed areas alternate with virtually normal areas. Patients with ulcerative colitis usually present with frequent bloody bowel movements with minimal abdominal pain, whereas patients with Crohn disease present with fewer bowel movements, less bleeding, and, more commonly, abdominal pain. Crohn disease is associated with intestinal fistula, fistula from the intestine to other organs, and perianal disease. Ulcerative colitis does not form fistulas, and perianal disease is uncommon. Strictures of the intestine are common with Crohn disease but rare in ulcerative colitis (when they are present, they suggest cancer).

- Ulcerative colitis involves only the colon.
- Crohn disease can involve the gastrointestinal tract anywhere from the esophagus through the anus.
- Ulcerative colitis is a continuous process.
- Crohn disease is a segmental inflammation.
- Ulcerative colitis is characterized by frequent, bloody bowel movements.
- Crohn disease is characterized by fewer bowel movements, less bleeding, and more abdominal pain.
- Crohn disease is associated with intestinal fistula, strictures, and perianal disease.

Extraintestinal Manifestations of Inflammatory Bowel Disease

Arthritis occurs in 10% to 20% of patients, usually monarticular or pauciarticular involvement of large joints. Peripheral joint symptoms mirror bowel activity: joint symptoms flare when colitis flares and joint symptoms improve as colitis improves. When axial joint symptoms develop, such as those of ankylosing spondylitis (which has a relationship with HLA-B27) and sacroiliitis, they are usually progressive and do not improve when colitis improves.

- Peripheral joint symptoms mirror bowel activity.
- Axial joint symptoms, such as those of ankylosing spondylitis and sacroiliitis, can develop and have a progressive course independent of bowel activity.

Skin lesions occur in 10% of patients. The 3 types of lesions are erythema nodosum, pyoderma gangrenosum, and aphthous ulcers of the mouth. Erythema nodosum and aphthous ulcers usually improve with treatment of colitis, whereas pyoderma gangrenosum has an independent course. Severe, refractory skin disease is an indication for surgical treatment.

- The skin lesions are erythema nodosum, pyoderma gangrenosum, and aphthous ulcers of the mouth.

Eye lesions occur in 5% of patients. The lesion is usually episcleritis or uveitis (or both). Episcleritis usually mirrors inflammatory bowel disease activity, but uveitis does not.

Liver disease also occurs in 5% of patients. Primary sclerosing cholangitis is more common in chronic ulcerative colitis than in Crohn disease. If the alkaline phosphatase level is increased in a patient with inflammatory bowel disease, the evaluation for primary sclerosing cholangitis includes ultrasonography, endoscopic retrograde cholangiopancreatography, and liver biopsy.

- If a patient's alkaline phosphatase level increases with inflammatory bowel disease, evaluate for primary sclerosing cholangitis.
- Central (axial) arthritis, pyoderma gangrenosum, primary sclerosing cholangitis, and uveitis usually follow a course independent of bowel disease activity.

Renal lithiasis occurs in 5% to 15% of patients. In Crohn disease with malabsorption, calcium oxalate stones occur. In chronic ulcerative colitis, uric acid stones are due to dehydration and loss of bicarbonate in the stool, leading to acidic urine.

Indications for Colonoscopy

Colonoscopy is indicated for evaluating the extent of the disease, performing biopsies, and evaluating strictures and filling defects. It is also indicated for differentiating Crohn disease from ulcerative colitis when they are otherwise indistinguishable. Another indication is for monitoring by random mucosal biopsy the development of dysplasia or cancer in patients who have had ulcerative colitis or Crohn colitis for more than 8 years.

- Colonoscopy and random mucosal biopsy are recommended for patients who have had ulcerative colitis or Crohn disease for >8 years.

Toxic Megacolon

In patients with active inflammation, avoid the causes of toxic megacolon, including opiates, anticholinergic agents, hypokalemia, and barium enema.

- In patients with active inflammation, avoid the causes of toxic megacolon.

Treatment of Ulcerative Colitis

Sulfasalazine and other aminosalicylates can induce remission in 80% of patients with mild or moderate ulcerative colitis and are effective maintenance therapy for 50% to 75% of patients with ulcerative colitis. The active agent of sulfasalazine, 5-aminosalicylic acid (5-ASA), is bound to sulfapyridine (the vehicle). Colonic bacteria break the bond and release 5-ASA, which is not absorbed but stays in contact with the mucosa and exerts its anti-inflammatory action. The efficacy of 5-ASA may be related to its ability to inhibit the lipoxygenase pathway of arachidonic acid metabolism or to function as an oxygen free radical scavenger (further studies are needed).

It is effective in acute disease and in maintaining remission. The side effects (male infertility, malaise, nausea, pancreatitis, rashes, headaches, hemolysis, impaired folate absorption, hepatitis, aplastic anemia, and exacerbation of colitis) are related to the sulfapyridine moiety and occur in 30% of patients who take sulfasalazine.

The 5-ASAs are a group of new drugs that deliver 5-ASA to the intestine in various ways. They eliminate sulfa toxicity but are more expensive than sulfasalazine. Two of these drugs are mesalamine and olsalazine. Mesalamine can be given topically (Rowasa suppositories and Rowasa enema) or orally (Asacol, which is 5-ASA coated with an acrylic polymer that releases 5-ASA in the terminal ileum, and Pentasa, which has an ethyl cellulose coating that releases 50% of the 5-ASA in the small bowel). Olsalazine consists of 2 molecules of 5-ASA conjugated with each other. Bacteria break the bond, releasing 5-ASA into the colon.

Aminosalicylates are used for mild to moderately active ulcerative colitis and for Crohn disease. Topical forms are useful for proctitis or left-sided colitis; systemic forms are used for pancolitis. Of the patients who do not tolerate sulfasalazine, 80% to 90% tolerate oral 5-ASA preparations. Side effects include hair loss, pancreatitis (often in patients who developed pancreatitis while taking sulfasalazine), reversible worsening of underlying renal disease, and exacerbation of colitis.

- Sulfasalazine and other aminosalicylates can induce remission in 80% of patients with mild or moderate ulcerative colitis and are effective maintenance therapy for 50%-75% of patients with ulcerative colitis.
- Sulfasalazine: side effects occur in 30% of patients.
- Other aminosalicylates are equally effective but more expensive; they are useful in 80%-90% of patients intolerant of sulfasalazine.

Topical corticosteroid preparations should be used twice daily by patients with active disease that is mild or moderate and is limited to the distal colon. Oral corticosteroids should be added to the regimen of patients with more proximal disease if sulfasalazine does not control the attacks. Up to 50% of the dose can be absorbed (depending on the preparation used and its vehicle). Oral preparations are indicated in active pancolonic disease of moderate severity in doses of 40 to 60 mg once daily or 20 to 40 mg daily in cases of mild disease that are unresponsive to topical corticosteroids and sulfasalazine. Prednisolone, the active metabolite, is the preferred form of drug for patients with cirrhosis (these patients may not be able to convert inactive prednisone to prednisolone). For patients who have a prompt response to oral corticosteroids, the dose may be tapered gradually at a rate not to exceed a 5-mg decrease in the total dose every 3 to 7 days. In severely ill patients, intravenous preparations should be given in large doses (prednisolone, 100 mg in divided doses) for up to 7 to 10 days. If improvement occurs at that time, therapy should be converted to oral corticosteroids (60-100 mg daily). If there is no improvement, surgical intervention (colectomy) is required. Because corticosteroids are not believed to prevent relapse, they should not be prescribed after the patient has complete remission and is symptom-free.

- Prescribe topical preparations twice daily for patients with active mild or moderate disease that is limited to the distal colon.
- Oral corticosteroids should be added to the regimen of patients with more proximal disease if topical steroids and sulfasalazine have not controlled the attacks.
- Oral preparations are useful in active pancolonic disease of moderate severity.
- Intravenous preparations are given to severely ill patients.
- Corticosteroids are useful in remission induction for ulcerative colitis but are not effective in maintenance of remission.

Total parenteral nutrition does not alter the clinical course of an ongoing attack. Indications for its use include severe dehydration and cachexia with marked fluid and nutrient deficits, excessive diarrhea that has not responded to standard therapy for chronic ulcerative colitis, and debilitated patients undergoing colectomy. Opiates (or their synthetic derivatives) and anticholinergic agents are contraindicated in chronic ulcerative colitis because they are ineffective and can contribute to the development of toxic megacolon.

- Total parenteral nutrition does not alter the clinical course of the ongoing attack.
- Use of opiates and anticholinergic agents is contraindicated in chronic ulcerative colitis.

Surgical treatment is curative in chronic ulcerative colitis. Indications for colectomy include severe intractable disease, acute life-threatening complications (perforation, hemorrhage, or toxic megacolon unresponsive to treatment), symptomatic colonic stricture, and suspected or documented colon cancer. Other indications are intractable moderate or severe colitis, refractory uveitis or pyoderma gangrenosum, growth retardation in pediatric patients, cancer prophylaxis, or inability to taper a regimen to low doses of corticosteroid (ie, <15 mg daily) over a period of 2 to 3 months. Procedures include proctocolectomy with ileoanal anastomosis and conventional Brooke ileostomy.

- Surgical treatment is curative in chronic ulcerative colitis.

Treatment of Crohn Disease

The use of sulfasalazine is discussed above (see "Treatment of Ulcerative Colitis" section). This drug is more effective for colonic disease than for small-bowel disease, although 5-ASA products designed to be released and activated in the small bowel may prove to be effective in the colon. Sulfasalazine does not have an additive effect or a steroid-sparing effect when given with corticosteroids, nor does it maintain remission in Crohn disease as it does in ulcerative colitis. None of the aminosalicylates are effective for the prophylaxis of Crohn disease.

- Sulfasalazine is more effective for colonic disease than for small-bowel disease.
- It does not have an additive effect or a sparing effect when given with corticosteroids.
- It does not maintain remission in Crohn disease.

The use of corticosteroids is discussed above (see "Treatment of Ulcerative Colitis" section). Corticosteroids are the agents that most quickly control an acute exacerbation of Crohn disease. They are the most useful drugs for treating acute small-bowel Crohn disease and for achieving rapid remission.

Azathioprine and 6-mercaptopurine (the active metabolite of azathioprine) have steroid-sparing effects. Their use should be reserved for patients with active disease who are taking steroids and whose corticosteroid dose needs to be reduced (or a given dose needs to be maintained in the face of worsening disease activity).

- 6-Mercaptopurine is the active metabolite of azathioprine.
- Azathioprine and 6-mercaptopurine are effective as maintenance therapy for Crohn disease.
- Both agents have a steroid-sparing effect.

Metronidazole (at a dose of 20 mg/kg) is effective for treating perianal disease. Six weeks may be needed for the therapeutic effect to become manifest. Recurrences are frequent when the drug dose is tapered or discontinued, leading to chronic therapy. It is less effective for colonic and small-bowel disease. Side effects include glossitis, metallic taste, vaginal and urethral burning sensation, neutropenia, dark urine, urticaria, disulfiram (Antabuse) effect, and paresthesias.

- Metronidazole is effective for treating perianal disease.
- Recurrences are frequent when the drug dose is tapered or discontinued.

Infliximab (Remicade) is a chimeric monoclonal antibody directed against tumor necrosis factor α. This intravenously administered anti-inflammatory agent is effective in treating moderately or severely active Crohn disease and ulcerative colitis that is refractory to conventional therapy and in treating fistulizing Crohn disease. Infliximab is a steroid-sparing agent that is effective in maintaining remission of Crohn disease. Infusion reactions consisting of pruritus, dyspnea, or chest pain may occur. The drug is associated with an increased risk of infection, including perianal abscesses, tuberculosis, and other respiratory infections. Rarely, subsequent infusions of infliximab may be associated with delayed hypersensitivity reactions.

- Infliximab is effective in treating moderately or severely active Crohn disease that is refractory to conventional therapy and in treating fistulizing Crohn disease.
- Infliximab is associated with acute infusion reactions, delayed hypersensitivity reactions, and an increased risk of infections.

Bowel rest per se does not have any role in achieving remission in Crohn disease. However, providing adequate nutritional support does help facilitate remission; any form of nutritional support is acceptable as long as the amount is adequate. Adequate nutrition can be essential in maintaining growth in children who have severe Crohn disease.

If Crohn disease is present during exploration for presumed appendicitis, the acute ileitis should be left alone (many of these patients do not develop chronic Crohn disease). Appendectomy can be performed if the cecum and appendix are free of disease. Of the patients with Crohn disease who have surgical treatment, 70% to 90% require reoperation within 15 years (many within the first 5 years after the initial operation). The anastomotic site is the most likely site for recurrence of disease. Indications for surgical treatment include intractable symptoms, acute life-threatening complications, obstruction, unhealed fistulas that cause complications, abscess formation, and malignancy.

- Of the patients with Crohn disease who are operated on, 70%-90% require reoperation within 15 years.
- The anastomotic site is the most likely site for disease recurrence.

Gastrointestinal Manifestations of AIDS

Gastrointestinal tract symptoms occur in 30% to 50% of North American and European patients with AIDS and in nearly 90% of patients in developing countries. The gastrointestinal tract in patients with AIDS is predisposed to a spectrum of viral, bacterial, fungal, and protozoan pathogens. The most frequent gastrointestinal tract symptom is diarrhea, which is often chronic, associated with weight loss, and usually caused by 1 or more identifiable pathogens. Dysphagia, odynophagia, abdominal pain, and jaundice are less frequent, and gastrointestinal tract bleeding is rare. The goal of evaluation is to identify treatable causes of infection or symptoms. When no cause is identified, the condition may be idiopathic AIDS enteropathy or it may be caused by as yet unidentified pathogens.

- The majority of AIDS patients with diarrhea have 1 or more identifiable pathogens.
- Some have no identifiable cause despite extensive evaluation. This may represent idiopathic AIDS enteropathy or as yet unidentified pathogens.

Viral

Cytomegalovirus

Cytomegalovirus is one of the most common and potentially serious opportunistic pathogens. It most commonly affects the colon and esophagus, although the entire gut, liver, biliary tract, and pancreas are susceptible. A patchy or diffuse colitis may progress to ischemic necrosis and perforation. Symptoms include watery diarrhea and fever and, less commonly, hematochezia and abdominal pain. Odynophagia may be present if the esophagus is involved. Diagnosis is based on biopsy specimens that show cytomegalic inclusion cells with surrounding inflammation ("owl's eye"). Treatment is ganciclovir, 5 mg/kg twice daily for 14 to 21 days. If the virus is resistant to ganciclovir, use foscarnet.

Herpes Simplex Virus

The 3 gastrointestinal tract manifestations of herpes simplex virus infection in patients with AIDS are perianal lesions (chronic cutaneous ulcers), proctitis, and esophagitis. The organs affected are the colon and esophagus. Symptoms include perianal lesions that are painful;

proctitis that causes tenesmus, constipation, and inguinal lymphadenopathy; and esophagitis that causes odynophagia, with or without dysphagia. Diagnosis is based on the cytologic identification of intranuclear (Cowdry type A) inclusions in multinucleated cells and is confirmed with viral cultures. Treatment is acyclovir given orally or intravenously.

Adenovirus

Adenovirus reportedly causes diarrhea. The organ affected is the colon. The main symptom is watery, nonbloody diarrhea. Diagnosis is based on culture and biopsy. There is no treatment.

Bacteria

Mycobacterium avium-intracellulare

Mycobacterium avium-intracellulare causes infection of the gut in patients with disseminated disease. The small intestine is affected more commonly than the colon. Symptoms include fever, weight loss, diarrhea, abdominal pain, and malabsorption. Diagnosis is based on finding acid-fast organisms in the stool and tissue, with confirmation from culture of stool and biopsy specimens. Treatment is multiple drug therapy with ethambutol, rifampin, ciprofloxacin, and clarithromycin.

Other Bacteria

Other important bacteria include the following:

Salmonella typhimurium and *Salmonella enteritidis*—Treatment is with amoxicillin, trimethoprim-sulfamethoxazole, or ciprofloxacin.

Shigella flexneri—Treatment is with trimethoprim-sulfamethoxazole, ampicillin, or ciprofloxacin.

Campylobacter jejuni—Treatment is with erythromycin or ciprofloxacin.

AIDS patients with *Salmonella*, *S flexneri*, or *C jejuni* have a substantially higher incidence of intestinal infection, bacteremia, and prolonged or recurrent infections because of antibiotic resistance or compromised immune function, or both.

Fungi

Candida albicans

In patients with AIDS, *Candida* causes locally invasive mucosal disease in the mouth and esophagus. Disseminated candidiasis is rare because neutrophil function remains relatively intact. The presence of oral candidiasis in persons at risk of AIDS should alert the physician to possible human immunodeficiency virus (HIV) infection. If oral candidiasis is present, endoscopy is required to confirm esophageal involvement. The symptoms of odynophagia suggest esophageal involvement. Diagnosis is based on histologic examination showing hyphae, pseudohyphae, or yeast forms. Treatment is with nystatin, ketoconazole, fluconazole, or amphotericin.

Histoplasma capsulatum

Histoplasma capsulatum causes an important opportunistic infection in AIDS patients who reside in endemic areas. Colonic involvement is more common than small-bowel involvement. Symptoms include diarrhea, weight loss, fever, and abdominal pain. Diagnosis is established by culture. Colonoscopy may show inflammation and ulcerations, and histologic examination with Giemsa stain shows intracellular yeast-like *H capsulatum* within lamina propria macrophages. Treatment is with amphotericin or itraconazole.

Protozoa

Cryptosporidium

Cryptosporidium is among the commonest enteric pathogens, occurring in 10% to 20% of patients with AIDS and diarrhea in the United States and in 50% of those in developing countries. The organs affected are the small and large intestines and the biliary tree. Symptoms include voluminous watery diarrhea, severe abdominal cramps, weight loss, anorexia, malaise, and low-grade fever. Biliary tract obstruction has been reported. Diagnosis is based on microscopic identification of organisms in stool specimens with modified acid-fast staining or stains specific for *Cryptosporidium*. Organisms may also be identified in biopsy specimens or in duodenal fluid aspirates. Treatment is with paromomycin, which reduces the diarrhea.

Isospora belli

Isospora belli is the more common cause of diarrhea in developing countries. The small intestine is primarily affected, but the organisms can be identified throughout the gut and in other organs. Symptoms include watery diarrhea, cramping abdominal pain, weight loss, anorexia, malaise, and fever. Diagnosis is based on identifying oval oocysts in stool with a modified Kinyoun carbolfuchsin stain. Biopsy specimens from the small intestine may show organisms in the lumen or within cytoplasmic vacuoles in enterocytes. Although *I belli* oocysts resemble *Cryptosporidium* oocysts, *I belli* oocysts contain 2 sporoblasts. *Cryptosporidium* oocysts are small and round and contain 4 sporozoites. Treatment is with trimethoprim-sulfamethoxazole.

Microsporida (Enterocytozoon bieneusi)

Organisms in the order Microsporida are emerging as important pathogens; they have been identified in up to 33% of AIDS patients who have diarrhea. The organ affected is the small intestine, and symptoms include watery diarrhea with gradual weight loss but no fever or anorexia. Diagnosis is based on electron microscopic identification of round or oval meront (proliferative) and sporont (spore-forming) stages of Microsporida in the villous but not crypt epithelial cells of the duodenum and jejunum. There are reports of positive stool specimens with Giemsa staining. There is no known treatment.

Other Protozoa

Entamoeba histolytica—Treatment is with metronidazole.

Giardia lamblia—Treatment is with metronidazole.

Blastocystis hominis—Because there is no evidence that *B hominis* is pathogenic, it does not need to be treated.

The rates of symptomatic infection with *E histolytica*, *G lamblia*, or *B hominis* are not markedly higher than in patients who do not have AIDS. *E histolytica* is a nonpathogenic commensal in most patients with AIDS. Giardiasis may require prolonged treatment, as in other immunocompetent persons.

Diagnostic Evaluation of Patients With AIDS Who Have Diarrhea

When patients with AIDS have diarrhea, initial studies include examination for stool leukocytes; stool cultures for *Salmonella* species, *Shigella flexneri*, and *Campylobacter jejuni* (≥3 specimens); stool examination for ova and parasites (using saline, iodine, trichrome, and acid-fast preparations); and stool assay for *Clostridium difficile* toxin. Additional studies include gastroscopy to inspect tissue, to aspirate luminal material, and to obtain biopsy specimens; examination of duodenal aspirate for parasites and culture; culture of duodenal biopsy specimens for cytomegalovirus and mycobacteria; colonoscopy to inspect tissue and to obtain biopsy specimens; culture of biopsy specimens for cytomegalovirus, adenovirus, mycobacteria, and herpes simplex virus; and staining biopsy specimens with hematoxylin-eosin for protozoa and viral inclusion cells, with methenamine silver or Giemsa stain for fungi, and with Fite method for mycobacteria.

Whether further evaluation is needed if the studies listed above do not yield a diagnosis is a matter of controversy. Most experts advocate empirical treatment with loperamide (Imodium). Others recommend that biopsy specimens from the duodenum be examined with electron microscopy for Microsporida or from the colon for adenovirus. Empirical treatment with loperamide is favored because there is no treatment for either Microsporida or adenovirus.

Colon

Pseudomembranous Enterocolitis

Pseudomembranous enterocolitis is a necrotizing inflammatory disease of the intestines characterized by the formation of a membrane-like collection of exudate overlying a degenerating mucosa. Precipitating factors include colon obstruction, uremia, ischemia, intestinal surgery, and all antibiotics (except vancomycin).

Antibiotic Colitis

The symptoms of antibiotic colitis are fever, abdominal pain, and diarrhea (mucus and blood), which usually occur 1 to 6 weeks after antibiotic therapy. Sigmoidoscopy shows pseudomembranes and friability. Biopsy specimens show inflammation and microulceration with exudation. The condition usually remits, but it recurs in 15% of patients. Complications include perforation and megacolon. The pathogenesis begins with the antibiotic altering the colonic flora, resulting in an overgrowth of *Clostridium difficile*. The toxin produced by *C difficile* is cytotoxic, causing necrosis of the epithelium and exudation (pseudomembranes). Diagnosis is based on a toxin assay, which is positive in 98% of patients, and on cultures, which are positive in about 75%. Radiography shows pseudomembranes. Proctoscopic findings may be normal or show classic pseudomembranes. The treatment is to discontinue the use of antibiotics and provide general supportive care (eg, fluids). Avoid use of antimotility agents. If there is no response, metronidazole (250 mg 3 times daily) is 80% effective and inexpensive. Vancomycin (125 mg 4 times daily) is also 80% effective but expensive. If the patient is very ill, cholestyramine binds

toxin. For a first recurrence, the same antibiotic can be used or the drug can be switched. For multiple recurrences, add cholestyramine and prolong the course of treatment with antibiotics.

- Antibiotic colitis: symptoms include fever, abdominal pain, and diarrhea 1-6 weeks after antibiotic therapy.
- A toxin assay is positive in 98% of patients.
- Cultures are positive in 75%.
- Metronidazole is the initial treatment.
- It recurs in 15% of patients.

Radiation Colitis

Irradiation injury usually affects both the colon and the small bowel. Endothelial cells of small submucosal arterioles are very radiosensitive and respond to large doses of irradiation by swelling, proliferating, and undergoing fibrinoid degeneration. The result is obliterative endarteritis.

Acute disease occurs during or immediately after irradiation; the mucosa fails to regenerate, and there is friability, hyperemia, and edema. *Subacute disease* occurs 2 to 12 months after irradiation. Obliterative endarteritis produces progressive inflammation and ulceration. *Chronic disease* consists of fistulas, abscesses, strictures, and bleeding from intestinal mucosal vessels. Predisposing factors include other diseases that produce microvascular insufficiency (eg, hypertension, diabetes mellitus, atherosclerosis, and heart failure) because they accelerate the development of vascular occlusion, total irradiation dose of 40 to 50 Gy, previous chemotherapy, adhesions, previous surgical procedure and pelvic inflammatory disease, and age (the elderly are more susceptible). Radiography of acute disease shows fine serrations of the bowel, and radiography of chronic disease shows stricture of the rectum, which is involved most commonly. Endoscopy shows atrophic mucosa with telangiectatic vessels. Endoscopic coagulation is effective treatment for bleeding, but surgery may be required for fistulas, strictures, or abscesses.

- Radiation colitis involves both the colon and the small bowel.
- The endothelial cells of the small submucosal arterioles are very radiosensitive.
- The result is obliterative endarteritis.
- Predisposing factors: hypertension, diabetes mellitus, atherosclerosis, chemotherapy, and >40 Gy of irradiation.
- The rectum is involved most commonly.

Ischemia

Review of Vascular Anatomy

The *celiac trunk* supplies the stomach and duodenum. The *superior mesenteric artery* supplies the jejunum, ileum, and right colon. The *inferior mesenteric artery* supplies the left colon and rectum.

Acute Ischemia

The symptoms of acute ischemia are sudden severe abdominal pain, vomiting, and diarrhea (with or without blood). Early in the course of ischemia, physical examination findings are normal despite complaints of severe abdominal pain, but later findings indicate peritonitis. Risk factors include severe atherosclerosis, congestive heart failure, atrial fibrillation (source of emboli), hypotension, and oral contraceptives.

There are several syndromes. *Acute mesenteric ischemia* is due to embolic obstruction of the superior mesenteric artery in 80% of patients. Most emboli (95%) lodge in this artery because of laminar flow, vessel caliber, and the angle it takes off from the aorta. The clue to search for emboli is atrial fibrillation. This syndrome results in a loss of small bowel and produces short-bowel syndrome. Radiography shows ileus, small-bowel obstruction, and, later, gas in the portal vein. The treatment is embolectomy. *Ischemic colitis* is due to a transient decrease in perfusion pressure in a setting of chronic, diffuse mesenteric vascular disease. This decrease occurs in severe dehydration or shock and results in ischemia of the gastrointestinal tract. It commonly involves areas of the colon between adjacent arteries, that is, "watershed areas," such as the splenic flexure and rectosigmoid. Patients with this syndrome present with abdominal pain and rectal bleeding. The characteristic radiographic feature is thumbprinting of watershed areas. The treatment is supportive, with administration of intravenous fluids to maintain adequate tissue perfusion and consideration of antibiotics if significant leukocytosis or fever is present. If the condition deteriorates, surgical resection may be necessary. *Nonocclusive ischemia* is due to poor tissue perfusion caused by inadequate cardiac output. It can involve both small and large bowels. Its distribution does not conform to an area supplied by a major vessel. It occurs in patients with cardiac failure or anoxia or in patients who are in shock.

* Ischemic colitis: diagnosis is based on the radiographic finding of thumbprinting of watershed areas.

Chronic Mesenteric Ischemia (Intestinal Angina)

Chronic mesenteric ischemia is uncommon. Symptoms include postprandial pain and fear of eating (weight loss). At least 2 of 3 major splanchnic vessels must be occluded. It is associated with hypertension, diabetes mellitus, and atherosclerosis. An abdominal bruit is a clue to the diagnosis. Angiography is diagnostic in about 50% of the cases and shows a stenotic area in 2 of 3 major vessels. The treatment is surgical revascularization.

Occlusion of the superior mesenteric vein accounts for approximately 10% of the cases of bowel ischemia. Risk factors include hypercoagulable states such as polycythemia vera, liver disease, pancreatic cancer, intra-abdominal abscess, and portal hypertension. Patients present with abdominal pain that gradually becomes severe. Diagnosis is based on angiographic findings. The treatment is surgical.

* Chronic mesenteric ischemia is associated with hypertension, diabetes mellitus, and atherosclerosis.
* Mesenteric venous thrombosis occurs with hypercoagulable states.

Amebic Colitis

The colon is the usual initial site of amebic colitis. Symptoms vary from none to explosive bloody diarrhea with fever, tenesmus, and abdominal cramps. Proctoscopy shows discrete ulcers with undermined edges and normal adjacent mucosa. If an exudate is present,

swab and make wet mount preparations for trophozoites. Indirect hemagglutination is useful for invasive disease. Radiography shows concentric narrowing of the cecum in 90% of the cases. Treat with metronidazole. *Entamoeba histolytica* is the only pathogenic ameba in humans.

* The colon is the initial site of disease.
* Proctoscopy shows discrete ulcers with undermined edges.
* Radiography shows concentric narrowing of the cecum in 90% of the cases.
* *E histolytica* is the only pathogenic ameba in humans.

Tuberculosis

Patients with tuberculosis present with diarrhea, a change in bowel habits, and rectal bleeding. The ileocecal area is the most commonly involved site. Radiography shows a contracted cecum and ascending colon and ulceration. Proctoscopy demonstrates deep and superficial ulcers. The rectum may be spared. A hypertrophic ulcerating mass may be seen. Biopsy samples stained with Ziehl-Neelsen stain are positive for acid-fast bacilli. All cases are associated with pulmonary or miliary tuberculosis.

* Tuberculosis is associated with diarrhea, change in bowel habits, and rectal bleeding.
* The ileocecal area is commonly involved.
* Deep and superficial ulcers are characteristic findings.
* All cases are associated with pulmonary or miliary tuberculosis.

Streptococcus bovis Endocarditis

Streptococcus bovis endocarditis is associated with colon disease (diverticulosis or cancer). The colon should be evaluated.

Irritable Bowel Syndrome

The term *irritable bowel syndrome* is used for symptoms that are presumed to arise from the small and large intestines. It refers to a well-recognized complex of symptoms arising from interactions of the intestine, the psyche, and, possibly, luminal factors. Most patients have abdominal pain that is relieved with defecation or associated with a change in the frequency or consistency of the stool. Other associated symptoms include abdominal bloating and passage of excessive mucus with the stool.

Patients with irritable bowel syndrome usually have a long duration of symptoms, symptoms associated with situations of stress, and no weight loss, no intestinal bleeding, and no associated organic symptoms (eg, arthritis or fever). Irritable bowel syndrome is a diagnosis of exclusion: the diagnosis is confirmed by an appropriate medical evaluation that does not reveal any organic illness. Always ask whether the patient's symptoms are related to ingestion of dairy foods because lactase deficiency must be ruled out. Patients who have upper abdominal discomfort and bloating may require an ultrasonographic examination of the abdomen and esophagogastroduodenoscopy. Patients with lower abdominal discomfort or with a change in bowel habits may require stool studies, proctoscopic examination, and colon radiography or colonoscopy.

The treatment of irritable bowel syndrome is reassurance, stress reduction, and a high-fiber diet or the use of fiber supplements. The use of antispasmodics to control abdominal pain or antimotility agents to control diarrhea should be reserved for patients who do not have a response to a high-fiber diet.

Nontoxic Megacolon (Pseudo-Obstruction)

Acute pseudo-obstruction of the colon occurs postoperatively (non-abdominal operations) and with spinal cord injury, sepsis, uremia, electrolyte imbalance, and drugs (narcotics, anticholinergics, and psychotropic agents). When the cecum is more than 13 or 14 cm in diameter, the risk of perforation increases. Obstruction should be ruled out with a Hypaque enema. Treatment includes placement of a nasogastric tube, discontinuation of drug therapy, correction of metabolic abnormalities, and, if needed, colonoscopic decompression or cecostomy.

Chronic pseudo-obstruction of the colon occurs with disorders that cause generalized intestinal pseudo-obstruction.

Congenital Megacolon

Congenital megacolon (Hirschsprung disease) occurs in 1 in 5,000 births. The incidence is increased with Down syndrome. Congenital megacolon usually becomes manifest in infancy; however, it can occur in adulthood. There is a variable length of aganglionic segment from the rectum to the proximal colon (usually confined to the rectum or rectosigmoid). The diagnosis is usually made at birth because of meconium ileus or obstipation. If the diagnosis is made when the patient is an adult, the patient has a history of chronic constipation. Colon radiography shows a characteristically narrowed distal segment and a dilated proximal colon. Rectal biopsy shows aganglionosis. Anorectal manometry shows loss of the anorectal inhibitory reflex. Treatment is with sphincter-saving operations.

- Congenital megacolon: increased incidence with Down syndrome.
- If the diagnosis is made when the patient is an adult, there is a history of chronic constipation.
- Colon radiography shows a characteristically narrowed distal segment and a dilated proximal colon.
- Rectal biopsy shows aganglionosis.
- Motility: absence of anorectal inhibitory reflex.

Lower Gastrointestinal Tract Bleeding

The evaluation of rectal bleeding should begin with a digital examination, anoscopy, and proctosigmoidoscopy. If a definitive diagnosis cannot be made, perform a barium enema or arteriography, depending on the nature of the bleeding. The inability to cleanse the colon appropriately during active bleeding makes the barium enema difficult to perform and interpret. Some advocate the use of nuclear scanning if the activity of the bleeding is uncertain. With active bleeding, angiography is the diagnostic procedure of choice. It is also indicated for patients with recurrent episodes of rectal bleeding who have had normal results on previous standard tests, that is, barium enema or colonoscopy. Colonoscopy is not useful if bleeding in the lower gastrointestinal tract is torrential, but it may be of some benefit if there is a slower rate of bleeding. Colonoscopy is valuable for evaluating patients who have unexplained rectal bleeding and persistently positive findings on tests for occult blood in the stool.

- Initial evaluation of rectal bleeding: digital examination, anoscopy, and proctosigmoidoscopy.
- If the activity of bleeding is uncertain, a nuclear scan may be the next best test.
- Colonoscopy is not useful if there is torrential bleeding in the lower gastrointestinal tract.
- Angiography is the procedure of choice with active bleeding.

The important causes of lower gastrointestinal tract bleeding are the following:

1. Angiodysplasia—usually involves the right colon and small bowel and may respond to endoscopic treatment
2. Diverticular disease—usually bleeding without other symptoms
3. Inflammatory bowel disease (colitis)—5% of patients present with it
4. Ischemic colitis—painful and bloody diarrhea
5. Cancer—rarely causes marked bleeding
6. Meckel diverticulum—the commonest cause of lower gastrointestinal tract bleeding in young patients; it is usually painless
7. Hemorrhoids—usually are present with rectal outlet bleeding

In the evaluation of lower gastrointestinal tract bleeding, stabilize the patient's condition, perform proctoscopy to rule out rectal outlet bleeding, and obtain a nasogastric tube aspirate or use esophagogastroduodenoscopy to rule out upper gastrointestinal tract bleeding. A radionuclide-tagged red blood cell scan may help determine whether bleeding is occurring, but it may not localize precisely the bleeding site. If there is active bleeding, perform angiography. If bleeding stops or occurs at a slow rate, perform colonoscopy. If the patient is young, perform a Meckel scan.

If angiography localizes the bleeding site, infusion of vasopressin or embolization may be useful. If colonoscopy demonstrates bleeding, injection of epinephrine, electrocoagulation, or laser coagulation may be useful. If bleeding is massive or if marked bleeding continues, surgical management is needed.

Angiodysplasia

Angiodysplasia is a common and increasingly recognized cause of lower gastrointestinal tract bleeding in elderly patients, usually involving the cecum and ascending colon. It is associated with cardiac disease, especially aortic stenosis. There are no associated skin or visceral lesions. Acquired vascular ectasias are believed to be associated with aging and to be due to chronic, partial, intermittent, and low-grade obstruction of submucosal veins where they penetrate the colon. Obstruction is from muscle contraction and distention of the cecum. Colon radiography is of no diagnostic value, but angiography localizes the extent of involvement. Colonoscopy may show lesions, and cautery application may be effective.

- Acquired vascular ectasias are associated with aging.
- Angiodysplasia is associated with cardiac disease, especially aortic stenosis.
- It usually involves the cecum and ascending colon.
- Colonoscopy may show lesions. Apply cautery.

Diverticular Disease of the Colon

Definitions

Diverticula are acquired herniations of the mucosa and submucosa through the muscular layers of the colonic wall. *Diverticulosis* is the mere presence of uninflamed diverticula of the colon. *Diverticulitis* is the inflammation of 1 or more diverticula. The diagnosis and management of the complications of diverticular disease are outlined in Table 7-13.

Diverticulitis

Microperforation or macroperforation of the diverticulum with subsequent peridiverticular inflammation is necessary to produce diverticulitis. The severity of the clinical symptoms depends on the extent of the inflammation. Free perforation is infrequent (diverticula are invested with longitudinal muscle and mesentery). Local perforations may dissect along the colon wall and form intramural fistulas. The clinical presentation is left lower quadrant pain, fever, abdominal distention, constipation, and, occasionally, a palpable tender mass. Treatment includes resting the bowel or using a low-fiber diet and antibiotics and obtaining an early surgical consultation. Indications for surgical treatment during the acute phase include the development of generalized peritonitis, an enlarging inflammatory mass, fistula formation, colonic obstruction, inability to rule out carcinoma in an area of stricture, or recurrent episodes of diverticulitis.

- Diverticulitis: the clinical symptoms depend on the extent of inflammation.

- Free perforation is infrequent.
- Clinical presentation: left lower quadrant pain, fever, abdominal distention, constipation, and, occasionally, a palpable tender mass.
- Treatment: bowel rest and antibiotics; obtain a surgical consultation.

Colon Polyps

Three types of epithelial polyps are benign: hyperplastic, hamartomatous, and inflammatory polyps. *Hyperplastic polyps* are metaplastic, completely differentiated glandular elements. *Hamartomatous polyps* are a mixture of normal tissues. *Inflammatory polyps* are an epithelial inflammatory reaction.

The fourth type of epithelial polyp is *adenomatous polyps*, which represent a failure of differentiation of glandular elements. They are the only neoplastic (premalignant) polyp. The 3 types of adenomatous polyps are tubular adenoma, mixed (tubulovillous) adenoma, and villous adenoma (syndrome of hypokalemia and profuse mucus). The risk of cancer with any adenomatous polyp depends on 2 features: size larger than 1 cm and the presence of villous elements. If a polyp is found on flexible sigmoidoscopy and biopsy shows a hyperplastic polyp, no further work-up is needed. If biopsy shows an adenomatous polyp, perform colonoscopy to look for additional polyps and to perform polypectomy.

- Adenomatous polyps are the only neoplastic (premalignant) polyp.
- The risk of cancer with any adenomatous polyp depends on size >1 cm and the presence of villous elements.
- If biopsy shows an adenomatous polyp, perform colonoscopy.

Table 7-13 Diagnosis and Management of Complications of Diverticular Disease

Complication	Signs and Symptoms	Findings	Treatment
Diverticulitis	Pain, fever, & constipation or diarrhea (or both)	Palpable tender colon, leukocytosis	Liquid diet, with or without antibiotics, or elective surgery
Pericolic abscess	Pain, fever (with or without tenderness), or pus in stools	Tender mass, guarding, leukocytosis, soft tissue mass on abdominal films or ultrasonograms	Nothing by mouth, intravenous fluids, antibiotics, early surgical treatment with colostomy
Fistula	Depends on site: dysuria, pneumaturia, fecal discharge on skin or vagina	Depends on site: fistulogram, methylene blue	Antibiotics, clear liquids, colostomy; later, resection
Perforation	Sudden severe pain, fever	Sepsis, leukocytosis, free air	Antibiotics, nothing by mouth, intravenous fluids, immediate surgical treatment
Liver abscess	Right upper quadrant pain, fever, weight loss	Tender liver, tender bowel or mass, leukocytosis, increased serum alkaline phosphatase, lumbosacral scan (filling defect)	Antibiotics, surgical drainage, operation for bowel disease
Bleeding	Bright red or maroon blood or clots	Blood on rectal examination, sigmoidoscopy, colonoscopy, angiography	Conservative: blood transfusion if needed, with or without operation

Hereditary Polyposis Syndromes Associated With Risk of Cancer

Only the polyposis syndromes associated with adenomatous polyps carry a risk of cancer.

Familial Adenomatous Polyposis

Familial adenomatous polyposis (FAP) is characterized by adenomatous polyps of the colon. Colorectal carcinoma develops in more than 95% of the patients. There are no extra-abdominal manifestations except for bilateral congenital hypertrophy of the retinal pigment epithelium. Diagnosis is based on family history and documentation of adenomatous polyps. Screening is indicated for all family members, and colectomy is indicated before malignancy develops. The inheritance is autosomal dominant; however, the phenotypic expression may vary considerably.

- Colorectal carcinoma develops in more than 95% of patients with FAP.
- There are no extra-abdominal manifestations except for bilateral congenital hypertrophy of the retinal pigment epithelium.
- Colectomy is indicated before malignancy develops.

Gardner Syndrome

In Gardner syndrome, adenomatous polyps involve the colon, although rarely the terminal ileum and proximal small bowel are involved. Colorectal cancer develops in more than 95% of patients. Extraintestinal manifestations include congenital hypertrophy of the retinal pigment epithelium; osteomas of the mandible, skull, and long bones; supernumerary teeth; soft tissue tumors; thyroid and adrenal tumors; and epidermoid and sebaceous cysts. Screening is indicated for family members, and colectomy should be performed before malignancy develops. The inheritance is autosomal dominant.

- Colorectal cancer develops in more than 95% of patients with Gardner syndrome.
- There are extraintestinal manifestations.
- Screening is indicated for family members.

Turcot Syndrome

In Turcot syndrome, adenomatous polyps of the colon are associated with malignant gliomas and other brain tumors. The inheritance is likely autosomal dominant but with variable penetrance.

- Only the polyposis syndromes associated with adenomatous polyps carry a risk of cancer.
- Perform colectomy for diffuse polyposis only if the polyps are adenomatous.
- Screening is indicated for patients with heritable polyposis syndromes only if the polyps are adenomatous.

Hereditary Polyposis Syndromes Not Associated With Risk of Cancer

Peutz-Jeghers Syndrome

In Peutz-Jeghers syndrome, hamartomas occur in the small intestine and, less commonly, in the stomach and colon. Pigmented lesions of the mouth, hands, and feet are associated with ovarian sex cord tumors and tumors of the proximal small bowel. The inheritance is autosomal dominant.

- Peutz-Jeghers syndrome: hamartomas of the small intestine.
- Pigmented lesions of the mouth, hands, and feet are associated with ovarian sex cord and proximal small bowel tumors.

Juvenile Polyposis

In juvenile polyposis, hyperplastic polyps involve the colon and, less commonly, the small intestine and stomach. Patients present with gastrointestinal tract bleeding or intussusception with obstruction.

- Polyposis syndromes are autosomal dominant.

Colorectal Cancer

Epidemiology

Epidemiology is important in etiologic theories. Colorectal carcinoma is the second most common cancer in the United States, with 100,000 new cases and 60,000 deaths annually. Colon cancer eventually develops in 6% of Americans, and the mortality rate has not decreased since the 1930s. The incidence, which varies widely among different populations, is highest in westernized countries. Compared with past rates, rates for cancer of the right colon and sigmoid colon have increased, but rates for cancer of the rectum have decreased: cecum or ascending colon, 25%; sigmoid, 25%; rectum, 20%; transverse colon, 12%; rectosigmoid, 10%; and descending colon, 6%.

- Colorectal cancer is the second most common cancer in the United States.
- Rates for cancer of the right colon and sigmoid colon have increased.

Etiology

The role of the environment as a cause of colorectal cancer is supported by regional differences and migrant studies of incidence. A high-fat diet increases the risk and may enhance the cholesterol and bile acid content of bile, which is converted by colonic bacteria to compounds that may promote tumors. A high-fiber diet is protective. Increased stool bulk may dilute carcinogens and promoters and decrease exposure by decreasing transit time. Fiber components may bind carcinogens or decrease bacterial enzymes that form toxic compounds. Charbroiled meat or fish and fried foods contain possible mutagens. Antioxidants (vitamins A and C), selenium, vitamin E, yellow-green vegetables, and calcium may protect against cancer.

- A high-fat diet increases the risk of colorectal cancer.
- A high-fiber diet has a protective effect.
- Charbroiled meat or fish and fried foods contain possible mutagens.

Genetic Factors

Certain oncogenes amplify or alter gene products in colon cancer cells. Aneuploidy is characteristic of more aggressive tumors. The carbohydrate structure of colonic mucus is altered in colon cancer.

Cell-cell interaction possibly has a role in cancer development. Also, genetic predisposition has a role in many patients with colon cancer. FAP syndromes are autosomal dominant. Most colon cancer arises in adenomatous polyps. Hereditary nonpolyposis colon cancer (Lynch syndrome) is an autosomal dominant disease that may account for up to 5% of cases of colon cancer. Genetic susceptibility in the general population also has a role; for example, there is a 3-fold increased risk of colorectal cancer in first-degree relatives of patients with sporadic colorectal cancer.

- Aneuploidy is characteristic of more aggressive tumors.
- Genetic predisposition to cancer exists in many patients with colon cancer.
- FAP is autosomal dominant.
- There is a 3-fold increased risk of colorectal cancer in first-degree relatives of patients with sporadic colorectal cancer.

Risk Factors for Colorectal Cancer

The risk factors for colorectal cancer include the following:

1. Age older than 40—The risk increases sharply at age 40, doubles each decade until age 60, and peaks at age 80.
2. Personal history of adenoma or colon cancer—The risk increases with the number of adenomas; from 2% to 6% of patients with colon cancer have synchronous colon cancer and 1.1% to 4.7% have metachronous colon cancer.
3. Inflammatory bowel disease—Dysplasia precedes cancer; the cancer rate begins to increase after 7 years of chronic ulcerative colitis and increases 10% per decade of disease. After 25 years, the risk is 30%. The risk is greatest for pancolitis. The risk is delayed a decade in left-sided-only colitis and is negligible in ulcerative proctitis.

Cancer risk is not related to the severity of the first attack, disease activity, or age at onset. The rate of colon cancer is also increased 4 to 20 times in Crohn disease or ileocolitis. A family history of colon cancer is a risk factor, and a personal history of female genital or breast cancer carries a 2-fold increased risk of colon cancer.

- Colorectal cancer risk factor: age older than 40.
- Risk increases with the number of adenomas.
- From 2%-6% of patients with colon cancer have synchronous colon cancer and 1.1%-4.7% have metachronous colon cancer.
- Cancer rate begins to increase after 7 years of chronic ulcerative colitis.
- After 25 years, the risk is 30%.
- The risk is greatest for pancolitis.
- Crohn disease: the rate of colon cancer is increased 4-20 times.

Pathology and Prognostic Indicators

Cancer arises in the epithelium and invades transmurally to penetrate the bowel wall; it then enters the regional lymphatics to reach distant nodes. Hematogenous spread is through the portal vein to the liver. The surgical-pathologic stage of the primary tumor describes the depth of invasion and the extent of regional lymph node involvement, which are important in determining prognosis.

Modified Dukes Classification

Survival is determined by the extent of the invasion, which is categorized according to the modified Dukes classification: A, mucosa, submucosa (5-year survival, 95%); B1, into, not through, the muscularis propria without nodal involvement (85%); B2, through the bowel wall without regional nodal involvement (70%-85%); C1, as in B1 but with regional nodes involved (45%-55%); C2, as in B2 but with regional nodes involved (20%-30%); and D, distant metastases (<1%).

Regional Node Involvement and Prognosis

The extent of regional node involvement and prognosis are as follows: 1 to 4 nodes, 35% recur; more than 4 nodes, 61% recur.

Other Pathologic Features and Prognosis

An ulcerating or infiltrating tumor is worse than an exophytic or polypoid tumor. Poorly differentiated histologic features are worse than highly differentiated ones. Venous or lymphatic invasion has a poor prognosis, as does aneuploidy.

Clinical Features and Prognosis

A high preoperative level of carcinoembryonic antigen is associated with a high recurrence rate and a shorter time before recurrence develops. The prognosis is poor if obstruction or perforation is present. The prognosis is worse for younger patients than older patients.

- The depth of invasion and the extent of regional lymph node involvement are important in determining prognosis.
- A high preoperative level of carcinoembryonic antigen is associated with a high recurrence rate and a shorter time before recurrence.
- The prognosis is poor if obstruction or perforation is present.
- The prognosis is worse for younger patients than for older patients.

Diagnosis

The clinical presentation is a slow growth pattern. Disease may be present for 5 years before symptoms appear. The symptoms depend on the location of the disease. Patients with a tumor in the proximal colon may present with symptoms of anemia, abdominal discomfort, or a mass. The left colon is narrower, and patients may present with obstructive symptoms, a change in bowel habits, and rectal bleeding.

If cancer is suspected, perform an air-contrast barium enema and flexible sigmoidoscopy or colonoscopy. If cancer is detected with an air-contrast barium enema or flexible sigmoidoscopy, colonoscopy is needed to rule out synchronous lesions.

A metastatic survey includes physical examination, evaluation of liver-associated enzymes, and chest radiography. Image the liver if the levels of liver-associated enzymes are abnormal. The preoperative level of carcinoembryonic antigen is helpful for assessing prognosis and for follow-up.

- Proximal colon disease: presenting symptoms may be related to anemia, abdominal discomfort, or a mass.
- Left colon disease: obstructive symptoms, change in bowel habits, and rectal bleeding.

- Preoperative level of carcinoembryonic antigen is helpful for assessing prognosis and for follow-up.

Treatment

For most cases, surgical resection is the treatment of choice. This includes wide resection of the involved segment (5-cm margins), with removal of lymphatic drainage. In rectal carcinoma, a low anterior resection is performed if an adequate distal margin of at least 2 cm can be achieved; this rectal sphincter–saving operation does not make the prognosis worse in comparison with abdominal perineal resection. The tumor may require resection to prevent obstruction or bleeding even if distant metastases are present.

- For most cases, surgical resection is the treatment of choice.

Postoperative Management—No Apparent Metastases

A single colonoscopy either preoperatively or within 6 to 12 months postoperatively is needed to exclude synchronous lesions. If the findings are negative, colonoscopy is repeated every 3 years.

Adjuvant chemotherapy with 5-fluorouracil and levamisole decreases recurrence by 41% and mortality by 33% in colonic stage C; it may be beneficial for stage B2. Radiotherapy plus 5-fluorouracil decreases the recurrence rate in rectal cancer stages B2 and C, but it is not clear whether there is any survival advantage.

- A single colonoscopy is preferred to exclude synchronous lesions; if the findings are negative, colonoscopy is performed every 3 years.
- 5-Fluorouracil and levamisole decrease recurrence by 41% and mortality by 33% in colonic stage C.

Prevention of Colorectal Carcinoma

Primary Prevention

The steps to be taken in primary prevention are not known, although epidemiologic data indicate that a high-fiber, low-fat diet is reasonable.

Secondary Prevention

Secondary prevention involves identifying and eradicating premalignant lesions and detecting cancer while it is still curable. Screening includes occult blood screening and endoscopy. With occult blood screening, earlier stage lesions are detected, but this has not decreased mortality. The Hemoccult test has a 20% to 30% positive predictive value for adenomas and 5% to 10% for carcinomas. With endoscopy, earlier stage lesions are detected, and the removal of adenomas results in a lower than expected incidence of rectosigmoid cancer but not in decreased mortality.

- Earlier stage lesions can be detected, but early detection has not been shown to decrease mortality.

Recommendations for Screening

Colon cancer screening recommendations are outlined in Tables 7-14 and 7-15. For average-risk patients (ie, anyone not in the high-risk group), colonoscopy every 10 years after age 50 has generally become the diagnostic standard; however, an annual occult blood test plus sigmoidoscopy every 3 to 5 years after age 50 is still an alternative. For patients with previous carcinoma or multiple adenomas, colonoscopy should be performed every 3 years until findings are normal (no polyps) and then every 5 years. For patients with a first-degree relative who has colorectal cancer, colonoscopy should be performed every 5 years beginning at age 40 or at the age that is 10 years before the youngest case in the family was diagnosed. For patients with hereditary nonpolyposis colorectal cancer (HNPCC) syndromes, colonoscopy should be performed at age 25 and then every 2 years until age 40 and then annually thereafter. For patients with FAP, annual sigmoidoscopy should be performed beginning at puberty until polyposis is diagnosed, and then colectomy should be performed. For patients with ulcerative colitis, annual colonoscopy and multiple biopsies should be performed starting after 8 years of pancolitis or after 15 years of left-sided-only chronic ulcerative colitis; dysplasia indicates the need for more frequent endoscopic follow-up and may lead to colectomy.

Pancreas

Embryology

The pancreas develops in the fourth week of gestation as a ventral and dorsal outpouching or bud from the duodenum. Each bud has its own duct. As the duodenum rotates, the buds appose and join, and the ducts anastomose. If the ducts of the dorsal and ventral pancreas do not fuse, the resulting anomaly is called *pancreatic ductus divisum*. It is debated whether this condition may predispose to acute or recurrent pancreatitis. If part of the ventral pancreas encircles the duodenum (usually the second part, proximal to the ampulla) and causes obstruction, the anomaly is called *annular pancreas*.

- Pancreatic ductus divisum: failure of the dorsal and ventral pancreas to fuse. May predispose to acute pancreatitis.
- Annular pancreas: part of the ventral pancreas encircles the duodenum (usually the second part, proximal to the ampulla) and causes obstruction.

Classification of Pancreatitis

Acute pancreatitis is a reversible inflammation. The 2 varieties are interstitial pancreatitis and necrotizing pancreatitis. *Interstitial pancreatitis*, in which perfusion of the pancreas is intact, accounts for 80% of the cases, with less than 1% mortality. *Necrotizing pancreatitis* is more severe and results when perfusion is compromised. It accounts for 20% of the cases, with 10% mortality if sterile and 30% if infected.

Chronic pancreatitis is irreversible (ie, there is structural disease, with endocrine or exocrine insufficiency). It is documented by pancreatic calcifications on abdominal radiography, parenchymal and ductal abnormalities on endoscopic ultrasonography (EUS), ductal abnormalities on endoscopic retrograde cholangiopancreatography (ERCP), scarring on pancreatic biopsy, endocrine insufficiency (diabetes mellitus), or exocrine insufficiency (malabsorption).

- Acute interstitial pancreatitis: perfusion is intact; mortality is <1%.
- Acute necrotizing pancreatitis: perfusion is compromised; mortality is 10% if sterile and 30% if infected.

Table 7-14 Colon Cancer Screening Recommendations: Routine Screening

Patient Risk	Age at Initial Screening	Frequency of Subsequent Screening If Findings Are Normal
Average risk	50 y	Every 10 y
Increased risk		
Family history of colon cancer when younger than 60 y	40 y or 10 y younger than age of relative at cancer diagnosis	Every 5 y
Risk of hereditary nonpolyposis colorectal cancer	25 y or 5 y younger than age of relative at diagnosis	Every 2 y until age 40 y; then annually
Risk of familial adenomatous polyposis	Flexible sigmoidoscopy at 10-12 y	Flexible sigmoidoscopy annually until age 40 y; then colonoscopy every 3-5 y
Ulcerative colitis or Crohn colitis	8-10 y after diagnosis of pancolitis or 15 y after left colitis only; if patient has primary sclerosing cholangitis, start immediately	Colonoscopy every 1-3 y

Data from ASGE guideline: colorectal cancer screening and surveillance. Gastrointest Endosc 2006;63:546-57 and Winawer SJ, Zauber AG, Fletcher RH, Stillman JS, O'Brien MJ, Levin B, et al. Guidelines for colonoscopy surveillance after polypectomy: a consensus update by the U.S. Multi-Society Task Force on Colorectal Cancer and the American Cancer Society. Gastroenterology. 2006;130:1872-85.

- Chronic pancreatitis is documented by pancreatic calcifications, ductal abnormalities, endocrine insufficiency (diabetes), or exocrine insufficiency (malabsorption).

Acute Pancreatitis

In acute pancreatitis, activation of pancreatic enzymes causes autodigestion of the gland. The clinical features are abdominal pain, nausea and vomiting ("too sick to eat"), ileus, peritoneal signs, hypotension, and abdominal mass.

Etiologic Factors

Alcohol is the most common cause and gallstones the second most

Table 7-15 Colon Cancer Screening Recommendations: Follow-up Intervals for Average-Risk Patients If Polyps Are Found

Finding	Next Colonoscopy
Hyperplastic polyps only	10 y
1 or 2 diminutive (<1 cm) tubular adenomas	5-10 y
≥3 diminutive polyps; any polyp ≥1 cm; any villous features; high-grade dysplasia	3 y (if normal findings at follow-up, increase interval to every 5 y)
>2 cm; piecemeal resection	2-6 mo

Modified from Winawer SJ, Zauber AG, Fletcher RH, Stillman JS, O'Brien MJ, Levin B, et al. Guidelines for colonoscopy surveillance after polypectomy: a consensus update by the U.S. Multi-Society Task Force on Colorectal Cancer and the American Cancer Society. Gastroenterology. 2006;130:1872-85. Used with permission.

common cause. The third most common cause is idiopathic (approximately 10% of cases). The following drugs cause pancreatitis: azathioprine, 6-mercaptopurine, L-asparaginase, hydrochlorothiazide diuretics, sulfonamides, sulfasalazine, tetracycline, furosemide, estrogens, valproic acid, pentamidine (both parenteral and aerosolized), and the antiretroviral drug didanosine (ddI).

The evidence that the following drugs may also cause pancreatitis is less convincing: corticosteroids, NSAIDs, methyldopa, procainamide, chlorthalidone, ethacrynic acid, phenformin, nitrofurantoin, enalapril, erythromycin, metronidazole, and nonsulfa-linked aminosalicylate derivates (such as 5-ASA and interleukin-2).

Other causes include hypertriglyceridemia, which may cause pancreatitis if the triglyceride level is usually greater than 1,000 mg/dL. Look for types I, IV, and V hyperlipoproteinemia and for associated oral contraceptive use. Hypertriglyceridemia may mask hyperamylasemia. Hypercalcemia may also cause pancreatitis; look for underlying multiple myeloma, hyperparathyroidism, or metastatic carcinoma. In immunocompetent patients, mumps and coxsackievirus cause acute pancreatitis. In AIDS patients, acute pancreatitis has been reported with cytomegalovirus infection. Pancreatic ductus divisum, or incomplete fusion of the dorsal and ventral pancreatic ducts, may predispose some people to acute pancreatitis, although this is a controversial matter.

- In nonalcoholic patients with acute pancreatitis, review all medications, check lipid and calcium levels, and rule out gallstones.
- Several medications definitely cause acute pancreatitis.

Clinical Presentation

Pain

Pain may be mild to severe; it is usually sudden in onset and persistent. The pain is located typically in the upper abdomen and radiates to the back. Relief may be obtained by bending forward or sitting up.

The ingestion of food or alcohol commonly exacerbates the pain. Patients without pain have a poor prognosis because they usually present with shock.

Fever

Fever, if present, is low grade, rarely exceeding 101°F in the absence of complications. (Fever >101°F suggests infection.)

Volume Depletion

Most patients are hypovolemic because fluid accumulates in the abdomen.

Jaundice

Patients with pancreatitis may have a mild increase in total bilirubin, but they usually are not clinically jaundiced. When jaundice is present, it generally results from obstruction of the common bile duct by stones, compression by pseudocyst, or inflamed pancreatic tissue.

Dyspnea

A wide range of pulmonary manifestations may occur. In more than half of all cases of acute pancreatitis, some degree of hypoxemia is present, usually from pulmonary shunting. Patients often have atelectasis and may have pleural effusions.

* Fever >101°F suggests infection.

Diagnosis of Acute Pancreatitis

Serum Amylase

Determining the serum level of amylase is the most useful test for acute pancreatitis. The level of amylase increases 2 or 3 hours after an attack and remains increased for 3 or 4 days. The magnitude of the increase does not correlate with the clinical severity of the attack. Serum amylase levels may be normal in some (<10%) patients because of alcohol or hypertriglyceridemia. A persistent increase suggests a complication, for example, pseudocyst, abscess, or ascites. Serum amylase is cleared by the kidney. The urinary amylase level remains elevated after the serum amylase level returns to normal. Isoenzyme identification may aid in distinguishing between salivary (nonpancreatic) and pancreatic sources. Serum lipase levels may help distinguish between pancreatic hyperamylasemia and an ectopic source (lung, ovarian, or esophageal carcinoma). Lipase levels are also increased for a longer time than amylase levels after acute pancreatitis. A CT scan of the abdomen may be useful. If the amylase level is mildly elevated and there is a history of vomiting but no signs of obstruction, one should consider performing an esophagogastroduodenoscopy to rule out a penetrating ulcer.

* If the presentation for pancreatitis is classic but the amylase value is normal, repeat the amylase test, check urinary amylase and serum lipase levels, and scan the abdomen.
* Persistent hyperamylasemia suggests a complication.
* If the amylase level is mildly elevated and there is a history of vomiting but no signs of obstruction, perform esophagogastroduodenoscopy to rule out a penetrating ulcer.

Nonpancreatic Hyperamylasemia

Nonpancreatic hyperamylasemia may result from parotitis; renal failure; macroamylasemia; intestinal obstruction, infarction, or perforation; ruptured ectopic pregnancy; diabetic ketoacidosis; drugs (such as morphine); burns; pregnancy; and neoplasms (lung, ovary, or esophagus).

Physical Findings

Physical findings include tachycardia, orthostasis, fat necrosis, and xanthelasmas of the skin. The Grey Turner sign (flank discoloration) and Cullen sign (periumbilical discoloration) suggest retroperitoneal hemorrhage. The abdominal findings often are less impressive than the amount of pain the patient is experiencing.

* Look for metastatic fat necrosis.
* The Grey Turner sign and Cullen sign suggest retroperitoneal hemorrhage.

Imaging Studies

Imaging considerations include the following:

Chest radiography—An isolated left pleural effusion strongly suggests pancreatitis; infiltrates may represent aspiration pneumonia or adult respiratory distress syndrome.

Abdominal plain film—Look for the sentinel loop sign (a dilated loop of bowel over the pancreatic area) and colon cutoff sign (abrupt cutoff of gas in the transverse colon); pancreatic calcifications indicate chronic pancreatitis.

Ultrasonography—The procedure of choice for acute pancreatitis is ultrasonography, although in the presence of ileus, air in the bowel may obscure visualization of the pancreas; ultrasonographic examination gives information about the pancreas and is the best method for delineating gallstones, but it is not a good method to use if the patient is obese.

CT—If visualization of the pancreas is poor with ultrasonography, CT is the next step; it gives the same information as ultrasonography, is slightly less sensitive in detecting stones and texture abnormalities, involves irradiation, and is more expensive; CT is indicated for critically ill patients to rule out necrotizing pancreatitis and is the better imaging choice for obese patients.

ERCP—ERCP has no role in the diagnosis of acute pancreatitis and should be avoided because it may cause infection.

Endoscopic papillotomy—Endoscopic papillotomy is indicated when acute pancreatitis is associated with jaundice and cholangitis.

* An isolated left pleural effusion on chest radiography is strongly suggestive of acute pancreatitis.
* On an abdominal plain film, look for the sentinel loop sign, colon cutoff sign, and pancreatic calcifications.
* Ultrasonography is the procedure of choice for patients with mild acute pancreatitis and for thin patients and to rule out gallstones.
* CT is indicated for obese patients and seriously ill patients to rule out necrotizing pancreatitis.
* ERCP has no role in the diagnosis of acute pancreatitis.

Treatment

Supportive care is the backbone of treatment, with monitoring for complications and treatment of them when they occur.

Fluids

Restore and maintain intravascular fluid volume; this usually can be accomplished with crystalloids and peripheral intravenous catheters. Monitor blood pressure, pulse, urine output, daily intake and output, and weight. Eliminate medications that may cause pancreatitis. The use of a nasogastric tube does not shorten the course or severity of pancreatitis, but it should be used in case of ileus or severe nausea and vomiting.

Analgesics

Meperidine (Demerol), 75 to 125 mg given intramuscularly every 3 or 4 hours, is preferred, especially over morphine, because it causes less spasm of the sphincter of Oddi. The efficacy of antisecretory drugs, such as H_2-blockers, anticholinergic agents, somatostatin, or glucagon, has not been documented. Total parenteral nutrition is unnecessary in most cases of pancreatitis. Peritoneal dialysis does not change the overall mortality, although it may decrease early mortality in severe pancreatitis.

- Supportive care is the backbone of treatment.
- Eliminate medications that may cause pancreatitis.
- The use of a nasogastric tube does not shorten the course or severity of pancreatitis.
- Meperidine (Demerol) is preferred because it causes less spasm of the sphincter of Oddi.

Complications

A local complication is phlegmon, a mass of inflamed pancreatic tissue. It may resolve. Pseudocysts, a fluid collection within a nonepithelial-lined cavity, should be expected if there is persistent pain and persistent hyperamylasemia. In 50% to 80% of patients, this resolves within 6 weeks without intervention. A pancreatic abscess develops usually 2 to 4 weeks after the acute episode and causes fever (>101°F), persistent abdominal pain, and persistent hyperamylasemia. If a pancreatic abscess is not drained surgically, the mortality rate is virtually 100%. Give antibiotics that are effective for gram-negative and anaerobic organisms. Jaundice is due to obstruction of the common bile duct. Pancreatic ascites results from disruption of the pancreatic duct or a leaking pseudocyst.

- A local complication of pancreatitis should be suspected if fever, persistent pain, or persistent hyperamylasemia occurs.

A systemic complication is respiratory distress syndrome, a well-recognized complication of acute pancreatitis. Circulating lecithinase probably splits fatty acids off lecithin, producing a faulty surfactant. Pleural effusions occur in approximately 20% of patients with acute pancreatitis. Aspirate analysis shows a high amylase content. Fat necrosis may be due to increased levels of serum lipase.

- Adult respiratory distress syndrome is a complication of acute pancreatitis.

- Pleural effusions occur in approximately 20% of patients with acute pancreatitis and have a high amylase content.

Assessment of Severity

Most patients with acute pancreatitis recover without any sequelae. The overall mortality rate of acute pancreatitis is 5% to 10%, and death is due most often to hypovolemia and shock, respiratory failure, pancreatic abscess, or systemic sepsis. The Ranson criteria and the Acute Physiology and Chronic Health Evaluation (APACHE) criteria are reliable for predicting mortality in acute pancreatitis (Table 7-16). Mortality is as follows: less than 3 Ranson criteria, 1%; 3 or 4 criteria, 15%; 5 or 6 criteria, 40%; and 7 or more criteria, more than 80%.

- Most patients with acute pancreatitis recover without any sequelae.

Chronic Pancreatitis

Chronic use of alcohol (≥10 years of heavy consumption) is the most common cause of chronic pancreatitis. Gallstones and hyperlipidemia usually do not cause chronic pancreatitis.

Hereditary pancreatitis is caused by a mutation in the cationic trypsinogen gene, which is inherited as an autosomal dominant trait with variable penetrance. Onset is before age 20, although 20% of patients may present later than this. Hereditary pancreatitis is marked by recurring abdominal pain, positive family history, and pancreatic calcifications. It may increase the risk of pancreatic cancer.

Trauma with pancreatic ductal disruption causes chronic pancreatitis. Protein calorie malnutrition is the commonest cause of chronic pancreatitis in Third World countries.

- Chronic pancreatitis is commonly caused by alcohol but seldom by gallstones or hyperlipidemia.
- Hereditary pancreatitis is seen in young people with a positive family history and pancreatic calcifications.
- Protein calorie malnutrition is the commonest cause of chronic pancreatitis in Third World countries.

Triad of Chronic Pancreatitis

The triad consists of pancreatic calcifications, steatorrhea, and diabetes mellitus. Diffuse calcification is due to heredity, alcohol, or malnutrition. Local calcification is due to trauma, islet cell tumor, or hypercalcemia. By the time steatorrhea occurs, 90% of the gland has been destroyed and lipase output has decreased by 90%.

- Patients with chronic pancreatitis present with abdominal pain, pancreatic calcification, steatorrhea, and diabetes mellitus.
- For steatorrhea to occur, 90% of the gland must be damaged.

Laboratory Diagnosis

Amylase and lipase levels may be normal, and stool fat may be normal. If malabsorption is present, stool fat is more than 10 g in 24 hours during a 48- to 72-hour stool collection while the patient is consuming a diet with 100 g of fat.

For the cholecystokinin (CCK)/secretin stimulation test of pancreatic function, secretin and CCK are injected intravenously

Table 7-16 Ranson Criteria

Admission	48 Hours
Age >55 y	PO$_2$ <60 mm Hg
Leukocyte count >15 × 10^9/L	Hematocrit decrease >10%
Glucose >200 mg/dL	Albumin <3.2 g/dL
Aspartate aminotransferase >250 U/L	Blood urea nitrogen increase >5 mg/dL
Lactate dehydrogenase >350 U/L	Calcium <8 mg/dL
	Estimated fluid sequestration >4 L

Abbreviation: U, units.
Modified from Ranson JHC. Acute pancreatitis: surgical management. In Go VLW, Gardner JD, Brooks FP, Lebenthal E, DiMagno EP, Scheele GA, editors. The exocrine pancreas: biology, pathobiology, and diseases. New York, Raven Press; 1986. p. 503-11. Used with permission.

and then the contents of the small bowel are aspirated and the concentration of pancreatic enzymes is determined.

In the bentiromide test, *para*-aminobenzoic acid (PABA) conjugated with *N*-benzoyl tyrosine (bentiromide) is given orally. If chymotrypsin activity is adequate, the molecule is cleaved and PABA is absorbed and excreted in the urine. This test requires a normal small intestine (normal D-xylose test) and is useful only in severe steatorrhea.

CT shows calcifications, irregular pancreatic contour, dilated duct system, or pseudocysts. ERCP shows protein plugs, segmental duct dilatation, and alternating stenosis and dilatation, with obliteration of branches of the main duct.

- Amylase and lipase levels may be normal, but evidence for structural disease or endocrine or exocrine insufficiency is present.

Pain

The mechanism for pain is not clearly defined; it may be due to ductular obstruction. One-third to one-half of patients have a decrease in pain after 5 years. The possibility of coexistent disease, such as peptic ulcer, should be considered. Abstinence from alcohol may relieve the pain. Analgesics, aspirin, or acetaminophen is used occasionally with the addition of codeine (narcotic addiction is a frequent complicating factor). Celiac plexus blocks relieve pain for 3 to 6 months, but long-term efficacy is less effective. A trial of pancreatic enzyme replacement for 1 or 2 months should be tried. Women with idiopathic chronic pancreatitis are most likely to have a response. Surgical treatment should be considered only after conservative measures have failed. Patients with a dilated pancreatic duct may have a favorable response to a longitudinal pancreatojejunostomy (Puestow procedure).

- Abstinence from alcohol may relieve pain.
- Narcotic addiction is a frequent complicating factor.
- A 1- or 2-month trial of pancreatic enzyme replacement is worthwhile. Women are more likely to have a response.
- Surgical treatment: only after conservative measures have failed.

Malabsorption

Patients have malabsorption not only of fat but also of essential fatty acids and fat-soluble vitamins. The goal of enzyme replacement is to maintain body weight. Diarrhea will not resolve. Enteric-coated or microsphere enzymes are designed to be released at an alkaline pH, thus avoiding degradation by stomach acid. The advantage is that they contain larger amounts of lipase. The disadvantages are that they are expensive and bioavailability is not always predictable.

Pancreatic Carcinoma

Pancreatic carcinoma is more common in men than in women. Patients usually present between the ages of 60 and 80 years. The 5-year survival rate is less than 2%. Risk factors include diabetes mellitus, chronic pancreatitis, hereditary pancreatitis, carcinogens, benzidine, cigarette smoking, and high-fat diet. Patients with pancreatic carcinoma usually present late in the course of the disease. They may have a vague prodrome of malaise, anorexia, and weight loss. Symptoms may be overlooked until pain or jaundice develop. Two signs associated with pancreatic cancer are the Courvosier sign (painless jaundice with a palpable gallbladder) and the Trousseau sign (recurrent migratory thrombophlebitis). Recent-onset diabetes and nonbacterial (thrombotic) *marantic endocarditis* may be associated with pancreatic cancer.

- Courvoisier sign: painless jaundice with a palpable gallbladder suggests pancreatic cancer.
- Trousseau sign: recurrent migratory thrombophlebitis is associated with pancreatic cancer.
- Recent-onset diabetes and nonbacterial (thrombotic) marantic endocarditis may be associated with pancreatic carcinoma.

Routine laboratory blood analysis has limited usefulness. Patients may have increased levels of liver enzymes, amylase, and lipase or anemia, although this is variable. Tumor markers are also nonspecific. Abdominal ultrasonography and CT are both approximately 80% sensitive in localizing pancreatic masses. Either imaging method may be used in conjunction with fine-needle aspiration or biopsy to make a tissue diagnosis. ERCP and EUS are used if the abdominal ultrasonographic or CT results are inconclusive. Both ERCP and EUS have a sensitivity greater than 90%. ERCP also allows aspiration of pancreatic secretions for cytologic analysis. The "double duct" sign is a classic presentation, with obstruction of both the pancreatic and the bile ducts. Biopsy specimens from suspect lymph nodes may be taken at EUS.

- Abdominal ultrasonography and CT are 80% sensitive in localizing pancreatic masses.
- ERCP and EUS have a sensitivity >90%.

Surgical treatment is the only hope for cure; however, most lesions are nonresectable. The criteria for resectability are a tumor smaller than 2 cm, absence of lymph node invasion, and absence of metastasis. Survival is the same for total pancreatectomy and the Whipple procedure: 3-year survival, 33%; 5-year survival, 1%; and operative mortality, 5%.

Radiotherapy may have a role as a radiosensitizer in unresectable cancer. However, survival is unchanged. The results of chemotherapy have been disappointing, and studies have not consistently shown improved survival.

Cystic Fibrosis

Because patients with cystic fibrosis are living longer, internists should know the common intestinal complications of this disease. Exocrine pancreatic insufficiency (malabsorption) is the common (85%-90% of patients) and most important complication. Endocrine pancreatic insufficiency (diabetes mellitus) occurs in 20% to 30% of patients. Rectal prolapse occurs in 20% of patients, and a distal small-bowel obstruction from thick secretions occurs in 15% to 20%. Focal biliary cirrhosis develops in 20% of patients.

- Exocrine pancreatic insufficiency occurs in 85%-90% of patients with cystic fibrosis.

Pancreatic Endocrine Tumors

Zollinger-Ellison syndrome is a non–beta cell islet tumor of the pancreas that produces gastrin and causes gastric acid hypersecretion. This results in peptic ulcer disease (see "Stomach and Duodenum" section).

Insulinoma is the most common islet cell tumor—a beta cell islet tumor that produces insulin, which causes hypoglycemia. The diagnosis is based on finding increased fasting plasma levels of insulin and hypoglycemia. CT, EUS, or arteriography may be useful in localizing the tumor.

Glucagonoma is an alpha cell islet tumor that produces glucagon. Patients present with diabetes, weight loss, and a classic skin rash (migratory necrolytic erythema). The diagnosis is based on finding increased glucagon levels and on the failure of blood glucose to increase after the injection of glucagon.

Pancreatic cholera is a pancreatic tumor that produces vasoactive intestinal polypeptide (VIP), which causes watery diarrhea (see "Secretory Diarrhea" subsection).

Somatostatinoma is a delta cell islet tumor that produces somatostatin, which inhibits insulin, gastrin, and pancreatic enzyme secretion. The result is diabetes mellitus and diarrhea. The diagnosis is based on finding increased plasma levels of somatostatin.

Octreotide is useful in treating pancreatic endocrine tumors except for somatostatinomas. Octreotide prevents the release of hormone and antagonizes target organ effects.

- Zollinger-Ellison syndrome: non–beta cell islet tumor of the pancreas.
- Insulinoma: commonest islet cell tumor.
- Pancreatic cholera: pancreatic tumor that produces VIP, which causes secretory diarrhea.
- Octreotide prevents hormone release and antagonizes hormone effects.

Part II
John J. Poterucha, MD

Interpretation of Abnormal Liver Test Results

The evaluation of patients who have abnormal liver test results includes many clinical factors: the chief complaints of the patient, patient age, risk factors for liver disease, personal or family history of liver disease, medications, and physical examination findings. Because of these many factors, designing a standard algorithm for the evaluation of abnormal liver test results is difficult and often inefficient. Nevertheless, with basic information, abnormalities can be evaluated in an efficient, cost-effective manner.

Commonly Used Liver Tests

Aminotransferases

Aminotransferases are found in hepatocytes and are markers of liver cell injury or hepatocellular disease. Hepatocellular injury causes these enzymes to "leak" out of the liver cells, and increased levels of these enzymes are detected in the serum within a few hours after liver injury. The aminotransferases consist of alanine aminotransferase (ALT), also known as serum glutamic-pyruvic transaminase (SGPT), and aspartate aminotransferase (AST), also known as serum glutamic-oxaloacetic transaminase (SGOT). ALT is more specific for liver injury than AST. Although AST is found not only in hepatocytes but also in skeletal and cardiac muscle, markedly increased levels of muscle enzymes may be accompanied by increased levels of both AST and ALT. Because ALT has a longer half-life, improvements in ALT lag behind improvements in AST.

Alkaline Phosphatase

Alkaline phosphatase is found on the hepatocyte membrane that borders the bile canaliculi (the smallest branches of the bile ducts). Because alkaline phosphatase is also found in bone and placenta, an isolated increase in the level of this enzyme should prompt further testing to determine whether the increase is from the liver or other tissues. Determination of alkaline phosphatase isoenzymes is one method of doing this. Another is the determination of γ-glutamyltransferase (GGT), an enzyme of intrahepatic biliary canaliculi that is more specific than alkaline phosphatase. Other than to confirm the hepatic origin of an increased level of alkaline phosphatase, GGT has little role in the diagnosis of diseases of the liver because its synthesis can be induced by many medications, thus reducing its specificity for *clinically important* liver disease.

Bilirubin

Bilirubin is the water-insoluble product of heme metabolism that is taken up by the hepatocyte and conjugated with glucuronic acid to form monoglucuronides and diglucuronides. Conjugation makes bilirubin water soluble, allowing it to be excreted in the bile. When bilirubin is measured in the serum, there are direct (conjugated) and indirect (unconjugated) fractions. Diseases characterized by over- production of bilirubin, such as hemolysis or resorption of a hematoma, are characterized by hyperbilirubinemia that is less than 20% conjugated. Hepatocyte dysfunction or impaired bile flow produces hyperbilirubinemia that is usually more than 50% conjugated. Because conjugated bilirubin is water soluble and may be excreted in the urine, patients with liver disease and hyperbilirubinemia have dark urine. In these patients, the stools have a lighter color because of the absence of bilirubin pigments.

Prothrombin Time and Albumin

Prothrombin time (PT) and serum level of albumin are markers of liver synthetic function. Abnormalities of PT and albumin imply severe liver disease and should prompt an immediate evaluation. PT is a measure of the activity of factors II, V, VII, and X, all of which are synthesized in the liver. Because these factors are also dependent on vitamin K for synthesis, deficiencies of vitamin K also produce abnormalities of PT. Vitamin K deficiency can result from the use of antibiotics during a period of prolonged fasting, small-bowel mucosal disorders such as celiac disease, and severe cholestasis, with an inability to absorb fat-soluble vitamins. True hepatocellular dysfunction is characterized by an inability to synthesize clotting factors even when stores of vitamin K are adequate. A simple way to distinguish between vitamin K deficiency and liver dysfunction in a patient with a prolonged PT is to administer vitamin K. A 10-mg dose of oral vitamin K for 3 days or 10 mg of subcutaneous vitamin K normalizes the PT within 48 hours in a vitamin K–deficient patient but has no effect on the PT in a patient with decreased liver synthetic function.

Because albumin has a half-life of 21 days, serum levels do not decrease suddenly from liver dysfunction. However, the serum level of albumin can decrease relatively quickly in a severe systemic illness such as bacteremia. This rapid decrease most likely results from the release of cytokines and the accelerated metabolism of albumin. A chronic decrease of albumin in a patient without overt liver disease should prompt a search for albumin in the urine.

Hepatocellular Disorders

Hepatocellular disorders are diseases that primarily affect hepatocytes and are characterized predominantly by increases in aminotransferases. The disorders are best considered as *acute* (generally <3 months) or *chronic*. Acute hepatitis may be accompanied by malaise, anorexia, abdominal pain, and jaundice. ALT and AST levels are usually greater than 500 U/L. Common causes of acute hepatitis are listed in Table 7-17.

The level and pattern of aminotransferase elevation may be helpful in the differential diagnosis of acute hepatitis. Acute hepatitis due to viruses or drugs generally produces markedly elevated levels of aminotransferases, often in the thousands (units per liter). In general, the concentration of ALT is more elevated than that of AST.

Table 7-17 Common Causes of Acute Hepatitis

Disease	Clinical Clue	Diagnostic Test
Hepatitis A	Exposure history	IgM anti-HAV
Hepatitis B	Risk factors	HBsAg, IgM anti-HBc
Drug-induced hepatitis	Compatible medication/timing	Improvement after withdrawal of the agent
Alcoholic hepatitis	History of alcohol excess, AST:ALT >2, AST <400 U/L	Liver biopsy, improvement with abstinence
Ischemic hepatitis	History of hypotension & heart disease	Rapid improvement of aminotransferase levels
Acute duct obstruction	Abdominal pain, fever	Cholangiography

Abbreviations: ALT, alanine aminotransferase; AST, aspartate aminotransferase; HAV, hepatitis A virus; HBc, hepatitis B core; HBsAg, hepatitis B surface antigen; U, units.

An ALT concentration greater than 5,000 U/L is usually due to acetaminophen hepatotoxicity, hepatic ischemia ("shock liver"), or unusual viruses such as herpes simplex. Hepatic ischemia typically occurs in patients with preexisting cardiac disease after an episode of hypotension. Aminotransferase levels are very high but decrease considerably within a few days. Another cause of transient elevations of aminotransferase levels is transient bile duct obstruction, usually due to a stone. These elevations can be as high as 1,000 U/L but decrease within 24 to 48 hours. In patients with pancreatitis, a transient increase in the AST or ALT concentration suggests gallstone pancreatitis. Alcoholic hepatitis is characterized by more modest increases in aminotransferase levels, which are always less than 400 U/L and, at times, near normal. In patients with alcoholic hepatitis, usually the AST:ALT ratio is greater than 2:1. Finally, patients with alcoholic hepatitis frequently have a markedly elevated level of bilirubin that is out of proportion to the aminotransferase elevations.

Diseases that produce a sustained (>3 months) increase in aminotransferase levels are in the category of chronic hepatitis. The increase (usually 2-fold to 5-fold) in aminotransferase levels is more modest than in acute hepatitis. Patients are usually asymptomatic but occasionally complain of fatigue and right upper quadrant pain. The differential diagnosis of chronic hepatitis is relatively lengthy; the more important and common disorders are listed in Table 7-18.

Cholestatic Disorders

Diseases that predominantly affect the biliary system are called cholestatic diseases. They can affect the microscopic ducts (eg, primary biliary cirrhosis) or the large bile ducts (eg, pancreatic cancer causing obstruction of the common bile duct), or both (eg, primary sclerosing cholangitis). Generally, the predominant abnormality in these disorders involves alkaline phosphatase. Although diseases that cause an increase in bilirubin are often referred to as *cholestatic*, severe hepatocellular injury, as in acute hepatitis, also produces hyperbilirubinemia because of hepatocellular dysfunction. The common causes of cholestasis are listed in Table 7-19.

Jaundice

Evaluation of a patient with jaundice is an important diagnostic skill (Figure 7-2). Jaundice is visibly evident hyperbilirubinemia, which occurs when the bilirubin concentration exceeds 2.5 mg/dL. It is important to differentiate conjugated from unconjugated hyperbilirubinemia. A common disorder that produces unconjugated hyperbilirubinemia is Gilbert syndrome. Total bilirubin is generally less than 3.0 mg/dL and direct bilirubin is 0.3 mg/dL or less. The concentration of bilirubin is generally higher in the fasting state or

Table 7-18 Common Causes of Chronic Hepatitis

Disease	Clinical Clue	Diagnostic Test
Hepatitis C	Risk factors	Anti-HCV, HCV RNA
Hepatitis B	Risk factors	HBsAg
Nonalcoholic steatohepatitis	Obesity, diabetes mellitus, hyperlipidemia	Ultrasonography, liver biopsy
Hemochromatosis	Arthritis, diabetes mellitus, family history	Iron studies, gene test, liver biopsy
Alcoholic liver disease	History, AST:ALT >2	Liver biopsy
Autoimmune hepatitis	ALT 200-1,500 U/L, usually female, other autoimmune disease	Antinuclear or anti–smooth muscle antibody, liver biopsy

Abbreviations: ALT, alanine aminotransferase; AST, aspartate aminotransferase; HBsAg, hepatitis B surface antigen; HCV, hepatitis C virus; U, units.

Table 7-19 Common Causes of Cholestasis

Disease	Clinical Clue	Diagnostic Test
Primary biliary cirrhosis	Middle-aged woman	Antimitochondrial antibody
Primary sclerosing cholangitis	Association with ulcerative colitis	Cholangiography (ERCP or MRCP)
Large bile duct obstruction	Jaundice & pain are common	Ultrasonography, ERCP, or MRCP
Drug-induced	Compatible medication/timing	Improvement after withdrawal of the agent
Infiltrative disorder or malignancy	Other clinical features of malignancy, sarcoidosis, amyloidosis	Ultrasonography, computed tomography
Inflammation-associated cholestasis	Symptoms of underlying inflammatory state	Blood cultures, appropriate antibody tests

Abbreviations: ERCP, endoscopic retrograde cholangiopancreatography; MRCP, magnetic resonance cholangiopancreatography.

when the patient is ill. A presumptive diagnosis of Gilbert syndrome can be made in an otherwise well person with unconjugated hyperbilirubinemia and normal levels of hemoglobin (to exclude hemolysis) and liver enzymes (to exclude liver disease).

Direct hyperbilirubinemia is a more common cause of jaundice than indirect hyperbilirubinemia. Patients with direct hyperbilirubinemia can be categorized as those with nonobstructive conditions and those with obstruction. Abdominal pain, fever, or a palpable gallbladder (or a combination of these) suggests obstruction. Risk factors for viral hepatitis, a bilirubin concentration greater than 15 mg/dL, and persistently high aminotransferase levels suggest that the jaundice is due to hepatocellular dysfunction. A sensitive, specific, and

noninvasive test to exclude obstructive causes of cholestasis is hepatic ultrasonography. With diseases characterized by obstruction of a large bile duct, generally ultrasonography demonstrates intrahepatic bile duct dilatation, especially if the bilirubin concentration is greater than 10 mg/dL and the patient has had jaundice for more than 2 weeks. Acute large bile duct obstruction, usually from a stone, may not allow time for the bile ducts to dilate. An important clue to the presence of an acute large duct obstruction is a marked but transient increase in the levels of aminotransferases. If the clinical suspicion for obstruction of the bile duct is still strong despite negative ultrasonographic results, magnetic resonance cholangiography should be considered. Uncomplicated gallbladder disease, such as cholelithiasis with

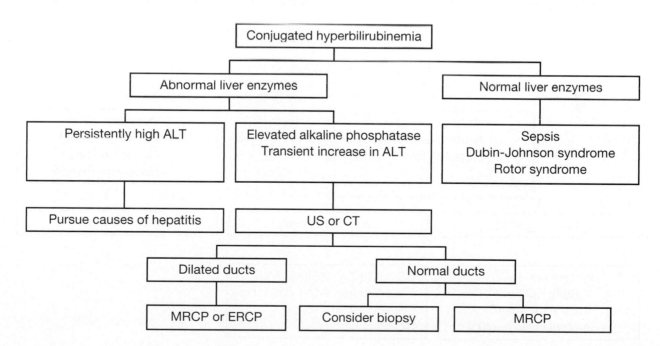

Figure 7-2. Evaluation of Conjugated Hyperbilirubinemia. ALT indicates alanine aminotransferase; CT, computed tomography; ERCP, endoscopic retrograde cholangiopancreatography; MRCP, magnetic resonance cholangiopancreatography; US, ultrasonography. (From Poterucha JJ. Approach to the patient with abnormal liver tests and fulminant liver failure. In Hauser SC, editor. Mayo Clinic gastroenterology and hepatology board review. 2nd ed. Rochester [MN]: Mayo Clinic Scientific Press and Boca Raton [FL]: Taylor & Francis Group; 2006. p. 263-70. Used with permission of Mayo Foundation for Medical Education and Research.)

or without cholecystitis, does not cause jaundice or abnormal liver test results unless a common bile duct stone or sepsis is present.

Algorithms for Patients With Abnormal Liver Test Results

Algorithms for patients with abnormal liver test results are at best only guidelines and at worst misleading. The patient's clinical presentation should be considered when interpreting abnormal results. In general, patients with abnormal liver test results that are less than 3 times the normal value can be observed unless the patient is symptomatic or the albumin level, PT, or bilirubin concentration is abnormal. Persistent abnormalities should be evaluated. Algorithms for the management of patients with increased levels of ALT or alkaline phosphatase are shown in Figures 7-3 and 7-4, respectively.

Specific Liver Diseases

Viral Hepatitis

Hepatitis A

With vaccination and improvements in food handling, hepatitis A virus (HAV) is becoming an unusual cause of acute hepatitis in the United States. The disease generally is transmitted by the fecal-oral route and has an incubation period of 15 to 50 days. Major routes of transmission of HAV are ingestion of contaminated food or water and contact with an infected person. Persons living in, or traveling to, developing countries, children in day care centers, and homosexual men are at highest risk of HAV infection. Hepatitis caused

by HAV is generally mild in children, who often have a subclinical or nonicteric illness. Infected adults are more ill and usually develop jaundice. The prognosis is excellent, although HAV can rarely cause fulminant hepatic failure. Chronic liver disease does not develop from HAV. Serum IgM anti-HAV is present during an acute illness and generally persists for 2 to 6 months. IgG anti-HAV appears slightly later, persists for life, and offers immunity from further infection. Immune serum globulin and HAV vaccine should be given to household contacts of infected patients and to those exposed to a known food-borne source. Hepatitis A vaccine is recommended for US citizens traveling to highly endemic areas, homosexual men, intravenous drug users, recipients of clotting factor concentrates, and patients with chronic liver disease.

- HAV is transmitted by ingestion of contaminated food or water or contact with an infected person.
- The incubation period is 15-50 days.
- IgM anti-HAV is present during the acute illness.
- The prognosis is excellent.
- Chronic liver disease does not develop.
- Immune serum globulin should be given to household contacts.
- Hepatitis A vaccine should be given to persons at high risk of infection and to patients with chronic liver disease.

Hepatitis B

Hepatitis B virus (HBV) is a DNA virus that is transmitted parenterally or by sexual contact. In high-prevalence areas (eg, certain areas of Asia and Africa), HBV is acquired perinatally or in early childhood. High-risk groups in the United States include persons

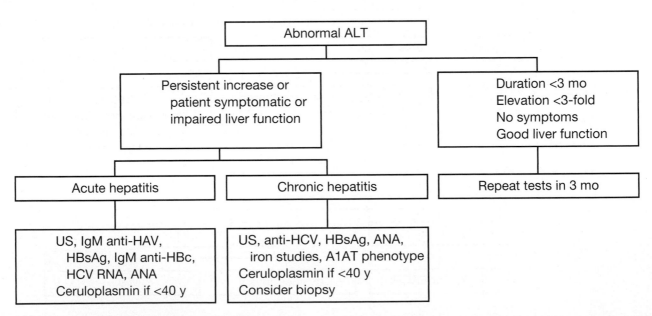

Figure 7-3. Evaluation of Abnormal Alanine Aminotransferase (ALT) Levels. A1AT indicates α_1-antitrypsin; ANA, antinuclear antibody; anti-HAV, hepatitis A virus antibody; anti-HBc, hepatitis B core antibody; anti-HCV, hepatitis C virus antibody; HBsAg, hepatitis B surface antigen; HCV, hepatitis C virus; US, ultrasonography. (From Poterucha JJ. Approach to the patient with abnormal liver tests and fulminant liver failure. In Hauser SC, editor. Mayo Clinic gastroenterology and hepatology board review. 2nd ed. Rochester [MN]: Mayo Clinic Scientific Press and Boca Raton [FL]: Taylor & Francis Group; 2006. p. 263-70. Used with permission of Mayo Foundation for Medical Education and Research.)

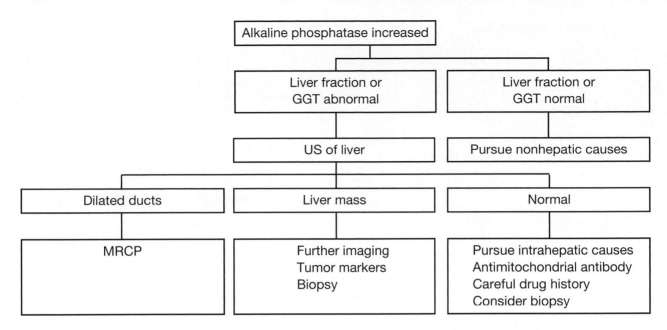

Figure 7-4. Evaluation of Increased Levels of Alkaline Phosphatase. GGT indicates γ-glutamyltransferase; MRCP, magnetic resonance cholangiopancreatography; US, ultrasonography. (From Poterucha JJ. Approach to the patient with abnormal liver tests and fulminant liver failure. In Hauser SC, editor. Mayo Clinic gastroenterology and hepatology board review. 2nd ed. Rochester [MN]: Mayo Clinic Scientific Press and Boca Raton [FL]: Taylor & Francis Group; 2006. p. 263-70. Used with permission of Mayo Foundation for Medical Education and Research.)

born in an area where HBV is endemic (eg, parts of Asia and Africa), injection drug users, and persons with multiple sexual contacts. The clinical course of HBV infection varies. Many acute infections in adults are subclinical, and even when symptomatic, the disease resolves within 6 months with subsequent development of immunity. During acute hepatitis, symptoms (when present) are generally more severe than those of HAV infection. Jaundice rarely lasts longer than 4 weeks. Some patients may have preicteric symptoms of serum sickness, including arthralgias and urticaria. These symptoms may be related to immune complexes, which can also cause polyarteritis and glomerulonephritis.

- HBV is transmitted parenterally or by sexual contact.
- Infants may acquire infection from the mother.
- High-risk groups: persons born in an area where HBV is endemic, injection drug users, and persons with multiple sexual contacts.
- Most infections in adults are subclinical.
- Jaundice rarely lasts >4 weeks.

A brief guide to the interpretation of serologic markers of hepatitis B is found in Table 7-20. Viral markers in the blood during a self-limited infection with HBV are shown in Figure 7-5. Note that IgM hepatitis B core antibody (anti-HBc) is nearly always present during acute hepatitis B. Some patients with acute hepatitis B, particularly those with fulminant hepatitis B, may lack hepatitis B surface antigen (HBsAg). Hepatitis B e antigen (HBeAg) and HBV DNA levels greater than 10^4 IU/mL correlate with ongoing viral replication and indicate high infectivity. Spontaneous conversion from an HBeAg-positive state to HBeAg-negativity with the appearance of hepatitis

B e antibody (anti-HBe) may be accompanied by an increase in the level of aminotransferases. Patients with hepatitis B variants in the precore or core promoter region of the genome may have high HBV DNA levels but lack HBeAg. Commonly encountered serologic patterns of HBV are shown in Table 7-21.

Five percent of patients who acquire HBV as adults and 90% of those infected as neonates do not clear HBsAg from the serum within 6 months and, thus, become chronically infected. Chronicity occurs more commonly in patients with a defect of the immune system. Patients who are infected perinatally or in early childhood generally go through a prolonged immune-tolerant phase. This phase is characterized by normal ALT, presence of HBeAg, and very high HBV DNA levels. Generally, liver biopsy in such individuals will show minimal changes with the exception of "ground glass" hepatocytes. The immune-tolerant phase can last up to the age of 40 years and generally evolves under immune pressure into the HBeAg-positive chronic hepatitis B phase, characterized by elevated ALT, the presence of HBeAg, more than 10^4 IU/mL of HBV DNA, and active inflammation and often fibrosis on liver biopsy. This phase is generally considered to lead to progressive liver damage, including cirrhosis and an increased risk of hepatocellular carcinoma. At a rate of about 10% per year, patients will mount an immune response that is sufficient to achieve a decrease in ALT, clearance of HBeAg, development of anti-HBe (seroconversion), and a decrease of HBV DNA levels to less than 2,000 IU/mL. This inactive carrier phase is generally not accompanied by progressive liver damage. Most patients remain in this phase for many years and have a better prognosis than patients with active liver inflammation and viral replication.

Table 7-20 Hepatitis B Serologic Markers

Test	Interpretation of Positive Results
Hepatitis B surface antigen (HBsAg)	Current infection
Antibody to hepatitis B surface (anti-HBs)	Immunity (immunization or resolved infection)
IgM antibody to hepatitis B core (IgM anti-HBc)	Recent infection or "reactivation" of chronic infection
IgG antibody to hepatitis B core (IgG anti-HBc)	Remote infection
Hepatitis B e antigen (HBeAg) &/or HBV DNA >10^4 IU/mL	Active viral replication
Antibody to hepatitis B e (anti-HBe)	Remote infection

Abbreviations: HBV, hepatitis B virus; IU, international units.
Modified from Poterucha JJ. Chronic viral hepatitis. In Hauser SC, editor. Mayo Clinic gastroenterology and hepatology board review. 2nd ed. Rochester (MN): Mayo Clinic Scientific Press and Boca Raton (FL): Taylor & Francis Group; 2006. p. 271-80. Used with permission of Mayo Foundation for Medical Education and Research.

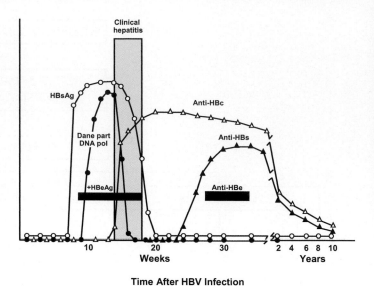

Figure 7-5. Viral Markers in Blood During Self-limited Hepatitis B Virus (HBV) Infection. Anti-HBc, hepatitis B core antibody; anti-HBe, hepatitis B e antibody; anti-HBs, hepatitis B surface antibody; HBeAg, hepatitis B e antigen; HBsAg, hepatitis B surface antigen; part, particle; pol, polymerase. (From Robinson WS. Biology of human hepatitis viruses. In Zakim D, Boyer TD, editors. Hepatology: a textbook of liver disease. Vol 2. 2nd ed. Philadelphia: WB Saunders Company; 1990. p. 890-945. Used with permission.)

About one-third of inactive carriers have a recurrence of chronic hepatitis characterized by an abnormal ALT level and an increased HBV DNA level. This may be associated with a recurrence of the HBeAg-positive state, although more commonly it is due to a precore or core promoter variant that produces HBeAg-negative chronic hepatitis B. This phase is associated with a progression of liver damage and, perhaps, an increased risk of hepatocellular carcinoma.

Patients with chronic hepatitis B and cirrhosis are at high risk of hepatocellular carcinoma, and liver ultrasonography should be performed every 6 to 12 months. Patients with neonatal acquisition of hepatitis B may develop hepatocellular carcinoma even in the absence of cirrhosis and surveillance is advised for the following patients without cirrhosis: Asian men older than 40 years, Asian women older than 50 years, Africans older than 20 years, patients with a family history of hepatocellular carcinoma, and patients with persistent elevations of ALT and HBV DNA.

* IgM anti-HBc is nearly always present during acute hepatitis B.
* HBV DNA level >10^4 IU/mL and HBeAg positivity correlate with ongoing viral replication and indicate high infectivity.
* HBsAg is not cleared in 5% of patients acquiring HBV as adults and in 90% of those infected as neonates.
* Inactive carriers of HBsAg have a liver that is essentially normal histologically and a good prognosis.
* Patients with HBV-induced cirrhosis are at high risk of hepatocellular carcinoma.

Patients with chronic hepatitis B, an abnormal ALT level, and active viral replication (HBV DNA level >10^4 IU/mL) are potential candidates for therapy. Treatment options are compared and contrasted in Table 7-22. Treatment with peginterferon alfa results in a 30% response rate as measured by the loss of HBeAg, and HBV DNA and the appearance of anti-HBe. Rarely, patients also clear HBsAg. Patients more likely to respond to peginterferon include those with high serum levels of aminotransferases, active hepatitis without evidence of cirrhosis on biopsy, and low serum levels of HBV DNA. Patients with HBV infection who have a response to peginterferon therapy may have a transient increase in aminotransferase levels after about 8 weeks of treatment. An acute hepatitis syndrome may be precipitated, and peginterferon is generally not given to patients with cirrhosis. Lamivudine, adefovir, entecavir, and telbivudine are oral agents that decrease HBV DNA levels and may result in clinical improvement, even in the presence of decompensation. The oral drugs are safer than peginterferon for patients with cirrhosis because flares of hepatitis and infectious complications are uncommon. Resistance is a concern with the oral agents; the highest rates of resistance occur with lamivudine, intermediate rates with adefovir and telbivudine, and low rates with entecavir.

Hepatitis B immune globulin should be given to household and sexual contacts of patients with acute hepatitis B. Infants and previously unvaccinated 10- to 12-year-old children (who are reaching the age when they will be at highest risk of acquiring the disease) should receive hepatitis B vaccine. The marker of immunity is hepatitis B surface antibody (anti-HBs). Neonates often acquire hepatitis B perinatally if the

Table 7-21 Interpretation of Hepatitis B Serologic Patterns

HBsAg	Anti-HBs	IgM Anti-HBc	IgG Anti-HBc	HBeAg	Anti-HBe	HBV DNA, IU/mL	Interpretation
+	−	+	−	+	−	>20,000	Acute infection; occasionally "reactivation" of chronic hepatitis B
−	+	−	+	−	−/+	−	Prior infection with immunity
−	+	−	−	−	−	−	Vaccination with immunity
+	−	−	+	−	+	<20,000	Chronic hepatitis B inactive carrier
+	−	−	+	+	−	>20,000	HBeAg-positive chronic hepatitis B
+	−	−	+	−	+	>20,000	HBeAg-negative chronic hepatitis B

Abbreviations: Anti-HBc, hepatitis B core antibody; anti-HBe, hepatitis B e antibody; anti-HBs, hepatitis B surface antibody; HBeAg, hepatitis B e antigen; HBsAg, hepatitis B surface antigen; HBV, hepatitis B virus; IU, international units.
Modified from Poterucha JJ. Chronic viral hepatitis. In Hauser SC, editor. Mayo Clinic gastroenterology and hepatology board review. 2nd ed. Rochester (MN): Mayo Clinic Scientific Press and Boca Raton (FL): Taylor & Francis Group; 2006. p. 271-80. Used with permission of Mayo Foundation for Medical Education and Research.

Table 7-22 Agents for Treatment of Hepatitis B Virus

Feature	Peginterferon	Lamivudine	Adefovir	Entecacvir	Telbivudine
Treatment duration	12 mo	Indefinite	Indefinite	Indefinite	Indefinite
Side effects	Many	Minimal	Rarely renal	Minimal	Minimal
Monthly charge, $	1,700	230	630	720	600
Disease flare	Common	Rare	Rare	Rare	Rare
HBeAg seroconversion, %	27	20	12	21	22
HBsAg seroconversion, %	3	<1	0	2	0
Resistance	None	12%-15%/y	1%-4%/y	1%-2%/y	22% at 2 y
Durability of response, %	90	50-80	~90	70	~80

Abbreviations: HBeAg, hepatitis B e antigen; HBsAg, hepatitis B surface antigen.

mother is infected. Because infected neonates are at high risk of chronic infection, all pregnant women should be tested for HBsAg. If a pregnant woman is HBsAg-positive, the infant should receive both hepatitis B immunoglobulin and hepatitis B vaccine.

Hepatitis D

Hepatitis D virus (HDV), or delta agent, is a small RNA particle that requires the presence of HBsAg to cause infection. HDV infection can occur simultaneously with acute HBV infection (coinfection) or HDV may infect a patient with chronic hepatitis B (superinfection). Infection with HDV should be considered only in patients with HBsAg; it is diagnosed by anti-HDV seroconversion.

* HDV requires the presence of HBsAg to cause infection.
* HDV infection is diagnosed by anti-HDV seroconversion.

Hepatitis C

Hepatitis C virus (HCV), an RNA virus, is the most common chronic blood-borne infection in the United States. Although the number of new cases of hepatitis C infection is decreasing, the propensity of the virus to cause chronic infection continues to result in an increasing number of deaths. HCV has a role in 40% of all cases of chronic liver disease and HCV infection is the number one indication for liver transplant. HCV is a parenterally transmitted virus. The most common risk factor is illicit drug use. Persons with a history of transfusion of blood products before 1990 (when routine testing of blood products for HCV was introduced) are also at considerable risk of infection with HCV. Sexual transmission of HCV occurs but seems to be inefficient. The risk of transmission of HCV to health care workers by percutaneous (needlestick) exposure is also low, approximately 2%. For a health care worker who has a needlestick exposure from a patient with hepatitis C, baseline testing for anti-HCV and ALT is recommended. Follow-up testing can be with HCV RNA at 4 to 6 weeks or anti-HCV and ALT at 4 to 6 months (or both). Prophylactic treatment with immune globulin or anti-hepatitis C therapy is not recommended.

Antibodies to HCV (anti-HCV) indicate exposure to the virus and are not protective. The presence of anti-HCV can indicate either current infection or a previous infection with subsequent clearance. The presence of anti-HCV in a patient with an abnormal ALT level and risk factors for hepatitis C acquisition is strongly suggestive of current HCV infection. The initial test used for anti-HCV determination is enzyme-linked immunosorbent assay (ELISA). Although this test is very sensitive (few false-negative results), false-positives occur. If the result for anti-HCV by ELISA is negative, the patient is unlikely to have hepatitis C. The specificity of ELISA is improved with the addition of the recombinant immunoblot assay (RIBA) for anti-HCV. A guide to the interpretation of anti-HCV test results is given in Table 7-23.

The diagnosis of HCV infection is made by the presence of HCV RNA, as determined with the polymerase chain reaction (PCR). HCV RNA levels do not correlate with disease severity and are mainly used to stratify the response to therapy. Hepatitis C genotypes similarly do not affect disease severity but do affect treatment response.

- HCV is a parenterally transmitted virus and a common cause of chronic hepatitis.
- Common modes of transmission are illicit drug use and transfusion of blood products before 1990.
- The presence of HCV RNA, determined by PCR, is used to make the diagnosis of HCV infection.

Patients with HCV infection rarely present with acute hepatitis. The natural history of hepatitis C is summarized in Figure 7-6. About 60% to 85% of persons acquiring hepatitis C develop a chronic infection, and subsequent spontaneous loss of the virus is rare. Consequently, most patients with hepatitis C present with chronic hepatitis with mild to moderate increases in ALT levels. Some patients have fatigue or vague right upper quadrant pain. Patients may also come to medical attention because of complications of end-stage liver disease or, rarely, extrahepatic complications such as cryoglobulinemia or porphyria cutanea tarda. Up to 30% of patients

chronically infected with HCV have a persistently normal ALT level. Because the majority of patients with hepatitis C are asymptomatic, treatment is generally aimed at preventing future complications of the disease. Patients with cirrhosis due to HCV generally have had HCV infection for more than 20 years.

Peginterferon alfa in combination with ribavirin is the current standard of care for patients with hepatitis C who are deemed candidates for treatment. This combination, given for 6 to 12 months (duration of treatment depends on genotype and rapidity of response), results in sustained clearance of HCV RNA from the serum in 60% of patients. Patients with genotype 2 or 3 and without clinical or biochemical evidence of advanced liver disease have an 80% to 90% chance of a sustained response to therapy and, thus, may be treated without liver biopsy. Patients with genotype 1 or 4 usually have a liver biopsy to aid in the decision about treatment because response rates are less than 50% and the potential risks of therapy may outweigh benefits. On the basis of the natural history of hepatitis C and the response to therapy, an algorithm for patients without any contraindication to treatment can be proposed, although deviations are common because of patient preference or transmission issues (Figure 7-7). These guidelines apply generally to the large percentage of patients with hepatitis C who are asymptomatic or who have nonspecific symptoms such as fatigue. Therapy should be recommended to patients with extrahepatic manifestations of hepatitis C, such as vasculitis related to cryoglobulinemia. Contraindications to the use of peginterferon alfa and ribavirin are advanced age, major comorbid illnesses, severe autoimmune disease, severe psychiatric disease, and uncontrolled substance abuse.

Patients who are not candidates for treatment should be evaluated annually with routine liver tests. Patients with cirrhosis are at increased risk of hepatocellular carcinoma, particularly if there is a history of alcohol excess. The risk of hepatocellular carcinoma complicating hepatitis C with cirrhosis is 1% to 4% per year. Surveillance with liver ultrasonography every 6 to 12 months is advised for patients who are potential candidates for treatment with liver transplant, percutaneous ablation, or transarterial chemoembolization. Patients with HCV infection and decompensated cirrhosis should be considered for liver transplant.

- Symptomatic, clinically recognized acute hepatitis C is unusual.
- Of the patients who acquire HCV, 60%-85% remain chronically infected.

Table 7-23　Interpretation of Anti-HCV Results

Anti-HCV by ELISA	Anti-HCV by RIBA	Interpretation
Positive	Negative	False-positive ELISA; patient does not have true antibody
Positive	Positive	Patient has antibody[a]
Positive	Indeterminate	Uncertain antibody status

Abbreviations: ELISA, enzyme-linked immunosorbent assay; HCV, hepatitis C virus; RIBA, recombinant immunoblot assay.
[a] Anti-HCV does not necessarily indicate current hepatitis C infection (see text).

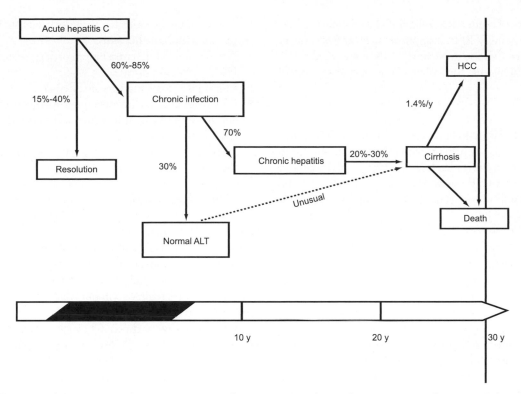

Figure 7-6. Natural History of Hepatitis C. Values are percentages of patients. ALT indicates alanine aminotransferase; HCC, hepatocellular carcinoma.

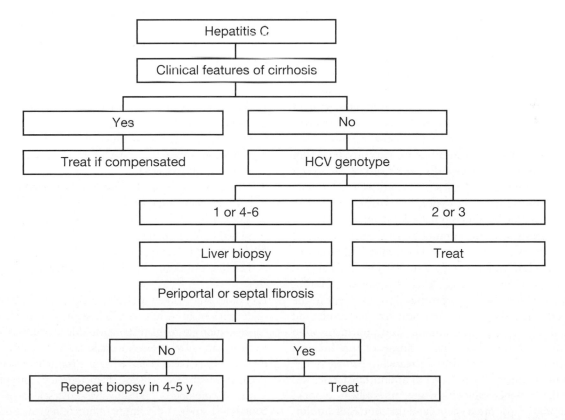

Figure 7-7. Treatment Algorithm for Patients With Hepatitis C and No Contraindications to Therapy. HCV indicates hepatitis C virus.

- The combination of peginterferon alfa and ribavirin results in sustained clearance of HCV RNA in approximately 60% of patients.
- Patients with cirrhosis due to hepatitis C are at increased risk of hepatocellular carcinoma, particularly if there is also a history of alcohol excess.

Hepatitis E
Hepatitis E virus (HEV) is an enterically transmitted RNA virus that causes acute hepatitis in patients who have lived or traveled in areas where HEV is endemic (India, Pakistan, Mexico, and Southeast Asia). Clinically, hepatitis E resembles hepatitis A. Women who acquire the infection during pregnancy have a high risk of fulminant hepatitis E.

- HEV is an enterically transmitted RNA virus that clinically resembles hepatitis A.
- Women who acquire the infection during pregnancy have a high risk of fulminant hepatitis E.

Miscellaneous
Epstein-Barr virus, cytomegalovirus, and herpesvirus may all result in hepatitis as part of a clinical syndrome. Infections with these agents are most serious in immunocompromised patients. Immunocompetent patients with infectious mononucleosis syndromes commonly have abnormal liver test results and mild increases in bilirubin levels, although clinically recognized jaundice is unusual. Herpes hepatitis generally occurs in immunosuppressed or pregnant patients and is characterized by fever, mental status changes, absence of jaundice, and AST and ALT levels greater than 5,000 U/L.

Autoimmune Hepatitis
Autoimmune hepatitis was previously called *autoimmune chronic active hepatitis* because the diagnosis required 3 to 6 months of abnormal liver enzyme test results. However, 40% of patients with autoimmune hepatitis present with acute hepatitis. Autoimmune hepatitis can affect patients of any age, predominantly females. The onset is usually insidious, and an initial liver biopsy specimen may show cirrhosis.

By definition, patients with autoimmune hepatitis should not have a history of drug-related hepatitis, HBV, HCV, or Wilson disease. Immunoserologic markers, such as antinuclear antibody (ANA), smooth muscle antibody, soluble liver antigen antibodies, or antibodies to liver-kidney microsomal (LKM) antigens, are usually detected. Patients with autoimmune hepatitis may have other autoimmune diseases, including Hashimoto thyroiditis. Aminotransferase levels are generally 4 to 20 times normal, and most patients have an increased level of gamma globulin. Corticosteroids (30-60 mg daily) produce improvement in the majority of patients, and the improvement in liver test results and gamma globulin levels is often dramatic. Azathioprine is often added to allow the use of lower doses of prednisone. Immunosuppressive doses should be decreased to control symptoms and to maintain the serum level of aminotransferases less than 5 times the reference value. Even after an excellent response to corticosteroids, relapse often occurs and the control of autoimmune hepatitis usually requires maintenance therapy.

- Autoimmune hepatitis is a chronic condition, but patients may present with acute hepatitis.
- Patients should not have a history of drug-related hepatitis, HBV, HCV, or Wilson disease.
- Immunoserologic markers are often detected.
- Most patients have improvement with corticosteroid therapy, and the improvement in liver test results and gamma globulin levels is often dramatic.
- The control of autoimmune hepatitis usually requires maintenance therapy.

Alcoholic Liver Disease

Alcoholic Hepatitis
Long-term, excessive use of alcohol (>20 g/d in women and >40 g/d in men) can produce advanced liver disease. Alcoholic hepatitis is characterized histologically by fatty change, degeneration and necrosis of hepatocytes (with or without Mallory bodies), and an inflammatory infiltrate of neutrophils. Almost all patients have fibrosis, and they may have cirrhosis. Clinically, patients may be asymptomatic or icteric and critically ill. Common symptoms include anorexia, nausea, vomiting, abdominal pain, and weight loss. The most common sign is hepatomegaly, which may be accompanied by ascites, jaundice, fever, splenomegaly, and encephalopathy. The level of AST is increased in 80% to 90% of patients, but it is almost always less than 400 U/L. Aminotransferase levels greater than 400 U/L are not a feature of alcoholic liver disease, and a search for other causes (eg, ingestion of acetaminophen) should be pursued. The AST:ALT ratio is frequently greater than 2. Leukocytosis is commonly present, particularly in severely ill patients. Although the constellation of symptoms may mimic biliary disease, the clinical features are characteristic in an alcoholic patient. Because cholecystectomy carries a high morbidity in patients with alcoholic hepatitis, the clinical distinction is important.

- Alcoholic hepatitis is characterized by fatty change, degeneration and necrosis of hepatocytes (with or without Mallory bodies), and an inflammatory infiltrate of neutrophils.
- Common symptoms include anorexia, nausea, vomiting, abdominal pain, and weight loss.
- Common signs are hepatomegaly, ascites, jaundice, fever, splenomegaly, and encephalopathy.
- The level of AST is increased (but is almost always <400 U/L) in 80%-90% of patients.
- The AST:ALT ratio is frequently >2.
- Leukocytosis occurs in severely ill patients.

Poor prognostic markers of alcoholic hepatitis include encephalopathy, spider angiomata, ascites, renal failure, prolonged PT, and a bilirubin concentration greater than 20 mg/dL. Many patients have disease progression, particularly if alcohol intake is not curtailed. Corticosteroid therapy may be beneficial as an acute treatment of alcoholic hepatitis in patients with severe disease characterized by encephalopathy and a markedly prolonged PT. Pentoxifylline is a safe agent that has shown benefit in 1 study. A discriminant function greater than 32 helps to identify patients with a poor prognosis.

Discriminant function = 4.6 (PT$_{patient}$ − PT$_{control}$) + bilirubin (mg/dL)

- Poor prognostic markers of alcoholic hepatitis: encephalopathy, ascites, renal failure, prolonged PT, and bilirubin >20 mg/dL.
- Corticosteroid therapy may be beneficial in severe disease.

Alcoholic Cirrhosis
Cirrhosis is defined histologically by septal fibrosis with nodular parenchymal regeneration. Only 60% of patients with alcoholic cirrhosis have signs or symptoms of liver disease, and most patients with cirrhosis have no clinical history of alcoholic hepatitis. Liver enzyme levels may be relatively normal in cirrhosis without alcoholic hepatitis. Concomitant HCV infection is common in patients with alcoholic liver disease. The prognosis of alcoholic cirrhosis depends on whether patients continue to consume alcohol and whether there are signs (jaundice, ascites, or gastrointestinal tract bleeding) of chronic liver disease. The 5-year survival rate for patients who have ascites, jaundice, or hematemesis and abstain from alcohol is 89% and for those who have signs and continue to consume alcohol, 34%. Liver transplant is an option for patients with end-stage alcoholic liver disease if they demonstrate that they can maintain abstinence from alcohol. The outcome of liver transplant for alcoholic liver disease is similar to that of transplant for other indications.

- Only 60% of patients with alcoholic cirrhosis have signs or symptoms of liver disease.
- Liver enzyme levels may be relatively normal.
- The 5-year survival for patients who have ascites, jaundice, or hematemesis and abstain from alcohol is 89%.
- The 5-year survival for those who have signs and continue to consume alcohol is 34%.
- Liver transplant is an option for patients who can demonstrate a pattern of abstinence from alcohol.

Nonalcoholic Fatty Liver Disease
Nonalcoholic fatty liver disease (NAFLD) is a common cause of abnormal levels of liver enzymes. A subset of NAFLD is nonalcoholic steatohepatitis (NASH), which is characterized histologically by fatty change and inflammation. Characteristically, patients with NAFLD have at least 1 of the following risk factors: obesity, hyperlipidemia, and diabetes. The aminotransferase levels are mildly abnormal, and the alkaline phosphatase level is increased in about one-third of patients. When advanced cirrhosis develops, fat may not be recognizable in liver tissue, and NASH most likely accounts for some cases of "cryptogenic" cirrhosis. The pathogenesis of NAFLD is unknown, and the effect of weight loss and control of hyperlipidemia and hyperglycemia is variable. In 10% of patients, NAFLD progresses to cirrhosis; the risk factors for more advanced disease are advanced age, marked obesity, and diabetes. Other than to control risk factors, there is no approved therapy for NAFLD. In patients with fat in the liver, it is important to rule out other diseases that result in steatosis, including hepatitis C, celiac disease, Wilson disease, alcoholic liver disease, and rapid weight loss.

Medical treatment of hyperlipidemia and diabetes are not contraindicated in patients with NAFLD. In fact, agents such as pioglitazone and rosiglitazone have resulted in biochemical and histologic improvement. For patients with NAFLD who are given potentially hepatotoxic medications, liver enzymes should be monitored regularly and medications can be continued as long as liver enzyme levels are less than 5-fold the reference value and liver function remains preserved.

Chronic Cholestatic Liver Diseases

Primary Biliary Cirrhosis
Primary biliary cirrhosis (PBC) is a chronic, progressive, cholestatic liver disease that primarily affects middle-aged women. Its cause is unknown but appears to involve an immunologic disturbance resulting in small bile duct destruction. In many patients, the disease is identified by an asymptomatic increase in alkaline phosphatase. Common early symptoms are pruritus and fatigue. Patients may have Hashimoto thyroiditis or sicca complex. Biochemical features include increased levels of alkaline phosphatase and IgM. When PBC is advanced, the concentration of bilirubin is high, the serum level of albumin is low, and PT is prolonged. Steatorrhea may occur because of progressive cholestasis. Fat-soluble vitamin deficiencies and metabolic bone disease are common.

Antimitochondrial antibodies are present in 90% to 95% of patients with PBC. The classic histologic lesion is granulomatous infiltration of septal bile ducts. Ursodiol treatment benefits patients who have this disease by improving survival and delaying the need for liver transplant. Cholestyramine and rifampin may be beneficial in the management of pruritus.

- PBC primarily affects middle-aged women.
- Common early symptoms: pruritus and fatigue.
- Alkaline phosphatase and IgM levels increase.
- Fat-soluble vitamin deficiencies and metabolic bone disease are common.
- Antimitochondrial antibodies are present in 90% to 95% of patients.
- Classic histologic lesion: granulomatous infiltration of septal bile ducts.
- Treatment: ursodiol.

Primary Sclerosing Cholangitis
Primary sclerosing cholangitis (PSC) is a chronic cholestatic liver disease characterized by obliterative inflammatory fibrosis of extrahepatic and intrahepatic bile ducts. An immune mechanism has been implicated. Patients may have an asymptomatic increase in the alkaline phosphatase level or progressive fatigue, pruritus, and jaundice. Bacterial cholangitis may occur in patients with dominant strictures or in whom instrumentation has been performed. Cholangiography, with either endoscopic retrograde cholangiopancreatography (ERCP) or magnetic resonance cholangiopancreatography (MRCP), establishes the diagnosis of PSC, showing short strictures of bile ducts with intervening segments of normal or slightly dilated ducts. This cholangiographic appearance

may be mimicked by acquired immunodeficiency syndrome (AIDS) cholangiopathy (due to cytomegalovirus or cryptosporidium), ischemic cholangiopathy after intra-arterial infusion of fluorodeoxyuridine, and IgG4-associated cholangitis.

- PSC: obliterative inflammatory fibrosis of extrahepatic and intrahepatic bile ducts.
- Asymptomatic increase in the alkaline phosphatase level.
- Cholangiography establishes the diagnosis.
- AIDS cholangiopathy mimics the cholangiographic appearance of PSC.

Seventy percent of patients with PSC have ulcerative colitis, which may antedate, accompany, or even follow the diagnosis of PSC. Treatment of ulcerative colitis has no effect on the development or clinical course of PSC. Patients with PSC are at higher risk of cholangiocarcinoma; its development may be manifested by rapid clinical deterioration, jaundice, weight loss, and abdominal pain. There is no effective medical therapy for PSC, and many patients have progressive liver disease and require liver transplant. Percutaneous or endoscopic balloon dilatation of bile duct strictures may offer palliation, especially in patients with recurrent cholangitis.

- Ulcerative colitis occurs in 70% of patients with PSC.
- Treatment of ulcerative colitis has no effect on the development of PSC.
- PSC patients are at higher risk of cholangiocarcinoma.
- Treatment of PSC is generally supportive.
- Many patients require liver transplant.

Hereditary Liver Diseases

Genetic Hemochromatosis

Genetic hemochromatosis is an autosomal recessively transmitted disorder characterized by iron overload. The physiologic defect appears to be an inappropriately high absorption of iron from the gastrointestinal tract. The *HFE* gene for genetic hemochromatosis has been identified. In the general population, the heterozygote frequency is 10%. Only homozygotes manifest progressive iron accumulation.

- Genetic hemochromatosis is a disorder of iron metabolism.
- Characteristic: high absorption of iron from the gastrointestinal tract.
- Autosomal recessive transmission.
- Only homozygotes have progressive iron accumulation.

Patients often present with end-stage disease, although an increased sensitivity to screening is aiding in earlier diagnosis. The peak incidence of clinical presentation is between the ages of 40 and 60 years. Iron overload is manifested more often and earlier in men than in women because women are protected by the iron losses of menstruation and pregnancy. Clinical features include arthropathy, hepatomegaly, skin pigmentation, diabetes mellitus, cardiac dysfunction, and hypogonadism. Hemochromatosis should be considered in patients presenting with symptoms or diseases such as arthritis,

diabetes, cardiac arrhythmias, or sexual dysfunction. Routine liver biochemistry studies generally show few abnormalities, and complications of portal hypertension are unusual. The serum level of iron is increased, the transferrin saturation is greater than 50%, and the serum levels of ferritin are high. Increased levels of iron and ferritin may occur in other liver diseases, particularly advanced cirrhosis. Testing for mutations in the *HFE* gene and liver biopsy with quantification of hepatic iron concentration are standard methods for diagnosing hemochromatosis. Of patients with hemochromatosis, 80% to 90% are homozygous for the C282Y mutation that is the basis for genetic testing. Generally, hepatic iron levels in hemochromatosis are greater than 10,000 mcg/g dry weight. A diagnostic algorithm is shown in Figure 7-8.

- Iron overload is more common in men.
- Clinical features: arthropathy, hepatomegaly, skin pigmentation, diabetes mellitus, cardiac dysfunction, and hypogonadism.
- Iron saturation and serum levels of ferritin are high.
- Standard tests for making the diagnosis: genetic testing and liver biopsy with quantification of hepatic iron concentration.

Hemochromatosis is treated with removal of iron by repeated phlebotomies. The standard recommendation is to remove 500 mL weekly to achieve a ferritin level less than 50 mcg/L or iron saturation less than 50%. A maintenance program of 4 to 8 phlebotomies annually is then required. When initiated in the precirrhotic stage, removal of iron can render the liver normal and may improve cardiac function and control of diabetes. Treatment does not reverse arthropathy or hypogonadism, nor does it eliminate the increased risk (30%) of hepatocellular carcinoma if cirrhosis has already developed. All first-degree relatives of patients should be evaluated for hemochromatosis.

- Hemochromatosis is treated with repeated phlebotomies.
- Treatment does not reverse arthropathy or hypogonadism or eliminate the increased risk of hepatocellular carcinoma.
- First-degree relatives should be tested for hemochromatosis.

Wilson Disease

Wilson disease is an autosomal recessive disorder characterized by increased amounts of copper in tissues. The basic defect involves an inability of the liver to prepare copper for biliary excretion. The liver is chiefly involved in children, whereas neuropsychiatric manifestations are more prominent in older patients. The Kayser-Fleischer ring is a brownish pigmented ring at the periphery of the cornea. It is not invariably present and is more frequent in patients with neurologic manifestations. Hepatic forms of Wilson disease include fulminant hepatitis (often accompanied by hemolysis and renal failure), chronic hepatitis, steatohepatitis, and insidiously developing cirrhosis. The development of hepatocellular carcinoma is rare. Neurologic signs include tremor, rigidity, altered speech, and changes in personality. Fanconi syndrome and premature arthritis may occur.

- Wilson disease: an autosomal recessive disorder characterized by increased copper in tissues.

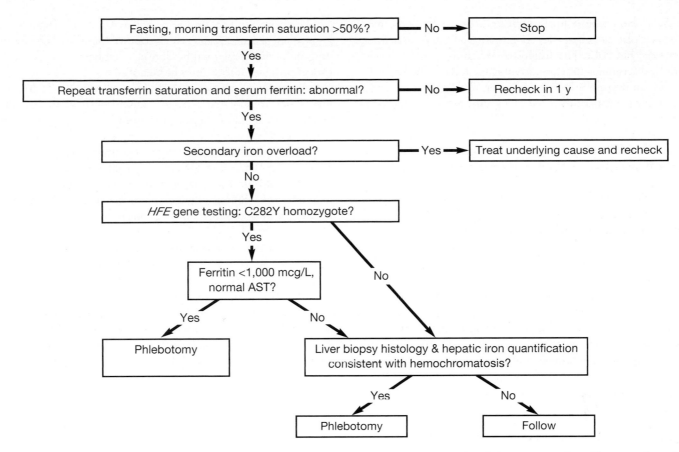

Figure 7-8. Diagnostic Algorithm for Genetic Hemochromatosis. Causes of secondary iron overload include anemias with ineffective erythropoiesis, multiple blood transfusions, and oral or parenteral iron supplementation. AST indicates aspartate aminotransferase. (From Brandhagen DJ, Gross JB Jr. Metabolic liver disease. In Hauser SC, editor. Mayo Clinic gastroenterology and hepatology board review. 2nd ed. Rochester [MN]: Mayo Clinic Scientific Press and Boca Raton [FL]: Taylor & Francis Group; 2006. p. 321-32. Used with permission of Mayo Foundation for Medical Education and Research.)

- Basic defect: inability of the liver to prepare copper for biliary excretion.
- Kayser-Fleischer ring: brownish pigmented ring at the periphery of the cornea.
- Hepatocellular carcinoma is rare.
- Neurologic signs: tremor, rigidity, altered speech, and changes in personality.

Evidence of hemolysis (total bilirubin increased out of proportion to direct bilirubin), a low or normal level of alkaline phosphatase, and a low serum level of uric acid (due to uricosuria) suggest Wilson disease. The diagnosis is established on the basis of a low level of ceruloplasmin and an increased urinary or hepatic concentration of copper. Ceruloplasmin levels may be misleading—they may be increased by inflammation or biliary obstruction and decreased by liver failure of any cause. High concentrations of copper in the liver are found in Wilson disease, although similarly high values can also occur in cholestatic syndromes. Genetic testing for Wilson disease is developing but is currently most reliable for screening among first-degree relatives when a specific mutation in the proband has been identified. Standard treatments for Wilson disease are penicillamine,

which chelates and increases the urinary excretion of copper, and trientine. Zinc inhibits absorption of copper by the gastrointestinal tract and can be used as adjunctive therapy. All siblings of patients should be evaluated for Wilson disease. Liver transplant corrects the metabolic defect of the disease.

- Diagnosis: low ceruloplasmin level and increased urinary or hepatic concentration of copper.
- Treatment: penicillamine or trientine; zinc.
- Liver transplant corrects the metabolic defect.

α_1-Antitrypsin Deficiency

α_1-Antitrypsin is synthesized in the liver. The gene is on chromosome 14. M is the common normal allele, and Z and S are abnormal alleles. Intrahepatic accumulation of α_1-antitrypsin in the ZZ phenotype causes liver disease; however, disease occurs in only 10% to 20% of patients with the ZZ phenotype. During the first 6 months of life, patients often have a history of cholestatic jaundice that resolves. In later childhood or adulthood, cirrhosis may develop. Patients with α_1-antitrypsin–induced liver disease often lack clinically important lung disease. The prevalence of cirrhosis in patients with the MZ phenotype is likely increased, but the risk is small. Hepatocellular carcinoma may complicate α_1-antitrypsin deficiency, especially in males. The diagnosis of α_1-antitrypsin deficiency is made by determining the α_1-antitrypsin phenotype. The serum levels of α_1-antitrypsin may vary and be unreliable. Liver transplant corrects the metabolic defect and changes the recipient's phenotype to that of the donor.

- Intrahepatic accumulation of α_1-antitrypsin causes liver disease.
- The diagnosis is made by determining the α_1-antitrypsin phenotype.
- Hepatocellular carcinoma can complicate α_1-antitrypsin deficiency, especially in males.
- Liver transplant corrects the metabolic defect.

Fulminant Hepatic Failure

Fulminant hepatic failure is defined as hepatic failure with encephalopathy developing less than 8 weeks after the onset of jaundice in patients with no history of liver disease. The common causes are listed in Table 7-24. Poor prognostic markers include a drug-induced cause (other than acetaminophen), older age, grade 3 or 4 encephalopathy, acidosis, and international normalized ratio (INR) greater than 3.5. Treatment is supportive, and patients should be transferred to a medical center where liver transplant is available.

- Fulminant hepatic failure: hepatic failure with encephalopathy developing <8 weeks after the onset of jaundice and in patients with no history of liver disease.
- Poor prognostic markers: drug-induced (not acetaminophen), older age, grade 3 or 4 encephalopathy, and INR >3.5.

Drug-Induced Liver Disease

Drugs cause toxic effects in the liver in different ways, often mimicking naturally occurring liver disease. Most drug-induced liver disorders

Table 7-24 Common Causes of Fulminant Hepatic Failure

Infective
    Hepatitis virus A, B, C (rare), D, & E
    Herpesvirus
Drug reactions & toxins
    Acetaminophen hepatotoxicity
    Idiosyncratic drug reaction
    Mushroom poisoning
Vascular
    Ischemic hepatitis ("shock" liver)
    Acute Budd-Chiari syndrome
Metabolic
    Wilson disease
    Fatty liver of pregnancy
Miscellaneous
    Massive malignant infiltration
    Autoimmune hepatitis

are idiosyncratic and not dose-related; 2% of the cases of jaundice in hospitalized patients and 40% of the cases of fulminant hepatitis are drug-induced. Consequently, all drugs that have been used by a patient with liver disease must be identified.

Acetaminophen toxicity is the most common cause of fulminant liver failure. Toxicity may occur at relatively low doses in alcoholics because alcohol induces hepatic microsomal P450 enzymes, which metabolize acetaminophen to its toxic metabolite. Acetaminophen hepatotoxicity is characterized by aminotransferase values greater than 5,000 U/L and often by renal failure. N-acetylcysteine should be given to any patient with acute liver failure in whom acetaminophen toxicity is suspected. Fulminant hepatic failure due to acetaminophen carries a better prognosis than that from other causes.

Valproic acid, tetracycline, and zidovudine may cause severe microvesicular steatosis associated with encephalopathy. Hepatotoxicity due to amiodarone may have histologic features that mimic those of alcoholic hepatitis or NASH. Methotrexate in a long-term, cumulative dose of more than 2 g may cause hepatic fibrosis; some physicians advocate periodic liver biopsy in patients receiving long-term methotrexate treatment for psoriasis or rheumatoid arthritis. Antituberculous agents, including isoniazid, rifampin, and ethambutol, may cause acute hepatitis. Antibiotics are frequently associated with acute hepatitis and may result in a prolonged cholestatic reaction. In some studies, amoxicillin-clavulanate is the most common antibiotic to cause hepatotoxicity. The chance of hepatotoxicity from lipid-lowering agents is extremely remote, even in patients with preexisting liver disease.

- Most drug-induced liver disorders are idiosyncratic, not dose-related.
- Drugs cause 2% of the cases of jaundice (in hospitalized patients) and 40% of the cases of fulminant hepatitis.
- In alcoholics, acetaminophen toxicity may occur at relatively low doses.
- Antibiotics are a common cause of drug-induced liver injury.
- Amiodarone may cause hepatotoxicity that histologically mimics alcoholic hepatitis or NASH.
- A long-term, cumulative oral dose of methotrexate >2 g may cause hepatic fibrosis.

Liver Tumors

Hepatocellular Carcinoma

The majority of hepatocellular carcinoma (HCC) cases occur with cirrhosis. The risk of HCC is increased in cirrhosis of nearly any cause but particularly if due to HBV, HCV, hemochromatosis, or alcohol. The level of α-fetoprotein is increased in only 50% of patients with HCC; however, a level of α-fetoprotein greater than 400 ng/mL in a cirrhotic patient with a liver mass is essentially diagnostic of HCC. A contrast-enhancing lesion on computed tomography (CT) or magnetic resonance imaging in a patient with cirrhosis is very suggestive of HCC, and biopsy is often not necessary for diagnosis. Common metastatic sites are lymph nodes, lung, bone, and brain. Liver transplant is an option for patients with 3 or fewer lesions (largest <3 cm) or a single lesion smaller than 5 cm.

Transplant is advised particularly for patients with cirrhosis who may not tolerate resection because of poor liver reserve. Transarterial chemoembolization, radioembolization, and percutaneous ablative techniques, such as alcohol injection or radiofrequency ablation, may be useful as primary treatment or neoadjuvant therapy for patients who are candidates for surgery or for liver transplant.

- The risk of HCC is increased in cirrhosis of nearly any cause.
- The α-fetoprotein level is increased in 50% of patients with HCC.
- Usually, imaging is characteristic and biopsy not necessary for diagnosis.
- Common metastatic sites: lymph nodes, lung, bone, and brain.
- Treatment options: liver transplant, hepatic resection, transarterial chemoembolization, radioembolization, and percutaneous ablation.

Cholangiocarcinoma

The incidence of cholangiocarcinoma is increasing in the United States. Recognized risk factors are PSC, *Opisthorchis* infection, and a history of choledochal cysts. Cholangiocarcinoma may be difficult to diagnose, especially in patients with PSC. For most patients, surgical resection is the treatment of choice, although resection is not possible in many patients. Liver transplant is an option in selected patients with cholangiocarcinoma.

Adenoma

Adenomas are associated with the use of oral contraceptives or estrogen. Patients most commonly present with incidentally discovered liver mass lesions, although they can present with acute right upper quadrant pain and hemodynamic compromise because of bleeding.

Cavernous Hemangioma

Cavernous hemangioma is the most common benign tumor of the liver. CT with contrast medium is often diagnostic, demonstrating peripheral enhancement of the lesion. Cavernous hemangiomas generally require no treatment and are not estrogen-dependent.

Focal Nodular Hyperplasia

Focal nodular hyperplasia (FNH) is a benign liver lesion that is probably a reaction to aberrant arterial flow to the liver. These lesions are typically discovered incidentally, although large lesions may cause abdominal pain. Diagnosis can usually be made with imaging; the characteristic findings are intense vascular enhancement and a central scar. Bleeding from FNH is rare and malignant transformation does not occur; therefore, resection is not necessary. Similar to cavernous hemangioma, FNH is not estrogen-dependent.

Metastases

Metastases are more common than primary tumors of the liver. Frequent primary sites are the colon, stomach, breast, lung, and pancreas. Surgical resection of isolated colon cancer metastases has a limited effect on long-term survival.

Complications of End-Stage Liver Disease

Most of the complications of cirrhosis are due to the development of portal hypertension. The mechanism of portal hypertension is related to increases in both portal vein blood flow and intrahepatic resistance to flow. Increased flow is related to splanchnic vasodilatation. Increased resistance is related to sinusoidal narrowing from fibrous tissue and regenerative nodules as well as active vasoconstriction from alterations in production of endothelin and nitric oxide.

Ascites

The pathogenesis of ascites involves stimulation of the renin-angiotensin-aldosterone system, resulting in inappropriate renal sodium retention with expansion of plasma volume. Pleural effusion (hepatic hydrothorax) occurs in 6% of patients with cirrhosis and is right-sided in 67%. Edema usually follows ascites and is related to hypoalbuminemia and possibly to increased pressure on the inferior vena cava by the intra-abdominal fluid. The sudden onset of ascites should raise the possibility of hepatic venous outflow obstruction (Budd-Chiari syndrome).

Paracentesis is indicated at presentation to confirm the cause of ascites. Tests most useful for determining the cause of ascites are measurements of total protein and the serum–ascitic fluid albumin gradient (SAAG), which is calculated as

$$SAAG = [serum\ albumin] - [ascitic\ fluid\ albumin]$$

A SAAG of 1.1 g/dL or more indicates portal hypertension. Ascites due to portal hypertension induced by congestive heart failure can be distinguished from cirrhotic ascites because congestive heart failure usually has an ascitic fluid protein level of 2.5 g/dL or more. Ascites from peritoneal carcinomatosis or tuberculosis generally has an ascitic fluid protein level of 2.5 g/dL or more and a SAAG of less than 1.1 g/dL (Table 7-25).

The treatment of ascites involves dietary sodium restriction and diuretics. Spironolactone (100-200 mg daily) and furosemide (20-40 mg) are usually used initially. The goal is to increase urinary sodium and to allow the loss of 1 L of ascitic fluid (1 kg of body weight) per day. Paracentesis should be performed therapeutically in patients with tense ascites or with respiratory compromise from abdominal distention. Large-volume or even total paracentesis in

Table 7-25 Use of the Serum-Ascites Albumin Gradient (SAAG) and Ascites Protein to Determine the Cause of Ascites

SAAG, g/dL	Ascites Protein <2.5 g/dL	Ascites Protein ≥2.5 g/dL
≥1.1	Portal hypertension due to cirrhosis	Portal hypertension due to hepatic venous outflow obstruction (including right heart failure)
<1.1	Nephrotic syndrome	Malignancy, tuberculosis

combination with 6 to 8 g of albumin for each liter of ascitic fluid removed is safe and well tolerated.

Refractory ascites is uncommon. Patients with refractory ascites have a low concentration of urinary sodium (<10 mEq/mL on a random specimen) despite maximal diuretic therapy. Those who are noncompliant with dietary sodium restriction excrete more than 80 mEq in 24 hours. For patients with refractory or resistant ascites, most physicians advocate therapeutic paracentesis as needed. A transjugular intrahepatic portosystemic shunt (TIPS) is effective in some patients with refractory ascites and is particularly useful for cirrhotic patients with pleural effusion as the main manifestation of fluid retention. Peritoneovenous shunts are complicated by disseminated intravascular coagulation and shunt malfunction and are rarely performed.

- The pathogenesis of ascites probably involves stimulation of the renin-angiotensin-aldosterone system, resulting in inappropriate renal sodium retention with expansion of plasma volume.
- Pleural effusion occurs in 6% of patients with cirrhosis and is right-sided in 67%.
- The sudden onset of ascites raises the possibility of hepatic venous outflow obstruction (Budd-Chiari syndrome).
- A SAAG ≥1.1 g/dL almost always indicates portal hypertension.
- Patients generally have a low urinary concentration of sodium.
- Treatment: sodium restriction and diuretics.
- Large-volume paracentesis is safe and well tolerated.

Spontaneous Bacterial Peritonitis

Spontaneous bacterial peritonitis (SBP) occurs in 10% to 20% of patients with cirrhosis who have ascites. *SBP is defined as a bacterial infection of ascitic fluid without an intra-abdominal source of infection.* Fever, abdominal pain, and abdominal tenderness are classic symptoms; however, many patients have few or no symptoms. SBP should be suspected in any patient with cirrhotic ascites. For all patients, diagnostic paracentesis is advisable as an initial step. Coagulopathy and thrombocytopenia are not contraindications for diagnostic paracentesis. A cell count and culture of ascitic fluid should be performed for all patients. Bedside inoculation of blood culture bottles with ascitic fluid increases the diagnostic yield. SBP is more common in patients with large-volume ascites and in patients with a low ascitic fluid protein concentration (<1.5 g/dL). Also, blood from all patients with SBP should be cultured because almost 50% of these cultures are positive. Variants of SBP are listed in Table 7-26.

SBP and culture-negative neutrocytic ascites should be treated, usually with a third-generation cephalosporin. Albumin should also be given (1.5 g/kg on day 1 and 1 g/kg on day 3). A polymicrobial infection of ascitic fluid should prompt a search for an intra-abdominal focus of infection; SBP nearly always involves only 1 organism. Patients with an episode of SBP are at high risk of recurrence, and prophylactic therapy with norfloxacin is recommended. Prophylactic therapy is also advised for any patient with cirrhosis who is hospitalized for gastrointestinal tract bleeding regardless of whether ascites or SBP is present.

- SBP occurs in 10%-20% of patients with cirrhosis who have ascites.

Table 7-26 Variants of Spontaneous Bacterial Peritonitis

Condition	Ascitic Fluid		Management
	Polymorpho-nuclear Cells/mL	Culture Results	
Spontaneous bacterial peritonitis	>250	Positive	Antibiotics
Culture-negative neutrocytic ascites	>250	Negative	Antibiotics
Bacterascites	<250	Positive	Treat if symptoms of infection are present; otherwise, repeat paracentesis for cell count & cultures

- Classic symptoms: fever, abdominal pain, and abdominal tenderness.
- Many patients have few or no symptoms.
- Bedside inoculation of blood culture bottles with ascitic fluid increases the diagnostic yield.
- SBP is more common in patients with large-volume ascites and in patients with low ascitic fluid protein (<1.5 g/dL).
- Prophylactic therapy is advised for patients with a previous episode of SBP and for cirrhotic patients with gastrointestinal tract bleeding.

Hepatorenal Syndrome

Hepatorenal syndrome, or functional renal failure, consists of renal failure in the absence of underlying renal pathologic abnormalities in patients with portal hypertension. The differential diagnosis is given in Table 7-27. Hepatorenal syndrome is difficult to differentiate from prerenal azotemia; thus, a brief trial of colloid expansion is indicated. Hepatorenal syndrome is often precipitated by vigorous diuretic therapy. Treatment is supportive, although the following may be useful: vasoconstrictors such as norepinephrine, vasopressin, or midodrine; octreotide with albumin infusion; and TIPS. After liver transplant is performed, renal function usually improves, although this is confounded by the renal toxicity of the antirejection drugs such as tacrolimus and cyclosporine.

- Hepatorenal syndrome: renal failure with normal tubular function in a patient with portal hypertension.
- It is difficult to differentiate from prerenal azotemia.
- It is often precipitated by vigorous diuretic therapy.
- After liver transplant, renal function usually improves.

Portal Systemic Encephalopathy

Portal systemic encephalopathy is a reversible decrease in the level of consciousness of patients with severe liver disease. Disturbed

Table 7-27 Differential Diagnosis for Hepatorenal Syndrome

Variable	Prerenal Azotemia	Hepatorenal Syndrome	Acute Renal Failure
Urinary sodium concentration, mEq/L	<10	<10	>30
Urine to plasma creatinine ratio	>30:1	>30:1	<20:1
Urine osmolality	At least 100 mOsm >plasma osmolality	At least 100 mOsm >plasma osmolality	Equal to plasma osmolality
Urine sediment	Normal	Unremarkable	Casts, debris

From Epstein M. Functional renal abnormalities in cirrhosis: pathophysiology and management. In Zakim D, Boyer TD, editors. Hepatology: a textbook of liver disease. Vol 2. 2nd ed. Philadelphia: WB Saunders Company; 1990. p. 493-512. Used with permission.

consciousness, personality change, intellectual deterioration, and slowed speech are common manifestations. The electroencephalogram is frequently abnormal, and patients often demonstrate asterixis (flapping tremor). The grading system commonly used for this condition is given in Table 7-28.

The sudden development of portal systemic encephalopathy in patients with stable cirrhosis should prompt a search for bleeding, infection (especially SBP), or electrolyte disturbances; however, simple precipitating events may include increased dietary protein, constipation, or sedatives. Serum and arterial levels of ammonia are usually increased. Lactulose decreases the nitrogenous compounds presented to the liver and is the first-line treatment for hepatic encephalopathy. Oral nonabsorbable antibiotics such as rifaximin or neomycin are given to patients with conditions refractory to lactulose. Dietary protein restriction is only advised for patients with no response to medical therapy.

- Portal systemic encephalopathy: reversible decrease in the level of consciousness of patients with severe liver disease.

Table 7-28 Grading System for Portal Systemic Encephalopathy

Grade of Encephalopathy	Level of Consciousnesss
0	Normal
1	Trivial lack of awareness Personality change Day-night reversal
2	Lethargic Inappropriate behavior
3	Asleep but arousable Confused when awake
4	Unarousable

Modified from Schafer DF, Jones EA. Hepatic encephalopathy. In Zakim D, Boyer TD, editors. Hepatology: a textbook of liver disease. Vol 1. 2nd ed. Philadelphia: WB Saunders Company; 1990. p. 447-60. Used with permission.

- Patients often have asterixis or flapping tremor.
- If portal systemic encephalopathy develops suddenly, look for bleeding, infection, or electrolyte disturbances.
- Treatment: lactulose.

Variceal Hemorrhage

Esophageal varices are collateral vessels that develop because of portal hypertension. Varices also can occur in other parts of the gut. Most patients with cirrhosis who have varices do not hemorrhage, but mortality among patients with a first hemorrhage is 10% to 30%. For patients who have cirrhosis but have not had bleeding, endoscopy to assess for the presence of varices is advised. Patients with moderate-sized or large varices, especially if there are red marks on the varices, should be treated with nadolol or propranolol to prevent bleeding. Endoscopic variceal ligation is used for patients who cannot tolerate β-blockers.

Bleeding from esophageal varices is generally massive. For patients with acute bleeding, early endoscopy is indicated for diagnosis and treatment. Endoscopic therapy consists of band ligation or, less commonly, sclerotherapy. Octreotide decreases portal venous pressure and may also be given for acute variceal bleeding.

- Esophageal varices are collateral vessels that result from portal hypertension.
- Most patients with cirrhosis who have varices do not hemorrhage.
- First hemorrhage: 10%-30% mortality.
- Bleeding is generally massive.
- Early endoscopy is indicated for diagnosis and treatment.

Of patients who bleed from esophageal varices, 80% to 100% have recurrent bleeding within 2 years after the first episode. Oral propranolol or nadolol may be used alone to prevent rebleeding in patients with preserved liver function, although most advocate serial endoscopic variceal ligation in combination with β-blockers until the varices have been obliterated. Patients with refractory bleeding are candidates for shunting procedures. TIPS is effective in controlling refractory variceal bleeding. The incidence of portal systemic encephalopathy after TIPS is 10% to 40%, but this complication usually can be controlled with medical therapy. Patients bleeding from gastric varices are more likely to require TIPS than those bleeding from esophageal varices.

Patients with cirrhosis may also have gastrointestinal tract bleeding from portal hypertensive gastropathy. Bleeding from this lesion is usually gradual, frequently presenting as iron deficiency anemia. Treatment is with nonselective β-blockers and administration of iron.

* Recurrent bleeding occurs in 80%-100% of patients.
* Patients with refractory bleeding are candidates for TIPS.
* The incidence of portal systemic encephalopathy after TIPS is 10%-40%.

Biliary Tract Disease

Gallstones and Cholecystitis

The 2 types of gallstones are cholesterol and pigment. Cholesterol gallstones occur when bile is supersaturated with cholesterol in relation to bile salts. Excessive cholesterol secretion (in females or with obesity or use of exogenous estrogens) or deficient bile acid secretion (bile acid sequestrant therapy) may lead to cholesterol gallstones. Pigment stones are a manifestation of hemolysis or cirrhosis, although there usually is no identifying cause. Gallstones can cause uncomplicated biliary pain, acute cholecystitis, common bile duct obstruction with cholangitis, and acute pancreatitis. Biliary pain is generally felt in the epigastrium or right upper quadrant and is usually severe and steady, lasting several hours. History is important; constant pain, food intolerance, and gaseousness are generally not features of biliary disease. Ultrasonography is 90% to 97% sensitive for detecting gallbladder stones. Cholecystitis may be suggested by gallbladder contraction, marked distention, surrounding fluid, or wall thickening. Ultrasonography also offers the opportunity to detect dilated bile ducts. If performed during an episode of pain, radionuclide biliary scanning is helpful in diagnosing cystic duct obstruction with cholecystitis. Positive test results are marked by nonvisualization of the gallbladder despite biliary excretion of radioisotope into the small intestine.

Asymptomatic gallstones require no therapy, even in high-risk patients. Acalculous cholecystitis, probably precipitated by prolonged fasting and gallbladder ischemia, generally only occurs in patients hospitalized with critical illnesses. Clinical manifestations are fever and abdominal pain; liver test results may not be abnormal. Diagnosis is made with ultrasonography or radionuclide biliary scan. Patients with episodes of biliary colic or acute cholecystitis should have cholecystectomy. Patients with high surgical risk may undergo percutaneous cholecystostomy.

Many patients without gallbladder stones have undergone cholecystectomy because of a decrease in gallbladder ejection fraction noted on radionuclide biliary scan. Most of these patients do not have resolution of pain, and therefore a decreased gallbladder ejec-

tion fraction should be interpreted with caution since often the patient's symptoms are unrelated to the finding.

* Cholesterol gallstones occur when bile is supersaturated with cholesterol.
* Pigment stones can occur with hemolysis or cirrhosis.
* Ultrasonography is 90%-97% sensitive for detecting gallstones.
* Radionuclide biliary scanning helps diagnose cystic duct obstruction with cholecystitis.
* Asymptomatic gallstones require no therapy.

Bile Duct Stones

Most bile duct stones originate in the gallbladder, although a few patients have primary duct stones. CT and ultrasonography are relatively insensitive for common bile duct stones, and diagnosis generally requires MRCP, ERCP, or endoscopic ultrasonography. ERCP also offers therapeutic potential for patients with bile duct stones and is the test of choice when clinical suspicion is high.

Patients with bile duct stones can have minimal or no symptoms, or they can have life-threatening cholangitis with abdominal pain, fever, and jaundice. Common bile duct stones should be removed. In 90% of patients, this can be performed with ERCP. The urgency of the procedure depends on the clinical presentation. Patients with minimal symptoms can have elective ERCP, but those with cholangitis and fever unresponsive to antibiotics should have urgent endoscopic treatment. Patients with gallbladder stones who have a sphincterotomy and clearance of their duct stones have only a 10% chance of having additional problems with their gallbladder stones; thus, cholecystectomy can be avoided in patients who are at high risk of complications with surgery.

* Most bile duct stones originate in the gallbladder.
* Diagnosis of common bile duct stones usually requires MRCP.
* Common bile duct stones should be removed.
* Urgent endoscopic treatment is needed if cholangitis and fever are unresponsive to antibiotics.

Malignant Biliary Obstruction

Malignant biliary obstruction is usually the result of carcinoma of the head of the pancreas, bile duct cancer, or metastatic malignancy to hilar nodes. If the disease is unresectable, palliative endoscopic or percutaneous stenting is as effective as surgical bypass. Patients with malignant biliary obstruction and impending duodenal obstruction are usually considered for palliative surgery, although endoscopic techniques can be attempted by expert endoscopists.

Gallbladder Carcinoma

Gallbladder carcinoma has a strong association with calcified (porcelain) gallbladder. For this reason, cholecystectomy is advised for patients with porcelain gallbladder.

Gastroenterology Pharmacy Review
Virginia H. Thompson, RPh, Alma N. Adrover, PharmD, MS

Review of H$_2$ Receptor Antagonists, Proton Pump Inhibitors, & Antacids

Drug	Indication	Dosage	Toxic/Adverse Effects	Comments
H$_2$ receptor antagonists[a]				
Cimetidine	Duodenal ulcer		Adjust dose in severe liver or renal disease	Absorption may be affected by antacids (avoid simultaneous administration)
	Active phase	800 mg po hs[b] × 4-6 wk	Reduces liver metabolism of drugs metabolized via cytochrome	Injectable form available
	Maintenance	400 mg po hs[b]	P450 pathway; multiple drug interactions; may cause CNS	
	Gastric ulcer		side effects	
	Active phase	800 mg po hs[b] × 6 wk *or* 300 mg po qid × 6 wk		
	Maintenance	400 mg po hs[b]		
	GERD	400-800 mg po bid × 12 wk		
	Heartburn (OTC)	100 mg po prn, max 400 mg daily		
Famotidine	Duodenal ulcer		Adjust dose in renal insufficiency (CrCl <50 mL/min)	Absorption may be affected by antacids (avoid simultaneous administration)
	Active phase	40 mg po hs[b] × 4-6 wk *or* 20 mg po bid × 4-6 wk		Does not inhibit cytochrome P450 pathway
	Maintenance	20 mg po hs[b]		Injectable form available
	Gastric ulcer			For heartburn, take 1 h before consuming foods or drinks suspected of causing GI distress
	Active phase	40 mg po hs[b] × 8 wk		
	Maintenance	20 mg po hs[b]		
	GERD	20 mg po bid × 6 wk		
	Heartburn (OTC)	10 mg po prn, max 20 mg daily		
Nizatidine	Duodenal ulcer		Adjust dose in moderate or severe renal disease	Absorption may be affected by antacids (avoid simultaneous administration)
	Active phase	300 mg po hs[b] *or* 150 mg po bid	May cause CNS side effects	Does not inhibit cytochrome P450 pathway; undergoes little hepatic metabolism
	Maintenance	150 mg po hs[b]		
	Benign gastric ulcer	300 mg po hs[b] *or* 150 mg po bid		For heartburn, take 1 h before consuming foods or drinks suspected of causing GI distress
	GERD	150 mg po bid × 6 wk		
	Heartburn (OTC)	75 mg po prn, max 150 mg daily		

Gastroenterology Pharmacy Review (continued)

Review of H$_2$ Receptor Antagonists, Proton Pump Inhibitors, & Antacids (continued)

Drug	Indication	Dosage	Toxic/Adverse Effects	Comments
H$_2$ receptor antagonists[a] (continued)				
Ranitidine	Duodenal ulcer		Adjust dose in renal insufficiency (CrCl <50 mL/min)	Zantac EFFERdose (effervescent formula) is available; dissolve tablets in 6-8 oz
	Active phase	150 mg po bid *or* 300 mg po hs[b]	May cause CNS side effects	(180-240 mL) water before drinking
	Maintenance	150 mg po hs[b]		Binds only weakly to cytochrome P450
				Injectable form available
	Gastric ulcer			
	Active	150 mg po bid		
	Maintenance	150 mg po hs[b]		
	GERD	150 mg po bid × 6 wk		
	Heartburn (OTC)	75 mg po prn, max 100 mg daily		
Proton pump inhibitors[c]				
Omeprazole	Duodenal ulcer	20 mg po daily × 4-8 wk	No dose adjustment needed in severe renal disease	Take 1 h before meals
	Helicobacter pylori	20 mg po daily[d]	Dose adjustment suggested in severe liver disease	Swallow whole; do not chew, crush, or split capsule
	Gastric ulcer	40 mg po qd × 4-8 wk	Inhibits metabolism of drugs metabolized by cytochrome	Available in generic form Omeprazole magnesium available OTC
	GERD/erosive esophagitis	20 mg po daily × 4-8 wk	P450 system	Available as immediate-release powder packets formulated with sodium bicarbonate to prevent acid degradation (Zegerid)
Esomeprazole	Gastric ulcer		Same as omeprazole	Isomer of omeprazole
	NSAID associated	20-40 mg po daily for up to 6 mo		Take 1 h before meals
	H pylori	40 mg po daily[d]		Swallow whole; do not chew or crush capsule
	GERD/erosive esophagitis	20 mg po daily × 4-8 wk		
Lansoprazole	Duodenal ulcer	15 mg po qd × 4 wk	Consider dose reduction in severe liver disease—primarily biliary elimination	Take 1 h before meals
	H pylori	30 mg po daily[d]		Swallow whole; do not chew or crush capsule
	Gastric ulcer	30 mg po daily for up to 8 wk		Oral suspension packets & orally disintegrating tablets available
	GERD/erosive esophagitis	15 mg po daily × 8-16 wk		Injectable form available
Rabeprazole	Duodenal ulcer	20 mg po daily after morning meal for up to 4 wk	Does not appear to interact with hepatic cytochrome P450	Swallow whole; do not chew, crush, or split tablet
	Gastric ulcer	20 mg po daily × 6 wk		May be taken with or without food
	H pylori	20 mg po bid × 7 d[d]		
	GERD/erosive esophagitis	20 mg po daily × 4-8 wk		

Gastroenterology Pharmacy Review (continued)

Review of H$_2$ Receptor Antagonists, Proton Pump Inhibitors, & Antacids (continued)

Drug	Indication	Dosage	Toxic/Adverse Effects	Comments
Proton pump inhibitors[c] (continued)				
Pantoprazole	Duodenal ulcer	40 mg po daily × 8 wk	Lowest potential for P450 metabolism & drug interactions	May be given with or without food
	Gastric ulcer	40 mg po daily × 8 wk		Swallow whole; do not chew, crush, or split tablet
	GERD/erosive esophagitis	40 mg po daily for up to 8 wk		Injectable form available
				May cause mild transient elevation of transaminases
Antacids[e]	Duodenal ulcer,			
Aluminum hydroxide	gastric ulcer, or GERD	500-1,500 mg po, 3-6 × daily	Binds with phosphate ions	May have cytoprotective effect
			May cause constipation	Useful in biliary reflux
			Use with caution in Alzheimer disease	
			Guard against accumulation in renal disease	
Calcium carbonate		500-1,500 mg po prn	Milk-alkali syndrome	40% elemental calcium
Magaldrate		30 mL po prn		Chemical entity of aluminum & magnesium hydroxide
Magnesium hydroxide		30 mL po prn	Cathartic effect at higher doses	May have cytoprotective effect
			Guard against accumulation in renal disease	
Sodium bicarbonate		300-2,000 mg po 1-4 × daily	Avoid sodium overload	Most rapidly acting antacid
			Milk-alkali syndrome	
Sodium citrate		30 mL po daily	Increases absorption of aluminum from aluminum-containing antacids, potentiating aluminum toxicity in renal disease	May chill & dilute with water before using
			Conversion to bicarbonate may be impaired in the presence of liver disease	

Abbreviations: bid, twice daily; CNS, central nervous system; CrCl, creatinine clearance; GERD, gastroesophageal reflux disease; GI, gastrointestinal tract; hs, at bedtime; max, maximal dosage; NSAID, nonsteroidal anti-inflammatory drug; OTC, over-the-counter (nonprescription); po, orally; prn, as needed; qid, 4 times daily.

[a] Indicated for phase 2 therapy in the treatment of reflux disease & for the prevention of bleeding associated with stress ulcers. Ineffective in preventing gastric ulcers & in decreasing the frequency of NSAID-induced mucosal erosions.

[b] Nocturnal acid secretion may be better controlled with administration at 6 PM instead of 10 PM because highest acid production starts at 7 PM.

[c] Indicated for healing & prevention of NSAID-induced gastric ulcers. This class of drugs provides the most complete control of acid production & better overall symptom control & mucosal healing. The class is most effective in treatment of GERD. Proton pump inhibitors may interact with drugs for which gastric pH is an important determinant of bioavailability, (ie, ketoconazole, ampicillin, iron, digoxin, cyanocobalamin).

[d] Used in combination as described in text in section on *H pylori* treatment.

[e] All antacids should be administered 30 minutes after meals & at bedtime. Coadministration of antacids with fluoroquinolones may result in crystalluria & nephrotoxicity. Give 2 hours before or 8 hours after antacid. Antacids reduce absorption of ketoconazole & tetracyclines. Do not give antacids within 3 hours of these drugs. Coadministration of enteric coated drugs (such as bisacodyl) & antacids may cause coating to dissolve too rapidly, resulting in gastric or duodenal irritation. Magnesium-containing antacids may cause diarrhea & hypermagnesemia—use with caution in patients with renal insufficiency. Antacids may also contain considerable amounts of sodium, causing overload in susceptible patients.

Gastroenterology Pharmacy Review (continued)

Review of Adjuvants for Treating Gastrointestinal Tract Disorders

Drug	Dosage	Toxic/Adverse Effects	Comments
Anticholinergics			
Atropine	0.4-0.6 mg po q 4-6 h prn	Drowsiness, dizziness, dry mouth, blurred vision, urinary retention	Take 30-60 min before meals
Hyoscyamine	0.125-0.25 mg po or SL tid-qid	Susceptibility to heat stroke	Increase dental hygiene because of decreased salivary secretion
Belladonna alkaloids	0.18-0.3 mg po tid-qid		
Scopolamine	0.4-0.8 mg po daily Patch: 1.5 mg q 3 d	Vision changes, drowsiness	Inhibits excessive GI motility Used for motion sickness
Glycopyrrolate	1-2 mg po bid-tid		
Antispasmodics			
Dicyclomine	20-40 mg po qid	Drowsiness, dizziness, dry mouth	Available for IM use
Antiflatulents			
Simethicone	40-120 mg po prn Maximum: 500 mg daily		Take after meals & before bedtime Defoaming action—chew tablets completely
Charcoal	520 mg after meals po prn	Can absorb other drugs in GI tract	Limit use to ≤2 d
Prokinetic			
Metoclopramide	10 mg po up to qid	Dopamine antagonist—increases LES Extrapyramidal symptoms may occur Dizziness, drowsiness, crosses BBB Avoid in depressed patients Avoid in epileptic patients	Take before meals & before bedtime Effective in decreasing symptoms but not in healing Injectable form available
Bethanechol	25 mg po qid after meals		Useful in combination with other agents Increases LES Increases esophageal clearance Injectable form available
Cytoprotective agents			
Misoprostol	200 mcg po qid with food	Diarrhea, cramping Do not use in pregnant women or women of childbearing age without prior pregnancy test	Abortifacient properties Used for prevention of NSAID-induced gastric ulcers & treatment of duodenal ulcers
Sucralfate	Active duodenal ulcer— 1 g po qid × 4-8 wk	Complexed with aluminum hydroxide—use with caution in renal failure (possible aluminum accumulation) Do not give antacids within 30 min of administration	Local action—not absorbed systemically Adheres to damaged mucosa & protects it against acid, pepsin, and bile salts Give 1 h before meals & before bedtime May decrease nosocomial pneumonia in ventilator-dependent patients

Abbreviations: BBB, blood-brain barrier; bid, twice daily; GI, gastrointestinal tract; IM, intramuscular; LES, lower esophageal sphincter tone; NSAID, nonsteroidal anti-inflammatory drug; po, orally; prn, as needed; q, every; qid, 4 times daily; SL, sublingually; tid, 3 times daily.

Gastroenterology Pharmacy Review (continued)

Review of Drugs for Treating Diarrhea, Constipation, Ulcerative Colitis, Crohn Disease, & Irritable Bowel Syndrome

Drug	Dosage	Toxic/Adverse Effects	Comments
Diarrhea			
Bismuth subsalicylate	2 tablets or 30 mL po prn up to 8 doses daily	Salicylate toxicity Decreases bioavailability of tetracycline Discoloration of tongue & stools Avoid in renal failure	Antacid & absorbent properties Used in prevention of traveler's diarrhea Do not use in patients with influenza or chicken pox because of risk of Reye syndrome Do not use in pregnancy (third trimester) Avoid in aspirin hypersensitivity
Diphenoxylate with atropine	2 tablets po qid for up to 2 d	Has central opiate effects & may cause cholinergic side effects: dizziness, drowsiness, dry mouth, miosis	Diphenoxylate is a meperidine congener without analgesic properties
Loperamide	4 mg po × 1, then 2 mg po prn; max 16 mg daily	Drowsiness	Slows intestinal motility Effective in treating traveler's diarrhea
Cholestyramine	4 g po daily to tid	Steatorrhea Long-term use may decrease absorption of iron, calcium, folic acid	Binds bile acids Mix powder with fluids Administer other medicines 1-2 h before or 6 h after
Octreotide[a]	50-250 mcg SQ tid	Flushing, bradycardia, dizziness	Somatostatin analogue Useful for secretory diarrhea
Constipation			

Fiber (bulk producing)
    Methylcellulose
    Polycarbophil
    Psyllium
	
	5 mL po up to tid
	2-4 tablets po daily
	5 mL po up to tid
		Bloating, flatulence, iron & calcium malabsorption
		Decreases effects of digoxin, warfarin, salicylates, tetracyclines, nitrofurantoin
		Watch for symptoms of esophageal obstruction in elderly patients
		Contraindicated in patients with intestinal ulceration & stenosis
			Recommended initial treatment for most forms of constipation
			Increases stool bulk
			Decreases transit time
			Drink a full glass of liquid with each dose

Stool softeners Docusate (sodium, calcium, potassium)	 100 mg po bid	Avoid taking with mineral oil	Best agent for constipation prevention Surfactant

Hyperosmolar agents
    Glycerin
    Lactulose[b]
    Sorbitol
	
	1 suppository per rectum prn
	30 mL po daily
	15-30 mL po daily
		Local irritation when used rectally
		Abdominal cramps (lactulose & sorbitol)
		Use with caution in patients with diabetes or renal impairment (lactulose & sorbitol)
			
			Sweet taste (lactulose & sorbitol)

Stimulants
    Bisacodyl
    Senna
    Castor oil
	
	10 mg po or per rectum daily
	2 tablets po daily
	30 mL po daily
		Rectal irritation (rectal bisacodyl)
		Avoid coadministration with antacids, H_2 receptor antagonists, & milk products (oral bisacodyl—enteric-coated)
		Urine discoloration (senna)
			Limit use to ≤1 wk

Gastroenterology Pharmacy Review (continued)

Review of Drugs for Treating Diarrhea, Constipation, Ulcerative Colitis, Crohn Disease, & Irritable Bowel Syndrome (continued)

Drug	Dosage	Toxic/Adverse Effects	Comments
Constipation (continued)			
Saline			
Milk of magnesia	30 mL po daily	Contraindicated in renal disease & CHF	Limit use to ≤1 wk
Magnesium citrate	30 mL po daily	Watch for symptoms of magnesium toxicity	
		May alter fluid & electrolyte balance	
Polyethylene glycol (PEG)	17 g po daily	Do not use in patients with suspected GI obstruction or perforation	For occasional use only. Dissolve in 8 oz of liquid before taking
Emollient/lubricant			
Mineral oil	15-45 mL po daily	Lipid pneumonia. Malabsorption of lipid-soluble vitamins. Reduces absorption of anticoagulants, oral contraceptives, & digoxin	Not for routine use
Lubiprostone	24 mcg po bid with food	For chronic idiopathic adult constipation	May cause diarrhea
Ulcerative Colitis & Crohn Disease			
Mesalamine (5-ASA)	2.4-4 g po daily in divided doses. 1 g daily per rectum (suppository or retention enema)	Overdose: symptoms of salicylate toxicity; if chest pain develops, consider pericarditis	Effective in treatment of mild or moderate active phases. Swallow tablets whole. May give oral & rectal therapy concurrently. Available as Asacol & Pentasa, which release 5-ASA in the terminal ileum & colon & in the small bowel & colon, respectively. Available in a new multimatrix (MMX) formulation: higher-dose tablets, delayed dissolution that allows exposure to colon, & better compliance
Olsalazine	1.5-3 g po daily in divided doses	Monitor for renal abnormalities. Causes diarrhea	Take with food. Bioconverted to 5-ASA in colon. Effective in treatment of mild or moderate active phases
Sulfasalazine	3-4 g po daily in divided doses	Use with caution in patients with asthma or glucose-6-phosphate dehydrogenase deficiency. Cross-sensitivity with sulfonamides. May impair folic acid absorption. Orange-yellow discoloration of the urine, skin, & soft contact lenses	Effective in treating acute disease & maintaining remission in ulcerative colitis. Does not maintain remission in Crohn disease. Swallow whole. Metabolized to sulfapyridine & 5-ASA by intestinal bacteria. Slow & fast acetylators exhibit differences in metabolism. Maintain adequate fluid intake

Gastroenterology Pharmacy Review (continued)

Review of Drugs for Treating Diarrhea, Constipation, Ulcerative Colitis, Crohn Disease, & Irritable Bowel Syndrome (continued)

Drug	Dosage	Toxic/Adverse Effects	Comments
Ulcerative Colitis & Crohn Disease (continued)			
Balsalazide	6.75 g po daily in divided doses	Monitor for renal abnormalities	Bioconverted to 5-ASA in colon
Prednisone	40-60 mg po daily Use topically for mild or moderate active disease in distal colon	Osteoporosis Cushingoid appearance Muscle weakness Adrenal suppression	Most effective in maintaining remission in ulcerative colitis Most effective in acute exacerbation of Crohn disease Use prednisolone in patients with cirrhosis
Azathioprine	2-5 mg/kg po daily	Immunosuppression	Metabolized to 6-mercaptopurine Drug interaction with allopurinol Injectable form available
6-Mercaptopurine	2.5-5 mg/kg po daily		Steroid-sparing effect
Metronidazole (perianal disease)	20 mg/kg po daily	Metallic taste, dark urine	Recurrence on discontinuation
Infliximab (Crohn disease)	5 mg/kg IV infusion over 2 h	Associated with severe acute infusion reaction, delayed hypersensitivity, & increased risk of infection Avoid in moderate or severe heart failure	For moderate or severe active Crohn disease refractory to conventional therapy & in fistulizing Crohn disease Perform tuberculosis test before therapy
Alosetron (IBS)	1 mg po daily; can be increased to 1 mg po bid after 4 wk	Associated with ischemic colitis	Returned to US market under tight controls after FDA removal Selective 5-HT3 antagonist For treatment of IBS in female patients, diarrhea predominant

Abbreviations: bid, twice daily; CHF, congestive heart failure; FDA, Food & Drug Administration; GI, gastrointestinal tract; 5-HT3, serotonin type 3; IBS, irritable bowel syndrome; IV, intravenous; max, maximal dosage; po, orally; prn, as needed; qid, 4 times daily; SQ, subcutaneously; tid, 3 times daily.

[a] Also indicated in the treatment of carcinoid syndrome.

[b] Also indicated in the treatment of portal systemic encephalopathy.

Gastroenterology Pharmacy Review (continued)

Review of *Helicobacter pylori* Treatment Regimens

Regimen	Drug Combination	Dosage Given Orally for 7 Days	Comment
1	PPI	Standard dose bid[a]	
	Clarithromycin	500 mg bid	Metallic taste
			Drug interaction with terfenadine, astemizole, & cisapride
	Amoxicillin[b]	1,000 mg bid	Be aware of penicillin allergy
			May cause nausea & diarrhea
2	PPI	Standard dose bid[a]	
	Tetracycline[b]	250 mg qid	Reduces effectiveness of oral contraceptives
			Absorption is reduced in presence of divalent & trivalent cations (calcium, magnesium, iron, aluminum)
			Photosensitivity—avoid exposure to sunlight
	Metronidazole[c]	500 mg bid	Avoid alcohol use
			May cause nausea & diarrhea
	Bismuth	2 tablets qid	Darkening of tongue & stools

Abbreviations: bid, twice daily; po, orally; PPI, proton pump inhibitor; qid, 4 times daily.

[a] Standard PPI doses: esomeprazole 40 mg, lansoprazole 30 mg, omeprazole 20 mg, pantoprazole 40 mg, or rabeprazole 20 mg.

[b] If unable to use amoxicillin or tetracycline, use metronidazole 500 mg po bid × 7 days.

[c] If resistant to metronidazole, use amoxicillin 1,000 mg po bid × 7 days.

Modified from Health care guideline: dyspepsia and GERD. 6th ed. Institute for Clinical Systems Improvement; ©July 2004 [cited 2006 Feb 22]. Available from: http://www.icsi.org. Used with permission.

Questions

Multiple Choice (choose the best answer)

1. A 55-year-old man presents with a 4-year history of progressive dysphagia with occasional regurgitation of food and liquids many hours after eating. Esophageal manometry reveals an absence of peristalsis and incomplete relaxation of the lower esophageal sphincter with swallowing. Which of the following is *not* true for this patient?

   a. A fundoplication is likely to resolve the regurgitation.
   b. Long-term pharmacologic therapy is unlikely to be effective.
   c. Pneumatic dilatation is an appropriate initial therapy.
   d. A parasitic infection can lead to a secondary form of this disorder.
   e. An upper gastrointestinal tract study is likely to reveal a dilated esophagus.

2. A 42-year-old man presents with an 8-week history of mild hoarseness and occasionally awakening at night with coughing spells. He is a nonsmoker with an 8-year history of asthma, which has worsened somewhat since he began taking theophylline 3 months ago. Which of the following treatment options is the most appropriate?

   a. Replace the theophylline with an oral, long-acting β-agonist.
   b. Replace the theophylline with an inhaled β-agonist.
   c. Replace the theophylline with a proton pump inhibitor (PPI).
   d. Increase the theophylline dose as needed.
   e. Perform chest radiography.

3. A 44-year-old man presents with intermittent dyspepsia that is relieved with antacids and eating. He experienced similar symptoms 2 years ago, when an ulcer was identified in his duodenal bulb on endoscopy. Those symptoms resolved with 1 month of PPI therapy. He has no other medical problems and does not take nonsteroidal anti-inflammatory drugs (NSAIDs). He does not smoke. His hemoglobin and gastrin levels are normal. Endoscopy shows a small duodenal bulb ulcer but no other abnormal findings. Antral biopsies show a chronic active gastritis. What would be the most appropriate treatment?

   a. Sucralfate therapy for 6 weeks
   b. PPI therapy for 6 weeks
   c. H$_2$-blocker therapy for 6 weeks, with discontinuation of smoking
   d. PPI therapy for 4 weeks, with 2 weeks of antibiotic therapy for *Helicobacter pylori*
   e. Billroth II antrectomy and truncal vagotomy

4. A 35-year-old woman with no prior medical problems presents with a 6-month history of dyspepsia and diarrhea. She takes no medications. On upper endoscopy, she is found to have multiple ulcerations from the bulb to the third portion of the duodenum. Duodenal and antral biopsy specimens show only acute inflammation. There is no family history of similar problems. Which of the following is most likely to confirm the diagnosis?

   a. Performing endoscopic ultrasonography of the pancreas and duodenum
   b. Checking serum salicylate levels to rule out surreptitious NSAID use
   c. Testing of serum antibodies for *H pylori*
   d. Performing a secretin test
   e. Repeating an upper endoscopy study after 6 weeks of PPI therapy.

5. A 32-year-old woman presents to your office with nonbloody diarrhea for 5 years. She states that she has 4 or 5 watery bowel movements per day and that several doctors have been unable to determine why she continues to have diarrhea. She has no other medical problems, takes no medications, and has no family history of similar problems. Colonoscopy and small-bowel radiographic findings are normal. Stool cultures, *Clostridium difficile* testing, ova and parasite examinations, and fecal leukocyte determinations are all negative. Serum chemistry results are all normal. Results from 72-hour stool collection are the following:

Component	Value
Fecal volume, g per day	350
Fecal fat, g per day	4
Stool sodium, mEq/L	75
Stool potassium, mEq/L	15
Measured stool osmolality, mOsm/kg	215

   Which of the following is the most likely diagnosis?

   a. Lactose intolerance
   b. Pancreatic insufficiency
   c. Factitious diarrhea
   d. Celiac disease
   e. Irritable bowel syndrome

6. A 55-year-old man with no past medical history presents with diarrhea for the past 6 months. He has also noted migratory arthralgias and has lost 9.1 kg. Stool fat is 35 g in 24 hours. After oral administration of 25 g of D-xylose, a 5-hour urine collection contains no D-xylose. What is the next step in evaluating and treating this patient?

   a. Empiric trial of pancreatic enzymes
   b. Prednisone

c. Small-bowel biopsy

d. Bone marrow biopsy

e. Stool examination for ova and parasites

7. A 34-year-old man with a history of ulcerative pancolitis for 10 years presents with left knee swelling and pain with a duration of 3 weeks. He also relates that he has had mildly increased stool frequency over the past 5 days. Examination reveals a healthy, afebrile man. Knee aspiration demonstrates sterile fluid with no crystals. Flexible sigmoidoscopy shows an acute exacerbation of ulcerative colitis. Laboratory evaluation shows the following: aspartate aminotransferase (AST) 33 U/L, alanine aminotransferase (ALT), 30 U/L, alkaline phosphatase 563 U/L, total bilirubin 1.9 mg/dL, and direct bilirubin 1.0 mg/dL. Treatment of the ulcerative colitis is initiated with mesalamine. Which of the following statements is *incorrect*?

a. He should undergo endoscopic retrograde cholangiopancreatography (ERCP).

b. The knee inflammation should resolve as the colitis improves.

c. His liver chemistry values should return to normal as the colitis improves.

d. The patient should undergo a full colonoscopy every 1 to 2 years.

e. His risk of colon cancer is greater than the risk for someone with chronic ulcerative proctitis.

8. A 41-year-old Asian woman presented to your office 1 week ago with complaints of diarrhea for 7 months and weight loss of 2.3 kg. She has 8 to 10 watery, explosive bowel movements daily with a large amount of flatus. She denies having blood or pain with bowel movements, fever, chills, or nausea. She returned today after completing several studies. Results of the following were normal: stool cultures, examination for ova and parasites, upper gastrointestinal tract and small-bowel follow-through radiography, barium enema study, and abdominal CT. Results of the following laboratory tests were normal: thyroid function test and levels of electrolytes, liver enzymes, albumin, amylase and lipase, iron, folate, vitamin B_{12}, gastrin, 5-hydroxy-indoleacetic acid, and vasoactive intestinal polypeptide. Results of 24-hour stool analysis showed the following: fecal fat 10 g in 24 hours, sodium 86 mEq/L, potassium 30 mEq/L, osmolality 300 mOsm/L, weight 800 g, and stool pH 4.0. What is the most appropriate next step for this patient?

a. Check for serum endomysial antibodies.

b. Recommend that she discontinue laxative use.

c. Recommend that she avoid dairy products.

d. Recommend that she add fiber to her diet.

e. Perform an esophagogastroduodenoscopy with small-bowel biopsies.

9. A 70-year-old man complains of diarrhea and 4 episodes of arthritis over the past 3 months. His family thinks he is becoming more forgetful. On examination, he appears hyperpigmented and has generalized lymphadenopathy. Stool fat is 20 g in 24 hours. Small-bowel biopsy shows periodic acid-Schiff (PAS)–positive/acid-fast–negative granules in macrophages in the lamina propria of the small intestine. What is the most likely cause of this patient's condition?

a. Topical sprue

b. Intestinal lymphangiectasia

c. β-Lipoproteinemia

d. Whipple disease

e. *Vibrio vulnificus* infection

10. A 51-year-old post menopausal woman presents to your clinic with complaints of bloating, flatus, and diarrhea for 4 years. She has seen 3 other physicians for this problem, but no diagnosis was made. She was advised to increase her intake of dietary fiber, try antidiarrheal drugs, and omit dairy products from her diet. None of these interventions has had any real benefit. She describes having 2 or 3 loose bowel movements daily without blood or cramping. Bloating is relieved temporarily with a bowel movement or passing of flatus. Physical examination findings are essentially normal. Laboratory evaluation of a fecal specimen shows negative stool cultures, ova or parasites, and no blood. The hemoglobin level is 9 g/dL, the mean corpuscular volume is 79 fL, and the serum iron level is 15 mg/dL. Serum electrolyte levels are normal as is a urinalysis. Which treatment is most likely to result in symptomatic relief?

a. An increase in dietary fiber and antidiarrheal agents

b. Oral iron supplementation

c. Treatment with metronidazole

d. Dietary modifications with removal of products containing gluten

e. A 2-week course of oral prednisone

11. The same patient in question 10 has been feeling well for 8 years but returns to your office with a recurrence of symptoms and mild epigastric discomfort for the past month. She has consistently followed a gluten-free diet. She also states that she has lost about 2.3 kg during the past month. What is the next most appropriate test?

a. Perform a CT scan of the abdomen.

b. Measure serum antiendomysial antibody levels.

c. Reassure her and reevaluate her diet to eliminate gluten.

d. Culture stool and examine stool for ova and parasites.

e. Perform colonoscopy with random biopsies.

12. A 32-year-old man is referred to you by a surgical colleague. The patient has had diffuse abdominal pain and diarrhea for 3 months. He has lost 4.6 kg during this period despite having a good appetite. His diarrhea is nonbloody but occurs 4 or 5 times per day with a small amount of bloating and gas. The surgeon had performed colonoscopy and esophagogastroduodenoscopy (EGD) and reported normal findings. Diarrhea has persisted despite

fasting for the test over the past 2 days. Stool cultures were negative 3 times. Endomysial antibody tests were also negative. Many fecal leukocytes were seen. What should you do next?

a. Perform CT of the abdomen.
b. Perform small-bowel radiography.
c. Perform capsule endoscopy.
d. Reassure the patient and prescribe antidiarrheal medication.
e. Start an empiric course of antibiotics for presumed infectious diarrhea.

13. A 41-year-old man with human immunodeficiency virus is seen in your outpatient clinic and has a history of diarrhea for 6 months. He has 5 or 6 watery bowel movements per day and has lost 3.6 kg during this time. He is reportedly taking his antiviral medications as prescribed and has been feeling well otherwise. The CD4 count is 150/mcL. You order stool cultures, examination for ova and parasites, *Giardia* antigen testing, and colonoscopy. Results of all these tests are negative. EGD with small-bowel biopsies shows no evidence of villous atrophy but does demonstrate small, round acid-fast organisms "carpeting" the duodenal epithelium. Which of the following is the most likely cause of his diarrhea?

a. *Clostridium difficile* colitis
b. Celiac disease
c. *Cryptosporidium*
d. Laxative abuse
e. Whipple disease

14. A 29-year-old woman presents to the emergency department with pain in her right flank radiating down to her right groin. For 12 years she has had severe Crohn disease, for which she has already undergone 3 surgical procedures, with a cumulative resection of 120 cm of her terminal ileum. Since her latest operation 2 years ago, she has had bloating, flatus, and persistently loose stools with an oily film in the toilet bowl water. Small-bowel follow-through radiography demonstrates no active inflammatory small-bowel disease or fistula. Urinalysis demonstrates many red blood cells. Over the next hour, with intravenous (IV) hydration, she gets spontaneous relief, but no urinary calculus is recovered. What therapy will most likely prevent a recurrence of similar episodes?

a. Increased oral fluids to prevent formation of kidney calculi
b. A low-fat diet and calcium supplementation with meals
c. Oral pancreatic enzyme supplementation
d. Daily citrate
e. Prednisone

15. A 76-year-old man presents to the emergency department with hematochezia. He had been feeling well until 3 days earlier, when left upper quadrant pain developed with subsequent nonbloody diarrhea. This morning, however, he noted that the diarrhea had become bloody. His symptoms have otherwise not changed. His history is significant only for a prior 3-vessel

coronary artery bypass graft and a cholecystectomy about 10 years ago. Blood pressure is 110/65 mm Hg, pulse is 85 beats per minute, temperature is 37.4°C, white blood cell count (WBC) is 10×10^9/L, and hemoglobin is 11.8 g/dL. What should you do next?

a. CT scan to rule out diverticulitis
b. IV hydration and bowel rest
c. Urgent angiograhy of the mesenteric vessels
d. Serum amylase and lipase level determination
e. Blood transfusion and urgent colonoscopy

16. While making rounds on the hospital service, your resident presents a 65-year-old man who was admitted through the emergency department with diarrhea for 3 days; the diarrhea was bloody for the past 2 days. He has remained hemodynamically stable overnight with IV hydration, and he is afebrile, but his diarrhea is no better. His laboratory test results are shown below:

Component	Yesterday	Today
WBC, $\times10^9$/L	18.0	19.5
Hemoglobin, g/dL	12.9	10.2
Platelet count, $\times10^9$/L	198	110
Sodium, mEq/L	143	139
Potassium, mEq/L	4.0	3.6
Creatinine, mg/dL	1.1	1.5
Serum urea nitrogen, mg/dL	31	45
AST, U/L	44	110
ALT, U/L	32	31
Lactate dehydrogenase, U/L (reference range, 112-257 U/L)	230	450

Which of the following organisms is most likely?

a. *Shigella* species
b. Toxigenic *Escherichia coli*
c. Norwalk-like virus (*Norovirus*)
d. *Clostridium difficile*
e. *Escherichia coli* O157:H7

17. A 23-year-old woman presents with diarrhea for 3 weeks and left lower quadrant discomfort. Her diarrhea is described as 3 or 4 loose, nonbloody stools per day. She denies fever, chills, nausea, or vomiting, and her appetite has been normal. Stool cultures are negative for pathogens, and no parasites are seen. She undergoes colonoscopy, which shows mild mucosal erythema and granularity that extends uninterrupted from the anal verge to the cecum. The terminal ileum is spared. Biopsy specimens demonstrate chronic crypt architectural changes as well as mild acute inflammation. What therapy should you recommend for this woman?

a. Oral mesalamine (Asacol)
b. Low-dose oral prednisone
c. Mesalamine enema (Rowasa)
d. IV infliximab
e. Oral azathioprine

18. A 19-year-old male high school track star presents to your office after seeing bright red blood on the toilet paper after a bowel movement. Physical examination findings are normal except for a small nodule approximately 5 cm from the anal verge. You refer him for flexible sigmoidoscopy, and nearly 100 polyps are noted. Biopsy findings are consistent with adenomatous polyps. He is adopted and has no knowledge of his family history. What should you recommend next?

a. Annual screening with flexible sigmoidoscopy
b. Colonoscopy with endoscopic removal of polyps if necessary, followed by annual screening with colonoscopy
c. Total proctocolectomy
d. Genetic testing for microsatellite instability
e. Abdominal CT scan to look for metastatic disease

19. A 64-year-old woman presents with left lower quadrant abdominal pain and constipation. On physical examination, her temperature is 38.3°C and a tender left lower quadrant abdominal mass is palpable. Laboratory studies include a normal abdominal radiograph and a complete blood cell count (CBC) showing a leukocyte count of 15.0×10^9/L with a left shift. What should you do next?

a. Obtain stool cultures and blood cultures and perform flexible sigmoidoscopy.
b. Obtain stool cultures and schedule a return visit in 2 days for review of the culture report.
c. Obtain stool cultures, begin oral antibiotic therapy, and instruct the patient to schedule a return appointment if her symptoms do not improve.
d. Admit her to the hospital, give her nothing by mouth, administer IV fluids and antibiotics, and obtain a surgical consultation.
e. Recommend emergency surgery.

20. A 44-year-old man presents to your office for a routine annual examination. His history is significant for 7 years of mild ulcerative colitis that has been well controlled with mesalamine alone. He has no family history of colon cancer or polyps. The patient is at increased risk of each of the following *except*:

a. Colon cancer
b. Primary sclerosing cholangitis
c. Pyoderma gangrenosum
d. Oxalate kidney stones
e. Ankylosing spondylitis

21. A 68-year-old man with a long history of alcohol abuse is referred to you by a colleague for evaluation of progressively loose stools over the past 2 years. The patient stopped drinking alcohol 5 years ago and feels well except for having diarrhea. He denies abdominal pain or nausea but does admit to a 4.1-kg weight loss over the past year. His physical examination findings are unremarkable. Laboratory findings are normal for iron, vitamin B_{12}, CBC, electrolytes, liver enzymes, amylase, and lipase. Stool studies show the following: sodium 100 mEq/L, potassium 45 mEq/L, pH 6.8, and fecal fat 55 g in 24 hours. Stool cultures and examination for ova and parasites are negative. CT scan of the abdomen does not demonstrate any masses or evidence of pancreatic inflammation. What should you recommend next?

a. Perform endoscopic ultrasonography to evaluate for chronic pancreatitis or malignancy.
b. Perform ERCP to evaluate for chronic pancreatitis or malignancy.
c. Reassure the patient and recommend an antidiarrheal agent.
d. Start an empiric trial of pancreatic replacement enzymes.
e. Reassure the patient and recommend a low-fat diet.

22. A 65-year-old man presents with abnormal liver test results. For the past 3 years, he has had an elevated level of alkaline phosphatase. He feels well and denies other medical problems or medications. Physical examination is notable for mild hepatomegaly and bibasilar pulmonary crackles. Cardiac examination findings are normal. Laboratory tests are notable for hemoglobin 14.3 g/dL, WBC $4,400 \times 10^9$/L, platelets 96×10^9/L, alkaline phosphatase (ALP) 533 U/L, AST 65 U/L, and ALT 76 U/L. Results are within the reference ranges for bilirubin, international normalized ratio (INR), and albumin. Chest radiography shows mild bilateral pulmonary infiltrates and prominence of the hilar areas consistent with adenopathy. Ultrasonography of the abdomen is notable for hepatomegaly, normal bile ducts, and mild splenic enlargement. What is the most likely diagnosis?

a. Congestive heart failure
b. Sarcoidosis
c. Amyloidosis
d. Lymphoma
e. Primary biliary cirrhosis

23. A 53-year-old woman presents with a 2-year history of fatigue, pruritus, and abnormal liver tests. She has a history of hypothyroidism, and her only medication is levothyroxine. She denies fever or weight loss. She drinks 2 glasses of wine per week. On physical examination, she has xanthomas, skin excoriations consistent with scratch marks, and hepatomegaly. Laboratory tests are notable for ALP 589 U/L, AST 65 U/L, ALT 76 U/L, and bilirubin 2.3 mg/dL. Results are within the reference ranges for INR, albumin, and gamma globulin. Ultrasonography of the abdomen shows hepatomegaly and normal-sized bile ducts. Which of the following tests is most likely to provide the diagnosis?

a. Antimitochondrial antibody
b. Antinuclear antibody

c. Endoscopic retrograde cholangiopancreatography
d. Angiotensin-converting enzyme level
e. Self-Administered Alcoholism Screening Test (SAAST)

24. A 63-year-old woman presents with fatigue and jaundice. Six weeks ago, she noted fatigue and 2 weeks ago, jaundice appeared. She has no history of liver disease. Medical history is notable for pernicious anemia, for which she takes monthly vitamin B_{12}. She denies fever or weight loss. She drinks 1 glass of wine per week and uses 2 g of acetaminophen daily. Physical examination shows jaundice and spider angiomata. Laboratory tests are notable for AST 643 U/L, ALT 789 U/L, ALP 120 U/L, bilirubin 7.3 mg/dL, INR 1.5, and gamma globulin 3.5 g/dL (reference range <1.6 g/dL). Abdominal ultrasonography reveals small gallbladder stones, normal-sized bile ducts, and splenomegaly. Which of the following is the most likely diagnosis?

a. Acute viral hepatitis
b. Primary biliary cirrhosis
c. Choledocholithiasis
d. Acetaminophen hepatotoxicity
e. Autoimmune hepatitis

25. A 46-year-old man presents with fatigue and weight loss. He has lost 9.1 kg in the past year despite an excellent appetite. He has 3 soft stools per day but denies melena or hematochezia. Because of iron deficiency anemia, he underwent a colonoscopy and EGD, the results of which were negative. No biopsy samples were obtained. He does not drink alcohol and his only medication is 1 ibuprofen tablet every 1 to 2 weeks. Physical examination shows muscle wasting in an otherwise well-appearing man who has a body mass index of 19 kg/m². Laboratory tests are notable for hemoglobin 9.8 g/dL, mean corpuscular volume 68, platelets 436 × 10⁹/L, AST 73 U/L, ALT 78 U/L, ALP 180 U/L, albumin 3.6 g/dL, and ferritin 8 mcg/L. Values for bilirubin and INR are within the reference ranges. Serologic tests for viral hepatitis and antinuclear antibody are negative. Liver ultrasonography shows an increased echogenicity consistent with fat. There is no bile duct dilatation. Which of the following would you advise at this time?

a. Liver biopsy
b. Serum ceruloplasmin
c. Tissue transglutaminase assay
d. Abdominal CT
e. Another colonoscopy

26. A 33-year-old woman presents for follow-up of a liver mass. Two weeks ago, left renal colic suddenly developed. CT of the abdomen showed a left renal stone, which later was passed. CT also showed a 3-cm liver mass; a subsequent contrast-enhanced CT showed that the 3-cm liver mass had the imaging characteristics of a cavernous hemangioma. The patient feels completely well and denies a prior history of liver problems. She does not drink alcohol, and her only medication is

an oral contraceptive. Results of the physical examination and CBC and the liver enzyme levels are all normal. Which of the following would you advise?

a. Perform a biopsy of the mass.
b. Repeat the CT in 6 months.
c. Stop the use of the oral contraceptive.
d. Perform liver MRI.
e. Do no further testing or evaluation.

27. A 63-year-old man is referred with a 3-month history of abdominal distention and peripheral edema. He was born in Laos and has a history of chronic hepatitis B. Physical examination shows jaundice, spider angiomata, muscle wasting, ascites, and peripheral edema. Laboratory tests are notable for hemoglobin 13.8 g/dL, WBC 4.8 × 10⁹/L, platelets 54 × 10⁹/L, AST 123 U/L, ALT 104 U/L, ALP 120 U/L, albumin 3.1 g/dL, bilirubin 4.2 mg/dL, and INR 1.5. The α-fetoprotein level is normal. Hepatitis B surface antigen, hepatitis B e antigen, and IgG antibody against hepatitis B core are positive, and the hepatitis B virus DNA level is 800,000 U/mL (4 million copies/mL). Liver Doppler ultrasonography shows ascites, a coarse echotexture of the liver, patent hepatic and portal veins, and splenomegaly. Analysis of the ascitic fluid shows WBC 50 cells/mm³, protein 1.9 g/dL, and albumin 1.0 g/dL. Which of the following would you advise at this time?

a. Administer peginterferon.
b. Administer entecavir.
c. Administer cefotaxime.
d. Perform echocardiography.
e. Use a transjugular intrahepatic portosystemic shunt.

28. A 36-year-old woman requests hepatitis C testing because she used illicit drugs intravenously 10 years ago. She is asymptomatic, has no medical history, and does not consume alcohol. Physical examination is notable for a body mass index of 35 kg/m². Laboratory tests are notable for hemoglobin 13.8 g/dL, WBC 4.8 × 10⁹/L, platelets 254 × 10⁹/L, AST 65 U/L, ALT 64 U/L, and ALP 120 U/L. Values for albumin, bilirubin, and INR are within the reference ranges. Results are positive for antibody to hepatitis C by enzyme immunoassay and recombinant immunoblot assay. Hepatitis C virus RNA is negative on 2 occasions. Hepatitis B surface antigen, antinuclear antibody, serum iron tests, and ceruloplasmin are negative or normal. Right upper quadrant ultrasonography is notable for a change in liver echotexture consistent with fat and cholelithiasis. Which of the following would you advise at this time?

a. Peginterferon and ribavirin
b. Weight loss and serial monitoring of liver tests
c. Referral for cholecystectomy and liver biopsy
d. Liver biopsy
e. Hepatitis C genotyping

Answers

1.   Answer a.

This patient has symptoms and manometric findings diagnostic of achalasia. This disorder commonly results in esophageal dilatation and does not respond to long-term medical therapy but will benefit from pneumatic dilation, botulinum toxin injection, or a surgical lower esophageal sphincter myotomy. Fundoplication will probably result in a significant worsening of symptoms and would be contraindicated in this patient. Achalasia is typically idiopathic, although secondary achalasia can result from a parasitic infection (*Trypanosoma cruzi* infection) seen in Central and South America.

2.   Answer c.

Atypical manifestations of gastroesophageal reflux disease include adult-onset asthma, hoarseness, coughing, chronic sinusitis, and noncardiac chest pain. These atypical symptoms are often made worse by traditional therapy with bronchodilators and smooth muscle relaxers since these cause relaxation of the lower esophageal sphincter and an exacerbation of the true primary problem.

3.   Answer d.

This patient has recurrent peptic ulcer disease. With evidence of chronic gastritis and with no NSAID use, this is most likely caused by *H pylori* infection. Although sucralfate or antisecretory therapy with H_2-blockers or PPIs may result in symptom resolution and ulcer healing, it does not address the primary problem and leaves the patient susceptible to ulcer recurrence. Surgery for recurrent peptic ulcer disease has been replaced almost entirely by medical therapy since the discovery of *H pylori*.

4.   Answer d.

Patients with Zollinger-Ellison (ZE) syndrome typically present with peptic ulcerations in unusual locations (such as beyond the duodenal bulb) as well as diarrhea due to acidic destruction of digestive enzymes and voluminous gastric fluid secretion. Diagnosis is made when gastrin levels are typically greater than 1,000 pg/mL in the absence of atrophic gastritis or PPI therapy. In ZE syndrome, gastrin levels paradoxically increase with IV administration of secretin, which is diagnostic. Since this patient does not have evidence of chronic gastritis on biopsy, atrophic gastritis and *H pylori* infection can be ruled out. Endoscopic ultrasonography is used to localize ZE tumors after the diagnosis has been made.

5.   Answer c.

The patient has long-standing symptoms suggestive of irritable bowel syndrome, but she clearly has an abnormal stool osmotic gap, which is compounded by the low stool osmolality. In both osmotic diarrhea and secretory diarrhea the measured stool osmolality should be in equilibrium with the serum osmolality (roughly 290 mOsm/kg for stool). The markedly low stool osmolality suggests that free water has been added to the stool sample after collection. Conversely, a markedly elevated stool osmolality (>400 mOsm/kg) suggests that the stool sample has been contaminated (either intentionally or inadvertently) with a hyperosmolar substance such as

urine. Fecal fermentation can occur after collection, which can result in increased osmolality if measurement is delayed. Only free water or other hypo-osmolar liquids, however, can cause stool osmolality to decrease.

6.   Answer c.

This patient has evidence of steatorrhea. Normally, D-xylose is absorbed in the small bowel but does not require pancreatic enzymes for absorption. Since D-xylose is not absorbed in this patient, small-bowel mucosal disease is the cause of the malabsorption. Histologic evaluation should rule out conditions such as sprue, Whipple disease, or lymphoma.

7.   Answer c.

This patient has 2 extraintestinal complications associated with chronic ulcerative colitis (CUC). The peripheral large-joint arthritis tends to follow colonic disease activity and should resolve as the colitis improves. The elevated alkaline phosphatase, however, should alert the physician to the possibility of primary sclerosing cholangitis (PSC). This should be diagnosed with ERCP, which would demonstrate characteristic narrowed irregularities of the biliary duct system. PSC runs a course independent of colitis disease activity. Routine screenng for CUC includes a full colonoscopy with random biopsies to screen for malignancies beginning 8 to 10 years after the diagnosis of pancolitis in CUC or beginning immediately after the diagnosis of PSC in a CUC patient. Screening in left-sided colitis alone can likely be delayed safely until 15 years after the initial diagnosis. The risk of malignancy with isolated proctitis is likely no higher than in the general population; hence, patients with proctitis do not require screening examinations different from those for the general population. After screening begins, a colonoscopy with biopsies every 10 cm should be performed every 1 to 2 years while there is no histologic evidence of dysplasia. If low-grade dysplasia or adenoma is seen in the affected colon, a colectomy is typically recommended. High-grade dysplasia warrants evaluation for ugent colectomy.

8.   Answer c.

This woman has an osmotic diarrhea as evidenced by the stool osmolar gap of 58, which is calculated as 290–2(86+30). This can be caused by laxative use or poorly absorbed anions. The key here is that the pH is less than 6, suggesting that the diarrhea is likely due to fermentation of a poorly absorbed carbohydrate in the colon. The most common cause of this type of carbohydrate malabsorption, especially in the Asian population, is lactase deficiency. Lactose intolerance can be treated effectively with dietary avoidance of lactose sugars (dairy products) or the addition of oral lactase supplements. Fecal fat may be mildly elevated simply because of rapid intestinal transit.

9.   Answer d.

Patients with Whipple disease may present with diarrhea, arthralgias, fever, and neurologic changes; 30% also have associated cardiac or pulmonary dysfunction. Patients with Whipple disease have PAS-positive granules in small-bowel biopsy specimens. *Mycobacterium avium-intracellulare* complex (MAC) is also a PAS-positive organism (the appearance can resemble the findings in Whipple disease). MAC, however, is also acid-fast–positive and the organism that causes Whipple disease is not. The diagnosis of Whipple disease is confirmed with use of a polymerase chain reaction test, which detects the organism in small-bowel biopsy material.

10. Answer d.

The diarrhea and flatus are suggestive of a possible malabsorptive process. Certainly irritable bowel syndrome is a possibility, but this is a diagnosis of exclusion. With the decreased iron stores but no source for bleeding, the likely cause of her iron deficiency is a malabsorptive process localized in the proximal small bowel. The malabsorptive diarrhea and iron deficiency are highly suggestive of celiac disease. Small-bowel biopsy is still considered the diagnostic standard because of the possibility of false-negative results on the serum antibody test, which can result from an IgA deficiency that is seen in up to 10% of patients with celiac disease. Steroids may give transient symptomatic relief, but a strict gluten-free diet is the only effective means to achieve long-term symptomatic relief.

11. Answer a.

The potential causes of symptomatic relapse in a patient with celiac disease need to be considered. The accidental ingestion of a gluten-containing product is the most common cause, but this woman has been doing well for years and seems motivated to keep gluten out of her diet. Other more serious complications need to be ruled out before simply resuming a gluten-free diet. The most important is the development of small-bowel lymphoma that can result from long-standing sprue. This would best be evaluated with an abdominal CT scan. Another possible cause of diarrhea is the development of lymphocytic colitis (microscopic colitis), which is more common in celiac disease. This should be excluded with colonoscopy, after exclusion of lymphoma.

12. Answer b.

The man has inflammatory enteritis as evidenced by the diarrhea with leukocytes, negative cultures, and apparent secretory diarrhea (it does not resolve with fasting). With the normal findings on colonoscopy, these findings suggest small-bowel disease such as Crohn enteritis. This disease would be identified best with small-bowel radiography. Although capsule endoscopy and CT may be used to identify small-bowel disease as well, the standard is a barium study (small-bowel radiography).

13. Answer c.

The patient has evidence of cryptosporidiosis involving the small bowel. With his low CD4 count, it is unlikely that he is taking his medications as prescribed. Primary therapy would be to improve his antiviral therapy compliance. Secondary treatment is controversial, but the combination of azithromycin and paromomycin has been shown to be effective. With normal villi, celiac disease and Whipple disease are unlikely.

14. Answer b.

The patient has had a large portion of her terminal ileum resected as a result of Crohn disease. She has had more than 100 cm removed, increasing her risk of bile acid depletion and subsequent steatorrhea, which she is demonstrating clinically. This excess of unabsorbed free fatty acids binds dietary calcium, which under normal conditions prevents excess oxalate absorption. Excess absorption leads to the formation of oxalate kidney stones. A low-fat diet and calcium supplementation with meals can help reduce the absorption of oxalate. In patients with less than 100 cm of small bowel resected, the primary cause of diarrhea is excess bile acids (more than what the small bowel can absorb), thus leading to bile acid–induced irritation of the colon and resultant diarrhea.

15. Answer b.

The history of pain and nonbloody diarrhea that turns bloody in a man with a history of vascular disease is a classic presentation for ischemic bowel disease. The most common areas are the watershed areas of the colon. The left upper quadrant pain is suggestive of splenic flexure involvement, which is a common site for this process. The patient has no fever or leukocytosis to suggest diverticulitis; he is not hemodynamically unstable, so a transfusion or urgent colonoscopy is not needed. Angiography is of little use in this setting since acute ischemic colitis is typically a small-vessel disease that is not apparent with interventional angiography or magnetic resonance angiography.

16. Answer e.

This constellation of symptoms and laboratory findings is most suggestive of hemolytic uremic syndrome (HUS), a complication of infection with *E coli* O157:H7. This occurs more commonly in the elderly or very young, and the risk may be increased with the administration of antibiotic therapy. *Shigella* is also invasive and can cause bloody diarrhea, but it is not associated with HUS. Infections with the other organisms listed typically result in watery diarrhea.

17. Answer a.

This woman has endoscopic and biopsy findings suggestive of CUC. The endoscopic changes and symptoms are rather mild and will likely respond to oral 5-aminosalicylic acid (5-ASA) therapy. Prednisone therapy is not indicated for mild symptoms unless they are refractory to 5-ASA compounds. An oral 5-ASA compound with colonic release is required because of the extent of the disease (ie, pancolitis), which would not be treated with enema or suppository therapy. IV infliximab is indicated for severe Crohn disease and not for CUC. Azathioprine is used as a steroid-sparing drug for long-term maintenance rather than as a remission-induction drug. 5-ASA compounds can be used for inducing remission of mild disease and for long-term maintenance therapy.

18. Answer c.

The patient has evidence of familial adenomatous polyposis, which results from the deletion of 1 copy of the *APC* gene from birth. In these patients, hundreds of adenomatous polyps develop in the early teen years and colon cancer almost uniformly develops by the age of 40. The recommendation is for a total proctocolectomy if the polyposis phenotype is already established. Microsatellite instability is an initial screen to look for genetic mutations associated with heredity nonpolyposis colon cancer.

19. Answer d.

The woman has a clinical history and examination findings that are classic for diverticulitis. Admit the patient to the hospital, give her nothing by mouth, administer IV fluids and antibiotics, and obtain a surgical consultation. Although her condition does not warrant emergent surgery, she may require surgery if her condition does not improve with hydration and antibiotics or she may need elective surgery after the condition resolves (especially if she has had multiple episodes).

20. Answer d.

All the factors listed are associated with higher risk for patients with ulcerative colitis except oxalate kidney stones, which occur in patients with Crohn disease after extensive terminal ileum resection and subsequent bile acid pool depletion and steatorrhea. Free fatty acids in the stool bind to calcium, thus freeing up dietary oxalate to be absorbed in excess.

21. Answer d.

The patient has definite risk factors for chronic pancreatitis. Although CT is sensitive for ruling out a pancreatic mass, sometimes it is not helpful for identifying changes of chronic pancreatitis. Endoscopic ultrasonography and ERCP are far more sensitive for identifying changes that are diagnostic for chronic pancreatitis, although in this patient the markedly elevated fecal fat is already rather specific for pancreatic insufficiency. A diagnostic and therapeutic trial of pancreatic enzymes is the most appropriate therapy.

22. Answer b.

The main differential diagnostic possibilities for an elevated ALP value are primary sclerosing cholangitis, primary biliary cirrhosis, drug-induced liver disease, large duct obstruction, or an infiltrative disorder such as amyloidosis, sarcoidosis, or malignancy. Chronically elevated ALP in an asymptomatic patient who has evidence of interstitial lung disease with hilar adenopathy and splenomegaly would be most consistent with sarcoidosis. Congestive heart failure would be expected to be accompanied by changes on cardiac examination and clinical evidence of fluid overload. Amyloidosis would cause symptoms due to renal or peripheral nerve involvement since the changes have been present for years. Lymphoma would also be associated with more symptoms because of the long duration of the alkaline phosphatase elevation. Primary biliary cirrhosis is more common in women and is not generally accompanied by pulmonary changes.

23. Answer a.

Diagnostic possibilities for a predominant elevation of ALP are primary sclerosing cholangitis (PSC), primary biliary cirrhosis (PBC), drug-induced liver disease, large duct obstruction, or an infiltrative disorder. In a middle-aged woman, the main diagnostic consideration is primary biliary cirrhosis, which could be confirmed with an antimitochondrial antibody test. Patients with PBC often have pruritus and xanthomas. The antinuclear antibody (ANA) may be positive in low titer in patients with PBC but would not confirm the diagnosis. Marked ANA elevations are more characteristic of autoimmune hepatitis, which would be characterized by predominant aminotransferase, rather than ALP, elevations. ERCP would be helpful to diagnose PSC or large bile duct obstruction. PSC is unlikely in a patient without ulcerative colitis, and longstanding bile duct obstruction usually results in dilated bile ducts apparent on ultrasonography. There are no pulmonary features to suggest sarcoidosis, so an angiotensin-converting enzyme level would not be helpful. The SAAST can be used to identify alcoholic patients, but patients with alcoholic liver disease ingest larger amounts of alcohol (>20 g/d). In addition, alcoholic liver disease usually results in an AST:ALT ratio greater than 2 and usually does not cause xanthomas.

24. Answer e.

This patient presents with symptoms and biochemical features of acute hepatitis; however, she also has evidence of chronic liver disease, including spider angiomata and splenomegaly. In a woman with a history of an autoimmune disease such as pernicious anemia, the most likely diagnosis is autoimmune hepatitis. At presentation, about 40% to 50% of patients with autoimmune hepatitis appear to have acute hepatitis, although most have clinical and histologic evidence of chronicity. Acute viral hepatitis would cause similar symptoms and liver enzyme levels but would not account for the changes of chronic liver disease. Primary biliary cirrhosis would result in a prominent elevation of ALP rather than aminotransferases. Choledocholithiasis would produce more abdominal pain and cause a more transient abnormality of liver tests. Acetaminophen hepatotoxicity would not occur with these doses of acetaminophen and is characterized by much higher aminotransferase levels.

25. Answer c.

Weight loss despite a good appetite and iron deficiency anemia without overt bleeding and with negative endoscopic studies are suggestive of malabsorption, and celiac disease should be excluded. Celiac disease can result in abnormal liver test results from steatosis or nonspecific hepatitis. Tissue transglutaminase assay is a good screening test for celiac disease and should be the next test. Liver biopsy would likely confirm steatosis but would not explain the underlying cause. Wilson disease can be a cause of otherwise unexplained steatosis but would not explain iron deficiency or weight loss, and therefore checking a serum ceruloplasmin would not be indicated. Abdominal CT would likely add little information to the examination and ultrasonographic findings. Another colonoscopy could be considered, although colon cancer is only rarely missed on initial colonoscopy and iron deficiency anemia and weight loss accompanying colon cancer are usually associated with anorexia.

26. Answer e.

Cavernous hemangiomas are found in about 5% of the general population and are therefore common incidental findings on cross-sectional abdominal imaging. Nearly all cavernous hemangiomas are asymptomatic. Rarely, lesions larger than 6 cm may cause pain and, even more rarely, bleeding. When radiologic features are consistent with an asymptomatic cavernous hemangioma, as in this case, no further testing or treatment is necessary. Biopsies of cavernous hemangiomas are safe but are only necessary if radiologic features are not consistent. Repeating the CT is necessary only if the lesion is atypical on imaging. The only benign liver lesion that is dependent on estrogen for growth is adenoma, and withdrawal of estrogens is not necessary for patients with cavernous hemangioma or focal nodular hyperplasia. Liver MRI is not necessary to confirm cavernous hemangioma when CT findings are characteristic.

27. Answer b.

The patient has evidence of cirrhotic stage hepatitis B with active viral replication; therefore, treatment with antiviral agents is indicated. Treatment can be with interferon or an oral agent such as entecavir. Interferon is contraindicated in patients with decompensated cirrhosis because of the risk of inducting a flare of the disease; therefore, the patient should receive an oral agent such as entecavir. Patients with decompensated hepatitis B who respond to treatment may also improve clinically, although this patient should also be referred for liver transplant. There is no evidence for spontaneous bacterial peritonitis or other infection; therefore, cefotaxime is not indicated. Because the fluid analysis results are consistent with cirrhotic ascites (serum–ascitic fluid albumin gradient >1.1 g/dL and ascites fluid protein <2.5 g/dL), echocardiography is not necessary. A transjugular intrahepatic portosystemic shunt is used only in patients with refractory bleeding or ascites due to portal hypertension.

28. Answer b.

The patient has a positive antibody test for hepatitis C. A positive enzyme immunoassay that is confirmed by recombinant immunoblot assay indicates prior exposure to the virus. This patient was most likely exposed during her prior intravenous drug use. Despite that exposure, the viral RNA tests were negative; therefore, she probably is 1 of the 15% to 40% of patients who clear hepatitis C after being acutely infected. Her abnormal liver test results are most likely due to nonalcoholic fatty liver disease. Weight loss with serial monitoring of liver tests would be advised at this time. Peginterferon and ribavirin are not necessary without an ongoing hepatitis C viral infection. Cholecystectomy is not necessary for asymptomatic cholelithiasis. Liver biopsy can be considered, but most would advise a trial of weight loss with monitoring of liver tests first. Hepatitis C genotyping can only be performed if patients have hepatitis C viremia.

8

General Internal Medicine

Scott C. Litin, MD
Karen F. Mauck, MD, MSc

The goal of this chapter is to discuss important topics that are not covered thoroughly in other chapters. The interpretation of diagnostic tests and results of therapy must be well understood by internists because these skills are used every day in practice. Frequently, internists are asked to make a preoperative risk assessment of a medical patient who is about to have a noncardiac operation. Managing anticoagulant therapy, assessing risk, treating patients who have hyperlipidemia, and managing other disorders frequently encountered in the office are also important. This chapter discusses these topics.

Interpretation of Diagnostic Tests

Diagnostic tests are tools that either increase or decrease the likelihood of disease. When a diagnostic test is applied to a population at risk of a particular disease, patients in the studied population can be assigned to 1 of 4 groups on the basis of disease status and the test result. Table 8-1 illustrates the concept.

By convention, the 4 groups are assigned the letters *a* for true-positive (TP), *b* for false-positive (FP), *c* for false-negative (FN), and *d* for true-negative (TN) (Table 8-2). On the basis of this table (called a *2×2 table*), the following test characteristics can be defined:
1. *Sensitivity*
   Positive (test) in disease (PID)
   True positivity rate—proportion of patients with the disease who have a positive test result

$$\text{Sensitivity} = \frac{TP}{TP+FN}$$

The 2×2 table definition: a/(a+c)
Rules to remember:
   SN out—if a test has 100% sensitivity, a negative test rules *out* the disorder
   Screening tests are used to maximize sensitivity and avoid missing a person who has the disease
   Characteristic of test—not affected by the prevalence of disease in the population

2. *Specificity*
   Negative (test) in health (NIH)
   True negativity rate—proportion of patients without the disease who have a negative test result

Table 8-2 2×2 Table

| | | Target Disorder | | |
		Present	Absent	
Diagnostic Test Result	Positive	True-positive a	False-positive b	a+b
	Negative	c False-negative	d True-negative	c+d
		a+c	b+d	a+b+c+d

Prevalence = (a+c)/(a+b+c+d)
Test characteristics
   Sensitivity = a/(a+c)
   Specificity = d/(b+d)
Frequency-dependent properties
   Positive predictive value = a/(a+b)
   Negative predictive value = d/(c+d)

Table 8-1 Four Outcomes of a Diagnostic Test

Outcome	Disease Status	Test Result
True-positive	Present	Abnormal
False-positive	Absent	Abnormal
False-negative	Present	Normal
True-negative	Absent	Normal

329

$$\text{Specificity} = \frac{TN}{TN+FP}$$

The 2×2 table definition: d/(b+d)

Rules to remember:

SP in—if a test has 100% specificity, a positive test rules *in* the disorder

Confirmatory tests are used in follow-up of screening to maximize specificity and avoid incorrectly labeling a healthy person as having disease

Characteristic of test—not affected by the prevalence of disease in the population

3. *Positive predictive value*

When a patient's illness is evaluated by interpreting a diagnostic test, the 2×2 table is read horizontally, not vertically. One really wants to know whether a patient with positive test results actually has the disease; that is, how well the test results predict a disease compared with the reference standard for that disease. Thus, in the 2 × 2 table, the horizontal rows for the diagnostic test result are of primary interest. Among all patients with a positive diagnostic test result (TP+FP), in what proportion, $\frac{TP}{TP+FP}$, has the diagnosis been predicted correctly or ruled in? This proportion is the *positive predictive value* (PPV).

* PPV is the proportion of patients who have the disease among all the patients who test positive for the disease.
* This provides information most useful in clinical practice.
* PPV is affected by the prevalence of the disease in the population.
* The 2×2 table definition: PPV = $\frac{TP}{TP+FP}$ = a/(a+b).

4. *Negative predictive value*

It is also important to know the percentage of patients with a negative test result (FN+TN) who actually do not have the disease. This proportion, $\frac{TN}{FN+TN}$, is the *negative predictive value* (NPV).

* NPV is the proportion of patients who do not have the disease of interest among all the patients who test negative for the disease.
* NPV is affected by the prevalence of disease in the population.
* The 2×2 table definition: NPV = $\frac{TN}{FN+TN}$ = d/(c+d).

5. *Prevalence*

Prevalence is defined as the proportion of persons with the disease in the population to whom the test has been applied. In terms of the 2×2 table, prevalence is written

$$\frac{TP+FN}{TP+FP+FN+TN} = \frac{a+c}{a+b+c+d}$$

How to Construct a 2×2 Table

The sensitivity, specificity, and predictive values of normal and abnormal test results can be calculated with even a limited amount of information. For example, assume that a new diagnostic test is positive in 90% of patients who have the disease and is negative in 95% of patients who are disease-free. The prevalence of the disease in the population to which the test is applied is 10%. This provides the following information:

Sensitivity = 90%
Specificity = 95%
Prevalence = 10%

This test is now ready to be applied to a group of patients by filling in a 2×2 table (Table 8-3). The calculation is often made easier if the test is applied to a large number of patients. For example, if it is applied to 1,000 patients, a+b+c+d = 1,000.

Because the prevalence of the disease is 10%, 100 patients have the disease (0.1×1,000 = 100, or a+c = 100). Of the patients, 90%, or 900, are disease-free (0.9×1,000 = 900, or b+d = 900).

Sensitivity of 90% means that 90% of the 100 patients with disease have a positive test result (a = 0.9×100 = 90) and 10% have a negative result (c = 0.1×100 = 10).

Specificity of 95% means that 95% of the 900 patients who are disease-free have a negative test result (d = 0.95×900 = 855) and 5% have a positive test result (b = 0.05×900 = 45).

The 2×2 table in Table 8-3 shows that 135 patients (a+b) have a positive test result; however, only 90 of these 135 patients actually have the disease. Therefore, the PPV of a positive test is $\frac{a}{a+b} = \frac{90}{135}$ = 66.7%. That is, only two-thirds of all patients with a positive test result will actually have the disease. Similarly, one can determine that 865 patients (c+d) have a negative test result; 855 of these 865 patients

Table 8-3   2×2 Table for Test With 90% Sensitivity, 95% Specificity, and 10% Prevalence

		Disease Present	Disease Absent	
Diagnostic Test Result	Positive	90 / a	45 / b	135 / a+b
	Negative	c / 10	d / 855	c+d / 865
		a+c	b+d	a+b+c+d
Total		100	900	1,000

Prevalence = (a+c)/(a+b+c+d) = 100/1,000 = 10%
Test characteristics
    Sensitivity = a/(a+c) = 90/100 = 90%
    Specificity = d/(b+d) = 855/900 = 95%
Frequency-dependent properties
    Positive predictive value = a/(a+b) = 90/135 = 66.7%
    Negative predictive value = d/(c+d) = 855/865 = 98.8%
Likelihood ratio (LR) for a positive test result:
    LR+ = Sensitivity/(1 − Specificity) = 90%/5% = 18
Likelihood ratio for a negative test result:
    LR− = (1 − Sensitivity)/Specificity = 10%/95% = 0.11
Pretest odds = Prevalence/(1 − Prevalence) = 10%/90% = 0.11
Posttest odds = Pretest odds × Likelihood ratio
Posttest probability = Posttest odds/(Posttest odds + 1)

are disease-free. Therefore, the NPV of the test is $\frac{d}{c+d} = \frac{855}{865} = 98.8\%$.

Clinicians should be able to perform these simple calculations. Clinical decision making by internists is more likely to depend on the PPV and NPV of test results for a given population than on the sensitivity or specificity of the test.

For example, if the prevalence of the disease in the clinician's population is 2% instead of 10%, the PPV and NPV can be recalculated. The PPV of abnormal test results decreases to 26.9%, which is quite different from 66.7% (based on a prevalence of 10%), although the sensitivity and specificity of the test (90% and 95%, respectively) have not changed (Table 8-4).

* An important factor in interpreting a patient's test result is knowledge of the prevalence of the disease in the population being tested.
* High-risk populations (high prevalence of disease) tend to improve the PPV of an abnormal test result.
* Low-risk populations (screening tests) make the NPV of a normal test result look impressive.

Use of Odds and Likelihood Ratios

Some physicians prefer interpreting diagnostic test results by using the likelihood ratio. This ratio takes properties of a diagnostic test (sensitivity and specificity) and makes them more helpful in clinical decision making. It helps the clinician determine the probability of disease in a specific patient after a diagnostic test has been performed.

The formula for a likelihood ratio for a positive test result (LR+) is

$$LR+ = \frac{\text{Positive test in disease}}{\text{Positive test in no disease}} = \frac{\text{Sensitivity}}{1 - \text{Specificity}}$$

Table 8-4   2×2 Table for Test With 90% Sensitivity, 95% Specificity, and 2% Prevalence

		Disease Present	Disease Absent	
Diagnostic Test Result	Positive	18 (a)	49 (b)	67 (a+b)
	Negative	2 (c)	931 (d)	933 (c+d)
		(a+c)	(b+d)	(a+b+c+d)
	Total	20	980	1,000

Prevalence = (a+c)/(a+b+c+d) = 20/1,000 = 2%
Test characteristics
    Sensitivity = a/(a+c) = 18/20 = 90%
    Specificity = d/(b+d) = 931/980 = 95%
Frequency-dependent properties
    Positive predictive value = a/(a+b) = 18/67 = 26.9%
    Negative predictive value = d/(c+d) = 931/933 = 99.8%

The formula for a likelihood ratio for a negative test result (LR−) is

$$LR- = \frac{\text{Negative test in disease}}{\text{Negative test in no disease}} = \frac{1 - \text{Sensitivity}}{\text{Specificity}}$$

For example, if test A has a sensitivity of 95% and a specificity of 90%,

$$LR+ = \frac{\text{Sensitivity}}{1 - \text{Specificity}} = 95/10 = 9.5$$

$$LR- = \frac{1 - \text{Sensitivity}}{\text{Specificity}} = \frac{5}{90} = 0.06$$

However, if test B has a sensitivity of 20% and a specificity of 80%, then

$$LR+ = \frac{\text{Sensitivity}}{1 - \text{Specificity}} = \frac{20}{20} = 1$$

$$LR- = \frac{1 - \text{Sensitivity}}{\text{Specificity}} = \frac{80}{80} = 1$$

As a general rule, diagnostic tests with an LR+ greater than 10 or an LR− less than 0.1 have a greater influence on the posttest probability of disease (ie, they are better tests) than diagnostic tests with likelihood ratios between 10 and 0.1. In the 2 examples above, test A is more likely to rule in or rule out disease than test B.

Sample likelihood ratios are provided in the example below and in Table 8-5.

Example

A 40-year-old white man is admitted to the hospital for pneumonia. He says that he consumes 2 six-packs of beer each week. On the basis of this history and your clinical judgment, you assume that he has a pretest probability of 20% for a diagnosis of alcoholism. You perform the CAGE questionnaire, and his responses are positive for all 4 questions. You notice that the LR+ for 3 or more CAGE questions is 250.

At this point, you have 2 choices. The first is to use a nomogram (Figure 8-1) and, with a straightedge, connect the pretest probability of 20% and the LR+ of 250 to the posttest probability. This shows that the posttest probability for a diagnosis of alcoholism is 99%.

The second option should be used when there is no nomogram for performing this simple calculation. Without a nomogram, the following must be done: 1) convert the pretest probability to pretest odds, 2) multiply the pretest odds by the likelihood ratio to obtain the posttest odds, and 3) convert the posttest odds to posttest probability.

Probability and odds can be converted somewhat interchangeably with the following formulas:

$$\text{Odds} = \frac{\text{Probability}}{1 - \text{Probability}}$$

$$\text{Probability} = \frac{\text{Odds}}{1 + \text{Odds}}$$

In the example, step 1 involves converting pretest probability to pretest odds. In this case, you estimated that the pretest probability

Table 8-5 Examples of Symptoms, Signs, and Tests and the Likelihood Ratio (LR)

Target Disorder	Patient Population	Health Care Setting	Symptom, Sign, Test	No. of Signs or Symptoms	LR
Alcohol abuse or dependency	Patients admitted to orthopedic or medical services over a 6-month period	US teaching hospital	Yes to ≥3 questions on CAGE		250
Sinusitis (by further investigation)	Patients with nasal complaints	US teaching hospital	Maxillary toothache, purulent nasal secretion, poor response to nasal decongestants, abnormal transillumination, or history of colored nasal discharge	≥4 3 2 1 0	6.4 2.6 1.1 0.5 0.1
Ascites	Male veteran patients	US veterans' hospital	Presence of fluid wave (done by internal medicine residents)		9.6

Data from Bush B, Shaw S, Cleary P, Delbanco TL, Aronson MD. Screening for alcohol abuse using the CAGE questionnaire. Am J Med. 1987;82:231-5; Williams JW Jr, Simel DL. Does this patient have sinusitis? Diagnosing acute sinusitis by history and physical examination. JAMA. 1993;270:1242-6; Williams JW Jr, Simel DL, Roberts L, Samsa GP. Clinical evaluation for sinusitis: making the diagnosis by history and physical examination. Ann Intern Med. 1992;117:705-10; Williams JW Jr, Simel DL. The rational clinical explanation: does this patient have ascites? How to divine fluid in the abdomen. JAMA. 1992;267:2645-8; Simel DL, Halvorsen RA Jr, Feussner JR. Quantitating bedside diagnosis: clinical evaluation of ascites. J Gen Intern Med. 1988;3:423-8.

of alcoholism is 20%. With the formulas above,

$$\text{Pretest odds} = \frac{0.20}{1 - 0.20} = 0.25$$

Therefore, 0.25 is the pretest odds of having the condition. Step 2 involves determining the posttest odds for a positive test. This can be determined by multiplying the pretest odds (0.25) by the LR+ for 3 or more positive questions on the CAGE questionnaire (250): 0.25×250 = 62.5. Step 3 allows conversion of posttest odds to posttest probability by placing the numbers in the following formula:

$$\text{Posttest probability} = \frac{\text{Odds}}{1 + \text{Odds}} = \frac{62.5}{63.5} = 98.4\%$$

In conclusion, the posttest probability for the diagnosis of alcoholism for this patient is 98.4%, which is close to the value obtained from the nomogram.

Interpretation of Therapeutic Results

Physicians often make treatment decisions on the basis of the results of randomized controlled trials (RCTs). To understand whether the results of such trials are impressive, the physician is required to translate these results into language understandable to both physicians and patients. This terminology can also be used to compare various therapies for the disease of interest. Several authors have coined terms and derived useful equations to help physicians make sense of RCTs concerned with therapy.

Relative Risk Reduction

The results of RCTs of anticoagulant therapy to prevent stroke in patients with atrial fibrillation have been published and summarized. In primary prevention studies, the average 1-year risk for stroke in the placebo group was 5% per year. Because no therapy was administered to that group, this can be called the *control event rate* (CER). In these studies of patients with atrial fibrillation treated with adjusted-dose warfarin (international normalized ratio [INR], 2.0-3.0), the approximate stroke risk was reduced to 2% per year. This can be called the *experimental event rate* (EER) because the patients received a particular therapy.

The traditional measure often used to report the difference between the treated and untreated groups is the *relative risk reduction* (RRR), which is calculated as $\frac{\text{CER-EER}}{\text{CER}}$. This measure relates the reduction in risk of the outcome event with the intervention compared with the baseline risk rate (CER). In this example, the RRR is $\frac{5\%-2\%}{5\%}$ = 60%. Therefore, anticoagulant therapy reduced the yearly risk of a stroke developing in patients with atrial fibrillation by 60% compared with the baseline risk of a stroke developing with no therapy. However, the RRR often is not clinically helpful because the number itself does not provide information about the baseline risk rate (ie, CER). For example, even if only a very small number of control patients (0.005%) and patients receiving anticoagulation (0.002%) experience stroke, the RRR is unchanged: $\frac{0.005\%-0.002\%}{0.005\%}$ = 60%. Therefore, the RRR often is not useful to the clinician or patient, although a large RRR can be used to make a dramatic endorsement for therapy by proponents of that therapy.

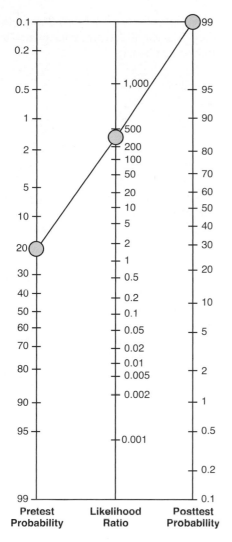

Figure 8-1. Nomogram.

* $RRR = \dfrac{CER-EER}{CER}$.
* Often RRR is not clinically useful because it does not provide information about the baseline risk rate.

Absolute Risk Reduction

In the example above, it would be useful for the physician and patient to know the absolute difference in rates of stroke between the control group and the atrial fibrillation group given anticoagulants (CER–EER). This measure is called the *absolute risk reduction* (ARR). In the combined Stroke Prevention in Atrial Fibrillation (SPAF) trials, the ARR or (CER–EER) = (5%–2%) = 3% per year.

* ARR = (CER–EER).
* ARR is clinically more useful for interpreting therapeutic results.

Number Needed to Treat

The physician and patient often want to know the number of patients needed to treat (NNT) with a therapy to prevent 1 additional bad

outcome. That number can be calculated as $\frac{1}{ARR}$. Therefore, the NNT to prevent 1 stroke by using the adjusted dose of warfarin in patients with atrial fibrillation would be $\frac{1}{0.03} = \frac{1}{3\%} = 33$. Therefore, the NNT would be 33 patients; that is, 33 patients would need to be treated with warfarin (INR, 2.0-3.0) for 1 year to prevent 1 additional stroke.

* NNT identifies the number of patients who need to be treated with a therapy to prevent 1 additional bad outcome.
* $NNT = \frac{1}{ARR}$.

Number Needed to Harm

Conversely, if the rate of adverse events caused by the experimental therapy is known and compared with the rate of adverse events in the placebo group, the number needed to harm (NNH) can be calculated. This useful number tells the physician how many treated patients it takes to produce 1 additional harmful event. In the studies dealing with stroke prevention in atrial fibrillation, the average risk of intracranial hemorrhage for the group given warfarin was 0.3% per year, compared with 0.1% per year for the placebo group. Therefore, the NNH can be calculated as the reciprocal of the absolute risk increase (ARI). The ARI can be calculated by subtracting the harm CER from the harm EER or, in this case, 0.3%–0.1% = 0.2%. In this example, NNH = $\frac{1}{0.2\%} = \frac{1}{0.002} = 500$. Therefore, 500 patients would need to be treated with anticoagulant for 1 year to cause 1 additional intracranial hemorrhage, compared with the control group.

* NNH identifies how many treated patients are needed to produce 1 additional harmful event.
* $NNH = \dfrac{1}{\text{Harm EER} - \text{Harm CER}}$.

Preoperative Medical Evaluation

More than 33 million US residents (about 10% of the US population) undergo surgery annually. This number is projected to increase substantially (by as much as 25% by 2020) as more baby boomers become eligible for Medicare. Internists are often expected to evaluate the fitness of patients for surgery and to help manage comorbidities in the perioperative period.

Goals of Preoperative Evaluation

The 2 main goals of a preoperative evaluation are the following:
1. To evaluate, assess, and quantify the risk of anesthesia and surgery and to communicate this risk to the patient, the anesthesiologist, and the surgeon to allow for informed decision making
2. To help appropriately direct perioperative care in an attempt to minimize this risk

Both patient-specific risks and surgery-specific risks contribute to overall perioperative risk. Although the most frequent types of major perioperative risks are cardiac, pulmonary, and thromboembolic, there are many other contributors of risk as well. The following sections cover what a perioperative evaluation should include, general risks of anesthesia and surgery, and more-specific risk assessment and management strategies. This review is not a comprehensive coverage of perioperative medicine, but it covers some of the most common and important issues to consider when evaluating perioperative risk.

Standard Aspects of the Preoperative Evaluation

History and Review of Systems

Include a careful cardiovascular history, focusing on clinical predictors outlined in the American College of Cardiology and American Heart Association (ACC/AHA) guidelines (Table 8-6). Functional status, based on the patient's report, can be estimated in metabolic equivalents (METs) (Table 8-7). A pulmonary, anesthesic, thrombotic, and bleeding history should also be reviewed. Document the presence and clinical status of any medical illnesses (eg, glaucoma, diabetes mellitus, hypertension, thyroid disease, sleep apnea, renal insufficiency, and cognitive impairment). Include a question about corticosteroid use in the past year and screening questions about potentially undiagnosed sleep apnea. Consider the possibility of pregnancy in any woman of childbearing age.

Past Medical, Surgical, Social, and Family History

Document all previous surgical procedures with approximate dates, type of anesthesia, and complications. Include a comprehensive list of the patient's past medical diagnoses. Include relevant smoking, alcohol, or drug history, including extent of past use and most recent use. Family history should be limited to first-degree relatives with serious anesthetic (eg, malignant hypertension) or bleeding complications.

Medications

Perhaps the greatest contribution that the internist can make to the preoperative assessment is the compilation of an accurate and complete medication list. Full dosing information should be included for all prescription and nonprescription drugs, dietary supplements, and herbs. Confirm the allergy list and ask about latex allergy.

Physical Examination

Include complete vital signs with manually measured blood pressure, temperature, and pulse and respiratory rates. The head and neck examination should include neck range of motion, an evaluation of the airway (Figure 8-2), carotid auscultation, and assessment of the jugular veins. The cardiopulmonary examination should focus on murmurs, gallops, rales, rhonchi, and wheezes. Include a brief abdominal examination for organomegaly or unexplained scars. Examine the extremities for palpable distal pulses and evidence of significant peripheral edema. When applicable, perform a limited neurologic examination that includes mental status and a gross sensory and motor evaluation (ie, baseline cognitive or neurologic problems).

Impression and Plan

This section should summarize your assessment of perioperative risk and any additional testing and management recommendations based on this risk. This usually includes the following statement: "The patient is medically optimized for planned surgical procedure." Avoid using the expression "cleared for surgery," which implies a guarantee

Table 8-6   Clinical Predictors of Increased Perioperative Cardiovascular Risk (Myocardial Infarction, Heart Failure, and Death)

Active cardiac conditions
  Unstable coronary syndromes
    Acute or recent MI with evidence of important ischemic risk by clinical symptoms or noninvasive study[a]
    Unstable or severe angina[b] (Canadian Class III or IV)[c]
  Significant arrhythmias
    High-grade atrioventricular block
    Symptomatic ventricular arrhythmias in the presence of underlying heart disease
    Supraventricular arrhythmias with unconrolled ventricular rate
  Severe valvular disease
  Decompensated heart failure
Clinical risk factors (from the revised cardiac risk index[d])
  History of ischemic heart disease (including patients with pathologic Q waves on ECG)
  History of compensated or prior heart failure (systolic or diastolic)
  History of cerebrovascular disease (TIA or stroke)
  Diabetes mellitus requiring insulin
  Renal insufficiency (preoperative serum creatinine >2 mg/dL)

Abbreviations: ECG, electrocardiogram; MI, myocardial infarction; TIA, transient ischemic attack.

[a] *Recent* MI means that MI occurred >7 days previously but ≤30 days; *acute* MI, ≤7 days.

[b] May include "stable" angina in patients who are unusually sedentary.

[c] Campeau L. Grading of angina pectoris. Circulation. 1976;54:522-523.

[d] Lee TH, Marcantonio ER, Mangione CM, Thomas EJ, Polanczyk CA, Cook EF, et al. Derivation and prospective validation of a simple index for prediction of cardiac risk of major noncardiac surgery. Circulation. 1999;100:1043-1049.

Modified from Fleisher LA, Beckman JA, Brown KA, Calkins H, Chaikof E, Fleischmann KE, et al. ACC/AHA 2007 guidelines on perioperative cardiovascular evaluation and care for noncardiac surgery: a report of the American College of Cardiology/American Heart Association Task Force on Practice Guidelines (Writing Committee to Revise the 2002 Guidelines on Perioperative Cardiovascular Evaluation for Noncardiac Surgery). J Am Coll Cardiol. 2007;50:e159-241. Used with permission.

of no problems and can be misinterpreted. For completeness, it is often helpful to divide this section into the following categories:

1. Cardiac risk—include important factors that led to your recommendations, such as active cardiac conditions, clinical risk factors, functional capacity, and the urgency and type of operation planned. Include your rationale and plan for additional testing if indicated and a plan for perioperative management and surveillance.

2. Pulmonary risk—include risk factors for perioperative pulmonary complications, the rationale for additional testing if indicated, and a plan for perioperative management for risk reduction.

Table 8-7   Estimated Energy Requirements for Various Activities

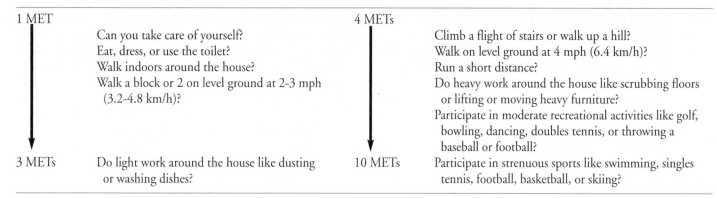

1 MET		4 METs	
	Can you take care of yourself?		Climb a flight of stairs or walk up a hill?
	Eat, dress, or use the toilet?		Walk on level ground at 4 mph (6.4 km/h)?
	Walk indoors around the house?		Run a short distance?
	Walk a block or 2 on level ground at 2-3 mph (3.2-4.8 km/h)?		Do heavy work around the house like scrubbing floors or lifting or moving heavy furniture?
			Participate in moderate recreational activities like golf, bowling, dancing, doubles tennis, or throwing a baseball or football?
3 METs	Do light work around the house like dusting or washing dishes?	10 METs	Participate in strenuous sports like swimming, singles tennis, football, basketball, or skiing?

Abbreviation: MET, metabolic equivalent.
Modified from Fleisher LA, Beckman JA, Brown KA, Calkins H, Chaikof E, Fleischmann KE, et al. ACC/AHA 2007 guidelines on perioperative cardiovascular evaluation and care for noncardiac surgery: a report of the American College of Cardiology/American Heart Association Task Force on Practice Guidelines (Writing Committee to Revise the 2002 Guidelines on Perioperative Cardiovascular Evaluation for Noncardiac Surgery). J Am Coll Cardiol. 2007;50:e159-241. Used with permission.

3. Deep venous thrombosis risk—include risk factors for deep venous thrombosis risk and the rationale for perioperative prophylaxis regimen.
4. Perioperative management of medical comorbidities—list other medical comorbidities that will affect perioperative care, and comment on management recommendations (for diabetes mellitus, seizure disorder, renal insufficiency, corticosteroid dependence, sleep apnea, hypertension, etc).
5. Perioperative management of medications—include a plan for continuing or discontinuing use of medications and a recommendation for the timing of the administration of the medications.
6. Perioperative alerts—include alerts for allergies, personal or family history of serious anesthetic complications, concern for difficult intubation, pacemaker dependence, defibrillator, known aortic stenosis, concern for neck instability in rheumatoid arthritis or Down syndrome patients, etc).

Risks of Anesthesia and Surgery

Mortality associated with anesthesia and surgery has markedly decreased in the past several decades. Today the overall mortality is 1:250,000 even though more complex surgical procedures are performed on sicker patients. The American Society of Anesthesiologists (ASA) classification, with broadly defined categories, is used to estimate overall risk of mortality within 48 hours postoperatively (Table 8-8). Although this classification system is quite subjective, it has stood the tests of time and reproducibility in broadly estimating overall risk.

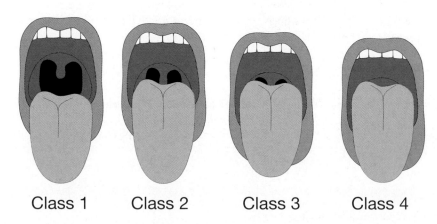

Class 1: soft palate, full uvula, tonsillar pillars

Class 2: soft palate, portion of uvula

Class 3: soft palate, base of uvula

Class 4: hard palate only

Figure 8-2. Mallampati Classification. The Mallampati Classification is based on the structures visualized with maximal mouth opening and tongue protrusion in the sitting position (originally described without phonation, but others have suggested minimum Mallampati Classification with or without phonation best correlates with intubation difficulty). (Modified from Mallampati SR, Gatt SP, Gugino LD, Desai SP, Waraksa B, Freiberger D, et al. A clinical sign to predict difficult tracheal intubation: a prospective study. Can Anaesth Soc J. 1985;32:429-34. Used with permission.)

Since the introduction of spinal anesthesia in the 1900s, many studies have compared the effects of neuraxial anesthesia with the effects of general anesthesia on surgical outcomes. A recent evidence review in 2005 highlighted the discrepancies in the literature surrounding this issue. Neuraxial anesthesia is probably associated with less blood loss and decreased maternal mortality and morbidity with cesarean delivery, but neuraxial anesthesia and general anesthesia are not associated with significantly different outcomes for mortality and cardiac events. However, patients who received a combination of general anesthesia with epidural analgesia had better pain control, decreased ileus, and fewer pulmonary complications. Many anesthesiologists recommend one type of anesthesia technique over another, but even though there are different risks and benefits of spinal, regional, and general anesthesia, the internist should not recommend a particular anesthetic technique or agent. This decision is best left to the anesthesia team at the time of surgery.

The type of operation performed is also an important determinant of cardiovascular morbidity and mortality (Table 8-9). However, the importance of associated disease in determining surgical risk may outweigh the nature of the procedure or the type of anesthesia used in predicting outcome. The following sections discuss cardiac and pulmonary risk assessment and management strategies.

Cardiac Risk Assessment and Risk Reduction Strategies

Coronary artery disease is a frequent cause of perioperative cardiac mortality and morbidity after noncardiac surgery. Perioperative myocardial infarction (MI) occurs in approximately 1% of general surgical procedures and in up to 3.2% of vascular surgical procedures. Among patients who have a perioperative MI, the hospital mortality rate is 15% to 25%, and those who survive to dismissal from the hospital have an increased risk of another MI and cardiovascular death during the ensuing 6 months postoperatively. Perioperative death attributed to cardiac causes is not as prevalent and occurs in 1% to 2% of all surgical procedures.

Cardiac Risk Assessment

Several cardiac risk assessment indices and guidelines are available. Choose one and become familiar with it, keeping in mind that there is no conclusive evidence that any risk-assessment method is without limitations. At Mayo Clinic, a stepwise approach is used for perioperative cardiac assessment as outlined in the "ACC/AHA 2007 Guidelines on Perioperative Cardiovascular Evaluation and Care for Noncardiac Surgery" (Figure 8-3). These guidelines present a framework for determining which patients are candidates for further testing on the basis of patient-related and surgery-related risk factors. When using these guidelines, keep in mind the following:

1. Surgical or percutaneous intervention is rarely necessary simply to lower the risk of surgery unless the intervention is indicated irrespective of the preoperative context.
2. No testing should be performed unless the results will probably influence patient treatment.
3. The guideline is intended to assist clinical decision making, not to replace clinical judgment.
4. The ultimate decision about the care of a particular patient must be made by the physician and the patient in light of all the specific clinical circumstances.

What information is needed for cardiac risk assessment? There are patient-specific factors and surgery-specifc factors that contribute to cardiac risk. The patient-specific risk factors are clinical predictors (including the patient's relevant clinical history) and the patient's functional status. The surgery-specific risks are most often related to urgency, duration, and type of surgery.

Assessing Patient-Specific Risk

Clinical predictors of increased perioperative risk of MI, heart failure, and death are classified into 2 categories (active cardiac conditions and clinical risk factors) on the basis of the pretest probability of cardiac disease (Table 8-6).

Functional capacity is estimated from the patient's history and is expressed in METs. One MET is a unit of sitting or resting oxygen uptake per kilogram of body weight per minute. Oxygen uptake is considered the best measure of cardiovascular fitness and exercise capacity. Table 8-7 outlines the estimated energy requirements for various activities. Functional capacity is classified as excellent (>10 METs), good (7-10 METs), moderate (4-7 METs), poor (<4 METs), or unknown. A clinically useful cutoff is 4 METs. Perioperative cardiac and long-term risks are increased in patients who are unable to meet a 4-MET demand during most normal daily activities.

Table 8-8   American Society of Anesthesiologists Classification of Anesthetic Mortality Within 48 Hours Postoperatively

Class	Physical Status	48-Hour Mortality
I	Healthy person younger than 80 y	0.07%
II	Mild systemic disease	0.24%
III	Severe but not incapacitating systemic disease	1.4%
IV	Incapacitating systemic disease that is a constant threat to life	7.5%
V	Moribund patient not expected to survive 24 hours, regardless of surgery	8.1%
E	Suffix added to any class to indicate emergency procedure	Doubles risk

From MKSAP IX: Part C, Book 4. American College of Physicians; 1991. Used with permission.

Table 8-9   Cardiac Risk Stratification for Noncardiac Surgical Procedures

Risk[a]	Procedure
High—reported cardiac risk often >5%	Emergent major operations, particularly in the elderly
	Aortic & other major vascular procedures
	Peripheral vascular procedures
	Anticipated prolonged surgical procedures associated with large fluid shifts or blood loss (or both)
Intermediate—reported cardiac risk generally <5%	Carotid endarterectomy
	Head & neck operations
	Intraperitoneal & intrathoracic procedures
	Orthopedic procedures
	Prostate operations
Low—reported cardiac risk generally <1%[b]	Endoscopic procedures
	Superficial procedures
	Cataract extraction
	Breast operation

[a] Combined incidence of cardiac death and nonfatal myocardial infarction.
[b] Further preoperative cardiac testing is not generally required.

From Fleisher LA, Beckman JA, Brown KA, Calkins H, Chaikof E, Fleischmann KE, et al. ACC/AHA 2007 guidelines on perioperative cardiovascular evaluation and care for noncardiac surgery: a report of the American College of Cardiology/American Heart Association Task Force on Practice Guidelines (Writing Committee to Revise the 2002 Guidelines on Perioperative Cardiovascular Evaluation for Noncardiac Surgery). J Am Coll Cardiol. 2007;50:e159-241. Used with permission.

Assessing Surgery Specific Risk

The surgery-specific cardiac risk of noncardiac surgery is related to 2 important factors. The first factor is the type of surgery itself, which may identify a patient with a greater likelihood of underlying heart disease (eg, vascular surgery). The second factor is the degree of hemodynamic cardiac stress associated with the surgery. Certain operations may be associated with, for example, pain, blood loss, and profound alterations in heart rate, blood pressure, and vascular volume. Types of procedures and their surgery-specific risks of cardiac death and nonfatal MI are outlined in Table 8-9.

A Stepwise Approach

With the above information, use the ACC/AHA guidelines in your decision process (Figure 8-3).

Step 1. Does the patient need emergency noncardiac surgery? If the answer is yes, the patient should be taken to the operating room without delay and risk stratification and surveillance should be done postoperatively.

Step 2. If there is no need for emergency surgery, consider whether the patient has an active cardiac condition as outlined above. If active cardiac conditions exist, the patient should be evaluated according to existing ACC/AHA guidelines. If there are no active cardiac conditions, proceed to step 3.

Step 3. Is the patient undergoing low-risk surgery? If so, the patient can proceed to the operating room without further cardiac evaluation.

Step 4. The patient is undergoing an intermediate- or high-risk procedure. Does the patient have a good functional capacity

(>4 METs) without symptoms? If yes, the patient should proceed to surgery without further evaluation. If the functional capacity is unknown or less than 4 METs, proceed to step 5.

Step 5. The patient is undergoing an intermediate- or high-risk procedure. Does the patient have any clinical risk factors?

1. With *no clinical risk factors*, the patient should proceed to surgery.

2. With *1 or 2 clinical risk factors*, the patient should proceed to surgery with a β-blocker dosage that controls the heart rate at less than 65 beats per minute. Noninvasive testing should be performed only if the results will change management.

3. With *3 or more risk factors*, the type of surgery needs to be considered.

   a. For an *intermediate-risk procedure*, the patient should proceed to surgery with a β-blocker dosage that controls the heart rate at less than 65 beats per minute. Noninvasive testing should be performed only if the results will change management.

   b. For *vascular surgery*, noninvasive or invasive testing should be considered if the results will change management. Often, heart rate control with β-blockers is the best course of action even in the highest-risk patients.

Choosing a Stress Test

If the decision has been made, based on risk assessment, that further cardiac testing is advisable, the next step is to choose the appropriate testing modality. There are many options for noninvasive testing, including exercise stress testing without imaging (not often used),

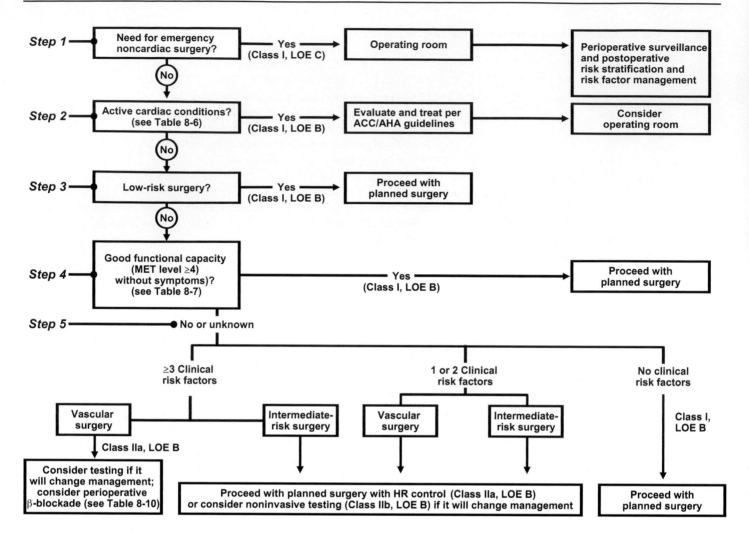

Figure 8-3. Stepwise Approach to Perioperative Cardiac Assessment. This cardiac evaluation and care algorithm for noncardiac surgery is based on active clinical conditions, known cardiovascular disease, and cardiac risk factors for patients 50 years or older as outlined in the American College of Cardiology and American Heart Association (ACC/AHA) 2007 Guidelines on Perioperative Cardiovascular Evaluation and Care for Noncardiac Surgery. *Clinical risk factors* include ischemic heart disease, compensated or prior heart failure, diabetes mellitus, renal insufficiency, and cerebrovascular disease. HR indicates heart rate; LOE, level of evidence; and MET, metabolic equivalent. (From Fleisher LA, Beckman JA, Brown KA, Calkins H, Chaikof E, Fleischmann KE, et al. ACC/AHA 2007 guidelines on perioperative cardiovascular evaluation and care for noncardiac surgery: a report of the American College of Cardiology/American Heart Association Task Force on Practice Guidelines [Writing Committee to Revise the 2002 Guidelines on Perioperative Cardiovascular Evaluation for Noncardiac Surgery]. J Am Coll Cardiol. 2007;50:e159-241. Used with permission.)

exercise testing with imaging (nuclear or echocardiographic), and pharmacologic stress testing with imaging (nuclear or echocardiographic). Some tests are contraindicated in certain populations; some tests may be more useful than others.

In general, if the patient can exercise without functional limitations and meet appropriate criteria (normal baseline electrocardiogram, no pacemaker, no digoxin, no history of percutaneous intervention or coronary artery bypass graft [CABG], and the physician thinks the patient will be able to achieve 85% of the maximal predicted heart rate), a regular Bruce exercise stress test is the most cost-effective test. However, most patients who meet these criteria usually do not require cardiac testing preoperatively. Furthermore, many patients cannot complete the test or do not

achieve 85% of their predicted maximal heart rate, which results in an inconclusive test.

If the patient can exercise and would likely be able to achieve more than 85% of the predicted maximal heart rate but does not meet the other appropriate criteria listed above, exercise testing with imaging would be necessary to give the additional information needed to interpret the test results. If the baseline electrocardiogram is abnormal (with the exception of left bundle branch block [LBBB]), if the patient is paced or is receiving digoxin, or if the patient has a history of previous intervention or CABG, an exercise stress test with imaging would be most appropriate. LBBB is the exception because tachycardia in patients with LBBB is associated with false-positive findings on nuclear and echocardiographic imaging in the area of the septum, even in the absence of left anterior descending coronary artery disease.

Pharmacologic stress, achieved with a vasodilatory agent (dipyridamole or adenosine) or an inotropic catecholamine (dobutamine), is used when the patient does not have the functional ability to exercise, cannot achieve 85% of the predicted maximal heart rate with regular exercise, or has LBBB on baseline electrocardiography. Pharmacologic stress is coupled with either nuclear imaging (sestamibi or thallium) or echocardiographic imaging.

Vasodilators such as dipyridamole and adenosine are contraindicated in patients with second or third degree heart block, sick sinus syndrome, symptomatic bradycardia, hypotension, critical carotid disease (cerebral ischemia), or bronchorestrictive or bronchospastic disease. The vasodilators are favored, however, in patients with LBBB, multiple wall motion abnormalities at baseline, severe hypertension, or symptomatic arrhythmias (atrial fibrillation with rapid ventricular response, paroxysmal supraventricular tachycardia, etc).

Dobutamine is contraindicated in patients with significant hypertension or hypotension or with LBBB (false-positives) but may be favored in patients with borderline-low or low blood pressure, bradycardia, bronchospastic or bronchorestrictive disease, or heart block.

Imaging can be achieved with nuclear agents (sestamibi or thallium) or with echocardiography. Nuclear imaging may be more appropriate in patients who have poor echocardiographic windows or multiple wall motion abnormalities. Echocardiographic imaging would be preferred in patients with valvular dysfunction, known decreased ejection fraction, or large breasts that might be associated with false-positive results in nuclear imaging studies.

In general, the diagnostic accuracy is similar between nuclear perfusion imaging and echocardiography. When feasible, echocardiographic imaging gives additional information beyond what nuclear imaging can and is generally more cost-effective.

- If the patient can exercise without functional limitations and meet appropriate criteria (normal baseline electrocardiogram, no pacemaker, no digoxin, no history of percutaneous intervention or CABG, and the physician thinks the patient will be able to achieve 85% of the maximal predicted heart rate), a regular Bruce exercise stress test is the most cost-effective test for preoperative cardiac risk stratification.
- In general, the diagnostic accuracy is similar between nuclear perfusion imaging and echocardiography. When feasible, echocardiographic imaging gives additional information beyond what nuclear imaging can, and is generally more cost effective.

Role of Preoperative Resting Echocardiography

Although routine perioperative evaluation of left ventricular function is not recommended, it is reasonable in some clinical situations to obtain a resting echocardiogram before planned elective surgery. These situations may include patients with dyspnea of unknown cause or patients with current heart failure or a prior history of heart failure who have worsening dyspnea or a change in clinical status. If patients are clinically stable, routine echocardiography is not recommended. A preoperative echocardiogram should be obtained, however, if a valvular abnormality or other clinically significant cardiac abnormality is suspected from the clinical examination.

Perioperative Cardiac Risk Reduction Strategies

Recent evidence suggests that surgical or percutaneous intervention is rarely necessary simply to decrease the surgical risk unless the intervention is indicated irrespective of the preoperative context. Because percutaneous or surgical intervention is also associated with risk of adverse cardiac outcomes, a morbidity and mortality advantage has not been shown for most patients when these interventions are performed before noncardiac surgery. The exception, however, is patients who would have been referred for intervention irrespective of the preoperative context (eg, left main coronary artery disease, severe 3-vessel disease).

β-Blockers have been reported to decrease the risk of perioperative cardiac complications in patients who are at risk. This subject is controversial because recent data have shown mixed results. However, until additional studies are completed, we recommend following the ACC/AHA guidelines published in 2007 (Table 8-10). Patients who are taking β-blockers already, regardless of the indication, should continue taking them in the perioperative period to avoid a rebound effect on blood pressure and pulse. Ideally, patients receiving β-blockers for perioperative cardiac risk reduction should begin taking them a few days preoperatively so the dose can be adjusted to achieve a resting heart rate of 55 to 65 beats per minute. The dose must be adjusted in the postoperative period (2-5 days) to keep the heart rate at 55 to 65 beats per minute and to achieve maximal benefit for risk reduction.

In the past, some physicians have avoided giving β-blockers to patients who have a diagnosis of chronic obstructive pulmonary disease. Recent data have not supported this practice, but instituting β-blockade in these patients must be done cautiously. For most patients, administration of a perioperative β-blocker is not associated with an increase in pulmonary symptoms.

There is insufficient evidence to suggest that the perioperative use of calcium channel blockers or nitrates reduces cardiac outcomes. Statins have been shown in several studies to improve perioperative outcomes in vascular surgery patients, but those studies were observational. There are not enough data to suggest that a statin administered in the perioperative period will decrease perioperative risk. However, it would be reasonable to continue the use of a statin perioperatively if the patient is currently taking one.

Monitoring for Perioperative Ischemia

Patients who have coronary artery disease or major risk factors for coronary artery disease are at higher risk of perioperative myocardial ischemia or MI. Although most perioperative ischemic events usually occur within 48 hours after surgery, many occur during anesthesia recovery or shortly thereafter owing to many ischemia-provoking stimuli (tachycardia, hypertension, hypercoagulability, sympathetic discharge, pain, etc).

Perioperative cardiac ischemia is often not associated with major or classic symptoms. Instead, it is usually associated with non–ST-segment elevation and non–Q-wave events. The most cost-effective approach to ischemia monitoring in high-risk patients is to evaluate serial electrocardiograms (ECGs) obtained preoperatively, immediately postoperatively, and on postoperative days 1 and 2. Patients who do have ST-segment changes suggestive of ischemia are at significantly increased risk of future MI and other adverse cardiac events. Diligent postoperative follow-up with additional testing and risk factor modification is indicated if perioperative ischemia or infarction is identified.

Biochemical evidence of myocardial injury is common in the perioperative period. Troponins are both sensitive and specific for myocardial injury, and troponin levels should be determined in patients who have signs, symptoms, or ECG evidence of ischemia. However, troponin determination as a surveillance method for perioperative ischemia is not cost-effective and should probably be reserved for patients who have a high risk of cardiac complications and who are undergoing a major surgical procedure.

Patients With Coronary Stents

The "ACC/AHA 2007 Guidelines on Perioperative Cardiovascular Evaluation and Care for Noncardiac Surgery" also recommend an approach to patients who have had coronary stent placement in the past. This has been an important issue since premature discontinuation of dual antiplatelet therapy markedly increases the risk of catastrophic stent thrombosis and death or MI. The approach is based on expert opinion; there are as yet no good studies to back it up.

For patients with bare metal stents, elective or nonurgent surgery should be delayed for 30 to 45 days after placement. After 30 to 45 days of dual antiplatelet therapy, surgery should be done with the patient receiving aspirin. Patients with drug-eluting stents should have elective or nonurgent surgery delayed at least 365 days after placement. After 1 year of dual antiplatelet therapy, surgery should be done with the patient receiving aspirin. If urgent or emergent surgery is needed within the required dual-antiplatelet therapy window, a difficult choice has to be made. If the surgery presents minimal

bleeding risk, some experts have advocated that the patient continue dual-antiplatelet therapy in the perioperative period. If the surgical bleeding risk is too high, the antiplatelet therapy can be stopped, but it should be resumed as soon as possible postoperatively (preferably requiring the patient to stop the antiplatelet therapy for only 5 days or less, if possible).

Stent thrombosis is a serious risk in the perioperative period, and any decision to stop dual antiplatelet therapy before the full recommended course should not be made until after a detailed discussion with the patient and the family about the risk of a potentially catastrophic outcome should stent thrombosis occur while antiplatelet therapy is interrupted. There is no evidence to support the efficacy of using anticoagulant-based medications (heparin, low-molecular-weight heparin, fondaparinux, etc) to "bridge" the patient while antiplatelet therapy is withheld.

Pulmonary Risk Assessment and Risk Reduction Strategies

Pulmonary complications (respiratory failure, atelectasis, and pneumonia) are as common as cardiac complications in patients undergoing noncardiothoracic surgery, with an overall rate of approximately 6%. These complications account for an increase in hospital length of stay as well as for an increase in perioperative morbidity and mortality.

Pulmonary Risk Assessment

Pulmonary risk can be divided into patient-related risk factors and procedure-related risk factors (Table 8-11). Although it seems intuitive that obesity, asthma, restrictive lung disease, and obstructive sleep apnea (OSA) would be associated with an increased incidence of perioperative pulmonary complications, there is not good evidence that this is the case. Clinical studies have not shown an increased risk of postoperative pulmonary complications in obese patients, even in patients with morbid obesity. Patients with mild

Table 8-10 Recommendations for Perioperative β-Blockade Based on Published Randomized Controlled Trials

Surgery	No Clinical Risk Factors[a]	≥1 Clinical Risk Factors[a]	CHD or High Cardiac Risk	Patients Currently Taking β-Blockers
Vascular	May consider	May consider	Yes[b]	Yes
			Reasonable to consider[c]	Yes
High-risk or intermediate-risk	Insufficient data	May consider	Reasonable to consider	
Low-risk	Insufficient data	Insufficient data	Insufficient data	Yes

Abbreviation: CHD, coronary heart disease.

[a] Clinical risk factors: history of ischemic heart disease (including those with pathologic Q waves on electrocardiography); history of compensated heart failure or prior heart failure (systolic or diastolic); history of cerebrovascular disease (transient ischemic attack or stroke); diabetes mellitus requiring insulin; or renal insufficiency (preoperative serum creatinine >2 mg/dL).

[b] For patients found to have coronary ischemia on preoperative testing or patients found to have CHD.

[c] For patients without ischemia or no previous testing.

Modified from Fleisher LA, Beckman JA, Brown KA, Calkins H, Chaikof E, Fleischmann KE, et al. ACC/AHA 2007 guidelines on perioperative cardiovascular evaluation and care for noncardiac surgery: a report of the American College of Cardiology/American Heart Association Task Force on Practice Guidelines (Writing Committee to Revise the 2002 Guidelines on Perioperative Cardiovascular Evaluation for Noncardiac Surgery). J Am Coll Cardiol. 2007;50:e159-241. Used with permission.

or moderate asthma have not been shown to have increased risk, nor have patients with chronic restrictive lung disease or restrictive physiologic characteristics (neuromuscular disease or chest wall deformities). OSA increases the risk of airway management problems, but its influence on postoperative pulmonary complications has not been well studied. OSA has been shown, however, to be associated with increases in the number of unplanned intensive care unit transfers, serious complications, and length of hospital stay in the postoperative period.

- Significant patient-related risk factors include chronic obstructive pulmonary disease (COPD), age older than 60 years, ASA class ≥II, functional dependence, congestive heart failure, and serum albumin <35 g/L.

Table 8-11 Risk Factors for Perioperative Pulmonary Complications

Risk Factors	Odds Ratio (95% CI)
Patient-related	
ASA class ≥II	4.9 (3.3-7.1)
Chronic obstructive pulmonary disease	2.4 (1.9-2.9)
Age, y	
50-59	1.5 (1.3-1.7)
60-69	2.3 (1.9-2.8)
70-79	3.9 (2.7-5.7)
≥80	5.6 (4.6-6.9)
Functional dependence	
Total dependence	2.5 (2.0-3.2)
Partial dependence	1.7 (1.4-2.0)
Congestive heart failure	2.9 (1.0-8.4)
Serum albumin <35 g/L	2.5 (2.0-2.6)
Impaired sensorium	1.4 (1.1-1.8)
Cigarette use	1.4 (1.2-1.7)
Procedure-related	
Surgical site or type of procedure	
Open abdominal aortic repair	6.9 (2.7-17.4)
Thoracic	4.2 (2.9-6.2)
Abdominal	3.1 (2.5-3.8)
Neurosurgical	2.5 (1.8-3.5)
Head and neck	2.2 (1.6-2.7)
Vascular	2.1 (0.8-5.4)
Emergency surgery	2.5 (1.7-3.8)
Prolonged surgery (>3 h)	2.3 (1.5-3.5)
General anesthesia	2.4 (1.8-3.1)
Transfusion >4 units	1.5 (1.3-1.7)

Abbreviations: ASA, American Society of Anesthesiologists; CI, confidence interval.
Modified from Smetana GW, Lawrence VA, Cornell JE. Preoperative pulmonary risk stratification for noncardiothoracic surgery: systematic review for the American College of Physicians. Ann Intern Med. 2006;144:581-595. Used with permission.

- Obesity, mild or moderate asthma, and restrictive lung disease are not significant risk factors for postoperative pulmonary complications.
- Procedure-related risk factors include prolonged surgery (>3 hours), open aortic aneurysm repair, abdominal surgery, thoracic surgery, head and neck surgery, vascular surgery, emergency surgery, and general anesthesia.

Pulmonary Testing

Historically, the common practice was to evaluate patients with spirometry testing and chest radiography during the routine preoperative evaluation as a way to predict the risk of pulmonary complications. Although consensus exists on the value of spirometry before lung resection or coronary artery bypass surgery, the value of spirometry before extrathoracic surgery has not been shown. Similarly, routine chest radiography has not been shown to influence perioperative management in patients undergoing nonthoracic surgery. Spirometry and chest radiography may be appropriate in patients undergoing extrathoracic surgery who have a previous diagnosis of COPD or asthma or who have respiratory symptoms identified during the preoperative evaluation. Additionally, some evidence suggests that chest radiography may be helpful if patients have cardiopulmonary disease or if they are older than 50 years and are undergoing upper abdominal, thoracic, or abdominal aortic aneurysm surgery. Although a low serum albumin level has been identified as a powerful predictor of risk of postoperative pulmonary complications, obtaining albumin levels routinely in the preoperative evaluation has not been the standard of care.

- Spirometry and chest radiography may be appropriate in patients undergoing extrathoracic surgery who have a previous diagnosis of COPD or asthma or who have respiratory symptoms identified during the preoperative evaluation.
- Some evidence suggests that chest radiography may be helpful if patients have cardiopulmonary disease or if they are older than 50 years and are undergoing upper abdominal, thoracic, or abdominal aortic aneurysm surgery.

Risk Reduction Strategies

All patients who are identified as having an increased risk of postoperative pulmonary complications should receive the following postoperatively: 1) deep breathing exercises or incentive spirometry (positive airway pressure for patients unable to perform these) and 2) selective use of a nasogastric tube (as needed for postoperative nausea and vomiting, inability to tolerate oral intake, or symptomatic abdominal distention). The following procedures should not be used for the purpose of reducing postoperative pulmonary complications: 1) right heart catheterization or 2) total parenteral or enteral nutrition (for patients who are malnourished or have low serum albumin levels).

- All patients who are identified as having an increased risk of postoperative pulmonary complications should receive the following postoperatively: 1) deep breathing exercises or incentive spirometry (positive airway pressure for patients unable to perform these) and 2) selective use of a nasogastric tube.

Venous Thromboembolic Prophylaxis

Although all surgical patients are at increased risk of venous thromboembolic (VTE) disease, certain patients form a high-risk subset, including those who are elderly and those who have prolonged anesthesia, previous VTE, hereditary disorders of thrombosis, prolonged immobilization or paralysis, malignancy, obesity, varicosities, or pharmacologic estrogen use. Reasonable guidelines for VTE prophylaxis in surgical patients are outlined in Table 8-12.

General principles to keep in mind include the following:

1. Aspirin alone is *not* recommended as prophylaxis against VTE for any patient group.
2. Hip and knee replacement surgeries and hip fracture surgeries are particularly high risk, as are malignancy surgeries. In these patient populations, the prophylaxis is more aggressive and data suggest that the prophylaxis should continue after hospital discharge (from 10 days to 1 month). (See Table 8-12 for details.)
3. Consider renal impairment when deciding on doses of LMWH, fondaparinux, and other antithrombotic drugs that are cleared by the kidneys, particularly in elderly patients and in those who are at high risk of bleeding. Many of these drugs are contraindicated in dialysis patients.
4. In all patients undergoing neuraxial anesthesia or analgesia, use special caution when using anticoagulant prophylaxis—it may be best to wait until the catheter is removed.

Perioperative Laboratory Testing

Results of routine laboratory and diagnostic tests, while often obtained, usually have little effect on perioperative management. Therefore, routine tests are often not necessary before many surgical procedures unless a specific indication is present. The following general recommendations are reasonable.

Coagulation Studies

Prothrombin time and international normalized ratio are recommended for patients who have a known coagulation abnormality or a history suggestive of coagulation problems (chronic liver disease, malnutrition, excessive bleeding with past procedures, etc). Additionally, patients who are taking anticoagulants or who will receive full doses of anticoagulants postoperatively should have coagulation studies preoperatively. Partial thromboplastin time and bleeding time are rarely indicated in this preoperative setting.

Complete Blood Cell Count

Hemoglobin measurement is recommended for patients with a history of anemia, diseases known to cause anemia, a history of recent blood loss, or physical signs suggestive of anemia (ie, tachycardia and pallor). Additionally, patients who are undergoing operations in which significant blood loss is anticipated (cardiac procedures, major vascular surgery, major spinal surgery, etc) should have a baseline hemoglobin measurement. Often, a hemoglobin is requested if the patient is being typed and crossed for blood products.

A *white blood cell count* is appropriate for patients who have conditions known to affect the white blood cell count, who are taking medications known to affect the white blood cell count, or who have symptoms of infection at the preoperative evaluation.

Platelet counts are recommended for patients with a history of platelet abnormalities or myeloproliferative disease and for patients who are taking medications known to alter platelet counts. Of course, if the history and physical examination identify concerns for altered hemostasis, platelet counts would also be indicated preoperatively.

Electrolytes

Potassium level measurement should be considered for patients who are taking digoxin, diuretics, angiotensin-converting enzyme inhibitors, angiotensin receptor blockers, or other medications known to alter electrolytes. It is recommended for any patient with a history of renal insufficiency or renal failure.

Sodium level measurement should be considered for patients who are undergoing urologic procedures that involve bladder irrigation or patients who have conditions associated with hyponatremia or hypernatremia (congestive heart failure, liver failure, syndrome of inappropriate secretion of antidiuretic hormone, etc).

Creatinine

Measurement of the creatinine level is recommended for patients with any of the following: renal insufficiency, age older than 50 years, diabetes, hypertension, cardiovascular disease, plans to undergo major surgery, or use of medications that may affect renal function.

Glucose

Glucose determination is recommended only for patients who have risk factors for diabetes or who are known to have diabetes and need to assess glucose control.

Liver Tests

Liver tests are rarely helpful preoperatively unless there is clinical concern that the test results might be relevant to the decision to proceed with surgery.

Urinalysis

Urinalysis is recommended only for patients with urologic symptoms at the preoperative evaluation or before a urologic procedure or certain orthopedic procedures. Orthopedic surgeons often request that a urinalysis be done before the placement of hardware to ensure that there is no potential focus of infection that could possibly seed the new hardware.

Electrocardiography

An ECG is recommended before intermediate- or high-risk surgery for men older than 40 years, or women older than 50. Additionally, an ECG is recommended for any patient (regardless of age) with known coronary artery disease or for those who are at increased risk of coronary artery disease because they have a history of diabetes, cerebrovascular disease, hypertension, chest pain, congestive heart failure, smoking, peripheral vascular disease, inability to exercise, or morbid obesity. An ECG is recommended for any patient with any new cardiovascular symptoms or with signs and symptoms of new or unstable cardiac disease. An ECG performed within 6 months

Table 8-12 Prevention of Venous Thromboembolism for Common Surgical Procedures

Type of Surgery	Recommended Therapy
General surgery	
Low-risk general surgery patient	Early ambulation
Moderate-risk general surgery patient	LDUH bid, LMWH
Higher-risk general surgery patient	LDUH tid, LMWH
High-risk general surgery patient prone to bleeding complications	IPC (ES is an alternative)
Very high-risk general surgery patient with multiple risk factors or malignancy surgery patient	LDUH tid or LMWH, combined with IPC & ES[a]
Vascular surgery	
Vascular surgery with no additional risk factors	Early ambulation
Major vascular surgery with additional VTE risk factors	LDUH, LMWH
Urologic surgery	
Transurethral or low-risk urologic surgery	Early ambulation
Major open urologic procedure	LDUH bid or tid, IPC or ES (or both), LMWH
Major open urologic procedure with additional risk factors	LDUH bid or tid, or LMWH, combined with IPC or ES (or both)
Urologic procedure with high bleeding risk or actively bleeding	IPC or ES (or both)
Orthopedic surgery	
Total hip replacement surgery	LMWH; warfarin or fondaparinux; possible adjuvant use of ES or IPC[b,c,d]
Total knee replacement surgery	LMWH, warfarin, or fondaparinux; optimal use of IPC is alternative[b,d]
Hip fracture surgery	Fondaparinux, LMWH, or warfarin[b,c,d]
Neurosurgery	
Intracranial neurosurgery	IPC or ES (or both); LMWH or LDUH may be acceptable alternative; consider IPC or ES in addition to LMWH or LDUH for high-risk patients
Trauma surgery	
Acute spinal cord injury	LMWH; although ES & IPC appear ineffective when used alone, ES & IPC may have benefit when used with LMWH, or if anticoagulants are contraindicated; during rehabilitation, consider continuation of LMWH or conversion to warfarin[d]
Trauma patient with an identifiable risk factor for DVT	LMWH as soon as considered safe; consider initial prophylaxis with IPC if administration of LMWH will be delayed or is contraindicated; in high-risk patients with suboptimal prophylaxis, consider screening with duplex ultrasonography
Neuraxial anesthesia	
Spinal puncture or use of epidural catheters	Anticoagulant-based prophylaxis should be used with caution until the catheter is removed

Abbreviations: bid, every 12 hours; CHF, congestive heart failure; DVT, deep venous thrombosis; ES, graduated elastic stockings; INR, international normalized ratio; IPC, intermittent pneumatic compression; LDUH, low-dose unfractionated heparin; LMWH, low-molecular-weight heparin; MI, myocardial infarction; tid, every 8 hours; VTE, venous thromboembolic prophylaxis.

[a] For patients undergoing surgery for malignancy, post-hospital prophylaxis with LMWH for 2 to 3 weeks after hospital discharge is recommended.

[b] Duration of 7 to 10 days is recommended with LMWH or warfarin; 29 to 35 days with LMWH may offer additional protection for patients undergoing hip surgery.

[c] LDUH, aspirin, dextran, and IPC reduce the overall incidence of venous thromboembolism but are less effective and are *not* recommended as the only form of prophylaxis in this population.

[d] Warfarin goal: INR, 2 to 3.

Data from Geerts WH, Pineo GF, Heit JA, Bergqvist D, Lassen MR, Colwell CW, et al. Prevention of venous thromboembolism: the Seventh ACCP Conference on Antithrombotic and Thrombolytic Therapy. Chest. 2004;126 Suppl 3:338S-400S. Used with permission.

preoperatively is adequate if clinical symptoms have not changed in the interim.

Chest Radiography

Chest radiography is recommended for patients older than 50 years, patients who have known cardiac or pulmonary disease, and patients who have symptoms or physical examination findings suggestive of new or unstable cardiopulmonary disease.

Current Concepts in Anticoagulant Therapy

INR

What Are the Recommended INR Therapeutic Ranges for Oral Anticoagulant Therapy?

The recommended INR therapeutic ranges are summarized in Table 8-13. In short, an INR of 2.0 to 3.0 is used for most indications except for the few high-risk conditions (eg, mechanical prosthetic heart valves) in which a slightly higher INR is suggested.

Antithrombotic Therapy for Venous Thromboembolic Disease

Guidelines for anticoagulation in patients with venous thromboembolic disease are summarized in Table 8-14.

Anticoagulation in Patients With Prosthetic Heart Valves

What Are the Recommendations for Anticoagulation in Patients With Mechanical Prosthetic Heart Valves?

It is strongly recommended that all patients with mechanical prosthetic heart valves receive warfarin. Levels of warfarin that maintain the INR at 2.5 to 3.5 are recommended in most situations. Patients with bileaflet valves in the aortic position and no other risk factors may have an INR of 2.0 to 3.0. Levels of warfarin producing an INR less than 1.8 result in a high risk of thromboembolic events, and levels that increase the INR to more than 4.5 result in a high risk of excessive bleeding. For high-risk patients with prosthetic heart valves, aspirin (80-100 mg daily) in addition to warfarin further decreases the risk of thromboembolism without increasing the risk of major bleeding, although minor bleeding is increased.

- All patients with mechanical prosthetic heart valves should receive warfarin.
- In most cases, use warfarin levels that maintain the INR at 2.5-3.5.
- Warfarin levels that decrease the INR to <1.8 result in a high risk of thromboembolic events, and warfarin levels that increase the INR to >4.5 result in a high risk of excessive bleeding.
- In patients with prosthetic heart valves, a low dose of aspirin plus warfarin may have an additive benefit without causing major bleeding (although minor bleeding may increase).

What Is Recommended if a Patient With a Prosthetic Heart Valve Has a Systemic Embolism Despite Adequate Therapy With Warfarin (INR, 2.5-3.5)?

If a patient with a prosthetic heart valve has a systemic embolism with adequate warfarin therapy, aspirin (80-100 mg daily) should

Table 8-13 Recommended Therapeutic Range for Oral Anticoagulant Therapy

Indication	INR
Prophylaxis for venous thrombosis (high-risk surgery)	2.0-3.0
Treatment of venous thrombosis	2.0-3.0
Treatment of pulmonary embolism	2.0-3.0
Prevention of systemic embolism	
Tissue heart valves[a]	2.0-3.0
Acute myocardial infarction (to prevent systemic embolism)[b]	2.0-3.0
Valvular heart disease	2.0-3.0
Atrial fibrillation	2.0-3.0
Mechanical prosthetic heart valves	
AVR & no risk factors[c]	
Bileaflet valve	2.0-3.0
Other disk valve or Starr-Edwards	2.5-3.5
AVR & risk factor[d]	2.5-3.5
MVR[d]	2.5-3.5

Abbreviations: AVR, aortic valve replacement; INR, international normalized ratio; MVR, mitral valve replacement.

[a] Treatment is usually for 3 months unless other risk factors continue.

[b] If oral anticoagulant therapy is elected to prevent recurrent myocardial infarction, an INR of 2.5 to 3.5 is recommended, consistent with Food and Drug Administration recommendations.

[c] Risk factors: atrial fibrillation, left ventricular dysfunction, previous thromboembolism, hypercoagulable state.

[d] Consider addition of aspirin, 80 to 100 mg once daily to decrease embolic risk.

Modified from Litin SC, Gastineau DA. Current concepts in anticoagulant therapy. Mayo Clin Proc. 1995;70:266-72. Used with permission of Mayo Foundation for Medical Education and Research, and data from Bonow RO, Carabello B, de Leon AC Jr, Edmunds LH Jr, Fedderly BJ, Freed MD, et al. Guidelines for the management of patients with valvular heart disease: executive summary. A report of the American College of Cardiology/American Heart Association Task Force on Practice Guidelines (Committee on Management of Patients With Valvular Heart Disease). Circulation. 1998;98:1949-84.

be added to the regimen. These patients may respond to a slight increase in the warfarin dose (increasing the INR to 3.5-4.5) if they are already taking a low dose of aspirin. However, no regimen completely eliminates the risk of systemic embolization or the risk of bleeding.

- No regimen ever totally eliminates the risk of systemic embolization or the risk of bleeding.

What Are the Recommendations for Anticoagulation in Patients With Bioprosthetic Heart Valves?

It is recommended that all patients with bioprosthetic valves in the mitral position receive warfarin therapy (INR, 2.0-3.0) for the first

Table 8-14 Guidelines for Anticoagulation in Adults With Venous Thromboembolic Disease

Deep Venous Thrombosis or Pulmonary Embolism	Guidelines for Anticoagulation
Suspected	Obtain baseline aPTT, PT, & CBC (& creatinine if LMWH is to be used) Check for contraindication to heparin therapy Give unfractionated heparin, 5,000 units IV, or weight-adjusted dose of LMWH SQ; order imaging study
Confirmed	Rebolus with heparin, 80 U/kg IV, and start maintenance infusion at 18 U/kg per hour[a] or use appropriate weight-adjusted dose of LMWH SQ Start warfarin therapy on first day at 5 mg & then administer warfarin daily at estimated maintenance dose Discontinue administration of LMWH or unfractionated heparin when it has been administered jointly with warfarin for at least 4 or 5 d & the INR ≥2.0 Anticoagulate with warfarin for at least 3 mo at an INR of 2.0-3.0 (longer treatment should be given to patients with ongoing risk factors or recurrent thrombosis)

Abbreviations: aPTT, activated partial thromboplastin time; CBC, complete blood cell count; INR, international normalized ratio; IV, intravenously; LMWH, low-molecular-weight heparin; PT, prothrombin time; SQ, subcutaneously; U, units.
[a] If unfractionated heparin is used, check aPTT at 6 hours to keep aPTT between 1.5 and 2.5 times control (anti-Xa heparin level of 0.3-0.7 IU/mL) and check platelet count daily.

3 months. Anticoagulant therapy is also reasonable during the first 3 months for patients with bioprosthetic valves in the aortic position who are in sinus rhythm. Certain patients with bioprosthetic valves have underlying conditions (ie, atrial fibrillation or left atrial thrombosis) that require long-term warfarin therapy to prevent systemic emboli. For patients with bioprosthetic heart valves who are in sinus rhythm, long-term therapy with aspirin (325 mg daily) may offer protection against thromboembolism and appears reasonable for those without contraindication.

* Patients with bioprosthetic valves receive warfarin therapy (INR, 2.0-3.0) for 3 months.
* Patients with bioprosthetic valves who have atrial fibrillation or left atrial thrombosis require long-term warfarin therapy to prevent systemic emboli.
* Long-term therapy with aspirin may provide protection against thromboembolism in patients with bioprosthetic heart valves who are in sinus rhythm.

Hemorrhagic Complications of Anticoagulation

When the Anticoagulant Effect of Warfarin Needs to Be Reversed, What Is the Best Way to Reverse It?

The anticoagulant effect of warfarin can be reversed by stopping treatment, administering vitamin K, or, in urgent situations with pronounced bleeding, replacing vitamin K–dependent coagulation factors with fresh frozen plasma. In urgent situations, fresh frozen plasma produces an immediate effect and is the treatment of choice. When warfarin therapy is discontinued, no marked effect on the INR is seen for 2 days or more because of the half-life of warfarin (36-42 hours) and the delay before newly synthesized functional coagulation factors replace dysfunctional coagulation factors.

Administering vitamin K rapidly lowers the INR, depending on the dosage of vitamin K and the severity of the anticoagulant effect. When high doses of vitamin K are administered, reversal occurs in about 6 hours. The disadvantage is that patients often remain resistant to warfarin for up to a week, making continued warfarin treatment difficult. This problem can be overcome by giving much lower doses of vitamin K (1-2.5 mg) orally, subcutaneously, or by slow intravenous infusion.

* The anticoagulant effect of warfarin can be reversed by stopping treatment, giving vitamin K, or replacing vitamin K–dependent coagulation factors with fresh frozen plasma.
* In cases of life-threatening bleeding or serious warfarin overdosages, replacement of vitamin K–dependent coagulation factors with fresh frozen plasma produces an immediate effect and is the treatment of choice.
* In nonurgent situations, a low dose of vitamin K (1-2.5 mg) may be given orally to decrease the INR and avoid warfarin resistance.

Are There Certain Patient Characteristics That Increase the Risk of Hemorrhagic Complications of Anticoagulant Treatment?

A strong relationship between the intensity of anticoagulant therapy and the risk of bleeding has been reported in patients receiving treatment for deep venous thrombosis and prosthetic heart valves. The concurrent use of drugs that interfere with hemostasis and produce gastric erosions (eg, aspirin and nonsteroidal anti-inflammatory drugs) increases the risk of serious upper gastrointestinal tract bleeding. Other drugs, such as trimethoprim-sulfamethoxazole, amiodarone, and omeprazole, inhibit the clearance of warfarin, thus potentiating its effect. Physicians should consider any medication a potential source of interaction until proved otherwise. Several existing disease states associated with increased bleeding during warfarin therapy include treated hypertension, renal insufficiency, hepatic insufficiency, and cerebrovascular disease.

* The relationship between the intensity of anticoagulant therapy and the risk of bleeding is strong.
* The concurrent use of drugs that interfere with hemostasis and produce gastric erosions increases the risk of serious upper gastrointestinal tract bleeding.
* Trimethoprim-sulfamethoxazole, amiodarone, and omeprazole potentiate the effect of warfarin and increase bleeding risk.

Common Clinical Problems in General Internal Medicine

Treatment of Hyperlipidemia

Case

A 55-year-old man with stable class II angina is referred for consideration of drug treatment for hyperlipidemia. He is otherwise healthy. He quit smoking cigarettes 2 years previously and has no other known risk factors for coronary artery disease (CAD). He has closely followed the advice of a dietitian for the past 6 months, but his cholesterol levels have not decreased markedly. His most recent values are total cholesterol 240 mg/dL, high-density lipoprotein cholesterol (HDL-C) 35 mg/dL, and triglycerides 75 mg/dL.

Discussion

Evidence has shown that lowering increased levels of low-density lipoprotein cholesterol (LDL-C) is associated with both primary and secondary prevention of coronary events. Moreover, several angiographic trials have shown consistent decreases in progression and increases in regression of atherosclerotic plaques that have been followed up for several years.

The third report of the National Cholesterol Education Program's Adult Treatment Panel (ATP III) identified patients with definite CAD or CAD risk equivalents (clinical atherosclerotic disease or diabetes mellitus) to be at very high risk (>20% chance of having cardiac events within 10 years) and suggested aggressive treatment.

In the second report (ATP II), the risk level was assigned by counting risk factors to identify patients with multiple (≥2) risk factors. The risk factors were those that are used to modify LDL-C goals. In ATP III, the risk level is assigned by means of counting risk factors and assessing a 10-year risk (Framingham risk scoring) for patients who have multiple risk factors. The risk factors used for modifying LDL-C goals include the following:

1. Cigarette smoking
2. Hypertension (blood pressure ≥140/90 mm Hg or taking antihypertensive medication)
3. Low HDL-C (<40 mg/dL)
4. Family history of premature CAD (CAD in male first-degree relative ≤55 years old; CAD in female first-degree relative ≤65 years old)
5. Age (men ≥45 years; women ≥55 years)
6. If patient has a high HDL-C (≥60 mg/dL), 1 risk factor is subtracted from the count

LDL-C is used to monitor patients with hypercholesterolemia and is calculated from the following formula:

$$LDL\text{-}C = Total\ cholesterol - HDL\text{-}C - \frac{Triglycerides}{5}$$

In this patient, LDL-C = 240 − 35 − (75/5) = 190 mg/dL.

Secondary causes of hyperlipidemia, such as the following, should be ruled out in all patients: diet (eg, alcohol abuse or increased saturated fats), diseases (eg, hypothyroidism, diabetes mellitus, nephrotic syndrome, renal failure, or obstructive liver disease), and drugs (eg, corticosteroids, progestins, thiazides, or β-blockers).

* Rule out secondary causes of hyperlipidemia in all patients: diet, diseases, and drugs.

The first line of therapy involves weight reduction for overweight patients, increased physical activity, and dietary therapy. Both weight reduction and exercise not only promote lowering of cholesterol levels but also provide other benefits, such as decreasing triglycerides, increasing HDL-C, decreasing blood pressure, decreasing the risk of diabetes mellitus, and prolonging life.

Therapeutic lifestyle changes (weight reduction, physical activity, and intensive diet therapy) are initiated for patients without CAD or risk equivalents if LDL-C is 160 mg/dL or more, for patients without CAD but who have at least 2 risk factors if LDL-C is 130 mg/dL or more, and for patients with CAD or CAD risk equivalents if LDL-C is more than 100 mg/dL. Strategies for LDL-C management by CAD risk are summarized in Table 8-15 and are modified from the ATP III goals on the basis of more recent clinical trial evidence.

If hypolipidemic drugs are prescribed, the choice of drug depends on the mechanism of action, side-effect profile, efficacy, and cost. The following discussion considers the most common classes of drugs used in the treatment of hyperlipidemia.

Bile acid sequestrants (eg, cholestyramine, colestipol, and colesevelam)—Clinical trials have documented their benefit and safety. Their mechanism of action involves removing plasma LDL-C by depleting the bile acid pool, which causes an increase in liver LDL-C receptors. These drugs are often given alone (to patients with mild increases in LDL-C levels) or in combination with other drugs (to patients with greater increases in LDL-C levels). Side effects include gastrointestinal tract symptoms, binding of other concurrently administered drugs, constipation, and increased triglyceride levels, especially in patients who begin with increased levels.

Nicotinic acid (niacin)—This agent is effective in decreasing total cholesterol and triglyceride levels as well as increasing HDL-C levels. Side effects are common and limit the use of this drug in many patients. Side effects include flushing, nausea, abdominal discomfort, and skin itching. Also, the levels of plasma glucose, uric acid, and liver enzymes may increase. Slow-release preparations reduce the side effect of flushing, but the incidence of liver dysfunction increases markedly, especially with higher doses. Small doses of aspirin taken before niacin may block flushing.

HMG-CoA reductase inhibitors, or statins (eg, lovastatin, pravastatin, simvastatin, atorvastatin, and rosuvastatin)—These drugs are highly effective in decreasing LDL-C by blocking liver cholesterol synthesis, which causes an increase in LDL-C liver receptors. They are the only drugs to consistently reduce mortality of subjects in both primary and secondary prevention studies. They have few side effects, although myalgias, myopathy, and an increase in liver enzymes may occur. Myopathy can increase with concurrent use of cyclosporine, niacin, erythromycin, and fibrates (fibric acid derivatives). Primary prevention studies have shown decreased mortality risks with the use of statins. In large secondary prevention trials, statin drugs have been shown to reduce total mortality, cardiac mortality, and the incidence of stroke. They are effective in treating severe forms of hypercholesterolemia.

Fibrates (eg, gemfibrozil and fenofibrate)—These are the drugs of choice for decreasing isolated increased levels of triglycerides. In some patients, these drugs slightly decrease LDL-C and increase HDL-C levels. Fenofibrate is more effective than gemfibrozil in decreasing LDL-C. Side effects are rare and related mostly to the gastrointestinal tract. These drugs also may increase the risk of gallstones. Therapeutically, they are most useful for disorders of hypertriglyceridemia, especially in patients with diabetes mellitus.

All the above-mentioned drugs have the potential to interact with warfarin (bile acid sequestrants can bind the drug, thus decreasing the INR, and the other hypolipidemic drugs may potentiate warfarin, thus increasing the INR). Therefore, when they are prescribed for patients taking anticoagulants, close monitoring is indicated.

Table 8-15 ATP III LDL-C Goals and Cutpoints for TLC and Drug Therapy in Different Risk Categories and Proposed Modifications Based on Recent Clinical Trial Evidence

Risk Category	LDL-C Goal	Initiate TLC	Consider Drug Therapy[a]
High risk: CHD[b] or CHD risk equivalents[c] (10-year risk >20%)	<100 mg/dL (optional goal: <70 mg/dL)[d]	≥100 mg/dL[e]	≥100 mg/dL (<100 mg/dL: consider drug options)[f]
Moderately high risk: ≥2 risk factors[g] (10-year risk 10%-20%)[h]	<130 mg/dL[i]	≥130 mg/dL[e]	≥130 mg/dL (100-129 mg/dL: consider drug options)[j]
Moderate risk: ≥2 risk factors[g] (10-year risk <10%)[h]	<130 mg/dL	≥130 mg/dL	≥160 mg/dL
Lower risk: 0 or 1 risk factor[k]	<160 mg/dL	≥160 mg/dL	≥190 mg/dL (160-189 mg/dL: LDL-C– lowering drug optional)

Abbreviations: ATP III, third report of the National Cholesterol Education Program Adult Treatment Panel; CHD, coronary heart disease; HDL-C, high-density lipoprotein cholesterol; LDL-C, low-density lipoprotein cholesterol; TLC, therapeutic lifestyle changes.

[a] When LDL-C–lowering drug therapy is used, the intensity of therapy should be sufficient to achieve at least a 30% to 40% reduction in LDL-C levels.

[b] CHD includes history of myocardial infarction, unstable angina, stable angina, coronary artery procedures (angioplasty or bypass surgery), or evidence of clinically significant myocardial ischemia.

[c] CHD risk equivalents include clinical manifestations of noncoronary forms of atherosclerotic disease (peripheral arterial disease, abdominal aortic aneurysm, and carotid artery disease [transient ischemia attacks or stroke of carotid origin or >50% obstruction of a carotid artery]), diabetes, and ≥2 risk factors with a 10-year risk of hard CHD >20%.

[d] Very high risk favors the optional LDL-C goal of <70 mg/dL, and in patients with high triglycerides, non–HDL-C <100 mg/dL.

[e] Any person at high risk or moderately high risk who has lifestyle-related risk factors (eg, obesity, physical inactivity, elevated triglycerides, low HDL-C, or metabolic syndrome) is a candidate for TLC to modify these risk factors regardless of LDL-C level.

[f] If baseline LDL-C is <100 mg/dL, institution of an LDL-C–lowering drug is a therapeutic option on the basis of available clinical trial results. If a high-risk person has high triglycerides or low HDL-C, combining a fibrate or nicotinic acid with an LDL-C–lowering drug can be considered.

[g] Risk factors include cigarette smoking, hypertension (blood pressure ≥140/90 mm Hg or taking antihypertensive medication), low HDL-C (<40 mg/dL), family history of premature CHD (CHD in male first-degree relative <55 years of age; CHD in female first-degree relative <65 years of age), and age (men ≥45 years; women ≥55 years).

[h] Electronic 10-year risk calculators are available at www.nhlbi.nih.gov/guidelines/cholesterol.

[i] Optional LDL-C goal <100 mg/dL.

[j] For moderately high-risk persons, when LDL-C level is 100 to 129 mg/dL, at baseline or with lifestyle therapy, initiation of an LDL-C–lowering drug to achieve an LDL-C level <100 mg/dL is a therapeutic option on the basis of available clinical trial results.

[k] Almost all people with ≤1 risk factor have a 10-year risk <10%, and 10-year risk assessment in people with ≤1 risk factor is thus not necessary.

From Grundy SM, Cleeman JI, Merz CNB, Brewer HB Jr, Clark LT, Hunninghake DB, et al. Implications of recent clinical trials for the National Cholesterol Education Program Adult Treatment Panel III Guidelines. Circulation. 2004;110:227-39. Used with permission.

Generally, the following drugs alone or sometimes in combination are recommended:

1. For patients with increased levels of LDL-C: HMG-CoA reductase inhibitors, bile acid sequestrants, and nicotinic acid
2. For patients with increased levels of LDL-C and triglycerides: HMG-CoA reductase inhibitors, nicotinic acid, and fibrates
3. For patients with isolated hypertriglyceridemia: therapeutic lifestyle change and, if drug treatment is indicated, fibrates and nicotinic acid

Drug therapy for hyperlipidemia must be individualized. In general, a positive effect is obtained and fewer side effects are experienced by starting therapy with low doses of medication and increasing the dose slowly, if necessary.

Tobacco Abuse

Case

A 60-year-old woman comes to your office for her annual mammogram, breast examination, and pelvic examination. You note from the preexamination questionnaire that she is a current smoker and has smoked one pack per day for 30 years. Examination of the lungs shows scattered rhonchi and wheezes with a prolonged expiratory phase. You broach the subject of smoking cessation with the patient, but she quickly and defensively counters with several statements, including "after 30 years of smoking, the damage is done" and "there's no sense quitting." The patient also fears gaining weight after quitting and says that when she did try to quit several years ago, she quickly became so nervous and edgy that she could not sleep and was unpleasant to be around. How might you devise a plan to deal effectively with this patient's tobacco abuse problem?

Discussion

Tobacco use is the leading cause of preventable premature death in the United States. It accounts for about 20% of all-cause mortality in the United States annually. In addition to being the causative factor for nearly 90% of all cases of lung cancer, smoking is associated with cancer of the oral cavity, larynx, esophagus, stomach, pancreas, uterine cervix, and genitourinary tract. However, among ex-smokers abstinent for 15 years or longer, the increase in lung cancer mortality is decreased to rates nearly those of nonsmokers.

Smokers are 2 to 6 times as likely to have an MI as nonsmokers, and 20% of all deaths due to cardiovascular disease are attributable to smoking. After several years of abstinence, the cardiovascular risk of ex-smokers is not significantly different from that of those who have never smoked.

Compared with smokers, ex-smokers have less phlegm production and wheezing, greater forced expiratory volume in 1 second (FEV$_1$) and vital capacity, better immune function, and lower mortality rates from pulmonary infections, bronchitis, and emphysema. Although some lung damage is irreversible, ex-smokers have a marked improvement in their pulmonary function during the first year of cessation. After that, the decline in lung function stabilizes at a non-smoker's rate. Smokers continue to show a decline in lung function at many times the rate of ex-smokers.

Often, one of the most compelling arguments for a patient to stop smoking is that it harms others. It is estimated that in the United States more than 50,000 people die annually of medical complications of passive smoking. Most of these deaths are from accelerated heart disease, although the number of lung cancer deaths is also substantial. Studies have estimated that nonsmoking spouses of smokers have an all-cancer risk about 1.5 times that of nonsmoking spouses of nonsmokers.

The Public Health Service Clinical Practice Guideline advises physicians to use an easy-to-remember 5-step approach for counseling their patients in smoking cessation.

1. *Ask*—Systematically identify all tobacco users at every visit. The physician should question patients about smoking at any new encounter, inquiring not only whether they smoke but how much they smoke. It is also helpful to ask whether they have ever tried to stop smoking, and if so, what happened.
2. *Advise* all smokers to quit. Make this a strong and personalized message. Fewer than two-thirds of physicians report advising their patients to stop smoking, and only two-thirds of patients report receiving smoking cessation advice from their physician. This counsel can often be an influential message to patients. The physician should state the advice clearly; for example, "As your physician, I must advise you to stop smoking now." It helps to personalize the "quit smoking" message by referring to other illnesses the patient has, family history, passive smoking issues, and so forth.
3. *Assess* each person's willingness to make a quit attempt. If a person is willing to make a quit attempt, move on to step 4 (*Assist*). If the patient desires intensive treatment, provide a referral. Some patients are unwilling to make a quit attempt. For them, provide a motivational intervention.
4. *Assist* the patient in stopping to smoke. Set a quit date with the patient. Try to do it within 4 weeks, acknowledging with the patient that the time is never ideal. Provide self-help materials. Recommend or prescribe nicotine gum, nicotine patches, intranasal nicotine spray, nicotine inhaler, or bupropion, especially for any patient who smokes more than 10 cigarettes daily and is motivated to attempt smoking cessation. Consider signing a stop-smoking contract with the patient.
5. *Arrange* follow-up visits. Set up a follow-up visit within 1 or 2 weeks after the quit date. Counseling programs and behavioral therapy programs can be effective in smoking cessation. A transdermal nicotine patch together with behavioral therapy results in significantly higher cessation rates than transdermal nicotine alone. If during follow-up visits you discover that the patient has had a relapse, explain that this is not uncommon. Encourage the patient to try again immediately.

Pharmacologic therapy to aid in smoking cessation should be recommended to most patients. In clinical trials, smoking cessation rates at 6 to 12 months are more than doubled among those using active therapy, as compared with placebo treatment. Two categories of pharmacologic smoking cessation treatment are available: nicotine replacement therapy and non-nicotine therapy. Nicotine replacement therapy is available in several forms. A transdermal nicotine patch releases nicotine at a steady rate for 16 to 24 hours and is associated with higher patient compliance because of its once-a-day dosing schedule. Nicotine gum, nicotine nasal spray, and nicotine inhaler are immediate-release forms of nicotine replacement and are effective in smoking cessation treatment but must be used several times each day. They have the advantage of allowing patients to use them in response to smoking urges. Currently, bupropion is the only non-nicotine therapy available that has proven efficacy for smoking cessation. It should not be used if the patient has seizure risk; otherwise, it is appropriate for any smoker who is motivated to stop smoking. Bupropion may have the added advantage of attenuating postcessation weight gain.

Several other important concerns of patients can be addressed and answered. For those who worry about weight gain with smoking cessation, it is useful to let them know that although the majority of patients do gain weight, the average is about 3 to 5 kg, and this can be anticipated and dealt with effectively. For patients who have noted difficulties with nervousness and poor sleep after smoking cessation, advise them that these symptoms are related to nicotine withdrawal and usually resolve after 2 or 3 weeks. Nicotine replacement therapies can often help control these symptoms. Some patients notice an increase in coughing after they stop smoking. This can be explained as a temporary response caused by an increase in the lung's ability to remove phlegm and, thus, represents recovery of the lung's own defense mechanisms. After cessation has been achieved, the patient should be advised to refrain from having even an occasional cigarette, because nicotine addiction seems to be triggered quickly in most ex-smokers.

Acute Low Back Pain

Case

A 55-year-old man comes to your office with a 3-day history of severe low back pain in the lumbosacral area. The patient does not recall any specific trauma, and the review of systems is negative for fever, weight loss, or other constitutional symptoms. The patient does not complain of numbness, tingling, or weakness in his legs, and he has no bladder or bowel symptoms. The patient works in a factory, and his job requires some minor lifting and bending. Make a diagnostic assessment, therapeutic plan, and suggestions about levels of activity.

Discussion

Acute low back problems are among the most common reasons for patients to visit a physician's office. Acute low back problems are defined as "activity intolerance due to lower back or back-related leg symptoms of less than 3 months' duration." It is important to know that 90% of patients with acute low back problems have a spontaneous recovery and return to previous levels of activity within 1 month. On the initial assessment of such a patient, a focused medical history and physical examination should be performed so that a potentially dangerous underlying condition is not overlooked. On the basis of this evaluation, low back symptoms can be classified into 1 of 3 working categories:

1. *Potentially serious spinal conditions*—This rare category includes tumor, infection, fracture, or major neurologic disorder. One should look for "red flags" in the history or examination that

would point to these conditions, that is, a history of trauma (fracture) or cancer (spinal epidural metastases), risk factors for spinal infection or for fever or chills (infection), and saddle anesthesia or bladder and bowel dysfunction (cauda equina syndrome).

2. *Sciatica*—This category includes back-related lower limb symptoms suggestive of lumbosacral nerve root compromise. Sciatica would be further suggested by a positive straight leg raise, as defined by pain below the knee at less than 70° of leg elevation, aggravated by dorsiflexion of the ankle. Crossover pain (ie, eliciting pain in the leg with sciatica by straight raising of the unaffected leg) is an even stronger indication of nerve root compression. Correlative findings on sensory examination, specific muscle strength loss, and reflex changes can be used to further diagnose sciatica and to localize the nerve root suspected to be involved.

3. *Nonspecific back symptoms*—This common category includes low back pain without signs or symptoms of a serious underlying condition or nerve root compression.

The patient in the case example appears to have nonspecific back discomfort. After this diagnosis is made, the physician could educate the patient about this problem, reassuring him that the evaluation results do not suggest a dangerous problem and that rapid recovery can be expected. Should the patient not recover within a month, a more extensive evaluation may be needed, including radiography and special studies.

In the interim, the physician must address the need for symptom control measures. This can include oral medications. The safest effective medication for acute low back problems appears to be acetaminophen, which has a low side-effect profile. Nonsteroidal anti-inflammatory drugs can also be prescribed, but the disadvantages are cost and side-effect profile (gastrointestinal tract irritation and ulceration). Muscle relaxants are reported to be no more effective than nonsteroidal anti-inflammatory drugs in treating low back symptoms, and they can produce marked drowsiness. A combination of relaxants and nonsteroidal anti-inflammatory drugs has not demonstrated an increased benefit. Opioids appear no more effective than safer analgesics and should be avoided if possible. If opioids are chosen, they should be prescribed for only short periods and the patient must be warned of the potential side effects of drowsiness, cloudy mentation, and constipation and the potential for dependency.

Physical methods are often used in the treatment of acute back problems; however, most of these methods, including traction, massage, ultrasound, and trigger point injections, have not been proved to be more effective than simple analgesics in studies of patients with acute symptoms. Spinal manipulation is safe and as effective as other commonly used treatments for patients who have acute low back symptoms in the absence of a radiculopathy.

Activity alteration is a balance between avoiding undue back irritation and preventing debility due to inactivity. Most patients do not require bed rest. In fact, it has been shown that patients with acute low back pain who continue ordinary activities within the limits permitted by the pain recover more rapidly than those treated with bed rest or back-mobilizing exercises. If bed rest is used, it should be used for only 2 or 3 days, because prolonged bed rest has a potentially debilitating effect and its efficacy in treatment is unproven. Generally, bed rest is reserved for patients with severe limitations caused by sciatica. Certain postures and activities can increase stress on the back and aggravate the symptoms. Patients must be taught to minimize the stress of lifting by keeping the lifted object close to the body at the level of the navel. Lifting with the legs as opposed to the back must be emphasized. Prolonged sitting sometimes aggravates problems, and patients should be encouraged to change their position frequently. Until the patient returns to normal activity, aerobic conditioning may be recommended to help avoid debilitation from inactivity. When requested, it may be appropriate for the physician to offer specific instructions about activity at work for patients with acute limitations due to low back symptoms. The physician should make it clear to both the patient and the employer that even moderately heavy unassisted lifting may aggravate back symptoms and that any restrictions are intended to allow for spontaneous recovery or for time to build activity tolerance through exercise.

General Internal Medicine Pharmacy Review
John G. O'Meara, PharmD

Antihyperlipidemic Agents

Drug (Trade Name)	Dose	No. of Doses per Day	Side Effects	Drug Interactions	Comments
Bile acid sequestrants			GI (bloating, constipation, flatulence)	Administer at least 4 h before or 2 h after other drugs	No systemic absorption; may be given to pregnant women Lipid effects: decrease LDL-C, increase or no change in HDL-C, & increase triglycerides
Cholestyramine (Questran, Prevalite, Locholest)	4-16 g	2			
Colestipol (Colestid)	2-16 g (tablets), 5-30 g (powder)	1 or 2			
Colesevelam (Welchol)	3.75 g	1 or 2	Fewer GI side effects than with cholestyramine & colestipol	Fewer drug interactions than with cholestyramine & colestipol	
HMG-CoA reductase inhibitors (statins)			Headache, myalgia, increased liver enzymes, diarrhea, rhabdomyolysis (rare)		Lipid effects: most potent agents for lowering LDL-C; also decrease triglycerides & modestly increase HDL-C All statins are contraindicated in pregnancy
Lovastatin (Mevacor)	20-80 mg	1 or 2		CYP3A4 inhibitors— increase serum levels of lovastatin, simvastatin, &, to lesser extent, atorvastatin (CYP3A4 inhibitors include azole antifungals [itraconazole, ketoconazole, voriconazole], macrolide antibiotics [erythromycin, clarithromycin], diltiazem, verapamil, cyclosporine, nefazodone, fluvoxamine, grapefruit juice, amprenavir, ritonavir, nelfinavir, & indinavir) Fibrates (increased risk of myopathy)	Lovastatin should be taken with evening meal

General Internal Medicine Pharmacy Review (continued)

Antihyperlipidemic Agents (continued)

Drug (Trade Name)	Dose	No. of Doses per Day	Side Effects	Drug Interactions	Comments
HMG-CoA reductase inhibitors (statins) (continued)					
Pravastatin (Pravachol)	40-80 mg	1		Cholestyramine, colestipol (decreased pravastatin absorption), amprenavir & cyclosporine (increased pravastatin serum levels), fibrates (increased risk of myopathy)	Not metabolized extensively by cytochrome system; therefore, reduced potential for drug interactions; administer at bedtime
Simvastatin (Zocor)	20-80 mg	1		Same as lovastatin, plus amiodarone	Administer at bedtime
Atorvastatin (Lipitor)	10-80 mg	1		Same as lovastatin	May take anytime during day (half-life ~14 h)
Fluvastatin (Lescol, Lescol XL)	20-80 mg	1		Potent inhibitor of CYP2C9; warfarin (increased hypoprothrombinemic effect by inhibition of warfarin metabolism)	Administer at bedtime; least potent of statins
Rosuvastatin (Crestor)	10-40 mg	1	Proteinuria & hematuria with higher doses	Minimal (~10%) hepatic metabolism (primarily CYP2C9 & CYP2C19), decreased potential for drug interactions	May take anytime during day Most potent statin, but increased risk of myopathy due to higher potency (myopathy is dose dependent)
Fibric acid derivatives			Dyspepsia, diarrhea, myopathy, hepatotoxicity, cholelithiasis		Lipid effects: most potent agents for decreasing triglycerides; also increase HDL-C
Gemfibrozil (Lopid)	1,200 mg	2		Warfarin (increased risk of bleeding), statins (increased risk of myopathy), sulfonylureas (increased risk of hypoglycemia)	Administer 30 min before morning & evening meals
Fenofibrate (Tricor)	54-160 mg	1		Same as gemfibrozil but with less risk of myopathy than with statins, cholestyramine, & colestipol (decreased fenofibrate absorption)	Give with a meal

General Internal Medicine Pharmacy Review (continued)

Antihyperlipidemic Agents (continued)

Drug (Trade Name)	Dose	No. of Doses per Day	Side Effects	Drug Interactions	Comments
Nicotinic acid (niacin)					Most effective agent in increasing HDL-C Aspirin (325 mg) 30 min before niacin may decrease flushing reaction (prostaglandin mediated) Immediate-release niacin: start low & titrate dose upward slowly to minimize side effects OTC formulations of immediate-release & extended-release niacin are available
Immediate-release (Niacor)	2-6 g	2 or 3	GI distress, skin flushing, tingling & warmth, headache, hypotension; hepatotoxicity (>2 g daily, increased risk with sustained-release formulation), hyperglycemia, hyperuricemia	Statins (increased risk of myopathy), cholestyramine, & colestipol (decreased niacin absorption)	
Extended-release (Niaspan)	1-2 g	1 at bedtime			
Cholesterol absorption inhibitor					
Ezetimibe (Zetia)	10 mg	1	Similar to placebo in clinical trials	Cholestyramine (decreased absorption of ezetimibe) Administer ezetimibe at least 2 h before or 4 h after a bile acid sequestrant Cyclosporine (increased ezetimibe levels)	Not recommended for patients with moderate or severe hepatic insufficiency No increase in myopathy or rhabdomyolysis when given with statins
Combination agents					
Extended-release niacin/lovastatin (Advicor)	Starting dose: 500/20 mg	1 at bedtime, maximum daily	See "Nicotinic acid" & "Lovastatin" entries	See "Nicotinic acid" & "Lovastatin" entries	See "Nicotinic acid" & "Lovastatin" entries
Ezetimibe/simvastatin (Vytorin)	Starting dose: 10/20 mg	1 in the evening	See "Ezetimibe" & "Simvastatin" entries	See "Ezetimibe" & "Simvastatin" entries	See "Ezetimibe" & "Simvastatin" entries
Omega-3 fatty acids					
Eicosapentaenoic acid (EPA) + docosahexaenoic acid (DHA)	CAD: ~1 g Increased triglycerides: 2-4 g	1 or 2	GI upset, fishy aftertaste	No increase in myopathy or rhabdomyolysis when given with statins	Give with a meal Decreases triglyceride levels by 20%-50% but also increases LDL-C Higher doses may interfere with platelet function & possibly cause bleeding

Abbreviations: CAD, coronary artery disease; GI, gastrointestinal tract; HDL-C, high-density lipoprotein cholesterol; LDL-C, low-density lipoprotein cholesterol; OTC, over-the-counter.

General Internal Medicine Pharmacy Review (continued)
Kari L. B. Matzek, PharmD

Summary of Drugs for Smoking Cessation

Drug	Side Effects	Drug Interactions	Comments
Nicotine replacement		Drug metabolism may be altered by use or nonuse of nicotine Monitor clinical outcomes	Do not smoke while taking nicotine replacement
Nicotine gum	Taste alteration, mouth & throat irritation, cough, headache		2-mg dose (NTE 30 pieces daily) 4-mg dose (NTE 20 pieces daily)
Nicotine inhaler	Taste alteration, mouth & throat irritation, cough, headache		Usual dose is 6-16 cartridges daily; do not use >6 mo
Nicotine lozenge	Taste alteration, nausea, heartburn, hiccups, cough, headache		Start with 2-mg lozenge if first cigarette is >30 min after waking Start with 4-mg lozenge if first cigarette is within 30 min of waking NTE 20 lozenges daily of either strength
Nicotine nasal spray	Nasal & throat irritation, runny nose, watery eyes, sneezing, congestion, taste alteration, headache	Nasal vasoconstrictors	Dose is 1 mg (2 sprays, 1/nostril), NTE 40 mg (80 sprays daily) Irritation decreases with use
Nicotine patch	Redness, itching, & burning at application site; nervousness, headache		Apply to clean, healthy, non-hairy skin; rotate sites of application every 24 h
Non-nicotine replacement			
Bupropion (Zyban)	Dry mouth, insomnia, headache, nausea, hypertension	MAOIs, TCAs, SSRIs, levodopa	Contraindicated in patients with previous seizure history May be taken with or without nicotine replacement Pregnancy category B
Varenicline (Chantix)	Nausea, vomiting, constipation, flatulence, sleep disturbance	No clinically significant drug interactions	Dose reduction should be considered for patients with intolerable nausea Incidence of side effects may be increased in patients using both varenicline Chantix and nicotine replacement Pregnancy category C

Abbreviations: MAOI, monoamine oxidase inhibitor; NTE, not to exceed; SSRI, selective serotonin reuptake inhibitor; TCA, tricyclic antidepressant.

General Internal Medicine Pharmacy Review (continued)
Magali P. Disdier, PharmD, PhD; Narith N. Ou, PharmD

Summary of Anticoagulants

Drug	Mechanism of Action	Side Effects	Drug Interactions	Comments
Warfarin	Inhibits synthesis of active coagulation factors Effects are delayed 2-3 d Liver metabolism	Bruising, bleeding Skin necrosis at initiation	Many CYP2C9[a] inhibitors, mainly amiodarone, sulfamethoxazole, quinolones, macrolides, metronidazole, fluconazole; high doses of acetaminophen; vitamin K–containing foods[b]	Monitor with INR; more frequent monitoring advised when administration of interacting medications is begun or stopped Lower dosing in liver failure & malnutrition & for elderly Effects can be reversed with vitamin K Pregnancy category X
Heparin	Inhibits thrombin action (main action) ATIII dependent Average half-life, 90 min Metabolism: liver & reticuloendohelial system	Bleeding, HIT/HITTS, bruise at SQ injection site	Other anticoagulants (LMWH, DTIs)	Weight-based dosing (continuous IV infusion), monitor with aPTT; effects are reversed by protamine SQ prophylaxis; preferred dosing, every 8 h Monitor hemoglobin & platelet count Anticoagulant of choice in pregnancy Long-term use may lead to osteoporosis
LMWH Enoxaparin (Lovenox) Dalteparin (Fragmin)	Inhibits Xa action ATIII dependent Half-life, up to 7 h Renal elimination	Bleeding, bruising at SQ injection site HIT (rare)	Other anticoagulants, thrombolytics	Weight-based dosing, once or twice daily May monitor & adjust dose using anti-Xa activity Caution in neuraxial anesthesia (risk of epidural hematoma) Caution in severe renal impairment (reduce dose of enoxaparin)
Fondaparinux (Arixtra)	Pentasaccharide Inhibits Xa action ATIII dependent Half-life, 17-21 h Renally excreted	Bleeding, bruising at SQ injection site Rare thrombocytopenia	Other anticoagulants (heparin, LMWH)	Weight-based dosing, once daily May monitor with anti-Xa activity Caution if body weight <50 kg (reduce therapeutic dosing, avoid prophylaxis) Caution in renal impairment

Abbreviations: aPTT, activated partial thromboplastin time; ATIII, antithrombin III; DTI, direct thrombin inhibitor; HIT, heparin-induced thrombocytopenia; HITTS, heparin-induced thrombocytopenia and thrombosis syndrome; INR, international normalized ratio; IV, intravenous; LMWH, low-molecular-weight heparin; SQ, subcutaneous.
[a] CYP2C9 is the cytochrome P450 2C9 isoenzyme. People with variations in the *CYP2C9* and *VKORC1* genes may require lower warfarin doses. Laboratory testing is now available.
[b] Vitamin K daily oral requirements are about 100 mcg for adults; low daily doses of 100 mcg can be used to stabilize an INR that is difficult to adjust.

General Internal Medicine Pharmacy Review (continued)
Magali P. Disdier, PharmD, PhD; Narith N. Ou, PharmD

Direct Thrombin Inhibitors[a]

Drug	Elimination	Side Effects	Drug Interactions	Comments
Lepirudin (Refludan)	Renally excreted Half-life, 0.8-2 h	Bleeding, anaphylaxis (on reexposure)	Thrombolytics (dose reduction suggested)	Weight-based dosing Monitor with aPTT Reduce dose in renal impairment Avoid if ARF or dialysis FDA-approved for anticoagulation in patients with HIT Risk of anti-lepirudin antibodies leading to increased effects
Bivalirudin (Angiomax)	Cleared through kidneys and proteolytic cleavage Half-life, 25 min	Increased bleeding	Thrombolytics, other anticoagulants, GPIs	FDA approved for patients undergoing PCI with or without GPIs Indicated for patients with HIT undergoing PCI Weight-based dosing; monitor with ACT or aPTT Reduce dosing in severe renal impairment
Argatroban	Hepatic metabolism Half-life, 39-51 min	Increased bleeding	Thrombolytics, other anticoagulants, GPIs	FDA approved for anticoagulation in patients with HIT Indicated as anticoagulant for patients with HIT undergoing PCI Weight-based dosing Monitor with aPTT or ACT Preferred DTI agent in renal impairment Dose requirement may be lower in severe renal impairment Falsely elevate INR when used with warfarin; consult package insert

Abbreviations: ACT, activated clotting time; aPTT, activated partial thromboplastin time; ARF, acute renal failure; DTI, direct thrombin inhibitor; FDA, Food & Drug Administration; GPIs, glycoprotein IIb/IIIa inhibitors; HIT, heparin-induced thrombocytopenia; INR, international normalized ratio; PCI, percutaneous coronary intervention.

[a] DTIs inhibit thrombin and block its thrombogenic activity. Their action is independent of antithrombin III. The only available DTIs are parenteral. They do not have an antidote; they are not to be used in conjunction with heparin, including low-molecular-weight heparin.

Questions

Multiple Choice (choose the best answer)

1. Your clinic has access to CT colonography. You know that the prevalence of colon lesions (adenomatous polyps ≥7 mm or cancers) in the elderly high-risk population that you screen is 10%. Recently you read an article stating that the use of CT colonography to identify lesions 7 mm or larger has a sensitivity of 60% and a specificity of 90%. If you use CT colonography in your high-risk elderly population to screen for lesions 7 mm or larger, what percentage of that group with a positive test will actually have an adenomatous polyp or cancer?

    a. 40%
    b. 60%
    c. 80%
    d. 90%
    e. 95%

2. On the basis of the sensitivity and specificity in question 1, what percentage of this group with negative findings on CT colonography will *not* have a lesion 7 mm or larger?

    a. 40%
    b. 60%
    c. 80%
    d. 90%
    e. 95%

3. You have recently read a randomized controlled trial assessing the efficacy of patient self-management of anticoagulation to reduce bleeding risks. In 1 group, patients were trained to adjust their own warfarin dosage according to the international normalized ratio (INR) results obtained using a home INR device. This group was compared with a clinic-based group of patients who visited their clinic every 4 weeks for INR checks. A physician then adjusted the dosage and arranged for the next INR check. At 1 year, the self-management group had a 2% risk of any (major or minor) bleeding events. The clinic-based group had a 7% risk of any bleeding events. On the basis of this information, how many patients need to be enrolled in a system of self-management of anticoagulants for a year to eliminate 1 adverse event of bleeding?

    a. 2
    b. 7
    c. 14
    d. 20
    e. 50

4. A 76-year-old woman is referred for a preoperative cardiac evaluation before a breast biopsy of a suspicious area of calcification identified on a screening mammogram. She has a complex medical history that includes insulin-dependent diabetes mellitus and an episode of heart failure 2 years ago. At that time, echocardiography demonstrated a left ventricular ejection fraction of 45%. Currently, she states that she has no symptoms of angina or congestive heart failure. Her medications include insulin, furosemide (40 mg daily), and lisinopril (20 mg daily). She does very little exertional activity. Chest radiography shows mild cardiomegaly, and no acute changes are noted on the electrocardiogram. What is the most appropriate next step in the perioperative evaluation and management of this patient?

    a. Perform a treadmill exercise test.
    b. Perform a pharmacologic stress test.
    c. Perform exercise echocardiography.
    d. Perform coronary angiography before the planned procedure.
    e. No further testing is needed, so the patient may proceed directly to the operating room for breast biopsy.

5. A 71-year-old man is referred for perioperative cardiac risk assessment. He is scheduled to have aortobifemoral vascular bypass grafting to correct symptoms of lower extremity claudication that forces him to stop after he walks half a block. He has a 50-pack-year smoking history and a history of emphysema. He continues to smoke, but he has no complaints of limiting respiratory symptoms. He has no history of angina, myocardial infarction, diabetes mellitus, or congestive heart failure. He has a sedentary lifestyle. His blood pressure is 145/85 mm Hg, and his pulse is 75 beats per minute. Medications include lisinopril (20 mg daily), pravastatin (40 mg daily), and aspirin (81 mg daily). His electrocardiogram (ECG) shows Q waves in the inferior leads. What should be the next step in perioperative evaluation and management of this patient?

    a. Perform a treadmill exercise test.
    b. Perform dobutamine stress echocardiography.
    c. Perform CT of the chest to assess for coronary calcification.
    d. Perform coronary angiography.
    e. No further testing is needed, so the patient may proceed directly to the operating room; no β-blockade should be used because of emphysema.

6. The patient in question 5 is found to have no stress-induced abnormalities on dobutamine echocardiography, but he does have a fixed inferior wall motion abnormality that does not change with stress. What would you recommend next?

    a. Proceed with surgery, but withhold all medications on the morning of surgery.
    b. Begin giving metoprolol, 25 mg orally twice daily; titrate to keep the pulse at 55 to 65 beats per minute throughout the perioperative period.

c. Begin giving a sustained-release formulation of diltiazem, 60 mg orally twice daily; titrate to keep the pulse at 55 to 65 beats per minute throughout the perioperative period.

d. Begin giving isosorbide dinitrate, 30 mg orally twice daily, and titrate to keep the blood pressure ≤140/80 mm Hg throughout the perioperative period.

e. Begin giving clonidine, 0.1 mg twice daily, to keep the blood pressure <140/90 mm Hg.

7. A 63-year-old woman is scheduled for a total hip arthroplasty. The orthopedic surgeon requests a preoperative evaluation for specific recommendations regarding prophylaxis for deep venous thrombosis (DVT). The patient has no history of DVT, increased bleeding, or a hypercoagulable state. She takes aspirin for osteoarthritis. What would you recommend for perioperative DVT prophylaxis for this patient?

a. Aspirin alone, continued indefinitely
b. Intermittent pneumatic compression stockings until hospital discharge
c. Fondaparinux, 2.5 mg daily, beginning 8 hours preoperatively and continuing until hospital discharge
d. Low-molecular-weight heparin (LMWH)—dalteparin, 2,500 units every 24 hours, beginning 12 hours postoperatively and continuing for 4 weeks
e. Adjusted-dose warfarin beginning the evening of surgery (goal INR, 2-3) and continuing for 4 weeks

8. A 66-year-old woman presents with acute pain in her left leg. Ultrasonography has confirmed a new thrombus in the left superficial femoral vein. Otherwise, she is healthy and states that she has not had recent trauma. Her creatinine is 1.4 mg/dL. She does not have a personal or family history of venous thromboembolism, and she has no major bleeding risks. She has a supportive husband at home who can help her with activities of daily living. She weighs 80 kg. What is the most appropriate next step in the management of this patient?

a. Leg elevation, elastic bandage wrap on leg, and anti-inflammatory drugs until she has recovered
b. Hospitalization and treatment with LMWH while initiating warfarin therapy
c. Hospitalization and treatment with unfractionated heparin while initiating warfarin therapy
d. Outpatient treatment with LMWH while initiating warfarin therapy
e. Request CT of the chest to look for pulmonary emboli before deciding on treatment choice.

9. A 54-year-old woman with diabetes mellitus who is receiving sulfonylurea therapy is referred for management of hyperlipidemia. Her total cholesterol is 220 mg/dL. High-density lipoprotein cholesterol (HDL-C) is 35 mg/dL, and the triglyceride level is 250 mg/dL. Similar values were noted 6 months ago when she met with a dietitian. She states that she has been compliant with diet therapy. The hemoglobin A_{1c} level is at the upper limit of the reference range. Which of the following is the most appropriate next step in the management of this patient's hyperlipidemia?

a. Continue the diet therapy and exercise; no drug therapy is needed.
b. Ask the dietitian to reinstruct this patient, and have the patient return in 6 months so the lipid values can be determined again.
c. Begin treatment with an HMG-CoA reductase inhibitor.
d. Begin treatment with gemfibrozil.
e. Begin treatment with nicotinic acid.

Answers

1. Answer a.

A 2×2 table must be constructed to determine the positive predictive value for the CT colonography test among high-risk patients being evaluated for colon polyps 7 mm or larger.

The correct answer is $\frac{a}{a+b}$ or 60/150 = 40%.

Diagnostic Test Result		Disease Present	Disease Absent	
	Positive	60 a	90 b	150 a+b
	Negative	c 40	d 810	c+d 850
		a+c 100	b+d 900	a+b+c+d 1,000

2. Answer e.

The negative predictive value of the CT colonography test is $\frac{d}{c+d}$ or 810/850 = 95%.

3. Answer d.

You are asked to determine the number needed to treat (NNT) in a randomized controlled trial showing that the self-management anticoagulant therapy group had a bleeding event rate of 2%; that is, the experimental event rate (EER) = 2%. The group receiving usual care group had an event rate of 7%; that is, the control event rate (CER) = 7%. NNT = 1/ARR, where ARR is the absolute risk reduction. ARR = (CER−EER). In this case, 7%−2% = 5%. Therefore, NNT = 1/.05 = 20.

4. Answer e.

Refer to Figure 8-3. The patient is scheduled for an elective procedure (step 1), has no active cardiac conditions (step 2), and is undergoing a low-risk operation (step 3). Therefore, according to the American College of Cardiology and American Heart Association (ACC/AHA) guidelines for perioperative cardiovascular evaluation, she can proceed to surgery without additional testing. Even though she has 2 clinical risk factors (diabetes and a history of heart failure) and she probably cannot achieve 4 metabolic equivalents (METs) on a regular basis, she does not need additional testing because of the low-risk nature of this surgical procedure from a cardiovascular standpoint.

5. Answer b.

This patient is scheduled for an elective surgery (step 1), he has no active cardiac conditions (step 2), this vascular surgery is not a low-risk surgery (step 3), he has poor functional capacity (step 4), and he has 1 clinical risk factor (probable past myocardial infarction on the ECG). According to the ACC/AHA guidelines for perioperative cardiovascular evaluation (Figure 8-3), this patient could either proceed to surgery with aggressive β-blockade or undergo noninvasive testing if it would change management (step 5). Since this patient has

not had a previous diagnosis of coronary artery disease and has ECG findings consistent with a prior myocardial infarction, it is certainly reasonable to perform a noninvasive study preoperatively to determine whether he has a continuing ischemic burden. If he did indeed have significant ischemia, consideration of revascularization could be entertained before this elective vascular surgery. The choice of stress test is simplified because he is limited in his ability to ambulate; therefore, an exercise test is not acceptable. Coronary CT has no role in preoperative cardiac risk assessment at this time. Coronary angiography is fairly invasive in this setting and would only be indicated if there were significant findings on the noninvasive stress test. The correct answer is dobutamine stress echocardiography.

6. Answer b.

This patient does have a fixed wall motion abnormality on stress testing, suggesting a previously undiagnosed inferior myocardial infarction. According to the ACC/AHA guidelines for perioperative β-blocker therapy, he would benefit from the use of β-blockade perioperatively to help reduce his risk of perioperative cardiac events. A diagnosis of chronic obstructive pulmonary disease is not a contraindication to the use of perioperative β-blockers; however, they should be instituted with careful attention to a change in respiratory symptoms. There are no data to suggest that the use of calcium channel blockers or nitrates reduces the risk of perioperative cardiac events. Use of aspirin would be stopped before the surgical procedure; however, this patient should take his lisinopril and pravastatin on the morning of surgery because blood pressure control is important as is the probable perioperative protective effect of perioperative statins in high-risk vascular surgery patients.

7. Answer c.

Patients who undergo a total hip replacement are at high risk of perioperative DVT. Observational studies suggest that 10% to 20% of these patients develop proximal DVTs and 4% to 10% develop clinical pulmonary embolism in the perioperative period. The American College of Chest Physicians guidelines suggest that there is good evidence to support 1 of the following options for DVT prophylaxis in this high-risk population: 1) dalteparin, 5,000 units subcutaneously every 24 hours, beginning 12 hours postoperatively (or 12 hours preoperatively) and continuing for 4 weeks; 2) fondaparinux, 2.5 mg subcutaneously every 24 hours, beginning 6 to 8 hours postoperatively and continuing for 4 weeks; or 3) adjusted-dose warfarin beginning the night before surgery (or the night of surgery) with a goal INR of 2 to 3, continuing for 4 weeks. The guidelines also specifically recommend *against* the use of aspirin, dextran, low-dose unfractionated heparin, compression stockings, pneumatic devices, or venous foot pumps as the *only* method of DVT prophylaxis in this high-risk population. There is also evidence to support prolonged prophylaxis (28-35 days postoperatively) for patients undergoing hip replacement or hip fracture surgery.

8. Answer d.

The superficial femoral vein is in the deep venous system; therefore, the patient needs to be treated with heparin and warfarin, overlapped for at least 4 to 5 days and until the INR is greater than 2.0. Outpatient LMWH has been approved by the US Food and Drug Administration for the treatment of DVT. The patient's estimated creatinine clearance is 50 mL/min, so she is a candidate to use LMWH. She has a good support system, and therefore it would be appropriate for her to be treated as an outpatient. She has no symptoms to suggest pulmonary embolism, and therefore CT of the chest is not indicated.

9. Answer c.

The patient has a coronary artery disease risk equivalent, that is, diabetes mellitus. In this circumstance, the low-density lipoprotein cholesterol (LDL-C) level at which to initiate drug therapy is 130 mg/dL or more, although many experts now suggest initiation if the LDL-C level is 100 mg/dL or more. Because her calculated LDL-C is 135 mg/dL, it is appropriate to initiate lipid-lowering drug therapy. An HMG-CoA reductase inhibitor is the drug of choice for patients with diabetes. Gemfibrozil is a consideration, but because of the potential drug interaction with sulfonylurea medications, it would not be a good choice. Nicotinic acid is a good medication for this lipid profile, but it increases blood glucose values in diabetic patients, and therefore it is not the best choice.

9

Genetics

Virginia V. Michels, MD

Genetic factors play a role in the development of many types of human disease. Genetic determinants may be chromosome abnormalities, single gene defects, mitochondrial mutations, or epigenetic or multifactorial factors.

Chromosome Abnormalities

Approximately a sixth of all birth defects and cases of congenitally determined mental retardation are due to chromosome abnormalities. Chromosome abnormalities occur in about 1 in 180 live births. One-third of these abnormalities involve an abnormal number (aneuploidy) of non-sex chromosomes (autosomes). Factors known to result in a higher-than-average risk for having a child with autosomal aneuploidy are maternal age 35 years or older and having previously had an affected child. Prenatal diagnosis by karyotyping of fetal cells obtained by amniocentesis or chorionic villus sampling can be offered to pregnant women who are at increased risk.

* Chromosome abnormalities occur in 1 in 180 live births.
* Risk factors for autosomal aneuploidy are maternal age ≥35 years and having had an affected child.

Down Syndrome

The most common autosomal aneuploidy syndrome in term infants is Down syndrome (incidence, 1 in 880). The most serious consequence of Down syndrome is mild-to-moderate mental retardation (average IQ, about 50). Forty percent of patients with Down syndrome have a congenital heart defect, most frequently ventricular septal defect or atrioventricular canal defect, although other congenital heart defects may occur. Median duration of survival is approximately 60 years. Thyroid disease, hearing loss, and celiac disease are common. Alzheimer disease develops in more than 40% by age 50 years. A few patients have hypoplasia of the odontoid process, which is important to diagnose before participation in certain sports. Males with Down syndrome are usually sterile, but affected females are fertile and have a very high risk of having an affected child. Most persons with Down syndrome have trisomy 21 as a result of a new mutation nondisjunctional event; in these cases, the risk to the parents of

having another affected child is 1% to 2% or higher, depending on maternal age. In 3% of persons with Down syndrome, a translocation chromosome abnormality is present, in which the extra chromosome 21 is attached to another chromosome, most commonly 14 (Figure 9-1). These translocation chromosomes may be inherited in an *unbalanced* form from a parent carrying a *balanced* form of the translocation; these parents have a 5% to 15% risk of having another affected child. Even if the parents have completed their childbearing, the karyotype of the affected individual should be determined so that other relatives (eg, adult siblings) can be counseled. The same principles are presumed to be true for other autosomal aneuploidy syndromes.

* The most serious consequence of Down syndrome is mild-to-moderate mental retardation.
* The most frequent heart defect in Down syndrome is ventricular septal defect or atrioventricular canal defect.
* Males with Down syndrome are usually sterile, but females are fertile.
* Most persons with Down syndrome have trisomy 21.
* Early-onset Alzheimer disease is common in adults with Down syndrome.

Sex Chromosome Aneuploidy Syndromes

Approximately 35% of chromosome abnormalities in live-born infants involve sex chromosome aneuploidy. Affected individuals may have an additional X or Y chromosome or be lacking one. Patients with 47,XXX or 47,XYY karyotypes usually have no major birth defects or mental retardation, although the mean IQ may be 90 rather than 100. Patients with a 47,XXY karyotype (Klinefelter syndrome) have a tall, eunuchoid body habitus, small testes, and infertility. However, reproduction sometimes can be achieved through in vitro techniques with intracytoplasmic sperm injection. They are at increased risk for breast cancer, nongonadal germ cell tumors, and leg ulcers.

Patients with a 45,X karyotype (Turner syndrome) or its variants—1 structurally abnormal X, such as 46,X,i(X)q (Figure 9-2)—or mosaicism for an X or Y chromosome—such as 45,X/46,XX—usually are mentally normal. Fluorescent in situ hybridization probes can be used to distinguish a marker X versus Y when it is so small that it

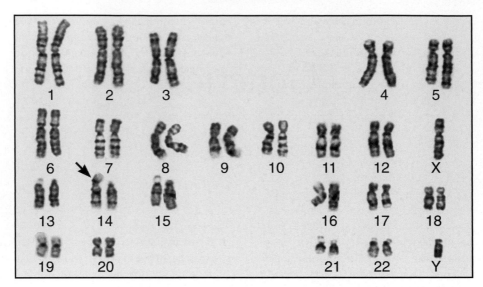

Figure 9-1. Karyotype 46,XY,-14,+t(14;21)(p11;q11) from patient with Down syndrome. Extra chromosome 21 material is translocated to chromosome 14 (arrow). Result is robertsonian translocation. The short arm, at the top of each chromosome, is referred to as the *p* arm; the long arm, at the bottom, is referred to as the *q* arm. (Karyotype courtesy of G. Dewald, Ph.D.)

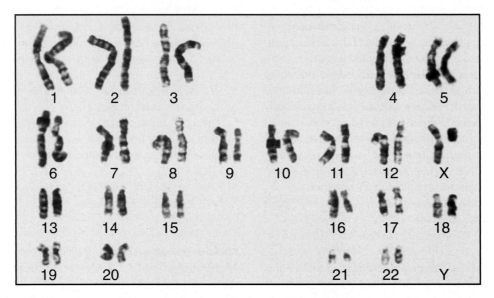

Figure 9-2. Karyotype 46,X,r(X) from patient with Turner syndrome. *r* is the designation for a ring chromosome. (Karyotype courtesy of G. Dewald, Ph.D.)

cannot be distinguished by karyotype analysis. This distinction is important for determining risk of gonadal malignancy (increased with Y chromosome material) and need for prophylactic gonadectomy. Streak gonads are usually present. Patients have a risk of approximately 30% for a bicuspid aortic valve with or without coarctation of the aorta. Women with Turner syndrome are at increased risk for ascending aortic aneurysm formation, and thus periodic echocardiographic monitoring is recommended. Short stature, webbed neck, increased number of pigmented nevi, failure to develop secondary sexual characteristics, short fourth or fifth metacarpals or metatarsals, renal malformations, and increased risk for thyroid disease are also variably present. Early diagnosis of sex chromosome aneuploidy is important for timely treatment with hormone replacement.

- Typical case of 47,XXY karyotype (Klinefelter syndrome): small testes, infertility, and tall, eunuchoid body habitus.
- Typical case of 45,X karyotype (Turner syndrome): short stature, lack of secondary sex characteristics, usually mentally normal, and 30% risk of bicuspid aortic valve or aortic coarctation.
- Risk for ascending aortic aneurysm is increased in Turner syndrome.

Other Chromosome Abnormalities
Thirty-four percent of chromosome abnormalities involve structural changes such as deletions, duplications, inversions, or translocations. They may be detected by peripheral blood karyotype, by subtelomeric fluorescent in situ hybridization probes for more subtle alterations

(Figure 9-3), or by array-based comparative genomic hybridization. The translocations may be balanced (no net loss or gain of genetic material) or unbalanced. People with balanced translocations are usually phenotypically normal and healthy but may be at increased risk for miscarriages or their children may have birth defects. Patients with net loss or gain of genetic material by any of the mechanisms listed above have phenotypic abnormalities that usually include mental subnormality and frequently other major or minor birth defects. Parents of all patients with a structural chromosome abnormality should have chromosome analyses to determine whether they are carriers of a balanced translocation.

* Parents of all patients with a structural chromosome abnormality should have chromosome analyses.

Fragile X-Linked Mental Retardation

The fragile X-linked mental retardation syndrome occurs in about 1 in 1,000 males. It is characterized by a visible fragile site on the long arm of an X chromosome at band q27 when the lymphocytes are cultured in media deficient in folic acid. The fragile site is never observed in all cells, and the frequency may be as low as 4%. Some carrier females do not express the fragile site cytogenetically. Molecular analysis for this disorder is more sensitive than cytogenetic analysis. Affected and carrier individuals have trinucleotide repeat (CGG) expansions within the *FMR1* gene. There are more than 200 repeats in mentally retarded males, and females with more than 200 repeats have a risk of mental subnormality of 50%. Patients with smaller repeat expansions of 55 to 200 are referred to as premutation carriers, and these men are at risk of a neurologic degenerative disorder even though they do not have mental retardation. Variable combinations of ataxia, intention tremor, dementia, parkinsonism, and peripheral or autonomic neuropathy may develop. These men, also referred to as transmitting males, have obligate carrier daughters who rarely show signs of the disease, who in turn may have mentally retarded sons, because the CGG repeat is more likely to expand when transmitted through a female. Affected males may be physically normal or have a long, thin face with prominent jaw, large simplified ears, and enlarged testes. Carrier females are phenotypically normal or mildly retarded and dysmorphic. The degree of mental retardation ranges from mild to profound.

* Males with fragile X may be physically normal or have a long, thin face, prominent jaw, large ears, enlarged testes, and mild to profound mental retardation.
* Molecular DNA analysis is the appropriate clinical test for fragile X.
* Premutation carriers are at risk for a neurodegenerative disorder.

Single Gene Defects

Autosomal Dominant

In autosomal dominant inheritance, the responsible gene is located on one of the autosomes and one copy of the gene is sufficient for the trait to be expressed or for the disease to be present (ie, heterozygotes have the disease). There is a 50% chance that any child born to an affected person will inherit the abnormal gene.

* In autosomal dominant inheritance, the responsible gene is located on one of the autosomes.

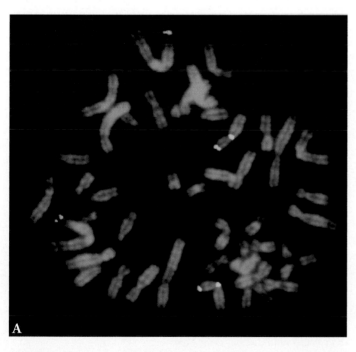
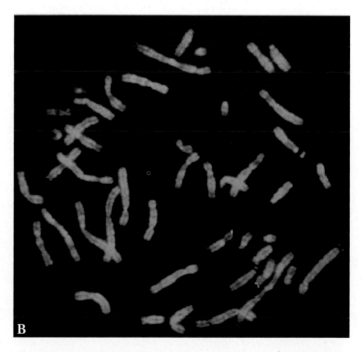

Figure 9-3. Fluorescent DNA probes for subtelomeres of each p and q arm of all chromosomes, except acrocentric p arms, are used to analyze a complete set of subtelomere regions. A, A normal pattern of 1p in green, 1q in red, Xp in yellow (fusion of green and orange), and X centromere in aqua (used as control). B, Chromosomes 16p in green and 16q in red have a normal pattern but, in addition, 16q probe is present on 4q. Thus, this chromosome 4 is derivative so that 4p probe is deleted (not shown) and 16q subtelomere region is duplicated. (Photograph courtesy of S. Jalal, Ph.D.)

- There is a 50% chance that a child of an affected person will inherit the abnormal gene.

The severity of the disease caused by the abnormal gene may be uniform for some conditions, such as achondroplasia, but the severity may be variable for other conditions, such as neurofibromatosis and Marfan syndrome. This difference of severity is referred to as *variable expression*. In contrast, *incomplete penetrance* means that some persons who have inherited the gene show no signs of it. Obviously, the clinical decision regarding whether a person has signs of the gene defect depends on the thoroughness of the examination and on the sensitivity of the investigative techniques. For example, many families with hypertrophic cardiomyopathy were thought to include members with incomplete penetrance until asymptomatic relatives were examined with echocardiography.

Although transmission of a disease through members of either sex through multiple generations of a family strongly suggests autosomal dominant inheritance, it is important to remember that autosomal dominant diseases can occur without a positive family history. This can occur because of incomplete penetrance, new mutation, somatic mosaicism, or incorrect assignment of paternity. New mutation events represent changes in the genetic material of the individual egg or sperm that give rise to the fetus. Although the risk for siblings of a person whose disease arose by new mutation is not increased over that of the general population, the risk for children still is 50%. Somatic mosaicism refers to the possibility that one of the parents has the gene defect in only some cells, including the reproductive cells (germinal mosaicism), such that the person has no or few signs of the disease but potentially can transmit the disease to one or more children.

- In autosomal dominant inheritance, disease severity may be uniform or variable.
- Incomplete penetrance: no signs of abnormal gene in a person who has inherited it.
- Somatic mosaicism: person has gene defect in only some cells.

Some of the diseases with autosomal dominant inheritance are listed in Table 9-1 and summarized on the following pages.

Imprinting is an epigenetic phenomenon that can influence the observed pattern of disease occurrence within families with single gene defects. For imprinted genes, the gene's activity (ie, expression) in an individual differs depending on which parent (mother or father) transmitted the gene. At the molecular level, these differences may result from methylation status and possibly other factors. An example of imprinting occurs in autosomal dominant familial paragangliomas due to *SDHD* gene mutations. Paragangliomas can develop in a person who inherits the defective gene from his or her father, but they do not develop in a person who inherits the defective gene from his or her mother. Regardless of whether or not a paraganglioma develops, the defective gene can be transmitted to the next generation.

Dilated Cardiomyopathy

The incidence of idiopathic dilated cardiomyopathy is approximately 6 in 100,000 and the prevalence 36 in 100,000. It is familial in at least 30% of cases, but the familial nature of the disease is often not apparent unless relatives undergo echocardiography. Penetrance is decreased and increases with advancing age, although children and young adults can be affected. Severity and mode of presentation, for example with heart failure or arrhythmia, can vary even within families. However, some families have a stronger predisposition to arrhythmias than others. In adults, the inheritance pattern is usually autosomal dominant, although X-linked inheritance and autosomal recessive inheritance also can occur. Mutations in more than 19 genes can cause dilated cardiomyopathy, including those that encode α-tropomyosin, α-actin, desmin, titin, δ-sarcoglycan, β-myosin heavy chain, cardiac troponin T, metavinculin, myosin-binding protein C, muscle LIM protein, α-actinin-2, phospholamban, cypher/LIM binding domain 3, α-myosin heavy chain, laminin A/C, SUR2A, cardiac troponin I, and cardiac sodium channel. The last is of interest because it also results in a strong likelihood of atrial fibrillation. Note that some of these genes also can be associated with hypertrophic cardiomyopathy, depending on where in the gene the mutation occurs. X-linked genes that can be involved in dilated cardiomyopathy include those encoding dystrophin, tafazzin and emerin (sometimes also associated with skeletal myopathy). Early diagnosis is important for treatment before refractory heart failure or undetected arrhythmia results in major morbidity or mortality.

Ehlers-Danlos Syndromes

There are at least 7 forms of Ehlers-Danlos syndrome. Type I, or gravis type, serves as a prototype for discussion of this group of genetically

Table 9-1   Examples of Diseases With Autosomal Dominant Inheritance

Achondroplasia
Amyloidosis (many types)
Dilated cardiomyopathy
Ehlers-Danlos syndrome, types I, II, III, IV, & some type VII
Hereditary spherocytosis, some types
Huntington disease
Hypertrophic cardiomyopathy
LEOPARD[a] syndrome
Low-density lipoprotein receptor deficiency (hypercholesterolemia)
Marfan syndrome
Multiple endocrine neoplasia, types 1, 2A, & 2B
Myotonic dystrophy
Neurofibromatosis, types 1 & 2
Noonan syndrome
Osler-Weber-Rendu disease (hereditary hemorrhagic telangiectasia)
Osteogenesis imperfecta, types I & IV, most type II
Polycystic kidney disease (some forms are autosomal recessive)
Porphyria (several types)
Tuberous sclerosis
Von Hippel-Lindau disease
Von Willebrand disease, some types

[a] Lentigenes (multiple), electrocardiographic conduction abnormalities, ocular hypertelorism, pulmonary stenosis, abnormalities of genitalia, retardation of growth, deafness.

heterogeneous disorders. The syndrome is inherited as an autosomal dominant condition. The basic defect in type I disease has been defined for some cases as a defect in the α-1 or α-2 chain of type V collagen. The disorder is characterized by velvety textured, hyperextensible, fragile skin that bruises and splits easily and heals poorly, resulting in wide, thin scars. Many tissues are friable, which is an important consideration when surgical procedures are needed. Even fetal membranes are affected and frequently rupture before term, resulting in premature birth. Wrinkled, redundant skin may develop over the knee and elbow joints. Small fat- or mucin-containing spherules may be present in the subcutaneous tissue and may be calcified. The joints are hyperextensible and prone to dislocations. Pes planus, scoliosis, degenerative arthritis, visceral diverticulosis, and spontaneous pneumothorax may occur. Mitral valve prolapse may occur in 50% of patients. Dilatation of the aortic root or pulmonary artery and prolapse of the tricuspid valve may occur. Vascular rupture is relatively rare. Type II Ehlers-Danlos syndrome is a milder form of type I. Type III Ehlers-Danlos syndrome is of unknown cause in most cases and is characterized by joint hyperextensibility with minimal skin involvement. Type IV Ehlers-Danlos syndrome is the most severe and is due to deficiency of type III collagen that results in tendency for arterial aneurysms and visceral organ rupture.

* Type I Ehlers-Danlos syndrome is an autosomal dominant condition.
* Features are velvety textured, hyperextensible, and fragile skin.
* Joints are hyperextensible and prone to dislocation.
* Associated conditions are pes planus, scoliosis, degenerative arthritis, visceral diverticulosis, and spontaneous pneumothorax.
* Mitral valve prolapse occurs in 50% of patients.
* Vascular rupture is relatively rare in types I and II.

Hypertrophic Cardiomyopathy

Hypertrophic cardiomyopathy frequently is inherited as an autosomal dominant disorder. The incidence is estimated to be 1 in 500, and it is one of the most common causes of sudden death in adolescents and young adults. Penetrance ranges from more than 60% to 100% in different families when relatives are studied with electrocardiography and echocardiography. Investigation of first-degree relatives is necessary. Even if parents are normal by echocardiography, the possibility of new mutation cannot be excluded; thus, children born to an affected parent must be considered at risk and should be evaluated to facilitate early diagnosis and treatment.

* Hypertrophic cardiomyopathy is autosomal dominant.
* Investigation of first-degree relatives is necessary.
* Children of affected parents are at risk.

The course of the disease may be variable, even within a family; therefore, the age at onset cannot be predicted precisely.

* The course of hypertrophic cardiomyopathy is variable.
* The age at onset cannot be predicted.

Molecular defects in more than 10 different genes can cause hypertrophic cardiomyopathy. These genes include the β cardiac myosin heavy-chain gene, cardiac troponin T, troponin I, α-tropomyosin, myosin-binding protein C, ventricular myosin essential light chain, ventricular myosin-regulating light chain, α-actin, titin, and α-myosin heavy chain. In addition, genes that encode the γ₂ regulatory subunit of adenosine monophosphate-activated kinase and the X-linked lysosome-associated membrane protein 2 can cause a glycogen storage disease of the heart that can mimic hypertrophic cardiomyopathy.

Marfan Syndrome

Marfan syndrome has an incidence of 1 in 10,000. It is an autosomal dominant disorder with variable expression, and approximately 20% of cases arise by new mutation. There are no well-documented instances of nonpenetrance.

* Marfan syndrome is relatively common—1 in 10,000.
* It is an autosomal dominant disorder.
* About 20% of cases arise by new mutation.

Marfan syndrome involves the musculoskeletal, ocular, and cardiovascular systems. Skeletal abnormalities include tall stature, a low upper:lower segment ratio, and increased arm span:height ratio of more than 1.05 (limbs are relatively long compared with the trunk), scoliosis or kyphosis, and pectus deformities. Increased joint laxity and hyperextensibility are common, but occasionally patients have limited extension of fingers and elbows. The face may be long and the palate highly arched. This marfanoid habitus may be present in patients with other disorders such as other connective tissue dysplasias, multiple endocrine neoplasia type 2B, Stickler syndrome, congenital contractural arachnodactyly, and homocystinuria. The characteristic body habitus is never sufficient evidence for making the diagnosis of Marfan syndrome in the absence of other criteria.

* Marfan syndrome involves the musculoskeletal, ocular, and cardiovascular systems.
* Typical case: tall stature, low upper:lower segment ratio >1.05, scoliosis or kyphosis, pectus deformities.

The ocular abnormalities associated with Marfan syndrome may include subluxation of the lenses, myopia, and retinal detachment. Dislocation of the lenses occurs in 50% to 80% of patients; the lens frequently is displaced upward. Gross dislocations may be evident without the aid of special equipment, but lesser degrees of dislocation may be evident only by slit-lamp examination. Therefore, all patients suspected of having Marfan syndrome must have a complete ophthalmologic evaluation. Patients with Marfan syndrome should have frequent ophthalmologic examinations to permit early detection of complications such as retinal detachment or glaucoma.

* Ocular abnormalities of Marfan syndrome: subluxation of lenses, myopia, retinal detachment.
* Dislocations of the lenses occur in 50%-80% of cases.
* All patients must have ophthalmologic evaluation.

The life expectancy of patients with Marfan syndrome is shortened because of cardiovascular disease. The most common manifestation is mitral valve prolapse with or without mitral regurgitation. Mitral valve prolapse in Marfan syndrome is progressive. Prophylactic antibiotic therapy for bacterial endocarditis is warranted. Acute onset of severe mitral regurgitation due to rupture of chordae tendineae may occur even in childhood. Mitral valve prolapse in a patient with a marfanoid body habitus is not a sufficient basis for the diagnosis of Marfan syndrome in the absence of a positive family history of Marfan syndrome or other characteristic findings. Patients with some forms of Ehlers-Danlos syndrome and nonspecific connective tissue dysplasias can have a similar body habitus, joint laxity, and mitral valve prolapse.

- Life expectancy in Marfan syndrome is shortened by cardiovascular disease.
- Mitral valve prolapse in Marfan syndrome is progressive.
- Prophylactic antibiotic for bacterial endocarditis is warranted.

Dilatation of the ascending aorta is the next most common cardiovascular disorder; it may lead to aortic regurgitation, aortic rupture, or dissecting aneurysm. More than 80% of patients have abnormalities found on echocardiography. Many patients have no evidence of cardiovascular disease on physical examination. The maximal aortic root diameter involves the region of the sinuses of Valsalva and sinotubular ridge. β-Adrenergic blockers appear to delay progressive dilatation.

- Most common cardiovascular manifestations are mitral valve prolapse and dilatation of ascending aorta.
- More than 80% of patients have abnormalities found on echocardiography.
- β-Adrenergic blockers might delay progressive dilatation.

Although surgical risks are increased in patients with Marfan syndrome because of tissue friability, surgical treatment frequently is successful for mitral and aortic regurgitation and for aortic dissection.

- Surgical risks are increased in Marfan syndrome.
- Surgical treatment is often successful for mitral and aortic regurgitation and aortic dissection.

Additional features sometimes associated with Marfan syndrome include decreased amounts of subcutaneous tissue, skin striae, inguinal hernias, pneumothorax, and degenerative joint disease.

Patients with Marfan syndrome are susceptible to traumatic aortic rupture; therefore, contact sports, strenuous physical exertion, and weight lifting should be restricted. Pregnancy poses significant risks for women with a dilated aorta.

The basic cause of Marfan syndrome is a defect in fibrillin; the gene encoding fibrillin is on chromosome 15q21. Mutations in the gene encoding transforming growth factor-β receptor 2 also can cause a marfan-like condition called Loeys-Dietz syndrome. Presymptomatic and prenatal diagnosis are possible in some families. However, because of limitations in molecular genetic testing, clinical criteria remain the appropriate basis for diagnosis. All first-degree relatives should be evaluated for signs of Marfan syndrome, including echocardiography and ophthalmologic examination.

- The cause of Marfan syndrome is a defect in fibrillin.
- Mutations in the gene encoding transforming growth factor-β receptor 2 also can cause a marfan-like condition.

Myotonic Dystrophy

Myotonic dystrophy, the most common form of muscular dystrophy in adults, has an incidence of approximately 1 per 8,000 to 20,000. The inheritance pattern is autosomal dominant with extremely variable expression. Although the average age at onset is in the second to third decade of life, the disease may be evident at birth or may first be noticed in the seventh decade. The disease is characterized by myotonia, muscle atrophy and weakness, ptosis of the eyelids, and expressionless facies resulting from particularly severe involvement of facial and temporal muscles. The rate of progression of the disease is variable, but disability is usually severe within 15 to 20 years after onset. Associated abnormalities may include premature frontal baldness, testicular atrophy or menstrual irregularities, gastrointestinal symptoms related to smooth muscle involvement, and cardiac disease. Distinctive refractile posterior subcapsular cataracts often are evident by slit-lamp examination. Although glucose intolerance is common, overt diabetes mellitus occurs in only about 6% of patients.

- Myotonic dystrophy is the most common form of muscular dystrophy in adults.
- The incidence is 1 in 8,000-20,000.
- The inheritance pattern is autosomal dominant with extremely variable expression.
- The age at onset is usually the second to third decade of life.
- Typical case: myotonia, muscle atrophy and weakness, ptosis of eyelids, expressionless facies, and premature frontal baldness.
- Disability is severe within 15-20 years after onset.
- Associated abnormalities: testicular atrophy or menstrual irregularities, gastrointestinal symptoms.
- Diabetes mellitus occurs in 6% of patients.

The diagnosis is based on clinical findings and a typical electromyographic pattern characterized by prolonged rhythmic discharges. The gene for myotonic dystrophy type 1 (*DMPK*) is located on chromosome 19q13, and genetic counseling is warranted for the patient and family. The molecular basis of most cases of myotonic dystrophy is expansion of a CTG trinucleotide repeat sequence affecting a gene encoding myotonin-protein kinase. Thus, direct DNA-based diagnosis of the disease is possible in most cases. The size of the trinucleotide repeat tends to increase as the genetic material is passed from one generation to the next. Increased repeat size tends to correlate with earlier onset and more severe disease, a phenomenon referred to as *anticipation*. First-degree relatives should be investigated. The risk for children born to an affected parent is 50%.

- The diagnosis of myotonic dystrophy is based on clinical and electromyographic findings or DNA analysis.
- Genetic counseling is warranted for patients and family members with myotonic dystrophy.
- First-degree relatives should be investigated.

Cardiac disease is present in approximately two-thirds of patients with myotonic dystrophy, and sudden death may occur as a result of conduction defects. Implantation of a pacemaker may be necessary. Central and alveolar hypoventilation is common and is a particular risk during recovery from anesthesia. Respiratory failure is a common cause of death.

- Cardiac disease occurs in two-thirds of patients with myotonic dystrophy, and sudden death may occur.
- Hypoventilation could complicate recovery from anesthesia.

Myotonic dystrophy type 2, sometimes referred to as proximal myotonic myopathy, is less common and is due to gene defects of zinc finger protein 9 on chromosome 3.

Neurofibromatosis

Type 1
Neurofibromatosis 1 is an autosomal dominant disorder with an incidence of 1 in 3,500. Approximately 50% of patients have the disease because of a new mutation. The disorder has markedly variable expression but very high penetrance. The diagnosis is based on 2 or more of the following clinical criteria: 6 or more café au lait macules of 1.5 cm or more in diameter, axillary or inguinal freckling, 2 or more Lisch nodules of the iris, 2 or more neurofibromas or 1 plexiform neurofibroma, a definitely positive family history, or 1 of these and 1 of the uncommon characteristic manifestations such as orbital or sphenoid wing dysplasia, optic or other central nervous system glioma, renal artery dysplasia with or without abdominal aortic coarctation, or tibial pseudofracture. Less specific signs of the disease may include pheochromocytoma and scoliosis. Malignancy, often neurofibrosarcoma, develops in fewer than 10% of patients. Patients should have, at minimum, an annual physical examination, including blood pressure check and thorough neurologic assessment. The gene has been identified and is a GTPase-activating protein involved in the ras signaling process. The gene is very large, and multiple different mutations have been identified. Therefore, DNA-based testing for direct diagnosis is difficult and usually not necessary unless prenatal diagnosis is desired.

- Neurofibromatosis 1 is autosomal dominant.
- The incidence is 1 in 3,500.
- The disorder has markedly variable expression but very high penetrance.
- Malignancy (often neurofibrosarcoma) develops in fewer than 10% of patients.
- Multiple different mutations have been identified.

Type 2
Neurofibromatosis 2 is an autosomal dominant disorder that is genetically distinct from neurofibromatosis 1. It is characterized by bilateral vestibular schwannomas (commonly referred to as *acoustic neuroma* in the past) or a family history of neurofibromatosis 2 with a unilateral vestibular schwannoma, or 2 of the following: meningioma, glioma, neurofibroma, schwannoma, or posterior subcapsular lenticular opacities. Spinal tumors occur in more than 60% of patients. Café au lait macules may or may not be present. The gene, referred to as *merlin*, is localized to chromosome 22q12. In addition to occurring in the germline of patients with neurofibromatosis 2, acquired mutations in this gene occur in some sporadic meningiomas and schwannomas. DNA-based diagnosis is available by direct mutation analysis in many patients. Patients should have an annual physical examination with thorough neurologic assessment, monitoring of hearing, and magnetic resonance imaging of the head with gadolinium. Magnetic resonance imaging of the spine should be done in patients with newly diagnosed disease or patients with symptoms referable to the spinal cord.

- Neurofibromatosis 2 is autosomal dominant.
- Characteristics: vestibular schwannomas, sometimes nervous system gliomas, subcapsular cataracts.

Osteogenesis Imperfecta
Osteogenesis imperfecta is characterized by multiple bone fractures. Multiple types exist, with defects in the α_1 or α_2 chains of type I collagen. The most common form is due to an autosomal dominant disorder with mild to moderate severity. Some patients have opalescent teeth, blue sclerae, hearing loss, and increased bruisability. Expression is extremely variable.

Tuberous Sclerosis
Tuberous sclerosis is an autosomal dominant disorder with variable expression and high penetrance. Approximately 50% of cases arise by new mutation. Tuberous sclerosis is characterized by subependymal nodules of the brain, cortical or retinal tubers, seizures, mental retardation in less than 50%, depigmented "ash leaf" or "confetti" macules, facial angiofibromas, dental pits, subungual or periungual fibromas, shagreen patches, and renal cysts or angiomyolipomas. Cardiac rhabdomyomas are more frequent in the fetus and infant and often resolve with age. Pulmonary fibrosis resulting in a honeycomb appearance on radiography or computed tomography is more frequent in young women and tends to progress rapidly. Central nervous system astrocytomas may occur. One gene defect that causes tuberous sclerosis is located on chromosome 9 (hamartin), and another is located on chromosome 16 (tuberin).

- Tuberous sclerosis is autosomal dominant and has high penetrance.
- About 50% of cases arise by new mutation.
- Typical case: cortical or retinal tubers, seizures, mental retardation in <50%, "ash leaf" macules, angiofibromas, subungual or periungual fibromas, shagreen patches, and renal cysts or angiomyolipomas.

Von Hippel-Lindau Disease
Von Hippel-Lindau disease is characterized by retinal, spinal cord, and cerebellar hemangioblastomas; cysts of the kidneys, pancreas, and epididymis; and renal cancers. Other manifestations include hemangioblastomas of the medulla oblongata, endolymphatic sac tumors, cysts and hemangiomas of other visceral organs, pancreatic cancer, and pheochromocytomas. Retinal hemangioblastomas may be the earliest manifestation. Annual ophthalmologic examination is important.

- Typical case: retinal, spinal cord, and cerebellar hemangioblastomas; cysts of kidneys, pancreas, and epididymis.
- Retinal hemangioblastomas may be the earliest manifestation of von Hippel-Lindau disease.

Hemangioblastomas of the central nervous system in von Hippel-Lindau disease are benign, and associated morbidity is due to space-occupying effects with associated cysts or syringomyelia. They occur most frequently in the cerebellum and spinal cord but also can be in the medulla oblongata and rarely in the cerebrum. Periodic magnetic resonance imaging with gadolinium is recommended.

Renal cysts, hemangiomas, and benign adenomas are usually asymptomatic but occasionally are extensive and mimic polycystic kidney disease. Renal clear cell cancers can develop within the cysts and are bilateral or multiple in 40% to 87% of cases. They are the leading cause of death, which occurs at a mean age of 44 years. Annual imaging of the kidneys is important. Solid tumors of 3 cm or larger should be removed with nephron-sparing and partial nephrectomy whenever possible.

- Renal cysts, hemangiomas, and benign adenomas are usually asymptomatic in von Hippel-Lindau disease.
- Renal cancer is a major cause of death.

Inheritance is autosomal dominant, and the risk for any child born to an affected person is 50%. Expression is variable, and penetrance is high in thoroughly evaluated families. Males and females are affected equally.

- Von Hippel-Lindau disease is autosomal dominant.

The gene that causes von Hippel-Lindau disease (*VHL*) is localized to chromosome 3p25-26. The normal gene has a key role in cellular response to hypoxia and acts as a tumor suppressor. Presymptomatic and prenatal diagnosis by direct mutation analysis is possible for most patients.

Autosomal Recessive

Autosomal recessive disease occurs because of abnormal genes that are located on the autosomes. However, 1 copy of the abnormal gene is not sufficient to cause disease, and heterozygotes (carriers) are not clinically different from the general population. When 2 persons who are heterozygotes for a given gene defect mate, the children are at 25% risk of inheriting the abnormal gene from both parents and, thus, of having the disease.

- Autosomal recessive inheritance: abnormal genes are located on autosomes, but 1 copy of the abnormal gene is not sufficient to cause disease.
- Heterozygotes (carriers) are not clinically different from the general population.

Because the heterozygous state may be transmitted silently through many generations before the chance mating of 2 heterozygotes occurs, it is not surprising that there rarely is a family history of the disease in previous generations. The occurrence of multiple affected siblings within a family suggests autosomal recessive inheritance; however, because of the small average family size in the United States, many autosomal recessive diseases seem to occur as isolated cases.

The risk for the children of a person who has an autosomal recessive disease depends on the frequency of the abnormal gene in the population. Except for common diseases such as cystic fibrosis or sickle cell anemia, the risk is usually small, provided that the person does not marry a relative or a person who has a family history of the same disease.

Many diseases that are caused by an identified metabolic defect, such as homocystinuria, are autosomal recessive diseases due to an enzyme deficiency. When the enzymatic or molecular defect is established, carrier testing and prenatal diagnosis sometimes are possible.

Some of the diseases with autosomal recessive inheritance are listed in Table 9-2 and summarized on the following pages.

Friedreich Ataxia

This is an autosomal recessive disorder. The first sign of the disease is ataxic gait. The mean age at onset is approximately 12 years. Dysarthria, hypotonic muscle weakness, loss of vibration and position senses, and loss of deep tendon reflexes develop subsequently. In some patients, diabetes mellitus, nystagmus, optic atrophy, dementia, respiratory dysfunction due to kyphoscoliosis, and decreased sensory nerve conduction velocities also develop. The major cause of death is cardiomyopathy. Since detection of the gene defect, many atypical cases have been recognized, such as older age at onset or preservation of deep tendon reflexes.

- Friedreich ataxia is autosomal recessive.
- Typical clinical scenario: A 12-year-old child presents with an ataxic gait, dysarthria, hypotonic muscle weakness, and loss of vibration and position senses, and loss of deep tendon reflexes develops subsequently.
- The major cause of death is cardiomyopathy.

In one series, 60 of 82 patients with Friedreich ataxia had clinical evidence of cardiac dysfunction 4 months to 4 years before death, and 56% died of heart failure. The mean age at death was 36.6 years. Cardiac arrhythmias, particularly atrial fibrillation, were common and occurred in 50% of fatal cases.

- Cardiac arrhythmias occur in 50% of fatal cases of Friedreich ataxia.

The risk for a sibling being affected is 25%. The gene involved, *FXN*, is localized to chromosome 9q13. The most frequent mechanism of mutation is expansion of a GAA trinucleotide repeat that results in abnormal accumulation of intramitochondrial iron.

- The risk of Friedreich ataxia in a sibling of an affected person is 25%.

Gaucher Disease

Gaucher disease is an autosomal recessive disorder due to deficiency of the enzyme glucocerebrosidase, which results in lipid storage in the spleen, liver, bone marrow, and other organs. Type 1 (nonneuronopathic) disease is most frequent in Ashkenazi Jews (carrier

Table 9-2   Examples of Diseases With Autosomal Recessive Inheritance

Alkaptonuria
α_1-Antitrypsin deficiency
Cystic fibrosis
Familial Mediterranean fever
Friedreich ataxia
Gaucher disease
Glycogen storage disease, types I, II, III, IV, V, VII
Hemochromatosis
Homocystinuria
Oculocutaneous albinism
Phenylketonuria
Pseudoxanthoma elasticum (some forms are autosomal dominant)
Refsum disease
Sickle cell disease
Tay-Sachs disease
α- and β-Thalassemia (severe forms)
Wilson disease

frequency, 1 in 10). The disease may be asymptomatic at any age or present in childhood or adulthood with splenomegaly, hepatosplenomegaly, thrombocytopenia, anemia, degenerative bone disease, osteoporosis, or pulmonary disease. Type 2 (infantile, neuronopathic) has no ethnic predisposition, and type 3 (juvenile form) has intermediate clinical signs. The first sign of neurologic involvement in types 2 and 3 is supranuclear ophthalmoplegia. Enzyme replacement therapy is effective for nonneuronopathic Gaucher disease.

- Gaucher disease is autosomal recessive.
- The disease is due to deficiency of the enzyme glucocerebrosidase.
- Type 1 is most frequent in Ashkenazi Jews.
- Type 2 has no ethnic predisposition.
- The first sign of neurologic involvement in types 2 and 3 is supranuclear ophthalmoplegia.
- Enzyme replacement therapy is effective for nonneuronopathic Gaucher disease.

Glycogen Storage Diseases
Glycogen storage disease type I is due to deficiency of the enzyme glucose-6-phosphatase. It is characterized by hypoglycemia, hypercholesterolemia, hyperuricemia, lactic acidosis, short stature, hepatomegaly, and delayed onset of puberty. In adults with this disease, malignant hepatomas, premature coronary disease, pancreatitis, gout, and renal disease may develop.

- Glycogen storage disease type I is due to deficiency of the enzyme glucose-6-phosphatase.
- Characteristics: hypoglycemia, hypercholesterolemia, hyperuricemia, lactic acidosis, short stature, hepatomegaly, delayed puberty.

Glycogen storage disease type II (Pompe disease) is an autosomal recessive disorder due to deficiency of the lysosomal enzyme α-1,4-glucosidase (acid maltase). The infantile form is characterized by hypotonia, macroglossia, and progressive cardiomyopathy resulting in death within the first year of life. Enzyme replacement therapy is available.

- Glycogen storage disease type II is autosomal recessive.
- The disease is due to deficiency of the enzyme α-1,4-glucosidase.
- Characteristics of infantile form: hypotonia, macroglossia, progressive cardiomyopathy.

Juvenile and adult forms of glycogen storage disease type II also exist. The presenting characteristic is skeletal muscle weakness, and cardiac involvement usually is absent or minimal.

- Characteristics of juvenile and adult forms of glycogen storage disease: skeletal muscle weakness, minimal or absent cardiac involvement.

Glycogen storage disease type III is due to an autosomal recessively inherited deficiency of amylo-1,6-glucosidase (debrancher) activity. The enzyme is deficient in the liver, and in some patients also in skeletal muscle, cultured skin fibroblasts, and leukocytes. Clinically, the disorder is characterized by hepatomegaly and growth retardation that resolves at puberty. There may be hypoglycemia and hyperlipidemia. Skeletal muscle weakness may develop in adult life. Cardiomyopathy, when present, may be life-threatening and mimic hypertrophic cardiomyopathy. However, histologic evaluation of cardiac tissue reveals increased intracellular glycogen with no disarray of myofibers or myofibrils. Deficiency of the enzyme has been documented in cardiac muscle.

- Glycogen storage disease type III is autosomal recessive.
- The disease is due to deficiency of amylo-1,6-glucosidase activity.
- Characteristics: hepatomegaly and growth retardation that resolves at puberty.

Homocystinuria
The classic form of homocystinuria is due to an autosomal recessively inherited deficiency of cystathionine β-synthase. The incidence of the disease is approximately 1 per 200,000. Clinically, it is characterized by tall stature with a low upper segment:lower segment ratio, pectus deformities, scoliosis, genu valgum, pes planus, and a highly arched palate. Lens dislocation is progressive, and the direction of displacement is usually, but not always, downward. Myopia, retinal detachment, secondary glaucoma, fair hair and skin, cutaneous flushing, and hernias may be present. Only 50% of affected persons have mental subnormality.

- The incidence of homocystinuria is about 1 per 200,000.
- Typical case: tall stature, pectus deformities, scoliosis, genu valgum, pes planus, highly arched palate, lens dislocation.
- Lens dislocation is progressive.

Cardiovascular abnormalities include arterial or venous thrombosis, coronary occlusions at a young age, renal artery narrowing resulting in hypertension and renal atrophy, cerebrovascular accidents, thrombophlebitis, and pulmonary emboli. Dilatation of the pulmonary artery and left atrial endocardial fibroelastosis have been reported. Thrombi are particularly likely to occur after operation, venipuncture, or catheterization, and they are more common in persons who also have factor V Leiden deficiency.

* Cardiovascular abnormalities of homocystinuria: arterial or venous thrombosis and coronary occlusions at a young age.
* Thrombi are likely after operation, venipuncture, or catheterization.

Histologic examination of the arteries shows marked fibrous thickening of the intima. Aortic intimal fibrosis may be severe enough to mimic coarctation. Medial changes consist of thrombosis and dilatation with widely spaced, frayed muscle fibers. The elastic fibers of the large arteries may be fragmented, and dilatation of the ascending aorta has been observed.

The disease sometimes may be diagnosed from positive results of urinary nitroprusside test and confirmed by quantitative urinary homocystine determination. Levels of plasma homocysteine and its precursor, methionine, are increased. Testing of the plasma homocysteine level is the most sensitive, with levels of 50 to 200 µmol/L. This should not be confused with the lesser increases that occur in hyperhomocysteinemia. The goal of treatment is to lower the plasma homocysteine level, which seems to result in slower progression and fewer symptoms of the disease; 50% of patients respond to pyridoxine therapy (25-1,000 mg/day). Supplemental folate also should be given because patients who are potentially capable of responding to pyridoxine may not do so in the presence of folate deficiency. A low-protein, low-methionine diet can be useful, but adults find it difficult to comply with this. For infants, a low-methionine formula is available. Betaine is of benefit for decreasing plasma homocysteine levels.

* In homocystinuria, levels of plasma homocysteine and its precursor, methionine, are increased.
* The goal of treatment is to lower the plasma homocysteine level.

Mild hyperhomocysteinemia, sometimes associated with polymorphisms in methylenetetrahydrofolate reductase, is believed to be a risk factor for atherosclerosis but is a different condition.

Pseudoxanthoma Elasticum

Pseudoxanthoma elasticum is usually autosomal recessive. It is characterized by yellowish skin papules, especially on the neck and flexural areas, angioid streaks and choroiditis of the retina, and vascular complications, including angina pectoris, claudication, calcification of peripheral arteries, and renal vascular hypertension. The defective gene is *ABCC6* located on chromosome 16p13.1.

* Characteristics of pseudoxanthoma elasticum: yellowish skin papules, angioid streaks and choroiditis of retina, and vascular complications.

Refsum Disease

Refsum disease is an autosomal recessive neurodegenerative disease characterized by cerebellar ataxia, hypertrophic polyneuropathy, and retinitis pigmentosa. Deafness, ichthyosis, and cardiac conduction defects are frequently present.

* Refsum disease is autosomal recessive.
* Typical case: cerebellar ataxia, hypertrophic polyneuropathy, retinitis pigmentosa.
* Frequently present: deafness, ichthyosis, cardiac conduction defects.

Phytanic acid is a fatty acid present in dairy products and fat from grazing animals. Patients with Refsum disease are deficient in the catabolic enzyme phytanic acid α-hydroxylase, which results in accumulation of ingested phytanic acid in fatty deposits in the involved organ systems.

* Patients with Refsum disease are deficient in phytanic acid α-hydroxylase.

Dietary restriction of phytanic acid results in clinical improvement and stabilization of the disease. Electrocardiographic changes sometimes resolve after treatment. Plasmapheresis removes phytanic acid from the body and may allow liberalization of the diet; it can be extremely valuable in the management of acutely ill patients.

Tay-Sachs Disease

Tay-Sachs disease is an autosomal recessive disease due to deficiency of hexosaminidase A. The classic infantile form of the disease is rapidly fatal and is due to storage of ganglioside GM_2 in neural tissue. It is particularly common in people of Ashkenazi Jewish ancestry; the carrier frequency is 1 in 30. Therefore, screening for carriers by determination of enzyme activity in serum (or leukocytes, particularly in pregnant women, in whom the serum level is unreliable) is recommended in this population. Prenatal diagnosis is available when both the mother and the father are carriers.

In late-onset disease, the mean age at onset is 18 years, and loss of balance is the most frequent chief complaint. Cerebellar atrophy is almost always present. Anterior motor neuron involvement and psychotic episodes are also common.

* Tay-Sachs disease is autosomal recessive.
* The disease is due to deficiency of hexosaminidase A.

X-Linked Recessive

X-linked recessive diseases are caused by abnormal genes located on the X chromosome. Female heterozygotes who have 1 abnormal gene on 1 X chromosome and 1 normal gene on the other X chromosome usually are clinically normal. Exceptions may occur because of the phenomenon of lyonization, in which one X chromosome is inactivated at random early in fetal life; if the normal gene is inactivated in a critical number of cells, the woman may have symptoms or clinical signs of the disease. However, the disease usually is less severe than in males. The likelihood of clinical signs of the disease developing in a female varies by disease. For example, it is rare for female carriers of hemophilia A (factor VIII deficiency) to have severe bleeding problems, but it is relatively common for carriers of ornithine carbamoyltransferase (ornithine transcarbamoylase) deficiency to have intermittent symptoms.

- X-linked recessive diseases are caused by abnormal genes on the X chromosome.
- The development of clinical signs of the disease in a female varies by disease.

Males who inherit the abnormal gene have no corresponding genetic loci on the Y chromosome and therefore are referred to as *hemizygotes*. Any male child born to a heterozygous female is at 50% risk for having the disease; female children are at 50% risk for inheriting the gene and being carriers. All the daughters of affected males are carriers, and all the sons are unaffected (ie, male-to-male transmission cannot occur).

- Males with the abnormal gene are called *hemizygotes*.
- A male child of a heterozygous female has a 50% risk of having the disease.
- A female child is at 50% risk of inheriting the gene.

X-linked recessive diseases also may arise by new mutation affecting either the mother or the afflicted son. Genetic counseling is difficult in these situations because if the mother represents the new mutation the risk for her future male children is 50%. However, if the child represents the new mutation, there is no significant risk for siblings of that child. DNA-based diagnosis allows for carrier detection for many diseases, which circumvents problems created by lyonization.

Some of the conditions with X-linked recessive inheritance are listed in Table 9-3 and summarized on the following pages.

Duchenne and Becker Muscular Dystrophies

Duchenne muscular dystrophy is one of the most common types of muscular dystrophy; its incidence is approximately 1 in 3,500 newborn males. Approximately a third of the cases arise by new mutation. Progressive skeletal weakness beginning at 2 to 5 years of age, with death in the late teens or 20s, is characteristic. Becker muscular dystrophy has later onset. The diagnosis is made on the basis of clinical findings and a markedly increased creatine kinase level. The muscle biopsy histologic findings are relatively nonspecific, but immunohistochemistry testing for dystrophin reveals deficiency.

- The incidence of Duchenne muscular dystrophy is 1 in 3,500 newborn males.
- Duchenne muscular dystrophy is X-linked recessive.
- Skeletal weakness at 2-5 years of age is characteristic.
- Becker muscular dystrophy has later onset.

The genetic defect that results in both Duchenne and Becker muscular dystrophies involves the dystrophin gene located on chromosome X at band p21. More than 85% of patients have a detectable gene abnormality on various molecular techniques. The dystrophin gene is very large, consisting of at least 60 exons and 1,800 kilobases. The protein product of this gene, dystrophin, is a rod-shaped cytoskeletal protein that is predominantly localized to the surface membrane of striated muscle cells. Identification of the molecular defect has resulted in improved ability to determine carrier status in female relatives by DNA analysis. This is a considerable improvement over carrier testing by measurement of creatine kinase levels, because levels are increased in only 70% of obligate carriers. DNA analysis also can be used for prenatal diagnosis. All males with Becker muscular dystrophy and the first-degree relatives of patients with Duchenne or Becker muscular dystrophy should have genetic counseling.

- Families in which Duchenne or Becker muscular dystrophy is present need genetic counseling.

The heart disease in patients with Duchenne or Becker muscular dystrophy is characterized by extensive changes in systolic time intervals, suggestive of compromised left ventricular function. There are histologic changes characterized by multifocal dystrophic areas with fibrosis and loss of myofilaments. These changes are most marked in the posterobasal segment and contiguous lateral and inferior walls of the left ventricle. Some families with dystrophin defects have dilated cardiomyopathy with or without serious skeletal muscle weakness.

- The heart disease in dystrophinopathies involves changes in systolic time intervals and dilated cardiomyopathy.

Fabry Disease

Fabry disease is a lysosomal storage disease due to deficiency of α-galactosidase A. Females may have less severe signs of the disease than males. Glycosphingolipids accumulate in the endothelium, perithelium (layers of connective tissue that surround the capillaries and small blood vessels), and smooth muscle of blood vessels. There is also accumulation in ganglion cells, myocardial cells, reticuloendothelial cells, and connective tissue cells.

- Fabry disease is due to deficiency of α-galactosidase A.
- The disease is X-linked recessive.
- Females may have less severe signs of the disease than males.

Acroparesthesias and episodes of severe burning pain in the palms and soles with proximal radiation may occur in childhood and adolescence. The first signs of the disease may be telangiectatic angiokeratomas

Table 9-3   Examples of Diseases With X-Linked Recessive Inheritance

Adrenoleukodystrophy (*ABCD1*: ATP-binding cassette subfamily D, member 1)
Chronic granulomatous disease (many cases; autosomal recessive forms are less common)
Color blindness
Duchenne & Becker muscular dystrophies
Fabry disease
Glucose-6-phosphate dehydrogenase deficiency
Hemophilia A & B
Ocular albinism
Rickets, hypophosphatemic
Testicular feminization

Abbreviation: ATP, adenosine triphosphate.

of the skin and mucous membranes. Sweating is impaired, and patients may have recurrent abdominal pain with fevers. Whorl-shaped corneal opacities and cataracts develop. In adulthood, cardiovascular and renal diseases are the major causes of morbidity and mortality. Enzyme replacement therapy is available.

- The first signs of Fabry disease may be telangiectatic angiokeratomas of skin and mucous membranes.
- Acroparesthesias may occur in childhood and adolescence.
- Whorl-shaped corneal opacities and cataracts develop.
- In adults, cardiovascular and renal diseases develop.

Mitochondrial Mutations

Mitochondria each contain several circular copies of their own genetic material, mitochondrial DNA. This mitochondrial DNA is approximately 16,000 base pairs in length and encodes for transfer RNAs and 13 protein subunits of the mitochondrial respiratory chain. Many mitochondrial enzymes, including most others of the respiratory chain complex, are encoded by nuclear DNA and transported into the mitochondria. Mitochondrial DNA mutations cause Leber optic atrophy and the multisystem syndromes of mitochondrial myopathy, encephalopathy, episodes of lactic acidosis, and stroke (MELAS), myoclonic epilepsy with ragged red fibers (MERRF), and neuropathy, ataxia, and retinitis pigmentosa (NARP). Many cases of Kearns-Sayre syndrome (cardiomyopathy and ophthalmoplegia) are due to mitochondrial deletions. Clinically, they are very diverse and do not always conform to these well-delineated syndromes. For example, diabetes mellitus type 2 with sensorineural hearing loss or cardiomyopathy also may occur with the classic MERRF mutation. Lactic acidosis in peripheral blood or cerebrospinal fluid and ragged red fibers may or may not be present in the mitochondrial disorders. Mitochondrial disorders can arise as new mutations or be maternally inherited; in most cases, only the egg contributes mitochondria that persist in the zygote, and the sperm usually does not. Mitochondrial mutations may be homoplasmic (present in all mitochondrial DNA) or heteroplasmic (present in only some of the mitochondrial DNA).

- Mitochondrial DNA mutations cause Leber optic atrophy and multisystem syndromes.
- Many cases of Kearns-Sayre syndrome are due to mitochondrial deletions.
- Usually, only the egg contributes mitochondria that persist in the zygote.

Multifactorial Causation

Multifactorial means that the disease or trait is determined by the interaction of environmental influences and a polygenic (many gene) predisposition. Human conditions that may have multifactorial causation include many common birth defects—such as congenital heart defects, cleft lip and palate, and neural tube defects—and many common diseases—such as diabetes mellitus, asthma, hypertension, and coronary artery atherosclerosis.

- Multifactorial causation: disease or trait is due to environmental influences and a polygenic predisposition.
- Birth defects that may have multifactorial causation: congenital heart defects, cleft lip and palate, neural tube defects.
- Diseases that may have multifactorial causation: diabetes mellitus, asthma, hypertension, coronary artery atherosclerosis.

The multifactorial model predicts that there will be a tendency for familial aggregation of the condition but without a strict mendelian pattern of inheritance. Familial aggregation also can be due to common environmental factors; thus, familial aggregation by itself is not sufficient to prove multifactorial causation.

Because familial aggregation exists for multifactorial disorders, it is implicit that the occurrence risk will be increased for members of an affected family over that of the general population. As expected, the risk is highest for first-degree relatives (parents, siblings, children), who have half of their genes in common. The risk is less for second-degree relatives (grandparents, aunts, uncles, grandchildren, nephews, nieces), who share one-quarter of their genes. The risk decreases exponentially thereafter; third-degree relatives (great-grandparents, cousins, great-grandchildren) share only one-eighth of their genes. Empiric (observed) risk figures for some well-studied multifactorial disorders fit well with the predicted risks.

The genetic liability in multifactorial causation is due to the cumulative effect of many genes, each having a small effect, rather than to the effect of one major gene. These genes create a liability that presumably is continuously distributed within the population. If the genetic liability is strong enough, under an unfortunate set of environmental circumstances the disorder will occur.

- Genetic liability in multifactorial causation is due to the cumulative effect of many genes.

For many multifactorial conditions, there is a difference in predilection between males and females which could result directly from genetic differences or from different internal (eg, hormonal) or external environmental factors. Furthermore, if a member of the less commonly affected sex has the condition, his or her genetic liability was probably greater and therefore the risk for his or her relatives is greater. Similarly, if a person has a more severe form of the disease, the risk for relatives is higher. For disorders in which disease frequency increases with age, earlier onset sometimes implies a greater risk for relatives. Finally, the greater the number of affected individuals within the family, the higher the risk for other relatives. There also are racial differences in the frequency of many disorders of multifactorial causation.

Premature coronary atherosclerosis provides a well-known example of these concepts and thus makes them easy to remember. Multiple genetic and environmental risk factors, such as high level of low-density lipoprotein cholesterol, low level of high-density lipoprotein cholesterol, obesity, diabetes, and smoking, predispose to atherosclerosis. The risk for coronary disease in the siblings of an affected 50-year-old woman is greater than that for a similarly affected man of the same age, particularly if the disease is severe in the 50-year-old woman. A positive family history, regardless of cholesterol levels, is also a risk factor, such that multiple affected relatives indicate a higher risk.

When the inheritance pattern of any disease is being determined, the possibility of genetic heterogeneity always must be considered. For example, there are both autosomal dominant and multifactorial causes of atrial septal defect which may be indistinguishable clinically. Failure to recognize that different genetic diseases can cause the same or similar clinical entities can result in confusion when determining risks.

Table 9-4 lists some conditions of multifactorial causation.

Diagnosis of Genetic Disease by DNA Analysis

Diagnosis of genetic diseases with peripheral blood specimens or specimens obtained by amniocentesis or chorionic villus sampling has become a routine part of clinical practice because of the identification of the basic genetic defect underlying numerous mendelian conditions and the capability for direct DNA diagnosis. Because individual genes are too small to be seen microscopically, standard chromosome analysis generally is not helpful even when the gene has been localized to a specific chromosome region.

Importance of an Accurate Clinical Diagnosis and Family History

Molecular genetic testing can be used for diagnosing a disorder in a patient who is suspected of having a specific disease. It also can be used for testing relatives who are at risk. The importance of a correct diagnosis in the index patient when diagnosis by DNA analysis for a relative is being contemplated cannot be overemphasized. This criterion is in contrast to many instances of genetic diagnosis by chromosome analysis in which the cytogeneticist usually can be relied on to note most abnormalities (fragile X and subtle deletions are examples of exceptions) regardless of the exact indication for the study. This approach is possible because the procedure of chromosome analysis involves examination of all 46 chromosomes in a given cell to look for gross structural changes. In contrast, it is impossible to systematically examine each of a person's 30,000 or more genes to detect all abnormalities.

* It is impossible to systematically examine each of a person's 30,000 genes.

The laboratory's process of detection of even one abnormal gene must be directed by the precise clinical diagnosis. The DNA-based assays are specific for the disease being studied, and abnormalities elsewhere in the genome will not be detected. Thus, if the incorrect assay is chosen because of an incorrect clinical diagnosis, the disease-causing mutation will not be detected. For example, if a patient is at risk for hypertrophic cardiomyopathy on the basis of a positive family history, it is important to know the exact molecular defect in an affected family member before molecular testing of the asymptomatic patient. Defects in multiple genes can cause hypertrophic cardiomyopathy, and others remain undiscovered. A normal result in an asymptomatic patient at risk, without the exact molecular diagnosis in the family, could mean either that the patient did not inherit the gene defect or that the gene defect in this particular family is not detectable by the selected tests.

In sporadic cases, the molecular diagnosis often can be established only for diseases for which direct DNA diagnosis is possible. In contrast, in families with multiple affected members, direct DNA diagnosis is the first choice when possible, followed by linkage analysis if the mutation cannot be directly identified. In these cases, an accurate family pedigree is essential. Diagnosis by linkage can be used only when there is no significant locus heterogeneity. For example, most patients with autosomal dominant polycystic kidney disease have a gene defect in *PKD1* on chromosome 16. However, up to 10% of families have a phenotypically similar disease due to a different, nonallelic genetic mutation. Thus, if a person who has a parent with polycystic kidney disease wants to know if he or she has inherited the gene defect, it should first be established whether the exact mutation can be found in the affected parent. There are numerous other examples of this type of genetic heterogeneity, including retinitis pigmentosa, spinocerebellar ataxias, and Charcot-Marie-Tooth disease.

Because of the rapid advances made in molecular genetics in the past several years, the genetic bases of many diseases are identified and new techniques for molecular diagnosis have become available. Therefore, linkage analysis now is rarely used for clinical diagnosis.

* Genetic heterogeneity can confound DNA studies.
* DNA-based diagnoses cannot be used for all families, even when DNA tests for a specific disease are available.

Southern Blot Procedure

After a patient's DNA has been extracted from peripheral blood lymphocytes, subjected to enzyme cutting, and electrophoresed to separate different sizes of DNA fragments, a radioactive probe for the disease gene or for the marker DNA segments is applied and hybridizes to the complementary DNA sequences of interest. The fragments then can be visualized on x-ray film. An example of linkage analysis by Southern blotting in a family with Duchenne muscular dystrophy is shown in Figure 9-4.

In addition to linkage analysis, Southern blotting can be used in some cases for direct detection of deletion or duplication types of mutations, or for single-base mutations if the enzyme restriction site is directly altered by the mutation. An example of direct detection of a deletion in a patient with Duchenne muscular dystrophy is shown in Figure 9-5.

Table 9-4   Conditions of Multifactorial Causation

Atherosclerosis
Atopic disease, allergy
Cancer
Cardiac malformations
Cleft lip & palate
Diabetes mellitus
Hypertension
Neural tube defects
Schizophrenia

Polymerase Chain Reaction

Polymerase chain reaction (PCR) has had great impact on clinical practice and involves replication of a specific, relatively small segment of DNA in an exponential fashion, so that up to a billion copies are produced. One uses known DNA sequences from within the area of interest, and these known DNA sequences allow creation of synthetic oligonucleotides that serve as primers to hybridize with the patient's DNA sequence to initiate the amplification process (Figure 9-6).

The multiple copies of the DNA segment that are produced by PCR then can be identified by various techniques, including direct visualization after gel electrophoresis. This allows detection of mutations in the patient's DNA. For example, PCR can be used for detection of mutations in specific regions of the dystrophin gene for the diagnosis of Duchenne muscular dystrophy and other diseases. Many automated DNA analysis techniques are available for more rapid clinical diagnosis.

Diseases Amenable to DNA Diagnosis

The number of diseases that can be diagnosed with DNA analysis is increasing as additional disease genes are localized or identified and cloned. The physician who encounters a clinical situation for the first time which may be amenable to DNA-based diagnosis should discuss the testing procedure and its limitations with the laboratory personnel or a geneticist familiar with the details of the specific disease testing before a detailed discussion of the presymptomatic or prenatal diagnosis with the patient. Ideally, these discussions should take place before a woman becomes pregnant.

Diagnosis by Fluorescent In Situ Hybridization

Fluorescent in situ hybridization (FISH) is a cytogenetic technique that is being used with increasing frequency for diagnosis of certain congenital and malignant disorders. The technique uses DNA probes homologous to the DNA area of interest within the chromosome so the probe binds the DNA segment of interest. The DNA probe is labeled with a fluorophore so it can be visualized under the microscope. The probe can be designed to bind to a discrete region of a chromosome, as in the case of Sphrintzen velocardiofacial syndrome. This syndrome is caused by a microdeletion (ie, a deletion otherwise too small to be seen under the microscope) (Figure 9-3). It is relatively common; the estimated frequency is approximately 1 in 4,000. This syndrome is characterized by a variable combination of subaverage intellect, a characteristic facial appearance, velopharyngeal incompetence resulting in nasal speech, cleft palate,

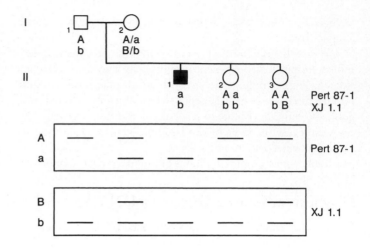

Figure 9-4. Representation of a family segregating for Duchenne muscular dystrophy and data for 2 probes that detect restriction fragment length polymorphism, Pert 87-1 and XJ 1.1. Bottom half of figure represents Southern blot analysis of these 2 probes with arbitrary designation of alleles A/a for Pert 87-1 and B/b for XJ 1.1. Square indicates normal male; circle, female; shaded symbol, affected individual. Sister II.3 of affected male II.1 inherited Ab haplotype from her father and AB haplotype from her mother. Because her brother has ab haplotype, it can be predicted that she is not a carrier and her fetus is not at increased risk. Although sister II.2 did inherit the ab haplotype, it cannot be determined with certainty that she is a carrier because it is not known whether the mutation arose in the brother or whether the mother is a carrier. Sister II.2 could elect prenatal diagnosis, with the realization that males who inherit the ab haplotype might be affected or unaffected, whereas those who inherit the Ab haplotype would most likely be unaffected.

mild-to-moderate hearing loss, predisposition to dental caries, congenital heart defect (especially tetralogy of Fallot), and increased risk for hypocalcemia. Many patients are so mildly affected that the syndrome is not diagnosed until they have a more severely affected child.

DNA probes also can be designed to "paint" an entire chromosome (whole chromosome paints) and are helpful for defining complex chromosome rearrangements, as can occur in some malignancies. Less commonly, DNA FISH probes can be used to identify single gene defects such as hereditary neuropathy with liability to pressure palsies due to deletion of peripheral myelin protein 22 on chromosome 17p11.2, or Charcot-Marie-Tooth disease type I due to a duplication of this gene.

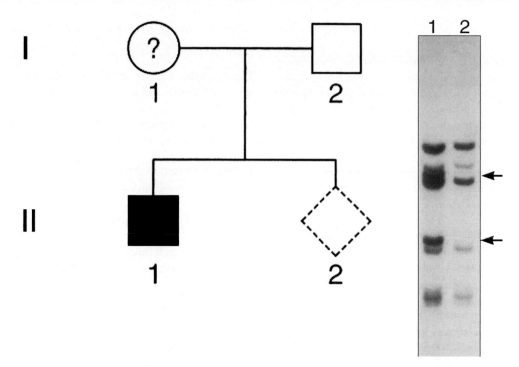

Figure 9-5. Mother (I.1) of this patient (II.1) with sporadic Duchenne muscular dystrophy wanted to know whether she was a carrier or whether a new mutation had occurred in her son because of her concern for the risk for future children. Southern blot analysis detected a deletion in her son (II.1) (lane 2 as compared with control in lane 1). By densitometry, the mother seemed to have less than the expected amount of DNA (not shown) corresponding to her son's deletion. Thus, she was determined to be a carrier for the dystrophy and can be offered specific prenatal diagnosis. If no deletion had been detectable (by various methods), then her carrier status could not have been determined.

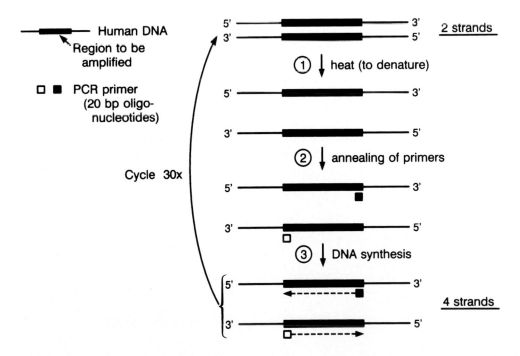

Figure 9-6. Polymerase chain reaction (PCR) is used to make multiple copies of a short segment of the DNA of interest. DNA from the patient is denatured to single-stranded DNA in the presence of oligonucleotide primers. DNA sequences of these primers are made to specification to anneal with DNA sequences on both sides of the DNA segment of interest. DNA between these primers is then synthesized, and the entire process can be repeated automatically.

Glossary

Array-based comparative genomic hybridization: Technique using microarrays of large insert clones that can detect deletions or duplications that are tens to hundreds of kilobases in size (ie, below the level of discrimination of a banded karyoptye).

Autosome: A chromosome other than a sex chromosome.

Chromosome: Long strands of double-stranded DNA that encode genes and that are associated with a protein framework. A normal human has 46 chromosomes per cell.

Deletion: Structural abnormality in which part of a chromosome is missing.

Duplication: Structural abnormality in which an extra copy of part of a chromosome is present.

Epigenetic: Effect on the phenotype or gene expression that does not involve the DNA sequence.

Gene: A portion of DNA molecule that codes for a specific RNA or protein product.

Hemizygote: A person who has a gene form on 1 chromosome but no homologous chromosome with a corresponding gene site. The term usually refers to males because they have only 1 X chromosome.

Heterozygote: A person who has different gene forms at a given site on 2 homologous chromosomes.

Homozygote: A person who has the same gene forms at a given site on 2 homologous chromosomes.

Inversion: Structural abnormality characterized by reversal of a segment within the chromosome.

Karyotype: The chromosome complement of an individual person.

Linkage (genetic linkage): Physical proximity of 2 gene loci on the same chromosome such that segregation is nonrandom.

Phenotype: The observable biochemical or physical characteristics of an individual as determined by genetic material and environment.

Proband: The index patient.

Recurrence: Occurrence of another case of a specific condition in the same family.

Translocation: Structural abnormality characterized by transfer of a piece of 1 chromosome to another chromosome.

Questions

Multiple Choice (choose the best answer)

1. An 18-year-old man is brought in by his parents for medical evaluation because he has mental subnormality (IQ 60) of unknown cause, and they want to seek legal guardianship. He has a maternal uncle who also is mentally subnormal and 2 healthy teenage sisters. His physical examination shows a long face with large ears and large testicles, but results of the rest of the examination are satisfactory. The parents think his mental deficiency is due to the umbilical cord being wrapped around his neck at birth, and he has had no other investigations to determine the cause. What is a reasonable course of action?

    a. Perform routine health maintenance evaluations only.
    b. Perform routine health maintenance evaluations and chromosome analysis only.
    c. Perform routine health maintenance evaluations and chromosome analysis and cytogenetic fragile X analysis.
    d. Perform routine health maintenance evaluations and chromosome analysis and molecular fragile X analysis.
    e. Perform routine health maintenance evaluations and linkage analysis involving the maternal uncle, parents, and patient.

2. A 24-year-old woman presents for evaluation after the birth of her first child, who was born hypotonic and has poor feeding. She reports that she is exhausted and that her hands cramp after holding and feeding the baby. What diagnosis is most important to make or exclude?

    a. Panic attacks
    b. Myotonic dystrophy
    c. Marfan syndrome
    d. Homocystinuria
    e. Von Hippel-Lindau disease

3. A healthy woman has a brother and son who both have Fabry disease. The level of her α-galactosidase is within normal limits. Select the appropriate explanation.

    a. The woman is an obligate heterozygote, and her normal enzyme level can be explained by X-chromosome lyonization.
    b. The woman's normal enzyme level proves that she is not heterozygous for Fabry disease.
    c. Fabry disease is autosomal dominant, and she represents an example of incomplete penetrance.
    d. Fabry disease is autosomal dominant, and she represents an example of variable penetrance.
    e. The woman has no clinical or biochemical signs of Fabry disease because a crossover event occurred during meiosis.

4. A 60-year-old woman presents with bone pains, splenomegaly, and thrombocytopenia. She is of Ashkenazi Jewish ancestry, and her enzyme level of glucocerebrosidase is deficient. The first treatment to be suggested should be:

    a. Splenectomy
    b. Splenectomy and enzyme therapy
    c. Enzyme therapy
    d. Enzyme and substrate reduction therapy
    e. Substrate reduction therapy

5. An 18-year-old woman with short stature presents with primary amenorrhea. To evaluate for possible Turner syndrome, the most appropriate genetic test is:

    a. Peripheral blood karyotype
    b. Peripheral blood fluorescent in situ hybridization (FISH)
    c. Bone marrow karyotype
    d. Skin fibroblast FISH
    e. Ovarian biopsy FISH

6. A 45-year-old man with von Hippel-Lindau disease has unilateral renal cancer. The tumor is 3.2 cm in size. The most appropriate treatment is:

    a. Unilateral nephrectomy
    b. Chemotherapy
    c. Radiation therapy
    d. Bilateral nephrectomy because additional renal cancers are almost certainly present
    e. Segmental nephrectomy

7. A 21-year-old man presents with painful paresthesias of the feet dating from late childhood. As part of his evaluation, you note that his creatinine level is increased to 1.9 mg/dL. What test would you consider first to make a diagnosis that explains these findings?

    a. Determination of serum iron with percentage saturation
    b. Mitochondrial DNA analysis
    c. DNA analysis for the Fabry gene
    d. DNA analysis for myotonic dystrophy
    e. Determination of serum α-galactosidase level

Answers

1. Answer d.

The mentally subnormal patient who has a similarly affected maternal uncle suggests, but does not prove, a pattern of X-linked inheritance. Chromosome analysis is indicated to look for a microscopically visible unbalanced chromosome abnormality that could be transmitted through a parent who is a carrier of a balanced form of the abnormality. The clinical abnormalities of fragile X are not specific enough to exclude some other type of chromosome abnormality. One of the most common causes of X-linked subnormality is fragile X-linked mental retardation. Although sometimes fragile sites can be seen on standard cytogenetic analysis, they are visible in only a small proportion of cells; depending on culture conditions, they may not always be evident. The more specific and sensitive test for fragile X-linked mental subnormality is molecular DNA analysis. Linkage studies would be inappropriate in this family 1) because of the small number of affected individuals and 2) because one would not know which locus to track. It is important to know the specific diagnosis in this family, in part because the healthy sisters could be carriers.

2. Answer b.

A consideration of panic attacks is reasonable, but first a diagnosis of myotonic dystrophy should be considered and can be easily tested for by determining whether percussion or grip myotonia is present. If there is any abnormality, the diagnosis can be confirmed in most cases by molecular analysis.

3. Answer a.

Fabry disease is X-linked. Heterozygous females may or may not have disease. If random X inactivation occurs in each cell (lyonization), a female may have symptoms or signs (although usually milder than males). Normal enzyme levels in blood do not completely exclude any manifestation of disease in a female, but they make it much less likely (hence, the usefulness of enzyme replacement therapy for Fabry disease).

4. Answer c.

Splenectomy removes a site for storage of material and therefore can worsen disease in other organs. Enzyme therapy is helpful for reducing storage in the spleen and improving platelet counts. Substrate reduction therapy with miglustat is approved by the US Food and Drug Administration only for persons who cannot tolerate enzyme therapy.

5. Answer a.

A peripheral blood chromosome analysis (karyotype) results in a diagnosis in the great majority of cases, without a need for more invasive testing. Karyotype is better than FISH because an abnormal X chromosome, such as an isoXq, can cause Turner syndrome and show an X signal by FISH, resulting in a missed diagnosis. FISH or analysis of other tissues may be helpful when karyotype on blood is normal and mosaicism is strongly suspected.

6. Answer e.

The renal cancers of von Hippel-Lindau disease are unlikely to metastasize when less than 3.0 cm in size. However, larger lesions can metastasize and should be definitively treated by surgical removal. Although subsequent renal cancers may develop, overall general health is best maintained by preserving renal function as long as possible, along with careful annual surveillance for new tumors.

7. Answer e.

A diagnosis of Fabry disease should be considered in a man with paresthesias or decreased renal function. A simple and quick enzyme assay can be used for diagnosis in males, who are hemizygotes for this gene on the X chromosome, and can allow for earlier initiation of treatment. Molecular analysis takes longer and is more expensive, but it may be a useful next step in the rare case of ambiguity by enzyme assay or for purposes of genetic counseling for female siblings, children, and other relatives.

10

Geriatrics

Margaret Beliveau Ficalora, MD

Geriatric Assessment

The assessment of elderly patients should differ from that of younger adults. The overall function of elderly patients is influenced by factors other than their medical diagnoses. When the medical problems of elderly patients are assessed, it is important to assess additional factors: functional status, cognitive capacity, financial resources, and the safety and appropriateness of their domicile. It also is wise to address advance directives with all geriatric patients. Appropriate preventive screening should be a part of the assessment of the elderly who are in good health.

In addition to an evaluation for conditions common to the geriatric population, such as heart disease, hypertension, diabetes mellitus, arthritis, and renal insufficiency, it is important to assess for conditions that can have a negative effect on function, such as impairment of vision or hearing (or both), mobility status, urinary incontinence, risk of falling, nutrition, and cognitive status. A thorough review of medications taken (prescription, herbal, and over-the-counter) is important.

- The overall function of elderly patients is influenced by factors other than medical problems.
- For elderly patients, it is important to assess functional status, cognitive capacity, financial resources, and the safety and appropriateness of their domicile.

Because the assessment of geriatric patients includes additional spheres of evaluation, the physician needs to become more efficient in the evaluation process. Previous medical records, paraprofessional interviews, screening tests, and patient questionnaires become valuable tools to expedite the history taking, thus allowing more time to focus on examining the patient and educating the patient on maintaining and improving function. These tools can decrease substantially the time required by the physician to obtain a thorough history, thus allowing the physician to concentrate on the physical examination and patient education about maintaining and improving function. A thorough geriatric assessment should include the following areas: vision, hearing, nutrition, continence, mobility and balance, medications, cognitive status, affect, functional status, frailty, social support, and advance directives.

Vision

Essentially all elderly patients have presbyopia, and the physician should determine whether the patient has access to proper assistive devices (reading glasses, magnifiers, and adequate light) to read. Assessment for other major eye diseases should be performed, including glaucoma, macular degeneration, and cataracts, because all these conditions increase in frequency with age and can markedly impair functional status.

Hearing

Impaired hearing is common among the elderly. In addition to periodic audiometric testing, it is important to ask the spouse or other family members if they are aware of the patient having any marked hearing loss. Patients often deny or minimize the symptoms of hearing impairment. Hearing impairment in the elderly is associated with decreased physical, social, and cognitive function. Improved hearing through the use of amplification devices improves the functional status of elderly persons. Only 50% of elderly patients who would benefit from hearing aids actually use them.

Nutrition

Both undernutrition and obesity are common nutritional problems among the elderly and increase the risk of morbidity, mortality, and reduced functional status. Elderly patients should be asked about any weight changes during the past 3 months, and they should be weighed at every physician visit. Height should be checked annually. These measurements allow calculation of body mass index (weight in kilograms/height in meters squared). Laboratory markers that reflect undernutrition and have been correlated with increased mortality among the elderly include hypoalbuminemia and low serum levels of cholesterol.

Continence

Urinary incontinence is common among the elderly, especially older women. Incontinence impairs social function and is a common reason for nursing home placement. Most elderly assume that incontinence is normal and will not bring up the issue of urinary incontinence with their physician. Therefore, it is important for physicians to ask patients about urinary incontinence.

Mobility and Balance
Impaired balance and mobility can reduce functional independence and are major risks for falls. Falls may also signify cardiac or neurologic dysfunction and may have serious sequelae. The patient should be asked about any recent falls and the circumstances surrounding them. The physician can perform simple tests of balance and gait. Lower extremity range of motion and strength should be assessed.

Medications
Polypharmacy is common among the elderly and can lead to serious drug-drug interactions and complications from adverse drug reactions. Patients should be asked about the medications they take, including prescription and nonprescription drugs and herbal products. Patients should be instructed to bring with them to the office all the medications they currently are taking or have taken recently so the physician can review them. The need for the medication, its dosage, and potential to cause harm or to interact with other medications should be assessed. Also, consideration should be given to whether 1 medication may be substituted for 2 or more drugs.

Cognitive Status
Although cognitive impairment is obvious in some elderly, it may be difficult to diagnose in others, especially when mild. Cognitive impairment is more common with advancing age, and the screening yield is highest among those older than 85 years, among whom the prevalence of Alzheimer disease can exceed 40%. Several screening tests are available. Most commonly used is the Mini-Mental State Examination, a 30-point assessment of several components of cognitive function. Other screening tests include clock drawing and making change. Because these are screening tests, a normal result does not definitively rule out the possibility of dementia (but makes it less likely that the patient has marked cognitive impairment). If cognitive impairment is suspected but the results of mental status testing are normal, the patient should have formal psychometric cognitive testing, which is more sensitive.

Affect
Depression is common among the elderly and potentially can reduce functional status. It also may result in considerable morbidity and mortality. Several effective screening tests, such as the Geriatric Depression Scale, are available. Unexplained weight loss may be a clue to depression.

Functional Status
How an elderly person functions in the environment is an important component of the assessment. Functional status represents a combination of the person's medical condition and his or her interactions with the social environment. It is important to remember that an elderly person's functional state may change quickly, and

various illnesses or prolonged hospitalization may cause a dramatic decline in functional status. The functional state is evaluated in 3 tiers: 1) the basic activities of daily living are the most simple activities required to remain independent, such as eating, bathing, dressing, transferring, and toileting; 2) the instrumental activities of daily living are the more complex activities required to maintain a household, such as shopping, driving, managing finances, and performing routine household chores; and 3) the advanced activities of daily living are the ability to function in the community and include the ability to hold a job or to participate in recreational activities. The environment of the patient should be assessed to determine whether the patient's functional state allows him or her to live safely in that environment.

Frailty
Frailty is difficult to define. It is a state between normal physical and social functioning and functional dependence. Frail elderly persons have limited capacity to respond to physical, emotional, or psychosocial stress. Objective criteria for the diagnosis include weight loss of more than 10 pounds in 1 year, loss of muscle mass and strength, decline in walking speed, exhaustion, and low physical activity. Pain and other comorbid conditions can limit a person's ability to exercise and predispose to frailty. Hypogonadism in men can lead to muscle wasting and fatigue. Diabetes is an important contributor to the development of frailty.

Weight loss may be multifactorial. Older patients with weight loss may have a physiologic anorexia of aging. They should also be screened for depression and other causes of cachexia. Weight loss can be associated with increased risk of hip fracture and death. Poor nutrition may lead to vitamin D deficiency.

- Diseases and other conditions predisposing to frailty should be identified and appropriately treated to prevent further functional decline.

Support Assessment
If an elderly patient has a compromised functional state, the degree of social support available for him or her should be determined. The physician needs to ascertain who is available to help with various tasks to keep the individual safe in an independent environment. Support usually includes family (most often an adult daughter), friends, and community services. A financial assessment should be made to determine whether the patient can afford treatments recommended by the physician or whether he or she qualifies for financial assistance from the government. A referral to social services may be needed to determine whether the patient meets the criteria for the benefits or services available.

Advance Directives
Advance directives should be discussed early with each elderly patient. It is important for the caregiver to know the patient's preferences should the patient become unable to make independent decisions because of an incapacitating illness. Living wills and a durable power of attorney for health care should be discussed and the directives reviewed periodically to determine whether the patient thinks they continue to reflect his or her wishes. These directives also should be

reviewed any time a major change occurs in the medical or functional status of the patient.

* A thorough geriatric assessment should include an assessment of vision, hearing, nutrition, continence, mobility and balance, medications, cognitive status, affect, functional status, frailty, social support, and advance directives.

Falls

Falls are a common cause of morbidity and an important contribution to mortality among the elderly. Because falls increase in frequency with advancing age, the likelihood of injury from falls also increases. It is estimated that three-fourths of all deaths related to falls occur in persons older than 65 years. The increased frequency of falls among the elderly reflects multiple age-related changes, including decreased strength from loss of muscle mass, decreased visual and hearing acuity, decreased proprioception, and slowed reaction time. These changes can produce an alteration of gait and decreased balance in an elderly person.

Most falls (70%) occur in the person's home. An accident, usually related to hazards in the environment (throw rugs, slippery floors, lack of grab bars in bathtubs, and inadequate lighting), is the most common cause of falls among the elderly who live independently. Most accidental falls occur while the person is performing typical daily activities such as walking or changing position (e.g., sitting to standing). An important percentage (10%) occur on stairs, more commonly while the person is descending the stairs. Falls that occur in nursing homes are more likely related to medical problems such as gait abnormalities, impaired balance, weakness, and confusion and are less likely to be caused by an environmental hazard. The common risk factors for injuries related to falls include weakness of the legs (stroke or neuropathy), gait instability (Parkinson disease), balance disorder (vertigo or orthostatism), cognitive impairment (dementia), and the use of multiple medications (Table 10-1). Medications that may contribute to falls include antihypertensive agents, diuretics, tricyclic antidepressants (which may produce orthostatic hypotension), sedative-hypnotics, ethanol, and neuroleptics (which may impair balance).

* Falls among the elderly usually reflect decreased strength from loss of muscle mass, decreased visual and hearing acuity, decreased proprioception, and slowed reaction time.
* Most falls (70%) occur in the person's home.
* Falls that occur in nursing homes are more likely related to medical problems.

Evaluation of Falls

A thorough medical history is the most important component of the assessment of a fall. If the reason for the fall is not known after the patient's history has been taken, it is unlikely that the cause will be found on physical examination or laboratory testing. The history should include the patient's perception of the cause of the fall, any warning symptoms the patient experienced before the fall, and any associated symptoms that occurred with the fall. The patient also

Table 10-1 Risk Factors for Falls

Lower extremity weakness
History of falls
Gait deficit
Balance deficit
Use of assistive device
Visual deficit
Arthritis
Impaired activities of daily living
Depression
Cognitive impairment
Age >80 years
Multiple medications

should be questioned about how he or she felt immediately after the fall. Loss of consciousness may suggest a cardiac or neurologic event (arrhythmia, seizure, or cerebrovascular event).

The physical examination should include a neurologic examination that tests gait, balance, reflexes, sensory impairment, and extremity strength. Any sensory impairment should be noted. Because falls may be associated with acute illnesses, patients should be assessed for infections, myocardial infarction, and gastrointestinal tract hemorrhage. Orthostatic hypotension, although common among the elderly, also may indicate a medication effect or hypovolemia from hemorrhage or dehydration.

* A thorough medical history is the most important component of the assessment of a fall.
* The physical examination should include a neurologic examination that tests gait, balance, reflexes, sensory impairment, and extremity strength.

Prevention and Treatment of Falls

The goal of the assessment of a fall is to decrease the likelihood of subsequent falls. The treatment plan is based on the findings of the assessment. However, more than 1 factor is often identified as contributing to falls. Potential interventions for the prevention of falls may include the following:

* Reduction in environmental hazards—provide adequate lighting, remove obstacles from floors, eliminate slippery floors, use appropriate footwear, eliminate bed side rails.
* Physical therapy—improve gait, balance, and strength, especially in the lower extremities.
* Assistive devices—improve gait and balance.
* Review of the medication program—avoid drug-drug interactions and eliminate potentially offending drugs.
* Treatment of medical problems that may contribute to falls (cataracts, postural hypotension, postprandial hypotension, Parkinson disease).
* The most effective management strategies are multidimensional and individualized.

Syncope

Syncope is defined as a transient loss of consciousness with loss of postural tone. It becomes more common with advancing age and has many causes. Although the cause of the syncopal spell itself is usually benign, several serious consequences can result from the fall, including bone fracture and subdural hematoma. Regardless of the cause of syncope, the underlying mechanism is inadequate cerebral blood perfusion. It has been estimated that as many as one-third of syncope cases have a cardiac cause. These include valvular heart disease (aortic stenosis, mitral regurgitation, and mitral stenosis), hypertrophic cardiomyopathy, myocardial infarction, or cardiac arrhythmias (tachyarrhythmias or bradyarrhythmias). An orthostatic decrease in blood pressure is also common in the elderly because of changes in baroreceptor function. In addition, several disease states can be associated with orthostatic hypotension, including peripheral neuropathy, Parkinson disease, and Shy-Drager syndrome. Also, various medications can produce hypotension, including antihypertensive agents, tricyclic antidepressants, neuroleptics, and diuretics. Although vasovagal syncope is more common in younger persons, it can occur in the elderly. Carotid sinus hypersensitivity, an exaggerated hypotensive reflex that occurs in response to carotid sinus massage, also can cause syncope. Other exaggerated cardiovascular reflexes that can result in syncope include micturition, defecation, and coughing. Seizures, hypoxemia (pulmonary embolism or respiratory failure), severe hypoglycemia, and anemia also can produce syncope.

The medical history is the most important part of the evaluation of syncope; the physical examination should focus on the signs related to cardiovascular or neurologic disease. Orthostatic blood pressure should be measured. Findings from the history and physical examination should guide the selection of tests to be performed. Tests that may be of value are electrocardiography and, occasionally, ambulatory cardiac monitoring when a cardiac arrhythmia is suspected. Rarely, electrophysiologic studies should be considered. When neurologic abnormalities are found on examination, an imaging study (computed tomography or magnetic resonance imaging) of the head may yield important information. Electroencephalography is useful when a seizure disorder is thought to cause syncope. Laboratory blood tests do not commonly reveal the cause of syncope; however, several of these tests may be helpful in certain circumstances. Blood count and electrolyte and creatinine determinations can give information about volume status. Measurement of cardiac enzymes may be useful if a recent myocardial infarction is suspected. Echocardiography should be performed if there is evidence of structural cardiac disease.

- It has been estimated that as many as one-third of the cases of syncope have a cardiac cause.
- Changes in baroreceptor function can result in an orthostatic decrease in blood pressure.
- The medical history is the most important part of the evaluation of syncope.

Vision Changes

A combination of anatomical and physiologic changes related to aging and various disease states common in the elderly frequently cause decreased vision. Vision loss increases with advancing age, and more than one-quarter of those older than 85 years report marked visual impairment. More than 90% of the elderly wear eyeglasses. It has been estimated that at least 25% of nursing home residents are legally blind. The most common eye problem in the elderly is presbyopia, difficulty with close focus. Presbyopia is the result of decreased lens flexibility, which occurs with aging. Cataracts are also more common with advancing age; they begin forming early in life, but the progression varies from person to person. The prevalence of cataracts is approximately 50% in those between 65 and 74 years old and up to 70% in those older than 75. Typically, cataracts produce a gradual reduction in visual acuity and represent opacities of the crystalline lens. In persons with early cataracts, near vision may actually improve; however, distant vision becomes blurred. This change occurs because of an increase in the convexity of the lens. Although cataracts are usually bilateral, one eye may be affected more than the other. Cataract surgery with intraocular lens implantation is effective for restoring visual acuity. The decision about the surgical treatment of cataracts should be individualized and based on the patient's disability.

Glaucoma is the most common cause of blindness worldwide and is characterized by increased intraocular pressure and associated optic nerve damage, manifested by cupping of the optic disk, atrophy of the optic nerve, and an associated reduction in the visual field. The 2 major types of glaucoma are chronic open-angle and angle-closure. Open-angle glaucoma is more common and occurs in up to 70% of adults with glaucoma. Chronic open-angle glaucoma produces a slow, progressive loss of peripheral vision that often is not appreciated by the patient until a considerable amount of vision is lost. Glaucoma is more common among African Americans than whites and is the most common cause of blindness in African Americans. In persons with the disease, a positive family history of glaucoma is very common. Open-angle glaucoma is associated with partial obstruction of aqueous humor flow through the trabecular meshwork. Funduscopic examination shows atrophy and cupping of the optic disk. Visual field testing documents typical peripheral field defects. A small number of patients with funduscopic or visual field changes of glaucoma have normal intraocular tension. If the physician routinely checks for glaucoma, it can be diagnosed and treated effectively before pronounced loss of vision occurs. The decision to treat glaucoma is not based only on the degree of increased ocular tension. Treatment is started when there is evidence of loss of vision or physical evidence of ocular damage.

Several options are available for the treatment of glaucoma, including surgery and medication. Medications are effective for decreasing the production of aqueous humor or for increasing its outflow. Pilocarpine causes pupillary constriction and opens the trabecular meshwork, resulting in increased flow of aqueous humor. β-Adrenergic blockers such as timolol decrease the production of aqueous humor, as do carbonic anhydrase inhibitors. Epinephrine decreases the production of aqueous humor and increases its flow. The goal of surgical treatment is to increase the flow of aqueous humor. Laser trabeculectomy is performed occasionally for open-angle glaucoma and usually is successful for increasing the outflow of aqueous humor.

Acute angle-closure glaucoma is much less common than chronic open-angle glaucoma and represents about 5% of glaucoma cases. It often presents after pupillary dilatation. It results from the obstruction of aqueous humor as it flows from the anterior chamber of the eye through the canal of Schlemm. This obstruction abruptly increases intraocular pressure. Patients with acute angle-closure glaucoma present with symptoms of intense eye pain, blurred vision with halos around lights, headache, and nausea. Physical examination reveals a slightly dilated pupil unresponsive to light. Urgent treatment is necessary to prevent permanent loss of vision.

Macular degeneration is the most important disease of the retina in the elderly. It is the leading cause of blindness in those older than 50. Macular degeneration is associated with the gradual and progressive loss of central vision, with sparing of peripheral vision. In addition to advanced age, macular degeneration has several risk factors, including a family history of macular degeneration, hyperopia, a light color of the iris, and chronic tobacco use. Although it initially tends to develop in 1 eye, it eventually becomes bilateral in many patients. It results in atrophy of the pigmented retinal epithelium. Impaired function of the photoreceptors eventually occurs, resulting in the characteristic loss of central vision and sparing of peripheral vision. The breakdown of the epithelium causes the deposition of drusen. The pathologic changes of macular degeneration generally can be seen on funduscopic examination. Laser treatment can be beneficial in some types of macular degeneration; however, the management of most patients with macular degeneration consists of devices used to assist vision, such as increased lighting and magnifying lenses.

* The most common eye problem in the elderly is presbyopia.
* Glaucoma is the most common cause of blindness worldwide. It is characterized by increased intraocular pressure and associated optic nerve damage.
* Chronic open-angle glaucoma is the most common form of glaucoma and produces a slow, progressive loss of peripheral vision.
* Macular degeneration is associated with the gradual and progressive loss of central vision and the sparing of peripheral vision.

Hearing Changes

Notable hearing loss in the elderly is common and usually due to a central auditory processing disorder, which causes difficulty with speech perception. The ability to discriminate speech is worse than predicted for the amount of pure tone lost. The prevalence of hearing loss, especially of high frequencies (presbycusis), increases markedly among persons older than 65 years and approaches 50% in those older than 80. Presbycusis is typically bilateral and associated with a high-frequency hearing loss. The cause is not known. Noise-induced hearing loss produces a similar high-frequency hearing loss. Elderly patients with a high-frequency hearing loss usually have the most difficulty with appreciating consonant sounds. A pronounced hearing

impairment is thought to be present when there is a loss of 25 decibels or more at 500, 1,000, or 2,000 Hz. Speech typically occurs between 1,000 and 3,000 Hz.

Causes of conductive hearing loss include cerumen impaction, perforation of the tympanic membrane, cholesteatoma, Paget disease, and otosclerosis. Hearing aids may be beneficial, and many improvements have been made in these devices. Some models of hearing aids are able to select the optimal frequency amplification for the specific environment, and others can be programmed to amplify the specific frequencies that the patient has lost. A less complex version amplifies the higher frequencies, the frequencies most commonly lost with aging. Hearing aids are most beneficial when used in an environment with minimal background noise, for example, a one-on-one conversation in a quiet room. They are least helpful when used in crowds with extensive background noise.

* The prevalence of hearing loss, especially of high frequencies (presbycusis), increases markedly in the elderly.
* Causes of conductive hearing loss include cerumen impaction, perforation of the tympanic membrane, cholesteatoma, Paget disease, and otosclerosis.

Rheumatologic Problems

Rheumatologic problems are among the commonest complaints of the elderly. These diseases tend to be chronic and often accumulate with time. Although most of these diseases are not life-threatening, they commonly cause an alteration in lifestyle and lead to substantial disability.

Osteoarthritis

Osteoarthritis is extremely common among the elderly and is present to some degree in more than 80%. It produces joint symptoms that vary with time and degree of activity. Osteoarthritis usually can be differentiated from rheumatoid arthritis by the medical history and physical examination findings (Table 10-2). Joint inflammation can occur in osteoarthritis, but it is more pronounced in rheumatoid arthritis. Although disease activity varies, acute worsening of a specific joint should make one suspicious of a superimposed crystalline arthritis (gout or pseudogout) or septic arthritis, which occasionally is found in patients with underlying chronic joint disease.

Osteoarthritis has a predilection for the hands (distal and proximal interphalangeal joints and first carpometacarpal joint of the thumb), knees, hips, and feet (first tarsometatarsal joint), with relative sparing of the elbow, wrist, metacarpophalangeal joints, and ankle. It has a typical radiographic appearance that includes asymmetrical narrowing of the joint space, presence of osteophytes, subchondral sclerosis, and cystic changes in the bone. Systemic symptoms do not occur. Joint pain is common with joint use and weight-bearing activity. Rest usually provides relief from the pain. The treatment of osteoarthritis includes adequate rest, local heat, and exercise to strengthen periarticular muscles, occasionally the injection of corticosteroids into the joint space when inflammation is present, and analgesics. Because joint inflammation is rarely marked in osteoarthritis, an analgesic such as acetaminophen should be tried initially for

Table 10-2 Comparison of Osteoarthritis and Rheumatoid Arthritis in the Elderly

Type of Arthritis	Systemic Symptoms	Joints Involved	Joint Findings	Radiographic Appearance	Initial Treatment
Osteoarthritis	No	Hands (DIPs > PIPs/MCPs), knees, feet	Marked joint inflammation uncommon	Asymmetric joint space narrowing, osteophytes, subchondral sclerosis, cystic changes	Rest, heat, exercise to strengthen periarticular muscles, occasional intra-articular corticosteroids, analgesics
Rheumatoid arthritis	Yes, plus extra-articular manifestations	Symmetric distal joints Hands (MCPs > DIPs/PIPs)	Inflammation common	Symmetric joint space narrowing	Nonsteroidal anti-inflammatory drugs

Abbreviations: DIP, distal interphalangeal; MCP, metacarpophalangeal; PIP, proximal interphalangeal.

pain relief. Once this has been tried and thought to be ineffective for managing the pain, more aggressive treatment should be used. Nonsteroidal anti-inflammatory drugs can be effective; however, they carry a risk of important adverse effects, especially when taken chronically. If nonsteroidal anti-inflammatory drugs are not tolerated or are ineffective, alternative treatment may include tramadol or codeine. Combinations of these drugs with low doses of acetaminophen may be helpful. Occasionally, corticosteroids may be injected into individual joints for temporary relief of pain. Some patients with knee osteoarthritis receive relief with injections of hyaluronic acid.

* Osteoarthritis usually can be differentiated from rheumatoid arthritis by the medical history and physical examination findings.
* Marked joint inflammation in osteoarthritis is uncommon.
* Radiographic findings in osteoarthritis include asymmetrical narrowing of the joint space, osteophytes, subchondral sclerosis, and cystic bone changes.

Rheumatoid Arthritis

Rheumatoid arthritis is often found in elderly patients, most commonly as a chronic disease that was acquired earlier in life. It also can develop later in life and has 2 presentations. As in younger persons, it may present with symmetric distal joint inflammation, positive rheumatoid factor, and a tendency to progress with time. The second presentation is common in the elderly and consists of the acute onset of proximal joint pain and stiffness, which can be very similar to polymyalgia rheumatica. Testing for rheumatoid factor often gives negative results, and rheumatoid nodules are often absent. In contrast to osteoarthritis, patients with rheumatoid arthritis have systemic symptoms. Extra-articular manifestations are occasionally present with rheumatoid arthritis and include potential involvement of the skin (rheumatoid nodules), lung (fibrosis, rheumatoid nodules, and pleural effusions), blood vessels (vasculitis), nervous system (mononeuritis multiplex), and hematologic system (Felty syndrome). Sjögren syndrome (splenomegaly and leukopenia) also occasionally

accompanies rheumatoid arthritis. Radiographs of joints involved by rheumatoid arthritis characteristically show symmetric narrowing of the joint space. Demonstrating inflammatory, symmetric arthritis on physical examination usually confirms the diagnosis. Laboratory test results often can be misleading in the elderly. Testing for rheumatoid factor is often negative in many elderly patients with rheumatoid arthritis. The test result can be false-positive in many elderly patients who do not have the disease, although the rheumatoid factor usually is of low titer. Anticyclic citrullinated peptide antibodies may be helpful in determining whether the positive rheumatoid factor actually represents disease. Elderly patients with rheumatoid arthritis receive the same therapeutic agents as younger patients: nonsteroidal anti-inflammatory drugs, chloroquine, methotrexate, gold, and low doses (5-7.5 mg daily) of corticosteroids.

* Patients with rheumatoid arthritis often have systemic symptoms.
* Extra-articular manifestations are occasionally present.
* Radiographically, rheumatoid arthritis characteristically shows symmetric narrowing of the joint space.
* The elderly with rheumatoid arthritis receive the same therapeutic agents as younger patients.

Total Joint Replacement for Osteoarthritis and Rheumatoid Arthritis

Total joint replacement is now one of the most commonly performed surgical procedures in the elderly. Total joint replacement is indicated for patients with osteoarthritis or rheumatoid arthritis who have failed conservative management. Ideal candidates are older patients who have persistent pain that interferes with their activities of daily living and negatively affects their quality of life. Although total joint replacement is indicated for anyone with a mature skeleton, it should be delayed as long as possible to minimize the risk of failure. Complications of total joint replacement include infection, dislocation, periprosthetic fracture, leg-length discrepancy, and loosening. However, about 90% of patients with total hip arthroplasties are pain-free and without complications 10 to 15 years postoperatively. Most patients who undergo total knee arthroplasty also report considerable pain relief, better function, and improved quality of life.

- Total joint replacement is effective for reducing pain and improving function for patients with advanced osteoarthritis or rheumatoid arthritis.

Crystalline Arthropathy

Crystalline arthropathy is common among the elderly (Table 10-3). Whereas gout tends to be more common in men and to involve more distal joints (especially the great toe), pseudogout is more common in women and tends to involve more proximal joints (especially the knee and wrist).

Gout is usually a monoarticular arthritis, although uncommonly presents as a polyarticular disease. It is caused by intra-articular deposition of uric acid crystals. It is associated with hyperuricemia, which may be produced by thiazide diuretics. Gouty attacks may be precipitated by stressful events such as surgery, severe illnesses, or trauma. Although gout usually is diagnosed on the basis of the medical history and physical examination, the diagnosis is confirmed by microscopic evaluation of the synovial fluid from an affected joint. Urate crystals are long and needle-shaped and negatively birefringent with polarizing microscopy. Treatment for an acute attack of gout includes nonsteroidal anti-inflammatory drugs. Colchicine, orally or intravenously, may be given to patients who should not receive nonsteroidal anti-inflammatory drugs. In some circumstances, intra-articular or systemic corticosteroids may be necessary. This therapy may be preferred for some elderly patients because of the high incidence of gastrointestinal or renal adverse effects. Long-term suppressive therapy usually is not initiated until several acute episodes of gout have occurred. Suppressive therapy may include allopurinol or probenecid daily or low doses of oral colchicine. Treatment of asymptomatic hyperuricemia is rarely necessary, although it is initiated in patients with uric acid renal stones or, occasionally, when starting chemotherapy for various hematologic malignancies.

- Gout tends to be more common in men and to involve more distal joints.

- Urate crystals are needle-shaped and negatively birefringent with polarizing microscopy.
- Treatment for an acute attack of gout includes nonsteroidal anti-inflammatory drugs, colchicine, or, in some cases, intra-articular or systemic corticosteroids.

Pseudogout (calcium pyrophosphate deposition disease) is usually a monoarticular arthritis that most frequently involves the knee or wrist. As with gout, an acute attack can occur with a stressful event such as surgery, trauma, or illness. Radiographs of joints with pseudogout often show linear articular calcification, although approximately 25% of the elderly have articular calcification with no clinical evidence of the disease. Calcium pyrophosphate crystals are rectangular and exhibit positive birefringence with polarizing microscopy. An acute attack is treated with nonsteroidal anti-inflammatory drugs or corticosteroids injected into the affected joints. Daily therapy with a low dose of colchicine may decrease the frequency of acute attacks.

- Pseudogout is usually a monoarticular arthritis, most commonly involving the knee or wrist.
- Calcium pyrophosphate crystals are rectangular and exhibit positive birefringence with polarizing microscopy.
- An acute attack is treated with nonsteroidal anti-inflammatory drugs or corticosteroids injected into the affected joints.

Polymyalgia Rheumatica and Temporal Arteritis

Polymyalgia rheumatica and temporal arteritis occur more commonly in women than in men and in persons older than 50 years. Patients with polymyalgia rheumatica describe stiffness, aching, and weakness of proximal muscles (shoulders and hips), especially in the morning. These symptoms are thought to be due to synovitis of the shoulder or hip joint (or both). The clinical presentation of polymyalgia rheumatica may be very similar to that of rheumatoid arthritis in the elderly. Patients also may complain of nonspecific malaise, fatigue, low-grade fever, and anorexia with weight loss. Although patients commonly describe weakness, muscle strength is normal when tested. The diagnosis usually is suspected from the classic history obtained from the patient; no specific laboratory test is diagnostic for the disease.

Table 10-3 Crystalline Arthritis

Crystalline Arthritis	Sex Distribution	Joint Involvement	Crystal	Crystal Characteristics	Initial Treatment
Gout	Male > female	Distal joints, expecially great toe	Uric acid	Long, needle-shaped, negative birefringence	NSAIDs ± intra-articular or systemic corticosteroids, colchicine
Calcium pyrophosphate deposition disease (pseudogout)	Female > male	Proximal joints, especially knee & wrist	Calcium pyrophosphate	Rectangular, positive birefringence	NSAIDs or intra-articular corticosteroids

Abbreviation: NSAID, nonsteroidal anti-inflammatory drug.

Patients usually have an increased erythrocyte sedimentation rate and, occasionally, mild anemia. The levels of muscle enzymes (creatine kinase and aspartate aminotransferase) are not increased. The response to treatment is very characteristic and often can be used to support the diagnosis. Treatment with low doses of oral corticosteroids (prednisone, 15-20 mg daily) produces dramatic improvement in symptoms, often within 24 hours. After treatment has been initiated, the corticosteroid dose can be tapered gradually, using the patient's clinical response and erythrocyte sedimentation rate as indicators of disease activity.

- Patients with polymyalgia rheumatica describe stiffness, aching, and weakness of proximal muscles.
- Patients usually have an increased erythrocyte sedimentation rate and, occasionally, mild anemia.
- Treatment with low doses of oral corticosteroids produces dramatic improvement in symptoms.

Temporal arteritis develops in about 15% of patients with polymyalgia rheumatica. Pathologically, there is inflammation of medium-sized arteries, which arise from the aortic arch. Systemic symptoms include low-grade fever and fatigue; anorexia with weight loss is also common. A majority of patients have a unilateral or bilateral headache, usually in the temporal area. Many also have scalp tenderness and jaw claudication due to facial artery involvement with disease. Loss of vision, including unilateral or bilateral visual blurring, visual field loss, diplopia, or blindness caused by ischemic optic neuritis, may occur and is the most worrisome symptom. As with polymyalgia rheumatica, temporal arteritis usually is suspected on the basis of the patient's description of the symptoms. Few findings are documented on physical examination. Some patients have tender, swollen, or pulseless temporal arteries. Rarely, bruits may be heard over medium-sized arteries involved by the disease. Although no diagnostic laboratory test is specific for temporal arteritis, almost all patients have a markedly increased erythrocyte sedimentation rate, often greater than 100 mm/h. Mild anemia also may be present. After temporal arteritis is suspected, the diagnosis should be confirmed with temporal artery biopsy. A 4- to 5-cm piece of temporal artery should be obtained, initially on the side of the patient's symptoms. If the pathologic findings are negative, a similar biopsy should be performed on the opposite side. The inflammatory changes in the artery may be spotty or confined to a small portion of the artery, occasionally causing difficulty in confirming the diagnosis pathologically. Temporal artery biopsy should not be performed routinely in patients with polymyalgia rheumatica who do not have symptoms of temporal arteritis. Treatment consists of prednisone, 60 mg daily, and may be started before the biopsy sample is obtained, assuming the biopsy is to be performed within 48 hours. The prednisone dose should be tapered on the basis of an assessment of the patient's clinical response to treatment and the response of the erythrocyte sedimentation rate.

- Temporal arteritis develops in about 15% of patients with polymyalgia rheumatica.
- Symptoms include low-grade fever, fatigue, anorexia with weight loss, unilateral or bilateral headache, scalp tenderness, and jaw claudication.

- The diagnosis should be confirmed with temporal artery biopsy.
- Treatment consists of high doses of corticosteroids.

Thyroid Disease

Thyroid disease becomes more common with advancing age. Most elderly patients with hyperthyroidism present with typical findings. A small but important percentage have atypical symptoms. Some elderly persons have anorexia with weight loss, altered stool frequency (either diarrhea or constipation), or cardiovascular abnormalities, including hypertension, increased angina, myocardial ischemia, congestive heart failure, and atrial fibrillation. Other symptoms that may develop include apathy, depression, tremor, and myopathy. Decrease in bone density is accelerated with hyperthyroidism. Ophthalmopathy, lid lag, tachycardia, and increased perspiration are relatively more uncommon in the elderly than in younger patients. The development of a goiter with hyperthyroidism is noted in about 60% of the elderly. The commonest cause of hyperthyroidism in the elderly is Graves disease. Radioiodine is the treatment of choice for hyperthyroidism in elderly patients.

- Most elderly patients with hyperthyroidism present with the typical findings, although apathy, depression, tremor, and myopathy may develop.
- The commonest cause of hyperthyroidism in the elderly is Graves disease.
- Radioiodine is the treatment of choice for hyperthyroidism.

The diagnosis of hypothyroidism in elderly patients is usually made by finding an increased level of sensitive thyroid-stimulating hormone (sTSH) on laboratory testing of asymptomatic patients. The common symptoms of hypothyroidism are vague (constipation, cold intolerance, and dry skin) and often attributed to the many "symptoms of aging." Almost all these cases of hypothyroidism are due to primary thyroid failure rather than to pituitary or hypothalamic insufficiency. The commonest cause of hypothyroidism in the elderly is Hashimoto thyroiditis. Treatment should begin with a low dose of thyroid supplement (25-50 micrograms daily) that is increased by 25 migrograms every 3 to 4 weeks. Patients with coronary artery disease should receive an even lower starting dose and more gradual dose increments because thyroid replacement that is too rapid can precipitate cardiac ischemia. It takes 6 to 8 weeks for a given dose of thyroid supplement to equilibrate; therefore, the sTSH values should not be checked before this time to assess whether the dose of thyroid supplement is correct. Thyroid hormone requirements decrease with advancing age, and most elderly require 75 to 100 micrograms daily; however, some require as little as 50 micrograms daily. Subclinical hypothyroidism can be found in approximately 15% of the elderly. These patients are clinically euthyroid and have a low-normal total (serum) thyroxine (T_4) level and a slightly increased sTSH level. Whether to treat these patients is a matter of controversy. Patients with an sTSH value less than 6 mIU/L and negative microsomal antibodies rarely have progression to clinical hypothyroidism. Most physicians choose to observe patients who have modest increases in sTSH (<10 mIU/L) unless symptoms of hypothyroidism develop or the sTSH level continues to increase.

- The common symptoms of hypothyroidism are vague and often attributed to symptoms of aging.
- The commonest cause of hypothyroidism in the elderly is Hashimoto thyroiditis.
- Treatment of hypothyroidism should begin with a low dose of thyroid supplement (25-50 micrograms daily) that is increased by 25 micrograms every 3 to 4 weeks.

Euthyroid sick syndrome is common in elderly hospitalized patients. Patients are clinically euthyroid but have low serum levels of tri-iodothyronine (T_3) and T_4 and a low-normal level of sTSH. Laboratory values tend to return to normal after the patient has recovered from the illness. The syndrome may be caused by a decreased amount of thyroid-binding protein and a substance that inhibits T_4 binding.

- Patients with euthyroid sick syndrome are clinically euthyroid but have low serum levels of T_3 and T_4 and a low-normal level of sTSH.

Sexual Function and Sexuality

Multiple physical and social changes occur with aging that can result in changes in the desire and capacity of an older person for sexual activity. Although there is evidence that interest in sexuality is retained well into older age, for several reasons the frequency of sexual activity tends to be reduced with aging. Whereas this is true for the elderly population in general, there is great variability in sexual interest and activity from one elderly person to another. One of the most important factors that may determine whether a person is sexually active is the availability of a partner who is capable of sexual activity. The setting in which the elderly live may also have a role in whether a person is sexually active. Many elderly live in an environment in which sexual activity is difficult or not condoned (eg, in a nursing home or in the home of their children). Because privacy may not be possible in these settings, intimacy is unlikely to occur.

Little is known about the influence of sex hormones on libido for either the male or the female. Although it is not thought that the presence of estrogen or progestin is primarily responsible for sexual desire in females, evidence suggests that androgens increase sexual interest. Lack of estrogen can produce reduced vaginal lubrication and mucosal atrophy, which can cause dyspareunia. Painful conditions such as osteoarthritis also may contribute to diminishing desire for sexual activity.

Erectile dysfunction increases in frequency with advancing age and is the most common reason for a man to reduce his degree of sexual activity. It may be related to psychosocial and physical factors. An erection is the result of a combination of neurologic and vascular activity, which may be impaired with aging.

With age, testosterone levels tend to decrease in males. This age-related change does not seem to be related to erectile dysfunction;

however, it may decrease interest in sexual activity. Many cases of erectile dysfunction are associated with complications of atherosclerotic disease such as coronary artery disease, peripheral arterial disease, and stroke. Hypertension and antihypertensive medications also have been associated with erectile dysfunction. Diabetes mellitus is associated with a high incidence of erectile dysfunction, which may be due to the vascular or neurologic complications (or both) of diabetes.

The evaluation of a patient with erectile dysfunction begins with a medical history. The patient's libido should be assessed, as should the frequency and quality of erections. Hypogonadism should be suspected when a marked reduction in libido has occurred. This also may be caused by depression. Critical to the evaluation of sexual dysfunction is a careful assessment of medications, alcohol intake, and a history of diseases that can cause erectile dysfunction. Medications that have been associated with erectile dysfunction include antihypertensive agents, phenothiazines, antidepressants, histamine$_2$-receptor antagonists, digoxin, and clofibrate. Symptoms of medical problems such as diabetes mellitus, peripheral neuropathy, peripheral arterial disease, hypertension, thyroid disease (both hypothyroidism and hyperthyroidism), and uremia should be sought. The physical examination should concentrate on findings that suggest the presence of hypogonadism, peripheral arterial disease, or peripheral neuropathy. Appropriate laboratory tests should include determination of sTSH, fasting blood glucose, and total and bioavailable testosterone levels. When hypogonadism is suspected, luteinizing hormone and prolactin levels should be determined. Nocturnal penile tumescence testing is considered unreliable and does not reliably distinguish between psychogenic and organic causes. A duplex scan of the penile arteries can be useful to assess blood flow to the penis. This test can be performed before and after vasodilator therapy and can predict the response to this therapy.

Treatment for erectile dysfunction includes both mechanical and pharmacologic therapies. Appropriate treatment for specific medical disorders that can be associated with erectile dysfunction should be started. Patients with hypogonadism should be given androgens. Androgens alone should not be expected to reverse erectile dysfunction. Vacuum devices are safe and relatively effective for any cause of erectile dysfunction. Intracorporeal injection of prostaglandin E_1 is also effective for producing a sustained erection. Patients tend to lose their enthusiasm for injections with time, probably because of the relatively invasive nature of the treatment. Sildenafil was the first oral medication approved for the treatment of erectile dysfunction. Currently, vardenafil and tadalafil are also available. They are effective in a majority of patients regardless of the underlying cause. They inhibit the breakdown of cyclic guanosine monophosphate and improve blood flow to the penis. Because of the potential for hypotension, they are contraindicated in persons receiving nitrate therapy. Vardenafil and tadalafil should not be used in individuals taking α-adrenergic antagonists because of a potential for hypotension. The risk of adverse effects associated with these medications may be increased in patients with coronary artery disease.

- One of the most important factors that may determine whether a person is sexually active is the availability of a partner.

- With age, testosterone levels tend to decrease in males and do not appear to be related to erectile dysfunction.
- Treatment for erectile dysfunction includes both mechanical and pharmacologic therapies.

Dementia

Dementia is an acquired cognitive impairment that affects all spheres of the intellect. It is a gradually progressive disorder and becomes more common with increasing age. Approximately 10% of the population older than 65 years has some degree of dementia. The number increases with age and has been reported to be as high as 50% among those older than 90 years. Dementia involves considerably more than the loss of memory. Other cognitive functions that are affected include judgment, abstract thinking, attention, ability to learn new material, and, eventually, the recognition and production of speech. Personality changes frequently accompany dementia. The commonest form of irreversible dementia is Alzheimer disease (50%-70% of cases), followed by vascular dementia (15%-25%). In the recent past, the prevalence of reversible dementias was thought to be as high as 30%. Currently, it is believed that in most patients with some reversibility in cognitive impairment, the improvement is only transient and in most of the patients irreversible dementia eventually develops. The prevalence of truly reversible dementia is low, from 1% to 2%. The most common causes of potentially reversible dementia include the following: depression, selected drugs, metabolic disorders (hypothyroidism, hyperthyroidism, hyperparathyroidism), toxic agents (heavy metals, pesticides, alcohol, various organic solvents), nutritional deficiencies (vitamin B$_{12}$, niacin, thiamine), normal-pressure hydrocephalus, subdural hematoma, central nervous system (CNS) tumors, and CNS infections (neurosyphilis, chronic fungal or bacterial meningitis, and human immunodeficiency virus [HIV] infection).

Mild Cognitive Impairment

Mild cognitive impairment (MCI) is dysfunction in some cognitive domains, but it is not severe enough to interfere with activities of daily life. MCI may be associated only with memory complaints (amnestic), or there may be impairments in multiple cognitive areas. MCI is a considerable risk factor for conversion to dementia (Alzheimer disease). Patients with MCI convert at a much higher rate than patients with normal cognition. These patients also are at increased risk for morbidity and mortality. Nursing home placement rates are 2 to 3 times higher for the elderly with MCI. Risk factors that predict progression include cerebrovascular disease and extrapyramidal signs. Brain imaging and genetic markers are being studied as predictors of future decline. No medications have been shown to decrease the rate of conversion to dementia.

- MCI is a risk factor for development of Alzheimer disease.

Alzheimer Disease

The diagnosis of Alzheimer disease cannot be confirmed until postmortem examination: no laboratory test or radiologic evaluation, including computed tomography or magnetic resonance imaging of the head, is specific for diagnosis of the disease. The diagnosis is made primarily on the basis of the history, usually from family members, and a determination of the cognitive status of the patient. The accuracy of clinicians for diagnosing Alzheimer disease is as high as 95%. The disease is a gradually progressive impairment of cognition. It is characterized by gradually progressive difficulty learning new tasks and information. Loss of memory begins with recent events and eventually includes memory of distant events. Both receptive and expressive language difficulty develop in which the patient has difficulty naming familiar objects and understanding language. Patients may easily become lost, even in familiar surroundings. Calculation skills decline, and patients may no longer be capable of such tasks as balancing a checkbook. Eventually behavioral problems develop in many patients, including the tendency to wander and to develop paranoia, agitation, delusions, or hallucinations (or a combination of these). Typically, patients with Alzheimer disease have little insight into the disease process and are often brought to the physician by a family member. Driving safety is often impaired in persons with dementia, and the physician should play a prominent role in discussing this with the patient and his or her family. At times the physician may need to take steps to prevent the patient from driving if safety is an issue.

Pathologically, the CNS findings include neuronal plaques, which represent extracellular deposits of protein containing amyloid, and neurofibrillary tangles, which are intracellular protein bound to microtubules. Neuronal plaques and neurofibrillary tangles are also found in nondemented persons but in much smaller amounts. Alzheimer disease is associated with a decreased amount of CNS neurotransmitters such as acetylcholine, norepinephrine, and serotonin. Acetylcholine deficiency is especially prominent, as is a decrease in choline acetyltransferase activity.

The evaluation of a demented patient establishes the existence and degree of cognitive impairment, ruling out reversible dementias. Screening mental status examinations (such as the Mini-Mental State Examination) often identify patients who may not have obvious cognitive impairment. If cognitive impairment is suspected but the mental status examination findings are normal, formal psychometric studies should be conducted. Normal findings on mental status examinations do not rule out dementia. The Mini-Mental State Examination is also used to follow future deterioration. The medical evaluation consists of a medical history and physical examination (including neurologic examination) and general laboratory tests. Accepted laboratory tests include a complete blood count; electrolyte panel; liver function tests; blood urea nitrogen; serum levels of creatinine, calcium, glucose, and vitamin B$_{12}$; thyroid function; syphilis serology; chest radiography; and electrocardiography. Although some form of brain imaging study (computed tomography or magnetic resonance imaging) is usually performed, there are arguments for and against this practice. An imaging study is performed to rule out various types of potentially reversible CNS lesions such as mass lesions, normal-pressure hydrocephalus, or previous strokes and not to examine for cerebral atrophy. If the patient has had dementia for an extended period, has no focal findings on neurologic examination, has no history of head trauma, and has no headache, an imaging study may not be cost-effective.

Electroencephalography, HIV testing, and lumbar puncture are performed only in unusual circumstances and are rarely necessary.

Until recently, the treatment of Alzheimer disease has been limited to controlling abnormal behavior (agitation, delusions, hallucinations, and paranoia) with various neuroleptic drugs (sedative-hypnotics and major tranquilizers). None of the neuroleptic medications commonly used improve cognitive function, and very often, they worsen memory and orientation. Major tranquilizers also may cause movement disorders (tardive dyskinesia) and can contribute to falls. The recent availability of acetylcholinesterase inhibitors (tacrine, donepezil, rivastigmine, and galantamine) has given clinicians the first real options for treating Alzheimer disease. Although acetylcholinesterase inhibitors are not considered disease-modifying drugs, they may transiently delay cognitive decline and should be considered for patients who have mild to moderate dementia. The major benefit of these drugs is their potential to delay institutionalization, although there have been reports of improvement in abnormal behaviors associated with dementia with the use of these drugs. The high prevalence of liver toxicity associated with tacrine has not been found with the other acetylcholinesterase inhibitors.

Memantine is a new and novel treatment for Alzheimer disease. It is neuroprotective and considered a disease-modifying agent. It can slow the progression of cognitive decline. This drug blocks the effect of glutamate, an excitatory neurotransmitter in CNS neurons. Glutamate stimulates N-methyl-D-aspartate receptors, which are commonly involved in memory and learning. Excessive receptor stimulation can result in damage to the receptor. Memantine inhibits the activity of glutamate, protecting the N-methyl-D-aspartate receptors from damage. Patients with Alzheimer disease can be given a combination of an anticholinesterase medication and memantine.

Evidence suggests that vitamin E and selegiline also may slow the progression of Alzheimer disease through their antioxidant activity. Nonsteroidal anti-inflammatory drugs may protect against the development of Alzheimer disease by suppressing the inflammation and immune response present in the brains of patients with Alzheimer disease. These agents are not given routinely for prevention because of the risk of adverse effects. Estrogen therapy has not been consistently shown to be of benefit in the prevention or treatment of Alzheimer disease. In the Women's Health Initiative Study, estrogen plus progestin did not improve cognitive function when compared with placebo, and a small increased risk of clinically meaningful cognitive decline occurred in the estrogen plus progestin group.

- The diagnosis of Alzheimer disease is established on the basis of the history, usually from family members, and a determination of the cognitive status of the patient.
- Screening mental status examinations often identify patients who may not have obvious cognitive impairment.
- Accepted laboratory tests include a complete blood count; electrolyte panel; liver function tests; blood urea nitrogen; serum levels of creatinine, calcium, glucose, and vitamin B₁₂; thyroid function; syphilis serology; chest radiography; and electrocardiography. A brain imaging study (computed tomography or magnetic resonance imaging) is usually performed.
- Acetylcholinesterase inhibitors may transiently delay cognitive decline.

Diseases other than Alzheimer disease may cause dementia. At times, it may be difficult to differentiate one from the other, although subtle differences often are present clinically.

Vascular Dementia

Vascular dementia tends to affect older persons and is due to repeated cerebral infarcts. It is the second most common cause of dementia and can be difficult to differentiate from Alzheimer disease. The patient usually has a stepwise progression of cognitive impairment consistent with the multiple ischemic infarcts, often with focal neurologic deficits also produced by the ischemic CNS events. Several types of vascular dementias are possible, including cortical multi-infarcts, subcortical multi-infarcts due to small-vessel thrombosis (lacunar strokes), and deep white matter small-vessel ischemia with demyelination (Binswanger disease). Amyloid angiopathy may cause cognitive impairment and is associated with cerebral hemorrhages. The presentation depends on which portion of the brain is affected by the ischemic insults. CNS imaging usually shows evidence of multiple strokes or white matter ischemia. Treatment consists of management of risk factors for cerebrovascular disease such as hypertension, diabetes mellitus, and hyperlipidemia. Also, antiplatelet therapy is usually given.

- Patients with vascular dementia usually have a stepwise progression of cognitive impairment.

Dementia With Lewy Bodies

Patients with this cortical dementia have cognitive impairments similar to those of Alzheimer disease. Pathologically, Lewy bodies are cytoplasmic inclusion bodies, and they can be found in subcortical brain tissue. Patients have findings of parkinsonism with bradykinesia, extremity rigidity, and postural instability. Absence of a resting tremor is common (unlike Parkinson disease). The ability of patients to maintain attention is poor. Also, they show marked day-to-day changes in cognitive status and may have hallucinations (visual and auditory). Patients are very sensitive to the effects of antipsychotic medications and frequently have adverse extrapyramidal reactions, which may be life-threatening.

- Dementia with Lewy bodies is associated with cognitive impairment and findings of parkinsonism.
- Patients typically show marked day-to-day changes.

Dementia With Parkinson Disease

Up to 40% of patients with Parkinson disease have development of dementia, and many are indistinguishable from those with Alzheimer disease. These patients have the features typical of Parkinson disease, including resting tremor, rigidity, and bradykinesia, in addition to the intellectual impairments of dementia, which tend to be very slowly progressive. For some patients, effective treatment of Parkinson disease with dopamine improves cognitive status, but not for those with more severe dementia.

- Up to 40% of patients with Parkinson disease have development of dementia.

Frontotemporal Dementia

Frontotemporal dementia is characterized by changes in personality and behavior due to prominent frontal lobe involvement. It has less effect on cognitive status and memory impairment. Onset of the disease tends to be somewhat earlier than for Alzheimer disease, often in the 50s and 60s. Patients frequently have poor personal hygiene and disinhibition and may demonstrate hypersexual behavior. Urinary incontinence is also common. Physical examination usually shows prominent frontal reflexes. CNS imaging shows the typical frontal and temporal lobe involvement. One type of frontotemporal dementia is Pick disease, characterized pathologically by intraneuronal inclusion bodies known as Pick bodies. Management of the behavioral disturbance is the most challenging aspect of the treatment of this condition.

* Pick disease is characterized by prominent changes in personality and behavior.

Creutzfeldt-Jakob Disease

Creutzfeldt-Jakob disease is an uncommon cause of dementia. It has an earlier onset than Alzheimer disease, usually in the sixth decade. The progression of the disease is rapid, eventually producing a vegetative state and the development of myoclonic jerks and seizures. Most patients die within 1 year after disease onset. The cause is thought to be infectious and due to prions.

* Creutzfeldt-Jakob disease is a rapidly progressive dementia associated with myoclonic jerks and seizures.

Other Dementias

Huntington disease is an autosomal dominant disorder with early onset of symptoms (usually in the fourth or fifth decade). Eventually, choreiform movements develop. Cognitive impairment is severe and progressive. Acquired immunodeficiency syndrome (AIDS) dementia affects up to 50% of persons with AIDS. It can produce a subcortical dementia, and it is gradually progressive. Currently, AIDS dementia is uncommon among the elderly. Also, dementia can occur as a chronic complication of Lyme disease years after onset of the infection.

Delirium

Delirium is an acute confusional disorder frequently mistaken for dementia. It is associated with a decreased level of consciousness, hallucinations, and delusions. Its several causes are listed in Table 10-4. It is important to differentiate delirium from dementia because of the potential for reversibility of cognitive impairment associated with delirium. Patients with delirium frequently have a preexisting mild (often unrecognized) dementia.

* Delirium is a reversible cause of cognitive impairment and may be related to medications or acute medical conditions.

Preoperative Assessment

Elderly patients commonly undergo anesthesia and surgery, and age alone should not be a contraindication for a surgical procedure. Most elderly persons have some increased risk of perioperative complications because of a combination of normal physiologic changes of aging and, more importantly, various disease states. Most perioperative deaths result from cardiac or respiratory complications. It can be difficult to determine preoperatively whether an elderly patient has marked cardiac or respiratory disease. The high prevalence of inactivity among the elderly commonly masks the presence of coronary or pulmonary disease because symptoms may be present only with exercise. Usually, an older patient who is active, without symptoms, at low risk for cardiorespiratory disease, and scheduled for a nonvascular operation does not require further testing. However, asymptomatic patients who are inactive and have several risk factors for cardiorespiratory disease may benefit from noninvasive cardiac or pulmonary testing (or both).

The patient's medications should be reviewed preoperatively. Because of the increased risk of postoperative bleeding, use of aspirin should be discontinued at least 1 week before the operation. Nonsteroidal anti-inflammatory drugs also can increase the risk of bleeding and their use should be discontinued preoperatively. Because of a shorter antiplatelet effect, nonsteroidal anti-inflammatory drugs may be taken up to 48 hours before the operation. Oral hypoglycemic medications should not be given the morning of the operation because of the risk of hypoglycemia. The blood glucose level can be managed by the administration of regular insulin if needed. Other medications that the patient takes daily should be given the morning of the operation. The use of cardiovascular medications, especially β-adrenergic blockers and clonidine, should not be discontinued abruptly. If corticosteroids have been taken recently in doses capable of suppressing adrenal function, they should be given preoperatively.

In addition to the questions typically asked of younger patients during a preoperative assessment, functional ability and cognitive status should be assessed in the elderly. The Mini-Mental State Examination is an adequate screening test for cognitive impairment. Patients with

Table 10-4 Causes of Delirium

Drugs
    Sedative-hypnotics
    Anticholinergic agents
    NSAIDs
    β-Adrenergic blockers
    Antipsychotic agents
Metabolic disturbances
    Hyperglycemia
    Hypoglycemia
    Hypercalcemia
Hypoxia
Hypotension
Common medical illnesses in patients with limited organ
  reserve function or organ failure
    Urinary tract infection
    Sepsis
    Pneumonia

Abbreviation: NSAID, nonsteroidal anti-inflammatory drug.

cognitive impairment preoperatively are at increased risk for postoperative delirium. Previous episodes of postoperative delirium are a substantial risk factor for recurrent episodes. They also may have difficulty completing a physical therapy program. It is not unusual for the functional status of an elderly person to deteriorate markedly after an operation, especially with a prolonged hospital stay. It is wise to prepare for assistance in the home or to consider temporary nursing home placement for possible strength rehabilitation to prevent even longer hospitalization.

- Most elderly persons have some increased risk of perioperative complications because of both normal physiologic changes of aging and various disease states.
- Most perioperative deaths result from cardiac or respiratory complications.

Preventive Geriatrics

For many disease states, there is evidence to recommend continuing screening tests with advancing age. In other areas, data are not sufficient about whether screening is beneficial for the elderly. In these situations, clinical judgment (taking into account the patient's functional status and estimated life expectancy) is important for deciding whether certain screening tests should be performed. Before a screening test is indicated, several basic principles must be considered, including the following: 1) the incidence of the disease is high enough to warrant performing screening tests, 2) there must be a period during which the disease is present but the patient is asymptomatic and the disease can be diagnosed with a screening test, 3) effective treatment is available for the disease, 4) early treatment of the disease has a better outcome than it would if the diagnosis is made after symptoms develop, and 5) the screening test has a reasonable sensitivity and specificity and is relatively inexpensive and safe.

Cardiovascular Disease
- High low-density lipoprotein cholesterol and low high-density lipoprotein cholesterol have predictive value in the elderly for coronary artery disease. Many organizations now recommend checking for hyperlipidemia in persons older than 65 years, especially those who have an established diagnosis of coronary artery disease or multiple risk factors.
- The risks of hypertension and the benefits of treatment extend to the elderly, and it is recommended that screening for hypertension be performed in the elderly.
- Routine screening for carotid artery disease in the elderly is not recommended.
- Routine screening with resting or exercise electrocardiography is not recommended for the elderly.

Malignancy
- Because breast cancer continues to increase in incidence with age, continued annual screening with mammography is recommended. For patients older than 75 years, clinical judgment should be used. If appropriate, it is reasonable to continue mammography as long as the patient's life expectancy exceeds 5 years.

- Although colon cancer is common among the elderly, screening recommendations require clinical judgment. Tests with an acceptable sensitivity and specificity (eg, colonoscopy) are difficult for many elderly and have some associated risks. Simple tests such as digital rectal examination or fecal occult blood tests have a low sensitivity and specificity. The American Cancer Society recommends several options for colon cancer screening. According to these recommendations, annual fecal occult blood testing and flexible sigmoidoscopy every 5 years are preferable. Colonoscopy should be performed if the results of either test are abnormal. For those at increased risk for colorectal cancer, such as a history of colorectal adenomatous polyps, screening with colonoscopy should be performed. The US Preventive Services Task Force recommends screening with fecal occult blood testing or sigmoidoscopy or both. Another option now available is computed tomography colography. This may be especially useful for persons receiving long-term anticoagulation with warfarin or those who have had difficulties or complications in the past with colonoscopy or flexible sigmoidoscopy.
- If cervical Papanicolaou smears have been performed appropriately at younger ages and the results have been negative, the US Preventive Services Task Force recommends discontinuing Papanicolaou smears at age 65 years. For the elderly who did not have regular screening with cervical Papanicolaou smears, the incidence of cervical cancer is notable. Screening is recommended for older women who have not previously had a screening test or if information about previous screening is unavailable or if screening is unlikely to have occurred in the past. Women who have had a hysterectomy with removal of the cervix for benign reasons and with no history of abnormal cancerous growth may discontinue routine cytologic testing. Women who have had a hysterectomy but who have a history of abnormal cell growth (cervical intraepithelial neoplasia, grade 2 or 3) should be screened annually until they have three consecutive negative vaginal cytologic tests. They may then discontinue routine cytologic surveillance.
- Although prostate cancer is common in males, screening tests are controversial. The US Preventive Services Task Force considers the evidence inadequate to recommend for or against screening for prostate cancer with the prostate-specific antigen test or digital rectal examination. The American Cancer Society recommends that a digital rectal examination and prostate-specific antigen test be offered annually to men older than 50 if they have a life expectancy of at least 10 years.
- Screening tests for lung cancer, including chest radiography, chest computed tomography, or sputum cytology, are not recommended for either smokers or nonsmokers.
- No screening test has been recommended for the early detection of ovarian cancer.

Pulmonary Changes

Pulmonary function decreases with advancing age, likely because of a combination of normal anatomical and physiologic changes, injury from exposure to various environmental toxins (tobacco and air pollution), and disease states that affect the lung. Changes in the shape of the thorax also contribute to changes in pulmonary physiology. The apical-to-base length of the lungs decreases as the anterior-to-posterior length increases with age. The bronchioles and alveolar ducts increase in diameter, decreasing alveolar surface area. The aging lungs also have reduced compliance because of decreased lung elasticity. These anatomical and physiologic changes result in reduced airflow rates, decreased efficiency of air exchange, and alterations in lung volumes. Changes that occur with aging in pulmonary physiology include a decrease in mucociliary clearance, vital capacity, 1-second forced expiratory volume (FEV_1), maximal breathing capacity, and diffusing capacity (DLCO). The lung residual volume and alveolar-arterial oxygen gradient (AaO_2) increase with age. Aging has no effect on total lung capacity.

- Pulmonary function decreases with advancing age because of a combination of anatomical and physiologic changes, exposure to environmental toxins, and disease states that affect the lung.

Respiratory Disease

Pneumonia is one of the top 10 causes of death among the elderly and is the cause of death of 15% of nursing home residents. The bacterial organisms that cause pneumonia change with advancing age. The elderly have an increased number of gram-negative bacteria as part of their normal oral flora. They also have an increased likelihood of aspirating oral secretions, which contributes to the increased incidence of pneumonia caused by gram-negative and anaerobic bacteria. The likely cause of pneumonia depends on the setting in which the elderly patient acquired the infection. Overall, *Streptococcus pneumoniae* is the most common etiologic organism. *Haemophilus influenzae*, other gram-negative bacteria, and anaerobes are common among the elderly in nursing homes and hospitals. Infections with anaerobe organisms must be considered if the patient is suspected of having an aspiration pneumonia. Organisms such as *Legionella*, *Chlamydia*, and *Moraxella catarrhalis* are also found occasionally in the elderly. Treatment for pneumonia should reflect the most likely etiologic agent (Table 10-5). Recently, a large percentage of *S pneumoniae* organisms have become penicillin-resistant. Nursing home-acquired pneumonia can be serious; however, if the patient's condition is not toxic and appears stable and the patient is able to take adequate oral fluids, the pneumonia can be treated in the nursing home if the patient is observed closely.

- The elderly have an increased number of gram-negative bacteria as part of their normal oral flora and an increased likelihood of aspirating oral secretions.
- *Streptococcus pneumoniae* is the most common etiologic organism of pneumonia.
- Pneumonia due to *Haemophilus influenzae*, other gram-negative bacteria, or anaerobes is common in nursing homes and hospitals.
- Infections with anaerobe organisms must be considered if the patient is suspected of having an aspiration pneumonia.

Tuberculosis, after decreasing in frequency for many years, is increasing in frequency. The number of reported cases has increased 20% during the past 10 years. Tuberculosis is more common with advancing age, with the elderly having 2 to 4 times the case rate of those younger than 65 years. Persons residing in nursing homes have from 2 to 6 times the case rate of the general population. Most cases of tuberculosis in the elderly are due to reactivation of a previous infection rather than to a newly acquired infection. It is thought that active tuberculosis eventually develops in about 10% of patients with a positive tuberculin skin test (PPD) (4% in the first 2 years). Tuberculosis is suspected on the basis of clinical findings, which can be subtle and include fatigue, anorexia with weight loss, and cough. Chest radiographic findings may be helpful in assessing whether disease is present. Confirmation of the disease requires evaluation of sputum and gastric washings for the presence of the acid-fast organisms. Although

Table 10-5 Empiric Management of Pneumonia in the Elderly

Patient Profile	Recommended Antibiotics
Community-acquired, treated as outpatient	PO quinolone with respiratory coverage (levofloxacin, moxifloxacin, gatifloxacin, gemifloxacin) or PO macrolide (azithromycin, clarithromycin) or PO doxycycline
Community-acquired, treated in hospital	IV quinolone with respiratory coverage (levofloxacin, moxifloxacin, gatifloxacin, gemifloxacin) or β-lactam (IV ceftriaxone, IV ampicillin-sulbactam) plus IV azithromycin
Nursing home-acquired, treated in nursing home	IV or PO quinolone with respiratory coverage (levofloxacin, moxifloxacin, gatifloxacin, gemifloxacin) or Macrolide (IV or PO azithromycin, PO clarithromycin) plus β-lactam (IV cefotaxime, IV or IM ceftriaxone, PO amoxicillin-clavulanate, IV ampicillin-sulbactam)
Nursing home-acquired, treated in hospital	IV quinolone with respiratory coverage (levofloxacin, moxifloxacin, gatifloxacin, gemifloxacin) or Macrolide (IV azithromycin) plus β-lactam (IV cefotaxime, IV ceftriaxone, IV ampicillin-sulbactam)

Abbreviations: IM, intramuscular; IV, intravenous; PO, oral.
Modified from Mandell LA, Bartlett JG, Dowell SF, File TM Jr, Musher DM, Whitney C. Update of practice guidelines for the management of community-acquired pneumonia in immunocompetent adults. Clin Infect Dis. 2003;37:1405-33. Used with permission.

culture results usually are available within 2 weeks, cultures may take up to 8 weeks to become positive. An increasing number of multidrug-resistant *Mycobacterium tuberculosis* organisms are being detected; however, these organisms are not common in the elderly because most cases are due to reactivation of the disease acquired many years ago when there were fewer drug-resistant organisms.

Without symptoms, the PPD is the best test available to determine the possibility of tuberculosis. Intermediate-strength tuberculin (5 tuberculin units) is administered intradermally, and the degree of induration (not erythema) is determined.

On admission to a nursing home, the patient should have a 2-stage PPD. The second test is administered on the seventh day if the patient has less than 10 mm of induration. The second test is interpreted 2 days after it is applied. Up to 15% of additional patients can be identified with this method. If the PPD is positive, chest radiography should be performed. If the findings are negative and the patient is asymptomatic, no treatment should be initiated unless it can be shown that the patient has had conversion to a positive PPD within the past 2 years. If the chest radiographic findings are abnormal, sputum and gastric washings should be obtained and cultured.

Up to one-third of all new patients admitted to a nursing home may have a positive PPD. Chemoprophylaxis is not recommended for all elderly patients with a positive PPD. Toxicity from isoniazid, especially hepatotoxicity, is very common in the elderly. Evidence of active tuberculosis should be excluded before chemoprophylaxis is given. Elderly patients receiving isoniazid treatment should have close follow-up for symptoms of hepatotoxicity. Isoniazid-induced hepatotoxicity is common with advancing age and develops in up to 5% of those older than 65 years. The baseline level of aspartate aminotransferase should be determined and checked periodically in elderly patients taking isoniazid. These patients also should receive vitamin B_6 (pyridoxine) supplements (10-25 mg daily) to prevent peripheral neuropathy.

Immunizations

Pneumococcal pneumonia vaccine is effective against 23 strains of *S pneumoniae*, which accounts for 80% of the strains that commonly cause pneumonia. Because of decreasing effectiveness, revaccination should be considered after 6 years for those who received their initial vaccination before age 65 years. The influenza vaccine is changed on a yearly basis, depending on the prevalent strain. It should be given in late autumn, and it should be given annually to high-risk persons, persons older than 65 years, and those in frequent close contact with the elderly. After the vaccine has been injected, it takes about 2 to 3 weeks before immunity to influenza develops. Any of the elderly who are unvaccinated during an influenza epidemic should be given amantadine or rimantadine. A new vaccine that has particular usefulness in elderly patients is the zoster vaccine. This is a live virus vaccine that has been shown to reduce the incidence of herpes zoster by about 60%. It has also been shown to decrease the incidence of postherpetic neuralgia. It is approved for use in patients older than 60 years.

- Pneumococcal pneumonia vaccine is effective against 80% of the bacterial strains that commonly cause pneumonia.

- Influenza vaccine should be given annually to high-risk persons, persons older than 65, and those in frequent close contact with the elderly.
- Zoster vaccine is indicated to reduce the risk of herpes zoster and postherpetic neuralgia.

Osteoporosis

Osteoporosis and its complications are extremely common among the elderly. Osteoporosis results in a loss of bone density, with preservation of a normal bone-to-mineral ratio. Hip, wrist, and vertebral compression fractures are common causes of morbidity and mortality. Peak bone density is achieved at about age 30 years; men have a greater bone density than women at all ages. After age 30 years, bone density gradually decreases. In women, loss of estrogen, either because of surgery (bilateral oophorectomy) or menopause, causes a more rapid decrease in bone density.

- Hip, wrist, and vertebral compression fractures are common causes of morbidity and mortality from osteoporosis.

The diagnosis of osteoporosis is usually made clinically. The World Health Organization uses T scores of bone mineral density. Osteopenia is defined as a T score between –1.0 and –2.5. Osteoporosis is defined as a T score of less than –2.5. The following help in establishing the diagnosis:

1. The presence of multiple risk factors, including advanced age, female sex, white, low calcium intake through much of one's lifetime, thin build, a history of corticosteroid or tobacco use, history of previous fracture (especially vertebral), northern European ancestry, prolonged inactivity, and family history positive for osteoporosis.
2. Ruling out secondary causes (glucocorticoid excess, hypogonadism, hyperthyroidism, hyperparathyroidism, osteomalacia, myeloma).
3. Physical examination findings (loss of height, increased thoracic kyphosis).
4. Radiographic findings of osteopenia or vertebral compression fractures.

- The diagnosis of osteoporosis is usually made clinically.

Bone density can be measured with several techniques, the most common of which is dual x-ray absorptiometry. Bone density is determined to assess the risk of fracture, to follow the progression of disease, or to evaluate the response to treatment.

- Bone density is determined to assess the risk of fracture, to follow the progression of disease, or to evaluate the response to treatment.

Previously, the treatment of osteoporosis was disappointing and was aimed at prevention. Currently, several options are available that can provide effective treatment for established osteoporosis. The initial treatment for osteoporosis in postmenopausal women should be adequate calcium intake, weight-bearing exercise, and adequate vitamin D (600-800 international units daily). Premenopausal women require 1,000 mg daily of elemental calcium, and postmenopausal women require 1,500 mg daily. Calcium carbonate is adequate for most, and it is the least expensive form of calcium supplementation. Calcium citrate should be used if the patient has a lack of gastric acid. Pharmacologic therapy is effective for increasing bone density as well as decreasing the risk of bone fractures. Although hormonal therapy has been shown to stabilize the decrease in bone density and, in some cases, to increase bone density slightly, it is no longer approved primarily for the prevention of osteoporosis on the basis of the Women's Health Initiative findings. The bisphosphonates alendronate and risedronate increase bone density and decrease the risk of hip and vertebral fractures. Compliance with these medications can be a problem, although both are now available in once-weekly dosing. They are poorly absorbed and bind to food and calcium and, thus, must be taken with tap water before food is ingested. Also, they have been associated with esophagitis. To minimize this, the patient must remain upright for at least 30 minutes after taking the medication.

Calcitonin increases vertebral bone density, but more data are needed to determine whether it decreases the risk of hip fracture. Calcitonin seems to have an analgesic effect and may be helpful in patients with painful osteoporotic vertebral compression fractures. Raloxifene is a selective estrogen receptor modulator that reduces bone resorption. Although it has estrogenlike effects on bone, it acts as an estrogen antagonist in the breast and uterus. It can cause a modest increase in bone mineral density in the hip and spine. Teriparatide is a synthetic polypeptide consisting of the biologically active N-terminal portion of human parathyroid hormone and is approved for the treatment of osteoporosis. Unlike all other treatment options for osteoporosis, parathyroid hormone increases bone formation rather than decreasing bone resorption. It seems to produce a greater increase in bone density than other pharmacologic treatments for osteoporosis; however, its high cost may be prohibitive for many patients. Also, it must be administered daily by subcutaneous injection. Hip protectors have been shown to reduce the risk of hip fractures in the elderly and should be considered for nursing home residents who have an increased risk of falling.

- Initial treatment of osteoporosis in postmenopausal women should be adequate calcium intake, weight-bearing exercise, adequate vitamin D (600-800 international units daily), and hormonal replacement therapy.
- Bisphosphonates increase bone density and decrease the rate of hip and vertebral fractures.
- Calcitonin appears to have an analgesic effect and may be helpful in patients with painful osteoporotic vertebral compression fractures.
- Raloxifene is a selective estrogen receptor modulator that reduces bone resorption and produces a modest increase in bone mineral density in the hip and spine.
- Teriparatide may be an option for a select group of patients with osteoporosis.

Osteomalacia

Osteomalacia is the result of defective bone mineralization and is caused most commonly by a deficiency of vitamin D. It may be due to inadequate intake of vitamin D, lack of exposure to the sun, malabsorption, chronic liver disease, or chronic renal disease. Radiographically, the bone appears osteopenic and can resemble osteoporosis. Unlike osteoporosis, several abnormal laboratory findings are associated with osteomalacia, including decreased levels of calcium, phosphorus, and 1,25-dihydroxyvitamin D and increased levels of alkaline phosphatase. Defective bone mineralization also may be caused by very low levels of phosphate. This can be due to excessive use of aluminum-containing antacids, tumor effect, or renal tubule disorders.

- Osteomalacia is the result of defective bone mineralization and is most commonly caused by a deficiency of vitamin D.
- Osteomalacia is associated with decreased levels of calcium, phosphorus, and 1,25-dihydroxyvitamin D and increased levels of alkaline phosphatase.

Pressure Ulcers

Seventy percent of pressure ulcers occur in persons older than 70 years. Approximately 60% of pressure ulcers develop during hospitalization, 18% in nursing homes, and the rest at home. They are especially common among the elderly in intensive care units. The most important risk factor for the development of a pressure ulcer is immobility. Nutritional deficiencies, age-related changes in the skin, and urinary incontinence are also contributing risk factors. Most pressure ulcers occur below the waist. The common sites include the sacrum, greater trochanter, ischial tuberosity, calcaneus, and lateral malleolus of the ankle. Four factors are thought to be important in the development of pressure ulcers: pressure, shearing force, friction, and moisture. When the persistent pressure of skin overlying a bony prominence exceeds the capillary pressure, the blood supply to the tissues is impaired. After approximately 2 hours, tissue ischemia can occur and result in skin ulceration. Friction and shearing forces are contributing factors when the patient is dragged across a bed or chair. This has the effect of causing angulation and occlusion of subcutaneous blood vessels and producing ischemia of the underlying tissue. Chronic skin moisture produces tissue maceration and promotes skin breakdown. This tends to magnify skin damage.

- Risk factors for the development of pressure ulcers are immobility, nutritional deficiencies, age-related changes in the skin, and urinary incontinence.

The most important component of pressure ulcer care is prevention. Preventive strategies include:

- Repositioning patients at least every 2 hours.
- Use of pressure-reducing mattresses.
- Minimizing head elevation.
- Lifting instead of dragging the patient.
- Keeping the patient as dry as possible when incontinent.
- Keeping the skin moisturized to help maintain skin integrity.

After a pressure ulcer has developed, the basic strategy for its treatment includes the following:

- Relieving pressure over the ulcer.
- Débridement of nonviable tissue.
- Optimizing the wound environment (preventing wound maceration and avoiding friction and shearing forces) to promote the formation of granulation tissue.
- Management of other conditions (malnutrition or infection when present) that may delay wound healing.

Pressure ulcers can be classified into one of 4 stages (I-IV). They tend to be understaged because often the underlying tissue damage is not immediately apparent.

Stage I: Nonblanchable erythema of intact skin. There may be associated edema.

Stage II: Partial-thickness skin loss involving the epidermis or dermis or both. The ulcer is superficial and may present as an abrasion, a blister, or a shallow crater.

Stage III: Full-thickness skin loss with damage or necrosis of subcutaneous tissue. The damage may extend to the fascia. The ulcer is a deep crater.

Stage IV: Full-thickness skin loss with extensive destruction, tissue necrosis, or involvement of muscle, bone, or tendons. Sinus tracts may be present.

Stages II, III, and IV pressure ulcers should be débrided of necrotic tissue when present. Stage II ulcers can be débrided mechanically with wet-to-wet (saline) gauze dressings changed every 6 hours. Also, several enzymatic débriding agents are available and effective. Surgical débridement may be useful, especially for deeper ulcers (stages III and IV). This should be done with caution in patients with lower extremity ulcers and arterial disease. Water débridement (whirlpool) is useful for larger ulcers. A moist wound environment is optimal for wound healing. Heat lamps dry the ulcer and should not be used. Several products are available to help maintain a moist wound environment, including semipermeable polyurethane films and foams, hydrocolloid dressings, and hydrophilic polymer gels. Topical iodine-povidone, hydrogen peroxide, and acetic acid compounds can impair wound healing and should not be used on pressure ulcers. Infection commonly complicates the healing of pressure ulcers. Infected ulcers require treatment with systemic antibiotics. Topical antibiotics have little penetration into deeper tissue and can promote the development of resistant bacteria. Culturing the surface of an ulcer does not represent accurately the bacteria involved in an infected ulcer; all skin ulcers develop surface bacterial colonization. An accurate determination of the bacteria involved requires deep tissue cultures.

An ulcer that does not heal should alert the physician to the presence of osteomyelitis. Bone radiography and bone scanning are often performed in patients with suspected osteomyelitis, but they have a rather high incidence of false-negative and false-positive results. Magnetic resonance imaging is an effective diagnostic test when osteomyelitis is suspected; however, bone biopsy with culture is the best confirmatory test.

Platelet-derived growth factor is occasionally useful for stimulating the healing of pressure ulcers. For large or very deep ulcers, surgical treatment may be necessary. The use of skin grafts or rotation flaps using neighboring subcutaneous tissue and muscle may be the best

option in these cases. Hyperbaric chamber pressure therapy may be useful in selected patients.

- Stages II, III, and IV pressure ulcers should be débrided of necrotic tissue.
- A moist wound environment is optimal for wound healing.
- Infected ulcers require treatment with systemic antibiotics.
- Bone biopsy with culture is the best confirmatory test for osteomyelitis.

Urinary Incontinence

Urinary incontinence is common among the elderly, affecting at least 15% of those living independently and about 50% of those in institutions. It is much more common in females than in males. It causes numerous medical, social, and economic complications and is a common reason for nursing home placement. The complications include urinary tract infection, skin breakdown, social isolation, and depression. Urinary incontinence also has been associated with an increased risk for falls in the elderly. Understanding urinary incontinence requires knowledge of the anatomy of the urinary tract and the physiology of normal micturition. Failure to appreciate this information can result in inaccurate diagnosis and ineffective treatment.

Anatomy

The detrusor muscle of the bladder consists of 3 muscular layers. Both sympathetic and parasympathetic nerves innervate the detrusor muscle. The internal sphincter is a smooth muscle under involuntary (sympathetic innervation) control. Stimulation of the sympathetic nerves results in contraction of the internal urinary sphincter and detrusor relaxation, promoting urine storage. Stimulation of the parasympathetic nerves produces contraction of the detrusor muscle and internal spincter relaxation, promoting bladder emptying. The external sphincter is striated muscle and under voluntary (pudendal innervation) control. It contracts in response to transient increases in intra-abdominal pressure (eg, cough or sneeze) to prevent urine loss, but it fatigues rapidly.

Stretch receptors in the wall of the detrusor muscle send information to the brain. The spinal cord carries sensory signals to the brain and motor signals to the bladder. The brain produces stimulation of the sympathetic nerves and inhibition of the parasympathetic nerves when urine storage is desired (relaxation of the detrusor muscle and contraction of the internal sphincter) and stimulation of the parasympathetic nerves and inhibition of the sympathetic nerves when bladder emptying is desired (contraction of the detrusor muscle and relaxation of the internal sphincter).

- Both sympathetic and parasympathetic nerves innervate the detrusor muscle.

Stimulation of the sympathetic nerves results in relaxation of the detrusor muscle, and stimulation of the parasympathetic nerves produces contraction of the detrusor muscle.

Effects of Age

Changes occur in the urinary system with aging, but these changes do not result in urinary incontinence. Incontinence is not a normal result of aging. However, the changes that occur can contribute to the problem of incontinence. These changes include smaller bladder capacity, early contractions of the detrusor muscle, decreased ability to suppress contractions of the detrusor muscle and to postpone urination, and increased nocturnal production of urine.

Medications Affecting Urination and Continence
Many medications can have an effect on urinary continence. They may alter the ability of the brain to appreciate bladder fullness or the ability of the internal sphincter to contract and relax, or they may interfere with the function of the bladder. These medications include potent diuretics that cause brisk filling of the bladder, anticholinergic agents, calcium channel antagonists or narcotics that can impair contraction of the detrusor muscle, sedative-hypnotics that may cause confusion, α-adrenergic agonists that increase internal sphincter tone, and α-adrenergic antagonists that decrease internal sphincter tone.

Established Incontinence
Patients are more likely to have reversible incontinence if the incontinence is of recent onset. Although established incontinence is more difficult to treat, it can be managed with substantial benefit to the patient. The 4 types of established incontinence are overactive bladder (urge incontinence), outlet incompetence (stress incontinence), overflow incontinence, and functional incontinence (Table 10-6). Functional or iatrogenic incontinence can occur in persons with mobility problems or as an adverse effect of medication.

Overactivity of the detrusor muscle (overactive bladder) is a common cause of established incontinence, accounting for 40% to 70% of cases. When overactive bladder results in incontinence, it is known as urge incontinence. Overactive bladder tends to be most common in middle-aged and older women and men. Although overactive bladder is equally common in men and women, urge incontinence is much more common in women. Overactive bladder causes early detrusor contractions at low bladder volumes. Symptoms include urinary frequency and urgency, with losses of small-to-moderate urine volumes. Nocturia often occurs. At times, detrusor overactivity occurs with CNS disease (mass lesions, Parkinson disease, stroke) or bladder irritation (urinary tract infection, benign prostatic hyperplasia, fecal impaction, atrophic urethritis). There is no association between chronic asymptomatic bacteriuria and urinary incontinence.

- Overactivity of the detrusor muscle is a common cause of established incontinence.
- Symptoms include urinary frequency and urgency, with losses of small-to-moderate urine volumes and nocturia.

Outlet incompetence (stress incontinence) is common in middle-aged women and rare in men (unless internal sphincter damage has occurred). It is caused by inadequate resistance of urinary outflow and worsened by laxity of pelvic floor musculature and lack of bladder support. This may be caused by hypermobility of the urethra or intrinsic urinary sphincter insufficiency. The symptoms include losses of small amounts of urine with transient increases in intra-abdominal

Table 10-6 Types of Established Urinary Incontinence

Type	Cause	Symptoms	Treatment Options
Urge incontinence	Detrusor overactivity	Urgency, frequency, nocturia. Loss of small to moderate volumes of urine	Behavioral: urge suppression, elimination of bladder irritants, timed voiding Pharmacologic: antimuscarinic medications (oxybutynin, tolterodine, trospium, darifenacin, folifenacin)
Stress incontinence	Urinary outlet incompetence from intrinsic urethral sphincter insufficiency or hypermobility of the bladder	Losses of small amounts of urine associated with transient increases in intra-abdominal pressure (eg, cough, sneeze, laugh)	Behavioral: continence tampons, vaginal cones, urethral plugs, continence pessaries, pelvic floor exercises Surgical: urethral sling, tension-free vaginal tape, bladder suspension, injection of periurethral bulking agents, artificial urinary sphincter
Overflow incontinence	Urinary outlet obstruction or detrusor underactivity	Difficulty emptying bladder, low urine flow, straining to void, urinary dribbling	Relief of bladder outlet obstruction (TURP), α-adrenergic antagonists, indwelling or intermittent bladder catheterization

Abbreviation: TURP, transurethral resection of prostate.

pressure (eg, cough, sneeze, laugh, or change in position). Some patients describe a combination of urge incontinence and stress incontinence. This is known as mixed urinary incontinence. In these patients, the history can be confusing because the patients describe symptoms of both urge incontinence and stress incontinence.

- Outlet incompetence (stress incontinence) is common in women.
- Symptoms include losses of small amounts of urine with transient increases in intra-abdominal pressure.

Overflow incontinence is uncommon. It occurs with urinary outflow obstruction (benign prostatic hyperplasia, prostate cancer, or pelvic tumor) or detrusor underactivity-hypotonic bladder (autonomic neuropathy). This often occurs transiently in the elderly after surgery. Symptoms include difficulty emptying the bladder, low urine flow, and frequent dribbling. Patients give a history of difficulty starting urination and a weak urinary stream, with stream hesitancy.

Functional incontinence is the inability of normally continent patients to reach toilet facilities in time. Often, it is due to various medications (eg, potent diuretics and α-adrenergic antagonists) and some limitation of mobility (restraint use, arthritis, or hemiparesis).

- Overflow incontinence is uncommon and due to urinary outflow obstruction or detrusor underactivity-hypotonic bladder.
- An atonic or hypotonic bladder often occurs transiently postoperatively.

Evaluation of Incontinence

The evaluation of urinary incontinence includes a thorough medical history, physical examination, and several simple selected laboratory tests. The history is most important and should include the amount of urine lost, duration of symptoms, precipitating factors, whether symptoms of obstruction exist, and the patient's functional status. Also, symptoms of neurologic disease, associated disease states, menstrual status and parity, and medications taken should be documented.

Physical examination of the abdomen should evaluate bladder distention and possible abdominal masses. Examination of the pelvis should include assessment for uterine, bladder, or rectal prolapse; atrophic vaginitis; and pelvic masses. The rectal examination should document any masses, fecal impaction, sphincter tone, and prostate enlargement or nodules. A neurologic examination should be performed to search for disease of the brain or spinal cord, autonomic nerves, or peripheral nerves. Patients should complete a voiding diary that records fluid intake, types of fluids ingested, and voidings (both continent and incontinent).

Laboratory tests commonly ordered in the investigation of urinary incontinence include urinalysis and urine culture to check for infection, pyuria, and hematuria; blood urea nitrogen and creatinine determination to assess renal function; and calcium and glucose measurements to assess polyuric states. Occasionally, intravenous pyelography or renal ultrasonography (or both) may be necessary to check for hydronephrosis, which may occur with chronic bladder outlet obstruction. A postvoid residual bladder volume test should be performed to determine the degree of bladder emptying when a patient describes symptoms of urinary outlet obstruction.

Urodynamic studies are occasionally necessary to establish the diagnosis of incontinence, but the results are not always consistent with the clinical picture and, thus, can be misleading. Urodynamic studies are indicated when patients have medically confusing histories or more than one type of urinary incontinence (mixed incontinence). Cystometry measures bladder volume and pressure and can be used to detect uninhibited detrusor muscle contractions, lack of bladder contractions, and bladder sensation. Voiding cystourethrography measures the urethrovesical angle and residual urine volume. Uroflow measures urinary flow rate, and electromyography evaluates the external sphincter and detects detrusor-sphincter dyssynergia.

- The medical history is the most important part of the incontinence evaluation.
- Urodynamic studies are occasionally necessary to establish the diagnosis of incontinence, but the results can be misleading in some patients.

Treatment of Incontinence

The treatment of urinary incontinence is usually successful to some degree. All patients should be encouraged to drink an adequate volume of fluid, 40 to 60 oz daily. The treatment of detrusor overactivity is aimed at suppressing the early contractions of the detrusor muscle. Behavioral training should be the initial treatment attempted. Often, it is successful for decreasing incontinent episodes. It includes eliminating bladder irritants (especially caffeine), urge suppression techniques (pelvic floor muscle contraction), scheduled toileting, and prompted voiding. When behavioral training is ineffective, pharmacologic therapy may be added. Medications that inhibit parasympathetic stimulation of the bladder muscle (antimuscarinics) are often effective. Drugs with antimuscarinic activity that are most commonly used include oxybutynin and tolterodine. Trospium, darifenacin, and solifenacin are also antimuscarinic medications that may have fewer peripheral anticholinergic adverse effects (dry mouth, constipation, blurred vision). Tricyclic antidepressants also have been used, but they have a higher risk of anticholinergic adverse effects. Topical estrogen therapy also may be effective in some women when atrophic urethritis is the cause of early contractions of the detrusor muscle.

- The treatment of detrusor overactivity is aimed at suppressing early detrusor contractions.
- Nonpharmacologic therapy should be attempted initially.
- Medications that inhibit parasympathetic stimulation of the bladder muscle (antimuscarinics) are often effective.
- Topical estrogen therapy may be effective in some women.

The treatment of outlet incompetence should also begin with behavioral therapy. Patients should be instructed in pelvic floor exercises (Kegel exercises). In some patients, this is more effective with the assistance of biofeedback. Although pelvic floor exercises are useful, they must be performed for several months before any benefit is recognized. Increasing the tone of the internal sphincter with α-adrenergic agonists (pseudoephedrine or imipramine) may be of limited short-term benefit. Tolerance to these medications develops quickly, and the beneficial effect disappears. Hormonal therapy (topical estrogen) has been used for outlet incompetence in an attempt to restore the mucosa of the urethra, increasing its resistance, but the results have been disappointing. Pessaries and continence tampons are occasionally used for outlet incompetence, but chronic use is difficult because of potential vaginal irritation. Urethral plugs are available and can provide temporary relief of symptoms. However, they potentially can produce urethral irritation.

For selected patients, surgical therapy may be effective. Internal sphincter bulking agents such as collagen may provide substantial benefit for up to 2 years. Occasionally a surgical procedure to provide an artificial urinary sphincter may be considered. For patients who have more severe symptoms of outlet incompetence, surgical suspension of the bladder and bladder neck sling therapy can restore continence. Tension-free vaginal tape is a relatively new procedure that provides a urethral sling and can be performed on an outpatient basis with the patient under local or regional anesthesia.

- Patients with outlet incompetence should be instructed in pelvic floor exercises.
- Pharmacologic treatment has limited short-term benefit.
- For selected patients, surgical therapy may be effective.

The treatment of overflow incontinence is aimed at providing complete drainage from a bladder that either is not contracting adequately or has marked outflow obstruction. For a hypotonic bladder, treatment can be tried with medications that increase the tone of the detrusor muscle, including the cholinergic agonist bethanechol. This may be effective for short-term use, for example, for a transient hypotonic bladder postoperatively; however, adverse effects are common in the elderly and limit its long-term use. Treatment of obstruction includes operation (transurethral resection of the prostate) and use of α-adrenergic antagonists (terazosin, doxazosin, or tamsulosin), which decrease the tone of the internal sphincter. An external (condom) urinary catheter is of little benefit because it does not provide adequate drainage of the bladder. Occasionally, an indwelling catheter or intermittent catheterization is necessary. When a patient is expected to regain contractile function of the bladder, intermittent catheterization is performed at a frequency determined by the residual urine volume. If outflow obstruction is a chronic condition and not expected to improve, indefinite self-catheterization or an indwelling catheter is usually necessary.

- Medications that increase the tone of the detrusor muscle can be tried for transient hypotonic bladder.
- Surgery is often necessary to relieve bladder outlet obstruction from benign prostatic hypertrophy.
- An indwelling catheter or indefinite catheterization is occasionally necessary.

Urologic Consultation

In most elderly patients, the diagnosis of urinary incontinence can be established without the need for evaluation by a urologist. The following conditions indicate the need for urologic evaluation: high postvoid residual urine volume, symptoms of urinary outflow obstruction, marked uterine or bladder prolapse, abnormal findings on prostate examination, recurrent urinary tract infection, hematuria, unknown diagnosis, or failure to improve with treatment.

Use of Urinary Catheters

External (condom) catheters have a slight risk of infection, and problems with penile skin breakdown limit long-term use. They also have minimal benefit in overflow incontinence. Intermittent catheterization has a small risk of infection with each catheter insertion (from 1% in persons who are ambulatory and otherwise healthy to 20% in those who are frail and have multiple chronic illnesses). It is useful for temporary incontinence, as in postoperative transient hypotonic bladder. Postvoid residual volumes should be used as a guide for determining the frequency of catheterization. Intermittent catheterization is of limited use in the management of chronic incontinence in nursing home patients because of catheter expense and in those living independently if they have limited manual dexterity or poor vision.

Essentially all patients with indwelling catheters eventually have development of marked bacteriuria, and the bacterial organisms typically change with time. Other than maintaining a closed urinary collection system, nothing has been found to prevent or even substantially delay the onset of bacteriuria. Neither urethral cleansing nor bladder irrigation has been shown to be effective. Routine surveillance cultures should not be performed, and the chronic use of suppressive antibiotics is not recommended. Antibiotic therapy does not prevent long-term colonization by bacteria and eventually results in infections caused by resistant organisms. Antibiotic treatment should be reserved for symptomatic infections only, although it may be difficult to determine when a symptomatic urinary tract infection is present in a catheterized elderly patient. In patients who have had urinary catheters removed, bacteriuria should be treated if the urine remains bacteriuric for more than 48 hours. In many cases, the bacteriuria will resolve with removal of the urinary catheter alone.

- Essentially all patients with indwelling catheters eventually have development of marked bacteriuria.
- Surveillance cultures should not be performed, and the bacteriuria should be treated only when it is symptomatic.
- Chronic use of suppressive antibiotics is not recommended.

Urinary Tract Infection

Urinary tract infection becomes more common with advancing age and causes a wide spectrum of disease. The prevalence in the elderly is much higher than in younger individuals. It is the most common infection in nursing home residents and the most common cause of sepsis in the elderly. Urosepsis is also a very common cause of delirium in the elderly. It also may produce the syndrome of asymptomatic bacteriuria. Incomplete emptying of the bladder, which is common in the elderly (cystocele, benign prostatic hyperplasia, or hypotonic bladder), urinary instrumentation, and chronic catheterization all predispose the elderly to urinary tract infection. The clinical presentation of bacteriuria in the elderly can vary tremendously. Many have no symptoms, and vague symptoms such as confusion, decreased appetite, and urinary incontinence commonly result in a delayed diagnosis. Pyuria is not a reliable indicator of bacteriuria in the elderly population, although the absence of pyuria is a reasonably good indicator of the absence of bacteriuria.

The elderly have various bacterial organisms that typically produce urinary tract infections, and these differ from younger patients. *Escherichia coli*, the most common organism to cause urinary tract infections in the younger population, causes about half to three-fourths of these infections in the elderly. Other gram-negative organisms such as *Enterococcus* sp, *Proteus* sp, *Klebsiella* sp, *Enterobacter* sp, *Serratia* sp, and *Pseudomonas* sp are frequent in the elderly. Polymicrobial infections and resistant organisms are also common. Because of the variety of organisms, the urine usually should be cultured when evaluating an elderly patient who has a urinary tract infection.

Asymptomatic bacteriuria becomes more common with age and has been associated with increased mortality; however, the mortality seems to be unrelated to the bacteriuria and is likely a marker for increased severity of illness, frailty, and debility. Asymptomatic bacteriuria should not be treated unless there is a history of chronic urinary obstruction or if bladder instrumentation is planned. Treatment is also advised prior to performing a transurethral resection of the prostate.

* Urinary tract infection is the most common infection in nursing home residents and the most common cause of sepsis in the elderly.
* Because of the variety of organisms, the urine should be cultured when evaluating an elderly patient who has a urinary tract infection.
* Asymptomatic bacteriuria should not be treated unless there is a history of chronic urinary obstruction, bladder instrumentation is planned, or a transurethral resection of the prostate is to be performed.

Use of Medications

More than 30% of all prescriptions are written for persons older than 65 years. Medications are a common cause of iatrogenic disease in the elderly and are handled differently in the elderly because of various changes in pharmacokinetics and pharmacodynamics. Overall, the activity of many drugs has a longer duration, lower doses often achieve desired therapeutic effects, adverse drug effects are more frequent, drug-drug interactions are more frequent, and the likelihood of drug toxicity is greater in the elderly.

Pharmacokinetics includes drug absorption, distribution, metabolism, and elimination. Age-related changes have an effect on each of these variables, affecting some more than others. Age-related changes that affect drug absorption include decreased blood supply to the small bowel (the site of most drug absorption), villous atrophy resulting in decreased surface area for the absorption of drugs, and decreased gastric acidity. Little evidence supports any marked reduction in drug absorption with increasing age. Drug absorption is the least important of the pharmacokinetic changes associated with aging. Drug distribution has a major role in altered pharmacokinetics and changes considerably with age. This is due to age-related alterations in the various volumes of distribution in the elderly. These changes include an increase in adipose tissue, a decrease in total body water and lean body mass, and, for many, a change in levels of plasma protein. The result of increased adipose tissue is an increase in the volume of distribution for lipid-soluble drugs, which can result in an increase in drug half-life (eg, highly lipid-soluble benzodiazepines). The decrease in body water creates a smaller volume of distribution for water-soluble drugs, potentially leading to a higher than expected drug concentration (eg, ethanol). A decrease in plasma protein (eg, albumin) results in less protein-bound (inactive) acidic drugs and a greater amount of free (active) drug. This can produce a greater than anticipated drug effect. α_1-Acid glycoproteins are acute-phase reactants that are increased in patients with inflammatory conditions. This can cause an increase in basic drug (lidocaine, propranolol) protein binding, thereby reducing the amount of bioavailable drug and possibly attenuating the drug effect.

Drug metabolism occurs primarily in the liver. With advanced age, the ability of the liver to metabolize drugs decreases because of various factors, including a decrease in the number of functioning hepatocytes, reduced hepatic blood flow, and reduced hepatic enzymatic activity. Phase I metabolism involves the oxidation or reduction of a drug by the cytochrome P450 system. This type of metabolism produces active metabolites and slows with age. Phase II metabolism involves acetylation and produces inactive metabolites. It shows no changes with advancing age. A patient's ability to metabolize a specific drug is extremely difficult to predict because no simple test is available that provides this information.

Drug elimination refers primarily to the ability of the renal system to excrete drugs from the circulation. Generally, renal function decreases with age, with both decreased renal plasma flow and glomerular filtration rate (up to 30%), although the variability among elderly persons is great. The serum level of creatinine is not a good measure of renal function in the elderly and tends to underestimate the degree of renal insufficiency. Creatinine is a product of muscle breakdown. Because lean body mass decreases with advancing age, less creatinine is produced. Thus, an elderly patient who has as much as a 30% reduction in renal function may have a normal serum level of creatinine. A more accurate estimate of renal function is the following:

$$\text{Creatinine clearance} = \frac{140 - \text{age} \times \text{weight (kg)}}{72 \times \text{creatinine}} = (\times 0.85 \text{ for women})$$

Age-related changes occur in pharmacokinetics involving drug absorption, distribution, metabolism, and elimination. Renal function is discussed further in the Nephrology chapter.

* Drug distribution has a major role in altered pharmacokinetics.
* The ability of the liver to metabolize drugs decreases in most elderly patients.
* Because of decreased renal function with age, elimination of many drugs is delayed in the elderly.
* Serum creatinine level may underestimate the degree of renal insufficiency.

Pharmacodynamic changes also occur with aging and have an effect on the action of medications. The term *pharmacodynamics* refers to drug sensitivity, which can change with age. These changes may reflect an alteration of receptor number or receptor sensitivity to a drug or an altered receptor response to a drug. Less is known about age-related altered pharmacodynamics than about pharmacokinetics; however, the pharmacodynamic changes for several drugs have been identified. There is a reduced responsiveness to β-adrenergic drugs (eg, less tachycardia with isoproterenol, less bradycardia with β-blockers), increased sedation with benzodiazepines, greater analgesia with opiates, and greater anticoagulant activity with warfarin.

Adverse drug effects are common in the elderly and frequently cause serious complications. Elderly patients often have limited organ reserve function and are unable to respond as younger persons can to an adverse effect. Drug-drug effects tend to occur more commonly in the elderly and tend to be more serious. The likelihood of a drug-drug effect is related to the number of medications taken.

- Pharmacodynamic changes result in an alteration in a given drug effect with age.
- Adverse drug effects tend to occur more often and are often more severe in the elderly, primarily because of reduced organ reserve capacity with age.

As a result of altered pharmacokinetics and pharmacodynamics with aging, medications need to be prescribed carefully for the elderly, avoiding polypharmacy whenever possible and watching for evidence of adverse drug effects and drug-drug interactions, both of which increase in frequency with age. Medications have been identified that have potentially greater risks in the elderly. These drugs should be prescribed with great caution for older patients. Some of these medications are discussed in the following paragraphs. See the Geriatrics Pharmacy Review for a more complete list of pharmacologic considerations in the elderly.

Long-acting benzodiazepines (diazepam, chlordiazepoxide, and flurazepam) are highly lipid-soluble and, thus, have a very long half-life in elderly patients. They also have active metabolites. These drugs can easily accumulate in the elderly and possibly produce drug toxicity. Barbiturates also are highly lipid-soluble and have very long half-lives in the elderly. Drug accumulation may occur; also, tolerance develops quickly to their sedating activity. Diphenhydramine is available over-the-counter and is often used to induce sleep. It potentially can cause cognitive impairment in the elderly. Propoxyphene is a weak analgesic with little therapeutic advantage over acetaminophen; yet, it has all the risks and adverse effects of narcotics. Pentazocine is a mixed agonist and antagonist oral narcotic that has significant potential for adverse effects on the CNS, including confusion and hallucinations.

Meperidine is a weak analgesic with an unpredictable rate of oral absorption. Its metabolites can accumulate in patients with renal insufficiency; seizures or respiratory depression may occur. Tricyclic antidepressants have the potential for various adverse effects because of their nonselective neurochemical blockade. α-Adrenergic antagonist activity can produce orthostatic hypotension, antihistamine activity can lead to sedation, and anticholinergic effects can cause urinary obstruction in men and delirium, constipation, and blurred vision. Monoamine oxidase inhibitors and antidepressants have marked potential for serious adverse effects, such as hypertension, when they interact with tyramine-containing products. Chlorpropamide, an oral hypoglycemic agent, is a first-generation sulfonylurea and has an extremely long half-life; thus, it has a substantial risk of causing prolonged hypoglycemia.

Geriatrics Pharmacy Review
Robert W. Hoel, RPh, PharmD

Drug	Toxic/Adverse Effects	Considerations in the Elderly
Antibiotics		
Nitrofurantoin	GI (nausea, vomiting), pulmonary fibrosis, peripheral neuropathy with long use	Requires clearance of ~60 mL/min for effective concentration in urine
Antihistamines	Anticholinergic: dry eyes & mouth, urine retention, constipation	Strongest anticholinergic agents are contraindicated because they cause confusion & a risk of falling
Older agents: diphenhydramine, hydroxyzine		Avoid older agents in the elderly. Newer agents are safer (loratadine, fexofenadine)
Iron products for anemia	Constipation, nausea, weight loss.	Anorexia & weight loss; elderly patients
Ferrous sulfate, gluconate, others	Ferrous sulfate (~30% elemental iron)	rarely tolerate more than once-daily dosing. Can alleviate anemia with ferrous gluconate, which is tolerated better than sulfate salt[1]
Endocrine agents		
Insulin, hypoglycemic, oral	Hypoglycemia is due to sulfonylureas & drug interactions	Administer carefully in anorexia. Avoid first-generation sulfonylureas (chlorpropamide) & glyburide (subject to hypoglycemia)
Metformin	Nausea, vomiting, diarrhea, life-threatening lactic acidosis	Lactic acidosis more likely with reduced renal clearance, acute or chronic
Rosiglitazone	Edema, weight gain. Can worsen heart failure	Visual deterioration may worsen; eye examination during treatment
Levothyroxine (Synthroid, Levothroid)	Dose is adjusted to results of thyroid laboratory studies. Excess dose worsens CHF, tachycardia, weight loss, palpitations, insomnia, sweating	Bioequivalence problems with switching between different products. Use of same brand should be continued
Psychotropics[a]		
Antipsychotics[b]		
Haloperidol	Tardive dyskinesia is common in elderly. Extrapyramidal or Parkinson disease-like symptoms, sedation	Consider atypical antipsychotic agents—less orthostasis & fewer dyskinetic effects
Phenothiazines (eg, chlorpromazine, thioridazine)	Sedation, orthostatic hypotension, dizziness, increased falls, anticholinergic & extrapyramidal effects. Dose-related prolongation of QTc interval	Consider atypical agents (less hypotension & fewer anticholinergic & extrapyramidal side effects)
Risperidone, olanzapine, quetiapine, ziprasidone	Weight gain, worsening hyperglycemia. Higher doses may prolong QTc interval	Reduce doses in problem renal or hepatic clearance. Risperidone has been associated with higher incidence of stroke & TIAs in trials
Antidepressants[c]		
Tricyclic agents (imipramine, amitriptyline)	Possible severe anticholinergic effects, dysrhythmias, drowsiness	Avoid due to strong anticholinergic effects, except for nortriptyline or desipramine, which have favorable side effect profiles
SSRI antidepressants	Fewer severe side effects than TCAs, but no more effective. Monitor for hyperserotonin effects	Adjust dose for renal & hepatic clearance; titrate dose gradually. Use with NSAIDs may increase incidence of GI bleeding. Taper gradually
Paroxetine, sertraline	Nausea, weight changes (loss), mental status changes (especially sedation), sexual dysfunction	Watch for weight loss
Fluoxetine	Hallucinations, anxiety	Often worsens anxious behavior
Nafazodone, trazodone	Sedation, anticholinergic effects, orthostasis, sexual dysfunction, agitation, or weight changes	Trazodone: sedation with lower dose, but weak antidepressant effect
Mirtazapine	Sedation, weight gain	Adjust dose for renal or hepatic clearance; titrate dose gradually

Geriatrics Pharmacy Review (continued)

Drug	Toxic/Adverse Effects	Considerations in the Elderly
Sedatives and hypnotics		
Benzodiazepines	Sedation, confusion, avoid old long-acting agents (ie, diazepam half-life 20-170 hours) & agents with active metabolites	Lorazepam & oxazepam may be preferred considering no phase 1 active metabolites
Zolpidem, zaleplon	Potential transient mental status issues	Use lowest doses in frail elderly; indicated only for short-term (7-10 day) treatment of insomnia. Recommend sleep hygiene
Diphenhydramine (in many OTC sleep aids)	Oversedation, CNS impairment, urinary retention, is due to strong anticholinergic effects	Higher incidence of delirium & confusion & should be avoided (see Beers lists)
Cognitive agents Donepezil, galantamine, memantine (NMDA)	Nausea, diarrhea, insomnia, fatigue. Donepezil better tolerated at usual dose of 5 mg daily, some may benefit at 10 mg daily	May temporarily slow progression of & may improve dementia-related uncontrolled behavior
Cardiovascular agents Digoxin	Dysrhythmias, confusion, visual disturbances, anorexia, nausea, vomiting, diarrhea at toxic levels	Avoid drugs that decrease clearance (NSAIDs). Monitor potassium & toxicity. Generally avoid doses more than 0.125 mg unless proven control of atrial fibrillation; adjust with renal decline
Nitrates	Tolerance to beneficial effects alleviated with 8- to 12-hour nitrate-free interval. Headaches	Hypotension & orthostasis, dizziness, syncope, falls
ACE inhibitors (or angiotensin receptor blocker)	Worsens renal function in artery stenosis, cough. Substitute ARB if ACE inhibitor not tolerated	ACE inhibitors have proven long-term benefits in CHF, proven renal benefit in diabetes
α-Adrenergic blockers	Syncope, orthostatic hypotension	Particular susceptibility to falls. Slower hepatic clearance
Calcium channel blockers	See Cardiovascular agents	Edema, constipation (verapamil), avoid short-acting nifedipine because of its tendency to cause hypotension
β-Adrenergic blockers	Bronchoconstriction with agents having B2 effect or in high doses of all agents, depression, orthostasis, glucose intolerance, blocks warning signs of hypoglycemia	Proven long-term benefits in CHF, MI
Diuretics (see Cardiovascular agents)	Electrolyte imbalances, dehydration, orthostasis	Especially prone to orthostasis, but low-dose thiazide is still first-line therapy in HTN
Antihypertensive agents (see Cardiovascular agents)	Additive orthostatic hypotension occurs with many common drugs	Orthostasis increases likelihood of falls & fractures
Anticoagulants Warfarin	Monitor INR (PT) & for bleeding. Review changes in entire drug regimen for interactions	Some elderly who are prone to fall may have risks of bleeding but show highest therapeutic benefit for stroke prevention
Gastrointestinal drugs H$_2$ antagonists	Confusion occasionally. Usually 12-week indication for ulcer treatment	Dose adjust to clearance. Do not necessarily prevent NSAID-induced GI ulcers
Proton pump inhibitors	Do not necessarily prevent NSAID-induced GI ulcers	No more side effects than in younger adults. Possible association with osteoporosis with years of use[2]

Geriatrics Pharmacy Review (continued)

Drug	Toxic/Adverse Effects	Considerations in the Elderly
Respiratory agents		
Metered-dose inhalers		Frequent inability to coordinate administration. Extended inhalation tube required
Theophylline	Tachycardia, insomnia, anxiety, narrow therapeutic index necessitates monitoring of drug levels	Side effects not tolerated well, sleeplessness, anxiety. Respiratory disease often controlled with other agents (ie, inhaler therapy)
Zafirlukast	Approved indication is asthma	Prolonged metabolism, indicating dose reduction
Osteoporosis agents[d]		
Calcium salts	Constipation. H_2 antagonists & proton pump inhibitors impair absorption of calcium salts, except calcium citrate	1,200-1,500 mg elemental calcium daily intake for all elderly, postmenopausal women. Add smoking cessation & weight-bearing exercise
Vitamin D	Many multivitamins have 400 units per dose	Recommend 800 IU vitamin D daily with calcium supplementation. Assess vitamin D status
Oral bisphosphonates: alendronate, risedronate	Erosive esophagitis	Take 30 min before meals & other medications with full glass of water & remain upright for 30 min
Calcitonin (salmon)	200 units per nasal spray. May help spine fracture-related pain	Efficacy data are weaker than with bisphosphonate or HRT
Hormone replacement therapy	Abnormal vaginal bleeding, thromboembolism, DVT	Estrogen with progestin to prevent endometrial cancer
Raloxifene	Thromboembolism, DVT, hot flashes	Effective osteoporosis prevention, but not menopausal symptoms
Incontinence agents[e]		
Oxybutynin, tolterodine	Drowsiness, anticholinergic effects; inhibits early detrusor contractions, hesitancy	Anticholinergic effects are poorly tolerated, leading to confusion, falls, constipation
Rheumatologic agents		
NSAIDs	Nausea, GI ulcers, fluid retention, nephrotoxicity	Use lowest dose possible. Avoid in kidney disease
COX-2 inhibitors	Nephrotoxicity, fluid retention, hypertension	Potentially fewer GI bleeds. GI bleeding occurs with other pro-ulcer agents (ie, aspirin, warfarin)
Hydroxychloroquine	Muscle weakness, retinal damage, visual disturbances, nausea	Long time to benefit; if no benefit in 6 months, stop use. Eye examinations every 6 mo
Methotrexate	Myelosuppression, nausea, hypotension (monitor CBC)	Start with lowest doses (given weekly for RA & prednisone sparing). Increase if needed & tolerated
Glucocorticoids	Nausea, weight gain, GI ulcers, hyperglycemia, osteoporosis, adrenal suppression	Taper to lowest effective dose. Consider prophylaxis for osteoporosis & *Pneumocystis carinii*
Colchicine	Nausea (diarrhea may indicate toxicity), myelosuppression	Must adjust dose for lower renal clearance in kidney disease & avoid in clearance less than ~20 mL/min due to toxicity potential

Geriatrics Pharmacy Review (continued)

Drug	Toxic/Adverse Effects	Considerations in the Elderly
Impotence agents		
Sildenafil, vardenafil	Headache, flushing, dyspepsia, hypotension, QTc prolongation (vardenafil), many drug-drug interactions	Contraindicated in patients receiving nitrate therapy, reduced renal & hepatic clearance (deccrease doses). Increase susceptibility to hypotension
Glaucoma agents		
Topical eyedrops	Burning, itching eyes	Many OTC ophthalmics may exacerbate narrow-angle glaucoma (oral decongestants, antihistamines)

[1] Rimon E, Kagansky N, Kagansky M, Mechnick L, Mashiah T, Namir M, et al. Are we giving too much iron? Low-dose iron therapy is effective in octogenarians. Am J Med. 2005;118(10):1142-7.

[2] Yang YX, Lewis JD, Epstein S, Metz DC. Long-term proton pump inhibitor therapy and risk of hip fracture. JAMA. 2006;296:2947-53.

Abbreviations: ACE, angiotensin-converting enzyme; ARB, angiotensin receptor blocker; CBC, complete blood count; CHF, congestive heart failure; CNS, central nervous system; COX, cyclooxygenase; DVT, deep vein thrombosis; GI, gastrointestinal; HRT, hormone replacement therapy; HTN, hypertension; INR, international normalized ratio; IU, international units; MI, myocardial infarction; NMDA, *N*-methyl-D-aspartate; NSAIDs, nonsteroidal anti-inflammatory drugs; OTC, over-the-counter; PT, prothrombin time; RA, rheumatoid arthritis; SSRI, selective serotonin reuptake inhibitor; TCA, tricyclic antidepressant; TIA, transient ischemic attack.

[a] Use of antipsychotics, sedatives and hypnotics, and anxiolytics in a nursing facility for treating behaviors associated with dementia is regulated and requires specific supporting documentation.

[b] Dementia is not a labeled indication for use of antipsychotics. They do not alter dementia but modify behavioral responses. In the elderly, dose should start at one-third of usual starting dose.

[c] Depression is the most common psychiatric diagnosis in the elderly.

[d] Osteoporosis is often an undertreated or preventable illness in the elderly.

[e] The cause should be assessed first & the appropriate agent given for urge, stress, or overflow incontinence (eg, benign prostatic hyperplasia).

Questions

Multiple Choice (choose the best answer)

1. A 68-year-old woman complains of a constant bilateral, high-pitched tone, especially when she is in bed at night or in other quiet surroundings. She also has noted gradually progressive difficulty over the years in hearing others, especially conversations in a crowded room. She has greater difficulty hearing and understanding women than men. Which of the following is true regarding this patient's problem?

   a. Most patients with this problem have a history of multiple ear infections as a child.
   b. This patient likely has greater difficulty understanding vowels rather than consonant sounds.
   c. The patient is unlikely to benefit from hearing amplification.
   d. This patient has a conductive hearing loss.
   e. A history of recurrent exposure to loud noise can cause similar symptoms at an early age.

2. A 72-year-old patient complains of left knee pain of 8 hours' duration. There is no history of preceding knee trauma. On physical examination, the patient has an obvious right knee effusion, which is slightly warm. Arthrocentesis was performed, and long, needle-shaped crystals were seen on microscopic examination of the synovial fluid. Which of the following statements is *not* true regarding the disease process in this patient?

   a. It is more common in men than women.
   b. This is usually a monoarticular disease, although multiple joints can be involved on occasion.
   c. The crystals exhibit positive birefringence under polarizing microscopy.
   d. An intra-articular corticosteroid injection may be appropriate treatment for selected patients with an acute attack.
   e. An attack after surgery or associated with a severe illness is not unusual.

3. An 85-year-old male nursing home resident describes urinary urgency with occasional urinary incontinence. He also has mild obstructive urinary symptoms including a slightly weak urinary stream and post-void dribbling. Which is the most appropriate initial treatment for this patient?

   a. Oxybutinin 5 mg taken twice daily
   b. Tolterodine LA 4 mg taken once daily
   c. Bladder catheterization
   d. Transurethral resection of the prostate
   e. Urge suppression by pelvic floor muscle contraction and timed voidings

4. An 84-year-old female nursing home resident with a history of advanced arterial occlusive disease with claudication, congestive heart failure, and moderate renal insufficiency has a pressure ulcer on the heel of her left foot. On examination, it is 2 by 3 cm in diameter and estimated to be stage II. Which of the following statements regarding this patient's ulcer is true?

   a. The tissue damage involves the full thickness of the skin and involvement of the subcutaneous tissue.
   b. The surface of the ulcer should be cultured for bacteria to determine whether the wound is infected.
   c. If the wound is thought to be infected, systemic antibiotics are more effective treatment than topical antibiotics.
   d. The ulcer should be débrided if an eschar forms over the surface of the wound.
   e. The ulcer will heal fastest if it is kept dry with the use of a heat lamp.

5. A 74-year-old man with chronic urinary retention is admitted to a nursing home for long-term care. He has an indwelling urinary catheter in place. A previous evaluation has shown that the patient has a large-volume, poorly contractile bladder, and it was recommended that the patient have the indwelling catheter in place indefinitely. Which of the following is true regarding the care of this patient?

   a. Chronic use of a daily, low-dose antibiotic can prevent the development of catheter-associated bacteriuria.
   b. The catheter should be changed monthly to prevent the development of bacteriuria.
   c. Monthly surveillance cultures of the urine should be done to determine the presence of bacteriuria.
   d. The urinary catheter should be changed before obtaining a specimen for urine culture.
   e. The catheter should be changed when the urine becomes cloudy or develops an abnormal odor.

6. Hypertension is diagnosed in a 65-year-old woman. An antihypertensive medication is thought to be warranted for her treatment. Her only other medical problem is urinary stress incontinence. Which of the following antihypertensive medications has the potential to worsen her incontinence?

   a. Atenolol
   b. Doxazosin
   c. Nifedipine
   d. Verapamil
   e. Hydrochlorothiazide

7. A 90-year-old woman presents to your office after a fall that happened about 2 weeks ago. The fall happened after she missed the curb and fell onto her right side. She has several ecchymoses on her right arm and is complaining about pain in her right hip. Radiographs of the hip performed at the time of the injury did not show a hip fracture, but the patient has been unable to walk since she fell. CT of the hip shows a minimally displaced trochanteric fracture. No operative intervention is planned, and the patient is dismissed to home. What is the most appropriate strategy to reduce her risk of further falls and injury?

a. Nursing home admission for 24-hour supervision and restriction of her physical activity.
b. Physical therapy assessment for gait and balance training and evaluation for appropriate assistive devices.
c. Cardiac work-up to determine whether she is having arrhythmias that might cause her to fall.
d. Hip protector pads for the patient to wear during the day.
e. Discontinue use of all her antihypertensive medications because they may cause orthostatic hypotension.

Answers

1. Answer e.

This patient is describing symptoms typical for presbycusis. This is a bilateral, symmetric, high-frequency hearing loss often associated with tinnitus. The tinnitus is most commonly appreciated in quiet surroundings. The hearing loss is often noticeable in crowded rooms and other environments with excessive background noise. Women's voices are typically more difficult to understand because they tend to be of a higher frequency than men's voices. Consonant sounds are more difficult to understand than vowel sounds, which tend to be a lower frequency. The findings are similar to those in individuals with previous exposure to loud noise. Presbycusis is a sensorineural hearing loss rather than a conductive hearing loss.

2. Answer c.

This patient likely has gout, although calcium pyrophosphate deposition disease (pseudogout) is also a possibility. Gout is more common in males, whereas pseudogout is more common in females. Gout is typically a monoarticular arthritis, although at times more than 1 joint can be involved. Either condition can follow a period of high stress, such as a surgical procedure. Treatment for an acute attack of either condition with a nonsteroidal anti-inflammatory drug is the usual initial therapy, although in selected patients an intra-articular corticosteroid can be effective treatment. The diagnosis in this patient is established by the patient's arthrocentesis results and synovial fluid evaluation. The synovial fluid in persons with gout contains long, needle-shaped crystals, which are negatively birefringent under polarized microscopy. Pseudogout is associated with rectangular crystals, which are positively refringent under polarized microscopy.

3. Answer e.

This patient has overactive bladder associated with urinary urge incontinence, a common form of urinary incontinence. Management of an 85-year-old patient with urinary incontinence should be with behavioral treatment initially, because medications can have potentially serious adverse effects in patients of this age group. Both oxybutynin and tolterodine LA would be effective for suppressing the premature detrusor contractions associated with overactive bladder. However, one needs to be careful in elderly men, who may have some degree of urinary outflow obstruction from an enlarged prostate. These antimuscarinic medications can produce or worsen urinary retention in these patients. A transurethral resection of the prostate would be expected to relieve the obstruction associated with benign prostatic hyperplasia, but it is not clear that this patient needs such a procedure. Bladder catheterization is not an appropriate treatment option for this patient because the bladder apparently contracts and empties adequately. Catheterization is also associated with bacteriuria, which can potentially result in urinary sepsis. Behavioral management should be initially tried in this patient and includes timed voiding, prompted voiding, and urge suppression techniques with pelvic floor muscle contraction.

4. Answer c.

Pressure sores are very common in frail elderly persons and can be classified into 4 stages depending on their depth of tissue involvement. A stage I pressure ulcer represents an area of nonblanchable erythema of intact skin. Stage II involves a partial-thickness skin loss involving the epidermis or dermis or both (a superficial ulcer). A stage III ulcer represents a full-thickness skin loss with damage or necrosis of subcutaneous tissue (a deep ulcer). Stage IV ulcers represent full-thickness skin loss with extensive tissue destruction, tissue necrosis, and possible involvement of muscle, bone, or tendons. Bacterial culture specimens taken from the surface of pressure ulcers will not give an accurate representation of the bacteria involved in an infected ulcer. A deep-tissue culture is required. If a pressure ulcer is infected, systemic antibiotics should be used rather than topical antibiotics. Topical antibiotics will not penetrate into the tissue adequately. Pressure ulcers heal fastest in a moist environment, and drying ulcers with heat lamps should be avoided. Nonviable tissue should usually be débrided unless it is present in an extremity with a compromised arterial supply, as in this case.

5.   Answer d.

Chronic indwelling catheters are associated with the development of bacteriuria. Nothing has been shown to prevent bacteriuria from occurring. Daily use of antibiotics will only result in bacteriuria resistant to the antibiotic used. Surveillance cultures will likely show that the bacteria present within the bladder changes with time. There is no evidence to suggest that changing urinary catheters routinely is beneficial to the patient. There is also no benefit to changing the catheter when the urine becomes cloudy or develops an abnormal odor. The catheter should be changed before checking a urine specimen for a urine culture because different bacteria may be present in the catheter than are present within the bladder. The catheter should also be changed if it obstructs.

6.   Answer b.

Urinary stress incontinence is associated with urethral sphincter incompetence. Doxazosin is an α-adrenergic antagonist and has the potential to relax the internal urinary sphincter, potentially worsening stress incontinence. Nifedipine and verapamil could theoretically have an effect on the urinary bladder. Because they are both smooth muscle relaxants, some patients may find their overactive bladder symptoms are somewhat improved with these medications. Neither is approved for treating overactive bladder, however. Neither atenolol nor hydrochlorothiazide would be expected to have any significant effects on the urinary bladder.

7.   Answer b.

This patient is undoubtedly at high risk for falls. She clearly remembered the fall and did not have a syncopal episode, thus cardiac monitoring would not be helpful. She also did not have symptoms of orthostatic hypotension, and there is no reason to discontinue her use of antihypertensive medications. Nursing home admission is not a foregone conclusion, because the patient may still be able to be at home safely. Restriction of her physical activity is likewise inappropriate, because this can lead to other problems such as depression and pressure sores. Hip protector pads may protect against hip fracture in certain patients, but they do not prevent falls. Physical therapy for gait training and an appropriate assistive device are the best way to prevent further falls.

11

Hematology

David P. Steensma, MD
Rajiv K. Pruthi, MBBS

Part I

David P. Steensma, MD
Rajiv K. Pruthi, MBBS

Benign Hematology

Anemias

Evaluation of Anemias

Anemia results from the inadequate production of red blood cells (RBCs) by the bone marrow (marrow failure), blood loss, or premature destruction of RBCs (hemolysis). In 1968, the World Health Organization (WHO) defined the lower limit of normal for venous hemoglobin concentration as 13 g/dL in males older than 14 years living at sea level and as 12 g/dL in nonpregnant females. However, accurate interpretation of an individual patient's hemoglobin level requires the use of an appropriate age-, sex-, and race-adjusted reference range.

An organized approach to the anemias is essential. After the history and physical examination, the initial evaluation of anemia begins with a complete blood cell count (CBC). With those results, anemias can be classified on the basis of mean corpuscular volume (MCV) as microcytic, macrocytic, or normocytic.

Microcytic Anemias

The most common forms of anemia are microcytic (Tables 11-1 and 11-2). The major causes of hypochromic microcytic anemias include iron deficiency, thalassemia syndromes, and the anemia of chronic disease. Less common causes of microcytosis include sideroblastic anemias, hemoglobin E or C, unstable hemoglobins, lead poisoning, vitamin C deficiency, copper deficiency, vitamin B_6 deficiency, treatment with sirolimus or mycophenolate, primary myelofibrosis, renal cell carcinoma, Hodgkin lymphoma, and Castleman disease. In the United States, iron deficiency is the cause of 80% to 90% of all hypochromic microcytic anemias (Figure 11-1). Of the remaining 10% to 20%, thalassemia syndromes and the anemia of chronic disease are much more common than the other rare forms of microcytic anemias. The CBC and other laboratory values provide additional information to aid in the differential diagnosis (Table 11-2). Blood loss should be considered in the differential diagnosis of any patient with anemia, especially microcytic anemia. Since the gastrointestinal tract is the most common site of occult blood loss, the evaluation of stool for blood loss is essential in the initial work-up of microcytic anemia.

Iron Deficiency

Iron deficiency is the most common cause of anemia in the world. In the United States, iron deficiency is still very common, especially in menstruating women and the elderly. Iron deficiency occurs in 11% of adolescent females and women of childbearing age, and iron deficiency severe enough to cause anemia occurs in 3% to 5%.

The causes of iron deficiency include blood loss, increased requirements relative to intake (as in pregnancy), and decreased absorption (partial gastrectomy and malabsorption syndromes). The following are associated with blood loss: gastrointestinal tract disorders (eg,

Table 11-1 Typical Features of Uncomplicated Microcytic Anemias (Decreased MCV)

Variable	Type of Anemia	
	Thalassemia	Iron Deficiency
RBC count, × 10^{12}/L	>5.0	<5.0
RBC distribution width, %	<16	>16

Abbreviations: MCV, mean corpuscular volume; RBC, red blood cell.

Table 11-2 Comparison of the Most Common Hypochromic Microcytic Anemias

Disease State	MCV	Red Blood Cell Count	TIBC	Transferrin Saturation	Serum Ferritin	Marrow Iron
Iron deficiency anemia	Decreased	Decreased	Increased	Low	Low	Absent
Anemia of chronic disease	Normal or decreased	Decreased	Normal	Normal or increased	Normal or increased	Normal or increased
Thalassemia minor	Decreased	Usually increased	Normal	Normal	Normal or increased	Normal

Abbreviations: MCV, mean corpuscular volume; TIBC, total iron-binding capacity.
Modified from Savage RA. Cost-effective laboratory diagnosis of microcytic anemias of complex origin. ASCP check sample H84-10(H-153). Used with permission.

ulcers, malignancy, telangiectasia, arteriovenous malformations, hiatal hernia, and long-distance runner's anemia), respiratory disorders (eg, malignancy and pulmonary hemosiderosis), menstruation, phlebotomy (eg, blood donor, diagnostic phlebotomy, treatment of polycythemia vera or hemochromatosis, and self-inflicted or factitious), trauma, and surgery. Although patients with advanced iron deficiency have microcytosis, a normal MCV is present in early iron deficiency or in combined anemia (eg, iron deficiency plus vitamin B_{12} deficiency).

The serum ferritin test is the most useful initial test for documenting iron deficiency, but even when there is true iron deficiency, the ferritin level may be increased in the presence of coexistent inflammatory states (eg, rheumatoid arthritis), liver disease, hepatocellular carcinoma, and malignancy. Even in the presence of inflammation, iron deficiency is very unlikely if the ferritin level is greater than 100 ng/mL. In contrast, a ferritin level less than 15 ng/mL almost always

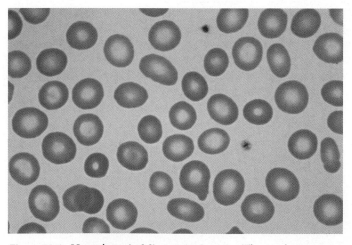

Figure 11-1. Hypochromic Microcytic Anemia. The erythrocytes are small with increased central pallor and assorted aberrations in size (anisocytosis) and shape (poikilocytosis). This pattern is characteristic of iron deficiency rather than thalassemia; in thalassemia, red blood cells are small but more uniform. If a mature lymphocyte is available for reference, the diameter of a normal erythrocyte (7 mcm) should be similar to the diameter of the nucleus of the lymphocyte. (Courtesy of Curtis A. Hanson, MD, Mayo Clinic.)

represents bona fide iron deficiency. The ferritin level is useful in assessment of iron stores in pregnant women, in whom the transferrin saturation is often elevated. Other laboratory tests consistent with iron deficiency include elevated total iron-binding capacity (TIBC), reduced transferrin saturation, elevated soluble transferrin receptor, and elevated zinc protoporphyrin.

Confusing problems in iron deficiency include patient compliance with iron treatment, inadequate doses of iron supplements, treatment with enteric-coated iron preparations that are poorly absorbed (since gastric acid is required for optimal absorption of elemental iron), diminished absorption (due to previous operation such as gastrectomy or intestinal bypass, or mucosal disease of the small bowel), use of antacids, ongoing blood loss in excess of iron replaced by treatment, other causes of anemia, and physician impatience with response. Oral replacement therapy is the treatment of choice for iron deficiency for most patients. The most cost-effective initial treatment is ferrous sulfate 3 times daily at a dose of 325 mg orally 1 hour before or 2 hours after meals (food may interfere with absorption). Reticulocytosis can be expected in about 4 to 7 days and some improvement in anemia should be seen by 3 to 4 weeks. Correction of the anemia would be expected in 6 weeks if the anemia is due solely to iron deficiency. Treatment with iron for another 6 months is necessary to replenish bone marrow reserves. Indications for intravenous iron therapy include patients on renal dialysis (in conjunction with recombinant erythropoietin) and patients who cannot tolerate or absorb enough iron orally. Four parenteral iron preparations are available in the United States: iron dextran with high-molecular-weight dextran (Dexferrum), which has a high rate of anaphylactoid reactions and should be avoided unless no other product is available; iron dextran with a lower-molecular-weight dextran (InFeD), which carries a smaller risk of anaphylactoid reactions and requires a test dose; iron sucrose; and ferric gluconate. Iron sucrose and ferric gluconate may be safer than iron dextran, but there is less experience giving "total replacement" doses with these preparations, and iron dextran is the only product compatible with total parenteral nutrition.

• Typical clinical scenario: An elderly patient with a history of abdominal pain and weakness is found to have a microcytic hypochromic anemia. The serum level of ferritin is low. The red blood cell (RBC) count is low. The RBC distribution width (RDW) index is increased. The diagnosis is iron deficiency anemia. A likely cause is colon cancer producing chronic blood loss. Endoscopy of the upper and lower gastrointestinal tract is indicated.

Thalassemia Syndromes

The thalassemias are probably the most common single-gene disorders in the world. β-Thalassemia results when β-globin chains are decreased or absent in relation to α-globin chains. In α-thalassemia, the converse is true: excess β-globin chains precipitate as tetramers called *hemoglobin H*, which can be detected by hemoglobin electrophoresis, chromatography, or supravital staining of a peripheral blood smear.

More than 50 different point mutations of β-globin genes or regulatory elements result in β-thalassemia of varying severity. Clinically, β-thalassemia is categorized into *β-thalassemia trait* (microcytosis and either normal hemoglobin or very mild anemia), *β-thalassemia intermedia* (microcytosis and moderate anemia without long-term transfusion dependence), and *β-thalassemia major* (profound anemia and lifelong transfusion dependence). β-Thalassemia can be identified with simple screening methods, including elevated hemoglobin A_2 level (Tables 11-1 and 11-2 and Figure 11-2). However, if iron deficiency coexists, the hemoglobin A_2 level may be normal because iron deficiency lowers the hemoglobin A_2 level.

Normally, individuals have 4 α-globin genes but only 2 β-chain loci. The absence of 1 or 2 of the 4 α-globin genes does not cause symptomatic abnormality (*α-thalassemia silent carrier, α-thalassemia minor*, α-thalassemia trait). Patients with α-thalassemia minor characteristically have a low-normal MCV and mean corpuscular hemoglobin (MCH), with a normal hemoglobin level. The absence of 1 or 2 α-globin genes cannot be diagnosed by simple hemoglobin assays; diagnosis requires molecular analysis, usually by Southern blotting. However, most cases may be managed without laboratory confirmation; if other causes of microcytic anemia have been ruled out and the patient has the appropriate ethnic background, α-thalassemia can be assumed. The absence of 3 α-globin genes causes hemoglobin H disease, a chronic hemolytic anemia of moderate severity. Patients with hemoglobin H disease may benefit from splenectomy if the hemolysis becomes problematic. Absence of all 4 α-globin genes is not compatible with life and results in stillbirth. Genetic counseling is indicated after the diagnosis of α- or β-thalassemia has been established.

- Typical clinical scenario: An African American person (or a person of Mediterranean or Southeast Asian ancestry) has mild anemia and is asymptomatic. The RBC count is normal or increased. The RDW is usually normal. The concentration of hemoglobin A_2 is increased (β-thalassemia) or normal (α-thalassemia).

Sideroblastic Anemias

The sideroblastic anemias are characterized by the presence of anemia (microcytic, normocytic, or macrocytic) and ring sideroblasts in the bone marrow, detectable by the Prussian blue reagent, which reacts with iron (Figure 11-3). Basophilic stippling or Pappenheimer bodies may be present in peripheral blood. Ring sideroblasts are abnormal

erythroid precursors that are full of iron-stuffed mitochondria that are ineffective at heme biosynthesis. Reactive causes include alcohol, zinc toxicity, and certain drugs such as isoniazid, pyrazinamide, and cycloserine. There are several forms of congenital sideroblastic anemia that may respond to vitamin B_6 (pyridoxine) therapy, and ring sideroblasts can also be seen in clonal myeloid disorders, especially myelodysplastic syndromes.

Vitamin C Deficiency (Scurvy)

Patients with vitamin C deficiency present with microcytic anemia and purpura, in addition to other signs such as gingival disease and peripheral edema. The areas of purpura may be large, with purpuric lesions centered on the hair follicles.

Macrocytic Anemias

The differential diagnosis of macrocytic anemias includes vitamin B_{12} deficiency, folate deficiency, drugs, myelodysplasia or other primary bone marrow disorders, liver disease, alcohol abuse, hypothyroidism, cold agglutinin disease (artifactual), heavy tobacco use, and reticulocytosis (eg, after hemolysis), since reticulocytes are larger than mature RBCs. A laboratory approach to macrocytic anemias is outlined in Figure 11-4. An MCV greater than

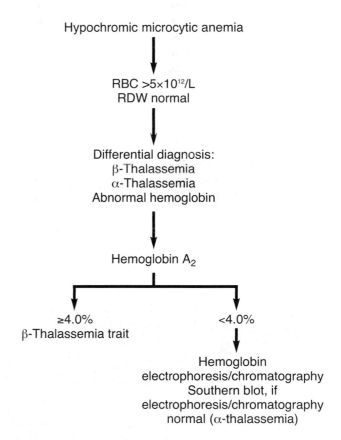

Figure 11-2. Algorithm for approach to diagnosis of hypochromic microcytic anemia with an increased total red blood cell (RBC) count and a normal RBC distribution width (RDW) index. (Modified from Savage RA. Cost-effective laboratory diagnosis of microcytic anemias of complex origin. ASCP check sample H84-10[H-153]. Used with permission.)

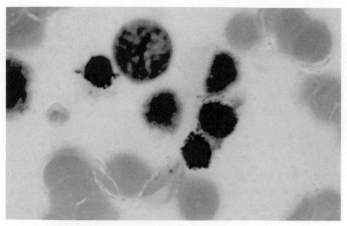

Figure 11-3. Ring Sideroblasts. Seen on iron staining of a bone marrow aspirate, ring sideroblasts can be reactive, congenital, or part of a myelodysplastic syndrome or other clonal myeloid disorder. (Courtesy of Curtis A. Hanson, MD, Mayo Clinic.)

115 fL is almost always a deficiency of either vitamin B_{12} or folate or an artifact due to RBC agglutination. Common drug-related causes of macrocytosis are chemotherapy drugs that inhibit purine or pyrimidine synthesis (azathioprine and 5-fluorouracil), deoxyribonucleotide synthesis (hydroxyurea and cytarabine [cytosine arabinoside]), and dihydrofolate reductase (methotrexate).

Vitamin B_{12} (Cyanocobalamin) Deficiency

Vitamin B_{12} is present in animal products and in small quantities in some plant-derived products such as ketchup because of contamination with insects during processing. Cobalamin is released from food by gastric enzymes, binds to R-binders released by the saliva and stomach, and then binds to intrinsic factor in the alkaline small bowel. Patients with achlorhydria of any cause do not absorb vitamin B_{12} because hydrochloric acid is required to free vitamin B_{12} from food. Additionally, sufficient mucosal surface in the ileum (where vitamin B_{12}–intrinsic factor complex is absorbed) and a normally functioning pancreas are required (pancreatic trypsin facilitates vitamin B_{12} release from R-binders). The many causes of vitamin B_{12} deficiency include pernicious anemia (defective production of intrinsic factor, usually due to an autoimmune process), atrophic gastritis (common in elderly persons), total or partial gastrectomy, ileal resection or Crohn disease involving the ileum, bacterial overgrowth syndromes, infection with *Diphyllobothrium latum* (a tapeworm acquired from consumption of raw fish), and pancreatic insufficiency (most commonly from chronic pancreatitis or cystic fibrosis). Vitamin B_{12} deficiency due to inadequate dietary intake is very rare. Nitrous oxide inactivates vitamin B_{12}, and abuse of this anesthetic (eg, by dentists) can lead to rapid development of severe vitamin B_{12} deficiency.

The symptoms and signs of vitamin B_{12} deficiency include a beefy and atrophic tongue, diarrhea, and neurologic signs (paresthesias, gait disturbance, mental status changes ["B_{12} madness"], vibratory/position sense impairment [dorsal column "dropout"], the absence of ankle reflexes, and extensor plantar responses).

The MCV is increased, and hypersegmented neutrophils are usually present (Figure 11-5). Neutropenia and thrombocytopenia are common, and giant platelets may be present. The serum and urinary levels of methylmalonic acid are increased (unlike folate deficiency)

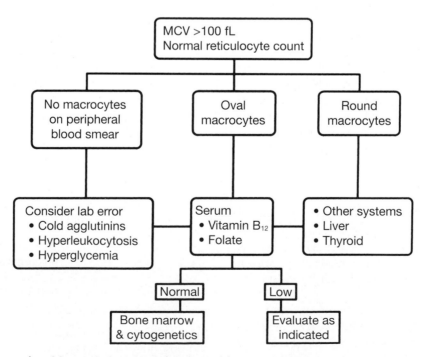

Figure 11-4. Laboratory Approach to Macrocytic Anemias. Lab indicates laboratory; MCV, mean corpuscular volume. (Modified from Colon-Otero G, Menke D, Hook CC. A practical approach to the differential diagnosis and evaluation of the adult patient with macrocytic anemia. Med Clin North Am. 1992 May;76:581-97. Used with permission.)

and serum homocysteine levels are increased (similar to folate deficiency). A serum level of vitamin B_{12} less than 200 pg/mL is strongly suggestive of the diagnosis of vitamin B_{12} deficiency, but vitamin B_{12} levels of 200 to 400 pg/mL (borderline or low-normal range) can also represent a deficiency state. When there is a strong suspicion of vitamin B_{12} deficiency but serum levels of vitamin B_{12} are borderline elevated, levels of urinary methylmalonic acid can help in making the diagnosis of vitamin B_{12} deficiency. An abnormal intrinsic factor antibody or parietal cell antibody is not always present but does help confirm the diagnosis of pernicious anemia as the cause of vitamin B_{12} deficiency. Of patients with pernicious anemia, about 90% have anti–parietal cell antibodies (compared with about 5% of the healthy population), and 60% to 70% have a positive intrinsic factor antibody test (rare in the healthy population). Serum gastrin levels are typically high.

The Schilling test is frequently described in textbooks but rarely performed anymore in clinical practice. It has largely been replaced by intrinsic factor antibody testing. The Schilling test confirms a defect in intestinal absorption and helps distinguish the cause of vitamin B_{12} deficiency. In part I of the test, radiolabeled vitamin B_{12} is administered orally, nonradioactive vitamin B_{12} is administered intramuscularly within 1 to 2 hours to saturate vitamin B_{12} binding sites, and the urinary and serum levels of radioactivity are measured. Normal urinary excretion rates after a flushing dose of nonradioactive vitamin B_{12} in the first 24 to 72 hours are greater than 7%. Low urine radioactivity with normal renal function means decreased absorption. The differential diagnosis of an abnormal finding in part I includes pernicious anemia, small-bowel disease interfering with absorption, and bacterial competition for vitamin B_{12}. In part II of the test, intrinsic factor is added to the radiolabeled vitamin B_{12}. Patients with pernicious anemia (intrinsic factor deficiency) will have normal results; if urinary excretion of radiolabeled vitamin B_{12} remains abnormally low, intestinal malabsorption or bacterial competition is suspected. Antibiotics are given in part III of

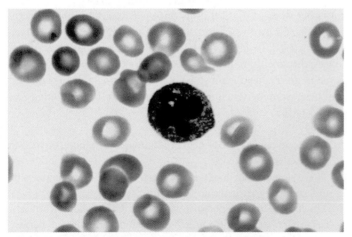

Figure 11-5. Hypersegmented Neutrophil. Polymorphonuclear leukocytes with 5 or more nuclear lobes are characteristic of vitamin B_{12} or folate deficiency and are not typically seen in other causes of macrocytic anemia.

the Schilling test, which helps distinguish between the causes of an abnormal result in part II of the test.

The treatment of pernicious anemia and other causes of vitamin B_{12} deficiency is vitamin B_{12}, typically at a dose of 1,000 mcg intramuscularly daily for 5 days, followed by 500 to 1,000 mcg intramuscularly every month. Alternatively, vitamin B_{12} may be given orally at a dose of 500 to 1,000 mcg daily, which is usually absorbed well enough to correct the deficiency even in patients with gastric resection, atrophic gastritis, or pernicious anemia. Lifelong maintenance treatment is required. Vitamin B_{12} levels are sometimes spuriously low in pregnancy and in persons receiving oral contraceptive treatment and are falsely elevated in patients with myeloproliferative disorders, due to alterations in levels of vitamin B_{12} binding proteins.

- Typical clinical scenario: An elderly patient has weakness and fatigue, perhaps with accompanying neurologic signs, and laboratory evaluation reveals macrocytic anemia. The vitamin B_{12} level is either frankly low or at the low end of the laboratory reference range. The serum level of methylmalonic acid is increased. Anti-intrinsic factor and anti-parietal cell antibody tests are positive.

Folate Deficiency

Megaloblastic anemia caused by folate deficiency develops quickly (within months) in patients with inadequate dietary intake of folic acid, in contrast to a period of more than 3 years for vitamin B_{12} deficiency to develop in patients with vitamin B_{12} malabsorption, because of the low storage levels of folic acid in tissues and the relatively high dietary requirement compared with vitamin B_{12}. Folate deficiency has become less common in the United States since fortification of grain products with folic acid was mandated in 1977. Folate is naturally present in leafy green vegetables and in some fruits such as bananas and lemons. Morphologically, anemia due to folate deficiency is indistinguishable from vitamin B_{12} deficiency. Folate is absorbed in the proximal small bowel (duodenum and proximal jejunum). Deficiency states are associated with increased requirements (pregnancy and hemolytic anemia), poor folate intake (alcoholics or persons following extremely restrictive diets), diseases of the small intestine that impair folate absorption (sprue or extensive inflammatory bowel disease), and interference with the recycling of folate from liver stores to tissue (alcohol). The possibility of concomitant vitamin B_{12} or iron deficiency (eg, due to malabsorption of both nutrients in sprue) should be considered if the response to replacement therapy is not optimal. The serum homocysteine level is increased in folate deficiency because of impaired folate-dependent conversion of homocysteine to methionine. In contrast to vitamin B_{12} deficiency, in folate deficiency the level of methylmalonic acid is normal. RBC folate levels are more accurate for detecting folate deficiency than serum folate levels, since serum folate levels fluctuate quickly with dietary changes. A single day of healthy meals in the hospital may normalize a patient's serum folate level and result in a false-negative result.

- Typical clinical scenario: A middle-aged alcoholic person presents with an MCV of 102 fL and normal vitamin B_{12} and serum folate levels. The homocysteine level is elevated.

Normocytic Anemias

The normochromic normocytic disorders present the greatest challenge in anemia diagnosis. Both iron and vitamin B_{12} deficiencies are possible causes and should be excluded. The differential diagnosis includes erythropoietic failure (aplastic anemia and RBC aplasia), marrow replacement (malignancy and fibrosis), kidney disease with lack of erythropoietin production, hemolysis, acute hemorrhage, mixed nutritional deficiency (eg, concomitant folate and iron deficiency), some myelodysplastic syndromes, chemotherapy, anemia of acute disease, and anemia of chronic disease (infections, neoplasia, rheumatoid arthritis, and other inflammatory rheumatologic conditions).

Anemia of Chronic Disease

Anemia of chronic disease is usually moderate (ie, hemoglobin 9-11 g/dL) with a low reticulocyte count, and the MCV is normal or modestly decreased. Anemia of chronic disease is sometimes called anemia of chronic inflammation, since it results from inhibitory effects on the bone marrow of inflammatory cytokines such as interferons, interleukin (IL)-1, IL-6, and tumor necrosis factor. More recently, hepcidin, a peptide produced by the liver in response to inflammatory elevation of IL-6, has been found to be elevated in anemia of chronic disease. Hepcidin causes macrophages to sequester iron and decreases iron absorption by enterocytes. As a consequence, serum iron levels are low in anemia of chronic disease, but unlike in iron deficiency, TIBC is also low and ferritin is usually normal or elevated (Table 11-2).

It is important to obtain a reticulocyte count to exclude hemolysis early in the evaluation of patients with normochromic normocytic anemia, and it is essential to exclude gastrointestinal tract blood loss that may be acute and not manifested by features of microcytic blood. No single blood test confirms anemia of chronic disease, but the presence of inflammatory markers (eg, elevated erythrocyte sedimentation rate or C-reactive protein, polyclonal hypergammaglobulinemia), typical iron studies, lack of another cause for the normocytic anemia, and the right clinical setting make the diagnosis likely. The soluble transferrin receptor concentration is helpful to differentiate iron deficiency anemia (the receptor level is usually increased in iron deficiency) from anemia of chronic disease (the receptor level is usually normal), since soluble transferrin receptor is not an acute-phase reactant (unlike ferritin). Patients with anemia of chronic disease do not benefit from iron therapy.

* Typical clinical scenario for anemia of chronic disease: The patient has human immunodeficiency virus (HIV) infection or other serious medical problems and moderate microcytic hypochromic anemia. The ferritin level is normal or high. The RBC count is low, and there is no evidence of hemolysis. The erythopoietin level may be within the normal range or even mildly elevated, but it is inappropriately low given the presence of anemia.

Erythropoietin

Erythropoietin is a glycoprotein that acts through specific receptors on RBC precursors in the marrow; 90% is produced in the kidneys and a small amount in the liver. Erythropoietin production increases with hypoxia. Hypoxic signals include anemia, hypoxemia, decreased oxygen release by RBCs (high oxygen-affinity hemoglobinopathies), and decreased renal blood flow (renal artery stenosis, hypoperfusion in congestive heart failure). Regulation is linked to an oxygen sensor in peritubular cells in the kidney. The serum levels of erythropoietin are not strongly influenced by age or sex. The higher hemoglobin value in men appears to be due to the effect of androgenic steroids on erythropoiesis, not erythropoietin. Recombinant human erythropoietins for therapeutic use have a protein sequence identical to that of native erythropoietin but a different glycosylation pattern. With erythropoietin therapy, hypertension may develop or progress in patients receiving renal dialysis. The risk of thrombosis is modestly increased. There may be a risk of cancer progression if patients with cancer who are not receiving chemotherapy get erythropoietin, or if higher goals are chosen for hemoglobin (eg, ≥12 g/dL).

The serum levels of erythropoietin are low—never absent—in chronic renal failure, polycythemia vera, rheumatoid arthritis and other inflammatory rheumatologic conditions, and HIV infection. High erythropoietin levels are present in persons with marrow hypofunction (pure red cell aplasia), nutritional deficiency states (iron deficiency), erythropoietin-producing tumors (rarely, hepatocellular carcinoma, cerebellar hemangioblastoma, or renal cell cancer); in persons living at high altitude; and in competitive athletes or others who abuse recombinant erythropoietin.

Approved indications for erythropoietin therapy include anemia caused by neoplastic agents (not anemia due solely to cancer), anemia caused by renal insufficiency, and anemia due to HIV infection in patients who are taking zidovudine. For patients undergoing an operation and donating autologous blood, erythropoietin may increase the amount of blood donated by about 40% but may increase the risk of thrombosis. Erythropoietin should not be used if anemia is due to iron deficiency, vitamin B_{12} deficiency, or another correctable cause. The erythropoietin level should be less than 500 U/L. Recombinant erythropoietin is recommended for chemotherapy patients when the hemoglobin level is less than 10 g/dL. Two preparations are available: epoetin alfa (typical dosage for patient with cancer or anemia of chronic disease, 150 U/kg 3 times per week or 40,000 units once per week) and darbepoetin alfa (200-300 mcg [2.25 mcg/kg] once every 2 weeks or 500 mcg every 3 weeks). Patients who have renal failure as the only cause of low erythropoeitin require lower doses. In a study of hemodialysis patients, an erythropoietin strategy with a hemoglobin goal of 11.3 g/dL resulted in better clinical outcomes than a strategy with a goal of 13.5 g/dL.

* Erythropoietin: a glycoprotein produced in the kidney; production increases with hypoxia.
* The erythropoietin level is low in renal failure, polycythemia vera, inflammatory arthritis, and HIV infection.
* The level is high in persons with pure RBC aplasia, iron deficiency, or certain erythropoietin-producing tumors and in persons at high altitude or those who abuse erythropoietin drugs.
* Indications for erythropoietin therapy include end-stage renal disease, anemia of HIV infection, and anemia due to treatment of cancer with antineoplastic agents.

The most common cause of failure to respond appropriately to erythropoietin (or loss of a previously satisfactory response) is iron deficiency. If erythropoietin is given to a healthy person, the hematocrit can increase dramatically. As the hematocrit increases above 50%, the viscosity of the blood rapidly increases. Thus, hypertension, myocardial infarction, or stroke may occur with the misuse of erythropoietin. Doping with erythropoietin for sporting events has been associated with cerebrovascular events due to marked increases in the hematocrit.

- Typical clinical scenario: A patient with lung cancer receiving chemotherapy presents to a primary care physician with a hemoglobin concentration of 8.5 g/dL. The serum erythropoietin level is normal or modestly higher than the laboratory reference range but lower than expected for the degree of anemia. Treatment with recombinant erythropoietin is indicated.

Aplastic Anemia

Aplastic anemia is an acquired disorder that may develop as a consequence of a defect in the stem cell population, defective marrow microenvironment, or immunologic factors. The immunologic factors include antibody-mediated bone marrow suppression, cellular cytolytic suppressive T-cell mechanisms, and bone marrow suppression by cytokines. Aplastic anemia is characterized by peripheral pancytopenia (the anemia is usually normocytic, sometimes macrocytic), bone marrow hypocellularity, and the absence of another disorder to explain the hypocellularity such as a neoplasm. The differential diagnosis of pancytopenia and hypocellular bone marrow includes aplastic anemia, myelodysplastic syndrome, T-cell clonal disorders (including T-cell large granular lymphocyte leukemia), paroxysmal nocturnal hemoglobinuria, and Fanconi anemia or other congenital bone marrow failure syndromes. The criteria for severe aplastic anemia include less than 25% of expected marrow cellularity and 2 of the following: 1) neutrophil count less than 0.5×10^9/L, 2) platelet count less than 20×10^9/L, and 3) a corrected reticulocyte count less than 1%.

Before the use of allogeneic bone marrow transplants and antithymocyte globulin, 80% of patients with severe aplastic anemia died within 2 years of diagnosis. Spontaneous recovery was rare (<20% of patients) and usually incomplete.

- Aplastic anemia: pancytopenia, hypocellular bone marrow, and absence of another cause of marrow hypoplasia.
- Full recovery is uncommon without treatment.

The clinical features of aplastic anemia relate to the cytopenias and include fatigue and dyspnea, easy bruising or bleeding, and infections. Lymphadenopathy and splenomegaly are uncommon. In most patients, the cause of aplastic anemia is idiopathic, especially in adults. Drugs and toxins are the second most common cause of aplastic anemia. Well-characterized suspects include chloramphenicol, phenylbutazone, methylphenylethylhydantoin (an old seizure medication), trimethadione (another older anticonvulsant), sulfonamides, gold salts, and aromatic hydrocarbons such as benzene. Paroxysmal nocturnal hemoglobinuria and infections are also associated with aplastic anemia. Infectious hepatitis is the most common infection to cause aplastic anemia. Hepatitis A and idiopathic hepatitis are the most common types of hepatitis to be associated with aplastic anemia. Hepatitis B only rarely causes aplastic anemia. Other infectious agents that are associated with aplastic anemia include Epstein-Barr virus, cytomegalovirus, influenza virus, HIV, parvovirus B19, and mycobacteria. Ionizing radiation also causes marrow aplasia.

Patients with aplastic anemia who are candidates for stem cell transplant should undergo HLA typing. Exposure to multiple transfusions may increase the risk of failure of a subsequent stem cell transplant. If transfusion is needed, select nonrelated donors and use cytomegalovirus-negative, leukocyte-poor RBC transfusions and single-donor platelet transfusions. Family members should not be donors because they are more likely to sensitize the patient to minor histocompatibility antigens present in the donor but absent in the patient. A search for unrelated HLA-matched donors should be considered for patients younger than 20 years without a sibling HLA match.

Immunosuppression is the treatment of choice for patients older than 40 years and includes antithymocyte globulin plus corticosteroids and cyclosporine. Up to 70% of patients respond, usually by 2 to 3 months. These agents are not usually curative. Even though blood cell count recovery usually is not complete, transfusions are not required, and the absolute neutrophil count is at a level sufficient to protect against infectious complications. About 30% of patients have relapse, and clonal myeloid disorders such as myelodysplastic syndrome (especially with monosomy 7) develop in 25% of patients. Toxic effects of antithymocyte globulin include anaphylaxis, fever, urticaria, rash, lung infiltrates, joint aches, thrombocytopenia, and fluid retention. Side effects of long-term cyclosporine therapy include hypertension, renal insufficiency, seizures, and hypomagnesemia.

Allogeneic hematopoietic stem cell transplant is the therapy of choice for patients with a syngeneic (identical) twin and should be considered for all patients younger than 20 years. It also should be considered for high-risk patients between the ages of 20 and 40 who have an HLA match. Graft failure rates are about 10%, and chronic graft-versus-host disease complicates 40% of cases.

- Common causes of aplastic anemia: autoimmune marrow suppression, idiopathic drug reaction, toxins, radiation, and viral infections.
- With severe aplastic anemia, when transplant is a consideration, transfuse judiciously.
- If the patient is younger than 20 years, or is younger than 40 years with high-risk features, and has an HLA-matched donor or identical twin, consider referral for allogeneic bone marrow transplant. If the patient is older than 40 or has no HLA match, treat with a combination of antithymocyte globulin, cyclosporine, and corticosteroids.

Hemolytic Anemias

There are many causes of hemolysis. The first priority in cases of suspected hemolytic anemia is to confirm that hemolysis is present; then the specific diagnosis can be pursued. Hemolytic anemias are characterized by increased RBC destruction, which may be compensated for by increased erythropoiesis. Laboratory evidence of increased erythropoiesis includes an increased reticulocyte count and marrow erythroid hyperplasia; evidence of increased RBC destruction includes an increase in indirect bilirubin and lactate dehydrogenase (LDH) and a decrease in the haptoglobin level (haptoglobin is a protein that is a scavenger of free hemoglobin released into the serum from burst red cells). If these tests suggest hemolytic anemia, specific causes should be sought.

There are several ways of classifying hemolytic anemias. These anemias may be acquired or hereditary. Red cells may be intrinsically defective or innocent bystanders in another pathologic process. Hemolytic anemias may be Coombs-negative or Coombs-positive. An aplastic crisis may occur in chronic hemolytic anemia and is usually due to development of folate deficiency or infection with parvovirus.

When hemolysis is suspected on the basis of potential evidence of increased RBC destruction, the initial evaluation includes a history and physical examination, CBC, assessment of RBC morphology (peripheral smear), and reticulocyte count. Conditions found during the work-up that can be mistaken for hemolysis include hemorrhage (particularly hematuria), recovery from deficiency states, metastatic carcinoma, and myoglobinuria. The differential diagnosis of hemolytic anemia is outlined in Figure 11-6.

- Hemolytic anemias may be hereditary or acquired.
- Evidence of increased RBC destruction includes elevated LDH, indirect hyperbilirubinemia, and low haptoglobin.
- Reticulocytosis is the normal marrow response to hemolysis.

Inheritance Patterns

Among the familial hemolytic anemias, RBC membrane defects and unstable hemoglobin diseases are usually autosomal dominant. Most enzymopathies are autosomal recessive. However, the most common enzymopathy, glucose-6-phosphate dehydrogenase (G6PD) deficiency, is sex-linked, as is phosphoglycerate kinase deficiency.

- Membrane defects and unstable hemoglobin diseases are autosomal dominant.
- Most enzymopathies are autosomal recessive.
- G6PD deficiency is sex-linked.

Laboratory Findings

The bilirubin value is usually 1 to 5 mg/dL and almost exclusively unconjugated or indirect. Direct bilirubin should be less than 15% of the total if the bilirubin value is greater than 4 mg/dL. Indirect bilirubinemia greater than 8 mg/dL suggests concomitant liver disease. The haptoglobin concentration is usually low and the LDH level is increased. Haptoglobin levels may also decrease transiently after RBC transfusion owing to free hemoglobin in the unit of blood cells. CBC abnormalities in autoimmune hemolytic anemia include anemia, thrombocytosis, and thrombocytopenia. The presence of autoimmune hemolytic anemia and autoimmune thrombocytopenia is called *Evans syndrome*. The reticulocyte value usually is persistently increased, reflecting an enhanced bone marrow response.

Peripheral Smear (Differential Diagnosis)

The peripheral smear may give clues to the cause of hemolytic anemia. Spherocytes (Figure 11-7) are associated with hereditary spherocytosis, alcohol, burns, *Clostridium* infections, autoimmune hemolytic anemia, and hypophosphatemia. Basophilic stippling occurs in lead poisoning, β-thalassemia, and arsenic poisoning. Hypochromia occurs in thalassemia, sideroblastic anemia, and lead poisoning. Target cells are present in thalassemia, hemoglobin C and E, obstructive jaundice, hepatitis, lecithin–cholesterol-acyltransferase deficiency (rare), and the splenectomized state (Figure 11-8). Agglutination is present in cold agglutinin disease (Figure 11-9). Stomatocytes are associated with acute alcoholism and also occur as an artifact. Spur

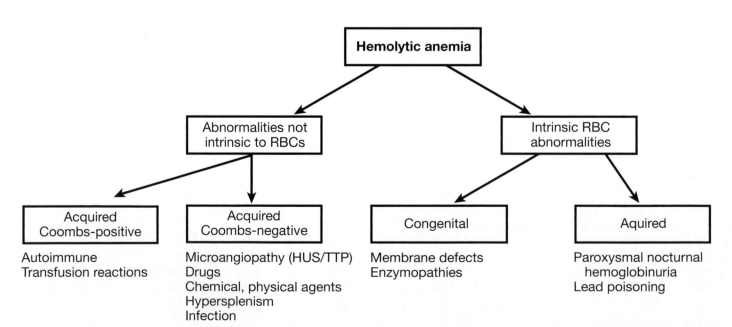

Figure 11-6. Differential Diagnosis of Hemolytic Anemia. HUS indicates hemolytic uremic syndrome; RBC, red blood cell; TTP, thrombotic thrombocytopenic purpura.

cells (acanthocytes) (Figure 11-10) are present in chronic liver disease, abetalipoproteinemia, malabsorption, and anorexia nervosa. Burr cells (echinocytes) occur in uremia (Figure 11-11). Heinz bodies are present in G6PD deficiency. Howell-Jolly bodies (the result of fragmentation of the nucleus) indicate hyposplenism and megaloblastic anemia (Figure 11-12). Polychromasia indicates reticulocytosis, which often accompanies recovery from blood loss or hemolysis (Figure 11-13). Intracellular parasitic inclusions may be seen in erythrocytes; these include the various stages of the malaria parasite and babesiosis (Figure 11-14).

Intravascular Hemolysis Versus Extravascular Hemolysis

Hemolysis may be extravascular, in which the red cells are lysed in the macrophages of the spleen and liver, or intravascular, in which the red cells are destroyed while still circulating within blood vessels. The differential diagnosis of intravascular hemolysis includes transfusion reactions from ABO antibodies, microangiopathic hemolytic anemia, paroxysmal nocturnal hemoglobinuria, paroxysmal cold hemoglobinuria, autoimmune hemolytic anemia (uncommon—in this condition the hemolysis is usually intravascular), cold agglutinin syndrome, immune-complex drug-induced hemolytic anemia, infections (including falciparum malaria and clostridial sepsis), and G6PD deficiency. All other forms of hemolysis are primarily extravascular.

* Most hemolysis is extravascular.

In intravascular hemolysis, hemoglobin is released into the plasma, where it combines rapidly with haptoglobin, which transports it to the liver. When haptoglobin is depleted, hemoglobinemia results and the plasma turns pink-red at free plasma hemoglobin concentrations of 50 to 100 mg/dL.

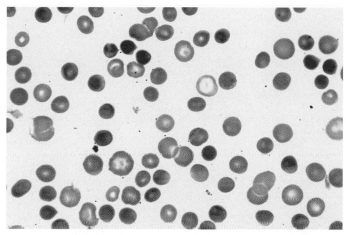

Figure 11-7. Spherocytes. Spherocytes are the smooth, small, and spheroidal darkly stained cells with minimal or no central pallor. They are most commonly seen in hereditary spherocytosis or autoimmune hemolytic anemia. (Courtesy of Curtis A. Hanson, MD, Mayo Clinic.)

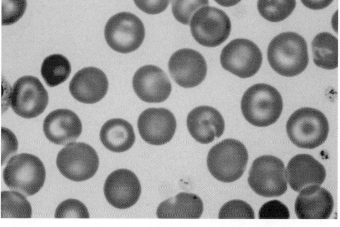

Figure 11-8. Target Cells. Target cells are the red blood cells with a broad diameter and dark center with a pale surrounding halo. They are most commonly seen in hemoglobin C disease, thalassemia, or liver disease or after splenectomy. (Courtesy of Curtis A. Hanson, MD, Mayo Clinic.)

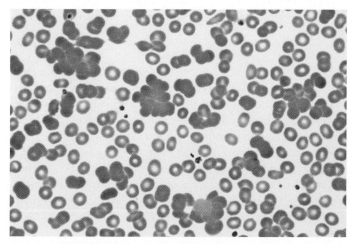

Figure 11-9. Agglutination. The random clumping of red blood cells is most commonly due to cold agglutinin disease or laboratory artifact. It is important to distinguish agglutination from rouleaux (see Figure 11-15).

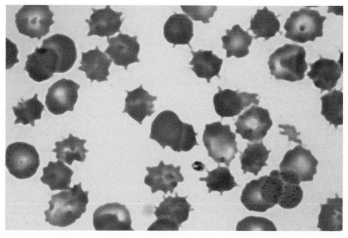

Figure 11-10. Spur Cells (Acanthocytes). Note the thin, thorny, or finger-like projections. Spur cells are characteristic of advanced liver disease and must be distinguished from burr cells (echinocytes) (see Figure 11-11). (Courtesy of Curtis A. Hanson, MD, Mayo Clinic.)

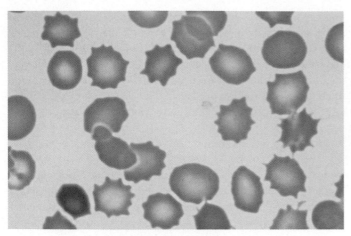

Figure 11-11. Burr Cells (Echinocytes). Burr cell projections are much smaller and more uniform in size than spur cell projections. Burr cells are characteristic of uremia, and the membrane abnormality is reversible with hemodialysis.

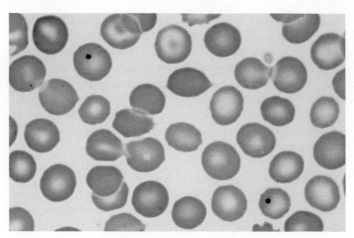

Figure 11-12. Howell-Jolly Bodies. These small, round blue inclusions are seen with Wright-Giemsa or a comparable stain. These are characteristic of hyposplenism due to splenectomy or to a functionally defective spleen. Howell-Jolly bodies should not be confused with Heinz bodies, which require a special preparation (Heinz body preparation) to observe and are not seen on a conventional peripheral smear.

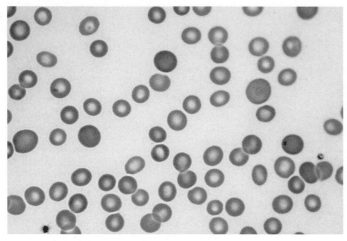

Figure 11-13. Polychromasia. The larger, bluish-tinged cells are reticulocytees. These are often seen in high numbers during recovery from blood loss or hemolysis.

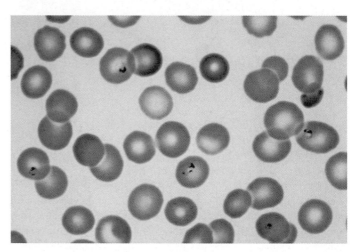

Figure 11-14. Intra-erythrocytic Ring-Shaped Parasites of Babesiosis. Malaria is the other common disease with an intra-erythrocytic parasite.

Hemoglobinuria occurs when the plasma hemoglobin exceeds 150 to 200 mg/dL and is seen only in intravascular hemolysis. The urine may become pink, red, brown, or black. Both hemoglobinuria and hematuria cause a positive urine chemical (dipstick) reaction for heme; urinalysis will show intact red cells in hematuria but not in hemoglobinuria. Other causes of red urine include beets, phenazopyridine (Pyridium), porphyrinuria, and myoglobinuria. Hemosiderin is an insoluble form of iron that accumulates in tissues in disease states. Hemosiderinuria is the result of desquamation of renal tubular cells that absorbed free hemoglobin in the urine several days to weeks earlier.

Coombs-Positive Hemolytic Anemia
Positive results with a direct Coombs test (a direct antiglobulin test) indicate the presence of C3 or IgG (or both) on the surface of RBCs. IgG may be alloantibodies or autoantibodies. The 3 most common causes of Coombs-positive hemolytic anemias are idiopathic (ie, autoimmune), drugs, and malignancy, including chronic lymphocytic leukemia, non-Hodgkin lymphoma, and ovarian carcinoma. The Coombs test gives positive results in up to 15% of all hospitalized patients, and studies have not demonstrated the cause in 95% of these patients. Hemolytic transfusion reactions are an uncommon but important cause of a positive direct Coombs test. The indirect Coombs test is used primarily in the blood bank to screen blood before transfusion.

- Direct Coombs test: detects the presence of C3 or IgG (or both) on RBCs.
- The cause of positive findings on the direct Coombs test is unknown for 95% of hospitalized patients.

- Transfusion-related and drug-related reactions are important causes of a positive direct Coombs test.

Mechanisms of Drug-Induced Hemolytic Anemia
There are several distinct mechanisms of drug-induced hemolytic anemia.

Autoantibody Mechanism
Methyldopa induces the formation of anti-Rh IgG antibodies that can induce hemolysis. The autoantibody mechanism associated with methyldopa is dose-related, and hemolysis develops in about 0.3% to 0.8% of patients who receive this drug. Hemolysis occurs 18 weeks to 4 years after first ingestion of the drug. The direct Coombs test becomes positive in 3 to 6 months, and the IgG level is high. There is no anamnestic response to rechallenge. Discontinuation of use of the drug usually leads to a rapid reversal in hemolysis. The mechanism of action is related to an altered cellular immune system, with a block in the activation of suppressor T cells. Other drugs with a similar mechanism known to cause autoimmune hemolytic anemia include procainamide, ibuprofen, and cimetidine.

Drug Adsorption Mechanism
In drug adsorption (hapten) immunohemolytic anemia (usually caused by a penicillin or cephalosporin), the drug binds to the RBC membrane and antibody forms against the drug membrane–antigen complex. Development of this complication requires high doses of drug for more than 7 days. The onset is subacute, with patients generally presenting at 7 to 10 days. A positive direct Coombs test develops in 3% of patients, and the response is dose-related in that 30% of patients have positive tests at 2 million units daily and 100% at 10 million units daily. Penicillin allergy is not necessarily present. Drug-adsorption immunohemolytic anemia may be fatal if not detected early. Other drugs, including tetracycline, quinidine, tolmetin, and cisplatin, may cause autoimmune hemolytic anemia through the same mechanism.

Immune-Complex Mechanism
In the immune-complex, or "innocent bystander," mechanism the antidrug antibody forms first and reacts with the drug to form an immune complex. The antidrug-antibody complex is then adsorbed on the RBCs. The cell-bound complex may activate complement, causing intravascular hemolysis. The direct Coombs test is positive because of the complement on the RBC surface. Clinically, a small quantity of drug is sufficient to cause autoimmune hemolytic anemia if there was previous exposure. Acute intravascular hemolysis with hemoglobinemia and hemoglobinuria is the usual clinical course. Drugs implicated in this type of autoimmune hemolytic anemia include quinidine, quinine, phenacetin, acetaminophen, para-aminosalicylate (PAS), isoniazid (INH), streptomycin, rifampin, methadone, probenecid, insulin, sulfonylureas, hydralazine, hydrochlorothiazide, stibophen (an antiparasitic), sulfa drugs, triamterene, and melphalan.

- Autoantibody mechanism: methyldopa.
- Drug adsorption (hapten) mechanism: penicillin.
- Immune-complex mechanism: quinine and quinidine.

- Typical clinical scenario: A patient has evidence of hemolysis (increased reticulocyte count, LDH, and indirect bilirubin), positive Coombs test with or without splenomegaly, and jaundice, with a history of exposure to 1 of the common offending drugs.

Warm Autoimmune Hemolytic Anemia
The first general principle in the treatment of warm autoimmune hemolytic anemia is to treat the underlying disease (if one can be identified) and to discontinue the use of drugs that have been implicated in hemolysis. If the patient's condition is clinically stable, do not transfuse blood. If transfusion is required, transfuse the most compatible RBCs by crossmatch with type-specific ABO and Rh blood. The major risk of transfusion is the formation of autoantibodies to foreign RBC antigens, which are more difficult for the blood bank to detect when an autoantibody is present.

Corticosteroids are indicated for the treatment of idiopathic autoimmune hemolytic anemia and are considered in the treatment of disease-associated autoimmune hemolytic anemia. In drug-related warm autoimmune hemolytic anemia, treatment usually is limited to discontinuing use of the implicated drug. The initial dosage of prednisone should be 1 mg/kg daily. Most patients have a response in 7 days. Patients should receive supplementation with oral folate (1 mg daily). If the patient has a relapse during tapering of the corticosteroid, return to the previous dose. Splenectomy is performed in steroid-refractory cases and will be required for about 60% of patients with idiopathic autoimmune hemolytic anemia. Rituximab or immunosuppressive drugs such as cyclophosphamide, danazol (400-800 mg daily), and high-dose intravenous gamma globulin are also effective in some cases.

Cold Agglutinin Syndrome (Primary Cold Agglutinin Disease)
Cold agglutinin syndrome is characterized by agglutination, chronic hemolytic anemia, and a positive direct Coombs test (anti-C3 monospecific only). Autoantibodies are IgM and are maximally reactive at low temperatures. The degree of hemolysis depends on the thermal amplitude of the antibody; antibodies that react not only at low temperatures but also at near-physiologic temperatures (eg, >33°C) cause more severe hemolysis. In addition, the higher the antibody titer, the more likely complement is to bind with subsequent hemolysis.

The clinical signs and symptoms are related to small-vessel occlusion and include acrocyanosis of the ears, tip of the nose, toes, and fingers. The skin is dusky blue and then turns normal or blanches. All digits may be affected equally. This should be differentiated from Raynaud phenomenon, in which the skin of 1 or 2 fingers turns white to blue to red.

The peripheral blood smear shows RBC agglutination that disappears if prepared at 37°C (Figure 11-9). Agglutinated RBCs clump together, spuriously elevating the MCV. Agglutination is commonly confused with rouleaux. In rouleaux, the cells stack in a linear pattern on one another (Figure 11-15); rouleaux is associated with monoclonal proteins. The anemia in cold agglutinin syndrome is usually mild to moderate. The cold agglutinin titer in cold agglutinin syndrome is typically greater than 1:1,000. Low titers of cold agglutinins (eg, 1:8) are common in general medical patients and are of no clinical significance. Therapy includes avoidance of the cold; patients may find it helpful to move to a warmer climate. Oral danazol (200 mg twice daily) or subcutaneous interferon alfa may be given as initial therapy. Some patients may respond to immunosuppressive drugs such as cyclophosphamide or chlorambucil or to rituximab (anti-CD20 antibody). Corticosteroids and splenectomy are ineffective. Plasma exchange is not very effective but can be considered if the patient is acutely ill, because IgM is intravascular.

- Cold agglutinin syndrome: agglutination and hemolytic anemia.
- Positive direct Coombs test (C3, not IgG) and cold agglutinin titer >1:1,000.
- Typical clinical scenario: The patient has acrocyanosis of the ears, tip of the nose, toes, and fingers. The diagnosis of cold agglutinin syndrome is made by finding, on a peripheral blood smear, RBC agglutination that disappears if the smear is prepared at 37°C rather than at room temperature (22°C). Differentiate from Raynaud phenomenon with Coombs-positive hemolytic anemia.

Immunology of Cold Agglutinins
An IgM antibody exhibits a reversible thermal-dependent equilibrium reaction, typically with the I or i antigen, which is related to the ABO blood group system of RBCs. Binding of antibody to antigen is favored at lower temperatures. Cold agglutinin syndrome is most commonly idiopathic, but it can also be secondary to malignancy or infection. A monoclonal κ protein can be found in cold agglutinin syndrome associated with chronic lymphocytic leukemia, multiple myeloma, lymphoma, and Waldenström macroglobulinemia. In secondary diseases, there is a polyclonal light chain reaction with a high thermal cold agglutinin of anti-I specificity (*Mycoplasma pneumoniae*) or anti-i specificity (infectious mononucleosis, cytomegalovirus, and lymphoma).

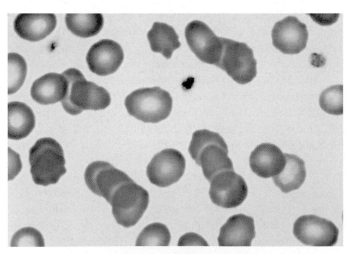

Figure 11-15. Rouleaux. Stacking of red blood cells in a linear pattern distinguishes this from agglutination (compare Figure 11-9). Rouleaux is most commonly associated with hypergammaglobulinemia, especially in human immunodeficiency virus infection or monoclonal plasma cell disorders. (Courtesy of Curtis A. Hanson, MD, Mayo Clinic.)

Mycoplasma pneumoniae (Anti-I)
Of the patients with *Mycoplasma pneumoniae*, 50% have cold agglutinin titers greater than 1:64, most have splenomegaly, and acrocyanosis is unusual. If cold agglutinin syndrome develops, this complication generally resolves in 2 or 3 weeks, but fatalities have been reported. Treatment includes keeping the patient warm and treating the infection with antibiotics.

Infectious Mononucleosis (Anti-i)
Of the patients with infectious mononucleosis, 40% to 50% have cold agglutinins and 3% have hemolytic anemia. The onset occurs by day 13 in 67% of patients. The duration of hemolysis is less than 1 month in 75% of patients and 1 to 2 months in 25%. Hepatosplenomegaly is present in most patients. Although corticosteroids are generally ineffective in idiopathic cold agglutinin syndrome, they may be useful for cold agglutinins associated with infectious mononucleosis.

Paroxysmal Cold Hemoglobinuria (Complement-Mediated Lysis)
Paroxysmal cold hemoglobinuria is the least common cause of autoimmune hemolytic anemia. Results of the Donath-Landsteiner test are positive. The Donath-Landsteiner antibody is an IgG antibody that binds to P antigen on erythrocytes at low temperatures in the periphery and then causes hemolysis at core physiologic temperatures. This condition can be idiopathic or secondary. The secondary causes include syphilis (congenital and late), mononucleosis, mycoplasma, chickenpox, mumps, and measles. Measles is the most common secondary cause now. Clinical manifestations include shaking chills, fever, malaise, abdominal pain, back pain, and leg pain. There is rapid evolution of severe anemia. The overall prognosis is good. This condition resolves after the infection clears. Treatment includes protection from the cold, treatment of the underlying disease, and possibly a short course of corticosteroids.

Coombs-Negative Hemolytic Anemias
The differential diagnosis of Coombs-negative hemolytic anemia is broad and includes hereditary red cell disorders such as enzymopathies (G6PD deficiency and pyruvate kinase deficiency), hemoglobinopathies, and membrane disorders; paroxysmal nocturnal hemoglobinuria; Wilson disease; and microangiopathic conditions including thrombotic thrombocytopenic purpura. Rarely, warm autoimmune hemolytic anemia is Coombs-negative owing to low antibody titers.

Glucose-6-Phosphate Dehydrogenase Deficiency
G6PD deficiency is the most common RBC enzyme deficiency. It causes decreased levels of glutathione, which is an antioxidant, making RBCs more sensitive to oxidative damage by infection (oxidative enzymes released by granulocytes), toxins (eg, naphthalene in mothballs), or drugs. G6PD is encoded on the X chromosome and is therefore sex-linked. All RBC enzymopathies are autosomal recessive except G6PD and phosphoglycerate kinase deficiencies, which are sex-linked. Rarely, females who are heterozygous for an abnormal G6PD are clinically affected owing to unfavorable lyonization.

There are more than 300 G6PD enzyme variants. The wild-type variant is called G6PD B. About 20% of African Americans have G6PD A+, which is functionally normal. The most common abnormal variants encountered in the United States are G6PD A– (in 11% of African American males) and G6PD Mediterranean, which is found primarily in persons of Mediterranean origin. This distinction is clinically important because G6PD A– is a milder variant that does not decay over the length of the RBC's life as fast as G6PD Mediterranean. Therefore, during an acute hemolytic crisis, G6PD assays may be falsely normal in patients with G6PD A–, since senescent RBCs with low G6PD activity levels will be preferentially destroyed, leaving only younger cells with normal levels. This is less likely with G6PD Mediterranean.

G6PD deficiency confers some protection against falciparum malaria. Protection extends to both males and heterozygous females. This selective advantage has been attributed to the inhibition of parasite growth and replication through the mechanism of increased oxidant stress.

The oxidation of hemoglobin leads to the formation of methemoglobin, and sulfhemoglobin may be a product, with precipitation, condensation, and attachment of the denatured portion to the inside of the membrane, forming Heinz bodies. There is individual variability to oxidant stress.

In the steady state, there is no anemia or RBC defect except with a few rare G6PD variants. There is an increased risk of hemolysis in patients with concurrent kidney or liver disease, viral or bacterial infection, diabetic acidosis, viral hepatitis, and low levels of blood glucose. Even a mild infection can produce hemolytic anemia; this is more common than hemolysis induced by drug provocation. *Favism* is sensitivity to fresh fava beans in patients with G6PD Mediterranean. Favism is not seen with G6PD A–. Drugs that commonly cause hemolytic anemia in G6PD deficiency include antimalarial agents (primaquine and chloroquine), dapsone, sulfonamides (sulfanilamide, sulfamethoxazole, sulfapyridine, and sulfasalazine), nitrofurantoin, diazoxide, high-dose aspirin, probenecid, and nitrites (which are derived from nitrates from nitroglycerin, fertilizer-contaminated home wells, and amyl nitrite).

Abnormal laboratory findings include intravascular hemolysis, methemoglobinemia, and methemalbuminemia (highly specific for intravascular hemolysis due to enzymopathy). Supravital staining for Heinz bodies is a good screening test, but their absence does not rule out the diagnosis. Heinz bodies are not seen on standard Wright-Giemsa–stained peripheral blood smears. The G6PD assay is the definitive test but should not be done during acute hemolysis in patients of African ancestry. Therapy includes treating the underlying infection and withdrawing use of the offending drug.

- G6PD deficiency: the most common RBC enzyme deficiency; it is inherited on the X chromosome.
- G6PD deficiency provides some protection against falciparum malaria.
- No anemia or RBC defect occurs in the steady state with the most common G6PD variants.
- Hemolysis is induced by infection more commonly than by drugs.
- A good screening test: Heinz bodies seen on supravital staining of the peripheral blood.
- Treat underlying infections and withdraw the use of offending drugs.

- Typical clinical scenario: Acute symptomatic anemia in an African American after infection or drug ingestion. There is evidence of intravascular hemolysis (including an increase in the LDH level), urinary hemoglobinuria, and hemosiderinuria and a decrease in haptoglobin levels. The Heinz body test is positive. The direct Coombs test is negative.

Other Enzymopathies

The most common RBC enzyme deficiency states are G6PD and pyruvate kinase deficiencies. Other enzymopathies are extremely rare. In a referral population, only 35% of the patients who were referred for an enzyme deficiency work-up had an identifiable enzyme deficiency. Many patients are inappropriately tested for enzyme deficiencies when another cause of hemolysis is more likely.

Hereditary Spherocytosis

Hereditary spherocytosis most commonly is an autosomal dominant disorder (75%) seen primarily in patients of northern European ancestry, but it can be autosomal recessive or sporadic. It is caused by an underlying defect in the RBC cytoskeleton owing to a partial deficiency in 1 or more of the components: ankyrin, spectrin, band 3, and protein 4.2. Osmotic fragility of RBCs is increased. The results of the incubated osmotic fragility test—the most reliable diagnostic test—are almost always abnormal. The clinical features include jaundice, splenomegaly, negative results on the direct Coombs test, abundant spherocytes, and increased osmotic fragility. Pigment gallstones are present in most patients by age 50. Treatment is splenectomy, which invariably causes a reduction in hemolysis. It should be performed after the first decade of life, since young children have high rates of postsplenectomy infection. Asymptomatic adults may be observed if they have a hemoglobin concentration greater than 11 g/dL and a reticulocyte count less than 6%.

- Hereditary spherocytosis: autosomal dominant (75%), autosomal recessive, or sporadic.
- Splenomegaly is invariably present and cholelithiasis is common.
- Other features: negative results on the Coombs test and increased osmotic fragility.
- Treatment: splenectomy after the first decade of life for patients with moderate or severe hemolysis. Asymptomatic adults with a hemoglobin concentration >11 g/dL and reticulocyte count <6% may be observed.
- Typical clinical scenario: A patient presents with extravascular hemolysis, spherocytosis, splenomegaly, and premature gallstones.

Paroxysmal Nocturnal Hemoglobinuria

Paroxysmal nocturnal hemoglobinuria (PNH) is an acquired clonal chronic hematologic stem cell disorder. Patients with this condition have a median survival of 10 years. Blood cells are unusually sensitive to activated complement and are lysed. Hemolysis occurs primarily at night because this is when plasma becomes more acidotic due to sleep-related physiologic changes (eg, relative hypoxia). The disorder is characterized by abnormal hematopoietic stem cells, reticulocytopenia, leukopenia, or thrombocytopenia due to lysis by complement. Normal and abnormal cells occur simultaneously in most patients.

A distinct class of membrane proteins is selectively deleted from the plasma membranes of maturing cells. The abnormal cells in PNH have decreased glycosylphosphatidylinositol (GPI)-linked proteins in erythroid, granulocytic, megakaryocytic, and, in some cases, lymphoid cells, which results from a somatic mutation in the *PIGA* gene. *PIGA* encodes an enzyme required for synthesis of GPI. Flow cytometric studies can detect the presence or absence of GPI-linked proteins, which include CD14, CD55, and CD59. This disease involves deficiencies in the surface molecules that normally regulate activation of C3B and C5 to C9 in the complement cascade. There is a decreased quantity of membrane proteins (decay-accelerating factor [CD55] and complement regulatory protein [CD59]) that regulate the alternate complement pathway on normal blood cells.

Clinically, PNH is characterized by a chronic hemolytic anemia with hemoglobinuria and hemoglobinemia (intravascular hemolysis). Venous thrombosis of the portal system, brain, and extremities is associated with 50% of the deaths in PNH. Episodes of severe pain may occur in the abdomen and back in conjunction with painful or difficult swallowing due to esophageal spastic dysphagia.

In up to 10% of patients, myelodysplasia or acute myeloid leukemia develops. PNH and aplastic anemia can coexist. There is a high risk of venous thrombosis for unclear reasons; Budd-Chiari syndrome is the main cause of death. Budd-Chiari syndrome (hepatic vein thrombosis) is manifested by abdominal pain, tender hepatomegaly, nausea, vomiting, fever, and increased serum levels of LDH and liver enzymes due to hepatocyte injury. Liver ultrasonography and venography help in making the diagnosis of Budd-Chiari syndrome. Treatment includes emergent heparinization, a long-term course of anticoagulation, and fibrinolytic therapy. Transplant or portocaval shunting may be necessary if portal hypertension develops.

The most useful assay for diagnosis of PNH is flow cytometry to establish the absence of the GPI-linked antigens. Flow cytometry has replaced the sucrose hemolysis test and the Ham test (acid hemolysis test).

Up to 60% of patients benefit from prednisone treatment. Prednisone may inhibit activation of complement. Prednisone does not help restore hematopoiesis if bone marrow failure is present. Eculizumab is a monoclonal antibody that inhibits terminal complement, and it is approved by the Food and Drug Administration (FDA) for long-term therapy of hemolysis in PNH. It also prevents thrombosis. Eculizumab is extremely expensive. Patients must have received quadrivalent meningococcal vaccine before receiving eculizumab, since terminal complement is important in defense against meningococcemia.

* PNH is a chronic disease.
* Venous thrombosis, especially Budd-Chiari syndrome, is associated with 50% of the deaths in PNH.
* Intravascular hemolysis occurs with hemoglobinuria and hemoglobinemia.
* Leukemia or myelodysplasia occurs in 5%-10%; aplastic anemia may coexist with PNH.
* Diagnosis: flow cytometry studies for GPI-linked proteins.
* Typical clinical scenario: A patient has pancytopenia, Coombs-negative anemia, dark urine, abdominal pain, absence of stainable iron in the marrow, and unusual venous thrombosis.

Thrombotic Microangiopathies: Differential Diagnosis

In microangiopathic hemolytic anemia, the RBCs are fragmented and deformed in the peripheral blood (Figure 11-16). The fragmentation is caused by fibrin deposits in small blood vessels, which lead to mechanical hemolysis. The results of the direct Coombs test are negative. Patients with microangiopathic hemolytic anemia are often thrombocytopenic. The associated disorders are characterized by widespread microvascular thrombosis leading to end-organ injury.

Microangiopathic hemolytic anemia is associated with thrombotic thrombocytopenic purpura, hemolytic uremic syndrome, malignant hypertension, pulmonary hypertension, acute glomerulonephritis, renal allograft rejection, obstetric catastrophes, HELLP syndrome (*h*emolysis, *e*levated *l*iver function tests, and *l*ow *p*latelet count), disseminated intravascular coagulopathy, collagen vascular diseases (scleroderma, systemic lupus erythematosus, Wegener syndrome, and periarteritis nodosa), carcinomatosis, vascular malformations including Kasabach-Merritt syndrome (giant hemangiomas that trap platelets), viral infections (HIV), bacterial infections (*Escherichia coli* O157:H7), drugs (mitomycin C, quinine, ticlopidine, tacrolimus, cisplatin, and cyclosporine), acute radiation nephropathy, bone marrow transplant (total body irradiation and allogeneic bone marrow transplant more commonly than autologous marrow transplant), and solid-organ transplant.

Thrombotic Thrombocytopenic Purpura

Thrombotic thrombocytopenic purpura (TTP) is characterized by the pentad of anemia, thrombocytopenia, neurologic signs, fever, and kidney abnormalities. Most patients do not manifest all 5 features before the diagnosis is made. The primary criteria are thrombocytopenia and microangiopathy, and these are sufficient to establish the diagnosis. The anemia is normochromic normocytic, with microangiopathic hemolytic features (Figure 11-16). The direct Coombs test gives negative results. The results of coagulation studies are normal or only mildly abnormal, in contrast to disseminated intravascular coagulopathy. The cause of this syndrome is unknown in more than 90% of the patients. TTP is associated with pregnancy and the use of oral contraceptives, HIV infection, cancer, bone marrow transplant, certain chemotherapy drugs (especially mitomycin C and bleomycin), and other drugs (crack cocaine, ticlopidine, and cyclosporine).

Clinically, thrombocytopenia is associated with bleeding in 96% of patients. Neurologic signs often wax and wane and include headache, coma, mental changes, paresis, seizure and coma, aphasia, syncope, visual symptoms, dysarthria, vertigo, agitation, confusion, and delirium. Kidney abnormalities include abnormal urinary sediment (common) and elevated creatinine (less common). Azotemia is an unfavorable prognostic sign.

The pathologic findings are characterized by widespread intraluminal hyaline vascular occlusions with platelet aggregates and fibrin, with no inflammatory changes in the microvasculature (terminal arterioles or capillaries). Microvascular changes can be found in virtually any organ. The preferred biopsy site is the bone marrow. Other sites to consider for biopsy are the gingiva, skin, petechial spot, muscle, and lymph nodes. Patients with TTP are deficient in the von Willebrand factor (vWF)-cleaving protease ADAMTS13 that

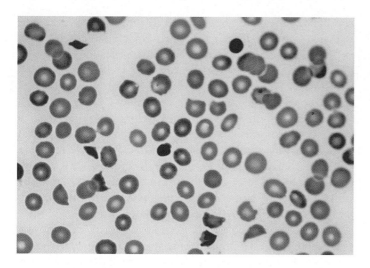
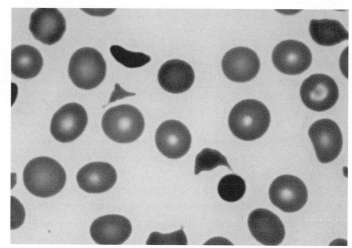

Figure 11-16. Schistocytes. Fragmented red blood cells are shaped like helmets, triangles, or kites. These are characteristic of any microangiopathic hemolytic process. (Courtesy of Curtis A. Hanson, MD, Mayo Clinic.)

normally reduces the size of the large vWF multimers. Large multimers of vWF appear to be the platelet-aggregating agents of TTP. An IgG antibody accounts for the lack of protease activity in the sporadic form of TTP.

Without treatment, more than 90% of patients die of multiorgan failure, but with treatment, 70% to 80% survive the disease and have few or no sequelae. The treatment of choice is *plasma exchange* (plasmapheresis with infusion of fresh frozen plasma or the supernatant fraction from cryoprecipitate preparations [*cryosupernatant*, also known as *cryo-poor plasma*]). Patients may need more than 10 treatments before a response is evident. The platelet count and LDH level track disease activity. Other ancillary treatments with unknown value include dipyridamole (400-600 mg daily), aspirin (dosages used range from 300 mg twice weekly to 600-1,200 mg daily), and prednisone (60 mg/kg daily). The overall response rate to plasma exchange therapy is 80% to 90%. The 10-year risk of relapse in the Canadian Apheresis Group Trial was 36%. Relapses are managed with plasma exchange. The management of refractory TTP includes intravenous vincristine, rituximab, splenectomy, or intravenous high-dose gamma globulin. Platelet transfusions should be used only when required for an invasive procedure since they can exacerbate the disease.

- TTP: the pentad of anemia, fever, thrombocytopenia, neurologic signs, and renal abnormalities.
- Cause is unknown in most cases.
- Features: Coombs test gives negative results, microangiopathy, ADAMTS13 deficiency, large vWF multimers.
- The treatment of choice is plasmapheresis with infusion of fresh frozen plasma (ie, plasma exchange).
- Typical clinical scenario: A patient presents with anemia, thrombocytopenia, neurologic signs and symptoms, renal abnormalities, or fever. Peripheral blood smear shows schistocytes. Clotting times (prothrombin time [PT] and activated partial thromboplastin time [aPTT]) are normal.

Hemolytic Uremic Syndrome

Hemolytic uremic syndrome is characterized by microangiopathic hemolytic anemia (anemia and thrombocytopenia) and renal microangiopathy, with a creatinine level greater than 3 mg/dL. Fever and neurologic signs are not a prominent part of this syndrome. The pathologic findings are similar to those in TTP but are limited to the kidneys. It is often preceded by an acute infectious process. Other associations include pregnancy, bone marrow transplant, chemotherapy, and immunosuppressive medications such as cyclosporine. The morbidity and mortality rates are much higher for adults than for children. A recurrent illness may be caused by defective production of the complement control protein factor H, similar to TTP. The syndrome may be associated with *E coli* O157:H7 diarrhea, as is the classic association in children. Other associations include various non-O157:H7 *E coli* serotypes and *Shigella dysenteriae*. Hemolytic uremic syndrome is usually not associated with a decrease in ADAMTS13 activity. The management of the hemolytic-uremic syndrome is supportive. Dialysis may be necessary, and corticosteroids may be incorporated in the management. Response to plasma exchange is variable, but in adults a trial is indicated.

Sickle Cell Disorders

Classification and Pathophysiology

The sickle cell disorders include sickle cell anemia (homozygous hemoglobin S), sickle cell trait (heterozygous hemoglobin S), and compound states (hemoglobin S along with thalassemia or other hemoglobinopathies (eg, sickle cell–hemoglobin C disease, sickle cell-β-thalassemia).

Sickle cell anemia occurs in patients of sub-Saharan African descent, and less commonly in patients of Middle Eastern or South Asian origin. About 8% of African Americans carry 1 copy of the sickle cell gene (trait), with sickle cell disease occurring in about 1 of 500 individuals. In the heterozygous state, hemoglobin S offers protection against severe falciparum malaria. In the homozygous state, sickle cell anemia is a serious, life-shortening disease. Hemoglobin S is different from hemoglobin A in the substitution of valine for glutamic acid at the sixth amino acid of the β chain. Deoxygenated hemoglobin S aggregates into rigid polymers that distort the cell into a sickle shape and injure the cell membrane (Figure 11-17). Vaso-occlusion is a function of decreased RBC deformability, increased viscosity, and increased RBC adherence to altered endothelium. Two-thirds of the RBCs are removed by extravascular mechanisms.

Vaso-occlusion occurs in arterioles and larger arteries, not capillaries. Polymorphonuclear leukocytes release activators that facilitate vaso-occlusion.

Sickling is inhibited by hemoglobin F, which is a potent inhibitor of polymerization. Sickling is promoted by low oxygen tension, low pH, high cellular concentration of hemoglobins, loss of cell water (a consequence of membrane injury), and coinheritance of hemoglobin D.

Prenatal diagnosis may be made by analysis of amniotic fluid or chorionic villi biopsy, which is preferred to fetal blood sampling.

Symptoms are not present until the patient is older than 6 months because of the high levels of fetal hemoglobin in early life. The first episode of vaso-occlusive disease typically develops between the ages of 12 months and 6 years. Acute crises result from obstruction of the microcirculation by intravascular sickling. Laboratory testing is not helpful in distinguishing a sickle cell crisis from other causes of pain.

Clinical Manifestations

Bone and joint pain crises are characterized by gnawing pain involving the trunk or extremities and swelling of the elbows and knees. Pain prevalence is highest between ages 19 and 39 years. The average duration of a painful crisis is 10 days. Radiographs may show bone infarcts and periostitis, but these do not appear until symptoms subside. Infarcts and periostitis may be documented with bone scans. Abdominal crises result from small infarcts of the mesentery and abdominal viscera, with symptoms lasting for 4 or 5 days. This is a

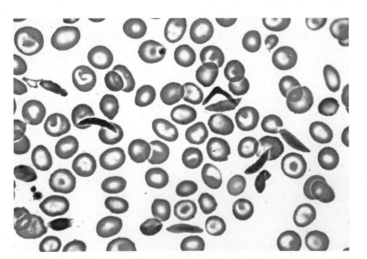

Figure 11-17. Sickle Cell Anemia. Several irreversibly sickled cells are seen. Abundant target cells indicate hyposplenism from autoinfarction of the spleen. Liver disease due to transfusional hemosiderosis was also a contributing factor to these target cells.

nonsurgical problem if bowel sounds are present. Associated signs and symptoms include fever, tenderness, hypertension, tachycardia, tachypnea, nausea, and vomiting. Splenic sequestration crisis is seen mostly in young children. Rapid enlargement of the spleen is caused by occlusion of sinusoids by sickled cells. Other vaso-occlusive crises include priapism and dactylitis.

The Cooperative Study of Sickle Cell Disease reported that the incidence of hemorrhagic stroke was highest among patients 20 to 29 years old, with a mortality rate of 26% in the first 2 weeks and no deaths after infarctive strokes. The frequency of stroke is 10% to 15% in the first 18 years of life. Transient ischemic attack is a strong risk factor for infarctive stroke, as is elevated flow in the middle cerebral artery as determined by Doppler ultrasonography.

Acute chest syndrome accounts for up to 25% of deaths in sickle cell disease. Clinical aspects include fever, chest pain, tachypnea, increased white blood cell (WBC) count, and pulmonary infiltrates. Sickling may be secondary or primary. When infection is present, causative organisms include pneumococcus, *Mycoplasma*, *Haemophilus*, *Salmonella*, and *E coli*. In a cooperative study, 13% of patients required ventilator support, 11% had simultaneous neurologic events, and the mortality rate was 9%. Thromboembolism and fat embolism can also precipitate acute chest syndrome. Chronic lung disease may result from sequelae of acute chest syndrome or chronic thromboembolic disease.

Aplastic crises usually follow a febrile illness, with the disappearance of reticulocytes and normoblasts. Infections from B19 parvovirus are more common in adults than in children and are self-limited. The aplastic crisis lasts 5 to 10 days. Chronic hemolysis can lead to folate deficiency.

Infections are the most frequent cause of death of patients younger than 5 years. The common organisms include *S pneumoniae* and *Haemophilus influenzae*. In patients older than 5 years, gram-negative bacteria predominate, with osteomyelitis caused by *Salmonella*, *Staphylococcus*, and pneumococci. Bone infarction is more common than osteomyelitis. In contrast to bone infarction, osteomyelitis manifests as high fever, a left shift with an increased leukocyte count, an increased erythrocyte sedimentation rate, and positive blood cultures. The challenge with *S pneumoniae* is not followed by appropriate opsonin production owing to hyposplenism. Preventive measures include prophylactic penicillin therapy and immunization.

The chronic manifestations of sickle cell anemia are multiple, but anemia is the most common. There is a progressive lag in growth and development after the first decade of life and a chronic destruction of bone and joints, with ischemia and infarction of the spongiosa. The vertebrae become "fish-mouthed." Avascular necrosis is common in multiple joints, and the incidence of femoral and humeral necrosis increases with advanced age. Ocular manifestations include retinopathy with stasis and occlusion of small vessels that is nonproliferative or proliferative. The small vessels may require laser photocoagulation.

Chronic cardiovascular manifestations include cardiomegaly, flow murmurs, and a pansystolic murmur with a click that mimics mitral regurgitation. Hepatobiliary manifestations include hepatomegaly with the pathologic features of distended sinusoids, periportal fibrosis, and hemosiderin pigment. Marked hyperbilirubinemia may be due to hepatitis, intrahepatic sickling, choledocholithiasis, or coexistent

G6PD deficiency. Hemochromatosis is a complication, especially in patients receiving frequent transfusions. There is an increased incidence of pigmented gallstones. Hepatic crises occur and resolve in 1 to 3 weeks. Renal manifestations include papillary necrosis, hyposthenuria by age 6 to 12 months (disruption of the countercurrent multiplier system, nocturia, and enuresis), hematuria (ulcer in renal pelvis and urate stones), nephrotic syndrome caused by focal segmental glomerulonephropathy, tubular damage from small infarcts, and priapism. Chronic renal insufficiency is common (25%-75% of patients). Leg ulcers are painful and may be complicated by infection.

Although disease manifestations do not increase during pregnancy, maternal mortality is 5% to 8% and fetal mortality 20%.

Laboratory findings include severe anemia (hemoglobin, 5.5-9.5 g/dL), sickled cells, cigar-shaped cells, ovalocytes, target cells, basophilic stippling, polychromatophilia, reticulocytosis (3%-12%), and hyposplenia with Howell-Jolly bodies (Figure 11-12). A persistent increase in the WBC count of $12 \times 10^9/L$ to $15 \times 10^9/L$ (in the absence of infection) with eosinophilia is characteristic. Evidence of chronic hemolysis may be present. Values on liver function tests are often increased. On cellulose acetate hemoglobin electrophoresis, hemoglobin S moves more slowly than hemoglobin A and is easily resolved. Routine diagnostic tests include the sickle solubility test, electrophoresis, and chromatography.

* Acute complications of sickle cell anemia include vaso-occlusive episodes, acute chest syndrome, dactylitis, splenic sequestration, aplastic crisis, infection, cholelithiasis, priapism, renal papillary necrosis, and cerebrovascular accidents.
* Chronic complications include hemolytic anemia, pulmonary hypertension, folate deficiency, retinopathy, chronic renal insufficiency, accelerated cardiovascular disease, transfusional hemosiderosis, nonhealing skin ulcers, osteopenia, and growth retardation.
* Acute chest syndrome is the leading cause of death in sickle cell anemia.
* Maternal and fetal mortality are increased.

Treatment

Many sickle cell crises can be prevented. Infection, fever, dehydration, acidosis, hypoxemia, cold, and high altitude should be avoided. Immunizations for encapsulated organisms, penicillin prophylaxis because of hyposplenism, and patient education about triggers of vaso-occlusion are essential. Acetaminophen is indicated for fever because aspirin contributes to an acid load. A temperature higher than 105°F (40.6°C) means infection rather than just infarction (infection is uncommon if the temperature is lower than 102°F [38.9°C]). Folate supplementation is indicated, especially during pregnancy. Iron chelation is recommended if the transfusion requirement is high and ferritin is elevated. Splenectomy is recommended for children who survive the initial splenic sequestration crisis. This is the only indication for splenectomy; most patients with sickle cell disease (hemoglobin SS) undergo autosplenectomy by means of recurrent infarction by age 5.

Blood transfusion and exchange transfusions are the most effective means of treatment available for severe complications. Hemoglobin S fractions of less than 30% have been recommended for life-threatening complications. It is easiest to achieve this goal with exchange transfusion. Posttransfusion increases in hemoglobin to more than 10 to 11 g/dL should be avoided except preoperatively. Exchange transfusion is indicated for stroke; prevention of cerebrovascular accidents in patients with a history of transient ischemic attack, stroke, or elevated middle cerebral artery flow rate; acute chest syndrome; priapism; and progressive retinopathy. Exchange transfusion may also be indicated in other situations such as protracted hematuria or chronic nonhealing skin ulcers. For elective surgery, simple transfusions should be used to achieve a hemoglobin concentration greater than 10 g/dL.

In vaso-occlusive crises, the cornerstone of treatment includes gentle hydration and pain control. Analgesics, including opioids, are essential and should not be withheld because of concern about drug-seeking behavior. Blood transfusions do not modify the course of vaso-occlusive episodes.

In the Multicenter Study of Hydroxyurea in Sickle Cell Anemia, which was a double-blind, placebo-controlled trial, hydroxyurea decreased the frequency of painful vaso-occlusive crises by about 50%. The frequency of the acute chest syndrome was also decreased and patients required fewer transfusions and hospitalizations. Hydroxyurea increases fetal hemoglobin and causes slight neutropenia, both of which may contribute to the efficacy of the drug. Hydroxyurea invariably increases the MCV, which can be used to monitor regimen adherence. Hydroxyurea is indicated for patients who have had severe complications such as acute chest syndrome and patients who have frequent painful crises.

Hematopoietic stem cell transplant with marrow or umbilical cord blood from HLA-identical siblings has demonstrated that sickle cell disease can be cured. The present indications for transplant include stroke and recurrent chest syndrome. Related umbilical cord blood transplant offers a good probability of success and has a low risk of graft-versus-host disease. Siblings with sickle cell trait are suitable donors.

With good management, 50% of patients with sickle cell anemia survive beyond the fifth decade. Few patients survive into their 60s, however, owing to chronic cardiac and cerebrovascular injury, hemosiderosis, and cumulative mortality from crises. Symptomatic patients die earlier. A high level of fetal hemoglobin predicts improved survival of young patients. Acute chest syndrome, renal failure, seizures, a baseline WBC count greater than $15 \times 10^9/L$, and a low level of fetal hemoglobin are associated with risk of early death. Most adult patients who die of sickle cell complications do so during an acute sickle cell crisis. Acute chest syndrome is the most common cause of death. Stroke is the next most common cause, followed by infection (*E coli*, *Staphylococcus aureus*, HIV, tuberculosis, malaria, pneumococci, and hepatitis).

Sickle Cell Trait and Compound States

Sickle cell trait (heterozygous hemoglobin S) is not associated with anemia, RBC abnormalities, increased risk of infections, or increased mortality. On electrophoresis or chromatography, 35% to 45% of hemoglobin is hemoglobin S. Associations with sickle cell trait include hematuria due to renal papillary necrosis, splenic infarction at high altitude (>10,000 feet [3,030 meters]), hyposthenuria, bacteriuria, pyelonephritis in pregnancy, pulmonary embolism, glaucoma, and decreased mortality from *Plasmodium falciparum* infection. There are reports of sudden death during strenuous exercise (eg, military boot camp) or scuba diving.

In sickle cell–hemoglobin C disease, patients have hemoglobin S and C, with an absence of hemoglobin A and normal or increased levels of hemoglobin F. Patients with sickle cell–hemoglobin C survive longer than those with sickle cell anemia. Sickle cell–hemoglobin C disorder is less severe than sickle cell disease, with preservation of the spleen into adulthood in many cases. However, patients have more retinal complications and a higher risk of aseptic necrosis of the femoral head and humeral head. There is mild anemia; in 10% of the patients, the hemoglobin concentration is less than 10 g/dL. Sickle cells are rare on the peripheral blood smear, and 50% of the cells in the peripheral blood are target cells.

The severity of hemoglobin S/β-thalassemia depends on the β-thalassemia allele. In β^0-thalassemia, in which no normal β-globin is made, the disease is similar to homozygous hemoglobin S. In β^+-thalassemia, in which some normal β-globin is produced, disease is less severe than sickle cell disease. Both affect the β chain. The spleen remains functional for longer than with homozygous hemoglobin S disease, but retinopathy is more common.

* Hydroxyurea decreases the frequency of painful vaso-occlusive crises by 50% and also decreases acute chest syndrome episodes.
* Acute chest syndrome, renal failure, seizures, a baseline WBC count $>15 \times 10^9$/L, and a low level of fetal hemoglobin are associated with the risk of early death in adults.
* Death is associated with acute pain and chest syndrome, stroke, and infection.
* Patients with sickle cell–hemoglobin C survive longer than those with homozygous sickle cell anemia.
* Achieving a hemoglobin S level of <30% with exchange transfusion is recommended for life-threatening complications, including acute chest syndrome and stroke.
* A posttransfusion increase in hemoglobin to >10 g/dL should be avoided except before elective surgery.
* Typical clinical scenario: An African American patient has pain, fever, stroke, or infection and evidence of Coombs-negative hemolytic anemia with Howell-Jolly bodies on a peripheral blood smear. The diagnosis is made with hemoglobin electrophoresis.

Neutropenia

The major causes of neutropenia include hematologic neoplasm, metastatic neoplasm involving the marrow, irradiation, vitamin B_{12} deficiency and folate deficiency, drugs, infections (HIV and hepatitis), congenital or acquired primary disorders of hematopoiesis (eg, cyclic neutropenia and aplastic anemia), autoimmune neutropenia (Felty syndrome, rheumatoid arthritis, systemic lupus erythematosus, and Sjögren syndrome), hypersplenism, hemodilution, and benign idiopathic neutropenia. Drug-induced neutropenia is associated with chemotherapeutic agents, sulfonamides, semisynthetic penicillins, phenothiazines, nonsteroidal anti-inflammatory drugs (indomethacin and phenylbutazone), antithyroid medications (propylthiouracil and methimazole), allopurinol, and anticonvulsants. Drug-induced neutropenia typically becomes manifest 1 to 2 weeks after initial drug exposure, or sooner following another exposure. The treatment of choice is to discontinue use of the offending drug. Corticosteroids offer no benefit in drug-induced neutropenia. Patients of African descent have a lower neutrophil count on average than patients of European descent, and some black patients have WBC counts below the laboratory reference ranges. If patients are asymptomatic and the neutropenia is nonprogressive, this need not be evaluated further.

The differential diagnosis of chronic neutropenia includes cyclic neutropenia, congenital neutropenia (eg, Kostmann syndrome), and chronic idiopathic neutropenia. In both congenital and cyclic neutropenia, mutations of the neutrophil elastase gene (*ELA2*) are common and are inherited in an autosomal dominant fashion. Cyclic neutropenia is characterized by oscillations in the neutrophil counts every 19 to 23 days. It is a disorder of neutrophil production. The typical clinical syndrome is manifested as furuncles, cellulitis, chronic gingivitis, and abscesses during neutrophil nadir. Patients can predict the timing of successive episodes. Treatment involves timely antibiotics, avoidance of dental and surgical work at neutrophil nadirs, good oral hygiene, and receiving recommended routine dental care. Granulocyte colony-stimulating factor (G-CSF) (filgrastim) may be effective in increasing the neutrophil count in cyclic neutropenia and chronic idiopathic neutropenia.

In the adult population, the recommended dosage of G-CSF is 5 mcg/kg daily subcutaneously. A single 6-mg dose of pegylated G-CSF (pegfilgrastim) 24 hours after chemotherapy is now the treatment of choice in most situations following chemotherapy outside of the transplant setting.

The 2006 American Society of Clinical Oncology recommendations for the use of WBC growth factors state that use of G-CSF is justified after cytotoxic chemotherapy when the risk of febrile neutropenia is approximately 20% and no other equally effective regimen that does not require colony-stimulating factors is available. Primary prophylaxis is recommended for the prevention of febrile neutropenia in patients who are at high risk of this complication because of age, disease characteristics, and myelotoxicity of the chemotherapy regimen. G-CSF use allows a modest to moderate increase in dose-intensity of chemotherapy regimens, which may improve outcomes in diseases such as breast cancer. Special circumstances for patients who might benefit from these agents include preexisting neutropenia due to disease, extensive previous chemotherapy, previous irradiation to the pelvis, a history of recurrent febrile neutropenia while receiving earlier chemotherapy, and conditions that potentially enhance the risk of infection (poor performance status, decreased immune function, open wounds, or active tissue infections). These agents are also effective adjuncts in progenitor-cell transplantation. Colony-stimulating factors should be given after the chemotherapy dosing or radiotherapy is completed. Granulocyte-macrophage colony-stimulating factor (GM-CSF) is another available growth factor, but the lack of randomized trials precludes definitive recommendations.

Transfusion Reactions

The primary cause of major transfusion reactions and transfusion-related deaths is medical error, which includes bypassed safeguards, similar patient names, and verbal or faxed communications. The major transfusion reactions include acute hemolytic transfusion reactions, transfusions associated with anti-IgA antibodies, transfusion-related acute lung injury (TRALI), adult respiratory distress syndrome, delayed hemolytic transfusion reactions, febrile transfusion reactions, urticarial (allergic) transfusion reactions, and circulatory overload (Table 11-3).

Acute Hemolytic Transfusion Reactions

Acute hemolytic transfusion reactions are the most life-threatening. They occur within minutes to hours. The recipient's preexisting RBC antibodies, usually IgM, against the donor's RBCs bind to the donor's RBCs and cause complement-mediated hemolysis. The most common cause is human error, especially when blood is released on an emergency basis. Of the fatal transfusion reactions, 85% involve ABO incompatibility. ABO compatibility is illustrated in Table 11-4. Other, nonclerical causes include antibodies not detected before transfusion, such as Kell, Duffy (Jk^a), and Kidd (Fy^a), which may have low titers at the time of crossmatching but upon reexposure result in a vigorous anamnestic response. Females are at greater risk than males, because sensitization through pregnancy leads to a higher frequency of preformed antibodies. Urgent transfusion of large amounts of blood products also increases the risk. Clinically, there is pain at the intravenous (IV) site, apprehension or a sense of impending doom, back pain, abdominal pain, fever, chills, chest pain, hypotension, nausea, flushing, and dyspnea. The direct Coombs test gives positive results in most cases.

Complications include oliguria, acute renal failure, and disseminated intravascular coagulation (DIC). The mortality rate is about 20%. Treatment includes immediate termination of the transfusion, vigorous administration of fluids, and furosemide to increase renal cortical blood flow. It is difficult to distinguish between an acute hemolytic transfusion reaction and a febrile nonhemolytic transfusion reaction when fever first occurs. Therefore, patients with fevers occurring during transfusion should be urgently evaluated.

Transfusion Reactions Associated With Anti-IgA Antibodies

Transfusion reactions can be associated with anti-IgA antibodies. These include anaphylactic reactions due to infusion of IgA-containing units of blood into a patient with IgA deficiency and preformed anti-IgA antibodies, the development of a class-specific anti-IgA antibody in patients with class-specific IgA deficiency, anti-IgA antibodies acquired through pregnancy or previous transfusions, and ataxia-telangiectasia, in which 44% of patients have class-specific anti-IgA antibodies. In each case, the pathogenesis of the transfusion reaction is due to anti-IgA antibodies of the IgG type that are capable of binding complement. Clinical features are similar to those of an acute hemolytic transfusion reaction. Treatment includes stopping the transfusion and giving antihistamines and conventional anti-anaphylactic drugs. Transfusion protocols for patients include use of washed RBCs and IgA-deficient plasma.

Transfusion-Related Acute Lung Injury

Transfusion-associated adult respiratory distress syndrome or TRALI is a complication of transfusion that is often unrecognized and ranks

Table 11-3   Risks of Complications From Transfusions in the United States

Complication	Risk Per Unit
Minor allergic reaction	3/100
Circulatory overload	Variable
Febrile, nonhemolytic	3/100
Delayed hemolytic transfusion reaction	1/4,000
Transfusion-related acute lung injury (TRALI)	1/10,000
Acute hemolytic transfusion reaction	$1/2.5 \times 10^4$ to $1/1.0 \times 10^6$
HIV infection	$1/2.1 \times 10^6$
Hepatitis B virus (HBV)	$1/2.0 \times 10^5$
Hepatitis C virus (HCV)	$1/1.9 \times 10^5$
HTLV I/II infection	$1/2.0 \times 10^5$
West Nile virus	Unknown
Bacterial infections	$1/2,000$ to $1/5.0 \times 10^5$
IgA-related anaphylaxis	$1/1.0 \times 10^5$
Graft-versus-host disease	Rare
Immunosuppression	Unknown
Posttransfusion purpura	Rare
Prion infection	Unknown

Abbreviations: HIV, human immunodeficiency virus; HTLV, human T-cell leukemia virus.

third among causes of transfusion-related deaths. It is characterized by acute respiratory distress during transfusion or within 6 hours after completion of transfusion, hypotension, bilateral pulmonary infiltrates, normal or low pulmonary capillary wedge pressure, no evidence of circulatory overload, and fever. Recovery is rapid with appropriate supportive care, occurring in 24 to 48 hours. The problem is with the blood donor, not the recipient. Most blood donors implicated in this complication have had multiple pregnancies. The pathogenesis relates to the interaction between donor-derived anti-WBC antibodies in the transfused blood and the WBCs in the transfusion recipient. Possible mechanisms include leukoagglutinins in plasma or HLA-specific lymphocytotoxic antibodies passively transfused from the donor to the recipient, resulting in polymorphonuclear leukocyte-complement–triggered microvascular injury that results in a leak into the pulmonary alveolar spaces and pulmonary edema and a white-out on the chest radiograph. The treatment is supportive. Essentially all patients require oxygen. Many patients require a ventilator with positive end-expiratory pressure and dopamine. This disorder may be misdiagnosed as circulatory overload. From 5% to 8% of patients die of complications of the pulmonary injury.

Delayed Hemolytic Transfusion Reactions

Delayed hemolytic transfusion reactions (1 in 4,000 transfusions) occur because of the inability to detect clinically significant recipient antibodies before transfusion. This transfusion reaction, which usually

Table 11-4   Blood Product Compatibility in the ABO System[a]

Recipient ABO Group	Acceptable Donor ABO Groups		
	Packed Red Blood Cells	Platelets and Fresh Frozen Plasma	Whole Blood (Rarely Used)
O	O	AB, A, B, or O	O
A	A or O	A or AB	A
B	B or O	B or AB	B
AB	AB, A, B, or O	AB	AB

[a] Natural alloimmunization against A and B antigens occurs in people lacking these antigens. Upon transfusion of ABO-incompatible blood, preformed antibodies serve as hemagglutinins, resulting in life-threatening acute hemolysis and complement activation. Hemagglutinins are found primarily in plasma; platelets are considered similar to plasma products with respect to ABO compatibility.

occurs 5 to 10 days after transfusion, is less dramatic and less dangerous than an acute hemolytic reaction. Delayed reactions are more common in females and in patients with sickle cell anemia who have received transfusions long-term. The recipient's plasma already contains antibody before transfusion because of previous transfusion or previous pregnancy. Delayed reactions usually involve the Rh or Kidd system. The antibodies become undetectable over time because of low antibody titers and increase quickly in titer on rapid stimulation by the transfusion; thus, they are detectable after the transfusion. Results of the direct Coombs test are positive. There is evidence of hemolysis. One-third of the patients are asymptomatic, and the reactions are detected by recurrence of laboratory-detected anemia without clear cause; the others present with symptoms of anemia, chills, jaundice, and fever. Management consists of monitoring hemoglobin concentration and renal output and avoiding use of units with the offending antigen in the future.

Urticarial (Allergic) Transfusion Reactions

Urticarial (allergic) transfusion reactions are a complication in 3% of transfusions. Glottal edema and asthma are rarely associated with urticarial transfusion reactions. The cause is an antibody in the recipient against foreign-donor serum proteins. Treatment consists of stopping the transfusion, which is not absolutely necessary, and giving antihistamines (premedicate with antihistamines if the patient had a previous reaction).

Febrile Transfusion Reactions

Febrile transfusion reactions are characterized by chills and fever usually about an hour after the transfusion starts, with accompanying flushing, headache, tachycardia, and generalized discomfort (eg, myalgias and arthralgias) lasting 8 to 10 hours. This occurs in 1% of all transfusions. The causes include cytokines from WBCs and platelets against donor antigens and antiserum protein antibodies. Treatment consists of stopping the transfusion to evaluate the problem further; initially, a febrile reaction cannot be distinguished from a hemolytic transfusion reaction because both conditions may present with fever. Preventive methods include leukoreduction.

Circulatory Overload

Circulatory overload may cause tightness in the chest, dry cough, and acute edema. This complication is seen in patients with an already increased intravascular volume or decreased cardiac reserve. This is a frequently overlooked diagnosis. Symptoms generally develop within several hours after transfusion. Management includes slowing the transfusion to 100 mL per hour, placing the patient in the sitting position, and giving diuretics.

Posttransfusion Purpura

Posttransfusion purpura is a rare syndrome characterized by the abrupt onset of severe thrombocytopenia 5 to 10 days after blood transfusion; the estimated mortality is 10% to 15%. Most cases involve patients whose platelets lack the HPA-1a antigen and who have an antibody from a previous pregnancy or transfusion. Intravenous immunoglobulin at a dose of 400 to 500 mg/kg is the treatment of choice.

Infection

Pathogen transmission may occur with transfusions. These risks and other risks of transfusion are summarized in Table 11-3.

Gaucher Disease

Gaucher disease is the most common of the lysosomal storage diseases. Adults with Gaucher disease most often have type 1 nonneuropathic Gaucher disease. Most patients are of Ashkenazi Jewish heritage. Massive splenomegaly and hepatomegaly are common, and owing to hypersplenism and marrow infiltration by Gaucher cells (Figure 11-18), 50% have anemia or thrombocytopenia. Bone lesions are present in 75% of patients, with the femur most commonly having an "Erlenmeyer flask" lytic deformity. Avascular necrosis and pathologic fractures may occur. The pathogenesis is related to an accumulation of glucocerebroside from deficient β-glucosidase. The Gaucher cells are large and have an eccentric nucleus and fibrillar cytoplasm that is wrinkled like tissue paper (Figure 11-18). Treatment options include recombinant β-glucosidase (imiglucerase) and, rarely, allogeneic bone marrow transplant.

Porphyria

The porphyrias are enzyme disorders that are autosomal dominant with low disease penetrance, except for congenital erythropoietic porphyria, which is autosomal recessive, and porphyria cutanea tarda, which may be acquired and is associated with hepatitis C and hemochromatosis. Most persons remain biochemically and clinically normal throughout the majority of their lives. Clinical expression is linked to environmental and acquired factors. Disease manifestations depend on the type of excess porphyrin intermediate. When there is an excess of the earlier precursor molecules (δ-aminolevulinic acid and porphobilinogen), the clinical manifestations are neuropsychiatric. These symptoms include autonomic dysfunction (abdominal pain, vomiting, constipation, tachycardia, and hypertension), psychiatric symptoms, fever, leukocytosis, syndrome of inappropriate antidiuresis, and neurologic symptoms (proximal paresis and paresthesias). If the excess is in the distal intermediates (uroporphyrins, coproporphyrins, and protoporphyrins), the manifestations are cutaneous (photosensitivity, blister formation, facial hypertrichosis, and hyperpigmentation). If the excess is of both early and late porphyrins, there are both neuropsychiatric and cutaneous manifestations.

Porphobilinogen production and excretion are invariably increased during marked symptoms caused by the 3 neuropathic porphyrias, which include acute intermittent porphyria, hereditary coproporphyria, and porphyria variegata. In hereditary coproporphyria and porphyria variegata, there is an accumulation of coproporphyrinogen/coproporphyrin or protoporphyrinogen/protoporphyrin and a concomitant increase in δ-aminolevulinic acid and porphobilinogen. In the acute porphyrias, urinary porphobilinogen is increased during the attacks. Patients with acute intermittent porphyria lack skin lesions. It is important to check fecal porphyrins in protoporphyria, porphyria variegata, and coproporphyria. The porphyrias are compared in Table 11-5. Secondary coproporphyrinuria has many causes, including impaired hepatobiliary transport of coproporphyrin (due to steroids) or increased liver or erythroid synthesis (due to alcohol, liver disease, or hemolytic anemia). An elevated coproporphyrin level alone, therefore, does not support a diagnosis of porphyria.

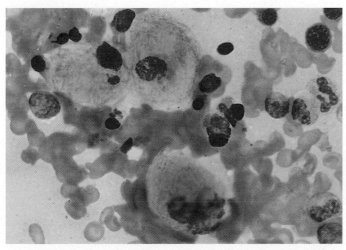

Figure 11-18. Gaucher Cells. These large cells have characteristic pale, foamy, and fibrillar cytoplasm. (Courtesy of Curtis A. Hanson, MD, Mayo Clinic.)

- In suspected acute porphyria, determine the 24-hour urinary porphobilinogen during the acute episode.
- Mild coproporphyrin elevation is nonspecific and not diagnostic of porphyria.
- Porphyria cutanea tarda is associated with chronic hepatitis C and with hemochromatosis.

Hematology of Acquired Immunodeficiency

Lymphocytopenias are the hallmark of AIDS. There is an absolute decrease of CD4 lymphocytes as the disease progresses, with a relative reduction of the CD4:CD8 ratio. Also, CD4 lymphocytes are functionally impaired. Whereas CD8 lymphocytes may increase in number early in the disease, they decrease late in the disease. Neutropenia occurs in 50% of the patients. Natural killer cells are normal in number but altered in function. Neutropenia may be due to autoimmune destruction with antigranulocyte antibodies in two-thirds of patients, decreased production, drugs (zidovudine [AZT], ganciclovir, trimethoprim-sulfamethoxazole, pentamidine), coexisting infections, or non-Hodgkin lymphoma. Neutrophil dysfunction is also manifested by decreased chemotaxis, granulation, and phagocytosis.

Anemia occurs in 70% of HIV-infected patients. Most commonly, the anemia is normochromic normocytic and similar to anemia of chronic disease. The degree of anemia is a prognostic factor. Many patients have inadequate erythropoietin levels and respond to recombinant erythropoietin therapy. Approximately 25% of patients have positive results on the direct Coombs test, but marked hemolysis is not common. Of patients treated with zidovudine, 30% develop pronounced anemia, which is characteristically macrocytic. Clinical studies have demonstrated that transfusions may decrease survival and increase the risk of cytomegalovirus infection. Anemia is also associated with infections from *Mycobacterium avium* complex, parvovirus B19, *Mycobacterium tuberculosis*, and *Histoplasma* species. Decreased vitamin B_{12} levels are detected in 20% of HIV-infected patients and are due to altered serum transport of vitamin B_{12} and not always to a deficiency in body stores. Microangiopathic hemolytic anemia may occur but is usually milder than with other causes of this disorder. Plasmapheresis with plasma exchange is the treatment of choice.

Thrombocytopenia occurs in 40% of HIV-infected patients and is often detected early in the disease. Platelet production and survival may be decreased in HIV-infected patients. ITP in HIV is usually accompanied by platelet-associated antibodies and responds to antiretroviral therapy (80% of patients), prednisone (90%), danazol, dapsone (60%), immunoglobulin given IV, and splenectomy (80%). Coagulation disorders may complicate HIV disorders. A lupus anticoagulant is present in 20% of HIV patients, usually in association with opportunistic infections, but is rarely associated with thrombosis or bleeding. Vitamin K deficiencies due to nutritional abnormalities, drugs, or liver dysfunction may occur. Other problems include increased level of vWF antigen (with a poor prognosis if >200%), increased level of tissue plasminogen activator (with a poor prognosis if >20 ng/mL), and increased level of fibrinogen.

Non-Hodgkin lymphoma is the second most common HIV-associated malignancy after Kaposi sarcoma, occurring in 2.9% of patients. Diffuse large B-cell lymphoma and Burkitt lymphoma are

Table 11-5   Comparison of Porphyrias

Porphyria Cutanea Tarda	Acute Intermittent Porphyria	Porphyria Variegata
Features		

Most common type of porphyria
Iron overload
Skin lesions on light-exposed areas
Hypertrichosis (usually mild)
Increased uroporphyrins in urine
No neuropathic features
	Increased urinary δ-aminolevulinic acid &
	  porphobilinogen during acute symptomatic
	  episodes; often normal levels between episodes
	Neurologic symptoms: abdominal pain of
	  3-5 days' duration without anatomical cause,
	  focal neurologic problems such as polyneuropathy
	  & motor paresis, psychiatric problems with
	  hallucinations, confusion, psychosis, seizures
	Decreased porphobilinogen deaminase activity
	Normal protoporphyrin & coproporphyrin in stool
		Clinically: photosensitivity, abdominal
		  pain, neurologic problems (similar to
		  acute intermittent porphyria)
		Increased protoporphyrin &
		  coproporphyrin in stool

Associations		

Alcoholic liver disease, chronic
  hepatitis C, hemochromatosis
Estrogens: females, males
  treated for prostatic carcinoma
Hexachlorobenzene
	Drugs that precipitate crises, including sulfonamides,
	  barbiturates, alcohol
	Menstrual cycle can exacerbate symptoms
	Infection or surgery can precipitate crisis
	Inadequate nutrition can precipitate crisis
		Common in South Africa (due to
		  founder effect), Holland

Treatment		

Phlebotomy to remove iron
Chloroquine
Low-dose antimalarials
	Avoid prolonged fasting & crash diets
	Large amounts of carbohydrate (400 g daily)
	Intravenous hematin
	Luteinizing hormone—releasing hormone agonists
	  for suppression of hormonal fluctuation
		Same as for acute intermittent
		  porphyria

the most characteristic histologic findings. Extranodal disease occurs in 66% of patients. Up to one-third of patients with HIV infection and lymphoma may have bone involvement. There is also an increased risk of Hodgkin lymphoma among HIV patients.

* Cytopenias are common in HIV infection and are multifactorial.
* Lupus anticoagulant is common but rarely causes thrombohemorrhagic complications.
* HIV-associated malignancies include non-Hodgkin lymphoma, especially diffuse large cell lymphoma, and Burkitt-like lymphoma.

Parvovirus Infection

Parvovirus infection (B19 virus), or fifth disease, is a highly contagious disease in children and causes a "slapped-cheeks" rash. Adults with this infection may develop a polyarthralgia syndrome or cytopenia. Abnormalities in the erythroid line include severe anemia, reticulocytopenia, and RBC hypoplasia in the bone marrow. Pancytopenia may occur. Immunoglobulin therapy administered IV is the treatment of choice. Complete recovery is the rule.

Massive Splenomegaly

The differential diagnosis of asymptomatic massive splenomegaly includes Gaucher disease, primary myelofibrosis, chronic myelogenous leukemia, portal hypertension, large splenic cyst, non-Hodgkin lymphoma, and hairy cell leukemia.

* Differential diagnosis of asymptomatic massive splenomegaly: Gaucher disease, primary myelofibrosis, chronic myelogenous leukemia, portal hypertension, splenic cyst, non-Hodgkin lymphoma, and hairy cell leukemia.

Spontaneous Splenic Ruptures

Spontaneous splenic ruptures have been reported to occur in infectious mononucleosis, cytomegalovirus infections, acute and chronic myelogenous leukemia, acute and chronic lymphocytic leukemia, myeloproliferative diseases, and non-Hodgkin lymphoma. Usually accompanied by hemorrhage, splenic rupture is a surgical emergency.

Part II

David P. Steensma, MD

Malignant Hematology

Malignancies

Chronic Lymphocytic Leukemia

Chronic lymphocytic leukemia (CLL) is a clonal lymphoproliferative disorder of mature lymphocytes (Figure 11-19) and is primarily seen in older patients (90% of patients are older than 50). The clinical diagnosis has classically required an absolute lymphocytosis with more than 5,000 mature-appearing lymphocytes per microliter and more than 30% lymphocytes in the bone marrow, but some patients now receive a diagnosis earlier with the detection of a mature B cell clone by flow cytometry testing. The characteristic immunophenotype is CD5+ (rare in other B-cell malignancies), CD20+, and CD23+; CD20+ and CD23+ are B-cell markers. CLL is more common in men than women and is rare in Asia. B-cell CLL, unlike many hematologic malignancies, is not associated with exposure to ionizing radiation, drugs, or chemicals. The 2 widely used staging classifications are outlined in Tables 11-6 and 11-7.

Low-risk patients have a normal hemoglobin level, low lymphocyte count, nondiffuse (nodular) bone marrow infiltration pattern by tumor cells, and a lymphocyte doubling time of more than 1 year. Newer prognostic factors that indicate a better prognosis include a normal karyotype, 13q deletion, hypermutated *IGVH* gene, high smudge cell index, and low expression of ZAP-70. The 2-year survival rate for patients with 13q deletion or normal karyotypes is 90% or more.

Poor risk factors include advanced-stage, unmutated *IGVH* genes, atypical lymphocyte morphology, trisomy 12, and deletion of

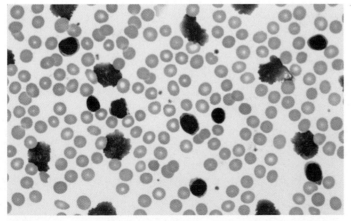

Figure 11-19. Chronic Lymphocytic Leukemia. There are a large number of small and mature lymphocytes with nuclei approximately the same size as red blood cells. Smudge cells are also characteristic of this disorder. (Courtesy of Curtis A. Hanson, MD, Mayo Clinic.)

17p, 11q, or 6q. Patients with a 17p deletion have a 2-year survival of 34% and do not respond to chemotherapy. Less than half of patients have a chromosomal abnormality detectable by karyotyping.

* Normal karyotype and 13q deletion predict a favorable prognosis, and 17p deletion predicts the most unfavorable outcome.
* Stage predicts survival.

The clinical course is chronic in most patients, and median survival exceeds 10 years. Complications include recurrent infection; 50% of patients have hypogammaglobulinemia, which is a contributing factor. Fever is due to infection and should not be attributed to CLL, except in Richter syndrome (transformation to large-cell lymphoma). Autoimmune and immunodeficiency complications include autoimmune hemolytic anemia (in 10% of the patients), monoclonal gammopathy (in 5%), immune-mediated thrombocytopenia (occurs in 2% and is IgG-mediated and treated with corticosteroids), pure RBC aplasia, hypogammaglobulinemia, impaired delayed-type hypersensitivity, increased susceptibility to microorganisms, and second malignancies. Prophylactic intravenous gamma globulin is indicated for gamma globulin levels less than 0.3 g/dL with or without previous infection.

* In CLL, fever is not related to the disease but to infection, except in Richter syndrome.
* Hypogammaglobulinemia occurs in 50% of the patients.
* Autoimmune hemolytic anemia occurs in 10%.
* Immune-mediated thrombocytopenia occurs in <5%.
* Prophylactic intravenous gamma globulin is indicated for gamma globulin levels <0.3 g/dL with or without previous infection.
* Typical clinical scenario: A middle-aged or older patient has an increased WBC count, lymphocytosis, and diffuse lymphadenopathy. Peripheral blood lymphocyte flow cytometry shows the presence of mature CD23+ B lymphocytes that aberrantly express the T-cell marker CD5. The cells are also "dimly" positive for surface immunoglobulin that is "light-chain restricted" (ie, almost all the cells express 1 type of light chain, either κ or λ).

CLL is associated with an increased incidence of solid tumors of the lung and skin (basal cell and squamous cell). Patients may develop secondary drug-induced myelodysplasia or acute myeloid leukemia. Infectious complications from various bacterial and viral organisms are frequent.

For patients with no adverse prognostic factors (Rai stage 0 or I, low lymphocyte count, and normal cytogenetics or 13q deletion), the standard practice is to withhold treatment until the disease is active or progressive. A French study of patients with early-stage disease found no difference in survival between groups that received treatment immediately or received treatment only after the disease had progressed. For patients with adverse prognostic factors (Rai

Table 11-6 Staging of Chronic Lymphocytic Leukemia: Rai Classification

Stage	Characteristics	Median Survival Time, mo
0	Peripheral lymphocytosis (>15 × 10^9/L), bone marrow lymphocytosis (>40%)	>150
I	Lymphocytosis, lymphadenopathy	101
II	Lymphocytosis, splenomegaly	71
III	Lymphocytosis, anemia with hemoglobin <11 g/dL excluding AIHA	19
IV	Lymphocytosis, thrombocytopenia	19

Abbreviation: AIHA, autoimmune hemolytic anemia.
Data from Rai KR, Sawitsky A, Cronkite EP, Chanana AD, Levy RN, Pasternack BS. Clinical staging of chronic lymphocytic leukemia. Blood. 1975;46:219-34.

Table 11-7 Staging of Chronic Lymphocytic Leukemia: International Workshop on Chronic Lymphocytic Leukemia Classification

Clinical Stage	Features
A	No anemia or thrombocytopenia and <3 areas of lymphoid enlargement (spleen, liver, & lymph nodes in cervical, axillary, & inguinal regions)
B	No anemia or thrombocytopenia but with ≥3 involved areas of lymphoid enlargement
C	Anemia (hemoglobin <10 g/dL) or thrombocytopenia (or both)

From International Workshop on CLL. Chronic lymphocytic leukaemia: proposals for a revised prognostic staging system. Br J Haematol. 1981;48:365-7. Used with permission.

stage III or IV, trisomy 12, or deletion of chromosome 11q and 17p), fludarabine-based chemotherapy is now the initial treatment of choice, with high rates for complete remission and molecular remission. The major toxic effects of fludarabine are myelosuppression and immunosuppression, which predispose to opportunistic infections due to a quantitative suppression in T-helper (CD4) lymphocytes. Chlorambucil with or without prednisone is still a reasonable treatment option in some elderly patients. Patients with refractory disease are often treated with alemtuzumab (anti-CD52 monoclonal antibody) or bendamustine. Bone marrow transplant is being evaluated in CLL but is not widely used, since most patients are elderly and not good candidates. Prednisone alone may be indicated for isolated immune-related anemia and thrombocytopenia.

Splenectomy may be indicated for patients with refractory immune anemia or thrombocytopenia, massive splenomegaly, and hypersplenism. With each relapse, the disease becomes more resistant to treatment.

- Observe asymptomatic patients who have low-risk disease.
- Treat patients who have advanced, high-risk disease.
- The optimal initial treatment is a fludarabine-based regimen.

Hairy Cell Leukemia

Hairy cell leukemia is characterized by an insidious onset of cytopenias without constitutional symptoms and is due to proliferation of clonal cells of B lymphocyte origin. Almost all patients have splenomegaly. The neoplastic cells have cytoplasmic projections that are "hairy,"

with multiple thin or blunt projections (Figure 11-20). Hairy cell leukemia is rare and accounts for less than 2% of all cases of leukemia. The male to female ratio is 4:1. The cause is not known.

The symptoms are related to cytopenias, infections, and splenomegaly. The bone marrow yields a "dry tap" (ie, no liquid marrow can be obtained) on attempted bone marrow aspiration; core biopsy specimens are hypercellular with diffuse infiltration by neoplastic cells and marrow fibrosis.

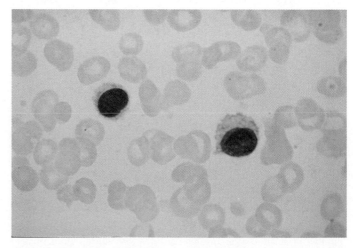

Figure 11-20. Hairy Cell Leukemia. These mature lymphocytes have eccentrically placed nuclei, pale cytoplasm, and characteristic projections.

- Cytopenias and splenomegaly are common.
- Hairy cells have cytoplasmic projections.
- Constitutes <2% of all cases of leukemia.
- Bone marrow aspirate: dry tap.
- Typical clinical scenario: A 50-year-old man has insidious onset of cytopenias and splenomegaly. Peripheral blood shows atypical WBCs with irregular projections. Bone marrow biopsy findings include malignant cells.

Infection is the major cause of death. Fever is not a manifestation of the disease but indicates an underlying infection. Impaired cell-mediated immunity predisposes patients to infections. The incidence of atypical mycobacterial infections is increased. There is a high incidence of viral infections, fungal infections, and parasitic diseases. Bleeding and vasculitis are other complications.

Observation alone may be indicated for patients who are asymptomatic with a normal CBC or very mild cytopenias. The treatment of choice for more severely affected patients is with 2-chlorodeoxyadenosine (also known as cladribine), which produces durable complete remission rates in 85% to 88% of patients after a single 7-day continuous, intravenous infusion. Other treatments include interferon and pentostatin, which produces complete remission in about 75% of patients. Most patients live for more than 10 years. Splenectomy improves peripheral blood cell counts but has no effect on the bone marrow.

- Hairy cell leukemia: infection is the major cause of death.
- Infection is related to granulocytopenia and impaired cell-mediated immunity.
- Fever denotes infection.
- Atypical mycobacterial infections are associated with the disease.
- 2 Chlorodeoxyadenosine (cladribine) is the treatment of choice for hairy cell leukemia. Other options include pentostatin and interferon.

Hodgkin Lymphoma

Treatment of Hodgkin lymphoma represents a major success of modern chemotherapy. With therapy, more than 80% of patients with Hodgkin lymphoma are cured. Untreated, the 5-year survival rate is less than 5%.

The age at presentation has a bimodal distribution, with the first peak at a median age of about 25 years and the second peak after age 60. Patients with Hodgkin lymphoma usually present with a locally limited disease that progresses in an orderly manner from a lymph node group to an adjacent region. The typical finding at presentation is lymph node enlargement, but virtually any organ or tissue may be involved (lung, bone marrow, liver, and bone). Less common presentations include generalized pruritus, cytopenias, abnormal findings on liver function tests, and jaundice (extrahepatic biliary obstruction, autoimmune hemolytic anemia, or, rarely, intrahepatic cholestasis). A small number of patients have pain in involved lymph nodes after alcohol consumption. Patients with Hodgkin lymphoma have impaired cell-mediated immunity and are predisposed to herpes zoster and cytomegalovirus infections. The most important unfavorable prognostic factors are hemoglobin concentration less than 11 g/dL, a serum level of albumin less than 4 g/dL,

male gender, age older than 45 years, stage IV disease (see Table 11-8 for definition), total WBC count greater than $15 \times 10^9/L$, and lymphocytopenia (lymphocyte count $<0.5 \times 10^9/L$).

The diagnosis of Hodgkin lymphoma is based on the presence of Reed-Sternberg cells, which typically have 2 or more nuclei with prominent nucleoli that give the cells the appearance of an owl's eyes (Figure 11-21). Polymerase chain reaction detects Epstein-Barr virus in lymph nodes in 60% to 80% of cases.

Disease stage is the principal factor in selecting treatment (Tables 11-8 and 11-9). The disease is routinely staged by use of computed tomographic (CT) scan of the chest, abdomen, and pelvis. Positron emission tomographic (PET) scans are also valuable in staging. Staging laparotomy is no longer performed.

Before treatment is started, male patients should be advised to store sperm if they intend to have children. Female patients should be advised not to become pregnant for 2 years after therapy because 75% of relapses occur during this period.

Radiotherapy is a consideration in the management of Hodgkin disease emergencies, including acute superior vena cava syndrome, airway obstruction, pericardial tamponade, and epidural spinal cord compression.

Currently, the treatment of choice for localized disease (stages IA and IIA) is a short course of chemotherapy with ABVD (doxorubicin [Adriamycin], bleomycin, vinblastine, and dacarbazine [DTIC]) and low doses of radiotherapy to the involved field. ABVD chemotherapy is administered for 2 cycles beyond a complete remission. The treatment of choice for advanced disease is combination chemotherapy. The cure rates are up to 65% for patients with advanced disease. There is less sterility and secondary leukemia with ABVD than with MOPP (mechlorethamine, vincristine [Oncovin], procarbazine, and prednisone) chemotherapy. The role of more aggressive combination therapies, such as Stanford V or dose-intensive BEACOPP (bleomycin, etoposide, doxorubicin [Adriamycin], cyclophosphamide, vincristine [Oncovin], procarbazine, prednisone), is being investigated.

Relapse patterns are relatively predictable in Hodgkin disease. After irradiation, relapse usually occurs in the first 2 years and involves

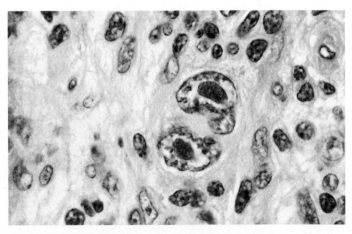

Figure 11-21. Hodgkin Disease. Reed-Sternberg cell is a large binuclear cell. (Courtesy of Curtis A. Hanson, MD, Mayo Clinic.)

Table 11-8 The Cotswolds Staging Classification of Hodgkin Lymphoma

Classification	Description
Stage I	Involvement of a single lymph node region or lymphoid structure
Stage II	Involvement of ≥2 lymph node regions on the same side of the diaphragm (the mediastinum is considered a single site, whereas hilar lymph nodes are considered bilaterally)
Stage III	Involvement of lymph node regions or structures on both sides of the diaphragm
Stage III-1	With or without involvement of splenic, hilar, celiac, or portal nodes
Stage III-2	With involvement of para-aortic, iliac, & mesenteric nodes
Stage IV	Involvement of 1 or more extranodal sites in addition to a site for which the designation "E" has been used
Designations applicable to any disease stage	
A	No symptoms
B	Fever (temperature >38°C), drenching night sweats, unexplained loss of >10% of body weight within the preceding 6 months
X	Bulky disease (a widening of the mediastinum by more than one-third or the presence of a nodal mass with a maximal dimension >10 cm)
E	Involvement of a single extranodal site that is contiguous or proximal to the known nodal site
CS	Clinical stage
PS	Pathologic stage (as determined by laparotomy)

From Lister TA, Crowther D. Staging for Hodgkin's disease. Semin Oncol. 1990;17:696-703. Used with permission.

nonirradiated sites adjacent to the treated fields. Relapse after chemotherapy occurs at sites of bulky disease. Patients who have relapse after radiotherapy still have about a 66% chance of cure with salvage chemotherapy. Those who have relapse after chemotherapy currently are offered autologous stem cell or bone marrow transplant. In a study that compared autologous bone marrow transplant with conventional chemotherapy for recurrent or refractory Hodgkin lymphoma, the 3-year event-free survival was 53% for the transplant group and 10% for the chemotherapy group.

Late complications of Hodgkin lymphoma therapy are substantial. The risks include infertility, amenorrhea, pneumococcal sepsis (in those who have undergone splenectomy), hypothyroidism, thyroid carcinoma, avascular necrosis of bone, cardiomyopathy due to

Table 11-9 Staging Procedures for Lymphoma

History and examination: identification of *B* symptoms (see designations in Table 11-8) & sites of palpable adenopathy
Imaging procedures: plain chest radiography; computed tomography of thorax, abdomen, & pelvis
Hematologic procedures: CBC with differential, determination of erythrocyte sedimentation rate, & bilateral bone marrow aspiration & biopsy (not always necessary in Hodgkin lymphoma)
Biochemical procedures: tests of liver function; measurement of serum albumin, lactate dehydrogenase, & calcium
Special procedures: PET scan

Abbreviations: CBC, complete blood cell count; PET, positron emission tomographic.

doxorubicin or radiotherapy, radiation pneumonitis, radiation-induced constrictive pericarditis, pulmonary fibrosis, and secondary malignancies. The secondary malignancies include acute myeloid leukemia, myelodysplastic syndromes, non-Hodgkin lymphoma, and solid tumors. ABVD is less leukemogenic than MOPP. Patients at highest risk are those who have received multiple courses of chemotherapy for relapsed disease. The risk of non-Hodgkin lymphoma is 4% at 10 years. Radiotherapy increases the risk of solid tumors (especially breast cancer) and hypothyroidism. After 15 years, the risk of secondary solid tumors is 13%; these tumors include malignancies of the stomach, breast, lung, thyroid, skin, and head and neck. Breast cancer is more likely in women treated for Hodgkin lymphoma at a very young age.

- Polymerase chain reaction detects Epstein-Barr virus in lymph nodes in 60%-80% of the cases of Hodgkin lymphoma.
- Disease stage is the principal factor in selecting treatment for Hodgkin disease.
- Of patients with relapse after radiotherapy, 66% are in long-term remission after chemotherapy.
- The treatment of choice for patients with advanced disease: ABVD chemotherapy.
- Autologous bone marrow or peripheral blood stem-cell transplant is indicated after a first relapse from any front-line chemotherapy for Hodgkin disease.
- Late complications of treatment include acute myeloid leukemia, solid tumors, hypothyroidism, and cardiomyopathy.
- Typical clinical scenario: A young patient has asymptomatic lymphadenopathy or mediastinal mass. Lymph node biopsy shows the presence of large binucleated or multinucleated cells with prominent nucleoli (Reed-Sternberg cells).

Non-Hodgkin Lymphomas

Non-Hodgkin lymphomas are clinically, pathologically, cytogenetically, and immunologically a diverse group of lymphoproliferative disorders. The frequency of non-Hodgkin lymphoma is increasing. The most recent classification is the WHO Classification of Neoplastic Diseases of the Hematopoietic and Lymphoid Tissues (Table 11-10).

The Ann Arbor Staging System (very similar to the staging system in Table 11-8) has traditionally been used for lymphoma. Low-grade (indolent) lymphomas may transform into aggressive lymphomas. The low-grade non-Hodgkin lymphomas, which include follicular histologic features, are a group of lymphoproliferative disorders that are not curable (unless pathologic stage I disease), most commonly present with advanced stage III or IV disease, are treatable with simple programs, occur in older patients, and have long survival (median, 8 years). The paradox of non-Hodgkin lymphomas is that most low-grade non-Hodgkin lymphomas are not curable, but patients live for a long time even after disease relapse. In contrast, the aggressive lymphomas are potentially curable, but the length of survival is short if the patient does not have remission.

Lymphoblastic lymphoma and Burkitt lymphoma have a higher risk of central nervous system involvement and tumor lysis syndrome.

Low-Grade (Indolent) Lymphomas

Because most low-grade non-Hodgkin lymphomas are not curable and relapse is almost inevitable, the most reliable end points are progression-free survival and overall survival, rather than achievement of complete remission. In patients who have been deemed to be in clinical complete remission, immunoglobulin κ/λ light-chain restriction studies of peripheral blood and bone marrow with flow cytometry still often demonstrate malignant cells in the peripheral blood, and polymerase chain reaction studies have also demonstrated persistent abnormal cell populations in patients believed to be in complete remission. Patients with follicular lymphoma, the most common type of indolent lymphoma, often have a t(14;18) translocation resulting in amplification of the anti-apoptotic *bcl-2* gene.

A few patients with localized non-Hodgkin lymphoma can be cured with involved field radiotherapy and rituximab. However, most patients with low-grade non-Hodgkin lymphoma have stage

Table 11-10 2001 World Health Organization Classification of Lymphoid Tissue Tumors

B-cell neoplasms
- Precursor B-cell neoplasm
  - Precursor B lymphoblastic leukemia/lymphoma
- Mature B-cell neoplasms
  - Chronic lymphocytic leukemia/small cell lymphocytic lymphoma
  - B-cell prolymphocytic leukemia
  - Lymphoplasmacytic lymphoma
  - Splenic marginal zone lymphoma
  - Hairy cell leukemia
  - Plasma cell myeloma
  - Solitary plasmacytoma of bone
  - Extraosseous plasmacytoma
  - Extranodal marginal zone B-cell lymphoma of mucosa-associated lymphoid tissue (MALT lymphoma)
  - Nodal marginal zone B-cell lymphoma
  - Follicular lymphoma
  - Mantle cell lymphoma
  - Diffuse large B-cell lymphoma
  - Mediastinal (thymic) large B-cell lymphoma
  - Intravascular large B-cell lymphoma
  - Primary effusion lymphoma
  - Burkitt lymphoma/leukemia
- B-cell proliferations of uncertain malignant potential
  - Lymphomatoid granulomatosis
  - Posttransplant lymphoproliferative disorder, polymorphic

T-cell & natural killer (NK)-cell neoplasms
- Precursor T-cell neoplasms
  - Precursor T lymphoblastic leukemia/lymphoma
  - Blastic NK-cell lymphoma
- Mature T-cell and NK-cell neoplasms
  - T-cell prolymphocytic leukemia
  - T-cell large granular lymphocytic leukemia
  - Aggressive NK-cell leukemia
  - Adult T-cell leukemia/lymphoma
  - Extranodal NK/T-cell lymphoma, nasal type
  - Enteropathy-type T-cell lymphoma
  - Hepatosplenic T-cell lymphoma
  - Subcutaneous panniculitis-like T-cell lymphoma
  - Mycosis fungoides
  - Sézary syndrome
  - Primary cutaneous anaplastic large cell lymphoma
  - Peripheral T-cell lymphoma, unspecified
  - Angioimmunoblastic T-cell lymphoma
  - Anaplastic large cell lymphoma
- T-cell proliferation of uncertain malignant potential
  - Lymphomatoid papulosis

Hodgkin lymphoma
- Nodular lymphocyte predominant Hodgkin lymphoma
- Classic Hodgkin lymphoma
  - Nodular sclerosis classic Hodgkin lymphoma
  - Lymphocyte-rich classic Hodgkin lymphoma
  - Mixed cellularity classic Hodgkin lymphoma
  - Lymphocyte-depleted classic Hodgkin lymphoma

Modified from Jaffe ES, Harris NL, Stein H, Vardiman JW, editors. World Health Organization Classification of Tumours. Pathology and genetics of tumours of haematopoietic and lymphoid tissues. Lyon: IARC Press; 2001. p. 120, 190, 238. Used with permission.

III or stage IV disease at diagnosis, which is not curable with standard treatment regimens. Observation (watchful waiting) is the initial treatment of choice for asymptomatic patients with no evidence of bulky disease. Early treatment or treatment with more aggressive regimens has not improved survival.

For patients with symptoms, bulky disease, or progressive disease, there are many therapeutic options. These include oral chlorambucil taken daily, intravenous CVP (cyclophosphamide, vincristine, and prednisone) with rituximab concomitantly or as maintenance therapy, rituximab, R-CHOP (rituximab with CHOP [cyclophosphamide, hydroxydaunomycin, vincristine, and prednisone]), radiolabeled anti–B-cell monoclonal antibodies, and nucleoside analogues such as fludaribine.

Anti-CD20 antibody therapy, rituximab, was initially approved for patients who have had relapse and is also effective when used as an initial treatment regimen. Rituximab is used with increasing frequency in other B-cell–mediated conditions, such as autoimmune disease. Anti-CD20 conjugated to yttrium 90 (Zevalin) and anti-CD20 conjugated to iodine 131 (Bexxar) produce high remission rates in patients with advanced follicular lymphoma who have had multiple relapses and are refractory to chemotherapy.

Gastric MALT lymphomas have clonal gene rearrangements and are associated with *Helicobacter pylori* infections. This is the first malignant lymphoproliferative disorder to respond to an antimicrobial approach. Up to 70% of patients have a response to a combination antibiotic and proton pump inhibitor regimen such as amoxicillin, metronidazole, and omeprazole. Other exceptions to the standard management programs for non-Hodgkin lymphoma include primary bone, isolated gastric, central nervous system, testicular, bowel, orbital, pulmonary, and cutaneous T-cell and B-cell lymphomas. Patients with HIV-related lymphoproliferative disorders with a CD4 count less than 200/mL have a poor response to standard treatment. Primary central nervous system lymphoma may be seen in association with HIV or without HIV infection. It has a poor prognosis and is currently treated with high-dose methotrexate with leucovorin rescue. Lymphoplasmacytic lymphoma is associated with Waldenström macroglobulinemia and is discussed in the "Monoclonal Gammopathies" subsection below.

Aggressive Lymphoma

In patients with the histologic features of diffuse large cell lymphoma, rituximab-plus-anthracycline–based combination chemotherapy (R-CHOP) regimens are the standard therapy (>50% are cured), with complete remission rates of 60% to 80% for stages II to IV disease. Long-term disease-free survival is predicted by the International Prognostic Factor Index.

For patients who had disease relapse after complete remission and who are sensitive to retreatment with standard chemotherapy regimens, autologous stem cell transplant is the standard therapy. The reported cure rates are 35% to 40%. Currently, the role of autologous bone marrow transplant as part of the initial management of high-risk patients with non-Hodgkin lymphomas is being evaluated in randomized studies.

Mantle cell lymphoma is characterized by a CD5+ (like CLL) and CD20+ immunophenotype and a t(11;14) translocation with overexpression of the cyclin D1 oncogene (unlike CLL; these abnormalities help define the disease as mantle cell lymphoma). It frequently involves blood and marrow in addition to lymph nodes and spleen, it may manifest in the gastrointestinal tract (lymphomatous polyposis), and it is refractory to chemotherapy. Stem cell transplant is usually incorporated early. Very aggressive lymphomas, such as Burkitt lymphoma and lymphoblastic lymphoma, are treated with regimens similar to those used for acute lymphoblastic leukemia.

The International Prognostic Factor Index is based on clinical pretreatment characteristics and predicts the relative risk of death. Clinical features that are associated with survival include age (≤60 vs >60 years); LDH (normal vs greater than normal); Eastern Cooperative Oncology Group (ECOG)/Zubrod performance status (0 or 1 vs 2-4); stage (I/II vs III/IV); and extranodal involvement (≤1 site vs >1 site). Patients are categorized into different risk groups based on the number of risk factors. Predicted 5-year survival in the low-risk group (with 0 or 1 adverse risk factor) is 73%; in the low-intermediate group (with 2 factors), 51%; in the high-intermediate group (with 3 factors), 43%; and in the high-risk group (with 4 or 5 factors), 26%.

- Non-Hodgkin lymphomas are diverse. The most common are follicular lymphoma and diffuse large B-cell lymphoma. Low-grade lymphomas respond to treatment but are incurable. Aggressive lymphomas are curable but cause death more quickly if they do not respond to treatment.
- The Ann Arbor Staging System has traditionally been used for non-Hodgkin lymphoma. It is similar to the staging system presented in Table 11-8.
- Currently, the most predictive pretreatment characteristics for the risk of death are age, LDH, performance status, stage, and extranodal involvement (the International Prognostic Factor Index).
- Exceptions to the standard management programs for non-Hodgkin lymphoma include MALT, primary bone, isolated gastric, central nervous system, testicular, bowel, orbital, pulmonary, and cutaneous T- and B-cell lymphomas.
- In most patients, low-grade lymphoma is not curable but survival time is long.
- Of patients with the histologic features of diffuse large cell advanced intermediate-grade non-Hodgkin lymphoma, R-CHOP with anti-CD20 monoclonal antibody therapy is superior to CHOP. About one-half of patients are cured.
- Patients with HIV-related lymphoproliferative disorders with a CD4 count <200/mL have a poor response to standard treatment.
- Low-grade, indolent lymphomas may transform into more aggressive lymphomas.
- Lymphoblastic lymphoma and Burkitt lymphoma have a higher risk of central nervous system involvement and tumor lysis syndrome.
- Typical clinical scenario for follicular lymphomas: A 65-year-old patient has asymptomatic cervical and axillary lymphadenopathy. Lymph node biopsy findings show involvement with lymphoma, predominantly small cells, with relative preservation of follicular architecture. Bone marrow is also found to be involved. In the absence of symptoms, observation is reasonable.
- Typical clinical scenario for diffuse large B-cell lymphoma: A patient with abdominal pain, fever, and weight loss is found to have

bulky retroperitoneal adenopathy. A biopsy specimen demonstrates diffuse replacement of the lymph node with large lymphoma cells. The usual treatment is staging evaluation, followed by chemotherapy such as R-CHOP.

Large Granular Lymphocyte Syndromes

Large granular lymphocytes (LGLs) are cytotoxic T cells or natural killer cells that have a pale blue cytoplasm containing scattered azurophilic granules (Figure 11-22). They normally represent about 5% of circulating lymphocytes. Viral infections, non-Hodgkin lymphoma, and connective tissue disorders can be associated with reactive, polyclonal expansion of LGLs. Clonal expansion of LGLs is called *T-cell LGL leukemia* or *LGL syndrome* and is associated with neutropenia, splenomegaly (and less commonly hepatomegaly), anemia, and moderate lymphocytosis. Up to one-third of T-cell LGL leukemia patients have rheumatoid arthritis (RA) and clinically have an overlap with Felty syndrome (triad of neutropenia, RA, and splenomegaly); more than half have detectable titers of rheumatoid factor. T-cell LGL is a chronic disorder than requires treatment only if symptoms are present. Immunosuppressive therapy with low-dose methotrexate or cyclosporine is often effective.

Monoclonal Gammopathies

In the monoclonal gammopathies, there is a monoclonal excess of 1 of the light chains due to a clonal plasma cell proliferation, resulting in abnormal κ:λ ratios. Serum free light-chain analysis is more sensitive than immunoelectrophoresis in identifying imbalance in these light chains. The differential diagnosis of monoclonal gammopathies includes monoclonal gammopathies of undetermined significance (MGUS) and malignant monoclonal gammopathies. The malignant gammopathies include multiple myeloma (IgG, IgA, IgD, IgE, and free light chain variants), plasma cell leukemia, plasmacytoma (solitary plasmacytoma of bone and extramedullary plasmacytoma), malignant lymphoproliferative diseases (Waldenström [primary] macroglobulinemia and malignant lymphoma), heavy chain diseases, and amyloidosis (primary or secondary to myeloma).

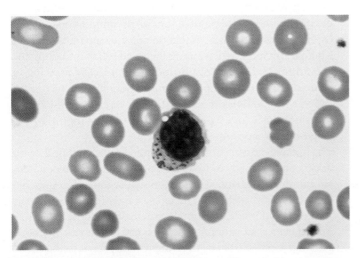

Figure 11-22. Large Granular Lymphocyte. The pale blue cytoplasm contains azurophilic granules.

Monoclonal Gammopathies of Undetermined Significance

In MGUS, the most common dysproteinemia, the monoclonal (M)-protein level is less than 3 g/dL in the serum and the percentage of plasma cells in the bone marrow is less than 10%. The serum level of creatinine is normal, and the urine has either no M protein or only a small amount. The serum levels of calcium and hemoglobin are normal. Anemia and osteolytic bone lesions are absent, and patients are usually asymptomatic, although a few may develop an MGUS-associated peripheral neuropathy that is difficult to distinguish from idiopathic peripheral neuropathy. MGUS may be a precursor to multiple myeloma. Of the patients with MGUS, about 1% per year experience progression to a malignant monoclonal gammopathy. Population-based studies have demonstrated that 3.2% of adults older than 50 years, 5.3% of those older than 70, and 7.5% of those 85 or older have an M protein in the serum. Of monoclonal gammopathies, 60% are IgG, 20% are IgM, 10% are IgA, and 7% are free light chains. IgD and IgE monoclonal gammopathies are very rare. In most patients, M-protein measurements are stable over time. Patients with MGUS should be observed. Serum protein electrophoresis should be repeated initially at 6 months and then at 12-month intervals indefinitely if there is no progression or symptoms. An abnormal κ:λ ratio on free light-chain analysis is a major independent risk factor for progression.

- MGUS is the most common dysproteinemia.
- Serum M protein <3 g/dL; <10% plasma cells in the bone marrow; normal concentrations of hemoglobin, creatinine, and calcium.
- Patients are usually asymptomatic.
- Patients are safely observed, with no chemotherapy.
- Typical clinical scenario: A patient without symptoms has a serum M-protein spike <3 g/dL and bone marrow plasma cells <10%. The CBC, serum creatinine level, and bone radiographs are normal. Observe, with no therapy.

Multiple Myeloma

Multiple myeloma is a result of the accumulation in the marrow of neoplastic plasma cells that produce homogeneous immunoglobulin or light chains in the serum or in the urine (or in both); it accounts for 1% of all malignancies. Osteoclast-activating activity due to exaggerated expression of specific cytokine results in osteolytic bone lesions. Interleukin-6 contributes to osteoclast activity and elevated C-reactive protein.

The median age at onset of multiple myeloma is 65 years. It is more common in males and African Americans. By definition, 10% or more plasma cells are found in the bone marrow (Figure 11-23). At least 1 of the following must be present: M protein in the serum greater than 3 g/dL by serum protein electrophoresis (in 80% of patients), M protein in the urine only (light-chain myeloma only; 20%), anemia, hypercalcemia, renal failure, or osteolytic bone lesions. M protein is detected in the serum or urine of 99% of patients with immunoelectrophoresis and free light-chain analysis.

Clinical features include weakness, fatigue, bone pain (66% of patients), anemia (initially about 66%, eventually all), renal insufficiency (50%), hypercalcemia (20%), and spinal cord compression

(5%). Back pain and chest pain are characteristically exacerbated by movement. Severe back pain may be a manifestation of spinal cord compression, requiring immediate magnetic resonance imaging (MRI) or CT, dexamethasone treatment, irradiation, and possible surgical decompression. Patients are at higher risk of infections with encapsulated gram-positive organisms such as *S pneumoniae* and *H influenzae*; so vaccination is recommended. The incidence of gram-negative infections and herpes zoster is also increased. The CBC findings are those of a normochromic normocytic anemia. The peripheral blood smear may show rouleaux. Radiographs show punched-out lytic lesions, osteoporosis, and fractures in 75% of patients at diagnosis. Bone scans are rarely helpful because the lytic lesions do not show up. MRI may be helpful if plain radiographs do not show abnormalities, especially spine lesions. Conventional cytogenetic assays are usually normal. There is growing use of fluorescence in situ hybridization (FISH) to detect chromosomal abnormalities in plasma cells, which is prognostically useful and helps determine initial therapy.

The median survival has been about 3 years. This is improving with peripheral blood stem cell transplant and newer treatment regimens. A β_2-microglobulin level greater than 2.7 mg/mL and a bone marrow plasma cell labeling index greater than 0.8% are adverse prognostic factors. If both values are low, the median survival is longer (about 6 years). Patients should be observed if they have *smoldering myeloma* (M protein >3 g/dL, >10% plasma cells in the bone marrow, no lytic bone lesions, and no other manifestations of myeloma).

Because multiple myeloma is not curable, treatment may be delayed until evidence of disease progression develops, the patient becomes symptomatic, or treatment is necessary to prevent imminent complications. Two randomized trials have demonstrated that patients with anemia only or small osteolytic lesions may be safely observed. The standard treatment of patients older than 70 years, poor performance status, pronounced renal failure, or other comorbid conditions is melphalan and prednisone given for 7 days every 6 weeks. The objective response rate is 50% to 60%; the median survival is

3 years. Palliative radiotherapy at a dose of 20 to 30 Gy is effective in the management of disabling focal pain that is due to lytic lesions and is unresponsive to analgesic therapy.

Autologous peripheral stem cell transplant is the initial treatment of choice for all other patients. Before an autologous peripheral stem cell harvest, treat with high-dose dexamethasone in combination with thalidomide or lenalidomide. These drugs do not have the toxic effects that melphalan has on stem cells. After a patient has received melphalan, it may be difficult to successfully harvest stem cells. Side effects of thalidomide include sedation, fatigue, constipation, and peripheral neuropathy. Use of lenalidomide has resulted in higher response rates with less severe peripheral neuropathy. Deep venous thrombosis (DVT) is a risk with these regimens. High-dose therapy followed by an autologous stem cell transplant improves the response rate and survival in patients with multiple myeloma, but the disease is still not curable. The overall response rates are 75% to 90%, and the complete response rate is 20% to 40%. Two transplants (*tandem transplant*) may be more effective than a single transplant, but this is controversial. The proteosome inhibitor bortezomib is effective in initial therapy, in pretreated patients with relapsed disease, and in patients with refractory multiple myeloma.

Anemia responds to erythropoietin in 50% of the patients. Bisphosphonate therapy, such as pamidronate and zoledronic acid, delays the onset of skeletal-related events, reduces bone pain, and modestly extends survival. The most worrisome side effect of bisphosphonate therapy is osteonecrosis of the jaw.

Renal failure may be caused by hypercalcemia, dehydration, or light chain nephropathy (myeloma kidney). Light chain nephropathy may respond to plasmapheresis.

* Plasma cells: <10% in MGUS and >10% in myeloma.
* Serum M protein: <3 g/dL in MGUS and usually >3 g/dL in myeloma.
* Multiple myeloma: usually M protein is in serum or urine (or both).
* Myeloma: bone pain (66% of patients), renal dysfunction (50%), hypercalcemia (20%), and spinal cord compression (5%).
* Severe back pain may be a manifestation of spinal cord compression, requiring immediate MRI or CT, dexamethasone treatment, irradiation, and possible surgical decompression.
* Myeloma: lytic bone lesions that do not show up on bone scan.
* Multiple myeloma patients are at increased risk of infections due to encapsulated organisms, including *S pneumoniae* owing to reduced production of normal gamma globulins.
* Patients with low-risk disease, including a plasma cell labeling index of ≤0.8% and β_2-microglobulin of ≤2.7 mg/mL, have longer overall survival.
* The initial treatment is now thalidomide or lenalidomide with dexamethasone followed by an autologous peripheral blood stem cell transplant. Patients who are too sick or too old to undergo transplant may benefit from melphalan and prednisone, with or without thalidomide, or from dexamethasone alone.
* Typical clinical scenario: A patient presents with back and bone pain that is exacerbated by movement. The patient is discovered to have anemia with or without renal insufficiency and hypercalcemia. A bone survey shows lytic bone lesions, and serum and

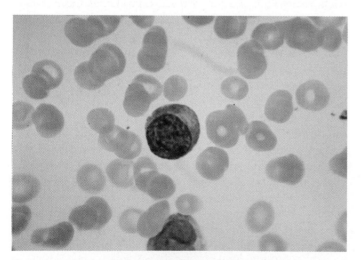

Figure 11-23. Plasma Cell. Note the eccentrically placed round nucleus; the copious, dark blue cytoplasm has a characteristic pale-staining area adjacent to the nucleus.

urine protein electrophoresis demonstrate M protein. Bone marrow biopsy specimens contain >10% plasma cells.

Solitary Plasmacytomas

Solitary plasmacytomas may occur without other evidence of multiple myeloma. These isolated extramedullary lesions are potentially curable with irradiation alone. If a serum monoclonal protein is present, it usually goes away after treatment.

Waldenström Macroglobulinemia

Waldenström macroglobulinemia is characterized by an IgM paraprotein that is usually greater than 3.0 g/dL, lymphadenopathy, anemia, or hepatosplenomegaly. Retinal vessel "sausage" formation may be present. The bone marrow is populated with well-differentiated plasmacytoid lymphocytes. Bence Jones proteinuria may be present in 80% of patients, and hyperviscosity syndrome occurs in 15%. Other features include cryoglobulinemia, sensorimotor peripheral neuropathy, cold agglutinin hemolytic anemia, and renal disease (nephrotic syndrome). Lymph node biopsy usually shows lymphoplasmacytic lymphoma.

Many patients have only an IgM MGUS, with no signs or symptoms, and should be observed without initial treatment. This is not the same as Waldenström macroglobulinemia.

Hyperviscosity syndrome is characterized by fatigue, dizziness, blurred vision, bleeding from mucous membranes, sausage-shaped retinal veins, and papilledema. The plasma volume is expanded, with an increase in serum viscosity. Because 80% of IgM is intravascular, the initial treatment of hyperviscosity is plasmapheresis with albumin and saline replacement, followed by chemotherapy. The treatment of choice is now rituximab in combination with cytotoxic agents. Transfusion with packed RBCs should not be given solely on the basis of the hemoglobin concentration, because the increased plasma volume produces spuriously low values and transfusion may worsen hyperviscosity.

- Waldenström macroglobulinemia: IgM paraprotein >3.0 g/dL.
- Hyperviscosity syndrome is treated initially with plasmapheresis.
- Treatment of choice is rituximab plus chemotherapy.
- Typical clinical scenario: A 65-year-old patient has fatigue, bleeding from oral and nasal areas, and visual and neurologic symptoms. Serum protein electrophoresis demonstrates an IgM M protein, and bone biopsy shows a lymphoplasmacytic infiltration.

Amyloidosis

Amyloidosis is a group of diseases with extracellular deposition of pathologic insoluble fibrillar proteins, which stain with Congo red, in organs and tissues. The amyloid fibrils in primary amyloidosis are fragments of the variable portions of the immunoglobulin light chains; in other forms of amyloidosis, the fibrils are made of other proteins. Patients with amyloidosis present with fatigue, weight loss, hepatomegaly, macroglossia, renal insufficiency, proteinuria, nephrotic syndrome, congestive heart failure, orthostatic hypotension, carpal tunnel syndrome, and peripheral neuropathy. Few patients have all these features; in most, involvement of 1 or 2 organ systems dominates the clinical picture. Amyloidosis is classified as primary (AL amyloidosis or light chain–related amyloidosis, which may be associated with multiple myeloma; 90% of patients in the United States), secondary (AA amyloidosis, due to chronic infections such as osteomyelitis, or autoimmune disease), familial (associated with mutations in transthyretin or other proteins), associated with aging (senile), localized (skin, bladder, or other organs), dialysis-associated (due to deposits of β_2-microglobulin), carpal tunnel syndrome (20% of patients), peripheral neuropathy, and orthostatic hypotension. Serum free light-chain analysis differentiates primary amyloidosis from other amyloid disorders.

Generally, the diagnosis of primary amyloidosis is first established by finding M protein in the serum or urine. The bone marrow usually has less than 20% plasma cells unless there is associated multiple myeloma, and there are no lytic bone lesions. Initial biopsies should include fat aspiration of the abdominal wall (80% positive), rectal biopsy (75%), or bone marrow biopsy (56%). Nearly 90% of patients with primary systemic amyloidosis have a detectable M protein in the serum or urine, which is λ in two-thirds of the patients. Serum free light-chain assays provide a quantitative measurement aid in assessing response to therapy since amyloid protein in tissue is broken down slowly, if at all. The bone marrow usually has plasma cells that have a clonal predominance of a light chain isotype.

Four of 10 patients present with nephrotic syndrome, 1 in 6 with right-sided congestive heart failure that worsens with calcium channel blockers, and about 1 in 7 with a sensorimotor peripheral neuropathy. Electrocardiography in patients with cardiac involvement may show low voltage or a pattern similar to that of myocardial infarction (Q waves). The echocardiogram is abnormal in 60% of patients, with concentrically thickened ventricles or a thickened intraventricular septum, or both. The neuropathy is usually progressive, painful, symmetrical, and demyelinating. Peripheral neuropathy is often associated with autonomic failure, as manifested by diarrhea, pseudo-obstruction of the bowel, or orthostatic syncope. About 50% of patients with amyloid neuropathy have carpal tunnel syndrome. Other symptoms and signs include fatigue, weight loss, change in voice, macroglossia, submandibular swelling, and postproctoscopic periorbital purpura. Acquired inhibitors of thrombin or factor X may occur.

The median survival for all patients with primary amyloidosis is 13 months; with overt congestive heart failure, less than 6 months; with nephrotic syndrome, 27 months; and with peripheral neuropathy, 42 months.

For light chain–related primary amyloidosis, treatment with melphalan and prednisone is modestly effective. Autologous stem cell transplant provides benefit in carefully selected patients, but some patients experience fluid retention and cardiac dysrhythmia during stem cell collection or transplant. Treatment of secondary (AA) amyloidosis involves correction of the underlying disease.

Patients with amyloidosis are unusually sensitive to digitalis. In congestive heart failure, salt restriction and diuretics are the mainstay of treatment.

The pathologic characteristics are as follows: primary amyloidosis involves the variable region of immunoglobulin light chains; secondary amyloidosis involves protein A.

- Amyloidosis: deposition of insoluble fibrils in tissues, leading to organ dysfunction.
- Primary (light chain) amyloidosis is the most common form and can be associated with multiple myeloma.
- Associated clinical features: fatigue, nephrotic syndrome, congestive heart failure with Q waves on electrocardiography and thickened intraventricular septum, sensorimotor, neuropathy, periorbital purpura, and macroglossia.
- Typical clinical scenario: A 64-year-old man with weakness, weight loss, congestive heart failure, carpal tunnel syndrome, peripheral neuropathy, and orthostatic hypotension has a λ light chain M spike detected on serum electrophoresis.

Acute Leukemias

Acute leukemia is defined by the presence of at least 20% undifferentiated blast cells in the bone marrow. The cause of acute leukemia is unknown in most cases, but there are many associations: previous diagnosis of myeloproliferative neoplasm or myelodysplastic syndromes; exposure to radiation or benzene; chemotherapy (alkylating agents, type II topoisomerase inhibitors [etoposide]); and congenital disorders such as Down syndrome, Fanconi syndrome (a DNA repair defect), and ataxia-telangiectasia. Patients who have been exposed to alkylating agents (eg, melphalan, cyclophosphamide, and chlorambucil) and who develop acute myelogenous leukemia (AML) typically do so 3 to 7 years later, usually with chromosome abnormalities involving chromosomes 5 and 7. Patients exposed to topoisomerase II inhibitors (eg, etoposide, doxorubicin) can develop secondary, treatment-related AML, usually less than 3 years after exposure and with abnormalities of chromosome 11q23 (*MLL* gene). Secondary AML is refractory to standard treatment regimens.

- Secondary AML due to alkylating agents often has abnormal chromosome 5 and 7 and is resistant to treatment.
- Secondary leukemia related to topoisomerase II inhibitors arises more quickly than that due to alkylating agents and has chromosome 11q23 rearrangements.

Acute Myelogenous Leukemia

The median age of patients with AML (Figure 11-24) is about 65. Fifty percent of patients have symptoms, especially fatigue, for more than 3 months before diagnosis. By definition, patients have 20% or more undifferentiated blasts with myeloid cell surface markers or cytochemical features in the bone marrow. Specific cytogenetic abnormalities predict outcome. Good prognostic signs include being younger than 40 years; having chromosomal abnormalities of t(8;21), t(15;17), or inv(16) or normal chromosomes (40%-50%); and achieving complete remission with 1 cycle of induction chemotherapy. Poor prognostic signs include age older than 40 years; an antecedent hematologic disorder, such as myelodysplastic syndrome, or a myeloproliferative neoplasm; previous treatment with alkylating agents or ionizing radiation; high-risk chromosomal abnormalities, including abnormalities involving chromosome 7, 5, or 11q23, or a complex karyotype; and poor general physical condition or underlying health problems.

For patients who present with extreme leukocytosis (WBC >80 × 10^9/L) with acute leukemia, the initial complication of most concern is cerebral hemorrhage due to leukostasis. Emergency treatment includes hydration, alkalinization of urine, allopurinol (600 mg loading dose and 300 mg daily thereafter), hydroxyurea (6-8 g orally), and leukapheresis, followed by the treatment of the specific type of leukemia. Leukapheresis reduces the blast count by about 50% and may need to be repeated. Cranial radiation is controversial and no longer widely performed.

Patients with acute promyelocytic leukemia (AML M3) (Figure 11-25) often present with DIC. These patients typically have t(15;17) (*PML-RARA* gene fusion). Involvement of the gingiva, central nervous system, sinuses, and testes is most common in AML M5 (monocytic) and AML M4 (myelomonocytic). Megakaryoblastic AML (AML M7) is rare and associated with Down syndrome.

- AML: median age of patients is 65 years.
- Good prognosis: patients <40 years old; chromosomal abnormalities t(8;21), t(15;17), or inv(16) or normal chromosomes; and achieving complete remission with 1 cycle of induction chemotherapy.
- Typical clinical scenario for acute leukemia: A 40-year-old patient has fever, sore throat, bleeding gums (thrombocytopenia), and anemia. The WBC count is 50 × 10^9/L. A peripheral blood smear shows numerous immature WBC precursors (blasts). Differentiation between AML and acute lymphoblastic leukemia requires evaluation of bone marrow biopsy specimens with special stains and immunophenotyping.
- Typical clinical scenario for acute promyelocytic leukemia (M3): A patient who has circulating blasts presents with disseminated intravascular coagulation. Cytogenetics show t(15;17).
- Typical clinical scenario for secondary, therapy-related AML: Cytopenias are demonstrated in a patient who has received chemotherapeutic agents for a previous malignancy. Cytogenetic studies show monosomy 5 or 7.

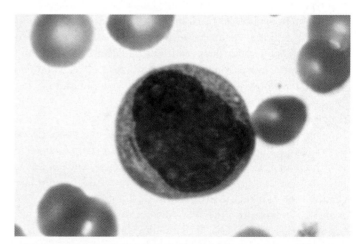

Figure 11-24. Acute Myelogenous Leukemia. Blast cells are large and have an open, granular nuclear chromatin, often with 1 or more nucleoli. The presence of an Auer rod means that the blast is myeloid rather than lymphoid.

Almost all patients will experience neutropenic fever during AML therapy, and rapid broad-spectrum antibiotic coverage for fever is essential. Treatment is divided into 1) induction therapy to reduce the leukemic burden and 2) consolidation therapy to maintain complete remission. There is no role for maintenance therapy in AML.

Induction chemotherapy includes cytarabine (also called ara-C or cytosine arabinoside) and an anthracycline agent (daunorubicin or idarubicin). The complete remission rate is about 80% for patients 60 years or younger and 35% to 50% for those older than 60 years, with the potential for cure in 20% of patients. Consolidation therapy is with 2 to 4 courses of high-dose cytarabine. High-dose cytarabine causes neurotoxicity (especially cerebellar) and chemical conjunctivitis that can be prevented and treated with corticosteroid eye drops. The 5-year survival for patients with good cytogenetics is 60%, but with poor cytogenetics, the 5-year survival is 10%. Intermediate-risk patients have a 5-year survival rate of 40%. Despite substantial recent advances, relapse occurs eventually in most patients with AML, usually within 3 years. Transfusion support is important; platelets are given for a platelet count less than $10 \times 10^9/L$ or signs of bleeding.

All-*trans*-retinoic acid (ATRA) is the treatment of choice in AML M3 (acute promyelocytic leukemia) (Figure 11-25) with t(15;17). Induction chemotherapy is with ATRA and an anthracycline-based program with idarubicin. Consolidation includes an anthracycline drug, and maintenance therapy includes ATRA for 1 to 2 years. Management of associated DIC includes aggressive platelet transfusions to maintain a platelet count of more than $50 \times 10^9/L$ and cryoprecipitate to maintain the fibrinogen at a level of 100 mg/dL or greater. Arsenic trioxide is the treatment of choice for relapsed AML M3, followed by transplant. Arsenic is also useful in consolidation therapy in higher-risk patients. Gemtuzumab, an anti-CD33 antibody conjugated to a toxin called calicheamicin, is approved for the treatment of CD33+ AML in patients older than 60 years experiencing a first relapse.

In patients with relapsed AML, reinduction of remission is followed by hematopoietic stem cell transplant, if feasible. Patients up to age 55 can be considered for myeloablative transplant, whereas those between ages 55 and 65 may still be eligible for allogeneic transplant after immunosuppressive reduced-intensity conditioning (so-called mini-transplant). The outcome is age-dependent: patients younger than 30 years have a better prognosis than those 30 or older. If the patient is younger than 55 years, stem cell transplant should be considered for those in first remission if they have an HLA-matched donor and poor prognostic factors, which include poor-risk cytogenetic features and antecedent hematologic disease. For patients without poor risk factors, transplant should be considered in early relapse or second remission. A rule of thumb for allogeneic transplant results in AML and myelodysplastic syndrome in patients over the age of 30 is the "rule of thirds": about one-third of the patients will die of complications, usually in the first 100 days; about one-third of the patients will be alive and disease-free 3 years later, albeit many with chronic graft-versus-host disease; and about one-third of the patients will survive transplant but will ultimately experience relapse.

Acute Lymphoblastic Leukemia

Acute lymphoblastic leukemia (ALL) is most common in children, for whom complete remission rates are greater than 90%, and 60%

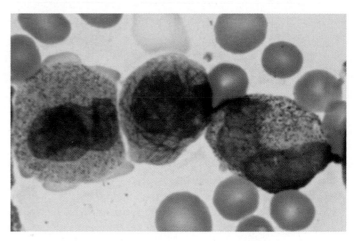

Figure 11-25. Leukemic Cells in Acute Promyelocytic Leukemia (AML M3). There are abundant cytoplasmic granules and Auer rods. (Courtesy of Curtis A. Hanson, MD, Mayo Clinic.)

to 70% of patients have long-term disease-free survival. In adults, however, ALL is less common and outcomes are much poorer. Remission rates are up to 75%; however, relapse occurs in most patients. Of ALL cases in adults, 80% are B cell in origin, 20% have T-cell markers, and 1% or 2% express surface immunoglobulin. Most B-cell leukemias express CD10, the common *ALL antigen* (CALLA). Patients with early pre–B-cell type acute lymphocytic leukemia, also called *null acute lymphocytic leukemia*, are CALLA negative.

One-third of the patients present with bleeding, and 25% have symptoms for more than 3 months. Bone pain, lymphadenopathy, splenomegaly, and hepatomegaly are more common in ALL than AML. Splenomegaly, lymphadenopathy, and hepatomegaly occur in three-fourths of the patients (compared with one-half of those with AML).

Survival decreases with increasing age, and the duration of complete remissions is also shorter in older patients. Poor prognostic factors include advanced age (especially >60), WBC count greater than $30 \times 10^9/L$, null cell phenotype, specific chromosomal abnormalities (see below), and failure to achieve remission within the first 4 weeks of intensive chemotherapy.

Most adults with ALL have chromosomal abnormalities. Those with normal chromosomes have the best prognosis. Those with the poorest prognosis have t(9;22), t(4;11), t(8;14), or t(1;19). These patients have lower complete remission rates, shorter duration of remission, and very poor survival.

ALL therapy is extremely complex. The 3 agents commonly used in induction therapy are vincristine, prednisone, and anthracyclines. Often other drugs are added such as L-asparaginase, cytarabine, methotrexate, and cyclophosphamide. The addition of L-asparaginase, cytarabine, or cyclophosphamide may improve the duration of remission but has not been shown to improve overall survival in adults. However, an intense cyclophosphamide regimen (*Hyper-CVAD*— cyclophosphamide, vincristine, Adriamycin, and dexamethasone) is growing in popularity because of high reported remission rates and ease of combining with imatinib in patients who have t(9;22).

Intensification or postinduction therapy is commonly used, followed by 2 to 3 years of maintenance therapy with low doses of methotrexate, 6-mercaptopurine, and intermittent pulses of corticosteroids and vincristine. All patients receive intrathecal therapy because of the high risk of relapse in the central nervous system (much higher than with AML). Males often get longer maintenance therapy because testes also serve as a "sanctuary site." Allogeneic transplant in first remission is recommended for patients with t(9;22) and t(4;11) because their prognosis with chemotherapy alone is so poor. For patients with relapsed disease, allogeneic transplant is the only potentially curative therapy.

In a study that compared bone marrow and peripheral blood allogeneic transplant in acute leukemia, myelodysplasia, and chronic myeloid leukemia, the use of peripheral blood led to faster hematologic recovery and improved survival. Bone marrow is harvested only to collect hematopoietic stem cells when a sufficient number cannot be obtained by peripheral blood leukapheresis. Umbilical cord blood represents a novel source of stem cells, but most adults are too large for a single unit of cord blood to fully reconstitute hematopoiesis and 2 units are needed.

Chronic Myeloid Disorders
Chronic myeloid disorders include myelodysplastic syndromes, chronic myeloid leukemia, myeloproliferative neoplasms, and atypical myeloid disorders. Patients with these disorders have less than 20% bone marrow blasts, which distinguishes them from AML. Chronic myeloid disorders often evolve into AML over time.

Myelodysplastic Syndromes
Myelodysplastic syndromes (MDS) are heterogeneous and share 3 common features: peripheral blood cytopenia, especially anemia; abnormal "dysplastic" bone marrow morphology; and a tendency to evolve to AML. Eight forms of MDS are described by WHO. Important prognostic factors include the proportion of bone marrow blasts, the karyotype (good risk, intermediate risk, and poor risk), and the number of blood lineages affected by cytopenias (0 or 1 is better than 2 or 3).

Transformation to acute leukemia occurs in about 25% to 30% of patients overall; patients with more than 10% marrow blasts have the highest risk. Infection is the most common cause of death, followed by complications of AML progression and hemorrhage. The risk of hemorrhage does not correlate well with the platelet count, probably because patients also have variable degrees of platelet dysfunction.

Clonal karyotypic abnormalities, predominantly chromosomal deletions, have been reported in 40% to 50% of patients with de novo disease and 70% to 80% of patients who have MDS as a consequence of prior chemotherapy or radiotherapy. By comparison, AML more commonly has balanced translocations, which are unusual in MDS. Del(5q), del(20q), and −Y chromosome confer a favorable prognosis. In contrast, a complex karyotype (ie, ≥3 chromosome abnormalities) or abnormality of chromosome 7 are associated with a poorer prognosis. Many patients with these poor-risk karyotypes have been exposed to DNA-damaging chemotherapy (eg, alkylating agents) or ionizing radiation.

The standard of care for most patients is supportive, with RBC transfusions, erythropoietin, and antibiotics for infection. G-CSF may decrease the risk of infections but does not improve survival.

Androgenic steroids such as danazol may improve the platelet count. Bleeding, especially chronic urinary bleeding, may be controlled with antifibrinolytic agents such as ε-aminocaproic acid. Patients with deletions of chromosome 5 involving band q31 respond well to lenalidomide treatment: two-thirds become transfusion independent, and some experience cytogenetic remission. Patients with other karyotypes do not respond as well. Myelosuppression is common and requires dose reduction. Patients younger than 55 years should be considered for conventional myeloablative allogeneic bone marrow transplant if the patient has an HLA match, and patients up to about age 66 can be considered for transplant with reduced-intensity conditioning. Decitabine and 5-azacytidine are DNA methyltransferase inhibitors recently approved by the FDA for use in MDS. They are also myelosuppressive, require prolonged therapy for response, and are usually reserved for patients who are transfusion dependent or have more than 5% blasts. Some patients with low-risk MDS respond to antithymocyte globulin.

- Patients with MDS present with cytopenias.
- The most common cause of death in MDS is infection. Only about 25% of patients progress to acute leukemia.
- Lenalidomide therapy is most effective in patients with del(5q) karyotype.

Chronic Myelogenous Leukemia
Chronic myelogenous leukemia (CML) constitutes 20% of all leukemias. The progeny of the leukemic stem cell retain some capacity for normal maturation (Figure 11-26). The Philadelphia chromosome, t(9;22), is the hallmark of this disease and is found by karyotyping in 90% to 95% of patients. The molecular equivalent of the Philadelphia chromosome, the abnormal BCR-ABL fusion, can be detected by FISH or polymerase chain reaction of peripheral blood or bone marrow specimens in the remainder of the patients. BCR-ABL fusion results in a constitutively active tyrosine kinase enzyme that signals cells to proliferate. With time, new chromosomal abnormalities appear. The disease terminates in a maturation block, evolving through an accelerated phase to a blast crisis after a variable length of time, usually 3 to 5 years. The presence of other chromosomal abnormalities in addition to t(9;22) is an adverse prognostic factor.

Symptoms include malaise, dyspnea, anorexia, fever, night sweats, weight loss, abdominal fullness, easy bruising, bleeding, gout, priapism, and hypermetabolism. Splenomegaly is present in 85% of patients.

Characteristic laboratory findings include leukocytosis, with less than 10% circulating blasts in the chronic phase of the disease. WBC counts of 100×10^9/L are common and urgent leukapheresis is not usually required since the leukocytes are mature and more deformable. Granulocytes in all stages of maturation are present on peripheral blood smear, with basophilia and eosinophilia and a characteristic myelocyte bulge (ie, increased numbers of myelocytes relative to other stages of granulocyte differentiation). The number of platelets is often increased, with large bizarre forms found in peripheral blood smears. The hemoglobin concentration ranges from 9 to 12 g/dL. The vitamin B_{12} level is increased because of increased

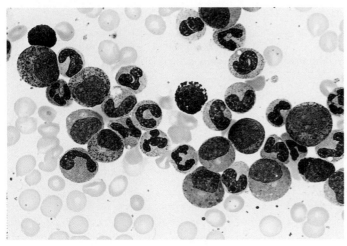

Figure 11-26. Chronic Myelogenous Leukemia. Normal-appearing myeloid cells represent all stages of maturation, with a decreased number of erythropoietic cells and 1 basophil precursor in the center. (Courtesy of Curtis A. Hanson, MD, Mayo Clinic.)

transcobalamin I, a vitamin B_{12} binding protein. Other findings may include pseudohyperkalemia and pseudohypoglycemia (in vitro artifacts due to the high WBC count), and a false-positive increase in the level of acid phosphatase in the serum. The bone marrow is hypercellular.

* CML: acquired defect of clonal origin due to abnormal *BCR-ABL* fusion.
* Philadelphia chromosome, t(9;22), is the hallmark of the disease.
* Increased WBC count; granulocytes in all stages of maturation.
* Typical clinical scenario: A patient without symptoms presents with a high WBC count, myelocyte bulge, basophilia, and splenomegaly. Cytogenetic studies show t(9;22).

The initial treatment of CML is imatinib mesylate. Imatinib is an oral agent that inhibits the *BCR-ABL* protein product. In a randomized trial that compared interferon and cytarabine versus imatinib, there were much higher hematologic response rates for imatinib. In addition, the cytogenetic response rates were superior (76% vs 12%). At 5 years, about 80% of the patients are still receiving imatinib and are in remission. Discontinuation of imatinib therapy is usually followed by relapse due to the persistence of leukemic stem cells. New and more potent *BCR-ABL* inhibitors have been developed for patients who are imatinib resistant; some inhibit other tyrosine kinases as well. These drugs include dasatinib and nilotinib. Most imatinib resistance is due to *BCR-ABL* mutations that impair imatinib binding. T315I is a *BCR-ABL* mutation that is not inhibited by any currently available drug. Patients who are resistant to tyrosine kinase inhibitors are eligible for allogeneic stem cell transplant.

Other treatments include hydroxyurea, interferon alfa and cytarabine, and allogeneic bone marrow transplant. Hydroxyurea is the treatment of choice for rapid lowering of high WBC counts and leukostasis. Recombinant interferon alfa-2a or alfa-2b suppresses the neoplastic clone with the Philadelphia chromosome. Interferon is usually combined with cytarabine. Hematologic responses are 40% to 80%, with cytogenetic remissions in the range of 10% to 40%.

Untreated, the chronic phase eventually progresses to the blast phase, which is characterized by blast counts greater than 20%; increases in anemia, thrombocytopenia, basophilia, and the leukocyte alkaline phosphatase score; splenomegaly; lymphadenopathy; and bone pain. Additional cytogenetic abnormalities are often present. Blast crisis is treated like AML.

* Imatinib is the treatment of choice. Resistance is usually due to *BCR-ABL* mutations that impair imatinib binding.
* The treatment of choice is imatinib. Imatinib-resistant patients are treated with dasatinib or nilotinib. Patients resistant to tyrosine kinase inhibitors can be treated with allogeneic transplant or interferon and cytarabine.

Philadelphia Chromosome–Negative Myeloproliferative Neoplasms

The classic myeloproliferative neoplasms include polycythemia vera, primary myelofibrosis, and essential thrombocythemia. CML was formerly considered a myeloproliferative neoplasm but is now usually discussed separately because of the disease-defining *BCR-ABL* fusion. Other common myeloproliferative neoplasms lack a disease-defining mutation. These are clonal processes that are characterized clinically by peripheral blood and bone marrow proliferation. Their characteristic features are listed in Table 11-11. These disorders are interrelated: polycythemia vera progresses to postpolycythemic myelofibrosis in 10% of patients, and essential thrombocythemia progresses to postthrombocythemic myelofibrosis in 5%. AML is a complication of polycythemia vera (10% of patients), essential thrombocythemia (<5%), and primary myelofibrosis (10%-20%). Each of these disorders carries a risk of thrombosis and hemorrhagic complications.

Recent studies have identified activating mutations of JAK2 tyrosine kinase in almost all patients with polycythemia vera and in about half of those with primary myelofibrosis and essential thrombocythemia. JAK2 V617F is the most frequent. JAK2 normally acts as the signal transduction molecule for the erythropoietin and thrombopoietin receptors.

* Myeloproliferative neoplasms include polycythemia vera, primary myelofibrosis, and essential thrombocythemia.
* JAK2 mutations are common and are universal in polycythemia vera.
* Polycythemia vera and essential thrombocythemia may progress to myelofibrosis. All myeloproliferative neoplasms can progress to AML, which is usually refractory to therapy.

Primary Myelofibrosis, Postpolycythemic Myelofibrosis, and Postthrombocythemic Myelofibrosis

Splenomegaly occurs in virtually 100% of the patients and is a hallmark of primary myelofibrosis. Other features are a leukoerythroblastic peripheral blood smear, including nucleated RBCs and dacrocytes (teardrop cells), and hypercellular marrow with megakaryocyte clustering and increased fibrosis (Figure 11-27). Myeloid cells are clonal, but fibroblasts in the marrow are reactive. Anemia may be

Table 11-11 Characteristic Features of Chronic Myeloproliferative Neoplasms

Characteristic	Polycythemia Vera	Primary Myelofibrosis	Essential Thrombocythemia	Chronic Myeloid Leukemia
Increased red cell mass	Yes	No	No	No
Myelofibrosis	Later	Yes	Rare	Later
Leukocytosis	Variable	Variable	Variable	Yes
Thrombocytosis	Variable	Variable	Yes	Variable
BCR-ABL oncogene	No	No	No	Yes
JAK2 V617F mutation	>95%	50%	50%	Never

caused by expanded plasma volume, ineffective erythropoiesis, blood loss, or hemolysis.

The spleen is characterized by extramedullary hematopoiesis in the sinusoids of red pulp. Hepatomegaly may occur in 70% of patients because of engorgement by blood, extramedullary hematopoiesis, or hemosiderosis. Foci of extramedullary hematopoiesis can occur in any area of the body but are most common in the spleen, liver, lung and pleural space, skin, eye, and central nervous system (spinal cord compression can result). The median survival is 3 to 5 years.

- The median survival is 3-5 years.
- Primary myelofibrosis: a hallmark is splenomegaly, often massive.
- Leukoerythroblastic peripheral blood smear includes teardrop cells.

Asymptomatic patients should be observed. Medical therapy for anemia with symptoms includes transfusion with packed RBCs, androgens (fluoxymesterone or danazol), or erythropoietin. Some patients respond to thalidomide or lenalidomide. In the evaluation of anemia, check the stool for occult blood loss from esophageal varices (due to portal hypertension from splenomegaly) and microinfarcts of the gut.

Symptoms related to the spleen, such as early satiety, infarcts, and pressure, can be treated with splenectomy, hydroxyurea, or splenic irradiation (for patients who are not surgical candidates). Splenectomy may be of benefit for mechanical symptoms, life-threatening thrombocytopenia, portal hypertension, and refractory thrombocytopenia. DIC is common and increases the risk of a complication at splenectomy. Hydroxyurea is indicated for symptomatic hepatosplenomegaly, leukocytosis, and thrombocytosis. Bone marrow transplant may be helpful in some young patients.

- Typical clinical scenario: A 58-year-old woman presents with fatigue, massive splenomegaly, and anemia. The differential blood cell count includes 2 nucleated RBCs, 4% myelocytes, and 2% metamyelocytes. RBC morphology demonstrates dacrocytes. The bone marrow is fibrotic.

Essential Thrombocythemia
Essential thrombocythemia (also called *essential thrombocytosis*) is a clonal hematologic disorder in which patients present with thrombocytosis and sometimes leukocytosis. Patients may be asymptomatic or may have thrombosis or hemorrhage. Patients have a relatively long life expectancy compared with that of patients who have other clonal myeloid disorders (>10 years). The overall risk of bleeding is 3% and of thrombosis, 20%. The risk factors for these events include age older than 60 and previous thrombosis. Young females with essential thrombocythemia have a higher risk of miscarriage. The risk of acute leukemic transformation is less than 2%.

The diagnosis of essential thrombocythemia includes a platelet count greater than 600×10^9/L, megakaryocytic hyperplasia, and absence of the Philadelphia chromosome or *BCR-ABL*. It may be challenging to distinguish essential thrombocythemia from reactive thrombocytosis or iron deficiency. Identification of JAK2 V617F supports the diagnosis of a clonal myeloproliferative neoplasm rather than reactive thrombocytosis.

Clinical findings that suggest reactive thrombocytosis include a recent normal platelet count, a clinical condition associated with reactive thrombocytosis (such as infection, cancer, asplenia, or an inflammatory disease), and no clinical features of a myeloproliferative neoplasm other than the high platelet count. An increased C-reactive protein level

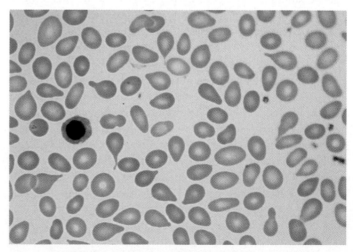

Figure 11-27. Leukoerythroblastic Blood Smear. The teardrop-shaped erythrocytes (dacrocytes) and nucleated red blood cell are characteristic of marrow fibrosis, whether due to primary myelofibrosis or a reactive cause.

in patients with thrombocytosis suggests a reactive process. Iron deficiency should also be excluded, since it may cause thrombocytosis.

Treatment depends on the clinical situation. All patients who can tolerate aspirin should receive low doses of aspirin. Platelet apheresis should be used only for emergent management of acute bleeding or thrombosis and is not indicated from the platelet count alone. Cytoreductive therapy is recommended for patients with acute thrombosis or a previous history of thrombotic events and those older than 60 years, who are at high risk of thrombohemorrhagic events. Currently, hydroxyurea is the cytoreductive treatment of choice for most patients. Anagrelide is a therapeutic alternative for patients who cannot tolerate hydroxyurea. Patients who are asymptomatic and young may be observed. Patients who are pregnant or want to become pregnant can be treated with interferon alfa since the other agents may be teratogenic. Patients with very high platelet counts ($>1,000 \times 10^9$/L) can develop acquired von Willebrand disease. For these patients, the bleeding risk is greater than the thrombotic risk.

* Essential thrombocythemia: elevated platelet count and secondary causes excluded. Half of the patients have JAK2 V617F, which confirms clonality and rules out reactive causes of thrombocytosis.
* Cytoreductive therapy is indicated for patients older than 60 years or those who have had prior thrombosis.
* Relatively benign prognosis with <5% leukemia transformation rate at 15 years.

Erythrocytosis

An increased hematocrit due to a decreased plasma cell volume and normal RBC mass is *relative polycythemia*. Relative polycythemia must be distinguished from a true elevation in the RBC mass. Absolute (true) erythrocytosis is almost always present when the hemoglobin concentration is greater than 18 g/dL in males and greater than 16.5 g/dL in females. The history, physical examination, CBC, oxygen saturation, erythropoietin level, and JAK2 V617F mutation status help distinguish reactive erythrocytosis from polycythemia vera. It is no longer necessary to measure the RBC mass with a nuclear medicine test. A high erythropoietin level indicates a secondary cause of erythrocytosis, such as a tumor (especially renal cell cancer, liver cancer, adrenal cancer, and cerebellar hemangioma); high altitude; chronic hypoxia (eg, lung disease from a cardiac shunt); cigarette smoking; or exogenous erythropoietin administration (eg, competitive cyclists).

The danger of erythrocytosis is hyperviscosity and vascular events. The cerebral blood flow decreases at a hematocrit greater than 45% to 50%. Thus, the goal of phlebotomy is to decrease the hematocrit to less than that level. Smoking 1.5 packs of cigarettes or more daily can increase the hematocrit to 60%. The RBC mass returns to normal when the person stops smoking, unless chronic lung disease has developed.

Polycythemia Vera

Polycythemia vera is a myeloproliferative disorder that results from activating mutations of JAK2 tyrosine kinase. Clinical features include postbathing pruritus, fatigue, erythromelalgia (acral dysesthesias and erythema), headache, dizziness, unexplained weight loss, joint symptoms, dyspnea, and epigastric distress. More than 50% of patients have

leukocytosis and thrombocytosis in addition to erythrocytosis. Polycythemia vera should be considered in the evaluation of an idiopathic thrombotic event, especially in an atypical site such as an abdominal vessel or dural sinus in the brain. Unfavorable prognostic signs are previous thrombotic disease, age older than 60 years, diabetes mellitus, vascular disease, and hypertension.

Bone marrow findings in polycythemia vera typically demonstrate trilineage hyperplasia. Most bone marrow specimens lack iron stores even if the patient is not phlebotomized, because the erythrocyte proliferation outstrips the available iron supply. Cytogenetic abnormalities are present in about 15% of patients. By definition, the bone marrow is negative for the Philadelphia chromosome and *BCR-ABL*. Morphologically, the bone marrow findings may resemble those of CML, so if there is leukocytosis it is important to exclude CML. The leukocyte alkaline phosphatase score is not often measured anymore, but it is increased in polycythemia vera and primary myelofibrosis and low in CML.

* Polycythemia vera: low or low-normal erythropoietin and universal finding of JAK2 mutation.
* Typical clinical scenario for polycythemia vera: A hemoglobin concentration >18 g/dL in a male or a persistent increase >2 g/dL from baseline, microcytosis, absence of iron stores, and splenomegaly. Other features include postbathing pruritus, unusual thrombosis, and erythromelalgia. The erythropoietin level is low.

The mainstay of therapy for all patients with polycythemia vera is phlebotomy. Treatment goals include maintaining the hematocrit below 45%. Low-dose aspirin therapy is indicated for all patients who do not have a contraindication to this therapy.

For patients who are older than 60 or have had prior thrombosis, cytoreductive therapy is indicated. Treatments include hydroxyurea, interferon alfa, and radiophosphorus (^{32}P). Hydroxyurea is the first choice. Interferon alfa is the treatment of choice for younger patients and women of childbearing age. Erythromelalgia is managed by using aspirin and by normalizing the platelet count. Radiophosphorus may be useful in older patients but increases the risk of AML 2.3-fold.

* For polycythemia vera, phlebotomy is the cornerstone of treatment.
* For patients older than 60 years or with a history of thrombosis, add hydroxyurea.

Atypical Myeloproliferative Neoplasms

Uncommon or atypical myeloproliferative neoplasms include hypereosinophilic syndrome, chronic eosinophilic leukemia, systemic mastocytosis, chronic myelomonocytic leukemia, and chronic neutrophilic leukemia. Patients with chronic eosinophilic leukemia have clonal blood eosinophilia and end-organ damage in sites such as the heart or the gut. Clonal eosinophilia is often characterized by rearrangements of PDGRFA tyrosine kinase, which responds well to imatinib therapy. When no clonal gene rearrangement is present but there is no other explanation for eosinophilia (eg, parasite or allergic disorder), the diagnosis of hypereosinophilic syndrome is given. Patients with systemic mastocytosis frequently present with skin lesions and allergic symptoms, they often have activating mutations for KIT tyrosine kinase, and they respond to imatinib. Chronic myelomonocytic leukemia (CMML) should not be confused with chronic myelogenous leukemia. CMML has features of both a myelodysplastic syndrome (cytopenias) and a myeloproliferative neoplasm (leukocytosis and frequent splenomegaly). CMML does not have *BCR-ABL* and does not respond to imatinib therapy. Chronic neutrophilic leukemia is rare and is characterized by proliferation of mature granulocytes in the absence of infection or other cause for reactive neutrophilia.

Oncogenesis

The hallmark of neoplastic disease is clonal proliferation of cells. Balanced reciprocal translocations affect specific sites on the genome (Table 11-12). Viral associations include HTLV-I in adult T-cell leukemia and Epstein-Barr virus in Burkitt lymphoma, Hodgkin disease, and posttransplant lymphoproliferative disorders.

- Viral associations with hematologic malignancies: HTLV-I in adult T-cell leukemia; Epstein-Barr virus in Burkitt lymphoma, Hodgkin disease, and posttransplant lymphoproliferative disorders.

Table 11-12 Common Chromosomal Rearrangements and Associated Specific Oncogenes in Hematologic Malignancy

Disease	Rearrangement	Oncogene	Gene Product
Burkitt lymphoma	t(8;14)	*C-MYC*	Cell cycle progression
	t(8;22)		Translocation into transcriptionally active immunoglobulin heavy or light chain loci
Chronic myelogenous leukemia	t(9;22)	*C-ABL*	Tyrosine kinase
Follicular small cleaved cell lymphoma	t(14;18)	*BCL-2*	Anti-apoptosis
Diffuse large cell non-Hodgkin lymphoma	...	*BCL-6*	Transcriptional repression
Mantle cell lymphoma	t(11;14)	*BCL-1*	Overexpression of PRAD1 Increase in cyclin D1
Promyelocytic leukemia	t(15;17)	*PML-RARA* fusion	Transcriptional corepressor
Acute myeloid leukemia	t(8;21)	*AML1 (CBFA)/ETO*	Part of transcription factor complex core binding factor
	inv(16)	*CBFB/MYH11*	Part of transcription factor complex core binding factor
	t(variable;11q23)	*MLL*	Zinc finger transcription factor

Part III

Rajiv K. Pruthi, MBBS

Coagulation (Hemostasis and Thrombosis)

Overview of Coagulation System

The coagulation system has 2 essential functions: to maintain hemostasis and to prevent and limit thrombosis. The procoagulant component of the hemostatic system prevents and controls hemorrhage. Vascular injury results in activation of hemostasis, which consists of vasospasm, platelet plug formation (platelet activation, adhesion, and aggregation), and fibrin clot formation (by activation of coagulation factors in the procoagulant system). The anticoagulant system prevents excessive formation of blood clots, and the fibrinolytic system breaks down and remodels blood clots. Quantitative abnormalities (deficiencies) and qualitative abnormalities of platelets and coagulation factors lead to bleeding disorders, whereas deficiencies of the anticoagulant system are risk factors for thrombosis.

The best screening tool to evaluate for a bleeding disorder is a thorough clinical evaluation that includes obtaining a detailed personal and family hemostatic history and performing a physical examination of the patient. Detailed inquiry into the presence and age at onset of spontaneous bleeding (epistaxis, easy bruising, joint bleeding, etc), unusual or unexpected posttraumatic or surgical bleeding (including dental extractions), and family history may suggest the presence of a bleeding disorder.

Laboratory Testing to Evaluate a Bleeding Patient

Initial tests include a complete blood count (CBC), prothrombin time (PT), activated partial thromboplastin time (aPTT), and fibrinogen. Additional testing includes assays for von Willebrand disease (vWD) coagulation factor assays, factor XIII assays, and platelet function tests.

Prothrombin Time (International Normalized Ratio)

The PT assesses the extrinsic and final common pathways of the procoagulant cascade (Figure 11-28). Deficiencies or inhibitors of clotting factors within the extrinsic and final common pathways result in prolongation of the PT. The main utility of the PT, from which the international normalized ratio (INR) is calculated, is for monitoring warfarin anticoagulation. The INR reduces interlaboratory variation of the PT and is calculated and reported by the laboratory.

Activated Partial Thromboplastin Time

The aPTT assesses the intrinsic and final common pathways (Figure 11-28); deficiencies or inhibitors of clotting factors within the intrinsic and final common pathways result in prolongation of the aPTT. The aPTT is commonly used to monitor unfractionated heparin therapy.

Bleeding Time

Originally introduced as a screening test for bleeding disorders, bleeding time (BT) has been used inappropriately for routine preoperative hemostatic assessment. It measures the time to stop bleeding from a standardized incision on the volar aspect of a patient's forearm and thus provides an estimate of the integrity of vascular, platelet, and fibrin clot formation. The multiple factors affecting the BT (inexperienced technologist, antiplatelet agents, fragile skin, quantitative or qualitative platelet disorders, or a bleeding disorder such as vWD) reduce the sensitivity and specificity of the test. A review of multiple studies led to the following conclusions: 1) In the absence of the clinical history of a bleeding disorder, the BT is not a useful predictor of risk of hemorrhage with surgical procedures. 2) Normal BT does not exclude the possibility of excessive hemorrhage with invasive procedures. 3) BT cannot reliably identify patients exposed to aspirin or nonsteroidal anti-inflammatory drugs. Thus, the BT has been discontinued in many institutions.

Approach to a Prolonged PT or aPTT

The PT and aPTT are screening tests to detect coagulation factor deficiencies or inhibitors. After excluding artifactual causes (elevated hematocrit, nonfasting sample, or heparin contamination of the specimen), the next step is to perform a mixing study in a 1:1 ratio with normal pooled plasma. Correction of the clotting time (ie, the clotting time shortens into the reference range) implies a coagulation factor deficiency, and inhibition of the clotting time (ie, it may shorten but

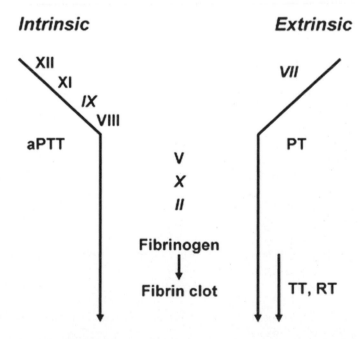

Figure 11-28. Coagulation Cascade.

not enough to be within the reference range) implies presence of an inhibitor. Types of inhibitors include 1) medications (eg, heparins and direct thrombin inhibitors); 2) inhibitors directed against specific clotting factors termed *specific factor inhibitors* (eg, factor VIII or factor V inhibitors); and 3) nonspecific inhibitors (eg, lupus anticoagulants). Additional testing such as clotting factor assays, inhibitor screening and titering assays, and tests for lupus anticoagulant typically lead to the diagnosis for the underlying cause of the prolongation of the PT and aPTT.

Bleeding Disorders Not Detected With PT and aPTT

Disorders that are not detected with the PT and aPTT include the following: 1) qualitative platelet defects, which require specialized platelet function testing; 2) vWD, which requires assays for vWF; 3) factor XIII deficiency, which requires specialized factor XIII screening or functional assays, and 4) deficiency of plasminogen activator inhibitor-1, which requires specific assays.

Overview of Bleeding Disorders

Bleeding disorders are broadly classified into congenital and acquired disorders. In turn, specific disorders include platelet disorders (quantitative and qualitative), factor deficiencies or inhibitors, and vascular bleeding disorders.

Congenital Plasmatic Bleeding Disorders (Factor Deficiencies)

Of the congenital plasmatic bleeding disorders, vWD is the most common. Others include hemophilia A, B, and C. Other factor deficiency states are rare (Table 11-13). All clotting factors are produced by the liver except vWF, which is produced by vascular endothelial cells and megakaryocytes.

von Willebrand Disease

Quantitative (types 1 and 3) and qualitative (types 2A, 2B, 2M, and 2N) abnormalities of vWF result in vWD. Endothelial cells and platelets store vWF. After secretion, the ultra-large-molecular-weight multimers of vWF, which are the most hemostatically active, are cleaved into multimers of smaller size by a protease, ADAMTS13. The 2 main functions of vWF are 1) to mediate platelet adhesion and aggregation and 2) to act as a carrier protein for factor VIII, protecting it from proteolytic inactivation.

Clinical Features—Depending on the severity of the deficiency, patients may be asymptomatic and bleed only when challenged with trauma or surgery (minor surgery, such as dental extraction, or major surgery). With more severe deficiency states, patients may have spontaneous bleeding symptoms. Spontaneous bleeding is typically mucocutaneous (bruising, epistaxis, hematuria, gastrointestinal tract hemorrhage); in type 3 vWD, bleeding occurs in joints and soft tissue. Bleeding may be exacerbated by the use of aspirin or nonsteroidal analgesics.

Laboratory Testing—Laboratory testing (Table 11-14) confirms the diagnosis. In type 1, there is a mild to moderate reduction in vWF antigen (vWF:Ag) and activity, whereas in type 3 vWD, vWF is absent. Type 2 variants are characterized by a disproportionate reduction in activity of the vWF called the *ristocetin cofactor* (RCoF) compared with vWF:Ag. Characteristically, high-molecular-weight-multimers are decreased in type 2 vWD, except for types 2M and 2N in which the multimers are normal. Healthy people with blood group O have vWF levels that are 25% to 30% lower than in people with blood groups A, B or AB; thus, they may receive a misdiagnosis of vWD. Therefore, ABO typing should be part of the initial testing. Acquired defects of vWF (*acquired von Willebrand syndrome*) may be seen in patients with aortic stenosis, myeloproliferative disorders, and monoclonal protein disorders. The syndrome mimics congenital

Table 11-13 Congenital Bleeding Disorders

Congenital Disorder	Deficient Factor	PT	aPTT	Prevalence	Mode of Inheritance
Hemophilia A	Factor VIII	NL	Prol	1:5,000[a]	X-linked recessive
Hemophilia B	Factor IX	NL	Prol	1:30,000[a]	X-linked recessive
Hemophilia C	Factor XI	NL	Prol	Up to 4%[b]	Autosomal
von Willebrand disease	von Willebrand factor	NL	NL/Prol	Up to 1%	Autosomal
Factor VII deficiency		Prol	NL	1:500,000	Autosomal
Rare coagulation factor deficiencies					
Factor V		Prol	Prol	1:1 million	Autosomal
Factor II		Prol	NL/Prol	Rare	Autosomal
Factor X		Prol	NL/Prol	1:500,000	Autosomal
Factor XIII		NL	NL	Rare	Autosomal
Combined factors VIII & V		Prol	Prol	Rare	Autosomal

Abbreviations: aPTT, activated partial thromboplastin time; NL, normal; Prol, prolonged; PT, prothrombin time.
[a] Live male births.
[b] Among Ashkenazi Jews.

Table 11-14 Approach to Assessment of von Willebrand Disease

1. Bleeding history
2. Complete blood cell count
3. vWD profile testing
   vWF:Ag
   RCoF
   FVIIIC
4. ABO blood group
5. Optional tests if initial data suggest vWD
   vWF multimers
   vWF:CBA
   vWF:FVIIIB
   RIPA
6. Genetic tests if indicated

Abbreviations: Ag, antigen; CBA, collagen-binding assay; FVIIIB, factor VIII binding assay; FVIIIC, factor VIII coagulant activity; RCoF, ristocetin cofactor; RIPA, ristocetin-induced platelet aggregation; vWD, von Willebrand disease; vWF, von Willebrand factor.

type 2 vWD. Acute physical exertion, inflammation, malignancy, hyperthyroidism, estrogens, and pregnancy increase vWF levels to normal and may mask a diagnosis of vWD. Hypothyroidism is associated with reduced vWF levels. Type 2B vWD is associated with thrombocytopenia; type 2N occurs as a result of mutations in the factor VIII binding domain of vWF. This subtype may be mistaken for mild hemophilia A.

Inheritance of von Willebrand Disease—Type 1 vWD is an autosomal dominant bleeding disorder with variable penetrance; type 3 vWD is autosomal recessive; types 2A, 2B, and 2M vWD are autosomal dominant; and type 2N (Normandy) vWD is autosomal recessive.

Management—Upon establishment of a diagnosis of vWD, a desmopressin (1-desamino-8-D-arginine vasopressin [DDAVP]) treatment trial should be performed for patients with types 1, 2A, or 2M vWD. Intravenous infusion of 0.3 mcg/kg body weight releases vWF from its storage sites; levels should be measured 60 minutes after infusion. Side effects include facial flushing, headache, mild decrease in blood pressure, mild tachycardia, and hyponatremia. Repeated doses at intervals shorter than 24 hours may result in a decrease or loss of response (tachyphylaxis) and syndrome of inappropriate antidiuresis (SIAD), leading to hyponatremia and seizures.

Desmopressin is generally not very helpful for patients with type 2B vWD since the release of endogenous vWF results in worsening of thrombocytopenia. Patients with type 3 vWD will not respond and should not undergo a desmopressin trial.

For patients who do respond, desmopressin is a reasonable alternative for prevention or treatment of minor bleeding, for minor procedures such as dental extraction, and for the management of menorrhagia in women with vWD. An intranasal formulation of desmopressin is also available. For patients who do not respond to desmopressin and for those in whom it is contraindicated, purified plasma-derived vWF concentrates are the therapy of choice.

The goals of management of vWD include prevention and treatment of hemorrhage. General measures include the following:
1. Patient education
2. Encouragement to wear a medical condition identification tag
3. Generation of treatment guidelines for management of bleeding
4. Referral to a comprehensive hemophilia treatment center for periodic follow-up

Specific measures include the following:
1. Desmopressin
2. Adjunctive ε-aminocaproic acid or vWF concentrates administered preoperatively to prevent bleeding or for management of bleeding
3. vWF concentrates

Hemophilia A and B

Hemophilia A and hemophilia B are clinically indistinguishable X-linked recessive bleeding disorders. Hemophilia A is due to a deficiency in blood coagulation factor VIII (FVIII), and hemophilia B is due to a deficiency in factor IX (FIX). On the basis of factor levels, the disease is classified as severe (<1%), moderate (1%-5%), or mild (>5%-40%).

Clinical Features—Patients with mild hemophilia seldom experience spontaneous hemorrhage but will bleed after trauma or surgery; rarely, they may not receive a diagnosis of hemophilia until adulthood. Patients with moderate disease experience infrequent spontaneous bleeding but typically bleed after minor trauma and surgery. Patients with severe disease experience frequent spontaneous bleeding, including hemarthrosis, soft tissue hematomas, and intracranial hemorrhage in addition to minor hemorrhage such as epistaxis and ecchymoses. Currently, regular prophylactic administration of factor concentrates to patients with severe disease has reduced chronic complications related to bleeding.

Management—At the initial diagnosis of mild and moderate hemophilia A, as with vWD, a desmopressin trial is performed with FVIII levels checked before and 1 hour after infusion of desmopressin. For patients who respond, desmopressin may be used for management of minor hemorrhage or for prophylaxis and treatment of minor surgical hemorrhage. Recombinant or plasma-derived FVIII concentrates are used to treat major hemorrhages and as prophylaxis for major surgery. Desmopressin is not used in patients with hemophilia B; instead, recombinant or plasma-derived FIX concentrates are used.

Inheritance of Hemophilia A and B—The hemophilias are X-linked recessive bleeding disorders. Typically, males are affected and females are asymptomatic carriers. Mothers and daughters of hemophilia patients are obligate carriers. Rarely, females may have extreme lyonization of their normal X chromosome, resulting in reduced factor levels and bleeding symptoms in carriers. Each male fetus of a carrier has a 50% risk of being affected, whereas each female fetus has a 50% risk of being a carrier.

Complications of Treatment of Hemophilia—There is a high prevalence of patients infected with transfusion-transmitted viruses such as hepatitis virus and HIV, although with contemporary clotting factor manufacturing processes, infection with these viruses is rare.

Recurrent hemarthrosis leads to premature degenerative joint disease. Currently, the most serious complication of hemophilia is the development of inhibitor antibodies, predominantly against FVIII and rarely against FIX. In these patients, standard FVIII and FIX concentrates are ineffective, and bypassing agents such as recombinant factor VIIa or prothrombin complex concentrates are used for management of surgery and hemorrhage.

Factor VII Deficiency

Factor VII (FVII) deficiency is typically a mild bleeding disorder, usually detected with a preoperative PT that is prolonged. Factor levels as low as 10% of normal may go undetected for many years. Bleeding symptoms are similar to those of hemophilia. Recombinant factor VIIa is the treatment of choice for prevention and treatment of hemorrhage; however, fresh frozen plasma is also an option.

Factor XI Deficiency (Hemophilia C)

Factor XI (FXI) deficiency is a rare autosomal recessive disorder that is prevalent in Ashkenazi Jews. This is a mild bleeding disorder that usually becomes manifest after surgery or trauma or with the initiation of treatment with antiplatelet agents or anticoagulants. Bleeding symptoms do not correlate well with FXI levels: Patients with mild deficiencies may have significant bleeding symptoms, whereas patients with more severe deficiencies may remain asymptomatic until they undergo surgery or are exposed to anticoagulant or antiplatelet agents. Fresh frozen plasma is the treatment of choice for prevention and treatment of hemorrhage. FXI concentrates are in clinical trials.

Factor XIII Deficiency

Severe factor XIII (FXIII) deficiency is characterized by significant bleeding but normal screening tests. Other characteristics include umbilical cord bleeding, delayed wound healing, delayed hemorrhage, and recurrent pregnancy loss. Its inheritance pattern is autosomal recessive. Cryoprecipitate is the treatment of choice for prevention and treatment of hemorrhage. FXIII concentrates are in clinical trials.

Factor Deficiencies That Prolong the aPTT But Do Not Result in Hemorrhage

Deficiencies of factor XII (FXII), high-molecular-weight-kininogen, and prekallikrein can result in a marked prolongation of the aPTT, yet even severe deficiencies are not risk factors for hemorrhage. Their role in hemostasis is being defined.

Acquired Bleeding Disorders

Acquired bleeding disorders can occur as a result of decreased production of clotting factors by the liver (as in liver disease) or increased consumption (as in DIC and fibrinolysis) (Table 11-15).

Liver Disease

Since most coagulation factors except for vWF are produced in the liver, hepatocellular damage and liver failure lead to a decreased production of clotting factors and a bleeding tendency. Supportive management includes replenishment of the deficient coagulation factors

with fresh frozen plasma (cryoprecipitate is a more concentrated form for fibrinogen and factor XIII) while the liver recovers or is transplanted.

Disseminated Intravascular Coagulation and Fibrinolysis

Disseminated intravascular coagulation and fibrinolysis (DIC/ICF) is a dynamic process with various causes (Table 11-16) resulting in microvascular thrombosis and consumption of clotting factors.

Clinical Features—DIC should be suspected in a patient presenting with underlying conditions known to predispose to DIC (Table 11-16). Most patients present with a new onset of bleeding; occasionally, patients present with thrombosis or both bleeding and thrombosis. Bleeding manifestations may include bleeding from surgical wounds and venipuncture sites, ecchymoses, petechiae, hematomas, vaginal bleeding, or hemorrhage from the gastrointestinal tract or

Table 11-15 Causes of Acquired Coagulation Factor Deficiencies

Cause of Deficiency	Deficient Factor
Warfarin	Vitamin K–dependent factors
Decreased nutritional intake or malabsorption	Vitamin K–dependent factors
Liver failure	Multiple factors
Amyloid	Factor X
Myeloproliferative disease	Factor V
Acquired von Willebrand syndrome	von Willebrand factor & factor VIII
Disseminated intravascular coagulation	Multiple factors

Table 11-16 Causes of DIC

Acute & Subacute DIC
  Malignancies (hematologic & solid organ)
  Infection or sepsis (bacterial)
  Obstetric complications (abruption, amniotic fluid embolism)
  Massive trauma
  Burns
  Advanced liver disease
  Snake bite
  Hemolytic transfusion reaction
Chronic DIC
  Solid tumors
  Obstetric complications (retained dead fetus)
  Advanced liver disease
Localized causes of systemic DIC
  Aortic aneurysm
  Giant hemangiomas

Abbreviation: DIC, disseminated intravascular coagulation.

genitourinary system. Thrombotic manifestations include necrotic skin lesions, venous thromboembolism (DVT and pulmonary embolism), and acute arterial occlusions (stroke and myocardial infarction), but they occur less frequently than bleeding.

Laboratory Testing in Suspected DIC—The laboratory findings vary and there is no single diagnostic laboratory test. Since this is a syndrome, clinical findings need to be interpreted along with laboratory data. An understanding of the pathophysiology of DIC helps with understanding laboratory testing and management. The underlying disease (Table 11-16) stimulates the procoagulant system to generate thrombin, resulting in consumption of the coagulation factors and platelets. The fibrinolytic system also gets activated, and plasminogen is converted to plasmin. Plasmin prevents stabilization of fibrin clots (resulting in circulating fibrin monomers) and degrades existing fibrin clots and fibrinogen-releasing cleavage products called D dimers. The circulating fibrin monomers are soluble and thus form weak clots. Typical laboratory findings in DIC include thrombocytopenia, prolonged PT and aPTT, low fibrinogen due to consumption, and increased D dimers and soluble fibrin monomer complexes.

Management—Principles of management include identifying and treating underlying disease while managing the coagulopathy.

Blood Component Replacement Therapy—For low-grade compensated DIC in which the patient is not bleeding and the coagulopathy is mild, observation may be reasonable. Transfusion of blood components is important for patients who have symptomatic hemorrhage or abnormal laboratory results and who are considered to be at risk of bleeding: cryoprecipitate for low fibrinogen (<100 mg/dL), fresh frozen plasma for markedly prolonged PT and aPTT (suggesting significant coagulation factor deficiency states), and platelet concentrates for thrombocytopenia (platelet count <30 × 10⁹/L or <50 × 10⁹/L for bleeding patients). It is important to monitor transfusion therapy with regular CBC, PT, aPTT, and fibrinogen levels 60 minutes after transfusions and every 6 to 8 hours after that. Thus, the target platelet count is more than 20 × 10⁹/L to 30 × 10⁹/L higher, especially if the patient is bleeding or undergoing procedures.

Ancillary Therapies for DIC—*Unfractionated heparin* has been used in selected circumstances. Its utility is based on the principle that it inhibits thrombin and interrupts the vicious circle of consumptive coagulopathy. Major risks include hemorrhage, including intracranial hemorrhage, and benefits are less clear because of the lack of randomized trials. Thus, heparin usually has a limited role, if any, in acute DIC (except with acute DIC associated with promyelocytic leukemia), but it may have a role in chronic DIC as seen with solid tumors, the retained dead fetus syndrome, aortic aneurysm, and giant hemangiomas. *Antithrombin* concentrate has not been shown to improve mortality among patients with DIC. *Recombinant activated protein C* improves mortality among patients with severe sepsis. *Fibrinolysis inhibitors*, such as ε-aminocaproic acid or tranexamic acid, are generally contraindicated in DIC.

Acquired von Willebrand Syndrome
Acquired von Willebrand syndrome is an acquired quantitative or qualitative abnormality of vWF that is associated with monoclonal protein disorders, myeloproliferative disease, hypothyroidism, and other malignancies. Occasionally no underlying disease is found.

Management consists of infusion of vWF concentrates to prevent and treat hemorrhage.

Acquired (Autoimmune) Hemophilia
In acquired (autoimmune) hemophilia, the development of FVIII inhibitors in previously healthy people results in a potentially life-threatening bleeding disorder. Management consists of maintaining hemostasis with special factor concentrates (prothrombin complex concentrates or recombinant FVIIa) and immunosuppression (glucocorticoids, cytotoxic chemotherapy, and anti-CD 20 antibody [rituximab]).

Platelet Disorders

Platelets are produced in the bone marrow and, after circulating for about 7 to 10 days, are destroyed in the reticuloendothelial system. Thrombocytopenia is most commonly acquired and is a risk of bleeding, and it commonly occurs as a result of decreased production or accelerated destruction. When thrombocytopenia occurs for the first time, the diagnosis of pseudothrombocytopenia should be excluded with examination of a peripheral blood smear. Rarely, thrombocytopenia is congenital.

Pseudothrombocytopenia
Pseudothrombocytopenia occurs as a result of EDTA-induced platelet clumping, so that platelets range from 50 × 10⁹/L to 100 × 10⁹/L. A peripheral blood smear is useful to detect clumping, and repeating the CBC with a specimen collected in citrate will clarify the situation. Platelet agglutination (Figure 11-29) is an antibody-mediated phenomenon caused by antibodies that bind to the patient's platelets after withdrawal of calcium in the test tube. The platelet count is spuriously low with automated techniques only; on the peripheral blood smear, the number is normal because the platelets are clumped or rarely adhere to neutrophils.

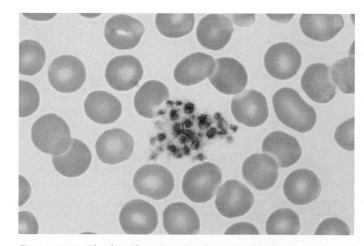

Figure 11-29. Platelet Clumping (Agglutination). This is a cause of artifactual thrombocytopenia. Drawing the blood in a citrate tube rather than an EDTA-anticoagulated tube usually eliminates this in vitro phenomenon. (Courtesy of Curtis A. Hanson, MD, Mayo Clinic.)

After exclusion of pseudothrombocytopenia, other causes are broadly classified as accelerated platelet destruction, decreased platelet production, or splenic sequestration (careful physical examination for splenomegaly will help exclude this possibility) (Table 11-17). Potentially serious causes for thrombocytopenia should be excluded, including heparin-induced thrombocytopenia (HIT), thrombotic thrombocytopenic purpura (TTP), and the HELLP syndrome (*h*emolysis, *e*levated *l*iver enzymes, and *l*ow *p*latelet count) seen in pregnancy.

Abormally large platelets (Figure 11-30) are seen in immune thrombocytopenia, clonal myeloid disorders (eg, essential thrombocythemia), and congenital disorders of platelet synthesis and function. These congenital disorders include conditions associated with mutations of the *MYH9* gene (eg, May-Heggelin anomaly) and Bernard-Soulier syndrome.

Thrombocytopenia Due to Increased Platelet Destruction

Idiopathic Thrombocytopenic Purpura

Idiopathic thrombocytopenic purpura (ITP) is an autoimmune disease characterized by thrombocytopenia, usually with a normal WBC count and hemoglobin concentration (Table 11-18). The diagnosis of ITP is a diagnosis of exclusion. Use of drugs associated with thrombocytopenia and heavy alcohol use should be excluded, and patients with risk factors should be tested for HIV. In adults, ITP has an insidious onset, with the diagnosis often incidentally established on a routine CBC. The clinical manifestations include petechiae and purpura, mucous membrane hemorrhage, and cerebromeningeal bleeding. Up to 60% of adults have progression to a chronic state

Table 11-17 Causes of Thrombocytopenia

Pseudothrombocytopenia
Dilutional
   Massive transfusion
   Pregnancy
Increased destruction
   Immune
      Autoimmune
      Idiopathic
      Secondary (drug-induced, connective tissue diseases)
   Nonimmune
      Consumptive (DIC)
      Sepsis
Decreased production
   Bone marrow failure syndromes
      Primary: Anaplastic anemia
      Secondary: Metastatic disease, hematologic malignancies
   Nutritional
      Vitamin B_{12} & folate deficiency
   Infections
      Viral (HIV, CMV, hepatitis)

Abbreviations: CMV, cytomegalovirus; DIC, disseminated intravascular coagulation; HIV, human immunodeficiency virus.

of ITP. In most patients, the platelet count is less than 50×10^9/L and in 30% it is less than 10×10^9/L (spontaneous bleeding may occur at this level). The mean platelet volume is increased. Only 10% of patients have splenomegaly. If splenomegaly is present, one should think of other causes. A bone marrow examination is appropriate to establish the diagnosis of ITP in patients older than 60 years, because the likelihood of another disorder causing thrombocytopenia (such as a myelodysplastic syndrome) is increased in older patients. Bone marrow examination in ITP shows a normal to increased number of megakaryocytes. Antibodies to specific platelet-membrane glycoproteins, usually the IIb/IIIa complex, and platelet-associated IgG can be detected in most patients but are not necessary for diagnosis or treatment.

The American Society of Hematology guidelines for treatment are as follows:

1. Patients with platelet counts of 50×10^9/L or higher do not routinely require treatment.
2. Patients with platelet counts less than 50×10^9/L but greater than 30×10^9/L should be treated if there is mucous membrane bleeding or risk factors for bleeding, including hypertension, peptic ulcer disease, and a vigorous lifestyle.
3. Patients with platelet counts less than 30×10^9/L should be treated.

Prednisone is the mainstay of initial treatment; initially, 70% of patients have a response, with about a 40% chance of long-term remission at the initial prednisone dosage of 1 mg/kg daily for up to 1 month. Patients with severe bleeding should be treated with intravenous immunoglobulin at a dosage of 1 g/kg per day for 2 days and platelets; high-dose intravenous corticosteroids can also be considered (eg, methylprednisolone, 1 g daily for 2-3 consecutive days; the initial response rate is 80%).

Splenectomy, the treatment of choice for steroid-refractory ITP, removes the predominant site of antibody production and platelet destruction; the likelihood of remission is 75%, with about 60% of patients remaining in long-term remission. Pneumococcal, meningococcal, and *H influenzae* vaccines should be administered

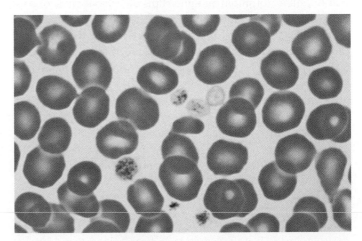

Figure 11-30. Giant Platelets. These may be associated with congenital platelet synthesis disorders, acquired clonal myeloid disorders, or immune thrombocytopenia. (Courtesy of Curtis A. Hanson, MD, Mayo Clinic.)

Table 11-18 Idiopathic Thrombocytopenic Purpura

Characteristic	Acute	Chronic
Presentation	Abrupt onset of petechiae, purpura, mucosal bleeding	Insidious petechiae, menorrhagia
Usual age	Children (2-6 y)	Adults (20-40 y)
Female to male ratio	1:1	3:1
Antecedent infection	Common (85%) Typically an upper respiratory tract infection	Uncommon
Platelet count, ×10⁹/L	<20	30-80
Duration	2-6 wk	Months to years
Spontaneous remission	80% within 6 mo	Uncommon, fluctuates

From Lee GR, Bithell TC, Foerster J, Athens JW, Lukens JN. Wintrobe's clinical hematology. Vol 2. 9th ed. Philadelphia: Lea & Febiger; 1993. p. 1331. Used with permission.

2 weeks before splenectomy. Absence of Howell-Jolly bodies on a postsplenectomy peripheral blood smear suggests an accessory spleen. Accessory splenectomy can result in remission. Pulsed dexamethasone (40 mg daily for 4 sequential days every 28 days for 12 months) is an option for the treatment of resistant ITP or disease relapse. Other agents used in refractory cases include azathioprine, cyclophosphamide, colchicine, cyclosporine, rituximab, vincristine, vinblastine, anti-Rh₀(D) immune globulin, danazol, and immunoadsorption apheresis on staphylococcal protein A columns.

- Spontaneous bleeding may occur with platelet counts <10 × 10⁹/L.
- ITP is a diagnosis of exclusion.
- Examine the peripheral blood smear (exclude microangiopathy).
- Consider discontinuing use of any drug that may cause the disease.
- A bone marrow examination is appropriate to establish the diagnosis of ITP in patients older than 60 years.
- In ITP with severe bleeding, intravenous immunoglobulin is the treatment of choice, with platelet transfusions and high-dose corticosteroids.
- Corticosteroids are the initial treatment, followed by splenectomy in relapsed or refractory cases.

Drug-Induced Thrombocytopenia
Rarely, drugs can cause thrombocytopenia as a result of immune-mediated mechanisms, direct platelet destruction, or bone marrow suppression. The pathophysiologic mechanism may be due to direct marrow toxicity or to haptens bound to a carrier protein. A thorough review of the patient's medication is essential. Drug-induced thrombocytopenia subsides in 4 to 14 days after use of the drug is discontinued—except for that caused by gold, which may take much longer. In contrast, viral-induced thrombocytopenia resolves in 2 weeks to 3 months. The drugs most commonly implicated include heparin, quinidine, quinine, valproic acid, gold, trimethoprim-sulfamethoxazole, amphotericin B, carbamazepine, chlorothiazide, chlorpropamide, procainamide, rifampin, and vancomycin. Glycoprotein IIb/IIIa antagonists, drugs that inhibit the interaction with fibrinogen and platelet interaction (abciximab [ReoPro], eptifibatide [Integrilin], and tirofiban [Aggrastat]), may cause thrombocytopenia and may cause acute (within 24 hours) or delayed (up to 14 days after initiating chronic therapy) thrombocytopenia secondary to antibodies in 0.5% to 2.0% of patients. HIT is one of the most lethal drug-induced thrombocytopenias.

Heparin-Induced Thrombocytopenia
HIT is a clinicopathologic syndrome that has a variable incidence of 1% to 7.8% with unfractionated heparin (UFH) (the incidence is lower with low-molecular-weight heparin [LMWH]). It can develop at any dose of heparin, including low-dose prophylaxis for venous thrombosis postoperatively. Type I HIT is of no clinical relevance. It is a common transient nonimmunologic event due to direct heparin-induced platelet aggregation occuring in the first 4 days of heparin therapy. In contrast, Type II HIT is clinically troublesome. It is an immunologic reaction usually occuring 4 to 14 days after heparin use (earlier in patients with recent heparin exposure) and is caused by IgG antibodies to a heparin-dependent antigen (ie, platelet factor 4 bound to heparin) that activates platelets through their Fc receptors. Platelet aggregation with thrombin formation and development of a clot may follow. Clinically, the predominant feature of type II HIT is thrombosis, not hemorrhage. The onset is at a median of 9 days with UFH and 14 days with LMWH. The platelet counts usually decrease 50% or more, and such a decrease in a patient receiving heparin should raise clinical suspicion, even if the count is still greater than 150 × 10⁹/L. The coagulation system may be activated, increasing the production of thrombin. HIT with thrombosis occurs in 10% of patients with type II HIT. Rapid-onset HIT may develop in patients who were exposed to heparin in the previous 120 days, with thrombocytopenia developing within hours after rechallenge. HIT thrombosis can occur up to 3 weeks after the cessation of heparin therapy. Venous thrombosis (DVT and pulmonary embolism) is more common than arterial thrombosis. Other clinical events include warfarin-induced venous gangrene with limb damage, acute platelet activation syndromes (fevers, chills, or transient amnesia) 5 to 30 minutes after an IV bolus of heparin, and skin lesions at the site of injection of heparin (necrosis or erythematous plaques).

The diagnosis is a clinical one that may be confirmed by functional assays (serotonin release assay) or antigen assays (heparin-dependent antibody against platelet factor 4).

The treatment of HIT is complex. The use of heparin in all forms must be discontinued, including line flushes and heparin-impregnated catheters. When HIT is due to UFH, LMWH is not used because of the high cross-reactivity of the antibody with an LMWH/platelet factor 4 complex. Alternatives to heparin include the direct thrombin inhibitors (eg, lepirudin or bivalirudin) or argatroban. Lepirudin, bivalirudin, and argatroban are monitored with the aPTT. For lepirudin and bivalirudin, the range is 1.5 to 2.5 times the baseline value and for argatroban, 1.5 to 3.0 times. Argatroban is the treatment of choice for patients on dialysis because it is not excreted by the kidneys. In contrast, for patients with hepatic failure, lepirudin (which is renally excreted) is preferred.

The risk of developing type II HIT varies with the dose of heparin, the type of heparin (UFH > LMWH) and clinical associations (higher risk for surgical than for medical patients).

- Drug-induced thrombocytopenia subsides in 4-14 days, except for that caused by gold.
- Viral-induced thrombocytopenia resolves in 2 weeks to 3 months.
- Heparin is the drug that most commonly causes thrombocytopenia. HIT requires discontinuation of the use of heparin; if there is a clotting risk, use an alternative anticoagulant that does not cross-react with heparin-induced antibodies.

Chemotherapy-Associated Thrombocytopenia

For chemotherapy-associated thrombocytopenia, the threshold for platelet transfusion is $10 \times 10^9/L$, unless other risk factors for bleeding (eg, fever, mucosal lesion) are present. Interleukin-11 (oprelvekin) is the only pharmacologic agent that is approved in the United States for chemotherapy-associated thrombocytopenia, but stimulators of the thrombopoietin receptor are likely to be approved soon. Interleukin-11 is modestly effective and is associated with cytokine toxicities such as fluid retention and atrial dysrhythmias. If refractoriness to platelet transfusion is suspected, a platelet count should be performed 1 hour after transfusion to assess response.

Thrombocytopenia Due to Decreased Platelet Production

Thrombocytopenia caused by decreased platelet production typically occurs as the result of a bone marrow–infiltrating malignancy (eg, solid tumor, leukemia, lymphoma), infections (eg, HIV, cytomegalovirus, sepsis), or bone marrow failure states such as myelodysplastic syndrome or aplastic anemia. Management consists of identifying and treating the underlying disease.

Congenital Platelet Disorders

Congenital abnormalities of the platelet receptor glycoproteins lead to platelet dysfunction and thrombocytopenia. Bernard-Soulier syndrome is due to abnormalities in the glycoprotein Ib/IX receptor and is characterized by large platelets; Glanzmann thrombasthenia is due to abnormalities in the glycoprotein IIb/IIIa; and Wiskott-Aldrich syndrome is associated with small platelets. Mucocutaneous bleeding and postoperative bleeding are typical. Platelet transfusions

are used for prevention and treatment of hemorrhage. A risk of frequent transfusions is platelet alloimmunization.

Thrombocytopenia in Pregnancy

From 6% to 8% of pregnant women at term and 25% of women with preeclampsia have mild thrombocytopenia (with platelets >70 $\times 10^9/L$). The most common causes of thrombocytopenia in pregnancy are physiologic gestational thrombocytopenia and nonphysiologic benign gestational thrombocytopenia, which account for 75% of cases and are not associated with adverse maternal or fetal outcomes. The diagnosis is one of exclusion. No treatment is required, and platelet recovery generally occurs within 72 hours after delivery.

Other common causes include preeclampsia (including the HELLP syndrome), idiopathic autoimmune thrombocytopenia (or ITP), DIC, acute fatty liver of pregnancy, HIV infection, antiphospholipid antibodies, drugs (quinine and quinidine, cocaine, and heparin), nutritional deficiency, and thrombotic thrombocytopenic purpura. The primary treatment of the HELLP syndrome is stabilization of the patient's condition and delivery of the fetus.

Thrombophilia: The Hypercoagulable States

Thrombophilia refers to the tendency for thromboembolism (ie, having risk factors for thromboembolism), which may be congenital or acquired (Table 11-19). The presence of increasing numbers of risk factors further increases the risk of venous thrombosis. Lupus anticoagulant and hyperhomocysteinemia are associated with arterial thrombosis. Thrombophilic defects can be broadly classified into abnormalities of the procoagulant system and abnormalities of the anticoagulant system.

Table 11-19 Inherited and Acquired Thrombophilias

Inherited thrombophilia
    Activated protein C resistance due to factor V Leiden mutation
    Prothrombin G20210A mutation
    Anticoagulant deficiencies: antithrombin, protein C, protein S
    Selected dysfibrinogenemia
Acquired thrombophilia
    Lupus anticoagulant or antiphospholipid antibody syndrome
    Pregnancy
    Immobilization (trauma, postoperative state)
    Estrogens (oral contraceptives, hormone replacement therapy)
    Solid organ malignancy
    Myeloproliferative diseases
    Paroxysmal nocturnal hemoglobinuria
    Prolonged travel
    Obesity
    Age
Mixed risk factors
    Hyperhomocysteinemia
    Elevated levels of factors VIII, IX, & XI

Defects in the Procoagulant System

Inherited Risk Factors

The most common inherited defect is activated protein C resistance due to the factor V Leiden mutation (R506Q). This mutation causes activated factor V (V$_a$) to be resistant to inactivation by activated protein C (hence the term *activated protein C resistance*, abbreviated as *APCR*). The heterozygous mutation has a prevalence of 5% to 7% in the healthy white population and 20% to 50% among persons with venous thromboembolism (VTE). Heterozygotes have an approximately 2- to 4-fold increased risk, whereas homozygotes have an 80-fold increased risk of VTE. An example of the interaction between genetic and acquired risk factors is heterozygous carriers of factor V Leiden who are taking estrogen-containing oral contraceptives. They have a 30-fold increased risk of VTE compared with the risk among oral contraceptive users without factor V Leiden.

The next most common defect is the prothrombin G20210A mutation, which results in an elevation in the plasma prothrombin level. The heterozygous mutation has a prevalence of approximately 3% in the healthy white population and 6% to 18% among persons with VTE. Heterozygotes have an approximately 2-fold increased risk of VTE. These defects are common among white people and rare among people of Asian or African ancestry.

Other Risk Factors

Additional abnormalities of procoagulant proteins that confer an increased risk of VTE include increased levels of FVIII, FIX, and FXI. Currently, there is no established cutoff for this increased risk and there is no known genetic basis for these abnormalities.

Defects in the Anticoagulant System

Congenital deficiencies of the anticoagulants antithrombin, protein C, and protein S confer an increased risk of VTE. In the majority of patients, VTE develops by 50 years of age. Rare congenital abnormalities of fibrinogen (dysfibrinogenemias) pose a risk of thrombosis rather than hemorrhage.

VTE (DVT and pulmonary embolism) affects 1:1,000 people in the Western Hemisphere and is a major cause of morbidity. The annual mortality rate is 50,000, higher than that for breast cancer.

Risk Factors for Venous Thromboembolism

Acquired Risk Factors

Antiphospholipid antibodies such as lupus anticoagulant, anticardiolipin antibodies, and anti-β_2-glycoprotein I antibodies pose a significant risk of both venous and arterial thrombosis. Antiphospholipid antibody syndrome is characterized by clinical and laboratory criteria that include vascular thrombosis (venous or arterial) or recurrent miscarriage, or both, and laboratory findings that show the presence and persistence (on subsequent testing after 12 weeks) of lupus anticoagulant or medium to high titers of anticardiolipin or β_2-glycoprotein I antibody. If testing of asymptomatic patients shows the presence of antiphospholipid antibodies, they do not need anticoagulant therapy. Patients with vascular thrombosis should be treated with long-term anticoagulation, and women with recurrent fetal loss benefit from heparin (UFH or LMWH) in combination with aspirin during pregnancy.

Other acquired risk factors for VTE include immobilization (hospitalization, paralysis, etc), orthopedic or general surgery, and estrogen-containing drugs, which pose a significant risk of VTE. When any of these risk factors is combined with an underlying inherited risk factor (eg, factor V Leiden), the chances of symptomatic VTE increase significantly.

Mixed Inherited and Acquired Risk Factors

In selected situations (eg, hyperhomocysteinemia), genetic determinants (eg, MTHFR C677T mutation) pose a risk that may be compounded by acquired determinants (eg, dietary deficiencies of folate and vitamins B$_6$ and B$_{12}$), resulting in an increased risk of VTE. Although patients with thrombosis may be considered to have a congenital or acquired thrombophilia, thrombosis is a multifactorial disease that results from an interaction between congenital and acquired risk factors. Patients with inherited risk factors have a baseline increased risk; symptomatic VTE develops when the inherited risk factors are present in combination with acquired risk factors, such as pregnancy, estrogen use, or surgery.

Prevention of Venous Thromboembolism

All hospitalized medical, surgical, and trauma patients should be assessed for risk of VTE and given appropriate prophylaxis. The risk of VTE must be balanced against the risk of hemorrhage and the presence of contraindications to anticoagulation (Table 11-20). Although the benefits of mechanical and pharmacologic prophylaxis have been demonstrated, no more than 30% of patients at risk receive some sort of prophylaxis. The risk of VTE in surgical patients varies with the site of surgery, surgical technique, duration, type of anesthesia, complications (infection, shock, etc), and degree of immobilization. High-risk surgical procedures include open abdominal or urologic surgery, neurosurgery, gynecologic surgery, and orthopedic surgery of the lower extremities (joint replacement and hip fracture repair). In addition, patient-related risk factors include intensive care unit admission, age, cardiac dysfunction, acute myocardial infarction, congestive heart failure, cancer and its treatment, paralysis, prolonged immobility, prior VTE, obesity, varicose veins, central venous catheters, inflammatory bowel disease, lobar pneumonia, nephrotic syndrome, pregnancy, and estrogen use.

Suggested Strategies for Prophylaxis

Education and Early Ambulation—All patients should be educated about the signs and symptoms of VTE and the role of prophylaxis. They should be encouraged to ambulate as early and as often as feasible.

Low-Risk Patients—The strategies focus on education and early ambulation.

Moderate-Risk or High-Risk Patients—The strategies are those for low-risk patients but with the following additions: elastic graded compression stockings (below-knee), intermittent pneumatic compression if immobilized, and pharmacologic prophylaxis (UFH and LMWH are equivalent).

Very High-Risk Patients—The strategies are those for moderate- or high-risk patients but with the following additions: UFH is not

Table 11-20 Risk Factors and Incidence of Venous Thromboembolism

Level of Risk	Surgery	Additional Risk Factors	Calf DVT, %	Proximal DVT, %	Clinical PE, %	Fatal PE, %
Low	Minor	None	2	0.4	0.2	0.002
Moderate	Minor	Yes	10-20	2-4	1-2	0.1-0.4
	Major	None				
High	Major	Yes	20-40	4-8	2-4	0.4-1.0
Very High	Major (hip or knee arthroplasty, hip fracture, major trauma, spinal cord injury)	Prior VTE, active malignancy	40-80	10-20	4-10	0.2-0.5

Abbreviations: DVT, deep venous thrombosis; PE, pulmonary embolism; VTE, venous thromboembolism.

recommended; LMWH, fondaparinux, and adjusted-dose warfarin are used to keep the INR between 2.0 and 3.0; and extended out-of-hospital prophylaxis may be needed.

Patients With a Previous History of VTE or Thrombophilia—The strategies are those for very high-risk patients.

Evaluation of the Patient With Venous Thromboembolism

A detailed history of the presence or absence of acquired risk factors for VTE should be obtained. A detailed family history of VTE may point to an underlying familial thrombophilia. In women, recurrent miscarriage may point to an underlying familial or acquired (eg, lupus anticoagulant) thrombophilia. A thorough physical examination should include evaluation for venous stasis and for detection of an underlying malignancy.

Although important, clinical findings alone are poor predictors of the presence or severity of VTE, and objective diagnostic testing is required. Initial steps include an estimation of the pretest probability of VTE and the use of the dimer with further diagnostic testing as indicated. Considerations in the clinical evaluation include patient and family history of VTE, pregnancy, estrogen use, recent trauma, surgery, hospitalization, malignancy, and travel. The most critical initial component of the examination is to determine the presence or absence of venous limb gangrene (phlegmasia cerulea dolens), in which severe obstruction of extremity venous drainage leads to congestion and eventual obstruction of arterial inflow. Thrombolytic therapy, fasciotomy, or thrombectomy may be indicated.

Step 1: Determine Clinical Pretest Probability—The Wells Model (Table 11-21) categorizes the pretest probability of DVT into high (≥3 points), moderate (1 or 2 points), and low (<1 point). In a study of 593 patients, 10 of 329 low-risk patients (3%), 32 of 193 moderate-risk patients (17%), and 53 of 71 high-risk patients (75%) had DVT diagnosed. The positive predictive value was 82%. For low-risk patients, the negative predictive value of ultrasonography was 99.7%; therefore, low-risk patients with normal ultrasonography results do not need further testing. However, for high-risk patients, the negative predictive value of ultrasonography was only 82%; therefore, further testing should be considered for high-risk patients. A similar model has been applied to pulmonary embolism (Table 11-22), which stratifies patients according to whether pulmonary embolism is less likely (≤4) or likely (>4).

Step 2: D-Dimer Levels—The level of D dimers, which are breakdown products from cross-linked stabilized fibrin clots, can be elevated in patients who have had thromboembolism, recent surgery, hemorrhage, or malignancies. Used in conjunction with evaluation of clinical pretest probability, a negative result for D dimer has a high negative predictive value for DVT, thus avoiding unnecessary diagnostic tests. It is most useful for ambulatory outpatients, and it should not be used to exclude VTE in hospitalized patients or patients with malignancy or recent trauma, surgery, or hemorrhage. In those patients, proceeding with imaging studies is appropriate.

Initial laboratory testing should include routine tests, such as CBC, blood smear, serum chemistry studies, baseline PT and aPTT (before initiation of anticoagulants), and urinalysis. Further investigations (eg, radiologic studies) should be reserved for further investigation of initial history and examination findings and patient risk factors (eg, smoking). Testing should also include age-appropriate cancer screening.

Thrombophilia Testing

It is reasonable to perform thrombophilia testing with the recognition that selected assays are affected by acute thrombotic events, heparin, and warfarin. Testing should be considered if results will affect long-term

Table 11-21 Wells Model for Predicting Clinical Pretest Probability of Deep Venous Thrombosis

Clinical Variable	Points
Active cancer	1
Paralysis or recent limb casting	1
Recent immobility >3 days	1
Local vein tenderness	1
Limb swelling	1
Lateral calf swelling >3 cm	1
Pitting edema	1
Collateral superficial vein	1
Alternative diagnoses likely	−2

Table 11-22 Wells Model for Predicting Clinical Pretest Probability of Pulmonary Embolism

Clinical Variable	Points
Clinical signs & symptoms of DVT	3
Alternative diagnoses less likely	3
Heart rate >100 beats per minute	1.5
Immobilization or surgery in previous 4 wk	1.5
Previous DVT or PE	1.5
Hemoptysis	1
Malignancy	1
Collateral superficial vein	1

Abbreviations: DVT, deep venous thrombosis; PE, pulmonary embolism.

management of anticoagulation (Table 11-19). Thrombophilia testing can be performed before initiation of anticoagulation or after completion of anticoagulation appropriate for a thrombotic event if certain caveats are recognized and appropriate follow-up testing is performed. DNA-based testing (factor V Leiden and prothrombin G20210A mutation) is not affected by acute thrombosis or anticoagulants. Anticoagulants can produce false-positive results for lupus anticoagulants and reduced protein C and protein S levels, and acute thrombosis can result in reduced levels of protein C, protein S, and antithrombin.

Thrombophilia does not alter acute management of VTE except in 2 circumstances. The prolonged baseline aPTT seen in association with lupus anticoagulants would make monitoring of UFH complex; however, use of heparin assay (anti-Xa levels) or use of LMWH, which requires no monitoring, could be considered. A congenital deficiency of protein C or protein S increases the risk of warfarin skin necrosis, especially if heparin therapy (with UFH or LMWH) is prematurely discontinued (see "Management of Venous Thromboembolism" section). Thrombophilia affects the duration of anticoagulation. For thrombophilic conditions that predict a high risk of recurrence, a longer duration of anticoagulation is needed.

Diagnostic Approach for Deep Venous Thrombosis
Low Clinical Pretest Probability Plus Negative D-Dimer Results—DVT is effectively ruled out and no further testing is needed, unless new or progressive symptoms occur. With this approach, VTE subsequently develops in less than 1% of patients.

Moderate or High Clinical Pretest Probability—patients in this category should have diagnostic imaging studies performed (eg, duplex ultrasonography with compression). If the imaging study results are negative, checking the D-dimer level is reasonable. If the level is elevated, further imaging studies are indicated.

Diagnostic Approach for Pulmonary Embolism
Pulmonary embolism should be considered in patients with dyspnea, pleuritic chest pain, and tachypnea. Initial assessment consists of assessing hemodynamic stability. Alternative therapies such as thrombolytic therapy or surgical thrombectomy may be indicated. If pulmonary embolism is less likely (score ≤4), the D-dimer level should be obtained;

if it is negative, alternative diagnoses should be considered, and if it is elevated, imaging studies should be performed. If pulmonary embolism is likely (score >4), proceeding directly to imaging studies is appropriate.

Treatment of Venous Thromboembolism
Acute Management of VTE—For established VTE, the aims of initial therapy include prevention of extension or embolization of the thrombus and reduction of postphlebitic syndrome, and the aim of long-term therapy is secondary prevention or reduction of the risk of recurrence. For patients who are hemodynamically unstable, hospitalization is critical; however, for most hemodynamically stable patients, outpatient anticoagulation is reasonable. After excluding contraindications to anticoagulation, initiate therapeutic doses of LMWH subcutaneously, and simultaneously initiate oral warfarin. LMWH does not need monitoring, but the INR is used to assess warfarin effect. The use of both agents is continued for at least 5 days or until the INR is in the therapeutic range (2-3) for at least 48 hours before the use of LMWH is discontinued. Use of knee-high compression stockings has been shown to reduce the incidence of postphlebitic syndrome.

Chronic Management of VTE—The use of warfarin is continued for an appropriate duration of therapy. INR is monitored every 4 to 6 weeks. Long-term outcomes have been shown to be superior when VTE is managed in anticoagulation clinics and with home INR devices.

Calf Vein Thrombosis—Asymptomatic calf vein thrombosis (CVT) can be observed if the patient is willing and able to return for follow-up compression ultrasonography to document stability or progression of the clot. For symptomatic or progressive CVT, anticoagulation should be initiated.

Proximal DVT—LMWH and warfarin should be administered as described above.

Pulmonary Embolism—Patients with pulmonary embolism should be hospitalized for at least 24 hours to assess stability. Selected asymptomatic, clinically stable patients may be treated as an outpatient with LMWH and warfarin as described above.

Duration of Warfarin Anticoagulation—For DVT and pulmonary embolism in association with a temporary (reversible) risk factor, 3 months of warfarin is sufficient. For DVT occurring with no apparent risk factor (idiopathic), warfarin is used for up to 6 months. For recurrent DVT, warfarin is used for at least 12 months. For hemodynamically significant or idiopathic pulmonary embolism, long-term warfarin is reasonable. Long-term warfarin is also reasonable for VTE in patients who have underlying thrombophilia from lupus anticoagulant or deficiency of protein C, protein S, or antithrombin or for patients who are compound heterozygous for factor V Leiden and prothrombin 20210A mutation. Continuing warfarin anticoagulation should be balanced with the risk of hemorrhage.

Anticoagulants

Anticoagulant drugs (antiplatelet agents, anticoagulants, and fibrinolytic agents) are used for prevention and treatment of venous and arterial thrombosis. Utility of specific agent is dictated by the pathophysiology of the thrombosis: antiplatelet agents are primarily used for arterial thrombosis, and anticoagulants that interfere with the procoagulant system are primarily used for VTE.

Mechanism of Action—The complexity of the coagulation system provides multiple potential targets for anticoagulants. Broadly considered, the mechanisms include depletion of procoagulant proteins (eg, warfarin) and inhibition of procoagulant proteins indirectly (eg, UFH, LMWH, and pentasaccharides such as fondaparinux) or directly (eg, direct thrombin inhibitors such as lepirudin, bivalirudin, and argatroban). The enhancement of the fibrinolytic system results in clot lysis (eg, thrombolytic therapy).

Warfarin

Mechanism of Action—Warfarin, a vitamin K antagonist, limits the γ-carboxylation of the vitamin K–dependent coagulation proteins II, VII, IX, and X and anticoagulant proteins C and S, impairing their biologic function in blood coagulation.

Plasma Half-Life—An oral dose is rapidly absorbed and has a high bioavailability. Although the half-life of the drug is 36 to 42 hours, recovery of vitamin K–dependent factors takes longer.

Clearance—Clearance is through the liver; thus, patients with liver disease, congestive heart failure, or metastatic cancers to the liver may have a reduced dosage requirement.

Dosing—A standard oral dose of 5 to 10 mg daily is initiated with dose adjustments of approximately 10% (increase or decrease), depending on the INR results.

Monitoring—The typical target INR is 2.5 (range 2-3) for most indications (eg, VTE, atrial fibrillation). Higher targets are recommended for prosthetic valves (INR, 2.5-3.5).

Clinical Use—Warfarin is used for primary treatment and secondary prophylaxis of venous and arterial thromboembolism and for prophylaxis in patients with mechanical heart valves.

Key Points About Warfarin

1. Drug interactions occur with various drugs. Herbal preparations either antagonize or exaggerate the warfarin effect. More frequent monitoring should be considered in such situations (eg, change in medication).
2. Vitamin K and vitamin K–rich foods antagonize the warfarin effect.
3. Upon discontinuation, it takes 4 to 5 days for the INR to normalize. It may take longer in the elderly or in those with congestive heart failure and metastatic cancers to the liver or other liver disease.
4. The variability in dose response between individuals is due to multiple causes (diet, pharmacogenetics, medication interaction, etc).
5. Warfarin failure is commonly due to subtherapeutic INRs.
6. Monitoring and follow-up in anticoagulation clinics and use of home INR monitoring results in superior outcomes (INR in the therapeutic range longer).
7. Patient education is critical.
8. Warfarin use in breastfeeding patients is safe.

Key Points About INR Monitoring

1. Although PT reagents contain a heparin neutralizer, the presence of excess heparin (eg, a sample collected shortly after administration of a bolus of UFH, or a sample collected through a heparin-coated catheter) will prolong the PT and thus the INR.
2. Direct thrombin inhibitors (lepirudin, aragatroban, and bivalirudin) may prolong the PT and INR.
3. Warfarin should be administered at night and INRs should be checked in the morning to allow FVII levels to stabilize. At least 16 hours should elapse between warfarin administration and specimen collection.
4. INR determinations should be obtained monthly in most hemodynamically stable patients, and no more than 6 weeks should elapse between determinations.

Key Points About Initiation of Warfarin Administration for VTE

1. Warfarin administration can be initiated simultaneously with heparin (UFH or LMWH) for the management of VTE.
2. Use of heparin and warfarin should be overlapped for at least 5 days or for at least 48 hours after a therapeutic INR is achieved.
3. Loading doses of warfarin provide no advantage over starting with typical maintenance doses of 5 mg.

Key Points About Toxicity and Management

1. If warfarin is taken in the first trimester of pregnancy, fetal hemorrhage and embryopathy can occur.
2. The average annual risk of bleeding is 3% to 9%.
3. Warfarin skin necrosis is a rare complication that can occur in patients with congenital protein C deficiency in whom heparin use has been discontinued prematurely and in patients with HIT type II who are receiving a direct thrombin inhibitor and warfarin and use of the direct thrombin inhibitor is discontinued prematurely.

Contraindications—Relative contraindications for warfarin include recent hemorrhage or a hemorrhagic tendency (eg, thrombocytopenia or coagulation factor abnormalities).

Key Points About Managing Supratherapeutic INRs
Nonbleeding patients

1. If the INR is greater than the therapeutic target but less than 5, lower or omit a warfarin dose, with a subsequent dose reduction (by about 10%).
2. If the INR is greater than 5 but less than 9, omit the next 1 or 2 doses of warfarin, monitor the INR daily, and resume warfarin at a lower dose.
3. If the INR is greater than 9, stop giving warfarin, give 1 to 2 mg vitamin K orally, and check the INR within 24 hours.

Patients with bleeding and any INR

1. Stop warfarin administration
2. Transfuse fresh frozen plasma
3. Give 1 mg vitamin K slowly intravenously (IV)

Patients with life-threatening bleeding

1. Stop warfarin administration
2. Transfuse fresh frozen plasma
3. Give 1 mg vitamin K slowly intravenously

4. Consider prothrombin complex concentrates or recombinant FVIIa

Unfractionated Heparin

Mechanism of Action—The essential pentasaccharide sequence on UFH binds to antithrombin, accelerating its inhibition of thrombin and factor Xa. It also increases the activity of tissue factor pathway inhibitor.

Plasma Half-Life and Clearance—UFH is cleared by the reticuloendothelial system. The anticoagulant effect wears off in 4 to 6 hours.

Clinical Use—UFH is used extensively in thromboprophylaxis, treatment of VTE, management of acute coronary syndromes, peripheral arterial surgery, artery bypass grafting, dialysis, and heparin flushes to maintain venous and arterial (peripheral and central) catheter patency.

Dosing—UFH can be administered IV or subcutaneously. Owing to extensive nonspecific plasma protein binding, an initial bolus of UFH (which saturates the nonspecific binding) is followed by continuous infusion.

Monitoring—There are 3 options for monitoring UFH:
1. aPTT—Therapeutic range, 1.5 to 2.5 times the control
2. Anti-Xa activity (heparin assay)—Therapeutic range, 0.4 to 0.7 IU/mL
3. Activated clotting time (ACT)—Restricted for use in cardiac bypass procedures

Pregnancy and Breast-feeding—UFH and LMWH do not cross the placenta and are not secreted in breast milk.

Heparin Resistance—Heparin resistance occurs in patients who require unusually high doses of heparin (eg, >40,000 units per 24 hours) to prolong their aPTT into a therapeutic range. The mechanism involves the following factors: 1) antithrombin deficiency, 2) increased heparin clearance, 3) elevations in heparin-binding proteins (acute-phase reactant proteins such as vWF), and 4) elevations in FVIII and fibrinogen levels. Heparin resistance is managed by targeting anti-factor Xa concentrations of 0.35 to 0.7 IU/mL, which results in an equivalent outcome in patients being treated for DVT who have heparin resistance.

Key Points About Use of UFH
1. Erratic bioavailability with subcutaneous administration
2. The need for IV administration
3. The need for frequent monitoring with aPTT
4. The risk of HIT
5. Risk of osteoporosis with long-term use

Toxicity and Management—The risk of hemorrhage increases with higher target aPTTs. Immune-mediated thrombocytopenia (HIT type II) occurs in up to 5% of patients receiving UFH (see the section on HIT). Hemorrhagic side effects resulting from excessive UFH can be treated with protamine; however, side effects include hypotension, bradycardia, and anaphylaxis.

Contraindications—Contraindications include a history of HIT type II, recent hemorrhage, and an underlying hemorrhagic tendency.

Low-Molecular-Weight Heparin (Dalteparin, Enoxaparin, and Tinzaparin)

Mechanism of Action—Like UFH, the essential pentasaccharide sequence of LMWH activates antithrombin, which in turn inhibits FXa. LMWH has a greater anti-Xa activity than anti-IIa activity.

Plasma Half-Life and Clearance—The half-life is 4 to 6 hours, and clearance is renal.

Monitoring—In general, monitoring is not required, but it is advisable in renal insufficiency (calculated creatinine clearance <30 mL/min), when the patient has low body weight (<50 kg) or obesity, and with prolonged use (eg, pregnancy). The anti-Xa assay (heparin assay) is used.

Therapeutic Range—The anti-Xa level measured 4 hours after the LMWH dose should be 0.6 to 1.0 IU/mL with twice-daily dosing and 1.0 to 2.0 IU/mL with once-daily dosing.

Clinical Use—Clinical indications are venous thromboprophylaxis and treatment of VTE.

Toxicity and Management—Hemorrhage may increase with higher doses. Rarely, immune-mediated thrombocytopenia (HIT type II) occurs in less than 1% of postsurgical patients. Hemorrhagic side effects can be partially reversed with protamine.

Contraindications—Contraindications include a history of HIT type II, recent hemorrhage, and an underlying hemorrhagic tendency. Dose adjustment is required for renal insufficiency.

Fondaparinux

Further depolymerization of LMWH results in isolation of the unique pentasaccharide sequence responsible for binding to antithrombin.

Mechanism of Action—The mechanism of action is similar to that of LMWH.

Plasma Half-Life and Clearance—The half-life is 17 hours. The clearance is renal, so dose modifications are necessary in renal disease, and fondaparinux is contraindicated in severe renal disease.

Monitoring—Assays specific for fondaparinux-mediated anti-Xa activity are available only in specialized laboratories.

Clinical Use of Fondaparinux—Fondaparinux is used to prevent and treat VTE.

Toxicity and Management—Hemorrhage may increase with higher doses. Protamine does *not* reverse hemorrhagic side effects. Although protamine is not effective for hemorrhage due to fondaparinux, administration of procoagulant agents such as recombinant factor VIIa (rFVIIa) has been shown to result in hemostasis. Since the patient probably has a thrombosis for which fondaparinux is being administered, use of rFVIIa may result in worsening of the thrombosis.

Contraindications—Contraindications include recent hemorrhage, underlying hemorrhagic tendency, and renal insufficiency.

Direct Thrombin Inhibitors (Lepirudin, Argatroban, and Bivalirudin)

Mechanism of Action—The mechanism of action is direct inhibition of thrombin. Key advantages of direct thrombin inhibitors are the following: 1) their ability to inhibit circulating and fibrin-bound thrombin, 2) the lack of nonspecific plasma protein binding (predictable anticoagulant activity), and 3) no risk of HIT.

Key Points About Plasma Half-Life and Clearance
1. Lepirudin—IV injection, 60 minutes; subcutaneous injection, 120 minutes; renal clearance
2. Argatroban—IV injection, 45 minutes; hepatic clearance
3. Bivalirudin—IV injection, 25 minutes; a fraction is excreted through the kidneys

Monitoring—The aPTT ratio target is 1.5 to 2.5. Monitor aPTT beginning 4 hours after initiation of the infusion and then daily thereafter. Recheck aPTT 4 hours after any dosage changes.

Clinical Use—Lepirudin and argatroban are used to prevent and treat HIT. Bivalirudin is used in acute coronary syndromes.

Toxicity and Management—Bleeding and rarely anaphylaxis can occur with lepirudin. There are no known reversal agents.

Thrombolytic Therapy (Streptokinase, Urokinase, and Recombinant Tissue-Type Plasminogen Activator)

Overview of Fibrinolysis—Plasminogen, the main fibrinolytic protein, is activated by plasminogen activators to plasmin, which cleaves fibrin clots, resulting in clot lysis.

Mechanism of Action—Thrombolytic agents are essentially plasminogen activators. Plasmin lyses fibrin clots into degradation products (D dimers, fibrin degradation products). The inability to distinguish pathologic thrombi from physiologic thrombi contributes to hemorrhagic complications common to all thrombolytic agents.

Clinical Utility of Thrombolytic Agents—Systemic or catheter-directed administration of thrombolytic agents is used to manage venous and arterial (myocardial infarction, stroke, and peripheral arterial) thrombosis that potentially threatens the patient's limb or life. These agents are also used for management of occluded central venous catheters and occasionally for catheter-associated thrombi. Although thrombolytic therapy has been used for iliofemoral vein thrombosis, its long-term benefit over standard anticoagulation has not been confirmed in randomized studies.

Laboratory Monitoring—Laboratory monitoring includes CBC, PT, aPTT, fibrinogen levels, and plasminogen levels.

Toxicity—Hemorrhage can occur. Streptokinase causes allergic reactions (about 6% of patients) and anaphylaxis (0.1%).

Management of Hemorrhage—Hemorrhage is managed with transfusion of cryoprecipitate to increase fibrinogen to approximately 100 mg/dL and platelet transfusion (platelets contain fibrinogen).

Antiplatelet Agents

Platelet plug formation is an initial hemostatic response, and the presence of multiple platelet receptors provides potential targets for antiplatelet agents.

Aspirin

Mechanism of Action—Inactivation of platelet prostaglandin H synthase (cyclooxygenase 1 and 2) leads to decreased production of thromboxane A_2, resulting in impairment of platelet activation. Absorption is rapid (<1 hour), and antiplatelet effects last for the duration of the platelet lifespan (1 week).

Clinical Use—Aspirin is used for primary prevention of myocardial infarction in patients older than 50 years (prevention of 4 events per 1,000 patients treated). Aspirin is used for secondary prevention of angina, acute myocardial infarction, transient ischemic attack, and thrombotic strokes and after coronary artery bypass surgery, peripheral arterial bypass surgery, and carotid endarterectomy. The dosage ranges from 75 to 325 mg daily.

Role in VTE Prophylaxis—Compared with heparin and warfarin, aspirin is inferior, so it should not be used in medical and surgical VTE prophylaxis.

Toxicities—Toxicities include gastric ulcerations and gastrointestinal tract blood loss. To account for the duration of its antiplatelet effect, aspirin use should be discontinued at least 5 to 7 days before major surgery.

Thienopyridines (Ticlopidine and Clopidogrel)

Mechanism of Action—The mechanism of action is inhibition of adenosine diphosphate receptors and thus inhibition of platelet activation. Clopidogrel is rapidly absorbed, and it inhibits platelets within 2 hours. As with aspirin, the inhibition effects last for 1 week.

Clinical Use—Currently, there are no data supporting the use of thienopyridines in primary prevention of cardiovascular events. The drugs are used in secondary prevention of thrombotic stroke, myocardial infarction, and symptomatic peripheral arterial disease in combination with aspirin for acute coronary syndromes.

Toxicities—Ticlopidine may cause bleeding and TTP; its use is declining. As with aspirin, use of clopidogrel should be discontinued at least 5 to 7 days before major surgery.

Glycoprotein IIb/IIIa Antagonists (Abciximab, Eptifibatide, and Tirofiban)

Mechanism of Action—Parenteral administration results in inhibition of the platelet receptor glycoprotein IIb/IIIa, resulting in platelet inhibition.

Clinical Use—These drugs are used for percutaneous coronary intervention, unstable angina, and non–Q-wave myocardial infarction. Oral glycoprotein IIb/IIIa inhibitors are not as effective for prevention of myocardial infarction.

Toxicity—Bleeding may occur. Severe thrombocytopenia may occur with abciximab.

Hematology Pharmacy Review
Scott E. Apelgren, MS, BCPS, BCOP, BCNSP, Robert C. Wolf, PharmD

Drug	Toxic/Adverse Effects	Comments
Alkylating agents		
Carmustine	Delayed marrow suppression, nausea, vomiting, pulmonary, hepatotoxicity, secondary leukemia	Cumulative marrow suppression, crosses blood-brain barrier
Busulfan	Pulmonary fibrosis, hepatic venoocclusive disease, skin hyperpigmentation	Liver metabolism, renal excretion
Carboplatin	Marrow suppression, nausea & vomiting, less nephrotoxicity & neurotoxicity than cisplatin	Renal excretion
Chlorambucil	Pulmonary, secondary leukemia, myelosuppression	Hepatic metabolism
Cisplatin	Nephrotoxicity, peripheral neuropathy, ototoxicity, magnesium depletion	Renal excretion, Raynaud phenomenon
Cyclophosphamide	Acute nonlymphocytic leukemia & dysmyelopoietic syndromes (monosomy 5 and 7), bladder cancer, leukopenia, hemorrhagic cystitis, pulmonary fibrosis, SIAD, alopecia, nausea, vomiting	Liver metabolism to active compound, renal excretion, lower dose with renal failure, late transitional cell carcinoma of bladder
Dacarbazine	Marrow suppression, flulike syndrome, severe nausea & vomiting, fever	
Melphalan	Marrow suppression, secondary leukemia, stomatitis (high dose)	Absence of renal clearance allows use of high-dose melphalan in patients with renal failure, erratic oral absorption
Nitrogen mustard	Marrow suppression, nausea & vomiting, sterility, secondary leukemia	
Streptozocin	Diabetes, marrow suppression, severe nausea & vomiting, renal	Leads to pancreatic & endocrine insufficiency
Procarbazine	Secondary leukemia, sterility	
Ifosfamide	Myelosuppression, CNS toxicity (lethargy, confusion), cystitis	Liver metabolism, renal elimination
Antibiotics		
Bleomycin	Pulmonary fibrosis (threshold 400 mcg/lifetime but may recur at lower doses), fever & chills, myalgias, skin pigmentation, alopecia, adult respiratory distress syndrome with oxygen	Lower dose with renal insufficiency
Dactinomycin	Marrow suppression, radiation recall, nausea & vomiting, mucositis, alopecia	
Daunorubicin	Marrow suppression, radiation recall, cardiomyopathy, mucositis, nausea & vomiting, alopecia, acute nonlymphocytic leukemia	Decrease dose by 50% if bilirubin >1.5 mg/dL or by 75% if bilirubin >3.0 mg/dL
Doxorubicin	Dose-related cardiomyopathy, marrow suppression, alopecia, nausea & vomiting, stomatitis, radiation recall, acute nonlymphocytic leukemia	Liver metabolism, biliary excretion, decrease dose by 50% if bilirubin >1.5 mg/dL or by 75% if bilirubin >3.0 mg/dL
Idarubicin	Myelosuppression, alopecia	
Mitomycin C	Delayed marrow suppression, nausea & vomiting, alopecia, hepatotoxicity, microangiopathic hemolytic anemia	Vesicant, alkylator, forms free radicals

Hematology Pharmacy Review (continued)

Drug	Toxic/Adverse Effects	Comments
	Antibiotics (continued)	
Mitoxantrone	Marrow suppression, cardiac toxicity, nausea & vomiting, mucositis, alopecia, blue sclera & urine	
	Hormones	
Corticosteroids	Diabetes, hepatotoxicity, aseptic necrosis, adrenal insufficiency, myopathy, infection, osteoporosis, peptic ulcer disease, hypokalemia, psychosis, cataract	
	Plant derivatives	
Etoposide (VP-16)	Acute nonlymphocytic leukemia, t(11q23), myelosuppression, hypotension, mucositis	
Vincristine	Neurotoxicity (peripheral, autonomic, cranial)	
Vinblastine	SIADH, myelosuppression	
	Antimetabolites	
2'-Deoxycoformycin	Myelosuppression & immunosuppression	
Fludarabine	Opportunistic infections	
2-Chlorodeoxyadenosine		
Cytarabine	Myelosuppression, neurotoxicity (high dose, conjunctivitis (high dose)	
Azacitidine	Myelosuppression, nausea, vomiting, diarrhea, constipation, fever, fatigue, elevated serum creatinine and hepatic enzymes, hypokalemia, renal tubular acidosis	Use with caution in patients with hepatic impairment
Decitabine	Myelosuppression, diarrhea, nausea, constipation, fever, peripheral edema	No dosing guidelines are available for patients with hepatic or renal impairment
Methotrexate	Myelosuppression, mucositis, hepatotoxicity	Drug interactions: NSAIDs, probenecid
Nelarabine	Anemia, leukopenia, neutropenia, thrombocytopenia, peripheral edema, headache, somnolence, peripheral neuropathy, neurotoxicity	Dose-limiting paresthesias, ataxia, confusion, convulsion, & coma have been reported
	Other agents	
Alemtuzumab	Fever, chills/rigors, opportunistic infections	Monoclonal antibody to CD52
Bortezomib	Sensory peripheral neuropathy, orthostatic hypertension, fever, thrombocytopenia, neutropenia	Proteasome inhibitor
Asparaginase	Hypersensitivity, hemorrhage/thrombosis,	
PEG-asparaginase	hyperglycemia, pancreatitis, increased LFTs, somnolence/confusion	
Hydroxyurea	Myelosuppression (rapid), anorexia, hyperpigmentation	
Lenalidomide	Anemia, neutropenia, thrombocytopenia, diarrhea, rash/pruritus, fatigue	Dose-dependent myelosuppression can be reversed by decreasing dose or briefly stopping treatment
Tretinoin	Retinoic acid syndrome; xerostomia, cheilitis; skin desquamation; dry, irritated eyes; myalgias; hyperleukocytosis; teratogenic; hypertriglyceridemia	Pulmonary infiltrates, fluid retention, hypotension (responsive/preventable with dexamethasone)

Hematology Pharmacy Review (continued)

Drug	Toxic/Adverse Effects	Comments
Other agents (continued)		
Thalidomide	Sedation, peripheral neuropathy, constipation, rash, teratogenic	
Arsenic trioxide	Acute promyelocytic leukemia differentiation syndrome, QT-interval prolongation, myelosuppression, targeted therapy	Fever, dyspnea, weight gain, pleural or pericardial effusion ± leukocytosis
Targeted therapy		
Dasatinib	Fluid retention, abdominal pain, diarrhea, nausea, vomiting, muscle pain, bleeding, myelosuppression, QT-interval prolongation, fever	Useful in patients who are intolerant of or refractory to imatinib
Imatinib (STI571)	Myelosuppression, fluid retention, nausea, muscle cramps, diarrhea, headache, myalgia, arthralgia	Tyrosine kinase inhibitor Multiple potential drug interactions via cytochrome P450-3A4 pathway
Rituximab	Fever, chills/rigors, headache, hypotension, anaphylactoid symptoms	Monoclonal antibody to CD20
Vorinostat	Fatigue, diarrhea, nausea, hyperglycemia, dysgeusia, anorexia, weight loss, thrombocytopenia, alopecia, muscle spasm	Oral histone deacetylase inhibitor
Immunotherapy		
Interferon alfa	Fatigue, flulike symptoms, myelosuppression, increased LFTs	Cytochrome P450 inhibitor (multiple potential drug interactions)
Filgrastim (G-CSF)	Bone pain, fever	
Sargramostim (GM-CSF)	Bone pain, fever	
Oprelvekin (interleukin 11)	Fluid retention, tachycardia, fatigue	
Gemtuzumab ozogamicin	Myelosuppression, fever, chills/rigors, hypotension, increased LFTs	Monoclonal antibody to CD33 conjugated to calicheamicin (antitumor antibiotic)

Abbreviations: CNS, central nervous system; G-CSF, granulocyte colony-stimulating factor; GM-CSF, granulocyte-macrophage colony-stimulating factor; LFT, liver function test; NSAID, nonsteroidal anti-inflammatory drug; SIAD, syndrome of inappropriate antidiuresis.

Hematologically Active Agents Used in Cardiology

Drug	Toxic/Adverse Effects	Hypersensitivity	Pregnancy Category
Argatroban	Hemorrhage, hypotension	Coughing, dyspnea, rash	B
Bivalirudin	Hemorrhage, GI symptoms	None	B
Lepirudin	Hemorrhage, heart failure	Anaphylactoid, angioedema (rare), cough, bronchial spasm, stridor, rash	B
Cilostazol	Headache, diarrhea, flushing, hypotension, tachycardia	Rash	C
Ximelagatran	Hemorrhage, elevated LFTs	Unknown	Unknown

Abbreviations: GI, gastrointestinal tract; LFT, liver function test.

Questions

Multiple Choice (choose the best answer)

Benign Hematology

1. A 67-year-old woman presents with a 4-month history of progressive dyspnea. Fourteen years ago, she received a diagnosis of diffuse large B-cell non-Hodgkin lymphoma involving the retroperitoneal lymph nodes and was treated with cyclophosphamide, hydroxydaunomycin, vincristine, and prednisone (CHOP) combination chemotherapy. Physical examination is remarkable for generalized pallor; there is no adenopathy or splenomegaly. The complete blood cell count (CBC) shows the following: hemoglobin 7.5 g/dL, mean corpuscular volume (MCV) 68.6 fL, and erythrocyte count 3.45 × 10^{12}/L. Which of the following is the next best test to evaluate the cause of the anemia?

    a. Ferritin level
    b. Vitamin B$_{12}$ level
    c. Folate level
    d. Peripheral blood smear
    e. Bone marrow examination with cytogenetics

2. A 73-year-old retired accountant seeks medical attention because of involuntary weight loss, increased abdominal girth, and progressive fatigue. Physical examination reveals a cachectic man with massive splenomegaly (the spleen is firm but not tender and extends to the pelvic brim), generalized pallor, and bilateral lower extremity pitting edema (2+). Laboratory studies indicate a hemoglobin of 6.5 g/dL with an MCV of 83 fL. The peripheral blood smear is shown. Which of the following is the most likely finding on bone marrow biopsy?

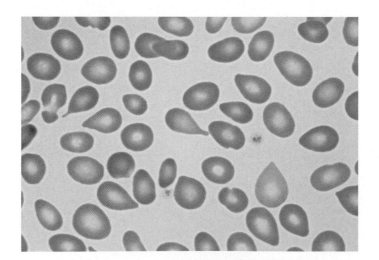

Question 2

a. Acellular marrow
b. Nodules of mature lymphocytes with λ light chain restriction
c. Replacement of the marrow by diffuse sheets of blasts containing Auer rods
d. Foci of atypical plasma cells
e. Hypercellular marrow with reticulin fibrosis

3. A 19-year-old man with β-thalassemia major broke his ankle in a skateboard accident and underwent surgical reduction of the fracture. Since childhood he has been treated with red blood cell (RBC) transfusions and iron chelation therapy. Preoperatively an RBC antibody screen was negative and he received a transfusion with 2 units of ABO/Rh-matched blood, owing to a hemoglobin of 8.3 g/dL. Surgical blood loss was minimal. Now, 8 days later, his hemoglobin is 8.1 g/dL, and he has mild painless jaundice. Antibody testing now shows an anti-Jk^a antibody. What is the most appropriate way to manage this complication?

    a. Intravenous gamma globulin
    b. Plasmapheresis
    c. Corticosteroids
    d. Epoetin alfa or darbepoietin alfa
    e. Transfusion of Jk^a-negative RBCs

4. A 67-year-old Sicilian woman presents with fatigue, low back pain, and a 9-kg weight loss. The physical examination findings are unremarkable. The hemoglobin concentration is 10.4 g/dL, the MCV is 78.4 fL, and the erythrocyte count is 4.10 × 10^{12}/L. The platelet count is 536 × 10^9/L. The erythrocyte sedimentation is 120 mm per hour and C-reactive protein is also elevated. The serum ferritin level is 357 ng/mL (reference range, 20-200 ng/mL). The total iron-binding capacity is 247 mcg/dL (240-450 mcg/dL) with 68% saturation. A peripheral smear shows moderate anisopoikilocytosis but is otherwise unremarkable. What is the most likely diagnosis?

    a. Iron deficiency
    b. Glucose-6-phosphate dehydrogenase (G6PD) deficiency
    c. Anemia of chronic disease
    d. Vitamin B$_{12}$ deficiency
    e. Lead poisoning

5. A 26-year-old previously healthy woman is referred for evaluation of abdominal distention, hepatomegaly, and anemia. A CBC demonstrates a hemoglobin concentration of 10.0 g/dL and an MCV of 97 fL. The white blood cell count (WBC) is 3.0 × 10^9/L. The platelet count is 98 × 10^9/L. The haptoglobin level is low. The total bilirubin is 4.0 mg/dL, with a direct bilirubin of 0.8 mg/dL. The peripheral smear shows polychromasia with no spherocytes. The reticulocyte count is 8.4%. A

Coombs test is negative. What is the next best test to evaluate the cause of her anemia?

a. Endoscopy to exclude a bleeding source
b. G6PD level
c. Flow cytometry for paroxysmal nocturnal hemoglobinuria
d. Antigliadin antibodies
e. Vitamin B_{12} level

6. A 68-year-old man presents for routine follow-up of insulin-requiring type 2 diabetes mellitus and autoimmune thyroid disease. A CBC shows a hemoglobin concentration of 10.5 g/dL, with an MCV of 108 fL. Ferritin is 206 ng/mL; bowel habits are normal and he has not had any blood in the stool. His weight has been stable over the past 3 visits. What is the most likely cause of the anemia?

a. Gastrointestinal tract bleeding
b. Alcoholism
c. Hypothyroidism
d. Celiac sprue
e. Pernicious anemia

7. A 53-year-old Lebanese-American restaurant owner takes a food-tasting tour to the Greek islands. On the last day of his trip, he partakes in a sumptuous feast including several regional delicacies. On the airplane home, he notices that his urine seems darker than normal, and his wife notices that his sclerae are yellow. His stool pattern is unchanged. The following day he visits his internist and is noted to be mildly icteric with normal vital signs; the spleen is nonpalpable. Examination is otherwise unremarkable. His hemoglobin is 10.8 g/dL, with a normal MCV. The total bilirubin is 5.7 mg/dL and the direct bilirubin is 0.3 mg/dL. A Coombs test is negative. Creatinine is 1.4 g/dL and a rapid urine dipstick test shows 3+ blood. The partial thromboplastin time (PTT) and international normalized ratio (INR) are normal. The peripheral blood smear is shown. What is the most likely diagnosis?

a. Enterotoxin-induced hemolytic uremic syndrome (HUS)
b. Hemolysis due to cocaine ingestion
c. Food poisoning–associated thrombotic thrombocytopenic purpura (TTP)
d. Hemolysis due to G6PD deficiency
e. Disseminated intravascular coagulation (DIC)

8. A 28-year-old internal medicine resident develops progressive confusion during overnight call. She is taken to the emergency department (ED) by 2 of her colleagues when they notice that she is acting strangely in the hospital cafeteria. While waiting to be seen by the ED staff, she has a brief generalized seizure. A CBC documents a hemoglobin concentration of 8.5 g/dL and a normal MCV. The platelet count is 8×10^9/L. The peripheral blood smear reveals a few schistocytes and a paucity of platelets. Prothrombin time and activated partial thromboplastin time are normal. The urinalysis reveals proteinuria (2+). A urine toxin screen shows only zolpidem, which the patient had been taking as a sleep aid. The serum creatinine is 3.0 mg/dL. What is the best initial treatment of this condition?

a. Heparin
b. Platelet transfusion
c. Plasma exchange
d. Rituximab
e. Corticosteroids

9. A 37-year-old homosexual man has a 2-year history of human immunodeficiency virus (HIV) infection and has been taking highly active antiretroviral therapy (HAART) since diagnosis. His current CD4 count is 565 cells/mcL. He has not yet had an AIDS-defining illness, and he remains active in his legal practice, although his general fatigue level has increased in the past 6 months. Over the past year, his hemoglobin has been decreasing slowly without evidence of blood loss or infection. Today a CBC shows a hemoglobin of 10.5 g/dL with a normal MCV, normal WBC, and a platelet count of 109×10^9/L. Which of the following is the most appropriate management of the anemia?

a. Iron supplementation
b. Vitamin B_{12} supplementation
c. Erythropoietin treatment
d. Corticosteroid treatment
e. Discontinuing HAART

10. A 19-year-old man presented with anemia (hemoglobin, 9.5 g/dL) and polyarthralgias soon after returning to college after Christmas break. A younger sibling at home just recovered from a febrile illness associated with a facial rash. The patient's father was an anxious hematologist, so a bone marrow examination was immediately performed. Bone marrow biopsy findings

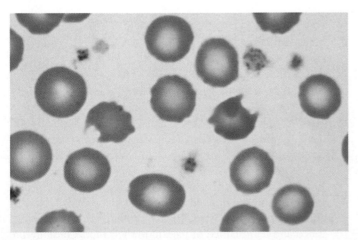

Question 7

showed RBC hypoplasia with giant pronormoblasts but was otherwise unremarkable. What is the treatment of choice for this condition?

a. Observation
b. Ganciclovir
c. Ciprofloxacin
d. Immunoglobulin therapy
e. Plasmapheresis

Malignant Hematology

11. A 69-year-old homemaker presents for follow-up of hypertension. She is asymptomatic. Physical examination is unremarkable. A CBC is performed, and her WBC is 22.5×10^9/L. Three years before, the WBC had been 10.4×10^9/L. The WBC differential now shows 84% lymphocytes. The peripheral blood smear reveals small mature-appearing lymphocytes and a few smudge cells. The platelet count is 180×10^9/L, and the hemoglobin is 13.4 g/dL. What is the best initial treatment of this patient?

a. Observation
b. Low-dose chemotherapy such as chlorambucil
c. Stem cell transplant
d. Rituximab
e. Combination chemotherapy

12. A 55-year-old engineer presents with a 5-day history of progressive costovertebral angle pain and mid-thoracic back pain. He has also noted increased fatigue in recent months, which he attributed to long hours at work. On physical examination, the spleen tip is palpable approximately 15 cm below the left costal margin in the nipple line. The WBC is 3.2×10^9/L, with an absolute neutrophil count of 800×10^9/L. The platelet count is 56×10^9/L. The hemoglobin is 11.9 g/dL. Bone marrow aspiration is difficult; the bone marrow biopsy shows a hypercellular marrow with increased reticulin fibrosis and abundant mature lymphocytes with cytoplasmic projections. Which of the following complications is this patient most at risk for?

a. Autoimmune hemolytic anemia
b. Superior vena cava syndrome
c. Infection with cytomegalovirus
d. Infection with atypical mycobacteria
e. Transformation to acute lymphoblastic leukemia

13. A 65-year-old retired welder has slowly progressive fatigue and dyspnea on exertion. He takes no medications, and his past medical history is remarkable only for a motor vehicle accident that caused multiple limb and rib fractures 10 years earlier. Physical examination shows generalized pallor but is otherwise unremarkable. A CBC reveals a hemoglobin of 9.8 g/dL with an MCV of 80 fL and a normal WBC and platelet count. Test

results of renal function, liver enzymes, and electrolytes are normal. Ferritin is elevated (588 ng/mL) and the peripheral blood smear shows only anisocytosis. The bone marrow aspirate is hypercellular; an iron-stained smear is shown. Which of the following is the most likely diagnosis?

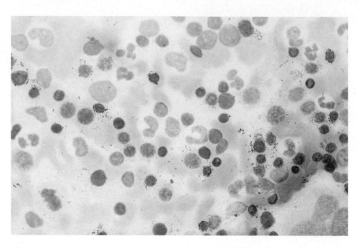

Question 13

a. Myelodysplastic syndrome
b. Chronic myeloid leukemia
c. Multiple myeloma
d. Vitamin E deficiency
e. Marijuana use

14. A 45-year-old accountant has dyspepsia. Physical examination is unremarkable. A CBC reveals a hemoglobin of 11.5 g/dL, with an MCV of 88 fL. The lactate dehydrogenase level is normal. Upper endoscopy reveals a small gastric nodule, which biopsy demonstrates is a MALToma. *Helicobacter pylori* is identified in the biopsy specimen. CT scans of the body show no areas of lymphadenopathy. What is the initial treatment of choice?

a. Observation
b. Rituximab
c. Radiation therapy
d. Combination therapy for *H pylori*
e. Gastrectomy with lymph node dissection

15. A 64-year-old woman received a diagnosis of multiple myeloma 4 months ago after presenting with anemia and renal insufficiency. Initial bone survey at that time showed a few scattered lytic lesions in her calvaria, 1 in the distal humerus, and 2 in the ribs. She is being treated with thalidomide and dexamethasone, and she has had a modest reduction (50%) in the amount of her monoclonal IgG κ protein. Earlier today she called and complained of pain in her left hip. A radiograph shows a large lytic lesion in the left greater trochanter with

impending fracture. Serum calcium level is 10.5 mg/dL. What is the most appropriate initial treatment?

a. A high-potency bisphosphonate such as pamidronate
b. Radiotherapy to the pelvis
c. Initiation of chemotherapy with melphalan and prednisone
d. Surgical stabilization of the femur
e. Immobilization of the patient to prevent fracture

16. A 71-year-old man presents with fatigue, weight loss, constipation, and dizziness when standing. On further rapid questioning, he also describes symptoms of a sensorimotor peripheral neuropathy. The physical examination reveals edema of the lower extremities (2+), diminished sensation, and absent ankle jerks. He is mildly anemic (hemoglobin, 11.3 g/dL) with an MCV of 86 fL; the WBC count and platelet count are normal. The creatinine is 3 mg/dL. One year ago the creatinine was 1.4 g/dL. A urinalysis shows proteinuria (4+). Serum protein electrophoresis shows a small IgG λ monoclonal protein (0.8 g/dL). What is the next best test?

a. CT of the abdomen
b. CT of the head
c. Fat aspirate with Congo red staining
d. Peripheral nerve biopsy
e. Small bowel radiography

17. A 38-year-old salesman presents with headaches, progressive fatigue, and intermittent blurry vision. Examination reveals generalized pallor and a palpable spleen tip. A CBC shows a hemoglobin of 8.9 g/dL, a WBC count of 156×10^9/L with 86% undifferentiated blasts, and a platelet count of 22×10^9/L. A serum chemistry panel shows the following: creatinine, 2.8 g/dL; potassium, 5.1 mEq/L; and uric acid, 11.8 mg/dL. Which of the following is the first telephone call you should make?

a. Radiation therapist to arrange for whole-brain irradiation
b. Blood bank to arrange for prompt RBC transfusion
c. Cell therapy technician to arrange for leukapheresis
d. Nephrologist to arrange hemodialysis
e. General surgeon to place Hickman catheter so that chemotherapy can begin

18. A 49-year-old woman presented with menorrhagia of 5 months' duration. The spleen was palpable 5 cm below the left costal margin. The leukocyte count was 56×10^9/L with 62% neutrophils, 11% lymphocytes, 12% basophils, 3% monocytes, 8% metamyelocytes, and 12% myelocytes. The platelet count was 100×10^9/L. Which test would most likely establish the correct diagnosis?

a. Fat aspirate
b. Imaging of the uterus
c. Flow cytometry
d. JAK2 mutation analysis
e. *BCR-ABL* molecular genetic studies

19. A 65-year-old woman who is taking a diuretic for hypertension presents with a transient ischemic attack. The platelet count is 690×10^9/L. The CBC reveals a normal hemoglobin level and normal MCV. Old records show that the platelet count was greater than 600×10^9/L for more than a year. C-reactive protein is normal. Ferritin is 38 ng/mL. A peripheral blood smear shows only an elevated platelet count. What is the most likely diagnosis?

a. Reactive thrombocytosis
b. Essential thrombocythemia
c. Early iron deficiency
d. Hyposplenism
e. Medication-induced thrombocytosis

20. A 60-year-old man with a history of hypertension and cigarette smoking presents with generalized pruritus that is most noticable after a warm bath. He is found to have moderate splenomegaly. Oxygen saturation is 94% on room air. A CBC shows the following: hemoglobin 17.6 g/dL, hematocrit 55%, MCV 79 fL, total erythrocytes 5.40×10^{12}/L, leukocytes 17×10^9/L, and platelet count 560×10^9/L. Serum erythropoietin is 2 IU/L. What is the most likely diagnosis?

a. Polycythemia vera
b. Stress erythrocytosis
c. Erythrocytosis due to hypoxia
d. Renal cell cancer
e. Renal insufficiency

21. A 36-year-old woman who has diffuse large cell non-Hodgkin lymphoma is being treated with CHOP chemotherapy plus rituximab. On the 11th day of the second cycle of treatment, a routine postchemotherapy CBC shows that the WBC is 0.5×10^9/L and the absolute neutrophil count is 250×10^9/L. The patient had been checking her temperature, and she is afebrile. She has symptoms of an upper respiratory tract infection and feels fatigued. What should be the management of this patient?

a. Observation
b. Levofloxacin
c. Trimethoprim-sulfamethoxazole
d. Granulocyte colony-stimulating factor (G-CSF)
e. Granulocyte transfusion

Coagulation

22. A 58-year-old man presented with melena. He has a history of a bleeding disorder. His maternal grandfather also had a bleeding disorder. Recently, his grandson received a diagnosis of a bleeding disorder after prolonged bleeding after dental extraction. The prothrombin time (PT) was normal. The activated partial thromboplastin time (aPTT) was 75 seconds (reference range, 23-33 seconds), which corrected to normal upon mixing with normal plasma. What is the next best test?

a. Factor VIII level
b. von Willebrand factor (vWF) antigen and ristocetin cofactor
c. Bleeding time
d. Platelet function studies
e. DIC work-up

23. A 28-year-old man bled after abdominal surgery. The aPTT was 49 seconds (reference range, 23-33 seconds). The PT was normal. The vWF antigen activity was 27%. The factor VIII activity was 23% (reference range, 55%-250%) and ristocetin cofactor activity was 24% (55%-200%). What is the treatment of choice for long-term management?

a. Humate-P
b. Recombinant factor VIII
c. Plasma-derived factor VIII concentrate
d. Recombinant factor IX
e. Fresh frozen plasma

24. An 80-year-old woman is admitted to the hospital for chronic cholecystitis. She underwent cholecystectomy and now, at postoperative day 8, she has a poor appetite. She continues to receive systemic antibiotics. Laboratory data (and reference ranges) are as follows: CBC, normal; PT, 16 seconds (8-12 seconds); aPTT, 40 seconds (23-33 seconds); and fibrinogen, 350 mg/dL (175-430 mg/dL). What is the most likely cause for her prolonged PT and aPTT?

a. Vitamin K deficiency
b. Platelet dysfunction
c. Factor XIII deficiency
d. Disseminated intravascular coagulation and fibrinolysis
e. Liver disease

25. A 68-year-old previously healthy woman recently underwent right total knee replacement. Now at postoperative day 7, she has begun ambulating. Her medications include narcotic analgesic and subcutaneous unfractionated heparin. Her physical examination findings are consistent with her postoperative state; she has no unusual bleeding or bruising. Her preoperative laboratory data were normal, and her current CBC shows a normal WBC and hemoglobin, but her platelet count is decreased to 50×10^9/L. What is the next most appropriate step in management?

a. Perform bone marrow aspiration and biopsy.
b. Discontinue heparin use and transfuse platelets.
c. Perform plasma exchange.
d. Discontinue heparin use and administer a direct thrombin inhibitor.
e. Start prednisone therapy.

26. A 62-year-old woman presents to the ED with diffuse abdominal pain and fatigue. At this time, the platelet count is 10×10^9/L. CT of the abdomen reveals retroperitoneal bleeding; the spleen is not enlarged. Coagulation studies (PT, PTT) are unremarkable, and the peripheral blood smear shows only thrombocytopenia. In addition to platelet transfusion, what is the best initial therapy?

a. Oral prednisone
b. Plasma exchange
c. Rituximab
d. Splenectomy
e. Interleukin-11 (oprelvekin)

27. A 32-year-old woman is referred to you because she has failed a life insurance screening examination owing to thrombocytopenia. She has a lifelong history of mild, easy bruising and bleeding, but she has never had a serious hemorrhagic episode. Her older sister underwent splenectomy for steroid-refractory immune thrombocytopenia at age 16 without any benefit. Her sister no longer believes in conventional physicians and instead treats her thrombocytopenia with an herbal preparation she obtains from Thailand over the Internet. The patient's father died after a motor vehicle accident; the mother is alive and healthy. Physical examination findings are unremarkable. A CBC shows a normal hemoglobin and WBC, but the platelet count is only 31×10^9/L. The peripheral blood smear is shown. What is the most appropriate management plan for this patient?

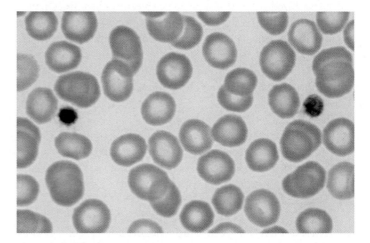

Question 27

a. Splenectomy
b. Rituximab
c. A trial of prednisone
d. Observation
e. Bone marrow examination

Answers

1. Answer a.
The low hemoglobin, low MCV, and decreased total erythrocyte count are consistent with iron deficiency. The leading causes of microcytic anemia are iron deficiency, anemia of chronic disease, and thalassemia. Although the patient's ethnic origin puts her at risk of thalassemia, the low erythrocyte count is more compatible with iron deficiency than thalassemia. Anemia of chronic disease does not result in severe microcytosis. The best initial test for evaluation of suspected iron deficiency is a ferritin level.

2. Answer e.
The peripheral blood smear shows numerous teardrop-shaped RBCs (dacrocytes). This finding is characteristic of marrow fibrosis from any cause, which in this case is most likely chronic idiopathic myelofibrosis, a myeloproliferative disorder. The patient has several other features of chronic idiopathic myelofibrosis, including massive splenomegaly and anemia.

3. Answer e.
The patient has experienced a delayed hemolytic transfusion reaction. He was probably sensitized to Jk^a (part of the Kidd group of erythrocyte antigens) by a previous transfusion, but the titer of the anti-Jk^a antibody was not high enough to be detected preoperatively. Rechallenge with Jk^a-positive cells led to increased antibody production and hemolysis. This complication is usually easily managed by transfusing with matched blood. Immunosuppression or techniques to suppress the antibody are not required. He is not likely to respond to recombinant erythropoietin given his severe intrinsic erythropoietic defect.

4. Answer c.
This picture is consistent with anemia of chronic disease. It is rare to have iron deficiency with a ferritin level greater than 100 ng/mL. Suppression of total iron-binding capacity is common in anemia of chronic disease and can render iron saturation unreliable. The sedimentation rate is quite elevated, suggesting an important inflammatory process. The Mediterranean type of G6PD deficiency usually does not cause anemia unless there is a provocative event such as an infection or exposure to an oxidative drug.

5. Answer c.
This patient has a macrocytic anemia; the macrocytosis is probably related to reticulocytosis, given the elevated reticulocyte proportion plus polychromasia on a peripheral blood smear. Coupled with the elevated indirect bilirubin and low haptoglobin, the overall picture is that of a Coombs-negative hemolytic anemia. Although G6PD deficiency can cause hemolysis, the patient is also leukopenic and thrombocytopenic. Pancytopenia and hemolysis make the diagnosis of paroxysmal nocturnal hemoglobinuria likely.

6. Answer e.
This patient has a macrocytic anemia. The most likely cause in this case is pernicious anemia, which is more common in patients with other autoimmune diseases such as hypothyroidism. Celiac sprue with folate malabsorption is also possible but less likely given the stable weight and normal bowel habits.

7. Answer d.
The peripheral blood smear shows "bite" cells, which are due to pitting of precipitated hemoglobin by the spleen. This is a finding that may be seen during a hemolytic crisis due to exposure to oxidative stress in a G6PD-deficient patient. The likely culprit here was fava beans in the feast that the patient enjoyed. The mild elevation in creatinine may have predated the illness or may be a result of hemoglobin-induced injury to the kidney. With a normal PTT, DIC is less likely. Food poisoning does not cause TTP.

8. Answer c.
This patient has TTP. She presents with classic findings, which include neurologic findings, renal findings, microangiopathic hemolytic anemia, and thrombocytopenia. Of the TTP pentad, only fever is not mentioned. The treatment of choice is plasma exchange. Platelets can make TTP worse, and there is no role for heparin. Rituximab and steroids have been used as adjuncts to therapy or for refractory TTP.

9. Answer c.
HIV infection and HIV therapy are associated with numerous hematologic complications, including anemia, thrombocytopenia, and an increased risk of lymphoproliferative disorders. The anemia often responds to erythropoietin treatment. There is no evidence that this patient is deficient in iron or vitamin B$_{12}$, and corticosteroids are of no value. Although discontinuation of HAART might be associated with improvement in anemia, it could lead to an increased viral load and declining CD4 counts, so it would be a bad idea.

10. Answer d.
This patient has parvovirus infection (B19 virus) or fifth disease. It is highly contagious in children. Adults with this infection may have a polyarthralgia syndrome with cytopenias, especially anemia and reticulocytopenia. Giant pronormoblasts are characteristic. However, bone marrow biopsy is not usually necessary. Serologic and PCR tests for parvovirus B19 virus are available. Intravenous immunoglobulin is the treatment of choice. Patients with chronic hemolytic anemia, such as sickle cell disease, may have profound aplasia after parvovirus infection and usually require transfusion support.

11. Answer a.
This patient has early (Rai Stage 0) chronic lymphocytic leukemia (CLL). In this setting, active treatment is not associated with improved outcome. Therefore, observation is appropriate. Treatment with chemotherapy or immunotherapy might be considered if the patient became symptomatic (eg, from progressive adenopathy or splenomegaly) or if anemia or thrombocytopenia developed. The role of stem cell transplantation in CLL is unclear, and this patient is too old to consider an allogeneic transplant.

12. Answer d.

The findings are most consistent with a diagnosis of hairy cell leukemia. Splenomegaly and cytopenias are the most characteristic presentation; bone marrow aspiration often results in a "dry tap." Patients with hairy cell leukemia are at increased risk of infection by bacteria and have a peculiar risk of atypical mycobacterial infection. Autoimmune hemolytic anemia can occur but is more characteristic of CLL. Superior vena cava syndrome occurs with lymphoproliferative disorders that involve the mediastinal nodes; in contrast, adenopathy is not a major feature of hairy cell leukemia.

13. Answer a.

The bone marrow aspirate smear shows ring sideroblasts, erythroid precursors with an excess of mitochondrial iron. Sideroblastic anemia can be congenital or reactive (eg, due to lead poisoning or isoniazid use), but in an older patient it is usually due to a myelodysplastic syndrome (refractory anemia with ring sideroblasts). Chronic myeloid leukemia is associated with a variable degree of anemia and a hypercellular marrow but not abundant ring sideroblasts. Marijuana, myeloma, and vitamin E deficiency are not associated with sideroblastic anemia.

14. Answer d.

H pylori is associated with gastric MALToma. The initial treatment of choice is an antibiotic and acid-suppression regimen. For patients who have more aggressive gastric lymphoma or for those with MALToma who have relapse or refractory disease, alternative treatments are required, usually including chemotherapy.

15. Answer d.

Bony lesions are a frequent complication of multiple myeloma and may result in pathologic fracture. Radiotherapy to the site of disease is appropriate, but if a fracture is impending (especially in a weight-bearing bone), immediate surgical stabilization is indicated. Bisphosphonates can lower the risk of such complications and can be used to treat hypercalcemia associated with myeloma, but they are of less value in the acute management of a painful lytic lesion.

16. Answer c.

The clinical presentation of postural hypotension, peripheral neuropathy, and nephrotic syndrome associated with a monoclonal protein is consistent with systemic amyloidosis. The gut may also be involved. There is an 80% yield in the diagnosis of primary systemic amyloidosis with a fat aspirate. Bone marrow biopsy may show a clonal plasma cell infiltrate.

17. Answer c.

The patient has acute leukemia and has presented in a blast crisis. He is at high risk of a stroke if the WBC count is not lowered urgently. Leukapheresis is indicated and should lower the WBC count by more than 50%. Oral hydroxyurea is also appropriate. The patient may ultimately require dialysis to address renal insufficiency associated with lysis of tumor cells, and he will need central venous access for definitive chemotherapy, but these are not emergent. RBC transfusion before addressing the leukemic cell burden will only increase blood viscosity and might worsen the situation.

18. Answer e.

This patient has a significant leukocytosis, a myelocyte "bulge," basophilia, and splenomegaly. This picture is consistent with chronic myeloid leukemia (CML). Cytogenetics would likely reveal a t(9;22) translocation (Philadelphia chromosome). The *BCR-ABL* rearrangement is assayed by polymerase chain reaction (PCR) or fluorescence in situ hybridization, with positive results in CML even when the Philadelphia chromosome is absent (<10% of cases). JAK2 mutation testing is abnormal in essentially all cases of polycythemia vera and half of the cases of essential thrombocytosis and chronic idiopathic myelofibrosis, but JAK2 is normal in CML.

19. Answer b.

Without evidence for inflammation or iron deficiency, the most likely diagnosis is essential thrombocythemia. The transient ischemic attack is probably related to the essential thrombocythemia. Hyposplenism is unlikely in the absence of Howell-Jolly bodies on the peripheral smear.

20. Answer a.

This patient has erythrocytosis. When erythrocytosis is associated with a low erythropoietin level, the diagnosis is almost certainly polycythemia vera. This patient has several other features that are also consistent with a myeloproliferative disorder (splenomegaly, aquagenic pruritus, leukocytosis, and thrombocytosis). A normal oxygen saturation makes chronic hypoxia less likely, and hypoxia would be associated with an erythropoietin level that was elevated, not suppressed.

21. Answer a.

This patient has neutropenia after chemotherapy but does not have a fever. Her upper respiratory illness is just as likely to be viral as bacterial. G-CSF could be used with subsequent cycles of chemotherapy to lower the risk of febrile neutropenia and allow full doses of chemotherapy to continue to be given, but it is of no proven value in this setting. Levofloxacin prevents infection in neutropenic patients with acute leukemia but is not routinely used in cancer patients. The treatment of choice is observation.

22. Answer a.

The patient's history is suggestive of an X-linked recessive bleeding disorder, and the prolonged aPTT, which corrects in the mixing study with normal plasma, suggests a coagulation factor deficiency state. Hemophilia A, factor VIII deficiency, is an X-linked recessive bleeding disorder. von Willebrand disease (deficiency of vWF) does not prolong the aPTT. The bleeding time will provide no information on why the aPTT is prolonged; furthermore, it is not available in many hospitals. Given that the PT was normal, it is unlikely this patient has DIC.

23. Answer b.

This patient has hemophilia A, for which recombinant factor VIII is a treatment of choice. Humate-P is used for von Willebrand disease, and recombinant factor IX is used for Hemophilia B. Fresh frozen plasma is seldom used.

24. Answer a.

Presumably, the patient had not eaten before surgery and has a poor appetite postoperatively. Vitamin K deficiency is extremely common and can prolong both the PT and the aPTT. Neither platelet dysfunction nor factor XIII deficiency is detected with PT and aPTT assays. Because the fibrinogen is normal, it is unlikely that this patient has DIC or liver disease.

25. Answer d.

This patient has heparin-induced thrombocytopenia (HIT). She is a high-risk patient (post–orthopedic surgery treatment with unfractionated heparin for deep venous thrombosis prophylaxis), and her platelet count has been low at 5 to 14 days after initiation of heparin. Because she has a high risk of thrombosis, stopping the use of heparin and administering a direct thrombin inhibitor is the treatment of choice. Bone marrow aspiration and biopsy will provide no additional diagnostic information, transfusion of platelets is contraindicated, there is no indication for plasma exchange in this situation, and prednisone therapy is not indicated in HIT.

26. Answer a.

This patient most likely has idiopathic thrombocytopenic purpura (ITP). The initial treatment of choice is oral corticosteroids. Intravenous gamma globulin can be used to increase the platelet count in the short term. Plasma exchange is of no proven value in ITP, and rituximab is usually used for steroid-unresponsive disease. Splenectomy would be considered for an ITP relapse after corticosteroid treatment or if it were refractory to corticosteroids. Thrombopoietin receptor stimulators have been useful in clinical trials in ITP but interleukin-11 is of no value.

27. Answer d.

This patient has large platelets and thrombocytopenia that is most likely congenital (her sister probably has the same syndrome). This is unlikely to be ITP; instead, it is more consistent with a disorder such as May-Hegglin anomaly or another macrothrombocytopenic disorder due to an *MYH9* mutation. Splenectomy is of no benefit, and corticosteroids and rituximab would be ineffective. Although the bleeding risk for this patient is elevated, no therapy is necessary or possible.

12

HIV Infection

Zelalem Temesgen, MD

Human immunodeficiency virus (HIV) belongs to the family Retroviridae, subfamily Lentiviridae. Retroviridae organisms share a distinct biologic characteristic: an initial stage of primary infection followed by a relatively asymptomatic period of months to years and a final stage of overt disease.

There are 2 types of HIV: HIV-1 and HIV-2. Most reported cases of HIV disease around the world are caused by HIV-1. HIV-1 is further classified into subtypes M, N, and O, referred to as clades. Subtype M (main) is the collective name for a group of clades designated A to K. For example, clade B is responsible for most HIV infections reported in the United States. HIV-2 is found predominantly in western Africa. Although HIV-1 and HIV-2 are clinically indistinguishable and have identical modes of transmission, HIV-2 appears to be less easily transmitted than HIV-1 and slower to progress to acquired immunodeficiency syndrome (AIDS).

* There are 2 types of HIV: HIV-1 and HIV-2.
* Most reported cases of HIV disease are caused by HIV-1.

Epidemiology

The AIDS epidemic is currently in its third decade and continues to affect a substantial number of people throughout the world. The number of people living with HIV continues to increase in every region in the world. According to the latest report from the World Health Organization (WHO), the total number of people in the world living with HIV is approximately 40 million. In more than 4 million of these people, HIV was diagnosed in 2006. Approximately 25 million have died of AIDS, 3 million in 2006 alone. More than 90% of all people living with HIV reside in developing countries where resources for diagnosis, prevention, and management of diseases are scarce. Among new infections, 2.8 million (65%) occurred in sub-Saharan Africa, where 59% of people living with HIV in 2006 were women and where 40% of new HIV infections were in young adults between 15 and 24 years of age. These disturbing trends have not been limited to sub-Saharan Africa. In Eastern Europe, East Asia, and Central Asia, the number of HIV infections in 2006 was 21% higher than that in 2004. In North America and Western

and Central Europe, the number of people living with HIV has increased as a result of both prolonged lifespans due to use of antiretroviral combination therapy and the steady number of new HIV infections. In the United States, 850,000 to 950,000 persons are living with HIV, including 180,000 to 280,000 who do not know they are infected. These latter persons are thought to account for 54% to 70% of all new sexually transmitted infections in the United States. The rate of new HIV or AIDS diagnoses in the United States is higher among African American men and women than among white men and women, 7 and 21 times, respectively.

Transmission

HIV is transmitted sexually, perinatally, by parenteral inoculation (eg, intravenous drug injection, occupational exposure), through blood products, and, less commonly, through donated organs or semen. Sexual transmission is the most common means of infection. Some of the conditions that may increase the risk of sexually acquiring HIV infection are traumatic intercourse (such as receptive anal); ulcerative genital infections such as syphilis, herpes simplex, and chancroid; and lack of circumcision. The use of latex condoms, especially if used properly, reduces the risk of HIV transmission. The mode of transmission of HIV infection varies from region to region. In North America, men who have sex with men make up the largest section of those living with HIV. In sub-Saharan Africa, heterosexual intercourse is the primary mode of transmission of HIV. In Eastern Europe and Central Asia, 67% prevalent HIV infections in 2005 were due to the use of nonsterile equipment used for injecting drugs.

* HIV is transmitted sexually, perinatally, by parenteral inoculation, through blood products, and through donated organs or semen.

In the United States, all blood donations have been routinely tested for HIV-1 antibody since early 1985. Since June 1, 1992, all US blood centers test for antibodies to both HIV-1 and HIV-2.

* In the United States, all blood donations have been routinely tested for HIV-1 antibody since early 1985.

Laboratory Diagnosis

The enzyme-linked immunosorbent assays and enzyme immunoassays are the most common assays used as a screening test for HIV-1 infection. They detect specific HIV antibodies. They have high (>99%) sensitivity and specificity but low positive predictive values in low-prevalence populations. For this reason, positive results require verification with an additional test. False-positive results can occur for several reasons. These include the presence of cross-reacting antibodies in certain patients (such as multiparous women, patients with multiple transfusions) and participation in HIV vaccine studies. Causes of false-negative results include testing during the pre-seroconversion (window) period, use of replacement transfusions, bone marrow transplantation, agammaglobulinemia, seroreversion in late-stage disease, unusual HIV subtypes (eg, HIV-2, clade O and N), and atypical immune response. Technical or laboratory error can be a cause of both false-positive and false-negative results. Rapid tests for HIV have been approved by the US Food and Drug Administration; they use whole-blood samples obtained from fingerstick, plasma, serum, or oral fluid specimens. Positive results of these tests are termed *preliminary positive* and also require confirmatory testing.

Individuals with positive or indeterminate results of enzyme-linked immunosorbent assay or enzyme immunoassay should have the test repeated. If results are repeatedly positive, the patient should undergo additional confirmatory testing, usually Western blot testing. The Western blot test detects specific viral proteins, such as Gag (p18, p24, p55), Pol (p31, p51, p66), and Env (gp41, gp120/gp160) gene products. The guidelines of the Centers for Disease Control and Prevention for interpretation of the Western blot are as follows: The presence of antibody against any 2 of the 3 major viral gene products (p24, gp41, or gp120/gp160) is classified as positive. A Western blot result is classified as negative if no bands are present. Results that cannot be classified as positive or negative on the basis of these criteria are categorized as indeterminate. If results are indeterminate, the clinician should assess the risk of HIV infection in the patient and retest in 3 to 6 months (Figure 12-1). HIV RNA assays may be of additional help in these cases. The risk of HIV infection is extremely low in patients with repeatedly indeterminate results of Western blot testing.

- Enzyme-linked immunosorbent assay or enzyme immunoassay should be repeated in persons with positive or indeterminate results.
- Western blot testing is used to confirm the results of enzyme-linked immunosorbent assay or enzyme immunoassay.

Pathogenesis

Contrary to previously held beliefs, HIV is not dormant during the so-called clinical latency period. There is active virus replication at all stages of disease. As many as 10 billion viral particles are produced and cleared daily in an HIV-infected person throughout all stages of disease. Concurrent with this rapid turnover of the HIV virus, more than 2 billion CD4 lymphocytes are produced every day.

- HIV is not dormant during the so-called clinical latency period.

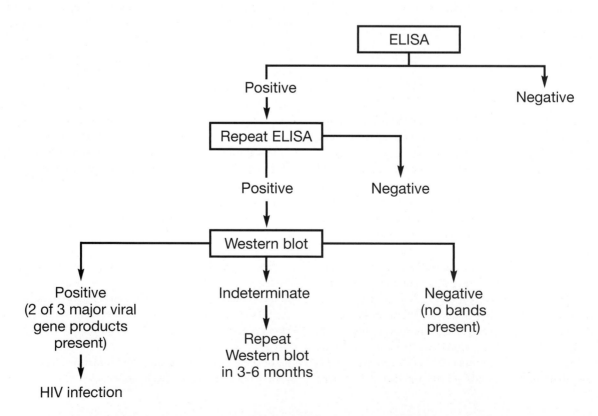

Figure 12-1. Testing for Human Immunodeficiency Virus (HIV). ELISA indicates enzyme-linked immunosorbent assay.

Synonyms for primary HIV infection syndrome are acute HIV infection and acute retroviral syndrome. Within days to weeks after exposure to HIV, upwards of 40% of infected individuals present with a brief illness that may last from a few days to a few weeks. This period of illness is associated with a huge amount of circulating virus, a rapid decline in the CD4 cell count, and a vigorous immune response. Patients usually present with a mononucleosis-like illness, but the clinical manifestations may be protean (Table 12-1). An atypical lymphocytosis is present in approximately 50% of patients. Results of enzyme-linked immunosorbent assay may be negative (window period), whereas p24 antigen, HIV culture, or polymerase chain reaction results may provide the diagnosis. The differential diagnosis includes infection due to Ebstein-Barr virus, cytomegalovirus, primary herpes simplex virus, toxoplasmosis, rubella, viral hepatitis, secondary syphilis, and drug reactions. Currently, treatment with the most potent antiretroviral combination regimen available is recommended with the hope of intervening before the HIV infection is fully established, when the viral population is relatively homogeneous and the host immune system is relatively intact.

* Acute HIV infection occurs within days to weeks after exposure to HIV.
* Patients usually present with a mononucleosis-type illness.
* Results of enzyme-linked immunosorbent assay may be negative for HIV.
* HIV p24 antigen, HIV culture, and HIV polymerase chain reaction results may provide the diagnosis.
* Treatment is with the most potent antiretroviral combination regimen.

Selected Infections and Conditions Associated With HIV Infection

Pneumocystis Pneumonia

Pneumocystis pneumonia is one of the most common opportunistic infections in patients with AIDS. It typically occurs in patients with CD4 counts less than 200 cells/mcL. Other factors associated with a higher risk of *Pneumocystis* pneumonia include CD4 percentage less than 15%, oral thrush, recurrent bacterial pneumonia, high HIV-1 RNA level, unintentional weight loss, and previous episodes of *Pneumocystis*

pneumonia. The onset of illness is insidious, with several days to weeks of fever, exertional dyspnea, chest discomfort, weight loss, malaise, and night sweats. Chest radiography typically shows bilateral interstitial pulmonary infiltrates, but a lobar distribution and spontaneous pneumothoraces may occur. Patients with early disease might have a normal chest radiograph. Pleural effusion is uncommon. Thin-section computed tomography usually shows patchy ground-glass infiltrates. Arterial blood gas analysis usually indicates hypoxemia and respiratory alkalosis. A wide A-a gradient (>35 mm Hg) and low PO_2 (<70 mm Hg) are associated with increased mortality. Increased lactate dehydrogenase level is common but is nonspecific. Several methods are used for the diagnosis of *Pneumocystis* pneumonia. Staining for *Pneumocystis* pneumonia in hypertonic saline-induced expectorated sputum is 30% to 85% sensitive. The sensitivity improves with liquefaction and the use of monoclonal antibody staining, and it may decrease with the use of prophylaxis for *Pneumocystis* pneumonia. Bronchoalveolar lavage is 85% to 90% sensitive. In rare circumstances, transbronchial lung biopsy may be needed to make the diagnosis. Open lung biopsy is even less commonly required. Extrapulmonary disease is uncommon but can be present in any organ.

* *Pneumocystis* pneumonia is one of the most common opportunistic infections in AIDS.
* Bronchoalveolar lavage is 85%-90% sensitive for the diagnosis of *Pneumocystis* pneumonia.

The treatment of choice for *Pneumocystis* pneumonia is trimethoprim-sulfamethoxazole. The usual recommended dosage is 15 mg/kg per day (trimethoprim component) in 3 or 4 equally divided doses for 21 days. If there is no improvement 4 to 8 days after treatment is begun, switching to or adding another drug should be considered. Alternative treatment options are listed in Table 12-2. Controlled studies have shown that adjunctive corticosteroid therapy increases survival in patients with moderate to severe disease, defined as room air PO_2 less than 70 mm Hg or an alveolar-arterial PO_2 difference (A-a gradient) more than 35 mm Hg. When indicated, adjunctive corticosteroid therapy should be started immediately; a delay may compromise its effectiveness.

* The treatment of choice for *Pneumocystis* pneumonia is trimethoprim-sulfamethoxazole.

Table 12-1 Clinical Manifestations of Primary Human Immunodeficiency Virus Infection

General	Neuropathic	Dermatologic	Gastrointestinal
Fever	Headache, retro-orbital pain	Maculopapular rash	Oral candidiasis
Pharyngitis	Meningoencephalitis	Roseola-like rash	Nausea, vomiting
Lymphadenopathy	Peripheral neuropathy	Diffuse urticaria	Diarrhea
Myalgia	Radiculopathy	Desquamation	
Lethargy	Guillain-Barré syndrome	Alopecia	
Anorexia, weight loss	Cognitive impairment	Mucocutaneous ulceration	

From Tindall B, Imrie A, Donovan B, Penny R, Cooper DA. Primary HIV infection. In: Sande MA, Volberding PA, editors. The medical management of AIDS. 3rd ed. Philadelphia: WB Saunders Company; 1992. p. 67-86. Used with permission.

- Adjunctive corticosteroid therapy increases survival in patients with moderate to severe disease.

Prophylaxis against *Pneumocystis* pneumonia is indicated in all HIV-infected patients with the previously detailed factors that are associated with a higher risk of *Pneumocystis* pneumonia. Drugs used for prophylaxis are listed in Table 12-3. The agent of choice is trimethoprim-sulfamethoxazole, which has the additional benefit of potential protection against other infectious agents (*Nocardia, Toxoplasma gondii, Staphylococcus aureus, Streptococcus pneumoniae, Haemophilus influenzae, Listeria monocytogenes, Isospora belli*) and prevention of extrapulmonary pneumocystosis. Secondary prophylaxis should be discontinued if patients have sustained a CD4 count of more than 200 cells/mcL for at least 3 months as a result of antiretroviral therapy. Prophylaxis should be reintroduced if the CD4 count declines to less than 200 cells/mcL or if *Pneumocystis* pneumonia recurs at a CD4 count of more than 200 cells/mcL.

- Typical clinical scenario: A 50-year-old patient with known HIV presents with shortness of breath and a 2-week history of fever and night sweats. Chest radiography shows bilateral pulmonary infiltrates. Arterial blood gas study reveals a room air PO_2 of 60 mm Hg. The A-a gradient is increased.
- *Pneumocystis* pneumonia prophylaxis is indicated with a CD4 count <200 cells/mcL, CD4 percentage <15%, oral thrush, recurrent bacterial pneumonia, high HIV-1 RNA level, unintentional weight loss, and previous episodes of *Pneumocystis* pneumonia.

Tuberculosis

The resurgence of tuberculosis in the United States is not entirely explained by the HIV epidemic. Factors such as socioeconomic conditions, immigration, breakdown of the public health infrastructure, and lack of interest of the medical and scientific community in tuberculosis all play a role. In addition to the impact of HIV on the incidence of tuberculosis, there are other important interactions between HIV infection and *Mycobacterium tuberculosis*: tuberculosis may accelerate the course of HIV infection; unlike many of the opportunistic infections in patients with HIV infection, tuberculosis can be cured if diagnosed promptly and treated appropriately; and tuberculosis can be prevented. Tuberculosis occurs among HIV-infected persons at all CD4 counts. However, its clinical manifestation may differ depending on the degree of immunosuppression. When tuberculosis occurs later in the course of HIV infection, it tends to have atypical features, such as extrapulmonary disease, disseminated disease, and unusual chest radiographic appearance (lower lung zone lesions, intrathoracic adenopathy, diffuse infiltrations, and lower frequency of cavitation). When tuberculosis occurs early in the course of HIV infection (CD4 count >350 cells/mcL), it tends to manifest with the classic presentation of upper lobe fibronodular infiltrates with cavitation. Outbreaks of multiple drug-resistant tuberculosis have been reported. Patients may have a fulminant course with high mortality (>70%) and a rapid course to death in 2 to 3 months.

- Tuberculosis can occur at all CD4 counts in HIV infection.
- Tuberculosis that occurs late in HIV infection tends to have atypical features.

The diagnosis of tuberculosis requires evaluation with a chest radiograph, sputum samples for acid-fast bacillus smear and culture, and aspiration or tissue biopsy if extrapulmonary disease is suspected. Mycobacterial blood cultures are useful in cases of disseminated disease. In patients with relatively intact immune function, the yield of sputum smear and culture is similar to that in HIV-negative patients.

The management of HIV-infected patients taking antiretroviral agents and undergoing treatment for active tuberculosis is complex. Treatment of tuberculosis in the setting of HIV should follow the general principles that apply to the treatment of non–HIV-infected patients; however, several issues require additional consideration. Protease inhibitors and nonnucleoside analogue reverse transcriptase inhibitors (NNRTIs) have substantive interactions with the rifamycins (rifampin, rifabutin, and rifapentine) used to treat mycobacterial

---

Table 12-2 Drugs for the Treatment of *Pneumocystis* Pneumonia

Drug
  Trimethoprim-sulfamethoxazole 15 mg/kg per day
  Trimethoprim PO 15 mg/kg per day + dapsone PO 100 mg per day
  Clindamycin IV 600 mg every 8 h (or PO 300-450 mg every 6 h) + primaquine PO 30 mg base per day
  Pentamidine IV 4 mg/kg per day
  Atovaquone suspension 750 mg twice daily
  Trimetrexate IV 45 mg/m^2 per day + leucovorin (folinic acid) IV 20 mg/m^2 every 6 h
  Prednisone[a] 40 mg PO twice daily for 5 days, followed by 40 mg PO daily for 5 days, then 20 mg PO daily until completion of therapy

Abbreviations: IV, intravenously; PO, orally.
[a] PaO_2 is less than 70 mm Hg or A-a gradient is more than 35 mm Hg.

Table 12-3 Drugs Used for Prophylaxis Against *Pneumocystis* Pneumonia

Drug
  Trimethoprim-sulfamethoxazole
    1 double-strength tablet daily
    1 double-strength tablet 3 times weekly
    1 single-strength tablet daily
  Dapsone 100 mg PO daily
  Aerosolized pentamidine 300 mg inhaled monthly via nebulizer
  Dapsone 50 mg PO daily + pyrimethamine[a] 50 mg PO 3 times a week
  Dapsone 200 mg PO weekly + pyrimethamine[a] 75 mg PO weekly
  Atovaquone 1,500 mg PO daily

Abbreviation: PO, orally.
[a] Plus leucovorin (folinic acid) 25 mg PO weekly.

infections. Protease inhibitors and NNRTIs not only are substrates for but also may inhibit or induce the cytochrome P450 system. Rifamycins, however, induce cytochrome P450 and may substantially decrease blood levels of the antiretroviral drugs. Compared with rifampin, rifabutin has substantially less activity as an inducer of cytochrome P450, and when used in appropriately modified doses it might not be associated with a clinically significant reduction of protease inhibitors or NNRTIs. Thus, the substitution of rifabutin for rifampin in treatment regimens for tuberculosis has been proposed as a practical choice for patients who are also undergoing therapy with protease inhibitors or with NNRTIs. A 6-month course may still be used for the treatment of tuberculosis that is susceptible to all first-line antituberculosis drugs. However, there is an increased risk for acquired rifamycin resistance that has led to specific recommendations about dosing schedules. Clinicians should also consider the factors that increase a person's risk for a poor clinical outcome (eg, lack of adherence to tuberculosis therapy, delayed conversion of *M tuberculosis* sputum cultures from positive to negative, and delayed clinical response) when deciding the total duration of tuberculosis therapy. Directly observed therapy should be strongly considered in all cases. Patients who have successfully completed a regimen of treatment for tuberculosis do not require secondary prophylaxis or chronic maintenance therapy. Patients with multiple drug-resistant tuberculosis are at high risk for relapse and treatment failure. Optimal regimens for these patients are unknown.

* Antituberculosis drugs interact with anti-HIV drugs.
* A 6-month course of treatment may be used for tuberculosis that is susceptible to all first-line antituberculosis drugs.
* Optimal regimens for multiple drug-resistant tuberculosis are unknown.

Recently, paradoxical reactions have been reported with the concurrent administration of antiretroviral and antituberculosis therapy. These reactions are attributed to recovery of the patient's delayed hypersensitivity response and include hectic fevers, lymphadenopathy, worsening of chest radiographic manifestations of tuberculosis (eg, miliary infiltrates, pleural effusions), and worsening of original tuberculous lesions (expanding central nervous system lesions). Changes in antituberculosis or antiretroviral therapy are rarely needed. If the symptoms are severe, a short course of steroids to suppress the enhanced immune response can be attempted while continuing with antituberculous and antiretroviral therapy.

HIV-positive patients who have skin reactions of more than 5 mm after administration of 5 tuberculin units of purified protein derivative and who do not have active tuberculosis are considered to have latent tuberculosis infection. Drug regimens recommended for treatment of latent tuberculosis infection are listed in Table 12-4. The use of pyrazinamide and rifampin together in a daily or twice-weekly regimen for the treatment of latent tuberculosis infection is no longer recommended because of high rates of hospitalization and death from liver injury associated with their use.

* Treatment of latent tuberculosis infection is recommended for all patients who are HIV-positive and have skin reactions of more

than 5 mm to 5 tuberculin units of purified protein derivative and who do not have active tuberculosis.

Mycobacterium avium Complex Infection

Organisms of the *Mycobacterium avium* complex are ubiquitous in the environment and include *M avium* and *Mycobacterium intracellulare*. They cause disseminated infection in HIV-infected persons, especially when immunosuppression is severe (CD4 count <50 cells/mcL). Disseminated *M avium* complex infection is the most common systemic bacterial infection in patients with HIV infection. Common presentations include low-grade fever, night sweats, weight loss, fatigue, abdominal pain, and diarrhea. Hepatomegaly, splenomegaly, and lymphadenopathy may be present. Common laboratory abnormalities include anemia and increased alkaline phosphatase levels. Blood cultures are usually positive; however, organisms can also be isolated from stool, respiratory tract secretions, bone marrow, liver, and other biopsy specimens.

* *M avium* complex causes infection when immunosuppression is severe (CD4 count <50 cells/mcL).
* *M avium* complex is the most common systemic bacterial infection in HIV-infected patients.

The organisms of *M avium* complex are resistant to conventional antimycobacterial agents. The current recommended treatment regimen includes one of the newer macrolides (eg, clarithromycin, azithromycin), ethambutol, and one or two additional drugs with activity against *M avium* complex. These include rifabutin, ciprofloxacin, amikacin, rifampin, and clofazimine. Rifabutin is thought to be the best option for a third agent and in randomized clinical trials has been shown to improve survival and to reduce the emergence of drug resistance. Similar to the paradoxical reactions with tuberculosis, an immune reconstitution and inflammatory syndrome of focal lymphadenitis and fever but without bacteremia has been noted. Treatment for *M avium* complex can be discontinued in patients who have completed more than 12 months of treatment, are asymptomatic, and have a sustained increase in their CD4 counts to more than 100 cells/mcL for at least 6 months after antiretroviral therapy. However, therapy will need to be resumed if CD4 counts decrease to less than 100 cells/mcL.

* *M avium* complex is resistant to conventional antimycobacterial drugs.

Table 12-4 Preferred Regimens for the Treatment of Latent Tuberculosis Infection

Isoniazid 300 mg PO daily + pyridoxine 50 mg PO daily for 9 mo
Isoniazid 900 mg twice weekly + pyridoxine 50 mg PO twice weekly for 9 mo
Rifampin 600 mg PO daily for 4 mo

Abbreviation: PO, orally.

For patients with AIDS whose CD4 count is less than 50 cells/mcL, prophylaxis with clarithromycin 500 mg twice daily or azithromycin 1,200 mg weekly is recommended. Rifabutin 300 mg daily is an alternative if these drugs are not tolerated. The detection of *M avium* complex organisms in the respiratory or gastrointestinal tract when a blood culture is negative is not, in itself, an indication for prophylaxis. Primary prophylaxis may be discontinued in patients with CD4 counts of more than 100 cells/mcL and a sustained suppression of HIV plasma RNA for more than 3 to 6 months.

* Prophylaxis for *M avium* complex is indicated for patients with AIDS whose CD4 count is <50 cells/mcL.

Cryptococcus neoformans Disease

Cryptococcus neoformans is a round or oval yeast that is acquired from the environment. It is inhaled into the lungs, where it usually causes asymptomatic infection, but it has a strong propensity for dissemination to the central nervous system. Other potential sites for dissemination include skin, bone, and the genitourinary tract. The most common manifestation of *C neoformans* disease is cryptococcal meningitis, which usually occurs when the CD4 count is less than 50 cells/mcL. The onset is insidious, symptoms are nonspecific (eg, fever, headache, malaise), and symptoms may have a waxing and waning course. Classic meningeal symptoms (eg, neck stiffness or photophobia) are present in only one-fourth to one-third of patients. Brain imaging findings are also nonspecific; cerebral atrophy and ventricular enlargement are the most common findings. Cerebrospinal fluid findings may be minimal or include an increased opening pressure, mild mononuclear pleocytosis, and increased protein value. Glucose levels may be normal or slightly low. The India ink preparation is positive in more than 70% of cases. The serum and cerebrospinal fluid cryptococcal antigen test has a sensitivity of 93% to 99%. Cultures of cerebrospinal fluid are usually positive. In up to 75% of patients, results of blood cultures are positive for *C neoformans*. Adverse prognostic factors include altered mental status on presentation and high fungal burden (positive result of India ink test, high antigen titers, and extraneural disease).

* *C neoformans* has a strong propensity for dissemination to the central nervous system.
* The most common manifestation of *C neoformans* disease is cryptococcal meningitis.
* The India ink preparation is positive in >70% of cases.

Initial therapy should include amphotericin B with flucytosine for 2 weeks, followed by fluconazole 400 mg daily for a total of 10 weeks. This initial therapy is followed by fluconazole (200 mg daily) for chronic suppression or maintenance therapy. Chronic suppression or maintenance therapy can be discontinued if patients remain asymptomatic and have a sustained increase in their CD4 counts of more than 100 to 200 cells/mcL for at least 6 months after antiretroviral therapy. However, chronic suppression or maintenance therapy needs to be reinitiated if the CD4 counts decrease to less than 100 to 200 cells/mcL. Although fluconazole and itraconazole can reduce the frequency of cryptococcal disease, routine primary prophylaxis is

not recommended for several reasons. These include cost, the relative infrequency of cryptococcosis, the possibility of drug interactions, and the potential for development of drug resistance.

* Typical clinical scenario: A patient with known HIV and a CD4 count of 20 cells/mcL presents with fever and headache. Computed tomography of the head shows mild cerebral atrophy but no specific lesions. Cerebrospinal fluid examination shows increased cerebrospinal fluid pressure, mild lymphocytosis, and increased protein concentration.
* Initial therapy for *C neoformans* infection in HIV includes amphotericin B with flucytosine followed by fluconazole.
* Routine primary prophylaxis for *C neoformans* disease is not recommended.

Cytomegalovirus

Cytomegalovirus disease usually affects persons with advanced HIV disease (CD4 count <50 cells/mcL). Other risk factors include previous opportunistic infections and high plasma HIV-1 RNA level (>100,000 copies/mL). Chorioretinitis is the most common clinical manifestation of cytomegalovirus disease. The usual symptoms are floaters, visual field deficits, and painless loss of vision. Funduscopic examination reveals yellowish white retinal infiltrates with or without intraretinal hemorrhage. Cytomegalovirus gastrointestinal disease most commonly involves the esophagus and colon and manifests with dysphagia, abdominal pain, and bloody diarrhea. Cytomegalovirus also can cause hepatitis, pneumonitis, sclerosing cholangitis, encephalitis, adrenalitis, polyradiculopathy, and myelopathy. Agents used for the treatment of cytomegalovirus disease and their general characteristics are listed in Table 12-5. After an induction course of therapy for 2 to 3 weeks or until clinical stability, maintenance therapy is continued with a reduced dose to prevent relapse. For gastrointestinal disease, maintenance therapy can be deferred until relapse is actually demonstrated. Relapses are generally treated with reinduction courses using the initial agent. If this approach fails or if the progression is rapid, treatment with an alternative agent or combination regimens (eg, ganciclovir plus foscarnet) should be considered.

Immune recovery uveitis, characterized by inflammation in the anterior chamber or vitreous, occurs in patients who experience a substantial increase in the CD4 count in the 4 to 12 weeks after antiretroviral therapy is started. Prophylaxis could be considered for cytomegalovirus-seropositive HIV-infected patients with a CD4 count of less than 50 cells/mcL. However, treatment-induced toxicities such as neutropenia, anemia, conflicting reports of efficacy, lack of proven survival benefit, and cost have precluded its routine use. Chronic maintenance therapy can be discontinued if patients remain asymptomatic and have a sustained increase in their CD4 counts to more than 100 to 150 cells/mcL for at least 6 months after antiretroviral therapy is completed. All patients whose maintenance therapy is discontinued should undergo regular ophthalmologic monitoring for detection of relapse and immune recovery uveitis. Chronic maintenance therapy will need to be reinitiated if there is ophthalmologic evidence of relapse or the CD4 counts decrease to less than 50 to 100 cells/mcL.

Table 12-5 Induction Treatment of Cytomegalovirus Retinitis

Drug	Dosage	Major Adverse Effect
Ganciclovir intraocular-release device (Vitrasert)[a]	Every 6 mo	Retinal detachment
Ganciclovir IV	5 mg/kg twice daily	Bone marrow suppression
Valganciclovir	900 mg PO twice daily	Bone marrow suppression
Foscarnet IV	60 mg/kg 3 times daily or 90 mg/kg twice daily	Renal toxicity
Cidofovir IV[b]	5 mg/kg weekly for 2 weeks, followed by 5 mg/kg every 2 weeks	Renal toxicity
Ganciclovir intravitreal injection[a]	2,000 mcg in 0.05-0.1 mL	Bone marrow suppression
Foscarnet intravitreal injection[a]	1.2-2.4 mg in 0.1 mL	Renal toxicity

Abbreviations: IV, intravenously; PO, orally.

[a] Local anti-cytomegalovirus therapy should be accompanied by systemic therapy, such as oral ganciclovir, to avoid the risk of development of extraocular diseases.

[b] Vigorous hydration and coadministration of probenecid are required to limit renal toxicity.

- Typical clinical scenario: A patient with known advanced HIV disease presents with painless loss of vision in both eyes. Fundal examination reveals yellowish white granules, exudates, and hemorrhages. Therapy with ganciclovir or other effective cytomegalovirus agents should be initiated promptly.
- Cytomegalovirus disease usually affects persons with advanced HIV disease.
- In HIV, cytomegalovirus can cause chorioretinitis, gastrointestinal disease, hepatitis, and other organ involvement.
- Maintenance therapy is indicated after treatment of initial cytomegalovirus infection.

Syphilis

Sexually transmitted diseases, including syphilis, that cause genital ulceration may be cofactors for acquiring HIV infection. In general, the clinical manifestations of syphilis are similar to those among non–HIV-infected persons. However, atypical presentations may occur. For example, in primary syphilis, multiple or atypical chancres can occur and primary lesions might be absent or missed. The manifestations of secondary syphilis are protean and might persist from a few days to several weeks before resolving or evolving to latent or later stages. The most common manifestations are macular, maculopapular, or pustular skin lesions characteristically involving the palms and soles and accompanied by generalized lymphadenopathy and constitutional symptoms of fever, malaise, anorexia, arthralgias, and headache. Manifestations of tertiary or late syphilis include neurosyphilis, cardiovascular syphilis, and gummatous syphilis. Neurosyphilis has been reported to occur earlier and more frequently and to progress more rapidly in patients with AIDS than in HIV-negative patients. Concomitant uveitis and meningitis also may be more common among HIV-1–infected patients with syphilis. There are reports of false-negative and false-positive serologic tests for syphilis in patients with HIV. However, serologic response to infection in general seems to be the same in HIV-positive and HIV-negative persons and there are no specific clinical manifestations of syphilis that are unique to HIV. Management of HIV-1–infected patients with syphilis is similar to the management of non–HIV-infected persons. However, HIV-infected patients require the following additional attention:

   Closer follow-up to detect potential treatment failures or disease progression

   Evaluation for clinical evidence of central nervous system or ocular involvement

   Penicillin-based regimens, whenever possible, for all stages of syphilis in HIV-infected persons

- In general, syphilis presents similarly in patients with AIDS and in HIV-negative patients.
- Syphilis can facilitate transmission of HIV.

Toxoplasmosis

Toxoplasma gondii, a protozoan, is the most common cause of focal central nervous system lesions in patients with AIDS. The most common symptoms of *Toxoplasma* encephalitis include headache and confusion; fever may be absent. Focal neurologic deficits occur in 69% of cases. The median CD4 count at diagnosis is 50 cells/mcL. Multiple ring-enhancing lesions with associated edema are usually noted on brain imaging studies. Magnetic resonance imaging is more sensitive than computed tomography for identifying lesions. The differential diagnosis of central nervous system mass lesions in patients with AIDS includes toxoplasmosis, lymphoma, and bacterial brain abscesses and infections caused by *C neoformans*, *Coccidioides immitis*, *M tuberculosis*, and *Nocardia asteroides*, among others.

- *T gondii* is the most common cause of focal central nervous system lesions in patients with AIDS.
- Multiple ring-enhancing lesions usually are noted on brain imaging studies.

Empiric antitoxoplasmosis therapy is indicated in patients with AIDS and positive *Toxoplasma* serologic testing who present with multiple intracranial lesions. The absence of antitoxoplasma IgG antibody makes a diagnosis of toxoplasmosis unlikely. The presence of only a single lesion on magnetic resonance imaging requires a more definitive diagnosis of toxoplasma encephalitis. Effective treatment should result not only in amelioration of symptoms but also in a reduction of the number, size, and contrast enhancement of the brain lesions. If the patient is seronegative for *Toxoplasma*, has a single mass lesion on both computed tomography and magnetic resonance imaging, or did not achieve the desired response after an empiric course of antitoxoplasmosis therapy for 10 to 14 days, the presumptive diagnosis of *Toxoplasma* encephalitis becomes doubtful and a diagnostic brain biopsy is indicated.

Drugs used for the treatment of HIV-associated toxoplasmosis are listed in Table 12-6. The initial regimen of choice is the combination of pyrimethamine plus sulfadiazine plus leucovorin. The preferred alternative regimen for patients unable to tolerate or who fail to respond to first-line therapy is pyrimethamine plus clindamycin plus leucovorin. Acute therapy should be continued for at least 6 weeks if there is clinical and radiologic improvement. Lifelong suppressive therapy (secondary prophylaxis), with the same agents used for acute therapy but at a reduced dose, is necessary to prevent relapse. Secondary prophylaxis can be discontinued in patients who successfully complete initial therapy, remain asymptomatic with respect to signs and symptoms of toxoplasmosis, and have a sustained (ie, >6 months) increase in their CD4 counts to more than 200 cells/mcL with antiretroviral therapy. Secondary prophylaxis should be started again if the CD4 count decreases to less than 200 cells/mcL. All HIV-infected persons with a CD4 count of less than 100 cells/mcL who are seropositive for *Toxoplasma* should receive primary prophylaxis against *Toxoplasma* encephalitis. The agent of choice for this is trimethoprim-sulfamethoxazole (1 double-strength tablet daily); dapsone plus

pyrimethamine is an alternative regimen. Atovaquone with or without pyrimethamine also may be considered.

- Lifelong suppressive therapy is needed to prevent relapse of HIV-associated toxoplasmosis.
- The agent of choice for primary prophylaxis against *Toxoplasma* encephalitis is trimethoprim-sulfamethoxazole.

HIV-infected patients should be tested for IgG antibody to *Toxoplasma* as part of their initial work-up; if the result is negative, they should be counseled about the various potential sources of *Toxoplasma* infection, such as raw or undercooked meat and handling of cat litter.

- Typical clinical scenario: A patient with known HIV disease presents with headache and confusion. There is evidence of upper and lower extremity weakness. Computed tomography shows multiple ring-enhancing lesions on brain imaging studies.

Progressive Multifocal Leukoencephalopathy

This is a demyelinating disease caused by the JC virus, a polyoma virus. Symptoms and signs are variable and consist of focal neurologic deficits without altered sensorium or a systemic toxic state. These symptoms include cognitive dysfunction, dementia, seizures, ataxia, aphasia, cranial nerve deficits, and hemiparesis or quadriparesis. Fever is usually absent. Symptoms evolve rapidly over weeks to months. Diagnosis is based on clinical findings and magnetic resonance imaging, which shows characteristic white matter changes (bright areas on T2-weighted images) without contrast enhancement or mass effect. Routine cerebrospinal fluid studies are generally nondiagnostic, but identification of JC virus DNA in the cerebrospinal fluid by polymerase chain reaction may confirm the diagnosis. Prognosis is poor, and there is no proven effective treatment. Neurologic improvement has been reported in some patients after the initiation of antiretroviral therapy.

- Progressive multifocal leukoencephalopathy is caused by the JC virus.
- The diagnosis is based on clinical findings and on white matter changes on magnetic resonance imaging.
- There is no proven effective therapy.

Mucocutaneous Candidiasis

Mucocutaneous disease, such as oral thrush, recurrent vaginitis, and candidal esophagitis, is common. The majority of infection is caused by *Candida albicans*. Candidal esophagitis is an AIDS-defining condition. Systemic candidal infection, including candidemia, is rare unless additional risk factors for disseminated fungal infection such as severe neutropenia and indwelling catheters are involved. Oropharyngeal candidiasis commonly presents with painless, creamy-white, plaquelike lesions of the buccal or oropharyngeal mucosa or tongue surface which can easily be scraped off with a tongue depressor. Less commonly, erythematous patches without white plaques or angular cheilosis can be noted. Esophageal candidiasis presents with retrosternal burning pain or discomfort and odynophagia. Endoscopic examination shows whitish plaques. Vulvovaginitis is characterized by a creamy to yellow-white adherent vaginal discharge associated with mucosal burning and itching.

Table 12-6 Drugs Used for the Treatment of HIV-Associated Toxoplasmosis

Preferred regimens
   Pyrimethamine[a] 200 mg PO loading dose followed by 50-75 mg PO daily + sulfadiazine 1,000-1,500 mg PO every 6 h + leucovorin 10-20 mg PO daily
   Pyrimethamine[a] 200 mg PO loading dose followed by 50-75 mg PO daily + clindamycin 600 mg IV or PO every 6 h
Alternative regimens
   Trimethoprim-sulfamethoxazole IV or PO 5 mg/kg trimethoprim + 25 mg/kg sulfamethoxazole every 12 h
   Pyrimethamine[a] 200 mg PO loading dose followed by 50-75 mg PO daily + clarithromycin 500 mg PO every 12 h
   Pyrimethamine[a] 200 mg PO loading dose followed by 50-75 mg PO daily + azithromycin 900-1,200 mg PO daily
   Atovaquone 1,500 mg PO twice daily + sulfadiazine 1,000-1,500 mg PO every 6 h
   Pyrimethamine[a] 200 mg PO loading dose followed by 75 mg PO daily + atovaquone 1,500 mg PO twice daily

---

Abbreviations: IV, intravenously; PO, oral, orally.
[a] With folinic acid 10 to 20 mg daily.

For mucocutaneous disease, initial treatment with clotrimazole troches or nystatin may be adequate. Fluconazole or itraconazole is used for the treatment of candidal esophagitis and topical treatment failures. Amphotericin B can be used for azole failures. Diagnosis of oropharyngeal candidiasis is usually clinical and is based on the appearance of lesions. Visualization of the organisms by microscopic examination of scrapings provides supportive diagnostic information.

The diagnosis of esophageal candidiasis is usually made presumptively on clinical grounds, but confirmation requires endoscopic visualization of lesions with histopathologic demonstration of the yeast forms in tissue. The diagnosis of vulvovaginal candidiasis is also based on the clinical presentation. Microscopic demonstration of the yeast forms in vaginal secretions supports the diagnosis.

Initial episodes of oropharyngeal candidiasis can be adequately treated topically, including clotrimazole troches or nystatin suspension or pastilles. However, oral fluconazole is as effective, more convenient, and generally better tolerated. Systemic therapy with a 14- to 21-day course of either fluconazole or itraconazole solution is required for effective treatment of esophageal candidiasis. Uncomplicated vulvovaginal candidiasis is effectively treated with short courses and responds readily to topical (clotrimazole, butaconazole, miconazole, ticonazole, terconazole, nystatin) or systemic (itraconazole oral solution, fluconazole) antifungals. Patients who have a history of 1 or more episodes of documented esophageal candidiasis should be considered candidates for secondary prophylaxis with fluconazole 100 to 200 mg daily.

Enteric Disease

Initial evaluation of patients with AIDS who have abdominal pain, diarrhea, and weight loss should include stool cultures for bacteria, 3 separate stool specimens for ova and parasites, and specific examination for cryptosporidiosis, isosporiasis, microsporidiosis, and *Cyclospora*, as indicated. *Cytomegalovirus* or *M avium-intracellulare* should be considered in the differential diagnosis, particularly in patients with advanced HIV infection. If no diagnosis is made, upper and lower gastrointestinal endoscopy and biopsy may yield pathogens that are treatable. The most common causes of bacterial diarrhea among patients with HIV-1 infection in the United States are *Salmonella*, *Campylobacter*, and *Shigella* species.

Salmonella *Infection*

In contrast to immunocompetent persons, HIV-infected persons are more likely to have *Salmonella* infection that is severe, invasive, and widespread. Bacteremia is common and constitutes an AIDS-defining diagnosis. The incidence of salmonellosis is 20- to 100-fold higher in HIV-infected persons than that in the general population. The source for *Salmonella* infection is ingestion of contaminated food, particularly undercooked poultry. Salmonellosis can present in 3 ways in HIV infection: a self-limited gastroenteritis; a more severe and prolonged diarrheal disease associated with fever, bloody diarrhea, and weight loss; and septicemia, with or without gastrointestinal symptoms. In the United States, the majority of cases of *Salmonella* septicemia are caused by nontyphoidal strains, in particular *Salmonella enteritidis* and *Salmonella typhimurium*. Bacteremia can occur with each of these syndromes and has a propensity for relapse.

Ciprofloxacin is the preferred agent for treatment. The treatment duration for mild gastroenteritis without bacteremia is 10 to 14 days. However, for patients with advanced HIV-1 disease (CD4 count <200 cells/mcL) or for those who have *Salmonella* bacteremia, treatment for at least 4 to 6 weeks is recommended. Alternatives to the fluoroquinolone antibiotics include trimethoprim-sulfamethoxazole or third-generation cephalosporins (eg, ceftriaxone or cefotaxime).

* HIV-infected persons are more likely to have *Salmonella* infection that is severe, invasive, and widespread.
* Ciprofloxacin is the preferred antibiotic for the treatment of salmonella infection.

Campylobacter *Infection*

The prevalence of *Campylobacter* infection seems to be higher in HIV-infected individuals. The incidence of *Campylobacter jejuni* is reported to be up to 39 times higher among HIV-1–infected persons, particularly men who have sex with men, than in the general population. Clinically, *Campylobacter* infection presents with a more prolonged diarrhea, invasive disease, bacteremia, and extraintestinal involvement (cellulitis, osteomyelitis, vasculitis, rheumatologic symptoms). In addition to stool and blood cultures, lower endoscopy for biopsy and histopathologic examination occasionally are required. For mild to moderate disease, a fluoroquinolone (ciprofloxacin) or a macrolide (azithromycin) for 7 days may be adequate, but patients with bacteremia should be treated for at least 2 weeks. A second active agent (eg, an aminoglycoside) might be required.

Shigellosis

Similar to *Campylobacter* and *Salmonella* infection, the risk for development of shigellosis is increased in persons with HIV-1 infection. In this setting, shigellosis presents as an acute, febrile, diarrheal illness with prominent upper and lower gastrointestinal symptoms. Bloody diarrhea and bacteremia also may be present. Relapses in gastroenteritis and bacteremia after appropriate treatment also have been reported. The recommended treatment is with a fluoroquinolone for 3 to 7 days. Alternatives to fluoroquinolones include trimethoprim-sulfamethoxazole or azithromycin. Treatment of bacteremia may require extension of treatment to 14 days or more.

Cryptosporidiosis

Cryptosporidium parvum is a protozoal organism that causes massive, watery diarrhea, crampy abdominal pain, anorexia, flatulence, and malaise. Fever and bloody diarrhea are uncommon, but malabsorption and dehydration are common. Cryptosporidiosis is diagnosed by identification of *C parvum* oocysts in fecal samples or biopsy specimens. The specimens are stained with either a modified acid-fast procedure or a fluorescent assay (immunofluorescent assay or enzyme immunoassay) that uses monoclonal antibodies to *Cryptosporidium* antigens. Biliary tract involvement may occur with cryptosporidiosis. If the CD4 count is more than 180 cells/mcL, cryptosporidium infection is usually self-limited (<4 weeks); if it is less than 140 cells/mcL, persistent disease develops in 80% to 90%. In adults, there are no proven regimens for the treatment of cryptosporidiosis, but paromomycin, a nonabsorbable aminoglycoside used for the treatment of *Entamoeba histolytica*, has been effective in some patients. Nitazoxanide has been approved by the US Food and Drug Administration for the treatment of diarrhea caused by *C parvum* and *Giardia lamblia* in pediatric patients 1 to 11 years of age.

- *C parvum* causes massive, watery diarrhea, crampy abdominal pain, anorexia, flatulence, and malaise.
- Cryptosporidiosis is diagnosed by identification of *C parvum* oocysts in fecal samples or biopsy specimens.
- Paromomycin has been effective in some patients.

Isosporiasis

Isospora belli causes illness similar to that caused by *C parvum*: profuse diarrhea without blood but accompanied by abdominal pain and malabsorption. Systemic symptoms, including fever, headache, and weight loss, also may be present. Isosporiasis is endemic in developing countries. The organism is identified with a modified acid-fast stain on fecal or biopsy specimens. Trimethoprim-sulfamethoxazole DS (160 mg of trimethoprim and 800 mg of sulfamethoxazole) 4 times daily for 10 days is effective for the treatment of *I belli* infections, but lifelong suppressive therapy may be required. Antiretroviral therapy has been associated with more rapid resolution of symptoms and fewer relapses.

- Isosporiasis causes profuse diarrhea without blood but accompanied by abdominal pain and malabsorption.
- Trimethoprim-sulfamethoxazole DS is effective treatment for isosporiasis.

Microsporidiosis

Two species of *Microsporidia*, *Enterocytozoon bieneusi* and *Encephalitozoon intestinalis*, cause enteric and biliary disease in patients with AIDS. Infection with these organisms resembles infection with *C parvum*, with perhaps less voluminous diarrhea. Extraintestinal manifestations include keratoconjunctivitis, disseminated disease, hepatitis, myositis, sinusitis, kidney and urogenital infection, ascites, and cholangitis. Gastrointestinal microsporidiosis is diagnosed by examination of stool specimens with light microscopy using selective stains that help differentiate the spores of the *Microsporidia* and the cells and debris in clinical samples. Ultrastructural examination with electron microscopy may be required for definitive diagnosis. The antiprotozoal agent albendazole has shown promise in the treatment of disease caused by *E intestinalis*. Another drug, fumagillin, has been reported to be effective for the treatment of intestinal microsporidiosis due to *E bieneusi* in patients with HIV infection.

- *Microsporidia* species cause enteric and biliary disease in patients with AIDS.
- Electron microscopy of biopsy specimens and special stains are required for diagnosis.

Cyclospora *Infection*

Cyclospora cayetanensis organisms are protozoal and cause gastrointestinal disease similar to cryptosporidiosis. Symptoms include watery diarrhea, fatigue, anorexia, myalgia, abdominal cramps, flatus, and nausea. Dehydration and weight loss are common. Biliary tract involvement is possible. In patients with AIDS, illness tends to be more severe and prolonged. Standard ova and parasite testing cannot detect the organisms; special staining techniques or electron microscopy may be required for diagnosis. Trimethoprim-sulfamethoxazole is effective for the treatment of *Cyclospora*. For patients with HIV infection, because relapse is common, the recommendation is 4 times daily dosing for 10 days followed by chronic suppression 3 times per week. Ciprofloxacin is an acceptable alternative for patients with sulfonamide allergy or intolerance.

- Symptoms of *Cyclospora* infection are watery diarrhea, fatigue, anorexia, myalgia, abdominal cramps, flatus, nausea, dehydration, and weight loss.
- Special staining or electron microscopy may be required for diagnosis.
- Trimethoprim-sulfamethoxazole is effective treatment.

Bacillary Angiomatosis

Bacillary angiomatosis was first described in 1983, and the causative organisms, *Bartonella quintana* and *Bartonella henselae*, were isolated for the first time in 1992. Bacillary angiomatosis is characterized by vascular proliferative lesions that can involve any organ in the body. The most commonly involved site is the skin, where it may present as nodules or plaques that are sometimes difficult to differentiate from those of Kaposi sarcoma. Other sites include bone, lymph nodes, brain, respiratory tract, and gastrointestinal tract. Characteristic fluid-filled spaces occasionally are noted in the liver and spleen and are called peliosis hepatis or peliosis splenis. Diagnosis is established by biopsy, demonstration of the organism on Warthin-Starry stain, and cultivation of the causative organism. Results of blood culture (lysis centrifugation technique) also may be positive if incubation is prolonged. Treatment is with erythromycin or doxycycline. Clarithromycin or azithromycin are considered second-line alternatives. The duration of treatment is at least 3 months.

- Bacillary angiomatosis is characterized by vascular proliferative lesions in skin and other organs.
- The differential diagnosis includes Kaposi sarcoma.
- The diagnosis is based on positive results of Warthin-Starry stain and cultivation of the causative organism.
- Treatment is with erythromycin or doxycycline.

AIDS-Associated Malignancies

Kaposi Sarcoma

Kaposi sarcoma is a tumor of uncertain origin; vascular proliferation is its most prominent feature. It is the most common neoplasm affecting HIV-infected persons. It is most common in the homosexual and bisexual population with AIDS. Herpeslike DNA sequences have been identified in AIDS-associated Kaposi sarcoma. These are thought to represent a new human herpesvirus, now designated human herpesvirus 8 (HHV-8). Seroepidemiologic studies have made a strong association between HHV-8 and Kaposi sarcoma. In addition, HHV-8 was found to be associated with all forms of

Kaposi sarcoma, and its seroconversion precedes the appearance of Kaposi sarcoma in HIV-infected persons. However, routine screening for HHV-8 with polymerase chain reaction or serologic testing is not indicated for HIV-1–infected persons. Clinical manifestations include nodules, plaques, lymph node enlargement, and signs and symptoms of visceral involvement. Skin, lung, and the gastrointestinal tract are the commonly affected organs. Lung involvement may mimic infection. Treatment options include local therapy (eg, radiotherapy, intralesional chemotherapy, cryotherapy) and systemic therapy (eg, chemotherapy, interferon-alfa). Liposome-encapsulated anthracycline chemotherapeutic agents recently have become available, potentially enabling delivery of higher doses of effective drug with fewer toxic side effects. Antiretroviral therapy also has resulted in a reduction in the frequency of occurrence of Kaposi sarcoma and a reduction in tumor burden and disease progression. Antiviral agents with in vitro activity against HHV-8—ganciclovir, foscarnet, and cidofovir—have been reported to reduce disease progression in limited studies. However, this effect remains to be confirmed in larger studies.

- Kaposi sarcoma is the most common neoplasm in HIV-infected persons.
- It is most common in the homosexual and bisexual population with AIDS.
- Kaposi sarcoma is possibly related to HHV-8 infection.
- Clinical manifestations include nodules, plaques, lymph node enlargement, and signs and symptoms of visceral involvement.

Non-Hodgkin Lymphoma

Non-Hodgkin lymphoma is much more common (as high as 200-fold increased risk) among HIV-infected patients than in the general population. It is a heterogeneous group of malignancies with varying biologic behavior and occurs in individuals with widely ranging levels of immune function. The vast majority of non-Hodgkin lymphomas in patients with HIV are of B-cell origin. Intermediate- or high-grade B-cell non-Hodgkin lymphoma is a Centers for Disease Control and Prevention-defined AIDS diagnosis. As patients with AIDS live longer, this complication will become more frequent. It commonly presents with constitutional symptoms (fever, night sweats, weight loss), lymphadenopathy, and involvement of extranodal sites such as the central nervous system, bone marrow, gastrointestinal tract, and liver. Involvement of the brain can be as an isolated disease (primary central nervous system lymphoma) or as leptomeningeal involvement in the context of spread of lymphoma elsewhere. The optimal treatment of HIV-associated non-Hodgkin lymphoma has not been well defined. Current recommendations suggest that most patients should receive standard-dose chemotherapy for *Pneumocystis* pneumonia prophylaxis (regardless of CD4 count) and growth factor support. Additionally, highly active antiretroviral therapy should be a component of the strategy.

- The vast majority of non-Hodgkin lymphomas in patients with HIV are of B-cell origin.
- Non-Hodgkin lymphoma in HIV commonly presents with constitutional symptoms (eg, fever, night sweats, weight loss), lymphadenopathy, and involvement of extranodal sites.

- Intermediate- or high-grade B-cell non-Hodgkin lymphoma is an AIDS-defining diagnosis.

Primary Central Nervous System Lymphoma

The incidence of primary central nervous system lymphoma in HIV-infected individuals is 1,000-fold higher than that in the general population. It occurs most often in the advanced stages of AIDS at a median CD4 count of less than 50 cells/mcL and is associated with Epstein-Barr virus in almost 100% of cases. The clinical presentation includes headache, confusion, lethargy, personality changes, memory loss, focal neurologic deficits, and seizure. Brain imaging studies show single or multiple contrast-enhancing lesions, often difficult to distinguish from those of toxoplasmosis. Biopsy is required for diagnosis. Whole-brain radiation has been the primary treatment of primary central nervous system lymphoma. Despite good initial radiographic response rates, the survival rate has remained dismal, with median survival times of 2 to 5 months. As has been the case with non-Hodgkin lymphoma, the advent of highly active antiretroviral therapy has rekindled interest in an aggressive approach to patients with primary central nervous system lymphoma. Whether the combination of radiotherapy or chemotherapy with highly active antiretroviral therapy will result in improved treatment outcome remains to be determined. Since the advent of highly active antiretroviral therapy, the incidence of primary central nervous system lymphoma has declined.

- Typical clinical scenario: A patient with known HIV disease and a CD4 count of 30 cells/mcL presents with headache and weakness of the right upper and lower extremities. Imaging shows 2 contrast-enhancing lesions in the left frontoparietal lobe.
- Primary central nervous system lymphoma is associated with Epstein-Barr virus.
- Clinical presentation includes headache, confusion, lethargy, personality changes, memory loss, focal neurologic deficits, and seizure.
- Biopsy is required for diagnosis.

Antiretroviral Agents

The Replication Cycle of HIV

A working knowledge of the HIV replication cycle is essential for understanding the mechanism of action of antiretroviral agents (Figure 12-2). The human immunodeficiency virus is an enveloped virus that contains 2 copies of viral genomic RNA and associated transfer RNA molecules in its core. In addition to the copies of RNA, the viral core also contains various Gag and Pol protein products. The first step in the HIV replication cycle is the interaction between the envelope proteins of the virus and specific surface receptors (eg, CD4 receptor) of the host cell, leading to the binding of the viral envelope and the host cytoplasmic membrane. Recently, additional cell surface proteins, so-called coreceptors, that are required for the virus entry into the host cell have been identified. After entry into the cell, the viral reverse transcriptase enzyme catalyzes the conversion of viral RNA into DNA. This viral DNA enters the nucleus and becomes inserted into the chromosomal DNA of the host cell (integration). This integrated

DNA may remain in an unexpressed form (eg, in resting lymphocytes) and persist in a latent state for a long period. In acutely infected cells, however, expression of the viral genes leads to production of viral proteins. The precursor Gag and Gag-Pol proteins, as well as viral RNA, are assembled at the cell surface into new viral particles and leave the host cell by a process called budding. During the process of budding, they acquire the outer layer and envelope. At this stage, the protease enzyme cleaves the precursor Gag and Gag-Pol proteins into their mature products. If this final phase of the replication cycle does not take place, the released viral particles are noninfectious and not competent to initiate the replication cycle in other susceptible cells.

The various steps in the HIV replication cycle (eg, viral entry, integration) are being investigated as potential sites of action for antiretroviral therapy.

Currently, 20 individual antiretroviral drugs and 4 coformulated products categorized in 4 classes have been approved by the US Food and Drug Administration for the treatment of HIV. The 4 classes of antiretroviral drugs are nucleoside/nucleotide analogue reverse transcriptase inhibitors, nonnucleoside analogue reverse transcriptase inhibitors, protease inhibitors, and fusion inhibitors.

Nucleoside and Nucleotide Analogue Reverse Transcriptase Inhibitors

Nucleoside and nucleotide analogue reverse transcriptase inhibitors (NRTIs) were the first agents to be developed as antiretrovirals. These agents are structurally similar to the building blocks of nucleic acids (RNA, DNA) but differ from their natural analogues by the replacement of the hydroxy (–OH) group in the 3′ position by another group that is unable to form the 5′ to 3′ phosphodiester linkage essential for DNA elongation. NRTIs block reverse transcriptase activity by competing with the natural substrates and incorporating into viral DNA to act as chain terminators in the synthesis of proviral DNA. To exert their antiviral activity, NRTIs must first be intracellularly phosphorylated to their active 5′-triphosphate forms by cellular kinases.

- NRTIs are structurally similar to the building blocks of nucleic acids.
- NRTIs block reverse transcriptase activity.

Resistance to NRTIs is associated with mutations in the *Pol* gene that codes for the enzyme reverse transcriptase. Specific mutations that confer resistance to individual agents have been identified. High-level zidovudine resistance has been associated with broad cross-resistance

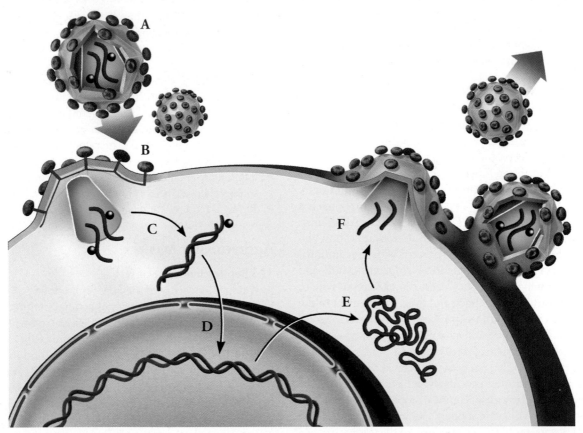

Figure 12-2. Life Cycle of Human Immunodeficiency Virus. A, The virus is an enveloped virus that contains viral genomic RNA and various Gag and Pol protein products. B, The interaction between the envelope proteins of the virus and CD4 receptor and other receptors of the host cell leads to the binding of the viral envelope and the host cytoplasmic membrane. C, The viral reverse transcriptase enzyme catalyzes the conversion of viral RNA into DNA. D, The viral DNA enters the nucleus and becomes inserted into the chromosomal DNA of the host cell. E, Expression of the viral genes leads to production of viral RNA and proteins. F, These viral proteins, as well as viral RNA, are assembled at the cell surface into new viral particles and leave the host cell by a process called budding. During the process of budding, they acquire the outer layer and envelope. At this stage, the protease enzyme cleaves the precursor Gag and Gag-Pol proteins into their mature products.

to other nucleoside analogues. Other mutations that confer cross-resistance to several agents also have been observed. The M184V mutation, associated with resistance to lamivudine, has a complex effect on other nucleoside analogues. This mutation may confer limited cross-resistance to didanosine and zalcitabine. It also may delay the development of zidovudine resistance and restore zidovudine activity once resistance emerges. This zidovudine resensitization effect also has been noted with the L74V mutation, selected for by didanosine.

* Resistance to NRTIs is associated with mutations in the *Pol* gene that codes for the enzyme reverse transcriptase.

There have been reports of a rare and potentially fatal syndrome consisting of severe hepatomegaly with steatosis and lactic acidosis in the absence of hypoxemia. Mitochondrial DNA depletion induced by NRTIs is responsible for this clinical syndrome. This syndrome is considered a classwide toxicity. However, stavudine (d4T), didanosine (ddI), and zalcitabine (ddC) are the drugs most frequently associated with it. Lamivudine (3TC), abacavir (ABC), tenofovir (TDF), and emtricitabine (FTC) are the NRTIs considered to have low mitochondrial toxicity potential.

Clinically, this syndrome has an insidious onset with gastrointestinal symptoms dominating initially (nausea, anorexia, abdominal pain, vomiting), but it can rapidly progress to involve additional systems, causing tachycardia, tachypnea, hyperventilation, jaundice, muscular weakness, and mental status changes. In some patients, the onset could be more dramatic with multiorgan failure. Associated laboratory abnormalities include increased lactate level, low arterial pH, increased anion gap, and increased liver enzyme values, including bilirubin. Lactate levels should be obtained only when patients' complaints are consistent with the presentation of this syndrome. Routine monitoring of the lactic acid level is not recommended. Once the presence of this syndrome is highly suspected, use of all antiretrovirals should be discontinued and symptomatic support with hydration instituted. Once lactate levels have returned to normal, antiretroviral drugs can be reintroduced, with use of NRTIs that have low potential for mitochondria toxicity for the nucleoside backbone of the antiretroviral regimen.

* A rare and potentially fatal syndrome of severe hepatomegaly with steatosis and lactic acidosis in the absence of hypoxemia has been reported in association with NRTIs.

Hypersensitivity reactions have been reported in approximately 5% of patients receiving abacavir. Symptoms consist of rash accompanied by systemic signs and symptoms such as fever, fatigue, nausea, vomiting, diarrhea, or abdominal pain. These symptoms usually appear within the first 6 weeks of treatment. The rash is usually maculopapular but can be variable in appearance. Hypersensitivity reactions also may occur without a rash. Symptoms usually resolve rapidly when use of the drug is discontinued. Once use of abacavir has been discontinued, it should not be reintroduced. More severe symptoms, including death, have been reported when use of abacavir is reinstituted. A genetic marker, HLA-B*5701, has been associated with an increased risk for development of a hypersensitivity reaction to abacavir.

Currently, 8 individual NRTIs are licensed for clinical use in the United States. Zalcitabine, because of its low potency, high pill burden, and adverse events, it is no longer used in clinical practice and its production has been discontinued. In addition to these individual drugs, there are 5 coformulated products that contain 2 or 3 reverse transcriptase inhibitors in a single pill. These coformulated products are zidovudine-lamivudine (Combivir), tenofovir/emtricitbine (Truvada), abacavir/lamivudine (Epzicom), zidovudine-lamivudine-abacavir (Trizivir), and tenofovir-emtricitabine efavirenz (Atripla).

General characteristics of currently available NRTIs are shown in Table 12-7.

Nonnucleoside Analogue Reverse Transcriptase Inhibitors

Nonnucleoside analogue reverse transcriptase inhibitors (NNRTIs) bind directly and noncompetitively to the enzyme reverse transcriptase. Although the drugs differ chemically from each other, they all bind to the same site, a site distinct from the substrate (dNTP) binding site. They block DNA polymerase activity by causing conformational change and disrupting the catalytic site of the enzyme. Unlike nucleoside analogues, NNRTIs do not require phosphorylation to become active and are not incorporated into viral DNA. They also have no activity against HIV-2.

* NNRTIs bind directly and noncompetitively to the enzyme reverse transcriptase.
* NNRTIs block DNA polymerase activity.
* NNRTIs do not require phosphorylation.
* NNRTIs are not active against HIV-2.

When NNRTIs are administered as a single agent or as a part of an inadequately suppressive treatment regimen, resistance emerges rapidly. Mutations conferring resistance to one drug in this class generally confer cross-resistance to most other NNRTIs. Cross-resistance to nucleoside analogues or protease inhibitors has not been observed. However, the Y181C mutation, selected for by nevirapine, reverses zidovudine resistance when introduced into isolates that carry the major zidovudine resistance mutations.

To date, 3 NNRTIs have been approved for the treatment of HIV: nevirapine, delavirdine, and efavirenz. Delavirdine is rarely used in clinical practice because of its low potency and large pill burden. Nevirapine and efavirenz are inducers of the hepatic cytochrome P450 system. Delavirdine, however, inhibits P450. Through this interaction with the P450 enzyme system, NNRTIs may change the metabolism of and thus lower (nevirapine, efavirenz) or increase (delavirdine) the plasma levels of coadministered drugs that are metabolized by the cytochrome P450 system. Similarly, drugs that induce or inhibit cytochrome P450 activity may have an effect on the plasma concentrations of NNRTIs. Malformations of the fetus have been noted in primates and humans exposed to efavirenz. Therefore, efavirenz is contraindicated in pregnant women.

* Mutations conferring resistance to one drug in NNRTIs generally confer cross-resistance to most other NNRTIs.

Table 12-7 Selected General Characteristics of Current Nucleoside and Nucleotide Analogue Reverse Transcriptase Inhibitors

NRTI	Dosage (All Oral)	Metabolism, Excretion[a]	Adverse Effects
Abacavir (ABC)	300 mg twice daily or 600 mg once daily	Hepatic via alcohol dehydrogenase & glucuronyl transferase; metabolites excreted renally	Diarrhea, anorexia, nausea, vomiting, headache, fatigue, hypersensitivity reaction[b]
Didanosine (ddI)	400 mg once daily If body weight <60 kg or if given with tenofovir: 250 mg once daily	50% renal excretion	Rash, abdominal pain, diarrhea, nausea and vomiting, asthenia, headache, fever, pancreatitis, peripheral neuropathy, lactic acidosis when used with stavudine)
Emtricitabine (FTC)	200 mg once daily	Metabolism, oxidation, & conjugation; renal excretion	Hyperpigmentation of skin, rash, diarrhea, nausea, vomiting, headache
Lamivudine (3TC)	300 mg once daily or 150 mg twice daily	5.6% to transsulfoxide metabolite; renal excretion	Decrease in appetite, nausea, vomiting, headache, fatigue, pancreatitis in children
Stavudine (d4T)	40 mg twice daily If body weight <60 kg: 30 mg twice daily	Renal excretion	Rash, diarrhea, nausea, vomiting, headache, lipoatrophy, hyperlipidemia, peripheral neuropathy, muscle weakness
Tenofovir (TDF)	300 mg once daily	Renal excretion	Diarrhea, flatulence, nausea, vomiting, osteopenia, renal impairment
Zidovudine (AZT, ZDV)	300 mg twice daily or 200 mg 3 times daily	Hepatic glucuronidation; renal excretion	Headache, nausea, anorexia, vomiting, macrocytic anemia, leukopenia, myopathy, lipoatrophy, hyperlipidemia

Abbreviation: NRTI, nucleoside and nucleotide analogue reverse transcriptase inhibitor.

[a] All NRTIs are excreted renally to varying extents, and dosage requirements are required with renal impairment.

[b] Occurs within days to 6 weeks of initiation of therapy. Can be severe or fatal. Rechallenge after a hypersensitivity reaction is contraindicated.

The general characteristics of the 3 NNRTIs currently approved for clinical use are listed in Table 12-8.

Protease Inhibitors

Protease inhibitors exert their antiviral effect by inhibiting HIV-1 protease. HIV-1 protease is a complex enzyme composed of 2 identical halves (ie, a symmetrical dimer) with an active site located at the base of the cleft. It is responsible for the cleavage of the large viral Gag and Gag-Pol polypeptide chains into smaller, functional proteins, thus allowing maturation of the HIV virion. This process takes place in the final stages of the HIV life cycle. Inhibition of the protease enzyme results in the release of structurally disorganized and noninfectious viral particles. Protease inhibitors have antiviral activity in both acutely and chronically infected cells. Protease inhibitors are metabolized by the cytochrome P450 system and are themselves, to varying degrees, inhibitors of this system. This leads to a considerable number of interactions with drugs that are inducers, inhibitors, or substrates of this system.

Currently, 10 protease inhibitors are approved for the treatment of HIV. General characteristics of currently available protease inhibitors are listed in Table 12-9.

- Protease inhibitors exert their antiviral effect by inhibiting HIV-1 protease.
- Protease inhibitors have antiviral activity in both acutely and chronically infected cells.
- Protease inhibitors have considerable interactions with drugs that are metabolized through the P450 system.

Protease inhibitors have shown potent antiretroviral, immunologic, and clinical benefits in HIV-infected persons, but their long-term efficacy and safety have not been completely elucidated. In fact, new side effects have become manifest with the continued widespread use of these drugs. Metabolic complications of these drugs have included hyperglycemia, frank diabetes mellitus, and abnormalities of lipid metabolism and lipid deposition. These complications have been noted

Table 12-8 Selected General Characteristics of Current Nonnucleoside Reverse Transcriptase Inhibitors

NNRTI	Dosage	Metabolism	Elimination[a]	Adverse Effects
Delavirdine (DLV)	400 mg 3 times daily	CYP substrate, CYP3A4 inhibitor	51% renal, as metabolites; <5% unchanged; 44% in feces	Rash, headache, hepatotoxicity
Efavirenz (EFV)	600 mg once daily	CYP3A4 substrate, mixed CYP3A4 inducer-inhibitor	14%-34% renal, as metabolites; 16%-61% in feces, primarily unchanged	Rash, CNS symptoms, teratogenicity, hepatotoxicity, dyslipidemia
Nevirapine (NVP)	200 mg twice daily after a lead-in period of 2 weeks at a dosage of 200 mg once daily	CYP3A4 substrate, CYP3A4 inhibitor	90% renal, as metabolites; <5% unchanged parent compound excreted renally; 10% in feces	Rash, hepatotoxicity,[b] dyslipidemia

Abbreviations: CNS, central nervous system; CYP, cytochrome P450; NNRTI, nonnucleoside reverse transcriptase inhibitors.

[a] A relatively low proportion of the parent compounds of current NNRTIs is excreted renally. Thus, no dose adjustment is necessary with renal impairment.

[b] The risk of nevirapine-associated hepatotoxicity is higher in women with CD4 counts more than 250 cells/mcL and in men with CD4 counts more than 400 cells/mcL.

even in patients who have responded well virologically to treatment and are otherwise in improved health. The biochemical and physiologic basis of protease inhibitor-related metabolic complications has, as of yet, not been adequately investigated and remains obscure. Of note, similar metabolic abnormalities have been reported in patients taking antiretroviral regimens that do not contain protease inhibitors.

* Metabolic complications of protease inhibitors have included hyperglycemia, frank diabetes mellitus, and abnormalities of lipid metabolism and lipid deposition.

Spontaneous bleeding has been reported in patients with hemophilia A and B treated with protease inhibitors, but a causal relationship between these incidents and protease inhibitor therapy has not been established.

The issue of resistance among protease inhibitors is complex and incompletely understood. Mutations that confer drug resistance have been identified in protease genes. Several of these mutations have been found to be key for individual protease inhibitors. Nevertheless, accumulation of several mutations is usually necessary for high-level resistance to occur, and cross-resistance is common among the various protease inhibitors that are currently in use. There is no cross-resistance between protease inhibitors and reverse transcriptase inhibitors.

The inhibitory effect of protease inhibitors on each other's metabolism has led to the common clinical practice of prescribing protease inhibitors with low-dose (100-400 mg daily) ritonavir. This enhances the pharmacokinetic profile of the protease inhibitors, allowing for dose reductions, more convenience (no food requirement), and less frequent dosing regimens. All currently licensed protease inhibitors are commonly prescribed as boosted agents, with the exception of nelfinavir, which is not well and reliably augmented by ritonavir. In fact, 4 protease inhibitors, darunavir, lopinavir, saquinavir, and tipranavir, should not be administered without con-

comitant ritonavir. Of these 4 drugs, lopinavir is the only drug that is produced coformulated with ritonavir. For the others, ritonavir has to be prescribed individually.

Fusion Inhibitors

Enfuvirtide (T-20) is the only fusion inhibitor that is currently approved by the US Food and Drug Administration. It binds a region of the HIV envelope glycoprotein gp41 and prevents viral fusion with the target cell membrane. Enfuvirtide is administered by subcutaneous injection. The standard dosage is 90 mg twice daily. Enfuvirtide is packaged in powder form in single-dose vials and must be reconstituted with sterile water. The current indication for enfuvirtide is for treatment in patients who have experienced multiple regimen failures. Three significant and noteworthy toxicities have been reported in clinical trials of enfuvirtide. Almost everyone experiences injection-site reactions that are typically erythematous nodules, are mild to moderate in severity, and rarely cause discontinuation of use of the drug. Much less frequent are hypersensitivity reactions. Bacterial pneumonia was noted at a higher frequency in enfuvirtide-treated patients than patients in the comparator arms. The explanation for this difference and its clinical significance are unknown. HIV can become resistant to enfuvirtide, but there is no cross-resistance to the other currently approved antiretroviral drugs.

Guidelines for Use of Antiretroviral Therapy for HIV Infection

Guidelines addressing the issue of antiretroviral therapy in different populations and situations have been developed and are updated regularly electronically as new information becomes available (http://www.aidsinfo.nih.gov).

Guidelines for Use of Antiretroviral Agents in HIV-Infected Adults

A panel of leading AIDS specialists, convened by the US Department of Health and Human Services in collaboration with the Henry J.

Table 12-9 General Characteristics of Current Protease Inhibitors

Name	Dosage	Metabolism	Adverse Effects

Atazanavir (ATV)	400 mg once daily
	If taken with efavirenz or tenofovir:
	  300 mg ATV with 100 mg
	  ritonavir once daily
		Hepatic, via multiple pathways CYP3A4	Rash, nausea, increased bilirubin, increased amylase, depression, diarrhea, increased liver enzymes, jaundice

Darunavir (DRV)	DRV 600 mg + ritonavir 100 mg twice daily	Hepatic, primarily CYP3A	Rash, hyperglycemia, hypertriglyceridemia, increased lipase, hypercholesterolemia, diarrhea, nausea, increased liver enzymes, headache, nasopharyngitis

Fosamprenavir (FPV)	Antiretroviral therapy-naive patients:
	  FPV 1,400 mg twice daily
	    or
	  FPV 1,400 mg + RTV 200 mg daily
	    or
	  FPV 700 mg + RTV 100 mg twice daily
	Protease inhibitor-experienced patients:
	  FPV 700 mg + RTV 100 mg twice daily
		Converted to amprenavir by cellular phosphatases, hepatically metabolized by CYP3A4	Stomach upset, rash, diarrhea, nausea, vomiting, increased liver function values

Indinavir (IDV)	800 mg every 8 hours
	  or
	IDV 800 mg + RTV 100 or 200 mg
	  twice daily
		Hepatic via CYP3A4	Kidney stones, nausea, vomiting, diarrhea, stomach upset, headache

Lopinavir-ritonavir (LPV/r)	400 mg LPV and 100 mg r twice daily
	  or
	800 mg LPV and 200 mg r once daily
	  (only in antiretroviral naive patients)
		Hepatic via CYP3A	Diarrhea, nausea, headache, fatigue

Nelfinavir (NFV)	1,250 mg twice daily or 750 mg 3 times daily	Hepatic via CYP2C19 & CYP3A4	Diarrhea, nausea, gas, rash
Ritonavir (RTV)	Used currently only as pharmacokinetic enhancer for other protease inhibitors at dosages of 100-400 mg daily & not for its own antiviral effect	Hepatic via CYP3A4 & CYP2D6 The most potent P450 inhibitor	Stomach upset, nausea, vomiting, diarrhea, taste disturbance, increased liver enzymes
Saquinavir (SQV)	Use only with ritonavir boosting: SQV 1,000 mg + RTV 100 mg twice daily	Hepatic via CYP3A4	Stomach upset, nausea, diarrhea, headache, abdominal pain, increased liver enzymes
Tipranavir (TPV)	Use only with ritonavir boosting: TPV 500 mg + RTV 200 mg twice daily	Hepatic via CYP3A4	Hypercholesterolemia, hypertriglyceridemia, diarrhea, transaminase increases, nausea, intracranial hemorrhage

Abbreviation: CYP, cytochrome P450.

Kaiser Family Foundation, has developed recommendations for use of antiretroviral agents in HIV-infected adults and adolescents. There is broad agreement that antiretroviral therapy should be initiated in patients with symptoms ascribed to HIV infection regardless of CD4 cell count. The optimal time to start antiretroviral therapy in asymptomatic patients is less clear. Current guidelines recommend initiating antiretroviral therapy in asymptomatic patients with less than 200 CD4 cells/mcL. For those with CD4 cell counts between 200 and 350 cells/mcL, many HIV clinicians prescribe antiretroviral therapy. Firm evidence for initiating antiretroviral therapy for patients who have CD4 cell counts of more than 350 cells/mcL is currently lacking, and many clinicians defer therapy in these patients.

The goal of treatment is maximal viral suppression for as long as possible. Response to treatment is evaluated with plasma HIV RNA (viral load) levels. HIV-1 RNA testing should be performed at baseline and repeated every 3 to 4 months during therapy, or at more frequent intervals if the situation warrants. A minimal change in plasma viremia is considered a 3-fold or $0.5\text{-}\log_{10}$ increase or decrease. A substantial decrease in CD4 count is a decrease of more than 30% from baseline for absolute cell numbers and a decrease of more than 3% from baseline in percentages of cells. In cases of therapy failures, a new regimen consisting of at least 2 new agents, without cross-resistance to the drugs in the failed regimen, should be substituted. Resistance testing (genotyping or phenotyping) has been found useful for making the appropriate drug selection for incorporation into a salvage treatment regimen.

Recommendations for Use of Antiretroviral Drugs in Pregnant Women

In the past few years, perinatal transmission of HIV has dramatically decreased in the United States. This decrease is a result of recommendations from the US Public Health Service for universal prenatal HIV counseling and testing with consent for all pregnant women and the use of zidovudine for reduction of perinatal HIV transmission. These recommendations were based on the results of Pediatric AIDS Clinical Trial Group Protocol 076. This trial demonstrated that zidovudine, when administered to the mother during the antepartum and intrapartum periods and to the newborn for the first 6 weeks of life, reduces the perinatal transmission of HIV by two-thirds. The advances in understanding the pathogenesis of HIV and the changes in antiretroviral therapy and monitoring of disease have made the establishment of new guidelines necessary. Consequently, the US Public Health Service has updated its recommendations for the use of antiretroviral drugs in pregnant women.

Health care providers of pregnant HIV-infected women must address 2 separate but related issues: treatment of the mother's HIV infection and reduction of the risk for HIV transmission to the fetus. The benefits of therapy must therefore be weighed against the potential risk for adverse events to the fetus or newborn. Decisions regarding initiation or alterations in therapy should involve the same factors as those used for women who are not pregnant, with the additional consideration of the potential impact of such therapy on the fetus and infant. HIV-infected pregnant women should be provided with the most complete and current information regarding the use of antiretroviral therapy, mode of delivery, and other issues and should be allowed to make their own decisions. The woman's autonomy in decision making should be respected. Antiretroviral therapy should be offered to all HIV-1–infected women during pregnancy, whether primarily for HIV-1 infection or for reduction of perinatal transmission or for both purposes. Additionally, to prevent perinatal transmission, zidovudine chemoprophylaxis should be incorporated into the antiretroviral regimen.

- Zidovudine administered to the mother during the antepartum and intrapartum periods and to the newborn for the first 6 weeks of life reduces perinatal transmission of HIV by two-thirds.

Recommendations for Postexposure Prophylaxis

Numerous studies have estimated that the average risk for HIV transmission is approximately 0.3% after percutaneous exposure to HIV-infected blood and 0.09% after mucous membrane exposure. A retrospective case-control study of health care workers documented that the use of zidovudine was associated with a 79% decrease in the risk for HIV transmission. Results of that study, as well as results from studies in animals and data from the Pediatric AIDS Clinical Trial Group on the efficacy of zidovudine for preventing perinatal transmission of HIV, prompted the US Public Health Service to issue recommendations for prophylaxis in health care workers after occupational exposure to HIV. With the availability of new drugs and the accumulation of more knowledge, these 1996 guidelines have recently been updated.

- In health care workers, the use of zidovudine is associated with a 79% decrease in the risk for HIV transmission.

The risk of infection is a function of the type of exposure and the infectivity of the exposure source. The guidelines provide an algorithm to guide clinicians in assessing risk and deciding when to offer postexposure prophylaxis. Systems, including written protocols, should be in place to prompt reporting and facilitate management of exposed health care workers. For most HIV exposures, a 4-week regimen of 2 antiretroviral drugs is recommended.

Combinations that can be considered for occupational postexposure prophylaxis include, 1) zidovudine plus lamivudine (or emtricitabine) or 2) tenofovir plus lamivudine (or emtricitabine). The addition of a protease inhibitor is recommended for exposures with an increased risk of transmission or when resistance to one of the recommended drugs is known or suspected. Current guidelines prefer lopinavir-ritonavir for use in expanded postexposure prophylaxis regimens. However, other protease inhibitors are also acceptable for use in these regimens.

Individual clinicians may, of course, prefer other antiretroviral drugs or combinations because of local knowledge and experience. These recommendations are based on information available at the time they were developed. A mechanism has been put in place, through the HIV/AIDS Treatment Information Service Web site, to regularly refine and update the recommendations in tandem with the evolution of knowledge about HIV infection.

- The risk of infection is a function of the type of exposure and the infectivity of the exposing source.

HIV Infection Pharmacy Review
Lynn L. Estes, PharmD

Nucleoside and Nucleotide Reverse Transcriptase Inhibitors: Select Characteristics

Drug Name and Aliases	Normal Adult Dose (Without Organ Dysfunction)	Dosing Instructions	Toxic/Adverse Effects	Metabolism or Excretion Route and Pharmacokinetic Drug Interaction Potential[a,b]
Abacavir (ABC, Ziagen)	300 mg twice daily or 600 mg once daily No dose adjustment needed for renal dysfunction	Take with or without food Alcohol increases abacavir levels	Hypersensitivity reaction can be severe or fatal (usually within days to 6 weeks of initiation). Symptoms may include fever, malaise, abdominal cramping, nausea, diarrhea, rash, increased transaminase & creatinine kinase levels, & respiratory symptoms Rechallenge after a hypersensitivity reaction is contraindicated & can have severe or fatal consequences GI intolerance, fever, malaise, headache, increased transaminase levels NRTI class side effects: fat redistribution; lactic acidosis & hepatomegaly with stenosis (infrequent) Pregnancy category C	Hepatic metabolism by alcohol dehydrogenase or glucuronyl transferase, with renal excretion of metabolites May inhibit or be affected by other drugs that inhibit alcohol dehydrogenase or UDPGT Alcohol increases abacavir levels
Abacavir 600 mg plus lamivudine 300 mg (coformulated; Epzicom)	1 tablet once daily CrCl <50 mL/min: give separately in dosing as per individual agents	Take with or without food	See individual agents	See individual agents
Abacavir 300 mg plus lamivudine 150 mg plus zidovudine 300 mg (coformulated; Trizivir)	>40 kg: 1 tablet twice daily CrCl <50 mL/min: give separately in dosing as per individual agents	Take with or without food	See individual agents	See individual agents

Didanosine (ddI, Videx EC)	≥60 kg:
	  EC capsules:
	    400 mg once daily
	  With tenofovir:
	    250 mg once daily
	
	<60 kg:
	  EC capsules:
	    250 mg once daily
	  With tenofovir:
	    200 mg once daily
	
	CrCl <60 mL/min: reduce dose
		Take on empty stomach	Pancreatitis, peripheral neuropathy, GI intolerance
			Fatal lactic acidosis reported in pregnant patients receiving a combination of stavudine & didanosine—avoid combination in pregnancy if possible
			NRTI class side effects: fat redistribution; lactic acidosis & hepatomegaly with steatosis (higher frequency with didanosine)
			Pregnancy category B
				50% renally cleared
				Tenofovir can substantially increase didanosine concentrations—reduce didanosine dose
				Ribavirin can increase didanosine exposure & risk of toxicity; use combination with caution
				Methadone can decrease didanosine levels; consider dose increase
				Hydroxyurea can increase potential for toxicity; avoid concomitant use

HIV Infection Pharmacy Review (continued)

Nucleoside and Nucleotide Reverse Transcriptase Inhibitors: Select Characteristics (continued)

Drug Name and Aliases	Normal Adult Dose (Without Organ Dysfunction)	Dosing Instructions	Toxic/Adverse Effects	Metabolism or Excretion Route and Pharmacokinetic Drug Interaction Potential[a,b]
Efavirenz 600 mg plus emtricitabine 200 mg plus tenofovir 300 mg (coformulated; Atripla)	1 tablet once daily CrCl <50 mL/min: give separately in dosing as per individual agents	Do not take with high-fat meal Take at bedtime to start with	See individual agents	See individual agents
Emtricitabine (FTC, Emtriva)	200 mg once daily CrCL <50 mL/min: reduce dose	Take with or without food	Generally well tolerated; headache, diarrhea, nausea, rash, generally mild skin discoloration (hyperpigmentation on palms or soles) Active against hepatitis B; flare may occur on discontinuation NRTI class side effects: fat redistribution; lactic acidosis & hepatomegaly with steatosis (infrequent) Pregnancy category B	Renal excretion
Emtricitabine 200 mg plus tenofovir 300 mg (coformulated; Truvada)	1 tablet once daily	Take with or without food	See individual agents	See individual agents
Lamivudine (3TC, Epivir)	≥50 kg: 150 mg twice daily or 300 mg once daily <50 kg: 2 mg/kg twice daily CrCl <50 mL/min: reduce dose	Take with or without food	Generally well tolerated; headache, nausea, diarrhea, abdominal pain, rash, pancreatitis in pediatric patients (rare in adults) Active against hepatitis B; flare may occur on discontinuation NRTI class side effects: fat redistribution; lactic acidosis & hepatomegaly with steatosis (infrequent) Pregnancy category C	Renal excretion
Lamivudine 150 mg plus zidovudine 300 mg (coformulated; Combivir)	1 tablet twice daily CrCl <50 mL/min: give separately in dosing as per individual agents	Take with or without food	See individual agents	See individual agents
Stavudine (d4t, Zerit)	≥60 kg: 40 mg twice daily <60 kg: 30 mg twice daily CrCl <50 mL/min: reduce dose	Take with or without food	Peripheral neuropathy, GI intolerance, headache, insomnia, pancreatitis, hyperlipidemia, ascending neuromuscular weakness Fatal lactic acidosis reported in pregnant patients receiving stavudine plus didanosine; avoid combination in pregnancy, if possible NRTI class side effects: fat redistribution; lactic acidosis & hepatomegaly with steatosis (higher frequency with stavudine) Pregnancy category C	50% renally cleared Possible increased risk of pancreatitis, neuropathy, hepatotoxicity, & lactic acidosis when combined with didanosine or hydroxyurea

HIV Infection Pharmacy Review (continued)

Nucleoside and Nucleotide Reverse Transcriptase Inhibitors: Select Characteristics (continued)

Drug Name and Aliases	Normal Adult Dose (Without Organ Dysfunction)	Dosing Instructions	Toxic/Adverse Effects	Metabolism or Excretion Route and Pharmacokinetic Drug Interaction Potential[a,b]
Tenofovir (TDF, Viread)	300 mg once daily CrCl <50 mL/min: reduce dose	Take with or without food	Mild GI complaints, asthenia, headache, renal dysfunction, osteomalacia Active against hepatitis B; flare may occur on discontinuation NRTI class side effects: fat redistribution; lactic acidosis & hepatomegaly with steatosis (infrequent) Pregnancy category B	Renally cleared Can substantially increase didanosine levels; reduce didanosine dose Can decrease atazanavir levels; use atazanavir in combination with ritonavir Concomitant therapy with ritonavir, lopinavir, atazanavir, or didanosine can increase tenofovir levels & toxicity; monitor closely Cidofovir, ganciclovir, & valganciclovir can compete for tubular secretion—monitor closely
Zidovudine (AZT, ZDV, Retrovir)	300 mg twice daily CrCl <15 mL/min: reduce dose	Take with or without food	Macrocytic anemia or neutropenia, malaise, GI intolerance, insomnia, asthenia, myopathy NRTI class side effects: fat redistribution; lactic acidosis & hepatomegaly with steatosis Pregnancy category C	Hepatic metabolism with renal clearance of metabolites Ribavirin can inhibit phosphorylation & activation of zidovudine

Abbreviations: CrCl, creatinine clearance; GI, gastrointestinal; NRTI, nucleoside and nucleotide reverse transcriptase inhibitor; UDPGT, uridine diphosphoglucuronyltransferase.

[a] Drug interactions listed are not all-inclusive and do not include drugs with overlapping toxicities.

[b] Package insert and other resources should be consulted for specific drug interactions.

From Wilson JW, Estes LL. Mayo Clinic antimicrobial therapy: quick guide. Rochester, MN: Mayo Clinic Scientific Press and New York, NY: Informa Healthcare USA, Inc; c2008.

HIV Infection Pharmacy Review (continued)

Nonnucleoside Reverse Transcriptase Inhibitors: Select Characteristics

Drug Name and Aliases	Normal Adult Dose	Dosing Instructions	Toxic/Adverse Effects	Metabolism or Excretion Route and Pharmacokinetic Drug Interaction Potential[a,b]
Delavirdine (DLV, Rescriptor)	400 mg 3 times daily	Take with or without food	Rash (common); can usually treat through but can be serious in some cases Mild headache, fatigue, GI complaints, increased transaminase levels Pregnancy category C	Hepatic metabolism Substrate for CYP3A4[c,d] & CYP2D6 Can inhibit CYP3A4,[e] CYP2D6, CYP2C9, & CYP2C19 Avoid H_2-receptor blockers or proton pump inhibitors
Efavirenz (EFV, Sustiva)	600 mg once daily (preferably at bedtime to start)	Take with or without food (a high-fat meal can increase bioavailability up to 50% & should be avoided)	Rash (can usually treat through if mild) CNS symptoms (eg, dizziness, light-headedness, nightmares, feeling of disengagement, impaired concentration, agitation) can be minimized by taking at bedtime & often subside after 2-4 weeks Case reports of psychosis, delusional thoughts, suicidal ideation, & depression (more frequent in patients with mental illness history) Increased transaminase levels, especially in patients with hepatitis Mild increase in cholesterol & triglyceride levels in some patients False-positive urine screening test for marijuana Pregnancy category D (avoid in pregnant patients)	Hepatic metabolism Substrate for CYP3A4[c,d] Can induce or inhibit CYP3A4[e] Can decrease methadone levels or effect; titrate dose
Efavirenz 600 mg plus emtricitabine 200 mg plus tenofovir 300 mg (coformulated; Atripla)	1 tablet once daily CrCl <50 mL/min: give separately in dosing as per individual agents	Take on an empty stomach (or at least not with a high-fat meal); take at bedtime to start with	See individual agents	See individual agents
Nevirapine (NVP, Viramune)	200 mg once daily for 14 days then 200 mg twice daily	Start with 2-week lead-in of reduced dose to reduce incidence of rash Autoinduction occurs & stabilizes at 2-4 weeks Take with or without food	Rash (can usually treat through if mild); rare serious cutaneous reactions (eg, Stevens-Johnson syndrome) Severe & fatal cases of hepatitis reported, particularly in first 18 weeks. Risk of hepatotoxicity may increase with increased transaminase levels, history of hepatitis B or C, CD4 >250/mcL in women & >400 mcL in men. If hepatitis occurs, discontinue nevirapine permanently. During first 8 weeks, monitor patients intensively for serious cutaneous reactions & signs of hepatotoxicity Nausea, headache, diarrhea Pregnancy category C	Hepatic metabolism Substrate for CYP3A4[c,d] Induces CYP3A4[e] Decreases methadone levels Decreases oral contraceptive levels; use alternative birth control

Abbreviations: CNS, central nervous system; CYP, cytochrome P450; GI, gastrointestinal.

HIV Infection Pharmacy Review (continued)

Nonnucleoside Reverse Transcriptase Inhibitors: Select Characteristics (continued)

^a Drug interactions listed are not all-inclusive and do not include drugs with overlapping toxicities.

^b Package insert and other resources should be consulted for specific drug interactions.

^c Abbreviated list of CYP3A4 **inducers** that can decrease serum levels of substrates for CYP3A4 (eg, protease inhibitors, nonnucleoside reverse transcriptase inhibitors): rifampin, rifabutin, rifapentine, carbamazepine, phenobarbital, phenytoin, nevirapine, efavirenz, St. John's wort.

^d Abbreviated list of CYP3A4 **inhibitors** that can potentially increase serum level of substrates for CYP3A4 (eg, protease inhibitors, nonnucleoside reverse transcriptase inhibitors): protease inhibitors, erythromycin, clarithromycin, azole antifungals, amiodarone, cimetidine, grapefruit juice.

^e Abbreviated list of CYP3A4 **substrates** (serum levels can be increased by CYP3A4 inhibitors such as protease inhibitors and decreased by CYP3A4 inducers such as nevirapine or efavirenz); benzodiazepines (avoid midazolam or triazolam; can use lorazepam with protease inhibitors); statins (avoid use of lovastatin or simvastatin with protease inhibitors; pravastatin and rosuvastatin do not substantially interact and atorvastatin can be used with caution and monitoring); dihydropyridine calcium channel blockers; ergot alkaloids (avoid with protease inhibitors); sildenafil, vardenafil, and tadalafil (dose reduction of erectile dysfunction drugs needed with protease inhibitors); some antiarrhythmics (eg, amiodarone, lidocaine, quinidine); warfarin; pimozide (avoid with protease inhibitors); rifabutin (may need dose alterations of one or both drugs); some antidepressants and anticonvulsants (eg, carbamazepine, phenytoin, phenobarbital); immunosuppressants (eg, cyclosporine, tacrolimus, sirolimus); azole antifungals.

From Wilson JW, Estes LL. Mayo Clinic antimicrobial therapy: quick guide. Rochester, MN: Mayo Clinic Scientific Press and New York, NY: Informa Healthcare USA, Inc; c2008.

HIV Infection Pharmacy Review (continued)

Protease Inhibitors: Select Characteristics

Drug Name and Aliases	Normal Adult Dose	Dosing Instructions	Toxic/Adverse Effects	Metabolism or Excretion Route and Pharmacokinetic Drug Interaction Potential[a,b]
Atazanavir (ATZ, Reyatez)	400 mg once daily; or 300 mg atazanavir plus 100 mg ritonavir, both once daily. Use boosted regimen with ritonavir when combined with tenofovir, efavirenz, or nevirapine	Take with food	Increased indirect bilirubin level (usually asymptomatic), jaundice, GI effects, rash. Prolonged PR interval, first-degree heart block in some patients. PI class side effects: increased lipid levels, lipodystrophy, hyperglycemia, hemolytic anemia, & spontaneous bleeding or hematomas with hemophilia; atazanavir has less effect on glucose & lipids than other PIs. Pregnancy category B	Hepatic metabolism. Substrate for CYP3A4[c,d]. Can inhibit CYP3A4,[e] CYP1A2, CYP2C9. Levels decreased by tenofovir; use atazanavir plus ritonavir; atazanavir can also increase tenofovir levels (monitor for adverse effects). Space apart from antacids, avoid use with H_2-receptor antagonists & proton pump inhibitors, if possible
Darunavir (DRV, Prezista)	600 mg with 100 mg ritonavir, both twice daily	Take with food	Diarrhea, nausea, headache, increased transaminase values, rash (contains a sulfonamide moiety—use with caution in patients with sulfonamide allergy). PI class side effects: increased lipid levels, lipodystrophy, hyperglycemia, hemolytic anemia, & spontaneous bleeding or hematomas in hemophilia. Pregnancy category B	Hepatic metabolism. Substrate for CYP3A4[c,d]. Inhibitor of CYP3A4[e]. Decreases oral contraceptive levels; use alternative method of birth control
Fosamprenavir (FPV, Lexiva)	PI-naive patients: fosamprenavir 1,400 mg twice daily or fosamprenavir 1,400 mg plus ritonavir 200 mg, both once daily; or fosamprenavir 700 mg, plus ritonavir 100 mg both twice daily. PI-experienced patients: fosamprenavir 700 mg plus ritonavir 100 mg, both twice daily. Coadministration with efavirenz: use boosted regimen with ritonavir	Take with or without food	Nausea, vomiting, diarrhea, headache, rash (including rare Stevens-Johnson syndrome); amprenavir is a sulfonamide & could theoretically have cross-allergenicity with other sulfonamides; increased transaminase levels. PI class side effects: increased lipid levels, lipodystrophy, hyperglycemia, hemolytic anemia, & spontaneous bleeding or hematomas in hemophilia. Pregnancy category C	Rapidly converted to amprenavir by cellular phosphatases in the gut. Amprenavir is a substrate for CYP3A4[c,d] & can inhibit CYP3A4

HIV Infection Pharmacy Review (continued)

Protease Inhibitors: Select Characteristics (continued)

Drug Name and Aliases	Normal Adult Dose	Dosing Instructions	Toxic/Adverse Effects	Metabolism or Excretion Route and Pharmacokinetic Drug Interaction Potential[a,b]
Indinavir (Crixivan)	800 mg q 8 h With ritonavir: indinavir 800 mg plus ritonavir 100 mg or 200 mg, both twice daily With efavirenz or nevirapine: 1,000 mg q 8 h	Take on empty stomach or with light meal, unless given with ritonavir Drink ≥48 ounces of water daily to decrease nephrolithiasis	Nephrolithiasis (can decrease risk by drinking ≥48 ounces of liquids daily) Increase bilirubin level (usually asymptomatic) Headache, nausea, vomiting, diarrhea, rash, increased hepatic transaminase levels, thrombocytopenia, dry skin & lips, ingrown toenails PI class side effects: increased lipid levels, lipodystrophy, hyperglycemia, hemolytic anemia, & spontaneous bleeding or hematomas in hemophilia Pregnancy category C	Hepatic metabolism Substrate for CYP3A4[c,d] Inhibits CYP3A4[e]
Lopinivir 200 mg plus ritonavir 50 mg (coformulated; rLPV, Kaletra)	Lopinavir 400 mg plus ritonavir 100 mg (2 tablets) twice daily; or lopinavir 800 mg plus ritonavir 200 mg (4 tablets once daily); use the once-daily regimen only in treatment-naive patients Treatment-experienced patients also on efavirenz or nevirapine: lopinavir 600 mg plus ritonavir 150 mg twice daily	Take with food	GI intolerance, diarrhea, headache, rash, asthenia Higher incidence of increased triglyceride & cholesterol levels than other PIs Increased transaminase levels PI class side effects: increased lipid levels, lipodystrophy, hyperglycemia, hemolytic anemia, & spontaneous bleeding or hematomas in hemophilia Pregnancy category C	Hepatic metabolism Substrate for CYP3A4[c,d] Both lopinivir & ritonavir are potent inhibitors of CYP3A4[e] Decreases methadone levels Decreases oral contraceptive levels; use alternative method of birth control Oral solution contains alcohol; avoid with metronidazole or disulfiram
Nelfinavir (NFV, Viracept)	1,250 mg twice daily or 750 mg 3 times daily	Take with food	Diarrhea, soft stool, nausea, flatulence, rash PI class side effects: increased lipid levels, lipodystrophy, hyperglycemia, hemolytic anemia, & spontaneous bleeding or hematomas in hemophilia Pregnancy category B	Hepatic metabolism Substrate for CP3A4[c,d]; Inhibits CYP3A4[e] (induces CYP3A4 occasionally) Decreases oral contraceptive levels; use alternative method of birth control

HIV Infection Pharmacy Review (continued)

Protease Inhibitors: Select Characteristics (continued)

Drug Name and Aliases	Normal Adult Dose	Dosing Instructions	Toxic/Adverse Effects	Metabolism or Excretion Route and Pharmacokinetic Drug Interaction Potential[a,b]
Ritonavir (RTV, Norvir)	When used as the only PI: 600 mg twice daily When used as a boosted agent with another PI: 100-400 mg in 1 or 2 divided doses	Take with meals when used as the sole PI	GI intolerance (dose-related; may resolve with continued therapy); less common when used in low-dose boosting regimen Taste changes, dizziness, headache, somnolence, paresthesias (circumoral and extremities), hepatotoxicity PI class side effects: increased lipid levels, lipodystrophy, hyperglycemia, hemolytic anemia, & spontaneous bleeding or hematomas in hemophilia. Increased lipid levels may be more severe with ritonavir than with other PIs Pregnancy category B	Hepatic metabolism Substrate for CYP3A4[c,d] Very potent inhibitor of CYP3A4[e] Inhibits or competes for CYP2C9, CYP2C19, & CYP2D6 Induces CYP1A2 (decreases theophylline levels) Decreases methadone levels Decreases oral contraceptive levels; use alternative method of birth control Space apart from didanosine
Saquinavir (SQV, Invirase)	Saquinavir 1,000 mg with ritonavir 100 mg, both twice daily	Take with a full meal (or within 2 hours of eating)	GI intolerance (may subside with continued therapy), diarrhea, headache, asthenia, rash, increased transaminase levels PI class side effects: increased lipid levels, lipodystrophy, hyperglycemia, hemolytic anemia, & spontaneous bleeding or hematomas in hemophilia Pregnancy category B	Hepatic metabolism Substrate for CYP3A4[c,d] Inhibits CYP3A4[e] Levels decreased by dexamethasone
Tipranavir (TPV, Aptivus)	Tipranavir 500 mg with ritonavir 200 mg, both twice daily	Take with food	Hypersensitivity (especially in young women); possible cross-allergy with sulfonamide Hepatotoxicity; contraindicated in patients with moderate or severe liver disease Fatal & nonfatal intracranial hemorrhages reported PI class side effects: increased lipid levels, lipodystrophy, hyperglycemia, hemolytic anemia, & spontaneous bleeding or hematomas in hemophilia Pregnancy category C	Substrate for CYP3A4[c,d] Net inhibitor or CYP3A4[e] Decreases oral contraceptive levels; use alternative method of birth control

Abbreviations: CYP, cytochrome P450; GI, gastrointestinal, PI, protease inhibitor.

[a] Drug interactions listed are not all-inclusive and do not include drugs with overlapping toxicities.

[b] Package insert and other resources should be consulted for specific drug interactions.

[c] Abbreviated list of CYP3A4 **inducers** that can decrease serum levels of substrates for CYP3A4 (eg, protease inhibitors, nonnucleoside reverse transcriptase inhibitors): rifampin, rifabutin, rifapentine, carbamazepine, phenobarbital, phenytoin, nevirapine, efavirenz, St. John's wort.

[d] Abbreviated list of CYP3A4 **inhibitors** that can potentially increase serum level of substrates for CYP3A4 (eg, protease inhibitors, nonnucleoside reverse transcriptase inhibitors): protease inhibitors, erythromycin, clarithromycin, azole antifungals, amiodarone, cimetidine, grapefruit juice.

[e] Abbreviated list of CYP3A4 **substrates** (serum levels can be increased by CYP3A4 inhibitors such as protease inhibitors and decreased by CYP3A4 inducers such as nevirapine or efavirenz); benzodiazepines (avoid midazolam or triazolam; can use lorazepam with protease inhibitors); statins (avoid use of lovastatin or simvastatin with protease inhibitors; pravastatin and rosuvastatin do not substantially interact and atorvastatin can be used with caution and monitoring); dihydropyridine calcium channel blockers; ergot alkaloids (avoid with protease inhibitors); sildenafil, vardenafil, and tadalafil (dose reduction of erectile dysfunction drugs needed with protease inhibitors); some antiarrhythmics (eg, amiodarone, lidocaine, quinidine); warfarin; pimozide (avoid with protease inhibitors); rifabutin (may need dose alterations of one or both drugs); some antidepressants and anticonvulsants (eg, carbamazepine, phenytoin, phenobarbital); immunosuppressants (eg, cyclosporine, tacrolimus, sirolimus); azole antifungals.

From Wilson JW, Estes LL. Mayo Clinic antimicrobial therapy: quick guide. Rochester, MN: Mayo Clinic Scientific Press and New York, NY: Informa Healthcare USA, Inc; c2008.

HIV Infection Pharmacy Review (continued)

Integrase Inhibitor: Select Characteristics

Drug Name	Normal Adult Dose	Dosing Instructions	Toxic/Adverse Effects	Metabolism or Excretion Route and Pharmacokinetic Drug Interaction Potential[a,b]
Raltegravir (Isentress)	400 mg twice daily	Take with or without food	Diarrhea, nausea, & headache were most commonly reported in studies Rare myopathy & rhabdomyolysis have been reported Rare hepatic toxicity has been reported, potentially preceded by symptoms of an allergic reaction	Metabolized by glucuronidation Does not affect cytochrome P450 enzymes Rifampin & other UGT1A1 inducers can decrease raltegravir levels; use with caution

Abbreviation: UGT1A1, uridine diphosphoglucuronosyltransferase 1A1.

[a] Drug interactions listed are not all-inclusive and do not include drugs with overlapping toxicities.

[b] Package insert and other resources should be consulted for specific drug interactions.

CCR5 Coreceptor Antagonist: Select Characteristics

Drug Name	Normal Adult Dose	Dosing Instructions	Toxic/Adverse Effects	Metabolism or Excretion Route and Pharmacokinetic Drug Interaction Potential[a,b]
Miraviroc (Selzentry)	300 mg twice daily For CCR5-tropic virus only: administer a tropism test before use	Take with or without food	Cough, fever, upper respiratory infections, rash, musculoskeletal symptoms, abdominal pain, & dizziness most commonly reported in studies Rare cardiovascular effects have been noted Rare hepatic toxicity has been reported, potentially preceded by symptoms of an allergic reaction	Substrate for CYP3A4 & P-glycoprotein

Abbreviations: CCR5, CC chemokine receptor 5; CYP, cytochrome P450.

[a] Drug interactions listed are not all-inclusive and do not include drugs with overlapping toxicities.

[b] Package insert and other resources should be consulted for specific drug interactions.

Chapter 12

HIV Infection Pharmacy Review (continued)

Fusion Inhibitor: Select Characteristics

Drug Name	Normal Adult Dose	Dosing Instructions	Toxic/Adverse Effects	Metabolism or Excretion Route and Pharmacokinetic Drug Interaction Potential[a,b]
Enfuvirtide (T-20, Fuzeon)	90 mg subcutaneously twice daily	Each 108-mg vial should be reconstituted 1:1 with sterile water before injection Reconstituted injection should be refrigerated & used within 24 hours	Local injection site reactions Possible increased rate of bacterial pneumonia Hypersensitivity reaction, nausea, vomiting, diarrhea, peripheral neuropathy Pregnancy category B	Thought to undergo catabolism to constituent amino acids Unlikely to have substantial cytochrome P450-related drug interactions

[a] Drug interactions listed are not all-inclusive and do not include drugs with overlapping toxicities.

[b] Package insert and other resources should be consulted for specific drug interactions.

Questions

Multiple Choice (choose the best answer)

1. A 30-year-old African American woman who is positive for human immunodeficiency virus (HIV) presents with waxing and waning headache, irritability, and malaise, which have been present during the past 4 weeks. She has received extensive treatment with antiretrovirals in the past, but all previous antiretroviral regimens have failed. She has a low-grade fever of 38.3° C and stable blood pressure and heart rate. She has no nuchal rigidity or neurologic deficits on examination. CT of the head shows no abnormalities except for mild cerebral atrophy. Her CD4 cell count is 75/mcL and HIV-1 RNA level is 100,000 copies/mL. The next most appropriate diagnostic test is:

    a. Stereotactic brain biopsy
    b. Positron emission tomography of the brain
    c. MRI of the brain
    d. Lumbar puncture and cerebrospinal fluid studies
    e. *Toxoplasma* serologic testing

2. A 29-year-old HIV-positive Hispanic man complains of shortness of breath, malaise, night sweats, and a nonproductive cough of 1 week in duration. He is currently not being treated with antiretrovirals. He has a temperature of 38.2°C. Examination of the heart, lungs, and abdomen is normal. There are no skin lesions. Chest radiography shows no abnormalities. On arterial blood gas analysis, the PO_2 is 70 mm Hg.

    Laboratory values are as follows:

    Hemoglobin: 12.5 g/dL
    Leukocyte count: 7,500/mcL
    Platelet count: 150,000/mcL
    Serum creatinine: 0.8 mg/dL
    CD4 cell count: 150/mcL

    What is the most appropriate next diagnostic step?

    a. Serum cryptococcal antigen test
    b. Tuberculin skin test
    c. *Legionella* urine antigen test
    d. CT of the chest
    e. Induced sputum with staining for *Pneumocystis*

3. A 40-year-old white woman presents with complaints of fatigue, malaise, and sore throat of 1 week in duration. She is concerned about HIV infection because it was diagnosed in her husband 7 years ago. She herself had been tested for HIV 6 months ago, and her test result was negative. The couple is sexually active and use condoms but not consistently. The husband is receiving antiretroviral therapy but there have been problems with suppressing his HIV. On physical examination, she has a temperature of 38.0°C, blood pressure 120/75 mm Hg, heart rate 80 beats per minute, and respiratory rate 20 breaths per minute. She has a macular erythematous rash on her trunk and swollen cervical lymph nodes. The rest of the examination, including lungs, heart, and abdomen, is unremarkable. Laboratory results are as follows: hemoglobin 12.5 g/dL, leukocyte count 8,000/mcL, and platelet count 200,000/mcL. Atypical lymphocytes are noted on peripheral smear. Serum creatinine level is normal at 1.0 mg/dL. Liver function test values (aspartate aminotransferase, alanine aminotransferase, bilirubin, and alkaline phosphatase) are all within normal range. The following statements about the diagnosis are true *except*:

    a. Results of HIV antibody testing may be negative.
    b. Antiretroviral therapy is indicated.
    c. P24 antigen may help in making the diagnosis.
    d. Polymerase chain reaction for HIV may help in making the diagnosis.
    e. This kind of presentation is rare.

4. A 35-year-old white man with a recent diagnosis of HIV comes to your office with his wife, who is not infected with HIV, and requests information about the risk of HIV transmission. They are interested in having children. Each of the following statements regarding HIV transmission is correct *except*:

    a. The proper use of condoms greatly reduces the risk of HIV transmission.
    b. Traumatic intercourse increases the risk of HIV transmission.
    c. Ulcerative genital infections increase the risk of HIV transmission.
    d. Kissing increases the risk of HIV transmission.
    e. Antiretrovirals decrease the rate of transmission from an HIV-infected pregnant mother to her fetus.

5. A nurse caring for an HIV-positive patient incurs a needle stick injury. Information pertinent to the proper management of this situation includes the following *except*:

    a. The average risk of HIV transmission from a needle stick is 0.3%.
    b. The HIV RNA value (viral load) influences the likelihood of transmission.
    c. Depth of injury influences the likelihood of transmission.
    d. Whether or not blood was visible on the needle or device influences the likelihood of transmission.
    e. If postexposure prophylaxis is initiated, it will need to be given for 12 weeks.

6. A 36-year-old white homeless man with a known diagnosis of acquired immunodeficiency syndrome (AIDS) presents with cough, night sweats, hemoptysis, and weight loss of several months in duration. On examination, he has a temperature of

38.7°C, blood pressure 135/80 mm Hg, heart rate 72 beats per minute, and respiratory rate 28 breaths per minute.

Laboratory values are as follows:

Hemoglobin: 11.6 g/dL
Leukocyte count: 7,500/mcL
Platelet count: 140,000/mcL
Serum creatinine: 1.0 mg/dL
CD4 cell count: 180/mcL
HIV-1 RNA: 150,000 copies/mL
Tuberculin skin test: 8 mm
Chest radiograph: bilateral lower lobe consolidations

You are asked about the likelihood of tuberculosis in this patient. Which of the following statements is correct?

a. The CD4 cell count is too high for tuberculosis to be likely.
b. The HIV-1 RNA value is too low for tuberculosis to be likely.
c. A tuberculin skin test result of 8 mm is considered negative.
d. The presence of abnormalities in the lower lung zones and the absence of cavities rule out tuberculosis.

e. Sputum samples for acid-fast bacilli smear and culture are indicated.

7. A 28-year-old white man with no significant previous medical history presents with a lesion on his penis. He denies discharge or other symptoms. He admits to unprotected sex with a prostitute approximately 3 weeks ago. On examination, he is afebrile and has normal vital signs. He has an indurated, clean-based, painless ulcer on the shaft of his penis. He also has bilateral enlarged inguinal lymph nodes. The rest of his examination is unremarkable.

The following statements about this infection are true *except*:

a. In general, the clinical manifestations of this infection are similar to those among HIV-uninfected persons.
b. In general, serologic response to this infection seems to be the same as that in HIV-positive and HIV-negative persons.
c. There are no specific clinical manifestations of this infection that are unique to HIV.
d. Closer follow-up of HIV-infected patients with this infection is not indicated.
e. Penicillin-based regimens, whenever possible, are preferred for all stages of this infection in HIV-infected persons.

Answers

1. Answer d.
The symptoms suggest a central nervous system process. In the absence of a focal mass on imaging studies, cryptococcal meningitis becomes prominent in the differential diagnosis and requires cerebrospinal fluid analysis for confirmation. Common cerebrospinal fluid findings include an increased opening pressure, mild mononuclear pleocytosis, and increased protein level. The India ink preparation is positive in more than 70% of cases. The serum and cerebrospinal fluid cryptococcal antigen test has a sensitivity of 93% to 99%. Cerebrospinal fluid cultures are the standard. Up to 75% of patients have blood cultures positive for *Cryptococcus neoformans*.

2. Answer e.
This patient's presentation is most consistent with *Pneumocystis* pneumonia. Staining for *Pneumocystis jiroveci*, the causative organism, in hypertonic saline-induced expectorated sputum is the initial diagnostic method of choice. If the result is negative, staining of specimens obtained through bronchoalveolar lavage should be attempted. Open lung biopsy is rarely needed.

3. Answer e.
The patient's presentation, a mononucleosis-like syndrome, is the most common presentation of acute HIV infection. Symptomatic acute HIV infection occurs in upward of 40% of HIV-infected individuals.

4. Answer d.
Kissing does not transmit HIV infection.

5. Answer e.
The recommended duration of postexposure prophylaxis is 4 weeks.

6. Answer e.
There are no CD4 or HIV-1 RNA cutoff values for tuberculosis. When tuberculosis occurs later (CD4 count <350/mcL) in the course of HIV infection, it tends to have atypical features, such as extrapulmonary disease, disseminated disease, and unusual chest radiographic appearance (lower lung zone lesions, intrathoracic adenopathy, diffuse infiltrations, and lower frequency of cavitation). HIV-positive patients who have skin reactions of more than 5 mm to 5 tuberculin units of purified protein derivative and who do not have active tuberculosis are considered to have latent tuberculous infection.

7. Answer d.
Although clinical presentation, serologic response, and general management of syphilis are similar in HIV-positive and HIV-negative persons, closer follow-up of HIV-positive patients who have syphilis is indicated to detect potential treatment failures or disease progression.

13

Hospital Medicine

James S. Newman, MD
David J. Rosenman, MD

Introduction

Hospitals in the United States have evolved substantially since the first one, the Pennsylvania Hospital, opened its doors in 1751. Technologic advancements and other innovative efforts to improve the quality of hospital-based care have resulted in large and complicated networks of personnel, information systems, devices, medications, and countless other resources. In parallel with these changes, the medical acuity of the hospitalized patient has generally increased. In addition, the professional demands on outpatient clinic–based physicians have made it increasingly difficult for them to maintain effective practices in the hospital. The field of hospital medicine emerged in response to this combination of increasing hospital complexity, patient acuity, and professional demands.

This chapter highlights several topics that may be unique to the hospital and are not discussed elsewhere in this textbook. They include practice management in hospital medicine, transitions to and from the hospital, hospital information systems, quality improvement in the hospital, patient safety and the complications of hospitalization, nutritional issues, approach to the elderly patient, medication safety, and several additional areas including medical care related to bioterrorism.

- Hospital medicine emerged in response to increasing hospital complexity, patient acuity, and professional demands.

Interfaces

Outpatient-to-Inpatient Interface

The potential for discontinuity of care exists at every point of transition. Although hospitalists may impart many benefits to the medical care of hospitalized patients, they can do this most effectively after information from the referring provider (whether in the emergency department or a clinic) has been provided. The hospitalist often must proactively seek this information. Clarification early in a patient's hospital stay helps to avoid medication errors, allergic reactions, and ignorance of patients' values and preferences.

Inpatient–Primary Hospitalist Interface

The hospital is designed uniquely to serve as a central venue for many types of therapies. Foremost and not to be underestimated is the value of a trusting and therapeutic relationship between the hospitalized patient and the physician. Ideally, patients should be full partners in therapeutic relationships, not passive recipients of treatment. The relationship between patient and physician can itself be therapeutic when it is rooted in trust, sensitivity, cultural awareness, mutual respect, and clear communication.

Primary Hospitalist–Consulting Specialist Interface

Consulting services are not always available to hospital-based internists. When consulting services are present, hospital-based physicians who seek the professional opinion of a specialist colleague should be specific in their request for consultation. This allows consulting services to optimize their time and provide more helpful consultative reports.

Comanagement Interface

The consulting hospitalist who participates in a comanagement model works in tandem with a second physician or service to provide collaborative care. Ideally, each contributor to a comanagement model works within a scope that is mutually agreed upon. In contrast to the purely consulting hospitalist who provides an opinion only, the comanager writes orders to carry out certain aspects of the management plan.

Professional Interfaces

Ideal care of the hospitalized patient results from a collaborative effort among people in dozens of professions. More than 100 unique human interactions are possible, for example, when a hospitalized patient has family members visiting and receives care that includes contributions by nurses, primary and consulting physicians, a clinical pharmacist, therapists (eg, respiratory, physical, occupational, speech), a social worker, a counselor, a dismissal planner, and a clinical dietitian. Taking into account shift work (rotating personnel) and the presence of learners and trainees from each of these fields, even a brief hospital stay leads to numerous professional interfaces. The quality of a patient's medical care and the experience in the hospital depend on the integrity of these many human interactions.

- The hospital is home to various professional interfaces, all of which contribute to the quality of patient care.

Hospital Dismissal

The process of dismissing a patient from a US hospital occurs more than 35 million times in a year. Most of these patients are older than 75 years; of those over 85 years, one-third go to long-term care facilities. A well-facilitated hospital dismissal promotes safety and decreases the likelihood of readmission.

Dismissal from the hospital marks a critical period of transition. The care setting changes from the hospital to home, assisted living, nursing home, hospice, or rehabilitation. Care providers change, as may the patient's diet, level of activity, and routes of medication administration. This culmination of the hospital stay brings with it the potential to affect patient satisfaction, safety, medical outcome, and cost of care. Patients at highest risk are the elderly and those with multiple medical conditions.

The discharge process should begin at admission. In an era of increasing costs and pressures to limit use of resources, a successful hospital discharge must be planned in detail and in advance. A premature discharge may lead to adverse drug events or other safety issues as well as to decreased satisfaction and an increased risk of readmission. Prolonged and unnecessary hospitalization may increase the risk of hospital-associated adverse outcomes such as hospital-acquired infections, falls, and debility as well as loss of independence and patient dissatisfaction. Approximately 20% of patients have adverse events after hospital discharge. At least one-third of these events are preventable and another third can be made less severe by timely intervention. Of these, adverse drug events are the most common.

- The hospital discharge is a critical transition.
- The discharge process should begin at admission.
- Elderly patients and those with complex medical issues are at highest risk.
- After discharge, 20% of patients have an adverse event, many of which are preventable.

The hallmark of a safe discharge is adequate communication. Education of the patient and the family is the first step since overcoming health illiteracy may be a barrier as well as dementia. The key to success is to ensure that patients understand their medications and the indications, the natural course of the disease, and the signs of deterioration of underlying disease processes. The patient with congestive heart failure who recognizes the early warning signs of exacerbation can seek care before reaching extremis. Often a surrogate, such as a family member, must learn on behalf of the patient. A properly written discharge summary can serve as an aid in the patient's recall of the events of the hospitalization as well as a reminder of further steps needed.

Another key communication interface is between the outpatient and inpatient providers. Just as the admitting physician would be hampered by a lack of past medical records, the outpatient physician is unable to properly care for a patient without accurate facts relating to the hospital stay. Many techniques are useful for improving this dialogue, including the premier tool: accurate and timely discharge summaries. In addition, the majority of outpatient physicians appreciate receiving a telephone update on their patient's condition upon discharge.

At discharge, an important patient handoff occurs, although many handoffs occur during hospitalization. A standardized handoff should include information about the patient's current condition, ongoing treatment, recent changes in condition, pending studies, and possible changes or complications for which to watch. Discharge instructions are a Joint Commission core performance measure.

- At any handoff, accurate information should be provided about a patient's care, treatment and services, current conditions, and any recent or anticipated changes.
- Discharge instructions are a Joint Commission core performance measure.

All patients should be discharged to a safe environment. Geriatric patients who have had long hospitalizations are frequently debilitated and require short-term rehabilitation. Assessment for the risk of falling should be part of this evaluation. Arrangements for home health care, home infusion therapy, or physical therapy should be made before discharge when indicated. Among the issues to consider at discharge are the patient's functional status (activities of daily living and instrumental activities of daily activity), cognitive status, caregiver capacity, knowledge deficits, and environmental factors. Preservation of independence and the ability to safely return home are important goals.

For certain disease states, there are guidelines that emphasize the discharged patient. For example, there are guidelines for initiation of β-blockers, statins, and angiotensin-converting enzyme (ACE) inhibitors at discharge in patients with myocardial infarction. No patient who smokes or uses tobacco in any form should be discharged from a hospital without an effort to initiate tobacco cessation.

Many medications carry a high risk of adverse events after hospital discharge (Table 13-1). Warfarin dosages can easily be subtherapeutic or supratherapeutic, depending on drug interactions, diet, and a patient's sensitivities. Educating the patient and communicating with the providers is essential in avoiding complications. Several other medications should be considered high risk at discharge. Drug side effects must be noted as well as guidelines for discontinuing use. Corticosteroids, for example, create short-term risks such as hypertension, delirium, and hyperglycemia as well as long-term effects such as osteoporosis and immunosuppression. Medication reconciliation is the process of making sure that the discharge medications are correct.

- Medication errors represent a significant source of adverse events at discharge.
- High-risk drugs require extended education and plans for follow-up and monitoring.
- Medication reconciliation is essential before discharge.

Table 13-1 High-Risk Drugs at Hospital Discharge

Antiarrhythmics
Antihypertensives
Corticosteroids
Diuretics
Narcotics
Oral hypoglycemic agents & insulin
Warfarin

Hospital Information Systems

Paralleling the growth of complexity of modern hospitals has been an equally impressive evolution in the management of medical information. Storing, retrieving, and managing massive quantities of increasingly complicated data have led to the development of computerized entry of physician orders and electronic clinical decision support systems. These applications, most of which undergo continuous refinement, have helped to bring order and efficiencies to the process of providing care in the hospital. They offer new opportunities for large-scale clinical research and help to ensure that standard-of-care therapies are provided dependably and consistently. The challenges that accompany these new technologies and the easy access to information they allow include protecting patient confidentiality and the security of private information. It is never ethical or proper to access a patient's confidential record unless it is required as part of one's job. The confidentiality of medical records is governed by the Health Insurance Portability and Accountability Act of 1996 (HIPAA).

Quality in the Hospital

Quality health care has been defined by the Agency for Healthcare Research and Quality as "doing the right thing, at the right time, in the right way, for the right person—and having the best possible results." Without a doubt, the complexity of health care delivery makes it impossible to be always certain of what "the right thing," "the right time," or "the right way" may be. The definitions of these goals will continue to evolve with our understanding of medicine. As a first step toward optimizing care of the hospitalized patient, though, organizations involved in inpatient quality assessment have defined several key measures believed to reflect the efficiency and effectiveness of care. Hospital-based physicians are widely expected to be aware of these goals and to work toward them (Table 13-2).

Achieving these quality-related goals in the hospital requires provider participation and, in anticipation of future goals, the practice of continuous quality improvement (CQI). CQI applies the scientific method to the clinical setting to test the implementation of changes in hospital care. It involves the repeating cycle of identifying a goal, defining a change that may help to achieve that goal, delineating indices to measure success, and then evaluating implementation of the change. CQI is 1 of several approaches that may help to optimize the performance of the hospital-based physician (Table 13-3).

Table 13-2 Selected Quality Measures

Clinical Condition	Selected Quality Measures
Acute coronary syndrome	Aspirin at arrival & discharge β-Blocker at arrival & discharge ACE inhibitor for LVSD
Congestive heart failure	Left ventricular function assessment ACE inhibitor for LVSD Smoking cessation advice & counseling
Community-acquired pneumonia	Oxygenation assessment within 24 h Pneumococcal screening & vaccination Antibiotic timing (first dose in <4 h) Smoking cessation advice & counseling

Abbreviations: ACE, angiotensin-converting enzyme; LVSD, left ventricular systolic dysfunction.

Patient Satisfaction

A patient's satisfaction with hospital care is a vital quality indicator that may have both financial and legal implications. Inpatient physicians should be aware of the patient satisfaction areas that increasingly are being assessed by oversight organizations. These include patients' perceptions of the frequency with which physicians and nurses treat them with courtesy and respect, listen carefully, respond promptly to a call light (particularly assistance with bed pans and other toileting needs), explain things clearly (including information about side effects and indications before medications are administered), clarify details of follow-up after hospital dismissal, and provide adequate pain control.

The communication skills of the hospital-based physician are paramount to providing optimal care in the hospital. During end-of-life care, communication is especially important. Frequent updates, culturally competent education, and empathy are essential to patients and families as they deal with impending death. The most important clinical elements of successful end-of-life care include control of pain, dyspnea, secretions, and anxiety.

- Patient satisfaction is a vital quality indicator.
- Patient satisfaction correlates with the communicative skills of the physician.

Table 13-3 Methods for Improving Physician-Related Elements of Hospital Care

Education—board recertification, guideline dissemination
Feedback—benchmarks & peer comparison
Regulation—required length of stay for childbirth
Financial—pay for performance
Provider-led initiative—continuous quality improvement
Informatics—computer-generated support

- Assistance with toileting needs is an important component of patient satisfaction.
- Satisfaction with end-of-life care depends on the response to clinical symptoms and the quality of communication.

Hospitals often mail written satisfaction surveys to patients after their stay. A commonly accepted goal is a response rate of at least 30%. The act of surveying may in itself demonstrate to the patient an interest in improving quality. The ideal survey questionnaire has 3 qualities: brevity, clarity, and consistency. A survey also may help to emphasize for physicians the importance of timely and efficient patient-centered care.

- A written survey can be a useful tool for assessing patient satisfaction.

Patient Safety

A report in 1999 from the Institute of Medicine highlighted the issue of patient safety in the hospital. Awareness of this issue has been raised by the often-quoted estimate of 44,000 to 98,000 deaths a year related to medical errors in US hospitals. Among hospitalized patients, 1% to 5% have a major injury related to their medical care.

The term *patient safety* refers to freedom from accidental or preventable injury. Errors in the hospital may result from failure to complete a planned action or, alternatively, from taking the wrong approach to achieve an aim. *Adverse events* are untoward incidents, therapeutic misadventures, iatrogenic injuries, or other adverse occurrences that result directly from care or services provided and not from the underlying disease or condition of the patient. A *near miss* (or *close call*) is an event or situation that could have resulted in an accident, injury, or illness but did not happen because of chance or a timely intervention. A *sentinel event*, as defined by the Joint Commission, is any unanticipated event in a health care setting resulting in death or serious physical or mental injury and not related to the natural course of the patient's disease. The most common reported sentinel events in 2006 were patient suicide, wrong-site surgery, postoperative complications, medication errors, delay in treatment, patient falls, death or injury from restraints, assault/rape/homicide, transfusion error, and infection-related events. Near misses are sentinel events.

- *Patient safety* refers to freedom from accidental or preventable injury.
- Adverse events are related to the delivery of care.
- A sentinel event is any unanticipated event in a health care setting resulting in death or serious physical or mental injury and not related to the natural course of the patient's disease.
- Common sentinel events include suicide, wrong-site surgery, medication errors, and delay in treatment.

A common method for identifying the source of an error is root cause analysis (RCA). RCA comprises a collection of problem-solving methods designed to isolate the root causes of untoward events. The hope in applying RCA is to learn from errors and avoid repeating them. RCA is an important tool of CQI.

- RCA is a common approach to identifying the source of error.

Several major national safety initiatives have targeted certain harmful events and called for increased efforts to eliminate them (Table 13-4).

Medication Safety

Initiation and withdrawal of medication administration can lead to drug errors, drug-drug and drug-disease interactions, and side effects. Adverse events related to the hospital environment itself include falls, thrombosis, debility, pressure ulcers, sleep deprivation, and aspiration pneumonia. Interventions such as surgery can lead to postoperative complications involving any organ system. Infections related to the hospital include health care–associated pneumonia, catheter-related bloodstream infections, *Clostridium difficile* colitis, and the development of resistant organisms. Discontinuity of care (at handoffs and discharges) and poor communication can lead to preventable injury and error. Paramount to navigating a patient successfully through the hospital maze is a keen awareness and understanding of these risks. In addition, health care workers may be injured in the hospital.

- Complications of hospitalization can arise from medications, environmental factors, procedures, infections, and miscommunication.

Adverse Drug Events

It has been estimated that adverse drug events (ADEs) affect 2% to 5% of hospitalized patients. ADEs not only are dangerous for patients, but they also are a financial burden on the health care system.

Table 13-4 Selected National Goals for Preventing Harm

Deploy rapid response teams
Deliver evidence-based care for acute MI
Prevent adverse drug events
Prevent central line infections
Prevent surgical site infections
Prevent ventilator-associated pneumonia
Use high-risk medications such as anticoagulatns & narcotics judiciously
Reduce surgical complications
Prevent pressure ulcers
Decrease spread of MRSA
Enhance use of evidence-based treatment of CHF & MI
Engage hospital leadership in safety issues
Prevent patient care errors related to handoffs
Prevent surgical errors related to wrong site, wrong procedure, or wrong person
Prevent continuity of medication errors
Prevent high-concentration drug errors
Promote effective hand hygiene practices

Abbreviations: CHF, congestive heart failure; MI, myocardial infarction; MRSA, methicillin-resistant *Staphylococcus aureus*.

Medication-related errors for hospitalized patients cost roughly $2 billion annually. Of the serious ADEs, 40% are preventable. About one-half of all medication errors occur with ordering and one-third with administration. Many of these errors can be prevented with implementation of certain hospital information systems.

* ADEs are frequent, expensive, dangerous, and often preventable.

Errors may involve the incorrect choice of medication for a condition: either the drug is prescribed inappropriately or the wrong drug is administered. Drug-drug interactions can cause error. Fluoroquinolones, for example, may inhibit the metabolism of warfarin and lead to an increase in the international normalized ratio. Missed drug allergies can lead to fatal consequences. Drug-disease interactions also are common; use of hepatically metabolized drugs, for example, should be avoided in patients with liver failure. Certain abbreviations, such as *QOD* (for *every other day*) and *U* (for *units*), may be misread and should not be used. An ADE resulting from drug administration started in the hospital may occur after the patient has been discharged.

Several drugs and drug classes are associated with a particularly high risk of adverse outcomes; these include narcotics, anticoagulants (including heparin and warfarin), sedatives, and insulin. Medications are often responsible for electrolyte and other pathophysiologic abnormalities (Table 13-5). A medication that is generally well tolerated by a patient in a healthy state may cause severe side effects if the person is ill or has related poor oral intake. Common culprits include long-acting oral hypoglycemic agents, diuretics, and other antihypertensives.

The interval history of drug side effects or allergy development should be obtained. A missed history of ACE inhibitor–induced cough or angioedema would be problematic for a patient admitted with congestive heart disease who might routinely be given ACE inhibitors. Certain supplements and over-the-counter medications may have clinically significant properties and side effects. Herbal remedies may affect coagulation (eg, dong quai, ginseng, and ginkgo), lead to hepatoxicity (eg, kava), or interact with warfarin. Frequently used over-the-counter medications can cause various unintended consequences, sometimes requiring hospitalization (eg, nonsteroidal anti-inflammatory drugs may cause gastrointestinal tract bleeding, and antihistamines may cause altered mental status and urinary retention).

* Medications such as long-acting oral hypoglycemic agents, diuretics, or antihypertensives may cause severe side effects such as hypoglycemia, renal failure, or hypotension in a patient with poor oral intake due to other unrelated acute medical issues.

A medication may be protean in its association with potential complications. Subtherapeutic dosing of heparin, for example, may potentiate thrombosis, whereas overdosage could lead to exsanguination. Appropriate dosing of heparin still could induce thrombocytopenia with associated paradoxical thrombosis. Heparin also may cause hyperkalemia by inhibiting aldosterone secretion. A key to providing safe pharmacologic treatment in the hospital lies in one's awareness of the potential complications associated with each drug's use. Commonly used drugs often associated with complications include narcotics, anticoagulants, sedatives, and insulin. Knowledge of cytochrome P450 interactions is increasingly important in polypharmaceutical management (Table 13-6).

Hospital Nutrition

Nutritional Assessment at Admission
As many as 40% of patients admitted to the hospital may be malnourished at admission. Hospitalization offers opportunities to correct this condition but also carries risks of further deterioration. The acute illness leading to hospitalization may itself trigger a hypermetabolic state. Catabolic hormones stimulate gluconeogenesis, induce glucose intolerance and insulin resistance, and increase net protein catabolism. Cytokines such as interleukins 1 and 6 and tumor necrosis factor may increase muscle proteolysis, increase metabolic rate, decrease hepatic protein synthesis, and stimulate the release of acute-phase reactants. These biochemical changes lead to impaired organ function and debility early in the course of hospitalization. Patients most at risk include patients with gastrointestinal tract dysfunction (eg, xerostomia, dysphagia, malabsorption, pancreatitis, diarrhea), malignancy, infection, chronic lung disease, alcoholism, and depression. Patients should be asked about functional barriers to oral intake, changes in appetite or bowel function, and unintentional weight loss. On physical examination a patient with severe malnutrition may have bitemporal muscle wasting, scaphoid abdomen, or anasarca, although the vast majority of undernourished patients will have more subtle findings. Malnourished patients frequently are vitamin deficient and may have related signs and symptoms (Table 13-7).

* As many as 40% of patients admitted to the hospital may be malnourished at admission.
* Patients most at risk include patients with gastrointestinal tract dysfunction (eg, xerostomia, dysphagia, malabsorption, pancreatitis diarrhea), malignancy, infection, chronic lung disease, alcoholism, and depression.

Nutritional Therapy in the Hospital
After a hospitalized patient has been identified as malnourished, the first question to ask is whether the digestive tract is functioning properly. If it is, and if the patient can eat, it must be determined whether the patient can eat enough to meet metabolic demands. If the patient can eat enough, malnourishment may have been the consequence of impaired access to enough food. The patient who cannot eat enough to satisfy metabolic demands should be evaluated further to distinguish a mechanical feeding problem from poor intake. Mechanical feeding problems may require alteration in the consistency of food or nutritional supplements (or both). Isolated poor intake may be treated with supplementation by the oral or nasogastric route. Patients unable to eat may benefit from placement of a nasogastric tube or (if there are problems with gastric emptying or aspiration) a nasojejunal feeding tube. A long-term need for enteral feeding may require percutaneous placement of a transabdominal gastric or jejunal tube. Circumstances in which the adequacy of gut function is uncertain

Table 13-5 Drug-Induced Pathophysiologic Changes

Drug	Change
Hypokalemia	
Diuretics	Urinary potassium wasting
Laxatives	Fecal potassium loss
Hyperkalemia	
β-Blocker, heparin	Hyporeninemic aldosterone synthesis
	Decreased cellular uptake of potassium
Cyclosporine	Hypoaldosteronism
Digoxin	Induced chloride shunt
	Impaired cellular uptake
	Reduced renal excretion
Pentamidine, trimethoprim	Altered sodium transport, increased in HIV+
NSAIDs	Hyporeninemic hypoaldosteronism
Succinylcholine	Intracellular leakage of potassium
Hyponatremia	
ACE inhibitor, amiodarone, chemotherapy, (vincristine, cisplatin, cyclophosphamide), ciprofloxacin, SSRIs	SIAD
Carbamazepine	Increased ADH sensitivity in renal tubules
Chlorpropamide	Increased number of ADH receptors
Thiazide diuretics	Distal renal tubular loss
Hypernatremia	
Amphotericin B, foscarnet	ADH deficiency
Cisplatin	
Carbamazepine, lithium	Suppressed ADH (drug-induced diabetes insipidus)
Hypocalcemia	
Biphosphonates	Inhibit osteoclastic activity
Citrate (transfusion plasma exchange)	Decreased ionized calcium from deposition
Foscarnet	Associated in patients with CMV and HSV
Phenytoin	Increased vitamin D metabolism
Phosphate enemas	Decreased ionized calcium from intravascular binding
Hypercalcemia	
Hypervitaminosis A, retinoic acid, levothyroxine	Increased bone resorption
Lithium	Altered PTH set point
Thiazide diuretics	Renal tubular calcium resorption
Hypomagnesemia	
Diuretics, cisplatin	Renal wasting

Abbreviations: ACE, angiotensin-converting enzyme; ADH, antidiuretic hormone; CMV, cytomegalovirus; HIV, human immunodeficiency virus; HSV, herpes simplex virus; NSAID, nonsteroidal anti-inflammatory drug; PTH, parathyroid hormone; SIAD, syndrome of inappropriate antidiuresis; SSRI, selective serotonin reuptake inhibitor.

may warrant parenteral nutrition, although such cases are relatively rare among nonsurgical patients.

The core components of parenteral nutrition are amino acids, vitamins, electrolytes, and fat. The electrolytes depleted most commonly in the hospital are magnesium, potassium, phosphorous, and calcium. When indicated, nutritional therapy may be provided through a peripheral (short-term) or central (long-term) intravenous catheter. In general, nutrition should be delivered to the digestive tract directly whenever possible. Enteral tube feedings have a dual benefit: they provide daily nutrient requirements and decrease the risk of stress ulcer bleeding.

- Malnourished patients should be assessed for the integrity of the gastrointestinal tract.
- Mechanical barriers to proper nutrition should be identified and the diet altered.
- A long-term need for enteral feeding may require percutaneous placement of a transabdominal gastric or jejunal tube.

Table 13-6 Frequently Encountered Cytochrome P450 Interactions

Cytochrome P450 Isoenzyme	Drug	Effect on Metabolism Increased	Decreased
1A2	Amitriptyline Cyclobenzaprine Haloperidol Acetaminophen Propranolol Verapamil Warfarin	Broccoli Charbroiled meat Brussels sprouts Nafcillin Insulin Omeprazole Tobacco	Amiodarone Fluoroquinolones
2C19	Proton pump inhibitors Phenytoin Propranolol Warfarin	Carbamazepine Prednisone Rifampin	Fluoxetine Ketoconazole Omeprazole
2C9	NSAIDs Glipizide ARBs Sulfonylureas Amitriptyline Celecoxib Fluoxetine Phenytoin Rosiglitazone Tamoxifen Warfarin	Rifampin	Amiodarone Fluconazole Isoniazid Sertraline Sulfamethoxazole Voriconazole
2D6	Carvedilol Metoprolol Amitriptyline Paroxetine Haloperidol Metoclopramide Ondasetron Oxycodone Tramadol	Dexamethasone Rifampin	Amiodarone Bupropion Citalopram Duloxetine Escitalopram Fluoxetine Metoclopramide Methadone Paroxetine Ranitidine Sertraline Diphenhydramine Hydroxyzine
3A4, 3A5, 3A7	Macrolides (excluding azithromycin) Benzodiazepines Cyclosporine Tacrolimus HIV antivirals Calcium channel blockers HMG-CoA reductase inhibitors (excluding pravastatin) Fentanyl Dapsone Dexamethasone Haloperidol Ondansteron Quetiapine Risperidone Trazodone Zolpidem	HIV antivirals Barbiturates Carbamazepine Glucocorticoids Phenytoin Rifampin St John's wort	HIV antivirals Amiodarone Macrolides (excluding azithromycin) Diltiazem Azole antifungals Verpamil

Abbreviations: ARB, angiotensin II receptor blocker; HIV, human immunodeficiency virus; NSAID, nonsteroidal anti-inflammatory drug.

Table 13-7 Nutritional Deficiencies

Nutrient	Signs, Symptoms, & Associated Conditions
Onset after short-term (weeks) deficiency	
Vitamin B$_1$ (thiamine)	Wet beriberi—congestive heart failure, edema
	Dry beriberi—neurologic disease
Vitamin B$_2$ (riboflavin)	Sore throat, hyperemic mucosae, normocytic normochromic anemia
	May be due to phenothiazines, tricyclic antidepressants
Vitamin B$_6$ (pyridoxine)	Seizures, glossitis, cheilosis
	May be due to isoniazid, cycloserine, penicillamine
Vitamin C	Petechial & gingival hemorrhage, corkscrew hair, spongy gums with tooth loss, poor wound healing
Magnesium	Muscle stiffness, tetany
Zinc	Acrodermatitis, poor wound healing
Essential fatty acids	Alopecia, thrombocytopenia, anemia, dermatitis
	Consider in patients receiving parenteral nutrition
Onset after mid-term (months) deficiency	
Copper	Hypochromic microcytic anemia
Vitamin K	Bleeding, high prothrombin time & international normalized ratio
Vitamin B$_3$ (niacin)	Pellagra (diarrhea, dermatitis, dementia)
Onset after long-term (years) deficiency	
Vitamin A	Night blindness (may progress to permanent blindness)
Vitamin D	Rickets, osteomalacia, elevated parathyroid hormone
	Calcium may initially be normal
Vitamin E	Areflexia, decreased vibrational & positional sense
Selenium	Myalgias, cardiomyopathy, hemolytic anemia
Chromium	Glucose intolerance, peripheral neuropathy
Iron	Anemia
Cobalt	Anemia
Vitamin B$_{12}$ (cobalamin)	Macrocytic anemia, smooth tongue, subacute combined degeneration of the spinal cord, bilateral paresthesias, impaired proprioception & vibrational sense, spastic ataxia, central scotomata, dementia, weakness, hyperreflexia, bilateral extensor plantar responses

Geriatric Assessment

The hospitalized geriatric patient requires special consideration for screening and prevention of complications. The broad topic of geriatric screening is covered in Chapter 10 ("Geriatrics") of this book. Several additional details are discussed here pertaining to function and safety, mobility and falls, neuropsychiatric issues, sensory function, urologic function, gastrointestinal tract issues, nutrition, and pain.

Functional assessment begins with evaluation of activities of daily living (ADL) and instrumental ADL (IADL) (Table 13-8). Safety assessment also includes questions related to the home environment, the presence of guns, use of a medical alert service, caregiver support systems, concerns about abuse and neglect, safe driving, and the presence of stairs, area rugs, or other barriers in the home.

Mobility and fall risk assessment should include the use of assistive devices such as walkers, toilet seats with arms, and footwear. The history of recent falls and the circumstances associated with them should be obtained. Physical therapy and occupational therapy guidance should be sought if needed. There are several simple mobility scales.

Neuropsychiatric evaluation should include screening for depression, delirium, and dementia. Delirium is common in hospitalized patients and results from various causes, including medication, infections, and opiates. Assessment can be performed using the Confusion Assessment Method (Table 13-9). Various tests are available to screen for dementia, including the Kokmen Short Test of Mental Status, the Mini-Cog assessment, and the Folstein Mini-Mental State Examination. Depression is a common problem and can be assessed using the Geriatric Depression Scale. Screening for alcoholism also is essential. Visual and auditory deficits may exacerbate cognitive problems, depression, and barriers to education.

Assessment for urinary incontinence, urinary retention, and problems with bowel function should occur at admission and before discharge. Nutritional issues specific to geriatric patients include problems related to dentition, dentures, the risk of dysphagia and aspiration, reduced appetite, and recent weight loss.

- Hospitalized geriatric patients should be evaluated for overall functional capacity, evidence of abuse, bowel and bladder problems, pain, and nutritional issues.

Table 13-8 Activities of Daily Living (ADL) and Instrumental Activities of Daily Living (IADL)

ADL	IADL
Bathing	Use of telephone
Dressing	Shopping
Use of toilet	Meal preparation
Mobility	Housekeeping
Continence	Laundry
Feeding self	Transportation
	Taking medicine
	Money management

* Functional assessment begins with evaluation of ADL and IADL.
* Home safety assessment should include consideration of the home environment, need for assistive devices, and evidence of abuse or neglect.

Polypharmacy

Polypharmacy, an individual's use of multiple medications, increases that person's risk of ADEs, including side effects and drug-drug interactions. It is especially common among geriatric hospitalized patients and patients treated for psychiatric conditions. In the United States, patients older than 65 years fill an average of 12 prescriptions per year—in addition to their use of nonprescription drugs and herbal medicines.

* In the United States, patients older than 65 years fill an average of 12 prescriptions per year.

The Complications of Hospitalization

Patients are admitted to the hospital to improve their health, but some diseases are the consequence of health care itself. Illness may be *iatrogenic* (caused by medical examination or treatment) or *nosocomial* (originating in the hospital). Hospitalized patients, already impaired by conditions that require hospitalization, are cared for in an unfamiliar environment, exposed to new medications, and subjected to the invasive placement of tubes and needles or other more involved procedures, leading to various adverse outcomes. Some of these adverse outcomes are predictable; others are not.

Pressure Ulcers

Pressure ulcers result from soft tissue being compressed between bone and an external surface, leading to tissue necrosis. Pressure ulcers are a very common complication of hospitalization. The damage occurs in a cone-shaped distribution, with the greatest damage adjacent to the bone. Dermal capillaries are coiled and relatively resistant to pressure; in contrast, the deeper subcutaneous capillaries run parallel to the fascial planes and are more sensitive to pressure injury. This combination may lead to deep necrosis with little external sign of injury. In addition to direct pressure, shearing force may potentiate the

development of skin ulceration. *Shearing force*, which occurs when a patient slides in a bed or chair, leads to stretching and angulation of the underlying subcutaneous tissue, and impairment in lymphatic and capillary flow. Other culprit external forces include friction and moisture. Patient-specific factors that may allow pressure ulcers to develop include immobility, incontinence, malnutrition, dehydration, circulatory dysfunction, impaired cognition, diabetes, sensory impairment, and neurologic disease such as paraplegia.

* Pressure ulcers are common and result both from external forces and from patient-specific factors.
* Patient-specific factors include immobility, malnutrition, and sensory impairment.
* External forces include pressure, shearing forces, friction, and moisture.

Prevention of ulcers is of utmost importance. The first step is to identify patients at risk and modify their risk factors. Frequent turning, maintaining skin hygiene, and maintaining nutritional integrity are essential. Sites most at risk are the heels and the sacrum. There are various pressure-relieving devices, including heel boots and specialty mattresses.

* The best treatment for pressure ulcers is prevention.

Ulcers can be staged according to their level of penetration. The most essential part of treatment is relieving the underlying pressure. The wound can be cleaned, débrided, and dressed. Eschar must be removed. The hallmark of ulcer treatment is maintaining a moist environment in the wound while keeping the surrounding intact epidermis dry. Superficial wounds are treated with semipermeable membranes; deeper wounds may require either hydrocolloids or hydrogels. Deep wounds may be treated surgically with skin grafts or flaps. Adjunctive therapy may include vacuum-assisted closure, larval therapy, or growth factors. Pressure ulcers may lead to infection and osteomyelitis, but routine antibiotics are not indicated.

* Ulcers are staged by degree of penetration.
* Ulcers should be kept moist while the surrounding skin is kept dry.
* The wound should be débrided by surgical, chemical, mechanical, or biotherapeutic means.
* Routine antibiotics are not indicated.

Table 13-9 Confusion Assessment Method[a]

1. Acute onset with fluctuating course
2. Inattention
3. Disorganized thinking
4. Altered level of consciousness

[a] Diagnosis of delirium requires the presence of 1 *and* 2 and either 3 *or* 4. Data from Inouye SK, van Dyck CH, Alessi CA, Balkin S, Siegal AP, Horwitz RI, et al. Clarifying confusion: the confusion assessment method. A new method for detection of delirium. Ann Intern Med. 1991;114(11):991-2.

Falls

Falls among hospitalized patients are common and may lead to serious injury or death. The outcome of a fall may be worse for a patient receiving anticoagulation. Risk factors for in-hospital falls include debility, toileting, orthostatic hypotension, altered mental status, sedation, history of previous falls, recent environmental changes, binders (such as urinary catheters), restraints, poor communication between providers, depression, sensory impairment, and incontinence. Falls tend to occur in periods of lower staffing such as nights and weekends. Interventions to prevent falls include identifying at-risk patients, avoiding excess binders, encouraging early mobilization, and providing physical therapy (Table 13-10).

- Falls in hospitalized patients are common and exacerbated by patient-specific and environmental factors.

Venous Thromboembolism

Venous thromboembolism (VTE) is a common complication of hospitalization. Even among patients receiving standard-of-care pharmacologic prophylaxis, the risk of VTE in some populations may be as high as 7% to 10%. That risk may be 15% or higher among patients not receiving appropriate prophylactic care. Unsuspected pulmonary embolism may be associated with 5% to 10% of hospital deaths. Conditions that predispose a patient to VTE include acute infectious disease, congestive heart failure, acute myocardial infarction, cerebrovascular accident, rheumatic disease, and inflammatory bowel disease. Clinical characteristics include age older than 75 years, previous VTE, immobility, recent trauma or surgery, estrogen use, obesity, and hypercoagulable states. Patients with malignancy—particularly pancreatic cancer and other mucin-positive adenocarcinomas—are at especially high risk. Patients with a cerebrovascular accident are also at higher risk but carry a putative increased risk of intracranial hemorrhage. This topic is discussed at greater length in Chapter 19 ("Neurology").

Prophylaxis for VTE can be accomplished by pharmacologic and nonpharmacologic means. Among the nonpharmacologic methods, ambulation is the most easily accomplished. In postoperative nonambulatory patients, graduated compression stockings reduced the rate of VTE by 50%. Isolated ankle exercises also are helpful in increasing lower extremity venous blood flow. These nonpharmacologic approaches are especially important among patients in whom anticoagulation is contraindicated.

Pharmacologic prevention with heparin, low-molecular-weight heparin, or fondaparinux (a factor Xa inhibitor) appears to be effective, although the rates of risk reduction and the rates of use vary by center.

Hospital-Acquired Infections

Catheter-Related Bloodstream Infections

It is the rare patient who is hospitalized without at least 1 intravascular catheter being placed either centrally or peripherally. Each year, 150 million central or peripheral intravenous catheters are placed (an averate of 5 per patient) and are related to 850,000 infections. Complications from these lines include local infection at the insertion site, bacteremia, septic thrombophlebitis, and endocarditis. Among the infections, 250,000 cause catheter-related bloodstream infections (CRBIs), which lead to increased morbidity, mortality, longer hospitalizations, and increased cost. The risk of infection is related to the type of catheter, who places the catheter, the technique, and the length of time the catheter remains in place. Specialized teams with a standardized approach diminish the infection rates. The highest risk is with peripheral catheters placed by surgical cutdown. The next highest risks are with use of peripheral steel needles, intra-aortic balloon pumps, and short-term hemodialysis catheters. Peripheral catheter sites commonly are changed every 72 to 96 hours to reduce the risk of infection and the patient discomfort associated with phlebitis. Nasal carriers of *Staphylococcus aureus* have a higher risk of CRBIs than do noncarriers. The recommended control and preventive guidelines from the Centers for Disease Control and Prevention (CDC) are listed in Table 13-11. Use of simple infection control procedures can reduce the risk of infection by 65%.

- Each year, 150 million intravenous catheters are placed (average, 5 per patient).
- Each year, there are 850,000 catheter-related infections, and 250,000 of these cause a CRBI.
- Risk is related to type of catheter and to the location and duration of placement; risk can be reduced by 65% with simple infection control procedures.

Table 13-10 Risk Factors for In-Hospital Falls and Prevention

Risk Factor	Assessment	Prevention
Debility	Functional musculoskeletal assessment	Physical therapy Early mobilization
Binders	Routinely assess need for urinary catheter, oxygen, & intravenous lines	Remove unneeded binders Avoid physical restraints
Delirium	Check medication list	Avoid psychotropics & unneeded medications
Inadequate records	Obtain fall history	Identify patients at risk
Undereducation	Assess patient's knowledge of call lights & assistive devices	Education of patients & families
Inadequate staff	Monitor ratio of number of staff to number of falls	Provide adequate staff for high-risk patients

Health Care–Associated Pneumonia

Health care–associated pneumonia (HCAP) is defined as pneumonia in a patient who has been hospitalized in an acute care facility for 2 or more days within the past 90 days, has resided in a nursing home or long-term care facility, has received recent intravenous antibiotic therapy or chemotherapy or wound care within 30 days of the current infection, or is receiving hemodialysis. The goals of treating HCAP should include recognition of HCAP, attempts at bacteriologic diagnosis while noting local variations, avoidance of the overuse of antibiotics, and application of prevention strategies.

Patients with HCAP are at risk of infection with multidrug-resistant (MDR) pathogens if any of the following risk factors are present: recent antibiotic therapy, current hospitalization of more than 5 days, high local resistance rates, and an immunosuppressed state. MDR pathogens are most frequent in intensive care units and transplant patients. Bacterial organisms frequently involved in HCAP include *Streptococcus pneumoniae*, methicillin-sensitive *S aureus* (MSSA) and methicillin-resistant *S aureus* (MRSA); antibiotic sensitive gram-negative bacilli, such as *Escherichia coli*, *Klebsiella pneumoniae*, *Enterobacter* species, *Proteus* species, and *Serratia marcescens*; and MDR enteric gram-negative bacilli such as *Pseudomonas aeruginosa* and *Acinetobacter*. Fungal pathogens such as *Candida* and *Aspergillus* may need to be considered in immunosuppressed patients. Although a viral pathogenesis is less frequent, the most common virus is *Influenza virus A*.

Hospitalized patients, especially those with impaired mentation or neuromotor deficits, may be at risk of aspiration. These patients should be kept in a semirecumbent position (30°-45°), especially when receiving enteral feeding. Enteral nutrition is preferable to the parenteral route for several reasons, including reducing the risk of central venous catheter infection and prevention of reflux villous atrophy of the intestinal mucosa. Antibiotic choice should reflect the potential pathogens.

- Treatment of HCAP should include early recognition, attempts at bacteriologic diagnosis, avoidance of the overuse of antibiotics, and application of prevention strategies.

Table 13-11   Control and Prevention Guidelines Recommended by the Centers for Disease Control and Prevention

Hand washing
Full barrier precautions when inserting central venous lines
Chlorhexidine for skin disinfection
Avoidance of a femoral insertion site
Timely removal of catheters

Data from Centers for Disease Control and Prevention. Guideline for hand hygiene in health-care settings: recommendations of the Healthcare Infection Control Practices Advisory Committee and the HICPAC/SHEA/APIC/IDSA Hand Hygiene Task Force. MMWR Recomm Rep. 2002;51(RR-16):1-45.

Hospital-Acquired Diarrhea

The most common cause of diarrhea in hospitalized patients is *Clostridium difficile*. It is 1 of the most common hospital-acquired infections and is a frequent cause of morbidity and mortality among elderly hospitalized patients. A patient may present as an asymptomatic carrier or with mild to moderate diarrhea, with pseudomembranous colitis, or with toxic megacolon. Symptoms usually occur after 5 to 10 days of antibiotic treatment, but they may develop as early as 1 day into treatment or as late as 10 weeks after its cessation. Presenting manifestations may include fever, abdominal pain, or a prominent leukocytosis. Diagnosis is made with demonstration of *C difficile* toxin in the stool, although patients may need to have direct colon imaging in unclear cases.

Treatment of *C difficile* colitis requires both nonpharmacologic and pharmacologic methods. Fluid losses and electrolyte imbalances should be corrected and antiperistaltic agents should be avoided. Strict observation of infection control policies for hospitalized patients is essential, as is hand washing with soap and water.

The preferred antibiotic treatment for this disease is metronidazole, although oral vancomycin is an alternative but more expensive option. Pregnant patients should be treated with oral vancomycin—*not* metronidazole.

Some patients do not respond to antibiotic therapy. Indications for surgical treatment include peritoneal signs, bacteremia, unresponsiveness to antibiotics, progressive fever, rigors, a persistently elevated white blood cell count, or computed tomographic (CT) scan showing evidence of significant pericolonic inflammation with increasing bowel wall edema. The recommended surgical procedure is subtotal colectomy with ileostomy, which may later be converted to an ileorectal anastomosis.

- *C difficile* is a common cause of diarrhea and can lead to increased morbidity and expense.
- Metronidazole is first-line treatment unless contraindicated, as in pregnancy.

Complications of Surgery

Preoperative assessment is covered at length in Chapter 8 ("General Internal Medicine") of this book. The following section deals with some of the common medical issues in postoperative patients, including ileus; delirium; alterations in pulmonary, renal, and cardiac function; and the complications of bariatric surgery.

Ileus

Postoperative ileus (POI) is a nonmechanical disruption of normal gastrointestinal tract motility. Physiologic dysmotility is generally of shorter duration than previously believed. Gastric motility and small-bowel motility normalize several hours postoperatively; colon motility normalizes at 24 to 48 hours. POI can cause patient discomfort, adversely affect nutrition, increase the risk of infection, compromise wound healing, increase catabolism, and increase the risk of need for parenteral nutrition by delaying oral feeding. The cause is most likely a combination of neurologic mechanisms, including inhibitory neural reflexes, inflammation from manipulation, and neurohumoral peptides. Signs include abdominal distention, diffuse abdominal pain, nausea and vomiting, absence of flatus, and inability to tolerate an oral diet. There are no standard preventive strategies, although limiting opiates, using minimally invasive surgery, and using epidural anesthesia may be of benefit.

Ischemia of the bowel or bowel perforation should be excluded; an elevated leukocyte count or metabolic acidosis would be suggestive. Liver function tests and pancreatic enzymes should be checked to exclude secondary causes such as pancreatitis. A flat and upright plain film of the abdomen may show multiple dilated loops of bowel, air fluid levels, and diminished colonic gas. CT scan of the abdomen can help differentiate ileus from small-bowel obstruction. If there is still doubt, consider CT enterography.

One form of ileus more common postoperatively is acute colonic pseudo-obstruction (Ogilvie syndrome). Plain radiography should be used to estimate cecal diameter; surgeons should be involved if this measurement exceeds 10 cm, the threshold for colonic perforation. Emergent decompressive colonoscopy also may be considered. Success has been reported with intravenous neostigmine, although mechanical obstruction must first be excluded, and cardiac monitoring is imperative. Pharmacologic treatment of ileus has not been proved to be of benefit nor has early ambulation, although it has other benefits. Appropriate measures include conservative management with bowel rest, maintenance of hydration, and minimal use of opiates.

- POI can cause pain, malnutrition, and infection.
- Evaluation of ileus should include blood cell counts, electrolytes, liver function testing, and radiologic imaging.
- Primary therapy should be aimed at bowel rest, hydration, and avoidance of drugs that have antiperistaltic effects such as opiates.

Postoperative Delirium

Elderly patients with postoperative delirium have generally poor outcomes, including poor cognitive and functional recovery, institutionalization, and death. In almost 25% of elderly patients, delirium develops during hospitalization, but the rate increases significantly with vascular surgery and may be as high as 60% with orthopedic surgery. An alteration in mentation may be from anesthesia, intraoperative hypoxia or hypotension, pain medications, or other nonoperative causes. Risk factors for postoperative delirium are listed in Table 13-12.

If a patient has been identified as delirious, a precipitating cause should be sought and treated. The search should include physical examination, laboratory examination, medication review, electrocardiography, and chest radiography. Nonpharmacologic management is the first step, including frequent orientation, quiet environment, and adequate hydration. The use of restraints or other binders should be avoided. Antipsychotic drugs such as haloperidol and olanzapine can be used.

- Initial treatment of delirium should be nonpharmacologic.
- Antipsychotic drugs such as haloperidol and olanzapine can be used.

Stress Gastrointestinal Tract Ulcers

Routine stress ulcer prophylaxis is not indicated. Certain conditions in critically ill patients carry a higher risk of upper gastrointestinal tract ulcers. These include thrombocytopenia, respiratory failure, liver failure, multisystem organ failure, and a previous history of ulcer and recent corticosteroid use.

Oliguria

Postoperative renal failure with acute oliguria (urine output <400 mL/day), is a common complication of surgical procedures and can be caused by various factors. Preload can be decreased by prerenal causes such as inadequate hydration, third spacing of fluid, and blood loss. Additionally, cardiac disease such as infarction may cause hypotension and decrease perfusion pressure. This same effect can result from vasodilation with sepsis, drugs, or anaphylaxis and from arterial obstruction with secondary thrombosis or emboli related to surgical procedures. Acute tubular necrosis from ischemia may occur. Also to be considered are contrast nephropathy, myoglobinuria after transfusion, and rhabdomyolysis and postrenal causes, such as urinary retention due to opiates, ureteral obstruction, or urethral obstruction from a dysfunctional urinary catheter.

Pulmonary Complications

Pulmonary complications of surgery are common. They include airway obstruction, atelectasis, bronchospasm, pleural effusions, pneumonitis, pneumonia, and pulmonary edema.

Upper airway obstruction can occur relatively early postoperatively. Causes include laryngeal edema, vocal cord injury, and obstruction by the tongue. The presence of stridor is a medical emergency.

Atelectasis and hypoxia are common postoperatively. The most clinically cost-effective treatment is use of incentive spirometry, although it is dependent on user compliance. Preoperative training can improve the efficacy of this treatment. Although pulmonary embolism should always be included in the differential diagnosis, a rush to a diagnostic test may be counterproductive in this situation. Treatments such as bronchoscopy and mucolytic therapy can be considered. Bronchospasm can be caused by aspiration, drug reactions, or activation of an underlying pulmonary disease. Treatment is similar to nonpostoperative management.

Table 13-12   Risk Factors for Postoperative Delirium

Geriatric patients
Preexisting cognitive impairment
Cerebrovascular & neurodegenerative disease
History of delirium
Alcohol abuse & withdrawal
Narcotic or benzodiazepine dependence
Anticholinergic medications
Hypoxia
Anemia
Hyperglycemia & hypoglycemia
Electrolyte abnormalities
Infection & sepsis
Myocardial ischemia

Pleural effusions are common in patients who have had abdominal surgery. Most are small and resolve spontaneously. If the effusion develops later in the hospital course, in combination with fever or leukocytosis, especially after abdominal surgery, the possibility of a subphrenic abscess should be considered. Chemical pneumonitis from aspiration of gastric contents is exacerbated by diminished upper airway reflexes perioperatively in combination with anesthetic medications. The radiographic presence of bibasilar infiltrates is suggestive.

Postoperative pneumonia, which is nosocomial by definition, raises the specter of a resistant organism. The most common organisms are *S pneumoniae* and *Haemophilus influenzae* in 20% to 30% of the patients. The risk of *S aureus*, which may be MRSA, is increased in neurosurgery patients, in patients with chronic renal failure or diabetes, and in intravenous drug abusers. *Pseudomonas* is more common in late infections after prolonged intubation. Other organisms to consider are *Acinetobacter* and anaerobes. Postoperative pneumonia should be treated as an HCAP.

- Pulmonary complications are common and include effusions, edema, atelectasis, pneumonia, and aspiration.
- Upper airway obstruction can be from laryngeal edema, vocal cord injury, or lingual obstruction.
- Atelectasis is best treated with incentive spirometry.
- Postoperative pneumonia should be treated as an HCAP.

Postoperative Fever

Most fever in the first days after surgery is related to inflammation. If the fever is persistent, a search is indicated for surgical site infections or other common hospital-related infections such as urinary tract infection, aspiration pneumonia, ventilator-related pneumonia, or line infection. Noninfectious causes include drug fever and, less commonly, deep venous thrombosis, malignant hyperthermia, gout, transfusion reactions, thyroid storm, and atelectasis. The type of fever and the timing may aid in the diagnosis. Neurosurgical procedures may cause meningitis. Abdominal surgery may result in deep abdominal abscess formation, and fever after transplant should lead to a search for unusual causes in a newly immunosuppressed patient.

- Persistent fever may be from surgical site infections, urinary tract infections, aspiration or ventilator-related pneumonia, or line infection.
- Noninfectious causes of fever include drug fever and, less commonly, deep venous thrombosis, malignant hyperthermia, gout, transfusion reactions, thyroid storm, and atelectasis.

Postoperative Myocardial Infarction

Postsurgical myocardial infarction carries a significant morbidity and mortality. Patients may present in an atypical fashion, without chest pain, secondary to concurrent pain medications or anesthetics. The infarction tends to occur within the first 5 days postoperatively and is diagnosed in the usual fashion. Serial electrocardiograms are not recommended postoperatively but may be warranted in patients at increased risk of ischemia. The use of preoperative β-blockers in patients at increased risk may decrease the risk of perioperative infarction.

Complications of Bariatric Surgery

Obesity has reached epidemic status in the United States, and patients are increasingly turning to bariatric surgery. Bariatric surgical procedures reduce caloric intake by modifying the anatomy and function of the gastrointestinal tract. The types of procedures can be characterized as restrictive or malabsorptive. Knowledge of the type of surgery will affect the medical management of complications. The most common restrictive procedures include gastroplasty and adjustable gastric banding; a malabsorptive procedure is biliopancreatic diversion. The Roux-en-Y gastric bypass is a combination of both. Relatively more complications occur in centers where the procedure is less frequently performed (Table 13-13). The mortality rate is 0.1% to 2%, depending on the facility, and is higher for the malabsorptive procedures. The most common causes of mortality are pulmonary embolism and anastomotic leaks. Nonfatal surgical complications include thromboembolism, anastomotic leaks, bleeding, incidental splenectomy, hernias, and small bowel obstruction. Nausea and vomiting occur in 50% of the patients with restrictive procedures. Dumping syndrome is common after the Roux-en-Y procedure, with a 70% incidence. This syndrome is characterized by facial flushing, light-headedness, palpitations, fatigue, and diarrhea; it is generally induced by a meal with a high glucose content. Nutritional complications and various gastrointestinal tract symptoms are common.

- Bariatric surgical procedures are restrictive, malabsorptive, or mixed.
- Complications can be classed as surgical, nutritional, and gastrointestinal.

Special Issues for Hospitalized Patients

Cultural Background

The US population increasingly is a blend of ethnic and genetic backgrounds. At least one-sixth of US residents speak a language other than English in their home. One out of every 5 young people (ages 16-25 years) in the United States has at least 1 parent who is an immigrant. This group comprises the most diverse generation in US history. The population of patients who will be hospitalized in the future will be drawn from this diversified pool. A patient's education level, social habits, employment and occupational history, and cultural background contribute to shaping the patient-physician relationship, the style of communication used, the risk of complications, and the management strategy.

As the diversity of the US population increases, the need to address racial and ethnic disparities in health care becomes essential. If language barriers are not addressed, a patient with limited English proficiency is at risk of medical error, resulting in a longer length of hospital stay for common admission diagnoses such as routine hip replacement, diabetes mellitus, stroke, and coronary artery disease. All facilities receiving federal health care dollars are obligated to provide interpreter services for patients who speak foreign languages and for patients who are deaf.

A patient's religious beliefs should be incorporated into the management plan. For example, in the case of a patient who is a Jehovah's

Table 13-13 Complications of Bariatric Surgery

Perioperative surgical complications
  Anastomotic leaks
  Pulmonary embolism
  Hemorrhage
  Incidental splenectomy
  Hernia
  Small-bowel obstruction
Nutritional complications
  With restrictive surgery
    Calcium
    Folate
    Vitamin B_{12}
  With malabsorptive surgery
    Protein malabsorption
    Fat-soluble vitamin deficiency (vitamins A, D, E, & K)
Gastrointestinal tract complications
  Dumping syndrome: flushing, palpitations, light-headedness,
    fatigue, & diarrhea
  Strictures
  Cholelithiasis
  Dehydration
  Ulcers

Witness, acknowledging, reconfirming, and abiding by a refusal to accept transfusion is essential to appropriate care.

- At least one-sixth of the people in the United States speak a language other than English in their home.
- All facilities receiving federal health care dollars are obligated to provide interpreter services.

Patients with Intellectual Disability

In relation to the general population, patients with intellectual disability (ID) are more likely to use the US health care system. Annually, 30% of patients with ID are seen in emergency departments, and 16% are hospitalized. Assessment of patients with ID may be complicated by their associated behavioral abnormalities or their impaired ability to communicate, making vigilance in observation and advocacy on their behalf all the more important. Patients with Down syndrome (trisomy 21) are more likely to have celiac disease, hypothyroidism, obstructive sleep apnea, seizures, and atlantoaxial instability (atlantoaxial stability may complicate endotracheal intubation). Patients with ID are at increased risk of aspiration due to neuromuscular dysfunction. Self-injurious behavior may be seen in nonverbal patients with pain. These patients should be checked for occult fractures, corneal abrasions, and other sources of pain. Many patients with ID have surrogate decision makers (relatives or court-appointed guardians); ethical issues arise frequently.

- Annually, 30% of patients with ID are seen in emergency departments; 16% are hospitalized.

- Patients with ID are at increased risk of aspiration due to neuromuscular dysfunction.

Treatment of Alcohol Withdrawal

The extent of alcohol abuse in hospitalized patients is underrecognized. Patients with alcohol withdrawal are best treated as inpatients, especially if they have a history of seizures, delirium tremens, psychiatric disease, or multiple medical comorbidities. Delirium tremens occurs in up to 20% of untreated patients.

Patients in *early withdrawal*, within 48 hours of the last drink, may have mild hypertension and tachycardia, mild hyperthermia, fine tremors, agitation, slightly impaired orientation, and early visual and auditory hallucinations. Seizures may occur during early withdrawal and may be the presenting complaint for admission. Seizures can occur in up to one-third of the patients and should be considered in patients who have had withdrawal seizures previously. Other causes or cofactors to exclude include hyponatremia, hypoglycemia, central nervous system trauma, and infection. Withdrawal seizures are best treated with benzodiazepines unless the patient is known to have a preexisting seizure disorder.

Some patients progress to *late withdrawal*, known classically as *delirium tremens*, but it is hard to predict which patients will progress to this stage. This condition is characterized by tachycardia, hyperthermia, gross tremors, delirium, disorientation, and hallucinations. Nausea and vomiting may lead to aspiration. Fluctuations in blood pressure may predispose the patient to cardiac and cerebrovascular events. A monitored bed is needed for patients with arrhythmias, and often a bed in the intensive care unit is required if the patient is severely affected and may need intubation.

Patients are monitored using the revised Clinical Institute Withdrawal Assessment (CIWA), a symptom-based point scale that measures the presence and extent of nausea and vomiting, tremulousness, diaphoresis, anxiety, agitation, paresthesias, auditory and visual hallucinations, headache, and disorientation. Most institutions have standardized scales for administering benzodiazepines, with a dosage system based on the CIWA score; this type of dosage system is also known as *symptom-triggered therapy*. Patients should receive aggressive treatment for withdrawal, especially if they have had severe withdrawal previously; initially, they should receive a loading dose of benzodiazepines. An alternative to the use of benzodiazepines, with their wide spectrum of effects is a barbiturate such as phenobarbital, which may be advantageous because it has a long half-life. Alcoholic patients should routinely receive chemical dependency counseling and psychiatric evaluation. They are at risk of Wernicke encephalopathy, which is seen in thiamine-deficient patients and is characterized by palsy of the abducens nerve (cranial nerve VI), nystagmus, ataxia, and disorientation. Thiamine, 100 mg per day, is the usual replacement dose. Hypomagnesemia should be treated; a low magnesium level may decrease the seizure threshold.

- The extent of alcohol abuse is often underrecognized.
- The CIWA is a symptom-based point scale that assesses nausea and vomiting, tremulousness, diaphoresis, anxiety, agitation, paresthesias, auditory and visual hallucinations, headache, and disorientation.

- Delirium tremens occurs in up to 20% of untreated patients.
- Wernicke encephalopathy, seen in thiamine-deficient patients, is characterized by palsy of the abducens nerve (cranial nerve VI), nystagmus, ataxia, and disorientation.

Treatment of Ethylene Glycol and Methanol Intoxication

Ingestion of methanol and ethylene glycol can be fatal; rapid response and recognition are essential. These common substances are found in antifreeze, solvents, cleaners, windshield wiper fluid, and other cleaning products. Methanol is also present in home-distilled alcohol (moonshine).

Alcohol dehydrogenase is involved in the metabolism of methanol to formaldehyde and formate and in the metabolism of ethylene glycol to glycolate, glyoxylate, and calcium oxalate. Formate causes retinal damage with optic disc hyperemia, edema, and eventually blindness. Concurrently, infarction or hemorrhage of the basal ganglia can occur. The ethylene glycol metabolites cause renal failure and hypocalcemia from calcium oxalate formation. Clinically, central nervous system depression is common. Both methanol and ethylene glycol cause severe metabolic acidosis with secondary hyperpnea and tachypnea; coma, seizures, and hypotension are late effects. Clinical signs of hypocalcemia may be present. Screening for concurrent overdosage of narcotics, salicylates, or acetaminophen should be a standard response. Methanol and ethylene glycol levels require gas chromatography and may not be readily available. Urinalysis may show calcium oxalate crystals in ethylene glycol poisoning.

The first step in management is standard airway and circulation support. Unless ingestion occurred within the previous 60 minutes, lavage of the stomach is unlikely to be of benefit because of rapid absorption. Sodium bicarbonate should be administered to correct the acidosis. Acidosis leads to protonation; alkalinization helps prevent penetration of metabolites into end organs. The most important step is the inhibition of alcohol dehydrogenase. This is done with either ethanol or fomepizole. Fomepizole, the preferred treatment, competitively inhibits alcohol dehydrogenase. Although costly, the long-term expense is less than that of untreated poisoning-related complications. Hemodialysis can remove toxic metabolites rapidly and should be considered for severe acidosis, elevated ethanol levels, or end-organ damage. Fomepizole is dialyzable and must be readministered accordingly.

- Methanol and ethylene glycol are found in antifreeze, solvents, cleaners, windshield wiper fluid, home-distilled alcohol, and other cleaning products.
- Ethylene glycol metabolites cause renal failure and hypocalcemia from calcium oxalate formation.
- Methanol is metabolized to formate, which causes retinal damage with optic disc hyperemia, edema, and eventually blindness; infarction or hemorrhage of the basal ganglia can occur.
- Treatment involves inhibition of alcohol dehydrogenase with either ethanol or fomepizole.

Bioterrorism

A terrorist attack might come in many forms: nuclear, biologic, or chemical. The hospital-based physician should be familiar with general management concepts in the event of a natural or man-made disaster. Chemical weapon release may cause mass casualties instantly; use of biologic weapons may take longer to become apparent.

Nuclear Agents

Exposure to radiation contamination can have serious health effects. A radiation release can contaminate the skin and clothing; removal and disposal of contaminated clothing in a safe and timely manner eliminates 90% of external contamination. The residual radiation on the clothing poses a hazard to health care workers. Internal contamination, through ingestion or inhalation cannot be removed, but it is not dangerous to health care workers. In the event of a nuclear explosion, patients may have radioactive shrapnel, which need to be surgically removed safely.

- Contamination can be external or internal or from shrapnel.
- Removal of contaminated clothing eliminates 90% of external contamination.
- Internal contamination occurs through inhalation or ingestion; it cannot be removed but is generally not hazardous to others.

Radiation can be ionizing or nonionizing. Nonionizing radiation, such as microwaves and infrared, causes thermal injury. The most familiar, common form is sunburn. Ionizing radiation comes from sources such as γ-rays and x-rays; it acts at the cellular level. The cells most critically affected by radiation are spermatocytes, bone marrow precursor cells, and crypt cells in the intestines.

- Ionizing radiation (eg, γ-rays, x-rays) acts at the cellular level.
- Nonionizing radiation (eg, microwaves, infrared) causes thermal injury.

There are several radiation syndromes. They involve the cerebrovascular system, the gastrointestinal tract, the bone marrow, and the skin. In the cerebrovascular syndrome, acute changes occur in the central nervous system. Capillary circulation is impaired, the blood-brain barrier is injured, interstitial edema occurs, and the meninges become inflamed. Edema can be seen on magnetic resonance imaging or CT, and electroencephalography may show spike-and-wave changes. The prodrome includes headache, nausea, fever, and hypotension. Severe and rapidly progressive prodromal symptoms suggest a significant and potentially fatal exposure.

Within 5 days of significant exposure, the gastrointestinal syndrome occurs. Early symptoms include nausea and vomiting. Later, crypt cell necrosis and epithelial cell death occur, with diarrhea, gastrointestinal tract bleeding, bowel necrosis, and bacteremia.

The hematopoietic syndrome is caused by destruction of bone marrow precursor cells. Initially, lymphopenia is predominant. The nadir of neutropenia and thrombocytopenia tends to occur at 2 to 4 weeks; late effects include hypoplasia or aplasia of the marrow. The cutaneous syndrome is a function of the localized dose and can occur both early and late. Early lesions at 1 to 2 days include erythema, edema, and desquamation.

- The cerebrovascular syndrome includes fever, hypotension, headache, cognitive dysfunction, cerebral edema, and death.

- The gastrointestinal syndrome occurs within 5 days of initial exposure, with early symptoms including nausea and vomiting; later, crypt cell destruction occurs with diarrhea, gastrointestinal tract bleeding, and bowel necrosis.
- In the hematopoetic syndrome, lymphopenia is predominant.
- The cutaneous syndrome is a function of the localized dose and can have early and late effects.

Biologic Agents

Various biologic agents can be used for terrorist purposes. This topic is covered at greater length in Chapter 15 ("Infectious Diseases") of this book. Biologic attacks can cause many deaths and create economic havoc. The release of a 100-kg anthrax spore device could lead to hundreds of thousands or millions of deaths. This would match the death toll from a nuclear weapon. CDC estimates that the cost would be $26 billion per 100,000 exposures.

- The death toll in a biologic attack can equal that of a nuclear attack.

Among the characteristics that make a biologic weapon more effective are ease of transmission, high mortality, effect on public perception, and the need for special public health requirements.

Chemical Agents

Chemical agents include nerve agents, toxic asphyxiants, pulmonary irritants, and blistering agents. Nerve agents (eg, sarin) have been used in warfare and terrorist attacks in public spaces such as on trains. These gases can either be absorbed through the skin and eyes or be inhaled. The effect is due to cholinesterase inhibition, which causes smooth muscle contraction, profuse secretions, small pupils, and clinical symptoms described as "runny nose, crying, drooling, defecating, urinating, and vomiting." Respiratory exposure can quickly lead to death (in 1-10 minutes) from respiratory failure. Contaminated clothing and jewelry should be removed. Contaminated skin should be washed with soap and water, and a skin decontamination lotion applied if available. Medical management of exposure includes use of pralidoxime and atropine, supportive care with fluid replacement, and respiratory support if needed.

- Nerve agents such as sarin can act through exposure to skin, lungs, or eyes.
- Nerve agents are cholinesterase inhibitors; symptoms include smooth muscle contraction, profuse secretions, and small pupils.
- Respiratory exposure can be fatal in 1-10 minutes.
- Cutaneous exposure can be treated with a skin decontamination lotion.
- Medical management includes atropine, pralidoxime, and supportive measures.

Toxic asphyxiants include cyanide and arsine. These agents affect mitochondrial function by reacting with the trivalent iron of cytochrome oxidase. Cyanide, which smells like bitter almond, has a rapid effect, starting with mucous membrane irritation and flushing. This is followed by tachypnea, tachycardia, and headache. The next stage includes nausea and vomiting, weakness, and tremors. Severe cases demonstrate acute lung injury and acute respiratory distress syndrome (ARDS), leading to cardiopulmonary arrest. Cyanide exposure can be treated initially with 100% oxygen therapy. Definitive therapy is with amyl nitrite inhalation or intravenous sodium nitrite. These nitrites form methemoglobin, which combines with cyanide to form cyanomethemoglobin, freeing cytochrome oxidase. An alternative is sodium thiosulfate, which enzymatically converts cyanide to the nontoxic compound thiocyanate. Arsine, which smells like garlic, causes similar symptoms, as well as the triad of hemolysis, hematuria, and abdominal pain. Hemodialysis is not of benefit, and there is no specific antidote.

- Cyanide and arsine are toxic asphyxiants that affect mitochondrial function through cytochrome oxidase inhibition.
- Symptoms of cyanide poisoning include mucous membrane irritation and flushing, followed by tachypnea and tachycardia.
- In severe cyanide poisoning, ARDS leads to cardiopulmonary arrest.
- Cyanide treatment includes oxygen supplementation, amyl or sodium nitrite, and sodium thiosulfate.
- Arsine poisoning leads to the triad of hemolysis, hematuria, and abdominal pain.

Pulmonary irritants are gases that can be common industrial chemicals and a source of accidental injury, but they can also be used for terrorist purposes. Examples include chlorine gas, ammonia, and phosgene. Exposure causes direct lung injury. If outdoors, exposed persons should go to higher ground. Early symptoms are nose and throat irritation, cough, and chest pain. Lung symptoms develop later. Acute lung injury is associated with a high mortalilty. Decontamination should include removal of clothes, decontamination of skin, and prolonged eye flush with water. Patients may present with acute respiratory distress. Chest radiography may demonstrate bilateral diffuse infiltrates.

- Pulmonary irritants include chlorine gas, ammonia, and phosgene.
- Early symptoms include mucous membrane irritation, cough, and chest pain.
- Acute lung injury is associated with a high mortality.
- Exposed persons should decontaminate clothing and skin and go to higher ground.

Vesicants, such as sulfur mustard, are blistering agents that interfere with DNA synthesis. In World War I, vesicants caused over 125,000 casualties. Early respiratory symptoms are related to upper respiratory tract irritation; at 12 hours, dyspnea occurs and may lead to pneumonia. Cutaneous symptoms include erythema, followed by pain and pruritus. Within 16 hours, blisters begin to form; they heal slowly, causing extensive scarring. Decontamination after exposure should include careful removal of clothing to avoid further exposure and application of a skin decontamination lotion. Ocular symptoms occur at about 12 hours. The cornea is injured and may scar; eye pain and eyelid swelling may occur.

- Vesicants are toxic to the eyes, skin, and lungs.

- Respiratory symptoms start with cough and hoarseness; at 12 hours dyspnea ensues and may lead to pneumonia.
- Cutaneous symptoms include erythema, pain, and pruritus; blisters form at 16 hours.
- Ocular symptoms occur after 12 hours, with corneal scarring.

Risks to Health Care Workers

Hospitals employ approximately 4.5 million of the 8 million health care workers in the United States or about 4% of the total US workforce. The hospital is a complex environment. Both students and experienced personnel function in a high-stress environment replete with various hazards, including radiation, toxic chemicals, biologic hazards, and needles. Needlestick injuries are a constant threat to hospital workers.

Health Care Workers and Needlestick Injuries

The hospital can be a dangerous place for health care workers. A 2004 CDC estimate is 385,000 needle stick injuries (NSIs) per year to health care workers (HCWs) in hospitals. The rate of NSI is higher in teaching hospitals; one-third occur in the operating room, and another one-fourth in the patient's room. The hollow bore syringe is the most frequent cause. Nurses have the highest rate among HCWs (approximately 35%), and residents and fellows have almost the same rate as attending physicians (10%). Phlebotomists have a fairly low rate (5%). There have been documented cases of transmission of viruses (eg, Ebola, herpes simplex virus, varicella-zoster virus) and of brucellosis, blastomycosis, leptospirosis, malaria, Rocky Mountain spotted fever, syphilis, toxoplasmosis, and tuberculosis. HCWs also have viral and bacterial exposures from animals in teaching institutions with research programs (herpesvirus B from primates, human T-lymphotropic virus, and various bacterial infections).

- NSIs are more frequent in teaching hospitals; one-third occur in the operating room and another one-fourth occur in the patient's room. The syringe is the most frequent cause.
- Nurses have the highest rate among HCWs (approximately 35%) and residents and fellows have almost the same rate as attending physicians (10%).

Before hepatitis B virus (HBV) vaccination, the rates of infection were more than 10,000 per year. The rate of infection in unvaccinated HCWs is 10% to 30%. Postexposure prophylaxis is required after HBV exposure from NSI or mucous membrane contact involving a patient with known or suspected hepatitis B surface antigen (HBsAg)-positive status. For an unvaccinated HCW, treatment with hepatitis B immunoglobulin (HBIG) and administration of HBV vaccination is indicated. An HCW who is a known responder to vaccine does not need treatment. An HCW who is a nonresponder (treated without an antibody response) should have HBIG or HBIG plus revaccination. For the HCW who has been vaccinated but has an unknown antibody response, test the status immediately and proceed accordingly.

- Hepatitis B exposure from NSI or mucous membrane contact involving a patient with known or suspected HBsAg-positive status requires evaluation for postexposure prophylaxis.
- For an unvaccinated HCW, treatment with HBIG and administration of HBV vaccination is indicated.
- An HCW who is a nonresponder (treated without an antibody response) should have HBIG or HBIG plus revaccination.

Hepatitis C virus (HCV) seroconversion after an NSI from an infected person is approximately 0% to 5%. No cases have been reported from blood exposure to intact skin, but cases have been reported from conjunctival exposure. Routine testing recommended after exposure includes 1) baseline testing for anti-HCV, HCV RNA, and alanine aminotransferase (ALT); 2) follow-up testing for HCV RNA at 4 to 6 weeks after exposure; and 3) follow-up testing for anti-HCV, HCV RNA, and ALT at 4 to 6 months after exposure. Treatment with immunoglobulin after exposure is not recommended; however, effective treatment is available for HCWs who have an acute HCV infection (pegylated interferon with an antiviral such as ribavirin).

- HCV seroconversion after an NSI from an infected person is approximately 0% to 5%.

Human immunodeficiency virus transmission is even less likely with exposure (0.3%); however, postexposure prophylaxis with a combination regimen of antiretroviral therapy is indicated.

Other Risks to Health Care Workers

Occupational exposures to antineoplastic and other hazardous drugs can occur at all stages of a drug's life cycle, from manufacture through administration and disposal. Hazardous drugs are those that have the following characteristics: carcinogenicity, teratogenicity, reproductive toxicity, organ toxicity, and genotoxicity. Health care–related injuries are a risk for many hospital employees. Maintenance workers may be exposed to solvents, asbestos, and electrical hazards. Housekeepers are exposed to detergents and disinfectants, NSIs and musculoskeletal injuries, and latex allergy from gloves (which is a problem for all hospital workers). Radiology technicians may be exposed to radiation and radioactive isotopes. Operating room workers may face the increased risk of reproductive problems due to exposure to waste anesthetic gases. Workplace stress, rotating shift work, long hours, sleep deprivation, and threat of physical violence (in emergency departments, psychiatric and dementia wards, etc) can also be of concern.

Questions

Multiple Choice (choose the best answer)

1. A 78-year-old man underwent surgical repair of a traumatic hip fracture without complications. In the afternoon of postoperative day 4 he reported abdominal discomfort, which was attributed to early ileus. The next morning the pain was worse and was localized to the right upper quadrant. The patient was then given nothing by mouth. Laboratory evaluation showed the following:

Component	Value
Hemoglobin, g/dL	11.7
Leukocytes × 10^9/L	21
Segmented neutrophils, %	70
Band forms, %	12
Lymphocytes, %	16
Monocytes, %	4
Platelets × 10^9/L	227
Alanine aminotransferase, U/L	53
Aspartate aminotransferase, U/L	43
Serum alkaline phosphatase, U/L	122
Serum total bilirubin, mg/dL	1.4
Serum amylase, U/L	80

Abdominal ultrasonography showed a dilated, thick-walled gallbladder with minimal pericholecystic fluid and no stones; the common bile duct and intrahepatic ducts appeared normal. A hepatobiliary iminodiacetic acid scan was suggestive of cholecystitis. Blood for cultures was drawn, and broad-spectrum antibiotic therapy was started. The patient has worsening symptoms this morning (day 6). Which of the following would be most appropriate at this point?

a. Endoscopic placement of a biliary stent
b. Cholecystectomy
c. Continued antibiotic therapy and bowel rest
d. Endoscopic retrograde cholangiopancreatography and sphincterotomy
e. Celiac artery angiography

2. A man is brought to the hospital with a depressed level of consciousness. He was found by the police beside a dumpster behind an automotive shop. He has no identification. On examination, his supine pulse rate is 108 beats per minute and supine blood pressure is 98/64 mm Hg; orthostatic changes cannot be determined because the patient cannot sit upright. His breath has a sweet, fruity odor. The optic fundi appear normal, and both pupils react briskly to light. Cardiovascular examination is unremarkable except for regular tachycardia. The abdomen is not tender. No peripheral edema is present. There are no suspicious skin lesions. Laboratory evaluation showed the following:

Component	Value
Plasma glucose, mg/dL	100
Blood urea nitrogen, mg/dL	16
Serum creatinine, mg/dL	1.0
Serum electrolytes	
Sodium, mEq/L	138
Potassium, mEq/L	3.9
Chloride, mEq/L	101
Bicarbonate, mEq/L	10
Arterial blood studies	
PO$_2$, mm Hg	134
PCO$_2$, mm Hg	28
pH	7.28

Urinalysis showed sheets of needle-shaped, monohydrate calcium oxalate crystals. Which of the following is the most likely diagnosis?

a. Methanol intoxication
b. Crystal methamphetamine overdosage
c. Ethylene glycol intoxication
d. Alcoholic ketoacidosis
e. Salicylate overdosage

3. A 72-year-old man is admitted to your service with symptoms of congestive heart failure after a recent colonoscopy. On physical examination he has hepatomegaly, periorbital purpura, and macroglossia with lateral scalloping. Which of these diagnostic tests is most likely to yield a diagnosis?

a. Antineutrophil cytoplasmic autoantibody test
b. Fat aspirate
c. Serum ferritin level
d. Serum copper level
e. Thiamine level

4. A 52-year-old man has nausea and abdominal distention 2 days after right total hip arthroplasty. Plain radiographs of the abdomen show normal-caliber loops of small intestine and a cecal diameter of 17 cm. Emergent decompressive colonoscopy relieves the patient's symptoms, although they recur the next day. The consulting service recommends a trial of neostigmine. Which of the following precautions would be most appropriate before initiating this therapy?

a. Cardiac monitoring
b. Electrocardiography to document the QT interval
c. Thyrotropin level
d. Fasting glucose level
e. Urinary sodium level

5. A 48-year-old man is admitted with severe fatigue, arthralgias, extensive bruising, leg edema, and a nonhealing wound of the

lower extremity. He describes a very poor diet, consisting mainly of bologna sandwiches and cupcakes, and states that he has not used heroin in "quite some time." On examination he has mild orthostatic hypotension, alopecia with corkscrew-shaped hair, gingival bleeding with tooth loss, pitting edema (2+), and a weeping 3-cm wound with surrounding erythema. Which of the following diagnoses would explain all of his symptoms?

a. Human immunodeficiency virus (HIV) infection
b. Hepatitis C
c. Abnormal collagen synthesis
d. Ketosis from heroin additives
e. Sarcoidosis

6. A 73-year-old woman is admitted for a humerus fracture, which is successfully repaired. Five days postoperatively, she has the following laboratory results:

Component	Value
Plasma glucose, mg/dL	110
Blood urea nitrogen, mg/dL	11
Serum creatinine, mg/dL	0.8
Serum electrolytes	
Sodium, mEq/L	138
Potassium, mEq/L	5.7
Chloride, mEq/L	101
Bicarbonate, mEq/L	28

Her medication list is reviewed. She is receiving the following medications:
Citalopram hydrobromide, 20 mg orally every 24 hours
Hydrochlorothiazide, 25 mg orally every 24 hours
Docusate sodium, 100 mg orally every 12 hours
Oxycodone, 5 mg orally every 6 hours as needed for pain
Acetaminophen, 500 mg orally every 6 hours
Heparin, 5,000 units subcutaneously every 8 hours
Levothyroxine, 25 mcg orally every morning
Fluids (5% dextrose in normal saline), 80 mL intravenously every hour

Her urinalysis results are as follows: pH 6.8, sodium 155 mEq/L, potassium 20 mEq/L. The laboratory profile is repeated, and the results are similar, without evidence of hemolysis.

Which of the following would be the most appropriate treatment of her hyperkalemia?

a. Give sodium polystyrene sulfonate, 30 g orally every 4 hours for 4 doses.
b. Give an enema with 60 g sodium polystyrene sulfonate.
c. Discontinue use of citalopram.
d. Discontinue use of oxycodone.
e. Discontinue use of heparin.

7. A 68-year-old man is admitted for gastrointestinal tract bleeding from a gastric ulcer. Twenty years ago, he had a similar event and required a transfusion. An intern is attempting to draw blood and, when you try to help, inadvertently punctures the skin of your hand with the needle. Which of the following is correct?

a. If you have had 3 doses of hepatitis B virus (HBV) vaccine, you need to do nothing else for HBV prophylaxis.
b. If the patient is HIV positive, your risk of seroconversion is 2.5%.
c. You are less likely to develop an infection from hepatitis C virus than from HIV.
d. The patient should be tested for HIV, and if the results are positive you should receive antiviral therapy.
e. Your chances of being stuck with a needle are smaller than those of a phlebotomist.

8. A 78-year-old woman is admitted to the hospital with urosepsis. She has a history of recurrent urinary tract infection. She was evaluated in an outpatient clinic 5 days before admission and began trimethoprim-sulfamethoxazole (TMP/SMX) therapy. Her past medical history includes chronic atrial fibrillation, gastroesophageal reflux disease, and osteoarthritis. Her medication at admission is as follows:
Double-strength TMP/SMX, 1 tablet orally every 12 hours
Metoprolol, 50 mg orally every 12 hours
Warfarin, 5 mg orally every 24 hours
Acetaminophen, 1 g orally every 6 hours as needed for pain

She complains of flank pain, lower abdominal pain, dysuria, fever, and chills. Urinalysis shows leukocytes (>100/high-power field), erythrocytes (5-10/high-power field), and gram-negative bacteria. Other laboratory results are as follows: hemoglobin 11.8 g/dL, leukocytes 14.7×10^9/L, and international normalized ratio (INR) 12.7. Which of the following would be appropriate?

a. Continue use of TMP/SMX, give 5 mg of vitamin K intravenously, and stop use of warfarin.
b. Discontinue use of TMP/SMX, administer a quinolone, reduce warfarin dosage, and give vitamin K 10 mg intravenously.
c. Discontinue use of TMP/SMX, administer a quinolone, reduce warfarin dosage, and do not give vitamin K.
d. Discontinue use of TMP/SMX, give no antibiotics until culture results are available, stop use of warfarin, and do not give vitamin K.
e. Discontinue use of TMP/SMX, administer a quinolone, stop use of warfarin, and give vitamin K 5 mg orally.

9. A 39-year-old woman is admitted after a motor vehicle accident. She sustained multiple compound fractures. She has a past medical history of hyperlipidemia; her only medications are a statin and oral contraceptive (doses are unknown). The

next morning she complains of chills. Her temperature is 38.2°C, her oxygen saturation is 92% on room air, and C-reactive protein (CRP) level is 49 mg/L (reference range <8 mg/L). Which of the following is least likely to be the cause of the patient's increased CRP level?

a. Trauma
b. Oral contraceptive
c. Wound infection
d. Statin
e. Pulmonary embolism

10. An unidentified man exposes patients in a waiting room to cyanide gas. You are called to help manage in the emergency. Which of the following is true of cyanide exposure?

a. Cyanide poisoning inhibits cholinesterase.
b. Cyanide gas has a strong garlic odor.
c. Definitive treatment involves hemodialysis.
d. Cyanide poisoning improves as methemoglobin is formed.
e. Cyanide gas is a vesicant.

11. A 37-year-old woman with trisomy 21 is admitted to your service with a humerus fracture after a fall. She has diarrhea. On the night of admission she has low oxygen saturation while sleeping. She refused all her medications for several days before the fall. Surgery will be required. Which of the following management issues related to patients with trisomy 21 is *false*?

a. The nighttime desaturation may be related to obstructive sleep apnea.
b. Routine preoperative radiography of the neck is not indicated.
c. The fall may have been caused by a seizure.
d. There is an increased incidence of celiac disease.
e. Thyroid function tests should be checked.

Answers

1. Answer b.
This patient has acute acalculous cholecystitis. He will require a cholecystectomy or be at risk of gallbladder gangrene and perforation. This form of cholecystitis can occur after any type of surgery, especially orthopedic and bowel surgery. Other risk factors for acalculous cholecystitis include the following: sepsis, hypotension, total parenteral nutrition, major trauma or burns, diabetes mellitus, infections, mechanical ventilation, use of opiates, cholesterol emboli, multiple transfusions, and childbirth.

2. Answer c.
This patient presents with altered mental status, mild tachycardia, and hypotension. A fruity odor is noted on his breath. His laboratory results are consistent with a high anion gap metabolic acidosis. Another clue is the presence of oxalate crystals in the urine. The differential diagnosis of this form of metabolic acidosis is the fodder for many mnemonics, such as SLUMPED (*s*alicylates, *l*actic acidosis, *u*remia, *m*ethanol/ethylene glycol, *p*araldehyde, *e*thanol, and *d*iabetic ketoacidosis). The fruity smell suggests ketosis. Oxalate crystals are a specific sign of ethylene glycol toxicity. Both methanol and ethylene glycol require the enzyme alcohol dehydrogenase for metabolism. Patients intoxicated with methanol or ethylene glycol can present with metabolic acidosis, hyperpnea and tachypnea, coma, seizures, and hypotension. Methanol leads to the formation of formate, which causes retinal damage with optic disc hypemia and edema, blindness, and basal ganglia infarcts. Ethylene glycol causes the formation of calcium oxalate crystals, leading to renal failure and hypocalcemia. Methanol and ethylene glycol intoxication are treated with fomepizole or ethanol, which inhibit alcohol dehydrogenase.

3. Answer b.
The spectrum of symptoms, including congestive heart failure, hepatomegaly, and macroglossia is suggestive of primary (AL) amyloidosis. AL amyloid is from deposition of protein derived from immunoglobulin light chain fragments. It is a plasma cell dyscrasia in which a monoclonal immunoglobulin is detectable in the serum or monoclonal light chains are detectable in the urine in approximately 80% of cases. AL amyloid can occur alone or in association with multiple myeloma or Waldenström macroglobulinemia. The deposits can infiltrate many organs, including the heart, liver, kidney, and skin. A fat aspirate stained with Congo red and examined with polarized light is the easiest diagnostic method, although rectal biopsy and scintigraphy with radioisotope-labeled serum amyloid P component are also options.

4. Answer a.
Acute colonic pseudo-obstruction (Ogilvie syndrome) is thought to be the consequence of impaired autonomic regulation postoperatively. The risk of colonic rupture increases significantly when the cecal diameter exceeds 10 cm. Emergent decompressive colonoscopy is an appropriate initial therapy. Neostigmine, which should be given only after mechanical obstruction has been ruled out, may lead to cardiac arrythmia; monitoring is warranted.

5. Answer c.
This patient presents with a spectrum of symptoms consistent with scurvy, or vitamin C deficiency, a condition related to malnutrition, especially in impoverished patients or substance abusers. Decreased vitamin C intake leads to unstable collagen synthesis resulting from

diminished hydroxylation of proline and lysine. A spectrum of cutaneous disease can be associated with hepatitis C, especially leukocytoclastic vasculitis due to cryoglobulinemia.

6.   Answer e.

This patient has hyperkalemia, but she has low urinary excretion of potassium and no evidence of acidosis. Many medications may cause hyperkalemia, most notably angiotensin-converting enzyme inhibitors, potassium-sparing diuretics, nonsteroidal anti-inflammatory drugs, and β-blockers. When an obvious cause is not present, such as over-supplementation of potassium chloride orally or intravenously, a search is warranted for less obvious causes such as renal tubular acidosis. In this patient, none of these is present. Heparin has many potential side effects, directly from anticoagulation (such as retroperitoneal hemorrhage) and immunologically (such as heparin-induced thrombocytopenia). In this case, the patient has heparin-induced hypoaldosteronism, which is causing secondary hyperkalemia. This can occur with all types of heparin, usually at doses greater than 5,000 U/day. The point to emphasize is that when an unexpected phenomenon is noted in a hospitalized patient, a search should always include medications and their side effects.

7.   Answer d.

Needlestick injuries are more common in teaching facilities and least common among phlebotomists. Hepatitis B seroconversion is more common than hepatitis C seroconversion, which is more common than HIV seroconversion. Vaccination with HBV vaccine does not assure immunity. Exposed health care workers should be checked for HBV antibodies, and nonresponders should receive hepatitis B immunoglobulin (HBIG) or HBIG and another vaccination. In this case, the provider should be tested for HBV antibodies; if results are positive, the provider should receive antiviral therapy.

8.   Answer e.

This patient appears to have had a large increase in INR related to a drug interaction between warfarin and TMP/SMX, leading to an INR greater than 9. This is a common complication of warfarin therapy. She is receiving warfarin for her atrial fibrillation and not for a hypercoagulable state or a recent venous thromboembolism, which would affect the approach toward reversal of anticoagulation. With the INR greater than 9 and no clinical evidence of bleeding, reversing anticoagulation with oral vitamin K and stopping the use of warfarin is appropriate. Oral and intravenous routes for administration of vitamin K are equal in efficacy, but the intravenous route carries the risk of anaphylaxis. This patient has a recurrent urinary tract infection with a high likelihood of antibiotic resistance since she continues to have symptoms despite antibiotic treatment. The use of a quinolone carries the risk of warfarin interactions as well. Other choices for antibiotic coverage might be considered. With an elevated white blood cell count and symptoms of pyelonephritis, antibiotic coverage is warranted. This case demonstrates the principle that hospitalized patients often have multiple disease processes that must be considered in making clinical decisions.

9.   Answer d.

CRP can be markedly elevated with various cardiac conditions, including trauma, pulmonary embolism, transplant rejection, infections, surgery, or neoplasm. Oral contraceptives may cause CRP elevation. Statins lower CRP levels. This patient has had significant trauma, and is at risk of myocardial injury or pulmonary embolism.

10.   Answer d.

Cyanide smells like bitter almond; arsine smells like garlic. Cyanide is a toxic asphyxiant not a vesicant, such as mustard gas. Nerve gas inhibits cholinesterase; arsenic inhibits mitochondrial function through inhibition of cytochrome oxidase. Treatment involves nitrites, which form methemoglobin that combines with cyanide to form cyanomethemoglobin, freeing cytochrome oxidase. An alternative is sodium thiosulfate, which enzymatically converts cyanide to the nontoxic compound thiocyanate. Hemodialysis is of no benefit.

11.   Answer b.

Patients with trisomy 21 have an increased incidence of atlantoaxial instability, and evaluation should occur preoperatively. The rates of hypothyroidism, sleep apnea, seizures, and celiac disease are all increased.

14

Hypertension

Gary L. Schwartz, MD

Hypertension

Definition

Because blood pressure is a continuously distributed trait in the population and the risk of cardiovascular disease associated with the level of blood pressure increases progressively as it exceeds 115 mm Hg systolic or 75 mm Hg diastolic, the definition of hypertension is somewhat arbitrary. Currently for adults, *hypertension* is defined as systolic blood pressure 140 mm Hg or higher or diastolic blood pressure 90 mm Hg or higher. Hypertension is further stratified into 2 stages on the basis of the highest level of either systolic or diastolic blood pressure (Table 14-1). Systolic blood pressure between 120 and 139 mm Hg or diastolic blood pressure between 80 and 89 mm Hg is considered *prehypertension*. Persons with prehypertension are at increased risk of cardiovascular disease and progression to hypertension over time compared with persons with normal blood pressure.

Table 14-1 Classification of Blood Pressure for Adults 18 Years or Older[a]

| Category | Blood Pressure Level, mm Hg | | |
	Systolic		Diastolic
Normal	<120	&	<80
Prehypertension	120-139	or	80-89
Hypertension			
Stage 1	140-159	or	90-99
Stage 2	≥160	or	≥100

[a] Not taking antihypertensive drugs and not acutely ill. When systolic and diastolic blood pressures are in different categories, the higher category should be selected to classify the person's blood pressure status. Modified from Chobian AV, Bakris GL, Black HR, Cushman WC, Green LA, Izzo JL Jr, et al. Seventh Report of the Joint National Committee on Prevention, Detection, Evaluation, and Treatment of High Blood Pressure. Hypertension. 2003;42:1206-52.

- *Hypertension* is defined as systolic blood pressure ≥140 mm Hg or diastolic blood pressure ≥90 mm Hg.
- *Prehypertension* is defined as systolic blood pressure 120-139 mm Hg or diastolic blood pressure 80-89 mm Hg.
- Prehypertension is associated with increased risk of cardiovascular disease and hypertension.

Isolated Systolic Hypertension

Isolated systolic hypertension, mainly a problem of people older than 55 years, is defined as systolic blood pressure 140 mm Hg or higher and diastolic blood pressure less than 90 mm Hg. Secondary causes include disorders associated with either increased cardiac output (eg, anemia, thyrotoxicosis, arteriovenous fistula, Paget disease of bone, and beriberi) or increased cardiac stroke volume (eg, aortic insufficiency and complete heart block).

- *Isolated systolic hypertension* is defined as systolic blood pressure ≥140 mm Hg with diastolic pressure <90 mm Hg.
- Isolated systolic hypertension mainly affects people older than 55 years.
- Secondary causes include increased cardiac output (eg, anemia, thyrotoxicosis, arteriovenous fistula, Paget disease of bone, and beriberi) and increased cardiac stroke volume (eg, aortic insufficiency and complete heart block).

Epidemiology

Blood pressure increases with age. Systolic blood pressure increases throughout life, but diastolic blood pressure plateaus in the fifth decade. Thus, both the incidence and prevalence of hypertension increase with age, and isolated systolic hypertension becomes the most common subtype in older persons. For a middle-aged person with normal blood pressure who lives to age 85 years, the residual lifetime risk of developing hypertension is 90%.

In addition to age, other nonreversible factors associated with increased risk of hypertension include being African American or having a family history of hypertension. Reversible factors include having a blood pressure level in the prehypertensive range, being overweight, having a sedentary lifestyle, ingesting a high-sodium–low-potassium diet, having excessive intake of alcohol, or having metabolic syndrome. *Metabolic syndrome* is defined by the presence of 3 or more of the following specific cardiovascular risk factors: abdominal obesity (waist circumference >40 inches [100 cm] in men or >35 inches [88 cm] in women), impaired fasting blood glucose (fasting glucose ≥100 mg/dL), blood pressure 130/85 mm Hg or higher, increased plasma level of triglycerides (≥150 mg/dL), or low high-density lipoprotein (HDL) cholesterol (<40 mg/dL in men or <50 mg/dL in women). It is hypothesized that insulin resistance may be an underlying pathophysiologic factor for metabolic syndrome. Correcting reversible factors can lower blood pressure and prevent the development of hypertension.

In young adulthood and early middle age, hypertension is more common in men than in women. In people older than 55 years, the reverse is true. Hypertension is more common in African Americans than in whites at all ages, and in both races it is more common in the economically disadvantaged.

Hypertension is a major risk factor for cardiovascular disease morbidity and mortality (eg, myocardial infarction, congestive heart failure, progressive atherosclerosis), chronic kidney disease, and dementia. It is the single most important risk factor for stroke. Although risk is continuous and proportionate over both systolic and diastolic blood pressure levels, diastolic blood pressure is the better predictor of risk in young people and systolic blood pressure is the dominant predictor of risk in people older than 60 years.

For any given level of blood pressure, the risk is greater in men than in women, in African Americans than in whites or other racial-ethnic groups, in older people than in younger people, and in those with longer duration of hypertension, additional risk factors for cardiovascular disease, or target organ injury. It is estimated that 72 million Americans have hypertension or are taking medication to decrease blood pressure. An additional 45 million Americans have prehypertension.

- Nonreversible risk factors for hypertension: older age, being African American, and having a family history of hypertension.
- Reversible risk factors for hypertension: prehypertension, overweight, sedentary lifestyle, high-sodium–low-potassium diet, excessive alcohol intake, and metabolic syndrome.
- Metabolic syndrome is defined by the presence of at least 3 of the following: abdominal obesity (waist circumference >40 inches [100 cm] in men or >35 inches [88 cm] in women), impaired fasting blood glucose (fasting glucose ≥100 mg/dL), blood pressure ≥130/85 mm Hg, plasma triglycerides ≥150 mg/dL, or HDL cholesterol <40 mg/dL in men or <50 mg/dL in women.
- Treatment of reversible risk factors can prevent or delay the development of hypertension and lower the risk of cardiovascular disease.
- Treatment of metabolic syndrome can prevent cardiovascular disease and the development of hypertension.
- Hypertension is a major risk factor for cardiovascular disease, renal disease, and dementia.
- Diastolic blood pressure is the best predictor of cardiovascular disease in young people.
- Systolic blood pressure is the dominant predictor of risk of cardiovascular disease in older people.

- Individual risk from hypertension is related to its level, duration, and the presence of other cardiovascular disease risk factors or target organ injury.
- At any given level of blood pressure, African Americans and men are at the greatest risk.

For persons with hypertension, death is most often due to complications of coronary artery disease. Factors that add to this risk are tobacco use, hyperlipidemia, diabetes mellitus, obesity, sedentary lifestyle, metabolic syndrome, gender (men and postmenopausal women), age older than 60 years, and a family history of premature cardiovascular disease (women <65 years, men <55 years). The presence of target organ damage (eg, stroke, left ventricular hypertrophy, ischemic heart disease, congestive heart failure, renal disease, retinopathy, peripheral vascular disease, and dementia) increases the risk of cardiovascular disease events even if blood pressure is subsequently controlled. This fact argues for early identification and prompt treatment of hypertension to avoid the development of target organ injury.

- The most common cause of death among persons with hypertension is coronary artery disease.
- Other risk factors for coronary artery disease include tobacco use, hyperlipidemia, diabetes mellitus, obesity, sedentary lifestyle, metabolic syndrome, male gender, postmenopausal state, older age, and family history of premature cardiovascular disease.
- Target organ damage increases the risk of cardiovascular disease events even if blood pressure is subsequently controlled.

Left ventricular hypertrophy is a strong predictor of sudden death and myocardial infarction in persons with hypertension. Other factors associated with increased left ventricular muscle mass include older age, obesity, and regular vigorous physical activity. Unlike increases in left ventricular mass associated with hypertension, obesity, and age, an increase due to vigorous physical activity is not associated with a higher risk of cardiovascular disease (athletic heart). Echocardiography is more sensitive than electrocardiography in detecting left ventricular hypertrophy.

- Left ventricular hypertrophy is a strong predictor of sudden death and myocardial infarction in persons with hypertension.
- Echocardiography is more sensitive than electrocardiography in detecting left ventricular hypertrophy.

Microalbuminuria is defined as a persistent urinary albumin excretion rate of 30 to 300 mg in 24 hours. In hypertensive persons, it is associated with an increased risk of cardiovascular disease and is a marker of vascular endothelial dysfunction. It is an early manifestation of nephropathy in type 1 diabetes mellitus but is often present at the time of diagnosis in type 2 diabetes mellitus and may simply reflect generalized vascular injury. In persons without diabetes, it is unclear whether microalbuminuria represents early kidney disease. Transient microalbuminuria can be due to fever, vigorous exercise, heart failure, or, in diabetic patients, poor glycemic control. Measurement of the albumin to creatinine ratio (milligrams of albumin divided by grams of creatinine) in an untimed urine specimen is a sensitive screening test. The range of the ratio associated with microalbuminuria is 20 to 200 in men and 30 to 300 in women. A 24-hour urine collection is the diagnostic standard. Testing for microalbuminuria is recommended in persons with diabetes and is elective to further define cardiovasular risk in persons without diabetes who have hypertension. In hypertensive persons it is unclear whether specific treatment (angiotensin-converting enzyme inhibitors [ACEIs] or angiotensin II receptor blockers [ARBs]) designed to reduce microalbuminuria is beneficial beyond effects on blood pressure control.

* Microalbuminuria is a persistent urinary albumin excretion rate of 30-300 mg in 24 hours.
* Transient microalbuminuria can be due to fever, vigorous exercise, heart failure, or, in diabetic patients, poor glycemic control.
* In hypertension, microalbuminuria is a marker of increased cardiovascular risk.
* In type 1 diabetes mellitus, microalbuminuria is an early manifestation of nephropathy.
* Measurement of the albumin to creatinine ratio in an untimed urine specimen is a sensitive screening method for microalbuminuria.
* The diagnostic standard for microalbuminuria is a 24-hour urine collection.

Diagnosis

The diagnosis of hypertension relies on several measures of blood pressure performed in a rigorous manner with a validated and well-maintained mercury or aneroid sphygmomanometer and with an appropriate-sized cuff (the bladder should encircle at least 80% of the arm). The person should be at rest in the seated position (back and feet supported) for at least 5 minutes before the measurement. Recent physical activity, use of tobacco or caffeine (within 30 minutes of the measurement), or a full urinary bladder can transiently increase blood pressure and should be avoided. The arm should be bare (no tight clothing constricting the upper arm) and positioned so the cuff is at the level of the heart. The cuff should be inflated to 20 to 30 mm Hg above the level that obliterates the palpable radial pulse. The cuff deflation rate should be 2 mm Hg per second. The systolic blood pressure is the point at which the first of 2 or more Korotkoff sounds is heard, and the diastolic blood pressure is the point at which the Korotkoff sounds are no longer heard. The diagnosis of hypertension in a person with an elevated blood pressure at screening is confirmed at 1 or more subsequent office visits. At least 2 standardized measures of blood pressure should be made at each visit and the results averaged. Appropriate timing of follow-up based on the screening blood pressure level is shown in Table 14-2. For most persons, confirmation can occur over 1 to 2 months. If initial blood pressure is severely elevated or if the patient has additional risk factors for cardiovascular disease or has clinical cardiovascular disease, confirmation should be made in a shorter time.

Some persons have elevated blood pressure when it is measured in the clinic environment but have normal blood pressure at all other times. This is called *office* or *white-coat hypertension*. In these individuals, the office blood pressure is an overestimate of the usual or average daily blood pressure level. There is no target organ injury despite persistently elevated office blood pressure readings. Self-measurement

Table 14-2 Follow-up Recommendations Based on Screening Blood Pressure Level in Adults

Screening Blood Pressure	Follow-up[a]
Normal	Recheck in 2 y
Prehypertension	Recheck in 1 y
Hypertension	
Stage 1	Confirm within 2 mo
Stage 2	Confirm within 1 mo; if blood pressure >180/110 mm Hg, confirm within 1 wk or treat immediately, depending on clinical situation

[a] Modify the follow-up schedule on the basis of knowledge of previous blood pressure measurement, other cardiovascular risk factors, or target organ disease.
Modified from Chobian AV, Bakris GL, Black HR, Cushman WC, Green LA, Izzo JL Jr, et al. Seventh Report of the Joint National Committee on Prevention, Detection, Evaluation, and Treatment of High Blood Pressure. Hypertension. 2003;42:1206-52.

of blood pressure outside the office setting can identify white-coat hypertension. In the absence of target organ disease, average self-measured blood pressure of less than 130/80 mm Hg confirms the diagnosis. If self-measured blood pressure is 130 to 140 mm Hg systolic or 80 to 90 mm Hg diastolic, the diagnosis is best confirmed with noninvasive, 24-hour ambulatory monitoring. In the short term, persons with white-coat hypertension are at low risk and do not require antihypertensive drug therapy; however, they are at increased risk of developing sustained hypertension and thus require long-term follow-up.

On average, self-recorded blood pressure or average awake blood pressure by ambulatory monitoring is 5 mm Hg lower than office blood pressure and, therefore, values greater than 135 mm Hg systolic or greater than 85 mm Hg diastolic are considered elevated (ie, hypertension is blood pressure ≥135/85 mm Hg by home or average awake ambulatory blood pressure). Blood pressure devices for home use need to be validated at regular intervals (twice yearly) by the health care provider.

Some persons present with findings of hypertensive target organ injury but have normal office blood pressure levels. Such individuals may have *masked hypertension*. This is the reverse of white-coat hypertension in that office blood pressure measures underestimate the usual or average daily blood pressure level. This diagnosis is suggested if self-measured blood pressure is elevated but is best confirmed with noninvasive, 24-hour ambulatory monitoring.

Older persons may have *pseudohypertension*, a falsely increased systolic and diastolic blood pressure when measured by the cuff method; it is the result of a stiff vascular tree caused by atherosclerosis. Similar to persons with white-coat hypertension, persons with pseudohypertension may have marked elevations of blood pressure but lack expected target organ injury. They may also complain of symptoms that suggest low blood pressure with treatment. Pseudohypertension may exist if the radial artery remains palpable after the brachial artery is occluded by cuff inflation (Osler maneuver). However, the Osler maneuver is not a very sensitive screening method for pseudohypertension. Confirmation requires intra-arterial blood pressure measurement.

- The diagnosis of hypertension requires several blood pressure measurements made in a standardized fashion on different occasions.
- Recent physical exercise, use of tobacco or caffeine, or a full urinary bladder can transiently elevate blood pressure.
- Hypertension by self-measurement or average awake ambulatory level is blood pressure ≥135/85 mm Hg.
- Office (white-coat) hypertension: elevated blood pressure only when measured in the clinic environment.
- Masked hypertension: elevated blood pressure only when measured outside the clinic environment.

- Pseudohypertension: inaccurately high cuff blood pressure as a result of a stiff vascular tree in older persons.

Evaluation

After the diagnosis of hypertension has been established, 1) identify lifestyle factors that contribute to higher blood pressure, 2) identify other risk factors for cardiovascular disease, 3) assess for target organ damage (Table 14-3), and 4) consider the possibility of secondary hypertension. Secondary hypertension accounts for approximately 5% to 10% of all cases of high blood pressure.

- Secondary hypertension accounts for 5%-10% of all cases of high blood pressure.

Clues to secondary hypertension are features that are inconsistent with essential hypertension. Classic features of essential hypertension

Table 14-3 Hypertensive Target Organ Injury

Target Organ	Injury	Clinical Marker/Diagnosis
Heart	Left ventricular hypertrophy	S_4 gallop
		Forceful & prolonged apical thrust
		Displacement of point of maximal intensity
		Chest x-ray film, electrocardiography, echocardiography
	Angina	History, electrocardiography
	Prior myocardial infarction	
	Prior revascularization	
	Heart failure (systolic or diastolic)	History
		Lung rales
		S_3 gallop
		Edema
		Chest x-ray film, echocardiography
Brain	Stroke	History
	Leukoaraiosis	Computed tomography or magnetic resonance imaging
	Transient ischemic attack	History
	Dementia	History
		Cognitive testing
Kidney	Chronic kidney disease	Creatinine, blood urea nitrogen, urinalysis, eGFR
Arteries	Peripheral artery disease	History of claudication
		Bruits
		Diminished pulses
Eye	Retinopathy	Funduscopic examination:
		Generalized & focal arteriolar narrowing[a]
		"Copper-wiring" of arterioles
		Arteriovenous nicking
		Cotton-wool spots[b]
		Microaneurysms & macroaneurysms[b]
		Flame & blot-shaped retinal hemorrhages[b]
		Retinal vein occlusion
		Optic disc swelling

Abbreviations: eGFR, estimated glomerular filtration rate; S_3, third heart sound; S_4, fourth heart sound.
[a] Feature predicts increased risk of coronary artery disease.
[b] Feature predicts increased risk of stroke.

are onset in the fourth or fifth decade of life, a positive family history for hypertension, initial blood pressure level categorized as stage 1 hypertension and easily controlled with 1 or 2 medications, no target organ damage, normal results of routine laboratory studies, and blood pressure that does not increase from an established level of control over a short period of time. Factors inconsistent with essential hypertension are listed in Table 14-4.

- Consider secondary hypertension if the presenting features are inconsistent with those of essential hypertension.

Drugs

Certain drugs can cause or aggravate hypertension or interfere with the action of antihypertensive medications. These drugs and their mechanisms of action are listed in Table 14-5.

- Oral contraceptives increase blood pressure by inducing sodium retention, increasing renin substrate, and facilitating the action of catecholamines.
- Nonsteroidal anti-inflammatory drugs block the formation of renal vasodilating, natriuretic prostaglandins, thus interfering

Table 14-4 Factors Inconsistent With Essential Hypertension

General
    Age at onset <30 y or >50 y
    Blood pressure >180/110 mm Hg at diagnosis
    Significant target organ damage at diagnosis
        Hemorrhages & exudates on retinal examination
        Renal insufficiency
        Cardiomegaly
        Left ventricular hypertrophy
    Poor response to an appropriate 3-drug program
Features suggesting specific secondary causes of hypertension
    Primary aldosteronism
        Unprovoked hypokalemia, Chvostek sign, Trousseau sign
    Pheochromocytoma
        Labile blood pressure with diaphoresis, tachycardia, headache, pallor, neurofibromas, orofacial neuromas (MEN-2)
    Renovascular disease
        Abdominal bruit
    Cushing disease
        Truncal obesity, pigmented striae, impaired fasting glucose, hypokalemia
    Coarctation of the aorta
        Delayed or absent femoral pulses
        "3" Sign & rib notching on chest x-ray film[a]
    Polycystic kidney disease
        Abdominal or flank mass, family history of renal disease

Abbreviation: MEN-2, multiple endocrine neoplasia type 2.
[a] See "Coarctation of the Aorta" subsection in the "Secondary Hypertension" section.

with the effectiveness of diuretics, β-blockers, and ACEIs and inducing sodium retention, which increases blood pressure.
- Tricyclic antidepressants inhibit the action of centrally acting agents (methyldopa and clonidine).

Laboratory Studies

Routine laboratory tests should include a complete blood count; measurements of sodium, potassium, glucose, creatinine (for estimation of glomerular filtration rate [GFR]), uric acid, calcium, cholesterol (total and HDL), and triglycerides; urinalysis; chest radiography; and electrocardiography. Urine albumin excretion or the albumin-creatinine ratio should be measured in patients who have diabetes mellitus or chronic kidney disease. Additional studies should not be performed unless abnormalities are identified on initial screening tests or the history or examination suggests a secondary form of hypertension.

Treatment

The goal of therapy is to eliminate the morbidity and mortality of cardiovascular disease attributable to hypertension by decreasing blood pressure to less than 140/90 mm Hg. A lower goal of less than 130/80 mm Hg is appropriate for persons with diabetes mellitus, established coronary artery disease, coronary artery disease risk equivalents (eg, carotid artery disease, peripheral arterial disease, and abdominal aortic aneurysm), those who are at high risk of coronary artery disease, and those with chronic kidney disease. An even lower goal of less than 120/80 mm Hg is advised for persons with reduced left ventricular function due to coronary artery disease.

Lifestyle Modifications

Lifestyle modifications lower blood pressure and should be encouraged for all persons with prehypertension (Table 14-6). The modifications may be sufficient as initial therapy for some persons with stage 1 hypertension. They are adjunctive therapy for those with more severe hypertension.

The Dietary Approaches to Stop Hypertension (DASH) eating plan is effective in lowering blood pressure in patients with prehypertension or stage 1 hypertension. The DASH eating plan includes consuming a diet rich in fruits, vegetables (high potassium), and low-fat dairy products (high calcium) with a reduced content of total and saturated fat.

The prevalence of hypertension is greater among persons who are obese. An increase in blood pressure often parallels weight gain, and numerous clinical trials have documented the effectiveness of weight loss to decrease blood pressure. Weight reduction to within the normal range (body mass index, 18.5-24.9) is the goal, although losses as small as 4.5 kg may decrease blood pressure.

Restriction of daily sodium intake to 100 mEq (2.4 g sodium or 6 g salt) decreases blood pressure in some but not all hypertensive persons. Although salt sensitivity is more common among persons who are African American, obese, or elderly or who have low-renin hypertension, higher blood pressure levels, or chronic kidney disease, the antihypertensive effect of many medications is enhanced by sodium restriction. Also, sodium restriction minimizes diuretic-induced potassium losses.

Table 14-5 Drugs That Can Increase Blood Pressure or Interfere With Antihypertensive Therapy

Drug	Mechanism
Oral contraceptives (with high estrogenic activity)	Induce sodium retention Increase renin substrate Facilitate action of catecholamines
Alcohol (>1 oz [30 mL] daily)	Activates sympathetic nervous system Increases cortisol secretion Increases intracellular calcium levels
Sympathomimetics & amphetamine-like substances (eg, cold formulas, allergy medications, diet pills)	Increase peripheral vascular resistance Interfere with action of guanethidine & guanadrel
Nonsteroidal anti-inflammatory drugs	Induce sodium retention by blocking formation of renal vasodilating, natriuretic prostaglandins, thus interfering with action of diuretics, β-blockers, & angiotensin-converting enzyme inhibitors
Corticosteroids, corticotropin	Iatrogenic Cushing disease
Tricyclic antidepressants	Block uptake of guanethidine Inhibit action of centrally acting drugs such as methyldopa & clonidine
Monoamine oxidase inhibitors (in combination with tyramine—found in aged cheeses & some red wines)	Prevent degradation & metabolism of norepinephrine released by tyramine-containing foods Increase blood pressure when combined with reserpine/guanethidine
Cocaine	Vasoconstriction Interferes with action of adrenergic inhibitors
Marijuana	Increases systolic blood pressure
Cyclosporine, tacrolimus	Renal & systemic vasoconstriction
Erythropoietin	Systemic vasoconstriction
Serotonin	Systemic vasoconstriction
Glycyrrhizinic acid (eg, chewing tobacco, imported licorice, health food products)	Inhibits renal cortisol catabolism

Regular aerobic exercise may decrease blood pressure directly and indirectly by facilitating weight loss. At least 30 minutes of daily aerobic activity, such as brisk walking, should be encouraged.

Restriction of daily alcohol intake to less than 1 oz (30 mL) of ethanol (<0.5 oz [15 mL] for women or lighter-weight men) is often associated with a decrease in blood pressure. Alcohol is a source of calories, and its use is often associated with poor compliance with antihypertensive therapy. Excessive alcohol intake may cause labile hypertension that is difficult to control in association with other symptoms (flushing and tachycardia) that suggest pheochromocytoma.

Because complications of coronary artery disease are the most common causes of death in hypertensive persons, all risks for cardiovascular disease must be addressed. The benefits of blood pressure reduction are diminished in smokers. Components of the metabolic syndrome coexist more often in hypertensive persons than in normotensive persons. Treatment of the metabolic syndrome decreases the risk of cardiovascular disease and the development of hypertension. It includes instruction in eating a low-fat, weight-loss diet; encouragement to exercise regularly; and use of medications to improve serum levels of lipids, blood pressure, and insulin sensitivity when appropriate.

Table 14-6 Effect of Lifestyle Modifications on Systolic Blood
Pressure

Modification	Recommendation	Expected Decrease in Systolic Blood Pressure, mm Hg[a]
Adopt DASH eating plan	Consume a diet rich in fruits, vegetables, & low-fat dairy products with a reduced content of saturated & total fat	8-14
Reduce weight	Normal body weight (BMI, 18.5-24.9)	5-20 (per 10 kg)
Restrict dietary sodium	Restrict daily sodium intake to ≤2.4 g (6 g sodium chloride)	2-8
Increase physical activity	Regular aerobic exercise (eg, brisk walking for 30 min) most days of the week	4-9
Limit alcohol intake	For most men: ≤2 drinks daily (1 oz [30 mL] alcohol) For women: ≤1 drink daily	2-4

Abbreviations: BMI, body mass index; DASH, Dietary Approaches to
Stop Hypertension.
[a] Effects on blood pressure may be greater in some individuals.
Modified from Chobian AV, Bakris GL, Black HR, Cushman WC,
Green LA, Izzo JL Jr, et al. Seventh Report of the Joint National
Committee on Prevention, Detection, Evaluation, and Treatment of
High Blood Pressure. Hypertension. 2003;42:1206-52.

* Follow the DASH eating plan.
* Reduce weight to within the normal range.
* Restrict daily sodium intake to 100 mEq.
* Exercise for at least 30 minutes daily.
* Restrict alcohol intake to <1 oz (30 mL) daily.
* Address all risk factors for cardiovascular disease.

A diet deficient in potassium may increase blood pressure; therefore,
an adequate intake of potassium should be encouraged. The DASH
eating plan is high in potassium. Studies do not support the use of
biofeedback or relaxation therapies for blood pressure control.

Encouragement of lifestyle modifications is appropriate treatment
for prehypertension. A trial of lifestyle modifications alone for up to
12 months is appropriate for patients with stage 1 hypertension who
do not have diabetes or other risk factors for cardiovascular disease,
target organ involvement, or clinical cardiovascular disease. If lifestyle
modifications fail to decrease blood pressure to less than 140/90 mm
Hg, drug treatment should be initiated. For patients at increased
risk because of additional risk factors for cardiovascular disease, drug

treatment should be started if lifestyle modifications are ineffective after
3 to 6 months. Drug treatment should be considered initially in addition to lifestyle modifications for patients with stage 2 hypertension or
for those with stage 1 hypertension who also have diabetes, target organ
involvement, or clinical cardiovascular disease. Successful changes in
lifestyle (eg, weight loss, reductions in salt and alcohol intake, and
increased exercise) may allow tapering of an established drug program.

* Lifestyle modifications are the treatment for prehypertension.
* A trial of lifestyle modifications alone for up to 12 months is
  appropriate initial therapy for stage 1 hypertension in the absence
  of diabetes, other risk factors, target organ involvement, or clinical
  cardiovascular disease.
* Stage 2 hypertension or stage 1 hypertension with concurrent
  diabetes, other risk factors, target organ damage, or clinical cardiovascular disease should be treated initially with both lifestyle
  modifications and drug therapy.

Pharmacologic Therapy
In more than 50% of persons with stage 1 hypertension, blood pressure can be controlled with single-drug therapy. Important factors to
consider when selecting a drug for initial therapy are its efficacy as
monotherapy, route of elimination, drug interactions, side effects,
and cost. Proper drug selection is important for maintaining long-
term compliance.

Patients with stage 2 hypertension, those with initial blood
pressure more than 20/10 mm Hg above the goal, and those targeted to lower blood pressure goals (ie, those with chronic kidney
disease, diabetes, or coronary artery disease) will often require 2 or
more drugs for blood pressure control. Consideration of initial therapy with a combination of 2 drugs (1 of which is a diuretic appropriate for the level of renal function) should be considered.

Drugs appropriate for monotherapy are thiazide-type diuretics, β-blockers (patients younger than 60 years), calcium channel
blockers (CCBs), ACEIs, and ARBs. Low-dose combinations may
also be used for initial therapy, as noted above. Thiazide diuretics
should be considered as the initial therapy of choice for most patients
with uncomplicated hypertension who lack clear indications for
other choices. Other classes of drugs should be considered if diuretics are ineffective or contraindicated or in settings in which the efficacy of an alternative drug has been established (eg, ACEIs in a
hypertensive person with congestive heart failure [see indications for
specific drugs below]). Centrally acting α-agonists (eg, clonidine, methyldopa, guanabenz, and guanfacine) and traditional vasodilators (eg,
hydralazine and minoxidil) may be associated with pseudotolerance.
Pseudotolerance is reflex stimulation of the renin-angiotensin-aldosterone system or the sympathetic nervous system (or both systems)
that results in fluid retention, an increase in vascular resistance, or
an increase in cardiac output with subsequent loss of efficacy with prolonged use. Therefore, these drugs are not ordinarily used as monotherapy. A centrally acting α-agonist is appropriate when given in
combination with a diuretic, whereas traditional vasodilators are best
as a third drug in combination with a diuretic and an adrenergic
inhibitor. Additional important factors influencing drug selection
include the recognition that certain drugs work better according to

a person's age and race (diuretics and CCBs are more effective in African Americans and the elderly; β-blockers, ACEIs, and ARBs are more effective in whites and younger patients). With combination therapy, make certain that the chosen drugs work in combination and that 2 drugs of the same class are not given simultaneously. Usually, 1 of the drugs in the combination should be a diuretic. Fatigue and impotence are potential side effects of all antihypertensive drugs.

- Drugs for monotherapy: diuretics, β-blockers, CCBs, ACEIs, and ARBs.
- Thiazide-type diuretics: the drugs of choice for most patients with uncomplicated hypertension.
- Combination therapy with 2 drugs should be considered for stage 2 hypertension or if initial blood pressure is >20/10 mm Hg above the goal.
- Centrally acting α-agonists are not ordinarily used as monotherapy but are appropriate in combination with a diuretic.
- Traditional vasodilators are best as a third drug in combination with a diuretic and an adrenergic inhibitor.

Thiazide Diuretics

Thiazide diuretics inhibit sodium reabsorption in the initial portion of the distal convoluted tubule of the nephron, where 5% to 8% of filtered sodium is reabsorbed. Acute effects to lower blood pressure are due to volume contraction and decreased cardiac output, but chronically they cause a reduction in peripheral vascular resistance through unknown mechanisms. The antihypertensive effect is limited by stimulation of the renin-angiotensin-aldosterone axis. In large group studies, diuretics are most effective in older persons and African Americans. They are also effective in the presence of obesity and diabetes. They are recommended for the initial treatment of uncomplicated hypertension and isolated systolic hypertension in the elderly. Concomitant diseases for which these drugs should be considered are edema states and heart failure associated with congestion. Thiazides have been shown to prevent first strokes and heart failure and to reduce cardiovascular mortality. They decrease the risk of osteoporotic fractures in postmenopausal women, lessen the risk of recurrent calcium nephrolithiasis, and are effective in lessening the risk of cardiovascular disease events in persons with diabetes or in those at high risk of coronary heart disease. They also are effective in the secondary prevention of stroke. In addition to their role as initial therapy, thiazide diuretics potentiate the effect of most other antihypertensive drugs. Metabolic disturbances associated with their use include hypokalemia, hyperuricemia, hypercalcemia (thiazides decrease urinary calcium excretion), hypomagnesemia, hyponatremia (more common in the elderly), fasting hyperglycemia (insulin resistance), hypochloremic metabolic alkalosis, and increased levels of low-density lipoprotein (LDL) cholesterol and triglycerides. Long-term therapy increases the risk of diabetes. Because of these potential adverse effects, relative contraindications to the use of thiazide diuretics include diet-controlled type 2 diabetes, gout, hyponatremia, hyperlipidemia, cardiac arrhythmias, and ischemic heart disease. The adverse metabolic effects of thiazide diuretics are dose-dependent and often of little consequence when currently recommended low doses are used (eg, 12.5-25 mg hydrochlorothiazide).

Drug interactions include potentiation of lithium toxicity (thiazides decrease the renal clearance of lithium), lessening of the anticoagulant effect of warfarin, and enhancement of digitalis toxicity and the effects of skeletal muscle relaxants. Nonsteroidal anti-inflammatory drugs and high dietary sodium decrease the antihypertensive effect of thiazide diuretics. They are usually ineffective when the serum creatinine level is greater than 1.5 to 2.0 mg/dL (estimated GFR <30 mL/min). Under these circumstances, a more potent loop diuretic or metolazone is more effective. Volume expansion is often etiologically important in hypertension accompanying chronic kidney disease with reduced GFR. Thiazide diuretics have been associated with volume depletion, pancreatitis, vasculitis, mesenteric infarction, hepatitis, intrahepatic cholestasis, interstitial nephritis, and photosensitivity. Rarely, they cause blood dyscrasias.

- Important indications for thiazide diuretics: uncomplicated hypertension, heart failure with congestion, edema states, isolated systolic hypertension in the elderly, high risk of coronary artery disease, or history of stroke.
- Thiazides increase the risk of diabetes developing but decrease the risk of cardiovascular events in persons with preexisting diabetes.
- Thiazides decrease the risk of osteoporosis-related fracture and recurrent calcium nephrolithiasis.
- Thiazides (except metolazone) are ineffective when estimated GFR is <30 mL/min.
- Metabolic disturbances: hypokalemia, hyperuricemia, hypercalcemia, hypomagnesemia, hyponatremia, fasting hyperglycemia, hypochloremic metabolic alkalosis, and increased levels of LDL cholesterol and triglycerides.
- Adverse effects: pancreatitis, vasculitis, mesenteric infarction, hepatitis, and photosensitivity.
- Drug interactions: thiazides potentiate lithium toxicity (they increase lithium levels by enhancing proximal tubular reabsorption of the drug) and enhance digitalis toxicity and the effects of skeletal muscle relaxants while lessening the anticoagulant effect of warfarin.

Loop Diuretics

Loop diuretics inhibit sodium reabsorption from the thick ascending portion of the loop of Henle in the nephron, where 35% to 45% of filtered sodium is reabsorbed.

Furosemide

The major indication for furosemide is hypertension associated with chronic kidney disease and an estimated GFR of less than 30 mL/min. Because of its short duration of action, furosemide must be given twice daily to maintain a reduced body fluid volume essential for an antihypertensive effect. Similar to thiazide diuretics, furosemide can cause volume depletion, hypokalemia, hyperuricemia, fasting hyperglycemia, and hypochloremic alkalosis. Unlike thiazide diuretics, furosemide increases urinary calcium excretion (which can cause hypocalcemia). Potential adverse effects include reversible deafness, postural hypotension (especially in older persons), photosensitivity, pancreatitis, blood dyscrasias, nephrocalcinosis, and interstitial nephritis. Furosemide enhances salicylate clearance and the effects of skeletal muscle relaxants but is not associated with an increase in lithium level. It is synergistic when used with metolazone, and the combination is effective in states of resistant edema. Avoid administration with aminoglycosides or other ototoxic drugs. Nonsteroidal anti-inflammatory drugs and high dietary sodium reduce the antihypertensive effect of all diuretics.

- Important indication for furosemide: hypertension associated with chronic kidney disease and estimated GFR <30 mL/min.
- Metabolic effects: hypokalemia, hyperuricemia, fasting hyperglycemia, hypochloremic alkalosis, and increased urinary calcium excretion (hypocalcemia).
- Adverse effects: reversible deafness and postural hypotension.

Bumetanide

The actions of bumetanide, including adverse effects, electrolyte alterations, and drug interactions, are identical to those of furosemide; however, bumetanide is a more potent diuretic on a milligram-per-milligram basis (1 mg is equivalent to 40 mg furosemide) and has twice the bioavailability of furosemide.

Ethacrynic Acid

The actions of ethacrynic acid are similar to those of furosemide. Although permanent hearing loss is a risk, ethacrynic acid is an alternative diuretic for patients with sulfa sensitivity because it is not a sulfonamide derivative.

Torsemide

Torsemide is different from the other loop diuretics in that it is eliminated mainly by liver metabolism, which prolongs its duration of action as long as 12 hours. Otherwise, its actions are similar to those of other loop agents.

Potassium-Sparing Diuretics

Spironolactone

Spironolactone is a mineralocorticoid receptor antagonist given specifically to persons who have primary aldosteronism or severe secondary aldosteronism. Use of this drug in severe heart failure has been shown to decrease the risk of morbidity and death. Its diuretic effect is antagonized by the concomitant use of salicylates. Adverse effects include hyponatremia, hyperkalemia, hyperchloremic acidosis, gynecomastia (but not breast cancer), mastodynia, menorrhagia, and skin rash. Spironolactone is often given in combination with thiazides to limit hypokalemia.

- Important indications for spironolactone: primary aldosteronism and states of secondary aldosteronism, especially severe heart failure.
- The diuretic effect is antagonized by the concomitant use of salicylates.
- Adverse effects: hyperkalemia, gynecomastia, mastodynia, menorrhagia, and skin rash.

Eplerenone

Eplerenone is a mineralocorticoid receptor antagonist similar to spironolactone, and its indications for use are generally the same as for spironolactone. This drug may lessen mortality among persons with heart failure following myocardial infarction. Eplerenone differs from spironolactone by having less affinity for progesterone and androgen receptors. Gynecomastia occurs less often; however, impotence and menstrual irregularities can occur. Hyperkalemia is the most common adverse effect. Inhibitors of the cytochrome P450 enzyme CYP3A4 may increase serum levels of eplerenone.

- Eplerenone may be better tolerated than spironolactone, primarily because of less risk of gynecomastia in men.

Triamterene

Triamterene inhibits renal potassium wasting by blocking the epithelial sodium channel in the distal tubule of the nephron. It is used most often in combination with thiazide diuretics to limit renal potassium wasting. Side effects include hyperkalemia and skin rash. Acute renal failure can occur if triamterene is used in combination with indomethacin. Triamterene may be excreted into the urine as crystals that can form stones, often containing calcium. The drug should not be used during pregnancy because it is a folic acid antagonist.

- Triamterene inhibits renal potassium wasting by blocking the epithelial sodium channel in the distal tubule of the nephron.
- Do not use in combination with indomethacin or during pregnancy.

Amiloride

Amiloride limits renal potassium wasting by the same mechanism as triamterene and is used most often in combination with thiazide diuretics. Its side effects are hyperkalemia, gastrointestinal distress, and skin rash.

Of the potassium-sparing diuretics, only spironolactone and eplerenone can cause gynecomastia. Except under special circumstances, potassium-sparing drugs should be avoided in cases of renal failure and when ACEIs or ARBs are used.

- In general, avoid potassium-sparing diuretics in renal failure and when ACEIs or ARBs are used.

Adrenergic Inhibitors

If a diuretic fails to control blood pressure, an adrenergic inhibitor can be added. Adrenergic inhibitors are divided into centrally acting and peripherally acting drugs.

Peripherally Acting Inhibitors

Reserpine—Reserpine blocks the transport of norepinephrine into storage granules in postganglionic sympathetic neurons, decreasing sympathetic nervous system tone. Side effects include depression, nasal congestion, and stimulation of gastric acid secretion; thus, contraindications for reserpine are a history of depression or peptic ulcer disease. Its use is also contraindicated in advanced renal insufficiency (GFR <10 mL/min). Reserpine is not commonly used in current practice; however, small doses (≤0.1 mg daily) in combination with a diuretic provide an inexpensive, well-tolerated, and effective combination for blood pressure control.

- Major side effects of reserpine: depression, nasal congestion, and stimulation of gastric acid secretion.
- Small dosages in combination with a diuretic provide an inexpensive, well-tolerated, and effective combination for blood pressure control.

Guanethidine—Guanethidine, which is used only as part of a combination drug program to treat resistant hypertension, is used uncommonly in current practice. It decreases blood pressure by causing degranulation of catecholamine storage granules in postganglionic sympathetic neurons. It does not enter the central nervous system. It has a long half-life. The maximal hypotensive effect of a given dose may not be manifested for 2 or 3 weeks. It should be given only once daily, and titration requires several weeks. Its major side effects are postural hypotension, fluid retention, diarrhea, and retrograde ejaculation. Tricyclic antidepressants, antihistamines, and ephedrine interfere with its action. Guanadrel sulfate, a short-acting form of guanethidine, is easier to titrate to an effective dose because it has a shorter half-life. Dose reductions are required in renal insufficiency.

- An important indication for guanethidine is resistant hypertension.
- Major side effects: postural hypotension, fluid retention, diarrhea, and retrograde ejaculation.
- Tricyclic antidepressants, antihistamines, and ephedrine interfere with its action.

α_1-*Receptor Blockers*—These drugs block α_1-adrenergic receptors on vascular smooth muscle cells, impairing catecholamine-induced vasoconstriction. They do not interfere with norepinephrine reuptake by peripheral sympathetic neurons; thus, there is no increase in levels of circulating catecholamines or heart rate. Because the initial dose can precipitate hypotension and syncope, it should be taken at bedtime. Longer-acting peripheral α_1-receptor blockers (doxazosin and terazosin) allow single daily dosing. Prazosin, an older drug, must be taken at least twice daily. These drugs may lessen voiding symptoms associated with benign prostatic hypertrophy. In elderly patients, the use of α_1-receptor blockers is frequently associated with orthostatic hypotension, but they do not have adverse metabolic side effects. Other side effects include gastrointestinal distress and, rarely, sedation, edema, and dry mouth. Because this class of drugs is less effective than diuretics in reducing the risk of congestive heart failure, it is no longer considered an option for the initial management of hypertension.

- α_1-Receptor blockers are no longer considered appropriate initial therapy for hypertension.
- Because the first dose can cause hypotension and syncope, it should be taken at bedtime.
- In elderly patients, these drugs are often associated with orthostatic hypotension, but they have no adverse metabolic side effects and may lessen symptoms of prostatism.

β-*Blockers*—Many β-blockers are available. They differ in cardioselectivity (affinity for cardiac β_1 receptors is greater than for noncardiac [vascular and bronchiolar] β_2 receptors), lipid solubility, and whether they have partial intrinsic (agonist) sympathomimetic activity (ISA). Non-ISA β-blockers lower blood pressure by reducing cardiac output and inhibiting both renin release and central sympathetic outflow. β-Blockers with ISA activity do not reduce cardiac output but cause mild peripheral vasodilatation. As lipid solubility increases (lipophilic), the liver metabolizes more of the drug, more of it enters the brain, and its duration of action is shorter. As lipid solubility decreases (hydrophilic), the drug is eliminated mainly by renal excretion, less of it enters the brain, and its duration of action is longer. The most lipid-soluble drugs are propranolol, penbutolol, and carvedilol. Intermediate lipid-soluble drugs are metoprolol, pindolol, and timolol. The least lipid-soluble drugs are atenolol, betaxolol, carteolol, celiprolol, esmolol, sotalol, and nadolol.

- β-Blockers differ by cardioselectivity, lipid solubility, and the presence or absence of ISA.
- As lipid solubility increases, the liver metabolizes more of the drug, more of the drug enters the brain, and its duration of action is shorter.
- As lipid solubility decreases, the drug is eliminated mainly by renal excretion, less of the drug enters the brain, and its duration of action is longer.
- The most lipid-soluble drugs (lipophilic): propranolol, penbutolol, and carvedilol (preferred in the presence of renal disease).
- The least lipid-soluble drugs (hydrophilic): atenolol, betaxolol, carteolol, celiprolol, esmolol, sotalol, and nadolol (preferred in the presence of liver disease).

β_1-Cardioselective β-blockers are acebutolol, atenolol, betaxolol, bisoprolol, celiprolol, esmolol, metoprolol, and nebivolol. Cardioselectivity is relative; at high doses, all β-blockers are nonselective (ie, they block both cardiac β_1 and noncardiac β_2 receptors). β-Blockers with ISA activity are pindolol, acebutolol, carteolol, celiprolol, and penbutolol. Cardioselectivity is not associated with a difference in blood pressure–lowering effect. However, it may be associated with less adverse effects on lipids (β-blockers can increase triglycerides and lower HDL cholesterol) and may allow quicker recovery from hypoglycemia in diabetic patients. Paradoxical increases in blood pressure under stress are also less likely with cardioselective drugs.

β-Blockers are appropriate initial therapy for hypertension in younger persons (<60 years old). For stroke prevention in persons 60 years or older, these drugs are less effective than alternative first-line agents and therefore should not be used as initial therapy in the absence of another indication. In large group studies, their antihypertensive effect is greatest in younger persons and whites. Certain comorbid conditions suggest the use of these drugs. Three β-blockers—propranolol, timolol, and metoprolol tartrate—prevent sudden death and recurrent myocardial infarction after an initial event. Most persons with congestive heart failure should be receiving a β-blocker (eg, metoprolol succinate, bisoprolol, or carvedilol). Also, these drugs should be considered for patients with hypertension who have concomitant angina or hypertrophic cardiomyopathy. Other concomitant conditions that may benefit from the use of these drugs are supraventricular arrhythmias, glaucoma, migraine headache, and essential tremor. Noncardioselective drugs may be effective in preventing migraines and inhibiting essential tremor. Given preoperatively, β-blockers (eg, atenolol or bisoprolol) decrease the risk of postoperative myocardial infarction in persons at increased risk of coronary artery disease. Although severe or poorly controlled asthma is a contraindication for β-blockers, many persons with well-controlled or mild asthma or mild chronic obstructive pulmonary disease can tolerate low doses of cardioselective agents. Contraindications to β-blocker therapy are conduction system disease of the heart, angina due to coronary vasospasm, Raynaud phenomenon, severe (but not mild) occlusive peripheral vascular disease, pheochromocytoma (in the absence of α-blockade), and depression. Because β-blockers may mask the symptoms of hypoglycemia and delay recovery from it, caution is required when these agents are given to patients with diabetes who are taking hypoglycemic drugs or insulin. Complete heart block can occur if a β-blocker is given in combination with verapamil. Side effects include cold extremities (non-ISA β-blockers), decreased exercise capacity, bronchospasm, dyslipidemia (elevated triglyceride level, lower HDL cholesterol [worse with lipid-soluble, non-ISA, noncardioselective drugs]), hyperkalemia (reduced aldosterone levels), worsening of psoriasis, fatigue, insomnia, nasal congestion, and possibly depression.

- Cardioselectivity is relative; all β-blockers are nonselective at high doses.
- Propranolol, timolol, and metoprolol tartrate prevent sudden death and recurrent myocardial infarction after an initial event.
- Most patients with congestive heart failure should be receiving a β-blocker.
- Contraindications: severe reactive airway disease, conduction system disease of the heart, angina due to coronary vasospasm, Raynaud phenomenon, severe occlusive peripheral vascular disease, pheochromocytoma (before α-blockade), and depression.
- β-Blockers (especially noncardioselective) may mask hypoglycemia and delay recovery from it, so they should be prescribed carefully for diabetics who take insulin or oral hypoglycemic drugs.
- Side effects: cold extremities, fatigue, impaired exercise tolerance, bronchospasm, dyslipidemia, insomnia, nasal congestion, and possibly depression.

Labetalol—Labetalol is the combination of a nonselective β-blocker and a postsynaptic α₁-receptor blocker. The ratio of α- to β-blocking action is 1:4. The drug lowers blood pressure primarily by decreasing peripheral vascular resistance. Labetalol can be given intravenously to treat hypertensive crisis. All the precautions applying to β-blockers apply to this drug. Labetalol can cause liver dysfunction and an increase in antinuclear antibody and antimitochondrial antibody titers. Common side effects are orthostatic hypotension and scalp itching. Labetalol may interfere with metanephrine and catecholamine assays, resulting in a false-positive test for pheochromocytoma.

- Labetalol can be given intravenously for hypertensive crisis.
- All precautions applying to β-blockers apply to labetalol.
- Labetalol can cause an increase in liver enzymes and in antinuclear and antimitochondrial antibody titers.
- Common side effects: orthostatic hypotension and scalp itching.
- Labetalol may result in a false-positive test for pheochromocytoma.

Carvedilol—Carvedilol is a weak β₁-selective blocker with α₁-blocking activity. This drug reduces the risk of death and hospitalization in persons with heart failure. It is also effective in the treatment of angina. Because the drug is mainly metabolized in the liver, reductions in dose are required in states of hepatic insufficiency. No dose adjustments are required in renal insufficiency.

- Carvedilol is beneficial in heart failure.

Centrally Acting α₂ₐ Agonists
These drugs stimulate central α receptors that exert an inhibitory effect on sympathetic outflow. Blood pressure is reduced because of a decrease in cardiac output and peripheral vascular resistance. Norepinephrine and renin levels decrease. Fluid retention occurs; thus, these agents should be used in combination with diuretics. Side effects common to all these agents are orthostatic hypotension, sedation, bradycardia, and dry mouth. Sudden discontinuation of any of these agents can cause a sudden rebound rise in blood pressure. This effect is augmented in the presence of concomitant β-blocker therapy.

- Common side effects of all centrally acting α₂ₐ agonists are sedation, dry mouth, bradycardia, and withdrawal hypertension.

Methyldopa—Daily doses should not exceed 3 g. Side effects include hepatitis, fever, positive Coombs test, hemolytic anemia, leukopenia, thrombocytopenia, and increased antinuclear antibody titers. Hemoglobin and liver enzymes should be checked periodically. Methyldopa potentiates lithium and haloperidol toxicity, increases prolactin levels with consequent breast stimulation, and interferes with metanephrine assays. Because newer centrally acting agents are safer, this drug should not be used often. Currently, a major use for this drug is in the treatment of hypertension in pregnancy, for which its safety has been established.

- An important indication for methyldopa is hypertension in pregnancy.
- Methyldopa side effects: hepatitis, fever, positive Coombs test, hemolytic anemia, leukopenia, thrombocytopenia, and antinuclear antibody positivity.
- It potentiates lithium and haloperidol toxicity and increases prolactin levels.

Clonidine—In contrast to methyldopa, clonidine is not associated with liver toxicity or hematologic abnormalities. Because of the possibility of rebound hypertension with sudden discontinuation, as with all central agents, the use of clonidine should be tapered and discontinued preoperatively if oral medications will not be allowed for several days postoperatively. Alternatively, with clonidine, conversion preoperatively to the transdermal form of the drug can be considered. The transdermal formulation takes 48 hours for therapeutic efficacy. Comorbid conditions that may benefit from clonidine include restless legs, menopausal hot flashes, and diabetic diarrhea.

- Clonidine is not associated with liver toxicity or hematologic abnormalities.

- An alternative to tapering the drug preoperatively is to switch to the transdermal form.
- Clonidine may help restless legs, menopausal hot flashes, and diabetic diarrhea.

Guanabenz—Guanabenz is similar in action to clonidine and methyldopa. It may also have weak peripheral neuronal blocking properties. Similar to clonidine and unlike methyldopa, it is not associated with liver toxicity or hematologic abnormalities. Also, unlike other central agents, guanabenz does not cause fluid retention.

- Guanabenz is not associated with liver toxicity or hematologic abnormalities.
- It is the only central α-agonist that does not cause fluid retention.

Guanfacine—Guanfacine, a newer clonidine-like drug, can be given once daily and may have fewer central nervous system side effects. Similar to guanabenz and clonidine, it is not associated with liver toxicity or a positive Coombs test.

- Guanfacine is not associated with liver toxicity or hematologic abnormalities.

Traditional Vasodilators

The traditional vasodilators are usually given as a third agent in combination with a diuretic and an adrenergic inhibitor to persons with severe or resistant hypertension. They are used most properly only in combination with a diuretic and an adrenergic inhibitor because they cause stimulation of the sympathetic nervous system (increase in heart rate and cardiac output) and renin release (fluid retention).

Hydralazine

Hydralazine decreases blood pressure by directly dilating arterioles. The daily dose should not exceed 200 mg. Its plasma half-life is prolonged in renal insufficiency. It can be used safely in pregnancy and is efficacious when used in combination with nitrates for congestive heart failure. Side effects include headache, palpitations, tachycardia, fluid retention, and a lupus-like syndrome (arthralgias, splenomegaly, and pleural or pericardial effusions). In addition, the drug can cause peripheral cytopenias (anemia, leukopenia, and thrombocytopenia), and peripheral neuropathy from pyridoxine deficiency. The liver enzyme *N*-acetyltransferase inactivates the drug. The level of this enzyme is genetically determined and persons are characterized as being "rapid acetylators" (high levels of the enzyme) or "slow acetylators" (low levels of the enzyme). Rapid acetylators require larger doses of the drug for an effect. Lupus-like syndrome is more common in slow acetylators. Hydralazine should not be used in the setting of recent cerebral hemorrhage, acute myocardial infarction, or a dissecting aortic aneurysm because of its tendency to increase cardiac output and cerebral blood flow.

- Hydralazine causes direct dilatation of arterioles.
- The daily dose should not exceed 200 mg.
- Side effects: headache, palpitations, tachycardia, fluid retention, lupus-like syndrome, cytopenias, and peripheral neuropathy.

- It can be used safely in pregnancy and in combination with nitrates for congestive heart failure.
- Do not use in the setting of recent cerebral hemorrhage, acute myocardial infarction, or dissecting aortic aneurysm.

Minoxidil

Minoxidil is a potent, direct vasodilator used to treat severe hypertension with or without renal insufficiency. Its side effects include substantial volume expansion with edema, hirsutism, and pericardial effusion. Often, high doses of both a loop diuretic and an adrenergic inhibitor are required to control reactive sympathetic stimulation and fluid retention.

- Minoxidil is a more potent vasodilator than hydralazine.
- Side effects: volume expansion with edema, hirsutism, and pericardial effusion.

Angiotensin-Converting Enzyme Inhibitors

ACEIs (eg, benazepril, captopril, enalapril, fosinopril, lisinopril, moexipril, perindopril, quinapril, ramipril, and trandolapril) decrease blood pressure by inhibiting the enzyme that converts angiotensin I to angiotensin II (angiotensin-converting enzyme [ACE]) and that causes the breakdown of bradykinin (kininase II). Pressor effects of angiotensin II that are reduced include direct vasoconstriction, stimulation of the sympathetic nervous system, thirst, renal sodium reabsorption, and antidiuretic hormone and aldosterone secretion. ACEIs also enhance the activity of bradykinin, a vasodilator. The effects of angiotensin II to promote cardiac and vascular smooth muscle hypertrophy are also reduced. Although they are vasodilators, ACEIs do not induce reactive fluid retention or sympathetic stimulation.

ACEIs are appropriate initial therapy for hypertension, and they work well in combination with other antihypertensive agents, particularly diuretics. In large group studies, ACEIs have been most effective in younger persons and whites. ACEIs retard progression of nephropathy in type 1 diabetes mellitus (captopril) and prevent the development of congestive heart failure and recurrent myocardial infarction in persons who have had an initial myocardial infarction complicated by reduced left ventricular function (eg, captopril, lisinopril, ramipril, and trandolapril). ACEIs are important in the treatment of established congestive heart failure (eg, captopril, enalapril, fosinopril, lisinopril, quinapril, ramipril, and trandolapril) and may induce regression of left ventricular hypertrophy more effectively than other antihypertensive agents. ACEIs are antiproteinuric and slow the progression of nondiabetic, proteinuric renal disease in both whites and African Americans. They may decrease the risk of nephropathy in patients who have type 2 diabetes mellitus with microalbuminuria. Also, they decrease the risk of death, myocardial infarction, and stroke in high-risk persons (ie, persons with known coronary artery disease, previous stroke, peripheral vascular disease, or diabetes with at least 1 additional risk factor) (eg, ramipril). The combination of an ACEI and a diuretic (eg, indapemide with perindopril) may prevent recurrent stroke. ACEIs are useful in the treatment of hypertensive crisis associated with scleroderma.

ACEIs increase insulin sensitivity and may lessen the risk of diabetes developing. Their use can be associated with hypoglycemia in diabetic patients. Captopril is the only sulfhydryl-containing ACEI. Unique side effects presumed to be due to the sulfhydryl group in captopril are skin rash, loss of taste, proteinuria with membranous glomerulonephropathy, and leukopenia. Leukopenia is more likely to occur in the presence of collagen vascular disease and renal insufficiency. Nonsulfhydryl-containing ACEIs are benazepril, enalapril, fosinopril, lisinopril, moexipril, perindopril, quinapril, ramipril, and trandolapril.

The side effects shared by all ACEIs are orthostatic hypotension (most common with concomitant diuretic therapy), hyperkalemia (most common with renal insufficiency or diabetes or with concomitant use of potassium-sparing diuretics, nonsteroidal anti-inflammatory drugs, β-blockers, or potassium supplements), cough (due to increased bradykinin levels; more common in women), bronchospasm, angioedema (more common in African Americans), and loss of renal function. Minor increases in creatinine are common after initiation of ACEI therapy. In persons with bilateral renal artery stenosis, ACEIs can cause acute renal failure because of disruption of autoregulation of glomerular filtration in the presence of severe renal ischemia. If serum creatinine increases by 20% or more from baseline with ACEI therapy, evaluation for bilateral renal artery stenosis should be considered. If creatinine increases by 30% or more, the drug should be stopped. Anaphylactic reactions can occur in patients during dialysis or apheresis.

All ACEIs except captopril and lisinopril are prodrugs and require conversion in the liver to the active form. This is only of concern in advanced liver disease. The kidneys eliminate all ACEIs except fosinopril and trandolapril, which have a balanced renal and hepatic elimination, with increased hepatic elimination in the setting of renal dysfunction. ACEIs differ in their ability to inhibit noncirculating ACE present in tissues (tissue ACE) and in lipophilicity, but these differences are of uncertain clinical significance. Drugs that inhibit tissue ACE include quinapril, benazapril, ramipril, perindopril, and trandolapril. The most lipophilic ACEIs are captopril, ramipril, fosinopril, trandolapril, and quinapril.

ACEIs are contraindicated in pregnancy because they can cause fetal toxicity. Fetal anomalies can occur during the first trimester of pregnancy; therefore, ACEIs should be generally avoided in sexually active women unless there is a concomitant medical condition that argues strongly for their use. If ACEIs are used, their use should be discontinued at the first sign of pregnancy.

- ACEIs inhibit the enzyme that converts angiotensin I to angiotensin II and is responsible for the metabolism of bradykinin.
- ACEIs are appropriate initial therapy for hypertension.
- ACEIs retard progression of nephropathy in patients with type 1 diabetes.
- ACEIs are antiproteinuric and slow the progression of nondiabetic proteinuric renal disease.
- ACEIs are important in the treatment of congestive heart failure.
- ACEIs prevent recurrent myocardial infarction and the development of congestive heart failure in persons who have had a myocardial infarction complicated by reduced left ventricular function.
- ACEIs may lessen the risk of death, myocardial infarction, and stroke in persons with known atherosclerotic vascular disease or diabetes and at least 1 additional risk factor.

- The combination of an ACEI and a diuretic may prevent recurrent stroke.
- Side effects of captopril: skin rash, loss of taste, proteinuria with membranous glomerulonephropathy, and leukopenia.
- Side effects of all ACEIs: orthostatic hypotension, hyperkalemia, cough, angioedema, and loss of renal function.
- ACEIs are contraindicated in pregnancy.

Angiotensin II Receptor Blockers

ARBs (eg, candesartan, eprosartan, irbesartan, losartan, olmesartan, telmisartan, and valsartan) lower blood pressure by blocking the cell surface receptors (AT_1) that angiotensin II interacts with to produce all its known pressor effects. Similar to ACEIs, ARBs increase plasma renin activity (PRA), but unlike ACEIs, ARBs also increase (not decrease) angiotensin II levels and ARBs do not increase bradykinin levels. Candesartan and olmesartan are prodrugs. Insurmountable antagonists of the AT_1 receptor are candesartan, irbesartan, olmesartan, telmisartan, and valsartan. The clinical importance of insurmountable antagonism of the receptor is uncertain.

ARBs are appropriate initial therapy for hypertension, and in large group studies, they have been most effective in younger persons and whites. ARBs are generally effective in the same clinical settings as ACEIs; thus, they are primarily alternatives to ACEIs when these agents are indicated but not tolerated. ARBs are antiproteinuric and have been shown to lessen the progression of nephropathy associated with type 2 diabetes mellitus (eg, losartan and irbesartan). The combination of ACEI and ARB therapy may have an additive antiproteinuric effect, but the role of combination therapy in retarding progression of renal disease is uncertain. Unlike with ACEIs, special benefits with ARBs after myocardial infarction or in congestive heart failure have not been established, with 2 exceptions: valsartan, which is indicated as an alternative drug for congestive heart failure in the presence of ACEI intolerance, and candesartan, which reduces heart failure mortality. ARBs (eg, losartan) decrease the risk of stroke in hypertensive persons with left ventricular hypertrophy.

The most common side effect of ARBs is dizziness. Diuretics or salt and volume depletion can potentiate their hypotensive effect. Similar to ACEIs, ARBs can cause fetal toxicity and should be avoided in pregnancy. They also can precipitate acute renal failure in persons with bilateral renal artery stenosis and can cause angioedema. In general, persons who experience angioedema with an ACEI should not be given an ARB. Unlike ACEIs, ARBs do not cause cough (cough may be due to high levels of bradykinin), and the risk of hyperkalemia may be less than with ACEIs. Losartan is the only ARB that is uricosuric. These drugs have no adverse effect on plasma lipids or glucose.

- ARBs inhibit the actions of angiotensin II by blocking its cell surface receptors.
- The major role for ARBs: a substitute for an ACEI when an ACEI is indicated but not tolerated.
- Side effects of ARBs: dizziness, hyperkalemia, acute renal failure, angioedema.
- ARBs do not cause cough but can cause angioedema.
- Avoid ARBs in pregnancy because of fetal toxicity.

Direct Renin Inhibitors

Aliskiren is the first and only Food and Drug Administration (FDA)-approved hypertension drug that acts by directly inhibiting renin. Consequently, plasma renin activity is reduced with concomitant reductions in circulating levels of both angiotensin I and angiotensin II. The exact role of this agent in the treatment of hypertension remains to be determined. There is limited experience with its use in cardiac or renal disease. Similar to ACEIs and ARBs, this drug is contraindicated in pregnancy, can cause angioedema, and is associated with increased risks of postural hypotension and hyperkalemia. Furosemide effectiveness is reduced with concomitant aliskiren therapy. A high-fat meal decreases the bioavailability of the drug. The most common side effect is diarrhea. Its use has been associated with skin rash, cough, and elevated creatine kinase levels.

- Aliskiren is a direct renin inhibitor; it reduces circulating levels of plasma renin activity and of both angiotensin I and II.
- The exact role of aliskiren in the treatment of hypertension is yet to be determined.
- Similar to ACEIs and ARBs, aliskiren is contraindicated in pregnancy and can be associated with angioedema and hyperkalemia.
- The most common side effect is diarrhea.

Calcium Channel Blockers

CCBs block the influx of calcium into vascular smooth muscle cells, causing vasodilation. They are divided into dihydropyridines (amlodipine, felodipine, isradipine, nicardipine, nifedipine, nisoldipine, and nitrendipine), benzothiazepines (diltiazem), and phenylalkylamines (verapamil). Only long-acting forms are approved for use in hypertension. The short-acting forms should not be used. Verapamil (and, to a lesser extent, diltiazem) slows the heart rate, depresses cardiac contractility, and inhibits cardiac atrioventricular nodal conduction. The dihydropyridines have less effect on cardiac conduction and heart contractility. CCBs are appropriate for initial therapy of hypertension.

Earlier studies suggested an increase in coronary heart disease events with the use of dihydropyridine CCBs, but more recent studies do not support this concern. In large group studies, CCBs have been most effective in older persons (especially with isolated systolic hypertension) and African Americans. They should be considered for persons with concomitant ischemic heart disease and chronic, stable angina (amlodipine, nicardipine, nifedipine, diltiazem, and verapamil); variant angina due to coronary vasospasm (amlodipine, nifedipine, and diltiazem); supraventricular arrhythmias (verapamil and diltiazem); Raynaud phenomenon (nifedipine); migraine headaches (verapamil); and esophageal spasm. Verapamil decreases the risk of a subsequent myocardial infarction if the first one was not associated with pulmonary congestion. Diltiazem decreases the risk of a subsequent myocardial infarction after a non–Q-wave infarction. The long-term use of nifedipine delays the need for valve replacement in chronic aortic insufficiency and may lower pressure in primary pulmonary hypertension. Dihydropyridine CCBs (eg, nitrendipine) lessen the risk of stroke in older persons with isolated systolic hypertension. Nondihydropyridines reduce proteinuria and have additive effects when used with ACEIs or ARBs. CCBs are helpful in cyclosporine-induced hypertension.

Use of all CCBs should be avoided in the setting of acute myocardial infarction. Verapamil and diltiazem should be avoided in the presence of cardiac conduction system disease (sick sinus syndrome and second degree or greater heart block) or when the left ventricular ejection fraction is less than 40%. All CCBs should be avoided in symptomatic heart failure, although dihydropyridine CCBs can be used safely in asymptomatic persons who require additional treatment to control blood pressure or angina. Verapamil in combination with β-blockers can lead to complete heart block and profound cardiodepression. Because it decreases the renal and nonrenal elimination of digoxin, verapamil increases the risk of digoxin toxicity. Quinidine and verapamil in combination can cause serious hypotension in persons with idiopathic hypertrophic subaortic stenosis.

- CCBs are direct vasodilators.
- Verapamil and diltiazem should not be used in sick sinus syndrome or heart block of second degree or greater.
- Avoid using verapamil in combination with β-blockers.
- Avoid verapamil and diltiazem if the left ventricular ejection fraction is <40%.
- Verapamil increases the risk of digoxin toxicity.
- All CCBs should be avoided in persons with symptomatic heart failure.

All CCBs can increase liver enzymes and cause hepatic necrosis. The most common side effect of verapamil is constipation, and the most serious side effect is heart block. Most of the side effects associated with dihydropyridine CCBs are related to peripheral vasodilation. These include headache, tachycardia, flushing, and dependent edema. The dependent edema associated with CCBs is not improved with diuretics but may be lessened by ACEIs. Gingival hyperplasia most commonly occurs with dihydropyridines but can occur with all CCBs. All CCBs can worsen esophageal reflux. Rarely, serious cutaneous eruptions can occur with CCBs. Cimetidine and other drugs that decrease blood flow to the liver may increase the biologic effects of CCBs. CCBs increase cyclosporine blood levels. Unlike other antihypertensive agents, nonsteroidal anti-inflammatory drugs do not interfere with the blood pressure–lowering effect of CCBs and a high-sodium diet may increase the blood pressure–lowering effect. The liver metabolizes all CCBs, and dose adjustments may be necessary if liver disease is present. CCBs can be used safely in renal insufficiency.

- The most common side effect of verapamil: constipation.
- The most serious side effect of verapamil: heart block.
- Common side effects: headache, tachycardia, flushing, and edema.
- CCBs can cause gingival hyperplasia.
- CCBs increase cyclosporine blood levels.
- CCBs can increase liver enzymes and cause hepatic necrosis.
- Nonsteroidal anti-inflammatory drugs and a high-salt diet do not lessen the blood pressure–lowering effect of CCBs.
- All CCBs are metabolized in the liver, so dose adjustments are necessary if liver disease is present.

Follow-up

After initiation of drug therapy, follow-up visits should be scheduled at monthly intervals until treatment goals are attained. For high-risk persons with stage 2 hypertension, follow-up intervals should be 1 to 2 weeks. If the first chosen drug fails to control blood pressure, but a response is observed and the drug is well tolerated, the dose can be increased or a second drug added. If no response is observed or severe side effects occur, the drug should be replaced with one from a different class. Serum creatinine and potassium levels should be checked within 1 to 2 weeks after initiation of ACEI or ARB therapy. Adverse metabolic effects of diuretics (ie, adverse effects on sodium, potassium, uric acid, glucose, cholesterol, and triglyceride levels) should be assessed after 1 month of therapy. When the blood pressure goal is achieved, follow-up visits should be considered at intervals of 3 to 6 months. Other comorbidities (eg, diabetes, coronary artery disease, heart failure, and renal disease) may influence the frequency of follow-up visits and laboratory tests. In addition to blood pressure control, other cardiovascular risk factors should be monitored and treatment initiated to achieve the appropriate goals. After blood pressure is controlled, the addition of low-dose aspirin (81 mg daily) should be considered because its use has been shown to lessen cardiovascular disease events in persons with controlled hypertension. In persons with inadequately controlled hypertension, aspirin use is associated with increased risk of hemorrhagic stroke.

Secondary Hypertension

Known secondary forms of hypertension account for approximately 10% of all cases of hypertension. Secondary forms are often considered in patients who have clinical features that are inconsistent with essential hypertension, as discussed earlier. Common general clinical clues are an unusual age at onset (younger or older than for essential hypertension), a sudden, unexplained increase in blood pressure from a previous state of control, or primary or acquired resistance to treatment. Common secondary causes include drugs (Table 14-5), increasing obesity, and obstructive sleep apnea. The traditional secondary causes are reviewed here. The clinical clues suggestive of secondary hypertension should be recognized, and when secondary hypertension is suspected, consultation with a subspecialist should be considered.

Renovascular Hypertension

Renovascular hypertension is one of the most common forms of potentially curable secondary hypertension. It occurs in 1% to 3% of the general hypertensive population, in 10% of persons with resistant hypertension, and in up to 30% of those with hypertensive crisis. It is less common in African Americans than in Caucasians. *Critical stenosis* of a renal artery (ie, ≥70% luminal narrowing) increases renin production from the ischemic kidney (Figure 14-1). Renin acts on circulating renin substrate (angiotensinogen) to produce angiotensin I, which is converted to angiotensin II (a potent vasoconstrictor) by angiotensin-converting enzyme in the lung and other tissues. In addition to vasoconstriction, angiotensin II directly increases renal sodium reabsorption and also stimulates aldosterone production, resulting in extracellular volume expansion. Angiotensin II also stimulates the sympathetic nervous system, contributing further to increased vascular resistance, and stimulates thirst and the release of vasopressin, contributing further to increased extracellular volume.

In unilateral disease, the nonischemic kidney is subjected to increased perfusion, resulting in higher sodium excretion and suppression of renin release. These effects lessen the degree of hypertension but perpetuate underperfusion of the ischemic kidney, which, in turn, perpetuates excess renin production. In bilateral disease, initial increases in renin cause extracellular volume expansion and volume-dependent hypertension, which persists because there is no contralateral normal kidney to excrete more sodium. In persons with bilateral disease, the hypertension is volume dependent but becomes renin dependent with extracellular volume depletion.

* Renovascular disease is the most common form of potentially curable secondary hypertension.
* Renal artery stenosis activates the renin-angiotensin system.
* Angiotensin II is a potent vasoconstrictor; it increases renal sodium reabsorption directly and through stimulation of aldosterone production, and also increases sympathetic nervous system activity, thirst, and vasopressin release.
* Renovascular hypertension is due to extracellular volume expansion and increased peripheral vascular resistance.
* Unilateral disease is associated with renin-dependent hypertension, whereas bilateral disease is associated with volume-dependent hypertension.

Correcting renal ischemia eliminates the stimulus for excess renin release and can cure or lessen hypertension. In unilateral renal artery stenosis, prolonged hypertension eventually causes nephrosclerosis in the nonischemic kidney (in combination with other cardiovascular risk factors) or ischemic injury to the involved kidney. If either occurs, relieving renal arterial stenosis may not cure hypertension. The longer the duration of hypertension before diagnosis, the greater the likelihood of these untoward renal outcomes and the less the likelihood of cure of hypertension with intervention.

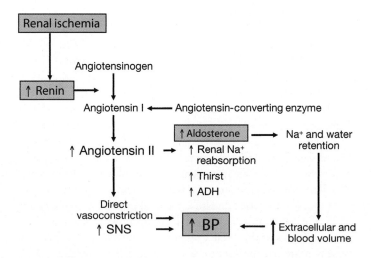

Figure 14-1. Stimulation of the Renin-Angiotensin-Aldosterone Axis in Renovascular Hypertension. ADH indicates vasopressin; BP, blood pressure; Na, sodium; SNS, sympathetic nervous system activity.

- Correcting renal ischemia eliminates excess renin release.
- The longer the duration of hypertension before diagnosis, the less likely that correction of renal ischemia will be beneficial.

Fibromuscular disease is the most common cause of renovascular hypertension in younger persons, especially women between 15 and 50 years old. Its cause remains unknown. It is more common in first-degree relatives of persons with the disease, but most cases are sporadic. It accounts for 15% of renovascular hypertension in the population. Lesions usually affect the middle and distal portions of the main renal vessels, often extending into branches. The disease more commonly affects the right renal artery and is bilateral in 35% of cases. Three major subtypes have been defined on the basis of the portion of the arterial wall involved: 1) intimal fibroplasia (1%-2% of cases), 2) medial fibromuscular dysplasia (95% of cases), and 3) periadventitial fibrosis (1%-2% of cases). Medial fibromuscular dysplasia, the most common subtype in adults, has a classic string-of-beads appearance (representing aneurysmal dilatations associated with intravascular webs) on angiography (Figure 14-2) and progresses in 30% of cases. Medial fibromuscular dysplasia may also occur in other vessels branching off the aorta (eg, carotid and celiac arteries) and rarely in other vessels (eg, vertebral, mesenteric, or coronary arteries). Carotid or vertebral artery involvement may be associated with intracranial aneurysms. The rare subtypes of intimal fibroplasia and periadventitial fibrosis can progress rapidly to severe stenoses. Dissection and thrombosis can occur and are seen more commonly with the rare subtypes. Occlusion of the renal artery is rare.

- Fibromuscular disease is the most common cause of renovascular hypertension in younger persons, especially women of child-bearing age.
- Medial fibromuscular dysplasia is the most common subtype and has a string-of-beads appearance on angiography.
- Dissection and thrombosis of a renal artery are complications most commonly seen with rare subtypes.
- Renal artery occlusion is rare.

Atheromatous disease is the most common cause of renovascular hypertension in middle-aged or older persons. It accounts for 85% of renovascular hypertension in the population and is more common in men than in women. The lesions usually are in the proximal third of the renal artery, often near or at the orifice (Figure 14-3). In many instances, renal artery obstruction is due to extension of aortic atheromatous disease across the orifice of the artery. Although atheromatous renal artery disease is common in older persons with hypertension (especially in diabetics or persons with evidence of atherosclerosis in other vascular beds), it causes or aggravates hypertension less often. The disease is bilateral in 30% of cases, and in 35% of cases it progresses even if blood pressure is controlled. Atherosclerosis of the renal artery can progress to occlusion of the vessel. Progressive disease can cause end-stage renal disease.

- Atheromatous disease is the most common cause of renovascular hypertension in middle-aged or older persons.

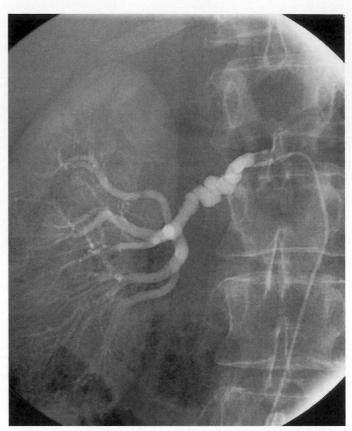

Figure 14-2. Fibromuscular Renal Vascular Disease (Medial Fibromuscular Dysplasia).

- The disease is bilateral in 30% of cases and progressive in 35%.
- It can cause renal artery occlusion.

Clues suggesting renovascular hypertension include lack of a family history of hypertension, onset of hypertension before age 30 (consider fibromuscular dysplasia, especially in a woman), onset of hypertension after age 50 (consider atherosclerotic renovascular disease, especially in a smoker or a person with coronary or peripheral arterial disease), presentation with accelerated or malignant hypertension, or sudden worsening of preexisting hypertension in a middle-aged or older person (renovascular hypertension superimposed on essential hypertension). Persons with cardiovascular risk factors (eg, tobacco use, hyperlipidemia, or diabetes) are at increased risk of atherosclerotic renal artery stenosis. The most important physical finding is an abdominal bruit, especially a high-pitched systolic-diastolic bruit in the upper abdomen or flank. However, 50% of persons with renovascular hypertension do not have this finding. Other physical clues are severe retinopathy of accelerated or malignant hypertension (eg, hemorrhages, exudates, and papilledema) or evidence of atherosclerotic occlusive disease in other vascular beds (atherosclerotic renal artery stenosis of >50% is observed in up to 20% of persons with coronary artery disease and in up to 50% of persons with peripheral arterial disease). Laboratory abnormalities are hypokalemia (due to secondary aldosteronism), an increased serum creatinine level,

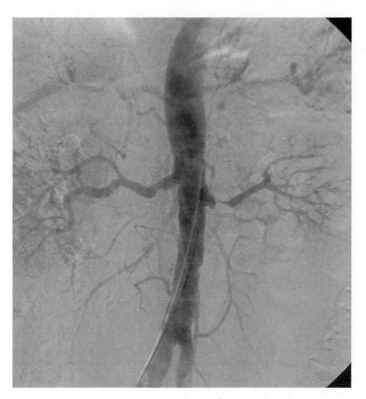

Figure 14-3. Atherosclerotic Renovascular Disease.

proteinuria (rarely in the nephrotic range), and a small kidney seen on an imaging study.

* For hypertension before age 30, especially in a woman, consider fibromuscular dysplasia.
* For hypertension after age 50, especially in a smoker or a person with coronary or peripheral arterial disease, consider atherosclerotic renovascular disease.
* The most important physical finding is an abdominal bruit; however, it is present in only 50% of cases.
* Laboratory abnormalities: hypokalemia, increased serum creatinine, proteinuria, and a small kidney seen on an imaging study.

Underlying bilateral renal artery stenosis may be indicated by an acute decline in renal function (≥20% increase in serum creatinine) either after the initiation of therapy with an ACEI or an ARB or after a drug-induced, sudden decrease in blood pressure. Other signs in patients presenting with bilateral renal artery stenosis (ie, ischemic nephropathy) include the sudden development of pulmonary edema accompanied by severe hypertension (ie, flash pulmonary edema), frequent episodes of symptomatic congestive heart failure accompanied by increases in blood pressure, or a subacute decline in renal function with or without worsening hypertension.

Patients with atheroembolic renal disease may also present with a sudden onset or worsening of hypertension and a subacute decline in renal function. Historical clues (eg, occurrence after angiography or vascular surgery), physical findings (eg, distal livedo reticularis and peripheral emboli), and laboratory abnormalities (eg, increased

erythrocyte sedimentation rate, anemia, hematuria, eosinophilia, and eosinophiluria) help identify this disorder.

* A sudden decline in renal function with the use of an ACEI or an ARB or an episode of unexplained pulmonary edema may indicate bilateral renal artery disease.
* The sudden onset or worsening of hypertension accompanied by a subacute decline in renal function may also be due to atheroembolic renal disease (especially if onset is after an angiogram or vascular surgery).

In young persons who have hypertension (even if not severe) of short duration and suggestive clinical features, evaluation for renovascular disease is indicated. Renal artery stenosis in these persons can be identified and corrected with a low risk of morbidity and mortality and a high probability of cure. Older persons should be evaluated for renovascular hypertension on a selective basis. In general, selection should be restricted to persons who have suggestive clinical features and blood pressure that cannot be controlled medically or who have an unexplained, observed decline in renal function or a cardiorenal syndrome (eg, recurrent flash pulmonary edema or resistant heart failure) and who are considered reasonable risks for (and are willing to undergo) interventional therapy.

* In young persons with hypertension of short duration, evaluate for renovascular disease.
* Older persons should be evaluated for renovascular hypertension on a selective basis.

Screening Tests

Although several tests are available to screen for renal artery stenosis, duplex renal ultrasonography, magnetic resonance angiography, and spiral computed tomographic (CT) angiography are considered the initial screening tests of choice. The major concern with all available screening tests is inadequate sensitivity leading to a missed opportunity to identify a correctable cause of hypertension.

Duplex Ultrasonography

Duplex ultrasonography is noninvasive and does not use contrast media. Its usefulness extends to persons who have renal insufficiency or a history of contrast allergy. Performance of the test does not require discontinuation of any antihypertensive drug. It identifies increases in blood flow velocity that occur with luminal narrowing of a renal artery. Criteria for a positive test are 1) a ratio of peak flow velocity in the involved renal artery to peak flow velocity in the aorta of more than 3.5 and 2) renal artery peak systolic flow of 180 cm/s or more. The resistive index in segmental vessels is a measure of small-vessel disease in the kidney and is calculated as

$$1 - (\text{end-diastolic velocity/peak systolic velocity}) \times 100$$

The resistive index is used to identify persons more (ie, a low resistive index) or less (ie, a high resistive index [>80]) likely to benefit from interventional therapy. Duplex ultrasonography also provides information on kidney size, screens for obstructive uropathy and aortic aneurysm, and identifies bilateral renal artery stenosis. Overlying bowel gas or other technical problems limit the complete study of both renal arteries in up to 50% of cases. Often, accessory or branch vessel disease is not identified. The sensitivity and specificity are 75% to 80%.

- Consider duplex ultrasonography in persons with renal insufficiency or a history of contrast allergy.
- Sensitivity and specificity are 75% to 80%.
- The resistive index can be used to determine the likelihood of benefit from intervention.
- Duplex ultrasonography also measures renal size and screens for obstructive uropathy and aortic aneurysm.
- In up to 50% of persons, 1 or both renal arteries cannot be studied adequately.
- Accessory or branch vessel disease may not be identified.

Magnetic Resonance Angiography

Magnetic resonance angiography (MRA) visualizes the main renal arteries without use of a radiocontrast agent or exposure to radiation. Its usefulness extends to persons with a history of radiocontrast allergy. Also, it is a reasonable choice for persons with a high likelihood of atherosclerotic renal artery disease but who have concomitant severe, diffuse atherosclerosis and, thus, are at high risk of atheroembolization with angiography.

MRA often uses gadolinium to enhance visualization of the renal circulation. Exposure to gadolinium from magnetic resonance imaging in patients with chronic kidney disease has been linked to the development of a debilitating and irreversible disease, *nephrogenic systemic fibrosis*, that is characterized by fibrosis of the skin, multiple organs (eg, liver, heart, lungs, and diaphragm), and skeletal muscle. At present, it is recommended not to use gadolinium in patients with an estimated GFR of less than 30 mL/min. MRA can be performed without gadolinium, but this results in reduced test performance.

Field limitations may decrease the ability to see lesions in the distal main renal arteries or lesions in branch vessels (common sites of fibromuscular disease). Accessory renal arteries may not be identified, the degree of arterial stenosis may be overestimated, and persons prone to claustrophobia may not tolerate being placed in the magnetic resonance equipment. Renal stents cause imaging artifacts, and persons with cardiac pacemakers, metallic artificial cardiac valves, or cerebral artery aneurysm clips cannot be imaged. Sensitivity is 80% to 90% (less for fibromuscular dysplasia), and specificity is 90%. This is an expensive screening test.

- MRA visualizes the renal arteries without a radiocontrast agent or radiation exposure.
- It is a good choice for persons with radiocontrast allergy.
- It is not a good test if fibromuscular disease is the concern.
- Renal stents cause imaging artifacts.
- Patients may feel claustrophobic.
- MRA cannot be used in persons with cardiac pacemakers or other metallic implants.
- Magnetic resonance imaging with gadolinium should not be used if the GFR is <30 mL/min.
- It is expensive.

Spiral Computed Tomographic Angiography

Spiral CT angiography offers excellent 3-dimensional images but requires a considerable amount of radiocontrast agent and patient cooperation. This is an option for persons with normal renal function who do not have a contrast allergy and in whom MRA is contraindicated. Renal stents do not cause imaging artifacts. Sensitivity and specificity are similar to those for MRA. It may be better than MRA for identification of fibromuscular disease, but it may miss lesions in segmental renal vessels. It is an excellent choice to assess for renal artery dissection. This is also an expensive test.

- Spiral CT angiography requires a considerable amount of radiocontrast agent.
- Consider spiral CT angiography for persons with normal renal function in whom MRA is contraindicated.
- It may be superior to MRA for identification of fibromuscular disease.

Other noninvasive tests are available to screen for renal artery stenosis; however, they are used less often because the test characteristics are inferior compared with those of duplex ultrasonography, MRA, and spiral CT angiography.

Historically, the intravenous pyelogram (IVP) was the mainstay screening test for renovascular hypertension. For screening, radiographs that are taken at 1-minute intervals for the first 5 minutes after injection of contrast medium are used to identify a delay in the appearance of contrast medium in the renal collecting system on the side of a renal artery stenosis. This is referred to as a *hypertensive IVP*. Characteristic findings on a hypertensive IVP suggesting renal artery stenosis are 1) unilateral reduction in renal size (≥1.5-cm decrease in pole-to-pole diameter of the smaller kidney); 2) delayed appearance of contrast medium in the collecting system of the ischemic kidney; 3) hyperconcentration of contrast medium in the ischemic kidney; 4) ureteral scalloping by collateral vessels; and 5) cortical thinning or irregularity. Sensitivity is 70% to 75%, and specificity is 85%.

Captopril Radionuclide Renal Scan

Some still consider the captopril radionuclide renal scan to be a useful screening test. However, recent reviews suggest a lower test sensitivity than was reported earlier. Currently, sensitivity is estimated at 75% and specificity at 85%. Pretest treatment of patients with captopril (25-50 mg given 1 hour before isotope injection) increases the sensitivity of the scan compared with that of standard renography. The rationale is that glomerular filtration in an ischemic kidney depends on the vasoconstricting effect of angiotensin II on the efferent arteriole of the nephron to maintain effective transglomerular filtration pressure. Treatment with an ACEI causes efferent arteriolar dilatation, with loss of filtration pressure in the nephron. This causes a decline of glomerular filtration in the ischemic kidney, with less of an effect on renal blood flow. These changes are identified with the scanning technique. The radionuclides used most commonly are iodine 131 orthoiodohippuric acid (OIH) and Tc-99m mercaptoacetyltriglycine (MAG3), which are markers for renal blood flow (they are excreted primarily by renal tubular secretion), and Tc-99m diethylenetriamine pentaacetic acid (DPTA), which is a marker for glomerular filtration rate (it is excreted primarily by glomerular filtration). Criteria for a positive test with DPTA are time to peak activity in the kidney of 11 minutes or more and a ratio of the glomerular filtration rate between the kidneys of 1.5 or more. The criterion for a positive test with OIH or MAG3 is residual cortical activity at 20 minutes of 30% or more of peak activity. The renal scan is safe for persons with a history of contrast allergy. The interpretive value is reduced by renal insufficiency (creatinine >2.0 mg/dL) or by bilateral or branch renal artery disease. Urinary outflow obstruction may mimic renal artery stenosis.

- Some consider the captopril radionuclide renal scan a useful screening test.
- Sensitivity is 75%, and specificity is 85%.
- It is safe for persons with a history of contrast allergy.
- It is ineffective in renal insufficiency.
- Findings with unilateral urinary outflow obstruction are similar to those with renal artery stenosis.

Captopril Test
Acute blockade of angiotensin II formation by ACEIs induces a reactive increase in PRA. The magnitude of this increase is usually greater in renovascular hypertension than in essential hypertension and is the basis for the captopril test. The use of antihypertensive drugs that influence the renin-angiotensin-aldosterone axis must be discontinued for several days before the test. PRA is measured at baseline and at 60 minutes after administering captopril orally. Criteria for a positive test are 1) PRA of more than 12 ng/mL per hour after administration of captopril, 2) absolute increase in PRA over baseline of at least 10 ng/mL per hour, and 3) increase in PRA of 150% or more if the baseline PRA is more than 3 ng/mL per hour or 400% or more if the baseline PRA is less than 3 ng/mL per hour. The results are compromised if the person has renal insufficiency. Sensitivity is 39% to 100%, and specificity is 72% to 100%. Because the results can be influenced by many factors that are difficult to identify and control, predictive accuracy is low.

- Captopril test: difficult to control all factors that influence test results.
- Sensitivity is 39%-100%, and specificity is 72%-100%.
- The test is unreliable in persons with renal insufficiency.

Renal Vein Renins
Lateralization of renal vein renins is a good predictor of a favorable outcome after intervention for unilateral renal artery stenosis; however, because many factors that influence renin secretion are difficult to identify and control (as noted for the captopril test), the predictive value of the test is low. It is invasive and expensive. Lateralization is present if the ratio of renin activity on the affected side compared with that on the normal side is 1.5:1.0 or more. Sensitivity is 63% to 77%, and specificity is 60% to 95%.

- Measurement of renal vein renin activity is an expensive and invasive test.

- Sensitivity is 63%-77%, and specificity is 60%-95%.
- Lateralization of renal vein renins is a good predictor of a favorable outcome after intervention for unilateral renal artery stenosis.

Digital Venous Subtraction Angiography
Digital venous subtraction angiography uses contrast media, but access to the circulation is through a peripheral vein. With the advent of newer screening tests, it is used less often. This technique provides adequate visualization of the proximal portion of the main renal arteries (the usual location of atherosclerotic disease) in 90% of persons but less effective visualization of the distal portions of the main renal arteries or branches (the usual location of fibromuscular dysplasia). This technique is expensive, and in 20% to 30% of persons, neither renal artery is identified because of superimposition of abdominal vessels or patient motion. Both the sensitivity and the specificity are 85% to 90%.

- In current practice, digital venous subtraction angiography is used less often.
- Both sensitivity and specificity are 85%-90%.
- The proximal portions of the main renal arteries are visualized in 90% of persons.
- It is less effective for assessing distal portions of the main renal arteries or branches.
- It is expensive.
- At least 1 renal artery is not identified in 20%-30% of cases.

Renal Arteriography
Conventional renal arteriography is the diagnostic standard to identify renal artery stenosis. In clinical situations in which the pretest likelihood is high (≥50%), a negative result from a screening test still leaves a significant posttest probability of disease (≥20%). Thus, in these settings, consideration should be given to performing renal angiography as the test of choice. Exceptions may be when patients have diabetes or severe generalized atherosclerosis with concomitant renal insufficiency and use of a noninvasive test initially, such as MRA (without gadolinium if GFR is <30 mL/min) or duplex ultrasonography, may be reasonable. This is because in these settings, the risk of contrast-induced acute renal failure or atheroembolism is significant. Contrast toxicity from angiography can be reduced with the use of alternative contrast agents such as carbon dioxide. However, the use of alternative contrast agents does not reduce the risk of atheroembolism.

- Renal arteriography: the diagnostic standard test for identifying renal artery stenosis.
- If pretest likelihood is high and the person is at low risk of contrast toxicity or atheroembolism, consider renal angiography as the initial test.

Therapy for Renovascular Hypertension
Options for the management of renovascular hypertension include medical and interventional therapies. Percutaneous balloon angioplasty, stent placement, and surgical procedures to relieve renal ischemia are the interventional treatments. Goals of interventional

therapy are to cure or improve hypertension or to preserve renal function. Medical therapy is reserved for persons who are not considered candidates for interventional therapy (because of the extent or location of the vascular lesions, high surgical risk, or uncertainty about the causative significance of the lesion) or who are unwilling to undergo interventional therapy. As noted earlier, selection of persons for screening excludes older persons with controlled hypertension and no evidence of progressive renal dysfunction even if renovascular disease is suspected. Indications for consideration of interventional therapy include recent onset of hypertension (especially in younger persons even if blood pressure is controlled), treatment-resistant hypertension, poorly controlled hypertension due to drug intolerance or noncompliance, and evidence of progressive renal dysfunction.

Percutaneous transluminal angioplasty is the treatment of choice for amenable lesions caused by fibromuscular dysplasia and is an option with or without stent placement in some cases of atherosclerotic renovascular disease. Hypertension is cured in 50% and improved in 35% of persons with fibromuscular dysplasia. The failure rate is 15%. In contrast, hypertension is cured in 20% and improved in 50%, with a failure rate of 30%, in persons with atherosclerotic renovascular disease. Complications of angioplasty include groin hematoma, dye-induced azotemia, dissection of the renal artery, renal infarction, and, rarely, rupture of the renal artery, with the potential for loss of the kidney and the need for immediate surgery. Atheroembolization is a risk in older persons with diffuse atherosclerosis.

- Angioplasty is the treatment of choice for amenable lesions caused by fibromuscular dysplasia and is an option for some lesions caused by atherosclerosis.
- Complications of angioplasty: groin hematoma, dye-induced azotemia, dissection of the renal artery, renal infarction, and, rarely, rupture of the renal artery.

Stent-supported angioplasty is an appropriate option for some persons with atherosclerotic renal artery stenosis, especially for orificial disease. In the presence of aneurysmal or severe atherosclerotic disease of the aorta requiring concomitant aortic reconstruction, or in persons in whom percutaneous intervention has failed, surgical intervention is the treatment of choice. Kidneys with a pole-to-pole length of 8 cm or less should be removed—not revascularized—if intervention is indicated and removal will not jeopardize overall renal function.

The role of interventional therapy for preservation of renal function in ischemic nephropathy is uncertain. In most cases, the underlying disease is atherosclerosis. Improvement in renal function, defined as a decrease in serum creatinine, occurs in 30% of cases. In approximately 50% of cases, the creatinine level does not decrease; however, benefit may be defined as stabilization of renal function. Of concern is that in 20% of cases, renal function deteriorates rapidly after the intervention, most likely from a combination of several factors, including contrast toxicity, acute renal artery thrombosis, or atheroembolization.

- Stent-supported angioplasty is an option for some patients with atherosclerotic renal artery stenosis.
- Surgical treatment is best for cases of atheromatous renal artery disease associated with aneurysmal or severe atherosclerotic disease of the aorta requiring concomitant aortic reconstruction and for percutaneous intervention failures.
- Intervention to preserve renal function in ischemic nephropathy is uncertain.

The medical treatment of renovascular hypertension is not different from that of essential hypertension. Both volume retention (due to aldosterone) and vasoconstriction (due to activation of the sympathetic nervous system and angiotensin II) contribute to the elevation of blood pressure. ACEIs and ARBs can precipitate acute renal failure in the presence of bilateral renal artery stenosis. Medical treatment does not correct the underlying ischemia of the affected kidney, and decreases in systemic blood pressure may further aggravate loss of renal function. Progression of atherosclerotic renal artery disease can be slowed by control of all modifiable risk factors, including the use of statin drugs for aggressive lowering of cholesterol. In medically managed persons, renal function should be followed carefully because deterioration may be a sign of progressive disease.

- The medical treatment of renovascular hypertension is similar to that of essential hypertension.
- If there is bilateral renal artery stenosis, ACEIs and ARBs can precipitate acute renal failure.
- Medical treatment does not correct the underlying ischemia of the affected kidney.
- Management of all modifiable cardiovascular risk factors can lessen the risk of progression of atherosclerotic renovascular disease.
- Typical clinical scenario for renovascular hypertension due to fibromuscular dysplasia: A 30-year-old woman complains of new-onset headaches for the past 2 months. She has no past history of hypertension. On examination, blood pressure is 180/110 mm Hg. On auscultation of the abdomen, a systolic-diastolic bruit is heard in the left upper quadrant.
- Typical clinical scenario for renovascular hypertension due to atherosclerosis: A 54-year-old man has a several-year history of mild hypertension that has been well controlled. He has a 30 pack-year history of cigarette smoking and hypercholesterolemia that is diet-controlled. He has a past history of coronary artery bypass graft surgery. Blood pressure suddenly worsens and is now 170/115 mm Hg. On auscultation of the abdomen, a systolic bruit is detected in the right upper quadrant. Bilateral femoral bruits are also noted.

Renal Parenchymal Disease

Renal parenchymal disease is the most common secondary cause of hypertension and is present in 2% to 5% of persons with elevated blood pressure. Also, hypertension is a common cause of chronic kidney disease and is the second most common cause of end-stage renal failure in the population. Persons with chronic kidney disease and hypertension are at high risk of cardiovascular disease. Contributing to this increased risk is a loss of the normal nocturnal decline in blood pressure ("non-dipper") in persons with renal disease.

Regardless of the cause of chronic kidney disease, hypertension is associated with a more rapid loss of renal function. This may be due to transmission of higher pressures into the glomerulus as afferent renal artery resistance fails to limit transmission of higher systemic pressures into the nephron. Higher glomerular transcapillary pressures and flows injure glomerular cells by several mechanisms, ultimately leading to glomerulosclerosis. In addition, the degree of proteinuria is an independent predictor of progressive loss of renal function.

At least 3 major mechanisms are involved in the hypertension of renal disease: volume expansion from impaired renal elimination of salt and water, oversecretion of renin, and decreased production of renal vasodilators (ie, prostaglandins, kallikrein, and kinin). In addition, accumulation of mediators of oxidative stress, reducing the availability of the vasodilator nitric oxide, and increased levels of the vasoconstrictor endothelin may also contribute.

The blood pressure goal in chronic kidney disease is less than 130/80 mm Hg. Achieving this goal lessens the risk of progressive loss of renal function and often requires the use of 3 or more antihypertensive drugs. Treatment should begin with dietary sodium restriction. In addition, diuretic therapy is often essential for blood pressure control. If serum creatinine is more than 2.0 mg/dL (GFR <30 mL/min), the more potent loop agents or metolazone is necessary. In diuretic-resistant persons, the combination of a loop agent with a thiazide may be required. Oversecretion of renin occurs in only a small proportion of persons with chronic kidney disease; however, ACEIs reduce proteinuria and high glomerular transcapillary pressures by decreasing resistance in the efferent arteriole of the nephron. These actions retard further loss of renal function in persons with diabetic or nondiabetic renal disease. ACEIs can cause hyperkalemia and an acute decline in renal function. Unless severe, modest acute declines in renal function (<30%) should be tolerated because the acute decline is often followed by stabilization and preservation of renal function chronically. An increase in serum levels of potassium of up to 5.5 mEq/L is usually well tolerated. An acute, severe decline in renal function with ACEI therapy (>30%) raises the possibility of bilateral renal artery stenosis. ARBs can be used if ACEIs are not tolerated and may be used instead of ACEIs in persons with type 2 diabetes and nephropathy. CCBs are effective blood pressure–lowering drugs in persons with chronic kidney disease. Nondihydropyridine CCBs reduce proteinuria, but dihydropyridine CCBs do not. In proteinuric renal disease not controlled with adequate doses of a diuretic and an ACEI, a nondihydropyridine CCB could be added as a third agent. β-Blockers should be considered if the person has angina or previously had a myocardial infarction. In advanced renal insufficiency, avoid the use of lipid-insoluble β-blockers, which rely on the kidney for excretion. Hydralazine or minoxidil should be considered for resistant hypertension (requires concomitant use of an adrenergic inhibitor and diuretic).

- Renal parenchymal disease: the most common secondary cause of hypertension.
- Hypertension: the second most common cause of end-stage renal disease.
- Treatment of hypertension in renal disease should include sodium restriction, diuretics appropriate to level of renal function, and ACEIs.
- ACEIs slow the progression of proteinuric renal disease.

- In chronic kidney disease, ACEI therapy can cause hyperkalemia and acute declines in renal function.
- ARBs are alternatives in ACEI-intolerant persons.
- Hydralazine or minoxidil should be considered for resistant hypertension.

Primary Aldosteronism

The syndrome of primary aldosteronism is characterized by the clinical and laboratory consequences of the autonomous overproduction of aldosterone by 1 or both adrenal glands. These consequences are hypertension, hypokalemia (with renal wasting of potassium and alkalosis), suppressed plasma renin activity, and increased aldosterone levels (Figure 14-4). Prevalence estimates range from 2% to 15% of the hypertensive population. Its main subtypes are unilateral aldosterone-producing adenoma (30%-40% of cases) and bilateral idiopathic zona granulosa adrenal hyperplasia (60%-70% of cases). Rarer subtypes are unilateral hyperplasia (2% of cases), glucocorticoid suppressible hyperplasia (familial hyperaldosteronism type 1, <1% of cases), and aldosterone-producing cortical carcinoma (<1% of cases). Primary aldosteronism should be suspected in any hypertensive person who presents with spontaneous hypokalemia or marked hypokalemia precipitated by usual doses of diuretics (potassium <3.0 mEq/L). Other causes of hypokalemic hypertensive syndromes should be considered: diuretics, renovascular hypertension, exogenous steroids, Cushing disease, excess deoxycorticosterone, Liddle syndrome, 11β-hydroxylase deficiency, and ingestion of licorice containing glycyrrhizinic acid (renal cortisol catabolism inhibitor). Primary aldosteronism may be the cause of resistant hypertension even in the absence of hypokalemia because approximately 30% of cases are not associated with spontaneous hypokalemia. It also should be considered in persons who have hypertension and a known adrenal mass (in addition to Cushing disease and pheochromocytoma) or in persons who have hypokalemia despite taking ACEIs or ARBs for treatment of hypertension (in the presence or absence of concomitant diuretic use).

- Primary aldosteronism: hypertension, hypokalemia (with renal wasting of potassium and alkalosis), suppressed plasma renin activity, and increased aldosterone.
- Main subtypes: unilateral aldosterone-producing adenoma and bilateral adrenal hyperplasia.
- Suspect primary aldosteronism in persons with spontaneous hypokalemia, marked hypokalemia precipitated by usual doses of diuretics, resistant hypertension, hypertension and an adrenal mass, or hypokalemia despite use of ACEIs or ARBs.

Clinical Features

Clinical symptoms are uncommon. Most persons with primary aldosteronism cannot be distinguished from those with essential hypertension. Rarely, severe hypokalemia may cause muscle weakness, cramps, headache, palpitations, polydipsia, polyuria, or nocturia. Hypertension is usually moderate, but it may be severe and resistant to control. Retinal vascular changes of severe hypertension may be present. Left ventricular hypertrophy and heart failure may be more common than with essential hypertension, in part because

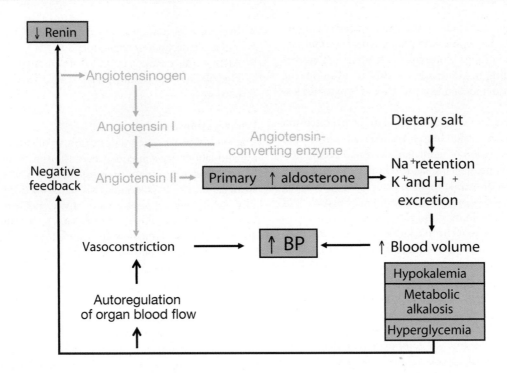

Figure 14-4. Clinical and Laboratory Consequences of the Autonomous Excess of Aldosterone. BP indicates blood pressure; H, hydrogen; K, potassium; Na, sodium.

of the profibrotic effects of aldosterone on the heart. Rarely, the sign of Trousseau or Chvostek may be present if marked alkalosis is associated with hypokalemia. Peripheral edema is rare.

- Clinical symptoms are uncommon.
- Severe hypokalemia may cause muscle weakness, cramps, headache, palpitations, polydipsia, polyuria, or nocturia.
- Peripheral edema is rare.

Laboratory Features

Characteristic laboratory abnormalities include hypokalemia, mild metabolic alkalosis (serum bicarbonate >31 mEq/L), and relative hypernatremia (serum sodium concentration >142 mEq/L). Relative hypernatremia is related to suppression of vasopressin from volume expansion, resetting of the central osmostat for vasopressin release, altered thirst, and hypokalemia-induced suppression of vasopressin release or action. A mild increase in the fasting blood glucose level is detected in 25% of persons (hypokalemia suppresses insulin release). The electrocardiogram may show changes of hypokalemia (ie, prolongation of the ST segment, U waves, and T-wave inversions) as well as left ventricular hypertrophy.

- Laboratory abnormalities in primary aldosteronism: hypokalemia, mild metabolic alkalosis, relative hypernatremia, and increased fasting glucose level.
- Electrocardiogram may show changes of hypokalemia (ie, prolongation of the ST segment, U waves, and T-wave inversions) or left ventricular hypertrophy.

Diagnosis

The investigation for primary aldosteronism is divided into 3 phases: 1) screening, 2) confirmation of the diagnosis, and 3) determination of the subtype.

Screening studies should include measurement of serum sodium, potassium, PRA, and bicarbonate. If the person is hypokalemic, a 24-hour urine collection for potassium should be performed initially to determine whether the hypokalemia is from renal potassium wasting (>30 mEq of potassium in a 24-hour collection in the presence of hypokalemia defines renal potassium wasting). A popular screening method is to simultaneously measure PRA and the plasma aldosterone concentration (PAC) and to calculate the PAC:PRA ratio. A ratio greater than 15 to 20 suggests the diagnosis of primary aldosteronism. The higher the ratio, the more likely the diagnosis. Ideally, PRA and PAC should be measured in the morning after discontinuing the use of drugs that could influence the measurements (eg, diuretics, β-blockers, ACEIs, ARBs, and spironolactone). Because PRA and PAC can vary significantly in persons with the disorder, a single normal value for the ratio does not exclude the diagnosis. Sensitivity of the ratio is 75% when measured with persons receiving antihypertensive medications and 85% when measured with persons not receiving antihypertensive drug therapy. Specificity is relatively low (75%) under either condition of measurement.

In persons with positive screening test results, 24-hour urinary aldosterone excretion should be measured during the fourth day of a high-salt diet. The diagnosis of primary aldosteronism rests on demonstrating renin suppression and inappropriately high aldosterone excretion in a sodium-replete state (24-hour sodium excretion >200-

250 mEq) in hypertensive persons. Before a diagnostic evaluation is initiated, the use of potentially interfering drugs must be discontinued and plasma volume status assessed. Spironolactone influences the renin-angiotensin-aldosterone axis and must be discontinued for at least 6 weeks before investigation. Diuretics, ACEIs, and ARBs may increase and β-blockers may decrease PRA levels in persons with primary aldosteronism. If hypertension must be treated in the interim, guanadrel, α-blockers, or CCBs may be used. After a high-salt diet for 3 days (and with concomitant vigorous potassium supplementation), a 24-hour urine specimen should be collected for measurement of sodium, potassium, creatinine, and aldosterone. PRA should also be measured. Creatinine can be used as an approximation of the adequacy of the collection. A 24-hour urine aldosterone greater than 12 to 14 mcg (when urinary sodium is >200-250 mEq) with a concomitant PRA less than 1.0 ng/mL per hour confirms the diagnosis of primary aldosteronism.

* In a hypokalemic, hypertensive person, a PAC:PRA ratio >15-20 suggests primary aldosteronism.
* Before diagnostic evaluation, discontinue the use of drugs that could influence PRA or PAC levels and assess plasma volume status.
* During the fourth day of a high-salt diet, measure PRA and collect a 24-hour urine specimen for measurement of sodium, potassium, creatinine, and aldosterone.
* A 24-hour urine aldosterone >12-14 mcg (with concomitant urinary sodium >200-250 mEq) along with a PRA <1.0 ng/mL per hour confirms the diagnosis of primary aldosteronism.

The major subtypes to distinguish are unilateral aldosterone-producing adenoma and bilateral adrenal hyperplasia. Removing an aldosterone-producing adenoma normalizes blood pressure in approximately 30% of cases and relieves hypokalemia in 100%. Unilateral or bilateral adrenalectomy seldom corrects hypertension when bilateral adrenal hyperplasia is present. CT or magnetic resonance imaging (MRI) of the adrenal glands is the initial study for distinguishing between subtypes. CT is effective in localizing adenomas larger than 1 cm in diameter when the adrenal glands are imaged at 0.3-cm intervals. Generally, if a single adenoma larger than 1 cm in diameter is clearly identified, surgical treatment is the choice. If no mass is identified, assume the diagnosis is bilateral hyperplasia and prescribe spironolactone, eplerenone, or other potassium-retaining diuretics. Often, additional medications are needed for blood pressure control.

* Removing an aldosterone-producing adenoma normalizes blood pressure in 30% of cases and hypokalemia in 100%.
* Unilateral or bilateral adrenalectomy seldom corrects hypertension in persons with bilateral adrenal hyperplasia.
* CT or MRI of the adrenal glands is the initial study for distinguishing between subtypes.
* If a single adenoma is >1 cm in diameter, the treatment is surgical.
* If no mass is detected, prescribe spironolactone, eplerenone, or other potassium-retaining diuretics and other medications as needed to control blood pressure.

If the results are equivocal or the gland opposite that containing the presumed adenoma is abnormal or if CT findings are normal in a person with severe hypertension, hypokalemia, and markedly elevated aldosterone (findings suggestive of an adenoma), sampling blood from the adrenal veins for aldosterone may identify the adrenal gland containing the functioning adenoma not clearly detected on imaging. In these situations, subspecialty consultation should be sought.

* If the results are equivocal, sampling blood from the adrenal veins for aldosterone may identify the adrenal gland containing the functioning adenoma.
* Typical clinical scenario for primary aldosteronism: A 42-year-old man is evaluated for resistant hypertension. The physical examination findings are normal except for an elevated blood pressure of 150/105 mm Hg despite treatment with an ACEI, a β-blocker, and a CCB. Initial laboratory values are sodium 144 mEq/L, potassium 2.9 mEq/L, glucose 110 mg/dL, and creatinine 1.0 mg/dL.

Pheochromocytoma

Pheochromocytomas are tumors of chromaffin cell origin (derived from the embryonic neural crest) that cause paroxysmal or sustained hypertension due to excess production of catecholamines. Tumors are present in the adrenal medulla (pheochromocytomas) or sympathetic ganglia (extra-adrenal pheochomocytomas or paragangliomas). Nonchromaffin paragangliomas (chemodectomas) arise from parasympathetic ganglia in the head and neck (carotid body and glomus jugulare [cranial nerves IX and X]). Patients with paragangliomas below the neck usually present with catecholamine excess, whereas patients with paragangliomas in the head or neck often present with clinical features associated with a mass effect (eg, cranial nerve palsies or tinnitus).

The incidence in the general population is 2 to 8 cases per million persons per year. The prevalence is 0.5% among persons with hypertension and suggestive symptoms and 4% among hypertensive persons with an adrenal tumor. A "rule of 10" is often quoted for pheochromocytoma: 10% are extra-adrenal (90% are located in 1 or both adrenal glands); 10% of extra-adrenal gland tumors are extra-abdominal (90% are located in the abdomen or pelvis); 10% occur in children (90% occur in adults between the third and fifth decades of life; equal occurrence in men and women); 10% are multiple or bilateral; 10% recur after the initial resection; 10% are malignant; 10% are found in persons without hypertension; and 10% are familial. Recent studies suggest that up to 11% of patients with presumed sporadic pheochromocytomas (eg, solitary adrenal tumor, negative family history, and no associated disease) may still have an inherited form of the disease. Thus, more than 10% of pheochromocytomas may actually be familial in origin.

Extra-adrenal pheochromocytomas may occur anywhere along the sympathetic chain (paragangliomas) and occasionally in aberrant sites (eg, superior abdominal para-aortic region [46%], glomus jugulare, inferior abdominal para-aortic region [29%], bladder [10%], thorax [10%], and head, neck, or pelvis [5%]). Chromaffin cells synthesize catecholamines from tyrosine. Norepinephrine is the end product in all sites except the adrenal medulla, where 75% of norepinephrine is metabolized to epinephrine. Extra-adrenal tumors produce only norepinephrine, whereas adrenal tumors may produce an excess of 1 or both catecholamines. A person with a tumor that secretes predominantly epinephrine has mainly systolic hypertension, tachycardia, sweating, flushing, and tremulousness and may present with hypotension. A person with a tumor that secretes mainly norepinephrine has both systolic and diastolic hypertension, less tachycardia, and fewer paroxysms of anxiety and palpitations.

- Pheochromocytoma: remember the "rule of 10."
- Ninety percent are in 1 or both adrenal glands.
- Tumors may occur anywhere along the sympathetic chain (paragangliomas).
- It is malignant in up to 10% of cases.
- An extra-adrenal tumor produces only norepinephrine.
- An adrenal tumor can produce an excess of epinephrine or norepinephrine (or both).

Pheochromocytomas associated with familial syndromes are more likely to be bilateral or extra-adrenal and occur at a young age. Familial syndromes have an inheritance pattern that is autosomal dominant with variable penetrance and include the following:

1. Multiple endocrine neoplasia type 2A (medullary carcinoma of the thyroid [increased plasma level of calcitonin], pheochromocytoma, and hyperparathyroidism due to primary hyperplasia) and type 2B (medullary carcinoma of the thyroid, pheochromocytoma, mucosal neuromas, thickened corneal nerves, intestinal ganglioneuromatosis, and marfanoid body habitus [Figures 14-5 and 14-6]). These are associated with activating mutations of the *RET* proto-oncogene. The risk of pheochromocytoma is 50%.
2. Neurofibromatosis (café au lait spots). The risk of pheochromocytoma, due to mutations in the *NF-I* gene, is 0.1% to 5.7%.
3. von Hippel-Lindau disease (pheochromocytoma, retinal hemangiomatosis, cerebellar hemangioblastomas, epididymal cystadenoma, renal and pancreatic cysts, and renal cell carcinoma). It is associated with loss-of-function mutations in the *VHL* tumor suppressor gene. The risk of pheochromocytoma is 10% to 20%.
4. Familial paraganglioma syndrome (tumors of the head or neck [glomus tumors] or carotid body). There is an association with mutations in the *SDHD* and *SDHB* genes. The risk of pheochromocytoma is 20%.
5. A simple form has no other glandular abnormalities.

Persons with a suspected familial pheochromocytoma should undergo genetic testing. This includes persons with a family history of pheochromocytoma and persons with an apparent sporadic tumor but with a presentation consistent with a familial tumor, such as young age (<21 years) and bilateral or extra-adrenal tumors. If a tumor is found, screening should be considered for first-degree relatives because of the autosomal dominant pattern of inheritance.

- Familial pheochromocytomas tend to be bilateral or extra-adrenal and occur at a young age.
- Pheochromocytoma is associated with neurofibromatosis, von

Hippel-Lindau disease, multiple endocrine neoplasia types 2A and 2B, and familial paraganglioma syndrome.
- Screening should be considered for first-degree relatives of persons with familial pheochromocytomas.

Signs and Symptoms

Symptomatic paroxysms of hypertension occur in less than 50% of persons; most have sustained hypertension. Paroxysms are characterized by the classic triad of headache, diaphoresis, and palpitations. A paroxysm is usually rapid in onset, rapid in offset, and may be triggered by exercise, bending, urination, defecation, induction of anesthesia, smoking, or infusion of intravenous contrast media. Some persons have unintended weight loss, hyperglycemia, and other signs and symptoms of hypermetabolism. Others have both hypertension and orthostatic hypotension. Rarely, persons may present with catecholamine-induced cardiomyopathy, secondary erythrocytosis, fever, or peripheral vasospasm. The hypertension can be severe, resistant to control, and associated with retinopathy of accelerated-malignant hypertension. With widespread use of imaging studies, a small number of asymptomatic persons with normal blood pressure are found to have pheochromocytoma. It should always

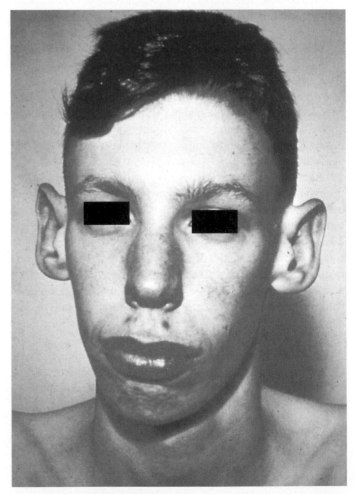

Figure 14-5. Marfanoid Appearance of a Patient With Multiple Endocrine Neoplasia Type 2B.

be considered when an incidental adrenal mass is noted on an imaging study.

- Classic triad of symptoms associated with pheochromocytoma: paroxysms of headache, diaphoresis, and palpitations.
- Paroxysms can be induced by exercise, bending, urination, defecation, induction of anesthesia, smoking, or infusion of contrast media.
- Some persons have unintended weight loss, hyperglycemia, or peripheral vasospasm; others have both hypertension and orthostatic hypotension.

Screening

Screening for pheochromocytoma should be selective. Candidates for screening are persons with paroxysmal hypertension with or without suggestive symptoms; an adrenal mass; refractory hypertension; concomitant diabetes mellitus; unintended weight loss and other features of hypermetabolism; marked hypertension in response to anesthesia induction, surgery, or angiography; onset of hypertension at a young age (<20 years); unexplained cardiomyopathy (chronic catecholamine excess is toxic to the heart); neurocutaneous lesions; retinal angiomas; orthostatic hypotension; or a family history of pheochromocytoma, medullary carcinoma of the thyroid, or hyperparathyroidism. States of sympathetic overactivity other than pheochromocytoma should be considered before screening. These include disorders associated with dysautonomia, significant physical or emotional stress, use of sympathomimetic drugs, coadministration of monoamine oxidase inhibitors and tyramine-containing foods ("cheese reaction"), acute withdrawal from alcohol, centrally acting antihypertensive drugs, or benzodiazepines.

Screening involves measurement of the O-methylated metabolites of catecholamines (metanephrine is the O-methylated metabolite of epinephrine, and normetanephrine is the O-methylated metabolite of norepinephrine). Plasma or urine measures of catecholamines alone lack diagnostic accuracy. Measurement of plasma free metanephrines (ie, metanephrine and normetanephrine) is considered the screening test of choice because of its high sensitivity. The largest source of free metanephrines is adrenal chromaffin cells. In persons with pheochromocytoma, free metanephrines are produced within the tumor cells from catecholamines that leak from storage vesicles. This process occurs continuously and is independent of catecholamine secretion by the tumor. Measurement of the 24-hour urinary excretion of total and fractionated metanephrines (ie, metanephrine and normetanephrine) and catecholamines is an alternative if the plasma test is unavailable. The urine test is less sensitive but more specific for pheochromocytoma (fewer false-positive results). Measurement of plasma free metanephrines should be strongly considered if a familial syndrome is suspected, if the person has a previous history of pheochromocytoma, or if clinical suspicion is high (eg, hypertension with a known vascular adrenal mass). A negative result for either the plasma test or the urine test excludes the diagnosis in most cases.

Because of the low prevalence of pheochromocytoma, false-positive results outnumber true-positive results among persons screened for this disorder. Dietary factors, drugs, and physiologic stresses can interfere with screening test results. Ideally, screening should be performed after discontinuing the use of drugs that are known to increase catecholamine levels or interfere with the analyses. Some of these are listed in Table 14-7. Phenoxybenzamine and tricyclic antidepressants can increase plasma and urinary normetanephrine. Buspirone can increase urinary metanephrine (but not plasma values). β-Blockers (including labetalol) can increase plasma metanephrine and urinary metanephrine and normetanephrine. Diuretics, CCBs, ACEIs, ARBs, and selective α_1-adrenergic receptor blockers do not interfere with plasma or urinary screening. Sympathomimetics can cause false-positive results for both plasma and urine tests. In those with marginally positive results, the factors noted in Table 14-7, if present, should be eliminated and the screening test repeated.

In persons with negative results from screening tests but who present with paroxysmal hypertension, other diagnoses should be considered. Many persons who have screening tests for pheochromocytoma have panic disorder or other undiagnosed disorders associated with emotional distress (pseudopheochromocytoma).

- Screening for pheochromocytoma: history of paroxysmal hypertension with or without suggestive symptoms, hypertension and an adrenal mass, refractory hypertension, hypertension with diabetes mellitus, hypermetabolism and unintended weight loss, or marked hypertension in response to anesthesia induction.
- The most sensitive screening test is plasma free metanephrines.
- Dietary factors, drugs, and physiologic stresses can interfere with screening test results.

Diagnosis and Treatment

CT or MRI of the abdomen and pelvis is the initial test used to locate a tumor (90% of all tumors are in 1 or both adrenal glands and 95% of all tumors are in the abdomen or pelvis) and should be performed only after biochemical testing has confirmed the presence of the disorder. The sensitivity for identifying a tumor that has a diameter of 1 cm or larger is 85% to 94% with CT and 90% with MRI. Total body MRI can be considered if a lesion is not found with abdominal imaging. Specialized studies are occasionally necessary to identify extra-adrenal tumors or small tumors not identified with CT or MRI

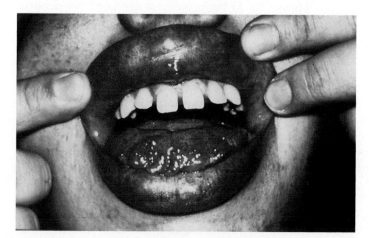

Figure 14-6. Oral Neuromas Associated With Multiple Endocrine Neoplasia Type 2B.

(ie, ^{123}I-metaiodobenzylguanidine [MIBG] scintigraphy or positron emission tomography using [^{18}F]fluorodeoxyglucose, [^{11}C]hydroxyephedrine, or 6-[^{18}F]fluorodopamine). If a large adrenal tumor or an extra-adrenal tumor is found on CT or MRI imaging, a subsequent MIBG scan should be considered. Large tumors are at increased risk of being malignant (with metastases), and extra-adrenal tumors may be multiple.

After the tumor has been identified, treatment is surgical. Preoperatively, administer α-blockers (phenoxybenzamine), followed by β-blockers if needed to control blood pressure and cardiac rhythm. Persons with hypertensive crisis can be given α-blockers or sodium nitroprusside intravenously. β-Blockers can be given if tachycardia is excessive. Because pheochromocytomas can recur in 10% of cases, long-term biochemical follow-up is required.

- Use CT or MRI of the abdomen and pelvis to locate the tumor.
- The treatment is surgical.
- Preoperatively, administer α-blockers, followed by β-blockers.
- Typical clinical scenario for pheochromocytoma: A 25-year-old college student is evaluated for spells. These are sudden in onset and offset and last 25 to 35 minutes. Symptoms include frontal headache, diaphoresis, pounding pulse, and nausea. According to persons witnessing a spell, the patient is pale. Since the onset of these spells, he has lost 9.0 kg. During a recent spell, his blood pressure was 220/160 mm Hg. He has no past history of hypertension. The examination findings are essentially normal except for evidence of weight loss, a resting pulse of 105 beats per minute, and blood pressure of 160/110 mm Hg.

Coarctation of the Aorta

Coarctation of the aorta is a constriction of the vessel, commonly just beyond the takeoff of the left subclavian artery (see Chapter 3, "Cardiology"). It usually is detected in childhood, but occasionally the diagnosis is not made until adulthood. It is more common in males. In up to 40% of cases, it is accompanied by a bicuspid aortic valve. Coarctation is also associated with an increased risk of intracranial aneurysms and can complicate Turner syndrome. The classic feature is increased blood pressure in the upper extremities, with low or unobtainable blood pressure in the lower extremities. The mechanism of hypertension involves both volume expansion and inappropriate renin secretion. Symptoms of coarctation include headache, cold feet, and exercise-induced leg pain (claudication). Clinical signs include elevated blood pressure in the arms, murmurs in the front or back of the chest (from collateral vessels), visible pulsations in the neck or chest wall (from collateral vessels), and weak femoral pulses or delay when the radial and femoral pulses are palpated simultaneously. A systolic ejection click and systolic ejection murmur may be heard if a bicuspid aortic valve is present. Chest radiography can be diagnostic. A characteristic "3 sign" is due to dilatation above and below the constriction plus notching of the ribs (Figure 14-7) by enlarged collateral vessels. The diagnosis is made with transesophageal echocardiography or MRI of the aorta.

Traditionally, treatment has been surgical repair of the aorta. Balloon angioplasty with or without stenting is becoming the treatment of choice. After repair, hypertension is usually transient and

Table 14-7 Causes of False-Positive Results From Plasma or Urine Screening Tests for Fractionated Metanephrines

Phenoxybenzamine
Tricyclic antidepressants
β-Blockers (including labetalol)
Buspirone
Drugs containing catecholamines (eg, decongestants)
Discontinuation of use of clonidine or related drugs
Discontinuation of use of benzodiazepine
Discontinuation of use of ethanol
Untreated obstructive sleep apnea

may be associated with mesenteric vasculitis and bowel infarction. Plasma renin activity levels are usually high. The recommended treatment for hypertension after repair is β-blockers or ACEIs.

- Coarctation of the aorta is usually just beyond the takeoff of the left subclavian artery.
- It usually is detected in childhood but may not be identified until adulthood.
- Classic feature: increased blood pressure in the upper extremities and low or unobtainable blood pressure in the lower extremities.
- Mechanism of hypertension: volume expansion and inappropriate renin secretion.
- Symptoms: headache, cold feet, and exercise-induced leg pain.
- Signs: murmurs in the front or back of the chest, visible pulsations in the neck or chest wall, and weak femoral pulses.
- Transesophageal echocardiography or MRI is used to make the diagnosis.
- Treatment is with balloon angioplasty or surgery.

Other Causes of Hypertension

Cushing syndrome (see Chapter 6, "Endocrinology") is often associated with hypertension and always should be considered in the hypertensive person who has impaired fasting glucose and unexplained hypokalemia. Hypothyroidism is associated with diastolic hypertension. It is a state of decreased cardiac output and contractility. Tissue perfusion is maintained by an increase in peripheral vascular resistance mediated by increased activity of the sympathetic nervous system. In contrast, hyperthyroidism is associated with systolic hypertension and a wide pulse pressure due to increased cardiac output and decreased peripheral vascular resistance.

Hyperparathyroidism may be associated with hypertension. Hypercalcemia may increase blood pressure directly by increasing peripheral vascular resistance and indirectly by increasing vascular sensitivity to catecholamines.

Approximately 35% of persons with acromegaly have hypertension, which is largely due to the sodium-retaining effects of growth hormone.

Obstructive sleep apnea is associated with hypertension that may be severe and resistant to control. Upper body obesity is a risk factor for obstructive sleep apnea and is common in hypertensive persons. Consider the diagnosis of obstructive sleep apnea in persons who are overweight, snore loudly, and complain of morning headaches and daytime sleepiness. Bed partners may observe breath-holding episodes at night. The mechanism of hypertension involves increased sympathetic nervous system activity. This condition can be associated with increased metanephrines.

Intracranial tumors, especially those occurring in the posterior fossa, may cause hypertension. Occasionally, hypertension is labile, with features suggesting pheochromocytoma.

Panic syndrome also may be associated with a labile increase in blood pressure and symptoms that suggest pheochromocytoma. Acute stress from various causes (emotional or physical) can increase blood pressure through intense stimulation of the sympathetic nervous system and the renin-angiotensin system (especially if volume contraction is present).

- Hypothyroidism can cause diastolic hypertension.
- Hyperthyroidism can cause systolic hypertension.
- Hyperparathyroidism and acromegaly may be associated with hypertension.
- Obstructive sleep apnea can cause hypertension and may increase metanephrines.
- Brain tumors in the posterior fossa and panic syndrome can cause labile hypertension, suggesting pheochromocytoma.
- Acute stress can increase blood pressure.

Hypertension in Pregnancy

Normally, blood pressure decreases early in pregnancy (first 16-18 weeks) and then gradually increases to the levels before pregnancy

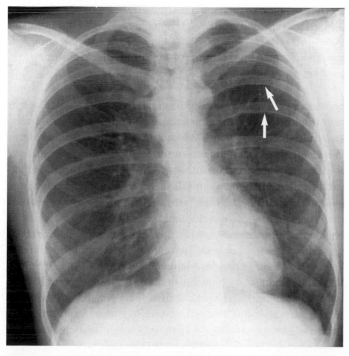

Figure 14-7. Coarctation of the Aorta. Chest radiograph showing notching (arrows) of ribs from collateral vessels.

(and plateaus at 36 weeks). Blood pressure decreases in normal pregnancy because of reduced peripheral vascular resistance. Systolic blood pressure is affected less than diastolic blood pressure because of increased cardiac output in response to vasodilatation. The usual nocturnal decrease in blood pressure is preserved during normal pregnancy.

During pregnancy, plasma angiotensinogen, renin activity, and aldosterone increase. Other substances that increase during normal pregnancy are estrogen, deoxycorticosterone, and vasodilating prostaglandins produced by the uteroplacental unit. Vessels are hyporesponsive to pressor agents, including norepinephrine and angiotensin II, in part because of the effect of prostaglandins and nitric oxide produced by the uteroplacental unit. Although aldosterone levels increase, renal sodium retention is not marked, probably because progesterone and prostaglandins are natriuretic. Progesterone is also a vasodilator. Plasma volume and cardiac output increase 50% to 60% from baseline during normal pregnancy, and renal blood flow and glomerular filtration rate increase by 35%.

- Blood pressure decreases early in pregnancy and gradually increases to the levels before pregnancy.
- Angiotensinogen, renin activity, and aldosterone increase.
- During pregnancy, vessels are hyporesponsive to norepinephrine and angiotensin II.
- Renal sodium retention is not marked, probably because progesterone and prostaglandins are natriuretic.
- In normal pregnancy, blood pressure decreases because of reduced peripheral vascular resistance.

Definition

Hypertension during pregnancy is defined as systolic blood pressure 140 mm Hg or greater or diastolic blood pressure 90 mm Hg or greater. The diagnosis is confirmed by documentation of elevated blood pressure on 2 determinations made 6 hours apart. Hypertensive disorders of pregnancy are associated with increased neonatal morbidity and mortality and account for 18% of maternal deaths.

Four major hypertensive syndromes in pregnancy are 1) *chronic hypertension*—hypertension known to be present before pregnancy or diagnosed before the 20th week of gestation (complicates 3% of pregnancies), 2) *preeclampsia-eclampsia* (described below; complicates 5%-8% of pregnancies), 3) *chronic hypertension with superimposed preeclampsia* (complicates 25% of pregnancies in hypertensive women), and 4) *gestational hypertension*—hypertension that develops for the first time after the 20th week of gestation without other findings of preeclampsia (complicates 6% of pregnancies), but it can evolve into preeclampsia. If gestational hypertension does not evolve into preeclampsia by delivery, and if blood pressure normalizes within 12 weeks post partum, the hypertension is called *transient hypertension of pregnancy*. This is a predictor of the future development of essential hypertension. If blood pressure remains elevated, it is recognized retrospectively as *chronic hypertension* that was previously undiagnosed and masked by the decrease in blood pressure that occurs during early pregnancy.

Women with hypertension developing before the 20th week of gestation or with early gestational hypertension are among a group more likely to have a secondary form (caused by renovascular disease, primary aldosteronism, Cushing syndrome, or pheochromocytoma). Further evaluation with noninvasive testing should be considered, especially if suggestive clinical clues are present.

* Hypertension during pregnancy: blood pressure ≥140 mm Hg systolic or ≥90 mm Hg diastolic.
* Transient hypertension is a predictor of the future development of essential hypertension.
* Consider secondary causes of hypertension in this age group.

The pregnancy-specific syndrome of preeclampsia is characterized by hypertension (blood pressure ≥140/90 mm Hg) and proteinuria (24-hour urine protein excretion ≥0.3 g) that develops after the 20th week of gestation. Eclampsia is defined by seizures that occur in the presence of preeclampsia which cannot be attributed to other causes. Findings that increase the certainty of the diagnosis of preeclampsia (and increase the risk of eclampsia) and the need for close monitoring and consideration for delivery include headache, blurring of vision and other cerebral symptoms, epigastric pain, nephrotic range proteinuria (≥3.5 g in 24 hours), oliguria, systolic blood pressure 160 mm Hg or higher or diastolic blood pressure 110 mm Hg or higher, creatinine level greater than 1.2 mg/dL, platelet count less than 100×10^9/L, evidence of microangiopathic hemolytic anemia (abnormal blood smear or increased lactate dehydrogenase), elevated liver enzymes (aspartate aminotransferase [AST] and alanine aminotransferase [ALT]), or pulmonary edema.

Preeclampsia occurs more commonly in African American women and in women who are relatively young or old to be pregnant (<18 years or >35 years), who are having their first pregnancy or a twin pregnancy, who are obese, who have diabetes mellitus or insulin resistance, who have a family history of preeclampsia in their mother, who have had preeclampsia with a previous pregnancy, or who have renal disease, chronic hypertension, a collagen vascular disease, or a congenital thrombophilia disorder. Preeclampsia that develops before the 20th week of gestation suggests molar pregnancy, fetal hydrops, α-thalassemia, or renal disease.

* Preeclampsia: hypertension and proteinuria after the 20th week of gestation.
* Eclampsia: preeclampsia with seizures.
* Risk factors for preeclampsia: African American race, relatively young or old for pregnancy, first or twin pregnancy, obesity, diabetes mellitus or insulin resistance, family history of preeclampsia in the mother, preeclampsia with a previous pregnancy, renal disease, chronic hypertension, collagen vascular disease, or congenital thrombophilia disorder.

In preeclampsia, the endovascular trophoblastic cells of the placenta do not adequately invade the uterine spiral arteries (abnormal placentation). Consequently, the normally thick-walled muscular spiral arteries are not transformed into saclike flaccid vessels capable of accommodating the 10-fold increase in uterine blood flow associated with normal pregnancy. This leads to underperfusion of the placenta (placental insufficiency). Circulating antiangiogenic proteins of placental origin (circulating soluble fms-like tyrosine kinase 1 [sFlt-1]

and soluble endoglin) have been identified and may have a role in the pathogenesis of preeclampsia. There is maternal intolerance to the fetal response to placental insufficiency, but this does not occur in all cases. Unknown maternal factors (genetic and environmental) are probably required. When present, circulating mediators produced by the hypoperfused placenta act on the common target organ in preeclampsia, the vascular endothelium. The altered vascular endothelial cells produce several factors (procoagulants, vasoconstrictors, and mitogens) that constrict and obstruct vascular beds, producing the characteristic pathologic changes (hemorrhage and necrosis) that may be seen in the brain, heart, and liver of women with preeclampsia. The characteristic glomerular lesion, glomerular endotheliosis, is characterized by endothelial cell swelling, subendothelial fibrinoid deposition, and mesangial cell interposition. Oxidative stress and inflammation are also important. Preeclampsia is a disorder of endothelial dysfunction and systemic vasoconstriction.

Unlike women with normal pregnancy, those with preeclampsia are sensitive to the pressor effects of norepinephrine and angiotensin II. Peripheral resistance markedly increases. Renal blood flow and glomerular filtration rate decrease (but may remain above the levels before pregnancy). Vascular volume decreases and is often associated with hemoconcentration. This hemoconcentration may result from extravasation of albumin into the interstitial space. Central venous pressure and pulmonary capillary wedge pressure are often low. Placental prostaglandin levels decrease. Renal fractional urate clearance decreases, and uric acid is most often increased. Hyperuricemia often distinguishes patients with preeclampsia from those with chronic hypertension in pregnancy. An increase in uric acid concentration and a decrease in the platelet count are the earliest laboratory findings associated with preeclampsia. The HELLP syndrome (hemolysis [elevated lactate dehydrogenase or bilirubin], elevated liver enzymes, and low platelet count) occurs when intravascular coagulation and liver ischemia develop in preeclampsia. The HELLP syndrome can rapidly develop into a life-threatening disorder of liver failure and worsening thrombocytopenia in the presence of only mild or moderate hypertension. The most serious complication of the HELLP syndrome is liver rupture (right upper quadrant abdominal pain), which is associated with high maternal and fetal mortality. The cause of seizures (eclampsia) is uncertain. Possibilities include cerebral vasospasm or cerebral edema due to severe elevations in blood pressure with disruption of cerebral autoregulation of blood flow.

Studies indicate that women who have had preeclampsia are more likely to have insulin resistance, altered endothelial function, and dyslipidemia than women who have had normal pregnancies.

* Women with preeclampsia are sensitive to the pressor effects of norepinephrine and angiotensin II.
* With preeclampsia, peripheral vascular resistance markedly increases.
* Uric acid is most often increased; this distinguishes women with preeclampsia from those with chronic hypertension in pregnancy.
* An increase in uric acid and a decrease in the platelet count are the earliest laboratory abnormalities in preeclampsia.
* Laboratory evaluation for hypertension developing after the 20th week of gestation: hemoglobin, hematocrit, platelet count,

24-hour urine protein, creatinine, uric acid level, AST and ALT, albumin, lactate dehydrogenase, blood smear, and coagulation profile.

Treatment of Chronic Hypertension in Pregnancy

Most women with stage 1 hypertension and normal renal function have good outcomes even without treatment. As blood pressure decreases in early pregnancy, previous drug therapy can often be reduced or discontinued. Lifestyle modifications (eg, mild weight loss, low-impact exercise, dietary salt restriction, and cessation of alcohol and tobacco use) should be recommended. For stage 1 hypertension, there is no evidence that drug therapy improves neonatal outcomes. Drug therapy should be considered if diastolic blood pressure is 100 mm Hg or higher, if systolic blood pressure is 150 mm Hg or higher in the second trimester or 160 mm Hg or higher in the third trimester, or if target organ injury occurs (left ventricular hypertrophy or increased creatinine level). Methyldopa (which has been studied most completely) is recommended as initial therapy. This is the only drug that has been shown to decrease perinatal mortality and for which long-term studies on the offspring are available.

If methyldopa is ineffective or not tolerated, other drugs can be considered. Except for ACEIs, ARBs, and direct renin inhibitors, none of the currently available drugs are known to increase perinatal morbidity or mortality. ACEIs, ARBs, and direct renin inhibitors are contraindicated because exposure to these agents anytime during pregnancy can cause serious fetal abnormalities (eg, limb defects, lung hypoplasia, craniofacial deformities, and renal dysplasia).

The use of β-blockers (atenolol) in the second trimester has been associated with intrauterine fetal growth retardation and low placental weight. Their use should be restricted to the third trimester. However, use in the third trimester can be associated with fetal bradycardia, impaired fetal compensatory response to hypoxia, and neonatal hypoglycemia. There is evidence that labetalol and pindolol are safe and effective for treating chronic hypertension in pregnancy.

Only limited data are available for CCBs, but they seem to be safe (nifedipine). They are potent tocolytics and can affect progression of labor. Their use can be associated with profound hypotension and circulatory collapse if magnesium sulfate is given concurrently for seizure prophylaxis in preeclampsia.

Because of theoretical concerns about diuretics decreasing vascular volume and placental blood flow, they are not considered first-line agents. However, if indicated (in salt-sensitive hypertension or in the presence of renal or cardiac disease), they are considered safe, and they can potentiate the effects of other agents to lower blood pressure. They are contraindicated in preeclampsia and intrauterine growth retardation.

- Lifestyle modifications can be used initially to treat mild hypertension.
- Use drug therapy if diastolic blood pressure is ≥100 mm Hg or systolic blood pressure is ≥150 mm Hg in the second trimester or ≥160 mm Hg in the third trimester.
- Recommended initial drug therapy: methyldopa.
- ACEIs, ARBs, and direct renin inhibitors are contraindicated during pregnancy.

Treatment of Preeclampsia-Eclampsia

Prevention strategies for preeclampsia have limited value. In recent studies calcium supplements have not been shown to lessen the risk. The use of low-dose aspirin early in pregnancy may reduce the risk, but this is controversial. It is important to identify the high-risk woman and to monitor her closely to identify preeclampsia early. Recent studies suggest that before the clinical onset of preeclampsia, increased levels of an antiangiogenic protein, sFlt-1, bind to the proangiogenic protein, placental growth factor (PIGF), causing its level to be reduced. Thus, increased sFlt-1 levels and decreased PIGF levels may be markers for increased risk of preeclampsia. The diagnostic accuracy of these tests has not been determined prospectively, and they are not currently available for clinical use. At present, early recognition of preeclampsia is based primarily on diagnostic blood pressure increases in the late second or early third trimester. Proteinuria is an important sign of progression and usually warrants hospitalization. The woman should be kept at rest in bed. Monitor blood pressure, urine output, and fluid retention (weigh the patient) daily. Periodically determine the platelet count, creatinine level, uric acid level, albumin level, and urinary protein excretion. Evidence of central nervous system involvement (eg, headache, disorientation, or visual symptoms) or liver distention (eg, abdominal pain or liver tenderness) are important findings that suggest progression of preeclampsia. Hepatic rupture is associated with 65% mortality and can be prevented only by delivery of the fetus. Evidence of progressive preeclampsia after the 34th week of gestation is an indication for delivery. When gestational age is critical (<34 weeks), worsening maternal symptoms, laboratory evidence of end-organ dysfunction, or deterioration of the fetal condition indicates delivery. If a fetus is immature and preeclampsia is nonprogressive, a period of observation is warranted. Hypertension should be treated with drugs if diastolic blood pressure is 100 mm Hg or greater. The oral agent of choice is methyldopa. Reasonable alternatives are α-β-blockers, CCBs, or hydralazine. Severe hypertension (ie, >160/110 mm Hg) is associated with increased risk of intracerebral hemorrhage and death and requires treatment. Persons with hypertensive encephalopathy or eclampsia require parenteral therapy to decrease blood pressure to less than 160/100 mm Hg (see below).

- Proteinuria is an important sign of progression and usually warrants hospitalization.
- Keep the woman at rest in bed.
- Central nervous system involvement or liver distention suggests progression of preeclampsia.
- Progressive preeclampsia after the 34th week of gestation is an indication for delivery.
- Before the 34th week of gestation, worsening maternal symptoms, laboratory evidence of end-organ dysfunction, or deterioration of the fetal condition indicates delivery.
- If diastolic blood pressure is ≥100 mm Hg, treat with drugs.
- Oral agent of choice: methyldopa.

Magnesium sulfate is the treatment of choice for impending eclampsia or for preventing recurrent seizures. It should be given as a continuous intravenous infusion during labor and delivery and for at least

24 hours post partum. Monitor the patient's patellar reflex, urine output, and respirations while giving magnesium. The usual loading dose can be given in the setting of marked renal dysfunction, but subsequent dosing must be guided by frequent monitoring of blood levels. Calcium gluconate is the treatment of choice for magnesium toxicity and should be kept at the bedside.

- Magnesium sulfate: treatment of choice for impending eclampsia or for preventing recurrent seizures.
- Calcium gluconate: treatment of choice for magnesium toxicity.

Treatment of Hypertensive Crisis

The drugs of choice for treatment of hypertensive crisis during pregnancy are intravenous labetalol or oral nifedipine. Treatment with labetalol can be initiated with a 20-mg intravenous bolus. If the response is inadequate, 40 mg can be given 10 minutes later and, if necessary, 80 mg can be given at 10-minute intervals for 2 additional doses (maximal dose, 220 mg). If blood pressure is not controlled, an alternative drug should be considered. Nifedipine tablets (10-20 mg every 30 minutes to a maximum of 50 mg) can be used, but remember the precautions with nifedipine (tocolytic; interaction with magnesium sulfate causes profound hypotension). It is important to note that the FDA has not approved rapidly acting nifedipine for the treatment of hypertension. Hydralazine can be used but is associated with more maternal and perinatal adverse effects than the other agents. Treatment can be initiated with a 5- to 10-mg bolus, followed by 5 to 10 mg every 20 to 30 minutes until control is achieved and then repeated as needed (usually every 3 hours). Side effects include tachycardia and headache. Avoid giving hydralazine to women with congestive heart failure or asthma. Generally, sodium nitroprusside should be avoided (cyanide poisoning in the fetus); rarely, however, it may be needed for hypertension that does not respond to the drugs mentioned above. An infusion can be started at a rate of 0.25 mcg/kg per minute and increased as needed to a maximal rate of 5 mcg/kg per minute. Risk of fetal toxicity increases with infusions that last longer than 4 hours.

- The drug of choice for treating hypertensive crisis: labetalol administered intravenously.
- For hypertension refractory to labetalol, consider oral nifedipine or hydralazine intravenously.
- Administer sodium nitroprusside only if blood pressure does not respond to other drugs.

Pregnancy, Hypertension, and Renal Disease

Renal disease is a risk factor for preeclampsia. The combination of mild renal disease (serum creatinine <1.4 mg/dL) and preexisting hypertension or hypertension occurring early in pregnancy is associated with increased maternal and fetal complications with a 10-fold increase in relative risk of fetal loss. The renal disease usually does not progress. Moderate or severe renal insufficiency often worsens during pregnancy and is associated with a risk of hypertension developing, if not present before conception, that is more than 50%. Risk of fetal loss is high. Hypertension in this setting often has a volume component requiring the use of loop diuretics. Magnesium sulfate is potentially hazardous with severe renal insufficiency, and maintenance

doses must be reduced. For women on long-term dialysis, conception is generally discouraged because of significant maternal morbidity and lower fetal survival. All pregnancies in renal transplant recipients are considered high risk. Pregnancy should not be considered until at least 1.5 to 2 years after transplant, and creatinine should be stable and no more than 2.0 mg/dL.

- Renal disease is a risk factor for hypertension and for preeclampsia.
- Renal disease increases the risk of maternal morbidity and fetal loss.
- Moderate or severe renal insufficiency may progress during pregnancy.
- Conception is discouraged for women on long-term hemodialysis.
- Conception can be considered in renal transplant recipients after 2 years if renal function is stable and creatinine ≤2.0 mg/dL.

Hypertension and Breast-feeding

Elevated blood pressure may persist for 6 to 12 weeks after delivery in preeclampsia or gestational hypertension. Most antihypertensive drugs are compatible with breast-feeding, and all studied drugs are excreted into breast milk. Methyldopa and hydralazine have been shown to be safe. Propranolol and labetalol are the preferred β-blockers. ACEIs and ARBs should be avoided because their use may be associated with adverse neonatal renal effects, and diuretics may suppress milk volume. Regardless of the drug chosen, the infant should be carefully monitored for adverse effects.

- Most antihypertensive drugs are compatible with breast-feeding.
- Avoid ACEIs or ARBs.
- Diuretics may suppress milk production.

Hypertensive Emergencies and Urgencies

Acute or severe increases in blood pressure are serious medical concerns; prompt therapy may be lifesaving. Clinically, these situations can be classified either as hypertensive urgencies or as hypertensive emergencies (crisis).

Definitions

Hypertensive Emergency

The term *hypertensive emergency* is defined as severe hypertension or a sudden increase in blood pressure with evidence of acute injury to target organs (eg, brain, heart, kidney, vasculature, and retina). It implies the need for hospitalization to immediately lower blood pressure with parenteral therapy. Examples include malignant hypertension, hypertensive encephalopathy, aortic dissection, unstable angina, acute myocardial infarction, eclampsia, pulmonary edema, and acute renal failure. *Malignant hypertension* is a clinical syndrome associated with severe elevation of blood pressure that is frequently fatal if not treated promptly. It is characterized by a marked increase in peripheral vascular resistance due to systemic (angiotensin II) or locally generated (endothelin) vasoconstrictor substances. Any form of hypertension can progress to the malignant phase. Clinical features include severe hypertension (diastolic blood pressure >130 mm Hg), retinal hemorrhages and exudates, papilledema, oliguria, azotemia, nausea and vomiting, findings of heart failure, and encephalopathy. *Hypertensive encephalopathy* is the result of cerebral edema due to breakthrough hyperperfusion of the brain caused by severely increased blood pressure. Manifestations include papilledema, headache, confusion, somnolence, stupor, gastrointestinal tract distress, visual loss, focal neurologic deficits, coma, and seizures.

Fibrinoid necrosis of arterioles is the characteristic vascular lesion of malignant hypertension. Arteriolar injury worsens ischemia and promotes further release of vasoactive substances, setting up a vicious cycle. Microangiopathic hemolysis with fragmentation of erythrocytes and intravascular coagulation may occur with fibrinoid necrosis.

- Hypertensive emergency: severely elevated or suddenly increased blood pressure associated with acute injury to target organs.
- Hospitalization and parenteral therapy to decrease blood pressure immediately are required.
- Hypertensive encephalopathy: papilledema, headache, somnolence, confusion, stupor, gastrointestinal tract distress, visual loss, focal neurologic deficits, coma, and seizures.
- Malignant hypertension: a rapidly progressive vasospastic disorder.
- Angiotensin II levels are increased.
- If not reversed, blood vessel walls undergo necrosis.

Hypertensive Urgency

The term *hypertensive urgency* is defined as severe hypertension without evidence of acute target organ injury but occurring in a setting in which it is important to decrease blood pressure to safer levels over a 24- to 48-hour period. Oral therapy in the outpatient setting is often adequate. Examples include severe hypertension in a person with known coronary artery disease, an aneurysm of the aorta (or other site), or a history of congestive heart failure or severe hypertension immediately following major surgery. *Accelerated hypertension* is a subacute, progressive increase in blood pressure associated with hemorrhages and exudates (but not papilledema) on retinal examination. If left untreated, it may progress to malignant hypertension.

- Hypertensive urgency: severe hypertension without acute target organ injury.
- Treatment is administered orally and hospitalization usually is not required.
- Accelerated hypertension may progress to malignant hypertension if not treated.

Causes

The causes of hypertensive urgencies and emergencies include the development of accelerated-malignant hypertension on the background of neglected essential hypertension (approximately 7% of cases of untreated hypertension progress to the malignant phase), sudden discontinuation of antihypertensive therapy (especially multidrug programs or programs containing clonidine and β-blockers), renovascular disease, collagen vascular diseases (especially scleroderma), eclampsia, acute glomerulonephritis, pheochromocytoma, monoamine oxidase inhibitors and tyramine-containing foods, intracerebral or subarachnoid hemorrhage, acute aortic dissection, acute head injury, and acute stroke. Approximately 50% of hypertensive crises occur in persons with preexisting hypertension.

- Common causes of hypertensive urgencies and emergencies: neglected essential hypertension, discontinuation of antihypertensive therapy, renovascular disease, scleroderma, pheochromocytoma, and stroke.

Evaluation and Management

Persons with hypertensive emergencies should be hospitalized in an intensive care unit. An arterial catheter should be inserted to monitor blood pressure continuously. In addition to a focused history (eg, compliance with previously prescribed medications, use of blood pressure–raising drugs) and examination (retinal examination is mandatory), initial laboratory studies should include chest radiography, electrocardiography, creatinine or blood urea nitrogen, urinalysis, glucose, sodium, potassium, hemoglobin, and blood smear (to look for fragmented erythrocytes). Studies to determine the underlying cause should be deferred. The challenge of treating hypertensive emergencies is to lower blood pressure promptly without compromising the function of vital organs. Blood pressure should be lowered quickly to a diastolic level of approximately 110 mm Hg (reduce mean blood pressure by 20%), followed by careful monitoring for evidence of worsening cerebral, renal, or cardiac function. Blood pressure is then gradually decreased to a diastolic level of 90 to 100 mm Hg. Ischemic pancreatitis and intestinal infarction are potential serious complications.

Generally, *sodium nitroprusside* is the drug of choice, but caution should be observed in states of increased intracranial pressure. It must be given in an intensive care setting, with an arterial catheter in place. This balanced arterial and venous dilator decreases both preload and afterload. The dose is 0.25 to 10.0 mcg/kg per minute by intravenous infusion. Adjustments in dose can be made at 5-minute intervals until the blood pressure goal is achieved. The infusion must be protected from light. Toxicity is related to the metabolism of nitroprusside to cyanide in erythrocytes (metabolic acidosis). Thus, thiocyanate levels should be monitored every 48 hours and therapy discontinued if the blood level is greater than 12 mg/dL. The risk is greater in the presence of renal disease. Sodium nitrite or hydroxocobalamin (25 mg per hour) can be infused in case of toxicity. Side effects of sodium nitroprusside include nausea, vomiting, agitation, disorientation, psychosis, muscular twitching, coarse tremor, and flushing. Frequently, patients with malignant hypertension are volume depleted because of pressure natriuresis. However, as blood pressure decreases, fluid retention occurs and the addition of a loop diuretic is often required.

- Sodium nitroprusside: the drug of choice for a hypertensive emergency.
- Toxicity is related to the metabolism of nitroprusside to cyanide in erythrocytes.
- Monitor thiocyanate levels every 48 hours.
- In case of toxicity, infuse sodium nitrite or hydroxocobalamin.
- Sodium nitroprusside side effects: nausea, vomiting, agitation, muscular twitching, coarse tremor, and flushing.

Several alternative parenteral agents are available for the management of hypertensive emergencies and urgencies.

Labetalol is a combination α-blocker and nonselective β-blocker with an onset of action of 5 to 10 minutes. It can be given in repetitive intravenous miniboluses of 20 to 80 mg or as a constant infusion at a dose of 0.5 to 2 mg per minute. Its duration of action is 3 to 6 hours. It can be used in most situations except acute heart failure. It is especially useful for postoperative hypertension, acute aortic dissection, and hypertensive crisis of pregnancy. The same cautions and contraindications apply to this drug as to other β-blockers (asthma and heart block). Adverse effects include scalp tingling, vomiting, heart block, and orthostatic hypotension.

Glyceryl trinitrate (nitroglycerin) is a direct arteriolar and venous vasodilator with an onset of action of 2 to 5 minutes and with a duration of action of 3 to 5 minutes. It is given as a constant infusion of 5 to 100 mcg per minute. This drug decreases myocardial oxygen demand by decreasing preload and afterload. It dilates epicardial coronary arteries and collaterals. Tolerance can develop with prolonged infusion. It is especially useful if acute coronary ischemia or acute congestive heart failure is present. Adverse effects include headache, flushing, nausea, and methemoglobinemia.

Hydralazine is a direct arteriolar vasodilator with an onset of action of 10 to 20 minutes if given intravenously and 20 to 30 minutes if given intramuscularly. The usual dose is 10 to 20 mg intravenously or 10 to 50 mg intramuscularly. Its duration of action is 3 to 8 hours. Hydralazine is used primarily to treat hypertensive crisis of pregnancy. Adverse effects include headache, flushing, nausea, vomiting, and myocardial ischemia (due to reflex increases in heart rate and stroke volume). Use of the drug should be avoided in acute aortic dissection and states of myocardial ischemia. Hydrozones form when hydralazine is mixed with dextrose.

Esmolol is a cardioselective β-blocker with an onset of action of 1 to 2 minutes and a duration of action of 10 to 20 minutes. It is given as a constant intravenous infusion in a dose of 50 to 300 mcg/kg per minute. Esmolol is useful in postoperative hypertension, aortic dissection, and ischemic heart disease. It is often used in combination with vasodilators for effective control of blood pressure. The cautions and contraindications that apply to β-blockers also apply to this drug. Adverse effects include nausea and bradycardia.

Enalaprilat is an ACEI with an onset of action of 15 minutes and a duration of action of 6 hours. It is given intravenously in doses of 1.25 to 5 mg every 6 hours, with a maximal dose of 20 mg in 24 hours or a smaller dose if renal disease is present. It is useful in postoperative hypertension and in settings of acute heart failure. Adverse effects include ACEI side effects, a precipitous decrease in blood pressure in high renin states (volume depletion), and an acute decline in renal function if renal artery disease is present. Its use should be avoided in pregnancy.

Nicardipine is a dihydropyridine CCB with an onset of action of 5 to 10 minutes and a duration of action of 1 to 4 hours. It is given as a constant intravenous infusion of 5 to 15 mg per hour. It is useful for postoperative hypertension. Nicardipine should not be given in the setting of acute heart failure. Adverse effects include headache, nausea, flushing, and phlebitis.

Phentolamine is an α-blocker that is administered intravenously in doses of 5 to 15 mg. The duration of action of a single bolus is approximately 15 minutes. It is most effective for states of catecholamine excess (discontinuation of use of clonidine, interaction between monoamine oxidase inhibitor and tyramine-containing food) and is the drug of choice if pheochromocytoma is suspected. Adverse effects include tachycardia and flushing.

Fenoldopam is a selective dopamine receptor (D_1) agonist that is given by constant intravenous infusion of 0.1 to 1.6 mg/kg per minute. It causes arteriolar vasodilatation. The onset of action is within 5 minutes and offset is over 30 to 60 minutes. This drug is useful with impaired renal function because it increases renal blood flow and sodium excretion. Side effects are nausea, vomiting, headache, and flushing.

Diazoxide is considered obsolete with the availability of newer and safer drugs.

- Glyceryl trinitrate (nitroglycerin) is useful in acute congestive heart failure or coronary ischemia.
- Tolerance can develop to glyceryl trinitrate.
- Labetalol and hydralazine are used for hypertensive crisis of pregnancy.
- Avoid use of hydralazine in acute myocardial infarction or angina and in dissecting aortic aneurysm.
- Esmolol, enalaprilat, and nicardipine are useful for postoperative hypertension.
- Phentolamine is the drug of choice if pheochromocytoma is suspected.
- Fenoldopam increases renal blood flow and sodium excretion.

As soon as possible, initiate regular oral treatment and taper intravenous treatment. After blood pressure has been controlled, search for the cause of the hypertensive crisis and consider secondary causes, especially renovascular disease, pheochromocytoma, and primary aldosteronism.

- Typical clinical scenario: A 54-year-old man has a 12-year history of hypertension. It was controlled with a combination of hydrochlorothiazide, clonidine, and amlodipine. Because of cost and side effects, the patient stopped all therapy abruptly 3 weeks ago. Over the past 2 days, a headache of increasing severity has developed. His wife has noted that he is confused and his speech is slurred; this prompted his visit to the office. On examination, the patient is stuporous and confused. His speech is slurred. Blood pressure is 230/140 mm Hg and the pulse is 115 beats per minute. Retinal hemorrhages and papilledema are noted. Rales are present in both lung bases. A third heart sound (S_3) gallop is noted. A chest radiograph shows findings of pulmonary edema. The creatinine level is 2.4 mg/dL. Erythrocytes are noted on urinalysis.

Hypertension Pharmacy Review
John G. O'Meara, PharmD

Drug (Trade Name)	Dose, mg	Frequency per Day	Toxic/Adverse Effects	Drug Interactions	Comments
Diuretics					
Thiazide-type (selected)			Glucose intolerance & insulin resistance, hyperlipidemia, hyperuricemia, hypokalemia, hyponatremia, hypomagnesemia	Lithium (increased lithium levels), NSAIDs (decreased diuretic effectiveness), bile acid sequestrants (decreased thiazide absorption)	Preferred in JNC 7 as the initial drug choice for most, either alone or in combination
Hydrochlorothiazide (HydroDIURIL, Esidrix)	12.5-50	1			Metolazone & indapamide may be effective in renally impaired patients
Chlorthalidone (Hygroton)	12.5-25	1			Lower doses avoid adverse metabolic effects
Indapamide (Lozol)	1.25-2.5	1			May be favorable for patients with concurrent osteoporosis (decreased renal calcium elimination)
Metolazone (Zaroxolyn, Diulo)	2.5-5	1			Effective for isolated hypertension in the elderly
Metolazone (Mykrox)	0.5-1	1			
Loop			Similar to thiazide-type agents except may cause hypocalcemia; monitor for dehydration, circulatory collapse, metabolic alkalosis	Similar to thiazides	Reserved for hypertensive patients with renal insufficiency
Bumetanide (Bumex)	0.5-2	2			
Ethacrynic acid (Edecrin)	25-100	2			
Furosemide (Lasix)	20-80	2			
Torsemide (Demadex)	2.5-10	1	Ototoxicity (usually associated with rapid IV injection, severe renal impairment, high doses, or concurrent use of other ototoxic drugs)		
Potassium-sparing			Hyperkalemia	Potassium supplements, ACEIs, ARBs (all increase risk of hyperkalemia); dofetilide (decreased renal elimination of dofetilide, with potential cardiac toxicity)	Weak diuretics alone; used in combination with other diuretics to avoid hypokalemia
Amiloride (Midamor)	5-10	1 or 2			
Triamterene (Dyrenium)	50-100	1 or 2			
Adrenergic inhibitors					
α_1-Blockers			Postural hypotension, tachycardia, dizziness, headache	Midodrine (decreased midodrine effectiveness)	Avoid "first-dose syncope" by starting with a low dose given at bedtime
Doxazosin (Cardura)	1-16	1			Not considered first-line agents because of negative ALLHAT trial outcomes with doxazosin
Prazosin (Minipress)	2-20	2 or 3			
Terazosin (Hytrin)	1-20	1 or 2			

Hypertension Pharmacy Review (continued)

Drug (Trade Name)	Dose, mg	Frequency per Day	Toxic/Adverse Effects	Drug Interactions	Comments
Adrenergic inhibitors (continued)					
β-Blockers (cardioselective)			Bronchospasm, brady-cardia, decreased exercise tolerance, may mask symptoms of insulin-induced hypoglycemia, im-paired peripheral circulation, insomnia, fatigue, decreased exercise tolerance, increased triglycerides (except agents with ISA), decreased HDL cholesterol	Non-DHP CCBs (heart block), sympathomimetics (unopposed α-adrenergic stimula-tion)	Acebutolol, carteolol, penbutolol, pindolol possess ISA
Acebutolol (Sectral)	200-800	2			Contraindications: sinus bradycardia, ≥2nd degree heart block, cardiogenic shock, & asthma/severe COPD
Atenolol (Tenormin)	25-100	1			
Betaxolol (Kerlone)	5-20	1			
Bisoprolol (Zebeta)	2.5-10	1			
Metoprolol (Lopressor, Toprol XL)	50-100	1 or 2			
β-Blockers (noncardioselective)					
Carteolol (Cartrol)	2.5-10	1			
Nadolol (Corgard)	40-120	1			
Penbutolol (Levatol)	10-40	1			
Pindolol (Visken)	10-40	2			
Propranolol (Inderal)	40-480	2			
Timolol (Blocadren)	20-60	2			
α-β-Blockers			Postural hypotension, bronchospasm, hepatotoxicity (labetolol)	Rifampin (decreased carvedilol plasma concentration)	
Carvedilol (Coreg)	12.5-50	2			
Labetolol (Trandate, Normodyne)	200-800	2			
Central α-agonists			Sedation, dry mouth, withdrawal hyperten-sion, depression Hepatic & autoim-mune disorders (methyldopa)	β-Blockers, tricyclic antidepressants (de-creased antihyper-tensive effectiveness)	Avoid abrupt withdrawal of clonidine (rebound hypertension) Methyldopa is the preferred antihypertensive in pregnancy
Clonidine (Catapres)	0.2-0.8	2 or 3			
Clonidine (Catapres-TTS)	0.1-0.3	Weekly (patch)			
Guanabenz (Wytensin)	8-32	2			
Guanfacine (Tenex)	0.5-2	1			
Methyldopa (Aldomet)	250-1,000	2			
Peripheral agents			Postural hypotension, diarrhea, depression, sedation, peptic ulcer	Tricyclic antidepres-sants (decreased antihypertensive effectiveness)	Reserpine contraindicated in depression, active peptic ulcer, ulcerative colitis
Guanadrel (Hylorel)	10-75	2			
Guanethidine (Ismelin)	10-150	1			
Reserpine (Serpasil)	0.05-0.25	1			

Hypertension Pharmacy Review (continued)

Drug (Trade Name)	Dose, mg	Frequency per Day	Toxic/Adverse Effects	Drug Interactions	Comments
Calcium channel antagonists					
DHPs			Edema, headache, flushing, postural dizziness, tachycardia, gingival hyperplasia	CYP3A4 inhibitors (may increase CCB plasma concentrations) CYP3A4 inducers (eg, rifampin, carbamazepine, barbiturates) may decrease plasma CCB concentrations	Immediate-release nifedipine not recommended for severe hypertension Long-acting DHPs effective for isolated systolic hypertension in the elderly
Nisoldipine (Sular)	10-40	1			
Nifedipine (Procardia XL, Adalat CC)	30-120	1			
Nicardipine (Cardene)	60-120	2			
Isradipine (DynaCirc)	2.5-10	2			
Felodipine (Plendil)	2.5-20	1			
Amlodipine (Norvasc)	2.5-10	1			
Non-DHPs			AV nodal block, brady-cardia, worsening systolic function; constipation (verapamil), rash (diltiazem)	Diltiazem & verapamil (CYP3A4 inhibitors) increase plasma levels of benzodiazepine, carbamazepine, tacrolimus, cyclo-sporine, lovastatin, simvastatin, pimozide, protease inhibitors, rifabutin, & ergot alkaloid	Non-DHPs contraindicated in ≥2nd degree AV block
Diltiazem (Cardizem, Tiamate, Tiazac, Dilacor, Diltia)	120-540	1 or 2			
Verapamil (Calan, Isoptin, Verelan, Covera HS)	120-480	1 or 2			
Direct vasodilators					
Hydralazine (Apresoline)	25-100	2	Headache, palpitations, tachycardia, angina, sodium & water retention, SLE (hydralazine), hyper-trichosis (minoxidil)	Diuretics, hypotensive agents, MAO inhibitors	Use both agents with a β-blocker & diuretic to minimize reflex tachy-cardia & fluid retention
Minoxidil (Loniten)	2.5-80	1 or 2			
ACEIs					
Benazepril (Lotensin)	10-40	1 or 2	Cough (~15%), dizzi-ness, rash, hyperka-lemia, angioedema (rare)	Potassium-sparing diuretics, potassium salts (increased risk of hyperkalemia), lithium (increased lithium levels), NSAIDs (decreased ACEI effectiveness)	Contraindicated in preg-nancy, renal artery stenosis (bilateral or solitary kidney) First-line agents for hyper-tensives with left ventricular dysfunction or heart failure Preferred in hypertensive diabetics with nephropathy
Captopril (Capoten)	12.5-100	2 or 3			
Enalapril (Vasotec)	2.5-40	1 or 2			
Fosinopril (Monopril)	10-40	1			
Lisinopril (Zestril, Prinivil)	10-40	1			
Moexipril (Univasc)	7.5-30	1			
Perindopril (Aceon)	4-8	1 or 2			
Quinapril (Accupril)	10-40	1			
Ramipril (Altace)	2.5-20	1			
Trandolapril (Mavik)	1-4	1			
Angiotensin II antagonists					
Losartan (Cozaar)	25-100	1 or 2	Similar to ACEIs but lower incidence of cough		Contraindicated in preg-nancy, renal artery stenosis (bilateral or solitary kidney); alternative for patients with ACEI-induced cough
Valsartan (Diovan)	80-320	1			
Irbesartan (Avapro)	150-300	1			
Candesartan (Atacand)	8-32	1			
Telmisartan (Micardis)	20-80	1			
Eprosartan (Teveten)	400-800	1 or 2			
Olmesartan (Benicar)	20-40	1			

Hypertension Pharmacy Review (continued)

Drug (Trade Name)	Dose, mg	Frequency per Day	Toxic/Adverse Effects	Drug Interactions	Comments
Aldosterone receptor antagonists					
Eplerenone (Inspra)	50-100	1 or 2	Hyperkalemia, hyper-triglyceridemia	ACEIs, ARBs, blockers, potassium supplements, & potassium-sparing diuretics (all increase risk of hyperkalemia), CYP3A4 inhibitors (increased levels of eplerenone)	Contraindications: serum potassium >5.5 mEq/L; type 2 diabetes with microalbuminuria; serum creatinine >2.0 mg/dL in males or >1.8 mg/dL in females; creatinine clearance <50 mL/min; concomitant use with potassium supplements or potassium-sparing diuretics, strong CYP3A4 inhibitors
Spironolactone (Aldactone)	25-50	1 or 2	Hyperkalemia, gynecomastia	Potassium supplements, ACEIs, ARBs, (all increase risk of hyperkalemia)	Avoid in renal impairment (serum creatinine >2.5 mg/dL)
Renin-angiotensin system antagonists					
Aliskiren (Tekturna)	150-300	1	Dose-related adverse effects (diarrhea), rash, angioedema (rare)	Furosemide (significantly decreased furosemide serum levels), ketoconazole (significantly increased aliskiren serum levels)	Contraindicated in pregnancy

Abbreviations: ACEI, angiotensin-converting enzyme inhibitor; ALLHAT, Antihypertensive and Lipid-Lowering Treatment to Prevent Heart Attack Trial; ARB, angiotensin II receptor blocker; AV, atrioventricular; CCB, calcium channel blocker; COPD, chronic obstructive pulmonary disease; DHP, dihydropyridine; HDL, high-density lipoprotein; ISA, intrinsic sympathomimetic activity; IV, intravenous; JNC 7, The Seventh Report of the Joint National Committee on Prevention, Detection, Evaluation, and Treatment of High Blood Pressure: the JNC 7 report (JAMA 2003;289:2560-72); MAO, monoamine oxidase; NSAID, nonsteroidal anti-inflammatory drug; SLE, systemic lupus erythematosus.

Questions

Multiple Choice (choose the best answer)

1. A 56-year-old man is referred for evaluation of treatment-resistant hypertension. He has a 9-year history of high blood pressure (BP). There is a family history of hypertension in his father. The patient's BP measured at home averages 160/94 mm Hg despite current therapy, which consists of hydrochlorothiazide 25 mg daily, losartan 100 mg daily, metoprolol tartrate 100 mg daily, and potassium chloride 40 mEq daily. He tolerates these medications well and is compliant with therapy. He attempts to eat a low-sodium diet but eats in restaurants 4 to 6 times per week. He is 4.5 kg overweight and sedentary. He denies use of excess alcohol or other drugs or herbal medications that might increase his BP or interfere with the actions of his medications. Examination is normal except for BP 165/96 mm Hg and pulse 52 beats per minute. Results of laboratory studies include the following: creatinine 1.2 mg/dL, sodium 144 mEq/L, potassium 3.6 mEq/L (reference range, 3.6-4.8 mEq/L), glucose 89 mg/dL, cholesterol 180 mg/dL, and triglycerides 160 mg/dL. The urinalysis is normal. Which is the next most appropriate step in the evaluation or treatment of this patient?

    a. Obtain a 24-hour ambulatory BP to exclude pseudoresistant hypertension from a white-coat effect.
    b. Optimize control of extracellular volume by increasing hydrochlorothiazide to 50 mg daily.
    c. Perform duplex ultrasonography of the renal arteries.
    d. Obtain plasma free metanephrines.
    e. Obtain plasma renin and aldosterone concentrations to screen for primary aldosteronism.

2. Over several office visits, a 34-year-old woman has an average BP of 145/102 mm Hg. Both of her parents and an older sibling have hypertension. She is a nonsmoker, and there is no history of diabetes mellitus or hyperlipidemia. Results of a physical examination and routine laboratory studies are normal. She is recently married and is actively trying to get pregnant. In addition to lifestyle recommendations, what is the most appropriate drug to consider for blood pressure reduction?

    a. Aliskiren
    b. Methyldopa
    c. Lisinopril
    d. Hydralazine
    e. Losartan

3. An 89-year-old man is sent to the emergency department from the local nursing home with complaints of headache, chest pain, and diaphoresis. Evaluation disclosed evidence of an acute inferior myocardial infarction. His BP is 210/115 mm Hg, and a loud epigastric bruit is heard over the epigastrium. He has a long-standing history of hypertension that had been previously well controlled. Other diagnoses include type 2 diabetes mellitus and dementia. He is admitted to the coronary care unit and has an uneventful hospital course. His BP is controlled with the addition of lisinopril (10 mg daily) to his program of hydrochlorothiazide (25 mg daily), atenolol (50 mg daily), and amlodipine (5 mg daily). His creatinine remains stable at 1.5 mg/dL, and his potassium remains normal with the use of lisinopril. What is the next most appropriate step in the management of this patient?

    a. Perform duplex ultrasonography of the renal arteries.
    b. Perform magnetic resonance angiography of the renal arteries.
    c. Measure plasma free metanephrines.
    d. Dismiss the patient to the nursing home with appropriate follow-up care.
    e. Perform renal angiography and consider angioplasty and stent placement.

4. A 78-year-old woman had total knee arthroplasty 2 days ago. She has a 35-year history of hypertension treated with hydrochlorothiazide (25 mg daily) and atenolol (50 mg daily). She complains of substernal chest pressure and dyspnea. An electrocardiogram shows ST-segment depression in the inferior leads. Her BP is 220/110 mm Hg, which is confirmed on subsequent measurement. What is the most appropriate parenteral antihypertensive drug to consider for this patient?

    a. Sodium nitroprusside
    b. Hydralazine
    c. Labetalol
    d. Nitroglycerin
    e. Nicardipine

5. A 56-year-old man has a history of hypertension for the past 16 years. He is currently taking atenolol (50 mg daily). Laboratory assessment reveals a creatinine of 1.8 mg/dL. A urinalysis shows evidence of proteinuria. Renal ultrasonography findings are normal. A 24-hour urine collection demonstrates 1.3 g of total protein. Urine and serum protein electrophoresis are negative for monoclonal protein. What is the most appropriate BP goal for this patient?

    a. Less than 120/80 mm Hg
    b. Less than 140/90 mm Hg
    c. Less than 130/80 mm Hg
    d. Less than 125/75 mm Hg
    e. Less than 135/85 mm Hg

6. You are evaluating a 54-year-old man for recently diagnosed hypertension. He donates blood regularly, and his BP had been 120/76 mm Hg consistently. However, a BP of 180/110 mm Hg was recorded recently, and several BP readings over the past 2 weeks have confirmed stage 2 hypertension. He is unaware of a family history of high blood pressure. He has had mild occipital headaches in the mornings, which are new, but he is otherwise asymptomatic. At present, he is taking no medications

and denies the use of over-the-counter medications or alcohol. He has a 30 pack-year history of smoking and a high cholesterol level that is diet managed. There is no history of diabetes mellitus. He has no history of coronary artery disease or stroke. Physical examination findings are normal except that his BP is 184/108 mm Hg. Results of routine laboratory studies are normal with the exception of an elevated total and low-density lipoprotein cholesterol. What is the most appropriate next step in the evaluation or management of this patient?

a. Discuss lifestyle modifications and closely follow the BP response over the next 3 months.
b. Begin antihypertensive drug therapy with hydrochlorothiazide (25 mg daily) and recheck BP in 4 weeks.
c. Discuss lifestyle recommendations and begin drug treatment with a 2-drug combination.
d. Begin treatment with lifestyle recommendations and a 2-drug combination that includes a diuretic, and consider evaluation for secondary hypertension.
e. Obtain a 24-hour ambulatory BP to confirm hypertension before initiating therapy.

7. A 61-year-old woman has a history of difficult-to-control hypertension that was brought under good control with the addition of captopril to her program of hydrochlorothiazide and amlodipine. However, 3 months later, the sudden onset of severe tongue, lip, and throat swelling required emergency resuscitation. A diagnosis was made of angioedema associated with angiotensin-converting enzyme inhibitor (ACEI). Symptoms did not recur after discontinuation of the drug, but her BP increased. She has no history of heart or renal disease. What is the most appropriate next step?

a. Given her good BP response to captopril, consider adding a non-sulfhydryl–containing ACEI to her program.
b. Avoid ACEIs, but consider the addition of an angiotensin II receptor blocker (ARB) to her program.
c. Avoid ACEIs and ARBs. Consider adding a β-blocker to her program.
d. Obtain a renal angiogram to assess for renovascular hypertension.
e. Switch her to a more potent loop diuretic for better BP control.

Answers

1.   Answer e.

Several considerations should be made when a patient presents with presumed treatment-resistant hypertension. Common causes are noncompliance with the treatment program (medications and dietary sodium intake) or the use of drugs that increase BP or interfere with the effectiveness of BP-lowering medications such as nonsteroidal anti-inflammatory drugs. This patient denies use of interfering drugs and does not provide any clues to suggest noncompliance with medication. The resting bradycardia suggests compliance with the β-blocker. Since he eats several meals weekly in restaurants, his dietary sodium intake is probably higher than ideal. Out-of-office measures of BP should be assessed to discriminate true resistant hypertension from a white-coat effect. In this case, home readings are elevated and similar to office BP measures. When these causes have been eliminated, the possibility of a secondary form of hypertension should be considered. Primary aldosteronism is now recognized as the most common treatable secondary cause of hypertension. This diagnosis should be considered in patients with hypokalemia regardless of presumed cause. The widespread use of ACEIs and ARBs has uncovered a group of patients at increased risk of this disorder. Because ACEIs and ARBs inhibit aldosterone production, their use is usually associated with an increase in plasma potassium level; thus, hypokalemia is quite uncommon. Therefore, low plasma potassium or the need for potassium supplements despite use of full doses of an ACEI or an ARB, with or without concomitant diuretic therapy as in this case, is a tip-off to the possibility of primary aldosteronism. If present, high dietary sodium intake worsens BP and potassium losses. Further evaluation of this patient should include screening for this disorder by determining the ratio of plasma aldosterone concentration to plasma renin activity, which has fair diagnostic accuracy. If the ratio is greater than 15 to 20, confirmatory testing should be performed. One of the most common issues accounting for poor control in treatment-resistant hypertension is lack of control of extracellular fluid volume. Full doses of a diuretic appropriate for the level of renal function are often needed to effectively decrease the BP. If a secondary cause of hypertension is not found in this patient, encouraging a low-sodium diet and increasing the diuretic dose would be appropriate steps in gaining BP control.

2.   Answer b.

Because this patient has stage 2 hypertension, drug therapy should be considered initially along with lifestyle modifications. She intends to become pregnant, so drug selection should be based on safety considerations for a fetus. Methyldopa is the most completely studied drug and is considered safe in pregnancy. Therefore, it is the drug of choice in this setting. Other drugs could be considered. The only classes of drugs that are absolutely contraindicated in pregnancy are ACEIs, ARBs, and direct renin inhibitors. These drugs can cause fetal growth retardation, fetal anomalies, and death. Recent studies suggest that these drugs can induce harm even during the first trimester. Therefore, they should not be given to a sexually active woman who is trying to become pregnant. Hydralazine is inappropriate as oral monotherapy for hypertension and is best used as a third agent in combination with a diuretic and an adrenergic inhibitor.

3.   Answer d.

This patient has a history consistent with essential hypertension. The presence of an abdominal bruit in combination with the apparent sudden worsening of his BP and good response to ACEI therapy suggests the possibility of superimposed renovascular hypertension. However, because correction of renovascular disease involves invasive procedures that are associated with significant potential risks (eg, atheroemboli, renal artery dissection or thrombosis, and contrast nephropathy), further evaluation in this setting should be limited to patients with refractory hypertension or progressive renal dysfunction. Because BP is well controlled and renal function is stable, no further evaluation for renovascular disease is necessary at this time. Pheochromocytoma is a rare condition that would not be a strong consideration in this patient. Screening in low-risk settings can be complicated by having to evaluate false-positive results.

4.   Answer d.

This represents a hypertensive emergency, which is defined as severe hypertension in the presence of acute target organ injury. Thus, immediately lowering her BP with a parenteral agent is indicated. Of the available agents, nitroglycerin is preferred in the setting of acute myocardial ischemia. It is a balanced arteriolar and venous dilator and lessens myocardial oxygen requirements by reducing both preload and afterload. Hydralazine is a direct arteriolar dilator and increases myocardial oxygen demand by increasing heart rate and stroke volume. Therefore, it is contraindicated in myocardial ischemia. The other options listed would be acceptable second-line agents. Of these, sodium nitroprusside is the most extensively studied.

5.   Answer c.

The primary goal of treating hypertension is to reduce cardiovascular, cerebrovascular, and renal morbidity and mortality. Treatment to a goal BP of less than 140/90 mm Hg has been associated in prospective trials with a lessening of cardiovascular and cerebrovascular events in the general hypertensive population. Because of greater risk relationships of BP with diabetes mellitus, chronic kidney disease, or coronary artery disease, a lower goal of less than 130/80 mm Hg is recommended in the presence of these comorbid conditions. An even lower goal of less than 120/80 mm Hg is advised if congestive heart failure is present. Evidence for the benefits of a lower BP goal in patients with chronic kidney disease is strongest in the subset with 24-hour protein excretion of 1 g or more.

6.   Answer d.

This patient has stage 2 hypertension. Current guidelines suggest initiating treatment with lifestyle modifications and 2 antihypertensive drugs, 1 of which should be a diuretic appropriate for the level of renal function. In addition, this patient has several features that are inconsistent with essential hypertension. These include onset after 50 years of age, stage 2 hypertension at diagnosis, and lack of a family history of hypertension. It would be appropriate to consider secondary causes. Renovascular disease and primary aldosteronism are the most common of the traditional secondary forms of hypertension. The presence of atherosclerotic risk factors (eg, tobacco use and elevated cholesterol) increases the risk of renovascular hypertension, which should be a strong consideration. In patients with renovascular hypertension, an audible bruit on abdominal examination is observed in only 50% of cases, so the lack of a bruit should not preclude further evaluation if other clinical predictors are present. White-coat hypertension is unlikely with the observation of elevated BP readings outside the clinic setting.

7.   Answer c.

Angioedema is a rare but potentially life-threatening complication of all ACEIs. This complication has also been observed with ARB and direct renin inhibitor (aliskiren) therapy. Thus, in general, patients who experience angioedema with ACEIs should not be given ARBs or direct renin inhibitor drugs. This is especially true if the episode of angioedema was severe and without an alternative cause or if the indication for the use of 1 of these agents is not compelling. The major indication for the use of loop diuretics in hypertension is the presence of renal insufficiency. Blood pressure response to a drug that inhibits the renin-angiotensin-aldosterone system by itself is not a strong predictor of the presence of underlying renovascular disease. β-Blockers suppress renin activity and may be a reasonable alternative choice in this situation.

15

Infectious Diseases

Abinash Virk, MD
Robert Orenstein, DO
Lynn L. Estes, PharmD
John W. Wilson, MD

Part I

Abinash Virk, MD

This chapter approaches the field of infectious diseases from 3 perspectives. The first section reviews the characteristics of specific pathogenic organisms, the second covers clinical syndromes associated with various infections, and the third section reviews the antimicrobial drugs.

Specific Microorganisms

Gram-Positive Cocci

Group A β-Hemolytic Streptococci: *Streptococcus pyogenes*

Infections
Group A streptococci are reemerging as an important cause of human disease. They are responsible for several different clinical syndromes. *Streptococcus pyogenes* is the most common cause of bacterial pharyngitis. Although the pharyngitis is usually self-limited, antibiotic therapy (penicillin) should be given to prevent acute rheumatic fever. Penicillin also will shorten the duration of symptoms if it is given within the first 24 hours of infection. Rapid diagnostic tests for streptococcal pharyngitis are easily administered and are specific but not as sensitive (50%-70%) as a throat culture for detecting *S pyogenes*. The sensitivity of a rapid polymerase chain reaction test (LightCycler) for group A streptococci is 93%. Common complications of streptococcal pharyngitis include paratonsillar abscesses, otitis media, and sinusitis.

- Common complications of streptococcal pharyngitis include paratonsillar abscesses, otitis media, and sinusitis.

Streptococcus pyogenes is a virulent organism that is responsible for many skin and soft tissue infections. Several terms are used to differentiate these by the depth of infection and resulting clinical appearance.

Impetigo describes a superficial skin infection (Figure 15-1). Historically, *S pyogenes* was the most common cause of impetigo. Since the 1980s, however, most cases of impetigo have been caused by *Staphylococcus aureus* or mixed infections with both *S aureus* and β-hemolytic streptococci.

Erysipelas is an infection of the skin with involvement of cutaneous lymphatic vessels. It often occurs on the face and produces a raised, violaceous rash with a well-demarcated border. This infection

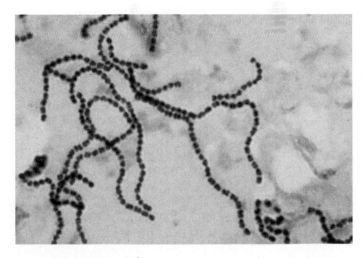

Figure 15-1. Chaining of β-Hemolytic *Streptococcus* in a Blood Culture (Gram Stain).

is painful and most often occurs in the elderly. Recent reports have associated erysipelas with "toxic strep" syndrome.

In *cellulitis*, the infection involves the skin and subcutaneous tissue. Cellulitis is most common in tissue damaged by trauma and in extremities with impaired venous or lymphatic drainage (eg, the arm after mastectomy or the leg after saphenous vein harvest for coronary artery bypass grafting). Minor inflammation or skin tears from tinea pedis may serve as a portal of entry for β-hemolytic streptococci. Recurrent cellulitis may develop in patients with history of dermatitis, malignancy, and a prior history of ipsilateral limb cellulitis.

Invasive Group A Streptococcal Infection

Since the mid 1980s, there have been increasing reports of severe group A streptococcal infection, including necrotizing fasciitis, myonecrosis, and a toxic shock–like syndrome. Suggested causes for the increase include the spread of virulent strains (especially M1 and M3), specific virulence factors (streptococcal pyogenic exotoxin and proteases), and a lack of immunity to these strains in the affected patients. In an outbreak of streptococcal necrotizing fasciitis in Minnesota, schoolchildren served as a reservoir for the responsible organism. Victims were mostly older and in poor health.

The overall mortality rate of streptococcal necrotizing fasciitis is 30%, even in previously healthy patients and with appropriate treatment. Many victims require amputation or extensive débridement of affected tissues. Effective treatment requires early recognition of the illness with prompt initiation of antibiotics, along with early and aggressive surgical débridement of devitalized tissue when indicated.

Unlike many other pathogens, group A streptococci remain exquisitely susceptible to the penicillins. The cephalosporins (first-generation) and vancomycin are effective alternative drugs. Erythromycin-resistant strains are reported but are so far uncommon in the United States. There is mounting evidence that clindamycin in combination with penicillin is the most effective antibiotic for treating streptococcal necrotizing fasciitis.

- Clindamycin in combination with penicillin is the most effective antibiotic for treating streptococcal necrotizing fasciitis.

Toxins

Group A streptococci produce many disease-causing exotoxins. Scarlet fever may develop in persons with no previous immunity to erythrogenic toxin. Production of hyaluronidase causes the rapidly advancing margins characteristic of cellulitis due to β-hemolytic streptococci. Streptococcal exotoxin A is similar to the toxin produced by *S aureus*, which causes toxic shock syndrome.

Nonsuppurative Complications

The nonsuppurative complications of group A streptococcal infection are *acute rheumatic fever* and *acute glomerulonephritis*. In the United States, there was a resurgence of acute rheumatic fever among children and military recruits during the 1980s. Treatment of group A streptococcal infection does not prevent poststreptococcal glomerulonephritis.

Rheumatic fever occurs only after streptococcal pharyngitis, never after skin infections. The diagnostic criteria for rheumatic fever

are described in Table 15-1. Decreasing inflammation with aspirin (or corticosteroids) is the main therapy for acute rheumatic fever, although it will not prevent the development of chronic rheumatic heart disease.

- There was a resurgence of acute rheumatic fever among children and military recruits in the 1980s.

The risk for recurrent episodes of acute rheumatic fever with subsequent streptococcal infection is extremely high. Continuous antibiotic prophylaxis is effective for preventing these recurrences. Monthly injections of benzathine penicillin G and orally administered penicillin, sulfonamides, and erythromycin are effective for preventing recurrences of rheumatic fever. If there was no carditis with the acute rheumatic fever episode and no attack within the previous 5 years, prophylaxis may be discontinued after the age of 25 years. For patients who had significant carditis with residual valvular disease, lifelong prophylaxis may be necessary. Endocarditis prophylaxis is a separate issue. New recommendations do not advise prophylaxis for endocarditis to this group unless the patient has had a prior endocarditis or has a prosthetic valve. The new endocarditis prophylaxis recommendations are provided in "Clinical Syndromes" (Part II of this chapter).

Table 15-1 Jones Criteria for Diagnosis of Initial Attack of Rheumatic Fever[a] (1992 Update)

Major manifestations
Carditis
Polyarthritis
Chorea
Erythema marginatum
Subcutaneous nodules
Minor manifestations
Clinical findings
Arthralgia
Fever
Laboratory findings
Elevated acute-phase reactants (erythrocyte sedimentation rate, C-reactive protein)
Prolonged PR interval
Supporting evidence of antecedent group A streptococcal infection
Positive throat culture or rapid diagnostic test
Elevated or rising streptococcal antibody titer

[a] If supported by evidence of recent *Streptococcus pyogenes* infection, then the presence of 2 major, or 1 major and 2 minor, criteria is enough for diagnosis. Exceptions in which the Jones criteria do not need to be fulfilled: 1) recurrent rheumatic fever (a single major or several minor criteria are sufficient if there is supporting evidence of a recent *S pyogenes* infection), 2) isolated chorea, and 3) indolent carditis.
From Special Writing Group of the Committee on Rheumatic Fever, Endocarditis, and Kawasaki Disease of the Council on Cardiovascular Disease in the Young of the American Heart Association. Guidelines for the diagnosis of rheumatic fever: Jones Criteria, 1992 update. JAMA. 1992;268:2069-73. Used with permission.

Acute glomerulonephritis may occur after infection with nephritogenic strains of *S pyogenes*. Both cutaneous infections and pharyngitis can result in acute glomerulonephritis.

- Continuous antibiotic prophylaxis is used to prevent recurrent acute rheumatic fever.
- Acute glomerulonephritis may occur after either streptococcal skin infections or pharyngitis.

Group B: *Streptococcus agalactiae*

This organism, part of the normal flora of the genital and gastrointestinal tracts, is an important cause of postpartum maternal and neonatal infections. The penicillins are the treatment of choice for infections caused by *S agalactiae*. Meningitis, which most commonly occurs in neonates, is best treated with penicillin or ampicillin plus gentamicin. Prepartum vaginal culture for group B streptococcus may identify persons at highest risk for infection and allow eradication of the organism before delivery.

Group D Streptococci

Streptococcus bovis is the most clinically important of the group D streptococci. There is an association between *S bovis* bacteremia and carcinoma of the colon or other colonic disease. *S bovis* is clinically similar to the viridans group of streptococci and is generally susceptible to penicillin and the cephalosporins.

- Typical clinical scenario: A 59-year-old man with bacteremia and *S bovis* endocarditis. Colonoscopy shows carcinoma of the colon. Penicillin (alone or with an aminoglycoside) is the treatment of choice for endocarditis caused by *S bovis*.

Enterococci

The enterococci are an important cause of nosocomial infections. All enterococci are intrinsically resistant to many antimicrobial agents, including all of the cephalosporins. This resistance allows the organisms to proliferate and cause infections in the hospital setting. In fact, the enterococci are only inhibited, not killed, by the penicillins or vancomycin alone. Strains that are resistant to both the penicillins and vancomycin (vancomycin-resistant enterococci) are spreading worldwide. Linezolid, dalfopristin/quinupristin, and a new antibiotic, daptomycin, inhibit the growth of vancomycin-resistant enterococci. Neither linezolid nor dalfopristin/quinupristin is bactericidal against the enterococci. Dalfopristin/quinupristin is active against only *Enterococcus faecium*.

To achieve the bactericidal activity necessary to cure endocarditis due to enterococci, a combination of penicillin (or ampicillin) plus gentamicin or streptomycin is required. The choice of aminoglycoside depends on the results of susceptibility testing. The duration of therapy depends on how long the patient has been ill with endocarditis. Four weeks of therapy is adequate if the illness has been present for less than 3 months. When a patient is symptomatic for longer than 3 months, there is an unacceptable failure rate with the 4-week regimen. Therefore, 6 weeks of therapy is recommended. Vancomycin should be used in place of penicillin only in the allergic patient, because it is considered less effective. Optimal regimens for isolates resistant to both gentamicin and streptomycin are unknown. A valve replacement procedure may increase the chance for successfully treating subacute bacterial endocarditis due to drug-resistant enterococci.

- Enterococcal endocarditis is best treated with a combination of penicillin (or ampicillin) plus streptomycin or gentamicin.

Enterococcal urinary tract infections or simple bacteremia usually respond to treatment with either a penicillin or vancomycin alone, as long as the strains are susceptible in vitro. Alternatives for treatment of uncomplicated urinary tract infections in penicillin-allergic patients include the fluoroquinolones, nitrofurantoin, or vancomycin.

Streptococcus pneumoniae

Streptococcus pneumoniae (pneumococcus) is a leading cause of community-acquired infections such as pneumonia, meningitis, otitis media, and sinusitis. Like many organisms, it is becoming increasingly resistant to traditional antibiotics. Potential complications of pneumococcal pneumonia include empyema and pericarditis from direct extension of infection. Empyema should be suspected when fever persists despite appropriate antibiotic therapy of pneumococcal pneumonia.

Streptococcus pneumoniae is the most common cause of bacterial meningitis in adults (Figure 15-2), including those with recurrent meningitis due to cerebrospinal fluid leaks. Meningitis due to susceptible *S pneumoniae* can still be treated successfully with high-dose penicillin G. However, given the spread of penicillin-resistant strains, meningitis should be treated with high-dose cefotaxime or ceftriaxone in combination with vancomycin while the results of susceptibility testing are awaited. Adjunctive treatment of meningitis with dexamethasone has been shown to be beneficial if started at the same time as the first dose of antibiotic.

- The most common cause of bacterial meningitis in adults is *S pneumoniae*.
- Consider the possibility of a cerebrospinal fluid leak in patients with recurrent *S pneumoniae* meningitis.

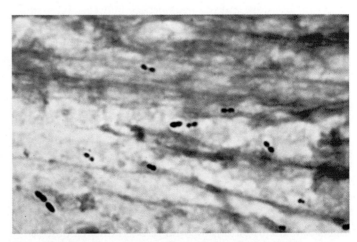

Figure 15-2. *Streptococcus pneumoniae* in Sputum (Gram Stain).

Asplenia predisposes individuals to severe infections with *S pneumoniae* (and other encapsulated organisms). After splenectomy, fulminant, often fatal, pneumococcal bacteremia with disseminated intravascular coagulation is more common. Similarly, *S pneumoniae* infections are more frequent and unusually severe in smokers, patients with asthma, and patients with sickle cell disease, multiple myeloma, alcoholism, or hypogammaglobulinemia.

Streptococcus pneumoniae is the leading cause of invasive bacterial respiratory disease in patients with human immunodeficiency virus (HIV) infection. Prophylaxis for *Pneumocystis jiroveci* pneumonia with trimethoprim-sulfamethoxazole may provide effective primary or secondary prophylaxis, but breakthrough infections with resistant organisms are not uncommon.

- Splenectomy predisposes to fulminant, often fatal, pneumococcal bacteremia with disseminated intravascular coagulation.
- *Streptococcus pneumoniae* infections are more frequent and unusually severe in smokers, patients with asthma, and patients with sickle cell disease, multiple myeloma, alcoholism, or hypogammaglobulinemia.
- *Streptococcus pneumoniae* is the leading cause of invasive bacterial respiratory disease in patients with HIV infection.

Infections due to *S pneumoniae* have traditionally been treated with penicillin. However, the rate of penicillin resistance (minimal inhibitory concentration, >2 mcg/mL) is increasing dramatically. According to the Active Bacterial Core Surveillance (ABCs) report, as of 2005, 9.9% of pneumococcal isolates in the United States had high-level resistance to penicillin. Penicillin-resistant strains are often resistant to the effects of other antibiotics such as the cephalosporins. Penicillin resistance is conferred by an alteration of the penicillin-binding proteins which results in a decreased affinity of these cell wall components for the penicillins. Risk factors for development of infection due to penicillin-resistant pneumococci include previous use of β-lactam antibiotics, nosocomial acquisition, and multiple previous hospitalizations.

Penicillin-resistant strains of *S pneumoniae* remain susceptible to vancomycin. High doses of cefotaxime, ceftriaxone, and imipenem also may be effective. Ciprofloxacin is usually not effective; however, the newer fluoroquinolones (levofloxacin, gatifloxacin, and moxifloxacin) are active against pneumococci. However, 0.9% of the strains are resistant to levofloxacin, as reported by the ABCs.

The pneumococcal vaccine is polyvalent, containing capsular polysaccharide from the 23 serotypes that most commonly cause pneumococcal infection. It is recommended for persons who are at an increased risk of invasive pneumococcal disease or complications. These include adults older than 65 years, patients of any age with chronic illness such as chronic cardiovascular disease (eg, congestive heart failure or cardiomyopathies), chronic pulmonary disease (eg, chronic obstructive pulmonary disease or emphysema), diabetes mellitus, alcoholism, chronic liver disease (cirrhosis), asplenia, or cerebrospinal fluid leaks. The vaccine can be given simultaneously with influenza virus vaccine. Pneumococcal vaccine booster is recommended 5 years after the initial dose in high-risk patients or in those who received the first dose before age 65 years.

- Typical clinical scenario: Pneumococcal infection in a splenectomized patient presents with fulminant bacteremia with disseminated intravascular coagulation. The diagnosis is *S pneumoniae* sepsis.

Viridans Streptococci

Several species of non-Lancefield typeable streptococci are referred to as the *viridans group of streptococci*. They are normal oral and enteric flora. This group of organisms is a common cause of subacute bacterial endocarditis, which should be suspected when viridans streptococci are found in blood cultures. Like the pneumococci, these organisms are increasingly likely to display resistance to penicillin. Viridans streptococcal bacteremia may be associated with shock and respiratory distress in neutropenic recipients of a bone marrow transplant.

Another streptococcal group known as the *Streptococcus anginosus* group (also known as the *Streptococcus intermedius* or the *Streptococcus milleri* group) is frequently associated with pyogenic abscesses. The *S anginosus* group consists of *S intermedius*, *Streptococcus constellatus*, and *S anginosus*. This is often a monomicrobial abscess and not necessarily associated with endocarditis.

- Typical clinical scenario: A 40-year-old man, 14 days after a bone marrow transplant, is neutropenic and has bacteremia with viridans streptococci, shock, and respiratory distress.

Staphylococci

Staphylococcus aureus (Coagulase-Positive *Staphylococcus*)

Toxins

Preformed enterotoxins produced by *S aureus* are a common cause of food poisoning in the United States. The toxin is heat stable and, therefore, is not destroyed by cooking contaminated foods. Exfoliatins are exotoxins produced by *S aureus* belonging to phage group II which cause scalded skin syndrome, an erythematous rash that progresses to bullous lesions, most commonly in children. It can be differentiated from toxic epidermal necrolysis by skin biopsy. Toxic shock syndrome is due to an exotoxin (TSST-1) produced by *S aureus* that may be causing an otherwise subclinical infection. Some *S aureus* strains (both methicillin-sensitive and -resistant) have been associated with production of exotoxins. One of these is the Panton-Valentine leukocidin toxin, which is produced in large quantities by the community-acquired strains of methicillin-resistant *S aureus*. This toxin is lethal to neutrophils and causes skin and soft tissue infections and severe necrotizing pneumonias. Hospital-acquired strains of MRSA generally do not contain this toxin.

- Preformed enterotoxins produced by *S aureus* are not destroyed by cooking food.
- Toxic shock syndrome is due to an exotoxin (TSST-1) produced by *S aureus* that may be causing an otherwise subclinical infection.

Clinical Syndromes

Staphylococcus aureus is the causative agent of several superficial infections, including folliculitis (infection of hair follicles without involvement of skin or subcutaneous tissues), furunculosis (a more extensive follicular infection often involving subcutaneous tissues), carbuncles (infection in thick inelastic tissues of the scalp or upper back), and impetigo (although this is most commonly caused by group A β-hemolytic streptococci). Surgical drainage of infected lesions occasionally is required.

Staphylococcus aureus is the most common cause of osteomyelitis in adults. It is the second most common cause of prosthetic joint infection, the coagulase-negative staphylococci being the most common.

- Staphylococcus aureus is a common cause of chronic osteomyelitis in adults.
- Staphylococcus aureus is the second most common cause of prosthetic joint infection.

Most cases of community-acquired S aureus bacteremia should be treated for 4 to 6 weeks with parenteral antibiotics because of the potential for metastatic abscesses and infective endocarditis. If nosocomial S aureus bacteremia is caused by a removable focus of infection (such as an intravenous catheter), 10 to 14 days of therapy is usually sufficient. Some experts recommend using transesophageal echocardiography to screen for endocarditis in all patients with S aureus bacteremia. Staphylococcus aureus infrequently causes community-acquired pneumonia, but it may develop as a complication of influenza. Staphylococcus aureus is a common cause of nosocomial infection, including postoperative wound infections, line-associated bacteremias, and ventilator-associated pneumonia. Detection of S aureus in the urine should raise concern for an underlying bacteremia with secondary seeding of the urinary tract.

- Cases of community-acquired S aureus bacteremia should be treated for 4-6 weeks with parenteral antibiotics.
- Staphylococcus aureus infrequently causes community-acquired pneumonia, but it may develop as a complication of influenza.

Mechanisms of Resistance
Most S aureus strains produce β-lactamase and thus are resistant to penicillin G. The semisynthetic penicillins (nafcillin, oxacillin) and first-generation cephalosporins remain active against such strains. Since first encountered in the 1970s, strains of S aureus with intrinsic resistance to the β-lactam antibiotics have spread worldwide. This resistance is caused by an alteration of the penicillin-binding proteins in the cell wall. These strains, referred to as MRSA (methicillin-resistant S aureus, or multiple drug-resistant S aureus), are resistant to all β-lactam drugs and often to other classes of antibiotics.

Community-Acquired MRSA
MRSA is a well-known nosocomial pathogen. However, new MRSA strains are now causing community-acquired infections. Genetic analyses show that these community-acquired MRSA (CA-MRSA) strains are not merely known nosocomial strains that have "escaped" from the hospital. Rather, they are unique new strains that are causing both sporadic infections and localized outbreaks. CA-MRSA may be more virulent than typical S aureus strains.

CA-MRSA is by definition resistant to the effects of all β-lactam antibiotics. Unlike nosocomial strains, CA-MRSA often remains susceptible to many other antibiotics, such as clindamycin, tetracyclines, and trimethoprim-sulfamethoxazole. Clinically, CA-MRSA infections may manifest as recurrent skin and soft tissue infections, necrotizing fasciitis, and hemorrhagic pneumonia. Outbreaks of skin infections among family members and within professional sports teams have been described.

Treatment
If S aureus is penicillin-susceptible (approximately 5% of clinical isolates), penicillin G is the most active agent. For penicillin-allergic patients, effective alternatives include cefazolin and vancomycin. If the isolate is methicillin-susceptible, then nafcillin, oxacillin, or cephalosporins (first-generation) are considered superior to drugs such as vancomycin. Vancomycin is the most reliably active drug for treating serious infections caused by MRSA. CA-MRSA is often susceptible to clindamycin, tetracylines, and trimethoprim-sulfamethoxazole. There should be a lower threshold for incision and debridement with CA-MRSA infections. Linezolid and dalfopristin/quinupristin, daptomycin, and tigecycline are newer drugs that are also active against MRSA. Occasional strains of MRSA may still be susceptible to trimethoprim-sulfamethoxazole, minocycline, or the macrolides. However, these antibiotics are mostly used for treatment of non–life-threatening infections.

Staphylococcus aureus organisms commonly colonize the nares, which may predispose to invasive infections. Subclinical nasal colonization can result in nosocomial transmission of MRSA. Topical mupirocin ointment or other therapies (such as trimethoprim-sulfamethoxazole with or without rifampin) may temporarily eradicate the nasal colonization, but relapse is common.

- Vancomycin is the most reliably active drug for treating serious infections caused by MRSA.
- CA-MRSA is often susceptible to clindamycin, tetracyclines, and trimethoprim-sulfamethoxazole.

Coagulase-Negative Staphylococci
Staphylococcus epidermidis is the most common of the coagulase-negative staphylococci, although many other staphylococcal species are included in this group. For clinical purposes, they are interchangeable. Coagulase-negative staphylococci are normal skin flora. They are opportunistic pathogens that commonly cause infections associated with medical devices. They rarely cause disease in otherwise healthy persons.

Clinical Syndromes
Coagulase-negative staphylococci are most commonly associated with intravascular device-related bacteremia, prosthetic valve endocarditis, osteomyelitis (usually after joint arthroplasty or other prosthetic implantations), and meningitis after neurosurgical procedures. Treatment usually requires removal of the foreign body and administration of appropriate antibiotics. Coagulase-negative staphylococci can cause peritonitis in patients undergoing chronic ambulatory peritoneal dialysis.

Staphylococcus saprophyticus is a unique species of coagulase-negative staphylococcus that is a common cause of urinary tract infections in young women.

Treatment

Coagulase-negative staphylococci are usually resistant to the β-lactam antibiotics. Unless in vitro susceptibility testing shows other active agents, infections due to coagulase-negative staphylococci should be treated with vancomycin. The fluoroquinolones may be active against some strains, but resistance may emerge rapidly. *Staphylococcus saprophyticus* is an exception because it is usually susceptible to the penicillins and many other antibiotics.

Determining the significance of blood cultures growing coagulase-negative staphylococci can be difficult. True infections generally result in multiple positive blood cultures, whereas one positive culture usually is considered to be contaminated.

A regimen of vancomycin plus rifampin for 6 weeks, with gentamicin added for the first 2 weeks, is recommended for the treatment of prosthetic valve endocarditis caused by coagulase-negative staphylococci. Valve replacement may be necessary in recalcitrant cases.

- Unless in vitro susceptibility testing shows other active agents, infections due to coagulase-negative staphylococci should be treated with vancomycin.
- Typical clinical scenario: A 29-year-old woman with an indwelling intravascular catheter has fever of 102°F. The diagnosis was infection with coagulase-negative *Staphylococcus*.

Gram-Negative Bacilli

Escherichia coli

Escherichia coli organisms cause invasive disease as a result of ascending infection (such as in the urinary tract) or a break in a mucosal barrier (such as intra-abdominal infection). *Escherichia coli* bacteremia is often related to focal infections such as intra-abdominal abscesses or pyelonephritis. *Escherichia coli* is the most common cause of urinary tract infections and spontaneous bacterial peritonitis. Like most gram-negative bacilli, *E coli* is variably susceptible to ampicillin (although resistance to ampicillin is increasing and susceptibility cannot be reliably predicted), the cephalosporins (including first-generation agents), trimethoprim-sulfamethoxazole, aminoglycosides, and the fluoroquinolones.

Escherichia coli O157:H7 produces a cytotoxic exotoxin that causes hemorrhagic colitis and may be complicated by hemolytic-uremic syndrome in approximately 10% of cases. This strain of *E coli* is a normal part of bovine fecal flora that can contaminate undercooked hamburger, unpasteurized apple cider, and other food products. Treatment of *E coli*-associated hemorrhagic colitis is supportive only. Antibiotics are actually contraindicated because their use may increase the risk for development of hemolytic uremic syndrome.

- Antibiotics are contraindicated in the treatment of *E coli* O157:H7-associated hemorrhagic colitis.

Klebsiella, Enterobacter, and Serratia

Klebsiella pneumoniae is an important cause of both community-acquired and nosocomial pneumonia and often is associated with alcoholism, diabetes mellitus, and chronic obstructive pulmonary disease. Red currant jelly-colored sputum is characteristic. Lung abscess and empyema are more frequent with *K pneumoniae* than with other pneumonia-causing organisms. Cephalosporins are the drugs of choice for treating most types of *Klebsiella*. Strains of *Klebsiella* resistant to ceftazidime have emerged. This resistance is caused by a broad-spectrum β-lactamase. Susceptibility testing results for such strains may erroneously report that they are susceptible to cefotaxime. If resistant to ceftazidime, consider them resistant to all cephalosporins.

- Lung abscess and empyema are more frequent with *K pneumoniae* than with other pneumonia-causing organisms.

Enterobacter and *Serratia* primarily are associated with nosocomial infections. *Enterobacter* species often are resistant to third-generation cephalosporins such as cefotaxime. Despite in vitro data suggesting susceptibility, β-lactamase production is induced when grown in the presence of cephalosporins. Carbapenems such as imipenem or meropenem, fluoroquinolones, cefepime, and trimethoprim-sulfamethoxazole are usually active against these strains.

- *Enterobacter* species often are resistant to third-generation cephalosporins such as cefotaxime, despite in vitro data suggesting susceptibility.

Pseudomonas aeruginosa

This organism predominantly causes nosocomial infection and is resistant to many common antibiotics. *Pseudomonas aeruginosa*, together with *S aureus*, is the most frequent cause of infections complicating severe burn injuries. Other infections caused by *P aeruginosa* include folliculitis associated with hot tubs, osteomyelitis (particularly in injection drug users), malignant otitis externa in patients with diabetes mellitus, complicated urinary tract infections, ventilator-associated pneumonia, and pulmonary infections in patients with cystic fibrosis. Patients with neutropenia are also at particularly high risk for *Pseudomonas* infection, especially bacteremia. Hence, the febrile neutropenic patient should be treated empirically with antipseudomonal antibiotics while culture results are awaited. Ecthyma gangrenosum is a necrotizing skin lesion that may develop in neutropenic patients with bacteremia due to *P aeruginosa*.

- *Pseudomonas aeruginosa*, together with *S aureus*, is the most frequent cause of infections complicating massive burns.
- Typical clinical scenarios: *P aeruginosa* causes malignant otitis externa in patients with diabetes mellitus. Ecthyma gangrenosum is a necrotizing skin lesion that develops in neutropenic patients with bacteremia due to *P aeruginosa*.

Agents active against most *P aeruginosa* organisms include the extended-spectrum penicillins (piperacillin, ticarcillin), aminoglycosides, ceftazidime and cefepime (the only cephalosporins reliably active against this organism), aztreonam, imipenem, and ciprofloxacin. Administering two active drugs, usually a β-lactam and an aminoglycoside, is recommended when treating serious infections caused by *P aeruginosa*. Antibiotic resistance frequently emerges during and after treatment.

Stenotrophomonas (Xanthomonas) maltophilia

This organism most commonly causes nosocomial infections. Its most notable trait is intrinsic resistance to imipenem and meropenem (as well as the aminoglycosides, quinolones, and most β-lactam drugs). *Stenotrophomonas maltophilia* usually is susceptible to trimethoprim-sulfamethoxazole and ticarcillin-clavulanate.

* *Stenotrophomonas maltophilia* is intrinsically resistant to imipenem and meropenem.

Salmonella

Salmonella infections are increasing in the United States. Well-identified outbreaks have been associated with food contamination. Undercooked chicken or eggs are often sources of infection. Other sources of infection include exposure to farm animals and also to pets such as turtles and reptiles. Gastroenteritis is the most common manifestation. However, more serious illnesses, including infections of atherosclerotic aortic aneurysms, may occur.

Salmonella typhi is rare in the United States. Patients with typhoid fever have relative bradycardia and rose spots (50%). The leukocyte count may be decreased. Blood cultures usually are positive within approximately 10 days of symptom onset, whereas stool cultures become positive later.

Salmonella choleraesuis causes chronic bacteremia and mycotic aneurysms. *Salmonella typhimurium* and *Salmonella enteritidis* produce gastroenteritis and occasionally bacteremia. Urinary tract infections caused by *Salmonella* occur in patients from the Middle East who are infected with *Schistosoma haematobium*.

* *Salmonella* causes infections of atherosclerotic aortic aneurysms.

As with many organisms, antimicrobial resistance is increasingly common with *Salmonella*. Most cases of *Salmonella* gastroenteritis resolve without therapy. In fact, treatment with antibiotics may actually prolong the duration of intestinal carriage and fecal shedding. Serious or invasive infections should be treated with a third-generation cephalosporin or fluoroquinolone while results of susceptibility testing are awaited.

* Most cases of *Salmonella* gastroenteritis should not be treated with antibiotics because treatment prolongs the carrier state.

Haemophilus influenzae

Widespread use of the vaccine against *H influenzae* B has dramatically reduced the incidence of invasive disease in children. Non-typeable strains of *H influenzae* more commonly cause disease in adults (primarily respiratory infection). Infections caused by *H influenzae* include pneumonia, meningitis, epiglottitis, and primary bacteremia. *Haemophilus influenzae* is associated with infectious exacerbations of chronic obstructive pulmonary disease and with sinusitis and otitis media. Chronic lung disease, pregnancy, HIV infection, splenectomy, and malignancy are risk factors for invasive disease.

* Chronic lung disease, pregnancy, HIV infection, splenectomy, and malignancy are risk factors for invasive disease due to *H influenzae*.

Up to 40% of *H influenzae* organisms recovered from adults with invasive disease are resistant to ampicillin by virtue of β-lactamase production. They can be treated with trimethoprim-sulfamethoxazole, third-generation cephalosporins, fluoroquinolones, or a β-lactam–β-lactamase inhibitor combination such as ampicillin-sulbactam.

* Approximately 40% of *H influenzae* clinical isolates are resistant to ampicillin.

Haemophilus influenzae is an uncommon cause of meningitis in adults, although it can occur with hypogammaglobulinemia, asplenia, or cerebrospinal fluid leak. Third-generation cephalosporins (cefotaxime or ceftriaxone) are the drugs of choice for *H influenzae* meningitis.

Other Haemophilus Species

Haemophilus parainfluenzae, *Haemophilus aphrophilus*, and *Haemophilus paraphrophilus* are normal oral flora. When these or other members of the HACEK (*Haemophilus aphrophilus*, *paraphrophilus*, and *parainfluenzae*; *Actinobacillus actinomycetemcomitans*; *Cardiobacterium hominis*; *Eikenella corrodens*; *Kingella* species) group of organisms are grown from blood cultures, their presence should always raise the suspicion for endocarditis. Large valvular vegetations with systemic emboli are common with HACEK endocarditis. Usual treatment is with ceftriaxone or ampicillin-sulbactam (if the organism is susceptible) for 4 weeks.

Bordetella pertussis

The incidence of whooping cough is increasing as the protection afforded by immunization declines with age. Twelve percent of cases now occur in persons older than 15 years. *Bordetella pertussis* infection often results in persistent coughing in older children and adults. As many as 50 million adults are now susceptible to infection as a result of waning immunity. Whooping cough may cause severe lymphocytosis (>100 lymphocytes × 10^9/L). Diagnosis of *B pertussis* infection may be difficult. Molecular testing (polymerase chain reaction) of a nasopharyngeal aspirate is more sensitive, rapid, and reliable than cultures. Early treatment of pertussis with a macrolide antibiotic is most effective. Newer macrolides (clarithromycin or azithromycin) are recommended for 5 days to close contacts of affected patients for prevention, irrespective of age or vaccination status. Aerosolized bronchodilators or corticosteroids may alleviate the persistent coughing. A new pertussis-containing tetanus-diphtheria vaccine is now available for use in adults. It is given as a single booster to replace a dose of tetanus-diphtheria booster. This approach is particularly emphasized for adults who have close contact with infants (eg, parents, health care workers, day care providers).

* *Bordetella pertussis* may cause severe lymphocytosis (>100 lymphocytes × 10^9/L).
* *Bordetella pertussis* can cause persistent coughing in older children and adults.

Brucella

Although rare (100-200 cases per year) in the United States, brucellosis may occur in meat handlers, persons exposed to livestock, or persons who drink unpasteurized milk. Most cases of brucellosis acquired in the United States occur in 4 states (Texas, California, Virginia, and Florida). However, brucellosis occurs most often in immigrants or ill travelers returning from developing countries. Brucellosis may cause a chronic granulomatous disease with caseating granulomas. Brucellosis (along with tuberculosis) is a cause of "sterile" pyuria. Chronic brucellosis is one of the infectious causes of fever of undetermined origin. Calcifications in the spleen may be an indication of the presence of infection (although histoplasmosis also causes splenic calcifications). Serologic testing, special blood cultures, and bone marrow cultures are helpful for making the diagnosis. Treatment is with doxycycline along with streptomycin or rifampin. Trimethoprim-sulfamethoxazole may be effective.

* Brucellosis may cause fever of unknown origin and is associated with animal exposures.

Legionella

Legionellae are fastidious gram-negative bacilli. *Legionella pneumophila* causes both community-acquired and nosocomial pneumonia, typically occurring in the summer months. Nosocomial legionellosis may be due to contaminated water supplies. Immunocompromised patients, especially those receiving chronic corticosteroid therapy, are especially susceptible to *Legionella* infections. Typical clinical features of legionellosis include weakness, malaise, fever, dry cough, diarrhea, pleuritic chest pain, relative bradycardia, diffuse rales bilaterally, and patchy bilateral pulmonary infiltrates.

Characteristic laboratory features of *Legionella* pneumonia include decreased sodium and phosphorus values, increased leukocyte level, and increased liver enzyme values. Legionellae organisms will not grow on standard media. Diagnosis depends on results of special culture, finding organisms by direct fluorescent antibody staining, or detecting an increase in anti-*Legionella* antibody titers. Urine antigen detection is a more sensitive (>80%) and simple diagnostic test for *L pneumophila* infections.

Legionellae are intracellular parasites. As such, they are resistant to all β-lactam drugs and aminoglycosides in vivo. Effective agents for treating *Legionella* include macrolides, fluoroquinolones, and, to a lesser extent, doxycycline. Fluoroquinolones are considered drugs of choice for therapy. Some authorities recommend adding rifampin for severe infection.

* Immunocompromised patients, especially those receiving chronic corticosteroid therapy, are especially susceptible to *Legionella* infections.
* Laboratory features of legionellosis include decreased serum sodium and phosphorus values, increased leukocyte level, and increased liver enzyme values.
* Typical clinical scenario: A 63-year-old man who is receiving chronic corticosteroid therapy presents with fever, dry cough, diarrhea, and patchy bilateral infiltrates on chest radiography. Laboratory tests show hyponatremia and increased liver function values. Diagnosis is *Legionella* infection and can be established by special *Legionella* culture, serologic tests, and urinary antigen detection. Therapy is with macrolides or fluoroquinolones.

Francisella tularensis

Francisella tularensis is spread by the bite of a tick or deer fly, by aerosol droplets, or by direct contact with tissues of infected animals (rabbits, muskrats, squirrels, beavers). Typically, infection causes an eschar at the site of inoculation, regional lymphadenopathy, and high fevers. Pneumonia also can occur. Streptomycin and gentamicin are the most effective therapies. Tetracycline is also active, but its use is associated with a 10% relapse rate. Tularemia has been identified as a potential bioterrorism agent.

* *Francisella tularensis* is spread by arthropod bite, aerosol droplets, or direct contact with tissues of infected animals.

Yersinia pestis

From 1950 to 1991, there were 336 cases of plague in the United States, and more than 50% of these occurred after 1980. Plague is enzootic in the southwestern United States. New Mexico had 56% of cases, and 29% of cases are among American Indians. Rats and fleas are the vectors. Clinical presentations include 1) lymphadenopathy with septicemia—the most common form—and 2) the pneumonic form (high case-fatality rate). Treatment is with streptomycin or tetracycline. As with tularemia, there is concern that plague could be used for bioterrorism.

Pasteurella multocida

Pasteurella multocida is a common cause of cutaneous infection after a cat or dog bite. Onset of illness is typically within 24 hours of the bite. It causes local inflammation, a rapidly progressing cellulitis, and bacteremia. *Pasteurella multocida* is susceptible to penicillin, amoxicillin, amoxicillin-clavulanate, tetracyclines, and fluoroquinolones. First-generation cephalosporins (cephalexin) and the antistaphylococcal penicillins (such as nafcillin and oxacillin) are not active against *P multocida* infections.

* Cephalexin and the antistaphylococcal penicillins should not be used to treat cat or dog bite wounds infected with *P multocida*.
* Typical clinical scenario: A 35-year-old man presents with cutaneous infection after a dog or cat bite. It rapidly progresses to cellulitis and bacteremia.

Capnocytophaga (Formerly DF-2)

These gram-negative bacilli are difficult to grow on routine culture media. They are normal oral flora of domestic animals (especially dogs) and humans. *Capnocytophaga* causes bacteremia and fulminant sepsis, primarily in splenectomized persons. Dog and cat bites are associated with 50% of cases. Occasionally, bacteremia with human oral *Capnocytophaga* species occurs in neutropenic patients with mucositis. Treatment with a penicillin or a cephalosporin is most effective.

* *Capnocytophaga* causes bacteremia and fulminant sepsis, primarily in splenectomized persons.
* Dog and cat bites are associated with 50% of cases.

Bartonella Species

Bartonella bacilliformis, Bartonella quintana, and Bartonella henselae are the most common Bartonella species that cause human disease. Bartonella bacilliformis causes Oroyo fever and is limited to the Andes region of South America. Bartonella henselae (formerly Rochalimaea henselae) is the primary causative agent of cat-scratch disease. The disease is characterized by a papule or pustule at the site of inoculation, followed by tender enlargement of the regional lymph nodes. Low-grade fever and malaise also may be present. Exposure to domestic cats (especially kittens) is the main risk factor. About 10% of patients may have extranodal manifestations. Disseminated infection with any of the Bartonella species can occur in patients with acquired immunodeficiency syndrome (AIDS). Bartonella quintana and B henselae infections in HIV or AIDS or other immunocompromised patients can present with cutaneous and visceral involvement, particularly the liver. Cutaneous neovascular proliferation causes skin lesions called bacillary angiomatosis, which appears like an angioma. This infection presents in the bones as lytic lesions. Bartonella henselae and B quintana can cause bacteremia and endocarditis. Bartonella henselae is associated with cat exposure, and B quintana occurs more often in alcoholic, homeless persons without specific cat exposure. Bartonella endocarditis usually presents subacutely and often requires surgical management.

Diagnosis of cat-scratch disease is based on the clinical picture and serologic evidence of antibodies to B henselae or other species. In biopsied tissue, the organisms can be seen with Warthin-Starry stain. Because cat-scratch disease is usually self-limited, treatment is indicated only for patients with significant symptoms or bothersome adenopathy. Azithromycin appears to be the most effective antibiotic for treatment of cat-scratch disease. For bacteremia or endocarditis, prolonged treatment with erythromycin, azithromycin, or doxycycline is given. For endocarditis, an aminoglycoside may be added for the first 2 weeks of the 8- to 12-week therapy.

- Bartonella henselae and B quintana can cause bacteremia and endocarditis. Bartonella henselae is associated with cat exposure, and B quintana occurs more often in alcoholic, homeless persons without specific cat exposure.

Vibrio Species

In the United States, consumption of raw or undercooked shellfish such as oysters is the most common source of infection with pathogenic vibrios (eg, Vibrio parahaemolyticus, Vibrio vulnificus). Disease usually manifests as self-limited enteritis. Cholera, caused by Vibrio cholerae, continues to cause periodic pandemics, the most recent affecting South and Central America. Although indigenous cases are rare in the United States and Canada, cholera has developed in travelers returning from affected areas.

Vibrio vulnificus is unique in that it causes a distinctive soft tissue infection in compromised hosts, especially those with underlying cirrhosis or hemochromatosis. Disease is usually acquired by the ingestion of raw oysters or through injury sustained in warm salt water. After the abrupt onset of fever and hypotension, multiple hemorrhagic bullae develop. Even with prompt therapy with ceftazidime or a tetracycline, mortality exceeds 30% for bacteremic V vulnificus infection.

- Consumption of raw oysters is the most common source of Vibrio infection in the United States.

Gram-Positive Bacilli

Listeria

Listeria monocytogenes is a small, motile, gram-positive, rod-shaped organism. Meningitis and bacteremia are the most common clinical manifestations of infection. Listeria may be difficult to visualize on Gram stain of spinal fluid. The elderly, neonates, pregnant women, and persons taking corticosteroids are at highest risk for disease due to Listeria. Epidemics have been associated with consumption of contaminated dairy products. Diarrhea may be a feature of epidemic listeriosis.

Penicillin and ampicillin are the most effective agents against Listeria. Antimicrobial coverage for Listeria (with ampicillin or trimethoprim-sulfamethoxazole) should always be included for bacterial meningitis in patients older than 50 years or if immunosuppressed. Combination with an aminoglycoside is often recommended for treatment of severe disease. Listeria is always resistant to the cephalosporins. Trimethoprim-sulfamethoxazole is an effective alternative for the penicillin-allergic patient. Treatment should be continued for 2 to 4 weeks to prevent relapse of disease.

- The elderly, neonates, pregnant women, and persons taking corticosteroids are at highest risk for disease due to Listeria.
- Epidemics mainly are associated with consumption of contaminated dairy products.
- Diarrhea may be a feature of epidemic listeriosis.

Corynebacterium diphtheriae

Diphtheria is a classic infectious disease that is easily prevented with vaccination. Epidemics of diphtheria recently occurred in states of the former Soviet Union. Diphtheria causes a focal infection of the respiratory tract (pharynx in 60%-70% of cases, larynx, nasal passages, or tracheobronchial tree). A tightly adherent, gray pseudomembrane is the hallmark of the disease, but disease can occur without pseudomembrane formation. Manifestations depend on the extent of involvement of the upper airway and the presence or absence of systemic complications due to toxin. Toxin-mediated complications include myocarditis (10%-25%), which causes congestive heart failure and arrhythmias, and polyneuritis (bulbar dysfunction followed by peripheral neuropathy). The respiratory muscles may be paralyzed.

- In diphtheria, toxin-mediated complications include myocarditis (10%-25%), which causes congestive heart failure and arrhythmias, and polyneuritis.
- Diphtheria may cause respiratory muscle paralysis.

The diagnosis of diphtheria is definitively established by culture with Löffler medium. Rapid diagnosis sometimes can be made with methylene blue stain or fluorescent antibody staining of pharyngeal swab specimens. Diphtheria is highly contagious. Equine antiserum is still the main therapy. Although there is no evidence that antimicrobial agents alter the course of disease, they may prevent transmission to susceptible hosts. Erythromycin and penicillin G are active against *C diphtheriae*. Nonimmune persons exposed to diphtheria should be evaluated and treated with erythromycin or penicillin G if culture results are positive. They should also be immunized with diphtheria-tetanus toxoid.

* Nonimmune persons exposed to diphtheria should be evaluated and treated with erythromycin or penicillin G if culture results are positive.

Cutaneous infection with *C diphtheriae* can occur in indigent persons and alcoholics. Preexisting dermatologic disease (most often in the lower extremities) is a risk factor. Lesions may appear "punched-out" and filled with a membrane, but they may be indistinguishable from other infected ulcers. Toxin-mediated complications (such as myocarditis and neuropathy) are uncommon. Diagnosis is established with methylene blue staining and culture of the lesion with Löffler medium.

* Cutaneous diphtheria is reported in indigent patients and alcoholics.

Bacillus Species

Bacillus species are increasingly recognized as causes of bacteremia in patients with indwelling catheters or prosthetic devices and in injection drug users. Other syndromes include ocular infections (posttraumatic endophthalmitis) and gastroenteritis. Anthrax (*Bacillus anthracis*) causes cutaneous disease in handlers of animal skins (also called woolsorters' disease).

Although many strains of *Bacillus* are susceptible to penicillins and cephalosporins, infection should be treated with vancomycin or clindamycin while the results of susceptibility tests are awaited.

In 2001, several cases of inhalational and cutaneous anthrax followed the deliberate dissemination of *B anthracis* spores through the mail. Inhalation anthrax is particularly deadly. It produces hemorrhagic mediastinitis, hemorrhagic meningitis, and bacteremia. A characteristic finding in inhalational anthrax is a widened mediastinum on chest radiography. Cutaneous anthrax usually manifests as a solitary papule that evolves into an eschar. Culture of blood, pleural fluid, cerebrospinal fluid, or a skin lesion confirms the diagnosis of anthrax. Sputum rarely reveals the organism. Nasal swab culture is useful for epidemiologic purposes but is not sufficiently sensitive to diagnose individual exposures.

Bacillus anthracis is usually susceptible to penicillins, tetracyclines, clindamycin, vancomycin, rifampin, and the fluoroquinolones. Inhalational exposures should be treated for at least 60 days. Combination therapy with multiple active drugs is preferred for inhalational anthrax.

Gram-Negative Cocci

Moraxella

Moraxella catarrhalis (*Branhamella catarrhalis*) is a respiratory tract pathogen primarily causing bronchitis and pneumonia in persons with chronic obstructive pulmonary disease. It also may cause otitis media, sinusitis, meningitis, bacteremia, and endocarditis in immunosuppressed patients. Ampicillin resistance through β-lactamase production is common. Trimethoprim-sulfamethoxazole, the fluoroquinolones, and amoxicillin-clavulanate are effective for therapy.

Neisseria

Neisseria meningitidis and *Neisseria gonorrhoeae* are discussed in "Clinical Syndromes" (Part II of this chapter).

Anaerobic Bacteria

Bacteroides and Prevotella

Bacteroides species are anaerobic gram-negative rods that are normal colonic flora (*Bacteroides fragilis* group). Related organisms also reside in the mouth (such as *Prevotella melaninogenica*). Infections caused by these organisms are often polymicrobial and result from disruption or perforation of mucosal surfaces. These anaerobes often produce abscesses containing foul-smelling pus. *Bacteroides* species also are associated with pelvic infections, particularly in women (eg, septic abortion, tubo-ovarian abscess, or endometritis). Anaerobic bacteremia usually is associated with focal infection elsewhere (such as intra-abdominal abscess). Osteomyelitis due to *Bacteroides* usually results from a contiguous source and is often polymicrobial (such as diabetic foot ulcer or osteomyelitis of the maxilla or mandible after dental infection). Pleuropulmonary infections include aspiration pneumonia and lung abscess, most commonly with *P melaninogenica* and other oral anaerobes.

* *Bacteroides* species are associated with intra-abdominal and pelvic abscesses.
* Anaerobic bacteremia usually is associated with focal infection elsewhere (such as intra-abdominal abscess).
* Pleuropulmonary infections caused by *Bacteroides* and *Prevotella* species include aspiration pneumonia and lung abscess.

Many strains of *Bacteroides* and *Prevotella* produce penicillinase, making them resistant to penicillin. Metronidazole, β-lactam–β-lactamase inhibitors such as ampicillin-sulbactam, piperacillin-tazobactam, and carbapenems such as imipenem or ertapenem are active against most anaerobic gram-negative rods. Resistance to clindamycin is increasingly common. The third-generation cephalosporins and fluoroquinolones have little activity against the anaerobic gram-negative bacilli.

Peptococcus and Peptostreptococcus

These anaerobic streptococci often are involved in polymicrobial infection. Like *Bacteroides*, they are part of the normal flora of the mouth and colon and are associated with anaerobic pleuropulmonary infection and intra-abdominal abscess.

Both *Peptococcus* and *Peptostreptococcus* are exquisitely sensitive to the penicillins. For patients allergic to penicillin, the effective alternative therapies include clindamycin, vancomycin, and cephalosporins.

Clostridia

Clostridium tetani

Clostridium tetani is a strictly anaerobic gram-positive rod that produces a neurotoxin (tetanospasmin). This neurotoxin, when produced by organisms in infected wounds, is responsible for the clinical manifestations of tetanus. Although rare in the United States, 200 to 300 cases still occur annually, mostly in elderly persons who have never been immunized.

The first muscles affected by tetanus are controlled by cranial nerves, resulting in trismus. Eye muscles (cranial nerves III, IV) rarely are involved. As the disease progresses, other muscles become involved (generalized rigidity, spasms, opisthotonos). Sympathetic overactivity is common (labile hypertension, hyperpyrexia, arrhythmias). The diagnosis of tetanus is based on clinical findings, although a characteristic electromyogram is suggestive.

* The diagnosis of tetanus is based primarily on clinical findings.

Treatment of tetanus includes supportive care, proper wound management, and administration of antiserum (human tetanus immune globulin). Penicillin G or metronidazole should be administered to eradicate vegetative organisms in the wound. Active tetanus does not induce protective immunity. Therefore, a primary tetanus immunization series should be given after an episode of tetanus.

* Active tetanus does not induce protective immunity to subsequent episodes of tetanus.

Clostridium botulinum

Clostridium botulinum produces a heat-labile neurotoxin that inhibits acetylcholine release from cholinergic terminals at the motor end plate. Botulism usually is caused by the ingestion of contaminated food (home-canned products and improperly prepared or handled commercial foods). Wound botulism results from contaminated traumatic wounds. Neonatal botulism can result from consumption of contaminated honey.

* Neurotoxin of *C botulinum* inhibits acetylcholine release from cholinergic terminals at the motor end plate.

The clinical symptoms of botulism include unexplained diplopia; fixed, dilated pupils; dry mouth; and descending flaccid paralysis with normal sensation. Patients are usually alert and oriented and have intact deep tendon reflexes. Fever is rare.

* Typical clinical scenario: In *C botulinum* infection (botulism), a patient presents with unexplained diplopia; fixed, dilated pupils; dry mouth; and descending flaccid paralysis with normal sensation.

Treatment of botulism is primarily supportive, although an equine antitoxin is available. In food-borne cases, purging the gut with cathartics, enemas, and emetics to remove unabsorbed toxin also may be of value. Antibiotic therapy does not affect the course of illness.

Other Clostridium Species

Clostridium perfringens is one of the causes of food poisoning. Illness usually develops 7 to 15 hours after ingestion and manifests as diarrhea with abdominal cramps. *Clostridium difficile* is the primary cause of antibiotic-associated pseudomembranous colitis (discussed

in detail in "Clinical Syndromes," Part II of this chapter). Bacteremia or soft tissue infection with *Clostridium septicum* indicates a high probability of coincident occult colonic malignancy.

* *Clostridium perfringens* may cause a food-associated illness.
* *Clostridium difficile* causes antibiotic-associated diarrhea.
* In patients with *C septicum* bacteremia, occult bowel carcinoma should be suspected.

Actinomycetes

Actinomyces israelii, an anaerobic, gram-positive, branching, filamentous organism, is the most common cause of human actinomycosis. *Actinomyces israelii* is part of the normal flora of the mouth. Infections are associated with any condition that creates an anaerobic environment (such as trauma with tissue necrosis, pus). The pathologic characteristic is formation of "sulfur granules," which are clumps of filaments. Infection is not characterized by granuloma formation.

* The pathologic characteristic of actinomycosis is "sulfur granules" (clumps of filaments).

Lumpy jaw is caused by a perimandibular infection with *A israelii*. It is characterized by a chronic draining sinus and may follow a dental extraction. Pulmonary actinomycosis develops when aspirated material reaches an area of lung with decreased oxygenation (such as in atelectasis). This condition often occurs in association with poor dental hygiene. A chronic suppurative pneumonitis may develop and eventually result in a sinus tract draining through the chest wall. There may be subsequent perforation into the esophagus, pericardium, ribs, and vertebrae. Ileocecal perforation from focal actinomycosis has been reported. Appendicitis may be a predisposing factor.

* Lumpy jaw is caused by a perimandibular infection with *A israelii*. It is characterized by a chronic draining sinus and may follow a dental extraction.

Actinomyces israelii also may be found in culture of tubo-ovarian abscesses and other pelvic infections. It is especially associated with pelvic inflammatory disease developing in a woman with an intrauterine device.

A prolonged course of penicillin is the preferred treatment of actinomycosis.

Mycobacteria

Mycobacterium tuberculosis

Clinical Disease

Pulmonary tuberculosis can manifest as primary infection, reactivation of previously latent infection, or reinfection. Primary infection involves continuous uninterrupted mycobacterial proliferation without a period of involution or quiescence. Primary disease commonly occurs in infants, children, and immunosuppressed adults. The radiographic findings of primary pulmonary disease include mid- or lower-zone parenchymal infiltrates with hilar adenopathy and pleural effusions. Reactivation-type pulmonary tuberculosis is the more common classic presentation in adults. Patients often present with symptoms such as prolonged cough (initially dry, later productive), fever, chills, night sweats, general fatigue, and weight loss. Hemoptysis and chest pain may occur. Chest radiographic abnormalities are variable but may include fibronodular infiltrates or cavitary disease, often found in the apical and posterior segments of the upper lobe or superior segments of the lower lobe. With cavitary disease, sputum samples are usually acid-fast bacillus smear-positive. Culture of respiratory specimens remains the standard for diagnosing tuberculosis and allows for drug susceptibility testing. However, in 10% to 15% of tuberculosis cases, the cultures are negative and diagnosis is dependent on radiographic or clinical findings. Nucleic acid amplification through polymerase chain reaction offers a more rapid means for identification of *M tuberculosis* than traditional culture. Tissue biopsy for histologic review often reveals classic caseating (necrotizing) granulomas with or without acid-fast organisms.

- In adults, reactivation-type pulmonary tuberculosis is the typical presentation.
- Symptoms of tuberculosis include prolonged cough, hemoptysis, fever, chills, night sweats, general fatigue, and weight loss.
- Chest radiographs may show fibronodular or cavitary disease in the apical and posterior segments of the upper lobe or superior segments of the lower lobe.
- Culture is important for *M tuberculosis* confirmation and susceptibility testing.

Treatment of Pulmonary Tuberculosis

Regimens for the treatment of pulmonary tuberculosis are outlined in Table 15-2. All 6-month regimens must contain isoniazid, rifampin, and an initial 2 months of therapy with pyrazinamide. All 9-month regimens must contain isoniazid and rifampin. Patient compliance is paramount to a successful treatment program, and directly observed therapy should be considered for all patients. Multidrug resistance is defined as resistance to both isoniazid and rifampin, although such strains also can be resistant to other drugs. Infections with multidrug-resistant tuberculosis are very difficult to treat and should be referred to an expert in tuberculosis management. Extensively drug-resistant tuberculosis is a relatively rare type of multidrug-resistant tuberculosis that is resistant to not only isoniazid and rifampin but also to the best second-line medications, including fluoroquinolones and at least 1 of 3 injectable drugs (ie, amikacin, kanamycin, or capreomycin).

- Directly observed therapy is strongly recommended for all patients with tuberculosis.

Extrapulmonary Tuberculosis

Lymphatic tuberculosis (scrofula) is most commonly found in the head and neck region, including posterior cervical and supraclavicular chains. Although most cases of mycobacterial lymphadenitis in children are caused by *Mycobacterium avium-intracellulare*, more than 90% of cases in adults are from *M tuberculosis* infection. Pleural

tuberculosis commonly presents with a unilateral effusion. Pleural fluid analysis shows a predominance of mononuclear cells and a low glucose level. Culture of the pleural fluid is usually negative, but pleural biopsy can increase the diagnostic yield to 90% to 95%. Genitourinary tuberculosis can involve the kidneys, ureters, bladder, and reproductive organs. Calcifications of renal parenchyma and ureteral strictures may occur. Vertebral infection with tuberculosis (Pott disease) causes an anterior wedging and collapse of the vertebral body, producing a gibbous deformity. Tuberculous infection of the central nervous system manifests as a chronic meningitis with basilar arachnoiditis, cranial nerve deficits, hydrocephalus, vascular thrombosis, and tissue necrosis. Findings on cerebrospinal fluid evaluation are mononuclear cell predominance, increased protein value, and decreased glucose value.

Miliary (disseminated) tuberculosis (simultaneous involvement of multiple organs) can be a progressive form of primary disease or a product of reactivating disease. Young children, the elderly, and immunosuppressed persons are most at risk. Chest radiography may show miliary shadows composed of 1- to 2-mm well-defined nodules throughout both lungs. Tuberculin skin testing commonly results in no reaction (cutaneous anergy), and the diagnosis of disseminated tuberculosis can be difficult. Extrapulmonary tuberculosis is adequately treated with the same regimens as those for pulmonary tuberculosis, with a few exceptions: an extended course of therapy is recommended for vertebral, central nervous system–meningeal, and disseminated tuberculosis. Adjunctive corticosteroids may be indicated in the management of meningeal and pericardial tuberculosis.

Table 15-2 Treatment of Pulmonary Tuberculosis[a]

Option 1
　Initiation: INH, RFP, PZA, EMB daily × 8 wk
　Continuation: INH, RFP daily or 2-3 times/wk DOT for 16 wk
Option 2
　Initiation: INH, RFP, PZA, EMB daily × 2 wk, then INH, RFP, PZA, EMB 2 times/wk DOT × 6 wk
　Continuation: INH, RFP 2 times/wk DOT × 16 wk
Option 3
　INH, RFP, PZA, EMB 3 times/wk DOT × 6 mo
Special circumstances
　Intolerant to PZA: INH, RFP × 9 mo[b]
　Pregnancy[c]: INH, RFP, EMB × 9 mo

Abbreviations: DOT, directly observed therapy; EMB, ethambutol; INH, isoniazid; PZA, pyrazinamide; RFP, rifampin.

[a] Ethambutol or streptomycin should be added to all regimens until susceptibility data are known or unless isoniazid resistance is less than 4% in the geographic area. Pyridoxine (vitamin B_6) should be given with all regimens containing isoniazid and during pregnancy.

[b] Twice per week dosing can be given after 1 to 2 months if isolate is sensitive.

[c] Streptomycin and pyrazinamide are not recommended during pregnancy; streptomycin may be harmful to the fetus, and pyrazinamide has not been well studied during pregnancy.

- Unlike in children, more than 90% of cases of mycobacterial lymphadenitis in adults are due to *M tuberculosis*.
- Adjunctive corticosteroids are beneficial in the management of meningeal and pericardial tuberculosis.
- A prolonged course of therapy is recommended for vertebral, central nervous system, and disseminated tuberculosis.

Screening for Tuberculosis

Current guidelines for detection of latent tuberculosis infection emphasize a targeted screening approach toward patients at risk for tuberculosis. Only persons at high risk for recent infection or with clinical conditions that increase the risk for tuberculosis should be screened. Criteria to identify persons with latent tuberculosis infection or high-risk contacts are listed in Table 15-3. Tuberculin skin test (TST) conversion is defined as an increase of 10 mm or more in induration within a 2-year period, regardless of age. All persons with a positive result of TST require chest radiography and evaluation to exclude clinical disease. For patients with chest radiographic findings consistent with prior or untreated tuberculosis, an evaluation for active disease, including sputum sample collection, should be performed before therapy is started. If chest radiography or clinical evaluation raises the suspicion for active disease, then combination chemotherapy should be initiated while culture results are awaited. Contacts of persons with infectious cases of tuberculosis should have a baseline TST. If the result is negative, a repeat TST is done 10 to 12 weeks later (a delayed-type hypersensitivity skin test response to

M tuberculosis is generally detectable 2-12 weeks after infection). Healthy immunocompetent adults may be observed without initiating medical therapy unless the initial TST result is 5 mm or more; however, immunosuppressed adults, HIV-infected persons, and children should start preventive therapy regardless of the initial TST. Treatment can be discontinued in children if repeat skin testing at 12 weeks is negative.

- Only persons at high risk for latent tuberculosis infection or with clinical conditions that increase the risk for tuberculosis should be screened, regardless of age.
- Tuberculin skin test (TST) conversion is defined as an increase of 10 mm or more in induration within a 2-year period, regardless of age.
- All persons with a positive result of TST require chest radiography and evaluation to exclude clinical disease.

Delayed-type hypersensitivity may wane over time in some individuals infected with *M tuberculosis*. In these persons, a TST many years after infection may be nonreactive; however, it can stimulate or "boost" hypersensitivity to subsequent skin tests and be misinterpreted as new infection. Two-step testing is designed to identify and distinguish between boosted reactions ("booster effect"), signifying previous infection, and reactions due to new or recent infection. If the first test result is positive, the patient should be considered infected (recent or remote). If the initial TST is negative, a positive repeat skin test 1 to 3 weeks later indicates previous rather than new infection. A negative

Table 15-3 Candidates for Treatment of Latent Tuberculosis Infection or Special Contacts,[a] by Diameter of Induration Produced by Tuberculin Skin Testing

<5 mm	≥5 mm	≥10 mm	≥15 mm
Child <5 y old & recent close contact HIV infection & recent close contact Immunosuppressed & recent close contact	HIV-infected persons Persons with organ transplants & other immunosuppressed patients (receiving the equivalent of ≥15 mg/day of prednisone for ≥1 mo) Recent contact with infectious tuberculosis Fibrotic changes on chest radiograph consistent with prior tuberculosis (if patient not previously fully treated)	Recent tuberculin skin test converters (within past 2 y) Injection drug users who are HIV-negative High-risk medical conditions[b] Residents & employees of high-risk congregate settings[c] Recent immigrants (within past 5 y) from areas where tuberculosis is common[d] Health care workers, depending on individual risk factors Children <4 y old Children or adolescents exposed to adults at high risk	No risk factors (tuberculin skin test not recommended)

Abbreviation: HIV, human immunodeficiency virus.
[a] Recent contacts who are initially negative on tuberculin skin testing should have a repeat test 10 to 12 weeks after last exposure to tuberculosis. Treatment can be discontinued if repeat result is negative.
[b] Gastrectomy, hematologic malignancies, reticuloendothelial diseases, renal failure, other malignancies, diabetes (insulin-dependent), silicosis, jejunoileal bypass.
[c] Nursing homes, long-term care facilities, prisons or jails, homeless shelters.
[d] Asia, Africa, Latin America.

TST *never* excludes tuberculosis. Although less common in otherwise healthy individuals, the TST result may be falsely negative in 20% to 25% of patients with active tuberculosis. In persons infected with both HIV and tuberculosis, the percentage of false-negative skin tests variably ranges between 30% and 80%, depending on the magnitude of cell-mediated immunity damage. Therefore, clinical judgment is always required when screening for tuberculosis.

* Two-step testing may help distinguish boosted reactions from new infection.
* If the first test result is positive, the patient should be considered infected (recent or remote).
* If the first test is negative and the repeat skin test 1-3 weeks later is positive (booster effect), the result most likely represents previous infection.

Outside the United States, the bacille Calmette-Guérin (BCG) vaccine is commonly administered to children and infants and can serve as a source of confusion in TST interpretation. Reactivity to the BCG vaccine by tuberculin skin testing generally decreases with time, and previous BCG vaccination generally should be disregarded in TST interpretation. Unless BCG vaccine was recently administered (ie, within the past year), significant TST reactions should not be attributable to BCG vaccine and probably indicate infection with *M tuberculosis*.

In 2005, the US Food and Drug Administration approved a new assay for the detection of *M tuberculosis* infection: the Quantiferon-TB Gold (QFT-G; Cellestis). The QFT-G assay measures the release of interferon-γ in fresh heparinized whole blood from sensitized persons when it is incubated with mixtures of synthetic peptides representing 2 proteins present in *M tuberculosis*: early secretory antigenic target-6 and culture filtrate protein-10. The sensitivity of the QFT-G assay is similar to that of TST, and the test is recommended for use in all circumstances in which the TST is currently used, as outlined above. Although the QFT-G assay can detect *M tuberculosis* infection with high specificity, it does not distinguish between active tuberculosis and latent tuberculosis infection. Its sensitivity for particular groups of patients with tuberculosis (eg, young children and immunocompromised patients) has not been determined. A recent study in San Francisco, California, evaluated the sensitivity of the QFT-G assay for the detection of tuberculosis among 242 persons with suspected tuberculosis. Thirty-seven subjects had culture-confirmed tuberculosis. Only 23 of 36 subjects (64%; 95% confidence interval, 48%-78%) had positive QFT-G assay results. Therefore, a negative QFT-G assay should not be used alone to exclude *M tuberculosis* infection in persons with symptoms or signs suggestive of tuberculosis.

* The QFT-G assay is similar to that of TST and is recommended to be used in all circumstances in which the TST is currently used.
* A negative QFT-G assay should not be used alone to exclude *M tuberculosis* infection in persons with symptoms or signs suggestive of tuberculosis.

Treatment of Latent Tuberculosis Infection

Administration of isoniazid for 9 months is preferred for treatment of latent tuberculosis infection for all patients, including those with HIV infection, chest radiographic lesions suggestive of prior inactive disease, and children and adolescents. Treatment with rifampin for 4 months is an alternative for patients intolerant to isoniazid or exposed to isoniazid-resistant tuberculosis. Rifampin plus pyrazinamide for 2 months is no longer recommended for therapy of latent tuberculosis infection because of an increased risk of hepatotoxicity. Completion of therapy is defined by the total number of doses administered and not on duration of therapy alone. Therefore, the 9-month daily isoniazid regimen should consist of at least 270 doses administered within 12 months, whereas the twice-weekly isoniazid regimen should consist of at least 76 doses administered within 12 months. Baseline and routine laboratory monitoring during treatment are generally not indicated, except for patients at increased risk of drug toxicity. Active hepatitis and end-stage liver disease are relative contraindications to use of isoniazid for treatment of latent tuberculosis infection. Contrary to the urgency for treatment of active tuberculosis in pregnant women, treatment of latent tuberculosis infection during pregnancy is usually less imperative and more controversial. Most authorities delay treatment of latent tuberculosis infection until after delivery; however, recently infected women and those with HIV coinfection should most likely be treated during pregnancy (preferably with isoniazid) and monitored closely.

* Isoniazid administration for 9 months is the preferred treatment for latent tuberculosis infection for all patients, including those with HIV infection, chest radiographic lesions suggestive of prior inactive disease, and children and adolescents.
* Baseline and routine laboratory monitoring during treatment of latent tuberculosis infection are generally not indicated, except for certain patients at increased risk of drug toxicity.

Diseases Other Than Tuberculosis Which Are Due to Mycobacteria

Mycobacterium marinum causes swimming pool granuloma and may occur after cleaning an aquarium. It presents with a chronic indurated nodule on the finger or hand. *Mycobacterium marinum* responds to therapy with rifampin plus ethambutol, doxycycline, or trimethoprim-sulfamethoxazole.

* *Mycobacterium marinum* causes swimming pool granuloma.

Mycobacterium kansasii produces a pulmonary disease resembling that caused by *M tuberculosis*. *Mycobacterium kansasii* is more resistant to isoniazid than is *M tuberculosis*. Standard treatment regimens include isoniazid, rifampin, and ethambutol and continue for 12 to 24 months.

* *Mycobacterium kansasii* pulmonary disease resembles tuberculosis.

Mycobacterium avium-intracellulare is an important cause of infection in advanced AIDS, in which disseminated disease is common. Although usually only a respiratory tract colonizer, *M avium-intracellulare* also may cause chronic pulmonary infections. There are 4 characteristic chest radiographic appearances for *M avium-intracellulare* pulmonary disease: multiple discrete nodules (71% of patients), bronchiectasis, upper lobe infiltrates, and diffuse infiltrates. The newer macrolides (clarithromycin and azithromycin) are the most active drugs against *M avium-intracellulare*.

- Chest radiographic findings with *M avium-intracellulare* pulmonary disease include multiple discrete nodules (71% of patients), bronchiectasis, upper lobe infiltrates, and diffuse infiltrates.

Rapid-growing mycobacteria include *Mycobacterium fortuitum* and *Mycobacterium chelonei*. Typically they cause indolent subcutaneous infections of an extremity. They also are associated with osteomyelitis and nosocomial infection (sternal osteomyelitis after cardiac operation, intramuscular injection). Treatment often requires surgical excision of the lesions. Although resistant to antituberculosis drugs, the rapid growers are usually susceptible to clarithromycin.

Spirochetes

Syphilis is discussed in Part II of this chapter in the section "Sexually Transmitted Diseases."

Leptospirosis

Leptospira interrogans infection is acquired by contact with urine from infected animals (rats, dogs), and it causes a biphasic disease. The infections occur more often after a rainy season. The organism can enter directly through the skin from contaminated water that contains animal urine. Leptospirosis can be diagnosed in persons exposed to contaminated freshwater and in persons who have fever on returning from traveling. The *first phase*, the leptospiremic phase, is characterized by abrupt-onset headache (98%), fever, chills, conjunctivitis, severe muscle aching, gastrointestinal symptoms (50%), changes in sensorium (25%), rash (7%), and hypotension. This phase lasts 3 to 7 days. Improvement in symptoms coincides with disappearance of *Leptospira* organisms from blood and cerebrospinal fluid. The *second phase*, immune stage, occurs after a relatively asymptomatic period of 1 to 3 days, when fever and generalized symptoms recur. Meningeal symptoms often develop during this period. The second phase is characterized by the appearance of immunoglobulin M antibodies. Most patients recover after 1 to 3 days. However, in serious cases, hepatic dysfunction and renal failure may develop. Death in patients with leptospirosis usually occurs in the second phase as a result of hepatic and renal failure.

- *Leptospira interrogans* infection is acquired by contact with urine from infected animals (rats, dogs).
- Leptospirosis is a biphasic disease.

The diagnosis of leptospirosis is established on the basis of clinical presentation and of cultures of blood and, rarely, cerebrospinal fluid in the first 7 to 10 days of infection. Urine cultures can remain positive in the second week of illness. Serologic testing by immunoglobulin M detection with enzyme-linked immunosorbent assay or microscopic agglutination test has a low sensitivity, especially in the acute phase, but it increases to 89% and 63% in the second phase of disease, respectively. The specificity of both tests is high (>94%) in all specimens. Treatment with penicillin G is effective *only* if given with-

in the first 1 to 5 days from onset of symptoms. Oral amoxicillin or doxycycline can be used for mild-moderate illness.

- Treatment of leptospirosis with penicillin G is effective only if given within the first 1-5 days from onset of symptoms.

Lyme Disease

Epidemiology

Lyme disease is the most common vector-borne (*Ixodes* ticks) disease reported in the United States. The incidence of disease is highest in the spring and summer, when exposure to the tick vector is most common. Experimental evidence suggests that ticks must be attached for more than 24 hours to transmit infection. Although Lyme disease has been reported from most states, it is most common in coastal New England and New York, the mid-Atlantic states, Oregon, northern California, and the Upper Midwest. The white-footed mouse and the white-tailed deer serve as zoonotic reservoirs for the etiologic agent *Borrelia burgdorferi*. Coinfections with *Babesia* or *Ehrlichia* species can occur in up to 15% and may increase the severity of symptoms.

- *Borrelia burgdorferi* is the etiologic agent of Lyme disease.

Clinical Syndromes

Stage 1 (early) occurs from 3 to 32 days after the tick bite. Erythema migrans (solitary or multiple lesions) is the hallmark of Lyme disease and occurs in 80% or more of infected persons. It can be associated with fever, lymphadenopathy, and meningismus. The rash of erythema migrans usually enlarges and resolves over 3 to 4 weeks. *Borrelia burgdorferi* disseminates hematogenously early in the course of the illness.

- Erythema migrans develops in ≥80% of patients with Lyme disease.

Stage 2 occurs weeks to months after stage 1. In 10% to 15% of cases, neurologic abnormalities develop (facial nerve palsy, lymphocytic meningitis, encephalitis, chorea, myelitis, radiculitis, and peripheral neuropathy). Carditis (reversible atrioventricular block) occurs in 5% to 10% of patients. Conduction abnormalities are mostly reversible, and permanent heart block is rare. Temporary pacing may be necessary in approximately 30% of patients. Dilated cardiomyopathy has been reported, and conjunctivitis and iritis also occur.

- During stage 2 of Lyme disease, 10%-15% of patients have neurologic abnormalities.
- Carditis occurs in 5%-10% of patients with Lyme disease.

Stage 3, although uncommon, can develop months to years after initial infection. Monarticular or oligoarticular arthritis occurs in 50% of patients who do not receive effective therapy. It becomes chronic in 10% to 20%. Chronic arthritis is more common in those with HLA-DR2 and HLA-DR4. Other manifestations are acrodermatitis chronica atrophicans (primarily with European strains), progressive, chronic encephalitis, and dementia (rare). Most patients will have detectable serum antibodies against *B burgdorferi*. Magnetic resonance imaging may show demyelination.

Diagnosis

Anti-*B burgdorferi* antibodies can be detected by enzyme-linked immunosorbent assay after the first 2 to 6 weeks of illness. Serologic testing is likely to be negative in the early stage (ie, with the erythema migrans rash). At this stage, a polymerase chain reaction test of the skin has a high yield, but this test in the blood is not sensitive and should not be used. Response may be diminished by antimicrobial therapy early in the course. Antibody testing is not standardized. False-positive results occur with infectious mononucleosis, rheumatoid arthritis, systemic lupus erythematosus, echovirus infection, and other spirochetal disease. The Western blot test is an adjunct in diagnosis when antibody response is equivocal or when a false-positive result is suspected. It is particularly useful in the first few months of illness.

Treatment

For stage 1 (early) Lyme disease in the absence of neurologic involvement or complete heart block, doxycycline (100 mg twice a day for 10-21 days), amoxicillin (500 mg 3 times a day for 10-21 days), and cefuroxime axetil (500 mg twice a day for 10-21 days) are effective therapeutic agents. Azithromycin, clarithromycin, or erythromycin is less effective than doxycycline or amoxicillin but can be used in penicillin-allergic patients. Because of the risk of vertical transmission, all pregnant women with active Lyme disease should be treated. Doxycycline is contraindicated in pregnant women and children younger than 8 years.

In Lyme carditis, the outcome is usually favorable. If first- or second-degree atrioventricular block is present, it should be treated with oral agents, whereas third-degree heart block should be treated with ceftriaxone, 2 g a day for 14 to 21 days, or penicillin G, 20 million units a day for 14 to 21 days. Lyme meningitis, radiculopathy, or encephalitis should be treated parenterally.

* In Lyme carditis, the outcome is usually favorable.

The outcome in patients with facial palsy is also usually favorable. In one series, 105 of 122 affected patients completely recovered. Corticosteroids have no role. If only facial nerve palsy is present (no symptoms of meningitis, radiculoneuritis), oral therapy with doxycycline or amoxicillin is used. The therapy used if other neurologic manifestations are present is described below.

* The outcome in patients with facial palsy due to Lyme disease is usually favorable.

If Lyme meningitis is present, ceftriaxone, 2 g a day for 14 to 28 days, or penicillin G, 20 million units a day for 14 to 28 days, should be given. Radiculoneuritis and peripheral neuropathy may have a greater tendency for chronicity and often occur with meningitis. Treatment is the same as that for Lyme-associated meningitis. The regimens for encephalopathy and encephalomyelitis are identical to those for meningitis.

* Radiculoneuritis and peripheral neuropathy may have a greater tendency for chronicity and often occur with meningitis.

Optimal regimens for Lyme arthritis (oral vs intravenous) are not established. Intra-articular corticosteroids may cause treatment failures. Joint rest and aspiration of reaccumulated joint fluid are often needed. Response to antibiotics may be delayed. If no neurologic disease is present, doxycycline is given (100 mg orally twice a day for 28 days). An alternative regimen is amoxicillin and probenecid (500 mg each, 4 times a day for 28 days) or ceftriaxone (2 g per day intravenously for 14-28 days).

Prevention

Prophylactic antibiotic therapy after a tick bite is not recommended. Use of single-dose doxycycline is recommended only if 1) the adult or nymphal *Ixodes scapularis* tick has been attached for 36 hours (as evidenced by engorgement of the tick or by certainty of time of exposure to tick), 2) prophylaxis can be started within 72 hours of tick removal, 3) the *B burgdorferi* prevalence rate is 20% among ticks within the region of the tick bite, and 4) doxycycline is not contraindicated. In the vast majority of tick bites, disease is not transmitted. Appropriate use of DEET (*N, N*-diethyl-3-methylbenzamide)- or picaridin-containing insect repellents and protective clothing are strongly recommended.

* Prophylactic antibiotic therapy after a tick bite is not recommended, unless 1) the adult or nymphal *I scapularis* tick has been attached for 36 hours (as evidenced by engorgement of the tick or by certainty of time of exposure to tick), 2) prophylaxis can be started within 72 hours of tick removal, 3) *B burgdorferi* prevalence rate is 20% among ticks within the region of the tick bite, and 4) doxycycline is not contraindicated.

Nocardia

Nocardia organisms are aerobic, gram-positive, filamentous, and branching and are visualized with a modified acid-fast stain. *Nocardia asteroides* is the cause of most human infections in the United States (Figure 15-3). *Nocardia brasiliensis* and *Nocardia madurae* cause mycetomas. Infections are most often opportunistic, occurring in immunosuppressed patients, including those with HIV or AIDS, but infections can occur in normal hosts also.

* *Nocardia* infections are most often opportunistic, occurring in immunosuppressed patients.

The respiratory tract is the usual portal of entry for *Nocardia* infection. Chronic pneumonitis and lung abscess are the most common findings. Hematogenous spread to the brain is relatively common. Computed tomography or magnetic resonance imaging of the head is advised in immunocompromised patients with pulmonary nocardiosis. Spread also can occur to the skin (12%) and joints (3%). In patients with chronic pneumonia who have neurologic symptoms or signs, *Nocardia* brain abscess should be considered.

* In patients with chronic pneumonia who have neurologic symptoms, *Nocardia* brain abscess should be considered.

Nocardiosis is not diagnosed until autopsy in up to 40% of cases. Antemortem diagnosis depends on obtaining appropriate stains and cultures (the organism will grow on fungal media). Because sputum culture is relatively insensitive, bronchoscopically obtained specimens or open lung biopsy may be needed to confirm the diagnosis. The disease must be differentiated from other causes of chronic pneumonia (such as bacterial, actinomycotic, tuberculosis, fungal infections).

Therapy involves drainage of abscesses and high doses of sulfonamide drugs (trimethoprim-sulfamethoxazole is the current drug of choice). Some species of *Nocardia* show evidence of sulfonamide resistance. Other antimicrobial agents used for nocardiosis include imipenem, amikacin, minocycline, and cephalosporins. Therapy depends on antimicrobial susceptibility patterns. Newer drugs such as linezolid have activity against *Nocardia* species.

- Nocardiosis is diagnosed at autopsy in up to 40% of cases.
- Trimethoprim-sulfamethoxazole is the current treatment of choice.

Rickettsiae

All rickettsial infections are transmitted by an insect vector except Q fever (respiratory spread). All are associated with a rash except Q fever and ehrlichiosis. The rash of Rocky Mountain spotted fever may be indistinguishable from that of meningococcemia. Rocky Mountain spotted fever rash begins on the extremities and moves centrally. The rash of typhus (both murine and endemic typhus) begins centrally and moves toward the extremities. Rocky Mountain spotted fever is most common in the mid-Atlantic states and Oklahoma, not the Rocky Mountain states. The pathophysiology of all rickettsial infections includes vasculitis and disseminated intravascular coagulation. Rickettsial pox is a common, although usually unrecognized, disease in urban areas of the United States. It is the only rickettsial disease characterized by vesicular rash. The mouse mite is the vector for rickettsial pox. A small eschar is present at the site of inoculation in 95% of patients.

- All rickettsial infections have an insect vector except Q fever.
- All are associated with a rash except Q fever and ehrlichiosis.

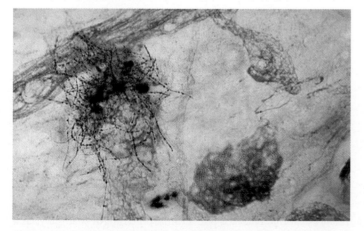

Figure 15-3. *Nocardia asteroides* (Modified Acid-Fast Stain, ×450).

- Rocky Mountain spotted fever rash begins on the extremities and moves centrally.
- Rocky Mountain spotted fever is most common in the mid-Atlantic states and Oklahoma, not the Rocky Mountain states.

Coxiella burnetii, the cause of Q fever, is acquired by inhalation of contaminated aerosol particles of dust, earth, or feces or after exposure to animal products, especially infected placentas. Sheep are common sources, but other animals, including cats, can harbor the disease (eg, a small outbreak occurred in a group of poker players after a cat gave birth beneath their card table). Disease manifests most commonly as an isolated febrile illness, most of those cases presenting with pneumonitis; 15% of patients have hepatitis (granulomatous), 1% have endocarditis, and some also present with central nervous system manifestations. Q fever is one of the causes of culture-negative endocarditis. It usually is diagnosed with serologic testing. Treatment is with tetracyclines or chloramphenicol.

- Among persons with Q fever, most have pneumonitis, and 15% have hepatitis.
- Q fever is one of the causes of culture-negative endocarditis.

Ehrlichia species are gram-negative intracellular bacteria that resemble rickettsial organisms and preferentially infect lymphocytes, monocytes, and neutrophils. The species that cause human ehrlichiosis are *E chaffeensis* (which infects monocytes), *E equi*, and *Anaplasma phagocytophilum* (which causes human granulocytic ehrlichiosis).

The disease is seasonal; the peak incidence is from May through July. The vectors are the common dog tick (*Dermacentor variabilis*), the lone star tick (*Amblyomma americanum*) for *E chaffeensis*, and *Ixodes* ticks for the agent of human granulocytic ehrlichiosis. The incubation period is approximately 7 days, followed by fever, chills, malaise, headache, and myalgia. Less than 50% of patients have a rash. Important laboratory features include leukopenia, thrombocytopenia, and increased levels of hepatic transaminases.

The severity of the disease is variable, but severe complications, including death, can occur. Coinfection with human granulocytic ehrlichiosis and *B burgdorferi* (Lyme disease) does occur and can be especially severe. Diagnosis depends on serologic analysis (indirect immunofluorescent assay) or detection by polymerase chain reaction amplification. Treatment is with doxycycline, 100 mg twice a day. Unlike the rickettsial diseases, chloramphenicol is often not effective against *Ehrlichia*.

Mycoplasma pneumoniae

This is one of the smallest microorganisms capable of extracellular replication. *Mycoplasma* organisms lack a cell wall. Therefore, cell-wall-active antibiotics such as penicillins are not effective treatment. *Mycoplasma* infection is spread by droplet inhalation. It primarily infects young, previously healthy persons and presents with rapid onset of headache, dry cough, and fever. Results of physical examination are often unremarkable, with the possible exception of bullous myringitis. Chest radiography usually shows bilateral, patchy pneumonitis. The chest radiographic findings are often out of proportion to the physical findings. Pleural effusion is present in 15% to 20% of cases. Neurologic complications include Guillain-Barré syndrome, cerebellar peripheral neuropathy, aseptic meningitis, and mononeuritis multiplex. Hemolytic anemia may occur late in the illness as a result of circulating cold hemagglutinins.

- Circulating cold hemagglutinins can cause hemolytic anemia.
- *Mycoplasma pneumoniae* infection is spread by droplet inhalation.
- Chest radiography usually shows bilateral, patchy pneumonitis.
- Pleural effusion is present in 15%-20% of cases.
- Neurologic complications include Guillain-Barré syndrome, cerebellar peripheral neuropathy, aseptic meningitis, and mononeuritis multiplex.

The diagnosis is established by specific complement fixation test. Cold agglutinins are nonspecific and unreliable for diagnosing *Mycoplasma* infections. Fluoroquinolones, macrolides, and tetracyclines are effective therapies. Because immunity to *Mycoplasma* infection is transient, reinfection may occur. Clinical relapse of pneumonia occurs in up to 10% of cases of *Mycoplasma* pneumonia.

Chlamydophila (Chlamydia) pneumoniae

Chlamydophila (Chlamydia) pneumoniae is a relatively newer *Chlamydophila (Chlamydia)* species known to be pathogenic to humans. *Chlamydia trachomatis* and *Chlamydophila psittaci* are the other 2 chlamydial species that cause human disease. In young adults, *C pneumoniae* causes 10% of cases of pneumonia and 5% of cases of bronchitis. It has been a cause of community outbreaks, and nosocomial transmission has occurred. Fifty percent of adults are seropositive for *C pneumoniae*. Birds are the source of infection with *C psittaci* (psittacosis), but there is no reservoir for *C pneumoniae*. Clinical manifestations of infection are usually mild and may resemble those caused by *M pneumoniae*. Pharyngitis occurs 1 to 3 weeks before the onset of pulmonary symptoms, and cough may last for weeks. The diagnosis is based on serologic testing. Treatment is with doxycycline or a macrolide. The newer fluoroquinolones such as levofloxacin and gatifloxacin have in vitro activity against *C pneumoniae*, but clinical efficacy studies are not available. Of note, trimethoprim-sulfamethoxazole and β-lactam antibiotics such as penicillins or cephalosporins are not active against chlamydial species.

- In young adults, *C pneumoniae* causes 10% of cases of pneumonia and 5% of cases of bronchitis.

Fungi

Coccidioidomycosis

Coccidioides immitis is a dimorphic fungus: in tissue it exists as a spherule, and in culture at room temperature it is mycelial (filamentous). It forms arthrospores that are highly infectious. *Coccidioides immitis* is endemic in the southwestern United States, especially the San Joaquin Valley of California and central Arizona. Disseminated disease is most likely to occur in males (especially Filipino and black), pregnant females, and immunocompromised hosts regardless of sex.

Nonpregnant white females seem to be more resistant to disseminated disease than white males.

- *Coccidioides immitis* is endemic in the southwestern United States.
- Disseminated disease is most likely to occur in males (especially Filipino and black), pregnant females, and immunocompromised hosts.

Half to two-thirds (~60%) of primary infections with *C immitis* are subclinical. The most common clinical manifestation is pneumonitis that is usually self-limited. Common manifestations are dry cough and fever (valley fever) that may resemble influenza. Associated findings include hilar adenopathy, pleural effusion (12%), thin-walled cavities (5%), and solid "coin" lesions. Disseminated infection predominantly affects the central nervous system, skin, bones, and joints.

- Primary infection with *C immitis* causes pneumonitis that is usually self-limited.

Coccidioidomycosis is one of the causes of erythema nodosum. When present, it usually indicates an active immune response that will control the infection. Erythema nodosum is more common in females and is often associated with arthralgias, especially of the knees and ankles.

- Coccidioidomycosis is one of the causes of erythema nodosum.

The diagnosis of coccidioidomycosis is based on detecting the organism by culture or biopsy with silver stains. A *C immitis* serologic (complement fixation) titer more than 1:4 is suggestive of infection. Skin testing is of epidemiologic value only. Detection of cerebrospinal fluid anticoccidioidal antibodies is the usual means for diagnosing coccidioidomycosis meningitis. A biopsy specimen may reveal a diagnostic *C immitis* spherule (Figure 15-4). Laboratory abnormalities may include eosinophilia and hypercalcemia.

Fluconazole, itraconazole, and amphotericin B are effective for therapy of coccidioidomycosis. The acute pulmonary form is usually self-limited and observation may be adequate. However, therapy is indicated if a patient is pregnant, is immunocompromised (patients with AIDS or receiving immunosuppressive regimens for organ transplantation or other medical reasons), or has worsening infection without therapy. Amphotericin B is the drug of choice for severe manifestations and for pregnant women with coccidioidomycosis. An alternative to fluconazole is itraconazole (200 mg twice daily). For meningitis, therapy with high-dose fluconazole is preferred and has largely replaced intrathecal amphotericin B. Because of the high relapse rate of *C immitis* meningitis, chronic suppressive therapy is necessary, usually with fluconazole. *Coccidioides* meningitis may be complicated by adhesive arachnoiditis. Newer antifungal medications such as voriconazole are active in vitro but clinical studies are not available, and caspofungin has limited in vitro activity against coccidioidomycosis.

Histoplasmosis

Histoplasma capsulatum is also a dimorphic fungus that grows as a small (3 mm in diameter) yeast in tissue. Culture at room temperature produces the mycelial form. Although present in many areas of the world, histoplasmosis is especially prevalent in the Ohio, Missouri, and Mississippi river valleys. Outbreaks have been associated with large construction projects and exposure to bird droppings. Histoplasmosis is acquired by inhalation of spores and also can be transmitted by organ transplantation from an infected donor. The risk of acquisition is increased with certain activities, including caving and bridge or other construction. Although healthy individuals may acquire histoplasmosis, patients with AIDS are particularly susceptible. *Histoplasma capsulatum* infection is one of the causes of caseating granulomata.

* Outbreaks of histoplasmosis have been associated with large construction projects and exposure to bird droppings.
* Although healthy individuals may acquire histoplasmosis, patients with AIDS are particularly susceptible.

Primary (acute) histoplasmosis may be clinically indistinguishable from influenza or other upper respiratory tract infections. After resolution, multiple small, calcified granulomas may be seen on subsequent chest radiography. The progressive (disseminated) form of histoplasmosis is uncommon but serious. The disseminated form and reactivation of prior disease are most likely to occur in infants, elderly men, and immunosuppressed persons, including those with HIV or AIDS and those receiving therapy with tumor necrosis factor-α inhibitor. Manifestations may resemble those of lymphoma, with weight loss, fever, anemia, increased erythrocyte sedimentation rate, and splenomegaly. Mucosal surface lesions, especially in the mouth, are not infrequent. As with tuberculosis, the adrenal glands may be infected, with resulting adrenal insufficiency. Chronic cavitary pulmonary disease due to *Histoplasma* may resemble tuberculosis.

* Primary (acute) histoplasmosis may be indistinguishable from influenza or other upper respiratory tract infections.
* As with tuberculosis, the adrenal glands may be infected by *H capsulatum*, with resulting adrenal insufficiency.

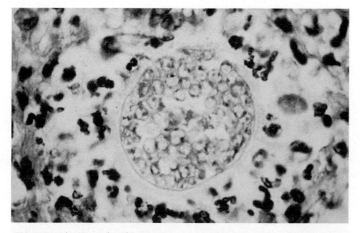

Figure 15-4. *Coccidioides immitis* Spherules in a Clinical Specimen (Grocott Methenamine-Silver Stain).

Serologic testing is of limited sensitivity and specificity and plays little role in the diagnosis of active infection unless increasing or markedly increased titers are detected. Biopsy, silver staining, and cultures of infected tissues are the best means of diagnosis. Bone marrow stains and cultures and fungal blood cultures are frequently helpful. Biopsy specimens of mouth lesions can be diagnostic. Detection of *Histoplasma* antigen in urine, cerebrospinal fluid, or serum is easily available as a diagnostic test, especially for disseminated disease.

The mild, acute forms of histoplasmosis are usually self-limited and do not require therapy. Amphotericin B in a *total* dose of 35 mg/kg (given over time as 0.5-1 mg/kg per day) is the drug of choice for all severe, life-threatening cases. Itraconazole is effective for most nonmeningeal, non–life-threatening cases and has largely replaced ketoconazole. Itraconazole dosage is 200 to 400 mg per day (guided by serum drug concentrations) for 6 to 12 months. Patients with AIDS require chronic maintenance therapy.

Blastomycosis
Yet another dimorphic fungal pathogen is *Blastomyces dermatitidis*. In tissue, the yeast forms are thick-walled and have broad-based buds (±10 µm in diameter) (Figure 15-5). In culture at room temperature, a mycelial form is found. Blastomycosis is endemic in the southeastern and upper midwestern United States. Primary pulmonary blastomycosis may be asymptomatic and may disseminate hematogenously to bone, skin, or prostate. Granulomas occur, but calcification is less frequent than with histoplasmosis or tuberculosis.

Blastomycosis affects lung, skin, bone (especially the vertebrae), male genitalia (prostate, epididymis, testis), and the central nervous system. The pulmonary form has no characteristic findings: pleural effusion is rare, hilar adenopathy develops occasionally, and cavitation is infrequent. It often mimics carcinoma of the lung. Cutaneous involvement with blastomycosis is common. Lesions, especially on the face, are characteristically painless and nonpruritic and have a sharp, spreading border. Chronic crusty lesions may occur.

* Blastomycosis affects lungs, skin, bone (especially the vertebrae), and male genitalia (prostate, epididymis, testis).
* The most common clinical forms of blastomycosis are pulmonary and cutaneous.

The diagnosis of blastomycosis is based on the results of biopsy, stains, and cultures. Serologic and skin testing are *rarely* helpful.

Amphotericin B (total dose is 20-25 mg/kg) or itraconazole (200-400 mg per day for 6 months) is effective as therapy for blastomycosis. Amphotericin B is reserved primarily for life-threatening infections. Mild-to-moderate nonmeningeal blastomycosis can be treated with itraconazole (200-400 mg/day) for 6 months.

Sporotrichosis
A fourth dimorphic fungal pathogen, *Sporothrix schenckii*, in tissue is a round, cigar-shaped yeast. In culture at room temperature it is mycelial. *Sporothrix schenckii* is most often found in soil, plants, or plant products such as straw, wood, and sphagnum moss, and thorny plants. Sporotrichosis is transmitted by cutaneous inoculation

(rose-gardener's disease) and, rarely, through inhalation. It manifests as a suppurative and granulomatous reaction.

Cutaneous infection produces characteristic crusty lesions ascending the lymphatics of the extremities from the initial site of infection. Similar lesions may be produced by infection with *M marinum*, *Nocardia*, or cutaneous leishmaniasis. Joint spaces rarely are involved. Sporotrichosis occasionally may cause chronic pneumonitis (with cavitation and empyema) or meningitis.

* Cutaneous sporotrichosis produces characteristic crusty lesions ascending the lymphatics of the extremities from the initial site of infection.
* Sporotrichosis occasionally may cause chronic pneumonitis (with cavitation and empyema) or meningitis.

The diagnosis of sporotrichosis may be difficult and depends on clinical recognition of the cutaneous lesions in most instances. Biopsy, culture, or serologic testing may aid in the diagnosis.

For the lymphocutaneous or cutaneous form, itraconazole is the therapy of choice. An effective alternative is supersaturated solution of potassium iodide. Amphotericin B is recommended for disseminated disease (pulmonary, joint), although it may respond poorly to therapy.

Aspergillosis

Aspergillus is an opportunistic pathogen that causes infection in immunocompromised persons, particularly those with prolonged neutropenia or steroid use. Although any species of *Aspergillus* can cause disease, *A fumigatus* is the most common pathogenic species. The organisms have large, septated hyphae (phycomycetes are nonseptated) branching at 45° angles (Figure 15-6). Especially in neutropenic hosts, they may invade blood vessels, producing a striking thrombotic angiitis similar to phycomycosis. Metastatic foci may cause suppurative abscess formation.

* *Aspergillus* organisms may invade blood vessels, producing a striking thrombotic angiitis.

The form of disease produced by aspergillosis primarily is determined by the nature of the immunologic deficit in the infected individual. Neutropenia predisposes to rapidly invasive bronchopulmonary disease with early dissemination to the brain and other tissues. The longer the duration of neutropenia, the higher the risk for invasive aspergillosis. Prompt therapy with high doses of amphotericin B and resolution of the neutropenia are necessary to control the disease. Diagnosis should be suspected when *Aspergillus* is isolated from any source in a susceptible individual.

T-cell deficiencies (primarily from corticosteroids) predispose to somewhat more indolent, although no less dangerous, forms of aspergillosis. Progressive pulmonary infiltrates, necrotic skin lesions, wound infections, and brain abscesses may result. Sinus infections with *Aspergillus* may be localized or invasive in patients with T-cell deficiencies.

Serologic testing is not helpful for diagnosing invasive *Aspergillus* in the compromised host.

* Neutropenia predisposes to rapidly invasive bronchopulmonary disease with early dissemination to the brain and other tissues.

Aspergillus also can cause localized disease in persons with normal immunologic function. Chronic necrotizing pulmonary aspergillosis occurs in patients with pulmonary emphysema. The chronic, progressive infiltrates of this condition often require tissue sampling for diagnosis. Treatment with surgical resection and systemic antifungal therapy is sometimes curative.

Aspergillus may produce a "fungus ball" in preexisting lung bullae (such as from ankylosing spondylitis, previous tuberculosis, or emphysema). Hemoptysis is the main symptom. Surgical excision may be necessary to prevent lethal hemorrhage.

Localized colonization with *Aspergillus* is common and usually does not produce disease. However, otitis externa (swimmer's ear) and allergic bronchopulmonary aspergillosis are exceptions. The symptoms of allergic bronchopulmonary aspergillosis resemble those of asthma. It is characterized by migratory pulmonary infiltrates, thick, brown, tenacious mucous plugs in the sputum, eosinophilia,

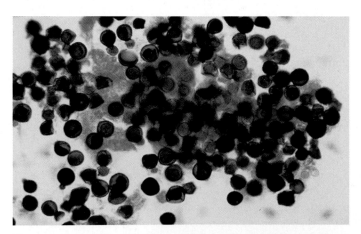

Figure 15-5. *Blastomyces dermatitidis* in Bronchoalveolar Lavage (Silver Stain, ×450).

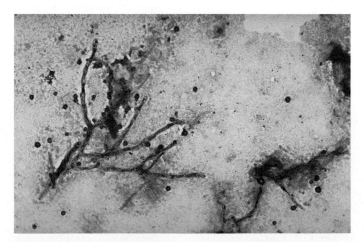

Figure 15-6. *Aspergillus fumigatus* in Bronchoalveolar Lavage (×450).

and high titers of anti-*Aspergillus* antibodies. Endophthalmitis due to *Aspergillus* may develop after ocular operation or trauma.

Aspergillus frequently colonizes the respiratory tract. Isolating the organism from the sputum of an immunocompetent host usually does not indicate disease and does not require treatment.

* Chronic necrotizing pulmonary aspergillosis occurs in patients with pulmonary emphysema.
* *Aspergillus* may produce a "fungus ball" in preexisting lung bullae (such as from ankylosing spondylitis, previous tuberculosis, or emphysema).

Aspergillus infections may respond poorly to currently available antifungal medications. Amphotericin B products are very effective, but they must be given in high doses. Lipid-based formulations of amphotericin B are advised for patients in whom nephrotoxicity develops with deoxycholate amphotericin B. Itraconazole was the first oral agent with substantial activity against *Aspergillus*. However, recently approved newer drugs such as voriconazole and caspofungin have potent in vitro and in vivo activity against *Aspergillus*. Intravenous voriconazole should be avoided in patients with severe renal insufficiency (glomerular filtration rate, <50 mL/min). Caspofungin is approved by the US Food and Drug Administration for refractory invasive aspergillosis. This has been used alone or in combination with amphotericin B products. Surgical debridement of infected tissues is often necessary for cure. Allergic bronchopulmonary aspergillosis responds to corticosteroid therapy, and itraconazole may be an important adjunctive therapy in decreasing or sparing the use of corticosteroids.

* Typical clinical scenario of *Aspergillus* infection: Fever and lung infiltrates occur in a patient with prolonged neutropenia.

Cryptococcosis

Cryptococcus neoformans is the only species of *Cryptococcus* that is pathogenic for humans. It is a yeast in both tissue and culture, is 4 to 7 mcm in diameter, and has thin-walled buds and a capsule (Figure 15-7). It is an opportunistic pathogen infecting persons with T-cell deficiencies or dysfunction (patients with Hodgkin disease, hematologic malignancy, organ transplantation, exogenous corticosteroids, chronic liver disease, and AIDS). The respiratory tract is the probable portal of entry. Cryptococcosis does not incite much inflammatory reaction, and calcification is rare.

* *Cryptococcus neoformans* is an opportunistic pathogen.
* *Cryptococcus* primarily infects persons with T-cell deficiencies or dysfunction (eg, Hodgkin disease, hematologic malignancy, organ transplant, exogenous corticosteroids, chronic liver disease, and AIDS).

Cryptococcus neoformans is acquired by inhalation. From the lungs it disseminates widely and easily crosses into the central nervous system. Pneumonia and meningitis are the most common forms of cryptococcosis. Meningitis may be insidious, with headache as the only symptom. Cranial nerve involvement may develop (including blindness with involvement of the optic nerve). *Cryptococcus* also may cause an indolent form of cellulitis.

* Pneumonia and meningitis are the most common forms of *C neoformans* infection.

Cryptococcal infection can be diagnosed with fungal culture (cerebrospinal fluid, blood, sputum, urine), silver staining of biopsy tissue, or detection of *Cryptococcus* antigen in body fluids. The cryptococcal antigen test is the most helpful of all fungal serologic tests. It measures capsular antigen, whereas most other fungal serologic tests measure antibody response. Remember that *Cryptococcus* very commonly spreads to the central nervous system. Therefore, if *C neoformans* is isolated from any source (such as sputum, urine, blood) in a susceptible patient, simultaneous meningitis should be suspected. India ink preparation largely has been replaced by antigen detection assay.

Cryptococcal infections respond to treatment with amphotericin B or fluconazole. Choice of therapy depends on extent of disease and host immune function. Mild to moderate noncentral nervous system cryptococcosis can be treated with fluconazole for 6 to 12 months. However, severe presentation, immunocompromised hosts, and central nervous system involvement should be treated with amphotericin B. Combining oral flucytosine (100-150 mg/kg per day) with amphotericin B for 6 weeks allows a lower dose of amphotericin to be used. Unfortunately, relapse rates are high regardless of the treatment regimen given. In a recent study comparing fluconazole (200 mg per day) with amphotericin B for 10 weeks, fluconazole was as effective as amphotericin B ("effective" is defined as clinical improvement or resolution of symptoms with negative results for culture of cerebrospinal fluid). However, mortality in the first 2 weeks of therapy was higher with fluconazole (15% vs 8%).

Cryptococcosis in patients with AIDS is difficult to cure; however, the advent of highly active antiretroviral therapy has improved outcomes. The goal of therapy is to control the infection and then suppress it with long-term antifungal agents. A common approach is to initiate therapy with amphotericin B (with or without flucytosine). Amphotericin therapy is continued until cerebrospinal fluid cultures are negative or there is unacceptable toxicity from the drug. Oral fluconazole (200-400 mg per day) is then given indefinitely.

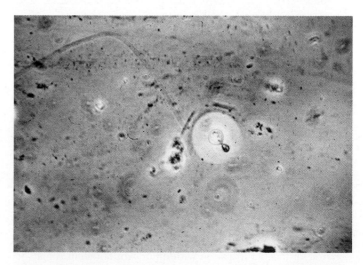

Figure 15-7. *Cryptococcus neoformans* in Cerebrospinal Fluid (×450).

Disappointingly, relapse remains frequent even with maintenance therapy. The newly approved caspofungin does not have any activity against *C neoformans*.

Candidiasis

Candida is a normal part of the human microflora. It grows as both yeast and hyphal forms simultaneously. Although *Candida albicans* is the most common species, numerous other species can cause human disease. *Candida* causes mucosal and cutaneous infections in both normal and immunocompromised hosts. Invasive disease primarily occurs in neutropenic hosts and as a nosocomial bloodstream infection.

Examples of candidiasis in the normal host include diaper rash and intertrigo, in which *Candida* growth on moist skin surfaces produces irritation. Vulvovaginal candidiasis is common, especially after a woman takes a course of antibiotics for an unrelated infection. Treatment with topical antifungal agents or a single dose of oral fluconazole is usually curative. Diabetes, corticosteroids, oral contraceptives, obesity, and HIV infection predispose to recurrent vulvovaginal candidiasis. Oral thrush may result from the same conditions.

Candida species cause 5% to 10% of nosocomial bloodstream infections. Candidemia most often occurs in critically ill patients receiving broad-spectrum antibiotics and parenteral nutrition. Neutropenia is another predisposing factor. Current blood culture techniques usually detect *Candida*, but culture results may be delayed. All intravenous catheters should always be removed or replaced when bloodstream infection with *Candida* is discovered. Metastatic abscesses can occur in any site after an episode of candidemia. *Candida* osteomyelitis or joint infections can occur as complications after an episode of line-related fungemia. Endophthalmitis may occur as long as 1 month after initial fungemia. For central venous catheter-related candidemias, catheter removal followed by amphotericin B (250-500 mg) or fluconazole is indicated.

Candida tropicalis, *Candida parapsilosis*, *Candida glabrata*, and multiple other species cause nosocomial illness, especially in immunocompromised patients. Note that these non-*albicans* species of *Candida* are more often resistant to fluconazole therapy.

Injection drug use is a risk factor for *Candida* endocarditis (and joint space infections, especially of the sternoclavicular joint). It is often caused by species other than *C albicans*.

* Fungemia develops from infected intravenous catheters, especially in the immunosuppressed host.
* Risk factors for *Candida* bloodstream infection include previous antibacterial therapy, cytotoxic or corticosteroid therapy, and parenteral nutrition.
* *Candida* endocarditis occurs most often in injection drug users.
* Diabetes, corticosteroids, oral contraceptives, obesity, and HIV infection predispose to recurrent vulvovaginal candidiasis.

Candida urinary tract infection is common in patients with urinary catheters and those receiving antibacterial drugs. Removal of the catheter is the primary therapy. If necessary, treatment with fluconazole or bladder irrigation with dilute amphotericin B may be curative, although recurrence is common.

Hepatosplenic candidiasis, also called chronic disseminated candidiasis, occurs in patients after prolonged chemotherapy-induced neutropenia. Symptoms of fever and increasing liver enzyme values manifest as the leukocyte count recovers. Typical "bull's-eye lesions" can be seen with ultrasonography, computed tomography, or magnetic resonance imaging of the infected liver. The preferred treatment is with at least 2 g of intravenous amphotericin B, but fluconazole or lipid complex amphotericin B also may be effective.

Candida esophagitis is a common cause of odynophagia in immunosuppressed patients, especially those with AIDS. Endoscopy is necessary to prove the diagnosis. *Candida* esophagitis is clinically indistinguishable from, and may coexist with, cytomegalovirus and herpes simplex virus esophagitis. Fluconazole is effective therapy for oral or esophageal candidiasis. Caspofungin is also active and is approved by the US Food and Drug Administration for treatment of candidemia or candidiasis caused by *Candida* species, including those that are resistant to azoles such as fluconazole. Caspofungin is available only as an intravenous drug.

* Hepatosplenic candidiasis typically develops as chemotherapy-induced neutropenia resolves.
* *Candida* esophagitis is clinically indistinguishable from, and may coexist with, cytomegalovirus and herpes simplex virus esophagitis.
* Typical clinical scenario for *hepatosplenic candidiasis*: A patient recovering from prolonged chemotherapy-induced neutropenia has fever and increasing liver enzyme values. The diagnosis is made with ultrasonography or computed tomography showing characteristic bull's-eye lesions.
* Typical clinical scenario for *Candida* esophagitis: Odynophagia in immunocompromised patients. Differential diagnosis is herpes simplex virus esophagitis. Diagnosis is made with endoscopy and culture.

Mucormycosis (*Rhizopus* Species, Zygomycetes)

Mucormycosis is a term used to describe infections caused by fungi of the order Mucorales. Older terms for this include *phycomycosis* and *zygomycosis*. There are many different fungi or Zygomycetes within this order that are pathogenic to humans. Of those, *Rhizopus* species are the most commonly isolated, followed by *Rhizomucor* and *Cunninghamella*. Mucormycosis is a disease of immunocompromised hosts. Pulmonary, nasal, and sinus infections are the most common. Facial pain, headache, and fever are common symptoms. Rhinocerebral mucormycosis results from direct extension into the brain. Diabetic ketoacidosis, neutropenia, renal failure, and deferoxamine therapy are all risk factors for this dreaded infection. The diagnosis of mucormycosis depends on finding the typical black necrotic lesions (usually in the nose or on the palate) and is confirmed by biopsy. Treatment involves reversing the predisposing condition as much as possible, surgical débridement of necrotic tissue, and amphotericin B.

* The diagnosis of mucormycosis depends on finding the typical black necrotic lesions (usually in the nose or on the palate) and is confirmed by biopsy.

- Diabetic ketoacidosis, neutropenia, renal failure, and deferoxamine therapy are all risk factors for mucormycosis.

Viruses

Herpesviruses

There are now 8 known herpesviruses: *herpes simplex virus* (HSV) *types 1 and 2*, *Epstein-Barr virus* (EBV), *cytomegalovirus* (CMV), *varicella-zoster virus* (VZV), *human herpesvirus 6* (HHV-6), *HHV-7* (not yet known to be associated with clinical disease), and *HHV-8*. All herpesviruses are DNA viruses that share the characteristic of establishing latency after primary infection, whether or not symptomatic.

Serologic evidence of infection is common by adulthood: HSV 1, 87%; HSV 2, 20%; EBV, 95%; CMV, 50%; and VZV, 90%. The rate of infection increases in populations of lower socioeconomic status.

Herpes Simplex Virus

Primary infection with HSV results from exposure of skin or mucous membranes to intact viral particles. Latent infection is then established in sensory nerve ganglia. Genital HSV infection is caused by HSV type 2 in 80% of cases and by HSV type 1 in the remaining 20%. The reverse is true for oral HSV. Genital HSV is more likely to recur when caused by HSV type 2. Recurrence rates can be decreased by 80% with chronic use of antiviral drugs. In normal hosts, this does not promote emergence of acyclovir-resistant strains.

Herpes simplex encephalitis is a nonseasonal, life-threatening illness usually caused by HSV type 1. Herpes simplex encephalitis causes confusion, fever, and, frequently, seizures. Simultaneous herpes labialis is present in 10% to 15% of cases. Antemortem diagnosis may be difficult. However, new techniques such as magnetic resonance imaging of the temporal lobes and amplification of HSV DNA from cerebrospinal fluid are extremely sensitive. Detecting periodic lateralized epileptiform discharges with electroencephalography is suggestive of herpes simplex encephalitis. Poor neurologic status, age older than 30 years, and encephalitis of more than 4 days in duration before initiation of therapy are associated with a poor outcome.

Neonatal HSV infection is acquired at the time of vaginal delivery. The mortality rate is high (20%) despite antiviral therapy. In neonates who survive, neurologic sequelae and recurrent HSV lesions are common. Cesarean section is recommended if a woman has active herpetic lesions at the time of delivery.

Acyclovir, famciclovir, valacyclovir, ganciclovir, foscarnet, and vidarabine inhibit replication of both HSV types 1 and 2. Acyclovir resistance may develop in patients with AIDS who are treated with multiple courses of acyclovir. Resistance usually is conferred by a mutation in the thymidine kinase gene, preventing phosphorylation of acyclovir to its active form.

- Recurrence rates of oral HSV can be decreased 80% with chronic suppressive therapy with acyclovir.
- Herpes simplex encephalitis can be diagnosed with magnetic resonance imaging and polymerase chain reaction amplification of HSV DNA from cerebrospinal fluid.

- Delivery by cesarean section is recommended if active genital lesions are present at the end of pregnancy.

HSV pneumonia is rare and usually occurs in immunosuppressed patients. When HSV is isolated from a respiratory source, it most commonly represents shedding from the oral mucosa rather than the lungs. HSV also is associated with visceral disease (such as esophagitis). Biopsy is required to reliably distinguish HSV from CMV or *Candida* esophagitis. *Eczema herpeticum* (Kaposi varicelliform eruption) occurs in areas of eczema. Large areas of skin are involved. *Herpetic whitlow* is a painful HSV infection of a finger, is most commonly acquired through contact with oral secretions (eg, in respiratory technicians, dentists, anesthesiologists), and occasionally is acquired through needle stick. Although nosocomial transmission of HSV is rare, recent reports stress the importance of mucous membrane precautions when treating all patients with HSV, particularly those with respiratory infection who undergo invasive procedures.

- *Herpetic whitlow* is a painful HSV infection of a finger, is most commonly acquired through contact with oral secretions (eg, in respiratory technicians, dentists, anesthesiologists), and occasionally is acquired through needle stick.

HSV can cause outbreaks among participants in contact sports (in wrestlers it is called *herpes gladiatorum*). The infection is transmitted by skin-to-skin contact. Lesions appear on the head (78%), trunk (28%), and extremities (42%). The rash may be atypical. Large, ulcerative perianal lesions can develop in patients with AIDS. Some of the lesions are mistaken for decubitus ulcers.

- HSV can cause outbreaks among participants in contact sports.
- Large, ulcerative perianal lesions can develop in patients with AIDS.

Epstein-Barr Virus

Most acute EBV infections are asymptomatic. Symptomatic *infectious mononucleosis* causes the clinical triad of fever, pharyngitis (80%), and adenopathy. Splenomegaly occurs in 50% of cases. One of the most serious complications of mononucleosis is splenic rupture. Other complications include hemolytic anemia, airway obstruction, encephalitis, and transverse myelitis. Associated laboratory abnormalities include atypical lymphocytosis, thrombocytopenia, and mild increases in liver enzyme values. Corticosteroids may be beneficial for treatment of hemolytic anemia and acute airway obstruction. Ampicillin or amoxicillin given during infectious mononucleosis commonly causes a diffuse macular rash.

Table 15-4 differentiates EBV from other causes of mononucleosis. The diagnosis of infectious mononucleosis depends on detection of heterophile antibodies (monospot test) or specific EBV immunoglobulin M antibodies. False-negative results of the monospot test are more likely with increasing age.

- Infectious mononucleosis has the clinical triad of fever, pharyngitis, and adenopathy.
- Splenomegaly occurs in 50% of cases of infectious mononucleosis.

- One of the most serious complications is splenic rupture.
- If ampicillin is given, a rash often develops.

Uncomplicated cases require symptomatic care only. The patient should not participate in contact sports for several months because of the risk for splenic rupture. Corticosteroids are not indicated for uncomplicated infection. Acyclovir and other antiviral drug therapy is not effective.

Chronic fatigue syndrome is a syndrome characterized by various nonspecific symptoms. Studies have definitively shown that EBV does not cause chronic fatigue syndrome.

- No therapy is indicated for uncomplicated cases of infectious mononucleosis.
- EBV does not cause chronic fatigue syndrome.

EBV infection in males with X-linked lymphoproliferative syndrome is a rare disorder of young boys in whom fulminant EBV infections develop and is associated with a 57% mortality rate. Complications include severe EBV hepatitis with liver failure and hemophagocytic syndrome with bleeding. In survivors, hypogammaglobulinemia, malignant lymphoma, aplastic anemia, and opportunistic infections develop. Death occurs by age 40 years in all cases. Acyclovir and corticosteroids do not seem to be beneficial.

In *EBV-associated Burkitt lymphoma and nasopharyngeal carcinoma,* patients have high titers of IgA antibodies to EBV. *Polyclonal and monoclonal B-cell lymphoproliferative syndromes* have been associated with EBV in patients who have had organ transplant and in patients with AIDS. Oral hairy leukoplakia in patients with AIDS is associated with EBV infection and responds to acyclovir therapy. EBV recently has been associated with leiomyosarcomas in transplant recipients.

- Polyclonal and monoclonal B-cell lymphoproliferative syndromes have been associated with EBV.

Cytomegalovirus

Primary CMV infection is usually asymptomatic in immunocompetent patients, but it can cause a heterophile-negative mononucleosis syndrome. It is a significant cause of neonatal disease. Perinatal infection can occur in utero, intra partum, or post partum and can cause congenital malformations. Primary infection of the mother during pregnancy results in a 15% chance of fetal cytomegalic inclusion disease. Young children in day-care centers commonly shed CMV in their urine and saliva. Their parents are at risk of acquiring primary infection from an asymptomatic child. CMV can cause fever of unknown origin in healthy adults, especially in those with day-care–aged children.

CMV can be transmitted by leukocytes in blood transfusions. Use of leukocyte-poor packed red blood cells or blood from CMV-seronegative donors decreases the risk of transmission via this route. Symptomatic infection develops about 4 weeks after transfusion and manifests as fever with atypical lymphocytes in the peripheral blood smear. Serologic testing confirms the diagnosis. Viral cultures are rarely helpful in diagnosing CMV disease in the noncompromised patient.

- CMV can cause heterophile-negative mononucleosis syndrome.
- CMV can be transmitted by blood transfusion.
- Fever and infectious mononucleosis-like picture on peripheral smear are characteristics in postoperative patients who have received blood transfusions.

In persons with impaired cellular immunity (such as those with AIDS or organ and bone marrow transplant recipients), CMV causes serious infections (CMV syndrome, retinitis, pneumonia, gastrointestinal ulcerations, encephalitis, adrenalitis). The diagnosis most often is established by isolation of CMV from blood or from culture, by histopathologic evidence of CMV infection in involved tissue (such as liver, lung, gastrointestinal tract), or from clinical findings alone (CMV retinitis).

- CMV causes serious infections (retinitis, pneumonia, gastrointestinal ulcerations, encephalitis, adrenalitis) in patients who have AIDS or take immunosuppressive medications.

The manifestations of CMV disease in persons with advanced AIDS are protean. Disease is almost always caused by reactivation of latent

Table 15-4 Infectious Mononucleosis-like Syndromes

Disease	Pharyngitis	Adenopathy	Splenomegaly	Atypical Lymphocytes	Heterophile	Other Test
Infectious mononucleosis	++++	++++	+++	+++	+	Specific EBV antibody + (VCA IgM)
CMV	−	−	+++	++	−	CMV IgM
Toxoplasmosis	−	++++	+++	++		Toxoplasmosis serology
HIV	+	+++	−	++	−	HIV serology (will likely be negative) HIV viral load HIV p24 antigen

Abbreviations and symbols: −, absent; +, ++, +++, and ++++, present to varying degrees; CMV, cytomegalovirus; EBV, Epstein-Barr virus; HIV, human immunodeficiency virus; IgM, immunoglobulin M; VCA, viral capsid antigen.

infection in this setting. Finding CMV in the blood or urine of patients with AIDS is common and has a low predictive value for symptomatic CMV disease. CMV retinitis occurs in 20% to 30% of patients with advanced AIDS. Diagnosis is based on ophthalmologic examination. The relapse rate for CMV retinitis in AIDS is high, even with chronic antiviral therapy.

Solid organ and bone marrow transplant recipients are another group of patients at risk for CMV disease. It is the most common infection after solid organ transplant (occurring primarily in the first 6 months after transplant). Those at highest risk are CMV seronegative before transplant and receive an organ from a seropositive donor. Latent virus is present in almost all tissues and begins replicating shortly after transplant. Symptomatic disease (CMV syndrome) usually develops in the first 4 to 8 weeks after a solid organ transplant and causes fever, leukopenia, increases in liver enzyme values, and end-organ involvement. CMV serum antigen testing or CMV detected in blood culture helps confirm the diagnosis. Patients who have had bone marrow transplant are especially at risk for CMV pneumonia. The mortality rate approaches 50% despite therapy. Prophylactic ganciclovir and, possibly, CMV immune globulin may decrease or delay posttransplant CMV disease.

* CMV retinitis occurs in 20%-30% of patients with advanced AIDS.
* CMV is the most common infectious complication of organ transplant.

Ganciclovir is the treatment of choice for most CMV infections in immunocompromised hosts. A randomized, placebo-controlled trial found that foscarnet and ganciclovir are equally efficacious for halting the progression of CMV retinitis in patients with AIDS but that patients taking foscarnet lived longer (12 vs 8 months). Both drugs are now approved for this indication. Full-dose induction therapy is given for 2 to 3 weeks, followed by chronic suppressive therapy indefinitely (usually as once-daily dosing). Oral valganciclovir has excellent bioavailability and can be used in select patients for suppression. Transplant recipients usually do not require suppressive medication after an episode of CMV disease. In patients with CMV pneumonia after bone marrow transplant, combining ganciclovir with intravenous immune globulin is more effective than ganciclovir alone. Nonimmunocompromised patients with CMV do not require treatment.

* Ganciclovir or foscarnet is the treatment of choice for most CMV infections.

Varicella-Zoster Virus
Primary infection with VZV usually occurs in childhood and causes chickenpox. Illness with chickenpox is more likely to be severe in adults and immunocompromised hosts. Varicella pneumonia occurs in 5% to 50% of cases. Pregnant women are especially vulnerable. They should be treated with high-dose acyclovir (10 mg/kg intravenously every 8 hours). Acyclovir is not associated with toxicity to the fetus. Pneumonia develops within 1 to 6 days after the onset of illness and usually recedes as the rash does. Encephalomyelitis is another serious complication of varicella infection, occurring predominantly in children. Onset is 3 to 14 days after the appearance of rash.

* Varicella pneumonia occurs in 5% to 50% of adults with chickenpox.
* Pneumonia begins to improve with disappearance of rash.

After primary infection, VZV DNA persists in a latent state in sensory neuron ganglia. Reactivated infection causes zoster (shingles), which manifests as a painful vesicular rash in a dermatomal distribution. Involvement of the fifth cranial nerve, especially the ophthalmic branch, may be sight-threatening. In nonimmune persons exposed to zoster, primary VZV infection may develop. Neurologic complications of herpes zoster include motor paralysis (localized to the dermatomal distribution of rash), encephalitis, and myelitis.

* Herpes zoster infection often involves the fifth cranial nerve, especially the ophthalmic branch.

Varicella immune globulin can prevent primary VZV infection, especially when given within 96 hours of exposure. It is indicated for 1) VZV-seronegative immunocompromised hosts who have had close contact with a person with chickenpox and 2) newborns of mothers with varicella infection that occurs 5 days before or 2 days after delivery.

Ten percent of mothers with active varicella will transmit the infection to the fetus. Infection during the first trimester may result in limb hypoplasia, cortical atrophy, and chorioretinitis. During the third trimester, multiple visceral abnormalities can occur, including pneumonia. The fetal and neonatal mortality rate is 31%.

* Among mothers with active varicella, 10% will transmit the infection to the fetus.

Treatment for varicella (*primary varicella-zoster*) infection is based on whether the patient is immunocompetent. Two recent randomized clinical trials showed that oral acyclovir (800 mg 5 times a day or equivalent) reduced the duration of skin lesions and viral shedding in adults and children. Its efficacy for reducing visceral complications (pneumonia) remains unknown. Early treatment (<24 hours) is necessary. The cost of therapy may limit its usefulness, but it is advocated by some to decrease the duration of illness. Acyclovir may reduce the risk of dissemination and of complications in immunocompromised patients. Treatment of zoster ophthalmicus reduces the incidence of uveitis and keratitis. For immunocompetent patients with zoster, 3 antiviral drugs (acyclovir, famciclovir, and valacyclovir) speed healing and reduce pain. Preliminary data suggest that the new antiviral agent famciclovir might decrease the duration of postherpetic neuralgia. Corticosteroids do not prevent postherpetic neuralgia. For disseminated infections (encephalitis, cranial neuritis), a recent controlled trial showed that high-dose intravenous acyclovir decreases the duration of hospitalization. Acyclovir-resistant VZV infection (which can occur in patients with AIDS) can be treated with intravenous foscarnet or cidofovir.

Two effective live virus vaccines for VZV are available. One VZV vaccine (Varivax) is for primary prevention, and a new, different (higher attenuated varicella colony-forming units per milliliter) vaccine (Zostavax) is now available for prevention of herpes zoster (shingles) and post-herpetic neuralgia in persons older than 60 years. VZV vaccine for primary prevention is recommended for children and VZV-seronegative adolescent and adult populations. It is contraindicated in pregnancy. Both vaccines are contraindicated in patients with impaired cellular immunity such as AIDS, leukemias, lymphoma, chemotherapy, transplant, chronic steroid therapy, or other cellular immunodeficiency states. Such immunocompromised patients should avoid contact with persons who have received the vaccine in the past month.

Human Herpesvirus 6
HHV-6 is a recently discovered lymphotropic virus. It causes the mild childhood infectious exanthem known as roseola infantum. Like CMV, reactivation of infection occurs after organ transplant. HHV-6 has been associated with pneumonitis after bone marrow transplant.

Human Herpesvirus 8
HHV-8 is also known as Kaposi sarcoma-associated virus. As the name implies, it is thought to be the causative agent of Kaposi sarcoma. It is related to EBV. Most recently, HHV-8 has been linked to body cavity-based lymphomas in patients with AIDS and Castleman disease.

Influenza
Type A is the most common. Epidemics occur every 2 to 4 years; pandemics occur every 20 to 30 years. Epidemics and pandemics are a result of a major antigenic shift in the influenza virus. About 80% to 90% of deaths due to influenza occur in persons older than 65 years. Complications include 1) primary influenza pneumonia (interstitial desquamative pneumonia) and 2) secondary bacterial infection, which usually is caused by S pneumoniae, Haemophilus, or S aureus. Rare cases of toxic shock syndrome have been reported when S aureus pneumonia complicates influenza.

* About 80%-90% of deaths due to influenza occur in persons older than 65 years.
* Secondary infection usually is caused by S pneumoniae or S aureus.
* Typical clinical scenario: An elderly patient, often with chronic obstructive lung disease, has influenza, which may or may not improve; then, the severity of symptoms increases substantially, with high fever, marked leukocytosis, and often respiratory failure.

Amantadine and rimantadine are effective against only influenza A virus, not influenza B. Therapy is most beneficial if begun within 48 hours of onset of symptoms. Vaccine, together with amantadine, can give about 95% protection against influenza A infection. Neuraminidase inhibitors (oseltamivir and zanamivir) are effective against uncomplicated disease caused by both influenza A and B. Both reduce the duration of symptoms by 1 day when started within 48 hours after onset of symptoms.

An inactivated influenza and live attenuated intranasal vaccine (recently approved by the US Food and Drug Administration) are used for the prevention of influenza. Target groups for vaccination are persons older than 50 years, residents of chronic care facilities, persons with cardiopulmonary disorders, healthy children between 6 and 23 months old, children 6 months to 18 years old receiving

long-term aspirin therapy (to prevent Reye syndrome), health care personnel, employees of chronic care facilities, providers of home health care, and those sharing the same household as high-risk persons. The live attenuated vaccine is approved only for healthy immunocompetent persons between the ages of 5 and 49 years. Adverse reactions to both vaccines include fever, myalgias, and hypersensitivity. For those who did not receive the vaccine, amantadine, rimantadine, or oseltamivir can be used for influenza prevention and are effective for prophylactic use after exposure to a patient with influenza. Amantadine is given at a dose of 200 mg per day; if the person is older than 65 years, only 100 mg per day is given to decrease the risk of side effects. The decreased dosage also is used for patients with impaired renal function or seizure disorders. Toxicity manifests as dizziness, restlessness, and insomnia. High-risk individuals who have not received the vaccine during the influenza season should be considered for chemoprophylaxis.

* Target groups for influenza vaccine are persons older than 50 years, residents of chronic care facilities, persons with cardiopulmonary disorders, healthy children between 6 and 23 months old, children 6 months to 18 years old receiving long-term aspirin therapy (to prevent Reye syndrome), health care personnel, employees of chronic care facilities, providers of home health care, and household members of high-risk persons.

Hantavirus Infection, Hantavirus Pulmonary Syndrome
In May 1993, an outbreak of an acute illness consisting of fever, rapidly progressive respiratory failure, and death was reported in the 4-state area of New Mexico, Arizona, Colorado, and Utah. Most of the initial cases occurred in young Navajo Indians. The causative agent is a virus belonging to the genus Hantavirus (family Bunyaviridae) and is now called the Sin Nombre virus. Infection is transmitted through inhalation of aerosolized secretions from the common deer mouse (Peromyscus maniculatus).

Since the early reports, cases also have been identified in most other states and Canada. The disease begins with a nonspecific prodrome (fever and generalized myalgia) followed in 4 to 5 days by respiratory symptoms (cough, dyspnea, and tachypnea). This progresses rapidly to an adult respiratory distress syndrome. Diagnosis is possible with serologic studies (such as enzyme-linked immunosorbent assay for antivirus immunoglobulin M and immunoglobulin G antibodies). Treatment is mainly supportive. Ribavirin, a guanosine analog, has been used effectively for treating hemorrhagic fever with renal syndrome caused by other related types of Hantavirus, but its efficacy in Hantavirus pulmonary syndrome is not yet established.

Poliovirus
Although wild-type polio has been eliminated from the Western Hemisphere, it remains endemic in parts of Asia and Africa. Disease still can be imported from these areas. There was a recent outbreak in the Netherlands among members of religious groups who were not vaccinated. Remember that polio is most often an asymptomatic infection. The virus affects the nuclei of cranial nerves and anterior motor neurons of the spinal cord, causing a flaccid paralysis. When paralysis develops, it is usually asymmetric. Vaccine-related polio,

although rare, can occur with the live virus vaccine. In July 2000, a vaccine-strain polio outbreak occurred in the Dominican Republic and Haiti. Patients traveling to these countries are advised to receive an injectable inactivated polio vaccine booster.

Rabies

Rabies is difficult to diagnose ante mortem. Manifestations are hydrophobia and copious salivation. It should be considered in any case of encephalitis or myelitis of unknown cause, especially in persons who have recently traveled outside the United States. The virus spreads along peripheral nerves to the central nervous system. The most common sources of exposure are dogs, cats, skunks, foxes, raccoons (Florida, Connecticut), wolves, and bats. Spread by other animals is *very rare*. Rodents rarely, if ever, transmit rabies. From 1980 to 1989, 9 of 13 cases in the United States were due to exposure to rabid animals outside the country. Rabies acquisition in the United States is predominantly related to bat exposure. Rabies also has been reported to occur in patients after corneal transplant. Aerosol spread is possible; it is most often due to exposure to bats during spelunking or in medical laboratories. The risk of nosocomial transmission is low. Definitive diagnosis is established by finding Negri bodies on biopsy of the hippocampus. Serum and cerebrospinal fluid can be tested for rabies antibodies when trying to diagnose the disease. Direct fluorescent antibody testing of a skin biopsy specimen from the nape of the neck is used to detect rabies antigen.

* Rabies should be considered in any case of encephalitis or myelitis of unknown cause.
* Most common sources of exposure are dogs, cats, skunks, foxes, raccoons, wolves, and bats.
* Definitive diagnosis is established by the presence of Negri bodies on biopsy of the hippocampus.

Postbite management includes observing the animal, if possible, immediate soap and water washing of the wound, getting rabies immunoglobulin (all injected into the site), and starting the rabies 5-dose postexposure vaccine schedule. Human diploid vaccine is more effective and less toxic than the older duck embryo vaccine. Human rabies immunoglobulin is now widely available, mitigating the need to use horse serum immunoglobulin. Human rabies immunoglobulin and vaccine are not of benefit after onset of clinical disease. Pre-exposure rabies vaccination is advised for patients likely to be in situations that put them at high risk for rabies, such as prolonged travel to rabies-endemic countries. Pre-exposure vaccination mitigates the need for rabies immunoglobulin and decreases the postexposure doses to only 2 (days 0 and 3 after bite).

Slow Viruses and Prion-Associated Central Nervous System Diseases

Progressive Multifocal Leukoencephalopathy

Progressive multifocal leukoencephalopathy is associated with AIDS, leukemia, lymphoma, and immunosuppression for organ transplant. It is caused by a papovavirus (JC virus). It can cause either diffuse or focal central nervous system abnormalities. Despite its name, progressive multifocal leukoencephalopathy usually causes solitary brain lesions, as seen on computed tomography or magnetic resonance imaging. Cerebrospinal fluid is normal in most cases. The diagnosis is based on brain biopsy, although detection of JC virus DNA in the cerebrospinal fluid is suggestive of progressive multifocal leukoencephalopathy. There is no proven effective therapy.

* Progressive multifocal leukoencephalopathy is associated with AIDS, leukemia, lymphoma, and immunosuppression for organ transplant.
* Progressive multifocal leukoencephalopathy is caused by a papovavirus (JC virus).

Subacute Sclerosing Panencephalitis (Inclusion Body Encephalitis)

This is a progressively fatal disease of children and adolescents. It is thought to be due to rubeola (measles) virus. Patients are younger than 11 years in 80% of cases. Onset is insidious, with progressive mental deterioration. Later, myoclonic jerks and diffuse abnormalities occur. Measles antibody levels in sera and cerebrospinal fluid are markedly increased. Brain biopsy is necessary for diagnosis (inclusion body encephalitis). There is no treatment. The disease is uniformly fatal.

Creutzfeldt-Jakob Disease

This is a rare, fatal, degenerative disease of the central nervous system. It occurs equally in both sexes, usually at older ages. There are both familial and sporadic forms of the disease. Creutzfeldt-Jakob disease usually presents as rapidly evolving dementia with myoclonic seizures. Prions (small proteinaceous infectious particles without nucleic acid) have been proposed as the cause of this disease. Nosocomial transmission of Creutzfeldt-Jakob disease can occur via corneal transplant recipients and exposure to cerebrospinal fluid. Several recent cases in Great Britain were linked to consumption of beef from cattle that had bovine spongiform encephalopathy. There is no treatment.

* Creutzfeldt-Jakob disease presents as rapidly evolving dementia with myoclonic seizures.

Measles (Rubeola)

There was a substantial increase in measles cases in the late 1980s and early 1990s in unvaccinated preschool children and vaccinated high school and college students (1990: 27,786 cases). Prodromal upper respiratory tract symptoms are prominent. Oral lesions (Koplik spots) precede the rash. Both measles infection and measles vaccine cause temporary cutaneous anergy (false-negative purified protein derivative test). Infection may cause more significant immunologic suppression, as exemplified by cases of reactivated tuberculosis in persons with measles.

* In measles, oral Koplik spots precede the rash.
* Measles vaccine may cause temporary cutaneous anergy.

Complications of measles include encephalitis and pneumonia. Encephalitis is often severe. It usually occurs after a period of apparent improvement of measles infection. In primary measles pneumonia, large, multinucleated cells (Warthin-Finkeldey cells) are found on lung biopsy. Secondary bacterial infection is more common than primary measles pneumonia. *S aureus* and *H influenzae* are the most common bacterial pathogens.

- Complications of measles include encephalitis.
- Secondary bacterial infection is more common than primary measles pneumonia.

Atypical measles occurs in patients vaccinated before 1968. After exposure to measles, atypical rash, fever, arthralgias, and headache (aseptic meningitis) may develop. The presence of a high titer of measles antibody in serum helps confirm the diagnosis.

Rubella

The prodromal symptoms of rubella are mild (unlike those of rubeola). Posterior cervical lymphadenopathy, arthralgia (70% in adults), transient erythematous rash, and fever are characteristic. Infection is subclinical in many cases. Central nervous system complications and thrombocytopenia are rare.

- Characteristics of rubella: posterior cervical lymphadenopathy, arthralgia (70% in adults), transient erythematous rash, and fever.

The greatest danger from rubella is to the fetus. When a pregnant female is exposed to rubella, rubella serologic testing should be done. If the titer indicates immunity, there is no danger and no further testing is indicated. If the titer indicates nonimmunity, the patient should be followed for evidence of clinical rubella. The serum titer should be checked again in 2 to 3 weeks to evaluate for evidence of asymptomatic infection. If the titer is not increased and there is no evidence of clinical rubella, then no intervention is indicated. If clinical rubella develops or seroconversion is demonstrated, there is a high risk of congenital abnormalities or spontaneous abortion. The risk varies from 40% to 60% if infection occurs during the first 2 months of gestation to 10% by the fourth month. Intravenous gamma globulin may mask symptoms of rubella, but it does not protect the fetus.

- Gamma globulin does not protect the fetus after exposure to rubella.

From 6% to 11% of young adults remain susceptible to rubella after receiving rubella vaccine. A pregnant female should not be given rubella vaccine because it can cause congenital abnormalities. Females of childbearing age should be warned not to become pregnant within 2 to 3 months from the time of immunization. Transient arthralgias develop in 25% of immunized women. Fever, rash, and lymphadenopathy also may develop. Symptoms may occur as long as 2 months after vaccination. They may be confused with other forms of arthritis.

Viral Meningoencephalitis

Etiologic agents of viral meningitis include mumps, enteroviruses, herpes simplex, and, in summer months, the equine encephalitis viruses.

Lymphocytic choriomeningitis is acquired by exposure to rodent urine. Lactate levels in cerebrospinal fluid are normal in viral meningitis. The lactate level usually is increased in bacterial meningitis.

Mumps

Mumps virus commonly affects glandular tissue. Parotitis, pancreatitis, and orchitis are characteristic manifestations. Orchitis occurs in 20% of males with mumps. It is unilateral in approximately 75%. Orchitis often is associated with recrudescence of malaise and chills, fever, headache, nausea, vomiting, and testicular pain. Sterility is uncommon, even after bilateral infection.

Although mumps cases are uncommon in the United States, in 2006 there was an outbreak of mumps. Approximately 5,000 cases were reported to the National Notifiable Diseases Surveillance System. Source of the initial cases was unknown. The median age of persons reported with mumps was 22 years, and the highest incidence was among the adults 18 to 24 years of age, many of whom were college students. Factors contributing to this outbreak included college campus environment, lack of a 2-dose measles-mumps-rubella college-entry requirement or lack of enforcement of a requirement, delayed recognition and diagnosis of mumps, mumps vaccine failure, vaccine that might be less effective in preventing asymptomatic infection or atypical mumps than in preventing parotitis, and waning immunity.

Clinical suspicion can be confirmed by serologic test (immunoglobulin M for mumps) within 5 days of illness onset or sending a parotid duct swab or other samples such as cerebrospinal fluid for viral cultures. If the initial immunoglobulin M antibody titer is negative, a second (convalescent) serum specimen for immunoglobulin M antibodies obtained 2 to 3 weeks after onset of the illness can be helpful for making the diagnosis. A 4-fold increase in immunoglobulin G antibodies compared with immunoglobulin G obtained initially can also help. Mumps virus can be transmitted by direct contact with respiratory droplets, saliva, or contaminated fomites. The incubation period is 16 to 18 days (range, 12-25 days) from exposure to onset of symptoms.

Mumps meningoencephalitis is one of the most common non-seasonal viral meningitides. It can cause low glucose values in the cerebrospinal fluid, mimicking bacterial meningitis. Deafness is a rare complication of mumps.

- Mumps meningoencephalitis is one of the most common non-seasonal viral meningitides.

Mumps polyarthritis is most common in men between the ages of 20 and 30 years. Joint symptoms begin 1 to 2 weeks after subsidence of parotitis, and large joints are involved. The condition lasts approximately 6 weeks, and complete recovery is usual. This condition may be confused with other forms of arthritis.

- Mumps polyarthritis is most common in men between the ages of 20 and 30 years.

Parvovirus B19

Parvovirus is a single-stranded DNA virus that infects the erythrocyte precursors in bone marrow, with resulting reticulocytopenia. It is the cause of erythema infectiosum (fifth disease) in children, transient arthritis in adults, and aplastic crisis in persons with hemolytic anemias. Infection during pregnancy results in a 5% chance of hydrops fetalis or fetal death. Serologic testing is the preferred diagnostic method in immunologically competent persons.

Parvovirus B19 infection may persist in immunosuppressed patients, resulting in red blood cell aplasia. Diagnosis is established by demonstration of giant pronormoblasts in bone marrow or identification of viral DNA in bone marrow or peripheral blood. Most patients respond to administration of commercial immune globulin infusions for 5 to 10 days. No treatment is recommended for parvovirus infections in the noncompromised host.

- Parvovirus B19 is the cause of erythema infectiosum (fifth disease) and transient arthritis.
- B19 virus can cause red blood cell aplasia in patients with AIDS.

Human T-Cell Lymphotropic Viruses

Human T-cell lymphotropic virus (HTLV)-I and -II are non-HIV human retroviruses. HTLV-I is endemic in parts of Japan, the Caribbean basin, South America, and Africa. It may be transmitted by sexual contact, infected cellular blood products (not clotting factor concentrates), and injection drug use. Vertical transmission (breast-feeding, transplacental) also occurs. HTLV-I is associated with human T-cell leukemia/lymphoma and tropical spastic paraparesis (also known as HTLV-I–associated myelopathy). However, clinical disease never develops in 96% of persons infected with HTLV-I. HTLV-II causes no known clinical disease. The seroprevalence of HTLV-I or -II is as high as 18% in certain high-risk groups (injection drug users, patients attending sexually transmitted disease clinics) (HTLV-II is 2.5 times more prevalent than HTLV-I). Among voluntary blood donors, the seroprevalence in the United States is estimated at 0.016%. With current screening practices, the risk of transmission of HTLV-I or -II through blood transfusion is estimated to be 0.0014% (1/70,000 units).

- HTLV-I may be transmitted by sexual contact, infected blood products, and injection drug use.
- HTLV-I infection is usually asymptomatic but is associated with human T-cell leukemia and chronic myelopathy.

Parasites

Helminths

Neurocysticercosis is an infection of the central nervous system with a larval stage of the pork tapeworm (*Taenia solium*). It is acquired by ingesting tapeworm eggs from fecally contaminated food. It is endemic in Latin America, Asia, and Africa. Recent cases have been reported among household contacts of foreign-born persons (working as domestic employees). The infected persons had not traveled to an affected area. The most common presentation is seizures. Brain imaging reveals cystic or calcified brain lesions. Serum or cerebrospinal fluid serologic testing can aid in the diagnosis. Treatment with praziquantel or albendazole may be beneficial. Albendazole is considered superior for neurocysticercosis because of better central nervous system penetration.

The coadministration of corticosteroids often is used to decrease cerebral inflammation associated with therapy.

- Neurocysticercosis is acquired by ingesting tapeworm eggs from fecally contaminated food.
- Seizures are the most common symptom of neurocysticercosis.

Strongyloides stercoralis is unique among the intestinal nematode infections. Unlike the other helminths, the larvae of this organism can mature in the human host (auto-infection). In immunocompromised hosts (neutropenia, steroids, AIDS, HTLV-I), a superinfection can develop with larval migration throughout the body. Gram-negative bacteremia is a common coinfection, resulting from disruption of the intestinal mucosa by the invasive larvae. Treatment is with ivermectin.

Trichinosis is acquired from eating undercooked meat, especially bear. Features include muscle pain (especially diaphragm, chest, and tongue), eosinophilia, and periorbital edema. Treatment is with mebendazole or albendazole.

Hookworm (*Necator americanus*) causes anemia. It is found mainly in tropical and subtropical regions. The larval form penetrates the skin. Walking barefoot is a risk factor. Treatment is with mebendazole or albendazole.

Ascariasis infection may cause intestinal obstruction or pancreatitis (worm migrates up the pancreatic duct). Treatment is with mebendazole or albendazole.

Schistosomiasis is a tropical disease that causes hepatic cirrhosis, hematuria, and carcinoma of the bladder. Transverse myelitis may develop as a result of schistosomiasis. It is acquired by direct penetration of the *Schistosoma* cercariae from contaminated water (lakes, rivers). Praziquantel is the drug of choice for schistosomiasis.

- Trichinosis is acquired from eating undercooked meat, especially bear.
- Transverse myelitis may develop as a result of schistosomiasis.

Protozoan Parasites

Acanthamoeba, a free-living ameba, causes amebic keratitis in persons swimming in fresh water while wearing soft contact lenses. The diagnosis is based on microscopic examination of scrapings of the cornea. Treatment is with topical antifungal agents. Patients often respond poorly to therapy and have progressive corneal destruction.

Symptomatic infection with *Entamoeba histolytica* (amebiasis) may cause diarrhea (often bloody), abdominal pain, and fever. Metronidazole, followed by a lumenocidal agent such as iodoquinol or paromomycin, is the preferred therapy (metronidazole does not kill amebae in the intestinal lumen). Asymptomatic carriage of amebic cysts should be treated with one of the lumenocidal agents.

- Metronidazole, followed by a lumenocidal agent such as iodoquinol or paromomycin, is the preferred therapy for symptomatic amebiasis.

Invasive amebiasis may lead to distant abscesses (primarily the liver, but other organs can be involved). An amebic liver abscess usually is single and is commonly located in the posterior portion of the right lobe of the liver. The anatomical location, the fact that it is usually a single abscess, and the absence of other signs of bacterial infection help to distinguish amebic hepatic abscess from bacterial abscess. Serologic tests (complement fixation) are positive in more than 90% of patients with amebic abscess. Hepatic abscess may rupture through the diaphragm into the right pleural cavity.

- Amebic liver abscess may rupture through the diaphragm into the right pleural cavity.

Giardia lamblia is the parasite most frequently detected in state parasitology laboratories. Infection characteristically produces sudden onset of watery diarrhea with malabsorption, bloating, and flatulence. Prolonged disease that is refractory to standard therapy may occur in patients with immunoglobulin A deficiency. The organism may be detected in stool specimens. Stool *Giardia* antigen testing by enzyme-linked immunosorbent assay is very sensitive and may obviate duodenal aspirates for diagnosis. Metronidazole, tinidazole, or nitazoxanide are effective for treating giardiasis.

- *Giardia lamblia* is the parasite most frequently detected in state parasitology laboratories.
- Giardiasis causes sudden onset of watery diarrhea and malabsorption, bloating, and flatulence.
- Prolonged giardiasis is particularly common in patients with immunoglobulin A deficiency.

Toxoplasma gondii is acquired from eating undercooked meat or exposure to cat feces. Primary toxoplasmosis is usually asymptomatic. In immunocompetent persons it may cause a heterophile-negative mononucleosis-like syndrome. Toxoplasmosis causes brain lesions and pneumonia in patients with AIDS. Immunocompromised patients with toxoplasmosis can be treated effectively with pyrimethamine in combination with either sulfadiazine or clindamycin.

- Toxoplasmosis is acquired from eating undercooked meat or exposure to cat feces.
- Toxoplasmosis may cause an infectious mononucleosis-like syndrome.

Malaria is endemic and spreading in many parts of the world. Spiking fevers, rigors, and headache are the hallmark of malaria. With falciparum malaria, the fevers may be irregular or continuous. *Plasmodium falciparum* is the most common cause of fever in a traveler returned from Africa. It is also more likely to cause malarial complications such as cerebral malaria, pulmonary edema, and death. *Plasmodium vivax* and *Plasmodium malariae* infections cause regular episodic fevers (malarial paroxysms). Malaria is diagnosed by examination of thick and thin blood smears (Figure 15-8).

- Diagnosis of malaria is based on examination of thick and thin blood smears.

Prophylaxis for malaria is increasingly difficult because of drug-resistant *P falciparum*. Personal protection should always be used (such as mosquito nets, insect repellents containing DEET [*N,N*-diethyl-3-methylbenzamide]). For travelers to chloroquine-sensitive areas (Central America [north of Panama], Mexico, Haiti, the Dominican Republic, and the Middle East), chloroquine phosphate is still effective. In chloroquine-resistant areas, mefloquine, doxycycline, or an atovaquone-proguanil hydrochloride combination tablet (Malarone) is suggested. Sulfadoxine-pyrimethamine (Fansidar) or a combination of chloroquine with proguanil is not recommended for prophylaxis for chloroquine-resistant falciparum malaria. Travelers to the mefloquine-resistant areas of the Thai-Myanmar and Thai-Cambodian borders should use doxycycline or atovaquone-proguanil hydrochloride. Mefloquine should be avoided in patients with cardiac conduction abnormalities, depression or other psychiatric disorder, or seizure disorder. No regimen guarantees 100% prophylaxis. While receiving mefloquine, patients should be advised not to take halofantrine for a febrile illness because of the risk of fatal cardiac arrhythmias. All patients should be advised to seek medical attention if fever develops within 1 year after return from an endemic area.

Chloroquine is the preferred treatment of infection caused by *P vivax*, *P malariae*, and known chloroquine-susceptible strains of *P falciparum*. Chloroquine-resistant strains may respond to quinine and doxycycline, atovaquone-proguanil hydrochloride, mefloquine, or artemether (this agent is not freely [see below] available in the United States). For severe *P falciparum* infections, intravenous quinidine is effective. In the United States, only parenteral quinidine along with doxycycline or clindamycin is available for severe malaria. Since July 2007, parenteral artesunate has been available in the United States through an Investigational New Drug Protocol from the Centers for Disease Control and Prevention. This drug should be used in combination with another antimalarial agent for severe malaria in concordance with malaria treatment guidelines of the World Health Organization. Exchange transfusion may be beneficial for severely ill patients with parasitemia of more than 10%.

Primaquine is used to eradicate the exoerythrocytic phase of *Plasmodium ovale* and *P vivax* infections, preventing later relapses. Primaquine can cause hemolysis in persons with glucose-6-phosphate dehydrogenase deficiency. Exchange transfusion may be beneficial as treatment for cases with overwhelming parasitemia.

Cryptosporidium parvum is an important cause of diarrhea, especially in persons with AIDS. Cryptosporidiosis is also a cause of self-limited diarrhea in otherwise healthy persons. Waterborne outbreaks (Georgia; Milwaukee, Wisconsin) have been reported. They occur most often in late summer or fall. Thirty-five percent of patients have another pathogen simultaneously, most often *Giardia*. The diagnosis may be missed on standard stool examination for ova and parasites. The stool *Cryptosporidium* enzyme-linked immunosorbent assay–based antigen test has sensitivity of 87%, specificity 99%, and positive predictive value 98%. It has to be ordered specifically if crytposporidoisis is in the differential diagnosis.

There is no effective therapy for *Cryptosporidium*. Paromomycin and nitazoxanide, a new drug, show some efficacy. Nitazoxanide has efficacy of 56% to 88% in immunocompetent patients.

- Cryptosporidiosis is an important cause of diarrhea in AIDS.

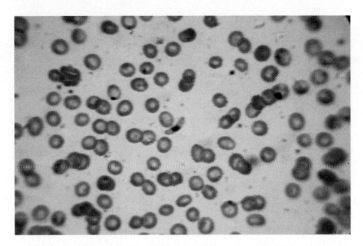

Figure 15-8. Banana-Shaped Gametocyte of *Plasmodium falciparum* in Thin Blood Smear.

Cyclospora cayetanensis is a recently described cause of persistent diarrhea, fever, and profound fatigue. First described in travelers to tropical areas of the world, disease due to *Cyclospora* also has been linked to consumption of contaminated food in the United States (raspberries from Guatemala). Like *Cryptosporidium*, the organism may not be detected on routine stool examinations. The illness can be effectively treated with trimethoprim-sulfamethoxazole.

* Infection with *C cayetanensis* causes persistent diarrhea, fever, and profound fatigue.

Leishmaniasis is a protozoan disease transmitted by the sand fly bite. Visceral leishmaniasis (kala-azar, caused by *Leishmania donovani*) causes fever, hepatosplenomegaly, hypergammaglobulinemia, cachexia, and pancytopenia. It has been reported in patients with AIDS in Spain. Bone marrow examination (Giemsa stain) is often diagnostic. Cutaneous leishmaniasis (caused by *Leishmania tropica*, *Leishmania major*, *Leishmania braziliensis*, and *Leishmania mexicana*) may be self-limited. Cutaneous leishmaniasis has occurred in military personnel returning from Iraq and Afghanistan. South and Central American forms of cutaneous leishmaniasis are often destructive and should be treated. Treatment is with antimony compounds or with amphotericin B or its liposomal formulations.

Babesia microti is a tick-borne (same vector as Lyme disease, *Ixodes scapularis*) parasite that infects erythrocytes and causes fever, myalgias, and hemolytic anemia. Often asymptomatic in normal hosts, severe disease may develop in asplenic individuals. Babesiosis is endemic in the northeastern United States, especially around Nantucket and Cape Cod. Cases of transfusion-transmitted babesiosis have been documented. The diagnosis is established with examination of peripheral blood smear or polymerase chain reaction amplification of *Babesia* DNA from peripheral blood. Treatment is with clindamycin and quinine or atovaquone plus azithromycin. Exchange transfusion has been needed in severely ill patients with high parasitemias. Simultaneous infection with babesiosis and Lyme disease may be especially severe.

* Babesiosis infects erythrocytes and causes fever, myalgias, and hemolytic anemia.

Part II

Robert Orenstein, DO

Clinical Syndromes

Infective Endocarditis

Native Valve Infective Endocarditis

Native valve infective endocarditis is more common in males and patients older than 65 years. The age- and sex-adjusted incidence rate of infective endocarditis is 5 to 7 cases per 100,000 person-years. Increasingly, degenerative valvular disease and mitral valve prolapse predominate as risks for development of endocarditis. However, endocarditis has developed in increasing numbers of patients without known cardiac disease. The mitral and aortic valves are most commonly involved. Mitral valve prolapse, bicuspid aortic valves, and aortic sclerosis now predominate as the underlying lesions in the absence of prosthetic materials.

Infective endocarditis may present with acute or subacute manifestations, depending on the virulence of the infecting organism. In 75% of patients with native valve infective endocarditis, the presentation is fever, often with other systemic signs and symptoms, including weight loss, skin lesions, and general malaise. Heart murmurs are noted in 85%, and one-third have a new murmur. Atypical presentations are more frequent in the elderly, and diagnosis requires a high index of suspicion. The diagnosis of infective endocarditis is often difficult and is based on clinical, microbiologic, and echocardiographic findings (Figure 15-9). Diagnostic criteria have been developed to aid the clinician in the diagnosis of infective endocarditis (Tables 15-5 and 15-6).

- Diagnostic criteria have been developed to aid in the diagnosis of infective endocarditis.

Microorganisms causing native valve infective endocarditis include viridans group streptococci (ie, *Streptococcus sanguis*, *Streptococcus mutans*, and *Streptococcus mitis*), 30% to 40% of cases; enterococci (ie, *Enterococcus faecalis* and *Enterococcus faecium*), 5% to 18%; other streptococci (ie, *Streptococcus bovis* and *Streptococcus pneumoniae*), 15% to 25%; *Staphylococcus aureus*, 10% to 27%; coagulase-negative staphylococci, 1% to 3%; gram-negative bacilli, 1.5% to 13%; fungi, 2% to 4%; miscellaneous bacteria, less than 5%; mixed infections, 1% to 2%; and culture-negative, less than 5% to 24%.

- The organisms most commonly involved in native valve infective endocarditis remain the viridans group streptococci.

Treatment of native valve infective endocarditis includes an emphasis on short-course therapy in patients with uncomplicated left-sided native valve infective endocarditis caused by penicillin-susceptible viridans group streptococci. For enterococcal endocarditis, combination therapy with penicillin G or ampicillin in addition to gentamicin

is recommended. Testing for high-level aminoglycoside resistance (gentamicin, >500 mcg/mL; streptomycin, >2,000 mcg/mL) and penicillin and vancomycin resistance is mandatory. The presence of high-level aminoglycoside resistance precludes use of this agent, and synergy may not be achieved.

Table 15-7 lists the recommended treatment regimens for native valve infective endocarditis.

Prosthetic Valve Infective Endocarditis

Prosthetic valve infective endocarditis accounts for 1% to 5% of all endocarditis cases. The increasing population of persons with prosthetic valves and pacemakers increases the population at risk. In contrast to native valve infective endocarditis, *S aureus* is the principal cause (23%) of prosthetic valve infective endocarditis, and the coagulase-negative staphylococci account for 17% (JAMA. 2007;297:1354-61). Most of these infections are diagnosed 60 days or more after valve replacement and 71% in the first year. Some studies suggest that the aortic valve is affected more often than the mitral valve. Early-onset endocarditis is defined as infection occurring 2 months or less after implantation, and late-onset endocarditis is infection occurring more than 2 months postoperatively. Early infection tends to have a more acute presentation. Microorganisms that cause prosthetic valve endocarditis are outlined in Table 15-8. Persistent bacteremia, congestive heart failure, abscess formation, and stroke are predictors of mortality in prosthetic valve infective endocarditis. Treatment regimens for prosthetic valve infective endocarditis are given in Table 15-9.

Additional Information About Infective Endocarditis

- Transthoracic echocardiography and transesophageal echocardiography visualize vegetations in approximately 60% and 90% of patients, respectively. Transesophageal echocardiography is superior to transthoracic for diagnosing complications of infective endocarditis such as cardiac abscesses and perivalvular extension.
- Infective endocarditis in injection drug users is caused by *S aureus* (60%), streptococci (16%), gram-negative bacilli (13.5%), polymicrobial infection (8.1%), and group JK corynebacterium (1.4%). *Candida* spp endocarditis also occurs in this patient population. Tricuspid valve involvement is common. Short-course (2 weeks) therapy with a penicillinase-resistant penicillin with or without an aminoglycoside or 4-week oral regimens with a fluoroquinolone and rifampin may be as effective as longer courses of therapy in uncomplicated right-sided endocarditis due to methicillin-susceptible *S aureus* in injection drug users, irrespective of whether the patient has human immunodeficiency virus (HIV).
- Culture-negative endocarditis may be the result of previous use of antibiotics (most common). The HACEK (*Haemophilus* spp, *Actinobacillus actinomycetemcomitans*, *Cardiobacterium hominis*, *Eikenella* spp, *Kingella kingae*) organisms are identified by newer culture methods and are less frequently associated with

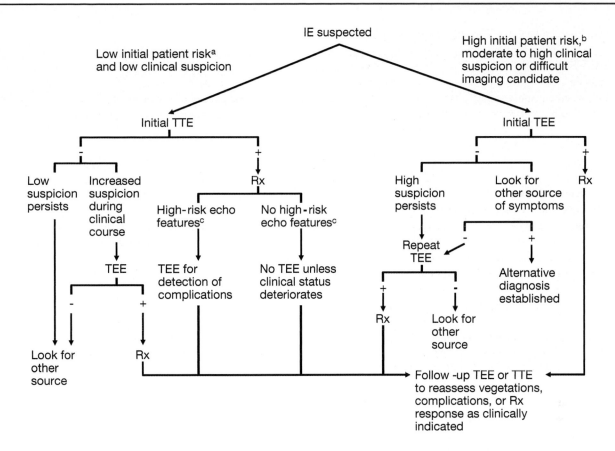

Figure 15-9. An approach to the use of echocardiography (echo) for the diagnosis of infective endocarditis (IE). [a]For example, a patient with fever and a previously known heart murmur and no other stigmata of IE. [b]High initial patient risks include prosthetic heart valves, many congenital heart diseases, previous endocarditis, new murmur, heart failure, or other stigmata of endocarditis. [c]High-risk echocardiographic features include large or mobile vegetations, valvular insufficiency, suggestion of perivalvular extension, or secondary ventricular dysfunction. Rx indicates antibiotic treatment for endocarditis; TEE, transesophageal echocardiography; TTE, transthoracic echocardiography. (From Bayer AS, Bolger AF, Taubert KA, Wilson W, Steckelberg J, Karchmer AW, et al. Diagnosis and management of infective endocarditis and its complications. Circulation. 1998;98:2936-48. Used with permission.)

culture-negative endocarditis. The most frequent causes of culture-negative endocarditis are listed in Table 15-10 . Several of these can be diagnosed with serologic or molecular tests in the absence of positive blood cultures.

Endocarditis Associated With Cardiac Devices

Pacemakers, implantable cardioverter-defibrillators, and other devices are increasingly associated with infectious complications. The incidence of pacemaker infections ranges from 0.13% to 19.9% and that for ICDs 0% to 0.8%; the mortality rate is 31% to 66% in the absence of removal. Table 15-11 and Figure 15-10 present helpful guidelines for the diagnosis and management of these.

Surgical Therapy

If cardiac valve replacement is needed, it should not be delayed to allow additional days of antimicrobial therapy. Surgical treatment is often indicated in cases of congestive heart failure refractory to medical management. Intractable congestive heart failure is the most common indication for cardiac valve replacement. Other generally accepted indications for cardiac valve replacement include evidence

of more than 1 serious systemic embolic episode, uncontrolled bacteremia despite effective antimicrobial therapy, and inadequate antimicrobial therapy. Other indications include invasive perivalvular infection as manifested by abscess or fistula on echocardiography, new or persistent electrocardiographic changes, persistent unexplained fever, fungal endocarditis, and relapse of appropriately treated prosthetic valve endocarditis due to penicillin-sensitive streptococci (Table 15-12).

- Surgical treatment is indicated in cases of congestive heart failure refractory to medical management.
- Intractable congestive heart failure is the most common indication for cardiac valve replacement.

Prevention

Recommendations for prevention of infective endocarditis have changed considerably. Recent reports have concluded that only a small number of cases of infective endocarditis can be prevented by prophylaxis for dental procedures (Circulation. 2007;116:1736-54). Prophylaxis for infective endocarditis is indicated only in patients with prosthetic cardiac valves, previous infective endocarditis, or

Table 15-5 Modified Duke Criteria for the Diagnosis of Infective Endocarditis

Definite infective endocarditis
  Pathologic criteria
    1. Microorganisms on culture or histologic examination of a vegetation, a vegetation that has embolized, or an intracardiac abscess specimen; *or*
    2. Pathologic lesions; vegetation or intracardiac abscess confirmed by histologic examination showing active endocarditis
  Clinical criteria[a]
    1. 2 major criteria, *or*
    2. 1 major criterion and 3 minor criteria, *or*
    3. 5 minor criteria
Possible infective endocarditis
    1. 1 major criterion and 1 minor criterion, *or*
    2. 3 minor criteria
Rejected
    1. Firm alternative diagnosis explaining evidence of infective endocarditis, *or*
    2. Resolution of infective endocarditis syndrome with antibiotic therapy for ≤4 days, *or*
    3. No pathologic evidence of infective endocarditis at surgery or autopsy, with antibiotic therapy for ≤4 days, *or*
    4. Does not meet criteria for possible infective endocarditis, as above.

[a] See Table 15-6 for definitions of major and minor criteria.
From Li SL, Sexton DJ, Mick N, Nettles R, Fowler VG Jr, Ryan T, et al. Proposed modifications to the Duke criteria for the diagnosis of infective endocarditis. Clin Infect Dis. 2000;30:633-8. Used with permission.

congenital heart disease and in recipients of a cardiac transplant who have cardiac valvulopathy (Table 15-13). For patients with these underlying cardiac disorders, prophylaxis is indicated before dental procedures, including manipulation of gingival tissue or periapical region of the teeth or perforation of oral mucosa. Current recommendations for antibiotic prophylaxis before a dental procedure are summarized in Table 15-14. Antibiotic prophylaxis is not indicated before genitourinary or gastroenterology procedures. Prophylaxis for infective endocarditis is currently not recommended on the basis of an increased lifetime risk of acquiring infective endocarditis.

* Routine prophylaxis for infective endocarditis is not recommended in patients with cardiac disorders.
* Prophylaxis for infective endocarditis is recommended only for patients with prosthetic cardiac valves, previous infective endocarditis, or congenital heart disease and in recipients of a cardiac transplant who have cardiac valvulopathy.

The changes in the recommendations for prophylaxis are summarized as follows:
* Bacteremia resulting from daily activities is much more likely to cause infective endocarditis than bacteremia associated with a dental procedure.
* Only an extremely small number of cases of infective endocarditis might be prevented by antibiotic prophylaxis even if prophylaxis is 100% effective.
* Antibiotic prophylaxis is not recommended based solely on an increased lifetime risk of acquisition of infective endocarditis.
* Limit recommendations for infective endocarditis prophylaxis to only those conditions listed in Table 15-13.
* Antibiotic prophylaxis is no longer recommended for any other

form of congenital heart disease except for the conditions listed in Table 15-13.
* Antibiotic prophylaxis is recommended for all dental procedures that involve manipulation of gingival tissues or periapical region of teeth or perforation of oral mucosa only for patients with underlying cardiac conditions associated with the highest risk of adverse outcome from infective endocarditis (Table 15-13).
* Antibiotic prophylaxis is recommended for procedures on respiratory tract or infected skin, skin structures, or musculoskeletal tissue only for patients with underlying cardiac conditions associated with the highest risk of adverse outcome from infective endocarditis (Table 15-13).
* Antibiotic prophylaxis solely to prevent infective endocarditis is not recommended for genitourinary or gastrointestinal tract procedures.
* The procedures noted in the 1997 prophylaxis guidelines for which endocarditis prophylaxis is not recommended are reaffirmed, and these are extended to other common procedures, including ear and body piercing, tattooing, and vaginal delivery and hysterectomy.

(Summary is from Circulation. 2007;116:1736-54.)

Meningitis

Bacterial Meningitis

The incidence of bacterial meningitis is estimated to be 3.0 cases per 100,000 person-years. The overall case fatality rate was 25% in a report of 443 cases of bacterial meningitis in adults between 1962 and 1988. Forty percent of cases were nosocomial. Common predisposing conditions for community-acquired meningitis include acute

Table 15-6 Definitions of Terminology Used in the Modified Duke Criteria for the Diagnosis of Infective Endocarditis

Major criteria

1. Blood culture positive for infective endocarditis
   a. Typical microorganisms consistent with infective endocarditis from 2 separate blood cultures
      1) Viridans streptococci, *Streptococcus bovis*, HACEK[a] group, *Staphylococcus aureus*, *or*
      2) Community-acquired enterococci, in the absence of a primary focus, *or*
   b. Microorganisms consistent with infective endocarditis from persistently positive blood cultures, defined as follows:
      1) At least 2 positive cultures of blood samples drawn more than 12 hours apart, *or*
      2) All of 3 or a majority of 4 or more separate blood cultures, with first & last samples drawn at least 1 hour apart
   c. Single blood culture positive for *Coxiella burnetii* or antiphase I immunoglobulin G antibody titer ≥1:800
2. Evidence of endocardial involvement
   a. Echocardiogram positive for infective endocarditis (TEE recommended in patients with prosthetic valves, rated at least "possible infective endocarditis" by clinical criteria, or complicated infective endocarditis [paravalvular abscess]; TTE as first test in other patients), defined as follows:
      1) Oscillating intracardiac mass on valve or supporting structures, in the path of regurgitant jets, or on implanted material in the absence of an alternative anatomical explanation, *or*
      2) Abscess, *or*
      3) New partial dehiscence of prosthetic valve
   b. New valvular regurgitation (worsening or changing of preexisting murmur not sufficient)

Minor criteria

1. Predisposition: predisposing heart condition or intravenous drug use
2. Fever: >38.0°C (100.4°F)
3. Vascular phenomena: major arterial emboli, septic pulmonary infarcts, mycotic aneurysm, intracranial hemorrhage, conjunctival hemorrhages, Janeway lesions
4. Immunologic phenomena: glomerulonephritis, Osler nodes, Roth spots, rheumatoid factor
5. Microbiologic evidence: positive blood culture but not meeting major criteria as noted previously[b] *or* serologic evidence of active infection with organisms consistent with infective endocarditis
6. Echocardiographic minor criteria eliminated

Abbreviations: TEE, transesophageal echocardiography; TTE, transthoracic echocardiography.
[a] HACEK, *Haemophilus* spp, *Actinobacillus actinomycetemcomitans*, *Cardiobacterium hominis*, *Eikenella* spp, and *Kingella kingae*.
[b] Excluding single positive cultures for coagulase-negative staphylococci and organisms that do not cause endocarditis.
From Li JS, Sexton DJ, Mick N, Nettles R, Fowler VG Jr., Ryan T, et al. Proposed modifications to the Duke criteria for the diagnosis of infective endocarditis. Clin Infect Dis. 2000;30:633-8. Used with permission.

otitis media, altered immune states, alcoholism, pneumonia, diabetes mellitus, sinusitis, and a cerebrospinal fluid leak. Risk factors for death among adults with community-acquired meningitis include age 60 years or older, obtundation on admission, and occurrence of seizures within 24 hours of symptom onset. In 66% of patients, fever, nuchal rigidity, and altered mental status are present (N Engl J Med. 1993;328:21-8).

Typical initial cerebrospinal fluid characteristics include a cell count of 1,000 to 5,000/mcL (range, <100-10,000) and a glucose value less than 40 mg/dL or a cerebrospinal fluid–serum glucose ratio less than 0.31. The leukocyte differential is more likely to show a predominance of polymorphonuclear neutrophils. The Gram stain is positive in 60% to 90% of cases. Countercurrent immunoelectrophoresis or latex agglutination tests may provide results in 15 minutes and are useful for the detection of *Haemophilus influenzae* type B, *S pneumoniae*, and *Neisseria meningitidis* types A, B, C, and Y, *Escherichia coli* K1, and group B streptococci in the absence of a positive Gram stain. Cerebrospinal fluid cultures are positive in 70%

to 85% of cases. Blood cultures may be positive. Polymerase chain reaction has been used to diagnose meningitis due to *S pneumoniae*, *H influenzae* type B, *Streptococcus agalactiae*, *Listeria monocytogenes*, and *N meningitidis*.

Organisms most commonly causing community-acquired meningitis in adults are *S pneumoniae* (38%), *N meningitidis* (14%), *L monocytogenes* (11%), streptococci (7%), *S aureus* (5%), *H influenzae* (4%), and gram-negative bacilli (4%). Management of suspected community-acquired bacterial meningitis is outlined in Figure 15-11, and recommendations for antimicrobial therapy are listed in Table 15-15.

Although still somewhat controversial in adults, recent guidelines (Clin Infect Dis. 2004;39:1267-84) do suggest a role for the use of dexamethasone in the early treatment of specific types of bacterial meningitis: suspected pneumococcal meningitis in adults and *H influenzae* type B meningitis in children. There is inadequate evidence to support dexamethasone use in other forms of bacterial meningitis. It is important to remember that the benefit occurs with administration before antibiotics. Thus the optimal approach is to

Table 15-7 Treatment of Native Valve Infective Endocarditis

Microorganisms	Therapy[a]	Alternative Therapy[a]
Penicillin-sensitive viridans group streptococci and *Streptococcus bovis* (MIC, ≤0.1 mcg/mL)	Aqueous crystalline penicillin G, 12-18 × 10⁶ U/24 h IV either continuously or in 6 equally divided doses for 4 wk *Or* Ceftriaxone sodium 2 g IV or IM for 4 wk[c] *Or* Aqueous penicillin G, 12-18 × 10⁶ U/24 h IV either continuously or in 6 equally divided doses for 2 wk *Plus* Gentamicin sulfate,[d] 1 mg/kg IV or IM every 8 h for 2 wk	Vancomycin,[b] 30 mg/kg IV in 2 equally divided doses, not to exceed 2 g/24 h unless serum levels are monitored for 4 wk Vancomycin therapy is recommended for patients allergic to β-lactams (immediate-type hypersensitivity); serum concentration of vancomycin should be obtained 1 h after completion of the infusion & should be in the range of 30-45 mcg/mL for twice-daily dosing
Relatively penicillin-resistant viridans group streptococci (MIC, >0.1 mcg/mL and <0.5 mcg/mL)	Aqueous crystalline penicillin G, 24 × 10⁶ U/24 h IV either continuously or in 4-6 equally divided doses for 4 wk *Plus* Gentamicin sulfate,[d] 1 mg/kg IV or IM every 8 h for 2 wk	Vancomycin,[b] 30 mg/kg IV in 2 equally divided doses, not to exceed 2 g/24 h unless serum levels are monitored for 4 wk Vancomycin therapy is recommended for patients allergic to β-lactams (immediate-type hypersensitivity); serum concentration of vancomycin should be obtained 1 h after completion of the infusion & should be in the range of 30-45 mcg/mL for twice-daily dosing
Enterococci (gentamicin- or vancomycin-susceptible) or viridans group streptococci with MIC ≥0.5 mcg/mL or nutritionally variant streptococci (All enterococci causing endocarditis must be tested for antimicrobial susceptibility in order to select optimal therapy) High-level aminoglycoside-resistant *Enterococcus faecalis*: ceftriaxone 2 g IV every 12 h *plus* ampicillin 2 g IV every 4 h for 4-6 wk	Aqueous crystalline penicillin G, 18-30 × 10⁶ U/24 h IV either continuously or in 6 equally divided doses for 4-6 wk *Or* Ampicillin sodium 12 g/24 h IV either continuously or in 6 equally divided doses *Plus* Gentamicin sulfate,[d] 1 mg/kg IV or IM every 8 h for 4-6 wk (4-wk therapy recommended for patients with symptoms ≤3 mo in duration; 6-wk therapy recommended for patients with symptoms >3 mo in duration)	Vancomycin,[b] 30 mg/kg IV in 2 equally divided doses, not to exceed 2 g/24 h unless serum levels are monitored for 4-6 wk *Plus* Gentamicin,[d] 1 mg/kg IV or IM every 8 h for 4-6 wk Vancomycin therapy is recommended for patients allergic to β-lactams (immediate-type hypersensitivity); serum concentration of vancomycin should be obtained 1 h after completion of the infusion & should be in the range of 30-45 mcg/mL for twice-daily dosing Cephalosporins are not acceptable alternatives for patients allergic to penicillin
Enterococcus faecium	Linezolid, 1,200 mg/24 h IV or PO in 2 divided doses for ≥8 wk *Or* Dalfopristin/quinupristin, 22.5 mg/kg per 24 h IV in 3 divided doses for ≥8 wk	Patients with endocarditis caused by these strains should be treated in consultation with an infectious diseases specialist Cardiac valve replacement may be necessary for bacteriologic cure Cure with antimicrobial therapy alone may be <50% Severe, usually reversible thrombocytopenia may occur with use of linezolid, especially after 2 wk of therapy Dalfopristin/quinupristin only effective against *E faecium* & can cause severe myalgias, which may require discontinuation of therapy Only small number of patients have reportedly been treated with imipenem/cilastatin-ampicillin or ceftriaxone + ampicillin

Table 15-7 (continued)

Microorganisms	Therapy[a]	Alternative Therapy[a]
Enterococcus faecalis	Imipenem/cilastatin, 2 g/24 h IV in 4 equally divided doses for ≥8 wk *Plus* Ampicillin sodium, 12 g/24 h IV in 6 divided doses for ≥8 wk *Or* Ceftriaxone sodium, 2 g/24 h IV or IM in 1 dose for ≥8 wk *Plus* Ampicillin sodium, 12 g/24 h IV in 6 divided doses for ≥8 wk *Pediatric dose* (should not exceed that of a normal adult): linezolid 30 mg/kg per 24 h IV or PO in 3 divided doses; dalfopristin/quinupristin 22.5 mg/kg per 24 h IV in 3 divided doses; imipenem/cilastatin 60-100 mg/kg per 24 h IV in 4 divided doses; ampicillin 300 mg/kg per 24 h IV in 4-6 divided doses; ceftriaxone 100 mg/kg per 24 h IV or IM once daily	
Staphylococcus aureus[c] Methicillin-sensitive	Nafcillin sodium or oxacillin sodium, 2.0 g IV every 4 h for 4-6 wk *Plus* Gentamicin sulfate (optional),[d] 1 mg/kg every 8 h IV or IM for first 3-5 days. Benefit of additional aminoglycoside has not been established	Cefazolin (or other first-generation cephalosporins in equivalent dosages), 2 g IV every 8 h for 4-6 wk *Plus* Gentamicin (optional),[d] 1 mg/kg every 8 h IV or IM for first 3-5 days Cephalosporins should be avoided in patients with immediate-type hypersensitivity to penicillin Vancomycin,[b] 30 mg/kg IV in 2 equally divided doses, not to exceed 2 g/24 h unless serum levels are monitored for 4-6 wk Vancomycin therapy is recommended for patients allergic to β-lactams (immediate-type hypersensitivity); serum concentration of vancomycin should be obtained 1 h after completion of the infusion & should be in the range of 30-45 mcg/mL for twice-daily dosing Daptomycin 6 mg/kg once daily may be used as an alternative in right-sided endocarditis due to MSSA or MRSA
Methicillin-resistant	Vancomycin,[b] 30 mg/kg IV in 2 equally divided doses, not to exceed 2 g/24 h unless serum levels are monitored for 4-6 wk	Consult infectious diseases specialist Daptomycin 6 mg/kg once daily may be used as an alternative in right-sided endocarditis due to MSSA or MRSA
HACEK group	Ceftriaxone sodium, 2 g IV or IM for 4 wk[c] *Or* Ampicillin[f]-sulbactam 12 g/24 h IV in 4 divided doses for 4 wk *Or* Ciprofloxacin 1,000 mg/24 h PO or 800 mg/24 h IV in 2 divided doses if unable to tolerate alternatives Cefotaxime sodium or other third-generation cephalosporins may be substituted	Consult infectious diseases specialist

Table 15-7 (continued)

Microorganisms	Therapy[a]	Alternative Therapy[a]
Neisseria gonorrhoeae	Ceftriaxone, 1-2 g every 24 h for ≥4 wk	Aqueous crystalline penicillin G, 20 × 10⁶ U/24 h IV either continuously or in 6 equally divided doses for 4 wk, for penicillin-susceptible isolates
Gram-negative bacilli	Most effective single drug or combination of drugs IV for 4-6 wk	
Urgent empiric treatment for culture-negative endocarditis	Vancomycin,[b] 30 mg/kg IV in 2 equally divided doses, not to exceed 2 g/24 h unless serum levels are monitored for 6 wk *Plus* Gentamicin sulfate,[d] 1.0 mg/kg IV every 8 h for 6 wk	
Fungal endocarditis	Amphotericin B *Plus* Flucytosine (optional) *Plus* Cardiac valve replacement (flucytosine levels should be monitored)	
Suspected *Bartonella*, culture negative	Ceftriaxone sodium, 2 g/24 h IV or IM in 1 dose for 6 wk *Plus* Gentamicin sulfate, 3 mg/kg per 24 h IV or IM in 3 divided doses for 2 wk *With or without* Doxycycline 200 mg/kg per 24 h IV or PO in 2 divided doses for 6 wk	Consult an infectious diseases specialist

Abbreviations: HACEK, *Haemophilus* spp, *Actinobacillus actinomycetemcomitans, Cardiobacterium hominis, Eikenella* spp, and *Kingella kingae*; IM, intramuscularly; IV, intravenously; MIC, minimal inhibitory concentration; MRSA, methicillin-resistant *Staphylococcus aureus*; MSSA, methicillin-sensitive *Staphylococcus aureus*; PO, orally.

[a] Dosages recommended are for patients with normal renal function.

[b] Vancomycin dosage should be reduced in patients with impaired renal function. Vancomycin given on an mg/kg basis produces higher serum concentrations in obese patients than in lean patients. Therefore, in obese patients, dosing should be based on ideal body weight. Each dose of vancomycin should be infused over at least 1 hour to reduce the risk of the histamine-release "red man" syndrome.

[c] Patients should be notified that IM injection of ceftriaxone is painful.

[d] Dosing of gentamicin on an mg/kg basis produces higher serum concentrations in obese patients than in lean patients. Therefore, in obese patients, dosing should be based on ideal body weight. (Ideal body weight for men is 50 kg + 2.3 kg per inch over 5 feet, and ideal body weight for women is 45.5 kg + 2.3 kg per inch over 5 feet.) Relative contraindications to the use of gentamicin are age older than 65 years, renal impairment, or impairment of the eighth nerve. Other potentially nephrotoxic agents (such as nonsteroidal anti-inflammatory drugs) should be used cautiously in patients receiving gentamicin.

[e] For treatment of endocarditis due to penicillin-susceptible staphylococci (MIC, <0.1 mcg/mL), aqueous crystalline penicillin G, 12-18 × 10⁶ U/24 h IV either continuously or in 6 equally divided doses for 4 to 6 weeks, can be used instead of nafcillin or oxacillin. Shorter antibiotic courses have been effective in some injection drug users with right-sided endocarditis due to *Staphylococcus aureus*. The routine use of rifampin is not recommended for the treatment of native valve staphylococcal endocarditis.

[f] Ampicillin should not be used if laboratory tests show β-lactamase production.

Data from Wilson WR, Karchmer AW, Dajani AS, Taubert KA, Bayer A, Kaye D, et al. Antibiotic treatment of adults with infective endocarditis due to streptococci, enterococci, staphylococci and HACEK microorganisms. JAMA. 1995;274:1706-13; modified from Steckelberg JM, Giuliani ER, Wilson WR. Infective endocarditis. In: Giuliani ER, Fuster V, Gersh BJ, McGoon MD, McGoon DC (editors). Cardiology: fundamentals and practice. Vol 2. 2nd ed. St. Louis: Mosby Year Book; 1991. p. 1739-72. Used with permission of Mayo Foundation; and modified from Baddour LM, Wilson WR, Bayer AS, Fowler VG Jr, Bolger AF, Levison ME, et al. Infective endocarditis: diagnosis, antimicrobial therapy, and management of complications. A statement for healthcare professionals from the Committee on Rheumatic Fever, Endocarditis, and Kawasaki Disease, Council on Cardiovascular Disease in the Young, and the Councils on Clinical Cardiology, Stroke, and Cardiovascular Surgery and Anesthesia, American Heart Association: executive summary. Circulation. 2005;111:3167-84. Used with permission.

Table 15-8 Causative Organisms for Prosthetic Valve Endocarditis (PVE) in 556 Patients

Causative Organism	Total, No. (%) (n=556)	Early PVE, No. (%) (n=53)	Late PVE, No. (%) (n=331)
Staphylococcus aureus	128 (23.0)	19 (35.9)	61 (18.4)
Methicillin-sensitive *S aureus*	82 (14.7)	8 (15.1)	43 (13.0)
Methicillin-resistant *S aureus*	36 (6.5)	10 (18.9)	11 (3.3)
Coagulase-negative staphylococci	94 (16.9)	9 (17.0)	66 (19.9)
Enterococcus spp	71 (12.8)	4 (7.5)	42 (12.7)
Viridans streptococci	67 (12.1)	1 (1.9)	34 (10.3)
Culture negative	62 (11.2)	9 (17.0)	41 (12.4)
Streptococcus bovis	29 (5.2)	1 (1.9)	22 (6.7)
Fungal	23 (4.1)	5 (9.4)	11 (3.3)
Polymicrobial	10 (1.8)	0	6 (1.8)
HACEK spp	8 (1.4)	0	7 (2.1)
Escherichia coli	7 (1.3)	1 (1.9)	3 (0.9)
Streptococcus agalactiae	5 (0.9)	0	3 (0.9)
Propionibacterium acnes	4 (0.7)	0	3 (0.9)
Streptococcus group G	4 (0.7)	0	3 (0.9)
Propionibacterium NOS	3 (0.5)	0	2 (0.6)
Pseudomonas aeruginosa	3 (0.5)	1 (1.9)	1 (0.3)
Streptococcus anginosus	3 (0.5)	0	2 (0.6)
Streptococcus NOS	3 (0.5)	0	2 (0.6)
Streptococcus pneumoniae	3 (0.5)	0	3 (0.9)
Listeria monocytogenes	2 (0.4)	0	2 (0.6)
Micromonas micros	2 (0.4)	0	2 (0.6)
Mycobacteria spp	2 (0.4)	0	1 (0.3)
Serratia marcescens	2 (0.4)	1 (1.9)	0
Streptococcus gallolyticus	2 (0.4)	0	0
Streptococcus group B	2 (0.4)	0	0
Streptococcus group C	2 (0.4)	0	1 (0.3)

Abbreviations: HACEK, *Haemophilus* spp, *Actinobacillus actinomycetemcomitans*, *Cardiobacterium hominis*, *Eikenella* spp, and *Kingella kingae*; NOS, not otherwise speciated.
From Wang A, Athan E, Pappas PA, Fowler VG Jr., Olaison L, Paré C, et al. Contemporary clinical profile and outcome of prosthetic valve endocarditis. JAMA. 2007;297:1354-61. Used with permission.

obtain a cerebrospinal fluid Gram stain and blood and cerebrospinal fluid cultures and administer dexamethasone and then the appropriate antibiotic. Dexamethasone 0.15 mg/kg should be given 10 to 20 minutes *before* the first dose of antibiotics and the dose repeated every 6 hours for the first 2 to 4 days. If subsequently it is determined that the patient does not have pneumococcal meningitis, use of dexamethasone should be stopped.

- Risk factors for death in bacterial meningitis: age 60 years or older, decreased mental status at admission, seizures within 24 hours of symptom onset.
- Gram stains of cerebrospinal fluid are positive in 60%-90% of cases.
- Organisms most commonly causing community-acquired infection in adults: *S pneumoniae*, *N meningitidis*, *H influenzae*, and *L monocytogenes*.

The causative organisms, affected age groups, and predisposing factors in bacterial meningitis are shown in Table 15-16, and empiric treatment in various age and patient groups is outlined in Table 15-17.

Although the *H influenzae* type B conjugate vaccine has clearly resulted in a decline in meningitis caused by this organism, and the same decline seems to be occurring with invasive pneumococcal disease in children, the impact of the 7-valent conjugate pneumococcal vaccine is not yet clear. Immunocompromised hosts, pregnant women, and elderly patients should receive an empiric antibiotic regimen that includes coverage for *L monocytogenes*. High-dose ampicillin is the treatment of choice. An aminoglycoside can be added to ampicillin if *L monocytogenes* meningitis is confirmed. High-dose intravenous trimethoprim-sulfamethoxazole can be used in patients with a penicillin allergy. *L monocytogenes* can be mistakenly reported as a diphtheroid on cerebrospinal fluid culture and labeled a contaminant.

Table 15-9 Treatment of Prosthetic Valve Infective Endocarditis

Organism	Therapy[a]	Alternative Therapy/Comments[a]
Staphylococcus aureus or coagulase-negative staphylococci: methicillin-resistant	Vancomycin,[b] 30 mg/kg IV in 2 equally divided doses, not to exceed 2 g/24 h unless serum levels are monitored for ≥6 wk *Plus* Rifampin,[c] 300 mg PO every 8 h for ≥6 wk *Plus* Gentamicin sulfate,[d] 1 mg/kg IV or IM every 8 h for first 2 wk of therapy. (If organism is not susceptible to gentamicin, ciprofloxacin may be substituted if the organism is susceptible in vitro)	Rifampin increases the amount of warfarin sodium required for antithrombotic therapy
Staphylococcus aureus or coagulase-negative staphylococci: methicillin-susceptible	Nafcillin sodium or oxacillin sodium, 2 g IV every 4 h for ≥6 wk *Plus* Rifampin,[c] 300 mg orally every 8 h for ≥6 wk *Plus* Gentamicin sulfate,[d] 1 mg/kg IV or IM every 8 h for first 2 wk of therapy. (If organism is not susceptible to gentamicin, ciprofloxacin may be substituted if the organism is susceptible in vitro)	Rifampin increases the amount of warfarin sodium required for antithrombotic therapy First-generation cephalosporins or vancomycin should be used in patients allergic to β-lactams Cephalosporins should be avoided in patients with immediate-type hypersensitivity to penicillin or to methicillin-resistant staphylococci
Enterococci (gentamicin- or vancomycin-susceptible) or viridans group streptococci or nutritionally variant streptococci or *Streptococcus bovis* (All streptococci causing endocarditis must be tested for antimicrobial susceptibility in order to select optimal therapy)	Aqueous crystalline penicillin G, 18-30×10^6 U/24 h IV either continuously or in 6 equally divided doses for 6 wk *Or* Ampicillin sodium, 12 g/24 h IV either continuously or in 6 equally divided doses *Plus* Gentamicin sulfate,[d] 1 mg/kg IV or IM every 8 h for 6 wk	Vancomycin,[b] 30 mg/kg IV in 2 equally divided doses, not to exceed 2 g/24 h unless serum levels are monitored for 4-6 wk *Plus* Gentamicin sulfate,[d] 1 mg/kg IV or IM every 8 h for 4-6 wk Vancomycin therapy is recommended for patients allergic to β-lactams (immediate-type hypersensitivity); serum concentration of vancomycin should be obtained 1 h after completion of the infusion & should be in the range of 30-45 mcg/mL for twice-daily dosing Cephalosporins are not acceptable alternatives for patients allergic to penicillin
Enterococcus faecium	Linezolid, 1,200 mg/24 h IV or PO in 2 divided doses for ≥8 wk *Or* Dalfopristin/quinupristin, 22.5 mg/kg per 24 h IV in 3 divided doses for ≥8 wk	Patients with endocarditis caused by these strains should be treated in consultation with an infectious diseases specialist Cardiac valve replacement may be necessary for bacteriologic cure Cure with antimicrobial therapy alone may be <50% Severe, usually reversible thrombocytopenia may occur with use of linezolid, especially after 2 wk of therapy Dalfopristin/quinupristin only effective against *E faecium* & can cause severe myalgias, which may require discontinuation of therapy Only small number of patients have reportedly been treated with imipenem/cilastatin-ampicillin or ceftriaxone + ampicillin

Table 15-9 (continued)

Organism	Therapy[a]	Alternative Therapy/Comments[a]
Enterococcus faecalis	Imipenem/cilastatin, 2 g/24 h IV in 4 equally divided doses for ≥8 wk *Plus* Ampicillin sodium, 12 g/24 h IV in 6 divided doses for ≥8 wk *Or* Ceftriaxone sodium, 2 g/24 h IV or IM in 1 dose for ≥8 wk *Plus* Ampicillin sodium, 12 g/24 h IV in 6 divided doses for ≥8 wk *Pediatric dose* (should not exceed that of a normal adult): linezolid 30 mg/kg per 24 h IV or PO in 3 divided doses; dalfopristin/quinupristin 22.5 mg/kg per 24 h IV in 3 divided doses; imipenem/cilastatin 60-100 mg/kg per 24 h IV in 4 divided doses; ampicillin 300 mg/kg per 24 h IV in 4-6 divided doses; ceftriaxone 100 mg/kg per 24 h IV or IM once daily	

Abbreviations: IM, intramuscularly; IV, intravenously; PO, orally.

[a] Dosages recommended are for patients with normal renal function.

[b] Vancomycin dosage should be reduced in patients with impaired renal function. Vancomycin given on an mg/kg basis produces higher serum concentrations in obese patients than in lean patients. Therefore, in obese patients, dosing should be based on ideal body weight. Each dose of vancomycin should be infused over at least 1 hour to reduce the risk of the histamine release "red man" syndrome.

[c] Rifampin plays a unique role in the eradication of staphylococcal infection involving prosthetic material; combination therapy is essential to prevent emergence of rifampin resistance.

[d] Dosing of gentamicin on an mg/kg basis will produce higher serum concentrations in obese patients than in lean patients. Therefore, in obese patients, dosing should be based on ideal body weight. (Ideal body weight for men is 50 kg + 2.3 kg per inch over 5 feet, and ideal body weight for women is 45.5 kg + 2.3 kg per inch over 5 feet.) Relative contraindications to the use of gentamicin are age older than 65 years, renal impairment, or impairment of the eighth nerve. Other potentially nephrotoxic agents (such as nonsteroidal anti-inflammatory drugs) should be used cautiously in patients receiving gentamicin.

Data from Wilson MR, Karchmer AW, Dajani AS, Taubert KA, Bayer A, Kaye D, et al. Antibiotic treatment of adults with infective endocarditis due to streptococci, enterococci, staphylococci, and HACEK microorganisms. JAMA. 1995;274:1706-13; and modified from Baddour LM, Wilson WR, Bayer AS, Fowler VG Jr, Bolger AF, Levison ME, et al. Infective endocarditis: diagnosis, antimicrobial therapy, and management of complications. A statement for healthcare professionals from the Committee on Rheumatic Fever, Endocarditis, and Kawasaki Disease, Council on Cardiovascular Disease in the Young, and the Councils on Clinical Cardiology, Stroke, and Cardiovascular Surgery and Anesthesia, American Heart Association: executive summary. Circulation. 2005;111:3167-84. Used with permission.

• Immunocompromised hosts, pregnant women, and the elderly should receive an empiric antibiotic regimen that includes high-dose ampicillin to cover *L monocytogenes*.

Meningococcal Meningitis

Meningitis often occurs in patients who are carriers of meningococci in the nasopharynx. Terminal component complement deficiencies predispose to repeated episodes of infection. Serotypes B, C, and Y cause most of the endemic disease in the United States. Many patients have a petechial rash. The pathogenesis of Waterhouse-Friderichsen syndrome (ie, acute hemorrhagic necrosis of the adrenal glands causing primary adrenocortical insufficiency) is related to disseminated intravascular coagulation. Treatment is with penicillin G if the minimal inhibitory concentration is <0.1 mcg/mL, otherwise high-dose ceftriaxone or cefotaxime is preferred. In close contacts of the index case (hospital workers with substantial respiratory exposure, roommates, household contacts, day-care center members, persons exposed to patient's oral secretions), chemoprophylaxis should be given within 24 hours of exposure, if possible. Rifampin, ceftriaxone, or ciprofloxacin (use only in patients 18 years or older) have been used. The carrier state is not eliminated by penicillin; thus, affected cases may require one of these drugs for eradication of carriage. Immunization of certain populations (eg, military recruits, college students living in dormitories, Hajj pilgrims, patients with terminal complement component deficiencies or asplenia) is also of benefit. The meningococcal vaccine contains polysaccharides of

Table 15-10 Causes of Culture-Negative Endocarditis

Previous use of antibiotics
HACEK organisms
  Haemophilus spp
  Actinobacillus actinomycetemcomitans
  Cardiobacterium hominis
  Eikenella spp
  Kingella kingae
Nutritionally variant streptococci (*Abiotrophia* spp)
Neisseria spp
Listeria monocytogenes
Brucella spp
Fungi
Mycobacteria
Legionella spp
Coxiella burnetii
Chlamydia spp
Mycoplasma spp
Nocardia spp
Rothia dentocariosa
Bartonella spp

groups A, C, Y, and W-135. A new meningococcal vaccine (Menactra) was recently approved and offers longer protection.

- In meningococcal meningitis, terminal component complement deficiencies predispose to repeated episodes of infection.
- If the risk of the carrier state is high (household contacts), rifampin, ceftriaxone, or ciprofloxacin should be used for prophylaxis.

The Acute Aseptic Meningitis Syndrome

This is a syndrome characterized by an acute onset of meningeal symptoms, fever, cerebrospinal fluid pleocytosis (usually lymphocytes), and negative bacterial cultures from the cerebrospinal fluid. A host of pathogens may cause this. Noninfectious causes of aseptic meningitis include medications, such as nonsteroidal anti-inflammatory drugs and trimethoprim-sulfamethoxazole; chemical meningitis; and neoplastic meningitis. Aseptic meningitis is most often caused by viruses. Despite the large number of potential agents, these cases often are differentiated by an accurate exposure history and seasonality. Cases occurring in spring may be associated with tick-borne diseases such as Lyme disease. Cases occurring in the late summer are most often associated with mosquito-borne arboviruses such as West Nile virus. The most frequent viral agents are the enteroviruses (most common in summer) and herpes simplex virus types 1 and 2 (often recurrent). Less frequent pathogens include mumps, lymphocytic choriomeningitis virus (rodents), other human herpesviruses, cytomegalovirus, HIV (acute retroviral syndrome), varicella-zoster virus, Epstein-Barr virus, and Colorado tick fever virus.

- Characteristics of aseptic meningitis: meningeal symptoms, fever, cerebrospinal fluid pleocytosis, negative bacterial cultures.
- The cause is most often viral.

Sexually Transmitted Diseases

New guidelines for the management of sexually transmitted diseases were issued in 2006 and can be found in their updated form at http://cdc.gov/std/treatment/.

Neisseria gonorrhoeae
Common uncomplicated infections include urethritis and cervicitis.

Table 15-11 Guidelines for the Diagnosis and Management of Cardiac Device Infections

1. All patients should have at least 2 blood specimens drawn for culture at initial evaluation
2. Generator tissue should be obtained for Gram stain & culture, & lead tip tissue should be obtained for culture
3. Patients who either have positive blood cultures or have negative blood cultures but had recently received antibiotics before blood cultures were done should have TEE to assess for device-related endocarditis
4. Sensitivity of TTE is low & is not recommended to evaluate for device-related endocarditis
5. Patients with negative blood cultures & recent prior use of antibiotics & valve vegetations on TEE should be managed in consultation with an infectious diseases expert
6. All patients with device infection should undergo complete device removal, regardless of clinical presentation
7. A large (>1 cm) lead vegetation is not a stand-alone indication for surgical lead removal
8. Blood cultures should be repeated in all patients after device explantation. Patients with persistently positive blood cultures should have treatment for at least 4 weeks with antimicrobials even if TEE is negative for vegetations or other evidence of infection
9. Duration of antimicrobial therapy should also be extended to ≥4 weeks in patients with complicated infection (endocarditis, septic venous thrombosis, osteomyelitis, metastatic seeding)
10. Adequate débridement & control of infection should be achieved at all sites before reimplantation of a new device
11. Reevaluation for continued need of the device should be performed before new device placement
12. If an infected cardiac device cannot be removed, then long-term suppressive antibiotic therapy should be administered after completing an initial course of treatment & securing a clinical response to therapy. Opinion of an infectious diseases expert should be sought

Abbreviations: TEE, transesophageal echocardiography; TTE, transthoracic echocardiography.
From Sohail MR, Uslan DZ, Khan AH, Friedman PA, Hayes DL, Wilson WR, et al. Management and outcome of permanent pacemaker and implantable cardioverter-defibrillator infections. J Am Coll Cardiol. 2007;49:1851-9. Used with permission.

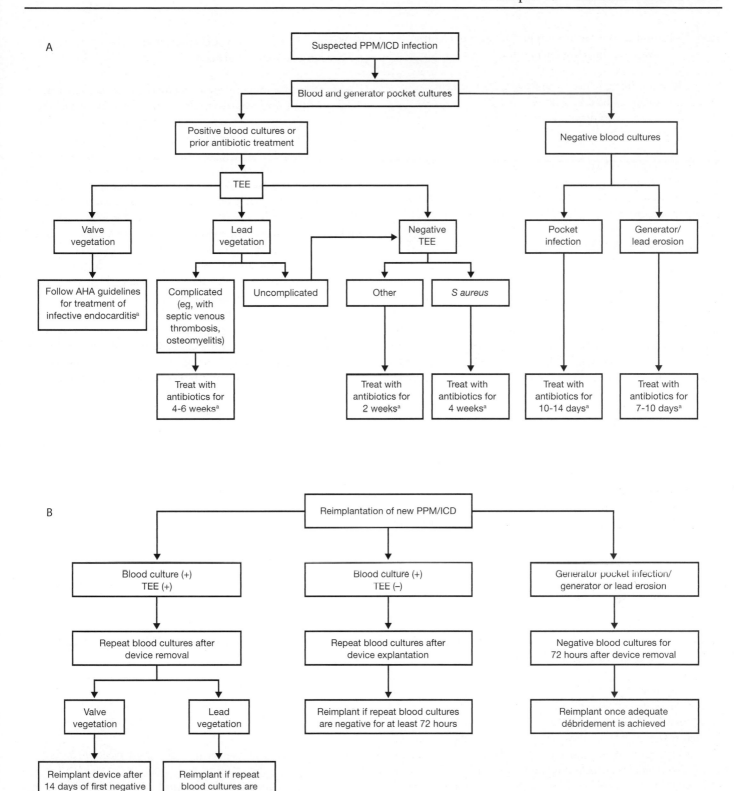

Figure 15-10. Algorithm for Management of Cardiac Device Infection. A, Approach to management of adults (also see Table 15-11). This algorithm applies only to patients with complete device explantation. B, Guidelines for reimplantation of new device (also see Table 15-11). [a]Duration of antibiotic treatment should be counted from the day of device explantation. AHA indicates American Heart Association; ICD, implantable cardioverter-defibrillator; PPM, permanent pacemaker; *S aureus, Staphylococcus aureus*; TEE, transesophageal echocardiography; +, positive; −, negative. (From Sohail MR, Uslan DZ, Khan AH, Friedman PA, Hayes DL, Wilson WR, et al. Management and outcome of permanent pacemaker and implantable cardioverter-defibrillator infections. J Am Coll Cardiol. 2007;49:1851-9. Used with permission.)

Table 15-12   Indications for Surgical Replacement of Cardiac Valves in Infective Endocarditis

Congestive heart failure refractory to medical management
>1 serious systemic embolic episode
Uncontrolled bacteremia despite antimicrobial therapy
Invasive perivalvular infection
New ECG changes
Persistent unexplained fever
Fungal endocarditis
Relapse of treated prosthetic valve endocarditis due to penicillin-sensitive streptococci

Abbreviation: ECG, electrocardiographic.

Symptoms are indistinguishable from those of nongonococcal disease. Gram stain and culture or molecular detection are required for diagnosis. Both men and women may be asymptomatic, but the asymptomatic carrier state is more common in females. Asymptomatic carriers are primarily responsible for transmission of the infection. In females, concomitant proctitis is common (rectal cultures should be done in all women). Gonococcal pharyngitis is often asymptomatic. Coexistence of chlamydial infection is common (both conditions should be treated). For diagnosis in males, a Gram stain of urethral exudate showing intracellular gram-negative diplococci has high sensitivity and specificity. Gram staining of cervical exudate has a sensitivity of only 50%, but the specificity is high. Definitive diagnosis requires culture on modified Thayer-Martin medium. Chlamydial infections and gonorrhea can be rapidly diagnosed with molecular diagnostic tests such as the ligase chain reaction or polymerase chain reaction assay on urine or swabs of genital secretions.

● *Neisseria gonorrhoeae* commonly causes urethritis, cervicitis, pharyngitis, and proctitis.

● Asymptomatic carrier state occurs in both males and females, but it is more common in females.

The prevalence of multiply resistant gonococcal strains is increasing. Resistance to penicillin and tetracycline is frequent. Because quinolone-resistant *N gonorrhoeae* has become common, quinolones are no longer recommended for empiric therapy of gonorrhea. Primary treatment is ceftriaxone (125 mg intramuscularly), plus doxycycline (100 mg orally twice daily for 7 days) or azithromycin (a single 1-g dose) to also treat *Chlamydia*. Alternative drugs include spectinomycin 2 g in a single intramuscular dose, ceftizoxime 500 mg in a single intramuscular dose, cefoxitin 2 g in a single intramuscular dose with probenecid 1 g orally, and cefotaxime 500 mg in a single intramuscular dose. There are no specifically recommended oral alternatives for gonorrhea. However, limited data suggest that cefpodoxime or high-dose azithromycin (2 g × 1 dose) might be options. Pharyngeal infection is best treated with ceftriaxone. Therapy recommended for pregnant women includes ceftriaxone (125 mg intramuscularly) plus erythromycin base (500 mg orally 4 times daily for 7 days). Erythromycin estolate is contraindicated during pregnancy because of drug-related hepatotoxicity. Cefixime, previously recommended as single-dose therapy for gonorrhea, is no longer available in tablet form but may be administered as 400 mg of the suspension (200 mg/5 mL). Alternatives include cefpodoxime 400 mg or cefuroxime axetil 1 g as single-dose therapy. Follow-up gonococcal cultures need to be performed only if nonstandard regimens are used. All patients with sexually transmitted diseases should be considered at risk for HIV infection, and testing should be offered. Sexual partners should be offered evaluation and treatment. A recent study suggested that partner-initiated treatment may reduce transmission rates. Table 15-18 outlines the treatment of gonococcal infections.

● Primary treatment of *N gonorrhoeae* includes ceftriaxone (125 mg intramuscularly) plus doxycycline (100 mg orally twice daily for 7 days) or azithromycin (single 1-g dose).

Table 15-13   Cardiac Conditions Associated With the Highest Risk of Adverse Outcome From Endocarditis for Which Prophylaxis With Dental Procedures Is Recommended

Prosthetic cardiac valve
Previous infective endocarditis
Congenital heart disease (CHD)[a]
 Unrepaired cyanotic CHD, including palliative shunts & conduits
 Completely repaired congenital heart defect with prosthetic material or device, whether placed by surgery or catheter intervention, during the first 6 months after the procedure[b]
 Repaired CHD with residual defects at the site or adjacent to the site of a prosthetic patch or prosthetic device (which inhibit endothelialization)
Cardiac transplant recipients who have cardiac valvulopathy

[a] Except for the conditions listed above, antibiotic prophylaxis is no longer recommended for any other form of CHD.
[b] Prophylaxis is recommended because endothelialization of prosthetic material occurs within 6 months after the procedure.
From Wilson W, Taubert KA, Gewitz M, Lockhart PB, Baddour LM, Levison M, et al. Prevention of infective endocarditis. Guidelines from the American Heart Association. A guideline from the American Heart Association Rheumatic Fever, Endocarditis, and Kawasaki Disease Committee, Council on Cardiovascular Disease in the Young, and the Council on Clinical Cardiology, Council on Cardiovascular Surgery and Anesthesia, and the Quality of Care and Outcomes Research Interdisciplinary Working Group. Circulation. 2007;116:1736-54. Used with permission.

Table 15-14 Regimens for a Dental Procedure

Situation	Agent	Regimen: Single Dose 30 to 60 min Before Procedure	
		Adults	Children
Oral	Amoxicillin	2 g	50 mg/kg
Unable to take oral medication	Ampicillin *Or*	2 g IM or IV	50 mg/kg IM or IV
	Cefazolin or ceftriaxone	1 g IM or IV	50 mg/kg IM or IV
Allergic to penicillins or ampicillin—oral	Cephalexin[a,b] *Or*	2 g	50 mg/kg
	Clindamycin *Or*	600 mg	20 mg/kg
	Azithromycin or clarithromycin	500 mg	15 mg/kg
Allergic to penicillins or ampicillin and unable to take oral medication	Cefazolin or ceftriaxone[b] *Or*	1 g IM or IV	50 mg/kg IM or IV
	Clindamycin	600 mg IM or IV	20 mg/kg IM or IV

Abbreviations: IM, intramuscularly; IV, intravenously.

[a] Or other first- or second-generation oral cephalosporin in equivalent adult or pediatric dosage.

[b] Cephalosporins should not be used in an individual with a history of anaphylaxis, angioedema, or urticaria with penicillins or ampicillin.

From Wilson W, Taubert KA, Gewitz M, Lockhart PB, Baddour LM, Levison M, et al. Prevention of infective endocarditis. Guidelines from the American Heart Association. A guideline from the American Heart Association Rheumatic Fever, Endocarditis, and Kawasaki Disease Committee, Council on Cardiovascular Disease in the Young, and the Council on Clinical Cardiology, Council on Cardiovascular Surgery and Anesthesia, and the Quality of Care and Outcomes Research Interdisciplinary Working Group. Circulation. 2007;116:1736-54. Used with permission.

- Fluoroquinolones are no longer recommended for treatment of gonorrhea.

Disseminated gonococcemia occurs in 1% to 3% of infected patients and is most likely to occur during menstruation (sloughing of endometrium allows access to blood supply, enhanced growth of gonococci due to necrotic tissue, and change in pH). There are 2 distinct phases. The bacteremic phase may manifest as tenosynovitis (often around the wrists or ankles), skin lesions (usually less than 30 in number), and polyarthralgia. Results of synovial fluid testing are usually negative. The nonbacteremic phase follows in approximately 1 week and may present as monarticular arthritis of the knee, wrist, and ankle; results of joint culture are positive in about 50%. Culture specimens should be obtained from the urethra, cervix, rectum, and pharynx.

- Disseminated gonococcemia is most likely to occur during menstruation.
- A bacteremic phase may manifest as tenosynovitis, skin lesions, and arthralgias; joint cultures are usually negative.
- A nonbacteremic phase may present as monarticular arthritis of the knee, wrist, and ankle; results of joint cultures are positive in about 50%.

Treatment is with ceftriaxone (1 g intravenously daily for 7-10 days); alternatives include ceftriaxone for 3 to 4 days or until clinical improvement followed by oral cefixime suspension 400 mg daily or

cefpodoxime 400 mg daily to complete a course of 7 to 10 days. If the strain is tested and found to be penicillin-susceptible, treatment includes penicillin G (10 million units intravenously daily) for 7 to 10 days or it is given for 3 or 4 days and then oral amoxicillin is used to finish a 7- to 10 day course. Chlamydial infection can coexist with gonococcal infection and should be treated. For meningitis, treatment includes ceftriaxone (1-2 g intravenously every 12 hours for at least 10-14 days). Alternative drugs are penicillin, if the strain is susceptible, or chloramphenicol. For endocarditis, ceftriaxone or penicillin is used for at least 28 days.

- Treatment of disseminated gonococcal infection is with ceftriaxone (1 g intravenously daily for 7-10 days).
- Chlamydial infections can coexist with gonococcal infection and should be treated.

Nongonococcal Urethritis and Cervicitis

The most common etiologic agent is *Chlamydia trachomatis*. Infection is often asymptomatic. Diagnosis can be made with culture, antigen detection, or molecular tests. Doxycycline (100 mg twice daily for 7 days) or azithromycin as a single 1-g dose is standard treatment. Women with *C trachomatis* cervicitis should be rescreened 3 to 4 months after treatment. *Ureaplasma urealyticum*, *Trichomonas vaginalis*, *Mycoplasma genitalium*, and herpes simplex virus are less common causes of nongonococcal urethritis. If urethritis does not resolve and reinfection or relapse of a chlamydial infection has been excluded, *Trichomonas* or

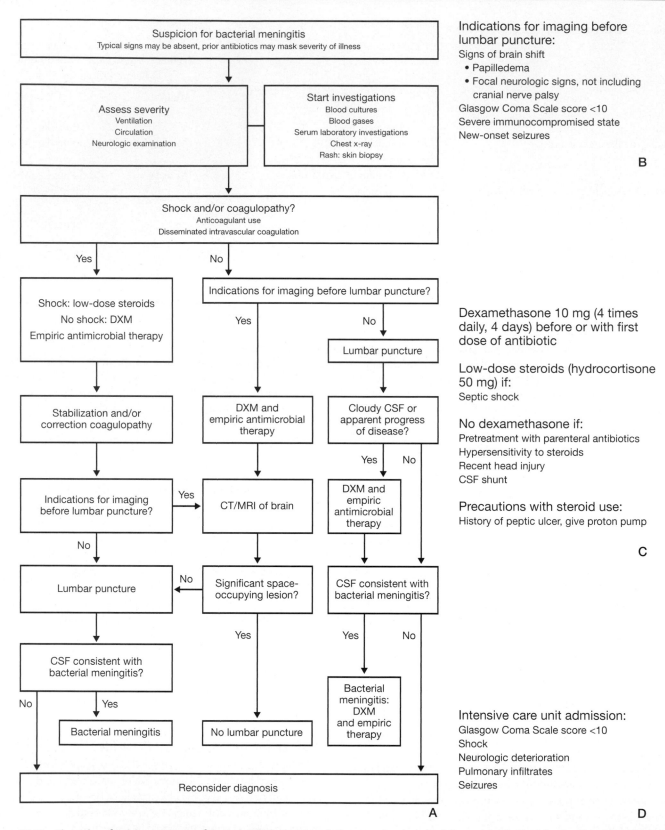

Suspicion for bacterial meningitis
Typical signs may be absent, prior antibiotics may mask severity of illness

Assess severity
Ventilation
Circulation
Neurologic examination

Start investigations
Blood cultures
Blood gases
Serum laboratory investigations
Chest x-ray
Rash: skin biopsy

Indications for imaging before lumbar puncture:
Signs of brain shift
• Papilledema
• Focal neurologic signs, not including cranial nerve palsy
Glasgow Coma Scale score <10
Severe immunocompromised state
New-onset seizures

B

Shock and/or coagulopathy?
Anticoagulant use
Disseminated intravascular coagulation

Yes — Shock: low-dose steroids / No shock: DXM / Empiric antimicrobial therapy

No — Indications for imaging before lumbar puncture?

Yes — DXM and empiric antimicrobial therapy

No — Lumbar puncture

Cloudy CSF or apparent progress of disease?

Stabilization and/or correction coagulopathy

Indications for imaging before lumbar puncture? — Yes → CT/MRI of brain

No — Lumbar puncture ← No — Significant space-occupying lesion?

CSF consistent with bacterial meningitis? — No / Yes — Bacterial meningitis

No lumbar puncture

Yes — DXM and empiric antimicrobial therapy

CSF consistent with bacterial meningitis? — Yes / No

Bacterial meningitis: DXM and empiric therapy

Dexamethasone 10 mg (4 times daily, 4 days) before or with first dose of antibiotic

Low-dose steroids (hydrocortisone 50 mg) if:
Septic shock

No dexamethasone if:
Pretreatment with parenteral antibiotics
Hypersensitivity to steroids
Recent head injury
CSF shunt

Precautions with steroid use:
History of peptic ulcer, give proton pump

C

Intensive care unit admission:
Glasgow Coma Scale score <10
Shock
Neurologic deterioration
Pulmonary infiltrates
Seizures

D

Reconsider diagnosis

A

Figure 15-11. Algorithm for Management of Patient With Suspected Community-Acquired Bacterial Meningitis. A, Algorithm for initial management of adults with bacterial meningitis. B, Indications for performing imaging before lumbar puncture. C, Recommendations for adjunctive dexamethasone therapy in adults with bacterial meningitis. D, Criteria for admission of patients with bacterial meningitis to the intensive care unit. CSF indicates cerebrospinal fluid; CT, computed tomography; DXM, dexamethasone; MRI, magnetic resonance imaging. (From van de Beek D, de Gans J, Tunkel AR, Wijdicks EFM. Community-acquired bacterial meningitis in adults. N Engl J Med. 2006;354:44-53. Used with permission.)

Table 15-15 Recommendations for Antimicrobial Therapy in Adults with Community-Acquired Bacterial Meningitis

	Empiric therapy	
Predisposing factor Age, y	**Common bacterial pathogens**	**Antimicrobial therapy**
16-50	*Neisseria meningitidis, Streptococcus pneumoniae*	Vancomycin plus a third-generation cephalosporin[a,b]
>50	*S pneumoniae, N meningitidis, Listeria monocytogenes*, aerobic gram-negative bacilli	Vancomycin plus a third-generation cephalosporin plus ampicillin[b,c]
With risk factor present[d]	*S pneumoniae, L monocytogenes, Haemophilus influenzae*	Vancomycin plus a third-generation cephalosporin plus ampicillin[b,c]

	Specific antimicrobial therapy	
Microorganism, susceptibility *S pneumoniae* Penicillin MIC	**Standard therapy**	**Alternative therapies**
<0.1 mg/L	Penicillin G or ampicillin	Third-generation cephalosporin,[b] chloramphenicol
0.1-1.0 mg/L	Third-generation cephalosporin[b]	Cefepime, meropenem
≥2.0 mg/L	Vancomycin plus a third-generation cephalosporin[b,e]	Fluroquinolone[f]
Cefotaxime or ceftriaxone MIC		
≥1.0 mg/L	Vancomycin plus a third-generation cephalosporin[b,g]	Fluoroquinolone[f]
N meningitidis Penicillin MIC		
<0.1 mg/L	Penicillin G or ampicillin	Third-generation cephalosporin,[b] chloramphenicol
0.1-1.0 mg/L	Third-generation cephalosporin[b]	Chloramphenicol, fluoroquinolone, meropenem
L monocytogenes	Penicillin G or ampicillin[h]	Trimethoprim-sulfamethoxazole, meropenem
Group B streptococcus	Penicillin G or ampicillin[h]	Third-generation cephalosporin[b]
Escheria coli & other Enterobacteriaceae	Third-generation cephalosporin[b]	Aztreonam, fluoroquinolone, meropenem, trimethoprim-sulfamethoxazole, ampicillin
Pseudomonas aeruginosa	Ceftazidime or cefepime[h]	Aztreonam,[h] ciprofloxacin,[h] meropenem[h]
H influenzae		
β-Lactamase negative	Ampicillin	Third-generation cephalosporin,[b] cefepime, chloramphenicol, fluoroquinolone
β-Lactamase positive	Third-generation cephalosporin[b]	Cefepime, chloramphenicol, fluoroquinolone
Chemoprophylaxis[i] *N meningitidis*	Rifampicin (rifampin), ceftriazone, ciprofloxacin, azithromycin	

Abbreviation: MIC, minimal inhibitory concentration.

[a] Only in areas with very low penicillin-resistance rates (<1%) should monotherapy with penicillin be considered, although many experts recommend combination therapy for all patients until results of in vitro susceptibility testing are known.

[b] Cefotaxime or ceftriaxone.

[c] Only in areas with very low penicillin-resistance and cephalosporin-resistance rates should combination therapy of amoxicillin (ampicillin) and a third-generation cephalosporin be considered.

[d] Alcoholism, altered immune status.

[e] Consider addition of rifampicin (rifampin) if dexamethasone is given.

[f] Gatifloxacin or moxifloxacin; no clinical data on use in patients with bacterial meningitis.

[g] Consider addition of rifampicin (rifampin) if the MIC of ceftriaxone is ≥2 mg/L.

[h] Consider addition of an aminoglycoside.

[i] Prophylaxis is indicated for close contacts (defined as those with intimate contact, which covers those eating and sleeping in the same dwelling and those having close social and kissing contacts) or health care workers who perform mouth-to-mouth resuscitation, endotracheal intubation, or endotracheal tube management. Patients with meningococcal meningitis who receive monotherapy with penicillin or amoxicillin (ampicillin) should also receive chemoprophylaxis, because carriage is not reliably eradicated by these drugs.

Table 15-15 (continued)

Note: The preferred intravenous doses in patients with normal renal and hepatic function: penicillin, 2 million units every 4 hours; amoxicillin or ampicillin, 2 g every 4 hours; vancomycin, 15 mg/kg every 8 to 12 hours; third-generation cephalosporin: ceftriaxone, 2 g every 12 hours, or cefotaxime, 2 g every 4 to 6 hours; cefepime 2 g every 8 hours; ceftazidime, 2 g every 8 hours; meropenem, 2 g every 8 hours; chloramphenicol, 1 to 1.5 g every 6 hours; fluoroquinolone: gatifloxacin, 400 mg every 24 hours, or moxifloxacin, 400 mg every 24 hours, although no data on optimal dose is needed in patients with bacterial meningitis; trimethoprim-sulfamethoxazole, 5 mg/kg every 6 to 12 hours; aztreonam, 2 g every 6 to 8 hours; ciprofloxacin, 400 mg every 8 to 12 hours; rifampicin (rifampin) 600 mg every 12 to 24 hours; aminoglycoside: gentamicin, 1.7 mg/kg every 8 hours. The preferred dose for chemoprophylaxis: rifampicin (rifampin), 600 mg orally twice daily for 2 days; ceftriaxone, 250 mg intramuscularly; ciprofloxacin, 500 mg orally; azithromycin, 500 mg orally.

The duration of therapy for patients with bacterial meningitis has often been based more on tradition than on evidence-based data and needs to be individualized on the basis of the patient's response. In general, antimicrobial therapy is given for 7 days for meningitis caused by *Neisseria meningitidis* and *Haemophylus influenzae*, 10 to 14 days for *Streptococcus pneumoniae*, and at least 21 days for *Listeria monocytogenes*.

From van de Beek D, de Gans J, Tunkel AR, Wijdicks EFM. Community-acquired bacterial meningitis in adults. N Engl J Med. 2006;354:44-53.

tetracycline-resistant *Ureaplasma* infection should be considered. Treatment consists of metronidazole (2 g orally in a single dose) plus erythromycin base (500 mg orally 4 times daily for 7 days) or erythromycin ethylsuccinate (800 mg orally 4 times daily for 7 days).

- Nongonococcal urethritis and cervicitis are most commonly caused by *C trachomatis*.

Herpes Genitalis

Seventy percent to 90% of cases of herpes genitalis are caused by herpes simplex virus type 2. Table 15-19 outlines the treatment of genital herpes.

Syphilis

The etiologic agent of syphilis is *Treponema pallidum*. It is estimated that half of cases are not reported. The incidence of syphilis is increased in large cities among sexually active persons, particularly among inner city minority populations and men who have sex with men.

Serologic tests for syphilis vary by institution. Some centers use the enzyme immunoassay for syphilis immunoglobulin M and G as a screen, followed by the rapid plasma reagin test to follow the treatment course. Other centers use the rapid plasma reagin test initially and confirm this with the fluorescent treponemal antibody test (FTA-ABS). This test is the most helpful serologic test for the diagnosis of syphilis (Table 15-20). Results of this test are positive before

Table 15-16 Organisms Involved, Affected Age Groups, and Predisposing Factors in Bacterial Meningitis

Organism	Age Group	Comment	Predisposing Factors
Streptococcus pneumoniae	Any age, but often elderly	Most common cause of recurrent meningitis in adults	Cerebrospinal fluid leak, alcoholism, splenectomy, functional asplenia, multiple myeloma, hypogammaglobulinemia, Hodgkin disease, HIV
Neisseria meningitidis	Infants to 40 y	Petechial rash is common Epidemics occur in closed populations	Terminal component complement deficiency
Haemophilus influenzae, type B	>Neonate to 6 y	Significant decrease in incidence since licensure of *H influenzae* B vaccine	Hypogammaglobulinemia in adults, HIV, splenectomy, functional asplenia
Escherichia coli, group B streptococci	Neonates		Maternal colonization
Gram-negative bacilli	Any age	*Staphylococcus aureus* & coagulase-negative staphylococci also common after neurosurgical procedure	Neurosurgical procedures, bacteremia due to urinary tract infection, pneumonia, etc, *Strongyloides* hyperinfection syndrome
Listeria monocytogenes	Neonates; immuno-suppressed		

Abbreviation: HIV, human immunodeficiency virus.

Table 15-17 Empiric Therapy for Bacterial Meningitis

Age Group/ Patient Group	Common Pathogens	Antimicrobial Therapy
Age		
0-4 wk	Group B streptococci, *Escherichia coli*, *Listeria monocytogenes*, *Klebsiella pneumoniae*, *Enterococcus* spp, *Salmonella* spp	Ampicillin plus cefotaxime or ampicillin plus an aminoglycoside
1-23 mo	Group B streptococci, *E coli*, *L monocytogenes*, *Haemophilus influenzae*, *Streptococcus pneumoniae*, *Neisseria meningitidis*	Vancomycin plus cefotaxime or ceftriaxone
2-50 y	*N meningitidis*, *S pneumoniae*	Vancomycin plus cefotaxime or ceftriaxone
>50 y	*S pneumoniae*, *L monocytogenes,* aerobic gram-negative bacilli	Vancomycin plus either cefotaxime or ceftriaxone plus ampicillin (cephalosporins have NO activity vs *Listeria*)
Basilar skull fracture	*S pneumoniae*, *H influenzae*, group A β-hemolytic streptococci	Vancomycin plus cefotaxime or ceftriaxone
Post-neurosurgery	Coagulase-negative staphylococci, *Staphylococcus aureus*, aerobic gram-negative bacilli (including *P aeruginosa*)	Vancomycin plus cefepime or ceftazidime or meropenem

Modified from Tunkel AR, Hartman BJ, Kaplan SL, Kaufman BA, Roos KL, Scheld WM, et al. Practice guidelines for the management of bacterial meningitis. Clin Infect Dis. 2004;39:1267-84. Used with permission.

Table 15-18 Treatment Regimens for Gonococcal Infections and Associated Conditions

Infection	Recommended Regimen	Alternative Regimen
Cervix, urethra, rectum[a]	Ceftriaxone 125 mg IM in a single dose *Or* Cefixime[c] 400 mg orally in a single dose or 400 mg by suspension (200 mg/5 mL) *Plus* Treatment for *Chlamydia* infection if not ruled out	Spectinomycin[b] 2 g IM in a single dose *Or* Single-dose cepholosporin regimen
Pharynx[a]	Ceftriaxone 125 mg IM in a single dose *Plus* Treatment for *Chlamydia* infection if not ruled out	
Disseminated gonococcal infection[d]	Ceftriaxone 1g IM or IV every 24 h	Cefotaxime 1g IV every 8 h *Or* Ceftizoxime 1 g IV every 8 h *Or* Spectinomycin[b] 2 g IM every 12 h After 24-48 h of clinical improvement, switch:[e] Cefixime 400 mg PO twice daily *Or* Cefixime[c] 400 mg by suspension (200 mg/5 mL) *Or* Cefpodoxime 400 mg orally twice daily
Pelvic inflammatory disease[f]	Parenteral A: Cefotetan 2 g IV every 12 h *Or* Cefoxitin 2 g IV every 6 h *Plus* Doxycycline 100 mg orally or IV every 12 h	Parenteral: Ampicillin-sulbactam 3 g IV every 6 h *Plus* Doxycycline 100 mg orally or IV every 12 h

Table 15-18 (continued)

Infection	Recommended Regimen	Alternative Regimen

Pelvic inflammatory disease[f] (continued)	Parenteral B:
	  Clindamycin 900 mg IV every 8 h
	  Plus
	  Gentamicin[g]
	Oral:[h]
	  Ceftriaxone 250 mg IM in a single dose
	  Plus
	  Doxycycline 100 mg orally twice daily for 14 d *with or without* metronidazole 500 mg orally twice daily for 14 d
	  Or
	  Cefoxitin 2 g IM in a single dose and probenecid 1g orally concurrently in a single dose
	  Plus
	  Doxycycline 100 mg orally twice daily for 14 d *with or without* metronidazole 500 mg orally twice daily for 14 d
	  Or
	  Other parenteral third-generation cephalosporin[j]
	  Plus
	  Doxycycline 100 mg orally twice daily for 14 d *with or without* metronidazole 500 mg orally twice daily for 14 d
		Fluoroquinolones:[i] levofloxacin 500 mg orally once daily or ofloxacin 400 mg twice daily for 14 d *with or without* metronidazole 500 mg orally twice daily for 14 d

Epididymitis	Ceftriaxone 250 mg IM in a single dose *Plus* Doxycycline 100 mg orally twice daily for 10 d Ofloxacin[k] 300 mg orally twice daily for 10 d *Or* Levofloxacin 500 mg orally once daily for 10 d	

Abbreviations: IM, intramuscularly; IV, intravenously; PO, orally.

[a] These regimens are recommended for all adult and adolescent patients, regardless of travel history or sexual behavior.

[b] Spectinomycin is currently not available in the United States.

[c] The tablet formulation of cefixime is currently not available in the United States.

[d] A cephalosporin-based intravenous regimen is recommended for the initial treatment of disseminated gonococcal infection. This is particularly important when gonorrhea is detected at mucosal sites by nonculture tests.

[e] Switch to 1 of the following regimens to complete at least 1 week of antimicrobial therapy. Cefixime[c] 400 mg orally twice daily *or* cefixime 400 mg by suspension (200 mg/5 ml) twice daily *or* cefpodoxime 400 mg orally twice daily.

[f] Parenteral and oral therapy seem to have similar clinical efficacy for women with pelvic inflammatory disease of mild or moderate severity. Clinical experience should guide decisions regarding transition to oral therapy, which usually can be initiated within 24 hours of clinical improvement.

[g] Loading dose intravenously or intramuscularly (2 mg/kg of body weight), followed by maintenance dose (1.5 mg/kg) every 8 hours. Single daily dosing may be substituted.

[h] Oral therapy can be considered for women with mild to moderately severe acute pelvic inflammatory disease because the clinical outcomes with oral therapy are similar to those with parenteral therapy. Women who do not respond to oral therapy within 72 hours should be reevaluated to confirm the diagnosis and should be administered parenteral therapy on either an outpatient or an inpatient basis.

[i] If parenteral cephalosporin therapy is not feasible, use of fluoroquinolones with or without metronidazole may be considered if the community prevalence and individual risk of gonorrhea are low. Tests for gonorrhea must be performed before instituting therapy.

[j] Ceftizoxime or cefotaxime.

[k] For acute epididymitis most likely caused by enteric organisms or with negative gonococcal culture or nucleic acid amplification test.

From Centers for Disease Control and Prevention. Updated recommended treatment regimens for gonococcal infections and associated conditions— United States, April 2007. Available from: http://www.cdc.gov/std/treatment/2006/updated-regimens.htm.

Table 15-19 Treatment of Genital Herpes

Reason for Treatment	Drug	Dosage
First episode	Acyclovir	400 mg PO 3 times daily for 7-10 d *Or* 200 mg PO 5 times daily for 7-10 d
	Or Famciclovir	250 mg PO 3 times daily for 7-10 d
	Or Valacyclovir	1 g PO twice daily for 7-10 d
Severe symptoms	Acyclovir	5 mg/kg IV every 8 h for 5-7 d
Recurrent episodes with severe symptoms[a]	Acyclovir	400 mg PO 3 times daily *Or* 200 mg PO 5 times daily *Or* 800 mg PO twice daily
	Or Famciclovir	125 mg PO twice daily *Or* 1g PO twice daily for 1 d
	Or Valacyclovir	500 mg-1 g PO daily for 5 d
Suppression (>6 recurrences a year)	Acyclovir[b]	400 mg PO twice daily
	Or Famciclovir	250 mg PO twice daily
	Or Valacyclovir	500 mg or 1 g PO once daily
Prevention	Valacyclovir[c]	500 mg PO daily

Abbreviations: IV, intravenously; PO, orally.

[a] For recurrent episodes with severe symptoms, therapy can be started at prodrome onset or within 1 day of onset of symptoms.

[b] Agents used for suppression are used for up to 1 year.

[c] Valacyclovir taken by the infected partner may prevent herpes simplex virus transmission among discordant sexual partners with herpes simplex virus.

those on VDRL testing, and thus they may be positive without a positive VDRL result in primary syphilis. VDRL results may be negative in 30% of patients with primary syphilis.

- FTA-ABS is the most helpful serologic test for the diagnosis of syphilis.
- VDRL results may be negative in 30% of patients with primary syphilis.

A chancre (clean, indurated ulcer) is the main manifestation of *primary syphilis*. It occurs at the site of inoculation and is usually painless. The incubation period is 3 to 90 days. It should be distinguished from herpes simplex virus and chancroid (painful exudative ulcer, *Haemophilus ducreyi*). Diagnosis is made by darkfield examination.

The manifestations of *secondary syphilis* result from hematogenous dissemination and usually occur 2 to 8 weeks after appearance of the chancre. Constitutional symptoms occur, in addition to rash, mucocutaneous lesions, alopecia, condylomata lata (ie, a broad and flat verrucous syphilitic lesion located in warm, moist intertriginous areas, especially about the anus and genitals), lymphadenopathy, and various other symptoms and signs. The diagnosis is based on the clinical picture and serologic testing. The condition resolves spontaneously without treatment.

Latent syphilis is the asymptomatic stage after symptoms of secondary syphilis subside. Those that occur after 1 year are classified as late. The diagnosis is based on serologic testing. For latent syphilis, a cerebrospinal fluid examination is indicated before treatment in patients with neurologic or ophthalmologic abnormalities, in patients with other evidence of active syphilis, at baseline in patients treated with a nonpenicillin regimen, before re-treatment of relapses, and in patients with HIV infection.

Tertiary syphilis can involve all body systems (cardiovascular—aortitis involving the ascending aorta, which can cause aneurysms and aortic regurgitation; gummatous osteomyelitis; hepatitis). However, neurosyphilis is the most common manifestation in the United States.

Neurosyphilis is often asymptomatic. Symptomatic disease is divided into several clinical syndromes that may overlap and occur

Table 15-20 Laboratory Diagnosis of Syphilis

Syphilis	Test, % Positive		
	VDRL	FTA-ABS	MHA-TP
Primary	70	85	50-60
Secondary	99	100	100
Tertiary	70	98	98

Abbreviations: FTA-ABS, fluorescent treponemal antibody absorption; MHA-TP, microhemagglutination assay for *Treponema pallidum*.
From Hook EW III. Syphilis. In: Bennett JE, Plum F, editors. Cecil textbook of internal medicine. 12th ed. Philadelphia: WB Saunders; 1996. p. 1705-14. Used with permission.

at any time after primary infection. The diagnosis is made from cerebrospinal fluid examination; abnormalities include mononuclear pleocytosis and an increased protein value. VDRL testing of cerebrospinal fluid is only 30% to 70% sensitive. The FTA-ABS test on cerebrospinal fluid is highly sensitive but not specific. Any cerebrospinal fluid abnormality in a patient who is seropositive for syphilis must be investigated. Syndromes include 1) meningovascular syphilis (occurs 4-7 years after infection and presents with focal central nervous system deficits such as stroke or cranial nerve abnormalities) and 2) parenchymatous syphilis (general paresis or tabes dorsalis). Parenchymatous syphilis occurs decades after infection and may present as general paresis (chronic progressive dementia) or as tabes dorsalis (sensory ataxia, lightning pains, autonomic dysfunction, and optic atrophy).

- Neurosyphilis is the most common manifestation in tertiary disease in the United States.
- The diagnosis is made from cerebrospinal fluid examination.
- VDRL testing of cerebrospinal fluid is only 30%-70% sensitive.

Treatment of syphilis is based on whether the disease is early or late. For early syphilis (primary, secondary, or early latent [<1 year]), benzathine penicillin G (LA only, not C-R—a mix of procaine and benzathine) is used—2.4 million units intramuscularly; follow-up serologic testing is done. (Some experts recommend completing 3 weekly 2.4 million-unit intramuscular doses in patients with HIV infection.) Alternatives are doxycycline (100 mg twice daily for 14 days) or tetracycline (500 mg orally 4 times daily for 14 days). Erythromycin (500 mg orally 4 times daily) is less effective.

Treatment for late disease (>1 year in duration, cardiovascular disease, gumma, late latent syphilis) is with benzathine penicillin, 2.4 million units intramuscularly weekly for 3 weeks. Alternatives are doxycycline (100 mg orally twice daily) or tetracycline (500 mg orally 4 times daily) for 4 weeks.

Treatment of neurosyphilis is with aqueous penicillin G (12-24 million units intravenously per day) for 10 to 14 days or procaine penicillin (2.4 million units intramuscularly per day) plus probenecid (500 mg 4 times daily) for 10 to 14 days.

Pregnant patients should receive a penicillin-based regimen for treatment of all stages of syphilis. If a pregnant patient has a penicillin allergy, she should be desensitized to penicillin.

For early and secondary syphilis, follow-up clinical and serologic testing should be performed at 6 and 12 months. Re-treatment with 3 weekly injections of 2.4 million units of benzathine penicillin G should be given to patients with signs or symptoms that persist or whose VDRL result has a sustained 4-fold increase in titer. HIV testing should be performed if not done previously. If the VDRL titer does not decrease 4-fold by 6 months, consideration also should be given to re-treatment.

Patients with latent syphilis should have a follow-up examination at 6, 12, and 24 months. If the VDRL result increases 4-fold, if a high titer (>1:32) fails to decrease 4-fold within 12 to 24 months, or if signs or symptoms attributable to syphilis occur, the patient should be examined for neurosyphilis and re-treated.

Follow-up in cases of neurosyphilis should include testing of cerebrospinal fluid every 6 months if cerebrospinal fluid pleocytosis was present initially; this testing is done until results are normal. If the cell count is not decreased at 6 months or if the cerebrospinal fluid is not entirely normal at 2 years, re-treatment should be considered.

Pelvic Inflammatory Disease

In this condition, proximal spread of infection from the endocervix causes endometritis, salpingitis, tubo-ovarian abscess, or pelvic peritonitis in various combinations. Organisms responsible are *N gonorrhoeae*, *C trachomatis*, *Mycoplasma hominis*, and various aerobic gram-negative rods and anaerobes. Fitz-Hugh-Curtis syndrome is an acute perihepatitis caused by direct extension of *N gonorrhoeae* or *C trachomatis* to the liver capsule. Occasionally, a friction rub can be auscultated over the liver and "violin string" adhesions between the liver capsule and parietal peritoneum can be observed with laparoscopy. *Actinomyces israelii* can be a pathogen in patients with an intrauterine device. Tuberculosis in older women, including postmenopausal women, should be considered. Clinical signs and symptoms include lower abdominal tenderness, adnexal tenderness, cervical motion tenderness, oral temperature more than 38.3°C, abnormal cervical discharge, increased erythrocyte sedimentation rate, and evidence of *N gonorrhoeae* or *C trachomatis* infection. Laboratory evidence includes laparoscopic or ultrasonographic documentation. The emphasis on early diagnosis is meant to decrease the incidence of infertility as a complication of pelvic inflammatory disease.

- In pelvic inflammatory disease, responsible organisms are *N gonorrhoeae*, *C trachomatis*, and anaerobes.
- Fitz-Hugh-Curtis syndrome is an acute perihepatitis caused by direct extension of *N gonorrhoeae* or *C trachomatis* to the liver capsule.
- The emphasis on early diagnosis is meant to decrease the incidence of infertility as a complication of pelvic inflammatory disease.

Treatment for inpatients includes cefoxitin (2 g intravenously every 6 hours) plus doxycycline (100 mg intravenously every 12 hours followed by 100 mg orally twice daily) for 14 days. Table 15-18 outlines the treatment of pelvic inflammatory diseases.

Hospitalization is indicated when the outpatient therapy is precluded by severe nausea and vomiting, the diagnosis is uncertain, pelvic abscess or peritonitis is present, the patient is pregnant, the patient is an adolescent, HIV infection is present, or noncompliance is suspected.

Tubo-ovarian abscess may be characterized by an adnexal mass on physical examination or radiographic examination or by failure of antimicrobial therapy. Most abscesses 4 to 6 cm in diameter respond to medical therapy alone with the preferred regimen of ampicillin, gentamicin, and clindamycin. Larger abscesses (>10 cm) most often necessitate operation.

- Tubo-ovarian abscess is characterized by an adnexal mass on physical examination or radiographic examination or by failure of antimicrobial therapy.

Trichomonas vaginalis
Vaginitis is usually characterized by a vaginal discharge or vulvar itching, odor, or irritation. The 3 entities most frequently associated with vaginal discharge are bacterial vaginosis (a replacement of the normal vaginal flora by an overgrowth of anaerobic microorganisms, mycoplasmas, and *Gardnerella vaginalis*), trichomoniasis (*T vaginalis*), and candidiasis.

Infection with *T vaginalis* produces a yellow, purulent discharge in 5% to 40% of cases. Dysuria and dyspareunia occur in 30% to 50% of cases. Petechial lesions on the cervix are noted with colposcopy (strawberry cervix) in 50% of cases. The vaginal pH is usually more than 4.5. The diagnosis is established with wet mount preparation of vaginal secretions (70%-80% sensitive). Other tests for trichomoniasis in women include an immunochromatographic assay (OSOM Trichomonas Rapid Test) and a nucleic acid probe test (Affirm VPIII) that evaluates for *T vaginalis*, *G vaginalis*, and *C albicans*. These tests are both performed on vaginal secretions and have a sensitivity of more than 83% and a specificity of more than 97%. Both tests are rapid, point-of-care tools. Culture is done in difficult cases. Treatment is with metronidazole (2 g as a single dose) or tinidazole (2 g: 4 500-mg tablets as a single dose). A 7-day course of metronidazole (500 mg twice daily) is an alternative. Gastrointestinal tolerance may be better with tinidazole, although there is less clinical experience with this agent. All partners should be examined and treated. Although treatment in asymptomatic pregnant women is controversial, treatment in symptomatic pregnant women should be a one-time dose of 2 g of metronidazole.

- Infection with *T vaginalis* often is characterized by yellow, purulent discharge.
- Diagnosis is established with wet mount or a rapid test of vaginal secretions.
- Treatment of *T vaginalis* is with metronidazole or tinidazole orally.

Gardnerella vaginalis (Bacterial Vaginosis)
This condition is characterized by a malodorous "fishy" smell and a grayish white discharge that is homogeneous and coats the vaginal walls. Dysuria and pain are relatively uncommon. Bacterial vaginosis is a polymicrobial syndrome due to replacement of vaginal lactobacilli with anaerobes and other organisms. Organisms associated with the syndrome are *Mobiluncus* spp, *M hominis*, *G vaginalis*, and

Prevotella spp. Risk factors for bacterial vaginosis include multiple sex partners, new partners, douching, and a lack of vaginal lactobacilli. The diagnosis is determined by excluding *Candida* and *Trichomonas* infections and other sexually transmitted diseases. The following are characteristics of the vaginal secretion: "clue" cells on wet mount examination, pH more than 4.5 and often more than 6.0, and a "fishy" smell when secretion is mixed with 10% KOH (positive "whiff" test). Recommended treatment regimens include metronidazole (500 mg orally twice daily for 7 days) or topical clindamycin cream or metronidazole gel (the clindamycin cream appears less efficacious than the metronidazole regimens). Single-dose metronidazole therapy has poor efficacy and clindamycin, 300 mg orally twice daily for 7 days, is an alternative. Bacterial vaginosis has been associated with adverse pregnancy outcomes. All symptomatic pregnant women should be treated. In pregnant patients, systemic therapy with metronidazole (500 mg twice daily for 7 days) or clindamycin (300 mg orally twice daily for 7 days) is recommended rather than topical agents in order to treat organisms in the upper genital tract. Treatment of asymptomatic nonpregnant carriers is not recommended. Some experts recommend treatment of asymptomatic pregnant women at high risk for preterm delivery. Routine treatment of sex partners is not recommended.

- Diagnosis of *G vaginalis* is established by excluding *Candida* and *Trichomonas* infections and other sexually transmitted diseases.
- Vaginal discharge has "clue" cells, a "fishy" smell when mixed with 10% KOH (positive "whiff" test), and a pH more than 4.5.
- Routine treatment of sex partners is not recommended.

Vulvovaginal Candidiasis
The predominant symptom of this condition is pruritus. It is typically caused by *C albicans*. Seventy-five percent of women will have 1 episode and 40% to 45%, 2 or more episodes. Usually there is no odor, and discharge is scant, watery, and white. "Cottage cheese curds" may adhere to the vaginal wall. The diagnosis is made by the addition of 10% KOH to the discharge to demonstrate pseudohyphae. Culture may detect an asymptomatic carrier. Treatment is with various topical agents from 1 to 7 days, depending on the dose and agent. Single-dose fluconazole (150 mg for 1 dose) therapy may be more convenient and less costly. Multiple-dose oral azole therapy also is used for severe, refractory cases. In severe or recurrent cases, consider HIV infection or drug-resistant candidal species.

- In vulvovaginal candidiasis, "cottage cheese curds" may adhere to the vaginal wall.
- In severe or recurrent cases, consider HIV infection.

Epididymitis
This condition usually presents as a unilateral, painful scrotal swelling. It should be distinguished from testicular torsion. In young, sexually active men, *C trachomatis* and *N gonorrhoeae* are the common pathogens. In older men, aerobic gram-negative rods and enterococci predominate. Urologic abnormality is more common in this population than in younger men. Doxycycline (100 mg orally twice daily for 7 days) plus ceftriaxone (250 mg intramuscularly)

Mayo Clinic Internal Medicine Review

is the treatment of choice in young males. In older men, treatment is individualized on the basis of results of urine Gram stain, results of culture, local susceptibility patterns, and presence of recent instrumentation.

- Epididymitis is usually unilateral; it should be distinguished from testicular torsion.
- In young, sexually active men, *C trachomatis* and *N gonorrhoeae* are the common pathogens.

Gastrointestinal Infection

Bacterial Diarrhea

The principal causes of toxigenic diarrhea are listed in Table 15-21, and those of invasive diarrhea are listed in Table 15-22. Fecal leukocytes usually are absent in toxigenic diarrhea. In invasive diarrhea, fecal leukocytes usually are present. The travel history is often important.

Campylobacter jejuni is being recognized with increasing frequency as a common cause of bacterial diarrhea. Approximately 10% to 30% of cases of Guillain-Barré syndrome are preceded by *C jejuni* infection. Outbreaks are associated with consumption of unpasteurized dairy products and undercooked poultry. The incidence of disease peaks in summer and early fall. Diarrhea may be bloody. Fever usually is present. The diagnosis is established by isolation of the organism from stool; a special medium is required. Treatment is with erythromycin. Alternatives are ciprofloxacin and norfloxacin (emergence of resistance to fluoroquinolones has been reported). Supportive care also is needed.

- Outbreaks of bacterial diarrhea caused by *C jejuni* are associated with consumption of unpasteurized milk and undercooked poultry.
- Approximately 10%-30% of cases of Guillain-Barré syndrome are preceded by *C jejuni* infection.

In bacterial diarrhea caused by *S aureus*, preformed toxin is ingested in contaminated food. Onset is abrupt, with severe vomiting (often predominates), diarrhea, and abdominal cramps. The duration of infection is 8 to 24 hours. Diagnosis is based on rapid onset, absence of fever, and history. Treatment is supportive.

- Bacterial diarrhea due to *S aureus* is caused by ingestion of preformed toxin in contaminated food.

Bacterial diarrhea caused by *Clostridium perfringens* is associated with ingestion of bacteria that produce toxin in vivo, often in improperly prepared or stored precooked foods (eg, meat and poultry products). Food is precooked and toxin is destroyed but spores survive; when food is rewarmed, spores germinate. When food is ingested, toxin is produced. Diarrhea is worse than vomiting, and abdominal cramping is prominent. Onset of symptoms is later than with *S aureus* infection. Duration of illness is 24 hours. The diagnosis is based on the later onset of symptoms, a typical history, and Gram staining or culture of incriminated foods. Treatment is supportive.

- In diarrhea caused by *C perfringens*, ingested bacteria produce toxin in vivo in precooked food.

Table 15-21 Bacterial Diarrhea: Toxigenic

Organism	Onset After Ingestion, h	Preformed Toxin	Fever Present	Vomiting Predominates
Staphylococcus aureus	2-6	Yes	No	Yes
Clostridium perfringens	8-16	No	No	No
Escherichia coli	12	No	No	No
Vibrio cholerae	12	No	Due to dehydration	No
Bacillus cereus				
a.	1-6	Yes	No	Yes
b.	8-16	No	No	No

Table 15-22 Bacterial Diarrhea: Invasive

Organism	Fever Present	Bloody Diarrhea Present	Antibiotics Effective
Shigella species	Yes	Yes	Yes
Salmonella (non-*typhi*)	Yes	No	No
Vibrio parahaemolyticus	Yes	Yes (occasional)	No
Escherichia coli O157:H7	Yes	Yes	No
Campylobacter	Yes	Yes	Yes
Yersinia	Yes	Yes (occasional)	±

* Diarrhea is worse than vomiting; abdominal cramping is prominent.

Two types of food poisoning are associated with *Bacillus cereus* infection. Profuse vomiting follows a short incubation period (1-6 hours); this is associated with the ingestion of a preformed toxin (usually in fried rice). A disease with a longer incubation occurs 8 to 16 hours after consumption; profound diarrhea develops and usually is associated with eating meat or vegetables. The diagnosis is confirmed by isolation of the organism from contaminated food. The illness is self-limited and treatment is supportive.

Diarrhea caused by *E coli* can be either enterotoxigenic (ETEC) or enterohemorrhagic. Enterohemorrhagic *E coli* should not be treated with antibiotics. Enterotoxigenic *E coli* is the most common etiologic agent in traveler's diarrhea. Treatment consists of fluid and electrolyte replacement along with loperamide plus a fluoroquinolone or rifaximin. Medical evaluation should be sought if fever and bloody diarrhea occur. For prophylaxis, water, fruits, and vegetables need to be chosen carefully. Routine prophylactic use of trimethoprim-sulfamethoxazole, ciprofloxacin, and doxycycline is not recommended because the risks outweigh the benefits in most travelers. Bismuth subsalicylate reduces the incidence of enterotoxigenic *E coli*-associated diarrhea by up to 60%.

* Enterotoxigenic *E coli* is the most common etiologic agent in traveler's diarrhea.

E coli O157:H7 causes a relatively uncommon form of bloody diarrhea. This agent has been identified as the cause of waterborne illness, outbreaks in nursing homes and child care centers, and sporadic cases. It also has been transmitted by eating undercooked beef and other contaminated food products. Bloody diarrhea, severe abdominal cramps, fever, and profound toxicity characterize this enterohemorrhagic illness. It may resemble ischemic colitis. At extremes of age (old and young), the infection may produce hemolytic uremic syndrome and death. This organism should be considered in all patients with hemolytic uremic syndrome. Antibiotics are not known to be effective and may increase the likelihood of hemolytic uremic syndrome.

* *E coli* O157:H7 has been identified as the cause of waterborne illness, outbreaks in nursing homes and child care centers, and sporadic cases.
* Eating undercooked beef also transmits *E coli* O157:H7.
* Bloody diarrhea, severe abdominal cramps, and profound toxicity characterize *E coli* O157:H7 infection; it may resemble ischemic colitis.
* Infection should be considered in all patients with hemolytic uremic syndrome.
* Antibiotic therapy is not recommended.

Vibrio cholerae causes a toxigenic bacterial diarrheal disease in which antibiotics (tetracycline) clearly shorten the duration of disease. However, fluid replacement therapy is the mainstay of management. It is associated with consumption of undercooked shellfish.

Diarrhea caused by *Shigella* species is often acquired outside the United States. It often is spread by person-to-person transmission but also has been associated with eating contaminated food or water. Bloody diarrhea is characteristic, bacteremia may occur, and fever is present. The diagnosis is based on results of stool culture and blood culture (occasionally positive). Treatment is with ampicillin (ampicillin-resistant strains are common), trimethoprim-sulfamethoxazole (in some countries, increasing resistance is being reported), norfloxacin, or ciprofloxacin. The illness may precede the onset of Reiter syndrome in persons with HLA-B2 and group B *Shigella flexneri*.

* Diarrhea caused by *Shigella* species is associated with person-to-person transmission and the consumption of contaminated food or water.
* Bloody diarrhea is characteristic, bacteremia may occur, and fever is present.
* Illness caused by *Shigella* species may precede the onset of Reiter syndrome.

Salmonella (non-*typhi*)-associated illness most commonly is caused by *Salmonella enteritidis* and *Salmonella typhimurium* in the United States. It is associated with consumption of contaminated foods or with exposure to reptiles and snakes, pet turtles, ducklings, and iguanas. *Salmonella* infection is a common cause of severe diarrhea and may cause septicemia in patients with sickle cell anemia or acquired immunodeficiency syndrome (AIDS). *Salmonella* bacteremia can lead to the seeding of abdominal aortic plaques resulting in mycotic aneurysms. In *Salmonella* enteritis, fever is usually present, and bloody diarrhea is often absent (a characteristic distinguishing it from *Shigella* infection). The diagnosis is based on stool culture. Treatment is supportive. Antibiotics only prolong the carrier state and do not affect the course of the disease. Antibiotics are used if results of blood culture are positive. Reactive arthritis may be a complication of this illness.

* *Salmonella* infection is a common cause of severe diarrhea.
* *Salmonella* infection may cause septicemia in patients with sickle cell anemia or AIDS.
* Bloody diarrhea is often absent (a feature distinguishing it from *Shigella* infection).

Vibrio parahaemolyticus infection is acquired by eating undercooked shellfish. It is a common bacterial cause of acute food-borne illness in Japan and is appearing with increasing frequency in the United States (Atlantic Gulf Coast and on cruise ships). Acute onset of explosive, watery diarrhea and fever are characteristic. The diagnosis is determined with stool culture. Antibiotic therapy is not required.

* Typical clinical scenario of *V. parahaemolyticus* infection: acute onset of watery diarrhea and fever after eating undercooked shellfish.
* Antibiotic therapy is not required.

Clinical syndromes associated with *Vibrio vulnificus* include bacteremia, gastroenteritis, and cellulitis. Most patients with bacteremia have distinctive bullous skin lesions and underlying hepatic disease (cirrhosis). The condition is associated with consumption of raw oysters. The mortality rate is high. Wound infections occur in patients who have had contact with seawater, such as with fishing injuries or contamination of a wound with seawater. Affected patients have intense pain and cellulitis in the extremities. Gastrointestinal illness is associated with consumption of raw oysters. The incubation period is approximately 18 hours. Vomiting, diarrhea, and severe abdominal cramps are features of this illness. Treatment of uncomplicated gastroenteritis is supportive. Bacteremia or cellulitis is treated with tetracycline, cefotaxime, or ciprofloxacin. *V vulnificus* is not uniformly susceptible to the aminoglycosides.

- *V vulnificus* bacteremia can cause distinctive bullous skin lesions and occurs in patients who are immunocompromised or have cirrhosis.
- It is associated with consumption of raw oysters or seawater contact.

Yersinia enterocolitica is the etiologic agent of several major clinical syndromes: enterocolitis, mesenteric adenitis, erythema nodosum, polyarthritis, Reiter syndrome, and bacteremia associated with contaminated blood products. Approximately 20% of infected patients have sore throat. Infection with *Y enterocolitica* causing mesenteric adenitis can mimic acute appendicitis. Acquisition of infection is thought to be associated with eating contaminated food products. The organism has been cultured from chocolate milk, meat, mussels, poultry, oysters, and cheese.

- In adults with *Y enterocolitica* infection, erythema nodosum, polyarthritis, and Reiter syndrome can develop.
- Infection with *Y enterocolitica* causing mesenteric adenitis can mimic acute appendicitis.

Colitis caused by *Clostridium difficile* should be distinguished from other forms of antibiotic-associated diarrhea (watery stools, no systemic symptoms, and negative tests for *C difficile* toxin). Symptoms often occur 2 to 4 weeks after stopping use of antibiotics. The illness is associated with antibiotic exposure in 99% of cases (any antibiotic can cause it). Nosocomial spread has been documented. Typical features are profuse, watery stools; crampy abdominal pain; constitutional illness; unexplained leukocytosis; the presence of fecal leukocytes; and a positive *C difficile* toxin. In toxin-negative disease, proctoscopy or flexible sigmoidoscopy can be used to look for pseudomembranes. Disease can be localized to the cecum (postoperative patient with ileus) and can present as fever of unknown origin. A recent toxigenic strain associated with a binary toxin has been associated with earlier onset, marked leukocytosis, and severe disease refractory to medical therapy, often requiring colectomy. Treatment in mild-moderate disease consists of metronidazole (250-500 mg orally 3 or 4 times daily for 7-10 days) or vancomycin (125 mg orally 4 times daily for 7-10 days). Metronidazole should be used as a first-line agent in mild to moderate disease. Oral vancomycin is preferred in cases of severe disease. Antiperistalsis drugs should not be used. If a patient is unable to take drugs orally, intravenous metronidazole (not vancomycin) or vancomycin enemas can be used. Relapse is frequent (about 15% of cases) and necessitates re-treatment. Treatment of asymptomatic carriers to decrease the nosocomial spread of infection or to reduce the risk of pseudomembranous colitis is not recommended.

- Colitis caused by *C difficile* often occurs 2-4 weeks after stopping use of antibiotics.
- Illness is associated with antibiotic exposure in 99% of cases (any antibiotic can cause it).
- Features of colitis caused by *C difficile* are profuse, watery stools; crampy abdominal pain; constitutional illness; fecal leukocytes; leukocytosis; and a positive *C difficile* toxin.
- Treatment of colitis caused by *C difficile* is with metronidazole (250-500 mg orally 3 or 4 times daily for 7-10 days) or vancomycin (125 mg orally 4 times daily for 7-10 days). Severe cases may require colectomy.
- Relapse is frequent (about 15% of cases).

Viral Diarrhea

Many types of viral diarrhea can be defined by their seasonal epidemiology. *Rotavirus infection* is the most common cause of sporadic mild diarrhea in children. It may be spread from children to adults. It usually occurs during the winter. Vomiting is a more common early manifestation than watery diarrhea. Hospitalization for dehydration is common in young children. Diagnosis is made by detection of antigen in stool. Treatment is symptomatic. A vaccine was available in the United States but was withdrawn from the market because of a temporal association between the use of the vaccine and the development of intussusception.

Noroviruses are a common cause of epidemic diarrhea and "winter vomiting disease" in older children and adults. They occur in families, communities, and institutions. Outbreaks have been associated with eating shellfish, undercooked fish, cake frosting, and salads and with drinking contaminated water. They are the cause of up to 10% of gastroenteritis outbreaks. These viruses have caused community-wide outbreaks and outbreaks of gastroenteritis on cruise ships. Nausea, vomiting, and watery diarrhea characterize this illness. It is a mild, self-limited (<36 hours) illness. Currently, no commercial diagnostic test is available. Treatment is symptomatic.

- Outbreaks of norovirus are associated with eating shellfish, undercooked fish, cake frosting, and salads and with drinking contaminated water.
- Numerous outbreaks of noroviruses have occurred on cruise ships.
- Illness is mild and self-limited (<36 hours).

Bacteremia, Sepsis, and Septic Shock

Bacteremia, or bloodstream infection in general, is defined as the presence of living bacteria or other organisms in the blood and is established by a positive blood culture or other microbiologic techniques. The systemic inflammatory response syndrome is characterized by a group of physiologic responses due to several infectious and noninfectious causes. If systemic inflammatory response syndrome is caused by an infection, then sepsis is said to be present. Some of the common manifestations of this syndrome or sepsis include tachypnea, tachycardia, irritability, lethargy, fever or hypothermia, hypoxemia, and leukocytosis. Septic shock is sepsis with hypotension (blood pressure <90 mm Hg or a reduction of 40 mm Hg from baseline) despite adequate fluid replacement.

Severe sepsis and septic shock are characterized by impaired tissue perfusion, hypotension, and multiorgan dysfunction in the setting of infection (blood cultures positive in 50%-60% of cases). Endotoxin activates endogenous mediators of inflammation with catastrophic consequences. The result can be increased vascular permeability, a decrease in peripheral vascular resistance, profound hypotension with progressive lactic acidosis, and death.

Common causative organisms of community-acquired bloodstream infections include *E coli*, *S aureus*, and *S pneumoniae*. Nosocomial infections most often are due to gram-negative aerobic bacilli, coagulase-negative staphylococci, *S aureus*, enterococci, and *Candida* spp. The frequency of any 1 organism depends on the host (ie, neutropenia is associated with *Pseudomonas aeruginosa*, central lines are associated with coagulase-negative staphylococci, *S aureus*, and *Candida* spp). The overall mortality rate is 20% to 30%. Management involves maintaining intravascular volume, administering appropriate bactericidal antimicrobials, and correcting any problems that lead to infection (such as draining abscesses). Adjunctive corticosteroids are of no proven benefit. Recombinant human activated protein C (drotrecogin alfa) has been approved by the US Food and Drug Administration for treatment of adults with septic shock.

* In septic shock, blood cultures are positive in 50%-60% of cases.
* Most frequent blood isolates: *E coli*, *S aureus*, *S pneumoniae*.
* Endotoxin activates endogenous mediators of inflammation with catastrophic consequences.

Neutropenia

This condition is characterized by an absolute polymorphonuclear neutrophil value less than 0.5×10^9/L, most often in the setting of chemotherapy for malignancy. Some high-risk patients with acute leukemia and expected prolonged neutropenia may benefit from prophylaxis with levofloxacin during the period of neutropenia. Bacteremia is documented in approximately 20% of neutropenic fever episodes. If ecthyma gangrenosum is present, *Pseudomonas* infection should be considered. Other gram-negative aerobic rods (such as *E coli*) also cause bacteremia. The frequency of bacteremia due to aerobic gram-positive organisms is increasing. Bloodstream infection with these organisms (*S aureus*, coagulase-negative staphylococci, enterococci, viridans streptococci, and *Corynebacterium jeikeium*) often is associated with central venous catheters or quinolone antibacterial prophylaxis. *Candida* species should be considered in cases associated with nodular skin lesions, fluffy white chorioretinal exudates, and fever unresponsive to empiric antibacterial agents. Anaerobic organisms are uncommon, except in cases of perirectal abscess and gingivitis. Empiric antimicrobial therapy after an attempt to identify the source of the infection is required for fever of 38.3°C or higher. Monotherapy with ceftazidime, cefepime, or imipenem alone is the preferred initial empiric antibacterial regimen. Alternative therapy with antipseudomonal penicillin plus an aminoglycoside is also acceptable. Vancomycin can be added to the initial regimen if there is severe mucositis, quinolone prophylaxis has been utilized, the patient is known to be colonized with methicillin-resistant *S aureus* or penicillin-resistant *S pneumoniae*, an obvious catheter-related infection is present, or the patient is hypotensive. If subsequent cultures show the presence of aerobic gram-positive organisms, vancomycin therapy can be continued. If there is no response after 5 to 7 days of treatment and the patient remains neutropenic, empiric therapy with an antifungal agent such as amphotericin, voriconazole, or caspofungin should be considered. Recent studies suggest benefit to the use of prophylaxis versus the filamentous fungi in high-risk neutropenic patients, including those with expected prolonged neutropenia, such as acute leukemia or myelodysplastic syndromes and bone marrow transplant recipients with graft-versus-host disease. In these groups, prophylaxis with posaconazole reduces mortality.

Urinary Tract Infection

Females

Because urethritis or cystitis can occur with low colony counts of bacteria (10^3 colony-forming units), routine urine cultures in young women with dysuria are not recommended. Urinalysis should be done with or without a Gram stain. If pyuria and uncomplicated urinary tract infection (UTI) are present, short-course treatment (3 days) should be initiated. Only if occult upper urinary tract disease, a complicated UTI, or sexually transmitted disease is suspected should appropriate culture and sensitivity testing be performed. Risk factors for occult infection and complications include emergency department presentation, low socioeconomic status, hospital-acquired infection, pregnancy, use of Foley catheter, recent instrumentation, known urologic abnormality, previous relapse, UTI at age less than 12 years, acute pyelonephritis or 3 or more UTIs in 1 year, symptoms for more than 7 days, recent antibiotic use, diabetes mellitus, and immunosuppression. Causative organisms include *E coli* and *Staphylococcus saprophyticus* (susceptible to ampicillin and trimethoprim-sulfamethoxazole), *Proteus mirabilis*, or *Klebsiella pneumoniae*. *Staphylococcus saprophyticus* may be reported on urine culture as "coagulase-negative staphylococcus."

* Routine urine cultures are not recommended in young women with dysuria.
* Associated organisms of UTI include: *E coli*, *S saprophyticus* (susceptible to ampicillin and trimethoprim-sulfamethoxazole), *P mirabilis*, or *K pneumoniae*.

For the first episode of cystitis or urethritis, treatment is given but no investigation is needed. Trimethoprim-sulfamethoxazole or an oral fluoroquinolone is more effective than ampicillin or other β-lactams. Short-course treatment (single-dose) has fewer side effects than standard (7-10 days) therapy, but the risk of relapse (due to retention of viable organisms in the vaginal or perivaginal area) is higher. Three-day therapy may be associated with relapse rates equal to those with treatment for 7 to 10 days and with less toxicity. In patients who fail to improve within 48 hours of treatment with trimethoprim or trimethoprim-sulfamethoxazole, drug resistance should be suspected and an oral fluoroquinolone should be considered. Rates of trimethoprim-sulfamethoxazole resistance may approach 20% in some communities. Because of this increase in drug resistance, patients treated with trimethoprim-sulfamethoxazole should be monitored closely for failure; alternative agents include a 7-day course of nitrofurantoin or a 3-day fluoroquinolone. If recurrence develops after 3-day therapy, subclinical pyelonephritis or resistance should be considered and treatment is then given for 14 days. Urologic evaluation is usually not necessary. It should be performed in patients with multiple relapses, painless hematuria, a history of childhood UTI, renal lithiasis, and recurrent pyelonephritis.

- For first episode of cystitis or urethritis, trimethoprim-sulfamethoxazole or an oral fluoroquinolone is more effective than ampicillin.
- Short-course treatment (3 days) has fewer side effects than standard (7-10 days) therapy, and risk of relapse of infection may be the same.
- Urologic evaluation should be pursued in patients with multiple relapses, painless hematuria, history of childhood UTI, renal lithiasis, and recurrent pyelonephritis.

For acute pyelonephritis, 2 weeks of therapy is equal in efficacy to 6 weeks of therapy. Recent data suggest that 1 week of treatment with a fluoroquinolone may be sufficient for uncomplicated pyelonephritis due to susceptible organisms in women. Most patients are sufficiently ill to require hospitalization. Many are bacteremic. Unless gram-positive cocci are seen on Gram stain (suggesting enterococci), a third-generation cephalosporin, trimethoprim-sulfamethoxazole, or a fluoroquinolone can be used as empiric therapy. If enterococci are suspected, ampicillin or piperacillin with or without gentamicin should be used. Enterococci are resistant to cephalosporins. Enterococci appear susceptible to trimethoprim-sulfamethoxazole in vitro (and may be reported as such on a susceptibility report), but trimethoprim-sulfamethoxazole fails in the therapy of enterococcal infections because the organism is able to circumvent the block of folate synthesis by using exogenous folinic acid, dihydrofolate, and tetrahydrofolate from the in vivo environment. Oral regimens can be substituted quickly as the patient improves. A urine culture is recommended 1 to 2 weeks after completion of therapy only in pregnant women, children, and patients with recurrent pyelonephritis in whom suppressive therapy is being considered. If relapse occurs, treatment is given for 6 weeks and a urologic evaluation is done. For recurrent lower UTI (more than 2 episodes per year), single-dose therapy, 3-day therapy, or 6-week therapy is used. For treatment failure, chronic suppressive therapy may be used; however, the risk of resistant organisms must be weighed. Asymptomatic bacteriuria (>10^5 colony-forming U/mL) in a midstream urine specimen should be treated only in pregnant women, patients undergoing urinary tract instrumentation, and renal transplant recipients.

- For acute pyelonephritis, 2 weeks of therapy is equal in efficacy to 6 weeks of therapy.
- A follow-up urine culture is not usually recommended.
- Cephalosporins and trimethoprim-sulfamethoxazole should not be used to treat enterococcal UTI.

Males

UTI is less common in males than females. Urologic abnormalities (such as benign prostatic hyperplasia) are common. Symptoms are unreliable for localization. Physical examination should include prostate examination, retraction of the foreskin to look for discharge, and palpation of the testicles and epididymis. When a UTI is suspected, urine culture and sensitivity testing should always be done. Causative organisms include *E coli* in 50% of cases, other gram-negative organisms in 25%, enterococci in 20%, and others in 5%. If signs and symptoms of epididymitis, acute prostatitis, and pyelonephritis are present, treat accordingly. If uncomplicated lower UTI is present, treatment duration is 10 to 14 days. If symptoms persist or relapse, the urine culture should be repeated. If results are positive, treat for a minimum of 6 weeks. If culture results are negative, consider further evaluation for 1 of the chronic prostatitis/chronic pelvic pain syndromes.

- Causes of UTI in males include *E coli* in 50%, other gram-negative organisms in 25%, enterococci in 20%, and others in 5%.
- Men with UTI should *not* receive short-course therapy.

Soft Tissue Infection

Cellulitis is a skin infection that involves the dermis and subcutaneous fat. The most common causes are β-hemolytic streptococci and *S aureus*. Community-acquired methicillin-resistant *S aureus* infections are an emerging problem. These infections are typically resistant to β-lactams and erythromycin but are susceptible to trimethoprim-sulfamethoxazole, rifampin, and sometimes clindamycin. These isolates have a different genetic mechanism of resistance (staphylococcal chromosomal cassette 4) from hospital-acquired methicillin-resistant *S aureus*. Many of the community-acquired methicillin-resistant *S aureus* isolates contain the Panton-Valentine leukocidin gene, which is associated with significant local toxicity. The optimal management of these community-acquired methicillin-resistant *S aureus* infections is not yet clear but agents such as dicloxacillin or cephalosporins are associated with clinical failure and should not be used. Abscesses, boils, or furuncles should be incised, drained, and sent for culture. Currently, combinations of trimethoprim-sulfamethoxazole or clindamycin with rifampin are recommended for outpatient therapy. Inpatients may be treated with these parenterally or with therapies including vancomycin, daptomycin, or linezolid.

Patients with lymphedema, patients who have had saphenous vein harvesting for coronary artery bypass grafting, or patients who have tinea pedis are predisposed to cellulitis, often due to streptococci. Recurrent leg cellulitis may be associated with pretibial location, prior malignancy, or local dermatitis. Treatment is typically with an antistaphylococcal penicillin or first-generation cephalosporin. Unusual causes of soft tissue infection are *Eikenella corrodens* and oral anaerobes after human bites, *Pasteurella multocida* after cat or dog bites, *Capnocytophaga canimorsus* after dog bites, *Aeromonas hydrophila* after freshwater exposure or exposure to leeches, *Vibrio vulnificus* after saltwater exposure, *Erysipelothrix rhusiopathiae* and *Streptococcus iniae* after fish exposure, and *P aeruginosa* after hot tub exposure.

Bone and Joint Infections

Acute Bacterial Arthritis (Nongonococcal)

This is most commonly due to hematogenous spread of bacteria. The hip and knee joints are commonly involved. Bacteria involved are gram-positive aerobic cocci (about 75% of cases): *S aureus* (most common) and β-hemolytic streptococci. Gram-negative aerobic bacilli also can cause infection (about 20% of cases); *P aeruginosa* is a common cause in injection drug users. Anaerobes, fungi, and mycobacteria are unusual. Clinical features include involvement usually of monarticular, large joints. Fever, pain, swelling, and restriction of motion are the most frequent signs and symptoms. The synovial fluid is usually turbid, and the leukocyte count generally exceeds 40×10^9/L (=75% polymorphonuclear neutrophils). The condition may overlap and be confused with other inflammatory arthropathies. Gram stain is 50% to 95% sensitive. Culture results are positive unless antibiotics have been used previously or the pathogen is unusual. Blood culture results are often positive. Radiographs are not helpful in routine cases because destructive changes have not had time to occur. Specific antimicrobial therapy is based on results of Gram stain, culture, and sensitivity testing. The duration of therapy is dependent on individual circumstances, such as the presence of complicating osteomyelitis. Usually, treatment is given for 2 to 4 weeks. Empiric therapy should include agents directed against *S aureus* and gram-negative bacilli. Drainage is essential. Percutaneous, arthroscopic, or open procedures are used. Hip, shoulder, and sternoclavicular joint involvement, development of loculations, and persistently positive culture results (not due to resistant organisms) are the usual indications for arthroscopy or open débridement.

* Acute bacterial arthritis (nongonococcal) is most commonly due to hematogenous spread of bacteria.
* Bacteria most commonly involved are gram-positive aerobic cocci (about 75% of cases): *S aureus* is most common.
* Monarticular, large joints usually are involved.
* Fever, pain, swelling, and restriction of motion are frequent.
* Synovial fluid is turbid; leukocyte count generally exceeds 40×10^9/L.
* Blood culture results are often positive.
* Drainage is essential.

Viral Arthritis

This is usually transient, self-limited polyarthritis. It may be caused by rubella (also may occur after vaccination), hepatitis B, mumps, coxsackievirus, adenovirus, parvovirus B19, and HIV, among others.

Chronic Monarticular Arthritis

Organisms involved include Mycobacteria (*Mycobacterium tuberculosis* is more common than *Mycobacterium avium-intracellulare*, *Mycobacterium kansasii*, *Mycobacterium marinum*), fungi (*Coccidioides immitis* and *Sporothrix schenckii* are more common than *Histoplasma capsulatum*, *Blastomyces dermatitidis*–acute, and *Candida* spp–acute), and others (*Brucella*, *Nocardia*).

* *Mycobacterium tuberculosis*, *C immitis*, and *S schenckii* often are involved in chronic monarticular arthritis.

Osteomyelitis

Acute *hematogenous osteomyelitis* is more common in infants and children than in adults. The metaphysis of long bones (femur, tibia) most commonly is affected. *Staphylococcus aureus* is the most common organism. Acute onset of pain and fever are typical features. The illness can present with pain only. Compatible radiographic changes and bone biopsy for culture and pathologic examination are used to establish the diagnosis. Results of blood culture may be positive. Specific parenteral antibiotic therapy is used for 3 to 6 weeks on the basis of culture and sensitivity test results. Débridement is usually not necessary unless a sequestrum is present.

* *Staphylococcus aureus* is the most common organism in acute hematogenous osteomyelitis.
* Acute onset of pain and fever are typical features.

Chronic osteomyelitis is more common in adults. It results from direct inoculation caused by trauma or adjacent soft tissue infection, for example. Open fractures and diabetic foot ulcers are common predisposing factors. *Staphylococcus aureus* is the most common organism. Coagulase-negative staphylococci are often pathogens if a foreign body (such as plate, screws) is present. Often, osteomyelitis complicating a foot ulcer is polymicrobial, including aerobic gram-positive and gram-negative organisms and anaerobes. Local pain, tenderness, erythema, and draining sinuses are common. Fever is atypical unless there is concurrent cellulitis. The condition can present with pain only. Compatible radiographic changes (often vague) and bone biopsy for culture and pathologic examination are used to establish the diagnosis. Results of blood culture are rarely positive. Adequate débridement, removal of dead space, soft tissue coverage, and fixation of infected fractures are essential. Specific parenteral antibiotic therapy is given for 4 to 6 weeks on the basis of culture and sensitivity test results.

* *Staphylococcus aureus* is the most common organism in chronic osteomyelitis.
* Coagulase-negative staphylococci are common pathogens if a foreign body is present.
* Local pain, tenderness, erythema, and draining sinuses are common.
* Specific parenteral antibiotic therapy is given for 4-6 weeks.

Diskitis and Vertebral Infections

Infection of the intervertebral disk and the adjacent vertebrae encompasses a broad spectrum of clinical entities referred to as *spondylodiskitis*, *disk space infection*, and *vertebral osteomyelitis*, all with or without associated epidural or psoas abscesses. These infections most often arise from hematogenous dissemination of infection from the skin and soft tissues, genitourinary tract, infective endocarditis, infected intravenous sites, injection drug use, or respiratory tract infection. Among all cases of osteomyelitis, 2% to 7% involve the vertebrae. Although rarely life-threatening, disk and vertebral infections may result in severe neurologic disability and disabling pain. Their incidence is greatest among males, peaks in the fifth decade of life, and is increasing, particularly among the elderly. Risk factors for spine infections include advanced age, immunocompromise, diabetes, intravenous drug use, renal failure, bacteremia, cancer, chronic corticosteroid use, intravascular devices, and recent instrumentation or spine surgery.

Diagnosis

The clinical presentation of vertebral osteomyelitis includes localized insidious pain and tenderness in the spine area in 90% of patients. Most commonly affected is the lumbar or lumbosacral region; cervical disease may occur in patients with head and neck infections or in injection drug users. The diagnosis of vertebral osteomyelitis requires a high index of suspicion in at-risk patients. Fever is present in less than half of cases. Because of the clinical uncertainty, a delay in diagnosis by weeks to months occurs, which can lead to motor and sensory deficits in 15% of patients. The goal of the diagnostic evaluation is to identify the organism and determine the site and extent of infection. The erythrocyte sedimentation rate is increased in more than 90% of cases, and the leukocyte count is increased in less than 50%. Blood cultures may be positive; if so, infective endocarditis may be present.

Diagnostic Imaging

Various imaging techniques can localize infection to the spine. Plain radiography may show vertebral endplate irregularity 2 to 8 weeks after the onset of symptoms, but it is neither sensitive nor specific. Gadolinium-enhanced magnetic resonance imaging is the most useful test for diagnosis because of its high sensitivity (96%), specificity (94%), and accuracy (92%). In patients who cannot undergo magnetic resonance imaging, nuclear scanning may help establish the diagnosis. A 3-phase technetium bone scanning is sensitive (87%-98%) for the presence of disk space infection. The best nuclear study for imaging disk space infections is technetium combined with gallium citrate scanning. Computed tomography-guided percutaneous aspiration or biopsy is often used to identify the causative organism. If the initial result is negative, the test should be repeated before proceeding to an open biopsy procedure.

Microbiology

Staphylococcus aureus and coagulase-negative staphylococci are the most common microorganisms cultured in vertebral osteomyelitis. *Mycobacterium tuberculosis* and *Brucella* are common in regions endemic for these organisms. Spine infections due to aerobic gram-negative bacteria such as *E coli* and *Candida* spp are more common in intravenous drug abusers, immunosuppressed patients, and postoperative patients.

Treatment

The goal of treatment is eradication of infection, restoration of function, and relief of pain. Most patients can be managed with antimicrobials, pain management, and external supportive bracing alone. Antimicrobial therapy should be directed by culture results. However, in culture-negative cases, empirical therapy should target methicillin-resistant *S aureus* and aerobic gram-negative bacilli with agents such as vancomycin plus a third- or fourth-generation cephalosporin. Antibiotics should be given parenterally for a minimum of 4 to 6 weeks or longer if there is extensive vertebral destruction or undrained collections. Surgical

interventions are limited to patients with progressive neurologic deterioration, spinal instability, progressive abscess, or failed medical therapy. The goals of surgery are to preserve neurologic function and facilitate bony fusion and stability.

Sinusitis in Adults

The physician's overall impression as to the presence or absence of sinusitis is the best clinical predictor of sinusitis. Independent clinical predictors of disease are maxillary toothache, poor transillumination, poor response to decongestants, and a history or examination finding of purulent discharge. Limited computed tomography scanning of the sinuses is the radiographic method of choice. Organisms that are usually involved are *H influenzae*, *S pneumoniae*, and oral anaerobes. Treatment is with oral trimethoprim-sulfamethoxazole, amoxicillin, amoxicillin-clavulanate, and levofloxacin, among other options.

- Organisms involved in sinusitis in adults are *H influenzae*, *S pneumoniae*, and oral anaerobes.

Hepatic (Bacterial) Abscess

Mechanisms of bacterial abscess include portal vein bacteremia resulting from, for example, appendicitis and diverticulitis, bacteremia caused by a primary focus elsewhere in the body, ascending cholangitis, direct extension (subphrenic abscess), or trauma. Fever is common. Right upper quadrant pain, tenderness on percussion, and increased values on liver function tests may or may not be present. Computed tomography and ultrasonography are helpful in diagnosis. Bacteriology depends on the mechanism of abscess formation. Infection is often polymicrobial and is due to aerobic gram-negative rods, anaerobic streptococci, and *Bacteroides* species. Blood cultures should be obtained, and empiric therapy should be initiated pending drainage. Drainage of the abscess usually can be performed percutaneously, and material is obtained for Gram stain, culture, and susceptibility testing. Empiric options include ampicillin plus gentamicin, a fluoroquinolone plus metronidazole, or a third-generation cephalosporin plus metronidazole, a β-lactam/β-lactamase inhibitor combination, or a carbapenem. If hematogenous route is suspected, an agent that is active against staphylococci should be used in the regimen.

Toxic Shock Syndrome

This syndrome is caused by the establishment or growth of a toxin-producing strain of *S aureus* in a nonimmune person. Clinical scenarios associated with this syndrome include young menstruating women with prolonged, continuous use of tampons, postoperative and nonoperative wound infections, localized abscesses, and *S aureus* pneumonia developing after influenza. It is a multisystem disease. Clinical criteria include fever, hypotension, erythroderma (often leads to desquamation, particularly on palms and soles), and involvement in 3 or more organ systems. Onset is acute; blood culture results are usually negative. The condition is caused by production of staphylococcal toxin (TSST-1). Treatment is supportive; subsequent episodes are treated with a β-lactam antibiotic, which decreases the frequency and severity of subsequent attacks. The relapse rate may be as high as 30% to 40% (menstruation-related disease). The mortality rate is 5% to 10%.

* Toxic shock syndrome is caused by a toxin-producing strain of *S aureus* in a nonimmune person.
* Toxic shock syndrome is a multisystem disease: fever, hypotension, erythroderma (often leads to desquamation, particularly on palms and soles).
* Onset is acute; results of blood culture are usually negative.
* Toxic shock syndrome is caused by production of staphylococcal toxin (TSST-1).

Streptococcal Toxic Shock Syndrome

This syndrome is similar to staphylococcal toxic shock syndrome. Patients have invasive group A streptococcal infections with associated hypotension and 2 of the following: renal impairment, coagulopathy, liver impairment, adult respiratory distress syndrome, rash (may desquamate), or soft tissue necrosis. Symptoms are caused by production of streptococcal toxin (pyrogenic exotoxin A). Most patients have skin or soft tissue infection, are younger than 50 years, and are otherwise healthy compared with patients with invasive group A streptococcal infections without the toxic streptococcal syndrome. Most patients are bacteremic (different from toxic shock syndrome due to *S aureus*). Treatment includes early aggressive antibiotic therapy, supportive care, and surgical débridement if needed. The case-fatality rate is 30%. Although there is no reported resistance to penicillin, clindamycin plus high-dose penicillin G is the preferred regimen because clindamycin may suppress exotoxin and M-protein production in addition to its activity against group A streptococci. In severe cases, consideration should be made for the use of early intravenous immunoglobulin therapy.

* Symptoms of toxic streptococcal syndrome are caused by production of streptococcal toxin.
* Most patients are bacteremic (different from toxic shock syndrome due to *S aureus*).
* Clindamycin plus high-dose penicillin G is the preferred antibiotic regimen.

Infections in Solid Organ Transplant and Immunodeficiency States

The spectrum of potential pathogens in patients after solid organ transplant is diverse. The individual risk of specific infection can be classified according to the following: symptoms and signs of illness at presentation (ie, meningitis vs pneumonia), posttransplant time course, serologic status of recipient and donor for certain infections (such as cytomegalovirus, toxoplasmosis), type of organ transplant, type and duration of immunosuppression, type of antimicrobial prophylaxis patient has received, and travel history and previous exposure to pathogens (such as tuberculosis, coccidioidomycosis).

The majority of infections in the first month after transplant are not opportunistic infections but instead are common nosocomial infections such as wound infections, UTIs, and line infections. Cytomegalovirus is an important pathogen in patients who have had transplant. Presentations can include febrile illness with viremia, hepatitis, colitis, gastritis, retinitis, myocarditis, and pneumonitis. Cytomegalovirus-seronegative recipients of organs from a seropositive donor are at highest risk for cytomegalovirus disease. The time of occurrence of opportunistic infections after solid organ transplant is given in Table 15-23. Pathogens associated with various immunodeficiency states are shown in Table 15-24.

* The majority of infections in the first month after transplant are not opportunistic infections but instead are common nosocomial infections such as wound infections, UTIs, and line infections.
* Cytomegalovirus is an important pathogen in patients who have had transplant. Presentations can include febrile illness with viremia, hepatitis, colitis, gastritis, retinitis, myocarditis, and pneumonitis. Cytomegalovirus-seronegative recipients of organs from a seropositive donor are at highest risk for cytomegalovirus disease.

Bioterrorism

After the September 11, 2001, terrorist attacks and the subsequent deaths from anthrax sent in the mail, it is imperative for physicians to be familiar with likely bioterrorism agents. The Centers for Disease Control and Prevention classified the following diseases as category A, high-priority diseases that pose a risk to national security: smallpox, anthrax, botulism, plague, tularemia, and viral hemorrhagic fevers.

The incubation period, lethality, chemotherapy, chemoprophylaxis, vaccine, and specimens that can be obtained for each agent are described in Table 15-25. These agents cause high mortality rates, can be easily disseminated or transmitted from person to person, and have the potential to have a major public health impact.

Severe Acute Respiratory Syndrome

Severe acute respiratory syndrome (SARS) is a rapidly progressive pneumonia that first developed in the Guangdong province of southern China in November 2002. The number of worldwide cases topped 8,000 by July 2003. The infection is caused by a novel coronavirus named SARS-associated coronavirus (SARS-CoV). Symptoms include fever often associated with myalgia, headache, dry cough, and dyspnea. The infection can progress to respiratory failure and death; the case fatality ratio is almost 10%.

The infection is suspected in a patient who has documented fever (>38°C) and lower respiratory tract symptoms and has had contact with a person believed to have had SARS or a history of travel to an area of documented transmission. Serum antibody tests and reverse-transcription polymerase chain reaction tests have been developed. The infection is highly contagious, and health care workers are particularly at risk of exposure. Infected patients must be isolated.

Table 15-23 Opportunistic Infections in Solid Organ Transplant

Month	Type of Infection After Transplant
1	Bacterial infections (related to wound, intravenous lines, urinary tract), herpes simplex virus, hepatitis B
1-4	Cytomegalovirus, *Pneumocystis carinii*, *Listeria monocytogenes*, *Mycobacterium tuberculosis*, *Aspergillus*, *Nocardia*, *Toxoplasma*, hepatitis B, *Legionella*
2-6	Epstein-Barr virus, varicella-zoster virus, hepatitis C, *Legionella*
>6	*Cryptococcus neoformans*, *Legionella*

Infection control precautions for hospitalized patients include standard precautions of good hand hygiene together with airborne isolation and the use of gowns, gloves, and eye protection. No specific treatment recommendations are available.

- SARS is a highly contagious, rapidly progressive respiratory infection caused by a novel coronavirus, SARS-associated coronavirus (SARS-CoV).
- No specific treatment is recommended, although infection control precautions need to be observed to minimize transmission.

Table 15-24 Pathogens Associated With Immunodeficiency

Immunodeficiency	Usual Conditions	Pathogens
Neutropenia (<0.5 × 10^9/L)	Cancer chemotherapy, adverse drug reaction, leukemia	**Bacteria:** Aerobic gram-negative bacilli (coliforms & pseudomonads, *Staphylococcus aureus, viridans streptococci*, coagulase-negative *Staphylococcus*) **Fungi:** *Aspergillus, Candida* spp
Cell-mediated immunity	Organ transplantation, human immunodeficiency virus infection, lymphoma (especially Hodgkin disease), corticosteroid therapy	**Bacteria:** *Listeria, Salmonella, Nocardia, Mycobacteria* (*M tuberculosis* and *M avium*), *Legionella* **Viruses:** CMV, *herpes simplex*, varicella-zoster, JC virus **Parasites:** *Toxoplasma, Strongyloides stercoralis, Cryptosporidium* **Fungi:** *Candida, Cryptococcus, Histoplasma, Coccidioides, Pneumocystis jiroveci* (PCP)
Hypogammaglobulinemia or dysgammaglobulinemia	Multiple myeloma, congenital or acquired deficiency, chronic lymphocytic leukemia	**Bacteria:** *Streptococcus pneumoniae, Haemophilus influenzae* (type B) **Parasites:** *Giardia* **Viruses:** Enteroviruses
Complement deficiencies C2, 3 C5 C6-8 Alternative pathway	Congenital	**Bacteria:** *S pneumoniae, H influenzae, S aureus,* Enterobacteriaceae *Neisseria meningitidis, S pneumoniae, H influenzae, Salmonella*
Hyposplenism	Splenectomy, hemolytic anemia	*S pneumoniae, H influenzae, Capnocytophaga canimorsus* (formerly known as CDC group DF-2)
Defective chemotaxis	Diabetes, alcoholism, renal failure, lazy leukocyte syndrome, trauma, SLE	*S aureus,* streptococci, *Candida*
Defective neutrophilic killing	Chronic granulomatous disease, myeloperoxidase deficiency	Catalase-positive bacteria: *S aureus, Escherichia coli, Candida* spp

Abbreviations: CMV, cytomegalovirus; PCP, pneumocystis pneumonia; SLE, systemic lupus erythematosus.
From Bartlett JG. Pocket book of infectious disease therapy. Baltimore: Williams & Wilkins; 1998. p. 236. Used with permission.

Table 15-25 Treatment for Infections Potentially Caused by Bioterrorism

Variable	Smallpox (Variola Major)	Anthrax (Bacillus anthracis)	Botulism Toxin (Clostridium botulinum)	Plague (Yersinia pestis)	Tularemia (Francisella tularensis)	Viral Hemorrhagic Fevers
Incubation period, days	7-17	1-14 (cutaneous); 1-42[a] (inhalational)	1-5	2-3	1-21	2-21
Lethality	High to moderate	Very high	High without respiratory support	High without treatment	Moderate if untreated	Variable
Chemotherapy[b]	Cidofovir (in vitro)	Cutaneous: Ciprofloxacin 500 mg PO every 12 h or Doxycycline 100 mg PO every 12 h Duration: 60 days Inhalational: Ciprofloxacin 500 mg IV every 12 h or Doxycycline 100 mg IV every 12 h Plus 1 or 2 antimicrobials with demonstrated susceptibility Duration: 60 days	CDC bivalent equine antitoxin for serotypes A, B (licensed) & monovalent for serotype E (investigational)	Streptomycin 1 g IM twice daily or gentamicin 5 mg/kg IV once daily or ciprofloxacin 400 mg IV every 12 h or 750 mg PO twice daily or chloramphenicol 25 mg/kg IV 4 times daily or doxycycline 100 mg IV twice daily Duration: 10 days	Streptomycin 1 g IM twice daily or gentamicin 5 mg/kg daily IV or ciprofloxacin 400 mg IV twice daily Duration: 10 days Doxycycline 100 mg IV twice daily or chloramphenicol 15 mg/kg IV 4 times daily Duration: 14-21 days	Supportive care. Ribavirin (arena viruses or bunyaviruses) 30 mg/kg IV initial dose, then 16 mg/kg every 6 h × 4 days, then 8 mg/kg every 8 h for 6 days. Passive antibody for AHF, BHF; Lassa fever, & CCHF
Chemoprophylaxis	Vaccinia immune globulin 0.6 mL/kg IM (within 3 d of exposure)	Ciprofloxacin 500 mg PO twice daily or Doxycycline 100 mg PO twice daily Duration: 60 days[c]	NA	Doxycycline 100 mg PO twice daily or Ciprofloxacin 500 mg PO twice daily or Chloramphenicol 25 mg/kg PO 4 times daily Duration: 7 days	Doxycycline 100 mg PO twice daily or Ciprofloxacin 500 mg PO twice daily Duration: 14 days	NA
Vaccine	Calf lymph vaccina vaccine: 1 dose by scarification	Anthrax vaccine: 0.5 mL SC at 0, 2, 4 wk, 6, 12, 18 mo, with annual boosters	DOD pentavalent toxoid for serotypes A-E (IND): 0.5 mL deep SC at 0, 2, 12 wk, then annual booster	Greer inactivated vaccine (FDA licensed) Not effective for aerosol exposure. No longer available	Live attenuated vaccine (IND). Recommended for laboratory personnel, not for postexposure prophylaxis	AHF candidate #1 vaccine (cross-protection for BHF) (IND). RVF inactivated vaccine (IND)

Table 15-25 (continued)

Variable	Disease					
	Smallpox (Variola Major)	Anthrax (Bacillus anthracis)	Botulism Toxin (Clostridium botulinum)	Plague (Yersinia pestis)	Tularemia (Francisella tularensis)	Viral Hemorrhagic Fevers
Specimen[d]						
Postexposure (0-24 h)	Nasal swab, sputum, induced sputum for culture & PCR	Nasal swab, sputum, induced sputum for culture, FA, & PCR	Nasal swabs, respiratory secretions for PCR & toxin assays. Serum for toxin assays	Nasal swab, sputum, induced sputum for culture, FA, & PCR	Nasal swab, sputum, induced sputum for culture, FA, & PCR	Nasal swabs & induced respiratory secretions for RT-PCR & viral culture
Clinical illness and convalescence	Serum for viral culture. Drainage from skin lesions, tissue scrapings, tissue for microscopy, EM, viral culture, PCR	Blood for culture & PCR. CSF for Gram stain, culture, & PCR. Tissue for Gram stain, culture, IHC, & PCR. Acute & convalescent sera for toxin & antibody studies	Nasal swabs, respiratory secretion for PCR & toxin assays. Usually no IgM or IgG	Blood, sputum, & tissue for Gram stain, culture, FA, F-1 antigen assays, IHC, & PCR. Acute & convalescent sera for antibody assays	Blood for culture & PCR. Sputum & tissue for Gram stain, culture, FA, IHC, & PCR. Acute & convalescent sera for antibody assays	Serum for viral culture, acute & convalescent antibody assays. Tissue for microscopy, EM, IHC, PCR

Abbreviations: AHF, Argentine hemorrhagic fever (Junin virus); BHF, Bolivian hemorrhagic fever; CCHF, Congo-Crimean hemorrhagic fever; CDC, Centers for Disease Control and Prevention; CSF, cerebrospinal fluid; DOD, US Department of Defense; EM, electron microscopy; FA, fluorescent antibody; FDA, US Food and Drug Administration; IgG, immunoglobulin G; IgM, immunoglobulin M; IHC, immunohistochemistry; IM, intramuscularly; IND, investigational drug; IV, intravenously; NA, not applicable; PO, orally; PCR, polymerase chain reaction; RT-PCR, reverse transcription-polymerase chain reaction; RVF, Rift Valley fever; SC, subcutaneously.

[a] A human case of inhalational anthrax developed at 42 days after exposure to the accidental release of *B anthracis* in Sverdlosk, Russia. This long incubation period may have been due, in part, to the use of postexposure prophylaxis in that setting or to inaccuracies in information regarding the date of the release (or if there was more than 1). The incubation period for inhalational cases acquired outside this setting (millworkers and others) ranges from 1 to 7 days.

[b] Dosages are for adult patients only. See agent-specific recommendations for children and immunocompromised populations.

[c] Increased duration because of possibility of concomitant aerosol exposure.

[d] Should be obtained only in coordination with infection control, public health, and Laboratory Response Network.

From Woods CW, Ashford D. Identifying and managing casualties of biological terrorism. In Rose BD, editor. UpToDate. Wellesley (MA): UpToDate; 2007. (http://www.uptodate.com). Used with permission.

Part III

Lynn L. Estes, PharmD

John W. Wilson, MD

Antimicrobials

The mechanisms of action, spectrum of activity, clinical uses, route of excretion, and toxic effects of various antimicrobial agents are emphasized. Some of this information is given in Tables 15-26 through 15-36.

Specific Antibacterial Agents

Penicillins

Natural Penicillins

Agents include penicillin G (intravenous [IV]), penicillin V (oral), procaine penicillin (intramuscular [IM]), and benzathine penicillin (IM, repository formulation).

Their **spectrum of activity** includes non–penicillinase-producing staphylococci (rare), β-hemolytic streptococci (group A, B, C, G), susceptible viridans streptococci, group D streptococci, penicillin-susceptible *Streptococcus pneumoniae* (incidence of penicillin resistance is increasing), most *Neisseria meningitidis* organisms, non–penicillinase-producing *Neisseria gonorrhoeae*, and susceptible anaerobes (*Clostridium* species, most oral *Bacteroides* and *Fusobacterium* species, and *Peptostreptococcus*). Susceptible enterococci are inhibited but not killed by the natural penicillins. Other microbes that these agents are active against include *Erysipelothrix*, *Listeria monocytogenes*, *Pasteurella multocida*, *Streptobacillus*, *Spirillum*, *Treponema pallidum*, *Borrelia burgdorferi*, and *Actinomyces israelii*. Most staphylococci and gram-negative organisms produce β-lactamase that inactivates the natural penicillins.

Pharmacokinetics: These agents have short half-lives necessitating frequent administration or continuous infusions (except long-acting IM formulations such as benzathine and procaine penicillin). They are renally eliminated and require dosage adjustment with renal dysfunction. IV penicillin penetrates the central nervous system when inflammation is present. Oral penicillin V is preferred to penicillin G because it is more acid-stable and attains higher systemic concentrations (but considerably lower than with IV penicillin).

Clinical uses of the natural penicillins include treatment of infections caused by group A streptococci, including streptococcal pharyngitis and skin or soft tissue infections (when staphylococci are not suspected). Additionally, these agents can be used to treat susceptible *S pneumoniae* infections (eg, respiratory tract infections) and susceptible enterococcal infections, often with an aminoglycoside if bactericidal activity is needed. Penicillin (benzathine or IV) is the drug of choice for all stages of syphilis. Less common uses of natural penicillins include treatment of Lyme disease (*Borrelia*) and IV penicillin for treatment of meningitis caused by *N meningitidis*, susceptible *S pneumoniae*, and *Listeria*. Table 15-28 lists the pathogens for which a penicillin is the drug of choice.

- Natural penicillins are effective treatment of infections caused by susceptible *S pneumoniae*, group A streptococci, and susceptible *Enterococcus*.

Aminopenicillins

Agents are ampicillin (IV and oral) and amoxicillin (oral). The advantages of amoxicillin over oral ampicillin are increased gastrointestinal absorption, decreased incidence of diarrhea, and dosing 3 times a day instead of 4.

Their **spectrum of activity** extends the antibacterial spectrum of the natural penicillins to include certain strains of *Escherichia coli*, *Proteus mirabilis*, *Salmonella*, *Shigella* (amoxicillin less active than ampicillin), β-lactamase–negative *Haemophilus influenzae* (60%-70%), and β-lactamase–negative *Moraxella catarrhalis* (<20%). Production of β-lactamase by the organism or alterations in binding to the penicillin-binding proteins has resulted in increasing resistance by some of these organisms.

Pharmacokinetics properties are similar to those of natural penicillins. These agents have short half-lives and are renally excreted.

Clinical uses of aminopenicillins include otitis media caused by *S pneumoniae* or β-lactamase–negative *Haemophilus*, infections caused by susceptible enterococci, endocarditis prophylaxis for gastrointestinal or genitourinary procedures, and *Listeria* meningitis (IV ampicillin). Aminopenicillins also can be used to treat susceptible *E coli* infections. However, resistance to this organism has increased to the extent that these agents are no longer empiric drugs of choice for the treatment of urinary tract infections.

- Aminopenicillins are front-line agents for treatment of otitis media, susceptible enterococcal infections, and *Listeria* meningitis.

Penicillinase-Resistant Penicillins

Agents include oxacillin (IV), nafcillin (IV), dicloxacillin (oral), and cloxacillin (oral).

The **spectrum of activity** is narrow and includes methicillin-susceptible *Staphylococcus aureus* and group A streptococci. Penicillinase-resistant penicillins have no gram-negative, enterococcal, or anaerobic activity.

The **pharmacokinetic properties** of these penicillins differ from the others in that they are the only penicillins that are not cleared renally. Nafcillin has hepatobiliary elimination and does not require dosage adjustment for renal function. Similar to the natural penicillins, they have short half-lives and require frequent administration or continuous infusions. The IV agents penetrate the central nervous system in the presence of inflammation.

Clinical uses include treatment of skin or soft tissue infections because of good activity for group A streptococci and methicillin-susceptible staphylococci. In addition, these are the drugs of choice for treatment of serious infections (eg, bacteremia, endocarditis)

Table 15-26 Routes of Elimination of Antimicrobial Agents

Antimicrobial	Major Route of Elimination
Acyclovir, valacyclovir, famciclovir	Renal
Amphotericin	Cellular
Anidulafungin	Nonrenal/nonliver
Azithromycin	Liver
Aztreonam	Renal
Carbapenems (imipenem, meropenem, ertapenem, doripenem)	Renal
Caspofungin	Liver
Cephalosporins[a]	Renal
Chloramphenicol	Liver
Clarithromycin	Liver/renal
Clindamycin	Liver
Cotrimoxazole (trimethoprim-sulfamethoxazole)	Renal
Cytomegalovirus agents: foscarnet, ganciclovir, valganciclovir, cidofovir	Renal
Dalfopristin/quinupristin (Synercid)	Liver
Daptomycin	Renal
Doxycycline	Liver/intestine
Erythromycin	Liver
Fluconazole	Renal
Flucytosine	Renal
Fluoroquinolones[b]	Renal
Itraconazole	Liver
Linezolid	Liver
Metronidazole	Liver
Micafungin	Liver
Oseltamivir	Liver
Penicillins[c]	Renal
Posaconazole	Liver
Rifamycins (rifampin, rifabutin, rifapentine)	Liver
Tetracycline	Renal
Tigecycline	Biliary
Vancomycin	Renal
Voriconazole	Liver

[a] Ceftriaxone has renal and biliary excretion; cefoperazone is excreted primarily in the bile.
[b] Moxifloxacin has liver metabolism; ciprofloxacin has hepatic and renal elimination.
[c] Nafcillin has hepatobiliary elimination.

caused by methicillin-susceptible staphylococci. They are more active than vancomycin in this setting.

- Penicillinase-resistant penicillins primarily are used for treatment of infections caused by group A streptococci and methicillin-susceptible S aureus. Thus, they are useful agents for skin or soft tissue infections caused by these organisms and also are used for treatment

of serious methicillin-susceptible staphylococcal infections (eg, endocarditis).

- These agents are more active than vancomycin for methicillin-sensitive staphylococci and are drugs of choice for infections caused by these organisms.

Carboxypenicillins and Ureidopenicillins

Agents include carbenicillin and ticarcillin (carboxypenicillins) and piperacillin (ureidopenicillin).

The carboxypenicillins have a broader gram-negative **spectrum of activity** than ampicillin. When used as antipseudomonal agents, they generally should be used in combination with an aminoglycoside or ciprofloxacin. They lack good activity against staphylococci and streptococci and have little or no activity against enterococci or *Klebsiella* species.

Piperacillin has a broad **spectrum of activity** against gram-negative bacteria. Compared with penicillin G and ampicillin, it is slightly less active against streptococci and enterococci but more active against *H influenzae* and *M catarrhalis*. Piperacillin is more active than carbenicillin and ticarcillin against Enterobacteriaceae, including most strains of *Klebsiella*. In addition, it is somewhat more active than ticarcillin against *Bacteroides fragilis*. Against *Pseudomonas aeruginosa*, piperacillin should be given in a higher dosing format, and combination therapy with an aminoglycoside or ciprofloxacin has been suggested for serious infections caused by *Pseudomonas* and *Enterobacter* species.

Clinical uses of carboxypenicillins and piperacillin include polymicrobial and nosocomial gram-negative infections.

- Carboxypenicillins have improved gram-negative activity compared with the natural penicillins or aminopenicillins. However, they lack good activity against staphylococci and streptococci and have little or no activity against enterococci or *Klebsiella* species.
- Piperacillin has good gram-negative activity that includes *Klebsiella* and other Enterobacteriaceae, *Pseudomonas*, some gram-positive activity (less than natural or aminopenicillins), and some anaerobic activity against *B fragilis*.

β-Lactamase Inhibitors

Agents in this group are amoxicillin-clavulanate (Augmentin), ampicillin-sulbactam (Unasyn), ticarcillin-clavulanate (Timentin), and piperacillin-tazobactam (Zosyn).

The **spectrum of activity** of the parent drug is increased by the addition of β-lactamase inhibitors. This results in enhanced activity against β-lactamase–producing organisms such as *S aureus* (methicillin-susceptible), *B fragilis*, most *Klebsiella pneumoniae*, *H influenzae*, and *M catarrhalis*. Similar to other β-lactam agents, they are not active against methicillin-resistant *S aureus*. The addition of the β-lactamase inhibitor usually does not change the activity of the parent compound against most strains of *Pseudomonas* or *Enterobacter*.

Because they have good activity against methicillin-susceptible staphylococci and group A streptococci, anaerobes, and some gram negative organisms, **clinical uses** of amoxicillin-clavulanate (Augmentin) and ampicillin-sulbactam (Unasyn) include polymicrobial skin or soft tissue infections (eg, bite wounds, infected

Table 15-27 Mechanisms of Action of Select Antimicrobials

Cell Wall	Protein Synthesis	Cell Membrane	Cell Synthesis	RNA Synthesis
Penicillins	Macrolides, ketolide	Amphotericin	Fluoroquinolones	Rifampin
Cephalosporins	Clindamycin	Azoles[a]		Rifabutin
	Aminoglycosides	Daptomycin	Flucytosine	Rifapentine
Carbapenems	Tetracyclines, tigecycline			
Vancomycin	Chloramphenicol			
Aztreonam	Metronidazole			
Echinocandins[b]	Linezolid			
	Dalfopristin/quinupristin			

[a] Ketoconazole, fluconazole, itraconazole, voriconazole, posaconazole.
[b] Caspofungin, micafungin, anidulafungin.

ulcers, cellulitis, and oropharyngeal infections). They also are used for treatment of otitis media, sinusitis, and aspiration pneumonia. They are alternatives for community-acquired pneumonia, community-acquired intra-abdominal infections, and urinary tract infections.

Clinical uses of piperacillin-tazobactam (Zosyn) and ticarcillin-clavulanate (Timentin) include coverage for mixed gram-negative, gram-positive, and anaerobic infections (including intra-abdominal infections, complicated skin or soft tissue infections, and nosocomial respiratory tract infections) and empiric broad-spectrum therapy for polymicrobial infections. Their activity against *Enterobacter, P aeruginosa*, and other gram-negative organisms provides enhanced coverage over ampicillin-sulbactam or amoxicillin-clavulanate for nosocomial infections.

- β-Lactamase inhibitors have good activity against β-lactamase–producing strains of *S aureus, B fragilis, K pneumoniae, H influenzae*, and *M catarrhalis*. Thus, their good gram-positive, gram-negative, and anaerobic activity provides good coverage for polymicrobial infections.

Table 15-28 Primary Antimicrobial Indications for Penicillins

Gram-positive cocci	Gram-positive bacilli
Enterococcus faecalis (non-penicillinase strains)[a]	*Clostridium perfringens*
E faecium[a]	*Clostridium tetani*
Staphylococcus aureus[b]	*Erysipelothrix rhusiopathiae*
Non-penicillinase strain (rare)	*Listeria monocytogenes*
Penicillinase-producing strain	Gram-negative bacilli
Streptococcus pyogenes (group A, B, C, G)	*Eikenella corrodens*
Viridans streptococci	*Leptotrichia buccalis*
Streptococcus bovis[c]	*Pasteurella multocida*
Anaerobic streptococci or peptostreptococci	*Spirillum* spp
Streptococcus pneumoniae (pneumococcus), "penicillin susceptible"[c]	*Streptobacillus moniliformis*
Gram-negative cocci	Other
Neisseria meningitidis[d]	*Actinomyces israelii*
	Leptospira spp
	Treponema pallidum (syphilis)
	T pallidum subsp *pertenue* (yaws)

[a] Aminoglycoside used in combination with penicillin for treatment of enterococcal endocarditis and other serious enterococcal bacteremias.
[b] Penicillins (and other β-lactams) are not active against methicillin-resistant *S aureus*. Penicillinase-resistant penicillins are drugs of choice for non–methicillin-resistant *S aureus* strains.
[c] Resistance to penicillin is increasing.
[d] Resistance to penicillin is uncommon but has been found (especially outside the United States).
Modified from Wright AJ. The penicillins. Mayo Clin Proc. 1999;74:290-307. Used with permission of Mayo Foundation for Medical Education and Research.

- The addition of the β-lactamase inhibitor usually does not change the activity of the parent compound against most strains of *Pseudomonas* or *Enterobacter*. Thus, piperacillin-tazobactam and ticarcillin-clavulanate have activity similar to that of piperacillin and ticarcillin, respectively. Ampicillin-sulbactam and amoxicillin-clavulanate do not have significant activity for these pathogens.
- β-Lactamase inhibitors are not active against methicillin-resistant staphylococci. No currently available β-lactam is active against these organisms.

Adverse Reactions to Penicillins

Hypersensitivity reactions are fairly common (3%-10% of cases). These reactions include maculopapular rash, urticaria, angioedema, serum sickness, and anaphylaxis. True anaphylaxis occurs in 0.004% to 0.015% of patients receiving penicillin. Skin testing in difficult cases can be used to predict subsequent severe (type I) penicillin allergy but will not predict maculopapular drug eruptions. Patients allergic to one penicillin agent should be considered allergic to all penicillins. Furthermore, there is a cross-allergenicity rate of 3% to 7% with cephalosporin compounds, and cross-allergenicity also may occur with the carbapenems. Cephalosporins and carbapenems should be avoided when possible in patients who have had a severe, immediate penicillin allergy (type I anaphylaxis or urticarial eruption). Rash is common when aminopenicillins (ampicillin and amoxicillin) are given to patients with infectious mononucleosis—this is usually not a true allergy.

Gastrointestinal side effects to penicillins include nausea, vomiting, and diarrhea—including *Clostridium difficile* colitis. The clavulanic acid component of amoxicillin-clavulanate (Augmentin) increases the incidence of diarrhea. Rare hematologic side effects include neutropenia, platelet dysfunction, and hemolytic anemia. Drug fever also can occur with penicillin therapy. Electrolyte disturbances, especially hyperkalemia, can occur when high doses of penicillin potassium are used in patients with renal dysfunction. Central nervous system side effects with penicillin G, when given in high doses, may include tremors, lowered seizure threshold, and neuromuscular irritability.

With penicillinase-resistant penicillins, interstitial nephritis, phlebitis, hepatitis, and transient neutropenia can occur with prolonged use.

Additional side effects for the carboxypenicillins include sodium overload, hypokalemia, and platelet dysfunction. These are more pronounced for carbenicillin than ticarcillin.

- A person who is allergic to one penicillin agent should be considered allergic to all penicillins. Additionally, there is a cross-allergenicity rate of 3%-7% with cephalosporin compounds and some cross-allergenicity with carbapenems.
- Transient neutropenia with prolonged use can occur with penicillinase-resistant penicillins (eg, nafcillin).
- Additional side effects for the carboxypenicillins (carbenicillin and ticarcillin) include sodium overload, hypokalemia, and platelet dysfunction. These occur less commonly with ureidopenicillins (piperacillin).

Cephalosporins

Cephalosporins have been divided into 4 generations according to spectrum of activity (Table 15-29). In general, first-generation agents have good gram-positive activity; second-generation agents have better gram-negative and somewhat less gram-positive activity; third-generation agents have improved gram-negative activity and variable gram-positive activity; and fourth-generation agents have good gram-negative and fairly good gram-positive activity.

First-Generation Cephalosporins

Representative agents include IV cefazolin and the oral agents cephalexin and cefadroxil.

The **spectrum of activity** of the first-generation agents includes good activity against methicillin-susceptible staphylococci, β-hemolytic streptococci, and many strains of *P mirabilis*, *E coli*, and *Klebsiella* species. Similar to all cephalosporins, the first-generation agents are not active against methicillin-resistant staphylococci, enterococci, *L monocytogenes*, *Legionella* species, *Chlamydophila pneumoniae*, *Mycoplasma pneumoniae*, and *C difficile*. These agents have fairly minimal gram-negative anaerobic activity.

Pharmacokinetics: The first-generation cephalosporins are renally eliminated and require dosage adjustment for renal dysfunction.

Table 15-29 The Cephalosporins

1st Generation	2nd Generation	3rd Generation	4th Generation
Cefazolin	Cefaclor	Cefotaxime	Cefepime
Cephalexin	Cefamandole	Ceftriaxone	
Cefadroxil	Cefmetazole	Ceftazidime	
Cephalothin	Cefonicid	Cefoperazone	
Cephradine	Cefotetan	Cefixime	
	Cefuroxime	Cefpodoxime	
	Cefprozil	Moxalactam	
	Loracarbef	Ceftizoxime	
	Cefoxitin	Ceftibuten	
		Cefdinir	
		Cefditoren	

They do not penetrate the blood-brain barrier and should not be used to treat meningitis or other central nervous system infections.

Clinical uses of the first-generation agents include activity for treatment of skin or soft tissue infections caused by most streptococci or methicillin-susceptible staphylococci. Similar to nafcillin, cefazolin is often used to treat serious infections caused by methicillin-susceptible staphylococci, including bacteremias and endocarditis. They are also commonly used for surgical prophylaxis and for community-acquired urinary tract infections caused by susceptible organisms. Currently available cephalosporins are not active against methicillin-resistant staphylococci or enterococci.

- First-generation cephalosporins are active against methicillin-susceptible staphylococci and most streptococci.
- Currently available cephalosporins are not active against methicillin-resistant staphylococci or enterococci.

Second-Generation Cephalosporins

Representative IV agents include cefamandole, cefoxitin, cefuroxime, cefmetazole, cefonicid, and cefotetan. Oral second-generation agents include cefuroxime, cefprozil, cefaclor, and loracarbef.

The **spectrum of activity** of the second-generation agents is, in general, improved gram-negative activity but slightly less gram-positive activity than the first-generation agents. Of the second-generation agents, cefuroxime has the best activity against *S aureus* and β-lactamase–producing *H influenzae* and *M catarrhalis*.

Cefamandole has limited advantage over cefazolin. It has some increase in activity against *E coli*, *Klebsiella*, indole-positive *Proteus*, *Enterobacter*, and non-β-lactamase–producing *H influenzae*. It contains the methylthiotetrazole (MTT) side chain, which can produce hypoprothrombinemia (increased international normalized ratio), resulting in bleeding problems and a disulfiram-like reaction when ethanol is consumed. Cephalosporins possessing an MTT side group are listed in Table 15-30.

Cefoxitin has some increase in activity over first-generation agents against *E coli*, *Klebsiella*, indole-positive *Proteus*, and *Serratia*. It is less active against *S aureus* and streptococci than first-generation cephalosporins. It is active against most strains of *B fragilis*.

The activity of cefotetan is fairly similar to that of cefoxitin. It has somewhat better activity than cefoxitin against aerobic gram-negative

Table 15-30 Cephalosporins With Methylthiotetrazole (MTT) Side Group

Agents:	Cefoperazone	Cefamandole
	Cefotetan	Cefmetazole
	Moxalactam (also decreased platelet aggregation)	
Effects:	1. Hypoprothrombinemia (↑INR) via competitive inhibition by MTT side group	
	2. Disulfiram-like reaction (with ethanol consumption)	

Abbreviation: INR, international normalized ratio.

rods. It also has a longer half-life so can be given less frequently than cefoxitin (every 12 hours, compared with every 6). It has the MTT side chain with the associated toxicities described for cefamandole.

The oral second-generation agents have improved gram-negative activity over first-generation agents. Their activity generally includes β-lactamase–producing *H influenzae* and *M catarrhalis*, penicillin-sensitive streptococci, and many community-acquired strains of *E coli*, *Klebsiella* species, and *P mirabilis*. Cefprozil and cefuroxime have the greatest gram-positive activity of the oral second-generation agents.

Pharmacokinetics: The second-generation cephalosporins are renally eliminated. Cefuroxime penetrates the central nervous system with inflammation but has been shown to be less effective for meningitis treatment than ceftriaxone or cefotaxime (slower activity and more long-term sequelae).

The most common **clinical uses** of cefuroxime, cefamandole, loracarbef, and cefonicid are for community-acquired respiratory tract infections and urinary tract infections. Cefotetan and cefoxitin have somewhat improved anaerobic activity and are used for community-acquired intra-abdominal infections, pelvic inflammatory infections (usually in combination with doxycycline), and surgical prophylaxis for obstetric, gynecologic, and colorectal procedures.

- Cefuroxime and the oral second-generation cephalosporins often are used for community-acquired respiratory tract infections.
- Cefoxitin and cefotetan have enhanced anaerobic and gram-negative activity. They are used for community-acquired intra-abdominal or pelvic inflammatory infections and surgical prophylaxis for obstetric, gynecologic, and colorectal procedures.
- Cefotetan and cefamandole have the MTT side chain, which is associated with hypoprothrombinemia (increased international normalized ratio), resulting in bleeding problems and a disulfiram-like reaction when ethanol is consumed.

Third-Generation Cephalosporins

Representative agents are IV cefotaxime, ceftizoxime, ceftriaxone, cefoperazone, and ceftazidime and oral cefixime, cefpodoxime, ceftibuten, and cefdinir.

Spectrum of activity: The third-generation cephalosporins have improved gram-negative activity versus the first- and second-generation agents. The gram-positive activity varies, as described below.

Some organisms, most notably *Enterobacter*, have developed an inducible resistance (AmpC β-lactamases) to these agents. Because resistance can occur during therapy, these agents generally should not be used alone for treatment of *Enterobacter* infections, even if shown to be susceptible initially. Extended-spectrum β-lactamases also have been found in some strains of *Klebsiella* and *E coli* and can cause resistance to most cephalosporins and penicillins. Widespread use of ceftazidime may be more likely to select for these resistant organisms. Some hospitals have had success in reducing resistance rates by restricting use of this agent.

Ceftazidime and cefoperazone are less active against staphylococci and streptococci than most other third-generation cephalosporins. However, they have activity against *P aeruginosa* (ceftazidime greater than cefoperazone). Penetration into cerebrospinal fluid for cefoperazone is less than that of other available third-generation cephalosporins, and it has the MTT side chain with the associated potential toxic effects. Thus, this agent is rarely used.

Cefotaxime, ceftriaxone, and ceftizoxime have very similar spectra. The primary difference among these agents is their pharmacokinetics. These agents have enhanced gram-negative activity compared with the second-generation agents but in contrast to ceftazidime and cefoperazone, they are not active against *Pseudomonas*. However, they have better activity against methicillin-susceptible staphylococci and streptococci (including *S pneumoniae* organisms, which are intermediately resistant to penicillin and viridans group streptococci) than ceftazidime and cefoperazone. Cefotaxime and ceftriaxone have good cerebrospinal fluid penetration in the presence of inflammation and have a primary role in the treatment of community-acquired bacterial meningitis and other central nervous system infections.

Oral agents in this class include cefpodoxime proxetil, cefdinir, cefixime, cefditoren, and ceftibuten. They have improved gram-negative activity over the second-generation oral cephalosporins, but they are not as active as the injectable third-generation agents against nosocomial gram-negative infections. None of the oral agents are effective against *Pseudomonas*. Cefixime and ceftibuten have the best gram-negative activity of any oral cephalosporins. However, neither is very active against staphylococci, and ceftibuten has poor streptococcal activity. Cefpodoxime proxetil, cefditoren, and cefdinir have better gram-positive activity than the other oral third-generation cephalosporins, particularly against staphylococci and streptococci. Although they have somewhat less gram-negative activity than cefixime or ceftibuten, they are active against *H influenzae*, *M catarrhalis*, *N gonorrhoeae*, and many other gram-negative organisms.

Pharmacokinetics: These agents are renally eliminated except ceftriaxone, which has dual renal and hepatobiliary elimination, and cefoperazone, which is primarily excreted in the bile. Cefotaxime, ceftazidime, and ceftizoxime are usually given every 8 hours, whereas the long half-life of ceftriaxone allows for dosing every 24 hours in most circumstances. Cefotaxime, ceftriaxone, and ceftazidime cross the blood-brain barrier in the presence of inflammation.

Clinical uses: Cefotaxime, ceftriaxone, and ceftizoxime are commonly used for community-acquired respiratory tract infections, urinary tract infections, and pyelonephritis. Cefotaxime and ceftriaxone are used for the treatment of community-acquired meningitis and other central nervous system infections. Additionally, ceftriaxone is used for the treatment of susceptible viridans group streptococcal endocarditis. The long half-life of ceftriaxone permits convenient treatment of susceptible outpatient infections that necessitate IV antibiotics.

The enhanced gram-negative activity of ceftazidime (and less commonly cefoperazone) makes this agent useful for the treatment of nosocomial gram-negative infections. Ceftazidime is useful for the treatment of pseudomonal infections—often in combination with another agent such as an aminoglycoside. Ceftazidime also has been used for the treatment of febrile neutropenia.

Third-generation cephalosporins can be used for nosocomial gram-negative infections or in combination with an anti-anaerobic agent (eg, metronidazole) for polymicrobial infections.

- Ceftazidime is more active than any other third-generation cephalosporin against *Pseudomonas* and is often used for nosocomial infections or treatment of febrile neutropenia.
- Cefotaxime, cefuroxime, ceftizoxime, and the oral third-generation agents provide good coverage of community-acquired respiratory and urinary tract pathogens.
- Third-generation cephalosporins can be used in combination with anti-anaerobic agents such as metronidazole for intra-abdominal and other polymicrobial infections.
- Inducible resistance to ceftazidime and other cephalosporins can develop in *Enterobacter* organisms, and extended-spectrum β-lactamase–producing *E coli* and *Klebsiella* are an increasing problem.

Fourth-Generation Cephalosporins

Cefepime is the first of the fourth-generation cephalosporins. Its **spectrum of activity** includes gram-positive activity (methicillin-susceptible *S aureus* and *Streptococcus* species) similar to that of cefotaxime. Its gram-negative activity (including *P aeruginosa*) is similar to or better than that of ceftazidime. In addition, cefepime has a lower potential for inducing resistance and may have more durable activity against some gram-negative organisms, such as *Enterobacter*, that may become resistant to third-generation agents. However, cefepime and other cephalosporin agents should not be used against extended-spectrum β-lactamase–producing gram-negative bacilli.

Pharmacokinetics: Cefepime is renally cleared and does penetrate into the cerebrospinal fluid in the presence of inflammation.

Clinical uses: Cefepime has gained widespread popularity because of a broadened spectrum of activity and decreased potential for development of resistance compared with ceftazidime. It is useful for the treatment of nosocomial infections, including respiratory tract, urinary tract, bloodstream, soft tissue, and intra-abdominal infections, in combination with an anaerobic agent. It is also a preferred agent for treatment of febrile neutropenia.

- Cefepime has gram-positive activity similar to cefotaxime and gram-negative activity similar to or better than ceftazidime. Its spectrum includes *Pseudomonas* and *Enterobacter* species.

Adverse Reactions to Cephalosporins

Cephalosporins usually are well tolerated. The most common **toxic effects** include adverse reactions related to the gastrointestinal tract (such as nausea, vomiting, diarrhea). Hypersensitivity reactions, primarily rashes, occur in 1% to 3% of patients taking cephalosporins. Anaphylaxis is rare. Cross-allergenicity may occur with penicillins. Other adverse reactions associated with cephalosporins include drug fever and *C difficile* colitis.

The MTT side chain can produce hypoprothrombinemia (increased international normalized ratio), resulting in bleeding problems and a disulfiram-like reaction when ethanol is consumed. Cephalosporins possessing an MTT side group are listed in Table 15-30.

Ceftriaxone has been reported to cause pseudocholelithiasis, cholelithiasis, biliary colic, and cholecystitis as a result of biliary precipitation of ceftriaxone as the calcium salt in up to 2% of cases, especially in children. This effect usually resolves with discontinuation of therapy. Ceftriaxone should not be administered with IV calcium, especially in neonates, because drug precipitation has been reported.

Carbapenems

Imipenem, Meropenem, and Ertapenem

Spectrum of activity: The carbapenems have the broadest antibacterial activity of any antibiotics currently available. The gram-positive spectrum includes β-hemolytic streptococci, *S pneumoniae*, and methicillin-susceptible *S aureus*. Imipenem and, to a lesser extent, meropenem provide coverage for susceptible *Enterococcus* species (inhibited only). However, ertapenem is not active against enterococci. These agents are more active than ceftriaxone or cefotaxime against *S pneumoniae* organisms, which have intermediate resistance to penicillin (minimal inhibitory concentration, 0.1-1.0 mcg/mL), and retain some activity against strains with high-level penicillin resistance (minimal inhibitory concentration, >2.0 mcg/mL). They are alternative agents against *Nocardia*.

Regarding gram-negative organisms, the carbapenems have good coverage for Enterobacteriaceae, *H influenzae*, and *M catarrhalis*. The carbapenems remain active against most extended-spectrum β-lactamase–producing *Klebsiella* species and *E coli* as well as ampC-producing organisms such as *Enterobacter*. Meropenem and imipenem cover most strains of *P aeruginosa* and *Acinetobacter* species; however, ertapenem lacks good coverage of these organisms.

The spectrum of each of these agents also includes excellent activity against anaerobes, including *Bacteroides*, *Clostridium*, *Eubacterium*, *Fusobacterium*, *Peptostreptococcus*, *Porphyromonas*, and *Prevotella* species.

Organisms to which carbapenems are not active include methicillin-resistant *Staphylococcus*, *Legionella*, *Chlamydophila* species, *Mycoplasma* species, *Pseudomonas cepacia*, and *Stenotrophomonas maltophilia*.

Differences in spectra between imipenem and meropenem are minimal but may include slightly better gram-positive activity for imipenem (probably only clinically significant for *Enterococcus faecalis*) and slightly better gram-negative activity for meropenem (including *P aeruginosa*). In contrast to imipenem and meropenem, ertapenem lacks good coverage for *Enterococcus*, *P aeruginosa*, and *Acinetobacter*.

Pharmacokinetics: Imipenem is administered intravenously and is hydrolyzed in the kidney by a peptidase located in the brush border of renal tubular cells. Administration with cilastatin, a dehydropeptidase inhibitor, solves this problem and allows imipenem to have activity in the urine. Meropenem and ertapenem do not require the addition of cilastatin. These agents are renally eliminated and require dosage adjustment for renal dysfunction. Ertapenem has a longer half-life than the other carbapenems and can be given once daily, which may be beneficial for outpatient therapy.

Clinical uses: Carbapenems are commonly used when broad-spectrum empiric therapy is needed in patients with sepsis and for treatment of polymicrobial infections, including intra-abdominal, pelvic, pulmonary, and necrotizing soft tissue infections. Additionally, carbapenems often can be used for the treatment of aerobic gram-negative bacilli that are resistant to the other β-lactam agents (including *Enterobacter* and extended-spectrum β-lactamase–producing Enterobacteriaceae). Imipenem and meropenem also are used for

febrile neutropenia, especially when anaerobic and antipseudomonal activity is needed. Ertapenem is considerably less costly than the other carbapenems and provides cost-effective therapy for mixed infections, for example, intra-abdominal, complicated respiratory tract, and complicated skin or soft tissue infections when *P aeruginosa*, *Acinetobacter* species, or *Enterococcus* are not likely to be serious pathogens. For mixed intra-abdominal infections, it is often not necessary to specifically cover *Enterococcus*.

Toxic effects of carbapenems include nausea and vomiting, diarrhea, hypersensitivity, drug fever, and overgrowth of resistant organisms (yeast, *S maltophilia*, *C difficile*). Seizures occur rarely with these agents; affected patients are those with a history of previous seizures, renal insufficiency without proper dosage adjustment, or structural central nervous system defects.

- The carbapenems have the broadest spectrum of activity of any antibiotic, including gram-positive, gram-negative, and anaerobic organisms. They commonly are used as broad-spectrum empiric therapy, but the spectrum often can be narrowed when results of cultures and sensitivities are known.
- Ertapenem is considerably less costly than the other carbapenems yet still provides a broad spectrum of activity. However, it does not provide good coverage of *Enterococcus*, *P aeruginosa*, or *Acinetobacter* species.

Aztreonam

Aztreonam is the only commercially available monobactam and is a derivative of naturally occurring monocyclic β-lactam compounds. Aztreonam is administered intravenously and is excreted by the kidneys. Unlike other β-lactams, cross-reactivity with aztreonam in patients with a penicillin or cephalosporin allergy is rare. However, because of a similar side chain, there may be some cross-allergenicity with ceftazidime.

Its **spectrum of activity** includes most aerobic gram-negative bacteria, including *P aeruginosa*. However, it has no activity against gram-positive anaerobic bacteria, and it is not synergistic with penicillins against the enterococci (in contrast to gentamicin and streptomycin). The **toxic effects** of aztreonam are similar to those of other β-lactams.

Clinical uses of aztreonam include the treatment (as an alternative agent) of aerobic gram-negative infections, especially in penicillin-allergic patients. It may be used in combination with other agents in the treatment of mixed polymicrobial infections.

- Aztreonam is active only against gram-negative aerobes.
- Aztreonam may be useful in cases of penicillin or cephalosporin allergy because cross-reactivity is uncommon.

Aminoglycosides

Agents in this group are gentamicin, tobramycin, amikacin, streptomycin, kanamycin, and neomycin.

The **spectrum of activity** of these agents includes most aerobic gram-negative bacilli, mycobacteria (*Mycobacterium tuberculosis*, streptomycin, amikacin, kanamycin; *Mycobacterium avium-intracellulare*, amikacin; *Mycobacterium chelonei*, amikacin; *Mycobacterium* *fortuitum*, tobramycin), *Brucella* (streptomycin), *Nocardia* (amikacin), *Francisella tularensis* (streptomycin), and *Yersinia pestis* (streptomycin). They are synergistic with certain β-lactams and vancomycin in the treatment of serious infections due to susceptible enterococci (gentamicin, streptomycin), staphylococci, and several aerobic gram-negative species.

Pharmacokinetics: The aminoglycosides are not absorbed orally and are therefore sometimes used for oral bowel decontamination. They are available as IV or IM preparations, except neomycin, which is available only as a bladder irrigant because of toxicities when given parenterally. Tobramycin is also available as an inhalation formulation for local bronchial distribution. They are renally eliminated through glomerular filtration, and the half-life in patients with normal renal function is 1.5 to 4 hours. These agents have minimal protein binding and are distributed to extracellular fluid. When administered systemically, they do not achieve adequate penetration to the central nervous system, lungs, eyes, or prostate. In addition, they are less active in a low pH environment (eg, abscess).

The major **adverse reactions** to aminoglycosides include nephrotoxicity and auditory or vestibular toxicity. Neuromuscular blockade is uncommon and can occur with rapid administration of large doses. The risk of nephrotoxicity varies among the different aminoglycosides; neomycin is the most nephrotoxic, and streptomycin is the least nephrotoxic. Risk factors include increased serum trough levels, total cumulative dose, advanced age, hypotension, concomitant use of other nephrotoxic drugs, and liver disease. Aminoglycoside nephrotoxicity is almost always reversible with discontinuation of the drug therapy, and it can be minimized if dosages are adjusted to achieve desired serum concentrations and if renal function is carefully monitored. Nephrotoxicity may be delayed or decreased when the entire daily dose is administered at once (single daily dosing of aminoglycosides). Other nephrotoxic drugs such as cisplatin, amphotericin B, vancomycin, and cyclosporine may potentiate nephrotoxicity.

Unlike nephrotoxicity, ototoxicity caused by aminoglycosides is almost always irreversible. Streptomycin, gentamicin, and tobramycin are preferentially toxic to the vestibular system, whereas amikacin and neomycin are primarily toxic to the auditory nerve. Advanced age and concomitant use of ethacrynic acid or furosemide seem to be risk factors for ototoxicity. Because of the imprecision of bedside testing for auditory and vestibular toxicity, routine audiologic and vestibular function evaluation should be considered when prolonged administration is anticipated and in patients predisposed to ototoxicity. Patients also should be routinely questioned about symptoms of ototoxicity.

Single daily dosing (also known as pulse dosing) is a simplified, efficacious, and cost-effective method of aminoglycoside administration. For most infections with gram-negative bacteria, single daily dosing is as effective as the more traditional multiple daily dosing format and may lower the risk of nephrotoxicity. Single daily dosing takes advantage of 3 basic principles: 1) aminoglycosides display concentration-dependent bactericidal action—that is, higher doses and serum concentrations result in more rapid bacterial killing; 2) aminoglycosides have a long post-antibiotic effect, resulting in persistent bacterial suppression even after serum concentrations decline below the minimal inhibitory concentration (allowing for less frequent drug administration); and 3) large, single daily doses result in periods with negligible serum concentrations, reducing renal cortical and auditory accumulation of the drug. Single daily dosing should not be used for enterococcal endocarditis and requires further evaluation in select patient groups, including pregnant women, children, and persons with cystic fibrosis, severe renal insufficiency, and neutropenic fever.

Although the **clinical uses** of aminoglycosides against gram-negative infections have largely been replaced with alternative, less toxic agents, the aminoglycosides continue to play an important role for some infections. They commonly are used in combination with other agents for the treatment of endocarditis caused by *Enterococcus* spp or viridans group streptococci. In addition, they may be used in combination for serious pseudomonal and other gram-negative infections, *Listeria*, mycobacterial infections, nocardiosis, and brucellosis. The aminoglycosides are first-line drugs to treat tularemia and *Yersinia* infections.

* Aminoglycosides are active against most aerobic gram-negative bacilli and are synergistic with β-lactams or vancomycin against susceptible enterococci.
* Major adverse reactions to aminoglycosides are nephrotoxicity and auditory or vestibular toxicity.
* Aminoglycoside nephrotoxicity is almost always reversible with discontinuation of the drug therapy.
* Ototoxicity is almost always irreversible.
* Single daily dosing is a cost-effective, efficacious, and potentially less toxic form of administration than traditional multiple daily dosing.

Tetracyclines

Agents are short-acting (tetracycline, chlortetracycline, oxytetracycline), intermediate-acting (demeclocycline, methacycline), and long-acting (doxycycline, minocycline).

In regard to **spectrum of activity**, these agents are drugs of choice for *Rickettsia*, *Chlamydia* species (including pelvic inflammatory disease), *M pneumoniae*, *Vibrio cholerae*, *Vibrio vulnificus*, *Brucella* species (with streptomycin or rifampin), *B burgdorferi* (early stages), and *Borrelia recurrentis*. These agents are also effective therapy or alternatives for *Actinomyces*, anthrax, *Campylobacter*, *P multocida*, *Spirillum minus*, *Streptobacillus moniliformis*, *T pallidum*, *F tularensis*, Whipple disease, *Y pestis*, *Nocardia* (minocycline), and *Mycobacterium marinum*. Minocycline also may be active against methicillin-resistant staphylococci (for mild disease in patients who cannot tolerate vancomycin) and *Stenotrophomonas*. The tetracyclines also may be used for the treatment of *Helicobacter pylori* infection (as part of combination therapy) and for respiratory tract infections with susceptible *S pneumoniae*. Although the tetracyclines are active in vitro against many other aerobic gram-positive and gram-negative organisms as well as some anaerobes, they are usually not the drugs of choice to treat the infections caused by these organisms because of the presence or emergence of resistant strains. Further information on the clinical indications for tetracyclines is given in Table 15-31.

Toxic effects include gastrointestinal upset, rash, and photosensitivity. The incidence of uremia may be increased in patients with renal failure. Other, more rare side effects include acute fatty liver of pregnancy, Fanconi syndrome (old tetracycline), or pseudotumor cerebri. The tetracyclines are not used in pregnant females or in children because they impair bone growth of the fetus and stain the teeth of children. Coadministration of milk, antacids, iron, calcium, or calcium-, magnesium-, or aluminum-containing compounds substantially decreases the enteric absorption of the tetracycline.

In addition to its **clinical use** in treating respiratory, genital, soft tissue, tick-borne, and systemic infections with the aforementioned organisms, the tetracyclines have certain non-antimicrobial therapeutic roles. Demeclocycline inhibits antidiuretic hormone-induced water reabsorption in the renal tubule and collecting duct and therefore is used in treatment of the syndrome of inappropriate antidiuretic hormone. The tetracyclines also are a useful sclerosing agent for the treatment of refractory or malignant pleural effusions.

* The tetracyclines should not be used during pregnancy or in children because they impair bone growth of the fetus and stain the teeth of children.

Table 15-31 Primary Clinical Indications for Tetracyclines

Genital infections or sexually transmitted diseases
　　Chlamydia trachomatis (nongonococcal urethritis, pelvic
　　　inflammatory disease, epididymitis, prostatitis, LGV)
　　Granuloma inguinale (donovanosis)
　　Alternative agent for *Ureaplasma urealyticum, Treponema
　　　pallidum* (syphilis)
Atypical respiratory tract pathogens
　　Mycoplasma pneumoniae
　　Chlamydophila pneumoniae
　　Chlamydophila psittaci (psittacosis)
　　Alternative agent for *Legionella pneumophila*
Systemic infections
　　Rickettsia spp (Rocky Mountain spotted fever, endemic &
　　　epidemic typhus, Q fever)
　　Brucellosis (in combination with rifampin or streptomycin)
　　Ehrlichiosis (HME, HGE)
　　Early Lyme disease
　　Vibrio infections
Other indications
　　Tularemia (*Francisella tularensis*)
　　Bacillary angiomatosis (*Bartonella* spp)
　　Leptospirosis
　　Helicobacter pylori (in combination therapy)
　　Mycobacterium marinum
　　Pasteurella multocida (in patients allergic to β-lactam agents)
　　As prophylaxis against mefloquine-resistant *Plasmodium
　　　falciparum* malaria

Abbreviations: HGE, human granulocytic ehrlichiosis; HME, human monocytic ehrlichiosis; LGV, lymphogranuloma venereum.

Tigecycline

Tigecycline is a novel glycylcycline antimicrobial that is structurally related to minocycline but with expanded activity. It is available only as an intravenous preparation.

The **spectrum of activity** of tigecycline is wide and includes several multidrug-resistant organisms, including those that are tetracycline-resistant. Its gram-positive activity includes methicillin-sensitive and methicillin-resistant staphylococci, streptococci (including tetracycline- and penicillin-resistant strains of *S pneumoniae*), and vancomycin-susceptible and vancomycin-resistant enterococci. Tigecycline also has broad gram-negative activity, including *E coli*, *Klebsiella* species, *Enterobacter*, *Citrobacter*, *Acinetobacter*, *Stenotrophomonas*, *Hemophilus*, and *Moraxella*. It does not have appreciable activity against *Proteus*, *Morganella*, or *Pseudomonas*. It seems to have good anaerobic activity and also displays good in vitro activity against rapid-growing mycobacterial organisms.

Pharmacokinetics: Tigecycline has a large volume of distribution, indicating extensive tissue distribution. It has a long half-life with a mean of 42 hours after multiple doses. It is primarily excreted into the bile, and renal clearance accounts for only 15% to 20% of total clearance. Dosage adjustment is not required for renal dysfunction, hemodialysis, or mild-moderate hepatic impairment.

The most pronounced **adverse effect** is a high incidence of nausea and vomiting. Similar to the tetracyclines, it can cause permanent tooth discoloration if given to children younger than 8 years.

Clinical uses: This agent currently is approved by the US Food and Drug Administration for complicated skin and intra-abdominal infections. It may be useful for use for multiresistant pathogens such as methicillin-resistant staphylococci, staphylococci with reduced susceptibility to vancomycin, vancomycin-resistant enterococci, and multidrug-resistant gram-negative organisms such as *Acinetobacter* or *Stenotrophomonas* and select rapidly growing mycobacteria. However, further clinical studies are needed to confirm efficacy for these pathogens.

Chloramphenicol

The **spectrum of activity** of this agent is broad and includes inhibition of most strains of clinically important aerobic and anaerobic bacteria. Exceptions are methicillin-resistant *S aureus*, many *Klebsiella* isolates, *Enterobacter*, *Serratia*, indole-positive *Proteus*, and *P aeruginosa*. It is active against *H influenzae*, *N meningitidis*, *N gonorrhoeae*, *Salmonella typhi*, *Brucella* species, and *Bordetella pertussis*. In addition, chloramphenicol is also active against *Rickettsia*, *Chlamydia*, *Mycoplasma*, and spirochetes.

Toxic effects include 2 types of hematologic manifestations: idiosyncratic aplastic anemia (dose-independent; severe, often fatal; incidence approximately 1/24,000 to 1/40,000) and dose-related, reversible bone marrow suppression (much more common, especially with a dose >4 g/day or increased serum levels). Gray baby syndrome (abdominal distention, cyanosis, vasomotor collapse) can occur in premature infants and possibly in patients with profound liver failure who cannot conjugate chloramphenicol and who have high serum levels. Rare toxic effects are hemolytic anemia, retrobulbar neuritis, peripheral neuritis, and potentiation of oral hypoglycemic agents.

The **clinical use** of chloramphenicol has largely been curbed by the availability of potent, less toxic alternative agents. Although chloramphenicol is no longer the drug of choice for any specific infection, it still remains widely used for typhoid fever in parts of the world where cost and availability limit other drug options. Chloramphenicol remains a useful alternative agent for central nervous system infections and rickettsial infections in patients allergic to β-lactams and tetracyclines, respectively.

* Toxicities with chloramphenicol include 2 main types of hematologic manifestations: idiosyncratic aplastic anemia (very rare and usually fatal) and dose-related bone marrow suppression.

Clindamycin

Clindamycin is active against aerobic and anaerobic gram-positive organisms. Its anaerobic activity includes *Actinomyces* species, *Clostridium* (except *C difficile*), *Peptococcus*, *Peptostreptococcus*, and most *Bacteroides* species. However, 10% to 20% of *B fragilis* organisms (a gram-negative anaerobe) are resistant. Clindamycin is active against gram-positive anaerobes such as staphylococci and group A streptococci, but emergence of resistance can occur during treatment. Double-disk diffusion testing is suggested for streptococcal or staphylococcal strains resistant to erythromycin to rule out inducible clindamycin resistance. Gram-negative aerobic bacteria and enterococci are resistant to clindamycin. Clindamycin does not penetrate well into the central nervous system.

Toxic effects most commonly include rash and gastrointestinal side effects. Antibiotic-associated diarrhea can occur in up to 20% of patients, and *C difficile* colitis occurs in 1% to 10%.

The **clinical uses** of clindamycin encompass the treatment of anaerobic infections and infections outside the central nervous system. Examples include anaerobic and mixed pulmonary, head and neck, and pelvic infections. For the treatment of polymicrobial infections, clindamycin is commonly combined with a gram-negative active agent. Because of increasing resistance with *Bacteroides* species, metronidazole may be a better choice for anaerobic activity in intra-abdominal infections. Clindamycin is a useful alternative in the treatment of soft tissue infections. Through the inhibition of protein synthesis, clindamycin may reduce pyogenic toxin production. The combination of clindamycin and penicillin for necrotizing group A streptococcal or clostridial infections may be superior to either drug alone.

* Clindamycin has activity against aerobic and anaerobic gram-positive organisms.
* About 10%-20% of *B fragilis* organisms are resistant to clindamycin.
* Antibiotic-associated diarrhea can occur in up to 20% of patients, including *C difficile* colitis in 1%-10% of patients.

Metronidazole

Metronidazole is quite active against most anaerobic microorganisms, including *Bacteroides* species. The exceptions include some anaerobic gram-positive organisms including *Peptostreptococcus*, *Actinomyces*, and *Propionibacterium acnes*. The agent is also effective against infections due to *Entamoeba histolytica*, *Giardia lamblia*, and *Gardnerella vaginalis*. Metronidazole is cleared hepatically.

Toxic effects include nausea, vomiting, reversible neutropenia, metallic taste, a disulfiram reaction when coadministered with alcohol,

and potentiation of the effects of oral anticoagulants. Major adverse reactions are rare and include central nervous system effects (seizures, cerebellar ataxia, peripheral neuropathy).

Clinical uses of metronidazole are broad because of its anaerobic bactericidal activity and excellent penetration into tissues (including the central nervous system). Metronidazole is an effective drug for the treatment of serious anaerobic and mixed infections (usually in combination with an agent active against aerobic organisms), including intra-abdominal infections, central nervous system abscesses, and some skin and soft tissue infections. Oral metronidazole is the treatment of choice for pseudomembranous colitis from *C difficile*, giardiasis, amebiasis (followed by a luminal agent), bacterial vaginosis, and trichomoniasis. For polymicrobial infections, additional agents may be necessary for coverage of aerobes and certain gram-positive anaerobes.

* Metronidazole is quite active against most anaerobic bacteria. It is often used in combination with agents active against aerobes for mixed infections including intra-abdominal infections.
* Oral metronidazole is the treatment of choice for pseudomembranous colitis from *C difficile*, giardiasis, amebiasis (followed by a luminal agent), bacterial vaginosis, and trichomoniasis.

Macrolides

Erythromycin

Erythromycin is available as IV and oral preparations and is active against group A β-hemolytic streptococci (macrolide resistance is increasing), most other β-hemolytic streptococci (including groups B, C, F, and G), and *S pneumoniae* (although resistance is increasing). Most methicillin-sensitive *S aureus* isolates are also sensitive to erythromycin, but resistance can develop. Additionally, erythromycin is active against *B pertussis*, *Campylobacter jejuni*, *T pallidum*, *Ureaplasma urealyticum*, *M pneumoniae*, *Legionella pneumophila*, and *Chlamydia* species.

Toxic effects include gastrointestinal upset (dose-related), cholestatic jaundice (especially the erythromycin estolate compound), and transitory deafness (especially with large doses, such as 4 g/day). Erythromycin is hepatically cleared and can increase the serum levels of several drugs that are metabolized through the cytochrome P450 system, including theophylline, carbamazepine, and cyclosporine. High doses (usually of the IV formulation) can prolong the QT interval. A recent study indicated an increased incidence of sudden cardiac death in patients taking erythromycin, especially in combination with another drug that inhibits the cytochrome P450 3A4 (CYP3A4) isoenzyme, thus decreasing the metabolism of erythromycin.

Clinical uses: Erythromycin is a drug of choice for *M pneumoniae* infections, diphtheria, pertussis, *C jejuni* gastroenteritis, and bacillary angiomatosis. It remains an active drug for pneumonia caused by *Chlamydia* and *Legionella* species. Erythromycin is an alternative agent for patients allergic to β-lactams for treatment of mild-to-moderate soft tissue infections caused by susceptible staphylococcal and nonenterococcal streptococcal infections. Additionally, erythromycin can treat and eradicate the carrier state of *Corynebacterium diphtheriae* and shorten the duration of *B pertussis* disease (whooping cough). Erythromycin is safe during pregnancy.

Erythromycin is commonly used as a promitility agent (unrelated to antimicrobial activity) in some gastrointestinal disorders.

- Erythromycin can increase the serum levels of several drugs that are metabolized through the hepatic cytochrome P450 system.
- Erythromycin, especially in combination with other drugs that can inhibit its metabolism, has been reported to increase risk of sudden cardiac death.
- Clinical uses include treatment of atypical respiratory pathogens (such as *Mycoplasma*, *Chlamydophila*, and *Legionella*), pertussis, diptheria, and *Campylobacter* gastroenteritis.

Clarithromycin

This agent provides good **activity** against most *S pneumoniae* (resistance is increasing), β-hemolytic streptococci, viridans streptococci, methicillin-sensitive *S aureus*, *M catarrhalis*, *L pneumophila*, *M pneumoniae*, *C pneumoniae*, *Chlamydia trachomatis*, *B burgdorferi*, and several non-tuberculosis mycobacterial species. It is superior to erythromycin for *S pneumoniae* and β-hemolytic streptococci. It is moderately effective against *H influenzae*.

In regard to **pharmacokinetics**, excellent concentrations are achieved in many body fluids. The drug penetrates macrophages and polymorphonuclear neutrophils. It is available only as an oral formulation, and food has no effect on absorption. Excretion is through the liver and kidneys.

Adverse effects include nausea and other gastrointestinal complaints (less often than erythromycin). As with erythromycin, reversible hearing loss may occur at high dosages. Similar to erythromycin, drug interactions due to inhibition of cytochrome P450 enzymes can occur and close scrutiny for possible drug interactions should be performed before prescribing this agent.

Clinical uses of clarithromycin include the treatment of mild to moderate upper and lower respiratory tract infections, including sinusitis, pharyngitis, acute and chronic bronchitis, and community-acquired pneumonia. Other indications include *M avium-intracellulare* complex and other atypical mycobacterial infections, in combination with other active agents.

Azithromycin

The **spectrum of activity** is similar to that of clarithromycin. However, it is more active against *H influenzae* than clarithromycin. Azithromycin is the most active macrolide against *Legionella* species and remains active against *M pneumoniae*, *C pneumoniae*, *C trachomatis*, and *U urealyticum*.

Pharmacokinetics: Oral bioavailability is approximately 37%. Azithromycin achieves excellent concentrations in many body fluids. The agent penetrates macrophages and polymorphonuclear neutrophils. Food decreases absorption of the capsules but not the tablets or suspension. Its half-life is 68 hours, which allows once-daily dosing. In addition, for many mild to moderate infections, a 5-day course of oral azithromycin is as effective as a 10-day course with an alternative drug. Additionally, a single-dose, extended-release formulation is now available. Azithromycin is hepatically metabolized.

Adverse effects are similar to those for clarithromycin. Intravenous azithromycin can cause pain at the injection site. Unlike erythromycin and clarithromycin, azithromycin has minimal drug interactions with the cytochrome P450 metabolic pathway.

Clinical uses of azithromycin include oral azithromycin for treatment of community-acquired mild to moderate upper and lower respiratory tract infections and skin and soft tissue infections. Because of activity against *Mycoplasma*, *Chlamydia*, and *Legionella* species and the availability in an intravenous form, azithromycin IV also is commonly used with a β-lactam agent as empiric therapy for severe community-acquired pneumonia. It is theorized that there may be beneficial anti-inflammatory activity of macrolides.

Azithromycin is a first-line sexually transmitted disease agent against *C trachomatis* and chancroid, and in high doses it has activity against *N gonorrhoeae*. It is also a first-line agent for prophylaxis (in patients with human immunodeficiency virus [HIV]) against *M avium* complex and is used as alternative treatment in combination therapy against *M avium* complex, other atypical *Mycobacteria*, and *Toxoplasma gondii* infections.

Ketolides

Telithromycin is the first ketolide antimicrobial agent and is available only as an oral formulation.

Spectrum of activity: The mechanism is similar to that of macrolidies; however, because of dual binding sites, it has improved activity against macrolide-resistant *S pneumoniae*. Telithromycin also has good activity against other community-acquired respiratory pathogens including *H influenzae*, *M catarrhalis*, *Mycoplasma*, *Legionella*, and *Chlamydia* pneumonia. It has similar activity to macrolides for *Staphylococcus*, *Bordetella*, and *Streptococccus pyogenes*.

Pharmacokinetics: About 70% of the dose is hepatically eliminated, with the CYP3A4 isoenzyme being responsible for about half. Telithromycin is also a potent inhibitor of CYP3A4, and concomitant administration results in increased plasma concentrations of other drugs metabolized by this pathway.

Adverse effects: Gastrointestinal effects may be more common than with clarithromycin, cephalosporins, or quinolones. Other adverse effects reported less frequently include vision problems, including blurred vision, difficulty focusing, and diploplia. Telithromycin can prolong the QT interval and should be avoided in patients with congenital QT prolongation, patients with ongoing proarrhythmic conditions, or patients receiving class IA or class III antiarrhythmic agents. It is not recommended unless no other therapeutic alternatives are available because of reports of severe hepatotoxicity and exacerbations of myasthenia gravis.

Clinical uses: Telithromycin is comparable to the macrolides in activity against respiratory pathogens but has enhanced activity against some penicillin- and erythromycin-resistant strains of *S pneumoniae*. It is as effective as other oral therapies routinely used for community-acquired pneumonia, acute exacerbation of chronic bronchitis, and acute sinusitis.

- Telithromycin is not recommended unless no other therapeutic alternatives are available because of reports of severe hepatotoxicity and exacerbations of myasthenia gravis.

Vancomycin

IV vancomycin, a glycopeptide antibiotic, has a **spectrum of activity** against most aerobic and anaerobic gram-positive organisms. However, it is not active against certain strains of *Lactobacillus, Leuconostoc, Actinomyces,* and vancomycin-resistant *Enterococcus* species. Vancomycin is a drug of choice for infections caused by methicillin-resistant *S aureus*, methicillin-resistant coagulase-negative staphylococci, highly penicillin-resistant *S pneumoniae, Bacillus* species, *Rhodococcus equi,* and other multiply resistant gram-positive organisms such as *Corynebacterium jeikeium.* It is also an alternative agent for infections caused by methicillin-sensitive staphylococci, enterococci (synergistic with aminoglycosides), or streptococci in patients intolerant of β-lactam antimicrobials. Although vancomycin is an active agent, it is less effective than antistaphylococcal β-lactams for treatment of methicillin-susceptible *S aureus* infections and is not the drug of choice in this setting.

Oral vancomycin is not systemically absorbed and is used for treatment of *C difficile* colitis.

Vancomycin-resistant strains of *Enterococcus* are becoming a serious problem. Additionally, of considerable concern is that staphylococcal organisms with reduced susceptibility or resistance to vancomycin have been reported. Fortunately, these are currently rare.

Pharmacokinetics: Vancomycin is renally eliminated and has a half-life of 4 to 6 hours in patients with normal renal function. Dosing nomograms are available for empiric dosage adjustment for renal function, and serum levels often are monitored for further adjustments. Vancomycin has been used for treatment of central nervous system infections, but its penetration is less than that of β-lactam agents. This agent is not orally absorbed.

Adverse effects: Although rare, ototoxicity is the major toxic effect with vancomycin. This side effect is more common in the elderly and when vancomycin and aminoglycosides are administered concurrently and may not readily be reversible. Infusion-related pruritus and the production of an erythematous rash or flushing reaction involving the face, neck, and upper body ("red man" or "red neck" syndrome) are due to a non–immunologic-related release of histamine. Its frequency can be reduced by slowing the rate of infusion and by the administration of antihistamines before vancomycin infusion. Nephrotoxicity can occasionally occur, and renal function should be monitored. Chemical thrombophlebitis, hypersensitivity, and reversible neutropenia are also known side effects.

The **clinical uses** for vancomycin outlined by the Centers for Disease Control and Prevention are listed in Table 15-32.

* Vancomycin is bactericidal against most aerobic and anaerobic gram-positive organisms.
* Vancomycin is a drug of choice for infections caused by methicillin-resistant *S aureus*, methicillin-resistant coagulase-negative staphylococci, ampicillin-resistant enterococci, highly penicillin-resistant *S pneumoniae*, and *Bacillus* sp.
* Oral vancomycin is not absorbed and should not be used to treat systemic infections.
* The major toxic effect is ototoxicity. Nephrotoxicity can occur when vancomycin is coadministered with other nephrotoxic agents.
* "Red man" syndrome is due to non–immunologic-related release of histamine. This is not a true allergy.

Cotrimoxazole (Trimethoprim-Sulfamethoxazole)

Cotrimoxazole consists of 2 separate antimicrobials, trimethoprim and sulfamethoxazole, combined in a fixed (1:5) ratio. Both trimethoprim and sulfamethoxazole inhibit microbial folic acid synthesis and act synergistically when used in combination.

The **spectrum of activity** of cotrimoxazole includes a wide variety of aerobic gram-positive cocci and gram-negative bacilli, including *S aureus* (moderate activity), many coagulase-negative staphylococci, most *S pneumoniae, H influenzae, M catarrhalis, L monocytogenes,* and many Enterobacteriaceae. It is active against *Pneumocystis jiroveci, S maltophilia,* and *Nocardia asteroides, Shigella* species (although resistant strains are reported), *Isospora belli,* and *Cyclospora cayetanensis.* It is not active against anaerobic bacteria, *P aeruginosa, Enterococcus,* or many strains of *Citrobacter freundii, Proteus vulgaris,* and *Providencia.*

Toxic effects with cotrimoxazole commonly include nausea and vomiting and rash. Hypersensitivity reactions are more common in patients with AIDS, but desensitization often can be done effectively for mild hypersensitivity. Nephrotoxicity, myelosuppression, hepatitis, and hyperkalemia are less frequent but may occur, especially when high-dose therapy (eg, 15-20 mg/kg per day of trimethoprim) is used for *Pneumocystis* or *Nocardia.* Caution or avoidance should be considered during the last trimester of pregnancy (to minimize risk of

---

Table 15-32 Therapeutic Indications for Vancomycin

* Serious infections caused by methicillin-resistant strains of *Staphylococcus aureus,* coagulase-negative staphylococci, & enterococci (resistant to penicillin/ampicillin)[a]
* Serious infections caused by *S aureus,* enterococci, or streptococci in patients intolerant of β-lactam antibiotics
* Infections caused by multiply resistant gram-positive organisms (eg, *Corynebacterium jeikeium* & resistant strains of *Streptococcus pneumoniae*)
* *Clostridium difficile* colitis (oral administration) only if metronidazole therapy fails or in seriously ill patients
* Surgical prophylaxis for major procedures involving implantation of prosthetic materials at institutions with high incidence of methicillin-resistant *S aureus* or methicillin-resistant *Staphylococcus epidermidis*

[a] Vancomycin may be less rapidly bactericidal than β-lactam agents for β-lactam–susceptible staphylococci.
Data from Centers for Disease Control and Prevention. Preventing the spread of vancomycin resistance. Fed Register. 1994;59:25758-63.

fetal kernicterus). Cotrimoxazole has several known drug interactions, including increasing the activity of oral anticoagulants, increasing plasma phenytoin concentrations, enhancing hypoglycemia in patients taking oral hypoglycemics, and contributing to myelosuppression when coadministered with immunosuppressive agents.

Clinical uses of cotrimoxazole include the treatment of selected opportunistic respiratory tract infections, urinary tract infections (although resistance for *E coli* is increasing), prostatitis, and gastrointestinal bacterial infections with susceptible organisms. It is the drug of choice for treatment of *P jiroveci* pneumonia, nocardiosis, and infections caused by *Stenotrophomonas*. It is also the drug of choice for prophylaxis against *P jiroveci* pneumonia and toxoplasmosis in HIV-infected patients. It is an alternative in penicillin-allergic patients with *Listeria* meningitis.

- The spectrum of activity of cotrimoxazole includes a wide variety of gram-positive and gram-negative aerobic organisms.
- It is the drug of choice for treatment of *P jiroveci* pneumonia, nocardiosis, and *Stenotrophomonas* infections and for prophylaxis against *P jiroveci* pneumonia and toxoplasmosis in HIV-infected patients.
- With cotrimoxazole, hypersensitivity reactions are common in patients with AIDS.

Fluoroquinolones

Agents include norfloxacin, ciprofloxacin, ofloxacin, levofloxacin, moxifloxacin, and gemifloxacin.

The **spectrum of activity** of fluoroquinolones varies from drug to drug. In general, they are active against most aerobic gram-negative bacilli, including the Enterobacteriaceae, *H influenzae*, and some staphylococci. Gram-positive and anaerobic activity varies. Of concern is that bacterial resistance to fluoroquinolones is increasing, particularly among *P aeruginosa*, staphylococci, and *N gonorrhoeae*.

The fluoroquinolone agents have been divided into "generations" on the basis of spectra and drug age. These vary slightly according to the reference source but are somewhat helpful for discussing the differences in spectra among the various agents.

The first-generation agent, nalidixic acid, is no longer used. Second-generation agents include ciprofloxacin, ofloxacin, and norfloxacin. Of these, ciprofloxacin is the primary agent used systemically. These agents achieve good tissue and fluid concentrations and can be used for infections at numerous sites. Ciprofloxacin has the best activity against *P aeruginosa* of the currently available fluoroquinolones. Ciprofloxacin does not have good activity against *S pneumoniae*, and clinical failures have been reported. Thus, it should not be used empirically for treatment of community-acquired respiratory tract infections.

The third-generation agent levofloxacin has improved activity against *S pneumoniae* and other gram-positive organisms. It also retains good gram-negative coverage. It has good activity against atypical pneumonia pathogens such as *C pneumoniae*, *M pneumoniae*, and *Legionella*.

The currently available fourth-generation agents include moxifloxacin and gemifloxacin. These agents have appreciable activity against anaerobes, including *B fragilis*, and enhanced activity against gram-positive organisms, such as *S pneumoniae*, other streptococcal species, and *Staphylococcus*. These agents also remain quite active against aerobic gram-negative bacilli and have enhanced activity against atypical pneumonia organisms (eg, *C pneumoniae*, *M pneumoniae*, and *Legionella*). However, they are less active than ciprofloxacin against *P aeruginosa*.

IV formulations of ciprofloxacin, ofloxacin, levofloxacin, and moxifloxacin are currently available. In general, oral formulations should be used whenever possible because they attain plasma levels similar to the IV formulations and are much less costly.

Clinical uses of the fluoroquinolones are quite broad. They are useful for treatment of gram-negative aerobic infections such as complicated urinary tract infections (not moxifloxacin because it does not achieve optimal urinary concentrations), prostatitis, and many resistant gram-negative organisms (eg, nosocomial pneumonia).

The newer agents, moxifloxacin, gemifloxacin, and levofloxacin, are particularly well suited to treatment of community-acquired respiratory tract infections. Other uses of fluoroquinolones include infectious diarrhea, osteomyelitis, and mycobacterial infections (second-line).

Pharmacokinetics: Fluoroquinolones are very well absorbed; thus, oral therapy often can be used in place of IV therapy. Norfloxacin, ofloxacin, levofloxacin, and ciprofloxacin are renally eliminated; doses should be adjusted for renal function. Moxifloxacin is primarily hepatically metabolized. Gemifloxacin has dual fecal and urinary elimination. The fluoroquinolones (except norfloxacin) generally penetrate well into most tissues and fluids.

Fluoroquinolones are generally fairly well tolerated. The more common **toxic effects** are gastrointestinal and include nausea, vomiting, abdominal pain, and diarrhea. *Clostridium difficile* colitis is rare. Rash appears to be most frequent with gemifloxacin.

Central nervous system effects are rare (incidence is somewhat variable among the agents) but can include headache, dizziness, lightheadedness, confusion, hallucinations, restlessness, tremors, and seizures. Seizures are uncommon and usually are associated with an underlying seizure disorder or central nervous system structural defect and high doses relative to organ function.

Fluoroquinolones can cause erosions in cartilage in animals and thus are not recommended in pregnant women or in patients younger than 18 years (exceptions exist where alternatives are scarce). Tendinitis and tendon rupture are rare complications of fluoroquinolones.

Levofloxacin, gemifloxacin, and moxifloxacin all have warnings about prolongation of the QT interval in their package inserts. This adverse effect is quite rare, but these agents generally should be avoided in patients at increased risk of arrhythmias.

There are several important **drug interactions** with fluoroquinolones. Gastrointestinal absorption of the fluoroquinolones is decreased by coadministration of divalent or trivalent cations, which are found in aluminum- and magnesium-containing antacids, multivitamin preparations that include zinc, and oral iron preparations. Calcium decreases absorption of norfloxacin, levofloxacin, and ciprofloxacin. Concurrent administration of sucralfate also inhibits their absorption. Spacing the administration of the fluoroquinolone and interacting drug by several hours can minimize these absorption interactions. Some fluoroquinolones, particularly ciprofloxacin and to a lesser extent, ofloxacin increase serum theophylline and caffeine concentrations. They can also enhance the effects of warfarin and close monitoring of the international normalized ratio is recommended if used in combination.

* Coadministration of aluminum-, calcium-, and magnesium-containing antacids, oral iron preparations, sucralfate, and multivitamin preparations with minerals decreases gastrointestinal absorption of the fluoroquinolones.
* Ciprofloxacin has the best activity against *Pseudomonas*, whereas moxifloxacin and gemifloxacin have enhanced activity against community-acquired respiratory pathogens.

Other Antibacterial Agents

Linezolid is an oxalodinone that possesses activity against gram-positive bacteria, including methicillin-resistant *S aureus*, methicillin-resistant *Staphylococcus epidermidis*, vancomycin-resistant enterococci (some resistance reported), and penicillin-resistant *S pneumoniae*. Additionally, it has activity against *Nocardia* (second line) and some *Mycobacterium* species, including *M tuberculosis* and many other mycobacterial species. Linezolid is not active against gram-negative bacteria.

Pharmacokinetics: Linezolid can be administered either orally or intravenously. Linezolid is rapidly and extensively absorbed after oral dosing; its bioavailability approaches 100%. Thus, oral administration is the preferred route whenever possible. It is well distributed throughout the body and penetrates into the cerebrospinal fluid. It is hepatically metabolized with predominantly inactive metabolites excreted through the kidneys.

Adverse effects include myelosuppression and peripheral neuropathy, especially with prolonged use. Headache, diarrhea, and optic neuropathy also can occur. Linezolid is also a weak monoamine oxidase inhibitor that can interact with some medications, such as selective serotonin reuptake inhibitor or monoamine oxidase inhibitor antidepressants. Rare cases of serotonin syndrome have been reported when linezolid is used in combination with antidepressants.

Clinical uses of linezolid include the treatment of infections caused by resistant gram-positive bacteria. Many clinicians advise cautious use of this agent because of its high cost and to preserve its activity against resistant gram-positive pathogens when there are few other available options. It is an attractive alternative agent for the treatment of susceptible gram-positive infections in patients intolerant to first-line agents.

Dalfopristin/quinupristin (Synercid) acts synergistically to produce good activity against gram-positive cocci, including vancomycin-resistant *E faecium*. However, activity against *E faecalis* is substantially decreased. This agent is also active against staphylococci, including methicillin-resistant strains.

Pharmacokinetics: Dalfopristin/quinupristin is available only for intravenous administration and is hepatically metabolized. Because it can inhibit the metabolism of other medications metabolized by way of the cytochrome P450 isoenzyme, close attention to potential drug interactions is advised.

Adverse reactions include a relatively high rate of inflammation and irritation at the infusion site, arthralgias, myalgias, and hyperbilirubinemia.

Daptomycin is a novel lipopeptide antibiotic. The **spectrum of activity** includes *S aureus* (including methicillin-resistant strains), *S pyogenes*, *Streptococcus agalactiae*, and *Enterococcus* (including vancomycin-resistant strains). It also has shown in vitro activity against *Corynebacterium* species, *Peptostreptococcus*, and *Eubacterium*, *Propionibacterium*, and *Clostridium* species.

Pharmacokinetics: Daptomycin is 92% bound to serum albumin in healthy adults. It has a 7- to 11-hour plasma elimination half-life. Excretion is primarily renal.

Toxicities of daptomycin include gastrointestinal effects, hypersensitivity reactions, headache, insomnia, myalgias, and rhabdomyolysis. The manufacturer suggests stopping use of statins during daptomycin therapy and monitoring creatine kinase values once weekly.

Clinical uses: This agent is used for complicated skin and skin structure infections and bloodstream infections caused by gram-positive pathogens. A recent study found non-inferiority for treatment of staphylococcal bacteremia and endocarditis. It may find use for treatment of vancomycin-resistant enterococci, but clinical data are currently scant. It should not be used for treating pneumonia because it may be inactivated by surfactant and has poor penetration.

* Daptomycin should not be used for treating pneumonia.

Antituberculosis Agents

First- and second-line drugs are summarized in Tables 15-33 and 15-34.

For the past 50 years, isoniazid (INH) has been the cornerstone of combination drug therapy against *M tuberculosis* and for treatment of latent tuberculosis infections. It is rapidly absorbed and readily diffuses across all body fluids and tissues. It penetrates into the cerebrospinal fluid and is effective for treatment of central nervous system disease. INH is metabolized by the liver and excreted in the urine, mostly as inactive metabolites. Although the rate of metabolism is determined by genetic acetylation phenotype, the acetylation status of an individual has not been shown to influence the outcome with daily therapy. INH is safe during pregnancy. Hepatitis is uncommon but is the most notable INH-related toxicity. When it occurs, it usually develops during the first 4 to 8 weeks of therapy. INH can increase the elimination of pyridoxine (vitamin B6), resulting in peripheral neuropathy. Malnutrition, alcoholism, diabetes, pregnancy, and uremia increase the risk of peripheral neuropathy. It usually develops in a "stocking-glove" fashion and can be prevented by adding supplemental pyridoxine 5 to 50 mg/day. Hypersensitivity reactions, positive antinuclear antibody titers, and lupuslike reactions also can occur with INH therapy.

* Hepatotoxicity is the most serious adverse effect of INH.
* Peripheral neuropathy can be prevented with the coadministration of pyridoxine.
* Hypersensitivity reactions, positive antinuclear antibody titers, and lupuslike reactions can occur with INH.

Rifampin is a potent, bactericidal antimycobacterial agent and a vital component in 6- and 9-month combination treatment regimens for active infection. It is rapidly absorbed and widely distributed

Table 15-33 First-Line Antituberculosis Medications

Variable	Isoniazid	Rifampin[a]	Pyrazinamide	Ethambutol
Dosage,[b] daily	5 mg/kg (300 mg)	10 mg/kg (600 mg)	15-30 mg/kg (2 g)	15-25 mg/kg
Dosage thrice weekly	15 mg/kg (900 mg)	10 mg/kg (600 mg)	50-70 mg/kg (3 g)	25-30 mg/kg
Dosage twice weekly	15 mg/kg (900 mg)	10 mg/kg (600 mg)	50-70 mg/kg (4 g)	50 mg/kg
Major toxic effects	Hepatitis	Drug interactions	Hepatitis	Optic neuritis (↓ red-green
	Peripheral neuropathy	Hepatitis	Hyperuricemia (gout	color discrimination;
		Cytopenias (↓ WBC, ↓ platelets)	is rare)	↓ visual acuity & fields)
	Hypersensitivity reactions	Orange discoloration of body	Arthalgias	
	(+ANA 25%; lupus-like	fluids (can permanently stain		
	reaction 10%)	soft contact lenses)		
	Mild CNS effects	Bleeding problems		
		Light-chain proteinuria		
		Hypersensitivity reactions		
		Rash		

Abbreviations: ANA, antinuclear antibody; CNS, central nervous system; WBC, white blood cell.
[a] Alternative rifamycins include rifabutin 300 mg daily (dose adjustment may be needed with some antiretroviral agents) and rifapentine 600 mg weekly.
[b] Dosing (daily and intermittent) is listed for adults only; maximum recommended doses in parentheses.

Table 15-34 Second-Line Antituberculosis Medications

	Drug							
Variable	Amikacin	Kinamycin	Capreomycin	Moxifloxacin	Levofloxacin	Ethionamide	Cycloserine	PAS
Major toxic effects	Auditory toxicity	Auditory toxicity	Vestibular toxicity	GI upset	GI upset	GI intolerance	Psychosis	GI intolerance
	Vestibular toxicity	Vestibular toxicity	Auditory toxicity	Prolonged QT interval	Dizziness	Hepatotoxicity	Convulsion	Rash
	Nephro-toxicity	Nephro-toxicity	Nephro-toxicity			Hypothyroidism	Depression	Hepatitis
Elimination	Renal	Renal	Renal	Hepatic	Renal	Hepatic & renal	Renal	Hepatic & renal

Abbreviations: GI, gastrointestinal; PAS, para-aminosalicylic acid.

throughout the body and achieves moderate cerebrospinal fluid penetration. It is predominantly hepatically metabolized with enterohepatic circulation; lesser amounts are excreted in the urine. It is safe in pregnancy. Hepatitis with an increase in transaminase value can occur with rifampin; however, increased bilirubin and alkaline phosphatase levels are more characteristic. Anemia, thrombocytopenia, orange discoloration of body fluids (including permanent staining of soft contact lenses), light-chain proteinuria, and hypersensitivity reactions can occur with rifampin. Rifampin will induce the hepatic cytochrome P450 metabolic pathway, causing a substantial decrease in the serum concentration of drugs metabolized by this pathway (Table 15-35). The maximal effect of these drug interactions may be delayed 1 to 2 weeks. Drug-to-drug interactions should be kept in mind when prescribing rifampin.

Rifabutin has activity similar to that of rifampin against *M tuberculosis*. Rifabutin induces the hepatic cytochrome P450 pathway to a lesser extent than rifampin. This allows for rifabutin use by HIV-coinfected patients taking certain protease inhibitors. Rifabutin has a side effect profile similar to that of rifampin and may additionally produce uveitis, arthritis or arthralgias, leukopenia, and bronze skin pigmentation. Of note, *M tuberculosis* isolates resistant to rifampin are usually resistant to rifabutin. Both rifampin and rifabutin have activity against *M avium* complex.

Rifapentine is another rifamycin antibacterial agent like rifampin and rifabutin but has a much longer half-life. This allows for less frequent dosing, reduced total number of doses to complete treatment, and easier administration of directly observed therapy. Once-weekly rifapentine and INH may be used in the continuation phase of therapy for select non-HIV infected patients.

Two fixed-dose combination drugs are currently available in the United States for the treatment of tuberculosis: INH plus rifampin (**Rifamate**) and INH plus rifampin plus pyrazinamide (**Rifater**).

Table 15-35 Drugs With Substantially Reduced Serum Concentrations in the Presence of Rifampin[a]

Azathioprine	Opioids/methadone
Azole antifungals	Oral contraceptives
Calcium channel blockers	Oral hypoglycemic agents
Corticosteroids	Phenytoin
Cyclosporine	Propranolol
Dapsone	Protease inhibitors
Diazepam	Quinidine
Digoxin	Theophylline
Efavirenz	Tolbutamide
Haloperidol	Warfarin
Imidazoles	

[a] The list is not all-inclusive; review drug interactions thoroughly when prescribing.

Typical daily doses are 2 tablets of Rifamate (300 mg INH, 600 mg rifampin) or 6 tablets of Rifater (300 mg INH, 720 mg rifampin, 1,800 mg pyrazinamide); however, individualized dosing adjustments may be needed.

* Increased bilirubin and alkaline phosphatase values may occur with rifampin.
* Rifampin and (to a lesser extent) rifabutin induce the hepatic cytochrome P450 system, decreasing the serum concentration of many coadministered drugs.
* Rifabutin may cause uveitis, arthritis or arthralgias, and bronze skin pigmentation.

Pyrazinamide (PZA) is more active in an acidic environment and exerts potent bactericidal activity within cavitary or suppurative disease. PZA is an essential initial component of a 6-month combination drug regimen; the benefit of PZA is less clear beyond the first 2 months of therapy. PZA is readily absorbed and diffuses throughout all body fluids and tissues. It achieves good cerebrospinal fluid penetration for the treatment of central nervous system disease. Because data are insufficient regarding the potential teratogenicity of PZA, the Centers for Disease Control and Prevention recommends it should generally be avoided during pregnancy. As with INH and rifampin, hepatitis also can occur with PZA. Hyperuricemia is common, although clinical gout is rare.

* PZA is most active during the first 2 months of therapy and within an acidic medium.
* Hepatitis and hyperuricemia may occur with PZA, but clinical gout is rare.
* PZA is an important initial component of a 6-month combination treatment program for active disease.

Ethambutol is readily absorbed, with variable cerebrospinal fluid penetration. It is predominantly excreted in the urine and is safe in pregnancy. Retrobulbar or optic neuritis is the most noteworthy toxic effect of ethambutol. It usually manifests as a decrease in red-green color discrimination, visual acuity, and visual field. Caution must be used in young children because visual testing may be unreliable.

Streptomycin is one of the oldest antituberculosis and aminoglycoside agents in use today. However, because of increased global resistance, streptomycin is no longer considered a first-line agent. It requires IV or IM injection and is renally excreted. Notable toxic effects are vestibular, auditory, and renal. Appropriate drug dosing should be based on serum drug concentrations. Vestibular, auditory, and renal function should be closely monitored.

* Retrobulbar or optic neuritis is the most noteworthy toxic effect of ethambutol.
* Vestibular, auditory, and renal toxicity can occur with streptomycin.

Drug intolerance and microbial resistance are common in the management of tuberculosis and may require the addition of one or more second-line antituberculosis agents (Table 15-34). The widespread use of these agents for mycobacterial disease is curbed by reduced activity or increased toxicity or both. **Amikacin**, **kanamycin**, and **capreomycin** are injectable agents with moderate antituberculosis activity. Auditory (high-frequency hearing loss), vestibular, and renal dysfunction are the most common toxic effects. Amikacin and kanamycin are aminoglycosides, whereas capreomycin is a polypeptide antibiotic. **Ethionamide** is highly absorbed and penetrates well into the cerebrospinal fluid. Its use is usually limited by gastrointestinal intolerance (nausea, vomiting, and dysgeusia). Additional side effects include arthralgias and certain endocrine disorders (hypothyroidism, glucose abnormalities, sexual and menstrual abnormalities). **Para-aminosalicylic acid** (PAS) has been in use for the past 50 years and is formulated in delayed-release granules with an acid-resistant outer coating (Paser granules). Rash is common with PAS use, as are gastrointestinal intolerance (nausea, vomiting, and abdominal discomfort), hepatitis, and hypothyroidism. Moxifloxacin, and levofloxacin are the preferred fluoroquinolones and are commonly used as second-line agents. They have moderate antituberculosis activity and are usually better tolerated than other second-line agents. **Cycloserine** is not as commonly used because of its high side-effect profile, but it has a role against multidrug-resistant tuberculosis. Notable side effects include psychosis, confusion, depression, and headaches. Coadministration of pyridoxine may help decrease the incidence of central nervous system-related side effects.

* Amikacin, streptomycin, kanamycin, capreomycin, levofloxacin, moxifloxacin, ethionamide, cycloserine, and PAS are second-line antituberculosis agents.
* They usually have reduced activity and increased toxicity.

Antifungal Therapy

Azole Antifungal Agents

The azole antifungal agents produce their fungistatic effect by interfering with the synthesis and permeability of fungal cell membranes.

They do this through inhibition of the fungal cytochrome P450 enzyme responsible for conversion of lanosterol to ergosterol, which is a major constituent of fungal cell membranes. The azole antifungal agents are less toxic alternatives to amphotericin for many types of fungal infections.

Selected pharmacologic properties of azole antifungal agents are listed in Table 15-36.

Fluconazole

Spectrum of activity: Fluconazole has good activity against most *Candida* species (less activity for *Candida glabrata* and *Candida krusei*), *Cryptococcus*, *Coccidioides*, *Histoplasma*, *Blastomyces*, and *Paracoccidioides* infections.

Pharmacokinetics: Because of the long half-life of fluconazole, it can be administered in a once-per-day dose. It is available in oral tablet, oral suspension, and IV formulations. Because of its excellent oral absorption and the considerably higher expense of IV therapy, fluconazole should be given orally whenever possible. Fluconazole achieves good penetration into the cerebrospinal fluid and is primarily renally eliminated.

Clinical uses include treatment of many types of susceptible candidal infections. The drug also may be used for prophylaxis of candidal infection in patients undergoing bone marrow transplantation and in AIDS patients with chronic, recurrent mucocutaneous candidiasis. A concern is emergence or selection of resistant fungi, such as *C krusei*, *C glabrata*, and more rarely, resistant *Candida albicans* (especially in HIV). In serious infections, speciation and susceptibility testing of candidal organisms should be considered.

Fluconazole is also used for treatment of cryptococcal meningitis. For this infection, most experts recommend initial therapy for serious infections with amphotericin B and flucytosine, followed by maintenance therapy with fluconazole. Additionally, fluconazole has been used successfully for treatment of *Coccidioides* meningitis. It is second-line therapy for non–life-threatening cases of histoplasmosis and blastomycosis (after itraconazole and amphotericin).

Adverse effects: This agent is generally well tolerated, and discontinuation of therapy is rarely necessary. The most common effects are gastrointestinal symptoms, rash, and headache. Mild increases in liver function values are occasionally found, but fatal hepatic necrosis is rare. There is no interference with adrenocortical function or synthesis of testosterone, which can occur with ketoconazole.

Drug interactions: Although to a lesser degree than other azoles, fluconazole, through inhibition of the CYP3A4, inhibits metabolism of several drugs, including phenytoin, oral hypoglycemic agents, carbamazepine, cyclosporine, tacrolimus, dihydropyridine calcium channel blockers, and warfarin. It also can increase concentrations of rifabutin, leading to potential uveitis. Coadministration with rifampin or INH decreases serum concentrations of fluconazole.

Itraconazole

Spectrum of activity: A major advantage of itraconazole over fluconazole is its greater activity against *Aspergillus*, *Sporothrix schenckii*, *Histoplasma capsulatum*, and *Blastomycosis dermatitidis*. It also has activity against *Coccidioides immitis* and *Candida* species (cross-resistance can occur).

Pharmacokinetics: Itraconazole is available in capsule and oral solution formulations and an IV preparation. The two oral formulations are not bioequivalent; the oral solution produces considerably higher serum concentrations and higher area under the curve. For optimal absorption, the capsule should be taken with food, and the liquid on an empty stomach. Because oral absorption (especially with the capsule formulation) is erratic, serum levels should be checked to document adequate systemic levels when itraconazole is used for serious infections. The IV formulation produces higher systemic levels than equivalent doses of oral itraconazole. Itraconazole is extensively metabolized and has an active metabolite, hydroxyitraconazole. The IV formulation was recently discontinued.

Clinical uses include mild-moderate histoplasmosis, blastomycosis, coccidioidomycosis, sporotricosis, invasive aspergillosis, and

Table 15-36 Selected Pharmacologic Properties of Azole Antifungal Agents

Factor	Antifungal Agent			
	Fluconazole	Itraconazole	Voriconazole	Posaconazole
Route of administration	Oral, IV	Oral, IV	Oral, IV	Oral
Requires gastric acidity for absorption	No	Yes for oral capsules	No	No
Food requirement	No	Yes with capsule	Empty stomach	Yes, high fat
Cerebrospinal fluid concentrations	High	Minimal (but some clinical efficacy noted)	High	Low
Half-life, h	25-30	24-64	6	20
Clearance route	Renal	Hepatic	Hepatic	Hepatic
Urinary levels of active drug	High	Low	Low	Low
Dose reduction for renal dysfunction	Yes	No for oral[a]	No for oral[a]	No

Abbreviation: IV, intravenous.

[a] The manufacturer warns against use of intravenous itraconazole in patients with creatinine clearance <30 mL/min and of voriconazole with creatinine clearance <50 mL/min because of the possible accumulation of the vehicle.

onychomycosis. Itraconazole is an alternative for treatment of many *Candida* species, although cross-resistance with fluconazole can occur. Itraconazole also has been studied as a corticosteroid-sparing agent in allergic bronchopulmonary aspergillosis.

The most common **side effects** involve the gastrointestinal tract and rash. Similar to fluconazole, hepatitis can occur but is rare. At lower doses, there is typically little or no effect on glucocorticoid or testosterone synthesis (as can be seen with ketoconazole). With higher doses or systemic levels, edema, hypokalemia, nausea, and vomiting can occur. Congestive heart failure has rarely been reported in patients with cardiac disease.

Drug interactions: Itraconazole inhibits metabolism and increases serum levels of many drugs, such as cyclosporine, tacrolimus, digoxin, midazolam, triazolam, and cisapride. Cyclosporine, tacrolimus, and digoxin levels should be monitored if concomitant therapy is used. Coadministration with rifampin, isoniazid, phenytoin, and carbamazepine can decrease itraconazole levels. Itraconazole capsules require gastric acid for absorption; thus, absorption is decreased with concomitant use of histamine$_2$ blockers, antacids, proton pump inhibitors, and didanosine chewable tablets (contain an antacid buffer). These gastric pH interactions are not substantial with the oral liquid formulation of itraconazole.

Voriconazole

Voriconazole has enhanced activity against *Aspergillus* species and *Scedosporium apiospermum* (*Pseudallescheria boydii*). It also has activity against *Candida* (including many fluconazole-resistant strains), *Fusarium* species, *Cryptococcus*, *Blastomyces*, and *Trichophyton*. It also has some activity against *Histoplasma*, but it is inactive against the Zygomycetes.

Pharmacokinetics: Voriconazole is well absorbed and penetrates tissues well (including central nervous system penetration with inflammation). It undergoes hepatic metabolism through cytochrome P450 enzymes. It inhibits the CYP3A4 enzyme and thus interacts with drugs metabolized through this pathway. In patients with creatinine clearance less than 50 mL/min, IV voriconazole should be used only if the benefit outweighs the risk because of potential accumulation of the intravenous vehicle (sulfobutyl ether β-cyclodextrin sodium). Similar to itraconazole, the clinical significance is unknown.

Clinical uses: Voriconazole has good activity against *Aspergillus* and *Candida* and is a welcome addition to the antifungal agents for immunocompromised patients. Voriconazole is not approved by the US Food and Drug Administration for the empiric treatment of neutropenic fever; however, its performance and measured outcomes were closely similar to those of amphotericin. Its activity against *Scedosporium*, *Fusarium*, and *Candida* species makes this agent a useful alternative in treating infections caused by these pathogens.

Toxic effects include transient visual disturbances, which have been reported in up to 10% to 20% of patients, and rash. Similar to other azoles, voriconazole can cause increased liver enzyme values and can cause hepatotoxicity.

* Voriconazole has good activity against *Aspergillus* and has become a drug of choice for this infection.
* Voriconazole frequently causes transient visual disturbances,

including blurred vision, changes in color vision, photophobia, and other visual perception changes. These are generally mild and typically do not cause discontinuation of therapy.

Posaconazole

Posaconazole is a new triazole antifungal that is structurally related to itraconazole. Posaconazole is approved for treatment of oropharyngeal candidiasis and for prophylaxis of invasive fungal disease in immunocompromised patients. It also may have a role in the treatment of invasive mold infections, including *Aspergillus*, *Fusarium*, and the Zygomycetes.

The **spectrum of activity** includes *Candida* (including species that are resistant to fluconazole), *Aspergillus*, *Histoplasma*, *Blastomyces*, *Coccidioides*, *Cryptococcus*, and *Scedosporium*. Importantly, it is the first azole antifungal to have activity against the Zygomycetes.

Pharmacokinetics: Posaconazole is available only as an oral suspension and absorption is significantly enhanced dependent on food, especially a high-fat meal. It has a half-life of about 20 hours and is extensively protein-bound with wide tissue distribution. It is metabolized primarily by glucuronidation, with elimination in feces. Unlike other azole antifungals, it is not a substrate of cytochrome P450 enzymes. However, it inhibits CYP3A4 and can decrease metabolism of other drugs metabolized by this isoenzyme so drug interactions should be reviewed prior to prescribing posaconazole.

Adverse reactions include gastrointestinal disturbances, dry mouth, headache, somnolence, increased liver function values, and possibly neutropenia.

* Posaconazole is the first azole antifungal to have significant activity against the Zygomycetes. It also has a wide spectrum of activity for other fungal pathogens.
* Posaconazole is available only as an oral preparation and absorption is enhanced by administration with food.

Ketoconazole

Ketoconazole was the first of the azole antifungals. It has a broad **spectrum of activity**; however, because of its toxicities and the improved pharmacologic characteristics of newer agents, ketoconazole is typically no longer an antifungal drug of choice.

Ketoconazole is available only as an oral agent and requires gastric acid for absorption. It has numerous drug interactions through inhibition of the cytochrome P450 system. The most common **toxic effect** of ketoconazole is dose-related gastrointestinal upset. Decreased synthesis of adrenal corticosteroids, most notably androgenic corticosteroids, is a dose-related effect that may occur with ketoconazole. This may lead to gynecomastia, menstrual irregularities, and loss of libido with impotence. A mineralocorticoid effect can occur, producing arterial hypertension, edema, and hypokalemia. This effect has been used therapeutically for treatment of Cushing syndrome.

Polyenes

Amphotericin B Products

Amphotericin binds to ergosterol in the cell membrane and alters permeability, resulting in leakage of select intracellular contents and cell death. The **spectrum of activity** of amphotericin is the broadest of currently available agents and includes most yeasts, *Aspergillus*, the Zygomycetes, dimorphic fungi, and most dematiaceous molds. It is commonly used for serious or life-threatening fungal infections, especially in immunocompromised patients. Organisms that might exhibit resistance include *P boydii*, *Candida lusitaniae*, *Candida guilliermondii*, *Fusarium* species, *Trichosporon* species, some of the species that cause chromoblastomycosis, and phaeohyphomycosis.

Toxic effects include infusion-related reactions such as fever, chills or rigors, nausea, and vomiting. Pretreatment options (such as diphenhydramine, acetaminophen, and meperidine) may lessen these adverse reactions if a patient experiences problems. Nephrotoxicity (usually reversible) is the other major side effect of amphotericin B. This can be reduced by saline hydration, every-other-day dosing, or use of a lipid formulation of amphotericin B. Nephrotoxicity is increased with concomitant use of cyclosporine or other nephrotoxic agents. Other adverse effects include hypokalemia, hypomagnesemia, reversible anemia, and phlebitis. More rarely, changes in blood pressure, bradycardia, neurologic effects, and pulmonary decompensation can occur.

Three lipid formulations of amphotericin B are available: amphotericin B lipid complex (Abelcet), amphotericin B cholesteryl sulfate (Amphotec), and liposomal amphotericin (AmBisome). These agents have considerably less renal toxicity than amphotericin B. The incidence of infusion-related adverse effects varies among these agents; liposomal amphotericin (AmBisome) seems to have the least infusion-related adverse effects and has a lower incidence of electrolyte disturbances. Unfortunately, lipid amphotericin preparations are very expensive; however they are increasingly prescribed because of improved patient tolerability.

Clinical uses of amphotericin include the treatment of deep-seated or life-threatening fungal infections. It is often used for serious candidal infections, fever not responding to antimicrobials in neutropenic patients, invasive *Aspergillus* infections, initial treatment of cryptococcal meningitis (often in combination with flucytosine), and life-threatening or disseminated histoplasmosis, blastomycosis, and coccidioidomycosis. It is the drug of choice for treatment of infections caused by the Zygomycetes.

* Amphotericin has a broad spectrum of activity against fungal pathogens including *Candida*, *Aspergillus*, and Zygomycetes.
* The most significant adverse effects are nephrotoxicity and electrolyte disturbances. The incidence of nephrotoxicity is less with the lipid formulations of amphotericin and liposomal amphotericin has a lower incidence of electrolyte abnormalities.

Echinocandins

Caspofungin

Caspofungin was the first agent available in the glucan synthesis inhibitor class of antifungal agents. These agents inhibit the synthesis of β-(1,3)-D-glucan, an integral part of the cell wall.

Spectrum of activity: Caspofungin has activity against *Aspergillus* and *Candida* species, including most azole-resistant strains. However, it has reduced activity against *Histoplasma*, *Blastomyces*, and possibly *Candida parapsilosis* and *C guilliermondii*. It is not active against *Cryptococcus*, *Fusarium*, or the Zygomycetes). Caspofungin is available only in an IV formulation and currently is not approved for use in patients younger than 18 years.

Pharmacokinetics: Caspofungin is slowly metabolized by hepatic acetylation and hydrolysis and also undergoes spontaneous chemical degradation. Only a small amount is excreted unchanged in the urine, and dose adjustment is not necessary for renal impairment.

Clinical uses: Caspofungin is a first-line antifungal agent for treatment of serious *Candida* infections and has activity at least equal to that of amphotericin. It is an alternative agent for treatment of *Aspergillus* infections and recently was approved for neutropenic fever not responding to antibacterial agents.

Adverse effects: Caspofungin is generally well tolerated. Possible histamine-mediated effects such as rash, facial swelling, a sensation of warmth, increased eosinophils, and, rarely, anaphylaxis have been reported. Other adverse effects that have uncommonly been reported include fever, phlebitis, gastrointestinal effects, flushing, increased liver function values, and hypokalemia. Concomitant cyclosporine therapy increases caspofungin serum levels and may result in transient increases in liver function values.

* Caspofungin is useful for serious candidal infections and is an alternative for treatment of aspergillosis and neutropenic fever.

Micafungin and Anidulafungin

Similar to caspofungin, these agents were available only as an intravenous preparation and share a similar **spectrum of activity** and **adverse effect** profile. Micafungin is metabolized by the liver but not significantly through the cytochrome P450 system. Anidulafungin undergoes cellular chemical degradation (nonrenal, nonhepatic). Neither agent appears to have significant drug interactions with tacrolimus or cyclosporine.

Clinical uses: The uses are similar to those of caspofungin.

Other Antifungal Agents

Flucytosine

The **modes of action** of this agent involve conversion to 5-fluorouracil triphosphate, intracellularly, which causes miscoding of fungal RNA, and the conversion to 5-fluorodeoxyuridine monophosphate, which inhibits DNA synthesis. It has **activity** against *Cryptococcus*, *Candida* species, and chromoblastomycosis.

Toxicity is often associated with high serum levels (>100 mcg/mL). Side effects include neutropenia, thrombocytopenia, diarrhea, nausea, gastrointestinal upset, and reversible increases in liver function values. Because flucytosine is eliminated renally, it requires dose adjustment with renal dysfunction. Serum levels should be monitored and appropriate dose adjustments made to minimize toxicity.

Clinical uses include combination therapy for cryptococcal meningitis (usually used in combination with amphotericin B), *Candida* meningitis, and disseminated candidal infections (usually in combination with amphotericin). Generally, flucytosine should not be used as monotherapy because of rapid development of resistance.

Antiviral Agents

Current agents are virustatic and have no activity against nonreplicating or latent viruses. Antiretroviral agents are discussed in the chapter on HIV infection, and agents used in treatment of hepatitis are discussed in the gastroenterology chapter. Other antiviral agents are discussed below.

Acyclovir

Acyclovir is a nucleoside analogue of guanosine. It is phosphorylated by virus-specific thymidine kinase to monophosphate and further phosphorylated to the triphosphate form by cellular enzymes. Acyclovir triphosphate inhibits viral DNA polymerase and also acts as a DNA chain terminator.

Acyclovir has good **activity** against herpes simplex viruses 1 and 2 and varicella-zoster virus. It has considerably less activity against Epstein-Barr virus and cytomegalovirus. Resistance to acyclovir can develop through mutations of either viral thymidine kinase or DNA polymerase.

Oral acyclovir is poorly absorbed (bioavailability of 15%-30%). Thus, patients with severe disease or who are immunocompromised should receive IV therapy. Acyclovir generally is well tolerated.

Toxic effects include gastrointestinal distress, headaches, and phlebitis (IV form). Reversible renal dysfunction resulting from crystalline nephropathy can occur with high-dose IV therapy. The risk can be decreased by saline hydration and appropriate dose adjustment for renal function. Confusion, delirium, lethargy, and seizures can occur with high-dose IV therapy in patients with high serum concentrations.

Clinical uses for acyclovir include herpes simplex virus infections (noncurative). It is effective for treatment of primary and recurrent episodes of herpes genitalis and for chronic suppression in patients with frequent recurrences. Topical acyclovir is less effective than oral therapy in genital herpes simplex virus infection. In immunocompromised patients, oral or IV acyclovir is effective in the suppression and treatment of oral-labial disease. High-dose IV acyclovir is the drug of choice for herpes simplex virus encephalitis.

Acyclovir also is used for varicella-zoster virus. In immunocompetent patients with primary varicella, it can shorten the healing time (about 1 day) and decrease the number of lesions if given early (within 24 hours). IV acyclovir in immunocompromised patients can halt progression and prevent dissemination of varicella-zoster. Varicella-zoster responds to oral acyclovir but at higher doses than those required for herpes simplex virus 1 or herpes simplex virus 2. Treatment of varicella-zoster virus decreases viral shedding and time to healing. However, it is effective only if given within 72 hours of the onset of symptoms. Early administration may also decrease postherpetic neuralgia.

* Crystalline nephropathy can occur with high-dose IV therapy. Its incidence can be reduced by saline hydration and appropriate dose adjustment for renal function.
* IV acyclovir is the drug of choice for herpes simplex virus encephalitis.
* Effective therapy of varicella-zoster virus requires higher doses of acyclovir than herpes simplex virus 1 or 2.

Valacyclovir

Valacyclovir is an oral prodrug of acyclovir that is converted extensively and almost completely to acyclovir (the active drug) and L-valine. Approximately 54% to 60% of the valacyclovir dose is available as active acyclovir, representing a 2-fold to 5-fold increase in bioavailability over that achieved after administration of oral acyclovir. The higher bioavailability of valacyclovir also allows for less frequent administration than with oral acyclovir. Like acyclovir, valacyclovir generally is well tolerated.

Toxic effects with valacyclovir are very similar to those with acyclovir. However, when valacyclovir was studied in very high doses (8 g/day) in immunosuppressed patients (patients who had transplant and patients with HIV), thrombotic thrombocytopenic purpura and hemolytic uremic syndrome were reported.

Clinical uses of valacyclovir include the treatment of varicella-zoster infections and the treatment and suppression of recurrent genital herpes infections (noncurative). Like acyclovir, valacyclovir may decrease postherpetic neuralgia.

* Valacyclovir is an oral prodrug of acyclovir that increases bioavailability 2-fold to 5-fold. For most indications it can be given less frequently than oral acyclovir.

Famciclovir

Famciclovir is an oral prodrug that is converted to its active form, penciclovir, through tissue and hepatic enzymatic processes. A prolonged intracellular half-life allows for dosing 3 times daily. It has good bioavailability and is well tolerated.

Clinical uses are similar to those of valacyclovir. It is useful for herpes simplex and varicella-zoster virus infections. It may reduce the duration of postherpetic neuralgia when given early in varicella-zoster infections. Similar to acyclovir and famciclovir, it is not effective against cytomegalovirus or Epstein-Barr virus.

Ganciclovir

This agent inhibits DNA polymerase and is dependent on phosphorylation by viral thymidine kinase. Like acyclovir, valacyclovir, and famciclovir, ganciclovir is active against herpes simplex viruses and varicella-zoster. However, it is about 10 times more potent than acyclovir against cytomegalovirus and Epstein-Barr virus and also has activity against human herpesvirus 6. It is available as oral, IV, and ocular preparations. The oral formulation is poorly absorbed, and thus IV therapy is needed for serious disease. Valganciclovir (see below) is an oral prodrug of ganciclovir that achieves significantly higher levels than oral ganciclovir.

Toxic effects include neutropenia and thrombocytopenia. The incidence of neutropenia may be increased when ganciclovir is used in combination with other immunosuppressive drugs. Cytopenias are reversible after use of the drug is stopped. It is teratogenic, carcinogenic, and mutagenic in animals. Less common side effects include fever, rash, anemia, and increased values on liver function tests. Like acyclovir, it is renally eliminated and close monitoring of renal function is required. Dosage adjustment for IV ganciclovir is needed even in the presence of mild renal impairment.

Clinical uses for ganciclovir include treatment of cytomegalovirus retinitis in patients with AIDS. Studies also have shown beneficial results in other cytomegalovirus infections (colitis, esophagitis, gastritis, and pneumonia) and in immunocompromised hosts. In patients with AIDS, maintenance therapy may be necessary to prevent relapse. Used in combination with hyperimmune globulin, ganciclovir reduces mortality from cytomegalovirus pneumonitis in patients who have had allogeneic bone marrow transplant. Oral and IV ganciclovir therapy may be given to at-risk patients before transplant to prevent cytomegalovirus infection.

Although in vitro activity is seen for Epstein-Barr virus and human herpesvirus 6, clinical efficacy remains unclear.

Oral ganciclovir is an alternative to IV maintenance therapy for cytomegalovirus retinitis in patients who have only peripheral cytomegalovirus lesions. Unfortunately, the oral formulation has poor bioavailability levels.

Ganciclovir ocular implants provide the drug directly to the site of the infection in patients with cytomegalovirus retinitis. Vitrasert implants are surgically implanted into the pars plana and deliver a slow release of drug over 7 to 8 months. Possible disadvantages include the spread of infection to the contralateral eye (thus it is often given with a systemic agent), a low incidence of endophthalmitis, and the need to replace the inserts.

* Ganciclovir is used for cytomegalovirus infections in immunocompromised patients.
* Bone marrow suppression is the most serious adverse effect. The incidence may be increased when ganciclovir is used in combination with other immunosuppressive drugs.

Valganciclovir

Valganciclovir is an oral prodrug of ganciclovir with 60% bioavailability. Once absorbed, it is rapidly converted to ganciclovir and achieves a similar area under the curve as IV ganciclovir. It is not a substitute on a "1-for-1" basis with ganciclovir (IV or oral) because valganciclovir has its own dosing platform. Its toxicity profile is similar to that of ganciclovir.

Clinical uses are directed against cytomegalovirus infection. It is approved for treatment of cytomegalovirus retinitis in HIV-infected patients, and the efficacy of valganciclovir has been shown to be similar to that of IV ganciclovir for induction therapy. Oral valganciclovir also has been used for treatment of cytomegalovirus disease in transplant and other immunocompromised patients.

Foscarnet

Foscarnet is a noncompetitive inhibitor of viral DNA polymerase and reverse transcriptase. It does not require phosphorylation and is often active against acyclovir-resistant and ganciclovir-resistant strains. It has in vitro activity against all human herpesviruses, HIV, and hepatitis B.

Toxic effects include nephrotoxicity, which usually develops during the second week and is reversible. Substantial renal impairment develops in about a third of patients. The risk of nephrotoxicity is increased with concurrent use of nephrotoxic drugs (eg, amphotericin B, aminoglycosides, and cyclosporine). Saline hydration may decrease the risk of nephrotoxicity.

Foscarnet is renally eliminated, and close renal monitoring is required to reduce adverse effects. Like IV ganciclovir, foscarnet requires dose adjustment with mild renal impairment.

Electrolyte disturbances, such as hypocalcemia, hyperphosphatemia, hypophosphatemia, hypokalemia, and hypomagnesemia, also commonly occur. Central nervous system side effects, fever, nausea, vomiting, anemia, fatigue, headache, leukopenia, pancreatitis, and genital ulceration also have been reported.

Clinical uses of foscarnet include treatment of ganciclovir-resistant cytomegalovirus disease and acyclovir-resistant herpes simplex virus or varicella-zoster virus. Occasionally, foscarnet has been used in combination with ganciclovir for severe cytomegalovirus retinitis.

* Foscarnet is effective for cytomegalovirus infections, including most strains that are resistant to ganciclovir.
* Nephrotoxicity is the major dose-limiting side effect. It usually develops during the second week and is reversible.

Cidofovir

Cidofovir is a nucleotide analogue with activity against herpesviruses, including cytomegalovirus, herpes simplex virus, varicella-zoster virus, and Epstein-Barr virus. Its US Food and Drug Administration indication is for the treatment of cytomegalovirus retinitis in patients with AIDS. Conversion of cidofovir to its active intracellular metabolite is performed by host (rather than viral) cellular phosphorylating enzymes. Thus, cidofovir may retain activity against ganciclovir-resistant strains of cytomegalovirus and acyclovir resistant strains of herpes simplex virus. The long intracellular half-life of cidofovir-active metabolites allows for weekly intravenous dosing during induction therapy and every-other-week IV administration during maintenance therapy.

The dose-limiting **toxic effect** of cidofovir is nephrotoxicity. Administration with probenecid and saline hydration decreases the incidence and severity of nephrotoxicity. Cidofovir is contraindicated in patients with preexisting renal dysfunction (serum creatinine >1.5 mg/dL, estimated creatinine clearance <55 mL/min, or urine protein ≥100 mg/dL), and renal function must be monitored closely during therapy. Optimally, it should not be given with other nephrotoxic drugs. Neutropenia also has been reported in up to 20% of patients. More rare adverse reactions include ocular hypotony and metabolic acidosis. Adverse effects to probenecid are also fairly common.

Amantadine and Rimantadine

Because of the high rates of resistance of influenza virus to amantadine and rimantadine, the Centers for Disease Control and Prevention no longer recommend use of these agents for treatment or prophylaxis of influenza virus.

Oseltamivir and Zanamivir

These agents are selective inhibitors of viral neuraminidase. Unlike amantadine and rimantadine, the newer agents—oseltamivir and zanamivir—have activity against both influenza A and influenza B viruses. They may convey some protective effect against avian flu, but they have not been highly tested for this use. Resistance is also much more difficult to induce with the newer agents than with amantadine or rimantadine.

Pharmacokinetics: Oseltamivir is available as oral tablets and is dosed twice daily. It is eliminated renally, and dose adjustment is necessary in patients with renal impairment. Zanamivir is available as an inhaled preparation and is dosed as 2 puffs given twice daily. It is dispensed with a special inhalation device called a Diskhaler. Demonstration of the use of this device needs to be provided to patients when this agent is prescribed. Some elderly patients or patients without good manual dexterity may find it difficult to use the device.

Oseltamivir is generally well tolerated. The primary **adverse effects** are nausea and vomiting. These occur in about 10% of patients and are usually not severe. Zanamivir is also generally well tolerated. However, it should not be prescribed for patients with underlying airway disease because they may experience bronchospasm or serious breathing problems. In addition, the drug has not been proved efficacious in this patient population. Elderly patients or patients with poor dexterity may have difficulty with the manipulation required for zanamivir inhalation.

Clinical uses for zanamivir and oseltamivir include the treatment and prophylaxis of influenza A virus and influenza B virus. They are considerably more expensive than amantadine or rimantadine. However, in comparison with the older agents, zanamivir and oseltamivir have the advantages of providing coverage against influenza B (which is less common than influenza A) and of having less resistance induction potential (clinical implications unclear). No studies have been done to compare these newer antiviral agents with the older agents. With both oseltamivir and zanamivir, treatment needs to be started very early after onset of symptoms (within 24-48 hours). These agents can reduce the severity and duration of symptoms (usually by about 1 day). They have not been highly tested in critically ill patients. Oseltamivir and zanamavir may convey some protective effect against avian flu.

Infectious Diseases Pharmacy Review
Lisa K. Buss, PharmD, Lynn L. Estes, PharmD

Drug	Primary Toxic/Adverse Effects	Primary Drug Interactions
Antibacterials		
Penicillins	Hypersensitivity reactions, GI effects (nausea, vomiting, diarrhea), interstitial nephritis, hematologic effects (anemia, neutropenia, thrombocytopenia, platelet dysfunction)	Probenecid
Natural penicillins		
Penicillin G		
Penicillin V		
Aminopenicillins		
Amoxicillin		
Amoxicillin-clavulanate	Clavulanate may cause diarrhea	
Ampicillin	Higher incidence of diarrhea than with amoxicillin	Allopurinol
Penicillinase-resistant penicillins		
Cloxacillin		
Dicloxacillin		
Nafcillin	Thrombophlebitis, hepatitis, neutropenia	
Oxacillin	Thrombophlebitis, hepatitis, neutropenia	
Extended-spectrum penicillins		
Ticarcillin	Hypokalemia, hypernatremia, bleeding	
Ticarcillin-clavulanate	Clavulanate may cause diarrhea, hypokalemia, hypernatremia, bleeding	
Piperacillin	Neutropenia, thrombocytopenia	
Piperacillin-tazobactam	Neutropenia, thrombocytopenia	
Cephalosporins	Hypersensitivity reactions, GI effects, hematologic effects, interstitial nephritis; cephalosporins with MTT side chains can cause hypoprothrombinemia & disulfiram-like reactions with alcohol	Probenecid
First-generation		
Cefadroxil		
Cefazolin		
Cephalexin		
Cephradine		
Second-generation		
Cefaclor		
Cefotetan	MTT side chain	Alcohol, warfarin
Cefoxitin		
Cefprozil		
Cefuroxime		
Cefuroxime axetil		Drugs that increase gastric pH
Third-generation		
Cefdinir		Antacids, iron supplements
Cefixime		
Cefoperazone	MTT side chain	Alcohol
Cefotaxime		
Cefpodoxime		Drugs that increase gastric pH
Ceftazidime		
Ceftibuten		
Ceftizoxime		
Ceftriaxone	Biliary sludge, gallstones	
Fourth-generation		
Cefepime		

Infectious Diseases Pharmacy Review (continued)

Drug	Primary Toxic/Adverse Effects	Primary Drug Interactions
Antibacterials (continued)		
Carbapenems	Nausea, vomiting, diarrhea, hypersensitivity reactions, injection site reaction, seizures (rare)	Probenecid
Ertapenem		
Imipenem-cilastatin		
Meropenem		
Aztreonam	Rash, diarrhea, nausea, vomiting	Probenecid
Aminoglycosides	Nephrotoxicity, auditory toxicity, vestibular toxicity, neuromuscular blockade	Other nephrotoxic or ototoxic drugs
Amikacin		
Gentamicin		
Kanamycin		
Neomycin		
Streptomycin		
Tobramycin		
Tetracyclines	Photosensitivity, permanent staining of developing teeth, GI upset, rash	Antacids, warfarin, digoxin, isotretinoin, iron
Demeclocycline		
Doxycycline		
Minocycline	Vestibular toxicity	
Tetracycline		
Tigecycline	Nausea, vomiting, diarrhea, staining of developing teeth	Warfarin
Chloramphenicol	Aplastic anemia, bone marrow suppression, gray baby syndrome, optic & peripheral neuritis	Phenytoin, rifampin
Clindamycin	Diarrhea, *Clostridium difficile* colitis, nausea, vomiting	Neuromuscular blockers
Metronidazole	Nausea, diarrhea, disulfiram-like reaction, metallic taste, reversible neutropenia	Alcohol, warfarin
Macrolides		
Azithromycin	Diarrhea, nausea	Warfarin, pimozide
Clarithromycin	Nausea, diarrhea, metallic taste	Similar to erythromycin
Erythromycin	GI effects, cholestatic jaundice, transient hearing loss, ventricular arrhythmias	Benzodiazepines, carbamazepine, cyclosporine, pimozide, theophylline, warfarin, digoxin, ergot alkaloids, cisapride, drugs that prolong QT interval
Ketolides		
Telithromycin	Prolong QTc interval, nausea, diarrhea, dizziness, headache, visual effects, loss of consciousness, hepatotoxicity, contraindicated in myesthenia gravis	Azole antifungals, rifampin, phenytoin, carbamazepine, phenobarbital, digoxin, lovastatin, atorvastatin, simvastatin, drugs that prolong QT interval, CYP3A4 inhibitor; prescribing info should be checked for full interactions
Vancomycin	Ototoxicity, red man syndrome, nephrotoxicity, chemical thrombophlebitis, reversible neutropenia	Aminoglycosides & other nephrotoxic or ototoxic drugs

Infectious Diseases Pharmacy Review (continued)

Drug	Primary Toxic/Adverse Effects	Primary Drug Interactions
Antibacterials (continued)		
Trimethoprim-sulfamethoxazole	Nausea, vomiting, hypersensitivity reactions (especially common in patients with AIDS)	Sulfonylureas, methotrexate, phenytoin, warfarin
Fluoroquinolones	GI effects, CNS effects, photosensitivity, arthropathy, tendon rupture, hypersensitivity	Antacids, calcium, iron, warfarin, sucralfate
Second-generation		
Ciprofloxacin		Theophylline, caffeine
Lomefloxacin		
Norfloxacin		
Ofloxacin		
Third-generation		
Levofloxacin	QT interval prolongation	Medications that can prolong the QT interval
Fourth-generation		
Moxifloxacin	QT interval prolongation	Medications that can prolong the QT interval
Gemifloxacin	QT interval prolongation	Medications that can prolong the QT interval
Trovafloxacin	Limited to inpatient use because of risk of hepatotoxicity	
Linezolid	Thrombocytopenia, diarrhea, nausea, optic neuritis, peripheral neuropathy, lactic acidosis	MAO inhibitors, tyramine-containing foods, pseudoephedrine, SSRI antidepressants, tramadol
Dalfopristin/quinupristin	Pain, edema, or inflammation at infusion site, arthralgia, myalgia, hyperbilirubinemia	Carbamazepine, cycloserine, delavirdine, diltiazem, HMG-CoA reductase inhibitors, methylprednisolone, midazolam, nevirapine, nifedipine, paclitaxel, tacrolimus, verapamil
Rifamixin	Nausea, vomiting, flatulence, rash	
Antituberculosis agents		
Isoniazid	Hepatitis, hypersensitivity reactions, lupus-like reactions, peripheral neuropathy	Carbamazepine, cycloserine, phenytoin, levodopa, prednisone, theophylline, warfarin
Rifampin & rifapentine	Orange discoloration of body fluids, leukopenia, thrombocytopenia, proteinuria, hypersensitivity reactions, hepatitis	Warfarin, azole antifungals, barbiturates, benzodiazepines, corticosteroids, cyclosporine, digoxin, estrogens, macrolides, protease inhibitors, tacrolimus, thyroid replacements, potent CYP inducer; prescribing info should be checked for full interactions

Infectious Diseases Pharmacy Review (continued)

Drug	Primary Toxic/Adverse Effects	Primary Drug Interactions
Antibacterials (continued)		
Antituberculosis agents (continued)		
Rifabutin	Neutropenia, body fluid discoloration, GI intolerance, rash, uveitis, increased values on liver function tests	Warfarin, azole antifungals, cyclosporine, hydantoins, macrolides, methadone, quinine, theophylline, protease inhibitors, CYP inducer; prescribing info should be checked for full interactions
Pyrazinamide	Hepatitis, hyperuricemia, nausea, anorexia, polyarthralgia	Ethionamide, probenecid
Ethambutol	Optic neuritis, hyperuricemia	Aluminum salts
Capreomycin	Ototoxicity, tinnitus, nephrotoxicity	Nephrotoxic agent such as aminoglycosides
Ethionamide	Anorexia, nausea, vomiting, gynecomastia, postural hypotension, drowsiness, asthenia, hepatitis, hypothyroidism	Isoniazid, cycloserine
Para-aminosalicylic acid	Rash, GI intolerance, hypersensitivity	
Cycloserine	CNS toxic effects (somnolence, headache, tremor, psychosis, seizures)	Ethionamide, isoniazid, alcohol
Antifungal agents		
Amphotericin B products	Infusion-related reactions (fever, chills, rigors, nausea, hypertension, hypotension), nephrotoxicity (less with lipid formulations), hypokalemia, hypomagnesemia	Other nephrotoxic agents
Flucytosine	Bone marrow suppression, GI effects, increased values on liver function tests	
Azole antifungals	GI upset, rash, pruritus, increased values on liver function tests, QT prolongation	Carbamazapine, cyclosporine, dihydropyridine, calcium channel blockers, barbiturates, phenytoin, rifampin, tacrolimus, warfarin, drugs that prolong the QT interval, potent CYP3A4 inhibitors & substrates; prescribing info should be checked for full interactions
Ketoconazole	Gynecomastia, diminished libido, impotence, menstrual irregularities, adrenal suppression, hypokalemia, edema	Antacids, corticosteroids, H$_2$-receptor blockers, HMG-CoA reductase inhibitors, proton pump inhibitors
Fluconazole	Headache	
Itraconazole	Headache, dizziness, hypokalemia, hypertension, edema, congestive heart failure	Antacids, corticosteroids, digoxin, H$_2$-receptor blockers, proton pump inhibitors, sucralfate
Posaconazole		
Voriconazole	Visual disturbances, nausea, vomiting	Sirolimus, tacrolimus, HMG-CoA reductase inhibitors, vinca alkaloids

Infectious Diseases Pharmacy Review (continued)

Drug	Primary Toxic/Adverse Effects	Primary Drug Interactions
Antifungal agents (continued)		
Echinocandins	Facial swelling, increased LFTs (rare) rash	
Caspofungin		Tacrolimus, cyclosporine,
Micafungin		sirolimus, nifedipine diluent
Anidulafungin		contains alcohol equivalent
		to about 1 drink per day
Antiviral agents		
Amantadine	Nausea, dizziness, light-headedness, insomnia, delirium	
Rimantadine	Insomnia, dizziness, nervousness, nausea, vomiting	
Oseltamivir	Nausea, vomiting, diarrhea, abdominal pain	
Zanamivir	Nausea, diarrhea, nasal symptoms, bronchospasm	
Acyclovir	Malaise, nausea, vomiting, diarrhea, phlebitis (IV), nephrotoxicity (IV)	
Famciclovir	Headache, nausea, diarrhea	
Ganciclovir	Diarrhea, nausea, anorexia, vomiting, leukopenia, neutropenia, anemia	Probenecid, zidovudine
Valacyclovir	Nausea, headache, diarrhea	
Valganciclovir	Headache, insomnia, diarrhea, nausea, leukopenia, neutropenia, anemia	Probenecid, zidovudine
Foscarnet	Renal impairment, leukopenia, electrolyte disturbances	Nephrotoxic drugs, medications that can prolong the QT interval
Cidofovir	Renal impairment, neutropenia, ocular hypotonia, headache, asthenia, alopecia, rash, GI distress	Nephrotoxic drugs
Ribavirin	Pruritus, nausea, headache, fatigue	Didanosine, abacavir, lamivudine, stavudine, zalcitabine, zidovudine
Adefovir	Stomach pain, weakness, headache, risk of hepatitis, nephrotoxicity, lactic acidosis	No known drug interactions
Entecavir	Headache, fatigue, dizziness, nausea, risk of hepatomegaly or lactic acidosis	No known drug interactions, administer 2 h before or after high-fat meals

Abbreviations: CNS, central nervous system; CYP, cytochrome P450; GI, gastrointestinal; H_2, histamine$_2$; HMG-CoA, 3-hydroxy-3-methylglutaryl coenzyme-A; IV, intravenous; LFT, liver function test (results); MAO, monoamine oxidase; MTT, methylthiotetrazole; SSRI, selective serotonin reuptake inhibitor.

Questions

Multiple Choice (choose the best answer)

1. A 57-year-old woman underwent transsphenoidal resection of a pituitary tumor 4 weeks ago. Her postoperative course was complicated by ongoing leakage of cerebrospinal fluid. Today she presents with new onset of fever, headache, and confusion. Meningeal signs are noted on examination. Which of the following bacteria will most likely grow from culture of this patient's spinal fluid?

   a. *Streptococcus pneumoniae*
   b. *Neisseria meningitidis*
   c. *Staphylococcus aureus*
   d. *Pseudomonas aeruginosa*
   e. *Listeria monocytogenes*

2. A 61-year-old woman presents with a 3-month history of low-grade fever and weight loss. A loud systolic murmur is found on cardiac auscultation. Two blood cultures yield *Enterococcus faecalis*. At echocardiography, a 9-mm vegetation is seen on a bicuspid aortic valve. Therapy is initiated with intravenous ampicillin, to which the *Enterococcus* is susceptible. The patient improves clinically during a 4-week course of antibiotic therapy. However, 2 weeks after the ampicillin therapy is stopped, the patient is again febrile. Blood cultures again yield *E faecalis* with the same susceptibility pattern. Which of the following interventions is indicated?

   a. Resume therapy with intravenous ampicillin and complete 6 weeks of therapy.
   b. Resume therapy with intravenous ampicillin, add intravenous gentamicin, and complete 6 weeks of therapy.
   c. Initiate therapy with intravenous ampicillin/sulbactam (Unasyn) and continue for 6 weeks.
   d. Resume therapy with intravenous ampicillin and recommend aortic valve replacement.
   e. Initiate therapy with intravenous vancomycin and intravenous gentamicin and continue for 6 weeks.

3. A 26-year-old sexually active woman presents to your office for counseling. She has had recurrent episodes of genital herpes for the past 3 years for which she has used self-treatment with acyclovir. She is now in a monogamous relationship with her fiancé, who is unaware of her history of genital herpes. They have consistently used latex condoms since being together but would like to get pregnant shortly after their marriage. She would like your advice on what to do to avoid infecting her new partner with herpes simplex virus. Which of the following should you advise?

   a. Tell her to have the fiancé tested because he is also probably positive for the virus.
   b. Tell her that infection of her future spouse is inevitable and she should tell him now.

   c. Tell her not to worry because genital herpes is not serious.
   d. Tell her that in 70% of cases transmission occurs during symptomatic outbreaks.
   e. Advise her that treatment with valacyclovir 500 mg daily may reduce her partner's risk of acquiring herpes simplex virus type 2 by approximately 50%.

4. A 71-year-old woman is brought to the emergency department after being found confused and disoriented at home by her family. She is febrile, disoriented, and aphasic and shortly thereafter has a seizure. She is stabilized. CT of the head excludes a hematoma. MRI of the head shows hemorrhagic changes in the right temporal lobe. The leukocyte count is $11,000 \times 10^9/L$, and results of routine biochemical analyses are normal. The total nucleated cell count in the cerebrospinal fluid sample is 35 cells/mm^3, erythrocytes 8,645/mm^3, glucose 45 mg/dL, and protein 170 mg/dL. Which of the following statements is true about this condition?

   a. Nucleic acid-based tests are inaccurate for making the diagnosis.
   b. Genital symptoms are common with this condition.
   c. Parenteral ganciclovir is the drug of choice.
   d. The mortality rate is approximately 30%.
   e. Administer parenteral thiamine followed by dextrose infusion.

5. A 57-year-old woman reports 3 days of dysuria and right-sided flank pain. In your office, her temperature is 38.4°C. On further questioning, she describes previous urinary tract infections with similar symptoms and a history of calcium oxalate renal stones in the right kidney and ureteral tract. Her most recent urinary infection was approximately 2 weeks ago, for which she received therapy with an antibiotic for 3 days. Her previous urine culture grew *Enterococcus faecalis* (>10^5 colony-forming units/mL). You are concerned that *Enterococcus* is again the most likely urinary pathogen. All of the following drugs are active against *E faecalis* except:

   a. Vancomycin
   b. Cefazolin
   c. Ampicillin
   d. Piperacillin/tazobactam
   e. Linezolid

6. A 77-year-old woman with severe osteoarthritis and a balance disorder comes to you for advice after receiving a letter from the blood bank. She was providing a directed blood donation for her husband, who has T-cell leukemia, but was told that one of *her* blood tests precluded her from donating. You review the test result and note that her syphilis immunoglobulin G (IgG) by enzyme-linked immunosorbent assay is positive. She states that she has been in a monogamous relationship with her husband, a retired military man,

since 1941. You request a rapid plasma reagin (RPR) test, the result of which is 1:32. Which of the following would you advise?

a. Advise her that the test result is false-positive and that she can donate.
b. Advise her to repeat the syphilis IgG test in 3 months.
c. Offer her treatment with 1 dose of benzathine penicillin.
d. Recommend she undergo a cerebrospinal fluid analysis and penicillin treatment on the basis of the results.
e. Tell her to divorce her husband because he has been cheating on her.

7. An 82-year-old diabetic woman receiving insulin therapy is brought to the emergency department by her family; she has had diarrhea and altered mentation for 1 day. Her family noticed her wandering around the apartment incoherently. In the emergency department, her temperature is 40°C and blood pressure is 92/60 mm Hg, and she is responsive only to sternal rub. CT of the head shows age-appropriate atrophy. A lumbar puncture is performed, and the cerebrospinal fluid leukocyte count is 110/mm^3, with 55% neutrophils, 25% monocytes, and 20% lymphocytes, glucose 60 mg/dL, and protein 90 mg/dL. Gram stain of the cerebrospinal fluid shows gram-positive rods. Which of the following antibiotics should be given in combination with gentamicin for treatment?

a. Ceftriaxone
b. Ampicillin
c. Vancomycin
d. Trimethoprim-sulfamethoxazole
e. Cefepime

8. A 53-year-old man presents to the emergency department with 2 days of pain and swelling in his left thigh. He has had 4 prior episodes of these lesions at other sites in the past 6 months. The lesion initially began as a small boil on the medial aspect of his thigh and has become increasingly swollen and painful. Today he has a temperature of 39.4°C and chills. The lesion is incised and drained, and Gram stain shows numerous gram-positive cocci in clusters. Which of the following antimicrobials would you recommend for management?

a. Cephalexin 500 mg orally 4 times daily for 7 days
b. Trimethoprim-sulfamethoxazole 1 tablet orally twice daily for 7 days
c. Cefadroxil 500 mg orally twice daily for 7 days
d. Levofloxacin 750 mg orally daily for 7 days
e. Azithromycin 500 mg orally then 250 mg daily for 4 days

9. An 82-year-old diabetic man with peripheral vascular disease presents to the office having had fever and malaise for 2 days. The plantar surface of his right foot has a 5 × 3-cm heaped-up ulcer with surrounding erythema. He has absent pulses in his right foot and ankle and has refused revascularization previously.

Plain radiography shows no bony erosions. Which of the following diagnostic studies would best establish the extent of his infection?

a. Three-phase bone scanning
b. Gallium scanning
c. Indium scanning
d. MRI
e. Angiography

10. A 29-year-old athletic woman suffers a cervical spine fracture and closed head injury after diving into a shallow pond. She has been mechanically ventilated in the surgical-trauma intensive care unit for 3 weeks. During her first week of hospitalization, hives developed while she was receiving vancomycin. Her tracheal aspirates have grown *Pseudomonas aeruginosa* and MRSA over the past week. She has been receiving meropenem for 10 days. Today a fever of 40°C develops and there are purulent secretions from her tracheostomy. A chest radiograph shows new diffuse infiltrates in the right upper and left lower lobes, and the tracheal aspirate Gram stain shows gram-negative rods and gram-positive cocci in clusters. Which antibiotic combination would be best while awaiting culture results?

a. Cefepime plus vancomycin
b. Meropenem plus colistin plus daptomycin
c. Piperacillin-tazobactam plus daptomycin
d. Ceftazidime plus colistin plus linezolid
e. Ertapenem plus linezolid

11. A 42-year-old power pole lineman from Hayward, Wisconsin, presents with a 3-week history of right knee pain and swelling. He has been sexually active with only his spouse and denies any known trauma or bites. He took a 1-week course of prednisone, which seemed to help his knee, but today he reports multiple nodular skin lesions on his arms, legs, and face. A Lyme disease antibody test and blood cultures are both negative. Which of the following antimicrobials would be most effective for his condition?

a. Ceftriaxone 1 g daily for 3 weeks
b. Doxycycline 100 mg orally twice daily for 3 weeks
c. Levofloxacin 500 mg orally daily for 3 weeks
d. Itraconazole 200 mg orally twice daily for 6 months
e. Fluconazole 400 mg orally daily for 6 months

12. A 66-year-old woman arrives in your office complaining of 1 week of crampy left lower abdominal pain and some loose stool. She has been well other than having an abscessed tooth, which she had extracted 5 weeks ago. She has a history of mitral valve prolapse and received a dose of amoxicillin before the extraction. A set of blood cultures obtained at a local emergency department are negative, and CT shows some thickening of the sigmoid colon. At the time of her examination you note a fever of 38.3°C, a soft midsystolic click without a

murmur, and left lower abdominal tenderness. Which of the following would you do next?

a. Obtain a transesophageal echocardiogram.
b. Repeat 3 sets of blood cultures.
c. Obtain a stool specimen to test for *Clostridium difficile* toxin.
d. Repeat the CT of the abdomen.
e. Start therapy with ciprofloxacin 500 mg twice daily and metronidazole 500 mg 3 times daily by mouth.

13. A 38-year-old Guatemalan man seeks your help because of a 2-week history of nausea and fever. Over the past week he has been having drenching night sweats. He was seen in the health department last month and had a positive result of purified protein derivative (PPD) skin test, and therapy with isoniazid was started. He had a normal chest radiograph at that time. His alanine aminotransferase value is 22 U/L, and ultrasonography of the right upper quadrant shows a normal gallbladder and large fluid density in the right lobe of the liver. Which of the following is the best test to establish a diagnosis?

a. CT or ultrasound-guided aspiration of the fluid collection
b. α-Fetoprotein test
c. QuantiFERON-TB Gold test for *Mycobacterium tuberculosis*
d. Serologic test for *Entamoeba histolytica*
e. Serologic test for *Echinococcus*

14. A 33-year-old schoolteacher is bitten by her neighbor's dog on her way to school. On arrival at the office of the school nurse her arm is warm, red, and swollen and she is referred to you. She has a history of frequent urinary tract infections, is 12 weeks pregnant, and has hives to penicillins, sulfonamides, and quinolone antibiotics. Which of the following would you recommend for management?

a. Ice packs and elevation
b. Amoxicillin/clavulanic acid 875 mg orally twice daily
c. Azithromycin 500 mg then 250 mg daily for 4 days
d. Doxycycline 100 mg twice daily for 7 days
e. Cephalexin 500 mg 4 times daily for 7 days

15. A 55-year-old farmer from South Dakota presents complaining of 3 days of fever and malaise severe enough that he was unable to complete his harvesting. When he awoke this morning, he could not move his right arm, and he comes to your office seeking help. His only prior medical problem was rheumatic fever as a child. Which of the following diagnostic tests would be most helpful to establish the cause of his symptoms?

a. MRI of the brain
b. Lumbar puncture and cerebrospinal fluid polymerase chain reaction test for herpes simplex virus type 1
c. Serum West Nile virus immunoglobulin M (IgM) antibody test.

d. Cerebral angiography
e. Transesophageal echocardiography

16. A 30-year-old previously healthy construction worker from northern Minnesota is brought to the emergency department after experiencing syncope. He had a low-grade fever in the past week, palpitations, and intermittent dizziness. He has 2 cats and a dog at home. He is unaware of any bites and has not traveled. He has had some intermittent skin problems and reports that he had a blotchy red rash on his back in August last year which resolved on its own. On examination, his temperature is 38.0°C, blood pressure 110/70 mm Hg, and pulse is 34 beats per minute and regular. Electrocardiography shows complete heart block. Blood and urine cultures are sent for analysis. Which of the following statements about his condition is true?

a. A permanent pacemaker is needed.
b. He will need ceftriaxone 2 g daily intravenously for 21 days.
c. Neurologic sequelae will ensue.
d. A urine test is diagnostic.
e. Person-to-person transmission is common.

17. A 39-year-old homosexual man hiking the Appalachian Trail in North Carolina in August is found by a fellow hiker to be disoriented and ill-appearing. He is brought to a local emergency department, where he reports 2 days of fever, chills, myalgias, and a severe frontal headache. At the time of his examination he appears ill, is febrile (temperature, 39°C), has meningismus and a diffuse petechial rash that includes the palms and soles of the feet, and a small nodule with a central blackish discoloration in his right groin. Laboratory values are leucocyte count 11.0 × 10^9/L, lymphocytes 4.0 × 10^9/L, platelets 85 × 10^9/L, and hemoglobin 11.6 g/dL. A lumbar puncture is done and the cerebrospinal fluid results are cell count of 230 cells mostly lymphocytes, protein 120 mg/dL, and glucose 34 mg/dL. What is the next best course of action?

a. Get a dermatology consultation for biopsy.
b. Start therapy with intramuscular benzathine penicillin.
c. Start therapy with intravenous doxycycline.
d. Start therapy with intravenous methylprednisolone.
e. Start antiretroviral therapy.

18. A 29-year-old medical student presents to your office complaining of persistent wheezing, shortness of breath, and a dry cough. These symptoms began during his 3-month global health elective rotation in Fiji, where he provided primary health care. While there, he ate at local restaurants, walked barefoot on the beach and grass, but drank only bottled water. He has a dog at home. His current chest radiograph shows right lower lobe interstitial infiltrates. Two months ago when the symptoms first started, a radiograph showed left upper lung infiltrates. Laboratory values are leukocytes 15 ¥ 109/L with 38% eosinophils. Which of the following is the most likely cause of his illness?

a. Pulmonary tuberculosis
b. Coccidioidomycosis
c. *Blastocystis hominis*
d. *Strongyloides stercoralis*
e. *Entamoeba histolytica*

19. A 20-year-old college student went on a diving trip to Belize with his environmental science class. During the trip, the students camped in the forest, swam and kayaked in caves, and went diving and snorkeling offshore. They took no special immunizations or medications before the trip. They ate the local food but drank only water that was run through a purification filter. Eight days after coming home to Iowa, the student complained of diarrhea and malaise. Ten days after her return, she felt worse and began having chills. She had no rash. Which of the following tests would *not* be recommended for her initial evaluation?

a. Blood cultures
b. Stool examination for ova and parasites, enteric pathogens culture
c. Dengue virus serologic test
d. Rabies antibody serologic test
e. Thick and thin blood smears for malaria

20. A 47-year-old Kuwaiti diplomat is admitted with a 1-day onset of dizziness, blurred vision, slurred speech, difficulty swallowing, and nausea. In the emergency department, he had a right eye ptosis, a fifth and seventh cranial nerve paralysis, palatal weakness, and impaired gag reflex. Respiratory distress developed, and he was intubated and sent to the intensive care unit where he required mechanical ventilation. He had no history of hypertension, diabetes, or heart disease. He recalled no tick bites. His only travel was 48 hours ago to meet with an Iraqi diplomat in New York. The 2 of them had lunch with 3 other members of their diplomatic entourage at a famous New York City restaurant. They had salad, a fondue, and crème brûlée. You receive a telephone call that the other 3 members of the Kuwaiti mission are hospitalized at different hospitals in New York City with similar symptoms. Which of the following diagnostic tests would best help explain his symptoms?

a. Western blot test positive for Lyme disease
b. Stool culture showing a large gram-positive rod
c. Stool culture showing a curved gram-negative rod
d. Positive cerebrospinal fluid cryptococcal antigen test
e. Toxin assay on the fondue

21. A 64-year-old postal worker complains of a painful ulcer on his left fifth finger. The lesion started 5 days ago as a small red spot but became increasingly swollen. Today, he noted soreness in his elbow and armpit and has a fever to 38.9°C. He is a widower and has 2 indoor, declawed cats at home. He traveled to Phoenix on vacation for 1 week last month. His chest radiograph is normal. Which of the following would be the most appropriate therapy for his illness?

a. Azithromycin 500 mg orally daily for 3 days
b. Streptomycin 1 g intramuscularly twice daily for 10 days
c. Ciprofloxacin 500 mg orally twice daily for 60 days
d. Amoxicillin/clavulanic acid 875 mg orally twice daily for 14 days
e. Fluconazole 400 mg orally daily for 6 months

22. A 24-year-old professional football player presents to the emergency department with nausea, fever, and a painful "spider bite" on his right shin; these symptoms began this morning. His temperature is 104°F, pulse is 138 beats per minute, and he is vomiting. His only medicine is sertraline (Zoloft), which he takes for depression. His serum creatinine value is 2.5 mg/dL. Blood cultures grow *Staphylococcus aureus* in 2/2 bottles which is resistant to oxacillin, cefazolin, erythromycin, and gentamicin but sensitive to clindamycin, trimethoprim-sulfamethoxazole, and linezolid. Which of the following treatment regimens is most appropriate?

a. Trimethoprim-sulfamethoxazole 1 double-strength tablet orally daily
b. Nafcillin 2 g every 6 hours intravenously
c. Clindamycin 300 mg 4 times daily orally
d. Vancomycin once daily intravenously
e. Linezolid 600 mg twice daily orally

23. A 51-year-old woman who had been receiving chemotherapy through a surgically placed central catheter for acute myelogenous leukemia was admitted to the hospital for management of a presumed line-related infection. Blood drawn for culture at the time of admission is now growing a gram-positive coccus resembling staphylococci; the organism is subsequently found to be resistant to penicillins and cephalosporins. Therapy with intravenous vancomycin is started, but approximately 20 minutes into the infusion of the first dose a diffuse "flushing-like" red rash develops over the patient's face, neck, and torso. The infusion is stopped and within an hour the rash has disappeared. What would you do next?

a. Discontinue use of vancomycin, and start therapy with chloramphenicol.
b. Discontinue use of vancomycin, and start therapy with nafcillin and rifampin.
c. Continue use of vancomycin but predose with antihistamine and corticosteroids.
d. Continue use of vancomycin but infuse at a slower rate.
e. Discontinue use of vancomycin, and observe the patient while not receiving antibiotics.

24. A 58-year-old woman was admitted to the hospital with a 2-week history of low-grade fever, fatigue, and progressive shortness of breath. A new systolic murmur over the mitral area is found on examination, and echocardiography shows a 5-mm vegetation on the anterior mitral valve leaflet. Both blood specimens drawn for culture on admission are positive for

Enterococcus faecalis. Which of the following antimicrobial regimens should be initiated?

a. Nafcillin
b. Ceftazidime and gentamicin
c. Ampicillin and gentamicin
d. Ceftriaxone and doxycycline
e. Penicillin G

25. A 45-year-old woman with Crohn disease and a chronic indwelling central venous catheter for total parenteral nutrition has blood cultures positive for *Staphylococcus aureus.* Antimicrobial susceptibility testing shows this organism to be methicillin-susceptible and penicillin-resistant. Which of the following antimicrobial regimens would you initiate?

a. Nafcillin
b. Vancomycin
c. Ampicillin and gentamicin
d. Imipenem
e. High-dose intravenous penicillin

26. A previously healthy 41-year-old man with a recent episode of sinusitis presents to the emergency department complaining of severe headache and fever. He appears quite ill, but no focal neurologic abnormalities are noted on examination. He does have some nuchal rigidity. Which would be the most appropriate *next step* in his management?

a. Have emergency CT of the head performed first, then initiate treatment with vancomycin and ceftriaxone and perform lumbar puncture for cerebrospinal fluid evaluation if no mass lesions are found.
b. Start cefazolin and ciprofloxacin therapy.
c. Start erythromycin and clindamycin therapy.
d. Start ampicillin and clarithromycin therapy.
e. Start cefotaxime and vancomycin therapy.

27. A 65-year-old man with a history of diabetic-associated nephropathy has been undergoing dialysis for the past 4 years. He has been hospitalized for management of cellulitis overlying an arteriovenous fistula in the right arm (used for dialysis). You would like to initiate therapy with an antimicrobial agent that does not require adjustment in renal failure. What would you use?

a. Meropenem
b. Cefazolin
c. Clindamycin
d. Piperacillin/tazobactam
e. Levofloxacin

28. A 55-year-old woman presents to your office complaining of a 5-week history of cough, night sweats, and a 10-lb weight loss. Chest radiography shows a fibronodular infiltrate in the right upper lobe with a small cavitary lesion. Collected sputum samples show the presence of acid-fast bacilli on smear. She is given a clinical diagnosis of pulmonary tuberculosis and, while culture results are pending, treatment is started with isoniazid, rifampin, pyrazinamide, and ethambutol. She was a former Peace Corps volunteer in Latin America and has a history of moderate alcohol consumption and non–insulin-dependent diabetes, for which she takes glyburide. While she is receiving therapy, numbness and tingling develop in both feet and lower aspect of the legs; these symptoms later become painful. What is the most likely cause for the patient's neuropathy?

a. Isoniazid
b. Rifampin
c. Pyrazinamide
d. Ethambutol
e. Spinal cord compression

29. During the first month of therapy in the patient described in question 28, you notice that her blood glucose levels are significantly higher than they had been 3 months ago. She has been taking all of her tuberculosis medications on a daily basis and glyburide for diabetes. She reports no dietary changes and has not started using any other additional medications during the past month. A few weeks after starting therapy, the patient reports decreased cough and improved energy levels. Which is the most likely explanation for this patient's hyperglycemia?

a. Isoniazid
b. Rifampin
c. Pyrazinamide
d. Ethambutol
e. Pancreatic tuberculosis

Answers

1. Answer a.

Streptococcus pneumoniae is the most common cause of meningitis associated with cerebrospinal fluid leaks. The organisms appear as gram-positive diplococci on Gram stain. The other organisms are far less common causes of meningitis in this setting.

2. Answer b.

Successful treatment of endocarditis caused by enterococci requires synergistic combination therapy with an aminoglycoside and penicillin. Penicillins used in combination with gentamicin or streptomycin are more effective than vancomycin-aminoglycoside combinations and are far less toxic. Adding sulbactam to ampicillin does not enhance efficacy because enterococci rarely produce β-lactamases. Valve replacement therapy may be indicated if hemodynamic decompensation develops from valvular dysfunction. However, the relapse of bacteremia after an inadequate course of therapy is not an indication for surgical intervention.

3. Answer e.

This young woman with recurrent herpes simplex virus type 2 would like advice on how to prevent transmission to her sexual partner. Recent studies suggest that there are 2 ways and that they are about 50% effective for reducing transmission: 1) the consistent use of latex condoms and 2) the use of valacyclovir 500 mg daily. Because she wants to get pregnant, use of condoms is not an option. Around 70% of transmission between partners occurs when the infected partner has asymptomatic viral shedding. Thus, simply avoiding intercourse in the absence of active lesions is not an adequate prevention strategy. Telling her spouse of her infection is reasonable but will not prevent transmission. It certainly is possible that her partner is already infected because genital herpes is the most prevalent sexually transmitted disease in the United States with over 45 million persons infected (ie, 1 in 4-5 adults is infected).

4. Answer d.

Herpes simplex encephalitis (HSE) is a nonseasonal, life-threatening illness usually caused by herpes simplex virus type 1. HSE causes confusion, fever, and, frequently, seizures. Simultaneous herpes labialis is present in 10% to 15% of cases. Genital lesions are not common. Amplification of HSV DNA (ie, HSV polymerase chain reaction) from cerebrospinal fluid is extremely sensitive (>95%) for diagnosis. HSE has a mortality rate of 70% if untreated and 20% to 30% if treated. Poor neurologic status, age older than 30 years, and encephalitis of more than 4 days in duration before initiation of therapy are associated with a poor outcome. Acyclovir remains the treatment of choice for HSE.

5. Answer b.

Ampicillin, piperacillin/tazobactam, linezolid, and vancomycin all provide excellent anti-enterococcal activity (for susceptible strains). The cephalosporins are not active against enterococci. Additionally, the quinolones do not generally produce reliable activity against *Enterococcus* sp.

6. Answer d.

This unfortunate elderly woman has been infected with *Treponema pallidum* at some time in the past and has either late latent syphilis or possible neurosyphilis. The test result is *not* false-positive, and she will be excluded from the blood donor pool. She needs further evaluation of her progressive gait disorder, and she should undergo a cerebrospinal fluid analysis to exclude neurosyphilis in order to determine the most appropriate therapy (either benzathine penicillin or intravenous penicillin). Her initial serologic test is a specific treponemal test and this was confirmed by the finding of the increased nontreponemal RPR titer of 1:32. An increased RPR titer in this setting suggests syphilis infection. Normally, the RPR is nonreactive unless there is a reason for cross-reactivity (false-positive). The measured titer of RPR is variable and may wane with time or, in some individuals, can remain serofast (no decrease to undetectable) even after treatment. However, a 1:32 titer suggests a 5-tube dilution from negative, and this patient has never been treated. Doing the specific treponemal assay first and finding the result to be positive eliminates the issues of having to confirm positive RPR titers, which are less specific. The patient should also be screened for other sexually transmitted diseases such as hepatitis B and human immunodeficiency virus (HIV). Interestingly, her husband has a T-cell leukemia, which could be associated with other sexually transmitted diseases such as HIV or human T-cell lymphotrophic virus (HTLV-1), and he should be tested for these and syphilis.

7. Answer b.

This elderly woman presented with altered mentation and fever after a brief gastrointestinal illness. Her cerebrospinal fluid shows a polymorphonuclear cell predominance, and Gram stain shows a gram-positive rod. All of these findings are consistent with a diagnosis of *Listeria monocytogenes* meningoencephalitis. Although vancomycin, ampicillin, and trimethoprim-sulfamethoxazole alone are all active against *Listeria*, the best choice for *Listeria* meningoencephalitis is the combination of ampicillin with an aminoglycoside (gentamicin). Ceftriaxone and cefepime, although active against most agents that cause bacterial meningitis, do not have activity against *Listeria*.

8. Answer b.

This man has had recurrent episodes of folliculitis and now has cellulitis with an abscess showing gram-positive cocci in clusters. The most likely cause of this is a community-acquired methicillin-resistant *Staphylococcus aureus* strain (CA-MRSA). These strains have rapidly become disseminated throughout much of the United States, in particular the USA 300 strain. These infections are most effectively managed by incision and drainage. Further antimicrobial therapy should be directed at this resistant pathogen. The cephalosporins and macrolides are ineffective against CA-MRSA. The treatment of uncomplicated skin and soft tissue infections is trimethoprim-sulfamethoxazole. Alternative oral agents potentially include clindamycin, tetracyclines, or linezolid.

9. Answer d.
This 82-year-old man has cellulitis surrounding a chronic neuropathic plantar ulcer in the setting of peripheral vascular disease and diabetes. To establish whether this is a cellulitis, soft tissue abscess, or osteomyelitis, the best study is MRI of the foot. Gallium, indium, and technetium bone scanning are not specific for the diagnosis of osteomyelitis and fail to provide evidence of deep soft tissue infection. Angiography may be useful for assessment of revascularization but does not aid in depth of diagnosis.

10. Answer d.
Ventilator-acquired pneumonia has developed in this unfortunate young athlete. She was known to be colonized with several multiresistant bacteria preceding the event and was receiving meropenem, which likely continued to select for multiresistant *Pseudomonas* and MRSA. In the setting of meropenem-resistant *P aeruginosa*, very few agents are effective. One strategy involves the combination of ceftazidime with colistin. To cover MRSA, a third agent would also be required. Because she had hives while receiving vancomycin, this agent would be avoided. Daptomycin fails to achieve adequate pulmonary concentrations and should be avoided in pneumonias. Linezolid has been as effective as vancomycin for treating nosocomial MRSA pneumonia and would be the third agent to use here.

11. Answer d.
The patient is a lineman from northern Wisconsin in whom a subacute monoarthritis of the right knee and multiple nodular skin lesions have developed. The differential diagnosis of infectious monoarthritis always includes gonorrhea, especially with a dermatitis arthritis syndrome. However, the patient has had no new sex partners and the chronicity of the knee swelling and the nodular lesions of the skin do not fit well with this diagnosis. Lyme disease can cause a monoarthritis, and he is from an endemic area. However, the cutaneous nodules do not fit this diagnosis. *Mycobacteria* and fungi may cause a subacute-chronic monoarthritis with negative bacterial cultures. Sporothrix may cause this picture but is not associated with the diffuse nodular lesions in a normal host. The most likely cause is the endemic fungus *Blastomyces dermatitidis*. This will cause a chronic monoarthritis, and the patient has a job which puts him at risk for it and he works in an area endemic for this. The nodular skin lesions are characteristic of blastomycosis. This infection should be treated with a prolonged course of itraconazole, which is more effective than fluconazole.

12. Answer c.
This 66-year-old woman had crampy lower abdominal pain and loose stools after receiving a brief course of amoxicillin. CT shows thickening of the sigmoid colon, which may occur with colitis rather than diverticulitis. Although she is at a slight risk for infective endocarditis, transesophageal echocardiography would not be recommended as part of her initial evaluation. Her original blood cultures were negative, and she has recently had abdominal CT. Initiation of ciprofloxacin and metronidazole would be reasonable for management of diverticulitis. However, the first step in a patient with left lower abdominal pain, sigmoid thickening, and diarrhea after receipt of antibiotics would be a stool test for *C difficile* toxin.

13. Answer d.
This immigrant from Guatemala has a focal lesion in the right lobe of the liver and has had fevers and sweats for 2 weeks. The most likely cause is a liver abscess. He has a history of tuberculosis exposure but has recently been receiving isoniazid preventive therapy. Hepatitis due to isonazid is unlikely in the setting of a normal alanine aminotransferase value. The QuantiFERON assay would add nothing to the PPD test, which was known to be positive. *Echinococcus* usually presents as a multicystic liver lesion. *Entamoeba histolytica* is endemic in Guatemala and is the likely cause of the liver abscess. The best test for diagnosis is the amebic serologic test; needle aspiration should be delayed until the results of this test are known. If the result is positive, he should receive treatment with metronidazole.

14. Answer c.
This pregnant schoolteacher has an infected dog bite with cellulitis. She has severe allergies to penicillins, sulfonamides, and quinolones. Cephalexin is not effective against *Pasteurella* in dog bites, and doxycycline needs to be avoided in this first-trimester pregnancy. Ice packs and elevation are not adequate, although they may be adjunctive. The best antibiotic to use is azithromycin.

15. Answer c.
The most appropriate diagnostic test is the serum West Nile virus IgM antibody test. The patient is a farmer from Iowa who has an acute febrile illness during the harvest season followed by the acute onset of limb motor weakness. These symptoms are most consistent with the poliolike illness observed in acute West Nile infection called acute flaccid paralysis. This illness seems to be more frequent in men between the ages of 45 and 55 years infected with the West Nile virus. Treatment is supportive, and the prognosis for recovery is slow and variable. MRI would not be helpful early in West Nile virus infection. The acute flaccid paralysis syndrome does not occur with herpes simplex virus encephalitis, and thus polymerase chain reaction for this virus on cerebrospinal fluid would not be helpful. Although cerebral angiography or echocardiography would be helpful to exclude endocarditis or a mycotic aneurysm, the brief febrile illness in the late summer months and the abrupt onset of single limb weakness do not fit with these entities.

16. Answer b.
Stage 2 of Lyme disease is associated carditis in 10% of patients. Atrioventricular conduction blocks are the most common manifestation of Lyme carditis. Electrocardiography may show variable atrioventricular conduction defects, ranging from first-degree atrioventricular block to complete heart block. Lyme carditis-related conduction defects are reversible with therapy and have a favorable outcome. Most patients may require only temporary pacing and do not need a permanent pacemaker. The drug of choice is either ceftriaxone 2 g every 24 hours for 14 to 21 days or penicillin G 20 million units per day for 14 to 21 days. Diagnosis is clinical and

supported by serologic evidence of Lyme disease. Neurologic sequelae are not expected in the absence of signs or symptoms of Lyme
meningoencephalitis. Transmission is by tick bite and not person-
to-person.

17. Answer c.

The diagnosis in this camper is Rocky Mountain spotted fever (RMSF)
caused by *Rickettsia rickettsii*. RMSF is acquired from a tick
(*Dermacentor* species) bite. The differential diagnosis includes secondary syphilis, acute human immunodeficiency virus (HIV),
meningococcemia, or pneumococcal meningitis. However, the history of camping, the season during presentation, the typical rash, the
presence of the eschar (uncommon in RMSF), and the cerebrospinal
fluid findings all make meningococcemia or pneumococcal meningitis less likely. Empirically, parenteral doxycycline therapy should be
started. The patient is reported to be healthy; therefore, *legionella* is
not a major concern in this situation and ampicillin would not be
the right choice. The diagnosis of RMSF is mostly clinical because
biopsy (sensitivity of 70%) and serologic testing may require more time.

18. Answer d.

Strongyloides stercoralis is ubiquitous, being much more common in
developing countries. It is acquired by direct penetration of skin,
such as when walking barefoot in areas with fecal contamination.
After the larvae penetrate the skin, they enter the venous circulation, travel to the lungs, penetrate the alveoli, and then travel along
the bronchi and trachea to be swallowed into the stomach and upper
intestine. While traveling in the lungs, the organism causes an
eosinophilic pneumonia that has fleeting infiltrates. In the intestine,
the larvae mature and penetrate the intestinal wall. Eggs deposited
in the mucosa by mature *Strongyloides* organisms mature into larvae and reinitiate the cycle. This process causes an "autoinfection" and
can be severe in immunocompromised hosts. In immunocompromised hosts (neutropenia, steroids, acquired immunodeficiency syndrome), a superinfection can develop with larval migration
throughout the body. Gram-negative bacteremia is a common coinfection, resulting from disruption of the intestinal mucosa by the
invasive larvae. Treatment is with ivermectin. Both tuberculosis and
coccidioidomycosis are associated with eosinophilia but of much
lower intensity and not likely to have fleeting infiltrates. Amebic
lung involvement is usually single abscess, mostly in the right and
without eosinophilia.

19. Answer d.

Vivax malaria is the most likely diagnosis. The tests that should be
performed for evaluation of undifferentiated fever in the returning
traveler from Central America include thick and thin smears for
malaria, blood cultures for typhoid and nontyphoidal *Salmonella*, and
stool examination for enteric pathogens and ova and parasites. With
the short incubation period and the location visited, dengue fever is
also a possibility, although an acute dengue IgM may be negative
early in the disease. A rabies antibody test would not be helpful
because the clinical scenario and time course do not fit. This test is
not used for diagnosis of rabies and is attainable only from the
Centers for Disease Control and Prevention.

20. Answer e.

Botulism is a paralytic illness resulting from a toxin produced under
anaerobic conditions by *Clostridium botulinum*. The diagnosis is
suggested by the clinical manifestations, which begin with cranial
nerve palsies (ptosis and extraocular palsies) and descending paralysis to involve the extremities. A good mnemonic is the 4 Ds: dry
mouth, dysphagia, diplopia, dysarthria, which occur in almost 90%
of cases. The incubation period is 18 to 36 hours. Patients presenting with clinical signs and symptoms of botulism should have serum
analysis for toxin by bioassay in mice, which can be obtained from
the health department. Analysis of stool, vomitus, and suspected
food items may also reveal toxin, which is diagnostic when coupled
with the appropriate clinical and neurologic findings. In the case
described, the heat-resistant *C botulinum* spores either survived the
initial cooking or were introduced afterward; the spores subsequently
germinated and produced toxin. The lid on a pot of gravy or stew
most likely produced the anaerobic environment necessary for toxin
production. Most outbreaks of foodborne botulism result from eating improperly preserved home-canned vegetables (especially aspara-
gus, green beans, and peppers). Treatment is administration of
antitoxin.

21. Answer c.

This postal worker has acquired cutaneous anthrax from handling
a contaminated piece of mail. This is a bioterrorist event and requires
activation of the local and national homeland security system. The
cutaneous lesions of anthrax present initially as a macule that then
develops edema, ulcerates, and often has surrounding satellite vesicles. Regional lymphadenopathy is common, and with bacteremic
spread pulmonary or central nervous system disease may develop.
Bacillus anthracis is a class A bioterror agent. Clues to bioterrorist
events include an increase in cases of an unusual disease, particularly outside the normal environs. The postal worker had not been
to any areas endemic for anthrax and thus was likely exposed from
a contaminated piece of mail. The diagnosis is made from a Gram
stain or punch biopsy of the skin lesion. This may be sent for a rapid
polymerase chain reaction. In severe cases of anthrax, combination
therapy is recommended and should be given parenterally. For localized treatment of cutaneous anthrax, the recommended treatment
is ciprofloxacin 500 mg twice daily for at least 60 days after the exposure. Ciprofloxacin 500 mg twice daily or doxycycline 100 mg twice
daily would also be recommended for 60 days to coworkers as prophylaxis after exposure.

22. Answer d.

This football player has a complicated skin infection due to one of
the community-acquired methicillin-resistant *Staphylococcus aureus*
isolates. These may present with what appears to be a "spider bite."
These isolates frequently possess a Panton-Valentine leukocidin gene
and are associated with significant local and systemic toxicity. These
community isolates often test susceptible to trimethoprim-sulfamethoxazole and clindamycin but are erythromycin-resistant and
resistant to β-lactams. Because of the severity of the infection and the
gastrointestinal symptoms, a parenteral agent is preferred—vancomycin. Linezolid should be avoided because of the difficulty with

oral medicines and the potential interaction with sertraline, causing a serotonergic syndrome.

23. Answer d.
"Red man" or "red neck" syndrome is an infusion-associated reaction that frequently is associated with vancomycin. Typical manifestations include an erythematous rash that involves the face, neck, and upper torso. Itching is common, and hypotension occasionally develops. The reaction can occur within a few minutes after initiation of vancomycin infusion or may develop soon after the infusion is complete. This peculiar syndrome is due to a nonimmunologic release of histamine and is related to the rate of vancomycin infusion. This complication can be avoided by slowing the infusion rate of vancomycin or administering vancomycin over at least 1 hour. Larger doses of vancomycin (eg, 1,500 mg) are typically infused over 1 hour. If slowing the rate of infusion does not prevent this reaction, addition of an antihistamine (eg, Benadryl) may be useful when given before the infusion of vancomycin.

24. Answer c.
Enterococcal endocarditis requires *2-drug* therapy to achieve bactericidal activity. Cell wall-active (β-lactam) antibiotics plus an aminoglycoside act synergistically to produce "cidal" activity against susceptible strains of enterococci. Nafcillin and the cephalosporins have negligible activity against enterococci. Penicillin monotherapy provides only bacteriostatic activity against enterococci, which would not be appropriate in the treatment of enterococcal endocarditis.

25. Answer a.
Nafcillin is the drug of choice for strains of *S aureus* that are susceptible to the semisynthetic penicillinase-resistant penicillins (ie, methicillin, nafcillin, oxacillin, cloxacillin, dicloxacillin). Strains resistant to these compounds (methicillin-resistant *S aureus*, or MRSA) remain susceptible to vancomycin; however, vancomycin is not as active as nafcillin against susceptible *S aureus*. Only a small percentage of *S aureus* isolates do not produce β-lactamase and remain sensitive to penicillin G. In this rare but fortunate situation, penicillin G would be the most active compound and the drug of choice.

26. Answer e.
This question addresses 3 important issues. First, if there is a clinical suspicion of bacterial meningitis, there should be no delay in starting antimicrobial therapy. If head CT is needed, appropriate empiric antimicrobial agents should be started *before* the patient undergoes CT. In the absence of focal neurologic findings, seizures, or papilledema, a cerebrospinal fluid examination can safely be done without a head CT. Second, before starting antimicrobial therapy, the physician needs to consider the most likely bacterial pathogens in

an otherwise healthy 41-year-old patient, namely, *Streptococcus pneumoniae* and *Neisseria meningitidis*. The recently diagnosed sinus infection is a clue that *S pneumoniae* may be the pathogen. Although *Listeria monocytogenes* is frequent in neonates, the elderly, and immunocompromised patients, it would be less likely in this patient. It would be prudent, however, to include ampicillin for empiric therapy in these high-risk patients. Third, the physician needs to prescribe antimicrobial agents that adequately penetrate the central nervous system blood-brain barrier to sterilize the cerebrospinal fluid. Of the listed agents, ceftriaxone, cefotaxime, ampicillin, and vancomycin penetrate the cerebrospinal fluid with concentrations high enough to sterilize it. Ciprofloxacin variably penetrates the cerebrospinal fluid and does not provide reliable activity against *S pneumoniae*. Ampicillin is appropriate for *Listeria* meningitis (with the addition of gentamicin), but clarithromycin does not adequately penetrate the cerebrospinal fluid. Cefotaxime (2 g every 4 hours or 3 g every 6 hours) or ceftriaxone (2 g every 12 hours) and vancomycin is a suitable initial antimicrobial program for this patient until culture results and drug susceptibilities are available.

27. Answer c.
Clindamycin is hepatically metabolized and requires no dose adjustment for renal insufficiency. Meropenem, cefazolin, piperacillin-tazobactam (Zosyn), and levofloxacin are all renally cleared and require dose adjustments with renal impairment.

28. Answer a.
Peripheral neuropathy has been described in 17% of recipients of isoniazid, 6 mg/kg per day. It is less common in patients taking the standard daily dose of 300 mg/day. Malnutrition, alcoholism, diabetes mellitus, uremia, and slow acetylators of isoniazid increase the risk of neuropathy. Isoniazid promotes the excretion of pyridoxine (vitamin B_6), and supplemental administration of 6 to 50 mg/day of pyridoxine can prevent this complication. Other side effects of isoniazid include hepatotoxicity, positive antinuclear antibody titer, lupuslike reaction, and drowsiness.

29. Answer b.
Rifampin induces hepatic microsomal cytochrome P450–mediated enzyme activity, which can profoundly decrease the serum levels of other drugs metabolized by this pathway. Rifampin interaction with more than 100 drugs, including oral hypoglycemic agents, has been described. In the treatment of human immunodeficiency virus and tuberculosis coinfection, rifampin induces the metabolism of protease inhibitors, reducing their antiviral activity. Other side effects of rifampin include hepatotoxicity, cytopenias (decreased leukocyte and platelet values), orange discoloration of body fluids, and hypersensitivity reactions.

16

Medical Ethics

C. Christopher Hook, MD
Paul S. Mueller, MD

Medicine is first and foremost a relationship. It is the coming together of one individual, the patient, who is ill or has specific needs and a second individual, the physician, whose goal is to help the patient and who possesses a unique set of knowledge and skills to pursue that goal. Because medicine is fundamentally a relationship, it is at heart an ethical endeavor. Physicians have a long history of creating codes or oaths to provide the ethical norms and framework to support and protect the underlying relationship. Medical ethics consists of a set of principles and systematic methods that attempt to guide physicians on how they ought to act in their relationships with patients and others. These principles and methods are based on moral values shared by both the lay society (which may vary from culture to culture) and the medical profession.

* Medical ethics consists of a set of principles and systematic methods that attempt to guide physicians on how they ought to act in their relationships with patients and others.

The Hippocratic Oath is foundational for much of Western medical ethics. Its principles form the framework for many of our current ethical standards, including beneficence and nonmaleficence (the duties to do good and avoid or prevent harm), confidentiality, and the prohibition of active euthanasia. Contemporary articulations of these core principles include the Declaration of Geneva (1983), World Medical Association International Code of Medical Ethics (1983), The American College of Physicians Ethics Manual (2005), and The American Medical Association Code of Medical Ethics (2004-2005).

Ethical Dilemmas

Advances in medical science and the ever-changing social and legal milieu are responsible for dynamic changes, challenges, and dilemmas in medical ethics. An ethical dilemma is a predicament caused by conflicting moral principles in which there is no clear course to resolve a problem (ie, credible evidence exists both for and against a certain action). Even when ethically challenging situations and dilemmas are resolved, physicians may still experience ethical distress due to conflicting values and personal conscience.

* Advances in medical science and the ever-changing social and legal milieu are responsible for dynamic changes, challenges, and dilemmas in medical ethics.
* Ethical dilemma: a predicament caused by conflicting moral principles in which there is no clear course to resolve a problem.

Principles of Medical Ethics

Today, there are several different philosophical frameworks for deriving the rules or particulars of medical ethics. Historically, and still today, the foremost ethical principle of medicine has been beneficence and its corollary, nonmaleficence, from which we understand our duty to do good for the patient and to avoid and prevent harm. If physicians were asked why each of us chose to practice medicine, almost universally our replies would be "to help others," or some similar sentiment. It is that desire to help that is the bedrock of medicine and medical ethics.

A formalized contemporary framework for medical ethics is called principalism. Proposed by Beauchamp and Childress, principalism, although not necessarily providing bedside guidance for each ethical dilemma, provides a useful delineation of 4 prima facie (at face value) principles that encompass most of the ethical concerns in the physician-patient relationship. These principles are (not necessarily in order of priority): 1) autonomy, 2) beneficence, 3) nonmaleficence, and 4) justice. We submit that although beneficence remains the core ethical principle, autonomy, nonmaleficence, and justice contextualize and inform our fundamental orientation to accomplish the good.

* Four prima facie principles of medical ethics: autonomy, beneficence, nonmaleficence, and justice.

Autonomy

Autonomy derives from the Greek words *autos* ("self") and *nomes* ("rule"). The principle of autonomy, or respect for persons, is the concept that persons have the right to establish, pursue, and maintain their values and goals (the right to self-determination). For autonomy to have meaningful expression, however, 2 requirements must be present: agency and liberty.

Agency is the capability to establish one's own values and goals and be able to make appropriate decisions based on those values and goals. From the requirement of agency derives the clinically important concept of decision-making capacity. Decision-making capacity is not the same as the legal term *competence*. Capacity is the physician's clinical determination of the patient's ability to understand his or her situation and make appropriate decisions for treatment, whereas competence is the legal determination and status that an individual has the right to make life-affecting decisions (not only health-related decisions but also, for example, financial decisions). Notably, judges' or courts' determination of competence is based in significant part on the clinical assessment of decision-making capacity.

- Autonomy, or respect for persons, is the concept that persons have the right to establish, pursue, and maintain their values and goals (the right to self-determination).
- Autonomy requires decision-making capacity.
- Competence is the legal determination and status that an individual has the right to make life-affecting decisions.

In clinical practice, the lack of decisional capability should be proved and not presumed. Confusion, disorientation, psychosis, and other cognitive changes caused by diseases, metabolic disturbances, and medical interventions can affect decision-making ability. Decisionally capable patients have the right to refuse all medical interventions, even at the risk of death.

- The lack of decisional capability should be proved and not presumed.

Several clinical standards are used to assess decision-making capacity: 1) the patient can make and communicate a choice; 2) the patient understands the medical situation and prognosis, the nature of the recommended care, available alternative options, and the risks, benefits, and consequences of each; 3) the patient's decisions are stable over time; 4) the decision is consistent with the patient's values and goals; and 5) the decision is not due to delusions.

Liberty, the second major element required in autonomy, allows the patient the freedom and opportunity to influence the course of his or her life and medical treatments. Recent court decisions, from the Quinlan case in 1976 to the Cruzan decision in 1990 (Table 16-1), along with strong support from the bioethical community, have established the right of patients to refuse any form of medical treatment, even if such refusal will lead to the patient's death.

- Liberty: the freedom and opportunity to influence the course of one's life and medical treatments.

The principle of autonomy, particularly as it affects the right of an individual to refuse life-sustaining treatments, has been affirmed by ethicists and the courts (Table 16-1). Nevertheless, a survey of physicians published in 1995 reported that 34% of physicians had, at least once in the preceding 12 months, declined to withdraw life-sustaining mechanical ventilation despite being requested to do so by a decisionally capable patient or by the surrogates of patients lacking decision-making capacity. Nearly 20% of physicians engaged in this practice because of the fear of malpractice litigation. Unfortunately, many physicians in the United States have a poor understanding of the laws regarding patient autonomy in the states in which they practice. For example, the 1995 survey found that 46% of the respondents from New York incorrectly believed that withdrawal of mechanical ventilation was illegal.

- Many physicians have a poor understanding of the laws regarding patient autonomy in the states in which they practice.

Preserving Patient Autonomy

It is not uncommon for physicians to care for patients who lack or lose decision-making capacity. Can a patient who now is unconscious or lacks decision-making capacity prevent unwanted treatment? Who speaks for the patient when he or she no longer possesses decision-making capacity? Because autonomy is based on a respect for persons, caregivers should endeavor to provide treatment in accordance with what the patient would have desired if he or she were still able to interact capably with the caregivers. To preserve their autonomy, patients may communicate through 2 means to express their wishes: advance directives and surrogate decision makers.

- The patient's autonomy is preserved by 1) advance directives and 2) surrogate decision makers.

Advance Directive

An advance directive is a document in which a person either states choices for medical treatments or designates an individual who should make treatment choices when the patient does not possess decision-making capacity. The term also can apply to oral statements from the patient to the caregivers, given at a time when the patient was decisionally capable. Advance directives can take several forms: 1) the living will, 2) the durable power of attorney for health care, 3) a document appointing a health care surrogate (in jurisdictions that do not formally recognize a durable power of attorney for health care), and 4) the advance medical care directive. Notably, the laws concerning advance directives vary from jurisdiction to jurisdiction (eg, the form of advance directive authorized and the required contents for the advance directive). It is therefore advised that each physician be familiar with the local statutes concerning advance directives.

- Advance directive: a document in which a person either states choices for medical treatments or designates an individual who should make treatment choices when the patient does not possess decision-making capacity.
- Legal requirements for advance directives vary from state to state.

Table 16-1 Pertinent Legal Rulings

Case, yr	Legal Issue	Court	Decision
Salgo, 1957	Informed consent	California Court of Appeals	First used term "informed consent"
Brooks, 1965	Jehovah's Witness refusal of blood	Illinois District Court	Patients have right to personal treatment on religious grounds
Canterbury, 1972	Degree of disclosure required for adequate informed consent	US District Court	Established "prudent patient test"
Quinlan, 1976	PVS—discontinuation of mechanical ventilation, previously articulated directive	New Jersey Supreme Court	Discontinuation (based on right to privacy)
Brophy, 1986	PVS—discontinuation of gastrostomy feedings, previously articulated directive	Massachusetts Supreme Court	Discontinue feedings (based on autonomy)
Bouvia, 1986	Severely impaired, refusal of nasogastric tube feedings by a decisionally capable patient	California Court of Appeals	Removal of nasogastric tube (based on autonomy)
Corbett, 1986	PVS—discontinuation of nasogastric tube feedings, no predefined directive(s)	Florida Court of Appeals	Discontinue feedings (based on right to privacy)
Cruzan, 1990	PVS—state of Missouri required "clear & convincing" evidence of individual's wishes before allowing withdrawal of life support	US Supreme Court	States have right to restrict exercise of right to refuse treatment by surrogates; decisionally capable patients may refuse life-sustaining therapy, including hydration, nutrition, & mechanical ventilation
Wanglie, 1991	PVS—family wished continued support despite objections to continue life-sustaining therapy by the physicians & institution	Minnesota District Court	Continuation (based on autonomy, substituted judgment)
Quill, Lee, 1997	Assisted suicide	US Supreme Court	States have the right to make laws prohibiting or allowing physician-assisted suicide & euthanasia
Schiavo, 2005	PVS—family conflict over withdrawal of feeding tube	Florida District Court of Appeals, Florida Supreme Court, US Supreme Cout	Upheld the right of surrogates to withdraw a feeding tube if acting in accord with patient's wishes
Gonzoles, 2006	Assisted suicide	US Supreme Court	Upheld the Constitutional legitimacy of the Oregon assisted suicide law

Abbreviation: PVS, persistent vegetative state.

Living Will: The traditional living will requires that 2 conditions be present before it takes effect: 1) the patient must be terminally ill, and 2) the patient must lack decision-making capacity. Like the laws concerning advance directives, the determination of terminally ill varies from jurisdiction to jurisdiction. Because of the requirement that the patient must be terminally ill, the living will is restricted in its use and may not be useful in many circumstances in which the patient lacks decision-making capacity but cannot necessarily be described as terminally ill. When activated, the living will provides guidance to the caregivers about what treatments the patient does or does not desire. It is, however, ineffective if vaguely written or applied to patients with uncertain prognoses.

- The living will requires that a patient be terminally ill before it takes effect.

Durable Power of Attorney for Health Care: The durable power of attorney for health care (DPAHC) is a document that designates a surrogate decision maker should the patient lose decision-making capacity. It does not require that the patient be terminally ill, and therefore it is an advance directive that is more useful. Within the DPAHC, the patient can make specific directives concerning different types of treatments such as cardiopulmonary resuscitation and artificial nutrition and hydration. The major value of the DPAHC, however, is that it identifies an individual who can dynamically interact with the health care team regarding the great breadth of medical decisions.

- DPAHC designates a surrogate decision maker should the patient lose decision-making capacity.

Specific Advance Medical Care Directive: Some patients have specific desires never to receive certain forms of therapy. For instance, many Jehovah's Witnesses do not want blood or blood products under any circumstances. Other individuals may refuse dialysis or some other intervention regardless of the circumstance. The advance medical care directive is a document that states this categorical refusal for a specific treatment. For example, it may take the form of a no-transfusion card or a MedicAlert bracelet or necklace.

- The specific advance medical care directive typically addresses 1 medical intervention.

The Patient Self-Determination Act of 1990: In response to the Cruzan decision (Table 16-1), the US Congress passed the Patient Self-Determination Act. This law attempts to ensure that patients are informed of their rights to accept or refuse medical interventions and to create and execute an advance directive. The Patient Self-Determination Act requires that hospitals, nursing homes, hospices, managed care organizations, and home health care agencies provide this information to patients at the time of admission or enrollment. The organizations are required to 1) document whether patients have advance directives, 2) establish policies to implement the advance directives, and 3) educate their staff and community about advance directives and these policies.

- The Patient Self-Determination Act requires that all health care providers, at the time of admission, dispense information to patients about their rights to accept or refuse interventions and to create an advance directive.

Surrogate Decision-Making

A surrogate is a person who represents the patient's interests and previously expressed wishes. The surrogate is optimally designated by the patient before critical illness. One type of surrogate is the durable power of attorney for health care, in which a legally binding proxy directive authorizes a designated individual to speak on behalf of the patient. The second type of surrogate is the patient's family or the court. The third type is a moral surrogate (usually a family member) who best knows the patient and has the patient's interests at heart. Difficulties may arise when the moral surrogate is not the legal surrogate.

- A surrogate represents the patient's interests and previously expressed wishes in the context of the medical issues.
- Optimally, a surrogate is designated by the patient before critical illness.

How should the surrogate make decisions for the patient's health care? If the patient has issued explicit directives (written or oral), the surrogate should follow those instructions, unless it clearly can be demonstrated that the patient did not understand the nature of the information or choices made in that explicit directive. This situation unfortunately occurs when advance directives are completed without discussing the nature of the questions addressed with a health care provider. In the absence of such directives, the surrogate should use substituted judgment, that is, the surrogate should decide to the best of his or her ability, based on the beliefs and values of the patient, what the choices would be if the patient were able to speak for himself or herself. In some circumstances the surrogate has not had enough communication about health care and life issues with the patient to be able to project how the patient would decide. There simply is not enough information to be able to specifically substitute for the patient. In these circumstances, the surrogate's obligation is to try to decide the best interests of the patient given the clinical scenario.

- In the absence of explicit directives (written or oral), surrogates should use substituted judgment (what the choices would be if the patient were able to speak for himself or herself).
- If substituted judgment is not possible, the surrogate should make choices in the best interest of the patient.

Several studies have shown that surrogates often choose courses that are not what patients would have chosen for themselves in specific circumstances. Because of this, physicians should stress the importance of having patients discuss their values and health care goals with their family members or surrogates. It is also the duty of each physician to discuss these issues with her or his patients. This practice allows physicians to understand their patients' values to ensure that their choices are not made on misinformation.

Although it is always helpful when the patient has an advance directive that appoints a surrogate, most patients do not have advance directives. If the patient lacks decision-making capacity and there is no advance directive, who speaks for the patient? The underlying principle is to find a person, or persons, who best knows and can share with the physician and other caregivers the patient's values and health care goals and how the patient would most likely choose if he or she could speak for himself or herself. The most common approach recognizes the following individuals in descending order of authority: 1) the spouse, 2) an adult child or the majority of adult children, 3) a parent or parents, 4) an adult sibling or the majority of adult siblings, 5) an adult relative who has exhibited special care and concern, and 6) if no relative can be located, a close friend. Notably, some jurisdictions may have different hierarchies of who may serve as surrogates (in this context, some states refer to surrogates as proxies), and some have none at all.

* A surrogate decision maker is helpful for directing or enforcing a specific advance directive.

Conflicts in Surrogate Decision Making: Situations may arise in which a surrogate's decisions or instructions to physicians conflict with the patient's previously expressed directive or with those of other family members. Because the primary responsibility of the physician is to the patient, the physician should determine as best as possible what the patient would choose for himself or herself. In these circumstances, it may be helpful to involve an independent third-party arbitrator, such as an ethics consultant or committee or legal counsel, to help work through the issues. This option is useful only if the physician is unable to resolve the conflict. Once it has been established what the patient would want, it is the obligation of the treating physician(s) to comply with those wishes, even in the face of disagreement with surrogates. Only if clear evidence can be provided that the advance directive does not reflect what the patient really desired can the directive be overruled.

* The primary responsibility of the physician is to serve the patient's interest.

Recently, the tragic case of Terri Schiavo, a young woman from Florida who had a cardiac arrest in 1990 which left her in a persistent vegetative state (PVS), and whose misfortunes propelled her family and the nation into a controversy that raged over several years, challenged the existing legal, ethical, and social framework concerning surrogate decision making. However, after 10 decisions by the Florida District Court of Appeals, 4 reviews by the Florida Supreme Court, and 4 appeals to the US Supreme Court, the authorization of surrogate decision makers to withhold or withdraw life-sustaining treatments was affirmed. (For a detailed analysis of the Schiavo case, please see Hook CC, Mueller, PS. The Terri Schiavo saga: the making of a tragedy and lessons learned. Mayo Clin Proc. 2005;80:1449-60.)

Informed Consent

A derivative of the principle of autonomy (and nonmaleficence) is informed consent. Informed consent is the voluntary acceptance of

physician recommendations for interventions (clinical and research settings) by decisionally capable patients, or their surrogates, who have been provided sufficient information regarding the risks, benefits, and alternatives of the proposed interventions. Hence, there are 3 required elements of informed consent: 1) patient decision-making capacity, 2) patient voluntariness, and 3) accurate and sufficient information. The amount of information shared with the patient should be guided not only by what the physician believes is adequate (professional practice standard) but also by that which the average, prudent person would need to have in order to make an appropriate decision (reasonable person standard). Included within this information is a discussion of available alternatives to the proposed treatment, including doing nothing. For example, a patient with a cancer amenable to surgical resection, chemotherapy, or radiation therapy, all associated with a similar long-term outcome, should receive a thorough discussion of each of the options and their potential complications and side effects, even if the physician may be biased toward 1 of the 3 treatments. It is the duty of the physician to set aside personal bias and provide detailed information on each treatment to allow the patient to make a well-informed decision. The patient can then take the information and consider it within the context of her or his own values, health care goals, and quality-of-life considerations.

* Informed consent requires patient decision-making capacity and voluntariness and accurate and sufficient information.
* Reasonable person standard: amount of information needed by a patient is that which the average prudent person would need to have in order to make a decision.

After a discussion of the available alternatives, the physician should present the patient with a single recommendation that the patient can accept or reject. Patients come to their physicians expecting the caregivers to use their knowledge and experience in providing them with a recommendation. Simply laying out a menu of choices before the patient may lead to confusion or the perception by the patient that the physician is unconcerned with his or her welfare. If the patient refuses the recommended treatment and chooses one of the alternatives, the physician should respect the patient's choice. The final plan should reflect an agreement between a well-informed patient and a well-informed, sympathetic, and unbiased physician.

In certain circumstances, a patient may require more information than what the average reasonable person might desire. For instance, some religious belief systems may specifically preclude certain forms of medical intervention that might not trouble another individual in the least. It is important to ensure that patients receive sufficient information within the context of the factors that are most important to them to help make an appropriate choice.

* The physician should provide all alternatives, followed by a single recommendation.
* If the patient refuses the recommended treatment, the physician should respect the patient's choice.

In rare exceptions, the physician can treat a patient without truly informed consent (eg, in an emotionally unstable patient who requires urgent treatment, when informing the patient of the details may produce further problems).

Informed consent from surrogates is necessary to perform an autopsy (except in certain instances such as coroners' cases, in which the decision is made by outside authorities) or to practice intubation, placement of intravascular lines, or other procedures on the newly dead.

* Informed consent from surrogates is necessary to perform an autopsy.

Implied Consent

The principle of implied consent is invoked when true informed consent is not possible because the patient (or surrogate) is unable to express a decision regarding treatment, specifically, in emergency situations in which physicians are compelled to provide medically necessary therapy, without which harm would result. This principle clarifies the duty to assist a person in urgent need of care. Implied consent has been legally accepted (eg, Good Samaritan laws) and provides the physician a legal defense against battery (although not negligence).

* Implied consent is invoked when true informed consent is not possible, such as in emergency situations.

Truth Telling

Truth telling is an integral aspect of autonomy. The physician must provide decisionally capable patients with truthful information on which to base medical decisions. Without the receipt of sufficient truthful information, patients cannot make truly autonomous decisions about their life plans. Occasionally, however, the physician may withhold part or all of the truth if it is believed that telling the truth is likely to cause significant injury. This is the concept of therapeutic privilege. For example, if it can be well ascertained that a patient will attempt harm to himself or herself or others if certain information is received, such as the diagnosis of cancer, then the information may be withheld. However, there is a *high* burden of proof on the withholding physician to establish the likelihood of injury. This decision for intentional nondisclosure must be fully recorded in the medical record.

Some decisionally capable patients may forgo complete disclosure, deferring the receipt of information and decision making to others. Forgoing complete disclosure may occur by individual preference or in the context of cultural norms. Regardless, this preference should be respected as the patient's autonomous choice.

* Truth telling on the part of the physician is an integral aspect of respecting patient autonomy.

Confidentiality

Privacy is an integral part of the respect for persons and protection of an individual's autonomy. Confidentiality respects that right to privacy and provides the patient the right to keep medical information solely within the realm of the physician-patient relationship. The physician is ethically and legally obliged to maintain a patient's medical information in strict confidence, a tradition dating back to the Hippocratic Oath. Ensuring confidentiality encourages complete communication of all relevant information that may affect the patient's health.

However, "the obligation to safeguard patient confidences is subject to certain exceptions that are justified because of overriding ethical and social concerns. When a patient threatens to inflict serious bodily harm on another individual, and there is reasonable probability that the patient will carry out the threat, the physician is obligated to take reasonable precautions for the protection of the intended victim, including notification of law enforcement authorities if necessary" (American Medical Association Council on Ethical and Judicial Affairs, 1997). Also, in some instances, a patient's data must be shared with public health care agencies, such as in the case of human immunodeficiency virus (HIV), *Mycobacterium* tuberculosis, and other infectious diseases and in cases of physical abuse, gunshot wounds, and other concerns to the public health and welfare. There are state to state differences in reporting requirements and each physician should be aware of local statutes.

A growing area of concern in maintaining confidentiality is in regard to heritable genetic traits. Currently, this concern is undergoing significant ethical and legal scrutiny.

An example that challenges the principle of confidentiality is the patient with HIV infection who refuses to inform third parties who have been or will be engaged in high-risk activities with the patient. A functional solution is the following: 1) attempt to persuade the infected patient to cease endangering the third party or to notify the third party of the risk; 2) if persuasion fails, notify an authority who can intervene; 3) if the authority takes no action or is not available (eg, the state does not pursue contact tracing after report of HIV), notify the endangered party of the risk (American Medical Association Council on Ethical and Judicial Affairs, 1988). It must be clearly stated that this approach still may be open to legal liabilities and is based on the medical profession's obligation to prevent harm. Public policy trends have been moving toward stronger protection of patient confidentiality.

* A physician is obliged to maintain medical information in strict confidence.
* The obligation to safeguard patient confidences is subject to certain exceptions that are justified because of overriding ethical and social concerns (eg, mandatory reporting requirements).

Futility

It has been clearly established, both ethically and legally, that patients have the right to refuse any and all medical therapies. But does the principle of autonomy give patients, or their surrogates, the right to demand treatments? This question particularly arises when patients or families request that cardiopulmonary resuscitation, mechanical ventilation, and other aggressive treatment be performed on patients with little chance of recovery or survival to dismissal. Can physicians unilaterally withhold or withdraw medical interventions if, in their opinion, the intervention is futile? The conflict seemingly is between the autonomy of the patients and the moral autonomy and integrity of the caregivers. Physicians are moral agents, just as much as patients, and should not be forced to violate their ethical beliefs and principles.

* Patients have the right to refuse any and all medical therapies.

The Oxford English Dictionary defines futility as "leaky, hence untrustworthy, vain, failing of the desired end through intrinsic defect." Therefore, a futile intervention is one that cannot achieve specified goals no matter how many times it is repeated. From this definition, it can clearly be stated that physicians are not required to provide treatments that have no pathophysiologic rationale, that have already failed in a given patient in the past, or that cannot achieve the goals of care already agreed on by the physician and patient or surrogate. However, many so-called futility conflicts arise in clinical situations in which an intervention is not impossible but is unlikely to benefit the patient or there is a conflict about the goals of treatment (such as maintaining physiologic life vs restoration of independent functioning or survival to dismissal). Many have tried to create functional definitions of futility that would cover these circumstances, but all have the flaw of establishing arbitrary thresholds that are value-laden in themselves.

* A futile intervention is one that cannot achieve the goals of intervention no matter how many times it is repeated.

When a futility conflict arises in a clinical situation, the approach to a solution should be one of due process, which attempts to negotiate consensus and resolve the conflict. The American Medical Association Council on Ethical and Judicial Affairs endorsed such a program ("Houston Policy," JAMA. 1996;276:571-4), which requires the following:

1. Earnest attempts to deliberate over and negotiate prior understanding among patient, surrogate, and physician about what constitutes "futile" care for the patient and what falls within acceptable limits for those involved. Many times the disagreement is based on inappropriate expectations of the patient or surrogate. When appropriate data about outcomes are shared, many requests for treatments such as cardiopulmonary resuscitation decrease.
2. Joint decision making should occur to the maximal extent possible.
3. Attempts should be made to negotiate and resolve disagreements (such as through ethics consultation).
4. If disagreements are irresolvable, a consultant or end-of-life decisions committee should become involved.
5. If the committee agrees with the patient and the physician remains unpersuaded, intra- or inter-institutional transfer may be arranged.
6. If the committee agrees with the physician and the patient or surrogate remains unpersuaded, intra- or inter-institutional transfer may be arranged.
7. If transfer is not possible, the intervention need not be offered.

Points 5 through 7 remain contested and controversial because of the potential unilateral overriding of the patient's or surrogate's wishes. At the time of this writing, the Houston Protocol (which is the basis for the futility statute of the state of Texas) has come under increasing criticism and legal challenge. In part, some of the problems have stemmed from situations in which patients have derived benefit from treatments previously declared futile. These situations illustrate the need for humility by physicians in prognostication. We serve our patients better when we identify situations as unlikely to improve rather than declaring absolute futility.

* As much as possible, resolution of futility conflicts should be attempted by using a due process approach.

Beneficence

Beneficence is acting to benefit patients by preserving life, restoring health, relieving suffering, and restoring or maintaining function. The physician (acting in good faith) is obligated to help patients attain their own interests and goals as determined by the patient, not the physician.

When we think of benefitting the patient, we must remember that there are several levels of defining benefit for a given situation, some objective and some subjective. The first level concerns the biomedical or physiologic benefit of a proposed intervention, is usually the least controversial area, and requires the most physician input. As physicians we often tend to stop at this first level, but the next 2 patient-defined levels are often of great importance to how a patient defines *benefit*.

The second level is personal benefit: how the patient interprets the situation in the context of her or his values and goals. This level may sometimes seem in conflict with the biomedical benefit. For example, a patient with end-stage cancer and ventilator-dependent respiratory failure will not derive any long-term biomedical benefit from continuing the intensive care. However, that patient may have the goal of living for another 48 hours in order to say good-bye to a child who is going to be arriving from a great distance. That specific goal enables the intervention to be understood as benefitting the patient.

The third level has been described as ultimate benefit, but it refers to the patient's belief system and world view. Does the patient's faith make claims as to the obligation to preserve life to the last breath? Here the patient's ultimate framework of beliefs may have a specific impact on the definition of benefit. As the patient's advocate, we must consider all 3 levels as we define benefit.

* Beneficence is acting to benefit patients by preserving life, restoring health, relieving suffering, and restoring or maintaining function.

Nonmaleficence

Nonmaleficence requires that one should not do evil or harm. This principle has roots in the statement of Hippocrates, "as to diseases, help, but at least do no harm." This principle also addresses unprofessional behavior, such as the verbal, physical, and sexual abuse of patients, or uninformed and undisclosed interventions or experimentation on patients.

* Nonmaleficence: "as to diseases, help, but at least do no harm."

Nonabandonment

Abandonment is the act of leaving the patient (for whom the physician has provided health care in the past) without providing for immediate or future medical care. This action has been "universally condemned as a serious and punishable infraction of both the legal and ethical obligations that physicians owe patients" (Ann Intern

Med. 1995;122:377-8). In contrast, nonabandonment denotes a requisite ethical obligation of physicians to provide ongoing medical care once the patient and physician mutually concur to enter into an alliance. Nonabandonment is closely related to the principles of beneficence and nonmaleficence and is fundamental to the long-term physician-patient relationship. This principle has several drawbacks and limitations. The degree of physician involvement in the relationship cannot be measured as to its quantity or quality. Furthermore, the extent of the relationship is dictated by the underlying medical condition. For instance, an annual examination may require a single visit to the physician, whereas a complicated disease process may bring the physician and patient closer to each other over a long period. It would be improper for the physician to force a patient to maintain a long-term physician-patient relationship if the latter is unwilling, for whatever reason. Noncompliance, in terms of taking medications or following a physician's instructions, by the patient is not grounds for abandonment. Physicians should strive to respond to the needs of their patients over time, but they should not trespass their own values in the process.

● Nonabandonment: a requisite ethical obligation of physicians to provide ongoing care once the patient and physician mutually concur to enter into an alliance.

Conflict of Interest
The principle of beneficence requires that the physician not engage in activities that are not in the patient's best interest. This is considered to be a significant problem in medicine today. Some studies have suggested that physicians' prescribing practices are influenced by financial and other significant rewards from drug companies. If the physician does not ardently avoid areas of potential conflict of interest (because of the principle of beneficence), the result may be maleficence. Authorship of scientific papers and editorials to promote drugs and appliances solely for immediate or future personal financial gains also constitutes conflict of interest (Ann Intern Med. 1997;126:986-8).

● Conflict of interest is contrary to the principle of beneficence.

The Impaired Physician
According to the American Medical Association, the impaired physician is one who is "unable to practice medicine with reasonable skill and safety to patients because of physical or mental illness, including deteriorations through the aging process, or loss of motor skill, or excessive use or abuse of drugs including alcohol." Impairment is distinct from competence, which specifically concerns the physician's knowledge and skills to adequately perform his or her duties as a physician. Impairment and incompetence both may seriously compromise patient care and safety. Under the obligation to protect patients from harm, physicians must protect patients from impaired and incompetent colleagues. Physicians have a moral, professional, and legal obligation to report impaired and incompetent colleagues to the appropriate authority. Different states vary in the specifics of reporting, but all have a reporting requirement. Typical authorities to contact include the institutional chief of staff or impairment program, local or state medical society impairment programs, or the state licensing body. It is important that reporting the behavior of a colleague be based on objective evidence rather than supposition.

● Physicians have an obligation to report impaired behavior in colleagues.

The Rule of Double Effect (Beneficence vs Nonmaleficence)
In the medical management of patients, sometimes the pursuit of a beneficent outcome risks the potential for serious injury or death. Consequently, the moral obligations for both beneficence and nonmaleficence conflict. The classic example of such a situation is the terminally ill patient who may require high doses of narcotics for adequate analgesia, but such doses also have the potential for respiratory depression and an earlier death. The rule of double effect is a means of trying to resolve the conflict. This principle states that 1) the act itself must be good or morally neutral, 2) the actor or agent intends only the good effect, 3) the bad effect must not be a means to the good effect (eg, death is the only way to achieve the desired outcome), and 4) the good effect must outweigh the bad effect. By the reasoning of double effect, and the high requirement of beneficence to address the suffering of patients, adequate analgesia for the relief of suffering should always be given even if death is hastened. The analgesics are to be given, however, in such a way as to relieve the pain and not specifically to hasten the death of patients, even terminally ill patients.

● Adequate analgesia, particularly in patients with incurable disease, is the responsibility of the physician.
● The physician has not performed immorally if death in a terminally ill patient is a result of respiratory depression from analgesic therapy; euthanasia is not the goal.

Justice
Every patient deserves and must be provided optimal care as warranted by the underlying medical condition. Allocation of medical resources fairly and according to medical need is the basis for this principle. The decision to provide optimal medical care should be based on the medical need of each patient and the perceived medical benefit to the patient. The patient's social status, ability to pay, or perceived social worth should not dictate the quality or quantity of medical care. The physician's clear-cut responsibility is to the patient's well-being (beneficence). Physicians should not make decisions about individual care of their patients based on larger societal needs. The bedside is not the place to make general policy decisions.

● Justice: allocation of medical resources fairly and according to medical need.
● Physicians should not make decisions about individual care of patients based on larger societal needs.

Ethical Considerations At the End of Life

Incurable Disease and Death
Probably the most distressing aspect of medical practice is the encounter with a patient who has an incurable disease and in whom

death is inevitable. The physician and patient (or surrogate) must formulate appropriate goals of therapy, choose what measures should be taken to maintain life, and decide how aggressive these measures ought to be. It is important to remind oneself that the patient is under enormous mental anguish and physical stress and that the ability to make solid decisions may be clouded. Furthermore, the decision(s) made by the patient may be guided by his or her understanding (whether adequate or not) of the medical condition and prognosis, religious beliefs, financial status, and other personal wishes. The patient may seek counsel from family, friends, and clergy as well as the attending physician.

- In incurable disease, recognize that the patient is under enormous mental anguish and physical stress.
- The ability of the patient to make solid decisions may be clouded.

The following guidelines are suggested in caring for patients with incurable diseases or who are dying. The patient and family (if the patient so desires) must be provided ample opportunity to talk with the physician and ask questions. An unhurried openness and willing-to-listen attitude on the part of the physician are critical for a positive outcome.

- The patient and family must be provided every opportunity to talk with the physician and ask questions.
- An unhurried openness and willing-to-listen attitude on the part of the physician are critical for a positive outcome.

The physician should assume the responsibility to furnish or arrange for physical, emotional, and spiritual support. Adequate control of pain, respect for human dignity, and close contact with the family are crucial. The emotional and spiritual support available through hospital chaplains or local clergy (as appropriate, given the patient's personal beliefs) should not be underestimated. At no other time in life is the reality of human mortality so real as in the terminal phases of disease. It is always preferable to allay the anxiety of the dying patient through adequate emotional and spiritual support rather than by sedation. The physician should constantly remind herself or himself that despite all the medical technology that surrounds the patient, the patient must not be dehumanized.

- Adequate pain control, respect for human dignity, and close contact with the family are crucial.
- It is better to allay the anxiety of the dying patient through adequate emotional and spiritual support rather than by sedation.

Physician-Assisted Death

All 4 principles of medical ethics have an impact on the issue of physician-assisted death, that is, physician-assisted suicide and euthanasia. Historically, the medical profession has taken a strong stand against physicians directly killing patients, but this prohibition has been challenged on the basis of patient autonomy, beneficence or compassion, and other grounds. Numerous opinion polls have shown that significant portions of the general population and the medical community now favor some legalization of physician-assisted sui-

cide, if not euthanasia. The American Medical Association and other large professional medical groups have maintained their stance against these practices.

In 1997, the US Supreme Court ruled that states may maintain laws prohibiting euthanasia and assisted suicide but may also pass laws allowing these practices. Although the Court did not find a right to physician-assisted death, it emphasized the patient's right to adequate, aggressive pain control, even if it might shorten the patient's life. In the election of 1997, the people of the state of Oregon reiterated their support for physician-assisted suicide by re-approving a referendum first passed in 1994 legalizing assisted suicide but still prohibiting euthanasia. The Oregon law requires that the patient 1) be terminal, 2) be decisionally capable, 3) has initiated 2 verbal requests and 1 written request for a prescription for a lethal overdose, 4) undergo a second-opinion consultation, 5) receive appropriate psychiatric intervention if perceived to be depressed, and 6) undergo a 15-day waiting period after the request has been made to allow the patient to change his or her mind. At this time, assisted suicide and euthanasia remain illegal in the other 49 states.

- Euthanasia and physician-assisted suicide are legally prohibited in the United States with the exception of the state of Oregon, which permits physician-assisted suicide.

Regardless of one's final position on this difficult issue, physicians are obligated to address the underlying concerns that lead patients and physicians to believe that assisted suicide and euthanasia are necessary (the New York State Task Force on Life and the Law, 1994). Physicians should be acquainted with appropriate means of pain management and palliative care and be willing to be aggressive in the relief of a patient's symptoms. Physicians also are obligated to recognize and appropriately treat depression. Furthermore, physicians should strive to address the other issues that may lead patients to desire assisted death, such as fear of abandonment and loss of control.

Withholding and Withdrawing Life-Sustaining Treatments

The decision to withhold or withdraw life-sustaining treatments may be compatible with beneficence, nonmaleficence, and autonomy. Granting patients' requests to withhold or withdraw unwanted medical treatments is legal and ethical. Granting a request to refuse or withdraw a medical intervention is not the same as physician-assisted suicide or euthanasia. In assisted suicide, the patient personally terminates his or her life by using an external means provided by a clinician (eg, lethal prescription). In euthanasia, the clinician directly terminates the patient's life (eg, lethal injection). In assisted suicide and euthanasia, a new intervention is introduced (eg, drug), the sole intent of which is the patient's death. In contrast, when a patient dies after an intervention is withheld or withdrawn, the underlying disease is the cause of death. The intent is freedom from interventions that are perceived as burdensome.

Notably, there is no ethical or legal distinction between withholding treatment in the first place, or choosing to withdraw a treatment once begun. The right of a decisionally capable person to refuse lifesaving hydration and nutrition was upheld by the US Supreme Court (Table 16-1), but a surrogate decision maker's right to refuse treatment for decisionally incapable persons has been restricted by some states. Currently, the states of New York, Missouri, and Florida require "clear and convincing evidence" that withdrawing and withholding of life-supporting treatment would be the patient's desire. Other states have lesser evidentiary standards for surrogates to withhold or withdraw life support. Brain death is not a necessary requirement for withdrawing or withholding life support. The value of each medical therapy (risk:benefit ratio) should be assessed for each patient. When appropriate, the withholding or withdrawal of life support is best accomplished with input from more than one experienced clinician.

- Withholding or withdrawing life support does not conflict with the principles of beneficence, nonmaleficence, and autonomy.
- Brain death is not a necessary requirement for withdrawing or withholding life support.

Do-Not-Resuscitate Orders

Do-not-resuscitate (DNR) orders affect administration of cardiopulmonary resuscitation (CPR) only; other therapeutic options should not be influenced by the DNR order. A DNR order can be compatible with maximal forms of treatment (eg, elective intubation, elective cardioversion, surgery). Every person whose medical history is unclear or unavailable should receive CPR in the event of cardiopulmonary arrest.

Of paramount importance are the patient's knowledge of the extent of disease and the prognosis, the physician's estimate of the potential efficacy of CPR, and the wishes of the patient (or surrogate) regarding CPR as a therapeutic tool. The appropriateness of a DNR order should be reviewed frequently because clinical circumstances may dictate other measures (eg, a patient with terminal cardiomyopathy who had initially turned down heart transplantation and wanted to be considered DNR may change her or his mind and now opt for the transplantation). Physicians should discuss the appropriateness of CPR or DNR with patients at high risk for cardiopulmonary arrest and with the terminally ill. The discussion should optimally take place in the outpatient setting, during the initial period of hospitalization, and periodically during hospitalization, if appropriate. DNR orders (and rationale) should be entered in the patient's medical records.

- DNR orders affect CPR only.
- A DNR order may be compatible with maximal forms of treatment.
- In the absence of a DNR order, universal consent for CPR is presumed.
- DNR orders should be reviewed frequently.

Persistent Vegetative State

Persistent vegetative state is a chronic state of unconsciousness (loss of self-awareness) lasting for more than a few weeks, characterized by the presence of wake-sleep cycles, but without behavioral or cerebral metabolic evidence of cognitive function or of being able to respond in a willful manner to external events or stimuli. The body retains functions necessary to sustain physiologic survival (eg, respiration, circulation, endocrine function) if provided nutritional and other supportive measures. Many patients in persistent vegetative state require only artificially administered nutrition and hydration, in addition to routine nursing care to continue to physically survive. The US Supreme Court has ruled that there is no distinction between artificially administered nutrition and hydration compared with mechanical ventilation or other interventions in terms of being medical treatments that can be withheld or withdrawn (Table 16-1).

- Persistent vegetative state: unconsciousness (loss of self-awareness) lasting for more than a few weeks.
- US Supreme Court ruling states that there is no distinction between artificially administered nutrition and hydration compared with mechanical ventilation or other interventions in terms of being medical treatments.

Definition of Death

Death is the irreversible cessation of circulatory and respiratory function or the irreversible cessation of all functions of the entire brain, including the brainstem. Clinical criteria (at times supported by electroencephalographic testing or assessment of cerebral perfusion) permit the reliable diagnosis of brain death.

The family should be informed of the brain death but should not be asked to decide whether further medical therapy should be continued. One exception is when the patient's surrogate (or the patient, via an advance directive) permits certain decisions, such as organ donation, in the case of brain death.

Once it is ascertained that the patient is "brain dead" and that no further therapy can be offered, the primary physician, preferably after consultation with another physician involved in the care of the patient, may withdraw supportive measures. This approach is accepted throughout the United States, with the exception of the states of New Jersey and New York, which have modified their definition of death statutes to allow a religious exemption for groups (such as Orthodox Jews) that do not accept brain death as a valid criterion for death. In these states, continued care may be requested of the caregivers until circulatory and respiratory function collapses.

The imminent possibility of harvesting organs for transplantation should in no way affect any of the aforementioned decisions. When organ and tissue donation is possible after the determination of brain death, the family should be approached, preferably before cessation of cardiac function, regarding organ donation.

- Death: irreversible cessation of circulatory and respiratory function or irreversible cessation of all functions of the entire brain, including the brainstem.

Authors' Note

Laws concerning ethical issues in medicine continue to evolve, reflecting changing attitudes of society. Certainly, legal decisions will continue to influence the practice of medicine. Many states have no directly applicable statutes or court cases relating to difficult ethical issues in medical practice. This review is meant as a guide; the individual practitioner is referred to the appropriate state medical society for further information regarding state-specific mandates.

Questions

Multiple Choice (choose the best answer)

1. An 83-year-old woman with advanced dementia is admitted to your hospital service because of failure to thrive, poor oral intake, and dehydration. Her advance directive, which was executed when she had decision-making capacity, states that under no circumstances is she to receive a feeding tube. The directive also names the patient's daughter, an attorney, as the surrogate decision maker. You review the advance directive with the daughter. Despite the specific instructions in the advance directive, the daughter demands that a feeding tube be inserted. In fact, she threatens to sue if the tube is not inserted promptly. Which of the following is the most appropriate next step?

   a. Insert a temporary nasogastric feeding tube and begin artificial hydration and nutrition in order to allow time for you to discuss the case with the hospital attorney.
   b. Explain to the daughter that it is your ethical and legal duty as the physician, and her duty as the surrogate, to comply with the patient's advance directive and not insert the feeding tube.
   c. Start intravenous fluids and nutrition.
   d. Honor the daughter's request and insert the feeding tube. Later, remove the tube after the daughter accepts the patient's terminal condition.
   e. Hydration and nutrition administered via a feeding tube are not medical treatments but rather are basic care akin to bathing, and cannot be refused by patients (or surrogates); hence, the tube must be inserted.

2. An 85-year-old woman with widely metastatic breast cancer who lives alone is admitted to your hospital service because of severe pain and a poor performance status. A concerned neighbor brought her to the hospital. The patient, who has been independent up to this point, has not told her 2 children, who live hundreds of miles away, of her recent problems. Currently, she is oriented, understands her prognosis, and indicates that she has an advance directive. The advance directive clearly lays out her refusal of any life-sustaining treatments and her desire for comfort care only. The neighbor, who brought the patient to the hospital, is named as the surrogate. The patient does not want her children to know her situation at all, not wanting to burden them. She specifically instructs you not to contact her children until after her death. One of the children, a daughter, who learns from another neighbor that her mother is in the hospital, calls and begs you to tell her about her mother's condition. She states that if her mother is seriously ill she needs to return home and reconcile some issues between them while there is still time. You should:

   a. Tell the daughter that you cannot provide any information regarding the patient without the patient's consent.
   b. Tell the daughter her mother's situation but request that she not divulge to the patient how she learned this information.

   c. Ask the neighbor surrogate to grant permission to disclose the patient's status to her children.
   d. Ask a hospital chaplain to convince the patient of the need to share her situation with her children.
   e. Refuse to speak to the daughter at all for fear that you would divulge too much about the patient's status.

3. A 75-year-old man is entering the final stages of metastatic renal cell carcinoma. His disease has progressed despite treatment with interleukin-2 and sunitinib. He is now admitted to the hospital with urosepsis. Given his overall poor prognosis and very low chance of surviving an arrest and cardiopulmonary resuscitation (CPR), his physician advises a do-not-resuscitate (DNR) order. Nevertheless, the patient requests that he receive all life-sustaining measures, including CPR if necessary, despite his poor prognosis. The physician should:

   a. Write a DNR order in the medical record and not tell the patient.
   b. Explain to the patient that CPR in this setting is futile and, hence, the physician cannot comply with the patient's request.
   c. Transfer the patient to a colleague who can deal better with irrational requests such as this one.
   d. So long as CPR is the default standard of care, it is better to comply with the patient's request than to overtly or surreptitiously override it. However, it is the physician's duty to ensure that the patient is informed of his very poor chances of survival after an arrest and CPR.
   e. Comply with the request but, should the patient have arrest, do a "slow" code.

4. You have been invited to attend a buffet luncheon at an exclusive restaurant sponsored by a pharmaceutical company. You know the cost of the luncheon is $40 per plate. It is also likely that company representatives will be giving away medical textbooks valued at more than $100 each. You should:

   a. Decline to attend because of potential conflicts of interest and the undue influence such gifts might have on your medical decision making.
   b. Attend the luncheon to get updated on the company's latest pharmaceuticals and, in turn, improve patient care.
   c. Attend the luncheon in order to obtain as much educational material as possible.
   d. Attend the luncheon because attending such events is widely accepted and practiced by physicians.
   e. Attend the luncheon because such gifts from pharmaceutical companies do not influence physician decision making.

5. While covering the hospital practice during a weekend, you discover that your partner prescribed azithromycin for a female patient with community-acquired pneumonia despite her having increased values on liver function tests. After you have

examined the patient, who is jaundiced, and discussed the plans for the day, the patient's clearly upset husband interrupts and asks, "Didn't Dr. Smith, your partner, mess something up here? Her cough is better, but she's weak and yellow and has no appetite. She should be going home, but she feels worse. Dr. Smith said, 'Everything's fine,' but I know something is wrong. What's going on?" You should:

a. Tell the husband to share his concerns with Dr. Smith on Monday when Dr. Smith will be making rounds again.
b. Ask the patient to sign a release form allowing you to discuss her care with her husband.
c. Describe the patient's condition, including the side effects of the medication she received, and what you propose to do to facilitate her recovery.
d. Excuse yourself from the room to "check on something," then call the hospital attorney for advice.
e. Tell the husband that given his lack of satisfaction with his wife's care, you would be happy to transfer her care to another physician or hospital.

6. Mr. White is a 60-year-old man with severe chronic obstructive pulmonary disease. He is a widower and has no children. He is admitted to the hospital with pneumonia and respiratory failure promptly develops. You tell him that he will die without intubation and mechanical ventilation. He does not have an advance directive, but he does have decision-making capacity. He tells you that he does not want mechanical ventilation, stating he is "at peace with God's will." He understands the consequences of his refusal, including death. Which of the following statements is true about the patient's decision?

a. It is ethically and legally permissible for a physician to override the patient's decision and intubate and mechanically ventilate him in order to keep him alive.

b. Because Mr. White doesn't have an advance directive, a court must affirm his decision.
c. His decision is inconsistent with standard medical practice and, hence, honoring his refusal of intubation and mechanical ventilation would be grounds for malpractice.
d. Patients with decision-making capacity have the right to refuse life-sustaining treatments even if such refusals result in death.
e. In cases such as these, hospital chaplains should be asked to convince patients to change their minds.

7. A 73-year-old man with metastatic pancreatic cancer is admitted to your hospital service because of intractable malignancy-associated pain. He also has a history of ischemic cardiomyopathy and has an implanted cardioverter-defibrillator (ICD). You give him intravenous morphine (morphine drip), and his pain improves. However, during the first day of his hospitalization, he experiences 4 uncomfortable ICD defibrillations; the defibrillations are appropriate (ie, because of ventricular dysrhythmias). Knowing that he is dying, the patient requests comfort care only. Furthermore, not wanting to experience more defibrillations, he requests deactivation of the ICD. He does not have an advance directive. Regarding the request to deactivate the ICD, you should:

a. Refuse to comply because doing so is the same as euthanasia.
b. Comply with the request.
c. Refuse to comply because he does not have an advance directive.
d. Refuse to comply because an ICD is not a life-sustaining treatment and deactivating an ICD is not a form of comfort care.
e. Although it is ethical and legal for a patient who has a medical indication for an ICD to refuse ICD implantation, it is unethical and illegal for a physician to deactivate an ICD after it is implanted.

Answers

1. Answer b.
Physicians and surrogate decision makers have ethical and legal duties to adhere to patients' advance directives so long as the instructions in the directives are reasonable and legal. In this case, the daughter cannot "trump" the advance directive. Rather, it is her duty to ensure that her mother's wishes are followed. Inserting a feeding tube (temporary or permanent) into this patient would violate the patient's previously expressed explicit wishes and therefore her autonomy. Finally, artificially administered (eg, via a feeding tube) hydration and nutrition are medical treatments, and, like other treatments, they can be refused by patients.

2. Answer a.
As much as one may disagree with the patient's choice to hide her situation from her children, she made it clear that she does not want her medical information shared with them. Providing the daughter information not only violates the ethical principle of respect for patient autonomy (ie, by breaching patient confidentiality) but also is against the law (Health Insurance portability and Accountability Act; HIPAA).

3. Answer d.
As long as CPR for cardiac arrest is the default standard of care, it is better to comply with such a request than to overtly or surreptitiously override it. In these situations, the physician's duty is to ensure that the patient understands the implications of the choice, especially the poor chance of surviving an arrest despite CPR. Doing a "slow" code after telling a patient that CPR according to standard protocol will be done is morally indefensible.

4. Answer a.
There is clear evidence that gifts from pharmaceutical companies (eg, lunches, books, pens), no matter how small, influence the prescribing habits of physicians. Furthermore, even though expenditures in research and development have remained stable in recent years, the investment in marketing by drug companies has increased dramatically, adding to the prices of new drugs. Physicians should avoid interacting with pharmaceutical company representatives because of duties to avoid conflicts of interest and to promote patients' just access to medical goods (eg, by not participating in activities that contribute to drug costs).

5. Answer c.
Physicians have an obligation to share the truth about errors or complications of interventions with patients. Patients must be informed about errors and complications in order to facilitate future decision making. Trying to skirt the issue may engender patient and family anger and increase the likelihood of legal misadventure. Alternatively, patients who are informed of errors and complications and receive sincere apologies and are made aware of efforts to correct the mistakes are more likely to work with rather than against the physician, a relationship that thereby reduces the risk of litigation. Certainly, in this case Dr. Smith needs to be held accountable for his mistake, but as the physician in charge at the moment you are obligated to address the concern as presented to you.

6. Answer d.
Patients with decision-making capacity have the right to refuse life-sustaining treatments even if such refusals result in death. These decisions do not need to be affirmed by ethics committees or courts, nor do they need to be in writing. The physician's obligation is to understand the rationale for such refusals and be certain the refusals are informed.

7. Answer b.
Dying patients with ICDs may experience uncomfortable defibrillations. As a result, to avoid defibrillations, many of these patients request ICD deactivation and withdrawal of other treatments (eg, mechanical ventilation, hemodialysis). Granting such requests is not the same as physician-assisted suicide or euthanasia. In physician-assisted suicide, the cause of death is the lethal agent prescribed by the physician. In euthanasia, the cause of death is the lethal agent administered by the physician. The cause of death after withholding or withdrawing a treatment is the underlying disease. Respect for patient autonomy underpins the right to refuse or request the withdrawal of treatments perceived by the patient as burdensome. Notably, there is no ethical or legal distinction between withholding a treatment and withdrawing a treatment after it has been initiated.

17

Men's Health

Thomas J. Beckman, MD
Haitham S. Abu-Lebdeh, MD

Benign prostatic hyperplasia (BPH) and erectile dysfunction are among the commonest diagnoses in a men's health practice.

Benign Prostatic Hyperplasia

BPH is common among older men. The prostate is the size of a walnut (20 cm3) in men younger than 30 years and it gradually increases in size, leading to BPH in most men older than 60 years. BPH results from epithelial and stromal cell growth, which begins in the transitional zone of the prostate and causes urinary outflow resistance. Over time, this resistance leads to detrusor muscle dysfunction, urinary retention, and lower urinary tract symptoms (LUTS). There is evidence that BPH progresses when left untreated. This progression is manifested as worsening prostate symptom scores, declining urinary flow rates, and increased risk of acute urinary retention. Other complications of BPH include urinary tract infections, obstructive nephropathy, and recurrent hematuria.

Diagnosing BPH is challenging because prostate size correlates poorly with LUTS and numerous conditions other than BPH cause LUTS (Table 17-1). Nonetheless, assessing symptom severity, identifying prostatic enlargement on digital rectal examination (DRE), and documenting decreased urinary flow rates with increased postvoid residuals yield accurate diagnoses in most cases.

- Clinical BPH exists in most men aged 60 or older.
- Prostate size correlates poorly with symptoms of BPH.
- Conditions other than BPH associated with LUTS include urinary tract infections, obstructive nephropathy, and recurrent hematuria.

History and Physical Examination

When obtaining a history, consider the patient's age. Because prostate size increases with age, LUTS are most likely due to BPH in men older than 50 years, and LUTS are most likely due to other conditions in men younger than 40 years. Reviewing medications is also essential because many medications cause LUTS by affecting detrusor muscle and urinary sphincter function: 1) anticholinergic and antimuscarinic medications decrease detrusor muscle tone; 2) sympathomimetic medications increase urethral sphincter tone; and 3) diuretics increase urinary frequency (Table 17-1). Additionally, over-the-counter cold medications may cause LUTS by various mechanisms. When older men with subclinical BPH simply discontinue taking new medications, LUTS often resolve. Finally, a focused review of systems should identify fever, hematuria (indicating urothelial malignancy), urethral instrumentation or sexually transmitted diseases (suggesting the possibility of urethral stricture), sleep disturbances, patterns of fluid intake, and use of alcohol and caffeine.

The American Urological Association International Prostate Symptom Score (AUA/IPSS) is an objective measure of LUTS associated with BPH. The AUA/IPSS aids in diagnosing BPH and following the progression of BPH over time (Figure 17-1). Numerous studies have shown the reliability and validity of the AUA/IPSS. The AUA/IPSS asks 7 questions about the following symptoms: frequency, nocturia, weak stream, hesitancy, intermittency, incomplete bladder emptying, and urgency. Each question is answered on a 5-point scale. When the responses to the 7 questions are summed, a score of 0 to 7 represents mild symptoms of BPH, 8 to 19 represents moderate symptoms, and 20 to 35 represents severe symptoms.

- Diuretics and sympathomimetic and anticholinergic medications cause LUTS.
- Numerous over-the-counter medications cause LUTS.
- The AUA/IPSS is a reliable and valid assessment of bothersome prostate symptoms.

For this chapter, the following sources were used with permission from Mayo Foundation for Medical Education and Research: Beckman TJ, Mynderse LA. Evaluation and medical management of benign prostatic hyperplasia. Mayo Clin Proc. 2005;80:1356-62; and Beckman TJ, Abu-Lebdeh HS, Mynderse LA. Evaluation and medical management of erectile dysfunction. Mayo Clin Proc. 2006;81:385-90.

Table 17-1 Differential Diagnosis for Benign Prostatic Hyperplasia

Category	Examples	Comments
Malignant	Adenocarcinoma of the prostate	Men should be offered PSA testing in conjunction with DRE
	Transitional cell carcinoma of the bladder	With microhematuria on urinalysis, consider urothelial
	Squamous cell carcinoma of the penis	malignancies
Infectious	Cystitis	Urinalysis & urinary Gram stain are useful in evaluating for cystitis
	Prostatitis	Prostatic massage specimens (VB3) assist in diagnosis of prostatitis
	Sexually transmitted diseases (eg, chlamydial	Sexually transmitted diseases may cause LUTS from urethral
	infection & gonorrhea)	scarring & stricture
Neurologic	Spinal cord injury	Primary mechanisms for neurologic causes of LUTS are detrusor
	Cauda equina syndrome	weakness or uninhibited detrusor contractions (or both)
	Stroke	Alzheimer disease can cause functional urinary incontinence
	Parkinsonism	
	Diabetic autonomic neuropathy	
	Multiple sclerosis	
	Alzheimer disease	
Medical	Poorly controlled diabetes mellitus	Medical conditions associated with urinary frequency are often
	Diabetes insipidus	overlooked causes of LUTS
	Congestive heart failure	
	Hypercalcemia	
	Obstructive sleep apnea	
Iatrogenic	Prostatectomy	Surgery sometimes causes neurologic impairment
	Cystectomy	Traumatic urethrocystoscopic procedures can cause scarring &
	Traumatic urethrocystoscopic procedures	urethral strictures
	Radiation cystitis	
Anatomical	Ureteral and bladder stones	Hematuria may be seen on urinalysis
		Consider urinary cytologic, cystoscopic, & renal imaging studies
Behavioral	Polydipsia	Consider assessing serum sodium
	Excessive alcohol or caffeine consumption	Voiding diary may provide useful information about fluid intake
Pharmacologic	Diuretics (eg, furosemide, hydrochlorothiazide)	Diuretics increase urinary frequency
	Sympathomimetics (eg, ephedrine, dextro-	Sympathomimetic medications increase urethral resistance
	amphetamine)	Anticholinergic & antimuscarinic medications decrease detrusor
	Anticholinergics (eg, oxybutynin, amantadine)	contractility
	Antimuscarinics (eg, diphenhydramine,	Over-the-counter medications may cause LUTS by various
	amitriptyline)	mechanisms
	Over-the-counter decongestants	
Other	Overactive bladder	UDS can help distinguish BPH from isolated detrusor dysfunction

Abbreviations: BPH, benign prostatic hyperplasia; DRE, digital rectal examination; LUTS, lower urinary tract symptoms; PSA, prostate-specific antigen; UDS, urodynamic studies; VB3, voiding bottle 3 (postprostatic massage) urine specimen.
From Beckman TJ, Mynderse LA. Evaluation and medical management of benign prostatic hyperplasia. Mayo Clin Proc. 2005;80:1356-62. Used with permission of Mayo Foundation for Medical Education and Research.

Patients with LUTS should be evaluated for neurologic deficits, especially if the patients have a history or presenting symptoms that suggest a neurologic disorder. In such cases, useful findings include saddle anesthesia, decreased rectal sphincter tone, absent cremasteric reflex, or lower extremity neurologic abnormalities. On examination of the abdomen, masses resulting from a renal tumor, hydronephrosis, or bladder distention may be detected. The penis should be examined for stricture or other pathologic changes. DRE findings most consistent with BPH are symmetric enlargement and firm consistency, often likened to the thenar muscle or the tip of the nose. In contrast, findings consistent with adenocarcinoma of the prostate are prostate asymmetry, induration, and nodularity, which is likened to the consistency of a knuckle or the forehead.

- Attempt to identify neurologic deficits on physical examination.
- Attempt to identify urethral stricture on physical examination.
- Prostate asymmetry, induration, and nodularity are consistent with prostate carcinoma.

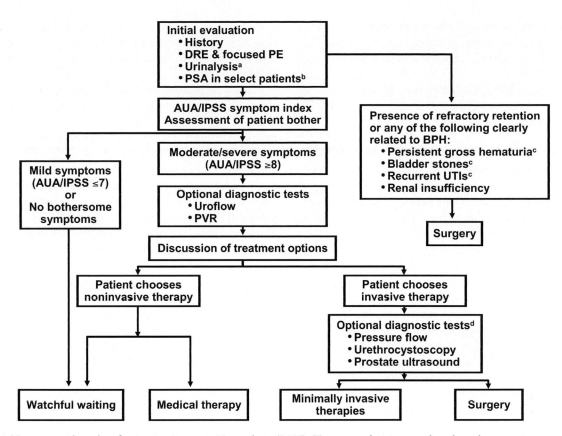

Figure 17-1. A Treatment Algorithm for Benign Prostatic Hyperplasia (BPH). Treatment decisions are based partly on patient symptom severity as determined with the American Urological Association International Prostate Symptom Score (AUA/IPSS). DRE indicates digital rectal examination; PE, physical examination; PSA, prostate-specific antigen; PVR, postvoid residual urine; UTI, urinary tract infection. [a]In patients with clinically significant prostatic bleeding, a course of a 5 α-reductase inhibitor may be used. If bleeding persists, tissue ablative surgery is indicated. [b]Patients with at least a 10-year life expectancy for whom knowledge of the presence of prostate cancer would change management or patients for whom the PSA measurement may change the management of voiding symptoms. [c]After exhausting other therapeutic options. [d]Some diagnostic tests are used in predicting response to therapy. Pressure-flow studies are most useful in men before surgery. (From AUA Practice Guidelines Committee. AUA guideline on management of benign prostatic hyperplasia [2003]. Chapter 1. Diagnosis and treatment recommendations. J Urol. 2003;170:530-47. Used with permission.)

Evaluation

A specimen for urinalysis should be obtained routinely when evaluating men with LUTS. Urinalysis findings may include pyuria and bacteriuria, which suggest infection; hematuria, which suggests inflammation or urothelial malignancy; and active urine sediment, which suggests a possible postobstructive nephropathy.

Optional studies include measuring serum creatinine and prostate-specific antigen (PSA) concentrations. The PSA measurement is optional because the results do not help discriminate BPH from adenocarcinoma of the prostate. Nevertheless, because LUTS may indicate prostate cancer, it is appropriate to routinely offer PSA testing. Additionally, annual screening for prostate cancer with DRE and PSA is appropriate for men aged 50 to 75 years, and sometimes older than 75, depending on the patient's preference and anticipated life expectancy.

- Urinalysis is routinely used to evaluate men with symptoms of BPH.
- Measurement of serum creatinine and PSA levels is optional.

Serum PSA levels strongly correlate with prostate volumes in men with BPH. Other causes of increased PSA levels are prostate carcinoma, bacterial prostatitis, acute urinary retention, instrumentation, prostate incision, and ejaculation. Conditions generally not believed to increase serum PSA levels are routine DRE, transrectal ultrasonography without biopsy, cystoscopy, and nontraumatic bladder catheterization.

- Other causes of increased PSA levels are prostate carcinoma, bacterial prostatitis, acute urinary retention, instrumentation, prostate incision, and ejaculation.
- Conditions that generally do not increase serum PSA levels are routine DRE, transrectal ultrasonography without biopsy, cystoscopy, and nontraumatic bladder catheterization.

There are different methods for interpreting serum PSA levels:
1. The traditional cutoff is 4 ng/mL.
2. Age-adjusted normal limits are commonly used because prostate volume increases with age.

3. The level of free (unbound) PSA is lower in men with adenocarcinoma of the prostate; therefore, a low ratio of free PSA to total PSA is more consistent with prostate carcinoma than with BPH.
4. A rapidly rising PSA is more suggestive of carcinoma than BPH; in particular, an annual PSA velocity greater than 0.75 ng/mL is considered abnormal.

A uroflow study with ultrasonographic measurement of residual urine volume is an objective, noninvasive way to evaluate men presenting with LUTS. An accurate study requires urine volumes of at least 150 mL. Men with BPH often have peak flow rates less than 15 mL/s and increased residual urine volume (Figure 17-2). Notably, men with detrusor dysfunction also have abnormal results. Consequently, as with any test, interpreting results of uroflow studies depends on the pretest probability of disease. If the pretest probability of BPH is high, an abnormal test result is useful for confirming the diagnosis. But if the pretest probability is intermediate, an abnormal uroflow result is less useful. In such cases, patients may need to undergo complete urodynamic studies to further distinguish BPH from other causes of LUTS.

* Different methods for assessing PSA include cutoff of 4 ng/mL, age-adjusted limits, free PSA to total PSA ratio, and PSA velocity.
* Uroflow is an objective, noninvasive assessment of LUTS.

Medical Management of Benign Prostatic Hyperplasia
Although this chapter focuses on the medical management of BPH, clinicians should recognize the indications for urologic referral and

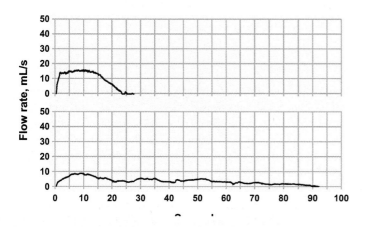

Figure 17-2. Top, Uroflow Tracing From a Young, Asymptomatic Male. Note the parabolic flow curve and peak flow rate >15 mL/s. This patient's ultrasonographically measured residual urine volume was 9 mL. Bottom, Uroflow tracing from an elderly man with benign prostatic hyperplasia. Note the prolonged voiding time and peak flow rate <10 mL/s. This patient's ultrasonographically measured residual urine volume was 100 mL. (From Beckman TJ, Mynderse LA. Evaluation and medical management of benign prostatic hyperplasia. Mayo Clin Proc. 2005;80:1356-62. Used with permission of Mayo Foundation for Medical Education and Research.)

consideration of invasive therapy. These indications are moderate or severe symptoms, persistent gross hematuria, urinary retention, renal insufficiency due to BPH, recurrent urinary tract infections, and bladder calculi.

Watchful waiting is reasonable for patients with mild or moderate symptoms. These patients are monitored at least yearly or when new symptoms arise. In addition, these patients may be advised to practice scheduled voiding (every 3 hours during the day), to avoid excess evening fluid intake, and to be aware of potential adverse effects of over-the-counter decongestants.

Nearly all patients presenting with BPH are candidates for medical therapy. Moreover, medical therapy has replaced interventional therapy as the most common treatment of BPH. Prescription medications available for treating BPH are α_1-adrenergic antagonists (eg, tamsulosin) and 5α-reductase inhibitors (eg, finasteride).

* Watchful waiting is reasonable for patients with mild or moderate BPH.
* Available prescription medications are α_1-adrenergic antagonists and 5α-reductase inhibitors.

The α_1-adrenergic antagonist medications work on the dynamic component of bladder outlet obstruction by decreasing prostatic smooth muscle tone. They are the first line of medical therapy for most men with BPH. Although all α_1-adrenergic antagonist medications are equally efficacious in treating BPH, terazosin and doxazosin are more likely to cause side effects (mainly orthostatic hypotension) than other medications in this class. Other common side effects of α_1-adrenergic antagonists include dizziness, hypotension, edema, palpitations, erectile dysfunction, and fatigue.

The second class of prescription medications for treating BPH, the 5α-reductase inhibitors, act on the static (anatomical) component of bladder outlet obstruction. These medications decrease the conversion of testosterone to dihydrotestosterone in the prostate, thereby limiting prostate growth. The two 5α-reductase inhibitors currently available are finasteride and dutasteride.

The following points about finasteride are important: it is most useful in men with severe BPH and large prostates (>40 cm^3), it may need to be taken for more than 6 months before an optimal drug effect is apparent, and it can significantly decrease serum PSA. For this reason, experts recommend correcting the serum PSA value in men taking finasteride by multiplying the value by 2. Side effects with finasteride are uncommon. The most frequent side effects are related to sexual dysfunction and include decreased libido, ejaculatory dysfunction, and erectile dysfunction. Finally, evidence supports the combined use of α_1-adrenergic antagonists and 5α-reductase inhibitors in men with inadequate responses to either drug alone.

* The α_1-adrenergic antagonists work on the dynamic component of bladder outlet obstruction.
* The 5α-reductase inhibitors work on the static component of bladder outlet obstruction.
* Combined use of α_1-adrenergic antagonists with 5α-reductase inhibitors is often effective in patients with inadequate responses to monotherapy.

- Correct the serum PSA value in patients taking finasteride by multiplying the value by 2.

Herbal medications used to treat BPH include derivatives from African star grass, African plum tree bark, rye grass pollens, stinging nettle, and cactus flower. The most commonly used alternative treatment for BPH is saw palmetto (*Serenoa repens*). Many mechanisms for saw palmetto have been entertained, yet none are proven. Saw palmetto is considered safe, and studies including randomized trials and a meta-analysis have shown that it compares favorably with finasteride and that, compared with placebo, saw palmetto improves flow and decreases symptoms.

Erectile Dysfunction

Male sexual dysfunction includes erectile dysfunction (ED), decreased libido, anatomical abnormalities (eg, Peyronie disease), and ejaculatory dysfunction. *ED*, defined as the inability to achieve erections firm enough for vaginal penetration, affects millions of men in the United States. The Massachusetts Male Aging Study showed that the prevalence of ED increased by age: approximately 50% of men experienced ED at age 50, and nearly 70% at age 70.

- *ED* is defined as the inability to achieve erections firm enough for vaginal penetration.

Erectile physiology includes hormonal, vascular, psychologic, neurologic, and cellular components. Testosterone is primarily responsible for maintaining sexual desire (libido), and hypogonadism is sometimes associated with ED. Other hormonal causes of ED include hyperthyroidism and prolactinomas. The penile blood supply begins at the internal pudendal artery, which branches into the penile artery, ultimately giving rise to the cavernous, dorsal, and bulbourethral arteries. Psychogenic erections, triggered by fantasy or visual stimulation, are mediated by sympathetic input from the thoracolumbar chain (T11-L2). Reflex erections are caused by tactile stimulation and are mediated by the parasympathetic nervous system (S2-S4). Overall, parasympathetic signals are responsible for erection, and sympathetic signals are responsible for ejaculation.

- Testosterone is primarily responsible for maintaining libido.
- Psychogenic erections are mediated by the thoracolumbar chain, whereas reflex erections are mediated by sacral nerve roots S2-S4.
- Parasympathetic signals control erection, and sympathetic signals control ejaculation.

Sexual arousal and parasympathetic signals to the penis initiate intracellular changes necessary for erection (Figure 17-3). Endothelial cells release nitric oxide, which in turn increases cyclic guanosine monophosphate (cGMP). Increased levels of cGMP cause relaxation of arterial and cavernosal smooth muscle and increased penile blood flow. As the intracavernosal pressure rises, penile emissary veins are compressed, thus restricting venous return from the penis. The combination of increased arterial flow and decreased venous return results in erection. This process is reversed by the activity of cGMP

phosphodiesterase (PDE) type 5, which breaks down cGMP, resulting in cessation of erection.

Although ED is rarely an indicator of serious diseases, it is strongly associated with cardiovascular risk factors. In fact, the Health Professionals Follow-up Study showed that risk factors for ED and cardiovascular disease were nearly identical and that physically active men had a 30% lower risk of ED than inactive men. Therefore, men with diabetes mellitus, hypertension, and coronary artery disease are at increased risk of ED. Not surprisingly, randomized controlled trial data show that erectile function significantly improves in obese men who lose weight through diet and exercise.

- Nitric oxide increases cGMP levels, which in turn causes cavernosal smooth muscle relaxation and erection.
- ED is strongly associated with cardiovascular risk factors.
- Weight loss may lead to improved erectile function.

Evaluating Patients With Erectile Dysfunction

History and Physical Examination

Certain questions should be asked routinely when taking a history from patients with ED (Table 17-2). Especially important are questions about common ED risk factors such as cardiovascular disease, smoking, diabetes mellitus, hypertension, hyperlipidemia, prescription medications, recreational drug use, and mood disorders. In addition, validated questionnaires, such as the International Index of Erectile Function (IIEF), are useful for monitoring patients' responses to ED treatments.

A complete multisystem examination may identify indicators of cardiovascular disease (eg, obesity, hypertension, or femoral arterial bruits), endocrinopathies (eg, visual field defects, thyromegaly, or

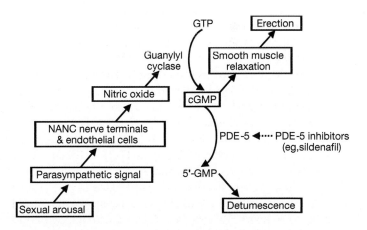

Figure 17-3. Mechanism for Penile Erection and the Molecular Activity of Phosphodiesterase Type 5 (PDE-5) Inhibitor Medications. cGMP indicates cyclic guanosine monophosphate; GMP, guanosine monophosphate; GTP, guanosine triphosphate; NANC, nonadrenergic noncholinergic. (From Beckman TJ, Abu-Lebdeh HS, Mynderse LA. Evaluation and medical management of erectile dysfunction. Mayo Clin Proc. 2006;81:385-90. Used with permission of Mayo Foundation for Medical Education and Research.)

gynecomastia), or neurologic abnormalities (eg, decreased sphincter tone, absent bulbocavernosus reflex, or saddle anesthesia). The penis should be palpated in the stretched position to detect fibrous plaques consistent with Peyronie disease, which may be present on the dorsum and base of the penis. The testicles should be evaluated for masses (indicating malignancy) and decreased size and soft consistency (indicating hypogonadism). Finally, examining patients with ED is often a good opportunity to screen for prostate cancer and to assess for benign glandular enlargement.

- A careful history should identify ED risk factors, including cardiovascular disease.
- Fibrous plaques in the penis most likely indicate Peyronie disease.
- Small, soft testicles may indicate hypogonadism.

Laboratory Testing

Although disease-specific testing is favored, serum testosterone levels are frequently measured in a men's health practice. If a patient is hypogonadal, serum prolactin and luteinizing hormone (LH) levels should be assessed. If the prolactin level is elevated or the LH level is not elevated, magnetic resonance imaging (MRI) of the brain should be used to rule out a pituitary adenoma. Additional useful testing that pertains to ED risk factors includes measuring the levels of fasting glucose, fasting lipids, and thyrotropin.

- If the prolactin level is elevated or the LH level is not elevated, MRI of the brain should be used to rule out a pituitary adenoma.

Medical Management of Erectile Dysfunction

Phosphodiesterase Type 5 Inhibitors

PDE-5 inhibitor medications are the first line of therapy for most men with ED. PDE-5 inhibitors have revolutionized the treatment of ED since the introduction of sildenafil in 1998, and experts have observed that these medications have considerably affected (both positively and negatively) the sexual culture of older people. After initial concerns about cardiovascular risks associated with PDE-5 inhibitors, studies have shown that these medications are generally safe, even in patients with stable coronary artery disease who are not taking nitrate therapy.

Three PDE-5 inhibitors are currently available: sildenafil (Viagra), vardenafil (Levitra), and tadalafil (Cialis). These medications inhibit cGMP PDE-5, thereby increasing cGMP levels and shifting the physiologic balance in favor of erection (Figure 17-3). In the absence of comparative clinical trials and meta-analyses, it appears that each of these medications is equally efficacious. Tadalafil has a longer half-life than sildenafil or vardenafil, which affords more spontaneity to tadalafil users (up to 36 hours). Patients should be instructed to take PDE-5 inhibitors at least 1 hour before sexual activity, and sildenafil should be taken on an empty stomach. Patients should also realize that PDE-5 inhibitors will not cause erections in the absence of sexual arousal (unlike intraurethral alprostadil and penile injection therapy).

- PPDE-5 inhibitors are safe in patients with stable coronary artery disease who are not taking nitrate therapy.
- The PDE-5 inhibitor medications are likely equally efficacious.

- PDE-5 inhibitors will not cause erections in the absence of sexual arousal.

Common side effects of the PDE-5 inhibitors, which are due to the presence of PDE throughout the body, are headache, flushing, gastric upset, diarrhea, nasal congestion, and light-headedness. A unique reaction to sildenafil is blue-tinged vision, probably related to the activity of sildenafil on PDE-6 in the retina. This reaction resolves with discontinuation of therapy. It is noteworthy that some varieties of retinitis pigmentosa have a PDE-6 gene defect. Consequently, patients with retinitis pigmentosa should not be prescribed medications from the PDE-5 inhibitor class.

- A unique reaction to sildenafil is blue-tinged vision, probably related to the activity of sildenafil on PDE-6 in the retina.
- Patients with retinitis pigmentosa should not be prescribed medications from the PDE-5 inhibitor class.
- Common side effects of PDE-5 inhibitors are due to the presence of PDE throughout the body.

A contraindication to use of PDE-5 inhibitors is nitrate therapy. Indeed, patients treated for acute coronary syndromes should not receive nitrate therapy within 24 hours of taking sildenafil or vardenafil and within 48 hours of taking tadalafil. Physicians should also be cautious about prescribing PDE-5 inhibitors for patients with poorly controlled blood pressure or multidrug antihypertensive regimens. In patients with known or suspected ischemic heart disease, cardiac stress testing is useful for stratifying the risk of PDE-5 inhibitor therapy; patients who achieve 5 to 6 metabolic equivalents without ischemia probably have low risk of complications from engaging in sexual activity.

- Nitrate therapy is an absolute contraindication to use of PDE-5 inhibitor medications.
- Cardiac stress testing helps stratify the risk of PDE-5 inhibitor therapy.

Treatment options for patients who have not had a response to PDE-5 inhibitors or who cannot take PDE-5 inhibitors include intraurethral alprostadil and penile injection therapy. These are generally more effective than PDE-5 inhibitors, but their obvious drawback is inconvenience. Contraindications for these treatments include blood cell dyscrasias (eg, sickle cell disease, leukemia, or multiple myeloma) and penile deformity, especially Peyronie disease. Anticoagulation is an additional contraindication to penile injection therapy. There is inadequate information on the safety of combining PDE-5 inhibitors and injection therapy, and hence, their coadministration is not advised.

Intraurethral Alprostadil

Intraurethral alprostadil (commercially available as MUSE, a medicated urethral system for erection) is effective in men of all ages who have various causes of ED. Intraurethral alprostadil is inserted into the tip of the penis with an applicator. Patients should be instructed on the application technique. Additionally, owing to the risk of syncope, administration of the first dose should be supervised by a health care provider. The most common side effect is urethral and genital

Table 17-2 Questions To Ask When Taking a History From Patients With Erectile Dysfunction

Question	Comment
Do you have difficulty achieving erections or difficulty with orgasms & ejaculation?	Sexual dysfunction includes various diagnoses, & it is important to determine whether the patient's primary complaint is ED
How often do you achieve erections? Are your erections firm enough for vaginal penetration?	Often patients are not satisfied with the quality of their erections, yet if patients can achieve erections adequately firm for vaginal penetration most of the time, their complaints are not classically defined as ED
Did your ED occur suddenly? Do you have nocturnal erections? Do you feel anxious or depressed? Do you & your partner have a satisfactory relationship?	The sudden onset of ED & the persistence of nocturnal erections indicate an inorganic (psychogenic) cause; in such cases, physicians should explore the psychosocial context of the patient's sexual history, such as whether the patient feels anxious or depressed or whether the patient is experiencing difficulties in his interpersonal relationship(s)
Do you have a desire to engage in sexual activity?	Decreased sexual desire may indicate hypogonadism; if patients are not interested in sexual activity, serum testosterone levels should be assessed & mood disorders should be considered
Do you have penile curvature or pain with erections?	A positive response to this question may indicate Peyronie disease, which is sometimes detected on physical examination; identifying Peyronie disease is important because it precludes intraurethral alprostadil & penile injection therapy
Can you engage in vigorous physical activity without chest pain or unusual dyspnea?	PDE-5 inhibitor medications will be considered in most patients, & sexual activity is associated with cardiovascular stress; hence, a history should be obtained to identify undiagnosed ischemic heart disease or to assess the stability of known ischemic heart disease
What medications are you taking?	Numerous medications are associated with ED, especially antihypertensives & psychotropics; identify medications inhibiting cytochrome P450 (eg, ritonavir) because these medications increase plasma levels of PDE-5 inhibitor medications; an absolute contraindication to PDE-5 inhibitor medications is the concurrent use of nitrates (eg, isosorbide mononitrate)
How much alcohol do you consume? Do you use illegal drugs?	Substance abuse, including alcoholism, is commonly overlooked as a cause of ED
Which treatments for ED have you already tried?	Knowing which medications patients have tried will help physicians decide the next best therapeutic plan
Do you have a history of diseases involving your heart, blood vessels, nervous system, or hormones? Do you have a history of hypertension, hyperlipidemia, diabetes mellitus, or tobacco abuse? Do you have a history of penile trauma or genitourinary surgery?	Identify common risk factors for ED
Do you ride a bicycle regularly?	Prolonged & frequent bicycle riding can cause excessive pudendal pressure, leading to ED

Abbreviations: ED, erectile dysfunction; PDE-5, phosphodiesterase type 5.
From Beckman TJ, Abu-Lebdeh HS, Mynderse LA. Evaluation and medical management of erectile dysfunction. Mayo Clin Proc. 2006;81:385-90. Used with permission of Mayo Foundation for Medical Education and Research.

burning, and hypotension can occur. As for all medical ED treatments, patients are educated about priapism, and they are instructed to go to an emergency department if they have erections for more than 4 hours.

- The most common side effect of intraurethral alprostadil is urethral and genital burning.
- Hypotension and syncope may occur with alprostadil.

Intracavernosal Penile Injections

Intracavernosal penile injection, an efficacious and generally safe therapy, is the most effective medical therapy for ED. In practice, a triple-therapy combination of alprostadil, papaverine, and phentolamine is usually used. The mechanism of action of these medications is to increase penile blood flow. Specifically, alprostadil and papaverine cause relaxation of cavernosal smooth muscle and penile blood vessels, and phentolamine antagonizes α-adrenoreceptors. The use of intraurethral alprostadil requires patient instruction, and the initial dose is administered under the supervision of a health care provider. Although many patients are hesitant to attempt penile injection, this method is associated with minimal discomfort.

- Intracavernosal injections are the most effective medical therapy for ED.
- Initial doses of intraurethral and intracavernosal injections should be supervised by a health care provider.

Testosterone

Various hormonal therapies, including testosterone, were once widely used to treat ED. The penile nitric oxide pathway is testosterone dependent, and for this reason it is necessary to screen for low serum testosterone in men who have no response to medical therapy with sildenafil or whose presentation suggests hypogonadism. Hypogonadism is diagnosed by the presence of hypogonadal symptoms (such as decreased libido, cognitive decline, and generalized muscle weakness), and by morning fasting total testosterone levels less than 200 ng/mL on at least 2 separate occasions. In hypogonadal men, combining PDE-5 inhibitor therapy with testosterone is often effective. Moreover, testosterone replacement alone increases sexual interest, nocturnal erections, and frequency of sexual intercourse. Nevertheless, testosterone replacement has not been shown to improve erectile function in men with normal serum testosterone levels.

- Hypogonadism is diagnosed by the presence of hypogonadal symptoms and morning fasting total testosterone levels <200 ng/mL on at least 2 separate occasions.
- Testosterone replacement has not been shown to improve erectile function in men with normal serum testosterone levels.

Testosterone is available by injection, skin patch, topical gel, or buccal oral tablets. Testosterone therapy is associated with potential risks. For example, prolonged use of high-dose, orally active 17α-alkyl androgens (eg, methyltestosterone) is associated with hepatic neoplasms, fulminant hepatitis, and cholestatic jaundice. Other risks of exogenous testosterone therapy include gynecomastia, alterations in the lipid profile (mainly decreased high-density lipoprotein cholesterol), ery-

thropoietin-mediated polycythemia, edema, sleep apnea, hypertension, infertility (through suppression of spermatogenesis), and benign prostatic hyperplasia. Exogenous testosterone also increases the risk of developing prostate carcinoma. Although testosterone replacement may not cause prostate carcinoma, it may stimulate the growth of existing occult prostate cancer. For this reason, all men should have screening for prostate cancer with DRE and serum PSA before beginning use of exogenous testosterone.

- Risks of testosterone therapy include hepatitis, cholestatic jaundice, hepatic neoplasms, gynecomastia, polycythemia, sleep apnea, and hypertension.
- Screening for prostate cancer is necessary before prescribing testosterone replacement.

The goal of testosterone replacement is to increase serum testosterone levels to the low or middle portion of the reference range. A recommended treatment is to apply topical testosterone, 1% gel at a starting dose of 5 g daily, to the shoulders, upper parts of the arms, or abdomen. A total testosterone level may be reassessed as soon as 14 days after starting treatment. The patient's therapeutic response and testosterone level are reassessed at 3 months, and decisions are then made about whether to continue using testosterone and whether to adjust the dose.

Although patients who receive testosterone replacement and have normal serum testosterone levels should not be at risk of adverse effects, monitoring patients during testosterone therapy is essential. Baseline determinations include whether the patient has a history of prostate cancer, benign prostatic hyperplasia, obstructive sleep apnea, liver disease, hypertension, or hyperlipidemia. Baseline testing includes a complete blood count and levels of serum PSA, lipids, and liver transaminases. PSA levels and prostate-related symptoms should be assessed at 6 months and then annually, and patients with elevated or increasing PSA levels should not be treated with testosterone. The hematocrit and levels of lipids should be monitored biannually for the first 18 months and annually thereafter; the testosterone dose should be decreased or therapy discontinued if hematocrit values are greater than 50%. Finally, patient response to therapy and side effects are monitored quarterly during the first year of treatment.

- Patients receiving testosterone replacement require regular monitoring.
- Elevated or increasing PSA levels are an indication to stop therapy.
- Hematocrit values >50% are an indication to decrease the dose of testosterone or stop therapy.

Nonmedical Treatments

Other treatments for ED include topical vacuum pump devices and surgically inserted inflatable penile implants. Penile pumps work by creating a vacuum around the penis, thus drawing blood into the penis. When the penis is engorged with blood, an elastic ring is placed over the base of the penis and the pump is removed. Importantly, patients should use vacuum pump devices with vacuum limiters, which prevent negative pressure injury to the penis. Penile implants are generally not offered unless patients have no response to medical treatments, including maximal-strength injection therapy.

Questions

Multiple Choice (choose the best answer)

1. A 75-year-old man complains of a weak urinary stream and nocturia. His only comorbidity is arthritis and his only medication is ibuprofen. On examination, the size of his prostate is normal. Which of the following is true?

    a. He should be reassured and dismissed.
    b. He does not have benign prostatic hypertrophy (BPH) because the size of his prostate is normal.
    c. He could not have BPH at his age.
    d. He should be offered medical therapy for BPH.
    e. He should be reassured that he does not have prostate cancer.

2. A 45-year-old man complains of sudden onset of a weak urinary stream. He has neuropathy, recently treated with nortriptyline. On examination, his prostate is enlarged (30 cm³). Which of the following is the best option?

    a. Perform electromyography and MRI of the spine to evaluate for neurologic causes of lower urinary tract symptoms (LUTS).
    b. Determine the prostate-specific antigen level.
    c. Discontinue nortriptyline therapy and recheck the patient in 1 month.
    d. Initiate medical therapy with an α-1-receptor blocker.
    e. Initiate medical therapy with a 5-α-reductase inhibitor.

3. A 65-year-old man complains of nocturia even though he is taking tamsulosin, 0.4 mg daily. Examination reveals an enlarged prostate (60 cm³). A uroflow study reveals a peak flow of 11 mL/s and a postvoid residual urine volume of 75 mL. Which of the following is the best treatment option?

    a. Increase tamsulosin to 0.8 mg daily.
    b. Continue use of tamsulosin and add finasteride.
    c. Discontinue use of tamsulosin and initiate use of finasteride.
    d. Recommend invasive therapy for BPH.
    e. All of the above.

4. A 60-year-old man complains of gradual-onset erectile dysfunction (ED). He worries that his ED indicates a serious health problem. Which of the following is the best option?

    a. Reassure the patient and explore potential causes of his ED.
    b. Recommend an extensive medical evaluation.
    c. Recommend a urologic consultation.
    d. Obtain a fasting morning total testosterone level.
    e. Question the diagnosis of ED and recommend nocturnal penile tumescence testing.

5. A 55-year-old man reports sudden onset of ED. He acknowledges having nocturnal erections. Which of the following is true?

    a. The sudden onset and nocturnal erections suggest a psychogenic cause.
    b. The sudden onset indicates a thromboembolic event.
    c. The sudden onset indicates hypogonadism from a pituitary hemorrhage.
    d. The patient's age indicates cardiovascular disease as the likely cause of ED.
    e. The patient is unlikely to have ED because he is younger than 60 years.

6. A 50-year-old smoker with diabetes mellitus and hypertension has not had an erection for more than 5 years. What is the most likely cause of his ED?

    a. Old age.
    b. Cardiovascular risk factors.
    c. Medications for cardiovascular disease.
    d. Depression.
    e. Hypogonadism.

7. A 70-year-old man has ED even after trying 100-mg doses of sildenafil, taken on an empty stomach 1 hour before sexual activity. Which of the following is the best option?

    a. Since the patient's ED did not improve with sildenafil, it is unlikely that he will ever have erections.
    b. The patient should consider surgical consultation regarding penile implants.
    c. The patient should be optimistic about success with penile injections.
    d. The patient should use a higher dose of sildenafil.
    e. The patient will likely benefit from a different phosphodiesterase type 5 (PDE-5) inhibitor medication.

Answers

1. Answer d.
Prostate size on digital rectal examination correlates poorly with clinical BPH. For this reason, patients older than 50 with LUTS should be offered medical therapy for BPH. However, LUTS may also result from disorders other than BPH, which should be considered within each clinical context. For example, consider the possibility of malignancy in elderly patients with voiding symptoms and no recent evaluation for prostate cancer. Of course, BPH is common after age 50, which is why answer *c* is incorrect.

2. Answer c.
Various medications with anticholinergic and sympathomimetic properties cause LUTS in elderly men, yet these medications are often overlooked as a cause of symptoms in men with subclinical BPH. Thus, the best option is to stop this patient's use of nortriptyline and reassess later. Evaluating for other conditions or starting medical therapy for BPH would be indicated only if the LUTS did not improve after discontinuing use of nortriptyline.

3. Answer b.
This patient clearly meets criteria for BPH given his LUTS, large prostate, reduced urinary flow rate, and increased postvoid residual urine volume. Evidence shows that men with large prostates (especially >40 cm³) and moderate to severe symptoms benefit from finasteride, and additional evidence shows that combination therapy is very effective in these patients. Consequently, this patient should benefit from the addition of finasteride. This scenario did not mention indications for immediate consideration of invasive therapy, so this option is incorrect.

4. Answer a.
Patients frequently express concern that ED represents a serious underlying disease. Although cardiovascular and other risk factors are associated with ED, ED is not usually the first presenting symptom. Educating patients and targeting these risk factors is a preferred approach. Since this patient described no other features to suggest hypogonadism, determination of the serum testosterone level would not be necessary. Nocturnal penile tumescence testing is rarely if ever required for evaluating patients with ED because a careful history, examination, and other testing (if necessary) usually provide enough information for diagnosis and treatment.

5. Answer a.
Suddenness of onset and nocturnal erections are very useful clues for psychogenic ED. Therefore, evaluation for organic causes (eg, vascular disease or cardiac risk factors) would be unnecessary and may cause anxiety. The last answer is incorrect because ED is common after the fifth decade of life.

6. Answer b.
Although old age, medications, and depression are common correlates of ED, as a rule of thumb, cardiovascular risk is the most important association to remember. Indeed, modifying cardiovascular risk by losing weight has been shown to improve erectile function in men with ED. Additionally, next to prostatectomy and other invasive urologic procedures, cardiovascular disease and risk factors are leading causes of ED. Hypogonadism is probably an uncommon cause of ED, especially in relatively young patients like the one described in this scenario.

7. Answer c.
The patient describes an inadequate treatment response to sildenafil, even after taking the maximal dose in an effective manner. Physicians often forget that penile injection therapy is more effective than medications at producing erections in men who are willing to try this approach. This patient is unlikely to benefit from another PDE-5 inhibitor medication because clinical experience indicates that all these medications are equally efficacious. Surgical consultation for consideration of penile implants is reserved for patients who have not had adequate responses from various medical treatments.

18

Nephrology

Fernando C. Fervenza, MD, PhD
Thomas R. Schwab, MD
Amy W. Williams, MD
Robert C. Albright, Jr., DO
Stephen B. Erickson, MD

Part I

Fernando C. Fervenza, MD, PhD
Thomas R. Schwab, MD

Glomerular Disease: Clinical Presentations

Clinical manifestations of glomerular injury can vary from the finding of isolated hematuria or proteinuria, or both, in an asymptomatic patient on a routine medical examination to the more florid presentation as nephritic syndrome, nephrotic syndrome, or rapidly progressive glomerulonephritis. In addition, some patients who present with advanced renal insufficiency, hypertension, and shrunken, smooth kidneys are presumed to have chronic glomerulonephritis. In this situation, renal biopsy is more likely to show nonspecific features of end-stage renal disease (ESRD).

Asymptomatic proteinuria is defined as urinary protein excretion of more than 300 mg/1.73 m^2 per 24 hours and less than 3.5 g/1.73 m^2 per 24 hours. *Normoalbuminuria* is defined as urinary albumin excretion of less than 30 mg/1.73 m^2 per 24 hours, *microalbuminuria* as urinary albumin of 30 to 300 mg/1.73 m^2 per 24 hours, and *overt proteinuria* as urinary albumin of more than 300 mg/1.73 m^2 per 24 hours. *Glomerular proteinuria* can be classified as *transient* or *hemodynamic* (functional) (eg, after fever, with exercise, or orthostatic) or as *persistent* (fixed). *Functional proteinuria* is benign. The diagnosis of orthostatic proteinuria can be made by obtaining two 12-hour urine collections for protein: 1 supine and 1 upright. In this condition, proteinuria is usually less than 1 g/1.73 m^2 per 24 hours. Fixed nonnephrotic proteinuria is usually secondary to glomerular diseases, but tubulointerstitial diseases can also be associated with proteinuria (usually <1,500 mg/1.73 m^2 per 24 hours). Overflow low-molecular-weight proteinuria is due to increased excretion of light chain (myeloma) or to lysozyme release (leukemic cells). The urine dipstick test (which detects albumin only) is negative when proteinuria is due to light chains, but proteinuria can

be detected easily by other tests, including the bedside sulfasalicylic acid test. *Hematuria* is defined as at least 3 red blood cells (RBCs) per high-power field in a centrifuged urinary sediment sample or RBCs more numerous than 10×10^6/L. *Glomerular hematuria* is characterized by the presence of dysmorphic RBCs or RBC casts (or both). *Macroscopic hematuria* due to glomerular disease is painless and often brown or a cola color rather than bright red; clots are rare. Other causes of brown urine include hemoglobinuria, myoglobinuria, and food or drug dyes (eg, beetroot).

Renal biopsy is often required if patients have active urinary sediment (dysmorphic RBCs, RBC casts, or white blood cell [WBC] casts), proteinuria of more than 1 g/1.73 m^2 per 24 hours, or renal insufficiency and if the diagnosis cannot be determined or the prognosis adequately predicted by a less invasive diagnostic procedure. Other indications for biopsy include acute renal failure lasting longer than 3 to 4 weeks, patients with an atypical course of diabetes mellitus, and systemic diseases in which the differential diagnosis includes amyloidosis, systemic lupus erythematosus (SLE), and systemic vasculitis. Percutaneous renal biopsy is contraindicated if the patient has uncontrolled hypertension, acute pyelonephritis, perinephric abscess, or renal neoplasm or if the patient is uncooperative. Patients with bleeding disorders, including severe thrombocytopenia, should be considered for a renal biopsy through a transjugular approach together with the use of fresh frozen plasma and platelet transfusion if indicated. A solitary kidney is not an absolute contraindication to biopsy. Complications include gross hematuria (<10%), arteriovenous fistula (<1%), need for nephrectomy (0.1%), and death (0.001%). A renal biopsy is rarely indicated in patients with small, shrunken kidneys because of the increased risk of bleeding and the low probability of providing a diagnosis.

- Clinical presentations of glomerular disease: asymptomatic hematuria or proteinuria, nephrotic syndrome, nephritic syndrome, rapidly progressive glomerulonephritis, or chronic glomerulonephritis.
- Renal biopsy: to determine the diagnosis and prognosis for patients with active urinary sediment, proteinuria >1 g/1.73 m^2 per 24 hours, or unexplained renal failure.
- Other indications: acute renal failure lasting >3-4 weeks, atypical course of diabetes mellitus, and undiagnosed systemic disease.
- Contraindications to percutaneous renal biopsy: bleeding disorders, uncontrolled hypertension, acute pyelonephritis, renal neoplasm, and uncooperative patients.

Nephrotic Syndrome

Nephrotic syndrome is defined as the presence of urinary protein greater than 3.5 g/1.73 m^2 per 24 hours, hypoalbuminemia (<3.0 g/dL), peripheral edema, hypercholesterolemia, and lipiduria. Edema can be prominent. Children usually manifest matinal periorbital edema that resolves during the day as the child stands upright. Severe hyperlipidemia can result in the development of xanthelasma. Urinalysis shows waxy casts, free fat, oval fat bodies, and lipiduria ("Maltese crosses"). Complications of nephrotic syndrome include hypogammaglobulinemia (which increases infection risk, especially cellulitis and spontaneous peritonitis), vitamin D deficiency due to loss of vitamin D–binding protein, and iron deficiency anemia due to hypotransferrinemia. Thrombotic complications are common (eg, renal vein thrombosis) and occur because of increased levels of prothrombotic factors (increased factor V, VIII, fibrinogen, and platelets and decreased antithrombin III and antiplasmin). Patients at increased risk include those with proteinuria greater than 10 g/1.73 m^2 per 24 hours and a serum albumin level less than 2 g/dL. Symptoms of renal vein thrombosis include flank pain and hematuria. In cases of bilateral renal vein thrombosis, patients may present with acute renal failure. Apart from renal vein thrombosis, in patients with nephrotic syndrome acute renal failure may develop from several mechanisms (eg, prerenal volume depletion, sepsis, interstitial nephritis, and drugs such as angiotensin-converting enzyme inhibitors [ACEIs] and nonsteroidal anti-inflammatory drugs [NSAIDs]). Management of nephrotic syndrome includes using diuretics, controlling blood pressure (ACEIs and angiotensin receptor blockers [ARBs] are preferred), and limiting the intake of protein (0.8 g/kg per day) and sodium (<4 g per day), and controlling lipid levels (with the use of HMG-CoA reductase inhibitors). Anticoagulation should be considered for patients at increased risk, (proteinuria >10g in 24 hours and serum albumin <2 g/dL), especially if the nephrotic syndrome is due to membranous nephropathy or amyloidosis.

- Nephrotic syndrome: urinary protein >3.5 g/1.73 m^2 per 24 hours.
- Other features: hypoalbuminemia, peripheral edema, hyperlipidemia, and lipiduria.

Nephritic Syndrome

Nephritic syndrome is characterized by oliguria, edema, hypertension, proteinuria (usually <3.5 g/1.73 m^2 per 24 hours), and the presence of an active urinary sediment with dysmorphic RBCs or RBC casts (or both). Because of methemoglobin formation in acidic urine, the urine has a cola or smoky appearance. The classic example is acute poststreptococcal glomerulonephritis in children.

- Nephritic syndrome: active urinary sediment (dysmorphic RBCs or RBC casts or both).
- Other features: oliguria, hypertension, edema, and proteinuria (usually <3.5 g/1.73 m^2 per 24 hours).

Glomerular Disease That Presents With Nephritic Syndrome

Poststreptococcal Glomerulonephritis

Poststreptococcal glomerulonephritis (PSGN) is an acute glomerulonephritis that develops 1 to 4 weeks after pharyngitis or skin infection with specific ("nephritogenic") strains of group A β-hemolytic streptococci. The latent period is 6 to 21 days (type 12 pharyngeal infection) or 14 to 28 days (type 49 skin infection). The disease, however, can occur after other infections (eg, staphylococcal, meningococcal, and pneumococcal infection). Thus, the name *postinfectious glomerulonephritis* would be more appropriate.

The typical presentation is the abrupt onset of nephritic syndrome. An active urinary sediment is present in almost all cases. Proteinuria is usually less than 3 g in 24 hours, but it may be in the nephrotic range in some cases. Cultures are usually negative, but titers for antistreptolysin O (ASO), antistreptokinase, antihyaluronidase, and antideoxyribonuclease (antiDNAse B) may provide evidence of recent streptococcal infection. ASO titers increase 10 to 14 days after infection and peak at 3 to 4 weeks, subsequently decreasing. Total hemolytic complement (CH50) and C3 levels are usually decreased (activation of the alternative complement pathway), but C4 levels are normal.

Light microscopy shows diffuse hypercellularity of the glomerular tufts, with mesangial and endothelial cell proliferation and infiltration of polymorphonuclear leukocytes (thus, the name *exudative*), monocytes or macrophages, and plasma cells. All glomeruli are affected in a homogeneous pattern. Early in the disease process, characteristic subepithelial "humps" can be detected with silver stain. Cellular crescents are uncommon and indicative of severe disease. Immunofluorescence shows granular deposition of immunoglobulin (Ig)G, C3, and occasionally IgM, which are distributed in 3 well-described patterns: "starry-sky," "mesangial," and "garland." With electron microscopy, small immune deposits are seen in the mesangial and subendothelial areas. Almost pathognomonic of PSGN is the presence of large "humps," which are dome-shaped subepithelial deposits in the glomerular basement membrane (GBM).

The treatment of PSGN is supportive. Appropriate antibiotic therapy is indicated for persistent infection and for persons who are contacts (to prevent new cases). Sodium restriction and the use of loop diuretics reduce the risk of fluid overload and help to control hypertension. For children, the prognosis is excellent, with most patients recovering renal function within 1 to 2 months after diagnosis. ASO titers assist in confirming resolution. In a few patients, especially adults, microscopic hematuria, proteinuria, hypertension, and renal dysfunction may persist for many years. Patients presenting with a crescentic nephritis have a poorer prognosis, with approximately 50% developing ESRD. Other forms of postinfectious glomerulonephritis include bacterial endocarditis and infected ventriculoatrial shunts.

- PSGN: usually due to group A β-hemolytic streptococcal infections.
- Active urinary sediment, with proteinuria <3 g/1.73 m^2 per 24 hours.
- Total and C3 complement levels are low.
- Light microscopy: diffuse hypercellularity of the glomerular tufts, with mesangial and endothelial cell proliferation, infiltration of polymorphonuclear leukocytes, and subepithelial "humps" with silver stain.
- Immunofluorescence: granular deposition of IgG and C3 in a "starry-sky," "mesangial," or "garland" pattern.
- AntiDNAse B confirms streptococcal infection, and serial ASO titers assist in confirming resolution.

IgA Nephropathy

IgA nephropathy (IgAN), or Berger disease, is a mesangial proliferative glomerulonephritis characterized by diffuse deposition of IgA in the mesangium. It is the most common glomerulopathy worldwide, with an incidence approaching 1:100 in some countries (eg, Japan). The typical presentation is with episodic macroscopic hematuria usually accompanying an intercurrent upper respiratory tract infection (synpharyngitic). This clinical pattern occurs most frequently in young adults in the second and third decades of life. Other patients are asymptomatic and may be identified when microscopic hematuria, with or without proteinuria, is found on routine urinalysis. Proteinuria is common, but nephrotic syndrome occurs in less than 10% of all cases. Patients with nephrotic syndrome may have minimal change disease superimposed on IgAN or other glomerulopathy. The pathogenesis has been linked to abnormal integrity of the intestinal mucosa, resulting in overexposure to ubiquitous environmental antigens. This leads to an exaggerated production of galactose-deficient (GD)-IgA1 by bone marrow–derived B cells. Undergalactosylation of the IgA1 molecules reduces their affinity to the clearance receptors on Kupffer cells in the liver and results in an increase in circulating GD-IgA1, formation of anti–GD-IgA1 autoantibodies, deposition of IgG or IgA anti–GD-IgA1 immune complexes in the mesangium, and activation of complement and cytokine cascades. Secondary causes include advanced chronic liver disease, celiac disease, dermatitis herpetiformis, and ankylosing spondylitis. With light microscopy, glomeruli may look normal or may show mesangial expansion. Immunofluorescence studies are diagnostic and demonstrate strong IgA staining within the mesangium. Electron microscopy shows electron-dense deposits in the mesangial cells that colocalize with the immune deposits.

The disease generally has a benign course, with patients maintaining a proteinuria less than 500 mg/1.73 m^2 per 24 hours and having preserved renal function. However, in 20% to 40% of patients, the disease progresses to ESRD within 10 to 25 years. Proteinuria of more than 1 g/1.73 m^2 per 24 hours, hypertension, impaired renal function at diagnosis, and glomerular or interstitial fibrosis identified in renal biopsy specimens are the most important predictors of a poor outcome. IgAN recurs in about 50% of patients after renal transplant, but loss of the allograft from recurrent disease is uncommon. Progression to ESRD in patients at high risk has been shown to be slowed by angiotensin II converting enzyme blockade (with ACEIs or ARBs or both), administration of high doses of corticosteroids, and fish oil capsules containing omega-3 fatty acids. Mycophenolate mofetil is a new immunosuppressive agent currently being studied in clinical trials, but results so far have been disappointing. Patients with IgAN and concomitant minimal change disease respond fully to corticosteroid therapy. For patients with rapidly progressive renal failure due to crescentic IgAN, a regimen of corticosteroids and cyclophosphamide, with the addition of plasma exchange or pulse methylprednisolone, has been tried with variable results. A few familial cases of IgAN have been described.

- IgAN: the most common glomerulopathy worldwide.
- Presentation: synpharyngitic hematuria, often with RBC casts.
- Secondary causes: advanced chronic liver disease, celiac disease, dermatitis herpetiformis, and ankylosing spondylitis.
- Prognosis: generally good in patients who are normotensive, with proteinuria <1 g/1.73 m^2 per 24 hours and serum creatinine <1.5 mg/dL.
- Treatment with combined ACEIs and ARBs, high-dose corticosteroids, and fish oil capsules containing omega-3 fatty acids slows the progression of the disease.

Henoch-Schönlein Purpura

Henoch-Schönlein purpura is the systemic form of IgAN. Patients usually present with microscopic or gross hematuria (or both) along with RBC casts, purpura, and abdominal pain. Renal biopsy findings are similar to those of IgAN with or without vasculitis. The prognosis generally is good for children and variable for adults. In patients with normal renal function, treatment is supportive only. Patients with progressive renal failure should be considered for treatment with high-dose corticosteroids with or without cytotoxic medication.

Membranoproliferative Glomerulonephritis

Membranoproliferative glomerulonephritis (MPGN) is defined as the diffuse proliferation of the mesangium and thickening of glomerular capillary walls, as seen with light microscopy. MPGN type I affects mainly children of both sexes between the ages of 8 and 16 years. MPGN type II is a rare disease (<1% of all renal biopsies). Secondary forms of MPGN tend to predominate in adults (>90%). The main cause of secondary MPGN type I is cryoglobulinemia in a patient with hepatitis C virus (HCV) infection. Other secondary causes include chronic infections, "shunt nephritis," malaria, SLE, congenital complement deficiency (C2 and C3), sickle cell disease, partial lipodystrophy (only type II), and α$_1$-antitrypsin deficiency. The clinical presentations of all forms of MPGN are variable and include nephrotic and nephritic features. Approximately one-third of the patients present with a combination of asymptomatic hematuria and proteinuria. Another third present with nephrotic syndrome and preserved renal function. Some patients (10%-20%) present with nephritic syndrome. Hypertension is common (50%-80% of patients). In MPGN type I and cryoglobulinemic MPGN, the levels of C3, C4, and CH50 are persistently low, reflecting activation of both complement pathways. In MPGN type II, the alternative pathway is activated, with patients having a persistently low level of C3 but a normal level of C4. A C3 nephritic factor is present in many cases. C3 nephritic factor is an autoantibody to alternative pathway C3 convertase, resulting in persistent breakdown of C3.

In MPGN type I, renal biopsy specimens show diffuse global thickening of capillary walls and endocapillary hypercellularity, giving the glomeruli a lobular appearance. The interposition of mesangium between the GBM and the endothelium triggers the production of neomembrane by the endothelial cells and results in glomerular capillaries developing a double contour or "tram-track" appearance, best seen with silver staining. Immunofluorescence shows the granular deposition of IgG and C3 in the mesangium and outlines the lobular contours. Electron microscopy shows immune deposits in the subendothelial space and mesangium. In MPGN type II, also known as *dense deposit disease*, electron-dense deposits replace the lamina densa and produce a smooth, ribbonlike thickening. Immunofluorescence shows intense capillary wall staining (linear to bandlike) for C3.

* MPGN: about one-third of the patients present with hematuria and proteinuria; about one-third present with nephrotic syndrome and preserved renal function. Nephritic syndrome is present in 10%-20%.
* Complement values are persistently low.
* C3 nephritic factor is often present.
* Secondary causes: hepatitis B and C, chronic infections, "shunt nephritis," SLE, and sickle cell disease.
* A "tram-track," or double contour, appearance is seen with silver staining.

In children, long-term corticosteroid therapy has been helpful. The use of dipyridamole (225 mg daily) and aspirin (975 mg daily) may temporarily slow the rate of progression of MPGN type I, but results are not lasting. Treatment in adults is unknown. MPGN type I usually has a slowly progressive course, with 40% to 50% of patients reaching ESRD in 10 years. Patients with MPGN type II have a worse prognosis, and clinical remission rates are less than 5%. Predictors of poor outcome include impaired renal function at presentation, nephrotic-range proteinuria (>3 g/1.73 m² per 24 hours), hypertension, the number of crescents (>50%), and the degree of tubulointerstitial damage. This disorder tends to recur in transplant recipients (type I, 30%; type II, 90%).

* Prognosis: worse with hypertension, poor renal function, and proteinuria >3 g/1.73 m² per 24 hours.

Rapidly Progressive Glomerulonephritis— Crescentic Glomerulonephritis

Rapidly progressive glomerulonephritis (RPGN) is defined as an acute, rapidly progressive (days to weeks to months) deterioration of renal function associated with an active urinary sediment and a focal necrotizing crescentic glomerulonephritis seen on light microscopic examination of renal biopsy specimens. A pulmonary-renal syndrome is frequent, and oliguria is not uncommon. Immunofluorescence

demonstrates 3 patterns: type I, linear IgG deposition (eg, Goodpasture disease or anti-GBM–mediated); type II, granular immune complexes (eg, SLE); and type III, pauci-immune (negative or weak immunofluorescence (eg, antineutrophil cytoplasmic autoantibody [ANCA] vasculitis) (Figure 18-1). *Goodpasture syndrome* indicates a pulmonary-renal syndrome and can be due to several conditions, including Goodpasture disease, ANCA vasculitis (microscopic polyangiitis or Wegener granulomatosis), SLE, cryoglobulinemia, and pulmonary edema.

* RPGN: acute (days to weeks to months) deterioration of renal function.
* Focal necrotizing crescentic glomerulonephritis seen in renal biopsy specimens.
* Pulmonary-renal syndrome (Goodpasture syndrome) is common and can be due to Goodpasture disease, ANCA vasculitis (microscopic polyangiitis or Wegener granulomatosis), SLE, cryoglobulinemia, pulmonary edema, and other conditions.

ANCA Vasculitides

In the Chapel Hill classification, systemic vasculitis can be classified according to the different vessels that are involved (Table 18-1). Of particular importance to nephrology are the ANCA vasculitides: microscopic polyangiitis, Wegener granulomatosis, and Churg-Strauss syndrome. This group is characterized by inflammation and necrosis of small blood vessels of the kidney and other organs that occur in association with autoantibodies against antigens present in lysosomal granules in the cytoplasm of neutrophils (ANCA). These antigens are myeloperoxidase (MPO) and proteinase-3 (PR3). On ethanol-fixed leukocytes examined with indirect immunofluorescence, anti-MPO antibodies frequently produce a perinuclear pattern (p-ANCA) and antibodies against PR3 form a cytoplasmic pattern (c-ANCA). Because nonspecific antibodies against other cytoplasmic antigens (eg, enolase, elastase, lactoferrin, and catalase) can also give a positive ANCA pattern on immunofluorescence, confirmation of the antibody specificity by enzyme-linked immunosorbent assay (ELISA) is required. Patients with ANCA vasculitis, which is the most common cause of RPGN in patients older than 60, have a wide range of signs and symptoms (Table 18-2).

Microscopic Polyangiitis

Microscopic polyangiitis is a necrotizing vasculitis with few or no immune deposits (pauci-immune) on immunofluorescence that affects small vessels (ie, capillaries, venules, and arterioles). A necrotizing arteritis involving small and medium-size arteries can be present. Necrotizing glomerulonephritis with crescents is common, and pulmonary capillaritis often occurs. Fifty percent of patients are MPO-ANCA–positive, 40% are PR3-ANCA–positive, and a few are ANCA-negative.

Wegener Granulomatosis

Wegener granulomatosis (WG) is a granulomatous inflammation involving the respiratory tract and necrotizing vasculitis affecting small and medium-size vessels (ie, capillaries, venules, arterioles, and arteries). In WG, as in microscopic polyangiitis, a necrotizing

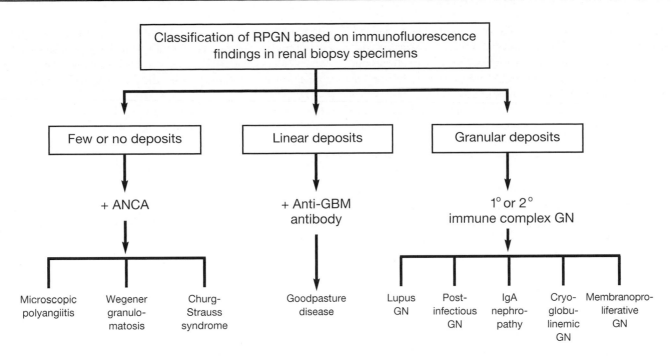

Figure 18-1. Rapidly Progressive Glomerulonephritis (RPGN). Classification according to immunofluorescence microscopy findings in renal biopsy specimens. ANCA indicates antineutrophil cytoplasmic autoantibody; GBM, glomerular basement membrane; GN, glomerulonephritis; GV, granulomatous vasculitis.

glomerulonephritis is common. Of the patients with WG, 75% are PR3-ANCA–positive, and 20% are MPO-ANCA–positive.

Churg-Strauss Syndrome

Churg-Strauss syndrome is characterized by peripheral blood eosinophilia, asthma or other form of atopy, an eosinophil-rich granulomatous inflammation involving the respiratory tract, and

a necrotizing vasculitis affecting small and medium-size vessels. Sixty percent of the patients are MPO-ANCA–positive.

ANCA vasculitis should be treated with a combination of high-dose corticosteroids and cyclophosphamide until remission is achieved (3-6 months). Patients with pulmonary hemorrhage or severe renal failure (serum creatinine >5.5 mg/dL or receiving dialysis) or both, should also receive plasma exchange. The prognosis in ANCA vasculitis is quite variable. According to recent reviews, 2 years after the diagnosis the mortality rate is 25% and the ESRD rate is 21%. However, with aggressive treatment up to 75% of patients may recover renal function, even if dialysis therapy was required at the start of treatment. ANCA vasculitides are associated with a high relapse rate (30%-50% within the first 5 years). Long-term treatment with low-dose corticosteroids in combination with azathioprine is beneficial in decreasing the frequency of relapses. Patients with WG who are nasal carriers of

Table 18-1 Chapel Hill Consensus on the Nomenclature of Systemic Vasculitis

Large-vessel vasculitis
  Giant cell (temporal) arteritis
  Takayasu arteritis
Medium-size vessel vasculitis
  Classic polyarteritis nodosa
  Kawasaki disease
Small-vessel vasculitis
  Microscopic polyangiitis[a]
  Wegener granulomatosis[a]
  Churg-Strauss syndrome[a]
  Henoch-Schönlein purpura
  Essential cryoglobulinemic vasculitis
  Cutaneous leukocytoclastic vasculitis
  Anti–glomerular basement membrane disease

[a] Strongly associated with antineutrophil cytoplasmic autoantibody (ANCA).

Table 18-2 Signs and Symptoms of ANCA Vasculitis

Cutaneous purpura, nodules, & ulcerations
Peripheral neuropathy (mononeuritis multiplex)
Abdominal pain & blood in stools
Hematuria, proteinuria, & renal failure
Hemoptysis & pulmonary infiltrates or nodules
Necrotizing (hemorrhagic) sinusitis
Myalgias & arthralgias
Muscle & pancreatic enzymes in blood

Abbreviation: NCA, antineutrophil cytoplasmic autoantibody.

Staphylococcus aureus benefit from long-term treatment with trimethoprim-sulfamethoxazole. The use of serial ANCA testing as a predictor of relapses has variable degrees of success. For making a therapeutic decision, the results of this test should not be taken in isolation but in the context of the patient's clinical history. Several medications (propylthiouracil, hydralazine, and penicillamine) and heavy silica exposure have been associated with the induction of ANCA and necrotizing glomerulonephritis.

Polyarteritis Nodosa

Polyarteritis nodosa is characterized by necrotizing inflammation of medium-size or small arteries without glomerulonephritis or vasculitis in arterioles, capillaries, or venules. Polyarteritis nodosa is ANCA-negative and associated with hepatitis B infection. The diagnosis is made by finding aneurysms on angiography or nerve biopsy (nerve biopsy alone may not be helpful because peripheral neuropathy also occurs in ANCA vasculitis).

* ANCA vasculitis: microscopic polyangiitis, WG, and Churg-Strauss syndrome.
* ANCA vasculitis: the most common cause of RPGN in patients older than 60 years.
* Renal biopsy: focal segmental necrotizing glomerulonephritis with crescents.
* Polyarteritis nodosa: ANCA-negative; associated with hepatitis B infection; normal glomeruli.
* "Drug-induced ANCA vasculitis": propylthiouracil, hydralazine, and penicillamine.
* Treatment: high-dose corticosteroids and cyclophosphamide.
* Plasmapheresis is also indicated for patients with ANCA vasculitis who have evidence of pulmonary hemorrhage or severe renal failure (serum creatinine >5.5 mg/dL or receiving dialysis).

Goodpasture Disease: Anti-GBM Antibody–Mediated Glomerulonephritis

Goodpasture disease is defined by a pulmonary-renal syndrome caused by circulating anti-GBM antibodies and linear staining seen along the GBM and alveolar basement membrane on immunofluorescence. The antibody is directed against the $\alpha 3$ chain of type IV collagen. Pulmonary hemorrhage may be absent or not clinically apparent. Other autoantibodies may coexist with anti-GBM antibodies (about 25%-30% of patients are also ANCA-positive). The treatment of Goodpasture disease is with high-dose corticosteroids (prednisone, 1 mg/kg daily up to 80 mg daily, or pulse methylprednisolone sodium succinate [Solu-Medrol], 1 g for 3 days) in combination with oral cyclophosphamide (2-3 mg/kg daily up to 200 mg daily; decrease the dose by 25% for patients older than 55 or with creatinine >5 mg/dL) and plasma exchange. The prognosis in patients with Goodpasture disease depends on the percentage of circumferential crescents of the renal biopsy specimen, the presence of oliguria, and the need for dialysis. Among patients with a serum creatinine level less than 5.0 mg/dL at the start of treatment, the probability of renal survival at 5 years is more than 90%. Patients who have 100% circumferential crescents and are receiving dialysis do not recover renal function and should not be treated with the immunosuppressive regimen outlined above, except in the presence of pulmonary hemorrhage. Goodpasture disease is a "single-hit disease"—it rarely recurs. Patients with ESRD are candidates for renal transplant after the antibody has disappeared (6-12 months).

* Goodpasture disease: pulmonary-renal syndrome, positive anti-GBM antibody, and linear staining of the GBM.

Glomerular Disease That Usually Presents as Nephrotic Syndrome

Minimal Change Nephropathy

Minimal change nephropathy (MCN) is defined by the absence of structural glomerular abnormalities, except for the widespread fusion of epithelial cell foot processes seen on electron microscopy, in a patient with nephrotic syndrome. MCN is the most common cause of nephrotic syndrome in children. Among patients with nephrotic syndrome, MCN is the cause in 70% to 90% of children younger than 10 years (although rarely before the first year of life), in 50% of adolescents and young adults, and in less than 20% of adults with primary nephrotic syndrome.

The pathogenesis of MCN is unknown. The association with Hodgkin lymphoma suggests that MCN may be a consequence of T-lymphocyte abnormalities, with T cells producing a lymphokine that is toxic to glomerular epithelial cells. This results in fusion of foot processes and detachment of podocytes, loss of the heparin sulfate negative-charge barrier of the basement membrane, and increased glomerular permeability to protein. There is a clear association with drugs, allergy, and malignancy. Children with the disease present with an abrupt onset of nephrotic syndrome. The presence of hematuria, hypertension, or impaired renal function is unusual in children. In adults, hypertension and renal insufficiency may be present. In children, the presence of nephrotic syndrome in a patient with normal urinalysis results indicates MCN until proven otherwise. If a child does not have a response to corticosteroid therapy, renal biopsy is justified. In adults, MCN accounts for less than 20% of the cases of patients presenting with a nephrotic syndrome, and renal biopsy is required to establish the diagnosis. The most important differential diagnosis is focal segmental glomerulosclerosis (FSGS).

In some patients, MCN may have a secondary cause. The most common secondary causes of MCN are the following:

1. Viral infections—mononucleosis and human immunodeficiency virus (HIV)
2. Drugs—NSAIDs (with interstitial nephritis)
3. Tumors—Hodgkin lymphoma and leukemia
4. Allergies—food, bee sting, and poison ivy

On light microscopic and immunofluorescence examination, the glomeruli are normal. Tubules may accumulate lipid droplets from absorbed lipoproteins. Occasionally, the findings are consistent with acute tubular necrosis. The presence of concomitant interstitial nephritis suggests drugs (eg, NSAIDs) as the cause of MCD. Electron microscopy shows effacement of the foot processes; however, this is a nonspecific finding that is also seen in patients with heavy proteinuria due to other glomerulopathies. In children, high-dose corticosteroid therapy is the cornerstone of treatment, with more than 90% of children achieving complete remission after 4 to 6 weeks of treatment. In adolescents and adults, the response to therapy is also high (>80%), but the response is slower and some patients may require up to 16 weeks of treatment to achieve remission. Generally, therapy is continued for 4 to 8 weeks after remission. Of the patients who have a response to corticosteroid therapy, 25% have a long-term remission. The others have at least 1 relapse. For patients who have frequent relapses, are steroid-dependent, or are resistant to steroids, alternative therapy includes the use of cyclophosphamide, chlorambucil, and cyclosporine. Overall, the prognosis is excellent, with patients maintaining renal function long-term. If there is no response to therapy or if progressive renal failure develops, an alternative diagnosis (such as FSGS) must be considered.

- MCN: abrupt nephrotic syndrome with normal renal function.
- It is the main cause of nephrotic syndrome in children. In adults, it accounts for <20% of cases of nephrotic syndrome.
- Secondary causes: viral, Hodgkin disease, and NSAIDs (with interstitial nephritis).
- MCN responds to corticosteroid treatment. Failure to respond to this therapy suggests an alternative diagnosis.

Focal Segmental Glomerulosclerosis

FSGS accounts for less than 15% of cases of idiopathic nephrotic syndrome in children. In adults, it accounts for approximately 25% of nephropathies. FSGS is the most common form of idiopathic nephrotic syndrome in African Americans. It may be idiopathic or due to different causes (eg, heroin abuse, HIV infection, sickle cell disease, obesity, vesicoureteral reflux, unilateral renal agenesis, remnant kidneys, and aging). The pathogenesis of idiopathic FSGS is unknown. In some patients, the presence of a circulating permeability factor has been demonstrated. Glomerular hypertension and hyperfiltration are thought to have a role in secondary causes of FSGS, as in patients with unilateral renal agenesis or remnant kidneys. Patients present with either asymptomatic proteinuria or full-blown nephrotic syndrome. Hypertension is found in 30% to 50% of patients, with microscopic hematuria in 25% to 75% of them. At presentation, the glomerular filtration rate is decreased in 20% to 30% of patients.

The pathologic diagnosis of FSGS is based on the identification in some glomeruli (focal) of areas of capillary obliteration, with increased mesangial matrix deposition and intracapillary hyalin deposits in parts of the glomerular tufts (segmental lesion). Interstitial fibrosis is a common finding. Immunofluorescence shows IgM and C3 deposition in the areas of glomerular scarring (nonspecific trapping). Electron microscopy demonstrates fusion of epithelial foot processes in the majority of the glomeruli, including those that appear normal on light microscopy. Four histologic variants of FSGS have been described. In the most common pattern, there is predilection for sclerosis in the perihilar regions. In the cellular/collapsing variant, hypertrophy and hyperplasia of the overlying epithelial cells result in global glomerular capillary collapse and sclerosis. The cellular/collapsing variant, which has the worst prognosis, is more common in African Americans and patients with HIV infection.

Prolonged (>4 months) high-dose corticosteroid therapy (prednisone, 1 mg/kg daily) has achieved up to a 40% to 60% remission rate of nephrotic syndrome, with preservation of long-term renal function. For patients who have a response to corticosteroids, alternative therapy includes the use of cytotoxic drugs, either alone or in combination with corticosteroids, and low-dose cyclosporine. Treatment options are limited for patients who do not have a response to corticosteroids. For these patients, the best evidence is for treatment with cyclosporine, but tacrolimus and mycophenolic acid have also been used with variable success. For patients who have protein excretion of less than 3 g daily, treatment with an ACEI or angiotensin II receptor antagonist (or both) may be sufficient to reduce proteinuria and improve renal survival. For patients with secondary forms of FSGS, treatment should target the primary cause, if possible. In all patients, treatment with an ACEI or an ARB, alone or in combination, may substantially reduce proteinuria and prolong renal survival. In an increasing number of cases (both familial and sporadic, in children and adults), the disease is associated with mutations in several podocyte-associated proteins (podocin, CD2-associated protein, and α-actinin-4). Patients who are homozygous for these mutations have no response to corticosteroid treatment.

Less than 5% of patients experience a spontaneous remission of proteinuria; in most patients who remain nephrotic, ESRD develops 5 to 20 years after presentation. The response to corticosteroid treatment and the degree of proteinuria are the best predictors of the long-term clinical outcome. Patients who have a non–nephrotic-range proteinuria have the best renal survival (>80% at 10 years). Patients who have the worst prognosis are those who have no response to treatment or who continue to have proteinuria of more than 10 g/1.73 m^2 per 24 hours regardless of the histologic variant; in the majority of them, ESRD develops within 3 years. Idiopathic FSGS may recur in a transplanted kidney.

- FSGS accounts for about 25% of cases of adult nephrotic syndrome.
- FSGS is the most common cause of nephrotic syndrome in African Americans.
- Patients present with hypertension, renal insufficiency, proteinuria, and hematuria.
- Secondary causes: HIV infection, heroin abuse, reflux nephropathy, and morbid obesity.
- Genetic mutations in podocyte-related proteins are increasingly recognized as causes of FSGS.
- Prolonged high-dose corticosteroid therapy: >40% of patients have a response.
- The cellular/collapsing variant has the worst prognosis.

HIV-Associated Nephropathy

HIV-associated nephropathy (HIV-AN) is characterized by progressive renal insufficiency in patients with nephrotic-range proteinuria (frequently massive) but often little edema. Large echogenic kidneys are seen on ultrasonography. Renal biopsy specimens show a collapsing form of FSGS. Tubules are often dilated, forming microcysts. With electron microscopy, numerous tubuloreticular inclusions (interferon fingerprints) are seen within the glomerular and vascular endothelial cells. HIV-AN is much more common, and clinically more severe, in African Americans than in whites. Other types of glomerulonephritis also encountered with some frequency in HIV-infected persons include IgAN, MPGN, MCN, membranous nephropathy (MN), and postinfectious glomerulonephritis. Thrombotic microangiopathy develops in some patients; it is not related to *Escherichia coli* O157:H7 and carries a high mortality. Treatment includes the use of antiretroviral agents, treatment of underlying infections, and use of ACEI to reduce proteinuria.

Membranous Nephropathy

MN is the leading cause of nephrotic syndrome in white adults. It occurs in persons of all ages and races but is most often diagnosed in middle age, with the incidence peaking during the fourth and fifth decades of life. The male to female ratio is 2:1. The pathogenic mechanisms that cause this immune complex localization and the subsequent development of proteinuria and the nephrotic syndrome are not completely understood, but in situ deposition of cationic antigens in the subepithelial space is thought to be involved. The nature of the antigen involved in the immune complex deposits of MN and its source are not known.

At presentation, proteinuria is greater than 2.0 g/1.73 m^2 per 24 hours in more than 80% of patients and more than 10 g/1.73 m^2 per 24 hours in as many as 30%. Initially, renal function is preserved in the majority of patients, and hypertension is present in less than 20% at diagnosis. A small proportion have microscopic hematuria. MN is an idiopathic (primary) or secondary disease (up to 30% of patients with biopsy-proven MN). Secondary MN is caused by autoimmune diseases (eg, SLE and autoimmune thyroiditis), infection (eg, hepatitis B and C), drugs (eg, penicillamine, gold, and NSAIDs), and malignancies (eg, colon cancer and lung cancer). MN is associated with malignancy in 7% to 15% of patients older than 60 years. Very early in the disease process, the glomeruli may appear normal in light microscopic preparations and the diagnosis can be made only with immunofluorescence or with electron microscopy to detect subepithelial deposits along the GBM. With more advanced lesions, capillary walls are thickened, and methenamine silver stain shows subepithelial projections ("spikes") along the capillary walls. The spikes represent deposition of new basement membrane material along the subepithelial deposits. Immunofluorescence microscopy shows marked granular deposition of IgG and C3 along the capillary walls.

Initial therapy for MN is generally supportive. The use of ACEIs and ARBs is recommended, but their effect in decreasing proteinuria is modest (about 40%). Therapies other than supportive care should be considered for patients who remain nephrotic after a trial of maximal angiotensin II blockade (6 months); they include a combination of corticosteroids and cytotoxic agents, and cyclosporine. Mycophenolate mofetil has been tried with success in some patients. Thrombotic complications (eg, renal vein thrombosis causes sudden loss of renal function in 25%-50% of patients) are frequent, and anticoagulation should be considered for patients with proteinuria greater than 10 g/1.73 m^2 per 24 hours and serum albumin less than 2 g/dL. Without treatment, nearly 25% of patients have spontaneous complete remission and 50% have partial remission. In patients who have spontaneous remission, it usually occurs within 6 to 12 months after

presentation. Spontaneous remission is less common in patients with proteinuria greater than 10 g in 24 hours. The probability of renal survival is more than 80% at 5 years and 60% at 15 years. The prognosis is worse in nephrotic patients. In 10% to 15% of patients the disease has an accelerated course, with ESRD occurring within 1 year after the diagnosis. In this last situation, superimposed anti-GBM disease, acute interstitial nephritis, and renal vein thrombosis should be ruled out.

- MN: the primary cause of idiopathic nephrotic syndrome in white adults.
- The peak incidence occurs during the fourth and fifth decades of life.
- Renal vein thrombosis causes sudden loss of renal function in 25%-50% of patients.
- Secondary causes: infections, multisystem disease, neoplasms, and medications.
- Spontaneous complete remission occurs in 25% of patients and partial remission in 50%.

Other Glomerular Disorders

Diabetic Nephropathy

Diabetic nephropathy (DN) is the commonest cause of ESRD in the United States (>50% of patients on dialysis; ≥80% have type 2 diabetes mellitus). DN occurs in both type 1 (30%-40% of cases) and type 2 (20%-30% of cases) diabetes mellitus. In type 1 diabetes mellitus, the peak onset of nephropathy is between 10 and 15 years after the initial presentation with diabetes. Patients who do not have proteinuria after 25 years of diabetes are unlikely to develop DN. A similar natural history is likely for patients with type 2 diabetes mellitus. The main risk factors for developing DN are a positive family history of DN, hypertension, and poor glycemic control. The risk may be greater in some racial groups (eg, Pima Indians and African Americans). The pathogenesis is secondary to increased glycosylation of proteins, with accumulation of advanced glycosylation end products that cross-link with collagen, in combination with glomerular hyperfiltration and hypertension.

DN is first manifested by the onset of microalbuminuria (defined as urinary albumin excretion of 20-200 mcg/min or 30-300 mg/1.73 m^2 per 24 hours). With time, microalbuminuria evolves into overt proteinuria (>300 mg/1.73 m^2 per 24 hours) and subsequent full-blown nephrotic syndrome. The presence of microalbuminuria is the primary predictor of renal disease (in 30%-45% of patients, microalbuminuria progresses to proteinuria after 10 years), with the degree of proteinuria correlating roughly with the renal prognosis. After overt proteinuria develops, the progression toward ESRD is relentless, although rates of decline vary among patients (5-15 years). In patients with type 1 diabetes, there is a strong correlation (95%) between the development of nephropathy and other signs of diabetic microvascular compromise, such as diabetic retinopathy and DN. This correlation is weaker for patients with type 2 diabetes, and up to one-third of these patients develop nephropathy without evidence of diabetic retinopathy. Hypertension occurs in about 75% of patients with proteinuria. Other renal manifestations of diabetes include frequent urinary tract infections, which may be complicated by the development of acute pyelonephritis and perinephric abscess, and papillary necrosis. A functional obstruction caused by neurogenic bladder may also occur. Because of the accelerated rate of atherosclerosis, diabetic patients also have a high incidence of cardiovascular disease, including renal artery stenosis. The stages of DN are listed in Table 18-3.

- DN occurs in 30%-40% of patients with type 1 diabetes mellitus and in 20%-30% of patients with type 2 diabetes mellitus.
- DN is the single most common cause of ESRD in the United States.
- Microalbuminuria is the primary predictor of renal disease.
- Other renal manifestations of diabetes are hypertension, recurrent urinary tract infections, acute pyelonephritis, perinephric abscess, papillary necrosis, and neurogenic bladder.

In the earliest stage of the disease, renal biopsy specimens show glomerular hypertrophy and thickening of the GBM. As the disease progresses, arteriolar hyalinosis and arteriosclerosis develop. This is followed by progressive mesangial expansion (diffuse diabetic glomerulosclerosis) and nodular formations (Kimmelstiel-Wilson nodules, which are pathognomonic for DN). Both the diffuse and the nodular mesangial expansions are composed of extracellular mesangial matrix and stain positive with silver and periodic acid–Schiff stain. Capsular drop lesions and fibrin cap lesions are also pathognomonic findings. Late in the disease, tubular atrophy and interstitial fibrosis occur. For patients with long-term diabetes, especially if retinopathy is present and other causes of proteinuria are excluded, renal biopsy may not be necessary. However, renal biopsy is indicated for patients with an atypical course of the disease (eg, nephrotic-range proteinuria within the first 10 years in type 1 diabetes or if loss of renal function is rapidly progressive). Start ACEI or ARB therapy in patients who have diabetes and microalbuminuria even if they are normotensive. The progression of DN can be retarded by tight glycemic control (glycated hemoglobin <7.0%) and the use of ACEIs or ARBs (target systolic blood pressure <125 mm Hg). Patients with diabetes who develop microalbuminuria should start ACEI or ARB therapy even if they are normotensive. Patients with ESRD due to diabetes mellitus are candidates for a solitary kidney or combined kidney-pancreas transplant. Hemodialysis and continuous ambulatory peritoneal dialysis are alternatives. Pancreatic islet cell transplant is a promising new therapy.

- Kimmelstiel-Wilson nodules are pathognomonic for DN.
- Aggressive glucose and blood pressure control slows progression.
- Diabetes mellitus is the most common cause of type IV renal tubular acidosis.
- Start ACEI or ARB therapy in patients who have diabetes and microalbuminuria even if they are normotensive.

Systemic Lupus Erythematosus Nephritis

Lupus nephritis (LN) is a major cause of morbidity and mortality in patients with SLE. Approximately 25% of patients with SLE have substantial renal involvement. If renal involvement occurs with SLE, it is usually early in the course of the disease, but rarely is renal involvement the sole manifestation of SLE. LN is more severe in children and in African Americans. The International Society of Nephrology/Renal Pathology Society (ISN/RPS) classification of LN recognizes 6 morphologic classes of renal involvement (Table 18-4). These patterns of LN are not static and may show a transition from 1 class to another either spontaneously or after treatment. A few patients may develop a necrotizing glomerulonephritis with crescents. Immunofluorescence shows glomerular deposition of

Table 18-3 Stages of Diabetic Nephropathy

Stage	Description
I	Hyperfiltration, glomerular filtration rate is 20%-50% above normal, microalbuminuria (30-300 mg/1.73 m^2 per 24 hours)
II	Normalization of glomerular filtration rate with early structural damage
III	Early hypertension
IV	Progression to proteinuria >500 mg/1.73 m^2 per 24 hours, hypertension, declining glomerular filtration rate (lasts 10-15 years)
V	Progression to ESRD (5-7 years); heavy proteinuria persists even to ESRD

Abbreviation: ESRD, end-stage renal disease.

Table 18-4 Abbreviated International Society of Nephrology/Renal Pathology Society (ISN/RPS) Classification of Lupus Nephritis (2003)

Morphologic Class	Renal Manifestation
I. Minimal mesangial lupus nephritis	Normal urinary sediment
II. Mesangial proliferative lupus nephritis	Low-grade hematuria &/or proteinuria Normal renal function
III. Focal lupus nephritis	Active sediment; proteinuria <3 g/1.73 m^2 per 24 hours
IV. Diffuse segmental (IV-S) or global (IV-G) lupus nephritis	Nephritic & nephrotic syndromes Hypertension; progressive renal failure
V. Membranous lupus nephritis	Nephrotic syndrome
VI. Advanced sclerosing lupus nephritis	Inactive urinary sediment Chronic renal failure

Modifed from Weening JJ, D'Agati VD, Schwartz MM, Seshan SV, Alpers CE, Appel GB, et al. The classification of glomerulonephritis in systemic lupus erythematosus revisited. J Am Soc Nephrol. 2004;15:241-50. Used with permission.

IgG, IgM, IgA, C1q, and C4 ("full-house" pattern). As seen with electron microscopy, immune deposits are localized to the glomerular capillary subendothelium (wire-loop) and a fingerprint-like pattern of tubuloreticular inclusions is common within glomerular and vascular endothelial cells. The type of renal lesion strongly influences the management of SLE, and kidney biopsy is indicated in patients with proteinuria and active urinary sediment, regardless of whether they have decreased glomerular function, to define the morphologic class. The histopathologic features correlate with the prognosis, with classes III and IV having the worst prognosis (5-year survival is about 80%). Immunosuppressive treatment is indicated for class III or IV LN. For patients with severe LN, the combination of high-dose corticosteroid (either orally or "pulse" intravenous methylprednisolone) with intravenous cyclophosphamide has produced the most effective therapeutic results, with improvement of serologic and clinical abnormalities. Recent studies suggest that the combination of mycophenolate mofetil plus oral prednisone is as effective as cyclophosphamide plus prednisone. Membranous LN is characterized by proteinuria, weakly positive or negative antinuclear antibody, and no erythrocyte casts. Initial therapy is supportive only. Patients who remain nephrotic should be considered for immunosuppressive treatment (eg, cyclosporine).

* Severe renal involvement occurs in 25% of patients with SLE.
* Focal or diffuse proliferative LN requires aggressive treatment with high-dose corticosteroids plus cyclophosphamide.
* Membranous LN (without proliferation) usually is not treatable with immunosuppressive agents unless nephrotic syndrome persists (>6 months).

Other manifestations of SLE include acute and chronic tubulointerstitial nephritis and glomerular capillary thrombi in patients with antiphospholipid antibodies. Drug-induced SLE rarely involves the kidney. SLE tends to flare during pregnancy, and pregnancy should be delayed until after SLE has been inactive for at least 1 year. SLE "burns out" with ESRD and generally does not recur in transplant recipients (recurrence rate, 2%-4%).

* Drug-induced SLE rarely involves the kidney.
* Pregnancy should be delayed until after SLE has been inactive.
* SLE "burns out" with ESRD and uncommonly (2%-4%) recurs in renal transplant recipients.

Monoclonal Gammopathies

Multiple Myeloma

The renal manifestation of multiple myeloma may be acute renal failure or a chronic progressive disease that may occur at any time during the course of the disease. Virtually all patients with multiple myeloma have monoclonal immunoglobulins or light chains in the serum and urine. Acute renal failure may occur as a result of intraluminal precipitation of multiple proteinaceous casts ("cast nephropathy") and the resulting acute noninflammatory interstitial nephritis (myeloma kidney). The casts are usually acellular with multiple fracture lines (broken casts), are seen mainly in the distal nephron, and

are the result of aggregates of light chains and Tamm-Horsfall glycoprotein. Coaggregation of Tamm-Horsfall glycoprotein with light chains is facilitated by increased concentrations of calcium, sodium, and chloride (such as after the use of a loop diuretic) in the urine; by conditions that reduce flow rates (such as intravascular depletion and the use of NSAIDs); or by the use of radiocontrast agents. Other renal manifestations include pseudohyponatremia, low anion gap, and type 2 renal tubular acidosis with Fanconi syndrome (low levels of phosphorus, urate, and potassium; glycosuria; and aminoaciduria). Ultrasonography shows normal-size or large kidneys. Treatment of cast nephropathy includes vigorous hydration, correction of hypercalcemia, and avoidance of nephrotoxic or precipitating agents. Alkalinizing the urine to keep the pH greater than 7 may be beneficial in some patients. Plasmapheresis can quickly remove light chains from the circulation and should be considered for patients with acute renal failure or hyperviscosity syndrome. Treatment with melphalan and prednisone decreases the circulating levels of light chains and stabilizes or improves renal function in two-thirds of patients with renal failure. Recent success has been achieved with myeloablative therapy followed by bone marrow transplant.

Amyloidosis

Amyloidosis is due to the systemic extracellular deposition of antiparallel, β-pleated sheet, nonbranching, 8- to 12-nm fibrils that stain positive with Congo red (green birefringence with polarized light) or thioflavin T. In primary (AL) amyloidosis, patients are typically older than 50 years, and the kidneys are affected in 50% of patients. Common renal manifestations include proteinuria, nephrotic syndrome (25% of patients), and renal failure. Immunofluorescence generally demonstrates λ light chains in the glomeruli (75% of patients). For patients with cardiac involvement, the prognosis is poor (median survival, <2 years). Treatment with prednisone and melphalan can be beneficial in some patients. In selected cases, high-dose melphalan followed by bone marrow transplant has led to resolution of the disease. Secondary (AA) amyloidosis is most common in patients with rheumatoid arthritis, inflammatory bowel disease, chronic infection, or familial Mediterranean fever and in subcutaneous drug users (heroin). Treatment of AA amyloidosis is directed at the underlying inflammatory process. Colchicine is helpful in patients with familial Mediterranean fever.

Light Chain Deposition Disease

In light chain deposition disease (LCDD), light chain is deposited along the GBM. LCDD is strongly associated with the development of myeloma, lymphoma, and Waldenström macroglobulinemia. Renal involvement is similar to that of amyloidosis, with proteinuria, nephrotic syndrome, and renal insufficiency. Renal biopsy specimens show acellular, eosinophilic mesangial nodules that stain strongly positive with periodic acid–Schiff, often mimicking diabetes mellitus. The deposited monoclonal proteins do not form fibrils and do not bind Congo red. Immunofluorescence microscopic findings are diagnostic, showing diffuse linear immunoglobulin light chain deposition (κ in 80% of cases) along the GBM and tubular basement membranes and in the nodules. As in amyloidosis, treatment with melphalan and prednisone has led to stabilization or improved renal function in some patients. At 5 years, patient survival is 50% to 70%, with renal survival ranging from 20% to 35%. Similar to AL amyloidosis, the disease recurs in transplant recipients.

Glomerulonephritis Associated With Hepatitis Infection

Cryoglobulinemic Glomerulonephritis

Type II or mixed essential cryoglobulins (Table 18-5) are commonly found in patients with HCV infection and contain HCV RNA and anti-HCV IgG. After they precipitate in the glomeruli, they bind complement, activate a cytokine cascade, and trigger an inflammatory response. Patients with this renal disease may present with proteinuria, microscopic hematuria, nephrotic syndrome, or renal impairment. Hypertension is common and may be severe, particularly in the presence of acute nephritic syndrome. Cryoglobulinemia is usually associated with low levels of C3 and C4. The cryocrits correlate poorly with disease activity (≥30%-40% of the patients do not have detectable cryoglobulins). On light microscopy, renal biopsy specimens show a membranoproliferative type I pattern of injury, with massive exudation of cells, mainly monocytic, and a double-contoured appearance of the GBM. Eosinophilic thrombi are often found in the capillary lumen and consist of cryoprecipitated immunoglobulins. On electron microscopy, diffuse, dense subendothelial deposits are seen occluding the glomerular capillary; some have a peculiar microtubular or crystalline appearance due to parallel fibrils. In some cases, a vasculitis affecting small and medium-size arteries may be seen. Combination treatment with interferon alfa and ribavirin is effective in clearing the virus from the circulation and results in improvement of proteinuria and renal function. However, relapses after discontinuation of the antiviral therapy are common. Treatment with prednisone, cytotoxic agents, and plasmapheresis is indicated in patients with acute nephritis. The renal prognosis is usually good, with few patients progressing to ESRD.

Hemolytic Uremic Syndrome and Thrombocytopenic Purpura

The 2 forms of hemolytic uremic syndrome (HUS) are a sporadic or diarrhea-associated form (D+HUS) and a non–diarrhea-associated form (D–HUS). The D+HUS is strongly linked to ingestion of meat contaminated with E $coli$ O157:H7. This bacterium produces a Shiga-like toxin that binds to a glycolipid receptor on renal endothelial cells and triggers endothelial damage. The D–HUS occurs in association with the use of oral contraceptives, cyclosporine, tacrolimus, mitomycin C, bleomycin, ticlopidine, or quinine or with antiphospholipid antibody syndrome (in the context of pregnancy), underlying malignancy, or radiotherapy. A familial recurrent form of D–HUS has also been described.

Thrombocytopenic purpura (TTP) occurs as an acute form or as a chronic (relapsing) form. It also occurs in association with some systemic diseases (SLE, scleroderma, or malignancy), drugs (cocaine, quinidine, or ticlopidine), and HIV infection. TTP occurs with a deficiency of the von Willebrand factor (vWF)-cleaving protease (chronic form) or with the development of an autoantibody against vWF-cleaving protease. Patients with HUS or TTP present with a microangiopathic hemolytic anemia and thrombocytopenia. HUS more commonly causes acute renal failure, and TTP is more commonly associated with fever, neurologic signs, and purpura. Markers of hemolysis are present and include low haptoglobin levels, increased levels of lactate dehydrogenase and unconjugated bilirubin, and a high reticulocyte count. Schistocytes are present in peripheral blood smears. In D+HUS, renal biopsy specimens show mainly capillary thrombosis, whereas in D–HUS there is predominant involvement of small arteries, with intimal mucoid proliferation and arterioles with onion-skinning and thrombosis.

Therapy for HUS is supportive. Plasma infusions, plasma exchange, and anticoagulation are ineffective. However, fresh frozen plasma infusions and plasma exchange are effective treatments for TTP. The transfusion of platelets should be avoided because of the risk of accelerating the process. Children with D+HUS have a good prognosis (90% recover renal function), but older patients have an increased mortality rate and unfavorable long-term renal survival.

- D+HUS: Shiga-like toxin production by E $coli$ O157:H7.
- Presentation of patients with HUS or TTP: microangiopathic hemolytic anemia and thrombocytopenia.
- Therapy: for HUS, supportive; for TTP, fresh frozen plasma infusion and plasmapheresis.
- D+HUS: good prognosis for children.

Table 18-5 Cryoglobulins and Associated Diseases

Cryoglobulin Type	Immunoglobulin Class	Associated Diseases
I. Monoclonal immunoglobulins	M>G>A>BJP	Myeloma, Waldenström macroglobulinemia
II. Mixed cryoglobulins with monoclonal immunoglobulins	M/G>>G/G	Sjögren syndrome, Waldenström macroglobulinemia, lymphoma, essential cryoglobulinemia
III. Mixed polyclonal immunoglobulins	M/G	Infection, SLE, vasculitis, neoplasia, essential cryoglobulinemia

Abbreviation: SLE, systemic lupus erythematosus.

Diseases with GBM Abnormalities: Alport Syndrome and Thin GBM Disease

Alport Syndrome

Alport syndrome is an inherited disorder of basement membranes. In more than half of the patients, the disease results from a mutation in the gene (*COL4A5*) that codes for the α5 chain of type IV collagen α5(IV). The syndrome is characterized by a progressive nephritis manifested by persistent or intermittent hematuria and is frequently associated with sensorineural hearing loss and ocular abnormalities. Most patients have mild proteinuria, which progresses with age; kidneys become nephrotic in approximately one-third of the patients. The disease is X-linked in at least 80% of the patients, but autosomal recessive and autosomal dominant patterns of inheritance have been described. In virtually all male patients, the syndrome progresses to ESRD, often by age 16 to 35. The disease is usually mild in heterozygous females, but some develop ESRD, usually after age 50. The rate of progression to ESRD is fairly constant among affected males within individual families, but it varies markedly from family to family. On light microscopy, the glomerular changes are nonspecific. Diagnostic features are usually seen on electron microscopy. At an early stage, thinning of the GBM may be the only visible abnormality and may suggest thin basement membrane disease. With time, the GBM thickens and the lamina densa splits into several irregular layers that may branch and rejoin, producing a characteristic "basket weave" appearance. Immunohistochemical studies of type IV collagen show the absence of α3(IV), α4(IV), and α5(IV) chains from the GBM and distal tubular basement membrane. This abnormality occurs only in patients with Alport syndrome and is diagnostic. In families with a previously defined mutation, molecular diagnosis of affected males or gene-carrying females is possible. For families in which mutations have not been defined, genetic linkage analysis can determine whether an at-risk person carries the mutant gene, provided that at least two other affected members are available for testing. No specific treatment is available for Alport syndrome. Tight control of blood pressure and moderate protein restriction are recommended to retard the progression of renal disease, but the benefit is unproven. Peritoneal dialysis, hemodialysis, and renal transplant are used successfully. Transplant recipients have a 5% to 10% risk of Goodpasture disease developing (because of the presence of Goodpasture antigen in the transplanted kidney).

Thin GBM Disease

Thin GBM disease, or thin basement membrane nephropathy, is a relatively common condition characterized by isolated glomerular hematuria associated with the renal biopsy finding of an excessively thin GBM. The pathogenesis is unclear. In contrast to patients with Alport syndrome, immunohistochemical studies of type IV collagen in the GBM of patients with thin GBM disease do not show abnormality in the distribution on any of the 6 chains. The clinical presentation includes persistent hematuria first detected in childhood. In some patients, hematuria is intermittent and may not be manifested until adulthood. Macroscopic hematuria is not uncommon and may occur in association with an upper respiratory tract infection. When first detected in young adults, 60% have proteinuria

less than 500 mg/1.73 m² per 24 hours. The glomeruli appear normal in light and immunofluorescence microscopic preparations of renal biopsy specimens. Electron microscopy shows diffuse thinning of the GBM. In adults, a GBM thickness less than 250 nm is strongly suggestive of thin GBM disease. The condition is usually benign and requires no specific treatment. For the majority of patients, the prognosis is excellent, with renal function preserved for a long time. However, a small proportion of patients have progressive renal disease that leads to ESRD.

Clinical Manifestations of Tubulointerstitial Renal Disease

Acute and chronic interstitial disease preferentially involves renal tubules. Some of the patterns of renal tubular injury are 1) tubular proteinuria (<1.5-2 g/1.73 m² per 24 hours), 2) proximal tubule dysfunction (hypokalemia, hypouricemia, hypophosphatemia, acidosis, glycosuria, and aminoaciduria), 3) distal tubule dysfunction (hyperchloremic acidosis, hyperkalemia or hypokalemia, and salt wasting), 4) medullary concentration dysfunction, nephrogenic diabetes insipidus with decreased urine-concentrating ability, 5) urinary sediment (pyuria, leukocyte casts, eosinophiluria, and hematuria), and 6) azotemia and renal insufficiency.

- Tubular proteinuria <1.5-2 g/1.73 m² per 24 hours.
- Proximal tubule dysfunction and distal tubule dysfunction.
- Medullary concentration dysfunction.

Acute Interstitial Nephritis

Acute interstitial nephritis (AIN) is an acute, usually reversible, inflammatory disease characterized by a mononuclear cellular infiltrate within the renal interstitium. AIN is relatively common (about 10%-15% of cases of acute renal failure) and occurs in any age group but is rare in children. AIN is most frequently associated with drugs, particularly antibiotics (such as methicillin, which interacts with anti–tubular basement membrane antibodies) and NSAIDs (which cause interstitial nephritis with nephrotic syndrome and renal insufficiency) (Table 18-6). Infections are the second most common cause. AIN also occurs in association with selected autoimmune systemic diseases and malignancies. In 10% to 20% of cases, AIN is idiopathic. Onset is sudden, with approximately 40% of patients having oliguria. In patients with drug-induced AIN, the systemic manifestations of a hypersensitivity reaction include fever (>50% of patients), maculopapular rash (40%), and arthralgias (25%). Flank pain is caused by distention of the renal capsule and occurs in approximately 50% of the patients. Renal impairment (60% of patients) varies from a mild increase in the serum level of creatinine to severe acute renal failure requiring dialysis. Tubular damage can impair the urinary concentration mechanism and result in the development of polyuria. Eosinophilia is common (50% of patients). Urinalysis demonstrates pyuria and hematuria in nearly 100% of the patients, but macroscopic hematuria is unusual. Rarely, RBC casts are seen in the urinary sediment. The presence of eosinophiluria (>1% of patients) is suggestive of AIN but is also seen in other unrelated renal

Table 18-6 Common Causes of Acute Interstitial Nephritis

Drugs

  Antibiotics—penicillin, methicillin (anti–tubular basement
    membrane antibodies), ampicillin, rifampin, sulfa drugs,
    ciprofloxacin, pentamidine

  NSAIDs—interstitial nephritis with nephrotic syndrome
    & renal insufficiency may have a latent period; not
    dose-dependent; recurs; possibly T-cell–mediated;
    allergic signs & symptoms are absent

  Diuretics—thiazides, furosemide, bumetanide (sulfa
    derivatives)

  Cimetidine

  Allopurinol, phenytoin, phenindione

  Cyclosporine

Infections

  Bacteria—*Legionella, Brucella, Streptococcus,*
    Staphylococcus, Pneumococcus

  Virus—Epstein-Barr, CMV, *Hantavirus,* HIV, hepatitis B,
    Polyomavirus

  Fungus—*Candida, Histoplasma*

  Parasites—*Plasmodium, Toxoplasma, Schistosoma,*
    Leishmania

Systemic diseases

  Systemic lupus erythematosus

  Sjögren syndrome

  Sarcoidosis

  Lymphoma, leukemic infiltration

  Renal transplant rejection

Idiopathic

Abbreviations: CMV, cytomegalovirus; HIV, human immunodeficiency virus; NSAID, nonsteroidal anti-inflammatory drug.

diseases. The absence of eosinophiluria does not exclude the diagnosis. Proteinuria is generally mild (<1 g/1.73 m² per 24 hours). The predictive value of gallium scanning is limited. Diagnosis sometimes requires renal biopsy. Therapy is primarily supportive. The likely inciting factor or factors need to be identified and eliminated. Treatment with prednisone (60 mg every other day) for 2 to 4 weeks may hasten the recovery of renal function and may be of benefit in patients who do not regain renal function within 1 week after discontinuing use of the offending agent. Corticosteroids are not indicated in infection-related AIN. Historically, drug-induced AIN has been considered a reversible process, with renal function returning to baseline values in the majority of patients. However, recent studies have shown that impaired renal function can persist long-term in up to 40% of the patients.

- AIN: nearly 100% of patients have pyuria; >50%, fever; 60%, renal insufficiency; 50%, eosinophilia; and 25%, arthralgias.
- Methicillin (anti–tubular basement membrane antibodies).
- NSAIDs: interstitial nephritis with nephrotic syndrome and renal insufficiency.

Analgesic Chronic Interstitial Nephritis

Analgesic nephropathy is a typical example of slowly progressive chronic interstitial nephritis due to the chronic consumption of mixed analgesic preparations, frequently complicated by papillary necrosis, and resulting in bilateral renal atrophy. It is responsible for 20% of cases of chronic tubulointerstitial nephritis and accounts for approximately 3% to 10% of patients reaching ESRD. There are major regional differences in its incidence, perhaps reflecting differences in consumption behavior, availability of phenacetin-containing analgesic mixtures, and medical awareness of the condition. Most of the initial cases of analgesic nephropathy were identified in patients who consumed large amounts of phenacetin, a fact that led to the removal of phenacetin from most markets around the world. More recently, it has been recognized that acetaminophen combined with acetylsalicylic acid can cause renal damage. Also, chronic use of NSAIDs can result in the development of analgesic nephropathy. The condition is 5 to 7 times more frequent in females than males. Besides having headaches, arthritis, muscular aches, and a history of peptic ulcer, patients usually have a history of chronic pain with the consumption of large amounts of analgesic mixtures over the years, but this can be difficult to ascertain in all patients, partly because of resistance to admit to analgesic abuse. The frequency of the diagnosis increases with age and is rare in patients younger than 30 years.

The early stages of the disease reflect abnormalities in tubular function, with impaired ability to acidify and concentrate the urine (polyuria). Hypertension occurs in 50% of patients, frequently in association with renal artery stenosis. Papillary necroses themselves usually do not cause symptoms. Renal colic and outflow obstruction can result from a sloughed papilla. Occasionally, the obstruction can be bilateral and patients may present with acute renal failure. Anemia is common and may be out of proportion to the degree of renal failure. Urinalysis shows sterile hematuria, pyuria, and mild proteinuria (<3 g/1.73 m² per 24 hours). Computed tomography without radiocontrast has become the standard method for making the diagnosis of analgesic nephropathy. The demonstration of a bilateral decrease in kidney size in combination with irregular ("bumpy") renal contours, especially papillary calcifications (92% positive predictive value), is considered diagnostic of analgesic nephropathy.

- Analgesic nephropathy: responsible for 20% of cases of chronic tubulointerstitial nephritis (3%-10% of patients have ESRD).
- It is 5 to 7 times more frequent in females than males.
- Characteristics include chronic pain, headaches, arthritis and muscular aches, and history of peptic ulcer.
- Patients generally do not admit to analgesic abuse.
- Computed tomography without contrast: small kidneys bilaterally, irregular ("bumpy") renal contours, and papillary calcifications are diagnostic of analgesic nephropathy.

Potential pathogenic mechanisms include direct drug toxicity to the renal papillae, hemodynamic factors, and genetic predisposition. Metabolism of phenacetin and acetaminophen results in increased concentration of highly reactive oxygen species in the renal papillae. These reactive radicals are normally "detoxified" by glutathione.

Depletion of medullary glutathione results in the binding of free reactive intermediates to lipids in the cell membranes and lipid peroxidation. Ultimately, a chain of oxidative damage results in cell death. Aspirin potentiates the toxicity of phenacetin and acetaminophen by depleting renal glutathione. NSAIDs contribute to the renal damage by inhibiting prostaglandin synthesis, which in turn leads to a decrease in renal papillary blood flow and papillary ischemia. The amount necessary to cause analgesic nephropathy is a total intake of 3 kg of phenacetin or 1 g daily for 3 years.

There is no specific form of treatment. Chronic consumption of analgesic medications, especially analgesic mixtures, must be discontinued, and if this is not possible, the regimen needs to be switched to single analgesic preparations. Other therapeutic maneuvers are similar to those for other forms of chronic renal failure.

The prognosis depends on whether analgesic misuse is stopped. Patients with analgesic nephropathy are at an increased risk of uroepithelial tumors, particularly transitional cell carcinomas (renal pelvis, ureter, bladder, and proximal urethra). Tumors frequently occur simultaneously at different sites in the urinary tract, and close follow-up with regular urinary cytologic examination is recommended. These patients are also at an increased risk of premature atherosclerosis and coronary artery disease.

- Phenacetin and its metabolites are concentrated in the renal papillae.
- Patients with analgesic nephropathy have an increased risk of premature atherosclerosis and coronary artery disease and of uroepithelial tumors.

Other causes of papillary necrosis can be remembered with the mnemonic *POSTCARD* (*p*yelonephritis, *o*bstruction, *s*ickle cell disease or trait, *t*uberculosis, *c*hronic *a*lcoholism with cirrhosis, analgesics, *r*enal vein thrombosis, and *d*iabetes mellitus).

Electrolyte- and Toxin-Induced Interstitial Nephritis

Acute uric acid nephropathy is associated with the tumor lysis syndrome that develops after chemotherapy, myeloproliferative disorders, heat stroke, status epilepticus, and Lesch-Nyhan syndrome. In acute uric acid nephropathy, intraluminal crystals cause intrarenal obstruction, the serum level of uric acid is often more than 15 mg, and 24-hour urinary uric acid is more than 1,000 mg. The spot urinary uric acid value divided by the spot urinary creatinine value is often greater than 1.0. Prevention requires alkaline diuresis, allopurinol, and, sometimes, hemodialysis. This disorder generally is completely reversible. Chronic uric acid nephropathy from saturnine gout (lead from moonshine or paint) or chronic tophaceous gout is due to interstitial crystal formation, that is, microtophi present in the renal parenchyma. It has only limited reversibility. In renal failure, de novo gout is rare; in this setting, it should be assumed that the patient has lead nephropathy until proved otherwise.

- Acute uric acid nephropathy is associated with tumor lysis syndrome and myeloproliferative disorders.

- Serum uric acid is >15 mg, and 24-hour urinary uric acid is >1,000 mg.
- The urinary uric acid–urinary creatinine ratio is >1.
- Prevention: alkaline diuresis and allopurinol.

Initially, hypercalcemia results in mitochondrial deposits of calcium in the proximal and distal tubules as well as in the collecting duct. Later, tubular degeneration with calcium deposition and obstruction occurs. Calcium inhibits sodium transport, induces nephrogenic diabetes insipidus, and causes intrarenal vasoconstriction. It also stimulates the release of renin and catecholamines, increasing blood pressure.

Hypokalemia has been associated with vascularization of the proximal and distal tubules and, possibly, chronic interstitial fibrosis. Nephrogenic diabetes insipidus is also associated with chronic hypokalemia.

Oxalate deposition from primary hyperoxaluria causes renal and extrarenal oxalate deposition. Extrarenal sites include the eyes, heart, bones, joints, and vascular system. Secondary causes of oxalate deposition include ethylene glycol, methoxyflurane, high doses of ascorbic acid, vitamin B_6 deficiency, and enteric hyperoxaluria.

Lithium induces nephrogenic diabetes insipidus and microcystic changes in the renal tubules. Interstitial fibrosis may be present.

Heavy metals such as cadmium, pigments, glass, plastic, metal alloys, electrical equipment manufacturing, and some cigarettes induce proximal renal tubular acidosis and tubulointerstitial nephritis. Lead intoxication can cause lead nephropathy, as mentioned above. The organic salt of mercury can induce chronic tubulointerstitial nephritis and membranous nephritis or acute tubular necrosis.

Cystic Renal Disease

Autosomal Dominant Polycystic Kidney Disease

Autosomal dominant polycystic kidney disease (ADPKD) is the most common hereditary renal disease, with a prevalence of 1:1,000 to 1:400. It is responsible for disease in about 10% of all patients who reach ESRD. In approximately 50% of patients, ESRD occurs by the age of 55 to 75 years. The disease is characterized by multiple, bilateral renal cysts in association with cysts in other organs such as the liver, spleen, and pancreas. Both males and females are affected. Mutations in at least 2 genes give rise to the disease. The *PKD1* gene is localized in the short arm of chromosome 16 and is responsible for 85% to 90% of cases of ADPKD. The *PKD2* gene maps to the long arm of chromosome 4. *PKD1* and *PKD2* encode for 2 distinct proteins: *PKD1* encodes for polycystin 1, and *PKD2,* polycystin 2. The molecular structure of polycystin 1 suggests that it may function as a cell membrane receptor involved in cell-cell or cell-matrix interactions, whereas polycystin 2 has similarities to a voltage-activated calcium channel.

Manifestations of renal involvement include pain, hematuria, hypertension, and renal insufficiency. Acute flank pain may occur as a result of cyst hemorrhage, infection, or stone. Macroscopic hematuria occurs in more than 40% of patients with ADPKD and may be the presenting symptom. Cyst hemorrhage is frequent, with macroscopic hematuria or with pain and fever simulating infection of the cyst. Urinary tract infection may occur as cystitis, pyelonephritis, cyst infection, or perinephric abscess. If cyst infection is suspected, aspiration of the cyst under ultrasonographic or computed tomographic guidance may be needed to confirm the diagnosis and to guide selection of appropriate antimicrobial therapy. Lipid-soluble antibiotics tend to penetrate the cysts well. Renal stones occur in approximately 20% of patients with ADPKD. In the majority of cases, the stones are composed of uric acid or calcium oxalate (or both). The diagnosis of renal stones can be difficult because of the distorted renal anatomy and the presence of calcifications in the cyst walls and parenchyma. Computed tomography is the procedure of choice to detect radiolucent stones and to differentiate stones from tumor or clots. The most common extrarenal manifestation of ADPKD is polycystic liver disease. Multiple cysts result in hepatomegaly. Females are affected more often than males. Other complications include cyst hemorrhage, infection, and rarely cyst rupture. Intracranial aneurysms are another important extrarenal manifestation of ADPKD. The incidence of the aneurysms varies between 5% and 22%, depending on whether the family history is negative or positive. The risk of rupture depends on the size of the aneurysm: minimal risk for aneurysms less than 5 mm in diameter but high risk for aneurysms more than 10 mm in diameter. Other associations are diverticulosis, cardiac valve myxomatous degeneration, and hypertension.

If the patient has a family history of ADPKD, the diagnosis can be established by using the following renal ultrasonographic criteria: 2 cysts arising unilaterally or bilaterally for persons younger than 30 years, 2 cysts in each kidney for those 30 to 59 years old, and at least 4 cysts in each kidney for those older than 60. Presymptomatic screening with ultrasonography before age 20 is not recommended because the results may not be conclusive. By age 25, cysts are usually seen with ultrasonography or computed tomography. Linkage genetic analysis can establish the diagnosis at the molecular level but requires testing other family members. It can also be used for prenatal diagnosis. Direct mutation analysis is possible in most families with

PKD2. In patients with *PKD1*, direct mutation analysis is difficult because of the larger size of the gene and because a large part of the gene is duplicated on chromosome 16. Therapy is directed at controlling hypertension and the renal and extrarenal complications of the disease. Lower urinary tract infection or asymptomatic bacteriuria should be treated to prevent retrograde infection of the kidney. Infected cysts may require percutaneous or surgical drainage. Screening for intracranial aneurysms is not routinely indicated. Transplant is the treatment of choice for patients who develop ESRD.

- ADPKD causes 10% of all cases of ESRD.
- By age 25, cysts are usually seen with ultrasonography or CT.
- Other cysts occur in the liver, spleen, and pancreas.
- Other associations are diverticulosis, cardiac valve myxomatous degeneration, intracranial aneurysms, and hypertension.

Medullary Sponge Kidney and Acquired Renal Cystic Disease

Medullary sponge kidney is characterized by dilated medullary and papillary collecting ducts. As a result, the renal medulla develops a "spongy" appearance on excretory urography. The disorder may be unilateral or bilateral or involve a single papilla. There is no known pattern of inheritance of this disorder. Medullary sponge kidney is clinically asymptomatic except for the development of nephrolithiasis, hematuria, and recurrent urinary tract infections.

Acquired renal cystic disease can affect up to 50% of long-term dialysis patients and may occur with hematuria and an increasing hematocrit. Although these cysts sometimes have neoplastic potential, they rarely metastasize. The disease regresses after transplant.

Congenital Nephrotic Syndrome

Congenital nephrotic syndrome refers to the presence of nephrotic syndrome at birth or in infants younger than 3 months. The Finnish type is the most common form. The disease is caused by mutation of the *NHPS1* gene that codes for nephrin. No treatment, other than kidney transplant, is effective.

Part II
Amy W. Williams, MD

Acute Renal Failure

Introduction

Acute renal failure (ARF) or acute kidney injury (AKI) is characterized by a rapid decline in renal function accompanied by retention of nitrogenous waste products and alterations in electrolyte balance and fluid balance. Many clinically accepted definitions are used to identify when an increase in serum creatinine should be classified as acute renal failure, including an increase in creatinine of 0.5 mg/dL in 24 hours or a doubling of creatinine in 1 to 3 days. Regardless of which criterion is used, it is important to recognize ARF early, identify the cause, and initiate treatment to avoid patient morbidity, mortality, and irreversible kidney damage.

After an acute decrease in renal function has been identified by comparing baseline and present creatinine values, the next steps are to determine whether the increased creatinine level truly reflects a decrease in the glomerular filtration rate (GFR) and whether the decrease in GFR is acute or chronic. A chronically increased level of creatinine usually indicates irreversible renal impairment. Drugs such as amiloride and trimethoprim interfere with creatinine secretion in the tubules, resulting in an increased serum level of creatinine without a decrease in GFR. Other causes of increased creatinine levels independent of GFR include other drugs (cefoxitin, cimetidine, and flucytosine), ketoacidosis (acetylacetate), and rhabdomyolysis. Blood urea nitrogen (BUN), a marker for nitrogenous waste retention, can be increased despite a normal GFR in patients with gastrointestinal tract bleeding, excessive protein intake, decreased urinary flow, or tissue trauma or from use of certain drugs (glucocorticoids or tetracycline). Another indicator of ARF or AKI is a change in urine flow. Oliguria (<400 mL per day), anuria (<50 mL per day), and polyuria (>3,000 mL per day) are all clues to the cause of renal dysfunction and help guide evaluation and treatment. For example, anuria may be due to complete urinary obstruction, rapidly progressive glomerulonephritis, cortical necrosis, or bilateral renal artery occlusion. Decreased kidney size indicates a chronic, irreversible component to the overall decrease in renal function. In selected circumstances, levels of creatinine or BUN (or both) that are within the reference range may be misleading. Patients who are elderly or who have severe muscle wasting may have a markedly decreased GFR even though they have a normal creatinine level. In severe liver dysfunction or protein malnutrition, the BUN level may be normal or minimally elevated even though GFR is markedly decreased. Therefore, it is important to know the baseline values for creatinine and BUN so that a change can be identified and, in these circumstances, to be alert for a decrease in GFR despite changes in the BUN or creatinine levels that are less than expected.

ARF is broadly classified into *prerenal*, *renal*, and *postrenal* causes. This classification facilitates the clinical evaluation and discovery of the cause from more than 100 potential causes. The incidence of ARF or AKI in hospitalized patients has increased over the years. The mortality rate for hospitalized patients with ARF or AKI has been reported to be as high as 37.8% for patients with sepsis and 19.4% for patients without sepsis. Thus, an understanding of the risks and potential causes of ARF, along with closely monitoring for evidence of ARF to enable early intervention, is important.

- Correlation of creatinine with GFR is less than precise because its excretion is dependent not only on GFR but also on tubular secretion.
- Causes of increased creatinine levels independent of GFR: ketoacidosis (acetylacetate), cefoxitin, cimetidine, trimethoprim, flucytosine, and rhabdomyolysis.
- Causes of an increase in BUN independent of GFR: gastrointestinal tract bleeding, tissue trauma, glucocorticoids, tetracycline.
- Anuria <50 mL per day: complete urinary obstruction, rapidly progressive glomerulonephritis, cortical necrosis, and bilateral renal artery occlusion.
- A chronically increased level of creatinine usually represents irreversible renal impairment.
- Decreased kidney size indicates a chronic, irreversible component to the overall decrease in renal function.

Prerenal Failure

Prerenal causes of ARF involve a decrease in effective renal blood flow leading to a decrease in GFR. If identified and treated, prerenal failure is usually reversible. Prerenal failure accounts for more than 50% of cases of ARF in hospitalized patients. All the following decrease renal blood flow: decreased cardiac output (as in congestive heart failure), decreased circulating volume due to hemorrhage, gastrointestinal tract blood losses, use of diuretics, burns and third spacing of fluid (pancreatitis, sepsis, crush injuries, or advanced cirrhosis), and renovascular disease leading to renal artery obstruction and arteriolar obstruction.

- Prerenal causes of ARF are due to a decrease in renal blood flow that leads to a decrease in GFR.
- Prerenal failure is usually reversible.

Many vasoactive drugs can cause a decrease in renal blood flow without a decrease in effective circulating volume or intravascular volume. Cyclosporine, an immunosuppressive used in transplant regimens and in treatment of immune-mediated diseases, causes renal vasoconstriction. In the setting of other renal or circulatory insults, cyclosporine can induce ARF. Nonsteroidal anti-inflammatory drugs (NSAIDs) decrease vasodilatory prostaglandin production by inhibiting cyclooxygenase. When renal blood flow is compromised, these vasodilatory prostaglandins maintain the GFR by inducing afferent arteriolar dilatation. Patients with underlying renal insufficiency, volume depletion, advanced liver disease, or congestive heart failure who take NSAIDs are at risk of ARF.

- Patients with underlying renal insufficiency, volume depletion, advanced liver disease, or congestive heart failure who take NSAIDs are at risk of ARF.

The intrarenal formation and action of angiotensin II helps maintain the GFR when renal perfusion is decreased. Medications that interfere with the action of angiotensin can induce ARF when renal blood flow is decreased. Angiotensin-converting enzyme inhibitors (ACEIs) and angiotensin receptor blockers (ARBs) increase the risk of an acute decrease in GFR in patients who have compromised intravascular volume, congestive heart failure, renal artery stenosis, or any type of chronic kidney disease. If these medications are indicated for treatment of hypertension, proteinuria, or cardiac disease, the patient's creatinine and potassium levels should be closely monitored. A slight increase in the creatinine level is expected, but use of the medication should be discontinued if there is a progressive increase in the creatinine level or evidence of ARF. If a patient taking an ACEI or ARB develops ARF due to any cause, prerenal or renal (acute tubular necrosis), use of the ACEI or ARB should be discontinued until renal function improves. Another prerenal cause of ARF is obstruction of the renal arteries or several intrarenal arteries. A rapid decline in renal function occurs with acute occlusion of the arteries supplying blood to the kidneys (thrombosis, stenosis, emboli, or vasculitis of the main renal arteries or several intrarenal arteries).

- Medications that interfere with the action of angiotensin can induce ARF when renal blood flow is decreased.
- Another prerenal cause of ARF is obstruction of the renal arteries or several intrarenal arteries.
- Rapid decline in renal function: thrombosis, stenosis, emboli, or vasculitis of the main renal arteries or several intrarenal arteries.

Renal Failure Due to Liver Disease

Hepatorenal syndrome is characterized by advanced liver disease and portal hypertension associated with ARF. The pathophysiologic mechanism is not completely understood, but splanchnic vasodilatation, an increase in cardiac output, a decrease in systemic resistance, and profound renovascular constriction occur. Early in the course of chronic liver disease or cirrhosis, there is a balance of intrarenal vasodilators and vasoconstrictors. As liver disease progresses, splanchnic dilatation increases, leading to severe renal vasoconstriction and ARF. This can happen with a sudden decrease in intravascular volume, as in spontaneous bacterial peritonitis, gastrointestinal tract hemorrhage, or aggressive diuresis, leading to a decrease in renal perfusion and an increase in renal vasoconstriction. Mediators proposed to have a role in the severe renal vasoconstriction include endothelin, vasoconstrictive prostaglandins, and an active renal sympathetic nervous system. Splanchnic arterial vasodilatation also induces the renin-angiotensin-aldosterone system and vasopressin, along with activation of the sympathetic nervous system, causing sodium and water retention. Patients are at increased risk of hepatorenal syndrome if they have severe liver disease associated with ascites, portal hypertension, jaundice, thrombocytopenia, hepatic encephalopathy, an increased prothrombin time, a baseline low level of urinary sodium, hyponatremia, or a mean arterial pressure less than 80 mm Hg.

The 2 types of hepatorenal syndrome have different prognoses and rates of progression. Type I has a much worse prognosis, with a rapid onset of ARF, and occurs with acute liver failure or chronic advanced liver disease. Type I hepatorenal syndrome usually follows an acute event that decreases effective circulating volume. Type II develops over a few weeks in persons with chronic liver disease who develop diuretic resistance and gradually develop ARF. The increase in the creatinine level in type II is much less than in type I, in which the creatinine level usually doubles in less than 2 weeks. Hyponatremia, hypokalemia, and hypoalbuminemia usually accompany the syndrome.

- Hepatorenal syndrome: severe liver disease associated with ARF.
- Type I: acute doubling of creatinine level with a poor prognosis.
- Type II: gradual worsening of renal function.

Careful review for possible precipitating events is important in the diagnosis and treatment of hepatorenal syndrome. Events that decrease intravascular volume can lead to ARF in patients with chronic liver disease or acute alcoholic hepatitis. Widely recognized precipitating events include gastrointestinal tract bleeding, spontaneous bacterial peritonitis, large-volume paracentesis (>5 L) without albumin infusion, systemic bacteremia, and hypovolemic shock. Overdiuresis can also lead to hepatorenal syndrome in patients with severe liver disease. Diuretics added to a treatment regimen can attenuate the already decreased renal blood flow by further decreasing intravascular volume.

When renal failure occurs in these patients, the diagnosis of hepatorenal syndrome is one of exclusion. Other causes of ARF, including volume depletion, need to be ruled out. This is often difficult when severe liver disease is associated with ascites, total body sodium, water overload, and oliguria. Urinalysis results are often suggestive of acute tubular necrosis, but urinary sediment can be benign. Urinary sodium less than 20 mEq/L, urine osmolality greater than 500 mOsm/L, and a low fractional excretion of sodium are consistent with a prerenal cause but can also be present in hepatorenal syndrome. A fluid challenge or central hemodynamic monitoring is used to determine intravascular volume status. The treatment of hepatorenal syndrome includes supportive measures until a liver transplant is available. Many other drugs have been used, with variable success, in an attempt to improve renal function: acetylcysteine, dopamine, albumin, misoprostol, and octreotide. The initial results of studies of the α_1-adrenergic agent midodrine and octreotide, a somatostatin analogue, have been promising. Several small trials have revealed that vasopressin or its analogue terlipressin reverses oliguria and ARF due to hepatorenal syndrome and improves survival. Current evidence recommends liver transplant as first-line therapy and albumin plus vasopressin or midodrine plus octreotide as preferred second-line therapy in hepatorenal syndrome. Therapy aimed at increasing circulating volumes and systemic vasoconstriction may prove to be effective in decreasing the stimuli for renovascular vasoconstriction and improving renal function until liver transplant. Another therapy used to support patients with hepatorenal syndrome while anticipating a liver transplant is transjugular intrahepatic portal systemic shunting. This procedure has been shown to decrease the activity of the renin-angiotensin system and its effect on the sympathetic nervous system, thus leading to an improvement in renal function.

- In patients with cirrhosis and severe liver disease who present with ARF, the intravascular volume status should be assessed to identify and treat any reversible prerenal component.
- Urinalysis results are often suggestive of acute tubular necrosis.
- The treatment of hepatorenal syndrome includes supportive measures until a liver transplant is available.

Many disease states that resemble hepatorenal syndrome need to be ruled out. Any condition that leads to a decrease in renal blood flow and is associated with liver dysfunction can resemble pseudohepatorenal syndrome (sepsis, hypotension, and congestive heart failure). Leptospirosis, acute Wilson syndrome, and immune-mediated diseases such as systemic lupus erythematosus, polyarteritis, and cryoglobulinemia can involve the liver and kidney. Ingestion of toxins or exposure to toxins (eg, methoxyflurane) that cause both liver and kidney dysfunction also need to be considered. Any patient with end-stage liver disease is at risk of acute prerenal failure due to severe systemic vasodilatation and intrarenal vasoconstriction.

Intrinsic Acute Renal Failure

Intrinsic or structural damage to the kidney that leads to ARF can be divided into 3 categories: *acute tubular necrosis, acute interstitial nephritis*, and *rapidly progressive glomerulonephritis*. (Rapidly progressive glomerulonephritis is discussed in Part I of this chapter.) Acute tubular necrosis injury can occur from a decrease in oxygen delivery to the kidney or from nephrotoxic injury. There is both a vascular component (involving intrarenal vasoconstriction and outer medullary vascular congestion) and a tubular component with tubular obstruction, back leak of filtrate, and interstitial inflammation. The most susceptible segments of the kidney are the medulla or S3 segment of the proximal tubule and the medullary thick ascending limb of the tubules owing to the high metabolic activity and the preferentially directed blood flow to the cortex.

The incidence of acute tubular necrosis in hospitalized patients is 5%. It occurs in 50% of patients undergoing emergency abdominal aortic aneurysm repair and in 20% undergoing cardiac surgery or operations related to trauma. Acute tubular necrosis occurs in 19% of patients with moderate sepsis, 23% with severe sepsis, and 51% with septic shock. In intensive care units, acute tubular necrosis is usually associated with multiorgan failure. In severely ill patients, the cause of acute tubular necrosis is usually multifactorial; for the recovery of the patient and kidneys, it is important that all causes are identified and corrected. The typical course of ARF due to acute tubular necrosis begins with a rapid increase in the serum creatinine level, accompanied by a decrease in urine output. The oliguric phase

lasts from 7 to 14 days if the initial insult is corrected and no further renal insult (eg, sepsis or hypotension) occurs. If the oliguric phase lasts longer than 4 weeks, other causes of ARF should be considered, and a renal biopsy may be required for further evaluation. The oliguric phase is followed by a diuretic phase, during which urine output increases, followed by delayed improvement in serum creatinine levels and GFR. The last phase occurs over 3 to 12 months as the GFR gradually improves. If the patient is oliguric for more than 16 days, renal function most likely will not return to baseline.

- The typical course of ARF due to acute tubular necrosis begins with a rapid increase in the serum level of creatinine, accompanied by a decrease in urine output.
- The oliguric phase is followed by a diuretic phase.

Many toxins, both endogenous (hemoglobinuria, myoglobinuria, calcium, uric acid, bilirubin, and bile salt) and exogenous (antibiotics, contrast dye, cyclosporine, acyclovir, and chemotherapeutic agents) can cause tubular damage. Retained bilirubin and bile salts as well as altered abdominal hemodynamics may contribute to the increased risk of acute tubular necrosis in patients undergoing biliary tract surgery. The length of time on cardiopulmonary bypass is related directly to the incidence of acute tubular necrosis. Hemoglobinuria and decreased renal blood flow may have a role in the development of acute tubular necrosis in these patients. Heme pigments (myoglobin and hemoglobin) cause intrarenal vasoconstriction and tubular obstruction that lead to ARF (Table 18-7).

Severe rhabdomyolysis is associated with ARF, hyperkalemia, hypocalcemia, hyperphosphatemia, and metabolic acidosis. Rigorous hydration with isotonic saline decreases the risk of acute renal injury.

- Many toxins, both endogenous and exogenous, can cause tubular damage.
- The length of time on cardiopulmonary bypass is related directly to the incidence of acute tubular necrosis.
- Acute tubular necrosis injury can occur from a decrease in oxygen delivery to the kidney or from nephrotoxic injury.

Another cause of intrinsic ARF is acute interstitial nephritis, which can be mediated by immunologic, infectious, or allergic reactions. Patients with ARF due to acute interstitial nephritis can present with various problems. Drug-induced acute tubular necrosis can be accompanied by any combination of fever, rash, urinary eosinophilia, and peripheral eosinophilia. Some drugs, such as NSAIDs, are usually not associated with eosinophiluria. The diagnostic value of eosinophiluria is poor

Table 18-7 Comparison of Heme Pigments

Pigment	Serum Color	Haptoglobin	CK	Heme Dipstick	Urine Benzidine
Hemoglobin	Red	Decreased	Normal	Positive	Negative
Myoglobin	Clear	Normal	Increased	Positive	Positive

Abbreviation: CK, creatine kinase.

(positive predictive value, 50%; negative predictive value, 90%). The most common cause of acute interstitial nephritis in hospitalized patients is an allergic reaction to a drug. Drugs associated with acute interstitial nephritis include β-lactam antibiotics, diuretics, allopurinol, NSAIDs, cimetidine, sulfonamides, rifampin, and phenytoin.

NSAIDs (cyclooxygenase [COX]-2 and COX-1 inhibitors) can cause ARF or AKI by various mechanisms. They block the production of vasodilatory prostaglandins, leading to intrarenal vasoconstriction and, when renal blood flow is compromised, reversible ARF. The decrease in vasodilatory prostaglandins allows angiotensin II–mediated constriction of different arterioles. NSAIDs are also associated with an acute tubulointerstitial nephritis (without eosinophils), acute nephrotic syndrome, hyperkalemia, hyponatremia, and an exacerbation of hypertension. These medications carry an increased risk of AKI in the elderly and in persons with chronic kidney disease.

* Patients with acute interstitial nephritis from NSAIDs usually present with proteinuria.
* The diagnostic value of eosinophiluria is poor; the positive predictive value is 50% and the negative predictive value is 90%.

Aminoglycoside renal toxicity occurs after 5 to 7 days of therapy and correlates with a cumulative dose received. Its effect on the tubules is reflected by the potassium and magnesium wasting in these patients. Despite having increased levels of creatinine, patients usually are nonoliguric. Aminoglycosides are freely filtered at the glomerulus and partially absorbed in the proximal tubule. The more amino groups on the aminoglycoside, the more toxic the agent (streptomycin is more toxic than gentamicin, which is more toxic than tobramycin). Once-daily dosing regimens have been shown to decrease the incidence of nephrotoxicity. Aminoglycoside levels should be monitored to decrease the risk of ototoxicity and nephrotoxicity.

* Aminoglycoside renal toxicity occurs after 5 to 7 days of therapy and correlates with a cumulative dose received.
* Aminoglycoside levels should be monitored to decrease the risk of ototoxicity and nephrotoxicity.

Amphotericin B is associated with distal tubule dysfunction. Findings include evidence of nephrogenic diabetes insipidus (nonoliguric) and type 4 renal tubular acidosis. Toxicity occurs after a dose of 2 to 3 g. Amphotericin B in liposomes may decrease its toxicity.

* Amphotericin B is associated with distal tubule dysfunction.

Cisplatin is associated with ARF and tubular dysfunction (hypomagnesemia and hypokalemia), with a cumulative dose of 50 to 75 mg/m². Forced diuresis while ensuring adequate hydration can prevent renal toxicity.

* Cisplatin is associated with ARF and tubular dysfunction.

Contrast-induced ARF is due to the multiple nephrotoxic effects of the contrast dye. Renal vasoconstriction, tubular obstruction, and direct tubular toxicity all negatively affect the GFR. Patients at risk of pronounced dye toxicity are those with diabetes mellitus, severe renal dysfunction (creatinine ≥2.0 mg/dL), congestive heart failure, acute myocardial infarction within 24 hours, peripheral vascular disease, or advanced age and those who receive a large dose or repeated doses of dye. The patient's urine output decreases and creatinine increases 24 to 48 hours after administration of the dye and returns to normal within 7 to 10 days. Clues to the diagnosis are a low fractional excretion of sodium and nephrotomograms revealing a renal outline enhanced by retained contrast dye. Intravenous administration of normal saline is the accepted preventive therapy. In high-risk patients, the use of low ionic contrast agents with lower osmolality, limiting the dose of the agent, and spacing repeated dye loads to allow for renal recovery are felt to be beneficial in reducing contrast nephropathy. The administration of drugs that either act as free radical scavengers, such as N-acetylcysteine, or prevent oxidant-mediated renal injury, such as sodium bicarbonate, have been shown in studies to prevent contrast-induced injury and ARF. The results of these studies, however, have not been consistent.

In patients at high risk of contrast nephropathy, withholding the use of medications, such as NSAIDs, that alter renal blood flow or intrarenal hemodynamics may help decrease the severity of the ischemic injury potentially caused by radiocontrast dye.

Cholesterol atheroembolic-induced renal failure is a cause of acute irreversible intrinsic renal failure. Atherosclerotic vascular disease, smoking, hyperlipidemia, hypertension, diabetes, and a high C-reactive protein increase the risk of ARF due to atheroemboli. It generally occurs in elderly patients, either spontaneously or after an invasive procedure. Atheroembolic disease and contrast nephropathy can occur in the same setting. Clinical findings may include livedo reticularis of the back, flank, abdomen, and extremities; emboli on funduscopic examination (Hollenhorst plaques); and evidence of microemboli of the digits and blue toe syndrome. Laboratory studies demonstrate an increased erythrocyte sedimentation rate, leukocytosis, eosinophiluria, peripheral eosinophilia, thrombocytopenia, and a low level of complement. Unlike in contrast nephropathy, recovery of renal function is rare, and if it does occur, it is gradual and incomplete. No treatment is known to reverse the microvascular occlusion and resulting inflammation. Patients often need support with renal replacement therapy.

* Cholesterol atheroembolic-induced renal failure is a cause of acute irreversible intrinsic renal failure.
* No treatment is known to reverse the microvascular occlusion and resulting inflammation.

Human Immunodeficiency Virus and AIDS Associated With Acute Renal Failure or Acute Kidney Injury

AKI in human immunodeficiency virus (HIV) infections can occur from various causes. Complications can be associated with the HIV infection, secondary infections, or therapeutic drug toxicities. AKI and Fanconi syndrome are associated with the antiviral tenofovir.

Postrenal Failure

Urine flow can be obstructed anywhere along the urinary tract. The pathogenesis of obstructive uropathy involves early vasoconstriction, followed by vasodilatation. Crystals can cause obstruction of the collecting system, leading to ARF. In tumor lysis syndrome and other disease states in which the serum concentration of uric acid is excessive (>15-20 mg/dL), uric acid crystals can cause acute obstruction and uric acid nephropathy. Methotrexate, intravenous acyclovir, and indinavir can precipitate in the tubules and cause ARF. Prevention includes maintaining adequate hydration in the patients when these medications are administered.

- Obstruction to urine flow can occur anywhere along the urinary tract.

Ureteral obstruction can occur from stone material, necrosed papillae, blood clots, or tumor. External compression and ureteral obstruction can occur from retroperitoneal fibrosis (idiopathic or from methysergide) or genitourinary tumors. Surgical ligation, an infrequent cause of ARF, needs to be considered in patients who have had retroperitoneal or genitourinary operations. Bladder outlet obstruction due to prostatic hypertrophy or cancer is a common cause of postrenal ARF in men, and genitourinary cancers are a common cause in women. Patterns of urine flow and symptoms may help distinguish between partial and complete obstruction. Wide fluctuations in urine volume may represent partial obstruction, whereas oliguria or anuria can occur with complete obstruction. Pain is more frequent with complete obstruction because of distention of the renal capsule, collecting system, or bladder. Acute obstruction is usually associated with pain, whereas slowly developing and partial obstruction can be painless. The location of the pain is a clue to the site of obstruction. A normal anion gap (hyperchloremia) acidosis can be present in cases of urinary obstruction. Type 1 renal tubular acidosis is also associated with hyperkalemia. The creatinine level is usually increased in bilateral or complete obstruction but can be normal or only slightly increased in partial or unilateral obstruction. Even though the creatinine level and urine output may be normal in partial obstruction, it is important to discover and correct the cause of the obstruction to avoid chronic tubular injury and irreversible renal injury. Hypertension can also accompany urinary tract obstruction. Acute unilateral obstruction induces activation of the renin-angiotensin system. Hypertension in bilateral or complete obstruction is related to volume expansion with normal renin and improves with correction of the obstruction and diuresis.

- The pathogenesis of obstructive uropathy involves early vasoconstriction, followed by vasodilatation.
- A normal anion gap acidosis can be present in cases of urinary obstruction.

Diagnosis and Evaluation of Acute Renal Failure

Often the differential diagnosis of the cause of ARF can be determined and narrowed considerably by obtaining a complete past medical history and a history of the present illness and by understanding the patient's risk factors for the different causes of ARF. Assessment of fluid balance is essential to distinguish between prerenal and intrinsic or postrenal causes. The presence of microinfarction and livedo reticularis suggests atheroemboli as the cause. A palpable bladder or flank tenderness is a clue that the cause is postrenal.

Laboratory studies are also critical for differentiating the causes of ARF. Findings on urinalysis can help to distinguish prerenal, intrinsic renal, and postrenal causes. Urinary osmolality is increased early in the course of prerenal azotemia and the sediment is usually benign, with only hyaline and occasional granular casts. Acute tubular necrosis is characterized by urine that is isosmotic with the serum and urinary sediment that may contain tubular epithelial cells, granular cells, and amorphous material. Urinary eosinophils and leukocytes are seen with acute interstitial nephritis. Erythrocyte casts indicate a rapidly progressive or acute glomerulonephritis. A normal urinary sediment and a dipstick test that is positive for blood are characteristic of ARF induced by heme pigments. In postrenal failure, urinalysis findings are often unremarkable. Crystalluria may be present in patients with urolithiasis, and hematuria may be a clue to a genitourinary cancer or to an obstructing lesion or a stone.

- Laboratory studies are critical for differentiating the causes of ARF.
- Findings on urinalysis can help distinguish prerenal, intrinsic renal, and postrenal causes.

Urinary chemistry tests or urinary indexes can also help distinguish among the 3 main categories of ARF (Table 18-8). During episodes of decreased renal blood flow (renal artery stenosis, decreased intravascular volume, congestive heart failure, or advanced cirrhosis), functional renal tubules reabsorb sodium, which helps to restore renal perfusion. Under these circumstances, urinary sodium excretion is low (<20 mEq/L) and the fractional excretion of sodium is less than 1%. Initially, in the continuum of prerenal failure, the fractional excretion of sodium is low, but as tubules are damaged by decreased oxygen delivery and acute tubular necrosis develops, the fractional excretion of sodium increases (>3%). Toxins (myoglobins, hemoglobin, and contrast media) and medications (ACEIs, ARBs, cyclosporine, and NSAIDs) that are vasoconstrictive, and thus decrease renal blood flow, are also associated with a low fractional excretion of sodium. Hepatorenal syndrome, early obstruction, cholesterol emboli, and acute glomerulonephritis are other causes of intrinsic

Table 18-8 Comparison of Urinary Indexes in Prerenal Failure and Acute Tubular Necrosis

Urinary Index	Prerenal Failure	Acute Tubular Necrosis
Urine osmolality, mOsm/L	≥500	≤350
Ratio of urinary creatinine to plasma creatinine	≥40	≤20
Ratio of BUN to plasma creatinine	>20	<15
FeNa, %[a]	<1	>3

Abbreviations: BUN, blood urea nitrogen; FeNa, fractional excretion of sodium; Na, sodium.

[a] $FeNa = \dfrac{[urinary\ Na] \times [plasma\ creatinine]}{[plasma\ Na] \times [urinary\ creatinine]} \times 100.$

renal failure that affect renal blood flow and are associated with a low fractional excretion of sodium.

It is well recognized that diuretic therapy induces natriuresis, which causes a high fractional excretion of sodium, even in prerenal azotemia. The fractional excretion of urea is not altered by diuretics. Fractional excretion of urea that is less than 35% indicates a prerenal state.

Postrenal failure due to obstruction can be determined with ultrasonography. Of these studies, however, 2% have false-negative results because of acute obstruction or retroperitoneal fibrosis and 26% have false-positive results. A combination of ultrasonography and computed tomography without contrast medium is 100% diagnostic for obstruction and can be used to determine the cause of obstruction in 84% of cases. Ultrasonography is the test of choice to determine whether hydronephrosis is present.

- Urinary chemistry tests or urinary indexes can help distinguish among the 3 main categories of ARF.
- Ultrasonography is the test of choice to determine whether hydronephrosis is present.
- Ultrasonography may not detect early obstruction.
- Fractional excretion of urea is reliable even in the setting of diuretic use.

Management of Acute Renal Failure or Acute Kidney Injury

Management of ARF or AKI begins by determining and managing the risk factors. Avoiding intravascular volume depletion, maximizing cardiac function, and avoiding nephrotoxic medications and intravenous contrast media are all essential in preventing an acute decline in renal function. It is also important to understand which medications affect renal blood flow and possibly withhold the use of these medications or carefully monitor for changes in renal function in AKI. These medications include ACEIs, ARBs, cyclosporine, tacrolimus, COX-2 inhibitors, and NSAIDs.

- Prevention of ARF begins by determining and managing the risk factors.

After ARF has occurred, the initial goal is to reverse any ongoing renal insults (restore intravascular volume, discontinue nephrotoxins, improve cardiac function, and relieve urinary obstruction) to prevent ongoing injury. In AKI due to urinary tract obstruction, relief of the obstruction is followed by polyuria. In this setting, therapy is aimed at preventing a new prerenal component to the ARF and correcting electrolyte disturbances by replacing two-thirds of the postobstructive diuresis volume. Fluid replacement often begins with 0.45 normal saline at 75 mL/h. Patients should be monitored for electrolyte disturbances and volume depletion. In patients with acute tubular necrosis or acute interstitial nephritis, diuretics have been used to maintain urine output, thus helping to maintain fluid balance and prevent hyperkalemia. It has not been proved that low-dose dopamine prevents ARF or restores renal function. If the patient becomes oliguric, despite improved hemodynamics or correction of the insult, renal replacement therapy should be considered.

- The initial goal is to reverse any ongoing renal insult.

- After the obstruction is relieved in patients with obstructive uropathy, replace two-thirds of the postobstructive diuresis volume to prevent adding a new prerenal component to the ARF.

Maintaining the nutritional requirements of patients with ARF is essential. Patients who are seriously ill are usually catabolic and require 35 to 45 kcal/kg daily and 1.5 g/kg of protein daily. Diets must be adjusted to limit potassium, sodium, magnesium, phosphorus, and fluid intake. If serum phosphorus levels increase despite dietary phosphorus restriction, phosphate binders should be added to the regimen.

- Maintaining the nutritional requirements of patients with ARF is essential.

As renal function changes, drug doses need to be adjusted and drug levels monitored. Be cautious prescribing medications that can accumulate and become toxic in patients with declining or low renal function (magnesium, aluminum-containing antacids, digoxin, renally cleared β-blockers, long-acting diltiazem preparations, and benzodiazepines). Administration of NSAIDs, COX-2 inhibitors, contrast agents, and other agents known to be nephrotoxic should be avoided.

- As renal function changes, drug doses need to be adjusted and drug levels monitored.

Dialysis

The goals of renal replacement therapy in ARF are to maintain fluid, electrolyte, acid-base, and solute balance; to prevent further insult; to promote healing; and to permit other support measures to be used (intravenous medications and parenteral nutrition). The indications for beginning renal replacement therapy for acute conditions are similar to those for chronic conditions. An increase in BUN indicates the accumulation of uremic toxins. In patients who are not receiving adequate protein nutrition or who have little muscle mass, the absolute value of BUN can underestimate the degree of renal failure and toxin accumulation. When the estimated GFR is less than 20 mL/min and immediate renal recovery is not anticipated, dialysis should be initiated before the BUN reaches 100 mg/dL. In acutely or critically ill patients, a BUN greater than 60 mg/dL may be an indication to begin dialysis. Hyperkalemia, acidosis, fluid overload not responsive to diuretics, evidence of central nervous system toxicity, pericardial rub, and gastrointestinal tract bleeding believed to be due to uremia are all indications to begin dialysis immediately.

- The goals of renal replacement therapy in ARF are to maintain fluid, electrolyte, acid-base, and solute balance; to prevent further insult; to promote healing; and to permit other support measures to be used.
- Hyperkalemia, acidosis, fluid overload not responsive to diuretics, evidence of central nervous system toxicity, pericardial rub, and gastrointestinal tract bleeding believed to be due to uremia are all indications to begin dialysis immediately.

The choice of renal replacement must be customized to the needs of the patient. Severe metabolic abnormalities requiring rapid correction (hyperkalemia with electrocardiographic [ECG] changes and severe acidosis) should be treated immediately with short high-flux hemodialysis. Patients with a stable hemodynamic condition able to tolerate rapid fluid and electrolyte shifts can undergo conventional high-flux, intermittent, dialysis 3 times per week. Severely ill catabolic patients requiring intravenous fluids for nutrition, continuous or frequent intravenous administration of medications, and intravenous fluid resuscitation are best dialyzed daily with intermittent dialysis or with continuous dialysis therapy to avoid large fluid gains and to maintain solute homeostasis. Patients with an unstable hemodynamic condition who require renal replacement therapy are best treated with a continuous dialysis modality (continuous venovenous hemodialysis [CVVHD], continuous venovenous diafiltration [CVVDF], or continuous venovenous hemodiafiltration [CVVHDF]). These methods with continuous gentle fluid and solute removal improve hemodynamic stability by decreasing osmolar and solute concentration changes as well as limiting fluid shifts.

Management of Chronic Kidney Disease

Chronic kidney disease (CKD), as defined by the National Kidney Foundation, has 5 stages, progressing from stage 1 (GFR is normal or >90 mL/min per 1.73 m^2) to stage 5 (GFR is <15 mL/min per 1.73 m^2). As in ARF, the initial steps in evaluating any patient with an increased level of creatinine or BUN are to determine whether the value represents a true decrease in GFR, whether the damage is chronic or acute, what the cause is, and whether there is a reversible component. The reversible causes of renal insufficiency are listed in Table 18-9.

The diagnosis of CKD is established by identifying comorbid illnesses known to lead to progressive renal insufficiency and documenting evidence of progressive renal dysfunction (Table 18-10).

Patients with irreversible CKD (GFR <33 mL/min per 1.73 m^2) usually have atrophic kidneys. Exceptions include patients with renal dysfunction due to amyloidosis, myeloma, diabetes mellitus, or polycystic kidney disease.

* Patients with CKD usually have small kidneys.

Table 18-9 Reversible Causes of Renal Insufficiency

Obstruction
Congestive heart failure
Medications
Hypertension
Infection
Volume loss
Hypothyroidism
Hypoadrenalism
Hypercalcemia
Hyperuricemia

The goal of identifying and treating CKD is to prevent progression of the disease, to avoid the morbidity and mortality of end-stage renal disease (ESRD), and to adequately prepare patients for eventual renal replacement therapy. This requires early intervention and adequate follow-up.

* The goal of identifying and treating CKD is to prevent progression of the disease, to avoid the morbidity and mortality of ESRD, and to adequately prepare patients for eventual renal replacement therapy.

Strict blood pressure control is essential to slow the progression of any renal disease. Blood pressure should be 130/80 mm Hg or less for those with CKD and 125/75 mm Hg or less if proteinuria is present. ACEIs and ARBs are the first-choice antihypertensive agents. They delay the progression of renal disease by lowering systemic blood pressure, by altering intrarenal hemodynamics, and by decreasing proteinuria. Diuretics are also useful in controlling blood pressure. Thiazide diuretics are useful until the GFR is less than 45 mL/min per 1.73 m^2. At that point, loop diuretics should be used. Fluid overload is often an important contributor to hypertension in persons with CKD. Electrolyte abnormalities (hyperkalemia with β-blockers, ACEIs, and ARBs) and conduction abnormalities (long-acting diltiazem and β-blockers that are renally excreted) need to be monitored. Hyperlipidemia, in addition to being associated with a higher risk of cardiovascular events in CKD, is also a risk factor for progression of CKD and should be aggressively treated with statins.

* Strict blood pressure control is essential to slow the progression of any renal disease.
* ACEIs and ARBs are the first-choice antihypertensive agents.

Proteinuria is a marker of renal dysfunction and is also a risk factor for progression of CKD. ACEIs and ARBs are beneficial in delaying the progression of disease not only by controlling blood pressure but also by decreasing proteinuria. The goal is to decrease proteinuria by 35% to 40% and to tightly control blood pressure.

* Proteinuria is a risk factor for progression of CKD.

Dietary adjustments are important for patients with CKD. As the GFR decreases, the ability of the nephron to handle potassium and phosphorus decreases. Patients should be monitored for hyperkalemia and hyperphosphatemia. Dietary potassium and phosphorus intake

Table 18-10 Causes of Chronic Kidney Disease

Cause	Cases, %
Diabetes mellitus	42
Hypertension	26
Glomerulonephritis	11
Other or unknown	20

should be restricted after the serum levels begin to increase. Hyperkalemia may occur with a GFR greater than 20 mL/min per 1.73 m² if distal tubular function is abnormal (type 4 renal tubular acidosis). Hyperphosphatemia, despite patient compliance with a low-phosphorus diet, requires the addition of a phosphate binder. Restriction of dietary protein decreases uremic symptoms (decrease in acid, sodium, oxalate, and nitrogen loads and nitrogen waste products). The benefits of protein restriction must be balanced against the morbidity and mortality associated with protein malnutrition. If the patient's protein stores are normal, a protein-restricted diet is recommended. After the serum level of albumin decreases, the protein restriction should be liberalized to prevent protein malnutrition.

* Dietary adjustments are important for patients with CKD.

After the GFR decreases to less than 33 mL/min per 1.73 m², erythropoietin production by the renal parenchyma is not sufficient to prevent anemia. The anemia of CKD is a normochromic normocytic anemia. Treatment with erythropoietin given subcutaneously should be started for all patients who develop anemia. Also, iron should be given orally to patients without a contraindication for supplemental iron. The target hemoglobin level is 11 to 12 g/dL. All patients should have iron stores and ferritin levels monitored. Resistance to erythropoietin can be caused by iron deficiency, inflammation, malignancy, secondary hyperparathyroidism, hematologic disorders, and increasing uremia. *Iron deficiency* is defined as a ferritin level less than 100 ng/mL and total saturation of less than 20%. Anemia in patients with CKD contributes to the development of left ventricular hypertrophy and progression of underlying renal disease.

* Treatment with erythropoietin given subcutaneously should be started for all patients who develop anemia.

Patients with stage 1 or 2 CKD should be referred to a nephrologist when blood pressure targets, anemia targets, or a decrease in proteinuria cannot be achieved. All patients with CKD that is stage 3 or above should be referred to a nephrologist. In addition to helping to maximize interventions to prevent further decline in renal function and to manage and treat the complications of CKD, referral to a nephrologist allows early education concerning renal replacement therapy options. These include in-center and home hemodialysis, peritoneal dialysis, and renal transplant.

End-Stage Renal Disease

The complications of progressive renal dysfunction and uremia involve all organ systems. Uremic symptoms and signs may occur at different levels of GFR depending on the patient's comorbid diseases and the management of the patient's condition preceding ESRD. Anemia of CKD is multifactorial; decreased erythropoietin production, hemolysis, and blood loss may all contribute to the low hemoglobin concentration. Anemia should be treated with erythropoietin and iron supplementation. Bleeding is common in CKD because of platelet dysfunction. Treatment with desmopressin is helpful in acutely reversing the bleeding tendency.

* Anemia of CKD is multifactorial.

The metabolic acidosis in early CKD is a non–anion gap acidosis due to decreased ammonium secretion. As renal dysfunction progresses and phosphates and sulfates accumulate, the acidosis becomes a high anion gap acidosis.

* The metabolic acidosis in early CKD is a non–anion gap acidosis.

Cardiovascular disease is a common cause of death among patients with ESRD and advanced renal insufficiency. In this population, hypertension is common and is associated with excess extracellular fluid volume and, in some cases, excess renin production. Hyperlipidemia and accelerated atherosclerosis contribute to the cardiovascular morbidity and mortality. As mentioned above, anemia can lead to left ventricular hypertrophy. Pericarditis may occur in 2 patterns. Pattern I is a hemorrhagic pericarditis that is treated with hemodialysis. Pattern II can occur in patients who are adequately dialyzed; it may be associated with hemorrhage and tamponade. A viral cause has been implicated, and corticosteroids often need to be given intrapericardially.

* Cardiovascular disease is a common cause of death among patients with ESRD.

Hyperkalemia can occur with a GFR less than 20 mL/min per 1.73 m² and oliguria, but distal tubular dysfunction (type 4 renal tubular acidosis or aldosterone deficiency) and medications (NSAIDs, ACEIs, ARBs, β-blockers, and potassium-sparing diuretics) that interfere with potassium handling can lead to hyperkalemia with a GFR greater than 20 mL/min per 1.73 m². Hyperkalemia associated with ECG changes should be treated emergently. Acute ECG changes due to hyperkalemia should be treated with an infusion of calcium to protect the myocardium, followed by an infusion of insulin to redistribute the potassium; however, with ECG changes and a low GFR, dialysis is indicated. Resins and dialysis are used to eliminate potassium. Chronic hyperkalemia can be treated with a scheduled dose of resins, a low-potassium diet, and the avoidance of medications that interfere with potassium handling.

* Hyperkalemia can occur with a GFR <20 mL/min per 1.73 m² and oliguria.

Through a complex feedback system, renal disease leads to phosphorus retention, hypocalcemia, acidosis, decreased 1,25-dihydroxyvitamin D production, and an increase in parathyroid hormone. Relatively early in advancing renal insufficiency (GFR, 30-40 mL/min per 1.73 m²), the development of hyperphosphatemia and decreased levels of 1,25-dihydroxyvitamin D begin the cascade leading to secondary hyperparathyroidism and the development of osteitis fibrosa cystica. This is the classic form of bone disease in ESRD, with overactive osteoclastic and osteoblastic activity. Osteomalacia (low-turnover bone disease) due to 1,25-dihydroxyvitamin D deficiency is characterized by an increase in osteoid and diminished or absent osteoclastic and osteoblastic activity. Osteoporosis also occurs with ESRD and chronic renal insufficiency. Aluminum bone disease can occur in CKD and ESRD in patients who ingest aluminum. These patients have low levels of parathyroid hormone and 1,25-dihydroxyvitamin D. They present with a microcytic anemia and frequent bone fractures. Aluminum osteodystrophy is diagnosed with an iliac crest bone biopsy and treated with deferoxamine chelation.

- Through a complex feedback system, renal disease leads to phosphorus retention, hypocalcemia, acidosis, decreased 1,25-dihydroxyvitamin D production, and an increase in parathyroid hormone.
- Osteoporosis also occurs with ESRD and chronic renal insufficiency.
- The classic form of bone disease in ESRD is osteitis fibrosa cystica, a disease with high bone turnover and high levels of parathyroid hormone.

Treatment and prevention of renal osteodystrophy focus on the suppression of parathyroid hormone production by maintaining a normal calcium and phosphorus balance. Treatment begins with a low-phosphorus diet. If the serum level of phosphorus remains elevated, enteric phosphate binders are needed. If the serum level of calcium remains low or parathyroid hormone levels remain high (or both), 1,25-dihydroxyvitamin D supplementation is added.

- Treatment and prevention of renal osteodystrophy focus on the suppression of parathyroid hormone production by maintaining a normal calcium and phosphorus balance.

β_2-Microglobulin deposition that occurs in CKD and ESRD can lead to carpal tunnel syndrome and debilitating arthritis. Pseudogout and periarthritis due to the deposition of hydroxyapatite in joint spaces are other musculoskeletal complications of uremia. Gastrointestinal tract complications of uremia include gastritis, colitis, ileitis, peptic ulcer disease, and constipation. Anorexia is a complication that is multifactorial but leads to protein and caloric malnutrition.

- Gastrointestinal tract complications of uremia include gastritis, colitis, ileitis, peptic ulcer disease, and constipation.

The neurologic complications of uremia range from peripheral neuropathy (sensory fibers affected more than motor fibers) to cognitive impairment and eventual central nervous system irritability associated with asterixis and seizures. Without treatment (dialysis or reversal of the renal failure), eventual coma and death occur.

- Neurologic complications of uremia range from peripheral neuropathy to cognitive impairment and eventual central nervous system irritability associated with asterixis and seizures.

Dialysis

Indications for dialysis include fluid overload, acidosis, hyperkalemia, hypernatremia, and uremic signs and symptoms. The choice of dialysis (hemodialysis or peritoneal dialysis) in chronic nonemergent renal failure depends on many clinical and mechanical factors as well as on patient choice. Both types of dialysis can be done in the home. Peritoneal dialysis offers a continuous ultrafiltration and solute clearance, avoiding rapid shifts and hemodynamic instability. Hemodialysis offers more efficient clearance of solutes. Selected patients who have poor hemodialysis access, cardiomyopathy, or a scheduled transplant may be candidates for peritoneal dialysis. The efficiency of peritoneal dialysis is low or inadequate in patients with a history of recurrent abdominal operations or diseases that lead to fibrosis of the peritoneal lining.

- Indications for dialysis include fluid overload, acidosis, hyperkalemia, hypernatremia, and uremic signs and symptoms.

Complications of Dialysis

All patients with ESRD who undergo hemodialysis in a center are at increased risk of hepatitis B and C. All of them should receive the hepatitis B vaccine.

Complications of hemodialysis include hemodialysis dysequilibrium due to brain edema and osmolar shifts with rapid dialysis and hemodynamic instability due to rapid fluctuations in potassium, calcium, and body osmoles and rapid fluid removal. These fluctuations are lessened as dialysis sessions are increased from 3 per week to 6 per week.

Infections involving central venous catheters or arteriovenous grafts can occur. Early detection and treatment with antibiotics are essential. If the catheter or graft remains contaminated, removal is required.

Complications of peritoneal dialysis include infections (peritonitis, exit site infections, and catheter tunnel infection), catheter leak, obesity, protein malnutrition, hyperlipidemia, and hyperglycemia. This form of dialysis is less efficient than high-flux hemodialysis.

Drugs removed or not removed with dialysis and drugs to be avoided if the patient receives dialysis are listed in Table 18-11.

Table 18-11 Dialysis and Overdoses

Drugs removed with dialysis	Drugs not removed with dialysis	Medications to avoid using in patients receiving dialysis
Methanol	Tetracycline	Tetracycline
Aspirin	Benzodiazepines	Nitrofurantoin
Ethylene glycol	Digoxin	Probenecid
Lithium	Phenytoin (Dilantin)	Neomycin
Sodium	Phenothiazines	Bacitracin
Mannitol		Methenamine
Theophylline		Nalidixic acid
		Clofibrate
		Lovastatin
		Magnesium
		Oral hypoglycemic agents
		Antiplatelet drugs
		Renally excreted β-blockers

Part III
Robert C. Albright, Jr., DO

Disorders of Water Balance

The most important principle in understanding disorders of water balance is that sodium balance is determined by the adequacy of the effective circulating volume, while water balance is determined by osmoregulation and the interplay between vasopressin activity, renal concentrating and diluting ability, and thirst. However, the serum level of sodium is not an index of effective circulating extracellular volume or total body sodium. Total body sodium, a surrogate for adequate effective circulating volume, can be estimated only by physical examination targeted to determine adequate tissue perfusion. Water balance is regulated by thirst, vasopressin, and the ability of the renal medulla to concentrate urine.

* The serum level of sodium by itself is not an index of extracellular volume or total body sodium.
* Water balance is regulated by thirst, vasopressin, and the ability of the renal medulla to concentrate urine.

Hyponatremia

Hyponatremia (plasma sodium <136 mEq/L) is the most common electrolyte abnormality in hospitalized patients. Its symptoms are protean and include lethargy, cramps, decreased deep tendon reflexes, and seizures. The diagnosis and management of hyponatremia are shown in Figure 18-2.

Diagnosis

The first step in evaluating patients with hyponatremia is to measure serum osmolality. Isosmotic hyponatremia may be caused by severe hypertriglyceridemia (>1,500 mg/dL; lipemia retinalis is always present), severe hyperproteinemia (>8.0 g/dL; Waldenström macroglobulinemia or myeloma), or isotonic infusions of glucose, mannitol, or glycine. Hyperosmotic hyponatremia may be due to severe hyperglycemia (sodium decreases 1.6 mEq/L for each 100 mg/dL increase in glucose) and to hypertonic infusions of glucose, mannitol, or glycine. The use of ion-selective sodium probes in many clinical chemistry laboratories has markedly decreased the incidence of "pseudohyponatremia."

The second step is to assess the extracellular fluid volume of the hypo-osmotic hyponatremic patient and to determine whether that patient is hypovolemic, euvolemic, or hypervolemic.

1. Hypo-osmotic *hypovolemic* hyponatremia—measure urine osmolality and sodium concentration (urinary spot sodium is often <20 mEq/L; fractional excretion of sodium <1%; urine osmolality ≥600 mOsm/kg); common causes are severe volume depletion, thiazide diuretics, and adrenal insufficiency.
2. Hypo-osmotic *hypervolemic* hyponatremia—measure urine osmolality and sodium concentration; edematous states and renal failure are common.
3. Hypo-osmotic *euvolemic* hyponatremia—measure cortisol and thyrotropin levels, urinary sodium level, and urine osmolality. Possible diagnoses include hypothyroidism, Addison disease, reset osmostat, psychogenic polydipsia, and the syndrome of inappropriate antidiuresis (SIAD).

The term *syndrome of inappropriate antidiuresis* has recently replaced the term *syndrome of inappropriate antidiuretic hormone* because up to 20% of patients who fulfill the criteria for SIAD do not have detectable circulating levels of vasopressin. SIAD is a diagnosis of exclusion. Patients must meet the following criteria: clinical euvolemia, hypotonic plasma, urine less than maximally dilute (urine osmolality in SIAD is greater than serum osmolality or >100-150 mOsm/kg), urinary sodium matches intake, absence of hypoadrenalism and hypothyroidism, and improvement with water restriction. Important clinical clues are low serum levels of uric acid, creatinine, and blood urea nitrogen (BUN). Some of the causes of SIAD include small cell carcinoma of the lung, central nervous system disorders, and drugs such as haloperidol, fluoxetine, and chlorpropamide.

Acute hyponatremia (<48 hours) has been described in several special clinical settings. Hyponatremia may occur in up to 5% of patients after surgery and anesthesia. Plasma vasopressin concentrations are increased because of nonosmolar stimuli such as pain, nausea, and the use of narcotics. Rarely, profound hyponatremia may occur. During transurethral prostatic resection, isotonic or hypotonic fluids containing glycine can be absorbed and depress the serum level of sodium. Schizophrenic patients with severe compulsive water drinking (>14 L daily) occasionally have acute hyponatremia. Also, infusions of oxytocin and cyclophosphamide may induce acute hyponatremia.

Chronic hyponatremia may be induced by the use of thiazides, chlorpropamide, carbamazepine, and nonsteroidal anti-inflammatory drugs (NSAIDs).

* The physical examination, osmolality of plasma and urine, and urinary sodium concentration provide important information for diagnosis.
* SIAD: serum levels of uric acid, creatinine, and BUN are low.

Therapy for Hyponatremia

A general tenet of therapy for hyponatremia is that the correction should occur at the rate at which it developed.

Hypovolemic Hyponatremia

Hypovolemic hyponatremia most often reflects volume depletion. The total sodium deficit can be calculated as follows:

Sodium deficit = total body water (lean body weight in kg × 0.5) × desired serum sodium (mEq/L) − current serum sodium (mEq/L)

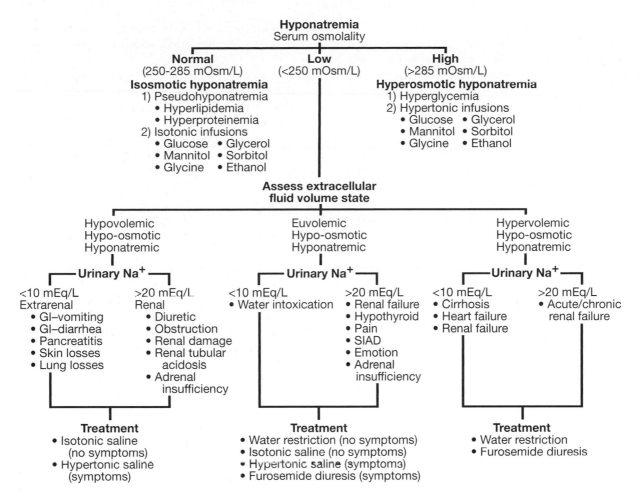

Figure 18-2. Diagnosis and Management of Hyponatremia. GI indicates gastrointestinal tract; Na, sodium; SIAD, syndrome of inappropriate antidiuresis.

Euvolemic Hyponatremia

As pointed out above, hyponatremia should be reversed cautiously, at a rate similar to that at which it developed, to avoid central pontine myelinolysis. However, the rate of onset often is unknown. Therefore, therapy is directed primarily by signs and symptoms. For patients with euvolemic hyponatremia who are asymptomatic, the treatment should be water restriction only. Patients with acute euvolemic hyponatremia who have neurologic symptoms require prompt therapy designed to facilitate the excretion of free water. Options include the infusion of hypertonic saline or the simultaneous infusion of isotonic saline and a loop diuretic. The amount of hypertonic saline required to increase the serum concentration of sodium to appropriate levels can be estimated roughly by calculating free water excess. However, these calculations assume steady-state urinary concentration, which may not occur as therapy is administered. Therefore, intense monitoring is needed, including hourly measurements of serum sodium, urinary sodium, and urine osmolality. In acute hyponatremia, the rate of correction should not exceed 8 to 12 mEq/L in the first 24 hours. In chronic hyponatremia, the rate of correction can be slow—fluid restriction is least harmful. Patients with chronic SIAD may benefit from treatment with demeclocycline.

Since the mid-1990s, there has been a steady accumulation of clinical data on the use of vasopressin receptor antagonists for treatment of hypervolemic hyponatremia (associated with cirrhosis or congestive heart failure) and euvolemic hyponatremia (associated with SIAD). These agents block either V_2 receptors (which are located on the renal tubular cells and stimulate aquaporin insertion and water retention) or V_{1a} and V_{1b} receptors (which stimulate vasoconstriction and adrenocorticotropin release). Lixivaptan, tolvaptan, and satavaptan are oral V_2-receptor–selective antagonists. Conivaptan is an intravenous formulation of a V_{1a}- and V_2-receptor antagonist, and, it is the only agent currently approved in the United States for euvolemic hyponatremia. These agents have been shown to be effective for mild hyponatremia in euvolemic and hypervolemic patients. However, there are no data as yet on the efficacy and safety of these agents for patients with severe hyponatremia (sodium <115 mEq/L) or patients with neurologic symptoms. These agents are contraindicated for patients with cirrhosis with variceal bleeding, since vasopressin is often an adjunct to control bleeding. Additionally, hypotension, as a result of nonselective V_{1a}-receptor blockade may complicate the use of conivaptan in the intensive care unit population. There is no role for these agents for patients with hypovolemic hyponatremia.

Hypervolemic Hyponatremia

Therapy for hypervolemic hyponatremia involves diuretics and correction or treatment of the underlying pathophysiologic state, which often involves liver, heart, or kidney disorders. Aquaretics, vasopressin V_2-receptor antagonists that are being used in clinical trials, may eventually be used in these settings.

Hypernatremia

As in hyponatremia, the symptoms of hypernatremia (plasma sodium >145 mEq/L) are often protean, with irritability, hyperreflexia, ataxia, and seizures. Because all forms of hypernatremia are associated with hypertonicity, there is no pseudohypernatremia. Hypernatremia is categorized as *hypovolemic, hypervolemic,* and *euvolemic.* The diagnosis and management of hypernatremia are outlined in Figure 18-3.

Hypovolemic hypernatremia often responds to saline, followed by a hypotonic solution. Hypervolemic hypernatremia responds to diuretics; rarely, dialysis may be needed. Euvolemic patients should receive free water, either orally or intravenously, to correct the serum level of sodium, generally no faster than 0.5 mEq per hour. A water deprivation test may be useful diagnostically.

The total free water deficit may be calculated as follows:

Total free water deficit = total body water (0.5 × lean body weight in kg) × [(current serum sodium in mEq/L ÷ desired serum sodium in mEq/L) – 1]

Additionally, obligate losses of free water (estimated to be 13 mL/kg daily) need to be considered in these calculations.

- Hypovolemic hypernatremia: check urinary sodium; the cause may be osmotic diuresis, excessive sweating, or diarrhea.
- Hypervolemic hypernatremia: may be caused by sodium poisoning.
- Euvolemic hypernatremia: loss of water, extrarenal (skin or lungs) or renal, diabetes insipidus (central or nephrogenic; water deprivation test).

Diabetes Insipidus

Polyuria

Polyuria is defined as urine output of more than 3 L per day. This may represent a solute or water diuresis. The normal daily required osmolar secretion is approximately 10 mOsm/kg. Therefore, water or solute diuresis may be distinguished by measuring urine osmolality and determining the total daily solute excretion. If osmotic diuresis is excluded, polyuria is often due to primary polydipsia or diabetes insipidus.

Central Diabetes Insipidus

An absence of circulating vasopressin (partial or complete) is due to destruction of the pituitary or to congenital causes (familial autosomal

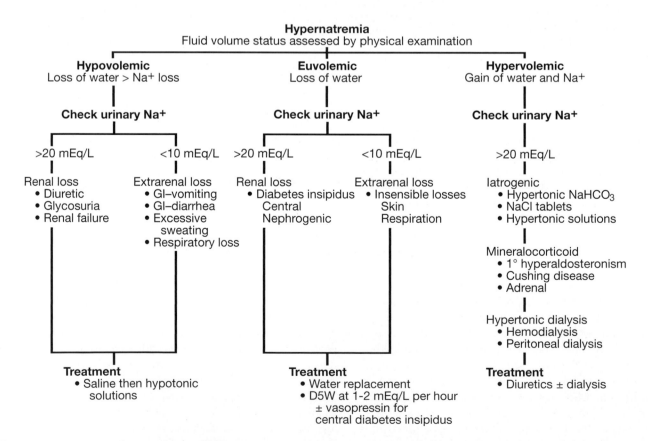

Figure 18-3. Diagnosis and Management of Hypernatremia. D5W indicates 5% dextrose in water; GI, gastrointestinal tract; NA, sodium; NaCl, sodium chloride; NaHCO3, sodium bicarbonate.

dominant central diabetes insipidus). This is a result of mutations in the prearginine-proarginine-vasopressin-neurophysin II gene.

Nephrogenic Diabetes Insipidus

A complete or partial resistance of the renal collecting duct cell to the actions of vasopressin may be the result of a familial X-linked disorder or, more commonly, an acquired lesion. Nephrogenic diabetes insipidus may be induced by lithium, demeclocycline, or amphotericin B (drug-induced nephrogenic diabetes insipidus). Occasionally, the concentrating defect involving lithium is not reversible. Renal diseases such as amyloidosis, sickle cell disease, light chain nephropathy, Sjögren syndrome, obstructive uropathy, and renal failure are common causes of nephrogenic diabetes insipidus.

Because of high levels of placenta-derived vasopressinase, a water diuresis may occur in pregnancy. Technically, this is not nephrogenic diabetes insipidus, though, because the women have a normal response to supplemental desmopressin, which is resistant to vasopressinase.

Hypercalcemia and hypokalemia also induce nephrogenic diabetes insipidus through multiple impaired intracellular pathways.

Patients with diabetes insipidus are symptomatic only if access to free water is restricted. This occurs primarily in very elderly, very young, or hospitalized patients or in institutional situations. Differentiating these polyuric states may be challenging. A detailed history of familial issues and use of medications is extremely important. Abrupt onset of polyuria is characteristic of acquired diabetes insipidus. A water deprivation test (or infusion of 5% saline) under closely supervised conditions often allows various polyuric states to be distinguished. The differentiation of diabetes insipidus from primary polydipsia with available laboratory tests is outlined in Table 18-12.

The serum concentration of sodium is often high-normal or increased in diabetes insipidus, whereas it is usually low-normal or low in primary polydipsia.

* Polyuria: urine output >3 L per day.
* Polyuric states are due to either water or solute diuresis.

* A closely supervised water deprivation test will differentiate most polyuric states.

Disorders of Sodium Balance

Disorders of sodium balance can be determined only by clinical examination. *Orthostatic hypotension* implies volume depletion and sodium deficiency. *Edema* implies volume excess and sodium excess.

Cerebral salt wasting has rarely been documented in situations of severe central nervous system injury. Differentiating this from SIAD may be difficult. A negative sodium balance that causes contraction of the extracellular fluid volume must be documented for cerebral salt wasting to be diagnosed. Often, the "sodium wasting" is physiologic in situations of severe central nervous system injury (such as subarachnoid hemorrhage), because high-volume therapy in the form of albumin and saline is often administered to prevent cerebral vasospasm. Hence, the apparently excessive urinary sodium levels are physiologic.

Disorders of Potassium Balance

Potassium is predominantly an intracellular cation. Total body potassium is approximately equal to 4,200 mEq, with only 60 mEq in the total volume of extracellular fluid. Gastric fluid contains 5 to 10 mEq of potassium/L and diarrheal fluid, 10 to 100 mEq/L. The intracellular balance of potassium is regulated by endogenous factors such as acidemia, sodium, adenosine triphosphatase, insulin, catecholamines, and aldosterone. The extracellular balance is regulated primarily by potassium excretion, which is regulated by urinary flow rate, aldosterone, vasopressin, and sodium delivery to the distal tubule.

Hypokalemia

Symptoms of hypokalemia include weakness, ileus, polyuria, and, sometimes, rhabdomyolysis. Hypokalemia also aggravates digoxin toxicity. A stepwise approach to the diagnosis of hypokalemia is given in Table 18-13 and outlined in Figure 18-4.

Table 18-12 Comparison of Diabetes Insipidus With Primary Polydipsia

Test	Normal	Complete CDI	Partial CDI	Nephrogenic DI	Primary Polydipsia
Urine osmolality with water deprivation,[a] mOsm/kg water	>800	<300	300-800	<300-500	>500
Increase urine osmolality with exogenous AVP,[b] mOsm/kg water	300	Dramatic	10% increase	0	0
Plasma AVP levels after dehydration, pg/mL	>2	Undetectable	<1.5	>5	<5

Abbreviations: AVP, arginine vasopressin; CDI, central diabetes insipidus; DI, diabetes insipidus.

[a] Water is restricted until patient loses 3.5% of body weight or urine osmolality does not change >10% over 2 hours.

[b] Aqueous AVP (5 units subcutaneously) is given, and urine osmolality is reversed in 60 minutes.

Table 18-13 Stepwise Approach to the Diagnosis of Hypokalemia

1. Exclude redistribution—β-agonists (albuterol & terbutaline for asthma & ritodrine for labor), acute alkalosis, vitamin B_{12} therapy for pernicious anemia (especially if thrombocytopenic), & barium carbonate
2. Determine whether potassium losses are renal or extrarenal—check urinary potassium level on high-sodium diet (Is potassium >20 mEq/d or <20 mEq/d?)
3. If loss is extrarenal, determine cause (laxative screen)—usually diarrhea, enemas, laxative abuse, villous adenomas, or ureterocolostomy
4. If loss is renal, determine whether hypertensive or normotensive (diuretic screen)
5. If hypertensive, check plasma renin & aldosterone levels, & check for primary aldosteronism or adrenal hyperplasia, exposure to glycyrrhizic acid in licorice or chewing tobacco, & adrenal abnormalities
6. If normotensive, check plasma bicarbonate levels & urinary chloride; the differential diagnosis includes renal tubular acidosis, vomiting, diuretic abuse, Bartter syndrome, & magnesium deficiency

• Hypokalemia symptoms: weakness, ileus, and polyuria.

Therapy for hypokalemia involves administration of potassium chloride. If the serum level of potassium is less than 2 mEq/L, the total potassium deficit is equal to 1,000 mEq; if the serum level of potassium is between 2 and 4 mEq/L, a decrease of 0.3 mEq/L is equivalent to a 100- to 500-mEq deficit (usually treat with potassium chloride, except that potassium phosphate is used in diabetic ketoacidosis and potassium citrate is used in severe acidosis). Do not give more than 10 mEq of potassium chloride per hour intravenously without the use of a central catheter and electrocardiographic monitoring. Dietary sodium restriction decreases the potassium-losing effects of diuretics. In patients with hypokalemia and hypomagnesemia, the magnesium levels need to be corrected.

Hyperkalemia

A stepwise approach to the diagnosis of hyperkalemia is given in Table 18-14 and outlined in Figure 18-5.

The goal of therapy for hyperkalemia is to antagonize the membrane effects and redistribute potassium. Treat, in the following order, with calcium, sodium bicarbonate, insulin, resins, and, finally, dialysis. For chronic therapy, use loop diuretics, sodium bicarbonate, resins, fludrocortisone, or dialysis.

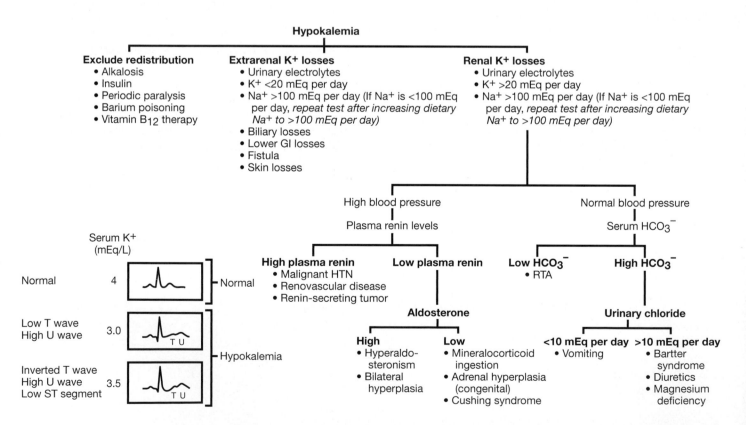

Figure 18-4. Diagnosis of Hypokalemia. GI indicates gastrointestinal tract; HCO_3, bicarbonate; HTN, hypertension; K, potassium; Na, sodium; RTA, renal tubular acidosis.

Table 18-14 Stepwise Approach to the Diagnosis of Hyperkalemia

1. Exclude pseudohyperkalemia (electrocardiogram is normal & heparinized plasma potassium is normal) caused by hemolysis of clotted blood (0.3-mEq/L increase), tourniquet ischemia, or severe leukocytosis or thrombocytosis
2. Determine cause based on redistribution or excess total body potassium (Figure 18-5)

Acid-Base Disorders

Clinically, it is absolutely critical that a stepwise approach to acid-base disorders be followed. The 6 steps listed in Table 18-15 should always be followed while interpreting an acid-base disorder.

Metabolic Acidosis

Metabolic acidosis is defined as a primary disturbance in which the retention of acid consumes endogenous alkali stores. This is reflected by a decrease in bicarbonate. The secondary response is increased ventilation, with a decrease in the partial pressure of carbon dioxide ($PaCO_2$). Metabolic acidosis can be caused by the overproduction of endogenous acid (diabetic ketoacidosis), loss of alkali stores (diarrhea or renal tubular acidosis), or failure of renal acid secretion or base resynthesis (renal failure).

- Metabolic acidosis: the primary disturbance is retention of acid or loss of bicarbonate.
- Secondary response: increased ventilation with decreased $PaCO_2$.

Some of the signs and symptoms of metabolic acidosis include fatigue, dyspnea, abdominal pain, vomiting, Kussmaul respiration, myocardial depression, hyperkalemia, leukemoid reaction, insulin resistance, and, when the pH is less than 7.1, arteriolar dilatation and hypotension.

Formulas for the predicted compensation of pure metabolic acidosis (which may take up to 24 hours) are listed in Table 18-16.

Metabolic acidoses are classified as either *normal anion gap* or *high anion gap*. Normal anion gap acidosis (*hyperchloremic metabolic acidosis*) may be the result of excessive bicarbonate losses from either gastrointestinal or renal sources. These may be discriminated by calculating a urinary net charge (or urinary anion gap). The appropriate titration of acidity involves the excretion of excess hydrogen ions as ammonium ions. Electroneutrality is preserved by coupling ammonium ion to chloride, forming ammonium chloride. Hence, appropriate titration of renal acidity should result in high levels of urinary chloride.

The *urinary net charge* (*urinary anion gap*) is calculated as follows (values are from random spot sample):

Urinary net charge = [sodium (mEq/L) + potassium (mEq/L)] − chloride (mEq/L)

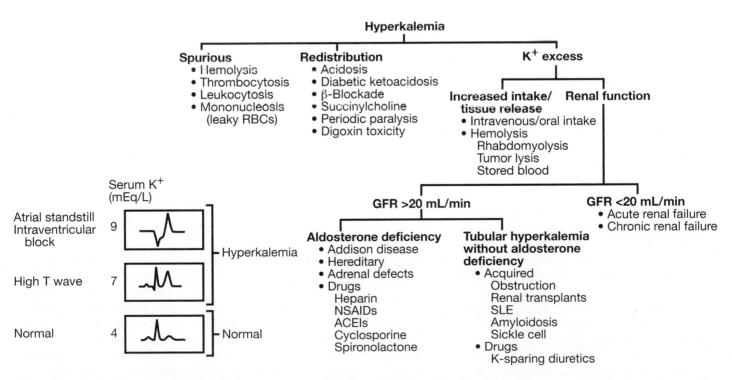

Figure 18-5. Diagnosis of Hyperkalemia. ACEI indicates angiotensin-converting enzyme inhibitor; GFR, glomerular filtration rate; K, potassium; NSAID, nonsteroidal anti-inflammatory drug; RBC, red blood cell; SLE, systemic lupus erythematosus.

Table 18-15 Six Steps for Interpreting Acid-Base Disorders

1. Note the clinical presentation
2. Always check the anion gap (hidden acidosis) & osmolar gap if possible

    Normal anion gap Na – (HCO$_3$ + Cl) = 8 to 12

        Cations = Na, gammaglobulins, Ca, Mg, K

        Anions = Cl, HCO$_3$, albumin, PO$_4$, SO$_4$, organic compounds

    High anion gap >12—MUDPILES (see text)

    Low anion gap <8—bromism, paraproteinemia, hypercalcemia/magnesemia, lithium toxicity, severe hypernatremia, severe hypoalbuminemia

    Osmolar gap >10 -ols—methanol, ethanol, ethylene glycol, isopropyl alcohol, mannitol

3. Use the Henderson equation to check the validity of the arterial blood gas values:

$$H^+ (nEq/L) = \frac{24 \times lungs\ (PCO_2)}{kidneys\ (HCO_3)}$$

pH	7.00	7.10	7.20	7.30	7.40	7.50	7.60	7.70
H$^+$	100	79	63	50	40	32	25	20

4. Is the pH high or low?
5. Is the primary disturbance metabolic (HCO$_3$) or respiratory (PCO$_2$)?
6. Is it simple or mixed?

Abbreviations: Ca, calcium; Cl, chloride; HCO$_3$, bicarbonate; K, potassium; Mg, magnesium; Na, sodium; PO$_4$, phosphate; SO$_4$, sulfate.

Table 18-16 Formulas for the Predicted Compensation of Metabolic Acidosis, Metabolic Alkalosis, Respiratory Acidosis, and Respiratory Alkalosis

Metabolic acidosis compensation

    PaCO$_2$ = last digits of pH

    PaCO$_2$ decreases by 1.0-1.3 mm Hg for each mEq decrease in bicarbonate

    Winter formula (favored formula):

        PaCO$_2$ = (1.5 × HCO$_3^-$) + 8 ± 2

Metabolic alkalosis compensation

    PaCO$_2$ = 0.9 (HCO$_3^-$) + 15 ± 5

    PaCO$_2$ = (HCO$_3^-$) + 15

    PaCO$_2$ increases 6 mm Hg for each 10-mEq/L increase in HCO$_3^-$

Respiratory acidosis compensation

    HCO$_3^-$ increases by 1 mEq/L for each 10–mm Hg increase in PaCO$_2$ (acute)

    HCO$_3^-$ increases by 3 mEq/L for each 10–mm Hg increase in PaCO$_2$ (chronic)

    Increase[a] in [H$^+$]= 0.75 × increase in PaCO$_2$ (mm Hg) from normal (acute)

    Increase[a] in [H$^+$] = 0.3 × increase in PaCO$_2$ (mm Hg) from normal (chronic)

Respiratory alkalosis compensation

    HCO$_3^-$ decreases by 2 mEq/L for each 10–mm Hg decrease in PaCO$_2$ (acute)

    HCO$_3^-$ decreases by 4 mEq/L for each 10–mm Hg decrease in PaCO$_2$ (chronic)

    Decrease[b] in [H$^+$] = 0.75 × decrease in PaCO$_2$ (mm Hg) from normal (acute)

    Decrease[b] in [H$^+$] = 0.2 × decrease in PaCO$_2$ (mm Hg) from normal (chronic)

Abbreviations: H, hydrogen; HCO$_3$, bicarbonate.
aDelta 0.01 pH = delta 1 nEq [H$^+$].
bpH 7.40 = 40 nEq [H$^+$].

The urinary net charge should result in values that are −8 or more negative in situations of hyperchloremic metabolic acidosis with appropriate renal titration. A positive value or a value less negative than −8 suggests renal tubular disorders (renal tubular acidosis).

Also, normal anion gap metabolic acidosis may be defined in terms of the serum concentration of potassium.

Hypokalemic normal anion gap metabolic acidosis can be associated with diarrhea, ureteral diversion, or the use of carbonic anhydrase inhibitors such as acetazolamide. Type 1 renal tubular acidosis, or classic renal tubular acidosis, is also a cause. This is associated with nephrocalcinosis and osteomalacia. The causes of type 1 renal tubular acidosis include glue sniffing (toluene effect), amphotericin B, lithium, Sjögren syndrome, hypergammaglobulinemia, and sickle cell disease. Type 2 renal tubular acidosis is also a hypokalemic normal anion gap metabolic acidosis. In adults, it is often associated with other proximal tubule defects, including glycosuria, uricosuria, phosphaturia, and aminoaciduria (Fanconi syndrome). Causes of type 2 renal tubular acidosis include myeloma, cystinosis (not cystinuria), lead, tetracycline, and acetazolamide.

The causes of hyperkalemic normal anion gap metabolic acidosis include acid loads such as ammonium chloride, arginine chloride,

lysine chloride, cholestyramine, total parenteral nutrition, hydrogen chloride, oral calcium chloride, obstructive uropathy, hypoaldosteronism (Addison disease), 21-hydroxylase deficiency, sulfur toxicity, and type 4 renal tubular acidosis. Type 4 renal tubular acidosis is associated with hyporeninemia and hypoaldosteronism, and it may be caused by diabetes mellitus, interstitial nephritis, spironolactone, amiloride, triamterene, or cyclosporine.

Patients in an intensive care unit often have normal anion gap acidosis because of "dilutional acidosis," which is due to large-volume saline resuscitation. The correction for hypoalbuminemia is necessary if the serum level of albumin is decreased. In this case, a correction factor of roughly 1.3 per gram of albumin below normal needs to be added to the anion gap calculation. Hence, in the intensive care unit or in cases of severe hypoalbuminemia, patients in whom hyperchloremic metabolic acidosis is suspected have high anion gap acidosis.

High anion gap metabolic acidosis has several causes. A common mnemonic is MUDPILES (methanol, uremia, diabetic ketoacidosis, paraldehyde, isoniazid, iron, lactic acidosis, ethanol, ethylene glycol, salicylates). An anion gap should prompt calculation of an osmolar gap: measured osmolar gap – calculated osmolar gap (normally, the result is <10).

Calculated osmolar gap = [Na+ (mEq/L) × 2] + (glucose/18 + BUN/2.8)

In chronic renal failure, the anion gap is usually less than 25. If the anion gap is greater than 25, one should think immediately of ingestion of a poison (generally a toxic alcohol: methanol, ethanol, ethylene glycol, or acetone). Isopropyl alcohol increases the osmolar gap but not the anion gap (acetone is not an anion).

- Dilutional acidosis often occurs in the intensive care unit.
- The anion gap needs to be corrected for hypoalbuminemia.
- In chronic renal failure, the anion gap is usually <25.
- An anion gap >25 suggests ingestion of a poison.

Metabolic acidosis is generally corrected by treating the underlying disorder, but the bicarbonate deficit can be determined by the following formula:

Bicarbonate deficit = 0.2 × body weight (kg) × [normal HCO3 (ie, 24) – measured HCO3]

Therapy for ingestion of a toxic alcohol (eg, methanol or ethylene glycol) involves inhibiting the metabolism of the relatively nontoxic parent compound to its toxic metabolite. Alcohol dehydrogenase has a much higher affinity for ethanol than for ethylene glycol or methanol. Therefore, if ethanol or another steric inhibitor (4-methylpyrazole) is available for alcohol dehydrogenase, the ingested substance can be excreted or cleared in its native form, thereby preventing toxicity. This is the rationale for administering either ethanol or 4-methylpyrazole after the ingestion of ethylene glycol or methanol. Clinically, patients who have ingested these compounds often present with very high anion gaps with osmolar gaps (a sign that inhibition of alcohol dehydrogenase is still worthwhile) and complex acid-base disorders. After the metabolism has been blocked, it is necessary to facilitate the removal of these compounds. Although hemodialysis efficiently removes them, supplemental ethanol is required during dialysis because this will be cleared also.

Aggressive supplementation of bicarbonate is rarely warranted except for cases of severe hemodynamic instability or pH levels less than 7.10. Treatment with bicarbonate may induce hypervolemia by the obligate infusion of sodium along with the bicarbonate (1 ampule of sodium bicarbonate = 50 mEq sodium and 50 mEq bicarbonate) and ultimately requires increased minute ventilation for appropriate buffering.

Metabolic Alkalosis

Metabolic alkalosis is defined as a primary disturbance in which plasma bicarbonate is increased. This can be caused by exogenous alkali, acid loss through the gastrointestinal tract or kidney, or loss of nonbicarbonate fluid causing contraction of remaining fluid around unchanged total body bicarbonate. The kidney must also be stimulated to sustain the high level of plasma bicarbonate. This can occur by contraction of extracellular fluid volume, hypercapnia, potassium depletion, steroid excess, hypercalcemia, or hypoparathyroidism. The secondary response is decreased ventilation with an increase in PaCO2. The signs and symptoms of metabolic alkalosis include weakness, muscle cramps, hyperreflexia, alveolar hypoventilation, and arrhythmias.

- Metabolic alkalosis: the primary disturbance is increased plasma bicarbonate.
- The kidney must be stimulated to sustain the high level of plasma bicarbonate.
- Secondary response: decreased ventilation with increased PaCO2.

The predicted compensation for pure renal metabolic alkalosis (which will take up to 24 hours) is presented in Table 18-16. Metabolic alkalosis can then be classified in terms of the spot urinary chloride and spot urinary potassium (Figure 18-6).

Respiratory Acidosis

The ventilatory system is responsible for maintaining PaCO2 within normal levels by adjustment of minute ventilation. Minute ventilation is controlled by tidal volume and respiratory rate. Normally, minute ventilation matches the production of carbon dioxide. When either carbon dioxide production exceeds the capacity of minute ventilation or respiratory physiology is deranged, carbon dioxide accumulates, causing respiratory acidosis. The kidneys compensate by retaining bicarbonate.

Pathophysiologic derangements may be divided into 2 basic components: 1) the respiratory pump, which generates the forces necessary for airflow, and 2) the loads opposing such forces.

- Respiratory acidosis: the primary disturbance is increased PaCO2.
- Compensation: renal retention of bicarbonate.
- Disorders are caused by either a defect in the respiratory pump or an increase in the opposing load.

Abnormalities of the respiratory pump (and examples of their causes) include acutely and chronically depressed central drive (medications, anatomical lesions, inflammatory or infectious conditions, and metabolic derangements such as hypothyroidism); abnormal neuromuscular transmission (medications such as succinylcholine and aminoglycosides and metabolic causes [eg, hypokalemia]); lesions of the nervous system (Guillain-Barré syndrome, myotonic dystrophy, multiple sclerosis, and amyotrophic lateral sclerosis); and muscle dysfunction (fatigue, hypokalemia, hypophosphatemia, hyperkalemia, malnutrition, and myopathic disease such as polymyositis).

Abnormalities of opposing forces under increased load (and examples of their causes) may be divided into lung stiffness (pneumonia, pulmonary edema, and acute respiratory distress syndrome), chest wall stiffness (flail chest, severe kyphoscoliosis, hemothorax, pneumothorax, obesity, peritoneal insufflation, and peritoneal dialysis), increased ventilatory demand (pulmonary embolism, sepsis, and overfeeding with carbohydrates), and high airflow resistance (upper and

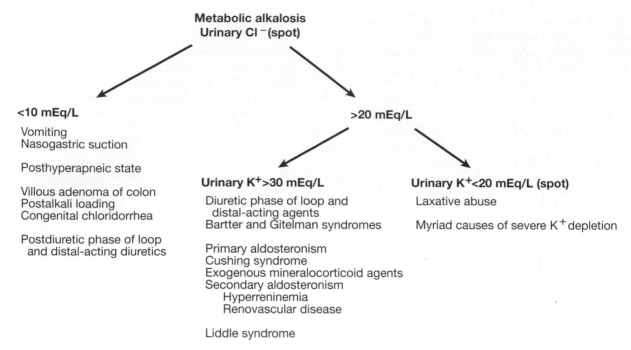

Figure 18-6. Metabolic Alkalosis Classified According to Spot Urinary Chloride and Spot Urinary Potassium. Cl indicates chloride; K, potassium.

lower airway obstruction, laryngospasm, aspiration, bronchospasm, edema, secretions, and chronic obstructive pulmonary disease).

Initially, evaluation of suspected respiratory acidosis requires simultaneous determination of arterial blood gas and electrolyte panel values. Immediate steps should focus on securing a patent airway and providing adequate oxygenation. Historical clues, physical examination findings, assessment of hemodynamics and gas exchange, and radiologic studies help to identify the cause.

Expected compensation for both acute and chronic respiratory acidosis is shown in Table 18-16.

Respiratory Alkalosis

Respiratory alkalosis (primary hypocapnia) results from either increased minute ventilation or decreased carbon dioxide production or both. The kidneys compensate by excreting bicarbonate over several days.

- Respiratory alkalosis: the primary disturbance is a decrease in arterial $PaCO_2$.
- Compensation: renal excretion of bicarbonate (over a period of days).

Broadly, disorders that cause primary respiratory alkalosis include hypoxemia, stimulation of ventilatory centers in the central nervous system, various drugs, pregnancy, sepsis, and liver failure (Table 18-17).

Therapy is directed at correcting the primary cause. Often sedation or a rebreathing apparatus may be required while the primary disorder is being treated. Occasionally it may be necessary to consider augmenting the renal excretion of bicarbonate. This can be achieved with acetazolamide (250-500 mg intravenously daily or every 12

hours). Rarely, supplemental hydrochloric acid may be needed in the form of 0.1 N hydrochloric acid. Expected metabolic compensation is indicated in Table 18-16.

- The primary causes of respiratory alkalosis include hypoxemia, stimulation of ventilatory centers in the central nervous system, pregnancy, sepsis, and liver failure.

Mixed Acid-Base Disorders

The coexistence of 2 primary acid-base disturbances (eg, metabolic acidosis and metabolic alkalosis) or 2 disturbances separated by time (eg, superimposed acute and chronic respiratory acidosis) or the presence of 2 forms of primary disorder (eg, metabolic acidosis with high anion gap and normal anion gap concomitantly) is commonly encountered in an acute care setting. These disorders can be differentiated and classified appropriately by applying the compensation formula, as guided by the medical history and physical examination findings. A cardinal tenet is that the pH deviates from normal toward the side of the primary acid-base derangement.

Delta Gap

In the presence of a high anion gap acidosis, the coexistence of nonanion gap acidosis or metabolic alkalosis may be detected by applying the delta gap formula, which is calculated as follows:

Delta gap = (current anion gap – normal anion gap) + serum bicarbonate level (mEq/L) = 24.

The delta gap should be calculated in all cases of increased anion gap metabolic acidosis.

The premise of the delta gap is based on the accumulation of each

Table 18-17 Disorders That Cause Primary Respiratory Alkalosis

Hypoxemia	Stimulation of chest receptors
Decreased FIO_2	Pneumonia
High altitude	Asthma
Laryngospasm	Pneumothorax
Cyanotic heart disease	ARDS
Severe circulatory failure	Pulmonary edema
Pneumonia	Pulmonary fibrosis
Pulmonary edema,	Pulmonary embolism
embolism	Other
CNS stimulation	Mechanical ventilation
Anxiety	(iatrogenic)
Pain	Pregnancy
Fever	Septicemia
Subarachnoid hemorrhage	Liver failure
Stroke	
Encephalitis	
Tumor	
Drugs or hormones	
Salicylates	
Xanthines	
Angiotensin II	
Catecholamines	
Progesterone	
Nicotine	

Abbreviations: ARDS, acute respiratory distress syndrome; CNS, central nervous system; FIO_2, fraction of inspired oxygen.

excess anion above the normal anion gap accounting for the titration of 1 mEq of bicarbonate per liter. Hence, a patient with an anion gap of 20 has an excess anion gap of 8 (assuming a normal anion gap of 12). Therefore, the expected bicarbonate level measured in the patient's serum is 16 mEq/L. A bicarbonate level less than this would suggest a coexisting nonanion gap metabolic acidosis (additional loss of bicarbonate). A serum bicarbonate level that is considerably higher than 16 mEq/L suggests a preexisting metabolic alkalosis (previous excess levels of bicarbonate). Arterial blood gas values may be normal, but a high anion gap indicates a mixed metabolic alkalosis and acidosis. In metabolic alkalosis and respiratory acidosis, bicarbonate is higher than predicted for acidosis.

Common complex mixed acid-base disorders include the following: 1) salicylate intoxication (high anion gap metabolic acidosis plus respiratory alkalosis)—PCO_2 is lower than predicted for acidosis; 2) chronic obstructive pulmonary disease with pneumonia (acute-on-chronic respiratory acidosis); 3) hyperemesis gravidarum (metabolic alkalosis superimposed on chronic respiratory alkalosis)—bicarbonate is higher and PCO_2 is lower than expected; 4) sepsis with liver failure (metabolic acidosis with respiratory alkalosis); and 5) metabolic acidosis, respiratory acidosis, and metabolic alkalosis (acute ingestion of toxic alcohol, aspiration pneumonia, and chronic vomiting).

- Bicarbonate <15 mEq/L is usually caused partly by a metabolic acidosis.
- Bicarbonate >45 mEq/L is usually caused partly by a metabolic alkalosis.
- Arterial blood gas values may be normal, but a high anion gap indicates a mixed metabolic alkalosis and acidosis.
- In metabolic acidosis and respiratory alkalosis, PCO_2 is lower than predicted for acidosis.
- In metabolic alkalosis and respiratory acidosis, bicarbonate is higher than predicted for acidosis.
- In mixed metabolic and respiratory alkalosis, bicarbonate is higher and PCO_2 is lower than expected.
- Triple disorders: diabetic/alcoholic (vomiting) + (ketoacidosis/lactic acidosis) + (pneumonia).
- Calculating the delta gap allows coexisting metabolic acid-base derangements to be differentiated.

Part IV

Stephen B. Erickson, MD

Urolithiasis

Genesis

It was previously assumed that all kidney stones crystallized as urine passed through the renal tubules and were retained by means of crystal-tubular cell interactions. Recently uroscopy with papillary biopsies has shown 2 different pathways for stone formation, both mediated by calcium phosphate crystals. Idiopathic calcium oxalate stones are induced to form on the outer surface of the papillary urothelium by calcium phosphate crystals that migrate from the loop of Henle through the medulla to the inner side of the urothelium. The earliest "stone" is called *Randall plaque*.

Cystine, brushite, apatite, and enteric hyperoxaluria stones form in the distal collecting duct in association with calcium phosphate crystals (Figure 18-7).

- Idiopathic calcium oxalate stones form as Randall plaques on urothelium.
- Other stones form in the distal collecting duct.

Epidemiology

The prevalence of urolithiasis in the United States is about 5% (and increasing) in women and 12% in men. Of patients with untreated urolithiasis, 30% to 75% have recurrence within 10 years because they have not mitigated their risk factors. Urolithiasis is strongly familial and related to diet and urine volume. Many patients have a metabolic disorder that can be demonstrated with further testing, but conservative treatment with diet and increased fluid intake eliminates the stone-forming tendency in 70% of patients. Among those for whom conservative therapy fails, medications are successful in most (Figures 18-7 and 18-8).

- The prevalence of urolithiasis in the United States is about 10%.
- It is strongly familial and related to diet and urine volume.

Risk Factors

Urine pH is important in the pathogenesis of some renal stones. Struvite and calcium phosphate stones tend to form in alkaline urine; uric acid and cystine stones form in acid urine. The most common stone type, calcium oxalate, is pH independent. Some anatomical factors that predispose to urolithiasis include medullary sponge kidney, polycystic kidney disease, and chronic obstruction. Historical factors include fluid intake, dietary intake, history of urinary tract infection, drugs, family history, and other illnesses. Laboratory studies should include reviewing earlier radiographic findings; stone protocol computed tomography (CT); stone analysis; serum calcium, phosphorus,

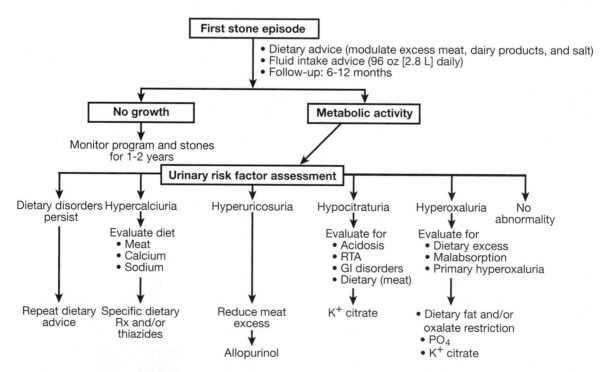

Figure 18-7. Approach to Therapy for Idiopathic Urolithiasis. GI indicates gastrointestinal tract; K, potassium; PO₄, phosphate; RTA, renal tubular acidosis; Rx, therapy. (Modified from MKSAP in the Subspecialty of Nephrology and Hypertension. Book 1 Syllabus and Questions, 1994. American College of Physicians. Used with permission.)

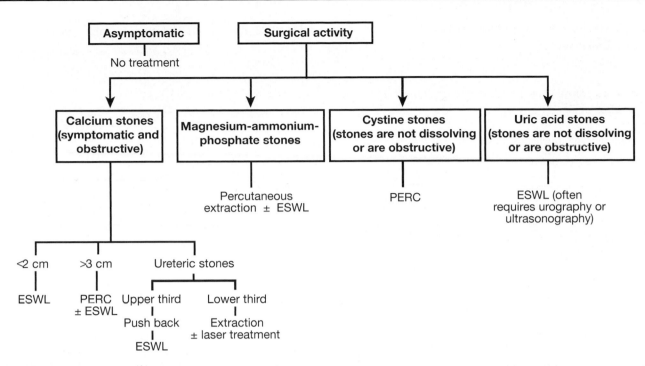

Figure 18-8. Algorithm for Surgical Treatment Choices Based on Size, Location, and Type of Kidney Stones. ESWL indicates extracorporeal shock-wave lithotripsy; PERC, percutaneous lithotripsy. (Modified from MKSAP in the Subspecialty of Nephrology and Hypertension. Book 1 Syllabus and Questions, 1994. American College of Physicians. Used with permission.)

potassium, and uric acid; urinalysis, urine culture, and 24-hour urine supersaturation, which includes volume, calcium, potassium, phosphorus, citrate, creatinine, oxalate, sodium, magnesium, uric acid, sulfate, and pH; and cystine analysis with the patient's usual diet. The characteristics of kidney stones are outlined in Table 18-18.

- Struvite and calcium phosphate stones form in alkaline urine.
- Uric acid and cystine stones form in acid urine.

Metabolic Activity and Surgical Activity
An evaluation of the disease activity to assess "surgical activity" and "metabolic activity" in patients who have urolithiasis is important for determining treatment. *Surgical activity* refers to unrelieved

hydronephrosis, unrelieved pain, or infection; *metabolic activity* refers to the formation of a new stone, growth of an existing stone, or passage of stones that were not identified by CT scan previously (Table 18-19).

Calcium Oxalate Stones
About 65% of all kidney stones are predominantly calcium oxalate. The risk factors for calcium oxalate stones are listed in Table 18-20. Causes include hypercalciuria, idiopathic hypercalciuria, other hypercalciuric states, hyperuricosuria, hyperoxaluria, and decreased excretion of inhibitors of crystallization. Conservative treatment includes correcting dietary stresses and increasing urine volume to more than 2.6 quarts (2.5 L) per day. Medications include potassium citrate

Table 18-18 Kidney Stone Characteristics

Type of Stone	Color	Shape	Frequency, %	Incident Male to Female Ratio	Urine pH
Calcium	White, tan, brown, black	Irregular	80	4:1	Oxalate—alkaline or acid Phosphate—relatively alkaline
Uric acid	Orange	Irregular or staghorn	10	10:1	Acid
Struvite	White, tan	Staghorn or irregular	10	1:10	Relatively alkaline
Cystine	Honey	Irregular or staghorn	1	1:1	Relatively acid

From Year 1 Renal Systems Syllabus for Mayo Clinic College of Medicine 2003 and 2004.

Table 18-19 Metabolic Activity and Surgical Activity in
           Urolithiasis

Metabolic
    New stones, growth of old stones, or passage of previously
    undetected stones
Surgical
    Unrelenting pain, unrelenting obstruction, or infection-related
    stones

Table 18-20 Risk Factors for Calcium Oxalate Stones

Family history
Hypercalciuria
Hyperoxaluria
Hyperuricosuria
Hypocitraturia
Low urine volume
Diet
    Low in fluids
    High in salt
    High in protein
    High or low in dairy products

for hypocitraturia, neutral phosphates for idiopathic calcium urolithiasis (but not in cases of urinary tract infection or renal insufficiency), thiazides for hypercalciuria (sodium must be restricted), and allopurinol for hyperuricosuria.

Primary hyperoxaluria is the most aggressive stone disease. Treatment includes fluids, pyridoxine (alters glycine metabolism, an oxalate precursor), neutral phosphates, or liver transplant.

- Calcium oxalate stones are the most common type.
- Calcium oxalate stones have diverse causes, including various metabolic abnormalities and dietary habits.

Calcium Phosphate Stones

Stones that are predominantly calcium phosphate comprise approximately 15% of kidney stones. The formation of calcium phosphate stones indicates a relatively alkaline urine pH.

Patients who have primary hyperparathyroidism typically have predominantly calcium phosphate stones. Parathyroid adenomas should be resected.

Some patients have renal tubular disorders associated with urolithiasis, including distal renal tubular acidosis (type 1). These patients often make pure calcium phosphate stones. They may also have nephrocalcinosis, a urine pH that is always greater than 5.3, and a hyperchloremic hypokalemic normal anion gap acidosis with a decreased level of urinary citrate (a stone inhibitor) and a high level of urinary calcium. The primary treatment is to correct the acidosis with alkali and to monitor urinary citrate excretion.

Other conditions associated with predominantly calcium phosphate stones are medullary sponge kidney and the use of absorbable alkalis (eg, Tums, Rolaids, Alka-Seltzer, and baking soda). Topiramate is an increasingly popular migraine treatment that causes calcium phosphate kidney stones in 1% to 2% of the people who use it. It acts by inhibiting carbonic anhydrase and creating renal tubular acidosis.

- The presence of calcium phosphate stones indicates a relatively alkaline urine pH.

Uric Acid Stones

Uric acid stones account for about 10% of all cases of nephrolithiasis. Of patients with uric acid urolithiasis, 75% have normal levels of uric acid in the serum and urine and 75% have persistently low urine pH. Patients with type 2 diabetes mellitus and stones are disproportionately represented; about 30% of their stones are uric acid. Of patients with primary gout, 25% form renal stones. An excess of

dietary protein also can predispose to uric acid stones, as can any cause of chronic diarrhea, including colectomy and ileostomy, because of decreased urine volume and hyperacidity. Uric acid urolithiasis is treated with preventive measures such as increased intake of fluid and decreased intake of protein. Alkalizing the urine to pH 6.5 not only helps prevent uric acid urolithiasis by treating the hyperaciduria, but it may also dissolve renal stones. Although the use of allopurinol usually is not as effective as alkalizing very acidic urine, it may be helpful for patients with hyperuricosuria and for dissolving stones.

- Of patients who form uric acid stones, 75% have persistently low urine pH.
- Renal stones form in 25% of patients with primary gout.
- Colectomy and ileostomy predispose to stones because the urine volume decreases and urine acidity increases.

Struvite Stones

Struvite stones comprise about 10% of all kidney stones. All patients who have magnesium-ammonium-phosphate stones are infected with urease-producing bacteria, which include *Proteus, Staphylococcus, Klebsiella, Enterobacter, Pseudomonas,* and, only rarely, *Escherichia coli.* The urine pH of these patients is alkaline, sometimes greater than the maximal physiologically achievable pH of approximately 8.0. Also, many of these patients have an underlying stone-forming tendency. Staghorn stones are not uncommon, and 50% occur bilaterally. Treatment includes giving antibiotics preoperatively and surgically removing all stone material, attempting to identify and treat the underlying stone-forming tendency, and giving bactericidal antibiotics postoperatively to eradicate infection. Failure to remove all stones requires indefinite antibiotic suppression.

- All patients with magnesium-ammonium-phosphate stones are infected with urease-producing bacteria.
- Urine pH is very alkaline.
- Staghorn stones: 50% occur bilaterally.
- Treatment: surgical removal and bactericidal antibiotics.

Cystine Stones

Only about 1% of patients with kidney stones have cystine stones.

Cystinuria is an autosomal recessive disorder in which homozygotes and some heterozygotes develop urolithiasis. Cystine crystalluria in routine urinalysis is diagnostic, as are positive findings on the nitroprusside test. These patients have a defect in the renal and intestinal absorption of *c*ystine, *o*rnithine, *l*ysine, and *a*rginine (mnemonic: *COLA*). The stones can be dissolved with urinary alkalization, cystine chelators such as tiopronin or penicillamine, and a high intake of fluid; however, urinary alkalization must be very intense, with urine pH maintained above 7.0. Adverse effects of penicillamine therapy include blood dyscrasias, gastrointestinal tract upset, membranous glomerulopathy, and a Goodpasture-like syndrome. Patients who have cystinuria often receive pyridoxine (25 mg daily) when taking penicillamine because cystine chelators indiscriminantly bind pyridoxine.

Inhibitors of Crystallization

Multiple inhibitors of calcium crystal formation and aggregation have been discovered. They are not routinely measured except for citrate and magnesium. Others include Tamm-Horsfall protein, nephrocalcin, osteopontin, pyrophosphate, and glycosaminoglycans. Patients who form calcium stones and who have no metabolic abnormality may be treated successfully with potassium citrate, phosphate, or magnesium salts to prevent further stones.

Drug-Induced Stone Disease

Medications that increase the tendency for stone formation include those listed in Table 18-21.

Urolithiasis and Bowel Disease

Enteric Hyperoxaluria

Patients must have an intact colon to absorb free oxalate. Free oxalate is overabsorbed when free fatty acids complex calcium and magnesium (the usual oxalate complexers). Fatty acids and bile acids also increase colonic permeability to oxalate. Other factors that increase oxalate supersaturation include decreased water absorption, decreased bicarbonate absorption, and decreased absorption of magnesium, phosphate, and pyrophosphate (inhibitors of crystallization). Treatment of this disorder includes correcting the underlying problem, increasing dietary calcium, decreasing dietary oxalate and fat, considering use of cholestyramine to bind bile acids, and increasing urine pH and inhibitors.

As bariatric surgery has become more common, hyperoxaluria is increasingly recognized by 1 year postoperatively with subsequent development of calcium oxalate stones. Hyperoxaluria is especially common in long loops in the Roux-en-Y gastric bypass.

- The absorption of free oxalate requires an intact colon.
- Bariatric surgery predisposes to oxalate stones.

Uric Acid Urolithiasis

Patients with bowel disease, especially those without a colon, may also develop uric acid urolithiasis. Ileostomy patients are frequently susceptible to these stones because of the loss of alkali and water. Treatment includes alkali and fluids.

- Patients with colectomies preferentially form uric acid stones.

Table 18-21 Medications Increasing the Tendency for Stone Formation

Calcium oxalate stones
    Calcium carbonate
    Vitamin C
    Vitamin D
    Steroids
    Loop diuretics
Calcium phosphate stones
    Acetazolamide
    Topiramate
    Zonisamide
Uric acid stones
    Chemotherapy
Other stones
    Allopurinol
    Triamterene
    Acyclovir
    Ephedra
    Guaifenesin
    Sulfonamides

Passing Stones

Expulsive therapy is gaining popularity on the basis of a few small controlled studies that used various dosages of prednisone to reduce ureteral edema and vasodilators (calcium channel blockers or α-blockers) to relax ureteral smooth muscle. Substantial improvement in the rate of stone passage has been reported. Traditional hydration therapy to promote stone passage remains popular but unproved.

Transplantation

Transplant is the treatment of choice for eligible patients who have end-stage renal disease (ESRD). More than 200,000 renal transplants have been performed; 17,093 kidney transplants were performed in 2006 (10,659 deceased and 6,434 living donors). More than 76,000 potential recipients are awaiting a kidney transplant, and the number increases annually. The main limitation is the small number of donor kidneys. Lifetime immunusuppression is required. Recipients range from younger than 1 year to older than 50 years. In 2006, there were 3,433 kidney tranplant recipients over 65 years. The recipient must not have cancer. Infections (including those of the teeth, sinuses, and bladder) need to be eradicated, and cholecystectomy for gallstones should be performed. Living donors must be 18 years or older and not have any systemic or renal disease. Cadaveric donors must be older than 6 months and not have infection or malignancy (except for nonmetastasizing brain cancer).

Recurrent Allograft Renal Disease

Causes of recurrent allograft renal disease include membranoproliferative glomerulonephritis, membranous nephropathy, focal segmental glomerulosclerosis, diabetes mellitus, primary hyperoxaluria, hemolytic-uremic syndrome, and IgA nephropathy (usually not clinically important).

Immunosuppression

Immunosuppression is usually achieved by depleting the lymphocytes, blocking lymphocyte response pathways, or changing the flow of lymphocytes. Immunosuppressive drugs have 3 effects: suppress rejection (a desired effect), cause infections or cancers (undesired effects), and affect other tissues by nonimmune mechanisms (an undesired effect). Immunosuppressive agents include prednisone, which blocks the production of interleukin 1 by macrophages and the production of cytokines (complications include cataracts, psychoses, peptic ulcer disease, infection, diverticulitis, and aseptic necrosis); azathioprine, which inhibits the proliferation of activated T cells (complications include bone marrow suppression, cholestasis, and infection; never treat with allopurinol); and cyclosporine, which inhibits the activation of helper T cells and the production of interleukins 2, 3, 4, and 5 and which is hydrophobic and lipophilic, requiring bile acids for absorption.

Cyclosporine levels are increased by ketoconazole, cimetidine, ranitidine, verapamil, diltiazem, and erythromycin. Cyclosporine levels are decreased by phenytoin, phenobarbital, ethambutol, sulfamethoxazole, ethanol, and cholestyramine. The adverse effects of cyclosporine include gum hyperplasia, hyperkalemia, hypertension, hemolytic uremic syndrome, and thrombotic thrombocytopenic purpura.

Several newer immunosuppressive drugs are used to prevent rejection. A complete description of each drug is beyond the scope of the chapter, but Tables 18-22 and 18-23 summarize the mechanism of action and nonimmune toxicity of these drugs.

Graft Failure (Most Commonly Chronic Rejection)

Graft failure is commonly due to chronic rejection. Acute tubular necrosis occurs after transplant in 20% to 50% of patients. The stages of rejection are hyperacute (hours), acute (days to years), and chronic (months to years). Recurrent disease occurs in 1% of patients. Surgical complications include renal artery stenosis, ureteral obstruction or leak, and lymphocele.

The medical complications of renal transplant are diverse and complex. Opportunistic infections are the most common cause of death, and the next most common cause is cardiovascular problems. Other complications are hyperlipidemia, malignancy (1%, including skin cancer, sarcomas, lymphomas [Epstein-Barr virus-associated], and solid tumors), polycythemia, proximal or distal renal tubular acidosis, and kidney stones (1%).

Pregnancy and the Kidney

Anatomical changes associated with pregnancy are renal enlargement (length may increase by 1 cm) and dilatation of the calyces, renal pelvis, and ureters. Physiologic changes include a 30% to 50% increase in glomerular filtration rate (GFR) and renal blood flow; a mean decrease of 0.5 mg/dL in the creatinine level and a mean decrease of 18 mg/dL in urea nitrogen; intermittent glycosuria independent of plasma glucose (<1 g per day); proteinuria (but <300 mg per day, sometimes postural); aminoaciduria (<2 g per day, involving most but not all amino acids); increased uric acid excretion; increased total body water (6-8 L), with osmostat resetting; 50% increase in plasma volume and cardiac output; and increased ureteral peristalsis. Bacterial growth in urine is promoted by the intermittent glycosuria and aminoaciduria. Hormonal effects include increased levels of renin, angiotensin II, aldosterone, cortisol, estrogens, prostaglandins (E_2 and I_2), and progesterone; insensitivity to the pressor effects of norepinephrine and angiotensin II; and progesterone counteracting the kaliuretic effects of aldosterone. Hypertension in pregnancy is discussed in Chapter 14 ("Hypertension").

Urinary Tract Infections

The prevalence of asymptomatic bacteriuria among pregnant women is similar to that among nonpregnant women, except that it is higher in those with diabetes mellitus and sickle cell trait. Asymptomatic urinary tract infections progress to pyelonephritis or cystitis in 40% of pregnant women. Recommendations include screening for asymptomatic bacteriuria monthly and treating asymptomatic bacteriuria (10-14 days). Symptomatic urinary tract infections frequently recur, and pyelonephritis occurs in 1% to 2% of patients. Symptomatic urinary tract infections should be treated aggressively with antibiotics (ampicillin or cephalosporins) for 6 weeks. Follow-up cultures are recommended every 2 weeks. Sulfa drugs near term and tetracyclines (because of fetal bone and tooth development and maternal liver failure) are contraindicated.

Acute Renal Failure in Pregnancy

Conditions that predispose to acute renal failure in pregnancy are sepsis, severe preeclampsia (HELLP syndrome [*h*emolysis, *e*levated *l*iver enzymes, and *l*ow *p*latelet count]), abruptio placentae, intrauterine fetal death, uterine hemorrhage, and presence of nephrotoxins. Cortical necrosis occurs in 10% to 30% of cases of gestational acute renal failure. Patients become anuric. Although patients may have partial recovery, they may have progression to ESRD years later. Postpartum hemolytic uremic syndrome (excluding retained placenta) may occur at 3 to 6 weeks postpartum. This is characterized by acute oliguria, uremia, severe hypertension, and microangiopathic hemolytic anemia. Disseminated intravascular coagulation and Shwartzman reaction occur, as in thrombotic thrombocytopenic purpura. Therapy includes dilatation and curettage, support, perhaps antiplatelet therapy (although the evidence is not strong), and plasma infusion. Acute renal failure and acute fatty liver of pregnancy (similar to hepatorenal syndrome) are caused by tetracyclines and possibly disseminated intravascular coagulation.

Parenchymal Renal Disease in Pregnancy

The outcome of lupus erythematosus depends on the clinical status prepartum. If the disease is quiescent 6 months before birth, 90% of the women have live births. If the disease is active prepartum, 50% have exacerbation and 35% have fetal loss. If the disease is stable prepartum, 30% of the women have reversible exacerbations. Congenital heart block may occur in the newborn. Glucocorticoids and cytotoxic agents have been used without causing teratogenic effects.

Table 18-22 Characteristics of Small-Molecule Immunosuppressive Drugs Used in Organ Transplantation or in Phase 2 or 3 Trials[a]

Drug	Description	Mechanism	Nonimmune Toxicity and Comments
Cyclosporine	11-Amino-acid cyclic peptide from *Tolypocladium inflatum*	Binds to cyclophilin; complex inhibits calcineurin phosphatase & T-cell activation	Nephrotoxicity, hemolytic-uremic syndrome, hypertension, neurotoxicity, gum hyperplasia, skin changes, hirsuitism, posttransplant diabetes mellitus, hyperlipidemia; trough monitoring or checking levels 2 h after administration required
Tacrolimus (FK506)	Macrolide antibiotic from *Streptomyces tsukubaensis*	Binds to FKBP12; complex inhibits calcineurin phosphatase & T-cell activation	Effects similar to those of cyclosporine but with a lower incidence of hypertension, hyperlipidemia, skin changes, hirsuitism, & gum hyperplasia & a higher incidence of posttransplant diabetes mellitus & neurotoxicity; trough monitoring required
Sirolimus (rapamycin)	Triene macrolide antibiotic from *S hygroscopicus* from Easter Island (Rapa Nui)	Binds to FKBP12; complex inhibits target of rapamycin & interleukin-2–driven T-cell proliferation	Hyperlipidemia, increased toxicity of calcineurin inhibitors, thrombocytopenia, delayed wound healing, delayed graft function, mouth ulcers, pneumonitis, interstitial lung disease; lipid monitoring required; recipients whose risk of rejection is low to moderate can stop cyclosporine treatment 2 to 4 mo after transplant
Everolimus	Derivative of sirolimus		
Mycophenolate mofetil & enteric-coated mycophenolate	Mycophenolic acid from penicillium molds	Inhibits synthesis of guanosine monophosphate nucleotides; blocks purine synthesis, preventing proliferation of T & B cells	Gastrointestinal tract symptoms (mainly diarrhea), neutropenia, mild anemia; blood-level monitoring not required but may improve efficacy; absorption reduced by cyclosporine
FK778 & malononitrilamide	Modification of A77 1726 (active derivative of leflunomide)	Inhibits pyrimidine synthesis, blocking proliferation of T & B cells	Anemia; other effects not known; in phase 2 trials
Azathioprine	Prodrug that releases 6-mercaptopurine	Converts 6-mercaptopurine to tissue inhibitor of metalloproteinase, which is converted to thioguanine nucleotides that interfere with DNA synthesis; thioguanine derviatives may inhibit purine synthesis	Leukopenia, bone marrow depression, macrocytosis, liver toxicity (uncommon); blood-count monitoring required
FTY720	Sphingosine-like derivative of myriocin from ascomycete fungus	Works as an antagonist for sphingosine-1-phosphate receptors on lymphocytes, enhancing homing to lymphoid tissues & preventing egress, causing lymphopenia	Reversible first-dose bradycardia, potentiated by general anesthetics & β-blockers; nausea, vomiting, diarrhea, increased levels of liver enzymes
CP-690,550 & Tyrphostin AG 490	Synthetic molecule	Binds cytoplasmic tyrosine kinase JAK3, inhibiting cytokine-induced signaling	Anemia caused by potential effects on JAK2

[a] Data about drugs come from the manufacturers' inserts for health care professionals and published articles.
From Halloran PF. Drug therapy: immunosuppressive drugs for kidney tranplantation. N Engl J Med. 2004;351:2715-29. Used with permission.

Table 18-23 Characteristics of Protein Immunosuppressive Drugs Used in Organ Transplantation or in Phase 2 or 3 Trials

Drug	Description	Mechanism	Toxicity and Comments[a]
Polyclonal antithymocyte globulin	Polyclonal IgG from horses or rabbits immunized with human thymocytes; absorbed to reduce unwanted antibodies	Blocks T-cell membrane proteins (CD2, CD3, CD45, etc), causing altered function, lysis, & prolonged T-cell depletion	The cytokine-release syndrome (fever, chills, hypotension), thrombocytopenia, leukopenia, serum sickness
Muromonab-CD3	Murine monoclonal antibody against CD3 component of T-cell–receptor signal-transduction complex	Binds to CD3 associated with T-cell receptor, leading to initial activation & cytokine release, followed by blockade of function, lysis, & T-cell depletion	Severe cytokine-release syndrome, pulmonary edema, acute renal failure, gastrointestinal tract disturbances, changes in central nervous system
Alemtuzumab	Humanized monoclonal antibody against CD52, a 25- to 29-kD membrane protein	Binds to CD52 on all B & T cells, most monocytes, macrophages, & natural killer cells, causing cell lysis & prolonged depletion	Mild cytokine-release syndrome, neutropenia, anemia, idiosyncratic pancytopenia, autoimmune thrombocytopenia, thyroid disease
Rituximab	Chimeric monocolonal antibody against membrane-spanning 4-domain protein CD20	Binds to CD20 on B cells & mediates B-cell lysis	Infusion reactions, hypersensitivity reactions (uncommon)
Basiliximab	Chimeric monoclonal antibody against CD25 (interleukin-2–receptor α chain)	Binds to & blocks the interleukin-2–receptor α chain (CD25 antigen) on activated T cells, depleting them & inhibiting interleukin-2–induced T-cell activation	Hypersensitivity reactions (uncommon); 2 doses required; no monitoring required
Daclizumab	Humanized monoclonal antibody against CD25 (interleukin-2–receptor α chain)	Has similar action to that of basiliximab	Hypersensitivity reactions (uncommon); 5 doses recommended but 2 may suffice; no monitoring required
LEA29Y	Protein combining B7-binding portion of CTLA-4 with IgG Fc region	Binds to B7 on T cells, preventing CD28 signaling & signal 2	Effects unknown; in phase 2 trials

[a] The toxic effects of alemtuzumab, rituximab, and LEA29Y in organ-transplant recipients must be established in phase 3 trials. The toxic effects of alemtuzumab are primarily those reported in nontransplant trials.

From Halloran PF. Drug therapy: immunosuppressive drugs for kidney tranplantation. N Engl J Med. 2004;351:2715-29. Used with permission.

Diabetes mellitus is associated with increased asymptomatic and symptomatic bacteriuria and increased preeclampsia. Proteinuria and hypertension may worsen, but renal function usually is stable.

Renal transplant recipients should postpone pregnancy for 2 years after transplant. Increased preeclampsia, infection, and adrenal insufficiency have been reported. Pregnancy is usually uncomplicated if the creatinine level is less than 1.5 mg/dL, blood pressure is normal, and the woman is receiving low-dose immunosuppressive therapy. Preeclampsia occurs in 25% of women, prematurity in 7%, and loss of renal function in 7%. Nonobstetrical abdominal pain indicates allograft stone or infection.

Evaluation of Kidney Function

Serum Creatinine

Creatinine is an end product of muscle catabolism and is commonly used as a filtration marker. Creatinine is released in the circulation at a steady rate. It is not protein bound, and it is filtered freely across the glomerulus and secreted by the tubules. Several medications, such as trimethoprim and cimetidine, inhibit creatinine secretion and increase the serum creatinine level. Other nonrenal factors that increase the serum creatinine level include race (African American), muscular build, and ingestion of creatine supplements. Factors that might decrease serum creatinine are older age, female sex, vegetarian diet, malnutrition, protein wasting, and being an amputee. Obesity does not affect serum creatinine.

There are problems with the current techniques used to measure serum creatinine and variability due to lack of standardization of the calibrations of these assays among different laboratories. The commonly used alkaline picrate (Jaffe) assay used to measure creatinine may be affected by noncreatinine chromagens (in some cases up to 20%).

The College of American Pathologists has attempted to minimize the heterogeneity among creatinine assays by preparing a fresh-frozen serum pool with a known creatinine level that is traceable to a primary reference at the US National Institute of Standards and Technology. This has been used to standardize creatinine measurements and calibrate equipment in various laboratories.

Urinalysis

The causes of urine discoloration are listed in Table 18-24. Dysmorphic erythrocytes (>80%) in the urinary sediment indicate upper urinary tract bleeding. The Hansel stain identifies urinary eosinophils.

Normal urine osmolality is 40 to 1,200 mOsm/kg, and the pH is 4 to 7.5. A pH less than 5.5 excludes type 1 renal tubular acidosis. A pH greater than 7 suggests infection. Acidic urine is indicative of a high-protein diet, acidosis, and potassium depletion. Alkaline urine is associated with a vegetarian diet, alkalosis (unless potassium depleted), and urease-producing bacteria.

Glycosuria in the absence of hyperglycemia suggests proximal tubule dysfunction.

Table 18-24 Causes of Urine Discoloration

Color	Cause
Dark yellow, brown	Bilirubin
Brown-black	Homogentisic acid (ochronosis)
	Melanin (melanoma)
	Metronidazole
	Methyldopa/levodopa
	Phenothiazine
Red	Beets
	Rifampin
	Porphyria
	Hemoglobinuria/myoglobinuria
	Phenazopyridine hydrochloride (Pyridium)
	Urates
Blue-green	Indomethacin
	Amitriptyline
Turbid white	Pyuria
	Chylous fistula
	Crystalluria

Renal Clearance

Clearance of *p*-aminohippurate is a measure of renal blood flow. Orthoiodohippurate is used in renal scans. The clearance rates of inulin, iothalamate, diethylenetriamine pentaacetic acid (DTPA), and creatinine are measures of the GFR. The Cockcroft-Gault estimation formula for males is

$$GFR = \frac{(140 - \text{age in years}) \times (\text{lean body weight in kg})}{S_{Cr} \times 72}$$

where S_{Cr} is the serum creatinine level. For females, the males' formula is multiplied by 0.85. Creatinine levels are increased independently of the GFR with ketoacidosis (acetoacetate), cefoxitin, cimetidine, trimethoprim, flucytosine, massive rhabdomyolysis, high intake of meat, and probenecid. Urea (blood urea nitrogen) levels are increased independently of the GFR with gastrointestinal tract bleeding, tissue trauma, glucocorticoids, and tetracyclines.

The Modification of Diet in Renal Disease (MDRD) Study equation is used to assess renal function. It is a 4-variable equation (plasma creatinine, age, race, and sex) that has been validated in African Americans, diabetic patients with renal disease, and kidney transplant recipients. The MDRD Study equation is

$$GFR = 186 \times (P_{cr})^{-1.154} \times (\text{age})^{-0.203} \times (0.742 \text{ if female}) \times (1.210 \text{ if African American})$$

where GFR is expressed in millimeters per minute per 1.73 m^2 and P_{cr} is the serum creatinine level.

The MDRD Study equation has been found to have greater precision and overall accuracy than the Cockcroft-Gault formula in the estimation of GFR, but it has not been validated in children, pregnant women, persons older than 70 years and other racial and ethnic groups. The equation also underestimates GFR in populations with higher GFRs, such as patients undergoing kidney transplant donor evaluation and patients with type 1 diabetes mellitus without microalbuminuria.

Neither equation works if patients have extreme creatinine generation (eg, patients with muscle-wasting conditions or very high or low protein intake, amputees, and large or small individuals).

Renal Imaging

Plain films magnify the kidneys 30%. Normal renal size is 3.5 times the height of vertebra L2 (>11 cm). The left kidney is up to 1.5 cm longer than the right one. An enlarged kidney indicates obstruction, infiltration (eg, amyloidosis, leukemia, or diabetes mellitus), acute glomerulonephritis, acute tubulointerstitial nephropathy, renal vein thrombosis, or polycystic kidney disease. Calcifications are associated with stone, tuberculosis, aneurysms, and necrosis of the papillary tips.

Excretory urography provides a detailed definition of the collecting system and can be used to assess renal size and contour and to detect and locate calculi. It is also used to assess renal function qualitatively. Rapid sequence excretory urography is a poor screening test for renovascular hypertension. Complications include a large osmotic load (congestive heart failure) and reactions (5%). An iodine load may occur and is a consideration if the patient has hyperthyroidism.

Ultrasonography is used to measure renal size (>9 cm) and to screen for obstruction, but the results may be negative early in the course of obstruction. Ultrasonography can be used to characterize mass lesions (eg, angiomyolipoma and solid versus cystic) and to screen for polycystic kidney disease. Ultrasonography may be used to assess for renal vein thrombosis, that is, to assess for the presence or absence of blood flow. Ultrasonography is not a screening test for renal artery stenosis.

CT demonstrates calcification patterns. It is used to stage neoplasms and as an adjunct to determine the cause of obstruction (without contrast medium). CT is used to assess cysts, abscesses, and hematomas.

Magnetic resonance imaging may be used to identify adrenal hemorrhage and to assess a mass in patients sensitive to contrast dyes. Magnetic resonance angiography is a promising screening method for renal artery stenosis. Extreme caution should be used to ensure that gadolinium-containing contrast material is not used in patients with stage 4 or 5 chronic kidney disease, renal and hepatic transplant recipients, patients with severe acute renal insufficiency or hepatorenal syndrome, and intensive care unit patients. More recently, more than 200 cases of nephrogenic systemic fibrosis (NSF) or

nephrogenic fibrosing dermopathy (NFD) have been directly associated with exposure to gadolinium-containing contrast material in patients with stage 4 or 5 chronic kidney disease.

NSF or NFD is a painful skin disease, characterized by thickening of the skin, that can involve the joints and cause significant limitation of motion within weeks to months. The National Kidney Foundation recommends that alternative imaging techniques be attempted if patients have an estimated GFR of 30 mL/min per 1.73 m^2 or less and that if patients need a gadolinium-based contrast material, the lowest possible dose should be used. In patients with stage 5 chronic kidney disease who are on dialysis, a reduced dose of gadolinium-based contrast material should be used only if absolutely unavoidable, and the patients should receive hemodialysis immediately afterward. Patients on peritoneal dialysis should not receive gadolinium.

Arteriography and venography are used to evaluate arterial stenosis, aneurysm, fistulas, vasculitis, and mass lesions and to assess living-related donor transplants.

Gallium and indium scans are used to evaluate acute interstitial nephritis, abscess, pyelonephritis, lymphoma, and leukemia.

DTPA and hippuran renal scanning are useful in assessing a transplanted kidney, obstruction (before and after furosemide), and infarct (presence or absence of blood flow).

Nephrology Pharmacy Review
Scott Luther Larson, PharmD

Drug (Trade Name)	Toxic/Adverse Effects	Comments
Hematopoietic agents		
Epoetin alfa (Epogen, Procrit)	Hypertension, CVA, CHF, local pain, iron deficiency, headache, edema, rarely seizures	Administration SQ or IV, usually 3 times weekly Maximize iron stores before & during therapy
Darbepoetin alfa (Aranesp)	Same as above	Administration SQ or IV, usually once weekly or every other week Maximize iron stores before & during therapy
Iron products		
Iron dextran (InFeD, Dexferrum)	Hypersensitivity reaction/anaphylaxis, bronchospasm, local pain, tissue staining, arthralgias, flushing, hypotension, rare seizures Risk decreased with dilution & slow infusion rate	Administration IV (slowly, to avoid tissue discoloration) or IM (as a Z-track injection) Requires test dose before administration (0.25-0.5 mL slow IV or deep IM)
Ferric gluconate (Ferrlecit)	Hypersensitivity reaction, hypotension, flushing, cramps Increased hypotension & flushing with rapid infusion	Less incidence of anaphylaxis than with iron dextran IV infusion route only Test dose recommended but not required
Iron sucrose (Venofer)	Hypotension, leg cramps, headache, nausea/vomiting, diarrhea, low risk of hypersensitivity reaction	Administration, only by slow IV push or injection No test dose needed before administration

Oral iron products
  Ferrous fumarate (33% elemental)
  Ferrous sulfate (20% elemental)
  Ferrous gluconate (11.6% elemental)
	GI upset, constipation, nausea/vomiting, dark stools	Best absorbed on an empty stomach
		Typically not adequate to replete iron stores in hemodialysis patient
		Iron absorption decreased with co-administration of antacids, calcium products, phosphorus binders
		Absorption of quinolone antibiotics decreased with coadministration of iron

Phosphorus-binding agents[a]		
Aluminum carbonate (Basaljel) Aluminum hydroxide (Amphojel, ALternaGEL)	Risk of aluminum accumulation/toxicity: encephalopathy, microcytic anemia, osteomalacia, seizures, dementia	Potent phosphorus binder Best for short-term use owing to toxicity Aluminum absorption increased with coadministration of citrate salts (ie, effervescent tablets & sodium citrate given with dialysis), resulting in increased risk of toxicity Decreased absorption of quinolone antibiotics & oral iron with coadministration
Calcium carbonate (Tums, Os-Cal)	Hypercalcemia, GI upset, constipation	Highest elemental calcium content Weakest elemental phosphorus binder Decreases absorption of quinolone antibiotics & oral iron with coadministration Absorption of digoxin may be decreased

Nephrology Pharmacy Review (continued)

Drug (Trade Name)	Toxic/Adverse Effects	Comments
Phosphorus-binding agents[a] (continued)		
Calcium acetate (PhosLo)	Same as above	More potent phosphorus binder than calcium carbonate
		Decreases absorption of quinolone antibiotics & oral iron with coadministration
		Absorption of digoxin may be decreased
Sevelamer HCl (Renagel)	Nausea/vomiting, diarrhea, constipation, dyspepsia	Non-elemental–based phosphorus binder
		May decrease LDL & total serum cholesterol levels
		Absorption of other medications may be decreased with coadministration
Lanthanum carbonate (Fosrenol)	Dyspepsia, diarrhea, nausea/vomiting; vascular dialysis graft occlusion	Expensive phosphorus binder
		Must be crushed or chewed
		May be given through feeding tubes
		Long-term effects on bone & other organs remain unknown
Vitamin D analogues		
Calcitriol (Calcijex [IV], Rocaltrol [PO])	Hypercalcemia, hyperphosphatemia, constipation, nausea/vomiting, headache, confusion, somnolence, dry mouth, myalgia	Increases absorption of calcium & phosphorus
		Directly suppresses PTH release
Paricalcitol (Zemplar [IV], [PO])	Same as above	More expensive than calcitriol
		Less absorption of calcium & phosphorus than calcitriol
		Directly suppresses PTH release
Doxercalciferol (Hectorol [IV], [PO])	Same as above	More expensive than calcitriol
		Less absorption of calcium & phosphorus than calcitriol
		Directly suppresses PTH release
Miscellaneous		
Cinacalcet (Sensipar)	Hypocalcemia, nausea/vomiting, diarrhea, myalgia	Mimics calcium on the parathyroid gland
		Acts quickly to suppress PTH release
Vitamins (Nephrocaps, Dialyvite, Nephro-Vite)	No important ones documented	Water-soluble vitamin replacement
Quinine sulfate (several)	Hypoglycemia, pancytopenia, tinnitus, nausea/vomiting, visual disturbances, headache, photosensitivity, rare DIC	Prevention or treatment of leg cramps
		Absorption of quinine may be decreased with coadministration of aluminum antacids
		Coadministration with digoxin may lead to increased digoxin levels
		Coadministration with warfarin may potentiate warfarin effects

Abbreviations: CHF, congestive heart failure; CVA, cerebrovascular accident; DIC, disseminated intravascular coagulation; GI, gastrointestinal tract; IM, intramuscular; IV, intravenous; LDL, low-density lipoprotein; PO, by mouth; PTH, parathyroid hormone; SQ, subcutaneous.
[a] All phosphorus-binding agents should be taken with food to enhance efficacy.

Nephrology Pharmacy Review (continued)

Drugs Associated With Acid-Base Disorders

Metabolic acidosis	Metabolic alkalosis
Acetaminophen OD	Bicarbonate
Acetazolamide	Citrate salts (especially with
Alcohol	abnormal renal function)
Amphetamine OD	Diuretics (loop & thiazides)
Cocaine	Phenolphthalein (laxative
Colchicine	abuse)
Cotrimoxazole	**Respiratory acidosis**
Ethylene glycol	Baclofen OD
Iron OD	Barbiturates
Isoniazid OD	Benzodiazepines
Mafenide	Opioids
Metformin	**Respiratory alkalosis**
Methanol	Salicylate OD (early)
Paraldehyde	
Propofol	
Salicylate OD (late)	
Spironolactone	

Abbreviation: OD, overdose.

Questions

Multiple Choice (choose the best answer)

1. A 65-year-old woman presents with a 3-month history of fatigue, weight loss, and arthralgias. One year ago, the serum creatinine level was normal, but now it is 2.8 mg/dL, and urinalysis demonstrates dysmorphic RBCs (red blood cells), proteinuria (2+), and RBC casts. Which diagnostic test is most likely to establish the diagnosis?

   a. Urine and serum protein electrophoresis
   b. Enzyme-linked immunosorbent assay (ELISA) for proteinase-3 (PR3) and myeloperoxidase (MPO), and immunofluorescence for antineutrophil cytoplasmic autoantibody (ANCA)
   c. Evaluation for urinary eosinophils
   d. Renal arteriography
   e. Erythrocyte sedimentation rate

2. A 35-year-old woman has a history of having type 1 diabetes mellitus, which has been well controlled, since age 20. She has no retinopathy. Six weeks ago, she had sudden onset of edema. Supine blood pressure is 140/80 mm Hg, serum creatinine 1.1 mg/dL, and 24-hour urinary protein 8 g. What is the most appropriate next step in the evaluation or management of this patient?

   a. Begin angiotensin-converting enzyme (ACE) inhibitor therapy.
   b. Limit dietary protein intake.
   c. Order antinuclear antibody (ANA), complement (C3 and C4), and anti–double-stranded DNA tests.
   d. Perform a renal biopsy.
   e. All of the above are correct.

3. A 35-year-old male smoker presents to the emergency department with a history of sudden onset of shortness of breath. Evaluation includes the following results: hemoglobin, 9 g/dL; serum creatinine, 3.8 mg/dL; urinalysis, proteinuria with RBC casts; chest radiographs, bilateral pulmonary infiltrates; ANCA testing, negative; and serum anti–glomerular basement membrane antibodies, positive. Which therapy is most likely to improve this patient's clinical course?

   a. Antibiotic therapy
   b. Oral prednisone and oral cyclophosphamide
   c. High-dose corticosteroids
   d. Intravenous cyclophosphamide
   e. Plasmapheresis, high-dose corticosteroids, and oral cyclophosphamide

4. A 30-year-old African American man presents for evaluation of edema. Evaluation includes the following findings: blood pressure 150/100 mm Hg, serum creatinine 1.3 mg/dL, glucose 98 mg/dL, serum albumin 2.8 g/dL, urinalysis with RBCs (1+) and proteinuria (3+), and 24-hour urinary protein 12 g. What is the most likely diagnosis?

   a. Focal segmental glomerulosclerosis
   b. Poststreptococcal glomerulonephritis
   c. Membranous nephropathy
   d. Interstitial nephritis
   e. Immunoglobulin (Ig)A nephropathy

5. A 70-year-old man comes for follow-up. He has a history of having Wegener granulomatosis since age 50, with multiple episodes of remission and relapses, and requiring treatment with prednisone and cyclophosphamide. His latest course of immunosuppressants was discontinued 2 years ago. He is currently taking no medication except for the occasional use of nonsteroidal anti-inflammatory drugs. He feels well. Results of laboratory studies include the following: serum creatinine, 1.2 mg/dL; complete blood cell count, normal; erythrocyte sedimentation rate, 5 mm in 1 hour; and ANCA testing, negative, but urinalysis shows more than 100 RBCs per high-power field (hpf). What would be your next step in managing this patient?

   a. Order renal ultrasonography.
   b. Perform a renal biopsy.
   c. Order excretory urography.
   d. Use prednisone and cyclophosphamide to treat another relapse.
   e. Perform cystoscopy.

6. A 50-year-old man presents with newly diagnosed nephrotic-range proteinuria. He felt well until 2 months ago, when bilateral ankle edema developed. Past medical history was unremarkable, except for a 35–pack-year history of cigarette smoking. The patient denies use of over-the-counter medications. He has no skin rashes, fever, or arthralgia. Apart from blood pressure of 145/90 mm Hg and bilateral ankle edema, the physical examination findings are unremarkable. Results of laboratory studies include the following: hemoglobin 14.8 g/dL, serum creatinine 1.5 mg/dL, total cholesterol 389 mg/dL, and 24-hour urinary protein 12 g. A renal biopsy specimen shows stage II membranous nephropathy. For this patient, all of the following recommendations are correct *except*:

   a. Test for hepatitis B and C.
   b. Perform chest radiography and guaiac testing of stool for occult blood.
   c. Test for ANA and anti–double-stranded DNA antibody.
   d. Obtain samples for blood cultures.
   e. Start protein and sodium restriction, start ACE inhibitor/ angiotensin II receptor blocker therapy, and start giving a statin.

7. Which of the following describes minimal change nephropathy?

    a. It is the commonest cause of nephrotic syndrome in adults.
    b. Patients do not have a relapse after remission.
    c. Proteinuria is nonselective.
    d. It does not depress serum complement levels.
    e. Confirmation by renal biopsy is always required.

8. A 60-year-old man is admitted from the emergency department to the intensive care unit with acute gastrointestinal tract bleeding due to esophageal varices. His blood pressure on arrival is 80/45 mm Hg and the hemoglobin level has decreased from 11 g/dL to 6 g/dL. He received 3 units of RBCs in the emergency department. Examination reveals a man appearing chronically ill with icteric sclerae. Abdominal examination shows marked ascites. His past medical history is significant for chronic liver disease with cirrhosis. You also note that his baseline level of creatinine was 1.2 mg/dL, baseline levels of serum sodium have been 128 to 132 mEq/L, and his spot urinary sodium 2 months ago (as an outpatient) was 10 mEq/L. His medications before admission were spironolactone and lactulose. He also recently completed a course of levofloxacin for community-acquired pneumonia. The patient's urine output since admission is less than 30 mL/h. Laboratory evaluation results from the emergency department include serum sodium 128 mEq/L, potassium 3.7 mEq/L, and creatinine 2.8 mg/dL. Urinalysis was unremarkable except for rare epithelial cells. On the basis of the initial examination and data, what is the most likely cause of the patient's renal failure?

    a. Acute hemolysis and heme pigment nephrotoxicity
    b. Hepatorenal syndrome type 1
    c. Prerenal azotemia
    d. Acute interstitial nephritis due to use of levofloxacin
    e. Abdominal compartment syndrome due to ascites

9. For the same 60-year-old man in question 8, what would be your first therapeutic intervention?

    a. Begin a dopamine infusion to increase renal perfusion.
    b. Administer octreotide.
    c. Administer hypertonic saline to gradually increase the serum level of sodium.
    d. Administer normal saline boluses to increase intravascular volume.
    e. Begin a furosemide drip to increase urine output.

10. A 76-year-old woman with a history of coronary artery disease, hypertension, and diabetes mellitus is admitted with chest pain. Increased troponin levels and the electrocardiogram confirm an acute myocardial infarction. She continues to have chest pain despite maximal medical therapy, and angiography is scheduled. Her medications include lisinopril, metoprolol, atorvastatin, insulin, and aspirin. Laboratory values include the following: creatinine 1.2 mg/dL, sodium 138 mEq/L, and potassium 4.5 mEq/L. Urinalysis showed a protein osmolality ratio of 0.87, an osmolality of 530 mOsm/L, and unremarkable microscopic findings. To prepare this patient for angiography, what would you do?

    a. Discontinue use of lisinopril and begin giving saline for hydration.
    b. Discontinue use of lisinopril and begin giving a bicarbonate infusion.
    c. Discontinue use of aspirin.
    d. Discontinue use of aspirin and begin giving a bicarbonate infusion.
    e. Discontinue use of lisinopril and aspirin and begin giving saline for hydration.

11. The same 76-year-old woman in question 10 undergoes angiography. Twenty-four hours after the angiography, her creatinine level increased from 1.2 mg/dL to 1.9 mg/dL. Forty-eight hours after the angiography, her creatinine level was 2.4 mg/dL and her urine output was markedly decreased. On physical examination, her blood pressure was 115/55 mm Hg and her pulse was 60 beats per minute. The patient is awake and alert. She has a 2/6 systolic murmur, minimal crackles in her lungs bilaterally at the bases, livedo reticularis over the mid abdomen and bilateral flanks, and trace edema in her extremities, with mottled toes and a dusky right first toe. Other laboratory findings 48 hours after the angiography include the following: urinalysis showing an osmolality of 320 mOsm/kg, 4 to 10 RBCs/hpf, 4 to 10 white blood cells (WBCs)/hpf, occasional granular casts, and occasional hyaline casts; serum sodium 138 mEq/L; potassium 4.3 mEq/L; and blood urea nitrogen (BUN) 43 mg/dL. In addition to the above laboratory findings, which findings would be most consistent with the cause of this patient's acute renal failure?

    a. Increased erythrocyte sedimentation rate (ESR), decreased levels of complement, and eosinophiluria
    b. Increased ESR, normal levels of complement, and increased ratio of BUN to creatinine
    c. Increased ESR, dysmorphic RBCs on urine microscopy, and decreased levels of complement
    d. Low fractional excretion of urea, normal levels of complement, and low level of spot urinary sodium
    e. Absence of eosinophiluria and peripheral eosinophilia; increased levels of creatine kinase and myoglobin.

12. A 34-year-old male weight lifter was involved in a motor vehicle accident and has multiple fractures of both legs from being trapped beneath his car. You are asked to evaluate his decreased urine output. On physical examination, the patient has been intubated, ventilated, and sedated. He has casts on both legs and a neck stabilizer. There are large ecchymoses along his left flank and chest. Present medications include ceftriaxone, famotidine, and a furosemide drip. Laboratory

values include the following: hemoglobin 10.2 g/dL, WBC count 10.9 × 10^9/L, platelets 192 × 10^9/L, creatinine 2.9 mg/dL, BUN 58 mg/dL, potassium 4.5 mEq/L, phosphorus 9 mg/dL, calcium 8.0 mg/dL, and creatine kinase 30,000 U/L. Urinalysis results were as follows: brown appearance, osmolality 300 mOsm/kg, pH 5.5, 21 to 30 RBCs/hpf, 4 to 11 WBCs/hpf, occasional granular casts, and occasional epithelial casts. What is the most likely cause of his acute renal failure?

a. Prerenal azotemia
b. Acute tubular necrosis
c. Acute tubular interstitial nephritis due to antibiotics
d. Acute glomerulonephritis
e. Rhabdomyolysis

13. A 66-year-old man is transferred for evaluation and treatment of acute pancreatitis. During the first 36 hours, he has required 10 L of normal saline to help stabilize his blood pressure. Despite fluid resuscitation and intravenous pressor support, his blood pressure remains 70/40 to 80/40 mm Hg. You are asked to evaluate his acute renal failure. On physical examination, the patient has been intubated, ventilated, and sedated. He has anasarca. On auscultation of his lungs and heart, he has bilateral rales and no rub. His abdomen is tender and distended. Laboratory test results include sodium 139 mEq/L, potassium 5.1 mEq/L, calcium 7.9 mg/dL, phosphorus 5.4 mg/dL, bicarbonate 17 mEq/L, creatinine 3.8 mg/dL, and BUN 82 mg/dL. Urinalysis showed osmolality of 320 mOsm/kg, pH 5.5, 1 to 3 RBCs, occasional granular casts, occasional epithelial casts, and occasional hyaline casts. Spot urinary sodium is 75 mEq/L. Fractional excretion of sodium is 3.6%. Which of the following would you recommend?

a. Give 1 ampule of bicarbonate.
b. Give a 1-L bolus of lactated Ringer solution.
c. Begin slow continuous venovenous hemodiafiltration.
d. Administer sodium polystyrene sulfonate, 30 g.
e. Begin intermittent high-flux dialysis to remove 1 L/h for 3.5 hours.

14. A 62-year-old woman with a history of urolithiasis, insulin-dependent diabetes mellitus for 20 years, and hypertension for 10 years returns to see you for a blood pressure check. Four weeks ago, furosemide, 10 mg daily, was added to her blood pressure therapy of metoprolol, 25 mg twice daily, and lisinopril, 20 mg daily. She now reports decreased urine output during the past week, nausea, and light-headedness whenever she stands up quickly. She also states that her chronic lower extremity edema has disappeared. On physical examination, she appears fatigued. On auscultation, her lungs are clear and she has a 1/6 systolic ejection murmur. In her abdomen, a midline bruit is present. Her extremities have no edema. She also states that she has begun taking ibuprofen for her low back pain. Clinical data are shown in the accompanying table.

Feature	1 Month Ago	Present
Weight, kg	75.3	70
Blood pressure, mm Hg	152/89	102/62
Pulse, per min	62	62
Creatinine, mg/dL	1.4	2
BUN, mg/dL	29	82
Potassium, mEq/L	4.4	5
Bicarbonate, mEq/L	24	24
Urine osmolality, mOsm/kg	360	570
Protein osmolality ratio	0.14	0.19
pH	5.4	5.4
Microscopy	Normal	Occasional hyaline casts
Urinary sodium, mEq/L	...	9

What is the most likely cause of her renal failure?

a. Obstruction due to ureteral calculi
b. Acute tubulointerstitial nephritis secondary to furosemide
c. Diabetic nephropathy
d. Type 4 renal tubular acidosis
e. Prerenal azotemia

15. A 74-year-old man has developed metabolic consequences while undergoing aggressive diuresis in the cardiac care unit for severe ischemic cardiomyopathy. He has lost more than 6 kg of weight since admission. Currently, his vital signs are stable, with a blood pressure of 100/60 mm Hg and a pulse rate of 100 beats per minute. His lungs are clear, and he no longer has a third heart sound (S$_3$) gallop. His extremities are not edematous. He is comfortable while receiving oxygen at 2 L/min, but he does complain of feeling fairly weak. Current laboratory test results are as follows: sodium 145 mEq/L, potassium 2.2 mEq/L, chloride 90 mEq/L, bicarbonate 36 mEq/L, BUN 88 mg/dL, creatinine 1.8 mg/dL, magnesium 1.7 mg/dL, urinary sodium <8 mEq/L, urinary chloride <15 mEq/L, arterial blood gas pH 7.55, PaO$_2$ 80 mm Hg, PaCO$_2$ 55 mm Hg, saturation 98%. What would you do next?

a. Give acetazolamide, 250 mg intravenously (IV), every 8 hours.
b. Give 0.1 normal hydrochloric acid, 20 mmol IV, immediately.
c. Give a bolus of 2 L 0.9% saline IV.
d. Aggressively correct the potassium chloride deficit to keep potassium >4 mEq/L, and consider IV magnesium supplementation.
e. Immediately arrange an endocrinology consultation to rule out hyperaldosteronism.

16. A 56-year-old diabetic woman with a history of stable angina and congestive heart failure presents with fatigue, malaise, and dyspnea. Her previous medication regimen included β-blockers, ACE inhibitors, spironolactone, NPH insulin, and digoxin.

She fell last week, resulting in low back pain for which she has been taking ibuprofen, 600 mg 3 times daily, for the past several days. While in the emergency department, she develops hypotension; the monitor shows a rather bizarre, wide-complex, bradycardiac rhythm. After ensuring airway and IV access, what is the most appropriate step?

a. Give calcium chloride or calcium gluconate IV immediately.
b. Give heparin IV, aspirin, and β-blocker IV.
c. Administer a sodium polystyrene sulfonate (Kayexalate) retention enema immediately.
d. Give digoxin IV.
e. Give amiodarone IV.

17. A 17-year-old male patient is noted to be polyuric (6 L urine daily) while recuperating from an emergency appendectomy. The operation was uncomplicated, and he is awake, alert, and oriented but very thirsty. His blood pressure is 90/60 mm Hg, and his pulse rate is 100 beats per minute. He has not had anything to eat or drink since he was admitted to the hospital. His mother says, "He seems to always be drinking at home." The patient's serum sodium level has increased from 144 mEq/L on admission to 155 mEq/L during the past 36 hours. He has been receiving 0.45% saline solution IV at 125 mL/h. Which of the following would be most consistent with this patient's clinical status?

a. Urine osmolality 50 mOsm/L, urinary sodium 10 mEq/L
b. Urine osmolality 250 mOsm/L, urinary sodium 75 mEq/L
c. Urine osmolality 450 mOsm/L, urinary sodium 75 mEq/L
d. Urine osmolality 500 mOsm/L, urinary sodium 150 mEq/L
e. Urine osmolality 800 mOsm/L, urinary sodium 400 mEq/L

18. A 28-year-old homeless man is found unconscious by the police near an abandoned apartment building. A jug containing greenish fluid is found near him. Test results from the emergency department are as follows: sodium 140 mEq/L, potassium 4.5 mEq/L, chloride 110 mEq/L, bicarbonate 8 mEq/L, BUN 38 mg/dL, creatinine 1.9 mg/dL, glucose 100 mg/dL, pH 7.22, $PaCO_2$ 22 mm Hg, PaO_2 89 mm Hg, and plasma osmolality 350 mOsm/L. Crystals are noted on urinalysis. What would you do next?

a. Begin infusion of an alcohol dehydrogenase competitive inhibitor (ethanol or fomepizole).
b. Begin preparation for emergency dialysis.
c. Begin infusion of an isotonic bicarbonate drip.
d. Order a toxin screen.
e. Administer activated charcoal via a nasogastric tube.

19. A 28-year-old nursing home assistant presents for evaluation of fatigue, malaise, and weakness. She has been unable to work due to weakness. She also reports thirst, aching joints, and a "gritty" sensation involving both eyes. Laboratory results are as follows: sodium 135 mEq/L, potassium 1.2 mEq/L, chloride 118 mEq/L, bicarbonate 10 mEq/L, BUN 12 mg/dL, and cre-

atinine 1.2 mg/dL. Arterial blood gas shows pH 7.28 and $PaCO_2$ 25 mm Hg. Urinalysis shows pH 6.6, urinary sodium 35 mEq/L, urinary potassium 30 mEq/L, and urinary chloride 50 mEq/L. What should be your next recommendation?

a. Order a diuretic screen.
b. Order a psychiatric consultation for bulimia.
c. Order stool electrolytes.
d. Begin giving sodium bicarbonate 450-mEq tablets, 2 by mouth 4 times daily.
e. Initiate potassium repletion followed by potassium citrate.

20. A 78-year-old woman has a subarachnoid hemorrhage and is admitted to the neurologic intensive care unit. Standard therapy has begun, including large volumes of isotonic crystalloid, dobutamine, and albumin infusions. She is provided with mechanical ventilation, sedated, and given intravenous nimodipine. Her serum sodium level steadily decreases from 138 mEq/L on admission to 108 mEq/L 60 hours later. This decrease has occurred despite large amounts of intravenous normal saline solution administered parenterally. Her vital signs are stable, with a blood pressure of 150/92 mm Hg and a pulse rate of 78 beats per minute. She has no signs of volume contraction, and her weight has increased 2 kg since admission. Her lungs are clear, and there is no peripheral edema. Laboratory results are as follows: serum osmolality 250 mOsm/L, urine osmolality 370 mOsm/L, urinary sodium 125 mEq/L, serum creatinine 0.5 mg/dL, and uric acid 1 mg/dL (reference range, 2.3-6 mg/dL). Serum cortisol and sensitive thyrotropin levels are within the reference ranges. What is the best therapeutic approach?

a. Calculate the sodium deficit, and plan replacement of 75% of the shortfall over 12 hours.
b. Discontinue use of all IV fluids.
c. Administer a vasopressin drip.
d. Calculate free water excess, with careful administration of hypertonic saline, and perhaps administer a loop diuretic.
e. Order a CT scan of the chest to rule out malignancy.

21. A 38-year-old woman presents to the emergency department with dyspnea and disorientation. She has a history of extensive small-bowel resections for recurrent enteric fistulas due to Crohn disease. She is currently taking prednisone, 10 mg daily, and azathioprine, 75 mg daily. No other medications or supplements have been used. On physical examination, her blood pressure is 130/70 mm Hg, her pulse rate is 90 beats per minute, her respiratory rate is 38 breaths per minute, and she is afebrile. Her lungs are clear. Cardiac examination findings are normal. Her abdomen is soft, and there are multiple scars across the abdomen, which are all well healed. She has an intact ileostomy. Examination of the lower extremities shows no cyanosis or trauma. Laboratory test results are as follows: sodium 135 mEq/L, potassium 4 mEq/L, chloride 110 mEq/L, bicarbonate 10 mEq/L, BUN 18 mg/dL, creatinine 0.8 mg/dL, and serum osmolality 286 mOsm/L. Serum lactate is normal. Arterial blood gas results are pH 7.19, PaO_2 100 mm Hg, $PaCO_2$ 23 mm Hg, and saturation

98%. Urinalysis shows no crystals or other abnormalities. A urinary drug screen is negative. What would you do next?

a. Infuse 3 ampules of sodium bicarbonate IV immediately, and seek a surgical consultation.
b. Administer norepinephrine to keep mean arterial pressure >120 mm Hg.
c. Give sodium citrate, 30 mmol 3 times daily by mouth.
d. Begin an oral bowel decontamination regimen.
e. Immediately seek a nephrology consultation for initiation of continuous venovenous hemodiafiltration for bicarbonate support.

22. A 38-year-old man with no prior history of kidney stones has Roux-en-Y bypass surgery to reduce his weight of 150 kg. One year later, he has lost 50 kg and has passed his first kidney stone. Which abnormality would you most expect to find in his 24-hour urine collection?

a. Hypercalciuria
b. Cystinuria
c. Hyperoxaluria
d. Hyperphosphaturia
e. Hyperuriocosuria

23. A 24-year-old man with recurrent idiopathic calcium oxalate kidney stones requires a percutaneous lithotripsy to remove kidney stones. Which anatomical abnormality would the urologist most likely see?

a. Benign cyst
b. Diffuse hemorrhage
c. Collecting duct stones
d. Papillary necrosis
e. Randall plaques

24. A 26-year-old female farmer has a solitary parathyroid adenoma surgically removed, followed by bilateral percutaneous stone removal. Postoperative radiographs show no residual stones. Nine months later she is shocked to learn that she has a large right renal staghorn calculus. The left kidney remains stone free. Urinalysis shows high urine pH, pyuria, and bacteriuria. What is the stone's composition?

a. Calcium oxalate
b. Calcium phosphate
c. Cystine
d. Struvite
e. Uric acid

25. A 52-year-old obese patient with type 2 diabetes mellitus begins passing multiple recurrent rust-colored stones from both kidneys. CT shows bilateral large stone, but radiography of the kidneys, ureters, and bladder (KUD) shows no stones. What is the best drug to treat this patient's stones?

a. Antibiotic
b. Potassium citrate
c. Magnesium
d. Neutral phosphate
e. Thiazide

26. A 17-year-old male student presents with his first renal colic. He reports a positive kidney stone history in multiple members of his father's family. His 24-hour urine supersaturation study shows supersaturation in the calcium oxalate crystal system. His urinary calcium excretion is 512 mg in 24 hours. In addition to diet and fluid changes, what stone preventive medication do you recommend?

a. Allopurinol
b. Potassium citrate
c. Magnesium
d. Neutral phosphate
e. Thiazide

27. A 34-year-old obese welfare recipient is disabled by multiple symptoms that do not suggest a single cause. She is referred to you for evaluation of chronic abdominal pain and a history of kidney stones. Analysis of a recently passed stone shows silica. What is your diagnosis?

a. Cystinuria
b. Enteric hyperoxaluria
c. Hypercalciuria
d. Malingering
e. Primary hyperoxaluria

28. A petite 27-year-old woman with recurrent kidney stones is referred to you for preventive therapy. Her 24-hour urine supersaturation study shows supersaturation in all crystal systems. What therapy do you recommend first?

a. Allopurinol
b. Hydration
c. Low-calcium diet
d. Potassium citrate
e. Thiazide

29. An 18-year-old woman has intractable migraine headaches. She is taking topiramate for prophylaxis. She presents to your office with her first calcium phosphate kidney stone. Her family history is negative for stones, and she is otherwise healthy. Her only other medication is an oral contraceptive. What stone prevention treatment do you recommend?

a. Calcium carbonate
b. Stopping use of the oral contraceptive
c. Potassium citrate
d. Stopping use of topiramate
e. Thiazide

Answers

1. Answer b.
This patient presents with rapidly progressive glomerulonephritis. In patients older than 60 years, the most common cause (80% of cases) is a pauci-immune crescentic glomerulonephritis (ie, ANCA-associated vasculitis). Myeloma kidney does not present with an active urinary sediment. Acute interstitial nephritis is a possibility, but there is no mention of drug intake or skin rash. Similarly, classical polyarteritis nodosa does not present with glomerulonephritis. Although systemic lupus erythematosus could be part of the differential diagnosis, this option is not included in the answers. Testing for ANCA is correct.

2. Answer e.
This 35-year-old patient with well-controlled type 1 diabetes mellitus and no retinopathy is very unlikely to have diabetic nephropathy. In addition, proteinuria correlates well with a decline in kidney function. Thus, if proteinuria of 8g in 24 hours was due to diabetic nephropathy, it would be unlikely that the serum creatinine level would be normal. Therefore, other causes of nephrotic syndrome must be ruled out. This includes performing a renal biopsy.

3. Answer e.
The patient presents with Goodpasture syndrome. Evidence clearly demonstrates that patients are most likely to have a response with the administration of high-dose corticosteroids, oral cyclophosphamide, and a course of plasmapheresis. Plasmapheresis is most useful in limiting the pulmonary hemorrhage and its sequelae.

4. Answer a.
The most common cause of nephrotic syndrome in African Americans is focal segmental glomerulosclerosis. In white adults, membranous nephropathy is the most common cause. IgA nephropathy is the most common cause worldwide of nephritic syndrome.

5. Answer e.
The aim is to identify long-term complications of immunosuppressive therapy such as, in this case, bladder cancer due to prolonged use of cyclophosphamide. Relapse of Wegener granulomatosis in the absence of positive ANCA testing (MPO/PR3) is extremely unusual.

6. Answer d.
Secondary causes of membranous nephropathy are detected in up to 30% of adult cases; hence, ruling out such cases is part of the standard of care in evaluating patients with newly diagnosed membranous nephropathy. The most common causes of secondary membranous nephropathy are carcinomas (lung, kidney, colon), autoimmune (systemic lupus erythematosus), infections (hepatitis B and C), and drugs (nonsteroidal anti-inflammatory drugs). Infectious endocarditis is not associated with membranous nephropathy.

7. Answer d.
Minimal change nephropathy is the commonest cause of nephrotic syndrome in children. Relapses are common and proteinuria is highly selective. In children, a confirmation renal biopsy is not required unless a patient has no response to corticosteroids. Serum complement levels are normal in minimal change disease.

8. Answer b.
The most likely diagnosis is hepatorenal syndrome. His risk factors include chronic liver disease with cirrhosis, low serum and urinary sodium levels at baseline, and hypotension. Most likely, his acute gastrointestinal tract bleeding was the precipitating factor leading to hepatorenal syndrome. Other causes such as prerenal azotemia need to be ruled out. His urinalysis results are not consistent with acute interstitial nephritis, acute hemolysis, or heme pigment nephrotoxicity. There is nothing to suggest acute hemolysis or heme pigment nephrotoxicity in his history. Abdominal compartment syndrome, when present, usually occurs with a very tense abdomen. Bladder pressures help rule out abdominal compartment syndrome.

9. Answer d.
The first line of treatment for hepatorenal syndrome is to ensure adequate intravascular volume. Fluid challenges are indicated and central hemodynamic monitoring can be helpful. After intravascular volume has been repleted, other drugs such as octreotide, N-acetylcystine, albumin, and terlipressin or misoprostol have been used to increase systemic vasoconstriction. Dopamine does not increase renal perfusion. Hypertonic saline is not indicated in this patient, and furosemide drip would be ineffective or, if effective, would further decrease intravascular volume.

10. Answer b.
The most appropriate recommendation would be to discontinue use of lisinopril and begin giving a bicarbonate infusion. There is no reason to stop use of aspirin. Certainly the patient should be well hydrated, but the patient's use of aspirin does not need to be discontinued and the patient should receive bicarbonate. Discontinuing use of β-blockers is not needed before administering the contrast dye.

11. Answer a.
This patient has had a shower of cholesterol emboli to her kidneys. Findings consistent with that cause of acute renal failure include an increased ESR, decreased levels of complement, eosinophiluria, and peripheral eosinophils. Renal injury from emboli is irreversible.

12. Answer e.
This patient is at high risk of rhabdomyolysis due to his crush injuries. Clues on examination, in addition to his multiple fractures, are the large ecchymoses along his right flank and chest. Classic electrolyte abnormalities with rhabdomyolysis include hyperkalemia, hyperphosphatemia, and hypocalcemia. Hypouricemia may develop and metabolic acidosis can occur. The findings on

urinalysis can be consistent with acute tubular interstitial nephritis, but no eosinophils were noted. Acute pyelonephritis can be associated with granular casts, WBCs, and RBCs on urinalysis, but there is nothing else in the history to indicate acute pyelonephritis. Prerenal azotemia is not consistent with a urine osmolality of only 300 mOsm/kg. This could be acute tubular necrosis, but the clinical presentation more strongly points to rhabdomyolysis.

13. Answer c.

This patient has acute renal failure most likely due to a systemic inflammatory response syndrome secondary to acute pancreatitis. This is associated with massive peripheral vasodilatation and third spacing of fluids. The patient would not tolerate intermittent dialysis because of his hemodynamic instability. Sodium polystyrene sulfonate would decrease his serum levels of potassium but would not improve his other electrolyte imbalances. Lactated Ringer solution should not be given because his potassium levels are increased. Bicarbonate infusion may temporarily improve his metabolic acidosis, but that is not indicated in this situation. The patient would benefit most from slow continuous venovenous hemodiafiltration, during which electrolyte disturbances can be corrected and the fluid gradually removed without large fluid shifts.

14. Answer e.

The patient's physical examination findings are consistent with intravascular volume depletion with a significant decrease in weight and blood pressure. The ratio of BUN to creatinine is increased. Urine osmolality is increased and the spot urinary sodium is very low. All these findings are consistent with prerenal azotemia. The urinalysis results are not consistent with acute tubular interstitial nephritis. There is nothing to indicate obstruction due to ureteral calculi. This decline in renal function is much too rapid to be attributed solely to diabetic nephropathy.

15. Answer d.

This patient has a classic case of contraction alkalosis. His CO_2 retention is expected as a result of his elevated bicarbonate levels. Treatment requires correction of his severe potassium deficiency with a chloride salt. This will facilitate tubular excretion of bicarbonate and restore homeostasis. Often in patients with severe potassium depletion, serum magnesium levels should be checked, and magnesium replaced as appropriate. Acetazolamide (a carbonic anhydrase inhibitor) may be necessary when further diuresis is required without correcting the primary problem (severe ischemic cardiomyopathy). However, in this case it is certainly appropriate to correct the electrolyte deficiencies as the initial step.

16. Answer a.

This patient has severe hyperkalemia, which needs to be treated immediately with IV calcium chloride to stabilize the cardiac conduction system. Next, IV furosemide, or perhaps Kayexalate, may be necessary. IV dextrose and insulin as well as bicarbonate may be of use. For anuria or renal failure, emergent initiation of dialysis may be preferable after immediate stabilization.

17. Answer a.

This patient has previously unrecognized diabetes insipidus. *Polyuria* is defined as urine output of more than 3 L daily. Since the body needs to excrete nearly 10 mOsm of solute per kilogram daily, one can quickly determine whether the diuresis is a solute or water diuresis. A water diuresis would suggest diabetes insipidus. Solute diuresis may be secondary to renal functional disorders or may be appropriate with massive amounts of retained solute (postobstructive renal failure). Repletion of the free water deficit is mandatory, and when the patient is able to take oral liquids, he should be able to keep up with his water losses.

18. Answer a.

This patient has ingested ethylene glycol, as evidenced by the high anion gap metabolic acidosis, the osmolar gap, and the crystalluria (calcium oxalate). The initial management step is to inhibit further metabolism of ethylene glycol into its toxic metabolite, glycolic acid. Forced diuresis and consideration of dialysis may then take place.

19. Answer e.

This patient has sicca complex and renal tubular acidosis, most likely due to Sjögren syndrome, as shown by the inappropriate positive urinary net charge (urinary anion gap). The urinary net charge is the sum of the urinary spot sodium and urinary potassium minus the urinary chloride. The urinary chloride concentration should be high in the case of a normally functioning nephron owing to the acid titration of hydrogen ions as ammonium ions (NH_4^+). Because ammonium has a positive charge, the ammonium is accompanied into the urine by chloride, maintaining electroneutrality. Repletion of potassium is foremost in these situations, however, because a potentially disastrous exacerbation of this patient's hypokalemia may occur with base supplementation alone. Note that diuretic abuse often leads to hypokalemia but not to metabolic acidosis, except in cases of carbonic anhydrase inhibitor ingestion.

20. Answer d.

This patient has syndrome of inappropriate antidiuresis. The seemingly elevated urinary sodium levels are explained by the patient's euvolemic condition: excess sodium is excreted in this euvolemic situation. Cerebral salt wasting is very rarely documented in patients with this syndrome and is differentiated by a consistently negative sodium balance inducing volume contraction and hypotension. Generally, it is prudent to correct hyponatremia at the rate at which it occurred; however, keeping the total daily correction less than 12 mEq/L daily is best. Because it is difficult to ascertain this patient's mental status, one must assume that the severe hyponatremia is causing cerebral manifestations and needs to be treated aggressively.

21. Answer d.

This patient has severe D-lactic acidosis. Note that standard serum lactate levels are not useful for detecting D-lactic acidosis. This condition is caused by overgrowth of small-bowel bacteria in blind loops. Decontamination of the small bowel, by oral or intravenous antimicrobial therapy, is the treatment of choice.

22. Answer c.

Bariatric surgery typically increases urinary oxalate by 1 year post-operatively. Excretion of other urinary analytes typically decreases owing to decreased intestinal absorption.

23. Answer e.

Randall plaques are the precursors of idiopathic calcium stones. Stones clogging the collecting duct openings on the renal papillae are seen in other stone-forming conditions.

24. Answer d.

The rapid unilateral recurrence of a staghorn stone is highly suggestive of struvite, especially in the presence of high urine pH and urinalysis sediment suggestive of a urinary tract infection. Recurrent hyperparathyroidism should cause bilateral stone formation without findings of infection.

25. Answer b.

Persons with type 2 diabetes mellitus form an unusually high percentage of uric acid stones. The characteristic finding is that uric acid stones are radiolucent on KUB radiography and radiodense on CT. Alkalizing the urine to pH 6.5 not only helps prevent uric acid urolithiasis by treating the hyperaciduria, but it may also dissolve renal stones. Although the use of allopurinol usually is not as effective as alkalizing very acidic urine, it may be helpful for patients with hyperuricosuria and for dissolving stones.

26. Answer e.

Severe familial hypercalciuria is most specifically treated with a thiazide. Other causes of calcium oxalate stones include hypercalciuria, idiopathic hypercalciuria, other hypercalciuric states, hyperuricosuria, hyperoxaluria, and decreased excretion of inhibitors of crystallization. Medications include potassium citrate for hypocitraturia, neutral phosphates for idiopathic calcium urolithiasis (but not in cases of urinary tract infection or renal insufficiency), thiazides for hypercalciuria (sodium must be restricted), and allopurinol for hyperuricosuria. Primary hyperoxaluria is the most aggressive stone disease. Treatment includes fluids, pyridoxine (alters glycine metabolism, an oxalate precursor), neutral phosphates, or liver transplant.

27. Answer d.

Silica, which occurs in sand, is not a component of human kidney stones.

28. Answer b.

When all the crystal systems are supersaturated, it is highly unlikely that multiple metabolic abnormalities exist. A simpler answer is that the patient has a very low urine volume; hence, increase the fluid intake to increase the urine output to more than 2.5 L daily.

29. Answer d.

Topiramate is an increasingly popular migraine treatment that causes calcium phosphate kidney stones in 1% to 2% of the people who use it. It acts by inhibiting carbonic anhydrase and creating renal tubular acidosis. Other causes of calcium phosphate stones include primary hyperparathyroidism, distal renal tubular acidosis, medullary sponge kidney, and the use of absorbable alkali.

19

Neurology

Brian A. Crum, MD
Eduardo E. Benarroch, MD
Robert D. Brown, Jr., MD

Part I—General Principles for Interpreting Neurologic Symptoms

Introduction

Neurologic disorders are commonly encountered in general clinical practice (about 10% of patients of primary care physicians in the United States have neurologic disorders, and about 25% of inpatients have a neurologic disorder as a primary or secondary problem). Because of the aging population, cerebrovascular disorders, dementias, and Parkinson disease are becoming more prevalent. Understanding a patient with neurologic disease depends on localizing the problem on the basis of the medical history and examination findings, considering a differential diagnosis, and correlating the clinical findings with abnormalities found on appropriate diagnostic testing.

* About 10% of patients of primary care physicians in the United States have neurologic disorders.
* About 25% of inpatients have a neurologic disorder as a primary or secondary problem.
* Primary care physicians should have a good working knowledge of common and emergency neurologic problems.

Neurologic Signs and Symptoms

General Categories

Neurologic signs and symptoms can be subdivided into 4 general categories:
1. Ill-defined, nonspecific, nonanatomical, and nonphysiologic regional or generalized symptoms
2. Diffuse cerebral symptoms
3. Positive focal symptoms (hyperactivity)
4. Negative focal symptoms (loss of function)

Ill-Defined Symptoms

Ill-defined symptoms include such things as vague dizziness, diffuse or unusual regional pain, diffuse and unusual numbness, vague memory problems, and unusual gait. Generally, no serious underlying neurologic problem is identified, especially if the symptoms are long-standing. Many patients have a serious underlying psychopathologic disorder, but often the patient either does not recognize this or denies it. However, remember that a psychiatric diagnosis should be made when psychologic factors are present and not because the physical examination and laboratory findings are normal.

* With ill-defined symptoms, no serious underlying problem is identified in most patients.
* Many of these patients have an underlying psychopathologic condition.
* Establish a psychiatric diagnosis on the basis of positive psychologic factors, not because the physical examination and laboratory findings are normal.

Diffuse Cerebral Symptoms

Diffuse cognitive problems occur in dementia and acute confusional states. Another common diffuse symptom is syncope or presyncope, which usually implies diffuse and not focal cerebral ischemia. Vasovagal syncope is the major culprit, especially in the young. Syncope is not a transient ischemic attack (TIA), which is a focal event. Most causes of syncope are systemic (ie, cardiogenic), not neurologic. In primary autonomic dysfunction, other neurologic signs and symptoms usually help make the diagnosis (eg, bladder or erectile dysfunction, peripheral neuropathy, sweating changes, parkinsonian features, and diabetes).

* Dementia and acute confusional states are due to diffuse cerebral disease.
* Syncope or presyncope implies diffuse, not focal, cerebral ischemia.
* Syncope is not a TIA.

- Systemic, not neurologic, problems usually cause syncope.

Positive Phenomena

Positive sensory phenomena include paresthesia (tingling or prickling) and pain. Positive motor phenomena include tremor and tonic or clonic movement of muscles. Lights, flashes, sparkles, and formed images are examples of positive visual phenomena. An example of a positive language phenomenon is unusual vocalization. Positive symptoms can be from central nervous system (CNS) disease such as seizures or migraine accompaniments (eg, flashing lights or squiggly lines). Positive phenomena occur from peripheral nervous system (PNS) disease due to nerve irritation, damage, and repair.

Negative Phenomena

Negative phenomena usually indicate damage to a specific area of the nervous system. Examples include weakness, numbness, speech difficulty, and blindness. TIAs and strokes usually produce negative phenomena; if there is more than 1 symptom, all the symptoms tend to appear at the same time. Migraines may have positive and negative phenomena; if there is more than 1 symptom, the symptoms tend to begin one after another and build up. Damage to the PNS leads to negative phenomena in regions supplied by the specific peripheral structure.

- TIAs and strokes produce negative phenomena.
- Migraines have positive and negative phenomena.

Localization

The neurologic history and examination findings are combined to clarify the localization of the disorder to the following 4 levels: supratentorial (cerebral cortex and subcortical regions, including the basal ganglia, hypothalamus, and thalamus); posterior fossa (cerebellum, brainstem, and cranial nerves); spinal cord (including extramedullary, intramedullary, cauda equina, and conus medullaris lesions); and peripheral (Table 19-1). Peripheral lesions may be localized further from proximal to distal: radiculopathy, plexopathy, peripheral neuropathy, neuromuscular junction, and muscle. Some disorders, however, are multifocal. From the signs and symptoms, the lesion is determined to be on the right or left side or bilateral. Next a determination is made of whether the process is diffuse (affecting a whole level), focal, or multifocal. Then the temporal profile is considered: acute (seconds to hours), subacute (days to weeks), or chronic (several months to years). In addition, the course is

Table 19-1 Localization of Neurologic Disorders

Level
Supratentorial
Posterior fossa
Spinal cord
Peripheral
Extent
Focal
Diffuse

important: progressive, static, improving, or relapsing. It is then possible to consider the most likely disease categories (vascular, infectious, inflammatory, neoplastic, etc) and to refine the differential diagnosis for the lesion and outline the diagnostic procedures, therapeutic options, and patient counseling.

- The history and examination dictate localization to the level and side of the nervous system.
- The temporal profile is then used to determine a differential diagnosis.

Findings in the Elderly

Examination of healthy elderly persons may show the following signs that cannot be considered pathologic when present in isolation:

1. Decreased acuity of the special senses: olfaction, audition, and vision
2. Decrease in upward gaze, visual pursuit, and saccadic function
3. Abnormal gait with reduced arm swinging, shorter steps, and slow walking speed
4. Difficulty with balance, with wider base and unsteady turns
5. Decreased vibratory sensation in the feet
6. Decreased pupillary response to light
7. Atrophy of the small muscles of the hand
8. Decreased or absent ankle reflexes

In addition, in most healthy elderly people some neurodiagnostic studies may appear abnormal, including spondylitic abnormalities visible on radiography, magnetic resonance imaging (MRI), or computed tomography (CT). White matter abnormalities on brain MRI are not uncommon. They are referred to as *leukoariosis* or *small vessel ischemic changes*. Slowing on electroencephalography (EEG) and slowing of nerve conduction velocities on electrophysiologic testing can occur.

- Age must be kept in mind when interpreting certain neurologic examination abnormalities.
- Most healthy elderly people have spondylitic abnormalities visible on plain cervical and lumbar radiographs and MRI as well as white matter changes on brain MRI.

General Principles of Neurologic Diagnostic Testing

CT and MRI

Vascular Diseases

CT is a good initial test for evaluating a patient with suspected TIA or stroke because it can quickly identify acute hemorrhage in brain parenchyma or the subarachnoid space (Table 19-2). CT (even with contrast enhancement) often gives equivocal or negative results in the first 24 to 48 hours after an ischemic cerebral infarction. In these situations, an MRI is the first neuroimaging test to show abnormalities during evolution of an ischemic cerebral infarct. With diffusion and perfusion MRI scanning, cerebral infarction or ischemia can be delineated early after the onset of symptoms, usually before CT shows any abnormality. In subacute and chronic stages of an ischemic cerebral infarction, MRI and CT provide equivalent information.

Table 19-2 Comparison of Computed Tomography (CT) and Magnetic Resonance Imaging (MRI) for Neurologic Imaging

CT Preferred	MRI Preferred
Evaluation of suspected acute hemorrhage	Evaluation of subacute & chronic hemorrhage
Evaluation of skull fractures	Evaluation of ischemic stroke
Evaluation of meningiomas	Evaluation of posterior fossa & brainstem tumors & lesions
Assessment of hydrocephalus	Diagnosis of multiple sclerosis
	Evaluation of the spinal cord

Vasculitic lesions or microinfarcts, as in systemic lupus erythematosus, are often seen on MRI but missed on CT. Subacute and chronic intracerebral hemorrhages are better defined by MRI, especially with gradient echo MRI, which is capable of identifying acute blood as well as old hemosiderin.

Magnetic resonance angiography (MRA) is not invasive and has replaced standard angiography for many indications. It is quite sensitive in defining the degree of stenosis in the carotid or vertebrobasilar system. However, MRA does not adequately evaluate more distal intracranial arteries, and arteriography is required for this indication. MRA is also used as a screening study for aneurysms. Arteriography still may be needed to examine the anatomical details of aneurysms or vascular malformations. CT angiography (CTA) has become another sensitive test for determination of vascular disease and anatomical features.

* For evaluating acute hemorrhage in the brain and subarachnoid space, CT is better than standard MRI.
* During evolution of an acute ischemic cerebral infarct, MRI is better than CT.
* For evaluating subacute and chronic stages of an ischemic cerebral infarct, CT and MRI are equivalent.
* MRA and CTA are useful noninvasive studies to evaluate for vascular pathology.

Trauma

MRI is competitive with but not comparable to CT for assessing the brain after craniocerebral trauma. Acutely after injury, CT is preferable because the examination time is shorter. Standard radiographic examination or CT is necessary to evaluate skull fractures because bone cortex is not visualized with MRI.

CT is highly dependable for demonstrating subdural hematomas, which are also visualized with MRI. Coronal MRI sections are usually best for visualizing the size, shape, location, and extent of subdural hematomas. MRI can show changes from diffuse axonal injury that are not visible on CT. This is often the pathologic substrate for mental status changes or coma after head trauma when intracerebral hemorrhage is excluded.

In adults and children with traumatic brain injury, recovery from unconsciousness is unlikely after 12 months. Recovery is rare after 3 months in adults and children with nontraumatic brain injury.

* Acutely after traumatic head injury, CT of the brain is recommended to exclude intracranial hemorrhage and skull fracture.
* CT is dependable for showing subdural hematomas.
* MRI, not CT, will detect diffuse axonal injury.

Intracranial Tumors

A wide spectrum of intracranial tumors is visualized with MRI and CT. Often MRI shows more extensive involvement (of 1 lesion or multiple smaller lesions) than CT, especially in gliomas or metastasis. CT with contrast and MRI with gadolinium are both excellent for detecting meningiomas. MRI is far superior to CT for identifying all types of posterior fossa tumors. It is the study of choice for identifying brainstem gliomas.

* MRI is favored over CT for the evaluation of tumors because it shows more anatomical detail and allows detection of smaller lesions.
* MRI is superior to CT for identifying posterior fossa tumors and brainstem gliomas.

White Matter Lesions

MRI is superior to CT in detecting abnormalities of the white matter. MRI is far superior to CT for identifying multiple sclerosis lesions (most commonly periventricular white matter lesions, often perpendicular to the lateral ventricles) and for assessing patients who have isolated optic neuritis. MRI shows that multi-infarct dementia (with multiple white matter infarcts) may be a common cause of adult-onset dementia. However, white matter changes in the elderly must be interpreted carefully because MRI shows changes in the white matter of most normal elderly persons.

* MRI is the test of choice in multiple sclerosis with periventricular white matter lesions, often perpendicular to the lateral ventricles, being the most common finding.
* MRI shows changes in the white matter of most normal elderly persons.

Spinal Cord

A wide spectrum of lesions at the cervicomedullary junction and in the spinal cord can be seen clearly with MRI because direct sagittal and coronal sections can be made with this imaging method. Thus, MRI is the study of choice for assessing the cervicomedullary junction and spinal cord. Generally, MRI is better than CT for identifying intramedullary and extramedullary lesions of the spinal cord. CT can be helpful if bony detail is important (eg, fractures and spurs).

* MRI is superior to CT for assessing the cervicomedullary junction and spinal cord lesions.

Dementia

In assessing dementia, either CT or MRI can demonstrate potentially fixable lesions (ie, subdural hematoma, brain tumor, or hydrocephalus), but MRI is more sensitive for determining the presence of multiple infacts in muti-infarct dementia. MRI can assess atrophy more accurately, especially in the mesial temporal lobes, a common finding in Alzheimer disease (AD). This is best viewed with a thin-slice coronal imaging technique.

Disk Disease
Protruding disks are well visualized on MRI sagittal sections, which show the relation of the disk to the spine and nerve roots. MRI is equal to CT myelography for evaluating herniated disks at cervical and thoracic levels, but at the lumbar level, MRI is better than CT myelography. In spinal stenosis, MRI and CT are roughly equivalent and less invasive than myelography.

* MRI sagittal sections show protruding disks.
* For evaluating cervical and thoracic herniated disks, MRI is equal to CT myelography, but MRI is better at the lumbar level.

Electromyography and Nerve Conduction Studies
Electromyography (EMG) and nerve conduction studies (NCS) should be performed by experts familiar with the intricacies of the procedure and who know its value and limitations. NCS involve shocking nerves and measuring certain electrophysiologic variables (amplitude of responses, conduction velocity, and distal latencies). EMG is performed by inserting a small needle into the muscle and recording electrical activity at rest and with light muscle contraction. These tests are excellent for detecting motor unit problems and, thus, are valuable for identifying diseases of the anterior horn cell, nerve root, peripheral nerve, neuromuscular junction, and muscle. They also assess the large-fiber sensory peripheral nervous system. They give no information, however, on small-fiber function, which requires specific testing of the autonomic nerves and sweating pathways. By helping to localize and to better define further diagnostic studies, EMG and NCS are an extension of the neurologic examination.

* NCS and EMG should be performed by experts.
* NCS and EMG are valuable for identifying motor unit problems—anterior horn cell, nerve root, neuromuscular junction, and muscle—as well as large-fiber sensory problems.
* NCS and EMG do not assess small-fiber function.

Electroencephalography
EEG is used mainly to study seizure disorders, but EEG is specific in only a few forms of epilepsy, such as typical absence epilepsy. A seizure disorder, or epilepsy, is a clinical diagnosis and not an EEG diagnosis, and a normal EEG does not rule out epilepsy. EEG has many nonspecific patterns that should not be overinterpreted.

Ambulatory EEG is available for detecting frequent unusual spells. EEG telemetry with video monitoring is helpful in defining epileptic surgical candidates, nonepileptic spells (pseudoseizures), and unusual seizures. EEG is imperative in diagnosing nonconvulsive status epilepticus.

* EEG is specific in only a few forms of epilepsy, including typical absence epilepsy.

* Epilepsy is a clinical diagnosis, not an EEG diagnosis.
* A normal EEG does not rule out epilepsy.
* EEG telemetry is helpful in defining epileptic surgical candidates, nonepileptic spells, and unusual seizures.

EEG is valuable for evaluating various encephalopathies. Many drugs cause an unusual fast pattern, and most metabolic encephalopathies cause a diffuse slow or triphasic pattern. Diffuse slow patterns are seen also in degenerative cerebral disease (AD). Unusual high-amplitude sharp wave activity helps define Creutzfeldt-Jakob disease and subacute sclerosing panencephalitis. EEG is often valuable in diagnosing certain infectious encephalopathies (eg, herpes simplex encephalitis).

EEG is essential for diagnosing various sleep disorders and is an *adjuvant* tool for diagnosing brain death. Brain death is a clinical diagnosis. EEG may be used as a monitoring device in surgery (eg, during carotid endarterectomy).

By 24 to 48 hours after a hypoxic insult, the EEG assists in predicting the likelihood of neurologic recovery. Poor outcome is seen with "alpha" coma, burst suppression, periodic patterns, and electrocerebral silence.

* EEG is valuable in diagnosing certain infectious encephalopathies (eg, herpes simplex encephalitis).
* EEG is an adjuvant tool for diagnosing brain death.
* Brain death is a clinical diagnosis.

Evoked Potentials
Evoked potentials indicate the intactness of various afferent pathways: visual evoked potentials, somatosensory evoked potentials, brainstem auditory evoked potentials, and motor evoked potentials. These tests have limited clinical use, mainly in multiple sclerosis and myelopathies. They are excellent monitoring devices for spinal surgery and posterior fossa surgery (monitoring spinal cord and cranial nerve function intraoperatively), and they may be useful for substantiating nonorganic disease, for example, hysterical paraplegia or hysterical blindness.

* Evoked potentials are used during intraoperative monitoring of neurologic function and also in some cases of multiple sclerosis and myelopathies.
* Evoked potentials may be useful for substantiating nonorganic disease (eg, hysterical paraplegia or hysterical blindness).

Lumbar Puncture and Cerebrospinal Fluid Analysis
Perform lumbar puncture only after a thorough clinical evaluation and after consideration of the potential value versus the hazards of the procedure. Imaging of the brain (CT or MRI) is mandatory if there is any suspicion of a CNS process.

Indications for Lumbar Puncture
Urgent lumbar puncture is performed for suspected acute meningitis, encephalitis, or subarachnoid hemorrhage (unless preceding CT findings indicate otherwise) and for fever (even without meningeal signs) in infancy, acute confusional states, and neurologic manifestations in immunocompromised patients. Other indications for

lumbar puncture are unexplained subacute dementia, multiple sclerosis, peripheral neuropathy, and headache.

When multiple sclerosis is suspected, if the cerebrospinal fluid (CSF) cell count is greater than 50/mcL, look for another disease (eg, sarcoidosis). Although IgG synthesis is increased in multiple sclerosis, this finding is nonspecific. The demonstration of oligoclonal bands is useful, but they also occur in other inflammatory diseases of the CNS.

Lumbar puncture is used to assess CSF pressure. High pressure occurs with pseudotumor cerebri (idiopathic intracranial hypertension) and low pressure with CSF hypovolemia from a CSF leak.

Lumbar puncture is indicated in cases of neurologic complications of infectious diseases, including acquired immunodeficiency syndrome (AIDS), Lyme disease, and any suspected acute, subacute, or chronic infection (viral, bacterial, or fungal).

Other indications for lumbar puncture are meningeal carcinomatosis, selected indications in non-Hodgkin lymphoma, and certain neuropathies (Guillain-Barré syndrome, acute inflammatory demyelinating polyneuropathy, and chronic inflammatory demyelinating polyradiculopathy).

There is no difference in headache frequency after immediate mobilization or after 4 hours of bed rest following lumbar puncture. Spinal headache depends on the size of the needle used and the leakage of CSF through a dural rent or tear. A 20-gauge needle is recommended.

Contraindications for Lumbar Puncture

Suppuration in the skin and deeper tissues overlying the spinal canal and anticoagulation therapy or bleeding diathesis are contraindications for lumbar puncture. A minimum of 1 or 2 hours should elapse between lumbar puncture and initiation of heparin therapy. If the platelet count is less than 20×10^9/L, transfuse platelets before performing a lumbar puncture. The use of aspirin is not a contraindication to lumbar puncture. Use of other antiplatelets, such as clopidogrel, may increase the risk of bleeding, and if it is possible to safely discontinue use of the drug for 5 to 7 days before performing the lumbar puncture, that is ideal.

Increased intracranial pressure due to a focal mass lesion is a contraindication. Lumbar puncture is dangerous when papilledema is due to an intracranial mass, but it is safe (and has been used therapeutically) in pseudotumor cerebri. In complete spinal block or stenosis, lumbar puncture may aggravate the signs of spinal cord disease.

- Perform lumbar puncture only after a thorough clinical evaluation.
- Increased IgG synthesis and oligoclonal banding in the CSF are nonspecific findings, but they are most suggestive of multiple sclerosis.
- CSF pressure is high in pseudotumor cerebri (idiopathic intracranial hypertension).
- CSF pressure is low with CSF hypovolemia.
- Lumbar puncture is dangerous when an intracranial mass is present, with or without papilledema.
- Lumbar puncture is safe in pseudotumor cerebri and it is therapeutic.

- Lumbar puncture aggravates the signs of spinal cord disease in complete spinal block.

Part II—General Principles From the Level of the Cerebral Cortex Through the Neuraxis to Muscle

Supratentorial Level: Symptoms and Clinical Correlations

The supratentorial region includes all levels of the nervous system inside the skull and above the tentorium cerebelli (ie, the top of the cerebellum). Symptoms and signs related to disorders of the cerebral cortex may lead to alterations in cognition and consciousness. Unilateral neurologic symptoms involving a single neurologic symptom (such as numbness [sensory system] or weakness [motor system]) commonly localize to the cerebral cortex. Abnormalities of speech and language are localized to the dominant cerebral hemisphere (typically the left side, even in most left-handers), whereas abnormalities of the nondominant hemisphere may lead to visuospatial deficits, confusion, or neglect of the contralateral side of the body. Abnormalities in the subcortical region may lead to weakness or numbness; they typically involve more than 1 limb. Abnormalities in the basal ganglia may lead to movement disorders, including tremor, bradykinesia (as in Parkinson disease), and chorea (as in Huntington disease). Disorders of the thalamus, another subcortical structure, typically cause unilateral sensory abnormalities, language problems, and cognitive changes. The hypothalamus is important in many functions that affect everyday steady-state conditions, including temperature, hunger, water regulation, sleep, endocrine functions, cardiovascular functions, and regulation of the autonomic nervous system. Cortical and subcortical abnormalities may also lead to visual system deficits, usually homonymous visual defects of the contralateral visual field.

Disorders of Consciousness

Consciousness has 2 dimensions: arousal and cognition. *Arousal* is a vegetative function maintained by the brainstem and medial diencephalic structures. *Cognition*—learning, memory, self-awareness, and adaptive behavior—depends on the functional integrity of the cerebral cortex and associated subcortical nuclei.

Coma or unconsciousness results from either bilateral dysfunction of the cerebral cortex or dysfunction of the reticular activating system in the upper brainstem (ie, above the middle level of the pons). *Unconsciousness* implies global or total unawareness; *coma* implies the lack of both wakefulness and awareness.

- Coma implies the lack of both wakefulness and awareness.

Brain Death

Brain death is the absence of function of the cerebral cortex and brainstem. This is diagnosed by showing lack of brainstem reflexes: pupillary response, corneal reflexes, oculocephalic (doll's eye) and oculovestibular (cold caloric) reflexes, gag reflex, and spontaneous respiration. Confirmatory tests include EEG, somatosensory evoked potentials, and angiography.

Minimally Conscious State

The minimally conscious state is a condition of severely altered consciousness in which minimal but definite behavioral evidence of self-awareness or environmental awareness is demonstrated. It is a disorder of limited responsiveness in which patients retain awareness, but their responses are so deficient that the evidence of their awareness may be difficult to detect. The minimally conscious state is distinguished from the vegetative state by the presence of behaviors associated with conscious awareness. The minimally conscious state may be a temporary state in a continuum from coma to vegetative state to minimally conscious state to normalcy, or, unfortunately, it may also be a permanent state. It is most important in young people with traumatic brain injury to recognize the minimally conscious state early in the course of the disease since it carries a better prognosis than the vegetative state. However, the prognosis of either of these conditions depends on the age of the patient, the duration of the condition, and the cause (traumatic brain injury in the young carries the best prognosis, whereas hypoxic/ischemic or hypoglycemic brain injury at any age carries the worst).

Persistent Vegetative State

Persistent vegetative state is the absence of cerebral cortex function with normal brainstem function (deafferentated state). The patient has no detectable awareness and no purposeful interaction with the environment but, unlike a patient in a coma, is wakeful and has sleep-wake cycles.

Locked-in Syndrome

Locked-in syndrome is normal cerebral cortex function with absence of brainstem function. The lesion usually is in the pons and causes quadriplegia and the inability to speak, swallow, and move the eyes horizontally (ie, the de-efferentated state). The patient, however, is wakeful and aware but is unable to communicate verbally because of the neurologic deficits. Often, though, these patients can communicate with eye blinks and vertical eye movements. This can also occur with severe neuromuscular weakness, such as in myasthenia gravis, Guillain-Barré syndrome, and botulism.

Stupor and Coma

For a person to stay awake, the cerebral hemispheres and reticular activating system must be intact. Patients with dysfunction of only 1 cerebral hemisphere have a focal neurologic deficit but are awake. Patients with a large unilateral cerebral lesion may go into stupor or coma if the lesion causes shifting and pressure changes in other parts of the brain, such as the opposite hemisphere or brainstem. These patients can have focal neurologic signs. Patients with brainstem lesions that directly affect the ascending reticular activating system are in coma but, again, have focal signs. Persons who feign coma have no focal signs, no abnormal reflexes, normal caloric responses, and a normal EEG. They account for a small percentage of patients with stupor and coma. The most common, potentially reversible causes of stupor and coma are toxic, metabolic, and infectious problems that affect both cerebral hemispheres diffusely (the famed "toxic/metabolic encephalopathy"). Thus, most patients in stupor or coma have an underlying systemic problem.

- Large unilateral cerebral lesions that cause a shift and pressure changes in the other hemisphere or brainstem produce focal neurologic signs together with coma.
- Brainstem lesions that cause coma also produce focal signs.
- Persons who feign coma have no focal signs, no abnormal reflexes, normal caloric responses, and a normal EEG.
- The most common reversible causes of stupor and coma are toxic, metabolic, and infectious diseases.

Patients with toxic/metabolic encephalopathies have changes in mental status and awareness before going into stupor or coma, but they typically have no focal neurologic signs. Corneal reflexes are lost early in the disease, but pupillary reflexes remain. Ocular motility tested by the doll's eye maneuver (oculocephalic reflexes) and the cold caloric response (oculovestibular reflex) are fully intact, at least early in the disease.

- Patients with systemic encephalopathies typically have no focal signs.

Acute Confusional States

Acute confusional state is malfunction of the cerebral cortex and reticular activating system. Acute confusional states are abrupt, of recent onset, and often associated with fluctuations in the state of awareness and cognition. They are manifested by confusion, inattention, disorientation, and delirium. Thus, patients may be inattentive, dazed, stuporous, restless, agitated, or excited and may have marked autonomic dysfunction and visual and tactile hallucinations. Abnormal motor manifestations are common, including paratonia, asterixis, tremor, and myoclonus. The usual etiologic factors of acute confusional states are toxic, metabolic, traumatic, infectious, organ failure of any sort, or ictal or postictal encephalopathies. Three large categories of primary causes for acute confusional states are systemic, neurologic, and psychophysiologic. Withdrawal states from alcohol, benzodiazepines, and barbiturates are also important causes of acute confusion or delirium.

- Three general causes of acute confusional states are systemic, neurologic, and psychophysiologic.

Dementia

Dementia is chronic malfunction of the cerebral cortex or subcortical structures (or both) with normal function of the brainstem. It is a clinical state characterized by a marked loss of function in multiple cognitive domains not due to an impaired level of arousal. Besides memory, other higher cognitive functions are impaired, including visuospatial, calculation, language, judgment, personality, and motor planning. The presence of dementia does not necessarily imply irreversibility, a progressive course, or any specific disease. Dementia is not a disease but an entity with various causes (Table 19-3).

A small percentage of patients have reversible causes of dementia. These include medication-induced causes, depression, thyroid disease, CNS infections, vitamin deficiencies, and structural brain lesions (eg, neoplasms, subdural hematomas, and symptomatic hydrocephalus).

● Dementia itself is not a disease; it is the potential result of many different diseases.

AD is the most common cause of dementia. It occurs in both young and old persons and is no longer subcategorized into "presenile" and "senile" types. Generally, patients present first with difficulties of memory, but eventually difficulties develop in several cognitive areas, including aphasia, apraxia, or agnosia. The patients also have various behavioral and psychiatric manifestations, and some may have myoclonus or akinesia. AD is not simply diffuse atrophy of the brain but a regionally specific illness that first affects hippocampal structures and acetylcholine-producing neurons.

Mild cognitive impairment (MCI) consists of memory loss that is clearly evident at bedside testing but does not interfere with everyday function. MCI represents a very early stage of dementia. In about 50% of patients, MCI progresses to AD over a 4-year period, and MCI progresses to AD in almost all patients eventually. MRI, with focus in the temporal lobes, may detect atrophy early in the mesial temporal lobe of patients with MCI at risk of AD. The apolipoprotein E (*APOE*) ε4 genotype also predicts a higher likelihood of AD, although the test is rarely done clinically since it adds little to a thorough history, examination, neuropyschometric testing, and MRI. In fact, most people with *APOE* ε4 will not end up having AD. Noncompetitive reversible cholinesterase inhibitors, such as donepezil (see below), may slow the progression and delay the onset of outright dementia in patients with MCI, most of whom have underlying AD pathology.

There is treatment for AD (Table 19-4). Some symptoms of AD are thought to be due to partial depletion of acetylcholine in the brain. Currently available, centrally active, noncompetitive reversible cholinesterase inhibitors, including donepezil, rivastigmine, and galantamine, may improve symptoms slightly and slow the decline of cognitive function. Donepezil is given once daily, whereas rivastigmine and galantamine are taken twice daily after meals. Tacrine, the first anticholinesterase agent used for the treatment of AD, may cause hepatotoxicity and is now rarely prescribed. The main side effects of these drugs are nausea, vomiting, and diarrhea. Donepezil is administered at bedtime but may cause vivid dreams, requiring that the dose be taken in the morning. Treatment with these drugs is continued until dementia reaches severe stages. The therapy should not be discontinued abruptly because the result may be abrupt cognitive deterioration. Vitamin E is also used in AD, although its efficacy in slowing the rate of progression is not clearly defined. Given the recent concern over increased mortality among patients taking vitamin E, some physicians have abandoned this treatment. A standard dose of 400 international units is probably safe.

Another mechanism for damage to neurons in AD is through excitotoxicity by glutamate. Memantine is an *N*-methyl-D-aspartate antagonist thought to reduce glutamate excitotoxicity, and it has been shown to slow the progression of cognitive dysfunction in AD. The combination of memantine and donepezil can slow the disease even more in severe AD. For donepezil, the usual dosage is 10 mg daily and for memantine, 10 mg twice daily.

Another common degenerative dementia is diffuse Lewy body disease. Patients with this disease typically exhibit parkinsonism, fluctuations of cognitive function, visual hallucinations, and rapid eye movement sleep behavior disorder. Antipsychotic medications may trigger a neuroleptic malignant-type syndrome in these patients. Cholinesterase inhibitors may improve hallucinations and other symptoms. Patients with a frontotemporal dementia such as Pick disease exhibit difficulties with executive function, inappropriate behavior, and aphasia.

Normal-pressure hydrocephalus (NPH) is a potentially reversible cause of cognitive dysfunction. The typical triad includes dementia, a

Table 19-3 Differential Diagnosis of Dementia

Potentially reversible dementias
   Metabolic-toxic disorders
      Vitamin B_{12} deficiency
      Hypothyroidism
      Alcoholism
   Structural lesions
      Normal-pressure hydrocephalus
      Subdural hematoma
      Neoplasm
      Vascular dementia
   Infections
      Chronic meningitis
      Neurosyphilis
      HIV dementia
Cryptococcal meningitis
   Inflammatory/immune disorders
      Vasculitis
      Limbic/paraneoplastic encephalitis
      Hashimoto/autoimmune encephalopathy
Gluten sensitivity
   Multiple sclerosis
Degenerative dementias
   Alzheimer disease
   Diffuse Lewy body disease
   Frontotemporal dementia (including Pick disease)
   Huntington disease
   Progressive supranuclear palsy
Prion-related disorders
   Creutzfeldt-Jakob disease

Abbreviation: HIV, human immunodeficiency virus.

Table 19-4 Pharmacologic Therapy in Alzheimer Disease

Cholinesterase inhibitors
   Donepezil, 5-10 mg daily
   Rivastigmine, 6 mg twice daily
   Galantamine, 12 mg twice daily
Glutamate antagonist
   Memantine, 10 mg twice daily

gait disorder, and urinary incontinence, although sometimes only the first 2 components are present. A shuffling, magnetic ("feet stuck to the floor") gait is most common. CT or MRI shows disproportionate enlargement of the ventricular system without any obstructive lesions. Removal of 30 mL of CSF, leading to improvement in the gait disorder, may predict a response to ventriculoperitoneal shunting, although through the years no clear predictive factors for shunting success have emerged. Unfortunately, shunting is not a benign procedure, and up to a third of patients eventually have complications, such as infection, hemorrhage, or failure of the shunt.

A typical diagnostic work-up for dementia may include a complete blood cell count, electrolyte survey and blood chemistry profile (including calcium, glucose, blood urea nitrogen, and creatinine), liver function tests, thyroid function tests, serum level of vitamin B_{12}, and serologic testing for syphilis. In selected patients, erythrocyte sedimentation rate, human immunodeficiency virus (HIV) testing, paraneoplastic antibody screening, chest radiography, urine collection for heavy metals, and toxicology screens should be performed. Also occasionally evaluated are antinuclear, extractable nuclear antigen, thyroid peroxidase (TPO), endomysial, and tissue transglutaminase antibodies. Neuroimaging should be done in all persons with dementia. MRI is preferred, although CT can exclude structural (and possibly reversible) causes of dementia (eg, NPH, tumor, subdural hematoma, and strokes). MRI has the advantage of detecting atrophy in mesial temporal lobes and hippocampal structures in AD. Neuropsychometric testing may also be considered, especially in mild or questionable cases. Lumbar puncture is indicated for persons who have had recent onset of symptoms, persons younger than 55 years who have dementia, and those with immunosuppression, possible CNS infection, reactive serum syphilis serologic findings, or metastatic cancer without findings on an imaging study. EEG may be useful in evaluating for Creutzfeldt-Jakob disease. In these patients, fluid-attenuated inversion recovery (FLAIR) MRI techniques can detect abnormalities in the cerebral cortex, basal ganglia, or thalamus when the findings of a standard MRI study are negative. The presence of increased levels of 14-3-3 protein in the CSF, although a nonspecific finding, strongly supports the diagnosis of Creutzfeldt-Jakob disease.

Typical Clinical Scenarios

* AD: A 70-year-old patient has had progressive loss of recent memory over the past 2 years. Mental status testing shows poor recall and learning with calculation, information, and language errors. The results of laboratory tests are normal. MRI shows moderate cerebral atrophy but no specific lesions.
* Multi-infarct dementia: An elderly patient with known coronary artery disease and hypertension has progressive memory loss, slowed movements and responses, and difficulty walking. Deep tendon reflexes of the left side are brisk. The results of routine laboratory tests and CSF examination are normal. MRI shows multiple infarcts in both cerebral hemispheres.
* Creutzfeldt-Jakob disease: A 60-year-old patient has had rapidly progressive dementia and myoclonic jerks over several months. The EEG shows unusual high-amplitude sharp waves. FLAIR MRI shows increased signal intensity in the cerebral cortex and basal

ganglia. The results of routine laboratory tests and CSF examination are normal, except for an increased level of 14-3-3 protein, which is highly supportive of the diagnosis.

Seizure Disorders

Seizure refers to electroclinical events, and *epilepsy* indicates a tendency for recurrent seizures. A classification of seizures is given in Table 19-5.

The proper treatment of epilepsy depends on accurate diagnosis of the seizure type, identification of the cause (if possible), and management of psychosocial problems. The EEG (preferably after the patient is sleep deprived) can be important in the classification of seizure type. MRI is also used to evaluate for focal or structural lesions. Much of the diagnosis rests on a supportive history. The presence of an aura and a period of altered mental status after the spell (postictal confusion) is highly suggestive of an epileptic seizure. The EEG is also important in deciding whether to treat a first unprovoked seizure. The risk of recurrent seizures is high if the initial EEG shows epileptiform activity and low if the EEG is normal.

Causes

Seizures occur at any age, but approximately 70% of all patients with epilepsy have their first seizure before age 20. Age distribution for the onset of epilepsy is bimodal, with the second most common group being the elderly population. Both the cause and the type of epilepsy are related to age at onset. However, the cause may not be

Table 19-5 Classification of Seizures

Partial (focal) seizures
    Simple partial seizures
        Partial simple sensory
        Partial simple motor
        Partial simple special sensory (unusual smells or tastes)
        Speech arrest or unusual vocalizations
    Complex partial seizures
        Consciousness impaired at onset
        Simple partial onset followed by impaired consciousness
    Evolving to generalized tonic-clonic convulsions (secondary generalized tonic-clonic seizures)
        Simple evolving to generalized tonic-clonic
        Complex evolving to generalized tonic-clonic (including those with simple partial onset)
    True auras—are actually simple partial seizures
Generalized seizures—convulsive or nonconvulsive (primary generalized seizures—generalized from onset)
    Absence and atypical absence
    Myoclonic
    Clonic
    Tonic
    Tonic-clonic
    Atonic
Unclassified epileptic seizures (includes some neonatal seizures)

found in many patients. Neonatal seizures are often due to congenital defects or prenatal injury, and head trauma is often the cause of focal seizures in young adults. Brain tumors and vascular disease are major known causes of seizures in later life. Seizures often occur during withdrawal from alcohol, barbiturates, or benzodiazepines in young and old adults. Seizures also occur with the use of drugs such as cocaine, usually in young adults. Metabolic derangements (eg, hypoglycemia, hypocalcemia, hyponatremia, and hypernatremia) can occur at any age, as can infections (eg, meningitis and encephalitis). Metabolic abnormalities usually cause primary generalized tonic-clonic seizures and rarely focal or multifocal seizures. CNS infections usually cause partial and secondary generalized tonic-clonic seizures.

Pseudoseizures (ie, psychogenic, nonepileptic seizures) are sudden changes in behavior or mentation not associated with any physiologic cause or abnormal paroxysmal discharge of electrical activity from the brain. They are often the cause of so-called intractable seizures. Effective treatment is elusive. A favorable outcome may be associated with an independent lifestyle, the absence of coexisting epilepsy, and a formal psychologic approach to therapy.

- Up to 70% of patients with epilepsy have their first seizure before age 20, although the fastest growing population with epilepsy is the elderly.
- The cause and type of epilepsy are related to age at onset.
- Head trauma is a major cause of focal seizures in young adults.
- Brain tumors and vascular disease are major causes of seizures in older persons.
- Seizures occur with withdrawal from alcohol, barbiturates, and benzodiazepines.
- Seizures occur during the use of cocaine (usually in young adults).
- Pseudoseizures are often the basis of so-called intractable seizures.

Anticonvulsant Therapy

Drugs used to treat seizures are listed in Table 19-6. Monotherapy is the treatment of choice. The dosage of the drug may be increased as high as necessary and to as much as can be tolerated. The coadministration of antiepileptic drugs has not been shown to have more antiseizure efficacy than the administration of only 1 drug without concurrently increasing toxicity. In studies of a large population, 1 particular drug may be shown to be more efficacious and less toxic, but for a given patient, an alternate drug may be more effective or have fewer side effects. The classic antiepileptic drugs are phenobarbital, phenytoin, carbamazepine, valproic acid, benzodiazepines, and ethosuximide. Simple and complex partial seizures are most likely to be controlled with phenytoin and carbamazepine, whereas secondary generalized tonic-clonic seizures respond equally well to carbamazepine, phenytoin, or valproic acid. Phenobarbital is equally efficacious but less well tolerated because of sedative side effects. Idiopathic generalized epilepsy with absence seizures is well controlled with ethosuximide. Valproic acid controls all forms of generalized seizures. Extended-release formulations are available for carbamazepine and valproic acid, and a rectal formulation is available for diazepam.

The newer anticonvulsant drugs include gabapentin, tiagabine, lamotrigine, topiramate, felbamate, zonisamide, oxcarbazepine, and levetiracetam. These agents generally have less potential for drug interactions and fewer side effects than the older drugs. They are indicated as add-on therapy for partial seizures. Felbamate, oxcarbazepine, and levetiracetam are also used as single-drug therapy for partial seizures. Felbamate, lamotrigine, and topiramate are also used as monotherapy for generalized seizures. Because the efficacy, high cost, and dosing schedule (twice daily) are similar for most of these new anticonvulsants, tolerability is frequently the major determinant in choosing a particular drug.

Anticonvulsants have both neurologic and systemic side effects. Dose-initiation side effects such as fatigue, dizziness, incoordination, and mental slowing are common in most patients and can be prevented with slow introduction of the drug. Dose-related side effects may limit the use of a particular drug in a given patient. A dose-related side effect common to most drugs is cognitive impairment. Other neurologic side effects include cerebellar ataxia (phenytoin), diplopia (carbamazepine), tremor (valproic acid), and chorea or myoclonus (phenytoin and carbamazepine). Idiosyncratic side effects are rare, unpredictable, severe, and sometimes life-threatening. Idiosyncratic and systemic side effects are listed in Table 19-7.

Table 19-6 Guidance for Use of Antiepileptic Drugs

Criteria	Possibilities	Drug
Type of seizures	GTCSs	PHT, CBZ, VPA, lamotrigine, topiramate
	Partial seizures with or without secondary GTCSs	PHT, CBZ, VPA, PB, lamotrigine, topiramate, zonisamide, levetiracetam
	Absence seizures	Ethosuximide, VPA, lamotrigine
	Myoclonic seizure	VPA, clonazepam, lamotrigine, zonisamide
	Atonic, akinetic, or mixed	VPA, felbamate, topiramate, lamotrigine
Use of other drugs metabolized in the liver	Use drugs that do not affect metabolism of other drugs	Gabapentin, tiagabine, lamotrigine, zonisamide, levetiracetam
Avoidance of oral contraceptive pill failure	Use drugs with no or minimal effect on contraceptive metabolism	VPA, clonazepam, gabapentin, tiagabine, lamotrigine, zonisamide, levetiracetam

Abbreviations: CBZ, carbamazepine; GTCS, generalized tonic-clonic seizure; PB, phenobarbital; PHT, phenytoin; VPA, valproic acid.

Many antiepileptic drugs are metabolized in the liver and are responsible for important drug interactions. Liver enzyme inducers such as carbamazepine, phenobarbital, phenytoin, primidone, oxcarbazepine, felbamate, and topiramate increase metabolism and decrease the efficacy of oral contraceptives in preventing pregnancy. Valproic acid and felbamate are enzyme inhibitors and increase the levels of other anticonvulsants. Gabapentin has the advantage of fewer drug interactions because it is eliminated primarily by renal excretion. It may be safer than other anticonvulsants in the management of seizures in patients with porphyria.

Special issues must be considered when managing epilepsy in pregnancy. Seizure control is attempted first with monotherapy, with the lowest possible dose of anticonvulsant and monitoring of drug levels. There is risk of fetal hemorrhage at delivery if the mother is taking phenytoin, phenobarbital, or carbamazepine. This risk can be minimized by administering vitamin K to the mother before delivery and to the fetus at delivery. Offspring of women with epilepsy are at increased risk of intrauterine growth retardation, minor abnormalities (eg, digit hypoplasia and craniofacial abnormalities), major malformations (eg, neural tube defects and cardiac malformations), microcephaly, cognitive dysfunction, and infant death. Various combinations of these findings, referred to as *fetal anticonvulsant syndrome*, have been described with virtually all anticonvulsants but most commonly with valproic acid. The risk of fetal malformation is about 2% in the general population, about 10% (with a risk of neural tube defects of 1%-2%) among patients receiving valproic acid, and about 3% among patients receiving other antiepileptic drugs. Multiple drugs at high doses generally are associated with a greater frequency of anomalies. Valproic acid and, to a lesser extent, carbamazepine are selectively associated with increased risk of neural tube defects. Valproic acid has also been associated with lower IQ in children exposed in utero during the first trimester.

All women with epilepsy and childbearing potential should receive folate supplementation of at least 0.4 mg daily (although dosages up to 4 mg daily have been recommended by some physicians, especially when there is a family history of newborns with neural tube defects). Prenatal screening should be offered to all women with epilepsy to detect any fetal malformation. The key is pregnancy planning. By the time a woman knows she is pregnant, any neural tube defect most likely already exists; thus, in most women with epilepsy of childbearing age, 2 forms of contraceptive are advocated. Before a woman attempts to get pregnant, folic acid supplementation is crucial and review of medications and optimal seizure control is vital. It is important to remember that for the vast majority of patients with epilepsy under treatment, the result of a pregnancy is a normal baby.

- The treatment of choice is monotherapy.
- Essentially all anticonvulsant drugs have the potential to cause developmental abnormalities.
- Valproic acid (and, to a lesser extent, carbamazepine) is associated with a higher likelihood of birth defects than the other anticonvulsants.

When to Start and When to Stop Anticonvulsant Therapy

Decisions about when to start and stop anticonvulsant therapy are difficult and there is simply no easy algorithm to rely on. The decision to begin anticonvulsant therapy after a first seizure should be individualized for each patient. The decision depends on the risk of additional seizures, the risk of seizure-related injury, the loss of employment or driving privileges, and other psychosocial factors.

Table 19-7 Systemic Side Effects of Antiepileptic Drugs

Side Effect	Drug Most Commonly Involved
Skin rash & Stevens-Johnson syndrome	10% risk with lamotrigine, CBZ, or PHT
	5% risk with other AEDs, least with VPA
	Topiramate & zonisamide are contraindicated for patients with allergy to sulfa drugs
Liver failure	Highest risk with VPA & felbamate
	Risk increased in infants with mental retardation & receiving polytherapy, with underlying metabolic disease or poor nutritional status
Bone marrow suppression	Highest risk with felbamate & CBZ
Gum hypertrophy, hirsutism, acne, osteoporosis	Phenytoin
Weight gain, hair loss, tremor	VPA
Weight loss	Felbamate, topiramate
Headache, insomnia	Felbamate
Behavioral & cognitive disturbances	Barbiturates, benzodiazepines, topiramate, levetiracetam
Kidney stones	Topiramate, zonisamide
Hyponatremia	CBZ or oxcarbazepine
Atrioventricular conduction defect	CBZ, PHT
Neural tube defect	VPA > CBZ, but all AEDs are potentially teratogenic

Abbreviations: AED, antiepileptic drug; CBZ, carbamazepine; PHT, phenytoin; VPA, valproic acid.

An important decision is whether a single generalized tonic seizure is provoked, for example, by sleep deprivation, alcohol, or concurrent illness. After the first seizure, the risk of recurrence ranges from 30% to 60%, with higher risks for patients with an abnormal EEG and a remote symptomatic cause (Table 19-8). After a second seizure, the risk of recurrence increases to 80% to 90%.

For many patients who have been seizure-free for 1 to 2 years, anticonvulsant therapy can be discontinued. The benefit of discontinuing therapy should be weighed against the possibility of seizure recurrence and its potential adverse consequences. In adults, relapse occurs in 26% to 63% of patients within 1 to 2 years after therapy is discontinued. Predictors of relapse are an abnormal EEG before or during medication withdrawal, abnormal findings on neurologic examination, frequent seizures before entering remission, or mental retardation. To lessen the chance of seizures after discontinuing therapy, withdrawal should not proceed faster than a 20% reduction in dose every 5 half-lives.

Typical Clinical Scenarios

- Absence seizures: A child has abrupt episodes of staring and unresponsiveness that last <10 seconds and are associated with complete recovery and no postictal abnormalities. These episodes occur several times a day, but otherwise the child appears normal. The diagnosis is absence seizure, for which ethosuximide or valproic acid is effective.
- Seizure due to an intracranial neoplasm: An elderly patient with a history of recent headaches has a generalized seizure. He has a 50-pack-year history of smoking but no previous history of a seizure disorder. Chest radiography shows a 2-cm mass in the left upper lobe of the lung. Brain metastases should be included in the differential diagnosis. Neuroimaging is indicated to establish the diagnosis.
- Drug-induced agranulocytosis: A neutropenic fever develops 1 month after a patient starts taking carbamazepine for a seizure disorder. The absolute neutrophil count is 1.0×10^9/L. Treatment is discontinuation of carbamazepine and use of an alternative anticonvulsant. The neutropenic fever should be managed with antibiotics.

Table 19-8 Risk Factors for Recurrence After the First Seizure

Age >60 y
No precipitating factor identified (eg, no sleep deprivation or
  alcohol use)
Partial seizure
Abnormal neurologic examination
Abnormal electroencephalogram (spikes or nonspecific)
Abnormal imaging study
Other factors
  Family history of seizures (in first-degree relative)
  History of febrile seizures
  Onset during sleep
  Postictal Todd paralysis
Occupational risk

- Interaction with oral contraceptives: A young woman with a chronic seizure disorder that has been well controlled with phenytoin for several years indicates that she has become pregnant despite taking birth control pills. The oral contraceptives have been rendered ineffective because of induction of liver enzymes by phenytoin. Lamotrigine, gabapentin, and levetiracetam do not induce liver enzymes as much and are good choices for women with a seizure disorder who take oral contraceptives.

Anticonvulsant Blood Levels

Measurement of anticonvulsant blood levels is readily available and helps attain the best control of seizures. It is extremely important to remember that therapeutic levels represent an average bell-shaped curve and that patients with well-controlled seizures are included under the bell-shaped curve. Seizures are well controlled in many patients who have anticonvulsant blood levels below or above the therapeutic range. The anticonvulsant dose should *never* be changed on the basis of blood levels alone. Remember, toxicity is a clinical phenomenon, *not* a laboratory phenomenon.

- Therapeutic levels represent an average bell-shaped curve.
- The dose of anticonvulsant should never be changed on the basis of blood levels alone.
- Toxicity is a clinical phenomenon, not a laboratory phenomenon.

If a patient with epilepsy under treatment has breakthrough seizures, several things need to be considered. These include compliance issues; excessive use of alcohol or other recreational drugs; psychologic and physiologic stress (eg, lack of sleep or anxiety); a combination of the preceding; systemic disease of any type, organ failure of any type, or systemic infection; a new cause of seizures (eg, neoplasm); newly prescribed medication, including other anticonvulsants (ie, polypharmacy) and over-the-counter drugs; toxic levels of anticonvulsants (with definite clinical toxicity); pseudoseizures; progressive CNS lesion not identified previously with neuroimaging or lumbar puncture; and no cause found. If no cause is found, anticonvulsant doses must be readjusted or the drug replaced with another one.

Surgery for Epilepsy

With improved technology, the anatomical site of seizure origin can be identified more accurately. Also, technical advances have made surgical management safer. Of the 150,000 patients in whom epilepsy develops each year, 10% to 20% have "medically intractable epilepsy."

Brain surgery is an alternative therapy if treatment with antiepileptic drugs fails. However, before seizures are deemed intractable, ascertain that the correct drugs have been given in the correct amounts. Anterior temporal lobe resection and other cortical resections involve removal of the epileptic focus. These operations are performed for complex partial seizures and are 80% to 90% effective in controlling seizures in the appropriate patients. If patients with complex partial seizures have treatment failure with 2 anticonvulsant drugs (or possibly even 1 drug), they should be referred for surgical evaluation.

Corpus callosotomy (ie, the severing of connections between the right and left cerebral hemispheres) is performed for some types of generalized epilepsy. Seizures that are medically refractory may respond to stimulation of the left vagus nerve with a permanent stimulator.

Deep brain stimulation is being studied for patients with intractable epilepsy. Stimulation of various structures, most commonly the anterior nucleus of the thalamus, is currently being studied in clinical trials.

- If treatment with antiepileptic drugs fails, vagal nerve stimulation and brain surgery are alternatives.
- Anterior temporal lobe operations and other cortical resections remove the epileptic focus.
- Resection operations are performed for complex partial seizures.
- Corpus callosotomy severs the connections between the left and right sides of the brain and is performed for generalized epilepsy.

Status Epilepticus

Status epilepticus is a medical emergency and a life-threatening condition. The seizure is prolonged, lasting more than 5 minutes, or there are repetitive seizures, without recovery between seizures. The most common causes of status epilepticus include stopping the use of an anticonvulsant agent or alcohol, recreational drug toxicity, and CNS trauma or infection. Rarely, status epilepticus is the initial presenting sign of epilepsy. The management of status epilepticus is summarized in Figure 19-1.

Nonconvulsive status epilepticus may cause an acute confusional state or stupor and coma, especially in the elderly. In these cases, there is often very subtle rhythmic motor activity in the limbs or face. EEG is a critical diagnostic tool in these cases because nonconvulsive status epilepticus must be treated as quickly and vigorously as convulsive status epilepticus.

- Status epilepticus is a life-threatening medical emergency.
- The seizure lasts >5 minutes, or there are repetitive seizures without recovery.
- Administer 50 mL of 50% dextrose with 100 mg thiamine intravenously.
- Slowly administer lorazepam intravenously.
- Antiepileptic treatment should begin with a loading dose of fosphenytoin.
- Cardiorespiratory monitoring is required if fosphenytoin or phenytoin is infused rapidly.

Headache and Facial Pain

Headache may indicate intracranial or systemic disease, a personality or situational problem, or a combination of these. Some headaches have a readily identified organic cause. Classic migraine and cluster headaches form distinctive, easily recognized clinical entities, although their pathophysiologic mechanisms are not fully understood. The major challenge is that often neither the location nor the intensity of the pain is a reliable clue to the nature of the problem. Episodic tension headache and migraine can be difficult to distinguish.

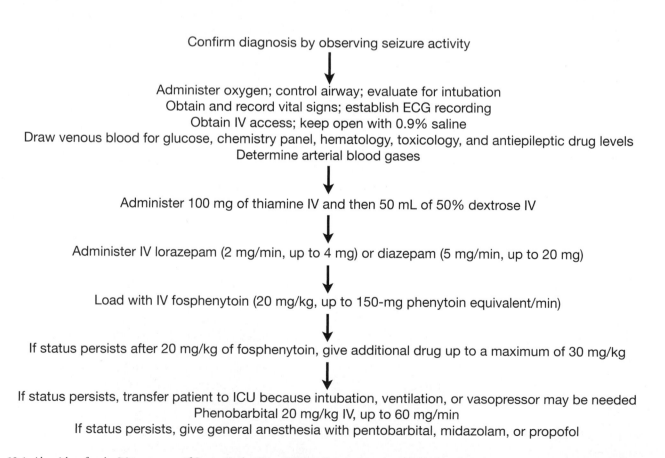

Confirm diagnosis by observing seizure activity

↓

Administer oxygen; control airway; evaluate for intubation
Obtain and record vital signs; establish ECG recording
Obtain IV access; keep open with 0.9% saline
Draw venous blood for glucose, chemistry panel, hematology, toxicology, and antiepileptic drug levels
Determine arterial blood gases

↓

Administer 100 mg of thiamine IV and then 50 mL of 50% dextrose IV

↓

Administer IV lorazepam (2 mg/min, up to 4 mg) or diazepam (5 mg/min, up to 20 mg)

↓

Load with IV fosphenytoin (20 mg/kg, up to 150-mg phenytoin equivalent/min)

↓

If status persists after 20 mg/kg of fosphenytoin, give additional drug up to a maximum of 30 mg/kg

↓

If status persists, transfer patient to ICU because intubation, ventilation, or vasopressor may be needed
Phenobarbital 20 mg/kg IV, up to 60 mg/min
If status persists, give general anesthesia with pentobarbital, midazolam, or propofol

Figure 19-1. Algorithm for the Management of Status Epilepticus. ECG indicates electrocardiographic; ICU, intensive care unit; IV, intravenous.

• Neither location nor intensity of headache pain is a reliable clue to the nature of the problem.

Conditions alerting physicians that a headache may have a serious cause are listed in Table 19-9. Chronic recurrent headaches are rarely, if ever, caused by eye strain, chronic sinusitis, dental problems, food allergies, high blood pressure, or temporomandibular joint syndrome. Headache without other neurologic signs or symptoms is rarely caused by a brain tumor. Serious causes of headache in which neuroimaging findings may be normal and lead to a false sense of security are listed in Table 19-10.

• "Worst headache of my life" is serious.
• Headache with abnormal neurologic findings, papilledema, obscuration of vision, or diplopia is serious.
• Most of the signs and symptoms in Table 19-9 can occur with chronic benign headache (tension-migraine headache).
• Headache without other neurologic signs or symptoms is rarely caused by a brain tumor.

Migraine and Tension Headache

Migraine is defined by multiple attacks of severe headache, often unilateral, which last several hours and are accompanied by photophobia, phonophobia, and osmophobia; nausea; a pounding quality to the headache; and an increase in the intensity with light activity. Most patients gravitate to a dark, quiet room and try to sleep. Many migraineurs experience an aura before the headache onset. The common auras are visual with flashing lights, jagged lines, or scintillating scotomas. Tension headaches can be severe but are often bilateral, squeezing or tight in quality, and lack all the other associated symptoms that occur in migraine.

Pharmacotherapy along with psychologic and physical therapy are components of an approach to treating headache. An overview of pharmacologic treatment is shown in Tables 19-11 and 19-12.

Table 19-9 Conditions Indicating That a Headache May Have a Serious Cause

"Worst headache of my life"
Headache in a person not prone to headache, especially a middle-aged or elderly patient
Headache associated with abnormal neurologic findings, papilledema, obscurations of vision, or diplopia
Headache that changes with different positions or increases with exertion, coughing, or sneezing
Changes in headache patterns—character, frequency, or severity—in someone who has had chronic recurring headaches
Headache that awakens one from sound sleep
Headache associated with trauma
Headache associated with systemic symptoms (eg, fever, malaise, or weight loss)
Most of the above signs & symptoms may occur in chronic benign headache (eg, tension-migraine)

Table 19-10 Serious Causes of Headache in Which Neuroimaging Findings May Be Normal

Giant cell or temporal arteritis
Glaucoma
Trigeminal or glossopharyngeal neuralgia
Lesions around sella turcica
Warning leak of aneurysm (sentinel bleed)
Inflammation, infection, or neoplastic invasion of leptomeninges
Cervical spondylosis
Pseudotumor cerebri
Low intracranial pressure syndromes (cerebrospinal fluid leaks)

Abortive headache medications may range from simple analgesics to anxiolytics, nonsteroidal anti-inflammatory drugs, ergots, and corticosteroids to major tranquilizers and narcotics. Dihydroergotamine mesylate (DHE 45) and sumatriptan, as well as related serotonin 1B/1D receptor agonists (the triptans: zolmitriptan, naratriptan, rizatriptan, almotriptan, eletriptan, and frovatriptan), are effective in aborting acute migraine attacks. Dihydroergotamine and sumatriptan can be administered parenterally or intranasally to patients who have severe nausea or vomiting. Sumatriptan and other vasoconstrictor drugs are contraindicated in patients with migraine associated with a focal neurologic deficit and in patients with symptomatic coronary artery disease.

Prophylactic medication should be given when the attacks occur more than 2 or 3 times a month or even less frequently if they are incapacitating, associated with focal neurologic signs, or of prolonged duration. When prophylactic medication is indicated, the following should be observed:

1. Begin with a low dose and increase it slowly
2. Perform an adequate trial of medication (1-2 months)
3. Confirm that the patient is not taking drugs that may interact with the headache agent (eg, vasodilators, estrogens, or oral contraceptives)
4. Determine that a female patient is not pregnant and that she is using effective contraception
5. Attempt to taper and discontinue use of prophylactic medication after the headaches are well controlled
6. Avoid polypharmacy
7. Establish a strong doctor-patient partnership; emphasize that management of headache is often a team effort, with the patient having a role equal to that of the physician
8. The best medication is *no* medication

Drugs used for prophylaxis include β-blockers, calcium channel blockers, amitriptyline or nortriptyline, valproic acid, and other anticonvulsants (gabapentin or topiramate). The most widely used β-blocker is propranolol; others are atenolol, metoprolol, and timolol. Valproic acid is an excellent preventive agent, but its use may be limited because of weight gain and hair loss. Amitriptyline is particularly useful in patients with migraine and chronic-type tension headache. Verapamil is a good alternative to β-blockers in athletes and is recommended for patients with suspected vasospasm as a cause of migrainous

Table 19-11 Treatment of Migraine

Abortive medications
    Triptans
    Ergotamine
    Nonsteroidal anti-inflammatory drugs
    Dihydroergotamine mesylate (DHE-45)
    Prochlorperazine, metoclopramide, chlorpromazine
    Magnesium sulfate (1.0 g intravenously)
    Methylprednisolone
Prophylactic medications
    β-Blockers
    Tricyclic antidepressants
    Valproic acid
    Topiramate
    Gabapentin
    Verapamil
    Botulinum toxin type A

Table 19-12 Choice of Triptan According to the Attack

Pattern	Drug of Choice[a]
Daytime attack, moderate to severe	Almotriptan (12.5 mg)
	Eletriptan (80 mg)
	Rizatriptan (10 mg)
Severe nausea or vomiting	Rizatriptan (10 mg)
	Zolmitriptan (2.5 mg)
	Zolmitriptan NS (5 mg)
Pain that awakens the patient	Sumatriptan SC (6 mg)
	Zolmitriptan NS (5 mg)
Frequent, long-duration attacks	Frovatriptan (2.5 mg bid)
	Naratriptan (1-2.5 mg bid)
	Zolmitriptan (2.5 mg bid)

Abbreviations: bid, twice daily; NS, nasal spray; SC, subcutaneously.
[a] If tolerance is a concern, choose almotriptan (12.5 mg) or naratriptan (2.5 mg).

infarction. There is excellent evidence that topiramate is effective in prevention of migraine at a dosage of 50 mg twice a day.

Naproxen and other nonsteroidal anti-inflammatory drugs produce analgesia through alternate pathways that do not appear to induce dependence. They may be useful for the following headaches: migraine, for both acute attacks and prophylaxis; menstrual migraine (especially naproxen); benign exertional migraine and sex-induced headache (especially indomethacin); cluster variants (eg, chronic paroxysmal hemicrania, episodic paroxysmal hemicrania, and hemicrania continua); idiopathic stabbing headache, jabs-and-jolts, needle-in-the-eye, and ice-pick headaches (indomethacin is often effective); muscle contraction headaches; mixed headaches; and ergotamine-induced headache.

Cluster Headache

Cluster headache, unlike migraine, predominantly affects men. Onset usually occurs in the late 20s but may occur at any age. The main feature is periodicity. On average, the cluster period lasts 2 to 3 months and typically occurs every 1 or 2 years. Attacks occur at a frequency of 1 to 3 times daily and tend to be nocturnal in more than 50% of patients. The average period of remission is about 2 years between clusters. Cluster is not associated with an aura. The pain reaches a peak in about 10 to 15 minutes and lasts 45 to 60 minutes. It is excruciating, penetrating, usually nonthrobbing, and maximal behind the eye and in the region of the supraorbital nerve and temples. Attacks of pain typically are unilateral. The autonomic features are both sympathetic paresis and parasympathetic overreaction. They may include 1) ipsilateral lacrimation, injection of the conjunctiva, and nasal stuffiness or rhinorrhea, and 2) ptosis and miosis (ptosis may become permanent), periorbital swelling, and bradycardia. The scalp, face, and carotid artery may be tender. In contrast to migraineurs, patients with cluster headaches tend to be hyperactive during a headache.

- Cluster headache affects mostly men, with onset in the 20s.

- Periodicity is the main feature.
- The cluster period lasts 2-3 months.
- Cluster headache is not associated with an aura.
- The pain peaks in 10-15 minutes and lasts 45-60 minutes.
- The pain typically is unilateral, excruciating, penetrating, nonthrobbing, and maximal behind the eye.
- In >50% of patients, the pain is nocturnal.
- Autonomic features are present.

Abortive therapy includes oxygen inhalation, 5 to 8 L/min for 10 minutes; sumatriptan; dihydroergotamine; ergotamine suppositories; corticosteroids (eg, 8 mg dexamethasone); local anesthesia (eg, intranasal 4% lidocaine); and capsaicin in the ipsilateral nostril. Sumatriptan is the drug of choice for management of an acute attack of cluster headache. Surgical intervention may be indicated under certain circumstances for chronic cluster headache but never for episodic headache.

Prophylactic treatment is the mainstay of cluster headache treatment. Calcium channel blockers (verapamil) are widely used. The usual daily dose of lithium is 600 to 900 mg in divided doses. Its effectiveness is known within 1 week. Topiramate has proved useful in cluster headache treatment. Methysergide is most effective in the early course of the disease and least effective in later years. Ergotamine at bedtime is particularly beneficial for nocturnal attacks. Corticosteroids are helpful for short-term treatment, especially for patients resistant to the above drugs or to a combination of the above. The usual dosage is 40 mg prednisone daily tapered over 3 weeks. An effective treatment for chronic cluster headache is the combination of verapamil and lithium. Valproic acid may also be useful.

- Prophylaxis of cluster headaches is the mainstay of treatment.
- Calcium channel blockers are widely used.
- Methysergide is effective early in the disease.
- Ergotamine is effective for nocturnal attacks.
- Corticosteroids are helpful short-term.

- The combination of verapamil and lithium is best for prophylaxis of chronic cluster headache.

Typical Clinical Scenarios

- Migraine: A young patient has recurrent, episodic (once a month or so), and severe headaches. Often, the headache is unilateral and associated with nausea, vomiting, and photophobia. MRI is normal.
- Tension headache: A young patient has a 3-year history of headaches, which occur almost every month and last several days. They are bilateral and are not associated with any neurologic deficit, nausea, or vomiting.
- Cluster headache: A 27-year-old man has a 1-month history of severe, excruciating headaches that occur daily and last for approximately 1 hour. He had a similar episode 1 year ago, in which the headache lasted 3 months and then resolved completely. The pain is unilateral and worse behind the right eye. The right eye becomes red and teary during the headache.

Medication-Overuse Headache

Chronic daily headache may occur de novo, probably as a form of tension headache or, more important, it may be part of an evolution from periodic migraine or tension headache. Chronic daily headache is often accompanied by sleep disturbances, depression, anxiety, and overuse of analgesics; most patients with this disorder have a family history of headache. Episodic migraine and other episodic benign headaches can evolve into a daily refractory, intense headache. This syndrome is usually due to the overuse (>2 days a week) of ergotamine tartrate, triptans, analgesics (especially analgesics combined with barbiturates), narcotics, and perhaps even benzodiazepines. To control the headache, the use of these medications has to be discontinued. Two points must be stressed: the overuse of these medications causes daily headache, and the daily use of these medications prevents other useful medications from working effectively.

The treatment of daily refractory headaches can require hospitalization and withdrawal of the overused medication, with repetitive intravenous administration of dihydroergotamine together with an antiemetic drug such as metoclopramide or prochlorperazine.

β-Blockers, calcium channel blockers, and tricyclic antidepressants do not cause transformation/withdrawal syndrome. Also, patients who do not have headache but who take large amounts of analgesics for other conditions (eg, arthritis) do not develop analgesic or rebound headache. Simple withdrawal of analgesics produces improvement in patients with chronic daily headache. A nonprescription medication can be withdrawn abruptly. However, prescription medications (eg, ergotamine tartrate, narcotics, and barbiturates) have to be withdrawn gradually. When narcotics or compounds containing codeine and ergotamine tartrate are withdrawn, clonidine may be helpful in repressing withdrawal symptoms. Some physicians think that even simple analgesics (eg, aspirin and acetaminophen) taken more than 2 days a week can cause daily headache syndrome. The overuse (>3 days a week for ≥2 weeks) of triptan drugs is now becoming a common cause of medication-overuse syndrome.

- Chronic daily headache is often accompanied by sleep disturbances, depression, anxiety, and analgesic overuse.

- Most patients with chronic daily headache have a family history of headache.
- Migraine and other headaches can become a refractory intense headache.
- Overuse of medications causes daily headache and prevents the effective action of other drugs.
- Hospitalization and withdrawal of overused drugs are usually required.
- Nonsteroidal anti-inflammatory drugs, β-blockers, calcium channel blockers, and tricyclic antidepressants do not cause transformation/withdrawal syndrome.
- There is improvement after withdrawal of analgesics.

Temporal Arteritis

In an elderly person, temporal arteritis (also called *cranial arteritis* or *giant cell arteritis*) should be in the differential diagnosis of any new temporal headache of mild to moderate severity. About 50% of persons with this diagnosis have headache or tender temporal arteries. Common additional symptoms include low-grade fever, jaw claudication, weight loss, anorexia, and other systemic symptoms. The erythrocyte sedimentation rate or the C-reactive protein concentration (or both) is consistently increased. If vision loss has already occurred, emergent therapy with high doses of corticosteroids is needed. To prevent vision loss in those who have no visual problem, prednisone therapy should be initiated immediately after the diagnosis has been made. Temporal artery biopsy is used to confirm the diagnosis before long-term treatment with prednisone is prescribed. However, if the biopsy cannot be performed, even for several days, prednisone therapy may be initiated until the biopsy is performed. The erythrocyte sedimentation rate may be followed to help gauge the response to treatment. The prednisone dose can be tapered slowly after several months of therapy, although long-term treatment with prednisone may be needed.

Polymyalgia rheumatica is another rheumatologic syndrome that is sometimes associated with cranial arteritis. It affects elderly patients and is associated with aching or pain and stiffness in the neck, upper back, shoulders, upper arms, and hip girdle. Systemic symptoms include various degrees of fever, anorexia, weight loss, apathy, and depression. True muscle weakness is not present except when attributed to pain.

Trigeminal Neuralgia

Patients with trigeminal neuralgia always have symptoms on the same side and usually in the second or third division of the trigeminal nerve. The idiopathic variety occurs in middle-aged and elderly patients and is heralded by a sharp, lancinating pain that usually can be triggered. Chewing, talking, or touching the skin or teeth often precipitates the pain of trigeminal neuralgia, and swallowing often precipitates the pain of glossopharyngeal neuralgia.

In the elderly, trigeminal neuralgia may be caused by an enlarged or tortuous artery (rarely a vein) that compresses the trigeminal nerve. This can be seen on MRI or MRA. Importantly, in idiopathic trigeminal neuralgia, sensory and motor functions of the trigeminal nerve are normal. If there are signs or symptoms other than pain, evaluate for other compressive lesions, for example, neoplasm. Consider the possibility of multiple sclerosis if trigeminal neuralgia occurs in a young person. Treatment options include carbamazepine, phenytoin, baclofen, gabapentin, and clonazepam. Carbamazepine is the most effective. Surgical treatment includes alcohol blocks, radiofrequency ablation of the gasserian ganglion (cranial nerve [CN] V), gamma knife radiosurgery, and an open craniotomy with microvascular decompression.

- Chewing, talking, or touching often precipitates pain in trigeminal neuralgia, as does swallowing in glossopharyngeal neuralgia.
- In idiopathic trigeminal neuralgia, there should be no other neurologic signs or symptoms when the patient is examined during an asymptomatic period.
- Consider multiple sclerosis if trigeminal neuralgia occurs in a young person.

Glossopharyngeal Neuralgia

The pain in glossopharyngeal neuralgia is similar to that in trigeminal neuralgia, but it occurs in the throat and neck and often radiates to the ear. Glossopharyngeal neuralgia may cause hypotension and syncope. It is usually idiopathic but has been reported with leptomeningeal metastasis or jugular foramen syndrome (head and neck malignancies). The treatment is the same as for trigeminal neuralgia (ie, carbamazepine and, occasionally, surgical management).

- Glossopharyngeal pain occurs in the throat and neck and radiates to the ear.

Intracranial Lesions

Leptomeningeal Lesions

Patients with inflammation, infection, or neoplastic invasion of the leptomeninges may present with similar signs and symptoms, as follows:

1. Cerebral—headache, seizures, and focal neurologic signs
2. Cranial nerve—any cranial nerve can be affected, especially CN III, IV, VI, and VII (CN VII is often affected in Lyme disease)
3. Radicular (radiculoneuropathy or radiculomyelopathy)—neck and back pain as well as radicular pain and spinal cord signs

Parasagittal Lesions

Because the cortical leg area and cortical area for control of the urinary bladder are located on the medial surface of each hemisphere, parasagittal lesions can cause spastic paraparesis with urinary problems and can, therefore, mimic a myelopathy. Meningioma is a common lesion in this location and may also cause seizures and headache.

- Parasagittal lesions may cause paraparesis with urinary problems.
- Meningioma may also cause seizures and headache.

Cortical Lesions

Cortical lesions produce focal signs. If the lesions are in the dominant hemisphere (usually the left), they cause language dysfunction, including problems of reading, writing, and speaking. Cortical lesions can also impair higher intellectual function, producing apraxia, agnosia, and neglect (ie, denial of illness or body parts), and they often impair cortical sensation (eg, joint position sense, traced figures, and stereognosis). A dense loss of primary sensation (eg, pinprick and touch) occurs with thalamic lesions.

- Cortical lesions may produce aphasia, apraxia, and agnosia.
- Thalamic lesions cause loss of primary sensation (eg, touch and pinprick).

Ventricular System

Hydrocephalus

A combination of signs and symptoms—impaired mental status, gait disturbance, and urinary problems—suggests hydrocephalus. If it is the obstructive type, signs of increased intracranial pressure may be present, including lethargy, nausea, vomiting, and headache; obscurations of vision are often associated with changes in position.

The following are types of hydrocephalus:

1. Communicating hydrocephalus
   a. Hydrocephalus ex vacuo—due to the loss of parenchyma, either gray or white matter, and not associated with the signs listed above (if the hydrocephalus is due to aging, the findings on neurologic examination are normal; if it is due to AD, clinical examination shows signs of dementia)
   b. Normal-pressure hydrocephalus—due to decreased reabsorption of CSF
   c. Hydrocephalus due to overproduction of CSF—rare and controversial; supposedly occurs with choroid plexus tumors
2. Obstructive (noncommunicating) hydrocephalus—due to an obstructive lesion anywhere in the ventricular system

- Normal-pressure hydrocephalus is due to decreased reabsorption of CSF and may be associated with urinary symptoms, gait disturbance, and memory dysfunction (see the "Dementia" subsection above).

Posterior Fossa Level: Symptoms and Clinical Correlations

Brainstem Lesions

Brainstem lesions can produce crossed neurologic syndromes; cranial nerve signs are ipsilateral to the lesion, but long-tract signs (ie, corticospinal) are usually contralateral (ie, crossed syndrome). Other symptoms associated with brainstem lesions include impairment of ocular motility; medial longitudinal fasciculus syndrome (ie, internuclear ophthalmoplegia); rotary, horizontal, and vertical nystagmus (downbeat nystagmus is highly suggestive of a lesion at the cervicomedullary junction); ataxia; dysarthria; diplopia; vertigo; and dysphagia.

- Long-tract signs are usually contralateral to the brainstem lesion.
- Downbeat nystagmus is highly suggestive of a lesion at the cervicomedullary junction.
- Cranial nerve signs are ipsilateral to the brainstem lesion.

Cerebellar Lesions

Problems with equilibrium and coordination suggest a cerebellar lesion. Lesions of the cerebellar hemisphere usually produce ipsilateral ataxia of the arm and leg. Lesions restricted to the anterior superior vermis, as in alcoholism, usually cause ataxia of gait (ie, a wide-based gait and heel-to-shin ataxia), with relative sparing of the arms, speech, and ocular motility. Lesions of the flocculonodular lobe cause marked difficulty with equilibrium and walking but not much difficulty with finger-to-nose and heel-to-shin tests if the patient is lying down.

Vertigo and Dizziness

Accurate visual, vestibular, proprioceptive, tactile, and auditory perceptions are necessary for normal spatial orientation. These inputs are integrated in the brainstem and cerebral hemispheres. The outputs are the cortical, brainstem, and cerebellar motor systems. The impairment of any of these functions or their input, integration, or output causes a complaint of "dizziness" (a sensation of altered orientation or space). Dizziness, vertigo, and dysequilibrium are common complaints. The results of diagnostic tests are often normal. Diagnosis depends mainly on the medical history, with physical examination findings in some cases. Vestibular tests rarely provide an exact diagnosis. The types of dizziness are listed in Table 19-13.

Vertigo

Vertigo is an illusion of movement (usually that of rotation) and the feeling of vertical or horizontal rotation of either the person or the environment around the person. Most patients report this as "spinning" or "rotational" feelings. Others experience mainly a sensation of staggering. In contrast to vertigo, "dysequilibrium" is a feeling of unsteadiness or insecurity about the environment, without a rotatory sensation. Vertigo occurs when there is imbalance, especially acute, between the left and right vestibular systems. The sudden unilateral loss of vestibular function is dramatic; the patient complains of severe vertigo and nausea and vomiting and is pale and diaphoretic. With acute vertigo, the patient also has problems with equilibrium and vision, often described as "blurred vision," or diplopia. Autonomic symptoms are common—sweating, pallor, nausea, and vomiting—and occasionally can cause vasovagal syncope.

Fluctuating hearing loss and tinnitus are characteristic of Ménière disease. Abrupt complete unilateral deafness and vertigo occur with viral involvement of the labyrinth or CN VIII (or both) and with vascular occlusion of the inner ear. Patients who slowly lose vestibular function bilaterally, as with ototoxic drugs, often do not complain of vertigo but have oscillopsia with head movements and instability with walking. Even with unilateral vestibular loss, if it is a slow process (eg, acoustic neuroma), patients usually do not complain of vertigo; they typically present with unilateral hearing loss and tinnitus. Vertigo invariably occurs in episodes. Common vestibular disorders with a genetic predisposition include migraine, Ménière disease, otosclerosis, neurofibromatosis, and spinocerebellar degeneration.

Benign positional vertigo (BPV) is the most common cause of vertigo. Symptoms include brief episodes of vertigo that usually last less than 30 seconds with positional change (eg, turning over in bed,

Table 19-13 Types of Dizziness

Vertigo
  Peripheral
  Central
Presyncopal light-headedness
  Orthostatic hypotension
  Vasovagal attacks
  Impaired cardiac output
  Hyperventilation
Psychophysiologic dizziness
  Acute anxiety
  Agoraphobia (fear & avoidance of being in public places)
  Chronic anxiety
Dysequilibrium
  Lesions of basal ganglia, frontal lobes, & white matter
  Hydrocephalus
  Cerebellar dysfunction
Ocular dizziness
  High magnification & lens implant
  Imbalance in extraocular muscles
  Oscillopsia
Multisensory dizziness
Physiologic dizziness
  Motion sickness
  Space sickness
  Height vertigo

getting in or out of bed, bending over and straightening up, and extending the neck to look up). The usual cause is a misplaced otolith in a semicircular canal. In about half of the patients who do not have BPV, no cause is found. For the other half, the most common causes are posttraumatic and postviral neurolabyrinthitis.

Typically, bouts of BPV are intermixed with variable periods of remission. Periods of vertigo rarely last longer than 1 minute, although after a flurry of episodes, patients may complain of more prolonged nonspecific dizziness that lasts hours to days (eg, a light-headedness or a swimming sensation associated with nausea). Management includes reassurance, positional exercises (ie, vestibular exercises), and the canalith repositioning maneuver. Drugs are not very useful, but meclizine and promethazine may help with the nausea and nonspecific dizziness. Rarely, in intractable cases, surgical treatment (section of the ampullary nerve) may be undertaken.

Vertigo of CNS origin is caused by acute cerebellar lesions (hemorrhages or infarcts) or acute brainstem lesions (especially the lateral medullary [Wallenberg] syndrome). Vertebrobasilar arterial disease is also a cause, but vertigo by itself is almost never a TIA. Other symptoms are necessary to make the diagnosis of vertebrobasilar insufficiency, such as dysarthria, dysphagia, diplopia, facial numbness, crossed syndromes, hemiparesis or alternating hemiparesis, ataxia, and visual field defects.

Presyncopal Light-headedness

Presyncopal light-headedness is best described as the *sensation of impending faint*. It results from pancerebral ischemia. Presyncopal light-headedness is not a symptom of focal occlusive cerebrovascular disease, but it may indicate orthostatic hypotension, usually due to decreased blood volume, chronic use of antihypertensive drugs, or autonomic dysfunction. Symptoms of vasovagal attacks are induced when emotions such as fear and anxiety activate medullary vasodepressor centers. Vasodepressor episodes can also be precipitated by acute visceral pain or sudden severe attacks of vertigo. Impaired cardiac output causes presyncopal light-headedness, as does hyperventilation. Chronic anxiety with associated hyperventilation is the most common cause of persistent presyncopal light-headedness in young patients. In most subjects, only a moderate increase in respiratory rate can decrease the $PaCO_2$ level to 25 mm Hg or less in a few minutes.

Five types of syncopal attacks especially common in the elderly are the following:

1. Orthostatic—multiple causes
2. Autonomic dysfunction due to peripheral (ie, postganglionic) or central (ie, preganglionic) involvement
3. Reflex—such as carotid sinus syncope or cough or micturition syncope
4. Vasovagal syncope—occurs less frequently in the elderly than in the young; however, the prognosis is worse in the elderly, with about 16% of them having major morbidity or mortality in the following 6 months compared with less than 1% of patients younger than 30 years; common precipitating events in the elderly include emotional stress, prolonged bed rest, prolonged standing, and painful stimuli
5. Cardiogenic (eg, from arrhythmias or valvular disease)

- Presyncopal light-headedness is the sensation of impending faint.
- It is not an isolated symptom of occlusive cerebrovascular disease.
- Vasovagal attacks occur less frequently in the elderly.
- In the young, a common cause of persistent presyncopal light-headedness is chronic anxiety with hyperventilation.
- The prognosis of vasovagal syncope is worse for the elderly; 16% have major morbidity or mortality within 6 months.
- In the elderly, vasovagal syncope may be precipitated by emotional stress, bed rest, prolonged standing, or pain.

Psychophysiologic Dizziness

Patients usually describe psychophysiologic dizziness as "floating," "swimming," or "giddiness." They also may report a feeling of imbalance, a rocking or falling sensation, or a spinning inside the head. The symptoms are not associated with an illusion of movement or movement of the environment or with nystagmus. Commonly associated symptoms include tension headache, heart palpitations, gastric distress, urinary frequency, backache, and a generalized feeling of weakness and fatigue. Psychophysiologic dizziness can also be associated with panic attacks.

Dysequilibrium

Patients who slowly lose vestibular function on 1 side, as with an acoustic neuroma, usually do not have vertigo but often describe a vague feeling of imbalance and unsteadiness on their feet. Dysequilibrium may be a presenting symptom of lesions involving motor centers of the basal ganglia and frontal lobe (eg, Parkinson disease, hydrocephalus, and multiple lacunar infarctions). The broad-based ataxic gait of cerebellar disorders is readily distinguished from milder gait disorders seen with vestibular or sensory loss or with senile gait.

- Dysequilibrium may be a presenting symptom of basal ganglia, frontal lobe, or cerebellar lesions.

Multifactorial Dizziness and Imbalance

Multifactorial dizziness and imbalance is common in the elderly and especially in patients with systemic disorders such as diabetes mellitus. A typical combination includes, for example, mild peripheral neuropathy that causes diminished touch and proprioceptive input, decreased visual acuity, impaired hearing, and decreased baroreceptor function. In these patients, an added vestibular impairment, as from an ototoxic drug, can be devastating.

The resulting sensation of dizziness and imbalance is usually present only when the patient walks or moves and not when supine or seated. There is a feeling of insecurity of gait and motion. The patient is usually helped by walking close to a wall, using a cane, or by holding on to another person. Drugs should not be prescribed for this disorder. Instead, the use of a cane or walker is important to improve support and to increase somatosensory signals.

- Multifactorial dizziness and imbalance is common in elderly diabetic patients.
- Added vestibular impairment can be devastating.
- Do not prescribe drugs for this disorder.

Spinal Level: Symptoms and Clinical Correlations

Sensory levels, signs of anterior horn cell involvement (ie, atrophy and fasciculations), and long-tract signs in the posterior columns, corticospinal tract, and spinothalamic tract suggest a spinal cord lesion. Extramedullary cord lesions are usually heralded by radicular pain. Intramedullary cord lesions are usually painless but may have an ill-described nonlocalizable pain, sensory dissociation, and sacral sparing. Conus medullaris lesions are often indicated by "saddle anesthesia" and early involvement of the urinary bladder.

- Extramedullary lesions are heralded by radicular pain.
- Intramedullary lesions are usually painless.
- Conus medullaris lesions are indicated by saddle anesthesia and early bladder involvement.

Causes of Myelopathy

A compressive or noncompressive spinal cord lesion may cause muscle weakness, which typically occurs in the arm and leg if the lesion is at the cervical level or only in the leg if the lesion is below the lower cervical level. The upper motor neuron pattern weakness is often bilateral and prominent in lower extremity flexors (iliopsoas, hamstrings, and anterior tibialis) and upper extremity extensors (triceps and wrist extensors). Bowel and bladder difficulties and numbness are frequently noted. The findings on examination include limb weakness, spasticity, and increased muscle stretch reflexes below the level of the lesion. Extensor plantar reflexes (Babinski signs) may also be elicited. Sensory findings are often noted.

The most common noncompressive lesion is transverse myelitis, usually of unknown cause. Some patients have a history of vaccination or symptoms suggestive of viral disease that usually precede the neurologic symptoms by a few days to 1 or 2 weeks. Up to 50% of these patients have antibodies, which were described in patients with neuromyelitis optica (NMO), to a water aquaporin channel (NMO IgG). They have recurrent episodes of severe myelitis and optic neuritis; consequently, long-term immunomodulatory therapy is usually indicated.

Compressive myelopathy is commonly due to degenerative spine or disk disease or to metastatic epidural neoplasm. The patients usually present with local vertebral column pain at the level of the spinal cord lesion. This symptom is present for weeks to months before the gross neurologic deficits occur, although occasionally bony pain may antedate other symptoms by only a few hours.

- Muscle weakness may be associated with a compressive or noncompressive spinal cord lesion.
- Transverse myelitis is the most common noncompressive lesion.

Motor Neuron Disease

Degenerative disorders that affect the motor neurons in the cerebral cortex and the anterior horn cells are called *motor neuron diseases*. The most common is amyotrophic lateral sclerosis (ALS). This disorder is the main cause of progressive, painless weakness. Typically, patients present with asymmetric weakness that usually begins distally and is associated with cramps and fasciculations. Footdrop and hand weakness are the most common first complaints. Often the initial, but incorrect, diagnosis is stroke, radiculopathy, carpal tunnel syndrome, or ulnar neuropathy. Some ALS patients have undergone unnecessary operations (eg, spinal or carpal tunnel procedures) before the correct diagnosis is made. Bulbar weakness (eg, dysarthria and dysphagia) can be the presenting problem and is always eventually present. Bowel and bladder difficulties are very uncommon, and sensory abnormalities are rare. Findings on examination include weakness, atrophy, fasciculations, and decreased or increased muscle stretch reflexes and extensor plantar responses. The hallmark is the mixture of both upper and lower motor neuron signs. Because of the progressive weakness affecting the limbs, bulbar muscles, and diaphragm, the disease is devastating, and patients have an average life span of 3 years after the onset of symptoms.

ALS is sporadic in 80% to 90% of cases. In those that are familial, 10% of the patients harbor a mutation in the oxygen radical detoxifying enzyme superoxide dismutase (SOD-1). No drug has been found to be effective in reversing the progressive course of this disease. Some beneficial effect has been noted with riluzole, especially in patients with bulbar onset of the disease. This drug prolongs ventilator-free survival by 3 months. Treating ALS with immunosuppression, such as by use of irradiation, corticosteroids, cyclophosphamide, or intravenous immunoglobulin (IVIG), is at best futile and at worst, costly and harmful. Recent failures include gabapentin, lamotrigine, and celecoxib. Treatment of ALS focuses on rehabilitation issues, nutrition, mobility, and communication in which a multidisciplinary approach is useful.

Multifocal motor neuropathy is a syndrome of purely lower motor neuron disease that can mimic ALS. Treatment for multifocal motor neuropathy with IVIG can be very effective. It is often distal and asymmetrical, accompanied by motor conduction block on NCS and EMG, and associated with high titers of serum antibodies to GM_1 gangliosides. Kennedy disease is a pure lower motor neuron degenerative process that is X-linked and caused by an excess of CAG repeats in the androgen receptor gene. This most commonly affects elderly men and also leads to gynecomastia, diabetes, and a sensory peripheral neuropathy. Genetic testing is widely available. There is no effective treatment, although the disease is much more slowly progressive than ALS.

Radiculopathy

Nerve root lesions usually are indicated by pain that is often sharp and lancinating, follows a dermatomal or myotomal pattern, and is increased by increasing intraspinal pressure (eg, sneezing and coughing) or by stretching of the nerve root. Paresthesias and pain occur in a dermatomal pattern. Findings are in the root distribution and include weakness, sensory impairment, and decreased muscle stretch reflexes. Radiculopathies have many causes, including compressive lesions (eg, osteophytes, ruptured disks, and neoplasms) and noncompressive lesions (eg, postinfectious and inflammatory radiculopathies and metabolic radiculopathies, as in diabetes). Indications for emergent neurologic and neurosurgical consultation are increasing weakness, bowel or bladder dysfunction, or intractable pain with an appropriate lesion seen on MRI. Large disk protrusions can cause minimal symptoms and are not by themselves grounds for urgent surgical intervention.

- Nerve root lesions are indicated by sharp, lancinating pain with a dermatomal or myotomal pattern.
- Pain is increased by sneezing and coughing.
- Pain often has a dermatomal pattern.
- Findings are weakness, sensory impairment, and decreased muscle stretch reflexes.
- Radiculopathies have many causes.
- Surgery is considered for increasing weakness, bowel or bladder dysfunction, or intractable pain with an appropriate lesion seen on MRI.

Degenerative Disease of the Spine

Cervical Spondylosis

MRI in combination with plain radiographs is the preferred approach for evaluating patients who have cervical spondylosis. Surgical results for the relief of symptoms of cervical radiculopathy are better when the cause is a soft disk herniation than when spondylitic radiculopathy and myelopathy are present. In fact, surgical treatment of cervical radiculopathy due to the herniation of a soft disk is so successful that most patients and doctors prefer surgical therapy to prolonged conservative treatment. Surgical treatment for cervical spondylitic myelopathy is much less successful, with fewer than two-thirds of patients having improvement, although the condition stabilizes in most. Cervical spondylitic myelopathy is a condition in which the spinal cord is damaged either directly by traumatic compression or indirectly by arterial deprivation or venous stasis as a consequence of proliferative bony changes in the cervical spine.

Lumbar Spine Disease

Bulging disks after the age of 30 years should be considered normal and are unlikely to cause nerve root compression. Bulging disks appear round and symmetrical compared with herniated disks, which appear angular and asymmetrical and extend outside the disk space. The criteria for surgical treatment of lumbar disk herniations include the presence of disk herniation on anatomical imaging; dermatome-specific reflex, sensory, or motor deficits; and failure of 6 to 8 weeks of conservative treatment.

The lateral recess syndrome is usually caused by an osteophyte on the superior articular facet and is characterized by the following: radicular pain that is unilateral or bilateral with paresthesias in the distribution of L5 or S1; the pain is provoked by standing and walking and is relieved by sitting; the results of the straight leg raising test are usually negative; and there is little or no back pain.

Lumbar stenosis is characterized by the following: most patients are older than 50 years; neurogenic intermittent claudication (pseudoclaudication) occurs; the symptoms are usually bilateral but can be asymmetrical or unilateral; the pain usually has a dull, aching quality; the whole lower extremity is generally involved; the pain is provoked while walking or standing; sitting or leaning forward provides relief; and there is often a "dead" feeling in the legs. Bicycling causes little or no pain. Decompressive operations for lumbar stenosis can be performed with low morbidity despite the advanced age of most patients. A very high initial success rate can be expected, although about 25% of patients become symptomatic again within 5 years. On reoperation, three-fourths of the patients ultimately have a successful outcome; failures result from progression of stenosis at levels not previously decompressed or restenosis at levels previously decompressed.

Musculoskeletal low back pain (without leg pain) is treated best with a formal program of physical therapy and exercise, weight reduction, and education on postural principles.

Peripheral Level: Symptoms and Clinical Correlations

Peripheral Neuropathy

Peripheral neuropathies are usually characterized by distal weakness and distal sensory changes. They are usually symmetrical and more severe in the legs than in the arms. Weakness related to peripheral nerve disorders is typically worse distally, occasionally with footdrop. Clumsy gait is often associated with distal numbness and paresthesias. Examination findings include distal weakness, sensory loss, atrophy, and, sometimes, fasciculations. Muscle stretch reflexes usually are decreased. If a single plexus (lumbosacral or brachial) is involved, the weakness may be isolated to a single limb. However, the findings still are consistent with a "lower motor neuron" lesion, with decreased reflexes, weakness, atrophy, and sensory loss. Neuropathy has many causes, and the pattern of the neuropathy might suggest its cause (Table 19-14). The evaluation of peripheral neuropathy is summarized in Table 19-15. An extensive search usually uncovers the cause in 70% to 80% of cases. A high percentage of the cases of "idiopathic neuropathy" referred to specialty centers are in fact hereditary neuropathies. On examination, the finding of high arches (ie, pes cavus) or fallen arches (ie, pes planus) with hammertoe deformities is a clue to a hereditary neuropathy.

* The pattern of neuropathy and time course suggest the cause.
* Peripheral neuropathy: distal weakness and sensory changes more in the legs than in the arms, usually symmetrical, and with distal muscle stretch reflexes impaired or absent.
* The cause of peripheral neuropathy is usually found in 70%-80% of cases.

Mononeuropathy

Mononeuropathy is characterized by sensory and motor impairment in a single nerve. The usual cause is compression, as in compressive ulnar neuropathy at the elbow, compressive median neuropathy in the carpal tunnel, and compression of the peroneal nerve as it winds around the fibular head. Diabetes mellitus is a common underlying disorder in patients with multiple compression mononeuropathies.

Mononeuropathy Multiplex

Mononeuropathy multiplex consists of asymmetrical involvement of several nerves either simultaneously or sequentially. It suggests such causes as trauma or compression, diabetes mellitus, vasculitis, Lyme disease, HIV neuropathy, sarcoidosis, leprosy, tumor infiltration, multifocal motor neuropathies, or hereditary neuropathy with predisposition to pressure palsies.

* Mononeuropathy multiplex: diabetes, vasculitis, leprosy, sarcoidosis, and Lyme disease.

Acute Inflammatory Polyradiculoneuropathy

A progressive neuropathy of rapid onset that affects both distal and proximal nerves suggests acute inflammatory demyelinating polyradiculoneuropathy (AIDP), or Guillain-Barré syndrome. The weakness and paresthesias ascend over several days, often accompanied by severe back pain. On examination, the reflexes are absent. There may also be respiratory muscle weakness, cranial neuropathy (particularly facial palsy, which can be bilateral), and autonomic instability. Typically, it is associated with an increased CSF protein concentration but no pleocytosis. There are characteristic NCS and EMG findings with conduction block and temporal dispersion. About 50% of patients have a mild respiratory or gastrointestinal tract infection 1 to 3 weeks before the neurologic symptoms appear. In the other patients, the syndrome may be preceded by surgery, viral exanthems, or vaccinations. Also, the syndrome may develop in patients who have autoimmune disease or a lymphoreticular malignancy. This syndrome has no particular seasonal, age, or sex predilection. Either plasma exchange or IVIG is effective in AIDP. Steroids are not effective. Attention must be paid

Table 19-14 Main Clinical Features and Differential Diagnosis of Peripheral Neuropathies

Pattern of Neuropathy	Common or Important Causes

Mononeuropathy	Compressive neuropathy
	    Idiopathic
	    Tumor
	    Trauma
	    Diabetes mellitus
	Hereditary neuropathy with liability to pressure palsies (HNPP)

Mononeuropathy multiplex	Diabetes mellitus Vasculitis Lyme disease HIV neuropathy Sarcoidosis Leprosy Multifocal motor neuropathy Hereditary neuropathy with predisposition to pressure palsies
Acute motor polyradiculoneuropathy	AIDP (Gullain-Barré syndrome) Lyme disease HIV neuropathy Porphyria Toxins (arsenic, thallium) Carcinomatous or lymphomatous meningitis
Chronic motor or sensorimotor polyradiculopathy	CIDP Paraproteinemia (eg, osteosclerotic myeloma) Hereditary neuropathy (eg, Charcot-Marie-Tooth disease) Lead toxicity Diabetes mellitus Amyloidosis
Length-dependent distal (stocking-&-glove) sensorimotor neuropathy	Diabetes mellitus Alcoholism Uremia Toxins (hexacarbons) Hereditary neuropathy Vitamin B_{12} deficiency Hypothyroidism Gluten sensitivity Copper deficiency
Sensory ataxic neuropathy	Sjögren syndrome Paraneoplastic disorder Diabetes mellitus Paraproteinemia Vitamin B_{12} deficiency HIV infection Cisplatin Vitamin B_6 excess Hereditary neuropathy
Painful peripheral neuropathy	Diabetes mellitus Vasculitis Hereditary amyloidosis Toxins (arsenic, thallium) Hepatitis C Cryoglobulinemia HIV neuropathy

Table 19-14 (continued)

Pattern of Neuropathy	Common or Important Causes
Painful peripheral neuropathy (continued)	CMV polyradiculoneuropathy in HIV-positive patients Alcoholism Fabry disease

Neuropathy with prominent autonomic involvement	Acute or subacute
	    Guillain-Barré syndrome
	    Subacute pandysautonomia
	    Paraneoplastic pandysautonomia
	    Porphyria
	    Vincristine neuropathy
	    Botulism
	Chronic
	    Diabetes mellitus
	    Amyloidosis
	    Sjögren syndrome

Abbreviations: AIDP, acute inflammatory demyelinating polyradiculopathy; CIDP, chronic inflammatory demyelinating polyradiculoneuropathy; CMV, cytomegalovirus; HIV, human immunodeficiency virus.

to other complications of the disease: deep venous thrombosis, constipation, back pain, tachyarrhythmias and hypertension, peptic ulcers, decubital ulcers, and accumulation of secretions in the respiratory tract and aspiration.

- In Guillain-Barré syndrome, 50% of patients have a mild respiratory or gastrointestinal tract infection 1-3 weeks before neurologic symptoms appear.
- Surgery, viral exanthems, or vaccinations may precede Guillain-Barré syndrome.
- The diagnosis is made clinically with support from NCS, EMG, and CSF analysis.
- Treatment is with either plasma exchange or IVIG.

Typical Clinical Scenarios
- Guillain-Barré syndrome: A 35-year-old patient has a fairly acute, 1-week history of weakness in both legs that is progressively worsening. The patient does not have any constitutional symptoms, and the results of routine laboratory testing are unremarkable. The patient has some tingling sensation in both feet. Neurologic examination shows mild sensory loss over the toes and generalized loss of deep tendon reflexes. The Babinski sign is not elicited. CSF analysis shows a high concentration of protein but no increase in cell count.
- Amyotrophic lateral sclerosis ("motor neuron disease"): A 50-year-old patient has a 6-month history of slowly progressive muscle weakness. Weakness involves all four extremities. It started with a left footdrop and now also involves proximal muscles. Physical examination demonstrates muscle wasting and fasciculations. The upper limb reflexes are absent, the lower limb reflexes are brisk, and the Babinski sign is elicited. No sensory abnormalities are detected on examination.

Other causes of subacute, predominantly motor neuropathy are Lyme disease, HIV- or cytomegalovirus-related polyradiculopathy, porphyria, organophosphate poisoning, hypoglycemia, toxins (arsenic and thallium), and paraneoplastic disease. Acute intermittent porphyria produces a severe, rapidly progressive, symmetrical polyneuropathy with or without psychosis, delirium, confusion, and convulsions. In most patients, weakness is most pronounced in the proximal muscles. Tick paralysis is a rapid, progressive ascending motor weakness caused by neurotoxin injected by the female wood tick. It occurs endemically in the southeastern and northwestern United States. After an asymptomatic period (about 1 week), symptoms develop, usually with leg weakness.

Chronic Inflammatory Neuropathies
Chronic, predominantly motor or sensorimotor neuropathies include chronic inflammatory demyelinating polyradiculoneuropathy (CIDP), paraproteinemic neuropathies (eg, associated with POEMS, amyloidosis, or osteosclerotic myeloma), hereditary neuropathies, lead toxicity, diabetes mellitus, and amyloidosis. Most neuropathies are distal, but occasionally there is predominant proximal weakness, which suggests AIDP, CIDP, porphyria, diabetic proximal motor neuropathy (also called diabetic amyotrophy), or idiopathic brachial plexopathy (Parsonage-Turner syndrome). In sharp contrast to its lack of success in AIDP, steroid therapy works in CIDP. Plasma exchange and IVIG are also effective. The other causes of a chronic neuropathy are numerous, with diabetes and hereditary neuropathies topping the list. Hereditary neuropathies are diagnosed with a thorough family history and close examination for signs of hereditary neuropathies, such as high arched feet and hammer toes. Connective tissue diseases, vasculitis, vitamin B_{12} deficiency, copper deficiency, sarcoidosis,

Table 19-15 Evaluation of Peripheral Neuropathy

Basic Laboratory Investigations	Special Investigations	Investigations in Selected Cases
CBC with platelets	Thyroid function test	Autonomic function tests
Erythrocyte sedimentation rate	Vitamin B_{12}	Cerebrospinal fluid analysis
Fasting blood glucose	Vitamin E	Sural nerve biopsy
Serum electrolytes	Cholesterol & triglycerides	Investigation for inborn errors of metabolism
Serum creatinine	HIV serology	Genetic studies
Liver function tests	Lyme serology	MRI of nerve roots or plexus
Serum & urine electrophoresis & immunoelectrophoresis	Hepatitis serology	
Urinalysis	Cryoglobulins	
Chest radiography	Angiotensin-converting enzyme	
Electromyography	Antineutrophil cytoplasmic antibodies	
	Antinuclear antibodies	
	Antibodies against extractable nuclear antigens	
	Gliadin antibodies, endomysial & tissue transglutaminase antibodies	
	Paraneoplastic antibodies	
	GM_1 antibodies	
	Porphyrins	
	Heavy metal screen	
	Serum copper & ceruloplasmin	

Abbreviations: CBC, complete blood cell count; HIV, human immunodeficiency virus; MRI, magnetic resonance imaging.

paraneoplastic syndromes, gluten sensitivity, and medications are other potential causes.

More than 60% of neuropathies associated with monoclonal gammopathy of undetermined significance are idiopathic, but some are associated with multiple myeloma, amyloidosis, lymphoma, or leukemia. The patients usually are older than 50 years and present early with symmetrical sensorimotor polyradiculoneuropathy. The CSF protein concentration is usually increased; IgM is more common than IgG or IgA. Plasma exchange can be effective therapy for patients with IgG or IgA neuropathy. They have a better response than those with IgM neuropathy. Other immunosuppressive therapy such as IVIG and perhaps rituximab may also be effective.

Sensory Ataxic Neuropathy

Sensory ataxic neuropathies are characterized by severe proprioceptive sensory loss, ataxia, and areflexia. Some neuropathies are due to peripheral nerve demyelination and others to involvement of large dorsal root ganglion neurons. A predominantly sensory polyneuropathy suggests paraneoplastic disorder, Sjögren syndrome, diabetes mellitus, paraproteinemias, HIV infection, vitamin B_{12} deficiency, cisplatin toxicity, vitamin B_6 excess, or hereditary neuropathy.

Painful Neuropathy

Some peripheral neuropathies affect predominantly the small-diameter nociceptive fibers or their dorsal root ganglion neurons and are characterized by severe burning pain distally in the extremities. The examination findings are normal except for the distal loss of pain and temperature sensation. Typical causes are diabetes mellitus, vasculitis, amyloidosis, toxins, hepatitis C, cryoglobulinemia, some HIV-associated neuropathies, and alcoholism. Randomized, double-blind, placebo-controlled studies in diabetic neuropathy have shown that the following medications are helpful: amitriptyline, tramadol, gabapentin, pregabalin, and duloxetine. Others that are useful when these agents are not useful or when they lead to side effects include carbamazepine, lidocaine patch (5%), narcotics, lamotrigine, mexiletine, and venlafaxine.

Autonomic Neuropathy

Neuropathy with autonomic dysfunction (eg, orthostatic hypotension, urinary bladder and bowel dysfunction, and impotence) suggests Guillain-Barré syndrome, acute pandysautonomia, paraneoplastic dysautonomia, porphyria, diabetes mellitus, amyloidosis, or familial neuropathy.

Acute pandysautonomia is a heterogeneous, monophasic, usually self-limiting disease that involves both the sympathetic and parasympathetic nervous systems. It may produce orthostatic hypotension, anhydrosis, diarrhea, constipation, urinary bladder atony, and impotence. The syndrome usually evolves over a few days to a few months, with recovery generally being prolonged and partial. This may be an immunologic disorder, but it is indistinguishable from paraneoplastic autonomic neuropathy. Some of the patients may have antibodies against the ganglion-type nicotinic acetylcholine receptor. IVIG treatment limits the duration and reduces the long-term disability of patients with acute pandysautonomia.

- Motor polyneuropathy: inflammatory demyelinating polyneuropathy, hereditary neuropathy, osteosclerotic myeloma, porphyria, lead poisoning, and organophosphate toxicity.
- Sensory polyneuropathy: diabetes, paraneoplastic, Sjögren syndrome, dysproteinemias, HIV infection, vitamin B_{12} deficiency, cisplatin toxicity, vitamin B_6 excess, and hereditary neuropathy.
- Neuropathy with autonomic dysfunction: amyloidosis, diabetes, Guillain-Barré syndrome, porphyria, and familial neuropathy.

Diabetic Neuropathy

Diabetes mellitus may cause CN III neuropathy. Affected patients usually present with sudden diplopia, eye pain, impairment of the muscles supplied by CN III, and relative sparing of the pupil. With compressive CN III lesions, the pupil usually is involved early. Painful diabetic neuropathies include CN III neuropathy, acute thoracoabdominal (ie, truncal) neuropathy, acute distal sensory neuropathy, acute lumbar radiculoplexopathy, and chronic distal small-fiber neuropathy.

- Diabetes may cause CN III neuropathy.
- The pupil is involved early in compression of CN III.

Acute or subacute muscle weakness can occur in various forms of diabetic neuropathy. Weakness, atrophy, and pain affect the pelvic girdle and thigh muscles (asymmetrical or unilateral—diabetic amyotrophy). This has been termed *diabetic polyradiculoplexus neuropathy* and is due to a microvasculitis of the nerve. Patients with diabetes (often mild and well controlled) may have bilateral proximal and pelvic girdle weakness, wasting, weight loss, and autonomic dysfunction. Intravenous steroids may speed the recovery.

Neuromuscular Transmission Disorders

Neuromuscular transmission disorders present with fluctuating weakness, with fatigable weakness in the limbs, eyelids (ie, ptosis), tongue and palate (ie, dysarthria and dysphagia), and extraocular muscles (ie, diplopia). Sensation, muscle tone, and reflexes usually are normal except in Lambert-Eaton myasthenic syndrome (LEMS), in which the weakness is more constant and reflexes are diminished. Drugs may cause problems at neuromuscular junctions; for example, penicillamine can cause a syndrome that appears similar to myasthenia gravis. Three major clinical syndromes of the neuromuscular junction are myasthenia gravis, LEMS, and botulism. Several drugs adversely affect neuromuscular transmission and may exacerbate weakness in these disorders. They include aminoglycoside antibiotics, quinine, quinidine, procainamide, propranolol, calcium channel blockers, and iodinated radiocontrast agents.

Myasthenia Gravis

Myasthenia gravis (MG) usually occurs in young women and older men and is often heralded by such cranial nerve findings as diplopia, dysarthria, dysphagia, and dyspnea. The deficits are usually fatigable, worsening with repetition or late in the day. However, muscle stretch reflexes, sensation, mentation, and sphincter function are normal. Because of remissions and exacerbations in this disease, patients can be considered "hysterical." The diagnosis of MG is based on the detection of nicotinic acetylcholine receptor antibodies and the presence of decremental responses to repetitive electrical stimulation of motor nerves. Administration of a short-acting acetylcholine esterase inhibitor (eg, edrophonium) can immediately reverse weakness due to MG; this can be used as a diagnostic test. Acetylcholine receptor antibodies are rare in conditions other than MG (ie, they do not occur in patients with congenital MG and in only about 50% of those with purely ocular MG). Striational antibodies are highly associated with thymoma and sometimes occur in LEMS or small cell lung carcinoma. They can occur in penicillamine recipients, bone marrow allografts, and autoimmune liver disorders. There are recent reports of antibodies to a muscle-specific kinase (MuSK) that are diagnostic for MG. These patients often have more severe weakness, often bulbar, and may be more resistant to treatments.

Treatment strategies for MG include anticholinesterase and immunomodulatory agents. Cholinesterase inhibitors, such as pyridostigmine bromide, are often given as initial therapy for MG. This therapy provides symptomatic improvement for most patients for a period of time. Thymectomy is indicated for selected patients younger than 60 years with generalized weakness and for all patients with thymoma. A CT chest scan should be performed in all patients with MG. Prednisone is the most commonly used immunomodulatory agent, but initial administration of high doses may exacerbate the weakness. Plasma exchange and IVIG are effective short-term therapies for patients with severe weakness and are particularly useful for a recent exacerbation, for preparation for surgery, or during the initiation of corticosteroid therapy. Other immunomodulatory agents include azathioprine, mycophenolate mofetil, cyclophosphamide, and cyclosporine. Rituximab and tacrolimus are being used more frequently in MG.

Lambert-Eaton Myasthenic Syndrome

Patients with LEMS often have proximal weakness in the legs and absent or decreased muscle stretch reflexes (sometimes reflexes are elicited after brief exercise). This syndrome usually is diagnosed in middle-aged men who often have vague complaints such as diplopia, impotence, urinary dysfunction, paresthesias, mouth dryness, and other autonomic dysfunctions (eg, orthostatic hypotension). LEMS is due to the presence of antibodies directed against presynaptic voltage-gated P/Q-type calcium channels. It often is associated with small-cell lung carcinoma. Treatment is focused on the cancer. Pyridostigmine can be helpful, like in MG, as can steroids.

Botulism

Botulism should be suspected when more than 1 person has a syndrome that resembles MG or when 1 person has abdominal and gastrointestinal tract symptoms that precede a syndrome that resembles MG. Bulbar and respiratory weakness is common, and pupillary abnormalities are distinctive compared with findings in MG. Botulism occurs after the ingestion of improperly canned vegetables, fruit, meat, or fish contaminated by the exotoxin of *Clostridium botulinum*. There is increased concern about the potential use of this toxin as a biologic weapon. Paralysis is caused by toxin-mediated inhibition of acetylcholine release from axon terminals at the neuromuscular junction. Although an antitoxin is available, treatment is mainly supportive, especially respiratory but also psychologic, because the signs and symptoms are reversible.

- Often, lesions of the neuromuscular junction are missed clinically.
- Onset of MG: diplopia, dysarthria, dysphagia, dyspnea, and fatigability, often in young women and older men.
- LEMS: proximal weakness in the legs and decreased or absent muscle stretch reflexes.
- LEMS occurs in middle-aged men who have vague complaints of diplopia, impotence, urinary dysfunction, and dry mouth.
- LEMS is often associated with small-cell lung carcinoma.
- Botulism should be suspected if more than 1 person has a syndrome that resembles MG.
- Ingestion of the exotoxin of *C botulinum* causes botulism.
- In botulism, the release of acetylcholine is inhibited at the neuromuscular junction.

Organophosphate Toxicity

Organophosphate toxicity causes the characteristic combination of miosis, excessive bodily secretions, and fasciculations. A key pathophysiologic factor is decreased acetylcholinesterase activity that causes the accumulation of excessive acetylcholine at the neuromuscular junction. The onset of symptoms varies from 5 minutes to 12 hours after exposure. Treatment is with atropine.

- In organophosphate toxicity, decreased acetylcholinesterase activity causes the accumulation of excessive acetylcholine at the neuromuscular junction.
- Atropine is used to treat organophosphate toxicity.

Muscle Disease

Patients with muscle disease typically present with symmetrical proximal weakness (legs more than arms) and weakness of neck flexors and, occasionally, of cardiac muscle. Muscle stretch reflexes and sensory examination findings are usually normal. Common patient complaints are difficulty arising from a chair or raising the arms over the head. Dysphagia is uncommon. There are rare myopathies with more predominant distal involvement (eg, myotonic dystrophy, inclusion body myositis, and distal muscular dystrophies). In myotonic dystrophy, atrophy and weakness begin distally and in the face and especially in the sternocleidomastoid muscles. An interesting feature of this dystrophy is myotonia, which is normal contraction of muscle with slow relaxation. Tests for myotonia include striking the thenar eminence with a reflex hammer and shaking the patient's hand, noting that the patient cannot let go quickly.

Muscle disease may be an acquired or progressive hereditary disease. *Myopathy* is a general term for muscle disease. If the disease is progressive and genetic, it is called *dystrophy*. However, patients with a muscular dystrophy may not have a positive family history. A classification of myopathies is given in Table 19-16. The diagnosis of myopathy is based on the history and physical examination, increased levels of creatine kinase, EMG, muscle biopsy results, and selected genetic testing. For many adults with acquired myopathy, no underlying cause is found.

Inflammatory Myopathy

Inflammatory myopathies include polymyositis, dermatomyositis, and inclusion body myositis. With inflammatory myopathies, especially dermatomyositis, an underlying cancer may also be present. Inclusion body myositis occurs mainly in men older than 60 years; they have asymmetrical weakness of proximal and distal muscles, with a predilection for quadriceps, biceps, and finger flexors (this pattern is highly suggestive of inclusion body myositis). Inclusion body myositis is not associated with collagen vascular diseases or neoplasms, and the creatine kinase level may be normal or slightly increased. Muscle biopsy should be used to confirm the diagnosis of an inflammatory myopathy, although it may be suggested by the history and examination findings, increased serum levels of creatine kinase, and EMG results.

Prednisone is the cornerstone for treatment of polymyositis and dermatomyositis. The most common pitfall in treating these conditions is not treating with high enough doses of prednisone for sufficient time. Dermatomyositis, unlike inclusion body myositis or polymyositis, responds to IVIG. In both polymyositis and dermatomyositis, other immunomodulatory agents, including azathioprine, methotrexate, mycophenolate mofetil, cyclosporine, cyclophosphamide, and chlorambucil, are indicated if relapse occurs during prednisone taper, if unacceptable side effects develop from prednisone, or if there is no response to prednisone or the response is slow. Plasma exchange is ineffective for polymyositis, dermatomyositis, and inclusion body myositis. Trials of immunosuppression in inclusion body myositis have been negative. A regular exercise program is important, and it has been shown that physical therapy and exercise are not detrimental to patients with myopathies.

- *Myopathy* refers to muscle disease.
- If the disease is progressive and genetic, it is called *dystrophy*.
- Myotonic dystrophy: atrophy and weakness begin in the face and sternocleidomastoid muscles.
- Myotonia (ie, normal contraction with slow relaxation) is a feature of myotonic dystrophy. With myotonia, the patient cannot let go quickly after a handshake.
- Acquired myopathy: no underlying cause is found in many adults.

Table 19-16 Classification of Myopathies

Dystrophies
Nonprogressive or relatively nonprogressive congenital myopathies
Inflammatory myopathies
    Infectious & viral—toxoplasmosis, trichinosis
    Granulomatous—sarcoidosis
    Idiopathic—polymyositis, dermatomyositis, IBM
    With collagen vascular disease
Metabolic myopathies
    Glycogenoses
    Mitochondrial disorders
    Endocrine
Periodic paralysis
Toxic—emetine, chloroquine, vincristine, statin drugs
Miscellaneous
    Amyloidosis

Abbreviation: IBM, inclusion body myositis.

- Patients with dermatomyositis: increased incidence of occult carcinoma.
- Causes of myopathies: collagen vascular disease, paraneoplastic changes, amyloidosis, endocrinopathy, sarcoidosis.

Acute Alcoholic Myopathy

Patients with acute alcoholic myopathy have acute pain, swelling, tenderness, and weakness of mainly proximal muscles. Gross myoglobinuria may cause renal failure.

- Gross myoglobinuria often occurs in acute alcoholic myopathy.

Toxic Myopathies

Statin drugs (HMG-CoA inhibitors) may produce an acute necrotizing myopathy characterized by myalgia, weakness, myoglobinuria, and a marked increase in creatine kinase. This toxic effect is potentiated by fibric acid–derivative drugs and cyclosporine. A more subacute to chronic myopathy can also occur with statins. Symptoms of cramps and myalgias can occur, occasionally with little or no muscle weakness or creatine kinase elevation. How soon symptoms abate after discontinuing the drug is unknown, although 3 to 6 months may be needed. It is also likely that in some patients statins unmask a presymptomatic acquired or genetic myopathy. In some patients, even after discontinuing the statin medication, the myopathic symptoms persist.

Electrolyte Imbalance

Severe hypokalemia (<2.5 mEq/L) and hyperkalemia (>7 mEq/L) produce muscle weakness, as do hypercalcemia, hypocalcemia, and hypophosphatemia. Familial periodic paralysis of hypokalemic-, hyperkalemic-, or normokalemic-type consists of episodes of acute paralysis that last 2 to 24 hours and can be precipitated by a carbohydrate-rich meal or strenuous exercise; cranial or respiratory muscle paralysis does not occur. The diagnosis is difficult to make and is based on the potassium levels during an attack, family history, EMG, and, occasionally, genetic testing for certain sodium and calcium channel mutations.

Endocrine Diseases

Hyperthyroidism and hypothyroidism, hyperadrenalism and hypoadrenalism, acromegaly, and primary and secondary hyperparathyroidism cause muscle weakness.

Acute Muscle Weakness

Physicians may overlook serious underlying diseases in patients whose chief or only complaint is weakness, especially if there are few or no obvious clinical signs. A delayed or missed diagnosis can lead to life-threatening complications such as respiratory failure, irreversible spinal cord dysfunction, and acute renal failure. In some patients with neuromuscular weakness, respiratory muscles may be affected, although strength in the extremities is relatively normal. Patients with early Guillain-Barré syndrome may have distal paresthesias and increased respiratory effort and be given the diagnosis of hysterical hyperventilation.

- A missed diagnosis can lead to life-threatening complications: respiratory failure, irreversible spinal cord dysfunction, and acute renal failure.

- Early Guillain-Barré syndrome may be misdiagnosed as hysterical hyperventilation.

Acute, diffuse muscle weakness can be classified into 5 groups according to the anatomical location of the disorder: disease of the brain, spinal cord, peripheral nerve, neuromuscular junction, or muscle. Causes of acute muscle weakness are summarized in Table 19-17.

Part III—Disorders by Mechanism

Cerebrovascular Disease

Ischemic Cerebrovascular Disease

Pathophysiologic Mechanisms

The causes of ischemic cerebrovascular disorders, including TIA and cerebral infarction, can be classified on the basis of the site of the source for the arterial blockage (eg, embolus from a proximal site or thrombosis in situ from distal causes) within the vascular system, starting from most proximal to distal. First, a cardiac source as the most proximal site includes both arrhythmias and structural disorders such as valve disease, dilated cardiomyopathy, recent myocardial infarction, and other cardiac structural disorders. Also, paradoxical emboli with a right-to-left shunt through a patent foramen ovale must be considered, although most patent foramen ovales are asymptomatic. Another potential proximal site of emboli is the aorta. The second site includes large-vessel disorders, with the most common cause being atherosclerosis or dissection in the carotid or vertebrobasilar system. The third site involves small-vessel occlusive disease caused by either inflammatory or noninflammatory arteriopathies (eg, hypertension-induced disease, isolated CNS angiitis, and systemic lupus erythematosus). The fourth source is hematologic disorders, including polycythemia, sickle cell anemia, thrombocytosis, severe leukocytosis (ie, acute leukemia), antithrombin III deficiency, protein C deficiency, protein S deficiency, hereditary resistance to activated protein C, factor V Leiden mutation, anticardiolipin antibody syndrome, lupus anticoagulant positivity, and hypercoagulable states caused by carcinoma. Illicit drug use is a common cause of stroke in young persons and results in arrhythmia, inflammatory arteriopathies, and a relative hypercoagulable state.

- Pathophysiologic mechanisms of ischemic cerebrovascular disease include a cardiac source, large-vessel disorders, small-vessel disorders, and hematologic causes.
- In young adults, recreational drugs are a major risk factor for stroke.

Risk Factors

Risk factors for atherosclerotic occlusive disease are similar to those predisposing to coronary artery disease: hypertension, male sex, advanced age, cigarette smoking, diabetes mellitus, and hypercholesterolemia. Emboli from intracardiac mural thrombi are also an important cause of TIA and cerebral infarction. Proven cardiac risk factors include persistent atrial fibrillation, paroxysmal atrial fibrillation, sustained atrial flutter, dilated cardiomyopathy, mechanical

Table 19-17 Important Causes of Acute Muscle Weakness

Cerebral disease
    Hemiparesis
    Paraparesis—anterior cerebral artery
Spinal cord disease
    Transverse myelitis
    Epidural abscess
    Extradural tumor
    Epidural hematoma
    Herniated intervertebral disk
    Spinal cord tumor
Peripheral nerve disease
    Guillain-Barré syndrome
    Acute intermittent porphyria
    Arsenic poisoning
    Toxic neuropathies
    Tick paralysis
Neuromuscular junction disease
    Myasthenia gravis
    Botulism
    Organophosphate poisoning
Muscle disease
    Polymyositis
    Rhabdomyolysis-myoglobinuria
    Acute alcoholic myopathy
    Electrolyte imbalances
    Endocrine disease

Modified from Karkal SS. Rapid accurate appraisal of acute muscular weakness. Updates Neurology. 1991, pp 31-39. Used with permission.

valve, rheumatic valve disease, recent myocardial infarction, and others, as outlined in Table 19-18. Other potential risk factors for cerebral infarction that are less well proven are also listed in the table.

Hypertension is the most powerful modifiable risk factor for stroke, but other modifiable risk factors include cigarette smoking, diabetes mellitus, elevated cholesterol, metabolic syndrome, sedentary lifestyle, obesity, obstructive sleep apnea, and, possibly, elevated homocysteine levels. Although low levels of alcohol consumption appear to have a protective effect for ischemic stroke, heavy alcohol consumption increases the risk of all types of stroke, particularly intra-cerebral and subarachnoid hemorrhage.

Transient Ischemic Attacks

TIAs place patients at high risk of subsequent cerebral infarctions: estimates are from 4% to 10% within 1 year to 33% within the patient's lifetime. Most TIAs are brief, usually lasting less than 10 to 15 minutes; 88% resolve within 1 hour. Patients with infarcts, hemorrhages, and mass lesions can present like patients with TIAs.

Amaurosis fugax is defined as temporary, partial, or complete monocular blindness and is a classic symptom of a carotid artery TIA. It can be mimicked by glaucoma, vitreous hemorrhage, retinal detachment, papilledema, migrainous aura, temporal arteritis, and even ectopic floaters.

The long-term prognosis for patients who have a TIA generally follows the rule of 3s: one-third will have cerebral infarction, one-third will have at least 1 more TIA, and one-third will have no more TIAs. The following features help to determine the risk of stroke after TIA: age over 60 years, hypertension, weakness or speech disturbance with the TIA, duration of TIA greater than 60 minutes, and diabetes mellitus.

- Most TIAs last less than 10-15 minutes.
- Patients with infarcts, hemorrhages, and mass lesions can present with symptoms like those of a TIA.
- Amaurosis fugax is a classic symptom of a carotid artery TIA.
- The rule of 3s for patients with TIA: one-third will have cerebral infarction, one-third will have at least 1 more TIA, one-third will have no more TIAs.

Carotid Endarterectomy

Carotid endarterectomy markedly decreases the risk of stroke and death of *symptomatic* patients who have a 70% to 99% stenosis of the carotid artery, as seen on angiography. For a 50% to 69% stenosis, carotid endarterectomy is moderately efficacious in selected symptomatic patients. Medical treatment alone is better than carotid endarterectomy for patients with a stenosis of 49% or less. Symptoms must be those of a carotid territory TIA or minor stroke and must be of recent onset (<4 months). To have a favorable risk-benefit ratio, the perioperative complication rate must be low (<6%). Carotid angioplasty with stent placement may be used as an alternative to

Table 19-18 Cardiac Risks for Cerebral Infarction or Transient Ischemic Attack

Proven cardiac risks
    Atrial fibrillation
    Paroxysmal atrial fibrillation
    Sustained atrial flutter
    Dilated cardiomyopathy
    Mechanical valve
    Rheumatic valve disease
    Recent (within 1 month) myocardial infarction
    Intracardiac thrombus
    Intracardiac mass (ie, atrial myxoma or papillary fibroelastoma)
    Infectious endocarditis
    Nonbacterial thrombotic endocarditis
Putative or uncertain cardiac risks
    Sick sinus syndrome
    Patent foramen ovale with or without atrial septal aneurysm
    Atherosclerotic debris in the thoracic aorta
    Spontaneous echocardiographic contrast
    Myocardial infarction 2-6 mo earlier
    Hypokinetic or akinetic left ventricular segment
    Calcification of mitral annulus

carotid endarterectomy, particularly for higher risk patients, such as those who previously had carotid endarterectomy, radiotherapy to the neck, or neck dissection; those with a stenosis high in the internal carotid artery; or those otherwise deemed at high risk for the operation. The safety and durability of the endovascular approach in comparison with those of carotid endarterectomy are not clear, and the available data are somewhat conflicting at this point.

Selected patients with an *asymptomatic* carotid stenosis of at least 60% benefit from carotid endarterectomy in terms of future risk of an ipsilateral stroke or death. In the Asymptomatic Carotid Atherosclerosis Study (ACAS), medical patients were treated with aspirin and risk-factor reduction. The risk of stroke was low for patients treated surgically and for those treated medically (5-year risk of ipsilateral stroke or death was 11% for those treated medically and 6% for those treated surgically). This amounted to approximately a 1% difference per year. No trend was noted on the basis of the various degrees of stenosis, but the number of events was small in each stenosis subdivision. Importantly, surgeons and hospitals were chosen particularly for having reported perioperative complication rates of less than 3% in asymptomatic patients. In the Asymptomatic Carotid Surgery Trial, the efficacy of surgery was similar to that of medical management. The primary end point was ipsilateral stroke or any perioperative stroke or death (within 30 days of the procedure or entry into the study). The risk was 11.8% over 5 years among the patients treated medically and 6.4% among patients receiving surgical management.

Patients with asymptomatic carotid occlusive disease who require an operation for some other reason (eg, coronary artery bypass graft or abdominal aortic aneurysm repair) usually can have that procedure performed without prophylactic carotid endarterectomy, because in this context the risk of stroke in asymptomatic persons is quite low. If a patient has recently had symptoms in the distribution of the stenotic carotid artery, the decision is more complicated. Generally, if a patient with an asymptomatic carotid stenosis is experiencing cardiac symptoms such as angina, coronary artery bypass graft is performed first and carotid endarterectomy may be considered later if the patient is otherwise an excellent surgical candidate.

Antiplatelet Agents

Aspirin, aspirin in combination with extended-release dipyridamole, clopidogrel, and ticlopidine are all effective for secondary prevention of stroke. The optimal dose of aspirin is uncertain, with ranges recommended from 30 to 1,300 mg daily. Clopidogrel is given as a single dose, 75 mg daily. A combination of low-dose aspirin and extended-release dipyridamole is well tolerated and provides another useful alternative to aspirin for prevention of stroke. The dosage of ticlopidine is 250 mg twice daily. Ticlopidine is now rarely given because of the associated neutropenia (thus, a complete blood cell count must be monitored every 2 weeks for the first 3 months of treatment) and thrombotic thrombocytopenic purpura, which also has rarely been reported with clopidogrel. There is evidence that the use of clopidogrel and aspirin does not provide more prevention for ischemic stroke but does increase the risk of significant bleeding; therefore, the combination for stroke prevention is discouraged.

Management of Acute Cerebral Infarction

If a patient has a severe neurologic deficit caused by an acute cerebral infarction, the immediate decision in the emergency department is whether the patient is a candidate for thrombolytic therapy (tissue plasminogen activator [TPA]). The initial therapeutic approach to ischemic infarction depends greatly on the time from the onset of symptoms to the presentation for emergency medical care. If the onset of symptoms was less than 3 hours before the evaluation, emergent thrombolytic therapy should be considered. If a patient awakens from sleep with the deficit, thrombolytic therapy should not be considered unless the duration of the deficit is clearly less than 3 hours.

The CT findings are important in selecting patients for TPA. CT should not show any evidence of intracranial hemorrhage, mass effect, early evidence of significant cerebral infarction (greater than one-third distribution of the cerebral hemisphere), or midline shift. Patients who may be excluded by clinical criteria are those with rapidly improving deficit, obtunded or comatose status or presentation with seizure, history of intracranial hemorrhage or bleeding diathesis, blood pressure elevation persistently greater than 185/110 mm Hg, gastrointestinal tract hemorrhage or urinary tract hemorrhage within the previous 21 days, traumatic brain injury or cerebral infarction within 3 months, or mild deficit. Eligible patients should have marked weakness in at least 1 limb or severe aphasia. Laboratory abnormalities that may preclude treatment are heparin use within the previous 48 hours with an increased activated partial thromboplastin time, international normalized ratio (INR) greater than 1.5, or blood glucose concentration less than 50 mg/dL.

In a treatment trial of intravenous TPA, the efficacy in improving neurologic status at 3 months was defined for TPA compared with placebo, with the agent administered within 3 hours after the onset of symptoms. Although there was a greater proportion (12% greater) of subjects with minimal or no deficit in the TPA group at 3 months after the event, there was no increase in the proportion of persons with severe deficits or disability. This is particularly important because there was an increased occurrence of symptomatic hemorrhage in the TPA group (6.4% compared with 0.6%).

Intravenous TPA should be given in a 0.9-mg/kg dose (maximum, 90 mg), with 10% given as a bolus and the rest over 60 minutes.

- Intravenous TPA should be considered for patients evaluated within 3 hours after the onset of symptoms of severe cerebral infarction.
- Do not treat with TPA if CT shows hemorrhage, mass effect, or midline shift.

A mechanical device approved for use in acute ischemic stroke up to 8 hours after symptom onset is the Merci Retriever. This device is used with endovascular access and has a tiny corkscrew-shaped portion designed to extract the occlusive clots from intracranial arteries, thereby minimizing ischemic damage. This is an option for ischemic stroke patients who are not eligible for TPA.

Stroke Risks With Nonvalvular Atrial Fibrillation

Atrial fibrillation is associated with up to 24% of ischemic strokes and 50% of embolic strokes. The stroke rate for the entire cohort of patients with chronic atrial fibrillation is generally about 5% per year. However, patients younger than 60 with "lone atrial fibrillation" have a lower risk of stroke than other patients with atrial fibrillation and are often treated with only aspirin. Stroke risk factors with atrial fibrillation include a history of hypertension, recent congestive heart failure, previous thromboembolism (including TIAs), left ventricular dysfunction identified on 2-dimensional echocardiography, and increased size of the left atrium identified on M-mode echocardiography. Patients with atrial fibrillation who have 1 or more risk factors generally should receive anticoagulation with warfarin (INR, 2.0-3.0) and those at low risk should receive aspirin.

For patients receiving anticoagulant therapy, the dominant risk factor for intracranial hemorrhage is the INR. Age is another risk factor for subdural hemorrhage. An INR of 2.0 to 3.0 is probably an adequate level of anticoagulation for nearly all warfarin indications except for preventing embolization from mechanical heart valves. Generally, the lowest effective intensity of anticoagulant therapy should be given.

- Atrial fibrillation is associated with 24% of ischemic strokes and 50% of embolic strokes.
- The stroke rate is about 5% per year.
- Patients with "lone atrial fibrillation" have a lower risk of stroke.

Hemorrhagic Cerebrovascular Disease

Intracerebral Hemorrhage
Hypertension commonly affects deep penetrating cerebral vessels, especially ones supplying the basal ganglia, cerebral white matter, thalamus, pons, and cerebellum. The following are common misconceptions of intracerebral hemorrhage: the onset is generally sudden and catastrophic, hypertension is invariably severe, headache is always present, reduced consciousness or coma is usually present, the CSF is always bloody, and the prognosis is poor and mortality is high. None of these features may be present, and the prognosis depends on the size and location of the hemorrhage. Amyloid angiopathy is the second most common cause of intracerebral hemorrhage in older persons and often causes recurrent lobar hemorrhages.

- With intracerebral hemorrhage, the prognosis depends on the size and site of the hemorrhage.

Surgical evacuation of intracerebral hematomas may be necessary for patients who have signs of increased intracranial pressure or for those whose condition is worsening.

Cerebellar Hemorrhage
It is important to recognize cerebellar hemorrhage because drainage may be lifesaving. The important clinical findings are vomiting and inability to walk. Long-tract signs usually are not present. Patients may have ipsilateral gaze palsy, ipsilateral CN VI palsy, or ipsilateral nuclear-type CN VII palsy (upper and lower facial weakness). They may or may not have headache, vertigo, and lethargy. Cerebellar hemorrhage may cause obstructive hydrocephalus.

- Vomiting and the inability to walk are important findings in cerebellar hemorrhage.
- Long-tract signs usually are not present.
- Cerebellar hemorrhage may cause obstructive hydrocephalus.

Subarachnoid Hemorrhage
Subarachnoid hemorrhage (SAH) accounts for about 5% of strokes, including about half of those in patients younger than 45, with a peak age range between 35 and 65 years. In up to 50% of cases, an alert patient with an aneurysm may have a small sentinel bleed with a warning headache, or the expansion of an aneurysm may cause focal neurologic signs or symptoms, for example, an incomplete CN III palsy. The prognosis is related directly to the state of consciousness at the time of intervention. The headache is characteristically sudden in onset, and although one-third of SAHs occur during exertion, one-third occur during rest, and one-third during sleep. The peak incidence of vasospasm associated with SAH occurs between days 4 and 12 after the initial hemorrhage. Other complications include 1) hemorrhagic infiltration into the brain, ventricles, and even subdural space, which requires evacuation; 2) hyponatremia associated with a cerebral salt-wasting syndrome or the syndrome of inappropriate secretion of antidiuretic hormone; and 3) communicating hydrocephalus.

In addition to the initial hemorrhage, vasospasm and rehemorrhaging are the leading causes of morbidity and mortality of patients who have an SAH.

The outpouring of catecholamines may cause myocardial damage, with accompanying electrocardiographic abnormalities, pulmonary edema, and arrhythmias. Arrhythmias can be both supraventricular and ventricular and are most likely to occur during the initial hours or days after a moderate-to-severe SAH.

Initial treatment is supportive, often in an intensive care unit. Prevention of vasospasm is best achieved with maintaining normal or increased blood pressure and intravascular volume as well as using the calcium channel blocker nimodipine. If the SAH is from a ruptured aneurysm, early intervention (surgical clipping or endovascular coiling) is often done by an experienced team.

- About 5% of strokes are an SAH.
- In 50% of cases, an alert patient with an aneurysm may have a small sentinel bleed.
- The prognosis is related directly to the state of consciousness at the time of intervention.
- Characteristically, the headache has a sudden onset.

The differential diagnosis of subtypes of hemorrhagic cerebrovascular disease is outlined in Table 19-19.

Neoplastic Disease

The most common neurologic symptoms of patients with systemic cancer are back pain, altered mental status, and headache. However, the most common neurologic complication of systemic cancer is metastatic disease, of which cerebral metastasis is most frequent. In patients with cancer and back pain, epidural metastasis and direct vertebral metastasis are common, but no malignant cause is found in about 15% to 20% of patients. Nonstructural causes are the most common reasons for headache. Some identified causes include fever, side effects of therapy, lumbar puncture, metastasis (cerebral, leptomeningeal, or base of skull), and intracranial hemorrhage (thrombocytopenia or hemorrhage due to intracranial metastasis). The most common cause of altered mental status is toxic-metabolic encephalopathy, which is also the most common nonmetastatic manifestation of systemic cancer. Less common causes include intracranial metastatic disease (parenchymal and meningeal), paraneoplastic limbic encephalitis, intracranial hemorrhage, primary dementia, cerebral infarction, psychiatric disorder, known primary brain tumor, bacterial meningitis, and transient global amnesia.

Neoplasms that commonly cause neurologic problems are those of the lung and breast, leukemia, lymphoma, and colorectal cancer. Breast, lung, and prostate cancer are most likely to spread to bone with epidural metastasis. The most common brain metastasis is from the lung. Meningeal metastases occur in lung and breast cancer, melanoma, leukemia, and lymphoma. Colorectal cancer causes local pelvic metastasis and is the most frequent cause of neoplastic plexopathy. Head cancer and neck cancer are the most frequent sources of metastasis to the base of the skull. Melanoma produces a disproportionate number of metastases in the CNS. Gastrointestinal tract tumors (eg, stomach, esophagus, and pancreas) have the least number of neurologic complications.

Many neurologic problems in patients with cancer can be diagnosed on the basis of the medical history and findings on neurologic examination and require knowledge of both nonmetastatic- and noncancer-related neurologic illness. Neurologic complications of systemic cancer can be divided generally into the following categories:

1. Metastatic—parenchymal, leptomeningeal, epidural, subdural, brachial and lumbosacral plexuses, and nerve infiltration; this is common
2. Infectious—unusual CNS infections because of immunosuppression
3. Complications of systemic metastases—hepatic encephalopathy
4. Vascular complications—cerebral infarction from hypercoagulable states, nonbacterial thrombotic endocarditis, and radiation damage to carotid arteries; cerebral hemorrhage from such entities as thrombocytopenia and hemorrhagic metastases
5. Toxic-metabolic encephalopathies—usually from multiple causes, hypercalcemia, syndrome of inappropriate secretion of antidiuretic hormone, medications, and systemic infections
6. Complications of treatment (irradiation, chemotherapy, or surgery)—radiation necrosis of the brain, radiation myelopathy, radiation plexopathy, fibrosis of the carotid arteries, neuropathies, encephalopathies, and cerebellar ataxia
7. Paraneoplastic (ie, nonmetastatic or "remote" effect of cancer)—syndromes have been described from the cerebral cortex through the central and peripheral neuraxes to muscle; they are rare
8. Miscellaneous—various systemic and neurologic illnesses having nothing to do with cancer

- Cerebral metastasis is the most common neurologic complication of systemic cancer.
- Toxic-metabolic encephalopathy is the most common nonmetastatic manifestation of cancer.
- Cancers commonly causing neurologic problems are lung, breast, and colorectal cancers, leukemia, and lymphoma.
- The most common source of brain metastasis is from lung and breast cancer, melanoma, leukemia, and lymphoma.
- The most frequent cause of tumor plexopathy is colorectal cancer.
- Melanoma produces a disproportionate number of metastases in the CNS.

Table 19-19 Differential Diagnosis of Subtypes of Hemorrhagic Cerebrovascular Disease

Hemorrhage into parenchyma
  Hypertension
  Amyloid angiopathy
  Aneurysm
  Vascular malformation
    Arteriovenous malformation
    Cavernous malformation
    Venous malformation (rare cause of hemorrhage)
  Trauma—primarily frontal & temporal
  Hemorrhagic infarction
  Secondary to brain tumors (primary & secondary neoplasms)
  Inflammatory diseases of vasculature
  Disorders of blood-forming organs (blood dyscrasia, especially leukemia & thrombocytopenic purpura)
  Anticoagulant or thrombolytic therapy
  Increased intracranial pressure (brainstem) (Duret hemorrhages)
  Illicit drug use (cocaine or amphetamines)
  Postsurgical
  Fat embolism (petechial)
  Hemorrhagic encephalitis (petechial)
  Undetermined cause (normal blood pressure & no other recognizable disorder)
Hemorrhage into subarachnoid space (subarachnoid hemorrhage)
  Trauma
  Aneurysm
    Saccular ("berry," "congenital")
    Fusiform (arteriosclerotic)—rarely causes hemorrhage
    Mycotic
  Arteriovenous malformation
  Many of the same causes listed under "Hemorrhage into parenchyma" above
Subdural & epidural hemorrhage (hematoma)
  Mainly traumatic (especially during anticoagulation)
  Many of the same causes listed under "Hemorrhage into parenchyma" above
Hemorrhage into pituitary (pituitary apoplexy)

- Common metastatic sites are the parenchyma of the cerebral hemispheres and cerebellum, leptomeninges, epidural and subdural spaces, brachial and lumbosacral plexuses, and nerve.

Radiosurgery (gamma knife and the linear accelerator [LINAC]-based systems) has been used to treat vascular malformations, acoustic neuromas, pituitary adenomas, and meningeal and (recently) metastatic tumors.

Primary CNS lymphoma is becoming more common in both AIDS and immunocompetent patients. Median survival has been increased with the combination of radiotherapy and chemotherapy, mainly intravenous methotrexate.

Paraneoplastic Disorders

The paraneoplastic disorders are associated with increased levels of circulating antibodies against membrane (eg, ion channels) or cytoplasmic components of neoplastic cells. The most common underlying malignancies are small cell lung carcinoma and breast cancer. Others include ovarian or testicular carcinoma, thymoma, Hodgkin disease, and parotid tumors. Paraneoplastic autoimmunity occurs with various neurologic syndromes, including limbic encephalitis (characterized by behavioral and memory abnormalities), brainstem encephalitis, opsoclonus-myoclonus, cerebellar ataxia, myelopathy, peripheral neuropathy, stiff-person syndrome (with axial and limb rigidity), sensory ganglionopathies, LEMS, dermatomyositis, and retinopathy. These syndromes are characterized by an acute or subacute onset and increased levels of 1 or more antibodies. Neither the neurologic syndrome nor the antibody is pathognomonic for a particular neoplasm, and many neurologic syndromes and antibodies may coexist in the same patient.

Among patients with LEMS, anti–calcium channel antibodies are present in 80% of the patients who have primary lung cancer (small cell, squamous cell, or adenocarcinoma) and in 36% of the patients who have no evidence of cancer. Those with LEMS who have cancer other than lung cancer usually are negative for these antibodies. Antineuronal nuclear antibodies (ANNA) type I (anti-Hu) are a marker of various neurologic disorders that occur with small cell lung cancer, and the ANNA type II (anti-Ri) antibodies occur in a spectrum of neurologic disorders associated with breast cancer, including cerebellar ataxia, myelopathy, opsoclonus, and other brainstem disorders. Purkinje cell antibodies (sometimes called "anti-Yo" antibodies) are detected in women with paraneoplastic cerebellar degeneration and are associated with ovarian, fallopian tube, endometrial, surface papillary, and breast carcinomas and occasionally with lymphoma. They are not found in men with paraneoplastic cerebellar degeneration or in women with gynecologic cancer without a neurologic syndrome. In a woman who does not have clinically known or laboratory-proven cancer but is positive for these antibodies, exploratory laparotomy probably is warranted. Amphiphysin antibodies occur in patients who have rigidity, peripheral neuropathy, and other neurologic syndromes generally associated with breast cancer. Antibodies to collapsin response mediator protein-5 (CRMP-5) are associated with several cancers (especially small cell carcinoma) and can lead to many neurologic complications, most notable of which is a movement disorder (ie, chorea) or optic neuropathy.

Movement Disorders

Tremor

Tremor is an oscillatory rhythmical movement disorder. A simple classification of tremor is rest tremor, postural tremor, and kinetic tremor (Table 19-20).

Rest tremor is observed with the arms lying in the patient's lap while he or she is sitting or with the arms at the patient's side while walking. Rest tremor occurs in Parkinson disease. *Postural tremor* is seen mainly with the arms outstretched, although there is often a kinetic component as well. Postural tremor is physiologic, but it is also noted pathologically in essential tremor. Drugs such as methylxanthines, β-adrenergic agonists, lithium, and amiodarone may produce postural tremor. *Kinetic tremor* is seen mainly in action, as in finger-to-nose testing. This type of tremor occurs with cerebellar disease and diseases of the cerebellar connections in the brainstem.

Essential Tremor

Essential tremor is the most common movement disorder. It is a monosymptomatic condition that is manifested as rhythmic oscillations of various parts of the body. Middle-aged and older persons are most commonly affected, and there is often a genetic component. The hands are affected most, with the tremor present in the postural position and often having a kinetic component. The head and voice can be affected. Head tremor can be either horizontal ("no-no") or vertical ("yes-yes"). Head tremor almost never occurs in Parkinson disease, but parkinsonian patients may have tremor of the mouth, lips, tongue, and jaw. The legs and trunk (orthostatic tremor) are affected less frequently in essential tremor. Essential tremor is a slowly progressive condition; its pathophysiologic mechanism is not known.

The agent most effective in decreasing essential tremor is alcohol. Alcoholic drinks substantially reduce the tremor for 45 to 60 minutes. However, the rate of alcoholism among patients with essential tremor is no different from that of the general population. Propranolol (80-320 mg daily), other β-blockers, and primidone (25-250 mg at bedtime) are effective. Other drugs that have been prescribed are clonazepam, gabapentin, and topiramate. Methazolamide has also been effective in some patients, especially for head tremor. Botulinum toxin has been used recently. Stereotactic thalamotomy can be effective for patients with severe functional disability whose tremor is unresponsive to drug therapy; surgery probably is underused. Thalamic stimulation (ie, deep brain stimulation) is effective for all types of tremor.

- Essential tremor occurs mostly in middle-aged and older persons.
- There is often a genetic component.
- The hands are affected most.
- Head tremor is almost never seen in Parkinson disease.

Parkinson Disease

Patients with Parkinson disease present with tremor (the initial symptom in 50%-70%, but 15% never have tremor), rigidity, and bradykinesia. Also, gait is unsteady—a slow, shuffling gait. Decreased blinking rate, lack of change in facial expression, small handwriting, and asymptomatic orthostatic hypotension are also common. Although

Table 19-20 Differential Diagnosis of Tremor

Feature	Parkinson Disease	Essential Tremor
Tremor type & frequency	Rest >> postural; 3-5 Hz	Postural, kinetic; 8-12 Hz
Affected by tremor	Hands, legs, chin, jaw	Hands, head, neck, voice
Rigidity & brady-kinesia	Yes	No
Family history	15%	60%
Alcohol response	Inconsistent	Consistent
Therapy	Levodopa, dopamine agonists, anticholinergics	Propranolol, primidone, gabapentin, botulinum toxin type A
Surgical treatment	Subthalamic stimulation	Thalamic (Vim) stimulation

Abbreviation: Vim, subnucleus ventralis intermedius.

dementia is more frequent among patients with Parkinson disease, it is noted in only about 25% of those in whom the disease develops after age 60. Other nonmotor manifestations of Parkinson disease are listed in Tables 19-21 through 19-23. The detection of cerebellar findings (ataxia), corticospinal signs (increased deep tendon reflexes, spasticity, or extensor plantar response), or lower motor neuron findings (decreased reflexes, flaccidity, or fasciculations) should each suggest a disorder other than Parkinson disease as a cause of parkinsonism. Parkinson-plus syndromes are frequently the diagnoses when any of these findings are present (Table 19-24). Several medications can lead to a parkinsonian presentation (Table 19-25).

* Tremor does not occur in 15% of patients with Parkinson disease.
* If ataxia, increased reflexes, spasticity, extensor plantar responses, or lower motor neuron findings are present, consider Parkinson-plus syndromes.

The treatment of Parkinson disease is summarized in Table 19-26. Initial treatment options include a combination of levodopa and carbidopa (Sinemet), anticholinergic agents, amantadine, or dopaminergic agonists. Anticholinergic agents should not be given to patients older than 65 because of the high incidence of side effects, such as memory loss, delirium, urinary hesitancy, and blurred vision. When given to a patient with newly diagnosed Parkinson disease, selegiline (a monoamine oxidase type B inhibitor) may delay the initiation of levodopa therapy as well as give mild symptomatic relief. Initial dosages of a combination of levodopa and carbidopa include a 25/100 tablet 3 times daily on an empty stomach. Side effects include nausea, hallucinations, confusion, dyskinesias, and orthostatic hypotension. Long-term high-dose levodopa monotherapy leads to dyskinesias and motor fluctuations. Management strategies include the use of smaller and more frequent doses of levodopa, long-acting levodopa preparations, dopaminergic agonists,

and inhibitors of catechol O-methyltransferase. A newer preparation of levodopa, apomorphine, can be administered subcutaneously for severe, hypomobile, "off" times. Unpredictable off periods may also be helped with the use of a protein restriction diet.

Dopaminergic agonists include the ergot derivatives bromocriptine and pergolide and the nonergot derivatives pramipexole and ropinirole. Although monotherapy with dopamine agonists carries a smaller risk of developing delayed motor complications than long-term levodopa therapy, these agents are less efficacious than levodopa. The use of dopaminergic agonists rather than levodopa for early treatment of Parkinson disease has been proposed. The rationale is that this will delay the potential toxic effects of dopamine metabolites in the brain. However, this point is controversial. Like levodopa, dopaminergic agonists may cause hallucinations, postural hypotension, and edema. An important side effect of all these agents is the development of unpredictable episodes of daytime sleepiness. Bromocriptine has been associated with pulmonary and retroperitoneal fibrosis. Reportedly, pergolide is associated potentially with valvular heart disease. New-generation antipsychotic drugs, such as clozapine, olanzapine, and quetiapine, can be used to manage drug-induced psychosis because they have a lower risk of exacerbating parkinsonism in these patients. Stereotactic pallidotomy and subthalamic nucleus stimulation are performed in patients with predominantly unilateral symptoms. These treatments are particularly effective for tremor and drug-induced dyskinesia.

Many patients with parkinsonism develop orthostatic hypotension, bladder dysfunction, and other autonomic manifestations. In these patients, Parkinson disease should be distinguished from multiple system atrophy. Findings suggestive of multiple system atrophy include lack of a predictable response to levodopa, the presence of cerebellar or pyramidal signs, severe orthostatic hypotension and urinary incontinence, sleep apnea, and laryngeal stridor. The management of orthostatic hypotension includes eliminating potentially offending drugs (eg, vasodilators, diuretics, dopaminergic agonists, and clozapine), increasing sodium and water intake, performing postural maneuvers, elevating the head of the bed, and wearing support stockings. Drug treatment includes fludrocortisone (0.1-1.0 mg daily) and vasoconstrictors such as midodrine (10-40 mg daily).

Table 19-21 Nonmotor Complications of Parkinson Disease

Complications
   Sleep disorders
   Autonomic involvement
   Hallucinations
   Depression
   Cognitive impairment
   Sensory symptoms
   Abnormal behavior
Management
   Complications tend to occur at late stages of the disease
   Always consider effect of medications as possible cause
   Treat only if disabling

Table 19-22 Neuropsychiatric Manifestations in Parkinson Disease

Problem	Possible Cause	Management

Hallucinations	Medication effect (exclude RBD)	Discontinue
		  Anticholinergics
		  MAO-B inhibitors
		  Amantadine
		Reduce or discontinue dopaminergic agonists
		Quetiapine (25-75 mg at bedtime)
		Cholinesterase inhibitors

Depression	Loss of serotonergic neurons	Optimize dopaminergic therapy SSRIs (may worsen symptoms or interact with selegiline)
Cognitive impairment	Bradyphrenia Dementia (consider DLB)	Optimize dopaminergic therapy Exclude treatable causes Cholinesterase inhibitors
Anxiety	Akathisia Stressors	Increase dopaminergic therapy

Abbreviations: DLB, dementia with Lewy bodies; MAO, monoamine oxidase; RBD, rapid eye movement sleep behavior disorder; SSRI, selective serotonin reuptake inhibitor.

Table 19-23 Other Manifestations in Parkinson Disease

Manifestation	Cause	Management
Pain	Early morning dystonia Motor fluctuations Mechanical	Increase levodopa dose Mobilization Physical therapy
Arm paresthesia	May reflect insufficient levodopa treatment	Increase levodopa dose Exclude other causes (carpal tunnel syndrome, etc)
Fatigue	Multifactorial	Stimulants (little help)
Diplopia	Medication effect Poor convergence	Consider reading glasses and prisms instead of bifocals
Pathologic gambling Hypersexuality	Activation of D3 receptors in limbic striatum	Warn patients before starting dopaminergic agonists Quetiapine or SSRI may help

Abbreviation: SSRI, selective serotonin reuptake inhibitor.

Pyridostigmine can also be used for orthostatic hypotension in dosages similar to those used in myasthenia gravis (30-60 mg 3 times daily).

Other Movement Disorders: Botulinum Toxin Therapy
Botulinum toxin, which blocks the neuromuscular junction, is effective therapy for cervical dystonia, blepharospasm, hemifacial spasm, spasmodic dysphonia, jaw-closing oromandibular dystonia, and limb dystonia, including occupational dystonias.

Inflammatory and Immune Disorders

Demyelinating Diseases
Idiopathic inflammatory demyelinating diseases of the CNS are as follows:

1. Multiple sclerosis
2. Isolated demyelinating syndromes—optic neuritis and transverse myelitis
3. Primary progressive demyelinating diseases—chronic progressive myelopathy and progressive cerebellar syndrome
4. Asymptomatic demyelinating diseases (noted on MRI or autopsy)

Multiple sclerosis is a common, disabling demyelinating CNS disorder of young adults, with an onset between 20 to 50 years of age. It affects women twice as often as men. Multiple sclerosis has a variable prognosis and an unpredictable course. Polygenetic and environmental (possibly viral) factors probably have a substantial effect on susceptibility to multiple sclerosis. The disease attacks white matter (and, later in the course, axons) of the cerebral hemispheres,

Table 19-24 Differential Diagnosis of Parkinson-Plus Syndromes

Manifestation	Suspect
Poor response to levodopa	Any parkinson-plus syndrome (MSA & PSP may respond)
Early falls	PSP or MSA
Severe OH & urologic Sx	MSA
Cerebellar signs	MSA or spinocerebellar degeneration
Vertical gaze palsy	PSP
Asymmetric apraxia	Corticobasal degeneration
Early dementia	Dementia with Lewy bodies of Creutzfeldt-Jakob disease

Abbreviations: MSA, multiple system atrophy; OH, orthostatic hypotension; PSP, progressive supranuclear palsy; Sx, symptoms.

Table 19-25 Drugs That Induce Parkinsonism or Tremor

Antagonist of D_2 receptors
  Neuroleptics (haloperidol, risperidone, resperine, etc)
  Antiemetics (metoclopramide, prochloperazine)
Other psychiatric drugs
  Selective serotonin reuptake inhibitors
  Tricyclics
  Lithium
Cardiovascular drugs
  Amiodarone
  Calcium channel blockers (flunarizine)
  Atorvastatin
Anticonvulsants
  Valproate
Others
  Cyclosporine
  Metronidazole
  Caffeine & other methylxanthines
  β-Adrenergic agonists
  Thyroxine
  Prednisone

brainstem, cerebellum, spinal cord, and optic nerve. Eighty percent to 85% of patients present with relapsing-remitting symptoms. In about 15% of patients, the disease is progressive from onset (primary progressive). Over time, 70% of patients with the relapsing-remitting form will develop secondary progressive multiple sclerosis. Symptoms reflect multiple white matter lesions "disseminated in space and time" and include spastic weakness of the limbs, ataxia, diplopia, sensory disturbances, loss of vision, and urinary bladder and bowel dysfunction. Other important symptoms include fatigue, subtle memory and cognitive dysfunction, and depression.

The diagnosis is based on established clinical criteria and supportive laboratory data. Abnormalities on MRI are most helpful and include multifocal lesions of various ages in the periventricular white matter, corpus callosum, brainstem, cerebellum, and spinal cord. Gadolinium-enhanced lesions are presumed to be active lesions of inflammatory demyelination. CSF findings include oligoclonal bands, increased IgG synthesis, and moderate lymphocytic pleocytosis (<50 mononuclear cells/mcL). Visual and somatosensory evoked potential studies are less helpful.

Predictors associated with a more favorable long-term course of multiple sclerosis include age younger than 40 at onset, female sex, optic neuritis or isolated sensory symptoms as the first clinical manifestation, and relatively infrequent attacks. Prognostic factors associated with a poor outcome include age older than 40 at onset, male sex, cerebellar or pyramidal tract findings at initial presentation, relatively frequent attacks during the first 2 years, incomplete remissions, and a chronically progressive course. However, no single clinical variable is sufficient to predict the course or outcome of this disease. Acute transverse myelopathy is usually a monophasic disorder and is rarely the first sign of multiple sclerosis. Abnormal MRI findings at presentation of a patient with a clinically isolated syndrome suggestive of multiple sclerosis (ie, isolated involvement of the optic nerve, brainstem, or spinal cord) are a strong predictor of the eventual clinical diagnosis of multiple sclerosis in the next 5 years. Interferon beta-1b, interferon beta-1a, and glatiramer acetate decrease the relapse rate and the intensity of relapse in patients with the relapsing-remitting type of multiple sclerosis. Evidence is mounting that these medications also reduce disability in the long run. They are expensive, however, and significant side effects can occur. There is evidence that a subset of multiple sclerosis patients has very benign disease; hence, not every patient with multiple sclerosis must receive long-term treatment.

A study of corticosteroid therapy for optic neuritis found that oral prednisone therapy was ineffective. The recommended therapy is a 3- to 5-day course of a high dose of intravenous methylprednisolone (1.0 g daily), which may be followed by a short oral prednisone taper, although tapering is not necessary. This 5-day intravenous steroid treatment is used in most multiple sclerosis exacerbations that are significant enough to impair a patient's function.

Several drugs are used to treat specific symptoms of multiple sclerosis. Trigeminal neuralgia, flexor spasms, and other paroxysmal symptoms respond to carbamazepine, and spasticity responds to baclofen and tizanidine. Fatigue, a disabling symptom of multiple sclerosis, occasionally responds to amantadine or modafinil.

- Typical clinical scenario for multiple sclerosis: A 35-year-old woman has a history of rapid loss of vision in the right eye, with pain on eye movement. A similar episode occurred 2 years ago and involved the same eye, and recovery was complete. She also has noticed weakness and paresthesias of both legs in the past 6 months. CSF analysis shows increased protein levels and oligoclonal bands on electrophoresis. Multiple T2 hyperintense areas consistent with demyelination are seen on MRI.

Neurologic Infectious Diseases

Infectious diseases of the nervous system are manifested in various combinations of meningitis, encephalitis, brain abscess, granulomas,

Table 19-26 Treatment of Parkinson Disease

Treatment	Indications	Caveats/Problems
Anticholinergic agent (eg, trihexyphenidyl)	Tremor predominant in young patients	Anticholinergic & cognitive side effects in patients older than 65 years
Amantadine	Early disease; adjuvant treatment for patients with dyskinesia	Dizziness, livedo reticularis, edema

Levodopa-carbidopa
    Sinemet 25/100
    Sinemet CR 50/200
	Most efficacious treatment; give early in disease to patients with marked impairment	Nausea, vomiting, orthostatic hypotension, hallucinations, motor fluctuations with chronic treatment

Dopaminergic agonists
    Bromocriptine
    Pergolide
    Pramipexole
    Ropinirole
	Motor fluctuations while taking Sinemet
	Some recommend use of these agonists early in course of disease
		As with Sinemet (except fluctuations), pleuro-pulmonary reaction & retroperitoneal fibrosis with ergots; patients may fall asleep while driving

COMT inhibitors Entacapone	Prolong duration of action of levodopa in patients with "wearing-off" effect	As with levodopa; diarrhea
MAO-B inhibitors Selegiline	Delay the need to start levodopa therapy; potential (not proven) neuroprotective effect	Insomnia

Atypical antipsychotics
    Clozapine
    Olanzapine
    Quetiapine
	Hallucinations; try to avoid extra-pyramidal side effects; may improve akathisia & dyskinesia	Risk of myelosuppression & orthostatic hypotension with clozapine

Surgical treatment
    Pallidotomy
    Subthalamic nucleus stimulation
	Prominent unilateral symptoms, particularly when associated with dyskinesia	Does not help axial problems or gait instability; risk of optic tract damage with pallidotomy; risk of paresis; speech or swallowing disturbances, particularly with bilateral pallidotomy

Abbreviations: COMT, catechol O methyltransferase; MAO, monoamine oxidase.

and vasculitis. The typical clinical and CSF findings and common causes of these diseases are summarized in Table 19-27. The most common causes and empirical treatment of bacterial meningitis are summarized in Table 19-28.

Lyme Disease—Multisystem Disorder

Stage I Lyme disease begins with the bite of an infected tick. Any body area may be bitten, but the thigh, groin, and axilla are common sites. Often, patients cannot recall the tick bite.

Stage II disease begins weeks to months after the initial infection and is characterized by neurologic, cardiac, and ophthalmic involvement. About 15% of the patients in the United States have neurologic involvement, usually meningoencephalitis, cranial neuritis, or radiculoneuropathy. Cranial neuropathies are common, most frequently with CN VII (bilaterally in one-third of patients). Thus, bilateral CN VII palsy in a patient from an endemic area is almost diagnostic of Lyme disease. Peripheral nervous system involvement can include the spinal roots, plexuses, and peripheral nerves.

Stage III disease marks the chronic phase and begins months to years after the initial infection. This stage is heralded by arthritic and neurologic symptoms. Any CNS symptom is possible, and there

may be psychiatric symptoms and cognitive impairment. Severe fatigue is a particularly prominent feature. Rarely, a multiple sclerosis–like demyelinating illness featuring gait disturbance, urinary bladder dysfunction, spastic paraparesis, and dysarthria may develop. These symptoms may have exacerbations and remissions; MRI shows multifocal white matter lesions.

- Lyme disease is a multisystem disorder.
- Patients often do not recall the tick bite.
- In the United States, 15% of patients have neurologic involvement.
- Cranial neuropathies, especially with CN VII, are common.
- Bilateral CN VII palsy in an endemic area is almost diagnostic of Lyme disease.
- In stage III disease, severe fatigue is prominent.

The longer the duration of symptoms before diagnosis and effective antibiotic treatment, the greater the risk that serious symptoms will outlast the period of acute infection. Laboratory diagnosis can be difficult; an enzyme-linked immunosorbent assay can be undependable both in identifying new cases and in distinguishing acute from remote healed infection. A confirmatory Western blot analysis

Table 19-27 Infectious Syndromes in the Central Nervous System

Syndrome	Clinical Features	CSF Analysis and Other Findings	Common or Important Causes
Aseptic meningitis	Headache, fever, neck stiffness for <4 wk	Mild to moderate mononuclear pleocytosis, normal glucose levels	Infectious—enteroviruses, arboviruses, HSV-2 and 6, HIV, mumps, *Borrelia burgdorferi*, *Treponema pallidum*, *Mycoplasma* Noninfectious—autoimmune disease, drug-induced
Bacterial meningitis	Headache, fever, neck stiffness for <4 wk	Moderate to marked polynuclear pleocytosis, low glucose levels	*Streptococcus pneumoniae*, *Neisseria meningitidis*, *Listeria monocytogenes*, *Haemophilus influenzae*
Recurrent meningitis	Multiple acute episodes for <4 wk	Mild to moderate mixed pleocytosis, variable glucose levels	Anatomical defects (*S pneumoniae*), HSV-2 autoimmune disease Chemical meningitis
Chronic meningitis	Chronic headache & cognitive, cranial nerve, or other focal symptoms for >4 wk	Mild to moderate mononuclear-pleocytosis, low glucose levels, meningeal enhancement or hydrocephalus on MRI	Infectious—*Mycobacterium tuberculosis*, fungal (eg, *Cryptococcus neoformans*) Noninfectious—sarcoidosis, neoplastic disease, vasculitis, autoimmune disorders
Acute encephalitis	Headache, fever, altered consciousness; frequently associated with seizures & focal or multifocal neurologic deficits	Mononuclear (occasionally polynuclear) pleocytosis, normal (occasionally low) glucose levels, abnormal EEG, high T2 signal lesions on MRI	HSV-1, La Crosse encephalitis, St Louis encephalitis, Rocky Mountain spotted fever VZV, EBV, CMV, HHV-6, & enteroviruses in immunosuppressed patients
Postinfectious encephalomyelitis	Fever, multifocal neurologic signs, altered consciousness	Multiple areas of hyperintense T2 signal consistent with multifocal demyelinating disease, lymphocytic pleocytosis	Postviral (varicella, mumps, measles, URTI), postimmunization

Abbreviations: CMV, cytomegalovirus; CSF, cerebrospinal fluid; EBV, Epstein-Barr virus; EEG, electroencephalography; HHV, human herpesvirus; HIV, human immunodeficiency virus; HSV, herpes simplex virus; MRI, magnetic resonance imaging; URTI, upper respiratory tract infection; VZV, varicella-zoster virus.

is recommended. Asymptomatic tick bites have a less than 1% chance of Lyme infection, and treating such patients for Lyme disease is not cost-effective. However, typical erythema migrans accompanying either a tick bite or other typical symptoms is sufficiently diagnostic to warrant treatment after exposure in an endemic area, even without abnormal serologic findings.

Neurologic Complications of AIDS

The nervous system is affected clinically in up to 40% of patients with HIV infection, and pathologic changes in the nervous system are found at autopsy in up to 90%. Neurologic features may be the presenting manifestation of the illness in 5% to 10% of patients. HIV infection is associated with various central and peripheral nervous system disorders, and multiple levels of the nervous system can be affected simultaneously. Therapy is available for many of these syndromes. The major HIV-related neurologic conditions include dementia, toxoplasmic encephalitis, CNS lymphoma, progressive multifocal leukoencephalopathy, cytomegalovirus encephalitis, cryptococcal meningitis, neurosyphilis, vacuolar myelopathy, distal symmetrical polyneuropathy, inflammatory demyelinating

polyradiculoneuropathy, mononeuropathy multiplex, progressive polyradiculopathy, and myopathy.

Patients with AIDS dementia complex have an increased concentration of CSF beta2-microglobulin, which may be a valuable marker for the severity of dementia and the response to treatment. Treatment with zidovudine markedly decreases the concentration of beta2-microglobulin. Other treatment considerations include the following:

1. Cytomegalovirus encephalitis is treated with ganciclovir.
2. A syndrome of lumbosacral polyradiculomyelopathy in patients presenting with progressive lumbosacral radicular symptoms (weakness, areflexia, and sensory loss in the legs) is often due to cytomegalovirus and, thus, is treated with ganciclovir.
3. Cryptococcal meningitis is treated with amphotericin B (also with flucytosine or fluconazole).
4. CNS lymphoma in AIDS patients is treated the same way as CNS lymphoma in immunocompetent patients, that is, with radiotherapy and chemotherapy.
5. Acute inflammatory demyelinating polyradiculoneuropathy responds well to plasma exchange or prednisone.

Table 19-28 Causes and Management of Bacterial Meningitis by Age

Age	Major Pathogens	Empirical Antibiotic Regimen	Pathogen	Specific Therapy
3 mo to 18 y	*Neisseria meningitidis, Streptococcus pneumoniae, Haemophilus influenzae*	Ceftriaxone (or cefotaxime); add vancomycin in areas with >2% incidence of highly drug-resistant *S pneumoniae*	*N meningitidis* *H influenzae*	Penicillin G or ampicillin for 7-10 d Ceftriaxone for 7-10 d
18-50 y	*S pneumoniae, N meningitidis*	Ceftriaxone (or cefotaxime); add vancomycin in areas with >2% incidence of highly drug-resistant *S pneumoniae*	*S pneumoniae* (MIC <0-0.1) *S pneumoniae* (MIC >0-0.1)	Ceftriaxone (or cefotaxime) for 10-14 d Vancomycin plus ceftriaxone for 10-14 d
>50 y	*S pneumoniae, Listeria monocytogenes,* gram-negative bacilli	Ampicillin plus ceftriaxone (or cefotaxime); add vancomycin if drug-resistant *S pneumoniae* is suspected	*L monocytogenes*	Ampicillin plus gentamicin for 14-21 d (for patients with major penicillin allergy, TMP-SMX may be substituted for ampicillin)

Abbreviations: MIC, minimal inhibitory concentration; TMP-SMX, trimethoprim-sulfamethoxazole.

6. Polymyositis is treated the same as it is in other patients, that is, with corticosteroid therapy.

Toxoplasmic encephalitis is a common opportunistic infection in AIDS patients. Treatment for this infection is with either pyrimethamine plus sulfadiazine or pyrimethamine plus clindamycin. However, CNS lymphoma and toxoplasmic encephalitis can be difficult to differentiate because they have similar clinical manifestations and CT and MRI characteristics. Therefore, patients with AIDS who present with a contrast-enhancing CNS mass lesion are treated empirically for toxoplasmic encephalitis, and they have follow-up CT or MRI scans to determine whether the lesion decreases in size. Patients whose lesions do not respond to medical treatment should have a stereotactic biopsy for diagnosis, especially for the diagnosis of lymphoma.

Current therapy for HIV and AIDS uses a "cocktail" of medications (highly active antiretroviral therapy [HAART]), some of which have their own neurologic complications. Zidovudine-induced myopathy responds to dose reduction or withdrawal of the medication. A painful, distal, sensory peripheral neuropathy occurs in patients receiving the nucleoside analogues zalcitabine (formerly called dideoxycytidine [ddC]), didanosine (formerly called dideoxyinosine [ddI]), and stavudine (d4T). The neuropathic symptoms may worsen after removal of the offending drug, the so-called coasting phenomenon.

Neurology of Sepsis

The nervous system is commonly affected in sepsis syndrome. The neurologic conditions encountered are septic encephalopathy, critical-illness polyneuropathy or myopathy (or both), cachexia, and panfascicular muscle necrosis. Neurologic complications also occur in intensive care units for critical medical illness. These complications include metabolic encephalopathy, seizures, hypoxic-ischemic encephalopathy, and stroke.

Septic Encephalopathy

Septic encephalopathy is brain dysfunction in association with systemic infection *without* overt infection of the brain or meninges. Early encephalopathy often begins before failure of other organs and is not due to single or multiple organ failure. Endotoxin does not cross the blood-brain barrier and so probably does not directly affect adult brains. Cytokines, important components of sepsis syndrome, may contribute to encephalopathy. Gegenhalten or paratonic rigidity occurs in more than 50% of patients, and tremor, asterixis, and multifocal myoclonus occur in about 25%. Seizures and focal neurologic signs are rare.

EEG is a sensitive indicator of encephalopathy. The mildest abnormality is diffuse excessive low-voltage theta activity (4-7 Hz). The next level of severity is intermittent rhythmic delta activity (<4 Hz). As the condition worsens, delta activity becomes arrhythmic and continuous. Typical triphasic waves occur in severe cases, especially in hepatic failure. In these cases, MRI and CT scans of the brain may be normal.

- Brain dysfunction is associated with systemic infection.
- Encephalopathy precedes failure of other organs.
- Cytokines are an important part of sepsis syndrome.
- More than 50% of patients have paratonic rigidity.
- Tremor, asterixis, and multifocal myoclonus occur in 25% of patients.
- EEG is a sensitive indicator of encephalopathy.

Critical Illness Polyneuropathy

Critical illness polyneuropathy occurs in 70% of the patients with sepsis and multiple organ failure. There is often an unexplained difficulty in weaning from mechanical ventilation. Nerve biopsy specimens show primary axonal degeneration of motor and sensory fibers without inflammation. Most patients also have concomitant myopathy.

Recovery from critical illness polyneuropathy is satisfactory if the patient survives sepsis and multiple organ failure.

- Nerve biopsy specimens show primary axonal degeneration of motor and sensory fibers without inflammation.
- Recovery from critical illness polyneuropathy is satisfactory.

Neurologic Complications of Organ Transplant

Because almost all organ transplant recipients require some degree of chronic, lifelong immunosuppressive therapy, the major neurologic complications of organ transplant are due to immunosuppression. These include the direct neurotoxic side effects of immunosuppressive drugs, infections, and the development of de novo malignancies. Direct neurologic side effects include the following:

1. Cyclosporine—Tremor is the most common side effect of cyclosporine, which also may produce various motor syndromes such as hemiparesis, paraparesis, and quadriparesis. Cyclosporine may cause encephalopathy and, less commonly, neuralgia and neuropathy; it is epileptogenic.
2. Corticosteroids—The side effects of corticosteroids include myopathy, steroid psychosis, withdrawal (including myalgias, arthralgias, headache, lethargy, and nausea), and spinal cord or cauda equina compression due to epidural lipomatosis.
3. Azathioprine—Azathioprine has no direct neurotoxic side effects.

CNS Infections

Infection of the CNS in immunosuppressed patients is relatively frequent and life-threatening. The 3 organisms that cause more than 80% of CNS infections are *Listeria monocytogenes*, *Cryptococcus neoformans*, and *Aspergillus fumigatus*. The greatest risk factor for CNS infection is the magnitude and duration of immunosuppression. Patients with severe and advanced CNS infections may present with little or no clinical evidence of infection. The period of the risk of infection is mainly from 1 to 6 months after transplant. Specific infections include 1) acute meningitis, most often due to *Listeria*; 2) subacute or chronic meningitis, generally due to *Cryptococcus*; 3) slowly progressive dementia, frequently due to progressive multifocal leukoencephalopathy (caused by the JC virus); and 4) focal brain abscess due to infection usually caused by *Aspergillus*, *Toxoplasma*, *Listeria*, or *Nocardia*.

CNS Involvement by De Novo Lymphoproliferative Diseases

There is an increase in non-Hodgkin lymphoma, especially primary CNS lymphomas. These lymphomas may be linked to infection with Epstein-Barr virus.

Other Neurologic Complications

Other complications affecting the nervous system after transplant can be classified as follows:

1. Complications arising from the underlying diseases
2. Problems resulting from the transplantation procedure
3. Side effects of immunosuppression
4. Posttransplant disorder peculiar to the specific type of transplant

The complications include compressive neuropathies, plexopathies, and radiculopathies; encephalopathy (especially with kidney, liver, and heart transplants); and cerebral infarctions (with bone marrow and heart transplants). Chronic graft-versus-host disease (especially with bone marrow transplants) involves the peripheral nervous system (but not the CNS), for example, polymyositis, myasthenia gravis, and peripheral neuropathy, including CIDP. A complication associated with liver transplant is central pontine myelinolysis, which is manifested as altered mental status or coma, pseudobulbar palsy, and quadriplegia.

Neurology Pharmacy Review
Anna C. Gunderson, PharmD, Sarah L. Clark, PharmD

Review of Drugs for Parkinson Disease, Alzheimer Disease, and Multiple Sclerosis

Drug (Trade Name)	Toxic/Adverse Effects	Drug Interactions	Comments
Parkinson disease			
Dopamine precursor Levodopa-carbidopa (Sinemet, Sinemet CR, Parcopa)	Contraindicated: narrow-angle glaucoma, MAO inhibitors used within previous 2 wk Dyskinesias, psychiatric disturbances, nausea/vomiting, orthostatic hypotension, loss of appetite	Decreased levodopa effect: antipsychotics, iron, prochlorperazine, pyridoxine (vitamin B_6), phenytoin, TCAs, isoniazid Increased levodopa effect: antacids, bupropion, metoclopramide Affected by levodopa: antihypertensives, MAO-A inhibitors	Carbidopa prevents dopadecarboxylase activity peripherally Regular release product *without* food; CR product *with* food Wearing off & on/off phenomena require adjustments in dose & administration schedule Taper dose over 3 days for discontinuation
Dopamine agonist Pramipexole (Mirapex)	Dyskinesias, psychiatric disturbances, nausea, constipation, orthostatic hypotension, syncope, confusion, hallucinations, sedation, sleep attacks, dizziness	Increased pramipexole effect: cimetidine Decreased pramipexole effect: DA antagonists[a]	First-line drug of choice Weekly titration to target dose Reduce pramipexole dose in renal impairment Take with food to decrease nausea/vomiting
Ropinirole (Requip)	Same as for pramipexole, more syncope, fewer hallucinations	Increased ropinirole effect: ciprofloxacin, estrogen Decreased ropinirole effect: smoking, DA antagonists[a]	Same as pramipexole No dose adjustment needed in renal impairment
Bromocriptine (Parlodel)	Same as for pramipexole; in addition, pleuropulmonary reaction, retroperitoneal fibrosis, erythromelalgia, pedal edema	Increased bromocriptine effect: clarithromycin, isometheptene, octreotide, phenylpropanolamine Increased effect by bromocriptine: cyclosporine, tacrolimus, sirolimus	If pleuropulmonary reaction, retroperitoneal fibrosis, or erythromelalgia occurs, must discontinue drug Take with food to decrease nausea/vomiting
Apomorphine (Apokyn)	Contraindicated: 5-HT3 antagonists (ondansetron, granisetron, etc) Severe nausea, headache, sedation, hallucinations, dizziness, bradycardia, hypotension, painful nodules with repeated SC administration Rarely: syncope & QT prolongation	Increased apomorphine effect: tolcapone, entacapone	Approved for acute treatment of "off" periods Give with an antiemetic Do not give IV; SC route recommended
MAO-B inhibitor Selegiline (Eldepryl, Emsam)	Contraindicated: methyldopa, dextromethorphan, duloxetine, isometheptene, meperidine, phenelzine, sibutramine, fluoxetine, bupropion, phenylephrine, phenylpropanolamine, pseudoephedrine, reserpine, sertraline, venlafaxine, methadone, propoxyphene, tramadol, TCAs, St John's wort If patch is used, additional contraindications: carbamazepine, oxcarbazepine, cyclobenzaprine, mirtazapine Exacerbates levodopa side effects, agitation, insomnia	Increased effect of selegiline: oral contraceptives, tramadol, amphetamine, sumatriptan, atomoxetine, buspirone, carbamazepine, cyclobenzaprine, oxycodone	Last oral dose given with lunch Hypertensive crises with tyramine foods a concern With oral selegiline dosages >10 mg daily & transdermal doses ≥9 mg daily, selegiline may cause hypocalcemia in diabetic patients

Neurology Pharmacy Review (continued)

Review of Drugs for Parkinson Disease, Alzheimer Disease, and Multiple Sclerosis (continued)

Drug (Trade Name)	Toxic/Adverse Effects	Drug Interactions	Comments
Parkinson disease (continued)			
MAO-B inhibitor (continued) Rasagiline (Azilect)	Same as selegiline	Increased rasagiline effects: ciprofloxacin, cyclobenzaprine, mirtazapine	Avoid foods containing thyamine
Anticholinergic Benztropine (Cogentin) Trihexyphenidyl (Artane)	Confusion, dry mouth, blurred vision, constipation, urinary retention	Decreased effect by anticholinergics: phenothiazines	Use with caution in BPH, elderly patients, & narrow-angle glaucoma Effective in only about 25% of patients Abrupt discontinuation causes rebound & withdrawal symptoms
COMT inhibitor Entacapone (Comtan)	Diarrhea, nausea, anorexia, orthostatic hypotension, dyskinesias, psychiatric disturbances, orange urine, severe explosive diarrhea	Increased effect by entacapone: COMT substrates (Epi, NE, dobutamine), nonselective MAO inhibitors, probenecid, cholestyramine, ampicillin, erythromycin, rifampin	COMT inhibitors are for adjunctive therapy to levodopa only Do not administer with nonselective MAO inhibitors
Tolcapone (Tasmar)	Same as for entacapone plus acute fulminant hepatic failure Contraindicated in liver disease	Increased effect by tolcapone: levodopa, COMT substrates	Requires written informed consent from patient Monitor LFTs q 2 wk × 1 y; then q 4 wk × 6 mo; then q 8 wk thereafter
Miscellaneous Amantadine (Symmetrel)	Dizziness, confusion, nausea, ankle edema, livedo reticularis, psychiatric disturbances, nausea, hypotension	Increased effect by amantadine: medications with anticholinergic properties Increased amantadine effect: triamterene, trimethoprim	Tolerance can develop in 6-12 wk Need to taper dose for discontinuation Adjust dose in renally impaired patients

Neurology Pharmacy Review (continued)

Review of Drugs for Parkinson Disease, Alzheimer Disease, and Multiple Sclerosis (continued)

Drug (Trade Name)	Toxic/Adverse Effects	Drug Interactions	Comments
Alzheimer disease			
Cholinesterase inhibitors[b]			
Donepezil (Aricept)	Nausea/vomiting, diarrhea, headache, insomnia	Possible increased donepezil effect: ketoconazole, quinidine	Fewer GI side effects Wait 4 wk before increasing dose
Rivastigmine (Exelon)	Nausea/vomiting, diarrhea, dizziness, headache, anorexia/weight loss	None known	Take with food Because of marked GI adverse reactions, start dosage at 1.5 mg twice daily & titrate to maintenance dosage If treatment is interrupted more than several days, start again with lowest daily dosage
Galantamine (Razadyne)	Nausea/vomiting, diarrhea, anorexia/weight loss, sleep disturbances	Increased galantamine levels: ketoconazole, paroxetine, fluvoxamine, amitriptyline, fluoxetine, quinidine	Take with food Dose reduction in renal or hepatic failure
Tacrine (Cognex)	Nausea/vomiting, diarrhea, dizziness, elevated LFTs, vivid dreams, agitation, confusion, ataxia, insomnia, myalgias	Increased effect by tacrine: theophylline Increased tacrine effect: cimetidine, estradiol, fluvoxamine, riluzole, levonorgestrel, norfloxacin	Monitor LFTs every other week for weeks 4-16, then q 3 mo Discontinue if jaundice, total bilirubin >3 mg/dL, or signs/symptoms or hypersensitivity in association with ALT elevation Recommended to take on an empty stomach; if significant stomach upset, take with meals
NMDA receptor antagonist			
Memantine (Namenda)	Dose dependent: dizziness, drowsiness, insomnia, headache, akathisia, nausea, hallucinations, confusion, constipation	Increased memantine effect: sodium bicarbonate, carbonic anhydrase inhibitors	Can be used with a cholinesterase inhibitor Decrease dose if renal impairment Takes 14 d for initial response Wait 1 wk between dose increases

Neurology Pharmacy Review (continued)

Review of Drugs for Parkinson Disease, Alzheimer Disease, and Multiple Sclerosis (continued)

Drug (Trade Name)	Toxic/Adverse Effects	Drug Interactions	Comments
	Multiple sclerosis		
Interferon beta-1a (Avonex, Rebif)	Contraindicated: pregnancy, albumin allergy, suicidal ideation, or severe depression Depression, anxiety, injection site reaction, flulike symptoms, photosensitivity, increased LFT, & leukopenia	Increased effect by interferon beta-1a: zidovudine Increased risk of infection with live vaccines	Avonex, weekly IM dosing; Rebif, 3 times weekly SC dosing Rebif & Avonex are not interchangeable For both interferon beta-1a & beta-1b: caution patients to immediately report depression or any thoughts of suicide; caution in preexisting seizure disorder Rebif: stop if jaundice or symptoms of liver dysfunction
Interferon beta-1b (Betaseron)	Same as for interferon beta-1a; side effects generally more severe with interferon beta-1b	Increased risk of infection with live vaccines	Every other day SC dosing Injection site rotation schedule Monitor WBCs, Plt, LFTs periodically
Glatiramer acetate (Copaxone)	Contraindicated: mannitol allergy Injection site reaction, flushing, palpitations, chest tightness, dyspnea	None reported	Daily SC dosing at bedtime Pregnancy category B
Natalizumab (Tysabri)	Contraindicated: PML Side effects: rash, increased LFTs, increased infection risk, arthralgia, headache, fatigue	None reported	Available only through TOUCH Prescribing Program because of risk of PML[c] IV infusion once monthly

Abbreviations: 5-HT3, serotonin type 3; ALT, alanine aminotransferase; BPH, benign prostatic hypertrophy; COMT, catechol O-methyltransferase; CR, continuous release; DA, dopamine; Epi, epinephrine; GI, gastrointestinal tract; IM, intramuscular; IV, intravenously; LFT, liver function test; MAO, monoamine oxidase; NE, norepinephrine; NMDA, N-methyl-D-aspartate; Plt, platelets; PML, progressive multifocal leukoencephalopathy; q, every; SC, subcutaneous; TCA, tricyclic antidepressant; WBC, white blood cell.

[a] Common DA antagonists include phenothiazines, droperidol, metoclopramide, and atypical antipsychotics.

[b] Antagonistic effects with anticholinergics; additive effects with cholinergics or other cholinesterase inhibitors.

[c] TOUCH (Tysabri Outreach: Unified Commitment to Health) Prescribing Program is a restricted distribution program (telephone: 800-456-2255).

Neurology Pharmacy Review (continued)

Review of Headache Drugs

Drug (Trade Name)	Toxic/Adverse Effects	Drug Interactions	Comments
	Immediate treatment		
Ergots Ergotamine tartrate (Ergostat) Ergotamine/caffeine (Cafergot, Ercaf) Dihydroergotamine (DHE 45, Migranal)	Contraindicated: pregnancy, PVD, CAD, sepsis, liver or renal disease, severe HTN, hemiplegic/basilar migraines, MI, stroke N/V, CNS, rebound headache, dependence, numbness/tingling of extremities Diarrhea with DHE 45	Protease inhibitors, macrolides, NNRT inhibitors decrease ergot metabolism Triptans add to vasospastic effects, avoid use within 24 h of ergots Sibutramine: could lead to serotonin syndrome β-Blockers: unopposed ergot action may lead to peripheral ischemia Nitrates: decreased ergot metabolism, decreased antianginal effects of nitrates	Avoid prolonged administration or excessive dose because of danger of gangrene Caffeine enhances intestinal absorption of ergotamine Most effective if given early in headache course DHE 45: used IM, IV, SC, or nasally; pretreat with antiemetic
Triptans Sumatriptan (Imitrex) Naratriptan (Amerge) Rizatriptan (Maxalt, Maxalt-MLT) Zolmitriptan (Zomig, Zomig-ZMT) Almotriptan (Axert) Frovatriptan (Frova) Eletriptan (Relpax)	Contraindicated: IHD, Prinzmetal angina, uncontrolled HTN, use with or within 24 h of ergots or other serotonin agonist, use with or within 2 wk of MAO inhibitors, hemiplegic or basilar migraine, stroke CNS, chest pain, GI, photo-sensitivity, headache recurrence	MAO-A inhibitors (but not MAO-B inhibitors) decrease metabolism of triptans. Nara-triptan is not metabolized by MAO-A & is less likely to interact with MAO inhibitors Ergots (see above) SSRIs, sibutramine: possible serotonin syndrome Propranolol increases rizatriptan by 70% & frovatriptan (in males) by 60% Almotriptan & eletriptan have important interactions with CYP3A4 inhibitors	Do not exceed recommended dose; each agent has specific requirements for daily maximum Imitrex: used SC or nasally but not IV Headache recurrence rate may be lower with naratriptan & frovatriptan (longer half-life) Eletriptan: caution in severe hepatic impairment Naratriptan: caution in severe hepatic & renal impairment
Analgesics Acetaminophen (Tylenol) NSAIDs Butorphanol nasal spray (Stadol)	Somnolence, dizziness, nasal congestion; may precipitate withdrawal in the opioid-dependent		Drugs of choice for menstrual migraine prophylaxis Ketorolac: given IV/IM for acute headache treatment Poor tolerance is often limiting factor for routine use
Midrin (isometheptene [sympathomimetic] + dichloralphenazone [mild sedative] + acetaminophen)	Contraindicated: glaucoma, severe renal disease, HTN, organic heart disease, liver disease, MAO inhibitor therapy CNS, agranulocytosis (dichloralphenazone)	MAO inhibitors with isometh-eptene may cause hypertensive crisis May potentiate effects of warfarin	Maximum: 5 capsules in 24 h

Neurology Pharmacy Review (continued)

Review of Headache Drugs (continued)

Drug (Trade Name)	Toxic/Adverse Effects	Drug Interactions	Comments
Immediate treatment (continued)			
Analgesics			
Meperidine (Demerol)	Contraindicated: concurrent MAO inhibitor, respiratory depression CNS, dependence Long-term use: rebound headache	MAO inhibitor: hypertensive crisis Ritonavir inhibits meperidine metabolism Sibutramine: possible serotonin syndrome	Give SC/IM for immediate headache treatment Metabolized to normeperidine, which accumulates with chronic dosing & renal dysfunction to cause CNS SEs
Butalbital products (Fiorinal, Fioricet)	Contraindicated: porphyria CNS, respiratory depression, tolerance/dependence, depression	Butalbital may increase metabolism of warfarin Avoid ethanol with butalbital	Fiorinal: butalbital + caffeine + aspirin Fioricet: butalbital + caffeine + acetaminophen
Corticosteroids			
Dexamethasone (Decadron)	Contraindicated: systemic fungal infection Peptic ulceration, immunosuppression, psychosis, HPA-axis suppression, fluid retention, osteoporosis, hyperglycemia	Anticholinesterases: steroids antagonize ACHE effects Rifamycins: increased metabolism of steroids	Give IV/IM for acute headache treatment Pretreat with antiemetic Limit to 1 dose
Prophylactic treatment[a]			
β-Blockers			
Propranolol (Inderal) Timolol (Blocadren) Metoprolol (Lopressor) Nadolol (Corgard) Atenolol (Tenormin)	Contraindicated: asthma or bronchospasm, sinus bradycardia, second or third degree heart block Fatigue, depression, blunting of hypoglycemic/hyperthyroid reactions, erectile dysfunction Abrupt withdrawal may precipitate angina or MI	Clonidine plus β-blocker: discontinue gradually & remove β-blocker first Epinephrine: initial hypertensive episode followed by bradycardia Verapamil: effects of both drugs are enhanced Ergots (see above)	Drugs of choice for migraine prophylaxis Avoid agents with ISA activity Failure of 1 agent does not preclude trial of another Several weeks before effects seen
Tricyclic antidepressants			
Amitriptyline (Elavil) Nortriptyline (Pamelor)	Contraindicated: avoid in acute recovery stage after MI Anticholinergic SE, cardiac abnormalities, decreased seizure threshold, CNS, photosensitivity	Clonidine: hypertensive crisis Sparfloxacin, grepafloxacin: risk of torsades de pointes MAO inhibitors: hypertensive crisis	Very toxic in overdose
Calcium channel blockers			
Verapamil (Calan, Isoptin) Nifedupine (Procardia, Adalat) Nimodupine (Nimotop)	Contraindicated: advanced heart failure, second or third degree AV block, LV dysfunction, sick sinus syndrome Arrhythmias, constipation	β-Blockers: increased effects of both drugs Digoxin: increased digoxin levels Use with dofetilide is contraindicated Prolongs half-life of quinidine No grapefruit juice with verapamil	Weak efficacy Tolerance may develop & may need to increase dose or change agents

Neurology Pharmacy Review (continued)

Review of Headache Drugs (continued)

Drug (Trade Name)	Toxic/Adverse Effects	Drug Interactions	Comments
	Prophylactic treatment[a] (continued)		
Anticonvulsants			
Divalproex sodium (Depakote ER)	See table for antiepileptic agents (valproic acid derivatives)	See table for antiepileptic agents (valproic acid derivatives)	
Gabapentin (Neurontin)	See table for antiepileptic agents	See table for antiepileptic agents	
Topiramate (Topamax)	See table for antiepileptic agents	See table for antiepileptic agents	
Lamotrigine (Lamictal)	See table for antiepileptic agents	See table for antiepileptic agents	
Miscellaneous			
Methysergide (Sansert)	Same as for ergots Retroperitoneal, pleuropulmonary, & cardiac fibrosis	Same as for ergots	Requires 3- to 4-wk drug holiday between each 6-mo treatment course Last-line agent because of severe SEs

Abbreviations: ACHE, acetylcholinesterase; AV, atrioventricular; CAD, coronary artery disease; CNS, central nervous system; GI, gastrointestinal tract; HPA, hypothalamo-pituitary-adrenocortical; HTN, hypertension; IHD, ischemic heart disease; IM, intramuscular; ISA, intrinsic sympathomimetic activity; IV, intravenous; LV, left ventricular; MAO, monoamine oxidase; MI, myocardial infarction; NNRT, nonnucleoside reverse transcriptase; NSAID, nonsteroidal anti-inflammatory drug; N/V, nausea and vomiting; PVD, peripheral vascular disease; SC, subcutaneous; SE, side effect; SSRI, selective serotonin reuptake inhibitor.

[a] Prophylaxis is indicated for patients with 1) prolonged aura, 2) >2 or 3 attacks per month in which abortive agents are ineffective or contraindicated, or 3) headache requiring daily symptomatic therapy.

Neurology Pharmacy Review (continued)

Review of Antiepileptic Drugs

Drug (Trade Name)	Toxic/Adverse Effects	Drug Interactions	Comments
Traditional AEDs[a]			
Phenytoin (Dilantin)	Contraindicated: sinus bradycardia, SA block, second or third degree AV block or Adams-Stokes syndrome Increased LFTs, nystagmus, gingival hyperplasia, folic acid deficiency, blood dyscrasias, hirsutism, metabolic bone disease, coarsening facial features, hyperglycemia IV: hypotension, bradycardia (monitor ECG), thrombocytopenia	IV administration of phenytoin during dopamine infusions may cause severe hypotension & cardiac arrest Liver enzyme inducer: causes increased metabolism of many other drugs (eg, cyclosporine, tacrolimus, theophyllines, oral contraceptives, itraconazole, antiarrhythmics, steroids, other AEDs) Rifampin, chemotherapy agents, theophyllines, steroids decrease phenytoin levels Phenytoin interacts with tube feedings, separate phenytoin & tube feeding by 2 h Cimetidine, fluconazole, sulfas, SSRIs, felbamate, topiramate increase phenytoin concentration	IV phenytoin precipitates in solution: give IV push Maximal rate: 50 mg/min; avoid IM use Metabolism is capacity-limited & shows saturability; avoid large dose changes Highly protein bound to albumin: may choose to check free phenytoin levels in hypoalbuminemic states Avoid frequent dose changes: steady state reached in 10-14 d
Fosphenytoin (Cerebyx)	Same as for phenytoin Groin paresthesia with IV administration	As for phenytoin	Antiepileptic activity is due to phenytoin (fosphenytoin is prodrug) Dose is expressed as PE IM product must be diluted before administration IV Maximal rate of IV infusion: 150 mg PE per minute Continuous monitoring of ECG, BP, & RR is essential during IV administration & for 10-20 min after end of infusion Avoid IM for treatment of status epilepticus

Neurology Pharmacy Review (continued)

Review of Antiepileptic Drugs (continued)

Drug (Trade Name)	Toxic/Adverse Effects	Drug Interactions	Comments
Traditional AEDs[a] (continued)			
Carbamazepine (Tegretol, Tegretol-XR, Carbatrol)	Contraindicated: bone marrow suppression, within 14 d of MAO inhibitors Blood dyscrasias: leukopenia (10%), aplastic anemia (rare), thrombocytopenia, agranulocytosis Hyponatremia Cholestatic jaundice Hepatitis Nausea/vomiting	Liver enzyme inducer: causes increased metabolism of other drugs (eg, warfarin, oral contraceptives, cyclosporine, TCAs, bupropion, other AEDs) Metabolized by CYP3A4 Macrolides, azole antifungals, grapefruit, fluoxetine, cimetidine, verapamil, propoxyphene, isoniazid increase carbamazepine concentrations Valproic acid increases carbamazepine epoxide (active metabolite) by 45% Felbamate, phenobarbital, phenytoin, rifampin decrease carbamazepine concentrations	Monitor CBC/DC at baseline, monthly ×2 mo, then every 12-24 mo (discontinue if WBC <3×10⁹/L or ANC <1.5×10⁹/L); LFTs at baseline & periodically, serum sodium periodically Structurally related to TCAs Carbamazepine induces its own metabolism, so true steady state may not be seen for 30 d even though half-life is short
Valproic acid derivatives (Depakote, Depakote Sprinkle, Depakote ER, Depakene, Depacon)	Contraindicated: liver disease/dysfunction Pancreatitis, rare fatal hepatotoxicity (risk greatest if age <2 y), GI, platelet aggregation inhibition, alopecia, thrombocytopenia (dose related), weight gain, hyperammonemia	Liver enzyme inhibitor: causes decreased metabolism of lamotrigine, phenobarbital, phenytoin, diazepam, & ethosuximide & increased levels of carbamazepine-epoxide Use caution in patients taking other agents affecting platelet function Carbamazepine, phenytoin, phenobarbital, rifampin decrease valproic acid concentrations Felbamate, salicylates, erythromycin increase valproic acid concentrations	Do not give injectable product IM Typical maximal infusion rate: 20 mg/min (some evidence that faster rate over 5-10 min is safe) Depakote tablets are not bioequivalent to Depakote ER tablets; do not crush any Depakote product
Phenobarbital	Contraindicated: respiratory disease when dyspnea or obstruction is present, porphyria Tolerance/dependence, hyperactivity in children, cognitive impairment, metabolic bone disease GI: marked liver dysfunction	Liver enzyme inducer: causes increased metabolism of other drugs (eg, warfarin, metronidazole, theophyllines, oral contraceptives, steroids, β-blockers) Felbamate, valproic acid, chloramphenicol decrease metabolism of phenobarbital Metabolized by CYP2C19	Maximal infusion rate: 60 mg/min; avoid intraarticular or SC injection
Primidone (Mysoline)	As for phenobarbital GI: nausea/vomiting	As for phenobarbital Phenytoin causes increased serum concentration of phenobarbital component	Metabolized by liver to phenylethyl-malonamide (active) & phenobarbital

Neurology Pharmacy Review (continued)

Review of Antiepileptic Drugs (continued)

Drug (Trade Name)	Toxic/Adverse Effects	Drug Interactions	Comments
Traditional AEDs[a] (continued)			
Felbamate (Felbatol)	Contraindicated: history of blood dyscrasias, liver dysfunction- Aplastic anemia, hepatotoxicity, photosensitivity, caution in renal impairment CNS, GI	Inducers (phenytoin, carbamazepine, phenobarbital) decrease felbamate concentrations Felbamate increases phenytoin, valproic acid, phenobarbital, carbamazepine-epoxide concentrations Metabolized by CYP3A4	Monitoring: CBC/DC at baseline & every 2-4 wk LFTs & bilirubin every 1-2 wk Recommended for use *only* in severe epilepsy refractory to all other treatment
Newer AEDs[b]			
Lamotrigine (Lamictal)	Photosensitivity Risk of severe, potentially life-threatening rash increases if age <16 y Risk *may* increase if lamotrigine is given concurrently with valproic acid, dose exceeds recommended dose, or dose is escalated faster than recommended GI	Valproic acid increases lamotrigine concentrations Lamotrigine decreases valproic acid concentrations Inducers (phenytoin, carbamazepine, phenobarbital) decrease lamotrigine concentrations Lamotrigine inhibits dihydrofolate reductase; be aware if administering other inhibitors of folate metabolism	*Must* use smaller doses of lamotrigine in combination with valproic acid Discontinue lamotrigine at the first sign of rash
Tiagabine (Gabitril)	GI (give with food) Weakness CNS	Inducers (phenytoin, carbamazepine, phenobarbital) decrease tiagabine concentration by 60% Metabolized by CYP3A4	Decrease dose &/or increase interval in hepatic insufficiency
Gabapentin (Neurontin)	GI CNS	Separate aluminum/magnesium antacids & gabapentin by 2 h	Renally eliminated, not metabolized; must be adjusted for renal insufficiency
Topiramate (Topamax, Topamax Sprinkle)	Nephrolithiasis Paresthesias Weight loss Metabolic acidosis	Inducers (phenytoin, carbamazepine, phenobarbital) may decrease topiramate concentrations Topiramate has additive effect with carbonic anhydrase inhibitors Topiramate decreases efficacy of estrogen component of oral contraceptives	70% of dose excreted unchanged in urine: use half the normal dose in patients with renal impairment Encourage fluid intake to avoid nephrolithiasis

Neurology Pharmacy Review (continued)

Review of Antiepileptic Drugs (continued)

Drug (Trade Name)	Toxic/Adverse Effects	Drug Interactions	Comments
Newer AEDs[b] (continued)			
Zonisamide (Zonegran)	Contraindicated: hypersensitivity to sulfa Do not use in renal failure (creatinine clearance <50 mL/min) Urolithiasis CNS GI	Inducers (phenytoin, carbamazepine, phenobarbital) may decrease zonisamide concentration Metabolized by CYP3A4 Zonisamide is not expected to interfere with metabolism of other drugs metabolized by cytochrome P450	Long half-life; may take up to 2 wk to reach steady state Encourage fluid intake to avoid urolithiasis Use caution in hepatic dysfunction
Newest AEDs			
Oxcarbazepine (Trileptal)	Hyponatremia 25%-30% of patients with hypersensitivity to carbamazepine have hypersensitivity to oxcarbazepine CNS GI	Oxcarbazepine inhibits CYP2C19, induces CYP3A4 Inducers (phenytoin, carbamazepine, phenobarbital) decrease 10-monohydroxy-carbazepine (active metabolite) levels Oxcarbazepine increases metabolism of oral contraceptives, felodipine	Initiate at half the normal dose if creatinine clearance <30 mL/min
Levetiracetam (Keppra)	Decreased erythrocytes, hemoglobin, hematocrit Infection Behavioral symptoms	Per clinical trials, levetiracetam does not appear to affect or be affected by other AEDs, but cases of increased phenytoin concentrations have been reported	Two-thirds of dose excreted unchanged in urine Must be adjusted for renal dysfunction IV: administer over 15 min IV indicated for NPO patients
Pregabalin (Lyrica)	Peripheral edema CNS Creatine kinase & rarely rhabdomyolysis	Pregabalin does not appear to affect or be affected by other AEDs	Dosing adjustments for renal dysfunction

Abbreviations: AED, antiepileptic drug; ANC, absolute neutrophil count; AV, atrioventricular; BP, blood pressure; CBC, complete blood count; CNS, central nervous system; DC, differential count; ECG, electrocardiography; GI, gastrointestinal tract; IM, intramuscular; IV, intravenous; LFT, liver function test; MAO, monoamine oxidase; NPO, nothing per os; PE, phenytoin equivalents; RR, respiratory rate; SA, sinoatrial; SC, subcutaneous; SSRI, selective serotonin reuptake inhibitor; TCA, tricyclic antidepressant; WBC, white blood cell count.

[a] For all AEDs, the most common side effects (SEs) are CNS effects (eg, drowsiness, dizziness, ataxia). With chronic administration, tolerance usually develops to these SEs. The general rule for dosing AEDs is "start low and go slow." Do not discontinue use of AEDs abruptly.

[b] Generally, the newer and newest AEDs tend to have fewer side effects than the older agents, tend to have fewer drug interactions than the older AEDs, and are approved as adjunctive agents with older AEDs. The value of blood level monitoring is undefined for the newer and newest AEDs.

Questions

Multiple Choice (choose the best answer)

1. A 77-year-old man is complaining of imbalance when walking. He also has an intermittent tremor of the right hand. He has slowed down a lot according to his wife. On examination, he is bradykinetic with a right hand rest tremor. Tone is increased in the right arm and leg. His walking is slow and shuffled and he falls backward when pulled from a neutral position. What is your most likely next suggestion?

    a. Perform autonomic reflex testing.
    b. Perform 4-hour neuropsychometric testing.
    c. Perfom MRI of the brain.
    d. Avoid carbidopa-levodopa because of concerns of toxicity in early Parkinson disease (PD).
    e. Prescribe a gradually increasing dose of carbidopa-levodopa.

2. A 62-year-old woman with a past history of breast cancer presents with right facial weakness and confusion of 2 weeks' duration. She also has left arm pain and weakness. She is confused with poor attention and recall. She is disoriented. There is weakness of the right face, both the forehead and the lower face. The left arm has weakness of triceps and an absent triceps reflex. This process localizes to all the following areas *except*:

    a. Left C7 nerve root
    b. Left motor cortex
    c. Right facial nerve
    d. Diffusely to the cerebral hemispheres
    e. It localizes to all the above areas.

3. A 23-year-old man presents to the emergency department after a presumed seizure. He is healthy and has no history or evidence of drug or alcohol use. Neurologic examination findings are normal. Which of the following would be *inappropriate*?

    a. CT of the brain
    b. MRI of the brain
    c. Counseling the patient that there is a high likelihood of another seizure and, therefore, he must take an antiepileptic drug
    d. Not prescribing an antiepileptic drug
    e. Electroencephalography (EEG)

4. A 66-year-old woman has sudden onset of right-sided weakness. She has a history of hypertension, diabetes mellitus, and hyperlipidemia. On examination, there is near paralysis of the right face and the arm (more than the leg) and loss of feeling and sensory neglect on the right side. There also appears to be right-sided visual field loss. All the following could be results of testing, *except*:

    a. Carotid ultrasonography with severe left carotid stenosis
    b. MRI showing a lacunar infarct in the left internal capsule

    c. Transesophageal echocardiogram (TEE) revealing atrial fibrillation and thrombus in the left atrium
    d. TEE showing atherosclerosis of the ascending aorta with mobile plaque
    e. MRA showing severe intracranial stenotic atherosclerotic disease

5. The wife of a 78-year-old man brings in her husband complaining that he is forgetful. He gets lost easily and is more quick-tempered than usual. He has slowed down quite a bit recently and is off balance when walking. He sometimes kicks, thrashes, or yells at night while sleeping. This has been going on for the past 2 years and is getting worse. He has a history of strokes. His examination shows some mild parkinsonian features (ie, rigidity, slow and shuffling gait but no tremor), and his mental status examination is diffusely abnormal. Which of the following would be *unlikely* to be results of the ensuing evaluation?

    a. Analysis of cerebrospinal fluid (CSF) shows increased 14-3-3 protein.
    b. MRI shows mesial temporal atrophy.
    c. MRI shows ventricular enlargement out of proportion to the degree of cerebral atrophy.
    d. Overnight sleep study shows rapid eye movement (REM) sleep behavior disorder.
    e. MRI shows multiple infarcts in cortical and subcortical areas.

6. A 55-year-old man has had an episode of loss of consciousness witnessed by a friend. Which of the following would *not* suggest an epileptic seizure as the cause of the episode?

    a. Total amnesia for the event
    b. A tongue bite
    c. A period of confusion after the event for 30 minutes
    d. No confusion after the event; back to normal immediately
    e. Repetitive movements of the extremities during the event

7. Which of the following is *unlikely* to be attributed to simply old age?

    a. Loss of vibration sensation in the toes
    b. Decreased hearing
    c. Parkinsonian tremor
    d. Gait unsteadiness
    e. Spondylitic changes on MRI of the lumbar spine

8. A 79-year-old man complained of headache and malaise for 1 week with significant proximal muscle achiness. He had an episode of transient monocular blindness in the right eye a few hours before the evaluation. Which of the following would be the most appropriate next step in his evaluation?

a. Carotid ultrasonography
b. Lumbar puncture
c. CT of the head
d. Erythrocyte sedimentation rate (ESR)
e. Magnetic resonance angiography (MRA)

9. In patients with diabetes mellitus, which of the following peripheral nervous system disorders would be *unlikely*?

a. Carpal tunnel syndrome
b. Mononeuritis multiplex
c. Pupil-sparing third nerve palsy
d. Myopathy
e. Lumbosacral plexopathy

10. A 65-year-old man presents with weakness that has progressed slowly during the past 2 years. He has trouble getting up out of a chair or out of bed. His grip is weaker. His right side seems to be worse than his left. There is no numbness, pain, or difficulty with speaking or swallowing. There are no visual complaints, such as double vision. On examination, he has asymmetric, mainly proximal weakness with the biceps and quadriceps being the weakest muscles. There is also weakness of the finger flexors. Sensory and cranial nerve examinations are normal. Reflexes are absent at the ankles and reduced elsewhere. Toes are downgoing. What is the most likely abnormal test result?

a. MRI showing cervical spinal stenosis
b. Positive acetylcholine receptor antibodies
c. Muscle biopsy showing congophilic inclusions and rimmed vacuoles
d. Electromyography (EMG) showing signs of motor neuron disease
e. Muscle biopsy showing inflammatory myopathy (polymyositis)

11. A 55-year-old woman complains of bilateral leg weakness with some bladder urgency and rare incontinence that have developed over 3 weeks. She has had no back or neck pain, although she does have some new holocephalic headaches. On examination, there is bilateral weakness of the iliopsoas, hamstrings, and anterior tibialis. Reflexes in the legs are brisk with upgoing toes bilaterally and clonus at the ankles. Sensory examination is normal. An MRI is ordered. What is the most likely MRI result?

a. MRI of the cervical spine shows a dorsal intramedullary lesion suggestive of demyelinating disease.
b. MRI of the thoracic spine shows a small bulging disk with no cord compression.
c. MRI of the lumbosacral spine shows a large herniated disk impinging on the L5 and S1 nerve roots bilaterally.

d. MRI of the brain shows a large frontal parasagittal extra-axial lesion most consistent with a meningioma.
e. MRI of the brain shows a new infarct in the left middle cerebral artery distribution.

12. A 42-year-old woman presents with acute onset of headache and neck pain, vertigo, nausea, and vomiting. Neurologic examination reveals left nystagmus, left Horner syndrome, absent left gag reflex, left appendicular ataxia, and anesthesia to pinprick in the left face and right arm and leg. Which of the following is the most likely diagnosis?

a. Complicated migraine
b. Vertebral artery dissection
c. Subarachnoid hemorrhage
d. Acute multiple sclerosis
e. Transverse sinus thrombosis

13. A 35-year-old woman has had mild bilateral lower extremity weakness for 5 days. She has a history of optic neuritis and other episodes of transient diplopia and dizziness. On examination, she has vision loss on the left and a mild spastic paraparesis. Which of the following is true?

a. This is typical of multiple sclerosis, and no treatment is necessary.
b. MRI of the head would probably show multiple infarcts.
c. Treatment with a 5-day course of intravenous steroids would be indicated to speed recovery.
d. CSF examination is mandatory.
e. Long-term treatment with an interferon will lead to disease remission.

14. A 65-year-old man presents with right facial weakness for 6 hours. This started with pain and numbness, which are better now. There are no ocular symptoms, rash, headache, or limb symptoms. On examination, there is weakness of eye closure and forehead wrinkling and movement of the lower face (smiling). Extraocular movements, facial sensation, gag, and tongue strength are normal. The patient has hypertension, diabetes mellitus, and atrial fibrillation. He is concerned about a stroke and inquires about tissue plasminogen activator (TPA). You decide which of the following?

a. This is a left middle cerebral artery (MCA) infarct, and TPA is indicated.
b. This is a left MCA infarct, but TPA is not indicated.
c. This is a lacunar infarct, and TPA is not indicated.
d. An MRI should be done first.
e. This is Bell palsy, and no testing needs to be done.

Answers

1. Answer e.

This patient has the typical symptoms and signs of PD. Although the autonomic nervous system can be involved in PD, there is no indication from the history to evaluate this further. Dementia can occur in PD but usually later in the disease course. MRI is unlikely to contribute additional diagnostic information when the cardinal clinical features of the disease are present—namely, bradykinesia, tremor, rigidity, and postural instability. Levodopa has not been proved to be toxic to neurons early in the disease course. It is, in fact, the most efficacious treatment and should be offered to all PD patients when symptoms affect the quality of life. The dosage is usually low initially (one-half of a 25-mg/100-mg carbidopa-levodopa tablet, 3 times daily on an empty stomach) and is gradually increased over several weeks to 25 mg/100 mg 3 times daily to reach symptomatic relief or side effects.

2. Answer b.

The disorientation and confusion localize most likely to the bilateral cerebral hemispheres. The right facial weakness must be a lower motor neuron process because the upper face is involved. Lesions above the facial nucleus level clinically spare the upper face because of the bilateral innervation of the facial nuclei. A left motor cortex lesion, therefore, would not produce these findings. The pain and weakness in the left arm suggest a cervical radiculopathy, likely C7. Metastatic breast cancer can produce this type of multifocal clinical picture with diffuse (encephalopathy) and focal (radiculopathy and cranial neuropathy) findings. Leptomeningeal involvement can lead to dysfunction of the underlying cerebral cortex and exiting cranial nerves and nerve roots during their course through the cerebrospinal fluid.

3. Answer c.

In an individual who is otherwise neurologically normal (normal findings on examination, imaging, and EEG), the risk of a second seizure after 1 isolated seizure is less than 50% (probably about 30%). Therefore, an antiepileptic medicine does not have to be used immediately. Administration of a medicine can lead to cost, side effects, and the social stigmata of treatment of epilepsy. The decision to use medicine can be postponed for the rest of the evaluation. In most cases, CT of the head is done immediately to exclude hemorrhage or a mass lesion. If there is a mass lesion, antiepileptic medication is warranted. MRI is reasonable for evaluating a possible cause since some structural lesions (ie, malformations of cortical development) can be seen only by MRI. EEG can help with seizure classification and prediction of recurrence risk.

4. Answer b.

The patient presented with motor, sensory, and visual deficits localized to the left cerebral hemisphere. This type of deficit indicates a large infarct with involvement of at least the frontal and parietal lobes. Internal capsule infarcts would produce more isolated motor deficits, usually with the face, arm, and leg affected to a similar degree. Sensory neglect is a sign that the cerebral cortex is involved. All the listed abnormalities are potential causes of an ischemic infarct.

5. Answer a.

The patient has a chronic, progressive cognitive disorder or dementia. MRI in Alzheimer disease may show generalized atrophy, although thin-slice coronal images often reveal more prominent mesial temporal/hippocampal atrophy. The patient also has a gait disorder, which in combination with dementia brings to mind normal-pressure hydrocephalus (NPH) as a possible diagnosis. Imaging in this disorder shows enlargement of the ventricles. Removal of large volumes of CSF and CSF shunting procedures can be beneficial. The level of 14-3-3 protein is most commonly elevated in Creutzfeldt-Jakob disease, which is a much more rapidly progressive disorder than what is described in the question. The acting out of dreams is common in neurodegenerative disorders, especially Parkinson disease and diffuse Lewy body disease, both of which can cause dementia and parkinsonian symptoms and signs. Overnight sleep studies show a loss of the usual atonia in REM sleep. Multi-infarct dementia is characterized by a history of strokes and a decline of cognitive function related to that. Both neurologic examination and imaging studies reveal residua of previous strokes.

6. Answer d.

An epileptic seizure is usually accompanied by total amnesia for the spell and a period of time after the spell (postictal confusion). If a patient has total awareness of the event and there is generalized motor seizure activity, a nonepileptic cause is almost assured. Tongue biting and urinary incontinence can occur during an epileptic seizure, although they are nonspecific. Repetitive or tonic-clonic movements of the limbs are common. Often, there is vocalization, and then breath holding. Forced eye closure is another sign of a nonepileptic event. Often, only inpatient EEG monitoring during a spell can accurately confirm whether an event is epileptic or not.

7. Answer c.

All the answers except *c* are common in elderly persons, especially those older than 70 years. Although tremor can be physiologic (everyone has a mild one, but some are worse than others), a rest tremor is not a normal finding in the elderly. A rest tremor, especially of 1 hand, is nearly pathognomonic for Parkinson disease.

8. Answer d.

The combination of headache preceding transient monocular loss of vision in an older person must suggest temporal arteritis until proved otherwise. Although headache and malaise are nonspecific, if the potential diagnosis of temporal arteritis is not considered and the condition is left untreated, permanent loss of vision could occur quickly. The condition often coexists with polymyalgia rheumatica—leading to muscle achiness and weakness. The ESR should be determined urgently and appropriate medical management with prednisone initiated. If the ESR result is negative, additional evaluation of the carotid artery with carotid ultrasonography or MRA would be appropriate. CT of the head is not clearly indicated. Lumbar puncture would not be part of the urgent evaluation.

9.   Answer d.

Diabetes mellitus can lead to multiple peripheral nervous system complications. Peripheral neuropathies of many types can occur (ie, length-dependent sensorimotor and small fiber sensory peripheral neuropathies). Compressive mononeuropathies affect the median nerve at the wrist and the ulnar nerve at the elbow and cause peroneal neuropathy at the knee. Lumbosacral plexopathy is usually a painful, unilateral or asymmetric condition of the leg, typically affecting the upper lumbar myotomes. Cranial neuropathies can occur, especially an ischemic third nerve palsy (which spares the pupil). Diabetes mellitus does not lead to a myopathy, other than an exceedingly rare muscle infarction.

10.   Answer c.

Inclusion body myositis is a late-onset, slowly progressive myopathy that has a predilection for certain muscles: biceps, quadriceps, and finger flexors. EMG shows evidence of a myopathic disorder, although occasionally neurogenic changes are also seen. Muscle biopsy is the diagnostic test of choice, often revealing rimmed vacuoles and congophilic inclusions. Treatment is supportive since most anti-inflammatory therapies are unsuccessful. Cervical spinal stenosis is unlikely with the lack of upper motor neuron signs. Acetylcholine receptor antibodies are present in myasthenia gravis, which clinically manifests most often with bulbar and limb weakness. Motor neuron disease is often confused clinically with inclusion body myositis, although an EMG showing only neurogenic changes should distinguish motor neuron disease. Polymyositis tends to cause more symmetric proximal weakness without the predilection for individual muscles such as the finger flexors.

11.   Answer d.

The examination suggests an isolated upper motor neuron process affecting both legs. This localizes to the spinal cord (cervical or thoracic) or to the bilateral motor cortex. A dorsal cervical spine lesion would be expected to result in sensory abnormalities. A mild thoracic disk protrusion without compression of the spinal cord would not produce this picture. A lumbosacral lesion would also not produce this type of abnormality unless it was in the upper lumbar spine at the level of the conus medullaris (L2 or higher). As shown on the mapping of the homunculus (which shows the cortical representation of motor and sensory function in the body), leg control is localized to the upper medial frontal lobes. A large frontal midline or parasagittal lesion, such as a meningioma, could compress both sides while sparing the sensory areas posteriorly. A unilateral cerebral stroke would not produce symmetric, bilateral lower extremity neurologic signs.

12.   Answer b.

The clinical findings (nystagmus, Horner syndrome, cerebellar abnormalities, and crossed sensory loss) suggest a brainstem localization. This is most consistent with Wallenberg syndrome (lateral medullary syndrome) due to damage to the lateral medullary region. The sudden onset of the deficit is most consistent with an ischemic or hemorrhagic process. Migraine is a very unusual cause of cerebral infarction and is more cortically based when it does occur. Subarachnoid hemorrhage usually does not cause sudden onset of focal findings in the brainstem. Although multiple sclerosis can develop suddenly, a gradual onset is more typical and is not associated with headache. Transverse sinus thrombosis can cause cerebral infarction but not infarction of the brainstem. The abrupt onset of pain in combination with a focal neurologic process would be more consistent with a vertebral artery dissection with resultant cerebral infarction.

13.   Answer c.

This is a typical scenario for multiple sclerosis. Episodes of demyelination lead to optic neuritis and vision loss; brainstem lesions cause diplopia, dizziness, and imbalance; spinal cord lesions cause paraparesis. MRI shows lesions in the periventricular white matter (often perpendicular to the ventricles), cerebellum, brainstem, and spinal cord. In a classic case, CSF examination is not mandatory. The main finding in CSF is the presence of unique immunoglobulin synthesis (oligoclonal bands). Treatment with intravenous steroids hastens recovery and is indicated for disabling attacks. Long-term treatment with interferon or glatiramer has been shown to reduce attack rates by one-third and reduce disability in the future.

14.   Answer e.

Facial weakness involving the upper and lower parts of the face suggests a peripheral cranial nerve VII process rather than a central cause. (A central process, such as one in the frontal lobe, causes weakness that is greater in the lower part of the face than in the upper part.) Bell palsy often begins with some pain or sensory symptoms. In this case, this is the diagnosis, given the pattern of facial weakness; an MRI is not necessary to make the diagnosis. An MCA infarction would be unlikely to cause only facial weakness. TPA is contraindicated after 3 hours. If diagnosed early (within the first 2 days or so), Bell palsy can be treated with prednisone and valacyclovir to speed recovery, although almost all patients recover with time.

20

Oncology

Timothy J. Moynihan, MD

Breast Cancer

Magnitude of the Problem

In the United States, around 200,000 new cases of breast cancer are diagnosed annually. Breast cancer will develop in approximately 1 in 8 women who achieve a normal life expectancy. Breast cancer is the second most common cause of cancer death among women in the United States (lung cancer is the most common). The incidence has decreased steadily during the past 3 years. The exact reason for this decrease is uncertain, but it may be due to prior mammography screening programs, some decline in recent use of mammography, a decrease in the use of postmenopausal estrogen after the results of the Women's Health Initiative study were released, or some other unknown factors. It is uncertain if this decline in new cases will be sustained.

* Breast cancer will develop in 1 in 8 American women.
* The incidence of breast cancer has decreased for the past 3 years, for uncertain reasons.
* Breast cancer is the second most common cause of cancer death in American women.

Risk Factors

The risk factors for breast cancer are outlined in Table 20-1. Breast cancer-associated genes (*BRCA1* and *BRCA2*) occur in fewer than 5% to 10% of cases of breast cancer, but those women who carry these genes may have up to a 50% to 80% chance for breast cancer developing in their lifetime. Less than 25% of women with breast cancer have known high-risk factors.

* Less than 25% of women with breast cancer have known high-risk factors.

Screening

The use of screening mammography in the age group 50 years or older has decreased breast cancer associated mortality by 20% to 30%. The use of screening mammography in the age group 40 to 50 years is controversial. There is general consensus that women 50 years or older should be screened with annual clinical examination and mammography. For women deemed at high risk for breast cancer, screening should be instituted at an appropriate earlier age, generally taken as 5 to 10 years before the earliest diagnosis of breast cancer in affected first-degree relatives. Currently, mammography misses about 10% of breast cancers detectable on physical examination. Thus, any palpable breast mass should be evaluated with ultrasonography. If ultrasonography shows a simple cyst, it can be either closely observed or aspirated. *For a palpable lesion that shows a solid component on ultrasonography, biopsy should be done, even in the presence of a normal mammogram.* Magnetic resonance imaging (MRI) recently was shown to be valuable for finding additional ipsilateral or contralateral lesions in women with newly diagnosed

Table 20-1 Risk Factors for Breast Cancer

High Risk: Relative Risk >4.0	Moderate Risk: Relative Risk 2-4	Low Risk: Relative Risk 1-2
Older age	Any first-degree relative with breast cancer	Menarche before age 12 y
Personal history of breast cancer	Personal history of ovarian or endometrial cancer	Menopause after age 55 y
Family history of premenopausal bilateral breast cancer or familial cancer syndrome	Age at first full-term pregnancy >30 y	Caucasian race
Breast biopsy showing proliferative disease with atypia	Nulliparous	Moderate alcohol intake
	Obesity in postmenopausal women	Long-duration (≥15 y)
	Upper socioeconomic class	estrogen replacement therapy

breast cancer. It is uncertain whether this finding will translate into improved outcomes. Current recommendations for MRI are confined to women at very high risk of breast cancer based on family history or prior exposure to radiation therapy (eg, upper mantle radiation for Hodgkin disease). One-time MRI is also recommended for women with newly diagnosed breast cancer. Women with very dense breast tissue on mammography also may benefit from MRI screening, because mammography is very insensitive in the setting of dense breasts and recent data show that breast density on mammography is an independent risk factor for the development of breast cancer.

- Screening for breast cancer can reduce mortality.
- Women 50 years or older need annual examinations and mammography.
- There is controversy about screening normal women who are 40 to 50 years old.
- Ten percent of breast cancers found on physical examination are missed by mammography.
- Ultrasonography is recommended for a suspicious palpable lump, even if mammography is negative.
- Biopsy should be done for lumps with a solid component on ultrasonography.
- MRI is recommended for women at very high risk for breast cancer, women with newly diagnosed breast cancer, and women with very dense breast tissue on mammography. These recommendations are currently controversial.

Pathology

Breast cancers are classified as ductal or lobular, corresponding to the ducts and lobules of the normal breast (Figure 20-1). Invasive (sometimes called infiltrating) breast cancer has the potential for systemic spread, as opposed to carcinoma in situ, which does not have metastatic potential because by definition it has not invaded through the basement membrane.

Ductal carcinoma in situ is noninvasive, does not have the potential for systemic spread, and is primarily treated locally only, including resection and breast irradiation. Use of selective estrogen receptor modulators (eg, tamoxifen, raloxifene) after resection of ductal carcinoma in situ is controversial. These drugs do decrease the risk of a subsequent breast event (defined as either recurrent carcinoma in situ or development of an invasive breast cancer in the ipsilateral or contralateral breast) in the subsequent 10 years from 13% to 8%; however, there is no evidence of a survival advantage and there are potential significant side effects with use of these medications.

Infiltrating ductal carcinoma is the most common histologic type (70% of breast cancers) of invasive breast cancer. Invasive lobular carcinoma makes up 25% of breast cancers, is more frequently multifocal and bilateral, and is less likely to be seen on mammography.

- Infiltrating ductal carcinoma is the most common histologic type of breast cancer.
- Lobular disease is more frequently multifocal and bilateral.
- Ductal carcinoma in situ is noninvasive and does not have the potential for systemic spread.

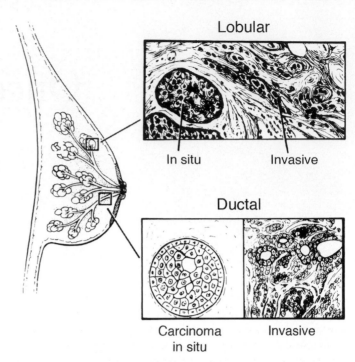

Figure 20-1. Breast Carcinomas: Ductal and Lobular, In Situ and Invasive.

- Use of selective estrogen receptor modulators after resection of ductal carcinoma in situ is controversial.

Staging

The staging system of the American Joint Committee on Cancer is shown in Table 20-2.

Natural History and Prognostic Factors

Nodal Status

The number of involved axillary nodes remains the most important predictor of outcome (Figure 20-2).

Tumor Size

After nodal status, tumor size is generally the most important prognostic factor (Table 20-3).

Hormone Receptor Status

In general, patients with estrogen-receptor–positive tumors have a better prognosis. However, the difference in recurrence rates at 5 years is only 8% to 10% when compared with receptor negative disease. Extent of hormone positivity may be very important in treatment outcome; patients with more than 90% of tumor cells staining positive for estrogen receptor respond very well to hormonal therapies and may be able to avoid adjuvant chemotherapy, whereas those whose tumors are only weakly positive for estrogen receptor may fare better with the use of chemotherapy.

Grade

Most breast cancers are high-grade. Patients with low-grade tumors have fewer recurrences and longer survival.

Table 20-2 Staging of Breast Cancer

Primary tumor (T)
  TIS Carcinoma in situ
  T1   T = ≤2 cm
  T2   T = 2.1-5 cm
  T3   T = >5 cm
  T4   T of any size with direct extension to chest wall or skin
Regional nodes (N)
  N0   No involved nodes
  N1   Movable ipsilateral axillary nodes
  N2   Matted or fixed nodes, or in clinically apparent ipsilateral internal mammary nodes in the absence of clinically evident axillary lymph node metastasis
  N3   Metastasis in ipsilateral infraclavicular lymph nodes
Distant metastasis (M)
  M0   None detected
  M1   Distant metastasis present (includes ipsilateral supraclavicular nodes)
Stage grouping

Stage I	T1 N0	
Stage IIA	T0 N1	
	T1 N1	
	T2 N0	= Operable disease
Stage IIB	T2 N1	
	T3 N0	
Stage IIIA	T0 N2	
	T1 N2	
	T2 N2	
	T3 N1,N2	= Locally advanced disease
Stage IIIB	T4, Any N	
Stage IIIC	Any T N3	= Advanced disease
Stage IV	Any T Any N M1	= Advanced or metastatic

Data from Singletary SE, Allred C, Ashley P, Bassett LW, Berry D, Bland KI, et al. Revision of the American Joint Committee on cancer staging system for breast cancer. J Clin Oncol. 2002;20:3628-36.

* The number of involved axillary nodes is the most important predictor of outcome.
* After nodal status, tumor size is the most important prognostic factor.
* Patients with receptor-positive tumors have a better prognosis.
* Patients with low-grade tumors have a better prognosis.

Treatment

Primary or Local-Regional Treatment

Primary local treatment for invasive breast cancer is either lumpectomy (also known as wide local excision or breast conservation) followed by radiation or mastectomy. Several randomized controlled clinical trials have shown therapeutic equivalence for breast conservation and mastectomy in terms of overall survival, whereas mastectomy has a slightly lower local recurrence rate. The outcome for women with invasive breast cancer depends on the presence of distant microscopic metastatic disease rather than on the treatment of local disease. The most important predictor for the presence of micrometastatic disease is involvement of axillary lymph nodes. All women with invasive breast cancer need to have the status of their axillary lymph nodes determined. This assessment can be accomplished by use of an axillary lymph node dissection or a newer procedure called a sentinel lymph node biopsy. Sentinel lymph node biopsy uses a radioactive tracer or a blue dye injected into the periareolar or peritumoral bed. The surgeon then is able to identify the first draining lymph node and remove it. If this sentinel lymph node shows histologic signs of cancer, then the patient should undergo a complete axillary lymph node dissection. If the sentinel lymph node does not have metastatic tumor cells, then the probability of other lymph nodes being affected is less than 5%. Sentinel lymph node biopsy decreases late complications such as lymphedema. Adequate surgical training is required to perform this procedure.

* Breast conservation plus radiation is equal to mastectomy in terms of overall survival.
* Sentinel lymph node biopsy carries less risk of arm lymphedema.
* Sentinel lymph node biopsy should be performed only by surgeons trained in this procedure.

Adjuvant Treatment

After primary treatment of the breast, additional systemic treatment (adjuvant) has been shown to decrease the risk of systemic recurrence and improve overall survival. The number of involved axillary lymph nodes is the single most important predictor of outcome. Women with metastatically involved axillary lymph nodes should be offered adjuvant treatment (Table 20-4): chemotherapy, hormonal therapy, or both. Women with negative lymph nodes have only a 25% or less chance of microscopic metastatic disease, and their risk of recurrence can be further estimated according to the data in Table 20-5. Adjuvant systemic treatment should be offered to women in the intermediate- and high-risk groups. Chemotherapy has been shown to decrease the risk of recurrence and improve overall survival in both node-negative and node-positive cancer, but it is associated with more toxicity than hormonal therapy. Sequential therapy with chemotherapy followed by hormonal therapy does offer additive effect against the cancer in women with hormonally sensitive disease. Women with node-positive cancers that overexpress the human epidermal growth factor receptor type 2 (HER2/neu) protein should also be offered adjuvant trastuzumab (Herceptin) therapy. Long term follow up of women with breast cancer is essential because only 17% of recurrences happen during the first 5 years after

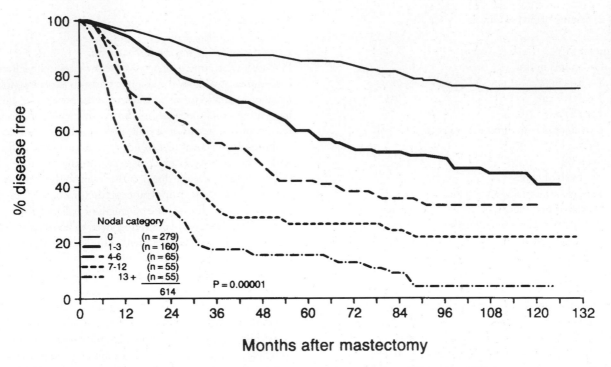

Figure 20-2. Relation of disease-free survival to numbers of nodal metastases in more than 600 women with breast cancer treated with radical mastectomy alone in the early 1970s. (From Fisher ER, Sass R, Fisher B. Pathologic findings from the National Surgical Adjuvant Project for Breast Cancers [protocol no. 4]. X. Discriminants for tenth year treatment failure. Cancer. 1984;53:712-23. Used with permission.)

initial diagnosis, and metastatic disease can develop 30 or more years later.

- Women with node-positive disease are at high risk of systemic disease and should be offered adjuvant treatment.
- Women with node-negative disease have a 25% or less chance of systemic disease.
- Adjuvant therapy decisions should be individualized on the basis of each person's risk of recurrence.

Table 20-3 Long-Term Results[a] in Patients With Node-Negative Breast Cancer Treated Surgically

Tumor Size, cm	No. of Patients	% Free of Recurrence	% Dead of Disease
<1	171	88	10
1.1-2.0	303	74	24
2.1-3.0	188	72	24
3.1-5.0	105	61	36

[a] Median duration of follow-up was 18 years.
Data from Rosen PP, Groshen S, Kinne DW. Survival and prognostic factors in node-negative breast cancer: results of long-term follow-up studies. Monogr Natl Cancer Inst. 1992;11:159-62.

Treatment of Advanced Disease

We currently lack curative therapy for recurrent or metastatic breast cancer. The median duration of survival for recurrent disease is 2.5 years. Survival is longer with bone only or soft tissue recurrence than with visceral recurrence. Because treatment is not curative, the initial systemic treatment for patients with estrogen-receptor–positive advanced disease is usually hormonal. Chemotherapy is used once disease has progressed while receiving hormonal therapy or in women with estrogen-receptor–negative breast cancer.

- There is no curative therapy for recurrent or metastatic breast cancer.
- The average survival with recurrent breast cancer is 2.5 years.

Chemotherapy

Active drugs against breast cancer include doxorubicin (Adriamycin, A), cyclophosphamide (C), methotrexate (M), 5-fluorouracil (F), paclitaxel (Taxol), docetaxel (Taxotere), capecitabine (Xeloda), vinorelbine (Navelbine), vincristine, vinblastine, mitomycin-C, etoposide, and cisplatin. Common combination regimens are CMF, CAF, and AC. The side effects of chemotherapy include reversible lowering of the blood counts and reversible hair loss. There appears to be a very small, but real, increase in the risk of secondary leukemias in women receiving adjuvant chemotherapy, especially anthracycline-based chemotherapy, and this may be increased in women who also receive growth factors such as filgrastim (Neupogen or Neulasta) to accelerate leukocyte recovery.

Table 20-4 Adjuvant Therapy: Node-Positive Breast Cancer[a]

	Estrogen-receptor Status	
	Positive	Negative
Premenopausal	Chemo + tam	Chemo
Postmenopausal	Chemo + hormones[b]	Chemo

Abbreviations: Chemo, combination chemotherapy; Tam, tamoxifen.
[a] One year of trastuzumb is added to chemotherapy or hormonal therapy for patients whose cancer is human epidermal growth factor receptor type 2.
[b] Hormonal therapy for postmenopausal women can be either tamoxifen or an aromatase inhibitor.

Hormonal Treatment

Tamoxifen is the most widely used hormonal agent in the treatment of patients with breast cancer. Tamoxifen is a nonsteroidal compound that on selected tissue acts like an antiestrogen (breast tissue) but on other tissue acts like an estrogen (bones, lipids, uterus). Its beneficial effects include 1) antitumor effects on breast cancer cells, 2) decreased risk (by 40%) of contralateral breast cancer, 3) improved bone density, and 4) favorable effects on lipid profiles. Tamoxifen also has side effects, including 1) vaginal dryness and hot flashes, 2) thromboembolic risk (1%-2%), 3) increased risk of endometrial cancer, and 4) increased risk of cataracts. Recent data show that women who experience hot flashes and other menopausal side effects from tamoxifen have a more favorable outcome with their breast cancer. The US Food and Drug Administration recently noted that women who are given tamoxifen should have testing of their CYP2D6 status, because this enzyme system is required for activation of tamoxifen to its active form. Women who have poor metabolizer status should not be treated with tamoxifen and those who are currently taking CYP2D6 inhibitors (such as paroxetine, cimetidine, citalopram) should not receive tamoxifen unless medications can be changed to eliminate drug interactions.

A newer class of hormonal agents, known as the aromatase inhibitors, is being used for treatment of postmenopausal women with breast cancer. These drugs include anastrozole (Arimidex), exemestane (Aromasin), and letrozole (Femara). These drugs show a slight superiority to tamoxifen in reducing the risk of recurrence of breast cancer, and they do not carry an increased risk of thrombotic or endometrial events. The aromatase inhibitors do increase the risk of osteoporosis and are considerably more expensive than tamoxifen. These drugs are useful only in women in a postmenopausal state, and premenopausal women who undergo chemotherapy-induced amenorrhea should not routinely receive these drugs because they have the ability to cause resumption of menstrual cycles.

- Tamoxifen has both antiestrogen and estrogenlike activity.
- Beneficial effects of tamoxifen: antitumor effects, increased bone density, improved lipid profile, and decreased risk of contralateral breast cancer.
- Side effects of tamoxifen: hot flashes, vaginal dryness, thromboembolic risk, and increased risk of endometrial cancer.
- Aromatase inhibitors are useful only for postmenopausal women.

- Aromatase inhibitors increase the risk of osteoporosis, but they do not increase thromboembolic risk or endometrial cancer risk.

Other hormonal agents used to treat advanced, hormone-sensitive breast cancer include megestrol acetate (Megace), a progestational agent; fluoxymesterone (Halotestin), an androgen; and the estrogen receptor antagonist fulvestrant (Faslodex).

Premenopausal women with hormonally sensitive disease may benefit from oophorectomy (either chemical or surgical).

Other Agents

Herceptin
About 25% of breast cancers overexpress the growth factor HER2. A monoclonal antibody directed against HER2 (trastuzumab, Herceptin) has been shown to have activity against breast cancers that overexpress HER2. Trastuzumab is synergistic with certain chemotherapy agents. Side effects of trastuzumab can include myocardial dysfunction, and it should not be used in conjunction with cardiotoxic chemotherapy agents such as doxorubicin. Used in the adjuvant setting, trastuzumab therapy of 1 year has shown a roughly 50% decrease in the risk of breast cancer recurrence in women with HER2-positive breast cancer.

Lapatinib
Lapatinib (Tykerb) is an oral agent that also interferes with the HER2 signaling pathway. As opposed to herceptin, which acts on the membrane-bound, extracellular domain of the HER2 pathway, lapatinib acts intracellularly and is effective in women with herceptin-refractory HER2-positive breast cancer. It is currently approved for use in women with recurrent herceptin-refractory breast cancer in combination with capecitabine chemotherapy.

Zoledronic Acid (Zometa) and Pamidronate (Aredia)
The use of the bisphosphonates can reduce the need for palliative radiation, bone fixation, and pain medicine in women with lytic bone metastases.

Patterns of Recurrence
Breast cancer tends to recur in bones, liver, lungs, or brain or locally in the chest wall or residual breast. Recurrences can occur decades

Table 20-5 Adjuvant Therapy: Node-Negative Breast Cancer[a]

	Risk		
	Low	Intermediate	High
Tumor size, cm	<1	1-2	>2
ER or PR	+	+	−
Grade	1	1-2	2-3

Abbreviations: ER, estrogen receptor; PR, progesterone receptor.
[a] Most oncologists would not treat tumors less than 1 cm.

after initial diagnosis, and this possibility must always be kept in mind in any patient with a history of breast cancer, no matter how distant.

Typical Clinical Scenarios

Localized node-positive breast cancer: A 40-year-old woman has a 3-cm mass in the right breast and 2 lymph nodes involved in the axilla. Biopsy shows adenocarcinoma that is hormone-receptor–negative but HER2/neu–positive. The diagnosis is node-positive adenocarcinoma of the right breast. Treatment is local therapy (modified radical mastectomy or lumpectomy plus radiation) followed by adjuvant chemotherapy plus trastuzumab for 1 year.

Metastatic breast carcinoma: A 65-year-old patient has a history of breast carcinoma treated 10 years earlier with operation and chemotherapy. The patient presents with back pain, and bone scanning shows multiple areas of increased uptake throughout the skeleton. Biopsy shows estrogen receptor- and progesterone receptor-positive adenocarcinoma consistent with breast primary tumor. There is no evidence of metastatic disease elsewhere. Initial therapy is focal radiation to painful sites, hormonal therapy, and use of bisphosphonates.

Cervical Cancer

Background

The incidence of and mortality from cervical cancer have decreased by 30% to 40% in recent decades, attributed to widespread use of Papanicolaou smear screening. Currently, 12,200 new cases of cervical cancer are diagnosed in US women each year, and there are 4,100 deaths annually. In addition, more than 50,000 cases of carcinoma in situ of the cervix are diagnosed annually. Risk factors for cervical cancer include first intercourse at an early age, a greater number of sexual partners, smoking, history of sexually transmitted disease, especially herpesvirus or human papillomavirus lesions, and lower socioeconomic class. It is now understood that human papillomavirus is an etiologic agent for cervical carcinogenesis.

If a cytologic smear shows dysplasia or malignant cells, colposcopy with directed biopsy should be done. The Papanicolaou smear has limited sensitivity; false-negative rates of 20% frequently are quoted. The American Cancer Society recommends that asymptomatic, low-risk women 20 years of age or older and those younger than 20 years who are sexually active have a Papanicolaou smear annually for 2 consecutive years and, if the results are negative, at least 1 every 3 years.

Treatment

Treatment for carcinoma in situ of the cervix is usually total hysterectomy. If additional childbearing is desired, a more conservative approach, such as a therapeutic conization, is another option. Early invasive carcinoma of the cervix is usually treated with total hysterectomy. For patients with higher-stage disease, a combination of chemotherapy (cisplatin-based) and radiation therapy is recommended.

Prevention

The majority of cases of cervical cancer are associated with human papillomavirus. A recently approved vaccine (Gardasil) can provide protection against the 4 most common strains of the virus and has shown efficacy in decreasing the risk of cervical cancer. The American Cancer Society currently recommends this vaccine for all females before onset of sexual activity (CA Cancer J Clin. 2007;57:7-28).

Other methods for prevention include decreasing high-risk behavior, such as limiting sexual partners and use of condoms.

Colorectal Cancer

Background

Colorectal cancer is diagnosed in approximately 148,000 Americans each year and causes 57,000 deaths. Colorectal cancer is the second most common cause of cancer death in North America and Europe. It is associated with high-fat, low-fiber diets. Population screening with fecal occult blood testing remains problematic. Although 1 study showed a reduction in mortality from colorectal cancer with fecal occult blood screening (N Engl J Med. 1993;328:1365-71), it should be noted that any participants who had positive results went on to have colonoscopy. Another study showed that fecal occult blood tests failed to detect 70% of colorectal cancers and 80% of large (≥2 cm) polyps (JAMA. 1993;269:1262-7). Although specific screening recommendations vary, some form of screening process should be initiated by age 50 years regardless of risk. For high-risk patients, such as those with a family history of colorectal cancer or a prior colorectal cancer, structural studies of the entire large bowel, such as colonoscopy or (less preferable) rectosigmoidoscopy plus barium enema, should be performed at appropriate intervals (such as every 1-3 years).

- Colorectal cancer is associated with high-fat, low-fiber diets.
- Although specific screening recommendations vary, some form of screening process should be initiated by age 50 years regardless of risk.
- For high-risk patients, the entire large bowel should be studied at appropriate intervals.

Risk Factors

High-risk groups include persons with 1) familial polyposis syndromes (familial adenomatous polyposis—for which a gene recently was identified on chromosome 5—and Gardner syndrome—gut polyps plus desmoid tumors, lipomas, sebaceous cysts, and other abnormalities), 2) familial cancer syndromes without polyps (hereditary nonpolyposis colorectal cancer or Lynch syndromes, which are marked by colon cancer with or without endometrial, breast, and other cancers), and 3) inflammatory bowel disease (incidence 12% after 25 years).

- High-risk factors for colorectal cancer are familial polyposis syndromes, including familial adenomatous polyposis and Gardner syndrome, both inherited as an autosomal dominant trait; select familial cancer syndromes without polyps; and inflammatory bowel disease.

Treatment

Surgery

Surgical resection is the preferred method of curative treatment for carcinomas of the colon or rectum. Surgical exploration and resection allows for pathologic determination of tumor depth of penetration through the bowel wall and assessment of regional lymph nodes. Prognosis is directly related to the stage of disease (Table 20-6), although rectal tumors tend to have a worse prognosis than colon carcinomas. Five-year survival rates for locoregional disease have improved in recent decades as a result of many factors, including improvements in preoperative staging, surgical technique, and adjuvant (postoperative) therapy.

* Surgical resection is the preferred treatment for colorectal cancer.
* Prognosis is directly related to the stage of disease.
* Five-year survival rates are improving.

Adjuvant Therapy

For colon cancers, adjuvant chemotherapy with a multidrug regimen that includes oxaliplatin, 5-fluorouracil (5-FU), and leucovorin, given for 6 months, is recommended for node-positive (stage III) disease. Controversy exists about standard recommendations for deeply invasive (stage II) colon carcinomas. For *rectal cancers*, a combination of chemotherapy (5-FU–based) and pelvic irradiation, preferably administered preoperatively (neoadjuvant), is standard for stage II and III disease.

* For stage III colon cancers, adjuvant chemotherapy includes oxaliplatin, 5-FU, and leucovorin.
* For rectal cancer, a combination of chemotherapy (5-FU–based) and radiotherapy is the standard recommendation.

Metastatic Disease

Certain patients with metastatic colorectal cancer may be candidates for an attempt at curative resection. Of carefully selected patients with minimal metastatic disease, limited to the liver or lung, approximately 30% survive beyond 5 years without further evidence of disease recurrence after resection of metastatic lesions and systemic chemotherapy (Ann Intern Med. 1998;129:27-35).

Palliative chemotherapy is the only option for the vast majority of patients with advanced metastatic colorectal cancer. The median duration of survival for patients given medical therapy is about 24 months. The combination of conventional chemotherapy (5-FU/leucovorin plus either irinotecan or oxaliplatin) plus bevacizumab (Avastin) is the standard treatment for metastatic disease. Capecitabine (Xeloda) can be used as an oral substitute for intravenous 5-FU. New, biologically targeted treatments such as bevacizumab (Avastin),

which targets new blood vessel formation, have been approved by the US Food and Drug Administration for patients with metastatic colon cancer as first-line therapy in combination with any 5-FU–based chemotherapy regimen. Cetuximab (Erbitux), a therapy targeted against the epidermal growth factor receptor, was approved in 2004 as combination treatment with irinotecan (or alone if irinotecan is not tolerated) for metastatic colon cancer. Panitumumab (Vectibix), a monoclonal antibody similar to cetuximab received US Food and Drug Administration approval in 2006 as therapy for patients with recurrent, advanced colorectal cancer.

* Surgical resection of metastatic disease can result in long-term disease-free survival in a select subset of patients.
* Palliative conventional chemotherapy options for advanced colorectal carcinoma include oxaliplatin, 5-FU, leucovorin, capecitabine, and irinotecan.
* The biologically targeted agents bevacizumab, cetuximab, and panitumumab are approved for treatment of metastatic colon cancer.

Carcinoembryonic Antigen

Until recently, routine use of carcinoembryonic antigen (CEA) to monitor patients after curative resection of colon cancer was not recommended. Current American Society of Clinical Oncology guidelines do recommend that the CEA level be checked preoperatively if it would assist in staging and surgical planning. After curative treatment for colon cancer, the guidelines recommend that the CEA level be checked every 3 months for at least 3 years in patients with stage II and III disease, as long as the patient's general medical condition is such that the patient would be a candidate for surgical intervention or chemotherapy. CEA may be useful for monitoring the response of metastatic disease to therapy.

Typical Clinical Scenarios

Node-positive colon cancer: A 60-year-old patient has a history of altered bowel habits over 3 months. Colonoscopy shows adenocarcinoma in the descending colon. The patient undergoes left hemicolectomy. Regional lymph nodes are found to be involved. In view of the positive lymph nodes, adjuvant chemotherapy with oxaliplatin, 5-FU and leucovorin is warranted.

Metastatic colon carcinoma: A 70-year-old patient with a history of colon carcinoma resected 10 years previously presents with increasing abdominal girth and jaundice. Computed tomography shows multiple nodules in the liver. The diagnosis is metastatic colon

Table 20-6 Staging of Colorectal Cancer and Survival

Dukes Stage	AJCC Stage	Depth of Penetration	Nodal Status	5-Year Survival, %
A	I	Submucosa or muscularis	Negative	90
B	II	Through muscularis or to other organs	Negative	60-80
C	III	Any	Positive	30-60

Abbreviation: AJCC, American Joint Committee on Cancer.

carcinoma, and therapy consists of palliative chemotherapy with oxaliplatin, 5-FU, leucovorin, and bevacizumab.

Localized ascending colon carcinoma: A 50-year-old patient has a new diagnosis of iron deficiency anemia. A mass in the ascending colon is found on a work-up for iron deficiency. The diagnosis is adenocarcinoma of the ascending colon. Resection shows no evidence of lymph node metastases, and no postoperative adjuvant chemotherapy is recommended.

Lung Cancer

Magnitude of the Problem
Approximately 172,000 new cases of lung cancer are diagnosed in the United States annually, resulting in approximately 157,000 deaths. Thus, only approximately 15% of patients with lung cancer survive the disease. Lung cancer is the leading cause of cancer mortality in both American men and women.

Risk Factors
About 95% of lung cancers in men and about 80% of lung cancers in women result from cigarette smoking. Men who smoke 1 to 2 packs per day have up to a 25-fold increase in lung cancer compared with those who have never smoked. The risk of lung cancer in an ex-smoker declines with time. Passive smoking is associated with an increased risk of lung cancer. Certain occupations (smelter workers, iron workers), chemicals (arsenic, methylethyl ether), and exposure to radioactive agents (radon, uranium) and asbestos have been associated with increased risks for development of lung cancer.

- 95% of lung cancers in men and 80% in women result from cigarette smoking.
- Men who smoke 1 to 2 packs a day have a 25-fold increase in lung cancer compared with those who have never smoked.
- Passive smoking is associated with an increased risk of lung cancer.

Screening
Several large, randomized trials have tested the utility of chest radiography and sputum cytology in screening for lung cancer. None of these studies have shown that either sputum cytology or regular chest radiography improves survival from lung cancer. Thus, screening is not currently standard. However, there are recognized methodologic problems with these studies, and some investigators believe that there is benefit to screening for this disease (Chest. 1995;107 Suppl 6:270S-279S). Several recent trials studying the use of computed tomography for early detection of lung cancer are highly controversial (JAMA. 2007;297:953-61 and N Engl J Med. 2006;355:1763-71). One trial does suggest that lung cancer cases found with screening computed tomography are more likely to be early stage and more amenable to surgical resection, but no survival advantage has yet been shown. A second trial that is still ongoing has shown that a very large number of false-positive results are found for every case of lung cancer, and these lead to the need for additional tests with considerable morbidity and expense. Furthermore, only a minority of patients who undergo screening for lung cancer actually stop smoking.

- Randomized trials have not shown a survival advantage to screening for lung cancer.

Histologic Types and Characteristics
Lung cancer is divided into small cell and non–small cell types. Small cell lung cancer occurs almost exclusively in smokers. The primary tumors are often small but are associated with bulky mediastinal adenopathy. They may be associated with paraneoplastic syndromes, including the syndrome of inappropriate secretion of antidiuretic hormone, and various neurologic abnormalities. Non–small cell lung cancers can be divided into squamous, adenocarcinoma, and large cell types. Squamous cell carcinomas may be associated with hypercalcemia due to the secretion of a parathyroid hormone-like peptide. Squamous carcinomas tend to occur centrally, whereas large cell and adenocarcinoma types tend to be more peripheral. Adenocarcinoma is the most frequent histologic subtype in nonsmokers. Bronchoalveolar carcinoma is a low-grade non–small cell carcinoma that frequently presents as a patchy infiltrate. It may be multifocal.

Staging
The classic *Tumor-Node-Metastasis* (TNM) system is simplified in Table 20-7.

Natural History
The natural history of surgically treated lung cancer, by stage, is shown in Figure 20-3.

Treatment

Non–Small Cell Lung Cancer
Resection is the treatment of choice for clinical stages I, II, and selected IIIA non–small cell lung cancer (NSCLC). The use of adjuvant chemotherapy recently was shown to improve survival by 10% to 12% compared with operation alone (N Engl J Med.

Table 20-7 Staging of Lung Cancer

	Non–small cell type
Stage I	Primary tumor >2 cm from carina; node negative
Stage II	Primary tumor >2 cm from carina; hilar nodes positive
Stage IIIA	Tumor <2 cm from carina, or invading a resectable structure, or ipsilateral mediastinal nodes positive
Stage IIIB	Tumor invading an unresectable structure, supraclavicular or contralateral mediastinal nodes positive or cytologically positive pleural effusion
Stage IV	Metastatic disease
	Small cell type
Limited	Limited to 1 hemithorax less supraclavicular lymph nodes. Can be encompassed within a tolerable radiation port
Extensive	All other disease (metastatic disease)

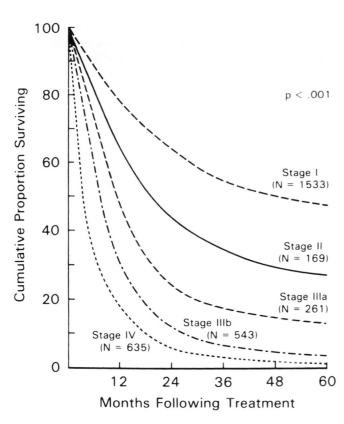

Figure 20-3. Survival Curves for Patients With Lung Cancer by Stage. (From Mountain CF. A new international staging system for lung cancer. Chest. 1986;89:225S-33S. Used with permission.)

2005;352:2589-97 and Lancet Oncol. 2006;7:719-27). The use of adjuvant radiation does not improve survival in resected stage II and III disease, but it is able to decrease the likelihood of local recurrence. In patients with locally advanced unresectable NSCLC, the use of concurrent chemotherapy and radiation improves the long-term survival compared with radiation alone. Although patients with metastatic disease are not cured, the use of chemotherapy has improved the overall survival by several weeks and the quality of life compared with best supportive care. These studies are hampered by lack of uniform definitions of what constitutes best supportive care.

- Operation is the treatment of choice for stages I and II and selected IIIA NSCLC.
- There is some improvement in survival with adjuvant chemotherapy.
- Chemotherapy is not curative for metastatic NSCLC.
- Chemotherapy improves the overall survival by several weeks and may improve quality of life for patients with metastatic NSCLC.

Chemotherapy for NSCLC
Active chemotherapy agents for NSCLC include etoposide, cisplatin, carboplatin, pemetrexed, cyclophosphamide, mitomycin-C, ifosfamide, gemcitabine, irinotecan, docetaxel, and paclitaxel. Recently, erlotinib, an inhibitor of the epidermal growth factor receptor, was shown to be superior to best supportive care for patients with metastatic NSCLC. Bevicizumab (Avastin), an angiogenesis inhibitor, has shown efficacy in NSCLC and is often included as part of the treatment regimen for patients with adenocarcinoma.

Small Cell Lung Cancer
Treatment of limited-stage small cell lung cancer consists of both chemotherapy and chest radiation. Surgical resection has not been shown to improve survival. For patients who have a complete response to chemotherapy and chest radiation therapy, prophylactic cranial irradiation is used to decrease the frequency of recurrence in the central nervous system. There is some controversy about whether this leads to improved overall survival. Prophylactic cranial irradiation is associated with the risk of a delayed leukoencephalopathy, but this risk can be reduced by the administration of radiation in small-dose fractions without concomitant chemotherapy. For limited-stage small cell disease, the median duration of survival is approximately 18 months; 30% to 40% of patients survive 2 years, and 10% to 20% survive 5 years.

- For small cell lung cancer, treatment of limited-stage disease consists of both chemotherapy and chest radiation.
- Prophylactic cranial irradiation decreases the frequency of recurrence in the central nervous system.
- Median survival is 18 months with limited-stage disease.

Chemotherapy is used for extensive-stage (stage IV) small cell lung cancer. Combination chemotherapy is favored over single-agent therapy. Active drugs include etoposide, cisplatin, cyclophosphamide, doxorubicin, and vincristine. High-dose chemotherapy with or without autologous bone marrow transplant or marrow colony-stimulating factors has not yet been proved superior to standard chemotherapy. The median duration of survival is approximately 9 months; about 10% of patients survive 2 years, and 1% or fewer survive 5 years.

- For extensive-stage small cell lung cancer, treatment is chemotherapy.
- High-dose chemotherapy has not yet been proved superior to standard chemotherapy.
- Median survival for patients with extensive-stage small cell lung cancer is 9 months.

Typical Clinical Scenarios
Localized lung cancer: A 60-year-old smoker presents with cough. On chest radiography and computed tomography, a 2-cm nodule is found in the right upper aspect of the chest without evidence of lymph node or metastatic disease. After the diagnosis of non–small cell lung carcinoma is confirmed, therapy is surgical resection.

Small cell lung carcinoma: This patient is similar to the one described above, but biopsy shows small cell lung carcinoma. Treatment consists of systemic chemotherapy plus radiation.

Melanoma

Background
Malignant melanoma is increasing at a rapid rate. If current trends continue, the lifetime risk for malignant melanoma to develop in

an American will be 1 in 75. Fortunately, the 5-year survival rate has doubled from approximately 40% in the 1940s to approximately 80% now, a change attributed to earlier detection. Melanoma is more common among fair-skinned people; people with a history of recurrent, blistering sunburns; persons with multiple atypical nevi; persons with freckling tendency; and certain families (first-degree relatives or persons with familial atypical mole/melanoma [FAMM] syndrome, formerly called the dysplastic nevus syndrome).

- The incidence of malignant melanoma is increasing rapidly.
- The 5-year survival rate has improved as a result of earlier detection.
- High-risk populations are identifiable.

Diagnosis ("ABCD") and Prognosis
Keys to the early diagnosis of malignant melanoma include the following:
    A: Asymmetry, especially a changing lesion
    B: Borders are irregular
    C: Color is variable, especially with blues, blacks, and tans dispersed throughout the lesion
    D: Diameter 6 mm or more
The Breslow microstaging method measures the thickness (ie, depth of penetration of the tumor from the epidermis into the dermis/subcutis) of a malignant melanoma and is the best independent predictor of survival (Table 20-8).

Management
Surgical excision to achieve a 1- to 3-cm margin around the lesion remains the principal treatment for primary malignant melanoma. In the absence of palpable adenopathy, an elective lymph node dissection is not routinely performed. With clinically palpable regional nodes, a node dissection is performed for curative intent and to achieve maximal local tumor control. For patients at high risk for recurrence (deep primary tumor >4.0 mm or resected node-positive disease), recent clinical trials have shown conflicting results, and therefore adjuvant therapy remains controversial.

Treatment for metastatic melanoma is primarily palliative. Surgical resection in selected patients (those with a long disease-free interval and limited disease at recurrence) can be considered. Systemic treatments commonly include immunotherapy (interleukin-2 or interferon), chemotherapy (temozolomide, dacarbazine, or nitrosoureas), or various combinations.

Typical Clinical Scenario
Malignant melanoma: A 60-year-old patient presents with a mole on the right leg that has been increasing in size during the past 3 months. Resection reveals malignant melanoma with a depth of invasion of 0.75 mm. Definitive therapy is reexcision to obtain a 1- to 3-cm margin around the lesion. No adjuvant therapy is recommended.

Ovarian Cancer

This disease is diagnosed annually in approximately 25,400 American women. It is the leading cause of death due to gynecologic cancer, resulting in 14,300 deaths annually. There are no early warning signs;

most patients present with vague gastrointestinal complaints such as bloating. Most patients (75%) present with advanced disease (ie, stages III and IV, disease spread beyond the pelvis). The term "ovarian cancer" refers to tumors derived from the ovarian surface epithelium, not germ cell tumors.

- Ovarian cancer is the leading cause of death due to gynecologic cancer.
- There are no early warning signs.
- Most patients (75%) present with advanced disease.

Staging
Stage I is confined to the ovary, stage II is confined to the pelvis, stage III includes spread to the upper abdomen, and stage IV includes spread to distant sites.

Cancer Antigen 125
Cancer antigen 125 (CA 125) is expressed by approximately 85% of epithelial ovarian tumors and released into the circulation. However, it is detectable in only 50% of patients with stage I disease. The highest serum levels of CA 125 are found in patients with ovarian cancer, but the serum CA 125 level also may be increased in other malignancies and in pregnancy, endometriosis, and menstruation. CA 125 is clearly of value for monitoring the course of ovarian cancer, but there is as yet no clear role for use of CA 125 for screening purposes.

- CA 125 is expressed by about 85% of epithelial ovarian tumors.
- The CA 125 level also may be increased in other malignancies and in pregnancy, endometriosis, and menstruation.
- CA 125 is useful for monitoring the course of ovarian cancer.

Screening
The tools evaluated thus far, namely, pelvic ultrasonography and determination of the serum CA 125 value, are inadequate for screening the general female population. Screening for this disease is difficult for several reasons. The incidence of ovarian cancer is relatively low, and there are no recognized pre-invasive lesions. Moreover, pelvic ultrasonography and CA 125 lack sufficient sensitivity and specificity. However, it seems reasonable to apply these techniques on a periodic basis to women at particularly high risk of ovarian cancer, for example, those with a strong family history of the disease (2 or more affected

Table 20-8 Ten-Year Survival in Melanoma, by Depth of Tumor

Depth, mm	% Alive
<0.85	96
0.85-1.69	87
1.7-3.6	66.5
>3.6	46

Data from Friedman RJ, Rigel DS, Silverman MK, Kopf AW, Vossaert KA. Malignant melanoma in the 1990s: the continued importance of early detection and the role of physician examination and self-examination of the skin. CA Cancer J Clin. 1991 July/Aug;41:201-26.

relatives) or known carriers of *BRCA* gene mutations. The cause of epithelial ovarian cancer is unknown. A small subset of patients (<5%) has an inherited predisposition to this disease. Generally, this occurs in families with both breast and ovarian cancer.

- Population screening for ovarian cancer is not recommended.
- Pelvic ultrasonography and CA 125 testing lack sufficient sensitivity and specificity to be routinely recommended.
- A small subset of patients (<5%) has an inherited predisposition to ovarian cancer and may benefit from screening.

Treatment

The initial management of patients with epithelial ovarian cancer includes a thorough surgical staging and debulking procedure. Outcome in this disease depends on the amount of tumor tissue remaining after initial operation. Patients with only microscopic residual disease fare better than those with less than optimally debulked tumors. Subsequently, patients are treated with 6 cycles of platinum- and paclitaxel-based chemotherapy. Recent studies have shown that the use of intraperitoneal cisplatin improves response rate and survival. This does require that a peritoneal catheter be placed at the time of the surgical debulking, and patients require hospitalization for each cycle of intraperitoneal chemotherapy.

- Management of ovarian cancer includes thorough surgical staging and debulking followed by chemotherapy, both systemic and intraperitoneal.
- The outcome depends on the amount of tumor tissue remaining after initial operation.
- Subsequent chemotherapy consists of a platinum compound and paclitaxel.

Outcome

Outcome depends on the stage of disease. Ninety percent of patients with stage I disease are alive at 5 years, versus 80% of those with stage II disease. Unfortunately, survival with advanced disease is poor: 15% to 20% of patients with stage III disease are alive at 5 years and only 5% of patients with stage IV disease are alive.

Typical Clinical Scenario

Ovarian cancer: A 50-year-old patient presents with ascites. Evaluation reveals a mass in the right ovary. Therapy consists of surgical debulking followed by chemotherapy, both systemic and intraperitoneal.

Prostate Cancer

Background

There are approximately 220,900 new cases of prostate cancer annually in the United States. It is the most common cancer in men in the United States and is the second leading cause of death from cancer in men in the United States (29,000 deaths annually). Identified risk factors for the development of prostate cancer include older age, race (African American), family history (first-degree relative), and possibly dietary fat. The American Cancer Society recommends a digital rectal examination in men 40 years or older and determination of the prostate-specific antigen (PSA) value in men 50 years or older. Use of PSA for prostate cancer screening is a controversial issue and has not been shown to reduce mortality. Screening in older men should be discontinued when they have a life expectancy of less than 10 years due to age or other comorbidities.

- Prostate cancer is the most common cancer among US men and the second leading cause of death from cancer in men.
- Risk factors include older age, race (African American), family history, and a high-fat diet.

Prostate-Specific Antigen

PSA is a serine protease produced by normal and neoplastic prostatic ductal epithelium. Its concentration is proportional to the total prostatic mass. The inability to differentiate benign prostatic hyperplasia from carcinoma on the basis of the PSA level renders it inadequate as the sole screening method for prostate cancer. PSA is useful for monitoring response to therapy in cases of known prostate cancer, particularly after radical prostatectomy, when PSA should be undetectable.

- The concentration of PSA is proportional to the total prostatic mass.
- The PSA test is inadequate as the sole screening test for prostate cancer.
- PSA is useful for monitoring response to therapy.

Prognostic factors for prostate cancer include stage of disease, grade of tumor, and pretreatment PSA level. Table 20-9 simplifies the staging of prostate cancer, including the TNM classification. Grading of tumors is performed by the pathologist with the Gleason scoring system. The surgical specimen is graded by the most predominant pattern of differentiation added to the secondary architectural pattern (eg, 3+5=8). Gleason grades 2 through 6 are associated with a better prognosis. Recent retrospective results indicate that the pretreatment PSA value is a strong predictor of disease outcome after operation or radiotherapy.

- Prognostic factors for the outcome of prostate cancer include tumor stage, grade, and pretreatment PSA value.
- Gleason grades 2 through 6 have a better prognosis.

Management

Management of Specific Stages

Significant controversy surrounds the primary treatment of prostate cancer in nearly all stages of the disease. Because this is a disease of older men, comorbid conditions, age, and performance status need to be considered when directing therapy because more men will die with prostate cancer than from prostate cancer. In general, patients with T1A prostate tumors are observed without treatment. For organ-confined prostate cancer (T1B, T1C, and T2 tumors), both radiation therapy and radical prostatectomy are equally viable options. Recently, some investigators have proposed observation alone and treatment with hormonal agents at the time of progression because

Table 20-9 Staging of Prostate Cancer

Whitmore	TNM[a]	Criteria
A1	T1A	Incidental focus of tumor in ≤5% of resected tissue
A2	T1B	Incidental tumor in >5% of resected tissue
B0	T1C	Tumor identified by needle biopsy (performed on basis of increased PSA value)
B1	T2A	Tumor ≤1/2 of 1 lobe
B2	T2B	Tumor >1/2 of 1 lobe but not both lobes
	T2C	Tumor involvement of both lobes
C	T3 or T4	Extracapsular local disease or local invasion
D1	N1	Pelvic node involvement
D2	M1	Distant disease

Abbreviation: PSA, prostate-specific antigen.
[a] *Tumor-Node-Metastasis* system.

the rate of death from prostate cancer is low for well-differentiated early-stage disease. A large trial is currently under way in the United States to test the value of operation compared with observation for organ-confined prostate cancer.

For stage C (T3 or T4) disease (locally advanced), radiotherapy is generally used. A trial combining androgen deprivation with local radiation therapy showed improved local control and overall survival in this patient cohort (N Engl J Med. 1997;337:295-300). Some centers use androgen deprivation to downstage tumors before an aggressive surgical approach.

For stage D1 disease (positive pelvic nodes), the management is controversial. Divergent approaches include androgen deprivation alone, x-ray therapy with or without androgen deprivation, close observation with androgen deprivation at progression, or, infrequently, prostatectomy with androgen deprivation. For advanced (D2) disease, androgen deprivation is the treatment of choice. Recent studies have shown that chemotherapy for metastatic, hormone-refractory disease does produce a modest survival advantage compared with observation only.

Prostatectomy

This is reserved for patients with localized disease. The 15-year disease-specific survival rate after prostatectomy is 85% to 90% for stage A2 or B disease. Nerve sparing prostatectomy is able to spare potency in 68% to 86% of patients. Risk of impotence increases with increasing age, size of tumor, extent of spread, and preoperative sexual function. Total urinary incontinence is rare (<2% of patients), although many men have some degree of incontinence after prostatectomy.

- Prostatectomy is used for localized disease.

- The 15-year survival rate is 85%-90% for stage A2 or B disease.
- Nerve sparing operations preserve sexual function in a majority of men.

Radiation Therapy

External beam radiotherapy is considered the equivalent of prostatectomy for overall survival. It is preferred for stage C disease at most centers. Impotence can occur, but less often than with prostatectomy. Chronic radiation proctitis is not uncommon. A concern related to radiotherapy is that repeat biopsies after treatment have shown apparently viable tumor in more than 35% of patients. The clinical importance of this residual tumor is unclear, but there may be a correlation with the subsequent appearance of distant metastasis, especially with a persistent, palpable abnormality in the gland.

Patients with organ-confined prostate cancer may also be candidates for brachytherapy. In this procedure, hundreds of radioactive seeds are placed in the prostate gland through a transrectal approach. This treatment works as well as external beam radiation therapy in appropriately selected patients, is less likely to cause radiation proctitis or impotence, but is less likely to adequately treat patients with extraprostatic spread of disease. Brachytherapy also requires fewer treatments and thus is often attractive to patients who live a long distance from the radiation center.

- External beam radiotherapy is considered the equivalent of prostatectomy for overall survival.
- Impotence is less frequent with radiotherapy than prostatectomy.

Androgen Deprivation

For advanced (D2) disease, bone is the most frequent site of metastatic disease. Hormonal therapy, although it is very effective and produces a response in most patients, is noncurative. The average duration of response to initial hormonal maneuver is 18 months. The average duration of survival is 2 to 3 years, but many patients live for years with metastatic prostate cancer. Once the disease progresses after the initial hormonal maneuver, it is typically less responsive to secondary hormonal therapy. Recent data have shown that prostate cancer is sensitive to chemotherapy and even can improve survival in men with androgen independent metastatic prostate cancer (N Engl J Med. 2004;351:1502-12).

- Bone is the most frequent site of metastatic disease from the prostate.
- Hormonal therapy is effective and produces a response, but it is noncurative.
- The average duration of survival with advanced prostatic cancer is 2-3 years.

The two sources of androgens in men are the testes (testosterone, 95%) and adrenal glands (5%). Androgen deprivation can be accomplished surgically with orchiectomy or medically. Potential agents include luteinizing hormone-releasing hormone (LHRH) agonists such as leuprolide, buserelin, and goserelin. They decrease androgen levels through continuous binding of the LHRH receptor and subsequent decrease of LH and thus testosterone. They are administered as a monthly injection of a depot preparation. A 3- or 4-month depot preparation is also available. LHRH agonists, on initial binding of the LHRH receptor, transiently stimulate LH release and thus cause an initial increase in the testosterone level. This explains the transient flare of prostate cancer that can occur in men with advanced disease when therapy with an LHRH agonist is initiated. This possibility must be considered in patients with impending spinal cord compression, urinary obstruction, or extensive painful bony metastases. Use of an antiandrogen such as bicalutamide (Casodex) before initiating LHRH antagonist therapy can block this flare.

* Androgen deprivation is accomplished with orchiectomy or medically.
* LHRH agonists decrease androgen levels.
* LHRH agonists initially stimulate a transient release of LH and testosterone.

Antiandrogens compete with androgens at the receptor level. These include flutamide, nilutamide, and bicalutamide. To effect total androgen blockade, an antiandrogen is added in patients who have had orchiectomy or who are receiving an LHRH agonist (these block testicular testosterone production but not adrenal androgen production). A prospective US study in which a combination of an LHRH analogue with flutamide was compared with placebo suggested an advantage for the addition of flutamide. However, other studies of total blockade have failed to show an advantage. A recent clinical trial comparing orchiectomy alone with orchiectomy plus flutamide failed to show a survival advantage for total androgen blockade. The antiandrogens may also block the "flare" induced by LHRH agonists.

* The use of an antiandrogen in combination with orchiectomy or an LHRH agonist to treat advanced prostate cancer remains controversial.
* Antiandrogens block the "flare" induced by LHRH agonists.

Chemotherapy
Prostate cancer had previously been considered refractory to most chemotherapy regimens. Newer combinations using paclitaxel (Taxol) and prednisone have shown not only significant responses but also improved survival in men with metastatic, hormone refractory prostate cancer.

Bisphosphonates
The use of bisphosphonates in men with bone metastasis remains very controversial and does not improve overall survival. Bisphosphonates can be a useful adjunct for treatment of painful metastases.

* Chemotherapy and bisphosphonates can be used for palliative effects in men with prostate cancer.

Follow-up Recommendations
After curative therapy with either definitive radiation or radical prostatectomy, PSA can be a sensitive marker for recurrence. PSA should be undetectable after successful primary surgical therapy, but some level

will persist after radiation treatment. After definitive local therapy, the median time between increased PSA level (biochemical recurrence) and development of symptoms from metastatic prostate cancer is 8 years, and median time to death from recurrent prostate cancer is 13 years. Thus, how closely any 1 patient is monitored depends on overall health, comorbid conditions, and overall life expectancy.

* After curative treatment of prostate cancer, the median time from biochemical recurrence of prostate cancer to first symptom from metastatic disease is 8 years and the median time to death from prostate cancer is 13 years.

Typical Clinical Scenario
Prostate cancer: A 70-year-old patient presents with back pain. The PSA value is markedly increased and the prostate is enlarged. Prostatic biopsy reveals prostatic carcinoma. On radiography and bone scanning multiple areas of increased uptake are found throughout the skeleton, consistent with metastatic disease. Therapy consists of hormonal manipulation, with either orchiectomy or LHRH agonists. If LHRH agonists are chosen, the patient should receive an antiandrogen for 1 month before initiating the LHRH agonist.

Testicular Cancer

Background
This cancer is diagnosed in 7,600 men annually. It is the most common carcinoma in males 15 to 35 years old. It is highly curable, even when metastatic. At high risk are males with cryptorchid testes (40-fold relative risk) or Klinefelter syndrome (also increased risk of breast cancer). Two broad categories are seminomas (40%) and nonseminomas. Types of nonseminomas include embryonal carcinoma, mature and immature teratoma, choriocarcinoma, yolk sac tumor, and endodermal sinus tumor. There is often an admixture of several cell types within nonseminomas. Any nonseminomatous component plus seminoma is treated as a nonseminoma.

* Testicular cancer is the most common carcinoma in males 15-35 years old.
* Testicular cancer is highly curable, even when metastatic.
* High-risk factors: cryptorchid testes, Klinefelter syndrome.
* Two categories: seminomas (40%) and nonseminomas.

Evaluation includes determination of β-human chorionic gonadotropin (hCG) and α-fetoprotein values and computed tomography of the abdomen (retroperitoneal nodes) and chest (mediastinal nodes or pulmonary nodules).

Staging
Stage I disease is confined to the testis, stage II includes infradiaphragmatic nodal metastases, and stage III is spread beyond retroperitoneal nodes. About 85% of nonseminomas are associated with an increased β-hCG or α-fetoprotein value. Approximately 10% of seminomas are associated with an increased β-hCG level. The α-fetoprotein value is never increased in pure seminoma; if it is increased, the tumor is not seminoma and should be treated as such.

- 85% of nonseminomas are associated with an increased β-hCG or α-fetoprotein value.
- 10% of seminomas are associated with an increased β-hCG value.
- The α-fetoprotein value is never increased in pure seminoma.

Management

Radical inguinal orchiectomy is the definitive procedure for both pathologic diagnosis and local control. Scrotal orchiectomy or biopsy is associated with a high incidence of local recurrence or spread to inguinal nodes. After orchiectomy, management depends on cell type (Table 20-10). Early-stage seminoma is treated with resection and radiation. Seminomas are exquisitely radiosensitive. For stage I and nonbulky stage II seminoma, infradiaphragmatic lymphatic irradiation is used. The 5-year disease-free survival rate is more than 95%. For bulky stage II disease and stage III disease, platinum-based chemotherapy is used. Approximately 85% of patients are cured. For stage I nonseminoma, close follow-up is often used rather than immediate retroperitoneal node dissection (a controversial issue). For stages II and III, platinum-based chemotherapy is given. Cure rates are more than 95% for minimal metastatic disease, 90% for moderate bulk disease, and about 50% for bulky disease (multiple pulmonary metastases, bulky abdominal masses, liver, bone, or central nervous system metastases).

- Radical inguinal orchiectomy is the definitive initial procedure for testicular cancer.
- Early-stage seminoma is treated with resection and radiation.
- Stage I nonseminoma may require no treatment after orchiectomy.
- Platinum-based chemotherapy is used for all other patients and results in high cure rates.

Extragonadal Germ Cell Tumor

This is uncommon. Patients present with increased β-hCG or α-fetoprotein values with midline mass lesions (retroperitoneum, mediastinum, or pineal gland). No gonadal primary tumor is identifiable on examination or ultrasonography. Cisplatin-based chemotherapy is frequently effective. Prognosis is not as favorable as with a testicular primary tumor.

Carcinoma of Unknown Primary Lesion

Background

Patients presenting with metastatic carcinoma with an unknown primary lesion make up 5% to 10% of general oncologic practice.

Table 20-10 Management of Testicular Cancer

| Stage | Treatment, by Cell Type | |
	Seminoma	Nonseminoma
I	XRT	? Observe
II	XRT	Chemo
III	Chemo	Chemo

Abbreviations: Chemo, chemotherapy; XRT, x-ray therapy.

The first principle of management is to establish the diagnosis with a sufficient histologic specimen. In general, open biopsy is preferable to fine-needle aspiration, because a larger specimen allows optimal histologic and immunohistochemical analysis. All patients should have a careful history and complete physical examination, including pelvic and rectal examinations. Most patients, approximately 60%, have an adenocarcinoma. In 35% of patients, poorly differentiated carcinoma will be diagnosed. Once a pathologic diagnosis is established, additional evaluation should be tailored according to the patient's risk factors (eg, smoking, breast cancer risk), symptoms and signs, sites of metastasis, and the histologic diagnosis. Special consideration should be given to rule out possible curable malignancies such as germ cell tumors or lymphoma or treatable malignancies such as breast, ovarian, or prostate cancer. Women presenting with axillary adenocarcinomas, with no clear breast primary lesion, should receive treatment for breast cancer. Women with peritoneal carcinomatosis generally have exploratory laparotomy with surgical cytoreduction, as for ovarian carcinoma. Men presenting with bone metastases, particularly osteoblastic metastases, should have a PSA test and their tumor material stained for PSA expression.

Treatment

If a potentially treatable neoplasm is ruled out, most patients with metastatic cancer of an unknown primary lesion have a very poor prognosis, with expected survival of 4 to 6 months. Some may benefit from palliative treatment (radiation or chemotherapy); many are managed best with supportive care and hospice care.

Paraneoplastic Syndromes

General

These conditions are the effects of a cancer occurring at a distance from the tumor; they are called *remote effects*. They do not necessarily indicate metastatic disease. Common paraneoplastic syndromes and associated tumor types are listed in Table 20-11.

Carcinoid Syndrome

This is caused by peptide mediators secreted by carcinoid tumors that most frequently arise in the small intestine and that may have metastasized to the liver. It is less frequent with primary carcinoid tumors arising from other sites such as lung, thymus, or ovary. The most common symptoms are episodic flushing and diarrhea; bronchospasm may occur. Flushing and diarrhea may occur spontaneously or be precipitated by emotional factors or ingestion of food or alcohol. Carcinoid heart disease (right-sided valvular disease) is a potential late complication.

Lambert-Eaton Syndrome

This consists of muscle weakness (proximal) and gait disturbance. Strength is increased with exercise. It is associated with small cell lung cancer.

Dermatomyositis

The female to male ratio is 2:1. Findings include muscle weakness (proximal), inflammatory myopathy, and increased creatine kinase values. Skin changes are variable and include heliotrope rash, periorbital edema, and Gottron papules. An underlying malignancy (lung, breast, gastrointestinal) is common in patients older than 50 years.

Chemotherapy

Basic Concepts

Currently, more than 70 cytotoxic agents are available for use in North America. Taken generally, chemotherapeutic agents impair the process of cell division. Cytotoxic chemotherapy drugs are not selective for cancer cells. These drugs have their predominant effect on cells that are more rapidly dividing, such as many forms of neoplastic cells. This selectivity for rapidly dividing cells explains the typical patterns of toxicity that occur with chemotherapy (ie, bone marrow, gastrointestinal mucosa, and hair follicles). The general classes and mechanisms of chemotherapeutic agents are shown in Figure 20-4 and the Oncology Pharmacy Review.

Biologically Targeted Agents

Newer therapeutic agents are now available that more specifically target abnormalities intrinsic to neoplastic cells and thus allow for more targeted therapy. Several biologically targeted agents were recently approved for cancer therapy. These drugs include monoclonal antibodies such as trastuzumab, bevacizumab, rituximab, and cetuximab and tyrosine kinase inhibitors gefitinib, erlotinib, and suitinib or temsirolimus (an inhibitor of the mammalian target of rapamycin) (Table 20-12). Tumor tissue can be tested to determine whether the specific target of interest is expressed. If so, these drugs can be used either alone or in combination with chemotherapy, radiation therapy, or other antitumor treatments. Of interest, response to some of the so-called targeted agents is not necessarily related to expression or staining of the target.

Toxicities associated with these new targeted agents tend to differ significantly from those of conventional chemotherapy; rash and diarrhea are the most common side effects. Each individual drug may have specific toxicities associated with it, but for the most part these are often better tolerated than those of conventional chemotherapy.

Applications

Chemotherapy can be used in the following settings: 1) advanced disease with palliative intent; 2) as adjuvant therapy after definitive local treatment to reduce risk of recurrence, thereby increasing the chance for cure; 3) as neoadjuvant (or preoperative) therapy; and 4) as primary therapy. Neoadjuvant therapy is used when patients present with a locally advanced malignancy and initial tumor reduction is needed before a primary treatment (such as operation or radiation)

Table 20-11 Classification of Paraneoplastic Syndromes

Syndrome	Mediator	Tumor Type
Endocrine		
Cushing syndrome[a]	ACTH	Small cell lung cancer
SIADH[a]	ADH	Lung, especially small cell
Hypercalcemia[a]	PTH-like peptide	Lung, especially squamous; breast; myeloma
Carcinoid syndrome	? Serotonin	Gut neuroendocrine tumors
	? Substance P	
Hypoglycemia	Insulin	Gut neuroendocrine tumors; other
	Insulin-like growth factors	
Neuromuscular		
Cerebellar degeneration	Anti-Purkinje cell antibodies	Lung, especially small cell; ovarian; breast
Dementia	?	Lung
Peripheral neuropathy[a]	Autoantibodies	Lung, gastrointestinal, breast
Lambert-Eaton	Antibodies to cholinergic receptor	Small cell lung cancer
Dermatomyositis	?	Lung, breast
Skin		
Dermatomyositis	?	Lung, breast
Acanthosis nigricans	? TGF-α	Intra-abdominal cancer, usually gastric
Hematologic		
Venous thrombosis[a]	Activators of clotting cascade & platelets	Various adenocarcinomas, especially pancreatic & gastric
Nonbacterial thrombotic endocarditis	Activators of clotting cascade & platelets	Various adenocarcinomas, especially pancreatic & gastric

Abbreviations: ACTH, adrenocorticotropic hormone; ADH, antidiuretic hormone; PTH, parathyroid hormone; SIADH, syndrome of inappropriate secretion of antidiuretic hormone; TGF-α, transforming growth factor-α.
[a] Most common types.

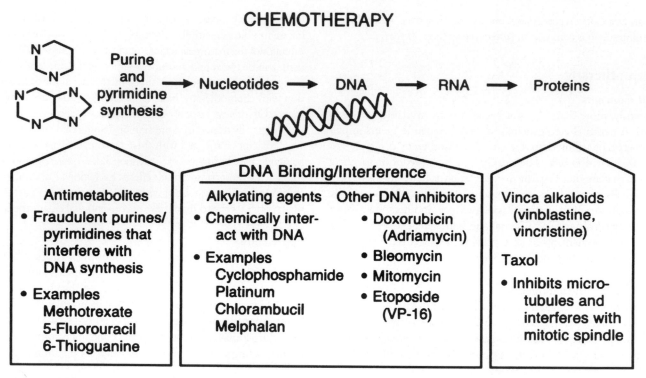

Figure 20-4. General Classes of Chemotherapeutic Agents.

can be applied. Adjuvant therapy is the use of chemotherapy when there is no known or observable residual tumor after primary treatment but there is a significant likelihood of recurrence. Many tumor types have shown benefit from an adjuvant chemotherapy approach, including breast, colon, and testicular.

Solid Tumors Sensitive to Chemotherapy
Germ cell tumors of the testis and ovary, choriocarcinomas, breast cancer, ovarian cancer, and small-cell lung cancer are sensitive to

chemotherapy. In recent years, combination chemotherapy regimens also have produced impressive tumor reductions in transitional cell carcinomas of the bladder, head and neck cancer, cervical cancer, colon cancer, and prostate cancer.

Why Chemotherapy Fails to Cure Most Advanced Solid Tumors
The reasons for failure are 1) tumor cell heterogeneity, including populations of cells resistant to cytotoxic agents; 2) large numbers of non-cycling or resting cells; and 3) pharmacologic sanctuaries—blood-tissue

Table 20-12 Biologically Targeted Therapies Currently Being Used for Cancer Treatment

Drug	Target	Drug Class	Type of Cancer Active Against
Trastuzumab	HER2/neu	Monoclonal antibody	Breast
Lapatinib	HER2/neu	Small molecule	Breast
Bevacizumab	Vascular endothelial growth factor receptor	Monoclonal antibody	Colon, lung, breast
Cetuximab	Epidermal growth factor receptor	Monoclonal antibody	Colon, head & neck
Rituximab	CD20	Monoclonal antibody	CD20-positive lymphomas
Gefitinib	Epidermal growth factor receptor	Tyrosine kinase inhibitor	Non–small cell lung
Erlotinib	Epidermal growth factor receptor	Tyrosine kinase inhibitor	Non–small cell lung, head & neck, renal cell
Suitinib	Epidermal growth factor receptor	Tyrosine kinase inhibitor	Renal cell
Temsirolimus	mTOR	Tyrosine kinase inhibitor	Renal cell

Abbreviations: HER2/neu, human epidermal growth factor receptor type 2; mTOR, mammalian target of rapamycin.

barriers and blood supply-tumor barriers. A recent concept of cancer stem cells is gaining popularity among cancer researchers.

Side Effects
The most common side effects of various chemotherapeutic agents are outlined in the Oncology Pharmacy Review.

Mechanisms of Tumor Cell Drug Resistance
Mechanisms include decreased drug uptake, increased drug efflux, decreased drug activation, increased drug inactivation, and increased production of a target enzyme.

Tumor cells may be resistant to a specific drug or they can have broad cross-resistance to structurally dissimilar drugs. This latter phenomenon is referred to as *multidrug resistance*. This seems to be mediated by a large plasma membrane glycoprotein, termed the *p-glycoprotein*, that functions as an energy-dependent drug-efflux pump.

- Tumor cells may be resistant to structurally dissimilar chemotherapy drugs (multidrug resistance).

Colony-Stimulating Factors
In recent years, bone marrow colony-stimulating factors have been isolated and are now available for clinical use. These naturally occurring glycoproteins stimulate the proliferation, differentiation, and function of specific cells in the bone marrow. They may act at the level of the earliest stem cell or at later mature functional cells. They differ in their specificity.

Granulocyte colony-stimulating factor (G-CSF), for example, acts fairly specifically to stimulate production of mature neutrophils; granulocyte-macrophage CSF (GM-CSF) acts more generally, stimulating several cell lineages, including monocytes, eosinophils, and neutrophils. Both CSFs have been used to stimulate leukocyte recovery after chemotherapy-induced myelosuppression. As a general rule, CSFs do not affect the depth of the leukocyte nadir but shorten the duration of neutropenia. Unfortunately, no currently available CSF reliably protects against thrombocytopenia. To be effective, use of a CSF should be initiated shortly after completion of chemotherapy (1-2 days) and delivered through the expected neutrophil nadir. Sustained release depot preparations are now available that can be administered once a week or less frequently. Once neutropenia has developed, use of growth factors does not enhance the recovery time, and they should only be used if the expected duration of neutropenia is more than 10 days to 2 weeks. Placebo-controlled studies examining the efficacy of G-CSF given at the start of a documented chemotherapy-induced neutropenia have failed to show clinical benefit in patients who are not at high risk. (See section below on febrile neutropenia.) The US Food and Drug Administration recently issued warnings about the use of G-CSF and what appears to be an increased risk of secondary leukemias. Furthermore, recent reports on the use of erythrocyte-stimulating agents such as erythropoietin (used to treat anemia associated with chemotherapy) have shown decreased tumor responsiveness to chemotherapy and increased risk of local recurrence. It is currently recommended that erythrocyte growth factors be used for as short a period as possible and only for symptomatic patients.

Oncologic Complications and Emergencies

Hypercalcemia
The most common underlying causes of hypercalcemia are malignancies and primary hyperparathyroidism. Patients with primary hyperparathyroidism have increased serum parathyroid hormone (PTH) values, but PTH is suppressed in cancer-associated hypercalcemia. Cancer-related hypercalcemia is often mediated by a PTH-related protein secreted by the tumor. This PTH-related protein can be detected with current assays. Tumors also can cause hypercalcemia by secreting other bone-resorbing substances or by enhancing conversion of 25-hydroxyvitamin D to 1,25-dihydroxyvitamin D. Local effects of osteolytic bone metastases are a relatively rare cause of hypercalcemia, but they can occur in prostate, breast, lung, or other cancers.

Effects on bone and kidney contribute to hypercalcemia. Accelerated bone resorption is due to activation of osteoclasts by various mediators, primarily the PTH-like peptide. The same factors that induce osteoclast-mediated bone resorption also stimulate renal tubular resorption of calcium. The hypercalcemic state interferes with renal resorption of sodium and water, leading to polyuria and eventual depletion of extracellular fluid volume. This reduces the glomerular filtration rate, further increasing the serum calcium level. Immobilization tips the balance toward bone resorption, worsening the hypercalcemia.

- PTH is suppressed in cancer-associated hypercalcemia.
- Malignancy-associated hypercalcemia is often mediated by PTH-related protein secreted by a tumor.
- Bone and kidney pathophysiologic effects lead to an increased calcium level.

Symptoms of hypercalcemia include gastrointestinal (anorexia, nausea, vomiting, constipation), renal (polyuria, polydipsia, dehydration), central nervous system (cognitive difficulties, apathy, somnolence, or even coma), and cardiovascular (hypertension, shortened QT interval, enhanced sensitivity to digitalis).

Cancers associated with hypercalcemia include lung (squamous cell), renal, myeloma, lymphoma, breast, and head and neck. Patients with breast cancer and those with myeloma are more likely to have bony involvement with their disease.

The magnitude of the hypercalcemia and the degree of symptoms are key considerations for the treatment of hypercalcemia. Generally, patients with a serum calcium value more than 14 mg/dL, mental status changes, or an inability to maintain adequate hydration should be hospitalized for immediate treatment. The serum calcium value should be adjusted if the serum albumin value is abnormal. The conversion formula is 0.8 mg/dL of serum total calcium for every 1 g of serum albumin more or less than 4 g/dL. If the serum albumin value is increased (as with dehydration), the total calcium value should be adjusted downward; if the serum albumin value is reduced (as in chronic illness), the total calcium value should be adjusted upward.

Patients with clinically symptomatic hypercalcemia are almost always intravascularly volume-depleted. Initial therapy therefore includes vigorous hydration with intravenously administered normal saline (200-400 mL/h). Loop diuretics are not used until *after* intravascular volume expansion has been completed. Furosemide facilitates urinary excretion of calcium by inhibiting calcium resorption in the thick ascending loop of Henle. A loop diuretic will help correct for volume overload once the patient has been rehydrated.

Bisphosphonates (pamidronate or zoledronic acid) are given intravenously (gastrointestinal absorption is poor). They bind to hydroxyapatite and inhibit osteoclasts. In addition to fluids, bisphosphonates have become the mainstay of treatment for hypercalcemia.

Gallium nitrate (200 mg/m^2 per day) is a highly effective inhibitor of bone resorption. It is administered as a continuous intravenous infusion for 5 days (unless normocalcemia is achieved earlier). Renal impairment limits its usefulness.

Mithramycin (25 mcg/kg) is given intravenously over 4 hours; this treatment can be repeated if necessary. Maximal hypocalcemic effect is reached at 48 to 72 hours. It is associated with hepatic and renal side effects and thrombocytopenia.

Glucocorticoids have an antitumor effect on neoplastic lymphoid tissue and are particularly useful in hypercalcemia associated with myeloma.

Calcitonin is given subcutaneously or intramuscularly. It has a rapid onset of action; thus, it is useful in immediate life-threatening situations. Calcitonin is a relatively weak agent with short-lived effect. Allergic reactions to salmon calcitonin are unusual, but an initial skin test with 1 unit is recommended before a full dose is given.

- Volume expansion *must* precede administration of furosemide.
- Furosemide inhibits calcium resorption in the thick ascending loop of Henle.
- Bisphosphonates bind to hydroxyapatite and inhibit osteoclasts.
- Mithramycin has hepatic and renal side effects.
- Calcitonin is a relatively weak agent with a rapid, short-lived effect.

Tumor Lysis Syndrome

This syndrome occurs as a result of the overwhelming release of tumor cell contents into the bloodstream such that concentrations of certain substances become life-threatening. It most commonly occurs in cancers with large tumor burdens and high proliferation rates which are exquisitely sensitive to chemotherapy. Tumor lysis syndrome can rarely occur spontaneously before antitumor therapy begins. Examples include high-grade lymphomas, leukemia, and, much less commonly, solid tumors (small cell lung cancer, anaplastic thyroid cancer, and germ cell tumors). The syndrome is characterized by an increased uric acid value, which leads to renal complications; acidosis; an increased potassium value, which can cause lethal cardiac arrhythmias; an increased phosphate value, which leads to acute renal failure; and a decreased calcium value, which causes muscle cramps, cardiac arrhythmias, and tetany. The syndrome can be prevented with adequate hydration, alkalinization, and administration of allopurinol before chemotherapy.

- Tumor lysis syndrome is a result of the overwhelming release of tumor cell contents into the bloodstream.
- It is most common in cancers with large tumor burdens and

high proliferation rates which are exquisitely sensitive to chemotherapy.
- It is characterized by increased uric acid, increased potassium, increased phosphate, acidosis, and decreased calcium.

Febrile Neutropenia

This is defined as a temperature of 38.5°C or more on 1 occasion or 3 episodes of 38°C or more plus an absolute neutrophil count of 500 × 10^9/L or less (or a total leukocyte count of 1,000 × 10^9/L or less). The risk of neutropenia is dependent on the type and dose of chemotherapy administered. Patients usually have no infection documented, but appropriate specimens for culture should be rapidly obtained before antibiotics are given. Until recently, management generally involved hospitalization and institution of parenteral broad-spectrum antibiotics. Recent extensive clinical experience and multiple randomized clinical trials have shown the safety and efficacy of outpatient therapy for select patients with febrile neutropenia. All patients need to be evaluated by a physician for both medical and social contraindications to outpatient treatment (Table 20-13). Patients who have no contraindication to outpatient treatment should be treated with oral amoxicillin/clavulanate (Augmentin) 875 mg twice daily and oral ciprofloxacin 500 mg every 8 hours. All patients should be reevaluated within 24 hours either by telephone contact or in person. Multiple randomized, placebo-controlled clinical trials have shown that the use of CSF at the time of febrile neutropenia is not indicated.

- Not all patients with febrile neutropenia need to be admitted to the hospital.
- Growth factors should not be used once neutropenia has developed.
- Growth factors may prevent the development of febrile neutropenia, but they must be used immediately after the chemotherapy.

Spinal Cord Compression

Acute cord compression is a neurologic emergency. It results most commonly from epidural extension of vertebral body metastases. The most common tumors include lung, breast, prostate, myeloma, and kidney. Occasionally, compression can occur from neighboring nodal involvement and tumor infiltration through intervertebral foramina (eg, lymphoma, sarcomas, lung cancer). The locations are cervical in 10% of cases, thoracic in 70%, and lumbar in 20%. Multiple noncontiguous levels are involved in 10% to 40%. The most important prognostic factor in preserving neurologic function is early diagnosis, before neurologic deficits have developed.

More than 90% of patients present with pain. Cervical pain may radiate down the arm. Thoracic pain radiates around the rib cage or abdominal wall; it may be described as a compressing band bilaterally around the chest or abdomen. Lumbar pain may radiate into the groin or down the leg. Pain may be aggravated by coughing, sneezing, or straight-leg raising. Focal neurologic signs depend on the level affected. Paresthesias (tingling, numbness), weakness, and altered reflexes also can be present (Table 20-14). Tenderness over the spine may help localize the level, but absence does not exclude the possibility of cord involvement. Autonomic changes of urinary or fecal retention or incontinence are very concerning and may predict for development of motor function loss in the near future.

Table 20-13 Medical and Social Contraindications to Outpatient Treatment of Febrile Neutropenia

Medical contraindications
    Anticipated duration of neutropenia of >7 days (typically patients with leukemia or lymphoma)
    Absolute neutrophil count $<100/10^9 \times L$
    Comorbid medical conditions
        Hypertension (systolic blood pressure <90 mm Hg)
        Hypoxia or tachypnea (respiratory rate >30 breaths/min)
        Altered mental status
        Renal insufficiency (creatinine >2.5 mg/dL)
        Hyponatremia (sodium <124 mg/dL)
        Bleeding
        Dehydration
        Poor oral intake
Social contraindications
    History of noncompliance or being unreliable with prior medical therapy follow-up
    Geographically remote (>30 miles from 24-hour emergency medical care)
    Unable to care for self & lack of reliable caregiver
    No telephone
    No transportation

Imaging studies include bone scanning or plain radiography, which reveal vertebral metastases in approximately 85% of patients with epidural compression. Magnetic resonance imaging of the entire spine is generally recommended. Computed tomographic myelography can be used in patients who cannot undergo magnetic resonance imaging.

Treatment usually includes an initial bolus of 10 to 100 mg of dexamethasone intravenously, depending on the severity of block. Thereafter, dexamethasone is given (4 mg 4 times daily), although some physicians favor higher doses for a few days followed by a rapid taper. Radiation therapy is applied to the involved area(s). Surgical resection and stabilization may lead to an increased chance at neurologic recovery in select patients who present with weakness or paralysis or in patients who present with no prior cancer diagnosis (Table 20-15). Patients with extensive organ involvement, progressive malignancies, or poor performance status are unlikely to be able to tolerate an extensive operative procedure and should be treated more conservatively.

- Early diagnosis of spinal cord compression, before development of neurologic deficit, improves outcome.
- Surgical therapy is indicated for select patients with neurologic deficit and spinal cord compression.

Palliative Care

Cancer Pain
More than 70% of patients with cancer have significant pain during the course of their disease. Multiple studies have shown that patients with cancer-related pain are not given adequate analgesic therapy. Barriers to optimal management of cancer pain include inadequate pain assessment by health care professionals, physician reluctance and inadequate knowledge of how to prescribe opioids, and patient reluctance to take opioids. Physician reluctance to prescribe opioids stems from concern about addiction, lack of familiarity with the agents, problems with management of side effects of opioids, and legal or regulatory concerns. Psychological addiction to opioids in cancer patients is very rare, occurring in less than 1% of patients.

Evaluation
Evaluation should include 1) a history regarding onset, quality, severity, and location of pain; exacerbating and relieving factors; and associated symptoms and 2) physical examination, which should include a complete neurologic examination. Diagnostic studies are determined by the results of the history and physical examination. Administration of analgesia should not be delayed while awaiting diagnostic studies or other tests.

Treatment

Three-Tiered Approach
Step 1: For mild pain, administer acetaminophen or a nonsteroidal anti-inflammatory drug around the clock. Studies of nonsteroidal anti-inflammatory drugs for cancer pain have shown that these agents are 1.5 to 2 times more effective than placebo.

Step 2: When step 1 fails to provide adequate analgesia, or for moderate pain, add codeine or oxycodone.

Step 3: For severe pain or inadequate pain relief with steps 1 and 2, agents include a strong opioid such as morphine, hydromorphone, oxycodone, methadone, and fentanyl (see the Oncology Pharmacy Review).

Table 20-14 Reflexes and Their Corresponding Roots and Muscles

Reflex	Root(s)	Muscle
Biceps	C5-6	Biceps
Triceps	C7-8	Triceps
Knee jerk	L2-4	Quadriceps
Ankle jerk	S1	Gastrocnemius

Table 20-15 Outcome of Patients With Spinal Cord Compression, by Neurologic Status

Status at Presentation	% Ambulatory After Radiation
Ambulatory	>80
Paraparetic	<50
Paraplegic	<10

General Principles

For most cancer pain, opioids are the main treatment approach. Mild to moderate pain (4-7 on a scale of 1-10) can often be effectively treated with oral medications. Severe pain (>7/10) should be treated with intravenous medications because they allow for much more rapid titration of dose and more prompt pain relief. If an intravenous access is not available, subcutaneous administration usually works well as long as the patient is reasonably well hydrated. Intramuscular administration is strongly discouraged because it is painful and absorption of drug is very erratic. Treatment should always begin with immediate-release oral or parenteral administration until the opioid requirements and effective dose for the individual patient are determined. Once the opioid dose required to relieve the pain is known, then a long-acting form should be added.

Dose of opioid used to treat pain is highly dependent on whether the patient is already using opioids, because many cancer patients do. Patients who are opioid-naïve should be treated with 5 to 15 mg of oral, immediate-release morphine, which is equianalgesic to 2 to 5 mg given intravenously. Other opioids are equally effective when compared with morphine. Equianalgesic tablets are readily available and should be used to calculate an equivalent dose. For patients already taking opioids, the total amount of opioids taken in the preceding 24 hours should be calculated. An immediate-release form of opioid equivalent to 10% to 20% of the 24-hour total dose should be administered as initial dose to try to relieve pain. Doses will then need to be adjusted to achieve adequate analgesia. Before adjusting the dose, one must wait until the time to peak effect has passed. For immediate-release oral agents, this is typically 1 hour, for intravenous agents, 6 to 10 minutes, and for subcutaneous agents, 20 to 30 minutes. Shortly after the time to peak effect, the patient should be reevaluated. If pain has decreased substantially, the same dose may be repeated on an as-needed basis, and the duration of the effect would be expected to be 3 to 4 hours for most immediate-release forms. If the pain has decreased only a small amount, then the same dose should be repeated and the patient reassessed after time to peak effect. If the pain has not changed at all, the next dose should be increased by 50% to 100% and the patient again reevaluated shortly after the time to peak effect has passed. Using such an algorithm has been shown to allow for rapid control of pain with minimal risk of adverse events (Figures 20-5 and 20-6).

There is no standard dosage. The dose must be increased until analgesia is achieved or side effects occur. Because the source of the pain is unlikely to be soon eliminated, scheduled, around-the-clock dosing is necessary. Once the effective dose is determined, then sustained-release or continuous-infusion intravenous opioid should be given. When the algorithms are followed, the last dose given that resulted in substantial diminishment of pain should be used. This is considered the effective 4-hour dose because the duration of analgesia (not to be confused with time to peak effect) would be expected to be 3 to 4 hours for both immediate-release oral and intravenous administration. The effective 4-hour dose should be used to calculate the 24-hour equivalent. This can then be given as either a continuous infusion intravenously or as a sustained-release oral form. An immediate-release form of an opioid should continue to be made available to the patient for unexpected exacerbations of pain. This "breakthrough" dose is calculated by using 10% to 20% of the total daily dose of opioid being given. Appropriate equianalgesic conversions should be made when changing the route or drug. Patients who require 4 or more breakthrough doses in a 24-hour period should have their long-acting opioid dose adjusted. Each time the 24-hour dose is adjusted, the breakthrough dose should likewise be adjusted by using 10% to 20% of the 24-hour total.

Adverse effects of opioids include sedation, nausea, constipation, respiratory depression, and myoclonus. Tolerance to opioid-induced sedation and nausea usually develops within a few days. For opioid-induced constipation, docusate sodium and senna should be used. Respiratory depression typically follows sedation; if a patient is excessively somnolent and has a very low respiratory rate, doses should be held. No narcotic is more or less likely to result in a particular side-effect profile. However, 1 narcotic may produce an adverse effect in a patient whereas another will not. Thus, sequential trials of different opioids may be needed to determine the 1 best suited for a patient. The fentanyl patch (a transdermal formulation) delivers drug continuously over 72 hours. It is especially useful for patients with poor tolerance of orally administered opioids or those unable to take medications orally. Because subcutaneous fat is required for absorption of the drug, this may not be a good choice in patients with severe cachexia. Likewise, patients who are severely dehydrated will not have adequate skin perfusion to absorb the drug.

- Pain is common in patients with cancer and is often undertreated.
- The appropriate opioid dose for any 1 patient is that which relieves pain without excessive side effects.
- Acute pain exacerbations should be treated with immediate release or parenteral opioids until the effective dose is determined.
- Once the effective opioid dose is known, scheduled, long-acting opioids should be given along with as-needed immediate-release opioids for breakthrough pain.
- Early referral to palliative care or hospice can improve quality of life.

Other Symptoms

Patients with cancer face numerous other symptoms and challenges as they progress through the course of their illness. Dyspnea, nausea, fatigue, weight loss, depression, difficulty concentrating or thinking, and sexual dysfunction are all common. Careful attention to symptoms and anticipation of expected symptoms can help alleviate many of these. Early referral to palliative care or hospice specialists can greatly enhance the patient's quality of life. Delineation of the patient's goals for care and development of advanced directives can allow the patient to remain in control and avoid unnecessary, painful, and, at times, harmful procedures.

Acknowledgment

The author gratefully acknowledges Lynn Hartmann, MD, and Scott Okuno, MD, for their extensive work on this chapter in previous editions and Julian Molina, MD, Axel Grothey, MD, and Thor Halfdanarson, MD, for their thoughtful comments and edits to the current edition.

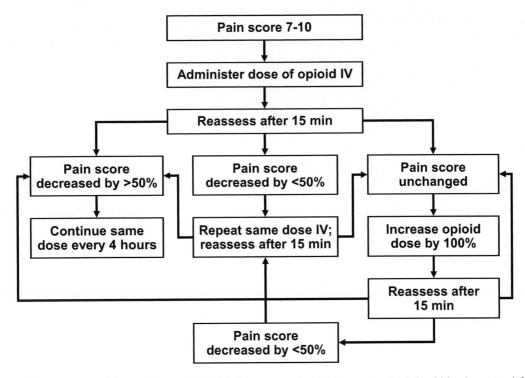

Figure 20-5. Algorithm for Treatment of Severe Cancer Pain With Intravenous Opioid. Dose of opioid should be determined from patient's status regarding pain and prior use of opioids. IV indicates intravenously.

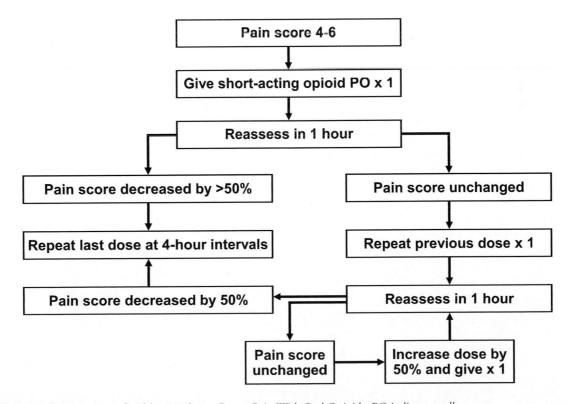

Figure 20-6. Algorithm for Treatment of Mild to Moderate Cancer Pain With Oral Opioids. PO indicates orally.

Oncology Pharmacy Review—Part I: General Classes of Agents
Scott E. Apelgren, MS, RPh

A. Alkylating Agents

Drug	Toxic/Adverse Effects	Comments
Carboplatin	Myelosuppression (especially thrombocytopenia)	Commonly dosed with the Calvert formula
Carmustine	Myelosuppression (delayed) Renal dysfunction Pulmonary fibrosis	Crosses blood-brain barrier Pain with infusion
Cisplatin	Nephrotoxicity Peripheral neuropathy Ototoxicity Anemia	Magnesium or potassium wasting is common Dose adjustment is needed for renal insufficiency Minimize concomitant nephrotoxins
Cyclophosphamide	Myelosuppression Hemorrhagic cystitis SIADH (high dose) Cardiomyopathy (high dose)	
Dacarbazine	Myelosuppression Flu-like symptoms Photosensitivity	Pain with infusion
Ifosfamide	Myelosuppression Hemorrhagic cystitis CNS toxicity	Mesna is used to prevent hemorrhagic cystitis Lethargy, confusion, seizures
Mechlorethamine	Myelosuppression Thrombosis Thrombophlebitis Vomiting	Nitrogen mustard
Oxaliplatin	Peripheral neuropathy Hypersensitivity Myelosuppression Diarrhea	Acute, transient, cold-exacerbated dysesthesia or delayed-onset, cumulative paresthesias
Streptozocin	Nephrotoxicity	Dose adjustment is needed for renal insufficiency Vesicant
Temozolomide	Myelosuppression Lethargy Ataxia Increased LFTs	

Abbreviations: CNS, central nervous system; LFTs, liver function test results; SIADH, syndrome of inappropriate secretion of antidiuretic hormone.

Oncology Pharmacy Review—Part I (continued)

B. Antimetabolites

Drug	Toxic/Adverse Effects	Comments
Capecitabine	Hand-foot syndrome Diarrhea Mucositis Fatigue	Oral prodrug of 5-fluorouracil Dose adjustment is needed for renal insufficiency Contraindicated in severe renal impairment

Fluorouracil	Diarrhea
	Mucositis
	Myelosuppression
	Ocular irritation
	Skin toxicity
	Myocardial ischemia
		Toxicity profile is dependent on administration
		  schedule
		  • Bolus—myelosuppression
		  • Continuous infusion—GI toxicity
		Leucovorin is concomitantly used to enhance
		  enzyme inhibition

Gemcitabine	Myelosuppression (especially thrombocytopenia) Increased LFTs Peripheral edema Flu-like symptoms Rash Anal pruritus Hemolytic uremic syndrome	

Methotrexate	Myelosuppression
	Mucositis
	Nephrotoxicity (high dose)
	CNS toxicity (high dose or IT)
	Hepatotoxicity
	Pulmonary fibrosis
		Leucovorin rescue for doses >100 mg/m^2 with
		  serum level monitoring
		Urinary alkalinization for high dose
		Distributes in "third-space" fluids, leading to
		  prolonged elimination & toxicity
		Drug interactions—NSAIDs, probenecid

Abbreviations: CNS, central nervous system; GI, gastrointestinal; IT, intrathecal; LFTs, liver function test results; NSAIDs, nonsteroidal anti-inflammatory drugs.

Oncology Pharmacy Review—Part I (continued)

C. Plant Derivatives

Drug	Toxic/Adverse Effects	Comments
Vincristine	Neurotoxicity (peripheral, autonomic, cranial) SIADH	Dose reduction for biliary dysfunction Vesicant
Vinblastine	Myelosuppression Neuromuscular (myalgias)	Dose reduction for biliary dysfunction Vesicant
Etoposide	Myelosuppression Alopecia Mucositis (high dose) Hypotension Secondary leukemia	Renal & hepatic elimination
Paclitaxel	Myelosuppression Peripheral neuropathy Alopecia Hypersensitivity Myalgias Bradycardia	Vesicant Dose adjustment for liver dysfunction Premedicate with dexamethasone & antihistamine (H1 & H2) Drug interaction (administer before cisplatin)
Docetaxel	Myelosuppression Fluid retention Peripheral neuropathy Skin reactions Hand-foot syndrome Hypersensitivity	Dose adjustment is needed for liver dysfunction Prevent fluid retention with dexamethasone 4 mg twice daily for 5 days (begin 1 day before docetaxel)
Irinotecan	Diarrhea (acute & delayed) Myelosuppression Abdominal cramping/pain	Dose adjustment is needed for liver dysfunction Loperamide ($\leq$24 mg/day) is used for delayed diarrhea
Topotecan	Myelosuppression Alopecia Mucositis (high dose)	Dose adjustment is needed for renal insufficiency

Abbreviation: SIADH, syndrome of inappropriate secretion of antidiuretic hormone.

Oncology Pharmacy Review—Part I (continued)

D. Antitumor Antibiotics

Drug	Toxic/Adverse Effects	Comments
Bleomycin	Pulmonary fibrosis (chronic) (>400 units) Febrile reaction Hyperpigmentation Mucositis	Dose adjustment is needed for severe renal insufficiency
Doxorubicin	Myelosuppression Cardiomyopathy (chronic) (>550 mg/m^2) Mucositis Alopecia Red-orange urine Secondary leukemia	Dose reduction is needed for biliary dysfunction Dexrazoxane may be used as cardioprotectant Vesicant Venous flare reaction on injection Radiation recall
Epirubicin	Myelosuppression Cardiomyopathy Mucositis Red-orange urine	Vesicant
Mitomycin	Myelosuppression (delayed) Blue-green urine Hemolytic uremic syndrome Pulmonary toxicity	Vesicant
Mitoxantrone	Myelosuppression Blue-green urine Cardiomyopathy	Vesicant

Oncology Pharmacy Review—Part I (continued)

E. Immunotherapy

Drug	Toxic/Adverse Effects	Comments
Aldesleukin (IL-2)	Capillary leak syndrome (fever, fluid retention, respiratory distress, hypotension) Myelosuppression Erythema	Concurrent corticosteroids may limit efficacy
Human papillomavirus vaccine	Injection site reactions (pain, swelling, erythema, pruritus), fever	Lifelong immunity without booster to be determined
Interferon-α	Flulike symptoms Fatigue Myelosuppression Increased LFTs	

Abbreviations: IL, interleukin; LFTs, liver function test results.

F. Targeted Therapy

Drug	Toxic/Adverse Effects	Comments
Bevacizumab	Bleeding Wound healing complications	Recombinant monoclonal antibody that inhibits vascular endothelial growth factor
Cetuximab (IMC-225)	Folliculitis	Monoclonal antibody against epidermal growth factor
Gefitinib	Diarrhea Rash (acne) Interstitial lung disease Ocular irritation	Inhibits the epidermal growth factor receptor tyrosine kinase
Panitumumab	Erythema, acneiform dermatitis, paronychia, pruritus, exfoliation, hypomagnesemia, fatigue, abdominal pain, nausea, diarrhea, constipation	Epidermal growth factor receptor inhibitor
Sorafenib	Diarrhea, fatigue, rash, hand-foot syndrome, hypophosphatemia, neutropenia, hypertension, increased serum amylase & lipase (but pancreatitis is rare), hemorrhagic complications	Dermatologic effects occur in about 40% of patients & may require dose adjustment
Sunitinib	Diarrhea, nausea, vomiting, anorexia, mucositis/stomatitis, bleeding events, neutropenia, hypertension, decreased left ejection fraction, hand-foot syndrome	Metabolized by CYP3A4, & drug interactions are possible
Trastuzumab	Fever Chills or rigors Cardiac dysfunction Diarrhea	Cardiac dysfunction most common when used in combination with doxorubicin

Abbreviation: CYP, cytochrome P450.

Oncology Pharmacy Review—Part I (continued)

G. Endocrine Therapy

Drug	Toxic/Adverse Effects	Comments
Tamoxifen	Hot flashes Vaginal dryness Endometrial cancer Thromboembolism	Antiestrogen
Anastrozole Letrozole Exemestane	Nausea (mild) Peripheral edema Diarrhea Asthenia Hot flashes	Aromatase inhibitors
Megestrol	Fluid retention Weight gain Thromboembolism	Progestin
Leuprolide Goserelin	Decreased libido Impotence Hot flashes Tumor flarc	LHRH agonists
Flutamide Bicalutamide Nilutamide	Gynecomastia Diarrhea Increased LFTs Impaired adaptation to dark (nilutamide) Pulmonary fibrosis (nilutamide)	Antiandrogens

Abbreviations: LFTs, liver function test results; LHRH, luteinizing hormone-releasing hormone.

H. Emetogenic Potential of Select Oncology Agents

High (Level 5)	Moderately High (Level 4)	Moderate (Level 3)	Mild (Level 2)	Low (Level 1)
Cisplatin	Carboplatin	Ifosfamide	Fluorouracil	Temozolomide
Carmustine	Cyclophosphamide	Gemcitabine	Methotrexate	Capecitabine
Mechlorethamine	Methotrexate[a]	Irinotecan	Etoposide	Vincristine
Dacarbazine	Doxorubicin	Epirubicin	Paclitaxel	Vinblastine
Streptozocin		Mitoxantrone	Docetaxel	Bleomycin
		Mitomycin	Topotecan	

[a] High-dose.

Oncology Pharmacy Review—Part II: Analgesics
Heidi D. Gunderson, PharmD, Robert C. Wolf, PharmD

A. Dosage Information: Common Opioid Agonists

Agonist	Dosage Form	Onset, min	Duration, h	Approximate Equianalgesic Dose, mg	
				Parenteral	Oral
Morphine	Tablet/capsule	15-60	4-12	10	30
	Solution	15-30	4-6		
	Suppository	30-60	4-6		
	Injection	IV: <5	4-6		
Oxycodone	Tablet/capsule	15-60	4-12	NA	20
	Solution	15-30	4-6		
Fentanyl	Transdermal patch	12 h	48-72	0.1	Patch: ~17 mcg/h
	Transmucosal lozenge	5-15	1-2		
	Injection	IV: <5	1-2		
Hydromorphone	Tablet	15-30	4-6	1.5	7.5
	Solution	15-30	4-6		
	Suppository	30-60	4-6		
	Injection	IV: <5	4-6		
Methadone	Tablet	30-60	4-12	a	a
	Solution	30-60	4-12		
	Injection	IV: <5	4-6		
Codeine	Tablet	30-60	4-6	120	200
	Solution	30-60	4-6		
	Injection	IM: 10-30	4-6		
Hydrocodone	Tablet/capsule	60	4-6	NA	30
	Solution	60	4-6		
Meperidine	Tablet	15-45	2-4	75	300
	Solution	15-45	2-4		
	Injection	IV: <5	2-4		

Abbreviations: IM, intramuscular; IV, intravenous; NA, not available.

[a] Equivalence ratios to methadone are dose-dependent. This ratio may range from 1:1 at low doses of oral morphine to as high as 20:1 for patients receiving oral morphine in excess of 300 mg daily. Methadone therapy should be started at lower doses and titrated up with adequate medication for breakthrough pain.

Oncology Pharmacy Review—Part II (continued)

B. Dosage Information: Common Nonopioid Analgesics

Analgesic	Dosage Form	Onset, min	Duration, h	Maximal Dose, mg/day
Miscellaneous				
Acetaminophen	Tablet	10-30	4-6	4,000
	Solution			
	Suppository			
Aspirin	Tablet	30	4-6	4,000
	Suppository			
Tramadol	Tablet	30-60	6-8	400
Nonsteroidal anti-inflammatory drugs				
Ibuprofen	Tablet	30	4-6	3,600
	Suspension			
Naproxen	Tablet	60	6-12	1,000
	Suspension			
Ketorolac	Tablet	30	4-6	40
	Injection	IV: 10	IV: 6	IV: 60-120
Cyclooxygenase-2 inhibitor				
Celecoxib	Capsule	45-60	8-12	400
Adjuvant analgesics				
Gabapentin	Tablet/capsule/solution	1-5 days	6-8	3,600
Pregabalin	Capsule	1-7 days	8-12	600
Amitriptyline	Tablet	3-14 days	12-24	200
Carbamazepine	Tablet	3-14 days	8-12	1,200
	Suspension			

Abbreviation: IV, intravenous.

Oncology Pharmacy Review—Part II (continued)

C. Effects and Other Considerations for Common Opioid Agonists and Nonopioid Analgesics

Drug	Toxic/Adverse Effects	Comments
Common opioid agonists		
Morphine	Sedation Respiratory depression	Morphine: orthostatic hypotension, use cautiously with hemodynamic instability; pruritus not uncommon (histamine-mediated)
Oxycodone	Nausea/vomiting Pruritus	Oxycodone: available orally only; often used in combination with a nonopioid analgesic. Cumulative dose of the nonopioid analgesic generally limits the ability to increase doses
Fentanyl	Euphoria	Fentanyl: delayed onset with the transdermal patch
Hydromorphone	Constipation Delirium	Hydromorphone: relatively short-acting; use in renal failure is safe because there are no active metabolites
Methadone	Hallucinations	Methadone: longer duration of effect with chronic use; cautious dose titration
Codeine	Dry mouth	Codeine: ceiling effect
Hydrocodone	Urinary retention	Hydrocodone: available only as oral agent in combination with a nonopioid analgesic. Cumulative dose of the nonopioid analgesic generally limits the ability to increase doses
Meperidine	Physical dependence	Meperidine: neuroexcitatory active metabolites accumulate with renal insufficiency; *not* recommended for chronic pain states; drug-drug interaction with MAO inhibitors There are many combination products that contain both an opioid agonist & nonopioid analgesic. The cumulative dose of the nonopioid analgesic generally limits the ability to increase doses
Common nonopioid analgesics		
Miscellaneous analgesics		
Acetaminophen	Hepatic dysfunction with higher doses or chronic use Renal tubular necrosis	Higher doses inhibit warfarin metabolism, which may prolong the INR
Aspirin	GI ulceration, inhibits platelet aggregation, renal insufficiency, tinnitus	
Tramadol	Dizziness, sedation, constipation, nausea or vomiting	Higher doses increase seizure potential
Nonsteroidal anti-inflammatory drugs/cyclooxygenase-2 inhibitors		
Ibuprofen	Dyspepsia	Class: use cautiously with other nephrotoxic agents
Naproxen	GI ulceration	
Ketorolac	Salt & water retention	Ketorolac: maximal duration of use is 5 days because of risk of GI or renal side effects
Celecoxib	Renal insufficiency Inhibition of platelet aggregation	Celecoxib has fewer GI side effects & does not inhibit platelet aggregation Increased risk of myocardial infarction/stroke (rofecoxib & valdecoxib were withdrawn from market)

Oncology Pharmacy Review—Part II (continued)

C. Effects and Other Considerations for Common Opioid Agonists and Nonopioid Analgesics (continued)

Drug	Toxic/Adverse Effects	Comments
Common opioid agonists (continued)		
Adjuvant analgesics		
Gabapentin	Sedation Dizziness Fatigue	Dose reduction is necessary with renal insufficiency Initiate at bedtime & titrate to effective dose (usually divided throughout day) Do not abruptly discontinue; taper over at least 1 wk
Pregabalin	Dizziness, sedation, blurred vision, tremor, peripheral edema	Dosage reduction is necessary with renal insufficiency Initiate at bedtime & titrate to effective dose (usually divided throughout day) Do not abruptly discontinue; taper over at least 1 wk
Amitriptyline	Sedation, dizziness, dry mouth, confusion, constipation, blurred vision, urinary retention, orthostatic hypotension	Administer at bedtime Other tricyclic antidepressants are also effective
Carbamazepine	Dizziness, sedation, nausea or vomiting, mild leukopenia, agranulocytosis (rare)	Erythromycin, clarithromycin, & propoxyphene inhibit carbamazepine metabolism

Abbreviations: GI, gastrointestinal; INR, international normalized ratio; MAO, monoamine oxidase.

Questions

Multiple Choice (choose the best answer)

1. A 35-year-old woman presents to you with questions about breast cancer screening. Her menses began at age 12 years; she is gravida 3, para 3; her first pregnancy was at age 22 years, she breastfed all of her children for 1 year; and she never took birth control pills or hormonal replacement therapy. She is concerned because her mother had breast cancer at age 35 years, her maternal aunt had ovarian cancer at age 40 years, and her grandmother died of breast cancer at age 48 years. At this time you should:

   a. Begin annual mammography and magnetic resonance imaging of both breasts and consider genetic testing to help determine her lifetime risk of breast and ovarian cancer.
   b. Defer screening mammography until age 50 years.
   c. Prescribe tamoxifen as a preventive agent.
   d. Recommend bilateral prophylactic mastectomies and oophorectomies.
   e. Perform screening colonoscopy.

2. An 82-year-old man is seen in your office for routine follow-up care. He has a prior history of chronic obstructive pulmonary disease, forced expiratory volume in the first second of expiration 25% of predicted, coronary artery disease with mild congestive heart failure, hypertension, and adult-onset diabetes. On rectal examination, the prostate is enlarged with a firm nodule. He denies any urinary symptoms. The prostate-specific antigen level is 8.5 ng/mL, and transrectal needle biopsy shows Gleason grade 6 adenocarcinoma. Bone scanning shows only some changes consistent with degenerative disease. At this time you can tell the patient that:

   a. Radical prostatectomy is likely to improve his overall survival and decrease his chance of death from prostate cancer.
   b. Given his lack of symptoms from prostate cancer and his comorbid conditions, a watchful waiting approach is reasonable.
   c. External beam radiation therapy is not effective against prostate cancer.
   d. Chemotherapy can be used to decrease his risk of recurrence of prostate cancer.
   e. Orchiectomy is the standard of care.

3. A healthy 42-year-old female executive presents to your office for a preemployment physical examination. She has no significant past medical illnesses and does not smoke or use any medications. She is in a stable, healthy marriage and she has 2 children, ages 18 and 20 years. She has not seen a physician for many years. Her family history is remarkable for an older brother having had colon cancer at age 50 years; he had resection and is doing well without evidence of recurrence 6 years later. There is no other significant family history. Routine cancer screening tests you would recommend for her at this time include:

   a. Chest radiography, mammography, and pelvic examination and Papanicolaou test
   b. Mammography, pelvic examination and Papanicolaou test, ovarian ultrasonography, and determination of the serum cancer antigen 125 level
   c. Clinical breast examination, mammography, pelvic examination and Papanicolaou test, digital rectal examination and fecal occult blood test, and colonoscopy
   d. Breast MRI, mammography, pelvic examination and Papanicolaou test
   e. Chest radiography, mammography and breast ultrasonography, pelvic examination and Papanicolaou test and pelvic ultrasonography, and colonoscopy

4. Risk factors for the development of colon cancer include:

   a. Prior history of polyps
   b. Family history of colon cancer
   c. Personal history of ulcerative colitis
   d. Age
   e. All of the above

5. A 67-year-old man with a history of stage II rectal cancer was treated with resection and combined chemotherapy and radiation 6 years ago. He has recovered well from the operations and treatments but still has some rectal and bladder urgency but no incontinence. He is concerned about late side effects of his prior therapy, specifically development of new cancers. You should tell him:

   a. He is at increased risk of secondary cancers of the bladder, prostate, and rectum, but the risk of this is only about 1 in 70 at 10 years.
   b. There is no need to worry because there is no increased risk for secondary malignancies in this setting.
   c. He is at high risk for lung cancer, so he should have routine screening chest radiography.
   d. He is right to worry because secondary cancers are very common in this setting, and he should have screening at regular intervals.
   e. There is no reason to screen for prostate cancer any longer because he has had radiation to this area.

6. A 74-year-old man presents to you with diffuse, severe bony pains. He has otherwise been healthy and has not seen a physician in many years. He takes no medications, and his past history is remarkable for an appendectomy in his 20s and some moderate alcohol use. Other than pain, his review of systems is noncontributory. Examination shows an elderly man who is obviously in pain. Neurologic examination is benign. There is

diffuse bony tenderness to spine, ribs, and multiple other bones. On rectal examination, the prostate is rock hard and nodular. Serum prostate-specific antigen level is 250 ng/mL, and bone scan shows the presence of diffuse metastases throughout the skeleton. Treatment options at this time include:

a. Systemic chemotherapy
b. Nonsteroidal anti-inflammatory agents and a luteinizing hormone-releasing hormone (LHRH) antagonist
c. LHRH antagonists alone
d. Strong, immediate-release opioids for the pain, titrated to pain relief, in combination with an anti-androgen before beginning therapy with an LHRH antagonist
e. Fentanyl patch for the pain and an orchiectomy

7. A 75-year-old man presents to you with a 6-month history of cough, anorexia, weight loss, and generalized decline in performance status. He has a prior history of adult-onset diabetes controlled with oral agents and diet, mild hypertension controlled with a thiazide diuretic, and a distant history of traumatic fracture of his humerus. He is a lifetime nonsmoker, worked as an attorney, has been married for 40 years, and has a family history that is not contributory. On physical examination, the man is cachectic and chronically ill. Findings include a 3-cm, hard right supraclavicular lymph node; diminished breath sounds at the right base; enlarged liver with firm, tender edge; Hemoccult-negative rectal examination; testes that are mildly atrophic but without masses; and normal prostate. Serum chemistry values show a normochromic-normocytic anemia, normal leukocyte count, and increased platelet count (350 × 10^9/L). The prostate-specific antigen level is 4.0 ng/mL, and the α-fetoprotein and β-human chorionic gonadotropin levels are normal. CT of the chest and abdomen shows diffuse pulmonary lesions; hilar, supraclavicular, and mediastinal lymphadenopathy; but no evidence of bowel obstruction. The liver has innumerable low-density lesions consistent with metastases. Biopsy of the supraclavicular lymph node shows a poorly differentiated carcinoma of uncertain primary tumor. Next steps in work-up include:

a. Positron emission tomography to look for the primary lesion
b. Colonoscopy, esophagogastroduodenoscopy, endoscopic retrograde cholangiopancreatography, and endoscopic ultrasonography to look for the primary lesion
c. Bone marrow biopsy to rule out lymphoma
d. Discussion of goals of care and referral to medical oncology
e. Molecular studies on the tumor to determine the site of origin

8. A 35-year-old woman presents to your office after noticing a nontender lump in the right breast. She has otherwise been healthy, and there is no family history of breast or any other cancer. Her history includes menarche at age 12 years; gravida 3, para 3, aborta 0; first pregnancy at age 22 years; no use of hormonal therapy of any kind; and no prior history of radiation exposure. On physical examination there is a palpable lesion

in the right breast at the 1-o'clock position that is freely mobile, firm, and 1 cm in largest diameter. Mammography shows dense breasts, no observable lesion, and no areas of abnormal microcalcifications. Next steps in the evaluation should include:

a. MRI of both breasts
b. Reassurance that normal results on mammography mean there is no problem
c. Ultrasonography of breast and palpable lesion, with biopsy if suspicious or solid
d. Genetic testing for *BRCA1* and *BRCA2*
e. Reassurance that because most breast cancer is inherited she should not be concerned

9. Factors important in the decision to use systemic adjuvant chemotherapy for breast cancer include:

a. Tumor size
b. Lymph node status
c. Hormone-receptor status of tumor
d. Age and comorbid medical conditions
e. All of the above

10. A 72-year-old woman with a 100 pack-year history of smoking presents to your office with a chronic cough and fatigue. Chest radiography shows a large, right lung mass; CT confirms the mass and also shows significant right hilar lymphadenopathy. You refer the patient to a local pulmonologist, who performs bronchoscopy and biopsy, which show a small cell carcinoma. Staging evaluation (including bone scanning and brain imaging) shows no disease outside the right hemithorax. The next step in management includes:

a. Referral to a medical oncologist and a radiation oncologist
b. Referral to a thoracic surgeon for consideration of resection
c. Bone marrow biopsy to complete staging evaluation
d. Advising the patient that there is no reason to stop smoking now that lung cancer has developed
e. Referring the patient to hospice

11. Risk factors for the development of cervical carcinoma include:

a. Early age at first intercourse
b. Number of sexual partners
c. Smoking
d. History of sexually transmitted disease
e. All of the above

12. A 26-year-old woman presents to your office after she noted a change in the size and shape of a mole on the left side of her scalp. Its diameter is 10 mm. The mole is shown here. Concerning features of this mole include:

a. Asymmetry
b. Irregular borders

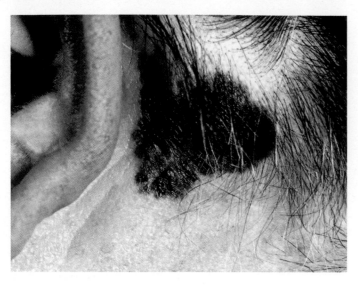

Question 12

c. Recent change in size and shape
d. Diameter of mole more than 6 mm
e. All of the above

13. A 54-year-old man presents to the emergency department with a complaint of fever to 102°F. He denies any other symptoms and maintains good oral intake. Ten days ago he received his third cycle of chemotherapy for non–small cell lung cancer, and he has been told that his cancer is responding well to this treatment. He lives with his wife and teenage son in town. On physical examination, he is a well-nourished man with total alopecia. He does not seem to be in any significant distress. Pulse is 68 beats per minute, respiratory rate is 16 breaths per minute, blood pressure is 134/85 mm Hg, and oral temperature is 102.5°F. The oropharynx is clear, lung examination is normal, and heart and abdominal examination is normal. Chest radiography shows a right lung mass that is smaller than shown on radiographs from 12 weeks ago. No infiltrates or other abnormalities are found. Results of electrolyte, liver function, and renal function tests are all normal. Results of complete blood count are hemoglobin 10.2 g/dL, platelet count 90×10^9/L, and leukocyte count 0.7 with an absolute neutrophil count of 0.2×10^9/L. Appropriate next steps in management include:

a. Reassurance and dismissal to home with close follow-up with his medical oncologist
b. Filgrastim (Neupogen) injection
c. Admission to the hospital and administration of broad-spectrum antibiotics, filgrastim, and erythropoietin
d. Blood and urine cultures, dismissal of the patient with ciprofloxacin and amoxicillin/clavulanate (Augmentin), and instructions to call his medical oncologist in the morning and to report any recurring fevers or worsening of symptoms
e. Admission for evaluation of bone marrow failure

14. A 65-year-old woman presents to your clinic with complaints of a red, swollen, and tender right breast. Her symptoms first developed 3 weeks ago, and she was given a course of antibiotics for mastitis. She denies ever having any fever or chills. Past medical history is remarkable for hypertension, hypercholesterolemia, and mild asthma. She has no prior history of any breast problems. The most recent mammogram, obtained 9 months ago, was normal. On examination, the patient is a well-nourished woman in no distress and her vital signs are unremarkable. There are no palpable lymph nodes in the supraclavicular or axillary regions. Lungs, heart, and abdominal examinations are benign. Examination of the left breast is benign. The right breast has marked erythema, edema of the skin, increased warmth, and diffuse enlargement compared with the left breast. No distinct masses are palpable. The nipple is inverted, which the patient reports is new. Appropriate next steps in the evaluation include:

a. Mammography and, if results are normal, treatment with repeat course of antibiotics
b. Mammography and, if results are normal, ultrasonography of breast; biopsy if any abnormality is found on mammography or ultrasonography. If ultrasonography does not show an abnormality, still proceed to biopsy of breast and skin
c. MRI of the breast
d. CT of chest and abdomen
e. Positron emission tomography

Answers

1. Answer a.
This woman's family history is highly suggestive of a dominant gene mutation such as *BRCA1* or *BRCA2*, and as such her risk for breast cancer is very high. In 2007, the American Cancer Society issued recommendations that women in such high risk groups be considered for MRI screening. In addition, the patient should be referred for genetic counseling and should consider breast and ovarian cancer gene testing. If the result is positive, her lifetime risk for breast or ovarian cancer may exceed 50%. Then it is reasonable to consider preventive treatments. Potential preventive treatments include prophylactic bilateral mastectomies and oophorectomies, chemoprevention with agents such as tamoxifen or raloxifene, or more frequent screening. MRI screening has been shown to detect more breast lesions, but it is not certain whether there is any survival or overall benefit, and there are certainly many false-positive results on MRI that do require further evaluation such as biopsy. In this setting, use of tamoxifen for prevention of breast cancer is highly controversial, but it should at least be discussed.

2. Answer b.
For patients older than 65 years, especially those with significant comorbid conditions, it is unclear whether radical prostatectomy improves the patient's survival, and it certainly has adverse effects on quality of life. Patients in good condition who are younger than 65 years do seem to have a survival advantage if treated with radical prostatectomy rather than watchful waiting. This elderly man with multiple other competing illnesses is unlikely to benefit from aggressive treatment. External beam radiation and brachytherapy both are reasonable treatment options, but they both do have a risk of impotence, rectal injury, and incontinence. Chemotherapy has no role outside of patients with metastatic disease. Orchiectomy or hormonal therapies are typically reserved for patients with metastatic disease.

3. Answer c.
Current American Cancer Society screening recommendations for otherwise healthy women include annual clinical breast examination and mammography beginning at age 40 years and pelvic examination and Papanicolau test for all sexually active women (can be done every 2-3 years after 3 successive annual examinations with normal results in low-risk women). In this woman, who has a first-degree relative who had colon cancer at age 50 years, current recommendations are for her to have her first colon cancer screening done at an age 10 years younger than the age at diagnosis of the affected relative. Normally, colon cancer screening is not begun until age 50 years, but the family history in this case should alter the recommendations. There is no standard role for chest radiography for screening, especially in a nonsmoker. Cancer antigen 125 is a serum marker for ovarian cancer and as yet has no role in screening, nor does routine ovarian or pelvic ultrasonography. Ultrasonography cannot currently be recommended for screening for breast cancer. Recent findings show that women who have a very high risk for breast cancer (>20% lifetime) should undergo screening MRI. These recommendations mostly include women who have an inherited gene mutation such as *BRCA1* or *BRCA2* or women who have had prior radiation to the breast region (most often for lymphoma).

4. Answer e.
The major risk factors for development of colon cancer include age; diet; prior history of polyps (adenomatous, not hyperplastic); prior history of colon, ovarian, uterine, or breast cancer; family history of colon cancer; and history of ulcerative colitis. Several familial syndromes increase the risk of colon cancer, including familial adenomatous polyposis, in which the colon is covered in thousands of polyps. Persons with this genetic defect have a virtually 100% chance for development of colon cancer by age 40 years. Hereditary nonpolyposis colon cancer (Lynch syndrome) is the other major hereditary condition that predisposes to colon cancer. Families with these syndromes have strong histories of ovarian, stomach, small bowel, pancreas, kidney, ureteral, bile duct, or bladder cancers.

5. Answer a.
Patients who have had pelvic radiation for rectal or prostate cancer are at increased risk for secondary malignancies in the area, but fortunately this risk is low (estimated to be 1 in 125 at 5 years, 1 in 70 at 10 years). Patients should still be screened for cancers for which they are at risk, as long as their general health and other medical conditions warrant screening. There is no increased risk for lung cancer per se in this patient, but lung metastases are a common type of recurrence of rectal cancer. The pattern of recurrence is different from that of colon cancer, which much more commonly metastasizes to the liver before traveling to the lung. The venous drainage of the rectum is into the inferior vena cava, whereas most of the venous drainage of the colon is to the portal system. Routine follow-up for otherwise healthy patients with colorectal cancers includes history and physical examination every 3 months for 2 years and then every 6 months for a total of 5 years; colonoscopy in 1 year, repeat colonoscopy in 1 year if results are abnormal, every 2 to 3 years if normal; carcinoembryonic antigen testing every 3 months for 2 years, then every 6 months for years 3 through 5; and chest, abdominal, and pelvic CT considered annually for 3 years if the patient is at high risk.

6. Answer d.
Systemic chemotherapy can be used to treat metastatic prostate cancer, but the toxicities are such that this is typically reserved for hormone-refractory, symptomatic disease only. Because this man has never had hormonal therapy, this would be the preferred treatment. Nonsteroidal anti-inflammatory agents are an effective analgesic, but this man is in a sufficient amount of pain that short-acting opioids should be used to control the pain while the underlying disease is treated. LHRH antagonists should never be used alone if there is symptomatic disease because an acute tumor flare often occurs when these are first used. An antiandrogen such as bicalutamide (Casodex) should be used for several weeks before the LHRH

antagonists to blunt this flare response. The fentanyl patch is a very good and effective long-acting opioid for patients with severe pain, but fentanyl should never be the first opioid used in an opioid-naive patient. Good pain management principles dictate that a short-acting opioid should be used and the doses adjusted until pain is controlled. Once opioid requirements are known, then longer-acting forms, given in a dose-equivalent manner, should be given. Orchiectomy is a reasonable first hormonal therapy for this man.

7. Answer d.

This patient has a carcinoma of unknown primary tumor with diffuse metastases and a very poor performance status. As such, his prognosis is extremely poor. Further evaluation in an attempt to define the primary lesion is unlikely to yield any information that will favorably affect the patient's course. Lymph node biopsy has confirmed that the patient has metastatic malignancy and thus positron emission tomography will add no useful information. Endoscopies to look for gastrointestinal or hepatobiliary primary lesions will not alter the outcome or treatment decisions as long as he has no signs or symptoms of bowel obstruction. If bowel obstruction is present, then palliative maneuvers would be appropriate. Because the lymph node biopsy shows a carcinoma, there is no need to consider lymphoma, and bone marrow biopsy will not be helpful. Molecular studies will not be helpful. Because the prognosis is very poor, discussions about goals of care are appropriate, as is referral to medical oncology for, at least, consideration of palliative chemotherapy or symptom management and hospice only.

8. Answer c.

Mammography is not very sensitive in young women because breast parenchyma tends to be very dense and often obscures any lesion. If mammography is suspicious in this setting, then biopsy should be done, but with normal mammographic results and a palpable mass further evaluation is still needed to exclude breast cancer. Studies released in the spring of 2007 suggested that once breast cancer is diagnosed, then MRI of the breast may be helpful to identify additional lesions in the ipsilateral or contralateral breast, but these recommendations are currently controversial. Because the patient has a palpable mass, this should first be evaluated; if invasive cancer is found, then MRI is reasonable. Given the absence of any family history, testing for the *BRCA1* or *BRCA2* gene is not recommended. The vast majority of breast cancers (90%-95%) occur in women with no significant family history. Ultrasonography should be done, and if this shows a suspicious lesion then biopsy is recommended. If ultrasonography has findings consistent with simple cyst, then close observation or aspiration is reasonable. Solid lesions on ultrasonography should be biopsied, with the possible exception of well-defined fibroadenomas, which do have a characteristic ultrasonographic appearance. If cancer is confirmed, then MRI is recommended as noted above. If ultrasonography does not show any lesion, palpable abnormalities should be either biopsied or observed very closely. MRI for further characterization is often recommended but is very controversial. Breast MRI should be performed at facilities with expertise in breast MRI and the capability of doing MRI-guided biopsies.

9. Answer e.

Postoperative adjuvant systemic therapy for breast cancer can significantly reduce the risk of recurrence and improve overall survival for many women. Treatment benefits depend in part on the risk for recurrence. In women with extremely favorable prognosis and a very low risk of recurrence, addition of a toxic therapy such as chemotherapy may add little benefit. However, for patients with a very high risk of recurrence, systemic treatments may have a very substantial impact on the likelihood of recurrence and survival, and patients may be willing to accept toxic effects in the short term for the long-term benefit. Elderly women with significant comorbid illnesses may experience excessive toxic effects, and this factor should also be considered.

10. Answer a.

Small cell lung cancer (with very rare exceptions) is not a surgical disease. Patients with limited-stage disease, as in this case, tend to be best served with use of a combination of chemotherapy and radiation. Bone marrow biopsies are no longer done as a routine part of staging evaluation for small cell lung cancer. Several studies show that patients with cancer who stop smoking do have a better response to therapy than those who continue to smoke. Although most patients with lung cancer do die of the disease, the median survival in patients with limited-stage small cell lung cancer is 1.5 to 2 years, and thus hospice referral is premature at this time.

11. Answer e.

The majority of cervical cancers are associated with human papillomavirus (HPV) infection. Risk factors for acquiring HPV include early age at first intercourse, number of sexual partners (women who have more than 8 sexual partners in a lifetime have an 80%-90% chance of having HPV in the cervix), lower socioeconomic status, smoking, and having had other sexually transmitted diseases. HPV vaccination may dramatically alter the risk for development of cervix cancer, especially in third-world countries, in which cervical cancer is the leading cause of cancer death in women. The US Food and Drug Administration recently approved the use of a vaccine against the 4 most common strains of HPV, and current recommendations are that all healthy females receive this vaccine before the initiation of sexual intercourse. The vaccine is administered in 3 separate injections. There is some controversy over the use of this vaccine.

12. Answer e.

This mole shows all the classic "ABCD" findings: *a*symmetry, irregular *b*orders, a recent *c*hange in size or shape, and *d*iameter of more than 6 mm. This lesion is very suspicious and should be removed without delay. Prognosis in melanoma is highly dependent on the thickness of the tumor, and the earlier it is found and removed, the better the outcome.

13. Answer d.

The patient has febrile neutropenia due to his recently administered chemotherapy. The vast majority of such patients can be safely managed on an outpatient basis provided they meet all criteria for outpatient treatment. He has minimal symptoms, is clinically stable, and has no social contraindications to outpatient therapy. Once patients are neutropenic, there is no role for growth factor support unless the expected duration of neutropenia is longer than 10 to 14 days; for most chemotherapy regimens with which that is likely to happen, patients are probably already receiving growth factor support. There is no reason to suspect primary bone marrow failure because his condition is temporally correlated with his chemotherapy.

14. Answer b.

This patient is presenting with classic findings of inflammatory breast cancer. Most patients with inflammatory breast cancer (which represents <10% of all breast cancer cases) present with an inflamed appearance to the breast, and most have had treatment with a course of antibiotics for presumed mastitis without improvement. Mammography may show an abnormality; if so, it should be biopsied. If mammography does not provide useful information, then ultrasonography with biopsy of any suspicious areas should be performed. If ultrasonography does not show any areas to biopsy, obtaining a core, blind biopsy of the breast and some skin is the next step. This often shows adenocarcinoma with dermal lymphatic invasion, which is the hallmark of inflammatory breast cancer. CT of the chest and abdomen is an appropriate part of the work-up but will not help to establish the diagnosis. Positron emission tomography will not differentiate between mastitis and cancer, and tissue biopsy is necessary for the diagnosis. MRI is being studied in this setting; it is not routinely recommended at this time, but it may prove to be helpful in select cases.

21

Preventive Medicine

Prathibha Varkey, MD, MPH
Martha P. Millman, MD, MPH

Definitions

Preventive medicine is the practice of medicine that detects and alters or ameliorates host susceptibility in a premorbid state (eg, immunization), risk factors for disease in a predisease state (eg, increased cholesterol level), and disease in the presymptomatic state (eg, in situ cervical cancer). Not all disease is preventable because not all risk factors (or all individuals at risk) are known, the cost of screening everyone is not feasible, barriers to medical access exist, interval disease occurs, characteristics of the target disease vary, and screening tests and treatments are imperfect.

Primary prevention is defined as the prevention of disease occurrence (eg, immunization to prevent infection and blood pressure control to prevent stroke). *Secondary prevention* is defined as the detection and amelioration of disease in a presymptomatic or preclinical stage (eg, initiation of statin therapy after the finding of coronary calcification). *Tertiary prevention* is defined as the prevention of future negative health effects of existing clinical disease (eg, use of aspirin and β-blockers after myocardial infarction to prevent recurrence).

Efficacy refers to the potential or maximal benefit derived from applying a test or procedure under ideal circumstances (eg, research studies with compliant patients and with ideal testing conditions and techniques). *Effectiveness* refers to the actual benefit derived from a test or procedure that is applied under usual—less than ideal—circumstances. Randomized trials in which results are analyzed by the *intention-to-treat* principle (ie, all members of a group are included in the analysis whether or not they complied) give a measure of effectiveness in a population. *Cost-effectiveness* refers to the cost incurred to achieve a given level of effectiveness. It is often expressed as the dollars spent per year of life saved. Often, the most cost-effective method of testing is not the most effective. For example, performing Papanicolaou (Pap) smears every 5 or 10 years is more cost-effective, but performing them every year is more effective.

* Cost-effectiveness: cost incurred to achieve a given level of effectiveness.
* The most cost-effective test may not be the most effective test.

Years of potential life lost describes a measure of the relative effect of a disease on society. This term usually refers to the years lost because of death from a disease before age 65 years (or sometimes 70). For example, colon cancer kills approximately 56,000 men and women annually and breast cancer kills approximately 41,000 women. However, on average, breast cancer kills at a younger age and so results in nearly 3 times as many years of potential life lost.

* Years of potential life lost: the years lost because of death from a disease before age 65 years (or sometimes 70).

Quality-adjusted life-years (QALYs) is a measure of the quality of life after a health care intervention. It is the product of life expectancy and quality of the remaining life-years. After the intervention, each year in perfect health is assigned the value of 1.0 and death is assigned a value of 0. If the years after the intervention are not lived in perfect health, the life-years are given a value between 0 and 1. For example, if after an intervention, 5 additional years of life are gained, during which the quality of life was 0.60, the intervention generated 3 QALYs.

Incidence (or *incidence rate*) refers to the number of new events (deaths or diagnoses) that occur in a population in a given time (eg, 188.6 cancer deaths per 100,000 people in the United States annually). *Prevalence* refers to the number of cases of a condition existing at a point in time in a population. Prevalence rate is directly related to disease duration. For example, about 944,306 people in the United States are currently infected with the human immunodeficiency virus (HIV).

Principles of Screening for Disease

The term *mass screening* is generally applied to the relatively indiscriminate testing of a population with the intent to improve the aggregate health of the population but not necessarily of every person in the population. An example is blood pressure or cholesterol testing in a public setting such as a shopping mall.

• Mass screening: indiscriminate testing of a population to improve the aggregate health of the population.

Case finding is the technical term often used for screening that is conducted in the office setting. The intent is to detect asymptomatic disease and to improve the health of the person. In testing asymptomatic persons, it is important to bear in mind the dictum "first do no harm."

• Case finding: screening conducted in the office setting to detect asymptomatic disease and to improve the health of a person.

Lead-Time Bias
Lead time is the period between early detection and the clinical presentation of disease. The inclusion of this period could result in falsely prolonged survival periods for patients screened as compared with those not screened even when the offered treatment has no benefit. This period must be excluded when evaluating methods of screening and treatment.

Length-Time Bias
Length-time bias is due to the variable rates of progression of diseases in patients. The slow progression of a disease could make it easier to detect by screening, which may result in overrepresentation of this type of disease in screening studies.

Desirable Screening Characteristics
The following disease, test, and host characteristics are desirable for screening:
1. Disease characteristics: The diseases screened should be common, cause substantial morbidity and mortality, have a long preclinical phase (during which the disease is curable or modifiable), have an effective treatment that is available to those screened, and have an acceptable treatment (ie, one that is not excessively painful or disfiguring).
2. Test characteristics: The tests should be inexpensive, safe, acceptable, easy to administer, technically easy to perform, and highly sensitive, and they should have a complementary, highly specific confirmatory test.
3. Host characteristics: The person should be at risk, have access to testing, be likely to comply with follow-up testing, and

have adequate overall life expectancy or functional life expectancy.

Burden of Disease in the United States
Diseases that cause the most morbidity and mortality in the United States may or may not be amenable to screening or case finding. Heart disease, cancer, and strokes are the leading causes of death (Tables 21-1 through 21-3). Mortality rates (Table 21-4) due to accidents, suicide, chronic liver disease, and assault are higher among men than women. Mortality rates due to diabetes, renal disease, septicemia, hypertension, and assault are higher among blacks. Mortality due to intentional self-harm is higher in the white population. The Hispanic population has higher mortality rates from assault, liver disease, and diabetes than the non-Hispanic white population. The mortality gaps between men and women and between blacks and whites have lessened slightly over time.

Cancer Prevention

In 2001, 37% of cancer deaths in high-income countries were attributed to the joint effect of the following risk factors: smoking (29%), excess alcohol use (4%), obesity (3%), low intake of fruits and vegetables (3%), physical inactivity (2%), sexual transmission of human papillomavirus (HPV) (1%), air pollution (1%), and contaminated injections in health care settings (0.5%). Compared with the nonobese, the risk of death due to cancer is 52% higher in obese men and 62% higher in obese women. Obesity has also been associated with higher death rates related to endometrial, cervical, breast, kidney, and colon cancers and multiple myeloma.

Lung Cancer
Lung cancer is a highly lethal form of cancer (it kills most of the people it afflicts) and is the leading cause of cancer death for men and women. The burden of disease (2007 estimates from the American Cancer Society) is 213,380 new cases and 160,390 deaths. The peak incidence occurs in men and women aged 60 to 79 years. Risk factors include the following:
1. Smoking—risk is 10 times greater for a smoker than for a nonsmoker
2. Age—risk at 70 years is 10 times greater than at 40 years

Table 21-1 Leading Causes of Death in the United States, 2003

	No. of Deaths	Death Rate (per 100,000 Population)	% of Total Deaths
Heart disease	685,089	235.6	28.0
Cancer	556,902	191.5	22.7
Cerebrovascular disease	157,689	54.2	6.4
Chronic lower respiratory tract disease	126,382	43.5	5.2
Accidents (unintentional injuries)	109,277	37.6	4.5

Modified from Heron MP, Smith BL. Deaths: leading causes for 2003. National vital statistics reports; vol 55 no 10. Hyattsville, MD: National Center for Health Statistics, 2007.

Table 21-2 Ten Leading Cancer Types for the Estimated New
Cancer Cases and Deaths in US Men, 2007[a]

Site or Type of Cancer	Cases in Men	
	No.	%
Estimated new cases		
Prostate	218,890	29
Lung & bronchus	114,890	15
Colon & rectum	79,130	10
Urinary bladder	50,040	7
Non-Hodgkin lymphoma	34,200	4
Melanoma of the skin	33,910	4
Kidney & renal pelvis	31,590	4
Leukemia	24,800	3
Oral cavity & pharynx	24,180	3
Pancreas	18,830	2
Total	766,860	100
Estimated deaths		
Lung & bronchus	89,510	31
Prostate	27,050	9
Colon & rectum	26,000	9
Pancreas	16,840	6
Leukemia	12,320	4
Liver & intrahepatic bile duct	11,280	4
Esophagus	10,900	4
Urinary bladder	9,630	3
Non-Hodgkin lymphoma	9,600	3
Kidney & renal pelvis	8,080	3
Total	289,550	100

[a] Excludes basal and squamous cell skin cancers and in situ carcinomas except urinary bladder. Estimates are rounded to the nearest 10.
Modified from Jemal A, Siegel R, Ward E, Murray T, Xu J, Thun MJ, et al. Cancer statistics 2007, CA Cancer J Clin. 2007;57:43-66. Used with permission.

Table 21-3 Ten Leading Cancer Types for the Estimated New
Cancer Cases and Deaths in US Women, 2007[a]

Site or Type of Cancer	Cases in Women	
	No.	%
Estimated new cases		
Breast	178,480	26
Lung & bronchus	98,620	15
Colon & rectum	74,630	11
Uterine corpus	39,080	6
Non-Hodgkin lymphoma	28,990	4
Melanoma of the skin	26,030	4
Thyroid	25,480	4
Ovary	22,430	3
Kidney & renal pelvis	19,600	3
Leukemia	19,440	3
Total	678,060	100
Estimated deaths		
Lung & bronchus	70,880	26
Breast	40,460	15
Colon & rectum	26,180	10
Pancreas	16,530	6
Ovary	15,280	6
Leukemia	9,470	4
Non-Hodgkin lymphoma	9,060	3
Uterine corpus	7,400	3
Brain & other nervous system	5,590	2
Liver & intrahepatic bile duct	5,500	2
Total	270,100	100

[a] Excludes basal and squamous cell skin cancers and in situ carcinomas except urinary bladder. Estimates are rounded to the nearest 10.
Modified from Jemal A, Siegel R, Ward E, Murray T, Xu J, Thun MJ, et al. Cancer statistics 2007, CA Cancer J Clin. 2007;57:43-66. Used with permission.

3. Sex—male to female ratio for lung cancer deaths is 1.24:1 and is related primarily to duration and intensity of smoking
4. Exposure to environmental, industrial, and occupational carcinogens—radon, asbestos, hydrocarbons, haloethers, nickel, arsenic, vinyl chloride, and ionizing radiation; risk of lung cancer increases with exposure to environmental tobacco smoke and varies with the duration and intensity of exposure

Screening tests include chest radiography and sputum cytology. Screening probably is not effective. Although the Mayo Clinic Lung Project detected more cases of cancer, mortality was not altered in approximately 12 years of follow-up study. This may have been because of "overdiagnosis" of clinically irrelevant lesions or lead-time bias. Annual chest radiography (or sputum cytology) solely to look for treatable-stage lung cancer should not be performed.

Studies are under way to evaluate newer imaging methods as well as cytologic and molecular evaluation of sputum for lung cancer screening. The International Early Lung Cancer Action Program

(I-ELCAP) reported an 88% 10-year survival for patients with stage I lung cancer, thus estimating that computed tomography (CT) screening of high-risk patients could prevent 80% of cancer deaths. However, analysis of other studies did not demonstrate a significant decline in advanced lung cancers or lung cancer death risk. Thus, the use of CT scans for lung cancer screening is not currently recommended.

Smoking is the leading preventable cause of cancer in the United States and a leading cause of heart disease and stroke. Physician advice to quit smoking and referral to smoking cessation programs are the most cost-effective preventive measures available. Smoking cessation decreases the risk of lung cancer, although the risk never returns to that of a nonsmoker.

- Lung cancer: the leading cause of cancer death for men and women.
- Risk factors for lung cancer: smoking, age, sex (male > female), environmental exposure to tobacco smoke and radon.

Table 21-4 Age-adjusted Death Rates by Race and Gender for 2004

| Rank | Cause of Death | | Age-Adjusted Death Rate Ratio | | |
			Male to Female	Black to White	Hispanic to Non-Hispanic White
...	All causes	800.8	1.4	1.3	0.7
1	Diseases of the heart	217.0	1.5	1.3	0.7
2	Malignant neoplasms	185.8	1.4	1.2	0.6
3	Cerebrovascular diseases	51.1	1.0	1.5	0.8
4	Chronic lower respiratory diseases	41.1	1.4	0.7	0.4
5	Accidents (unintentional injuries)	37.7	2.1	0.9	0.8
6	Diabetes mellitus	24.5	1.3	2.2	1.5
7	Alzheimer disease	21.8	0.7	0.8	0.6
8	Influenza & pneumonia	19.8	1.4	1.1	0.9
9	Nephritis, nephrotic syndrome, & nephrosis	14.2	1.4	2.3	0.9
10	Septicemia	11.2	1.2	2.2	0.8
11	Intentional self-harm (suicide)	10.9	4.0	0.4	0.5
12	Chronic liver disease & cirrhosis	9.0	2.2	0.9	1.6
13	Primary hypertension & hypertensive renal disease	7.7	1.0	2.8	1.0
14	Parkinson disease	6.1	2.3	0.4	0.6
15	Assault (homicide)	5.9	3.7	5.6	2.7

Data from Heron MP, Smith BL. Deaths: leading causes for 2004. National vital statistics reports; vol 56 no 5. Hyattsville, MD: National Center for Health Statistics, 2007.

- Annual chest radiography or sputum cytology solely to look for treatable stage lung cancer should not be performed.
- Smoking is the leading preventable cause of cancer in the United States.

Breast Cancer

Breast cancer is the second leading cause of cancer death for women. The lifetime risk is estimated at 1 in 8 women. The burden of disease (2007 estimates from the American Cancer Society) is 178,480 new cases and 40,460 deaths. Thus, breast cancer is moderately lethal (it kills many but not most of the people it afflicts). Risk factors include the following:

1. Age—risk increases throughout life, and the risk for an 80-year-old woman is 12 times that for a 30-year-old woman
2. Family history—10% to 15% of women with breast cancer have a first-degree relative who had breast cancer. Thus, the risk increases from 1.8 to 2.9 times in women with 1 or 2 first-degree female relatives with breast cancer. This risk is increased if the relative was premenopausal and decreased if the relative was postmenopausal
3. Socioeconomic status—if high, risk is increased 2 times
4. Nulliparity or older than 30 years at first full-term pregnancy—risk is increased 2 times
5. Obesity—relative risk for postmenopausal women with a body mass index (BMI) greater than 30 compared with those with a BMI less than 25 ranges from 1.31 to 1.45

Additional risk factors include younger age at menarche, older age at menopause, prolonged postmenopausal hormone therapy, dense tissue within the breast, moderate or high alcohol intake, and, possibly, cigarette smoking.

- Breast cancer: the second leading cause of cancer death for women.
- Lifetime risk: 1 in 8 women.
- Among women with breast cancer, 10% to 15% have a first-degree relative who had breast cancer. If a woman is a *BRCA1* or *BRCA2* carrier, she has a 50% to 85% lifetime risk of breast cancer.

Screening procedures include the following:

1. Breast self-examination—no demonstrated effectiveness
2. Clinical breast examination—sensitivity is about 50% to 70% and specificity is greater than 90%
3. Mammography—sensitivity is 75% to 95% for women 50 or older. Sensitivity is lower for women who are younger than 50, have dense breast tissue, or take hormone replacement therapy. Specificity is 95% to 99%. Positive predictive values (PPVs) are about 5% to 10%, with 20% to 50% of biopsy examinations finding cancer, depending on age (higher percentages in older women). Randomized controlled trials worldwide have examined the effectiveness of mammography. They showed an approximate 30% decrease in mortality, but only 2 trials showed statistical significance.

Data are conflicting or inconclusive for women younger than 50 or older than 70 years.

4. As of 2007, the American Cancer Society recommends annual magnetic resonance imaging (MRI) screening as an adjunct to mammography for women who are *BRCA* mutation positive, for women with a first-degree relative with *BRCA*, and for women with a lifetime risk of at least 20% to 25% of developing breast cancer. MRI has a sensitivity of 71% to 100% in these high-risk populations. Positive predictive values are currently not available owing to lack of follow-up. Current evidence is inadequate to recommend for or against MRI screening among women with a personal history of breast cancer, carcinoma in situ, atypical hyperplasia, or dense breast tissue on mammogram.

* Breast physical examination has a sensitivity of 50%-70% and a specificity >90%.
* Mammography has a sensitivity of 75%-95% and a specificity of 95%-99%.
* Studies are inconclusive about the benefit of mammography for women younger than 50 or older than 70.

Screening Risks

Radiation is estimated to produce 80 additional radiation-induced breast cancer deaths among 1,000,000 women screened annually for 10 years, compared with more than 90,000 breast cancers expected to be detected.

* Radiation produces 80 additional cases of breast cancer among 1,000,000 women screened.

Cost-effectiveness

If 25% of women 40 to 75 years old in the United States were screened annually, 11,000,000 per year would be screened at a cost of $1.3 billion annually for physical examination and mammography. The cost of screening and the work-up would be 100 times as expensive as the cost saved by reduced treatment. Cost per year of life saved ranges from about $9,000 to $12,000, with lower costs for women 50 to 69 years old and higher costs in both younger and older age groups. The cost per year of life saved for women aged 50 to 79 years by biennial screening mammography is around $17,269. A recent retrospective cost-effectiveness analysis showed a gain of 947.5 million QALYs at the cost of $166 billion for mammography over the lifetimes of screened women. This was a gain of 1.7 million QALYs for an additional cost of $62.5 billion when compared with women without screening. Screening women aged 40 to 80 years was the most expensive option. A US Preventive Services Task Force (USPSTF) study showed additional costs of $34,000 to $80,000 per year of life saved and found it cost-effective to screen women after 65 years of age if they had not been screened regularly in the past.

Recommendations

Current recommendations are as follows:

1. There is general agreement to recommend clinical breast examination and mammography every 1 to 2 years for women 50 to 69 years old. Otherwise, recommendations vary.

2. The American Cancer Society and several other groups recommend screening with mammography and clinical breast examination beginning at age 40. Recommendations for screening intervals differ among organizations.

3. The American Cancer Society recommends annual MRI screening as an adjunct to mammography in women with *BRCA* mutation, women with a first-degree relative with *BRCA*, and those with a lifetime risk of 20% to 25% or more of developing breast cancer.

4. The USPSTF recommends screening mammography alone or clinical breast examination and mammography every 1 to 2 years for women 40 or older.

Colorectal Cancer

Colorectal cancer is the second leading cause of cancer death in the United States. The burden of disease (2007 estimates from the American Cancer Society) is 112,340 new cases of colorectal cancer and 52,180 deaths due to colorectal cancer. The lifetime risk of developing this cancer is approximately 5% to 6%. Less than 2% of these cancers occur in people younger than 40, and 90% occur in those older than 50. The risk of developing colorectal cancer is approximately 2 times greater than the risk of dying of it (which reflects the potential survivability of colorectal cancer and the age of the population involved; ie, there are competing causes of death). Colorectal cancer is now the second cancer for which randomized controlled trial evidence has demonstrated decreased mortality because of screening.

* Colorectal cancer is the second leading cause of cancer death.
* Lifetime risk is 5%-6%.
* Colorectal cancers: 90% occur in patients older than 50.

Natural History

Cancer may develop de novo in the colon, but most tumors probably develop from adenomatous polyps. The risk of a polyp becoming malignant appears to be related to its histologic characteristics and size. Polyps that are histologically villous or tubulovillous increase the risk of colorectal cancer. Clinically significant polyps are ones larger than 10 mm. In addition, the presence of multiple polyps increases risk. The average time from formation to malignant transformation for a polyp is 7 to 10 years.

* The risk of a polyp becoming malignant appears to be related to its histologic characteristics and size.
* Clinically significant polyps are >10 mm.
* The time from polyp formation to malignant transformation is 7-10 years.

Risk Factors

Risk factors for colorectal cancer include the following:

1. Age—risk doubles every 7 years after age 50
2. Family history—if a first-degree relative has disease, the risk increases 2 times to 3 times; for multiple prior adenomatous polyps, the risk increases 2 times to 4 times

3. History of endometrial, ovarian, or breast cancer—risk increases 2 times
4. Familial adenomatous polyposis (Gardner syndrome)—risk is approximately 100% by age 40 to 45
5. Inflammatory bowel disease (ulcerative colitis and Crohn colitis)—risk is approximately 30% with a 30- to 40-year history of disease
6. Hereditary nonpolyposis cancer syndrome (adenocarcinoma at various locations at an early age in multiple siblings)—risk is approximately 50%

- Risk for colorectal cancer doubles every 7 years after age 50.
- If a first-degree relative has colorectal cancer, the risk increases 2 to 3 times.
- Previous adenomatous polyps—risk increases 2 to 4 times.
- History of endometrial, ovarian, or breast cancer—risk increases 2 times.
- Familial adenomatous polyposis (Gardner syndrome)—risk is nearly 100% by age 40-45.
- Inflammatory bowel disease—about a 30% risk with a 30- to 40-year history of chronic colitis.

Tests

The fecal occult blood test (FOBT) is 30% to 50% sensitive and does not detect polyps well. Proctoscopy is more than 90% sensitive for the area of the colon visualized; in studies, it detected about 30% of cancers. Flexible sigmoidoscopy is also more than 90% sensitive for the area of the colon visualized; in studies, it detected about 60% of cancers. With barium enema and colonoscopy, the entire colon may be visualized, with 85% to 95% sensitivity.

- FOBT is 30% to 50% sensitive.
- Proctoscopy and flexible sigmoidoscopy are >90% sensitive for the area of colon visualized.
- With barium enema and colonoscopy, the entire colon may be visualized, with 85%-95% sensitivity.

Recommendations

An algorithm for colorectal cancer screening is shown in Figure 21-1. The available randomized controlled trial data show about a 30% decrease in mortality for persons older than 50 who have an annual FOBT. For persons with average risk, the American Cancer Society recommends that screening begin at age 50 with FOBT annually, flexible sigmoidoscopy or double-contrast barium enema every 5 years, or colonoscopy every 10 years.

The USPSTF strongly recommends colorectal cancer screening for men and women 50 years or older. Screening options include FOBT, flexible sigmoidoscopy, colonoscopy, and double-contrast barium enema. The guidelines also recommend that persons with a family history of hereditary syndromes associated with a high risk of colon cancer should be referred for diagnosis and management. Patients with a family history of colon polyps or cancer should undergo screening for colorectal cancer at least 10 years before the age of the index case at diagnosis or at age 40 (whichever age is younger). Earlier screening is advised for patients with inflammatory bowel disease, family history of hereditary polyposis, and cancer syndromes.

- Screening patients with average risk of colorectal cancer is recommended at the age of 50.
- Patients with a family history of colon polyps or cancer should undergo screening for colorectal cancer at least 10 years before the age of the index case at diagnosis or at age 40.
- Earlier screening is advised for patients with inflammatory bowel disease, family history of hereditary polyposis, and cancer syndromes.

Prostate Cancer

For the purposes of screening, prostate cancer is a troublesome disease, primarily because of the great difference between the burden of prevalent disease and the burden of clinical disease. The 2007 estimates from the American Cancer Society are 218,890 new cases of prostate cancer and 27,050 deaths. Pathology studies show that a small focus of prostate cancer is found in 30% to 40% of 60-year-old men. Prostate cancer is diagnosed in only 8% to 9% of the men, with many cases diagnosed incidentally at transurethral resection of the prostate. Currently, 80% of diagnoses are made in men older than 65. Although prostate cancer is the leading cancer diagnosis and ranked second in male cancer mortality, a man's risk of dying of prostate cancer is estimated to be 3% to 4%.

- Prostate cancer is diagnosed in 8%-9% of US men.
- Only 3%-4% of US men die of prostate cancer.
- Currently, 80% of the diagnoses are made in men older than 65 years.

Natural History

Prostate cancer is a hormonally induced cancer that is generally slow growing. In most host males, it does not alter the life span or lifestyle. Growth of a tiny nidus of cancerous cells into a clinically important cancer takes 10 to 15 years. In elderly hosts, this process is usually halted by intervening causes of death. Aggressiveness and morbidity are related to size, grade, and ploidy.

- Prostate cancer is a hormonally induced cancer.
- It does not alter the life span or lifestyle of most host males.
- Growth into a clinically important cancer takes 10-15 years.

Risk Factors

Risk factors for prostate cancer include the following:
1. Age—risk increases exponentially after age 50
2. Race—in the United States, African-American men have 2 times the risk of whites, and whites have 2 times the risk of Asians
3. Family history—having a first-degree relative with prostate cancer increases the risk 3 times, having a brother with prostate cancer before age 63 increases the risk 4 times, and having a sister with breast cancer increases the risk 2 times

Additional risk factors include *BRCA1* or *BRCA2* mutations, dietary factors (eg, high intake of animal fat or low intake of vegetables),

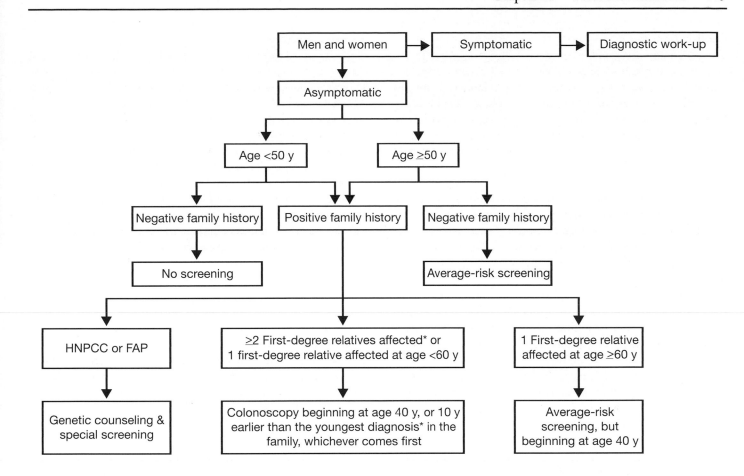

Figure 21-1. Algorithm for Colorectal Cancer Screening. See text for description of average-risk screening. Asterisk indicates either colorectal cancer or adenomatous polyp. FAP indicates familial adenomatous polyposis; HNPCC, hereditary nonpolyposis colorectal cancer. (From Winawer S, Fletcher R, Rex D, Bond J, Burt R, Ferrucci J, et al. Colorectal cancer screening and surveillance: clinical guidelines and rationale—update based on new evidence. Gastroenterology. 2003;124:544-60. Used with permission.)

prior prostatitis, and higher serum testosterone and insulin-like growth factor 1 concentrations.

- For prostate cancer in the United States, African-American men have twice the risk of whites, who have twice the risk of Asians.

Tests

A digital rectal examination has a PPV of 6% to 33%. Transrectal ultrasonography has a PPV of about 10% to 20% (values vary depending on population and previous screening). The prostate-specific antigen (PSA) test has a PPV of 25% to 35% for a PSA between 4 and 10 mg/mL. Use of the PSA velocity (change in PSA over time) or the free PSA to total PSA ratio (or both) may improve screening accuracy, but further study is needed. Because there is much undetected disease, PPV values do not have the usual meaning.

Recommendations

No good data are available from population-based randomized controlled trials on the effect of early detection and treatment on survival. There is little agreement on recommendations for screening. Aggressive screening for prostate cancer would uncover many new cases (causing a surge in incidence) and result in many additional treatments. However, because of the natural history of the disease, screening may have minimal effect in decreasing mortality, the desired benefit. The American Cancer Society recommends that a digital rectal examination and the PSA test be offered annually to men older than 50 who have a life expectancy of at least 10 years. The USPSTF guidelines conclude that there is insufficient evidence to recommend for or against routine screening for prostate cancer with a digital rectal examination or PSA test.

- There is little agreement on recommendations for prostate cancer screening.

Some authorities have recommended against any form of screening—digital rectal examination, ultrasonography, or PSA—primarily because of concern that the effect on survival would be minimal and would not warrant the risk of morbidity of treatment (ie, surgical risk, posttreatment risk of urinary incontinence, or loss of erectile function). Screening, if performed, should be done in men likely to have a 10-year survival.

Cervical Cancer

The 2007 estimates from the American Cancer Society are 11,150 new cases of cervical cancer and 3,670 deaths. Cervical cancer has a bimodal risk curve divided between in situ carcinoma and invasive carcinoma. This cancer has a long preclinical phase, and progression from dysplasia to invasive cancer may take 10 to 15 years or more. A strong association exists between HPV infection (types 16, 18, and others) and cervical cancer. Cervical cancer is largely a sexually transmitted disease.

- Cervical cancer: bimodal risk curve divided between in situ carcinoma and invasive carcinoma.
- It has a long preclinical phase.
- Cervical cancer is strongly associated with HPV infection.

Risk Factors

Risk factors for cervical cancer include the following: 1) age—the risk of invasive carcinoma increases throughout life; 2) sexual activity—early age at onset; 3) multiple sexual partners; 4) a history of sexually transmitted disease, especially HIV infection; and 5) smoking.

- Cervical cancer risk factors: early age at onset of sexual activity, multiple sexual partners, a history of sexually transmitted disease, and smoking.

Tests

The Pap smear has a sensitivity of 55% to 80% and a specificity of 90% to 99%. The expertise of the cytologists and pathologists as well as the clinician's sampling technique are important for test effectiveness.

Liquid-based cytology (LBC) is a newer method of preparing cervical cells. LBC has the potential advantages of better slide preparation with fewer unsatisfactory smears, more uniform samples, and improved laboratory efficiency. In a meta-analysis, the sensitivity of LBC was 12% to 17% higher in the general population and 12% to 15% higher in the high-risk population when compared with the traditional Pap smear. A pilot study in the United Kingdom showed an 87% reduction in the number of inadequate samples with LBC when compared with the traditional Pap smear.

The USPSTF has concluded that the evidence is insufficient to recommend for or against routine use of new technologies (LBC, computerized rescreening, and algorithm-based screening) to screen for cervical cancer. No current guidelines recommend using HPV testing for cervical cancer screening.

- Pap smear: 55%-80% sensitivity and 90%-99% specificity.

Screening Effectiveness

No randomized controlled trial of screening has been conducted in a general population. However, evidence from case-control studies and observational studies suggests effectiveness. The estimated overall effect of screening with a Pap smear every 10 years is a 64% reduction in invasive cancer; every 5 years, an 84% reduction; every 3 years, a 91% reduction; every 2 years, a 92.5% reduction; and every year, a 93.5% reduction.

Recommendations

There is general agreement to start screening at the onset of sexual activity and every 1 to 3 years thereafter, depending on risk. The USPSTF guidelines recommend routine screening for all women who have been sexually active and who have a cervix. Screening should begin with the onset of sexual activity and should be repeated at least every 3 years. The American Cancer Society recommends that cervical cancer screening start 3 years after onset of sexual activity, but no later than age 21. Also, it recommends annual screening with a conventional Pap test, or every 2 years if liquid-based cytology is used, until age 30. The recommendation permits less frequent testing after age 30 (every 2-3 years), based on past screening results and risk factors. The recommendation suggests offering women the option to discontinue screening after age 65 to 70 if there is evidence of adequate past screening.

- General recommendation: screen at the onset of sexual activity and every 1-3 years thereafter, depending on risk.

Ovarian Cancer

Ovarian cancer is the fifth leading cause of cancer death in women. The burden of disease (2007 estimates from the American Cancer Society) is 22,430 new cases of ovarian cancer and 16,210 deaths. Ovarian cancer is the leading cause of gynecologic cancer death. Age-adjusted death rates have been increasing slowly in the past 25 years.

- Ovarian cancer is the fifth leading cause of cancer death in women.
- Age-adjusted death rates have been increasing slowly.

Risk Factors

With a history of at least 1 term pregnancy, the relative risk is 0.6 to 0.8. With the use of oral contraceptives for 3 to 6 months, the relative risk is 0.6; if oral contraceptives are used more than 10 years, the relative risk is 0.2. Tubal ligation may also reduce risk.

Family history of ovarian cancer can increase a woman's lifetime risk of ovarian cancer from 1.6% to 5%. Those who are BRCA1 or BRCA2 carriers have a lifetime risk of 15% to 50%. Long duration of ovulatory years (ie, early menarche or late menopause) is a risk factor. High-fat diet and endometriosis may also increase risk.

- Only 4%-5% of ovarian cancers are familial.

Screening Tests

Bimanual examination is insensitive. Ultrasonography, either transvaginal or transabdominal, is more sensitive than bimanual examination but has a poor PPV. The cancer antigen 125 (CA 125) assay is more sensitive than bimanual examination but also has a poor PPV. Ultrasonography and the CA 125 assay have a significant false-positive rate. It is estimated that 10 to 60 abdominal operations would have to be performed for every 1 cancer detected, at a cost of more than $13 billion annually, to screen the 43 million women older than 45. An adequate study of efficacy, even with a highly sensitive and specific test, would require tens of thousands of participants.

- For ovarian cancer, bimanual examination is insensitive.
- Ultrasonography and the CA 125 assay are more sensitive than bimanual examination, but both have a poor PPV.
- For every 1 ovarian cancer detected, 10-60 abdominal operations would have to be performed.

Recommendations

The USPSTF and American Cancer Society do not recommend screening for ovarian cancer. Women with a family history of cancer syndromes should be offered a referral to a genetics counselor. The data on the utility of intensive screening protocols in these women are conflicting.

Table 21-5 summarizes cancer screening of proven benefit for average-risk persons. Table 21-6 summarizes cancer prevention of proven benefit.

Prevention of Infectious Diseases

Tuberculosis Prevention

Burden of Disease

In 1997, the worldwide prevalence of tuberculosis (TB) infection (latent or active) was estimated to be 1.86 billion cases, with an annual incidence rate of about 8 million. Approximately 2,000,000 people worldwide die annually of TB. The US incidence is approximately 15,000 cases per year, with fewer than 1,000 deaths per year. The incidence decreased from 1953 to 1985, and then TB made a resurgence because of immigration from endemic areas, HIV infection, and increased use of immunosuppressive drugs. Since 1993, the incidence has consistently decreased.

- TB: the US incidence is approximately 15,000 cases and fewer than 1,000 deaths annually.

Natural History

Infection occurs through inhalation of droplets bearing *Mycobacterium tuberculosis*. After being infected, healthy persons are usually asymptomatic. However, it is believed that the tubercle bacillus remains viable in granulomata for many years. The risk of reactivation after asymptomatic infection (purified protein derivative [PPD] conversion) is 5% for the first 1 or 2 years after infection. In another 5%, disease develops later in life.

- The tubercle bacillus remains viable in granulomata for many years.
- The risk of reactivation (after PPD conversion) is 5% for the first 1-2 years after infection.
- In another 5%, disease develops later in life.

Persons at higher risk of TB infection include those with close contact with a person with active TB, foreign-born persons from areas of high prevalence, residents and employees of high-risk congregate settings (eg, nursing homes and prisons), health care workers, medically underserved low-income populations, high-risk racial or ethnic minority populations, and persons who inject illicit drugs.

Table 21-5 Cancer Screening Tests With Proven Benefit[a]

Type of Cancer	Recommendation
Cervical	Sexually active women (all ages): cervical Pap smear every 1-3 y
Breast	Normal-risk women 40 years or older: screening mammograms with or without clinical breast examination every 1-2 y
	High risk women: screening MRI as an adjunct to mammography
Colon	Normal-risk persons 50 years or older—1 or both of the following: 1) Fecal occult blood test 3 times yearly 2) Flexible sigmoidoscopy or double-contrast barium enema every 5 y or colonoscopy every 10 y

Abbreviations: MRI, magnetic resonance imaging; Pap, Papanicolaou.
[a] Secondary prevention.

Table 21-6 Cancer Prevention[a]

Type of Cancer	Recommendation
Lung	Smoking cessation counseling
Ovarian	Oral contraceptive use

[a] Primary prevention.

Persons at higher risk of active TB developing after infection include HIV-infected persons (7%-10% risk each year), persons recently infected with TB (5% risk for the first 1-2 years after infection), persons with certain medical conditions (eg, diabetes mellitus and end-stage renal disease), persons who inject illicit drugs, and persons with a history of inadequately treated TB.

- Persons infected with both *M tuberculosis* and HIV have a 7%-10% risk each year of active TB developing.

Testing

The PPD (Mantoux) test is a 5–tuberculin-unit intradermal skin test. The area of induration (not erythema) is measured at 48 to 72 hours. All persons with a positive PPD test should have chest radiography and clinical evaluation for active TB. Targeted skin testing is recommended for high-risk groups.

In low-risk persons, consider the reaction positive if it is larger than 15 mm. A 10-mm reaction is considered positive for the following groups: recent arrivals from countries of high prevalence, persons who inject illicit drugs, residents and employees of high-risk congregate settings, mycobacteriology laboratory personnel, and persons with medical conditions that increase the risk of TB. A 5-mm reaction is considered positive for HIV-positive persons, recent contacts of a person with active TB, persons with fibrotic changes on chest radiographs consistent with old healed TB, and immunosuppressed patients.

Persons exposed in the past may be relatively anergic, but the response can be boosted by repeating the test (2-step PPD testing procedure). Previous bacille Calmette-Guérin (BCG) vaccination may produce skin reactivity, but positive reactors should be considered to have true infection and be given appropriate follow-up care. Recent measles-mumps-rubella (MMR) and oral polio vaccine (OPV) vaccination (within 6 weeks) may diminish skin reactivity, and testing should be avoided during this interval. Chest radiography and sputum are not useful screening tests for conversion but may detect active disease in high-risk persons.

* Chest radiography and sputum are not useful screening tests for TB.

In 2005, the Food and Drug Administration (FDA) approved the QuantiFERON-TB Gold (QFT-G) test, which uses ESAT-6 and CFP-10 protein mixtures, as an option for the diagnosis of latent tuberculosis infection (LTBI) and TB. Interferon-γ released by sensitized lymphocytes is detected by an enzyme-linked immunosorbent assay (ELISA). The limitations of QFT-G have not been studied conclusively. QFT-G has 80% sensitivity in detecting culture-confirmed, untreated TB. Sensitivity in children and immunocompromised individuals with TB has not been ascertained. No confirmatory test for LTBI exists, so assessing the sensitivity of QFT-G has been difficult. The predictive value of QFT-G depends on the prevalence of *Mycobacterium tuberculosis* infection in the tested population.

Preventive Measures

Primary prevention is with BCG vaccine, an attenuated species of *Mycobacterium bovis*. The efficacy of BCG vaccine ranges from 0% to 80%. It is appropriate in high-risk areas because it is inexpensive, requires a single dose, and has a low risk (only 100 fatalities in 2 billion administrations). BCG vaccine is not indicated in areas of low prevalence because it confuses interpretation of the PPD response. Currently, BCG vaccination is not recommended for any adult in the United States. Another primary preventive measure is environmental controls, especially in a health care environment, with respiratory isolation, high-efficiency filter masks, and special venting of rooms and wards with TB cases.

* BCG vaccine efficacy ranges from 0%-80%.
* Its use is not indicated in low-prevalence areas.

Secondary prevention is with isoniazid treatment. Its use is indicated for recent converters (<2 years), contacts of infected persons with a PPD reaction of 5 mm or more, history of TB with inadequate treatment, positive skin test with abnormal but stable chest radiographic findings, and positive PPD test (of any duration). The dosage is 5 to 10 mg/kg daily, up to a maximum of 300 mg daily (the usual adult dose), given as a single oral dose. Treatment should continue for 9

months. Primary side effects are liver toxicity and peripheral neuropathy. Peak toxicity is in persons older than 50 years (2%-3%). Monitoring for side effects is generally through symptoms only. Baseline laboratory testing and periodic monitoring of liver transaminase (aspartate aminotransferase [AST] or alanine aminotransferase [ALT]) levels is not routinely recommended. Testing should be considered for pregnant or postpartum women, persons with liver disease or other chronic medical conditions, and those taking other medications.

Alternative treatment regimens for latent TB infection include rifampin and pyrazinamide daily for 2 months or rifampin alone for 4 months.

* Isoniazid: 5-10 mg/kg daily, up to a maximum of 300 mg daily.
* Treatment should continue for 9 months.
* Peak toxicity is in persons older than 50 (2%-3%).

Immunizations

One of the greatest successes of modern medicine for preventing disease and extending life has been immunization. Adults have continuing needs for immunization throughout life. Physicians who administer vaccines are required by law to keep permanent vaccine records (National Childhood Vaccine Act of 1986) and to report adverse events through the Vaccine Adverse Event Reporting System (VAERS). Service in the US military may be considered verification of vaccination for measles, rubella, tetanus, diphtheria, and polio. Providers are now required to give patients vaccine information pamphlets before vaccination as a mechanism for informed consent.

Immunity may be of 2 types: 1) In passive immunity, preformed antibodies are provided in large quantities to prevent or diminish the effect of infection or associated toxins (eg, tetanus immune globulin [TIG] and hepatitis B immune globulin [HBIG]). Passive immunity lasts for only several months. 2) In active immunity, an antigen is presented to the host immune system, which in turn develops antibodies (eg, hepatitis or tetanus) or specific immune cells (eg, BCG). Active immunity generally lasts from years to a lifetime. Active immunity may be induced by live virus vaccines (eg, measles), killed virus vaccines (eg, influenza), or refined antigen vaccines (eg, pneumococcal).

Live virus vaccines are contraindicated in some persons. In general, pregnant women, people with immunodeficiency diseases, leukemia, lymphoma, generalized malignancy, or those who are immunosuppressed because of therapy with corticosteroids, alkylating drugs, antimetabolites, or radiation should *not* be given live virus vaccines. HIV-infected persons who are immunocompetent and leukemia patients who have been in remission for 3 months or more after chemotherapy generally may be vaccinated with *some* live virus vaccines. Live virus vaccines include measles, mumps, rubella, smallpox, varicella, yellow fever, and OPV.

Inactivated virus vaccines include enhanced inactivated polio (eIPV), hepatitis A, hepatitis B, influenza, and rabies. Inactivated bacterial vaccines include cholera, typhoid, meningococcal, plague, and pneumococcal.

An adult immunization schedule has been developed and endorsed by several groups (Figure 21-2).

Anthrax

Anthrax is primarily a zoonosis that develops after contact with infected animals, hides, meat, and wool. Cutaneous anthrax is the most common form of the disease, which manifests as an ulceration of the skin and fever. The intentional spread of anthrax spores in 2001 led to an outbreak of anthrax that resulted in 5 deaths.

In 1970 a vaccine for anthrax was licensed for use in select populations. It was recommended for laboratory personnel who work directly with the organism, people who work with imported animal hides or furs, people who handle potentially infected animal products (eg, veterinarians who work in countries with a high incidence of anthrax), and military personnel in areas with high risk of exposure to the organism.

Currently aluminum hydroxide adsorbed cell-free anthrax vaccine (Anthrax Vaccine Adsorbed [AVA]) is available for preexposure prophylaxis. The vaccine is administered in 6 doses; the first 3 doses are given at 2-week intervals and the other 3 doses are given at 6, 12, and 18 months after the first dose. Side effects are generally mild and include mild erythema and pruritus at the injection site.

Diphtheria

Diphtheria is a rare disease primarily because of vaccination. However, up to 40% of adults may lack protective antibody levels.

Recommendations

Vaccinate with a combination of tetanus and diphtheria toxoids (Td) (see "Tetanus" subsection below). The diphtheria-tetanus-pertussis (DTP) preparation recommended for children should not be used for adults.

Hepatitis A

In the United States, the rate of hepatitis A infection tends to vary from year to year. In 2001, the infection rate was 4 per 100,000 population. Clinical disease develops in more than 70% of infected older children and adults. Also, more than 10,000 infected persons are hospitalized yearly, and approximately 80 deaths are due to fulminant hepatitis. Signs and symptoms usually last less than 2 months. However, 10% to 15% of patients have prolonged or relapsing illness, which may last up to 6 months.

Spread of hepatitis A virus (HAV) occurs by the fecal-oral route, most commonly within households. Common-source outbreaks due to contaminated food and water supplies have occurred. Blood-borne transmission is uncommon but can occur through blood transfusion and contaminated blood products and from needles shared with an infected viremic person. Sexual transmission has also been reported.

Vaccine	Age group		
	19-49 years	50-64 years	65 years
Tetanus, diptheria, pertussis (Td/Tdap)[a]	1 dose Td booster every 10 y / Substitute 1 dose of Tdap for Td		
Human papillomavirus (HPV)[a]	3 doses (females) (0, 2, 6 mo)		
Measles, mumps, rubella (MMR)[a]	1 or 2 doses	1 dose	
Varicella[a]	2 doses (0, 4-8 wk)		
Influenza[a]		1 dose annually	
Pneumococcal (polysaccharide)	1-2 doses		1 dose
Hepatitis A[a]	2 doses (0, 6-12 mo or 0, 6-18 mo)		
Hepatitis B[a]	3 doses (0, 1-2, 4-6 mo)		
Meningococcal[a]	1 or more doses		
Zoster		1 dose	

[a] Covered by the Vaccine Injury Compensation Program.

☐ For all persons in this category who meet the age requirements and who lack evidence of immunity (eg, lack documentation of vaccination or have no evidence of prior infection)

▨ Recommended if some other risk factor is present (eg, on the basis of medical, occupational, lifestyle, or other indications)

Figure 21-2. Recommended Adult Immunization Schedule, United States 2007-2008, by Age Group. Detailed footnotes accompanying this figure are published at http://www.cdc.gov/vaccines/recs/schedules/adult-schedule.htm.

Hepatitis A vaccination provides an opportunity to lower the disease incidence and ultimately to eradicate infection because humans are the only natural reservoir of the virus. A single dose of hepatitis A vaccine induces a protective antibody level within 4 weeks after vaccination. A second dose of vaccine 6 to 12 months later induces long-lasting immunity. Target groups for immunization include persons traveling to or working in countries that have high or intermediate HAV endemicity; men who have sex with men; illicit drug users; persons who have an occupational risk of infection (those who work with HAV-infected primates or with HAV in a research laboratory), chronic liver disease, or clotting-factor disorders; and some food handlers. Hepatitis A vaccination of children has been used effectively to control outbreaks in communities that have high rates of hepatitis A.

Travelers who are allergic to a vaccine component or who elect not to receive vaccine should be encouraged to get immune globulin (0.02-0.06 mL/kg provides protection for 3-5 months). Immune globulin should also be given to travelers leaving on short notice, and it can be given concomitantly with vaccine, using separate sites and syringes.

Postexposure prophylaxis with immune globulin, along with hepatitis A vaccination, is appropriate for household, sexual, and drug-using contacts of patients with hepatitis A infection.

Prevaccination serologic testing may be cost-effective for adults who were born or lived for extended periods in areas of high HAV endemicity and for men who have sex with men. Postvaccination testing is not necessary because of the high rate of vaccine response.

Hepatitis B

The lifetime risk of acquiring hepatitis B is 5% for the general population; 150,000 cases occur annually in the United States, resulting in 8,000 hospitalizations and 200 deaths. Of the patients affected, 90% are 20 years or older; 5% to 10% become carriers, and one-fourth of these develop chronic active hepatitis. Annually, 4,000 persons die of hepatitis B virus-related cirrhosis and 1,500 die of hepatitis B virus-related liver cancer.

- The lifetime risk of acquiring hepatitis B is 5% for the general population.
- Of affected patients, 5%-10% become carriers.
- Annually, 4,000 persons die of hepatitis B virus-related cirrhosis and 1,500 die of hepatitis B virus-related liver cancer.

The current vaccine is yeast recombinant, developed from the insertion of a plasmid into *Saccharomyces cerevisiae*, which produces the copies of the surface antigen. Human plasma–derived vaccine is no longer made. The target population includes adults at increased risk, that is, men who have sex with men, intravenous drug users, heterosexual persons with multiple sexual partners, and those with a history of other sexually transmitted diseases; household and sexual contacts of hepatitis B virus carriers; workers in health-related and public safety occupations involving exposure to blood or body fluids; hemodialysis patients; recipients of concentrates of clotting factors VIII and IX; morticians and their assistants; and travelers who will be living for extended periods in high-prevalence areas or who are likely to have sexual contacts or contact with blood in the endemic areas (especially in eastern Asia and sub-Saharan Africa).

Vaccination

Normally, vaccination consists of 3 doses, given at 0, 1, and 6 months. An alternative dosing schedule to induce immunity more rapidly (eg, after exposure) involves 4 doses, the first 3 given 1 month apart and a fourth dose at 12 months. Postexposure prophylaxis consists of HBIG given in a single dose of 0.06 mL/kg or 5 mL for adults. It should be administered along with the vaccine in separate syringes at separate sites, but they may be administered at the same time. Current evidence suggests that for most vaccinees the vaccination has a duration of 7 years or more. Currently, revaccination is not routinely recommended. For persons who received the vaccine in the buttock or whose management depends on knowledge of immune status (eg, surgeons or venipuncturists), periodic serologic testing may be valuable. Those with antibody to hepatitis B surface antigen (anti-HBsAg) titers less than 10 mIU/mL should be revaccinated. Revaccination with a single dose is usually effective.

- Currently, revaccination for hepatitis B is not routinely recommended.

The most common side effect of hepatitis B vaccination is localized soreness. Guillain-Barré syndrome (0.5 per 100,000) has been associated with human plasma–derived hepatitis B vaccine. Comparable information is not available for the recombinant vaccines. Vaccination during pregnancy is considered advisable for women who are at risk of hepatitis B infection. The risk of association with hepatitis B virus infection in pregnancy far outweighs the risk of vaccine-associated problems.

- Guillain-Barré syndrome (0.5 per 100,000) has been associated with human plasma–derived hepatitis B vaccine.

Human Papillomavirus

More than 20 million people are infected with HPV and about 80% of women are infected by age 50. More than 50% of sexually active individuals have HPV. An HPV vaccine (Gardasil) was approved by the FDA in 2006 for the prevention of HPV infection among females aged 9 to 26 years. In clinical trials it was 100% effective against HPV strains 16 and 18, which are responsible for about 70% of cases of cervical cancer. It was also 99% effective against strains 6 and 11, which are responsible for 90% of the cases of genital warts. It is given in a 3-dose series; the second dose is given 2 months after the first dose, and the third dose is given 6 months after the first dose. Contraindications include anaphylaxis to yeast or to components of the vaccine. Common side effects include pain, erythema, and pruritus at the injection site and, less commonly, fever.

Influenza

During the 20th century, influenza pandemics occurred in 1918, 1957, and 1968, and each one resulted in a large number of deaths worldwide. Epidemics of influenza occur in the United States almost annually and are caused primarily by influenza A viruses and occasionally by influenza B viruses or both. The incidence peaks in mid to late winter—earlier in recent years. Influenza A is classified by 2 surface antigens: hemagglutinin (subtypes H1, H2, and H3) and neuraminidase (subtypes N1 and N2). Because of differing subtypes and antigenic drift, infection or vaccination more than 1 year previously may not give protection the following year. Influenza B is antigenically more stable but still has moderate drift. Control of both influenza A and B is with vaccination or chemoprophylaxis or both.

The vaccine is an inactivated (killed) virus vaccine (virus grown in egg culture) containing viral strains that circulated during the previous season. Each year it contains 3 viruses: 2 influenza A viruses and 1 influenza B virus. Vaccines may contain whole virus or split virus (subvirion). Split-virus vaccines are used in children to decrease febrile reaction. All forms may be used in adults. Ideally, vaccination should occur in October or November.

The side effects include local soreness; fever, malaise, and myalgia (which occur 6-12 hours after vaccination and may last 1-2 days); and anaphylactic reaction (probably due to egg protein). The target populations include persons 65 or older, especially those who reside in a nursing home or long-term care facility; persons with chronic pulmonary or cardiovascular disease, including asthma, chronic metabolic disease such as diabetes mellitus, renal dysfunction, or immunosuppression; health care workers; and women in the second or third trimester of pregnancy during influenza season (November-March). Consideration may be given to persons in vital roles, to those in institutional settings, and to travelers. The only contraindication is egg allergy.

FluMist, a live attenuated nasal spray influenza vaccine was licensed in 2003 and is approved for use in healthy people between the ages of 5 and 49 years. In 1 large study, it reduced the chance of influenza by 92% compared with placebo. Common side effects include rhinorrhea, headache, sore throat, and cough in adults.

Chemoprophylaxis for influenza A has been available for many years, with either amantadine hydrochloride or rimantadine hydrochloride. These drugs interfere with the replication cycle of influenza A. In healthy populations, they are 70% to 90% effective if given daily throughout an epidemic. For treatment of disease, they decrease fever and other symptoms if given within 48 hours of disease onset. These agents are used to control influenza outbreaks, usually in institutions, and are given to all unvaccinated workers and residents. They may be given regardless of vaccination status to persons at high risk. Workers should continue taking the medication until 2 weeks after vaccination or indefinitely during the period of risk if the vaccine is contraindicated. The drug dosage (100-200 mg daily) varies with age. Owing to the recent high levels of resistance to amantadine hydrochloride and rimantadine hydrochloride, the Centers for Disease Control and Prevention has recommended that neither of these 2 drugs be used for prophylaxis until susceptibility has been reestablished in circulating influenza A viruses. Oseltamivir or zanamivir can be prescribed if antiviral treatment for influenza is indicated.

- Amantadine and rimantadine are 70%-90% effective against influenza A only.
- Currently they are not recommended for prophylaxis owing to widespread resistance.

The side effects are usually minor, occurring in 5% to 10% of recipients, and may abate with continued use. Central nervous system side effects—nervousness, anxiety, insomnia, and decreased concentration—occur less frequently with rimantadine than with amantadine. Digestive system side effects include anorexia and nausea. Serious side effects are seizure and confusion, usually seen in the elderly or in those with kidney or liver disease. In these groups, the dose should be decreased in accordance with the recommendations made in the package inserts.

Chemoprophylaxis using the neuraminidase inhibitors oseltamivir and zanamivir has been shown to be effective in preventing influenza A and B. Oseltamivir given in a dosage of 75 mg daily for up to 6 weeks during an influenza outbreak has a protective efficacy of 74%. The most common side effects of oseltamivir are nausea and vomiting. Zanamivir, an orally inhaled powder, is recommended for children older than 7 years and adults. When given in a dosage of 10 mg daily it showed a protective efficacy of 78% for influenza A and 85% for influenza B. Zanamivir can cause rare bronchospasm and oropharyngeal edema and is not recommended for individuals with underlying airway problems.

Measles

Vaccination decreased the number of cases of measles from 500,000 yearly (with 500 deaths) to 3,500 yearly in the mid-1980s. A disease resurgence occurred in 1989 to 1991, with a peak incidence of more than 27,000 cases in 1990. Since 1993, fewer than 500 cases have been reported in most years. Measles is no longer considered to be endemic in the United States. All cases appear to be the result of importation, with limited spread among US residents. Measles is often more severe in adults. Complications include pneumonia, laryngotracheobronchitis, hepatitis, and bacterial superinfection. The risk of encephalitis with measles infection in an adult is approximately 1 in 1,000. Infection during pregnancy may result in spontaneous abortion or premature labor and low birth weight. Malformation does not appear to be as much of a problem as with rubella.

- The risk of encephalitis with measles infection in an adult is approximately 1 in 1,000.

Target

Adults born after 1956 who have no medical contraindication should be vaccinated if they have no dated documentation of at least 1 dose of live measles vaccine on or after their first birthday, physician-documented disease, or documented immune titer. Persons with expected exposure to measles should consider revaccination or titer measurement because up to 10% of persons born before 1957 may not be immune. Persons at risk include travelers to endemic areas, those in school settings, and health care workers. They should have 2 doses of measles vaccine documented on or after their first birthday. MMR is the preferred vaccine. If they have never been vaccinated, they should receive 2 doses given at least 1 month apart.

Exposure Precautions

If an exposed person is unvaccinated, vaccinate within 72 hours if possible or give immune globulin (up to 6 days after exposure) if the person is not a vaccine candidate (0.25-0.5 mL/kg body weight, up to 15 mL—the dose depends on immunocompetence). Health care workers should remain away from work for 5 to 21 days after exposure if they are not immune.

Side effects include fever higher than 39.4°C (usually occurs on days 5 to 12) in 5% to 15% of those vaccinated and a rash in 5%. Encephalitis is rare (1 case per 1 million immunizations). No apparent increase in side effects occurs with a second vaccination. Contraindications are immune globulin or blood products given within the previous 3 to 12 months, pregnancy, gelatin or neomycin allergy, and others as noted above for live virus vaccines.

Meningococcal Meningitis

Approximately 3,000 cases of meningococcal meningitis were reported in 2005. Of these cases, 13% occurred in children younger than 1 year and 20% occurred in adolescents and young adults (14-24 years). Meningococcal meningitis has a case fatality rate of 10% to 14%. Among the survivors, 11% to 19% develop long-term sequelae, including deafness, limb loss, and neurologic deficit.

The 2 vaccines effective against *Neisseria meningitidis* are the polysaccharide vaccine (MPSV4 or Menomune) and the conjugate vaccine (MCV4 or Menactra). Both prevent meningitis caused by serogroups A, C, Y, and W135. MCV4 is recommended for all children at their preadolescent visit (11-12 years of age) or at high school entry if they have not received a vaccination. Routine vaccination is also recommended for college freshmen living in dormitories, microbiologists routinely exposed to *N meningitidis*, US military personnel, and persons who have a history of functional or anatomical asplenia, a terminal complement component deficiency, or an increased risk of contracting *N meningitidis*. The vaccine is also recommended for postexposure prophylaxis and for persons traveling to a country with an outbreak of meningococcal disease.

The vaccine is administered subcutaneously as a single 0.5-mL dose. Adverse reactions are mild and infrequent and consiste principally of localized erythema.

Antimicrobial chemoprophylaxis with rifampicin (600 mg every 12 hours for 2 days) is the major preventive measure in sporadic cases of *N meningitidis*. Because systemic antimicrobial therapy does not eradicate nasopharyngeal carriage of *N meningitidis*, it is important to give chemoprophylaxis to the index patient before hospital discharge.

Mumps

A highly effective vaccination program decreased the number of cases of mumps from approximately 200,000 yearly to less than 1,000 yearly during the 1990s. Vaccine side effects of fever, rash, pruritus, and purpura are uncommon, and central nervous system problems and parotitis are rare. There is no increased risk with revaccination. The contraindications are the same as for measles.

Pneumococcal Pneumonia

Pneumococcal pneumonia is an important cause of death among older persons. The overall case fatality rate is 5% to 10%, but it is higher (20%-40%) among persons with underlying disease or alcoholism. The risk of bacteremia for persons 65 years or older with *Streptococcus pneumoniae* infection is 50 per 100,000. Two-thirds of persons with

serious pneumococcal disease have been hospitalized in the previous 5 years, which represents a missed opportunity for vaccination.

The current adult vaccine contains purified capsular polysaccharide of 23 pneumococcal serotypes that cause approximately 90% of the bacteremic pneumococcal infections in the United States. After a single dose of vaccine, the titers persist for 5 years or more in healthy adults. Side effects of vaccination include localized erythema and pain, which occur in about 50% of all vaccinees. Other side effects, which occur in less than 1% of persons vaccinated, include fever, myalgia, and severe local reactions. Anaphylaxis occurs in 5 per 1,000,000 of those vaccinated. Revaccination within approximately 1 year is associated with increased local reactions. The target population for vaccination includes persons 65 or older, adults with chronic cardiovascular or pulmonary disease, diabetics, and persons at higher risk of pneumococcal infection because of, for example, alcoholism or cerebrospinal fluid leak. The target population also includes immunocompromised persons (eg, those who are asplenic) and patients with Hodgkin disease, lymphoma, multiple myeloma, chronic renal failure, nephrotic syndrome, HIV infection, or organ transplant.

It is not necessary to revaccinate persons who received the original 14-valent pneumococcal vaccine. However, persons at highest risk of pneumococcal infections, especially immunocompromised persons, should be revaccinated with the 23-valent vaccine. Revaccination once after 5 years should be considered for adults with conditions associated with rapid antibody decline after initial immunization, especially those with nephrotic syndrome, renal failure, or renal transplant. Persons 65 or older should be given a second dose of vaccine if they received an original dose more than 5 years previously and were younger than 65 at the time of primary immunization.

- The target population is persons at least 65 years old or adults with chronic disease.
- Pneumococcal vaccination should be repeated for persons 65 or older if they received their initial vaccine more than 5 years earlier and before 65 years of age.

Polio

Polio has been eradicated from the entire Western Hemisphere. The few cases that occur in the Western Hemisphere are due to the oral vaccine virus strain. There are OPV (live virus) and eIPV (killed virus) vaccines. A primary series with either one has more than 95% effectiveness. Polio vaccination is not recommended for persons older than 18 unless they plan to travel to an endemic area and have no history of a previous primary series. For these persons, eIPV is recommended because of the lower risk of paralysis. The primary series consists of 3 doses of eIPV, given at 0, 1, and 6 to 12 months. If the person will be traveling in less than 4 weeks, a single dose of eIPV should be given. If the primary series is incomplete, it should be completed regardless of the interval since the last dose. If the person previously received OPV, 1 dose of eIPV should be given. For OPV, the risk of paralysis is approximately 1 in 1,000,000 after the first dose, and for susceptible household contacts, it is approximately 1 in 2,000,000.

- Polio vaccination is not recommended for persons older than 18 unless they plan to travel to an endemic area.

Rabies

Preexposure prophylactic vaccination is recommended for animal handlers, laboratory workers, persons traveling to hyperendemic areas for more than 1 month, and those with vocations or avocations with exposure to skunks, raccoons, bats, and other animals. In the United States, the reservoir of infection includes carnivorous animals, particularly skunks, raccoons, foxes, and bats. Except for woodchucks, rodents are rarely infected. Preexposure vaccination consists of 3 doses of rabies vaccine, given on days 0, 7, and 21 or 28. Ideally, preexposure vaccination should be completed at least 1 month before travel or potential exposure.

Following a potential or known rabies exposure (eg, animal bite or bat contact), a person who has had preexposure vaccination needs only 2 doses of rabies vaccine: 1 immediately and another 3 days later. Appropriate postexposure treatment for unimmunized persons includes administration of rabies immune globulin (part of it infiltrated in and around the bite and the rest given intramuscularly) and 5 doses of rabies vaccine. The first dose of vaccine should be given as soon as possible after exposure and additional doses on days 3, 7, 14, and 28 to 35 after the first dose. Local wound care, tetanus prophylaxis, and combined postexposure treatment with rabies immune globulin and 5 doses of rabies vaccine are recommended for all severe exposures. Use of postexposure treatment depends on many factors, including type of contact, animal involved, availability of the animal for observation or testing, and rabies endemicity in the area. The decision is best made with input from local public health authorities.

Rubella

Infection with rubella in the first trimester results in congenital rubella syndrome in up to 85% of infected fetuses. The goal of vaccination is to prevent the occurrence of this disease. Vaccination is highly effective, and there is no evidence of transmission of vaccine virus to close household contacts. The target population includes all women of childbearing age, all health care workers, and travelers to endemic areas. The side effects include arthralgias in 25% and transient arthritis in 10%, usually 1 to 3 weeks after vaccination. Vaccination rarely causes chronic joint problems, certainly much less frequently than natural infection. Contraindications are immune globulin given within the previous 3 months (but not blood products, eg, Rh$_0$(D) immune globulin [RhoGAM]), pregnancy or likely pregnancy within 3 months (although there are no documented cases of congenital rubella syndrome in vaccinated pregnant women), and allergy to neomycin but not to egg (because it is prepared in a diploid cell culture).

Smallpox (Vaccinia)

The World Health Organization declared the world free of smallpox in May 1980. Smallpox vaccination subsequently was given only to laboratory personnel working directly with orthopoxviruses. During 2002, preparations began for the use of smallpox vaccine for bioterrorism preparedness. Vaccination of health care workers started in 2003. Seven individuals developed cardiac complications (myocardial infarction, angina, and myopericarditis) following vaccination. No causal association has been established between the vaccine and cardiac problems thus far.

The Advisory Committee on Immunization Practices of the Centers for Disease Control and Prevention has released detailed recommendations for preexposure vaccination and for use of smallpox vaccine if a smallpox emergency occurs. The live virus smallpox vaccine is highly effective in inducing immunity that lasts for up to 5 years after primary vaccination. Additional doses may confer long-term immunity, possibly for a decade or more. Side effects include fever, skin rash, eczema vaccinatum, generalized vaccinia, and post-vaccinal encephalitis. Inadvertent inoculation at other sites may occur.

Transmission of vaccine virus to close contacts has been documented. Contraindications include pregnancy, history or presence of eczema, HIV infection, altered immunocompetence, and known allergy to a vaccine component. Vaccinia immune globulin can be given to persons with complications of vaccination.

Tetanus

Approximately 50 cases of tetanus are reported each year. Most cases occur in adults who are either unvaccinated or inadequately vaccinated. Vaccination is nearly 100% effective.

Recommendations

The primary series, a 3-dose series, should be completed before adulthood, usually in early childhood. The primary series consists of Td (DTP in childhood). The last childhood dose is usually a booster at age 15 years. Tdap (tetanus toxoid, diphtheria low dose, and acellular pertussis) is recommended as a booster dose for adolescents (11-18 years) who received DTaP (Diphtheria, Tetanus, and acellular pertussis) or DTP as children but have not received a booster dose of Td. Those who have received a booster of Td are still encouraged to receive Tdap for protection against pertussis. A combination series of Td and Tdap is recommended for those who have not completed their primary series. Adults in close contact with infants are advised to get Tdap to prevent pertussis in the infant.

Adults who have had a primary series should be vaccinated every 10 years (eg, mid decade is easy to remember; if the last childhood dose was at 15 years, vaccinate at ages 25, 35, 45, etc). Clean, minor wounds during the 10-year interval require no further vaccination. However, for a contaminated wound, the patient should receive a Td booster if it has been more than 5 years since the last booster. If immune status is unknown or lacking (specifically, no primary series), both toxoid (ie, Td) and immune globulin (ie, TIG), 250 units intramuscularly, should be given. Td is the preferred toxoid for an emergency as well as for routine vaccination. When Td and TIG are given in an emergency setting, they should be given in separate syringes at separate locations, but they may be given at the same time.

- Tetanus vaccination: the primary series is a 3-dose series.
- Adults who have had a primary series should receive a booster every 10 years.
- For a contaminated wound, the patient should receive a Td booster if it has been more than 5 years since the last booster.

● A patient with a contaminated wound and unknown or incomplete primary vaccination should receive both Td and TIG.

Side Effects
Td may be given in pregnancy, although it is desirable to wait until the second trimester. Maternal antibodies are passed to the infant transplacentally and confer passive immunity for several months after birth.

● Maternal antibodies are passed to the infant transplacentally.

A history of neurologic reaction, urticaria, anaphylaxis, or other severe hypersensitivity reaction is a contraindication to the readministration of toxoids. Skin testing may be performed if necessary. In the emergency setting, TIG may be used when tetanus toxoid or Td is contraindicated if other than a clean minor wound is sustained. Arthus-type hypersensitivity, a severe local reaction starting 2 to 8 hours after injection, often with fever and malaise, may occur in persons who have received multiple boosters. These people have very high levels of antitoxin and do not need boosters more frequently than every 10 years, even in the emergency setting.

Varicella
Primary infection with varicella zoster virus (VZV) results in chickenpox, and recurrent infection produces herpes zoster or shingles. Factors associated with recurrent disease include aging, immunosuppression, and intrauterine exposure to VZV and varicella at a young age (<18 months).

Complications of VZV infection, which occur more commonly in older children and adults, include bacterial infection of lesions, viral or secondary bacterial pneumonia, central nervous system manifestations (aseptic meningitis and encephalitis), hospitalization, and death.

Varicella vaccination is recommended for all children between 12 and 18 months old. It is also recommended for nonimmune adolescents and adults who are at highest risk of exposure and those most likely to transmit varicella to others. These groups include health care workers, family members of immunocompromised persons, teachers of young children, women of childbearing age, military personnel, persons working in institutional settings, and international travelers.

Persons older than 13 should receive 2 doses of varicella vaccine 4 to 8 weeks apart. Vaccine contraindications include severe allergy to neomycin, moderate or severe illness, immunosuppression, pregnancy, and recent receipt of a blood product. Adverse events following vaccination include injection site lesions, swelling, or pain; generalized varicella-like rash; and systemic reaction with fever. There is a risk of transmission of vaccine virus from a vaccinated person, especially with vaccine-associated rash, to a susceptible contact. However, this potential risk is low, and the benefits of vaccinating susceptible health care workers are thought to outweigh this risk. Protection of high-risk individuals who cannot be vaccinated (eg, an adult with immunodeficiency disease) involves vaccination of household and other close contacts.

Prevaccination serologic testing of adolescents and adults is probably cost-effective. Postvaccination testing is not necessary because of the high rate of seropositivity after 2 doses of vaccine (>99%).

Postexposure use of varicella vaccine is effective in preventing or modifying disease when given up to 3 to 5 days after exposure. Antiviral medication (acyclovir) is thought to be effective for preventing or modifying disease when started within a week of exposure. In 2006, the FDA licensed Zostavax, a live attenuated VZV vaccine for the prevention of herpes zoster (shingles) in individuals 60 years or older. It is contraindicated in pregnant women; individuals with a history of anaphylactic or anaphylactoid reactions to gelatin, neomycin, or other components of the vaccine; those with a history of primary or secondary immunodeficiency states or active tuberculosis; and those receiving immunosuppressive therapy. In a large study, vaccination with Zostavax prevented shingles in 50% of the subjects and reduced the incidence of postherpetic neuralgia in 67% of the study participants. Common side effects include inflammation, erythema, and soreness at the injection site.

Prevention of Chronic Diseases

Cardiovascular Disease
Cardiovascular mortality in the United States has decreased approximately 25% since 1975. Of this decrease, 45% is attributed to improvements in cardiovascular disease treatment and 55% to cardiovascular risk reduction, particularly the decline in smoking and the more aggressive treatment of hypertension. Despite advances in cardiovascular disease treatment and risk reduction strategies, cardiovascular disease remains the leading cause of death in most countries. The INTERHEART Study, a case-controlled study that evaluated risk factors in an international population of patients who experienced an acute myocardial infarction (MI) identified the following as contributing to 80% of this population's attributable risk: current smoking, elevated lipoprotein B levels (correlated to elevated low-density lipoprotein [LDL] cholesterol levels), type 2 diabetes mellitus, hypertension, and psychosocial stressors. Most of the cardiovascular risk (90% in men and 94% in women) was deemed to be due to potentially modifiable lifestyle factors. Cardiovascular risk reduction was correlated with daily consumption of fruits and vegetables, moderate to strenuous physical activity, and modest alcohol consumption.

● Modifiable lifestyle risk factors contribute up to 90% of the population attributable cardiovascular risk.

Risk Factors

Smoking
Smoking is a significant risk factor for cancer and cardiovascular disease. In the INTERHEART Study, 36% of the population risk for a first MI was attributed to smoking. A meta-analysis identified a 36% reduction in cardiac mortality among smokers with coronary heart disease who had quit smoking for at least 2 years. After smokers quit, the risk of a recurrent cardiac event decreases to that of nonsmokers within 3 years. Screening for nicotine use and a patient's readiness to quit should be verified at least annually on patient health care visits. Counseling strategies based on the Agency

for Health Care Policy and Research clinical practice guidelines use the mnemonic *5 As* (*a*sk, *a*dvise, *a*ssess attempts to quit, *a*ssist, and *a*rrange). (Please refer to Chapter 8, "General Internal Medicine," for details.)

- The risk of a cardiovascular event in a former smoker approaches that of a nonsmoker after 3 years of smoking abstinence.

Lipids

In the INTERHEART Study, 49% of the population risk for a first MI was attributed to dyslipidemia. Several primary prevention trials have demonstrated the effectiveness of lipid modification therapy on decreasing LDL cholesterol and triglycerides and increasing high-density lipoprotein (HDL) cholesterol, thus decreasing cardiovascular and cerebrovascular events. The West of Scotland Coronary Prevention Study demonstrated a 31% to 38% cardiovascular event reduction in patients treated with a statin. The number needed to treat ranged from 17 to 66, according to the baseline cardiovascular risk. The estimated cost published in 1999 was $25,000 per life-years gained.

The USPSTF recommends lipid screening for men aged 35 or older, for women aged 45 or older, and for any adult aged 20 or older who has additional cardiovascular disease risk factors (eg, diabetes mellitus, family history of premature cardiovascular disease or dyslipidemia, hypertension, or smoking). National Cholesterol Education Program Third Adult Treatment Panel (NCEP ATP III) guidelines of 2001 recommend screening adults age 20 or older every 5 years. Cholesterol target goals for high-risk populations were modified in 2004. Additional discussion on cardiovascular risk stratification, identification of lipid targets, and treatment strategies are provided in other chapters of this book (Chapter 3, "Cardiology"; Chapter 6, "Endocrinology"; and Chapter 8, "General Internal Medicine"). The National Heart Lung and Blood Institute Web site provides an interactive, 10-year acute coronary death or MI risk calculator.

- Primary prevention trials demonstrate an approximately 35% reduction in cardiovascular events with statin therapy.

Diabetes Mellitus

The USPSTF recommends fasting blood glucose screening for diabetes mellitus in adults who have hypertension or hyperlipidemia. Gestational diabetes glucose tolerance screening is recommended during pregnancy. Screening for diabetes mellitus in others should be based on assessment of individual risk factors. The American Diabetes Association recommends screening every 3 years. Strategies to reduce or delay progression to overt diabetes mellitus should be reviewed with the at-risk patient, particularly if impaired fasting glucose (ie, range, 101-125 mg/dL) is evident. Risk reduction strategies, which included weight loss, dietary modification, and exercise, demonstrated a 58% reduction in progression to overt diabetes mellitus during 4 years of follow-up in an at-risk population in the Diabetes Prevention Program. The number needed to treat in this trial was 6.9.

In the INTERHEART Study, 10% of the population risk for a first MI was attributed to diabetes. The Diabetes Control and Complications Trial demonstrated that, compared with conventional treatment of type 1 diabetes mellitus, intensive treatment reduced fatal and serious nonfatal cardiovascular events by 57%.

The data from similar clinical trials involving patients with type 2 diabetes mellitus are variable in supporting a positive effect of intense glucose management on cardiovascular risk. Additional discussion of the diagnosis and treatment of diabetes is provided in Chapter 6 ("Endocrinology").

- Dietary modification, exercise, and weight loss can reduce the risk of diabetes mellitus in an at-risk population by up to 58%.

Hypertension

The relationship between blood pressure and cardiovascular risk is continuous. Adverse sequelae due to elevated blood pressure are noted in an incrementally increasing rate at blood pressure values above 115/75 mm Hg. In the INTERHEART Study, 18% of the population risk for first MI was attributed to hypertension. A reduction of 30% to 39% in strokes and a reduction of 20% to 28% in cardiac events in patients whose hypertension was treated to reach target values were reported by the Blood Pressure Lowering Treatment Trialists' Collaboration. The calculated number needed to treat was 11 men and 21 women to prevent 1 coronary heart disease event.

Blood pressure screening recommendations, diagnosis, and treatment are outlined in detail in Chapter 14 ("Hypertension"). *The Seventh Report of the Joint National Committee on Prevention, Detection, Evaluation, and Treatment of High Blood Pressure (JNC7)* guidelines recommend blood pressure measurement at least every 2 years in adults who have a blood pressure of 120/80 or lower. More frequent blood pressure measurements, perhaps leading to diagnostic tests and treatment strategies through lifestyle modification or medication, are indicated at higher values.

- Adverse sequelae due to high blood pressure are noted incrementally at blood pressure values above 115/75 mm Hg.

Psychosocial Stressors

Psychosocial stressors have been correlated with cardiovascular risk, but data quantifying this risk vary. Psychosocial stressors were identified as contributing to 33% of the population attributable risk in the INTERHEART Study. The USPSTF recommends screening for depression if follow-up intervention can be arranged. Screening can be simplified into 2 questions:

1. During the past 2 weeks have you persistently felt down, depressed, or hopeless?
2. During the past 2 weeks have you had little pleasure or interest in doing things?

An expanded discussion on the diagnosis and treatment of mood disorders is provided in Chapter 22 ("Psychiatry").

Obesity

According to the INTERHEART Study, for the first MI, abdominal obesity correlates with a population attributable risk of 21% and lack of daily intake of fruits and vegetables, 13.7%. In the Framingham Study population, the risk of heart failure was 2.1 in obese men and 1.5 in obese women over a 14-year time frame. The risk of atrial fibrillation was 1.5 in the same study population. The estimates of obesity-correlated stroke risk were 2.0 for men and

2.4 for women. Both obesity and weight gain in adulthood were strongly correlated with an increased risk of type 2 diabetes mellitus. Years of life lost due to obesity were 5 in young black women, 8 in young white women, 13 in young black men, and 20 in young white men.

Intentional weight loss improves lipid levels, lowers high blood pressure, and reduces the risk of diabetes. Intentional weight loss in women with obesity-related health conditions has been associated with a 40% to 50% reduction in cancer mortality, a 30% to 40% reduction in diabetes-related mortality, and a 20% reduction in all-cause mortality. In those with no preexisting illness, a 9-kg intentional weight loss was correlated with a 25% reduction in all-cause mortality. The USPSTF recommends intensive dietary counseling for those who have hyperlipidemia or risk factors for cardiovascular or other diet-related chronic disease.

The USPSTF recommends screening all adults for obesity. Typically, weight and BMI are used on the basis of their ease of measurement. However, an elevated waist circumference or a waist to hip ratio is more closely correlated with cardiovascular and diabetes risk. Targets are a BMI less than 25, a wasit to hip ratio less than 0.9 in men and less than 0.8 in women, and a waist circumference less than 40 inches (100 cm) in men and 35 inches (88 cm) in women. The USPSTF recommends that intensive counseling ($\geq$2 sessions per month) and behavior intervention be offered to obese patients. Counseling strategies may incorporate the 5 A's behavior counseling framework described in Chapter 8 ("General Internal Medicine").

- Obesity increases the risk of diabetes, cardiovascular events, heart failure, atrial fibrillation, and many cancers.

Physical Activity

Both obesity and physical inactivity are correlated with increased cardiovascular risk. Approximately 200,000 deaths per year in the United States are attributed to a sedentary lifestyle. Lack of cardiovascular fitness has been associated with an all-cause mortality of 2.76 and a cardiovascular mortality of 3.09. Physical activity has an integral role in reducing one's risk of cardiovascular disease, type 2 diabetes, and obesity. A 12.2% reduction in first MI risk was identified in the INTER-HEART Study population among those who were physically active 4 or more hours a week. The percentage of Americans who participated in light to vigorous physical activity for at least 20 minutes at least 3 times a week decreased from 31.2% to 29.7% between 2000 and 2005. However, thus far there is a lack of data indicating a positive effect of counseling on patient activity behavior. Healthy People 2010 targets include a reduction in the physically inactive US population to 20% or less and an increase to more than 30% in the population of those who exercise at least 20 minutes at least 3 times a week.

- Lack of cardiovascular fitness is correlated with cardiovascular and all-cause mortality.

Screening Tests

Novel Cardiovascular Risk Markers
Since 30% of acute cardiac events occur in people without readily apparent cardiovascular risk factors, there has been an ongoing impetus to identify additional cardiovascular risk markers. Lipoprotein (a) cholesterol, LDL cholesterol particle concentration analysis, and apolipoprotein B are testing strategies to identify an elevation in the atherogenic component of LDL cholesterol. Elevations of lipoprotein (a) and lipoprotein (a) cholesterol, which are often familial, have been correlated with an increased cardiovascular risk in some studies of dyslipidemia. Elevated small dense LDL particle concentration and elevated apolipoprotein B, which often are evident in patients with diabetes or metabolic syndrome, have been correlated with increased cardiovascular risk. High-sensitivity C-reactive protein, an inflammatory marker, has been identified as a moderate predictor of coronary artery disease, particularly in women. Statin therapy lowers both the high-sensitivity C-reactive protein and the LDL cholesterol

Thus far, screening for these markers has not been supported as a population screening modality. However, patients with an intermediate cardiovascular risk (ie, 10%-20% according to the Framingham Study assessment) might be screened to assess the need for intensification of cardiovascular risk reduction strategies.

Coronary Artery Calcification
Calcium is progressively incorporated in atherosclerotic plaques. The presence of calcium in coronary arteries as identified by coronary artery CT is an indicator of developing coronary artery disease. For identifying more than 50% stenosis in age- and gender-ranked patients, coronary artery CT has a sensitivity of 81% in men and 76% in women and a specificity of 77% in men and 77% in women. However, cholesterol plaque that does not yet contain calcium is not identified on CT without intravenous contrast media. Typically, less coronary artery calcium is identified in blacks who have significant cardiovascular risk factors. The MESA (Multi-Ethnic Study of Atherosclerosis) Web site provides a risk calculator to estimate risk based on gender, ethnicity, and coronary artery CT scan score. Although acute coronary events are due to rupture of an unstable plaque that might not contain calcium, patients who have calcium-containing plaques typically have additional noncalcium plaques. Some studies indicate that the calcium score provides additional identification of high-risk individuals beyond that proved by the Framingham risk score. However, data on the effect of the calcium score on patient treatment and outcomes are conflicting.

Thus far, screening for coronary artery calcium is not recommended for the general population. However, the discussion on coronary artery CT scanning in the asymptomatic patient continues.

Twelve-Lead Resting Electrocardiography and Exercise Stress Test
A relative risk range of 2 to 4 for a cardiac event has been associated with an abnormal resting electrocardiogram (ECG). The 12-lead ECG has a sensitivity of 32% and a specificity of 87%. Thus the 12-lead ECG has limited utility in screening an asymptomatic person who has no significant cardiovascular risk factors.

The exercise treadmill stress test has a sensitivity of 68% and a specificity of 77%. The PPV of an abnormal stress test for a cardiac event ranges from 6% to 48%. The use of a treadmill stress test for screening purposes in an asymptomatic person with no significant cardiovascular risk factors is not supported by the USPSTF or the

American College of Cardiology and American Heart Association. However, screening may be considered for a patient who has significant cardiovascular risk factors and plans to embark on a vigorous exercise program or for a patient who would put others at risk if a sudden cardiac event occurred (eg, a bus driver).

Chemoprophylaxis

Aspirin

Daily low-dose aspirin prophylaxis results in a 44% reduction in MI and a 17% reduction in strokes in women. The USPSTF recommends that men aged 40 or older and postmenopausal women consider low-dose aspirin prophylaxis if the individual's calculated 10-year Framingham risk is 6% or more. The potential benefits in cardiovascular risk reduction should be weighed against the risk of gastrointestinal tract or intracranial bleeding. An aspirin dose of 75 to 81 mg is sufficient.

* Daily low-dose aspirin prophylaxis is recommended for men aged 40 or older and for postmenopausal women who have an estimated 10-year cardiovascular or cerebrovascular event risk of ≥6%.

ω-3 Fatty Acids

ω-3 Fatty acids supplementation has been shown to lower triglycerides by 10% to 33% in a dose-dependent manner. In addition, the Kuopio Ischemic Heart Disease Risk Factor Study demonstrated a 44% risk reduction in acute coronary events in a prospective population study of men with no known cardiovascular disease.

Vitamins

In general the use of vitamins, including vitamin E, folate, and antioxidants, has not been proved to be of benefit in cardiovascular or cancer risk reduction. However, folic acid supplementation in women who could become pregnant reduces infant neural tube defects by an estimated 41% to 85%. Niacin can increase HDL cholesterol by 20% to 35% in a dose-dependent fashion. In the Age-Related Eye Disease Study, antioxidants and zinc supplementation reduced progression to advanced age-related macular degeneration and vision loss in patients who had developing macular degeneration. Targeted vitamin supplementation should be considered for those at risk of deficiency (eg, related to alcoholism, bariatric surgery, and chronic renal insufficiency). A target of 5 servings of vegetables and fruit per day is the preferred recommendation for the general population.

* Women who can become pregnant should take folic acid supplementation to decrease the risk of fetal neural tube defects.

Osteoporosis

Screening, diagnosis, and treatment are discussed in Chapter 6 ("Endocrinology") and Chapter 10 ("Geriatrics"). The USPSTF recommends screening all women at age 65 and those at increased risk between ages 60 and 64. Risk factors include weight less than 127 lb (58 kg), corticosteroid use (>7.5 mg prednisolone for >3 months), family history, chronically low levels of estradiol in women or testosterone in men, and chronically low calcium and vitamin D intake. Medicare currently partially covers bone mineral density screening in women and men who are at risk.

A target of a daily vitamin D intake of 400 international units has not clearly shown benefit in fracture risk reduction. However, a target of a vitamin D intake of 800 international units has been shown to reduce the risk of hip fracture by 26% and the risk of falls by 22% in an elderly ambulatory population. Calcium supplementation attenuates menopausal and age-related bone density loss.

* Osteoporosis screening is recommended for women at age 65 or at age 60 and older if additional risk factors are present.

Abdominal Aortic Aneurysm

Abdominal aortic aneurysm risks include male gender, age older than 65, personal history of smoking, and family history involving a first-degree relative. The USPSTF recommends a 1-time abdominal aortic aneurysm screening in men aged 65 to 75 who have ever smoked. Abdominal ultrasonography for abdominal aortic aneurysm screening has a sensitivity of 95% and a specificity of nearly 100%. Among men who have smoked, the number needed to screen is 500. Surgical repair of a 5.5-cm abdominal aortic aneurysm results in an estimated 43% reduction in abdominal aortic aneurysm–specific mortality.

* One-time abdominal aortic aneurysm screening is recommended for men age 65 or older who have smoked.

Injury Prevention

Unintentional injuries were the fifth leading cause of death among adults and infants in the United States in 2004. They were the leading cause of death among persons aged 1 to 39 years, the second leading cause of death among persons aged 40 to 44 years, and the third leading cause of death among males and among Hispanics as a whole. Although motor vehicle crashes were the leading cause of injury, the number of accident-related deaths has declined since 1990. Presumed factors include child safety seats, seat belts, air bags, reduction in alcohol-impaired driving (attributed to public safety campaigns and law enforcement strategies), and changes in vehicle and roadway design.

In 2004, 39% of fatal traffic crashes were alcohol related, accounting for the loss of 40 years of potential life. Nonalcohol-related fatal traffic crashes resulted in the loss of 38 to 39 years of potential life. The USPSTF recommends screening for alcohol misuse and behavioral counseling to reduce alcohol misuse in adults. Additional information on screening and management of alcohol dependence is provided in Chapter 22 ("Psychiatry").

Age-related deaths due to firearms and poisoning, which includes illicit drug use, were the second and third leading causes, respectively, of accidental deaths in the United States in 2004. Assault was the fourth leading cause of death among children aged 1 to 14 years, and the second leading cause of death among persons aged 15 to 29. Suicide was the third leading cause of death among persons aged 10 to 29 and the second leading cause of death among persons aged 30 to 34.

- Unintentional injuries, assault, and suicide are significant health issues.

Acknowledgments

Sudhakar P. Karlapudi, MBBS, is acknowledged for background research on this chapter. Sally J. Trippel, MD, MPH, is acknowledged for her extensive work on this chapter in previous editions.

Questions

Multiple Choice (choose the best answer)

1. Which of these patients should be advised to have a screening colonoscopy?

   1. Patient 1—a 48-year-old asymptomatic man with no personal or family history of colon cancer or colon polyps
   2. Patient 2—a 48-year-old woman whose 52-year-old brother had an adenomatous colon polyp diagnosed last year
   3. Patient 3—a 48-year-old man whose paternal grandfather died of colon cancer at age 55
   4. Patient 4—a 48-year-old woman whose brother had an adenomatous polyp at age 60 and whose father died of colon cancer at age 65

   a. Patients 1 and 4
   b. Patients 2 and 3
   c. Patients 3 and 4
   d. Patients 2 and 4
   e. Patients 1 and 2

2. A 55-year-old man comes into the urgent care clinic at your medical facility with a hand laceration. He accidentally cut his finger with a kitchen knife while preparing to slice vegetables. He has a 1.5-cm laceration on the palmar surface of his left middle finger, overlying the proximal phalanx. Flexor tendon and vascular structures are intact. He has no record of prior tetanus vaccinations but believes that he probably had "baby shots" because his mother was a nurse. He served in the US Army during the Vietnam War and recalls getting many vaccinations while in basic training. He cannot recall getting any vaccinations since leaving military service. You clean and suture the laceration. Which of the following do you recommend for tetanus prophylaxis?

   a. No tetanus prophylaxis because this is a clean, minor wound
   b. Tetanus-diphtheria (Td) booster injection
   c. Tetanus immune globulin (TIG)
   d. TIG and Td booster injection

   e. No tetanus prophylaxis because he should have had a primary series while in military service and possibly also during infancy

3. A 28-year-old Somali woman comes into your office for a refugee health evaluation. A tuberculin (PPD) skin test shows 10 mm of induration after 48 hours. She spent 1 year in a refugee camp in northern Kenya and then 5 years in a private residence in Nairobi, Kenya, before immigrating to the United States. She is not aware of exposure to anyone with active pulmonary tuberculosis (TB). She denies TB symptoms. Physical examination findings are normal. Chest radiography shows fibrotic changes in both upper lobes and a nodule in the right upper lobe. What do you recommend?

   a. No further evaluation or treatment
   b. PPD skin test repeated in 2 weeks
   c. Chest radiography repeated in 12 months
   d. Induced sputum specimens for mycobacterial smear and culture daily for 3 days
   e. Isoniazid (INH), 300 mg daily for 9 months

4. A 35-year-old man is concerned about possible rabies exposure. Approximately 3 months ago he was staying in a cabin in northern Minnesota and awoke during the night with a bat flying around the bedroom. He killed the bat with a tennis racket, picked it up with his hands, and disposed of it in a garbage can. He recently spoke with a friend about the incident, and his friend mentioned that bats can carry rabies. He cannot recall if he had any cuts, abrasions, or other skin breaks on his hands when he handled the bat. He is currently asymptomatic. What do you recommend?

   a. No further evaluation or treatment because he has remained healthy for 3 months after exposure
   b. Rabies immune globulin administered intramuscularly in the buttocks
   c. Three doses of rabies vaccine: the first dose today and additional doses in 7 and 21 or 28 days

d. Five doses of rabies vaccine: the first dose today and additional doses in 3, 7, 14, and 28 to 35 days

e. Rabies immune globulin administered intramuscularly in the buttocks and 5 doses of rabies vaccine: the first dose today and additional doses in 3, 7, 14, and 28 to 35 days

5. A 28-year-old woman is concerned about possible exposure to chickenpox. She has never had chickenpox. Varicella serology was negative 1 year ago. She did not receive varicella vaccine because she was trying to become pregnant when the serology results were available. Three days ago she visited a family that recently immigrated to the United States. A child in the family had an illness with skin lesions, which was subsequently diagnosed as chickenpox. The patient had a couple of days of spotting at her last 2 menstrual periods instead of her usual 5- to 7-day menstrual flow. A urine pregnancy test is positive. What do you recommend?

a. A second varicella serology

b. Postexposure varicella vaccination

c. Varicella zoster immune globulin (VZIG)

d. Acyclovir immediately (80 mg/kg daily in 4 divided doses)

e. No further evaluation or treatment

6. A 65-year-old man requests the following tests to screen for cardiovascular disease: an exercise treadmill cardiac stress test, carotid ultrasonography, a screening coronary artery CT scan, and abdominal aorta aneurysm ultrasonography. He had a 40-pack-year smoking history, having quit smoking at age 55. His body mass index is 24. His blood pressure is 118/72 mm Hg without antihypertensive medication. He exercises 60 minutes 4 times a week. Which screening test is currently recommended by the US Preventive Services Task Force?

a. Carotid ultrasonography

b. Coronary artery CT scan

c. Abdominal aorta ultrasonography

d. Cardiac treadmill stress test

e. Serum homocysteine estimation

7. A 38-year-old man comes in for further evaluation of several episodes of dysuria. He completed a 7-day course of doxycycline (100 mg twice daily) for chlamydial urethritis 6 weeks ago. He admits to having vaginal intercourse with a new female sexual partner 7 to 8 weeks ago. He admits to having 3 other female sexual partners during the past 5 years. Genital examination findings are unremarkable. Voided urinalysis shows 20 to 30 white blood cells and no bacteria. Gram stain and culture of a urine specimen are negative. A first-voided urine specimen is negative for *Chlamydia trachomatis* and *Neisseria gonorrhoeae* by amplified DNA testing. A subsequent urethral swab specimen is negative for *C trachomatis* and *N gonorrhoeae* as well as for herpes simplex virus (on polymerase chain reaction testing). Prostatic fluid culture is positive for *Ureaplasma urealyticum*. You recommend treatment for *Ureaplasma* prostatitis with a course of ofloxacin. What else do you recommend?

a. No further testing or treatment

b. Human immunodeficiency virus (HIV)-1 and HIV-2 antibody test and syphilis serology

c. HIV-1 and HIV-2 antibody test, syphilis serology, and hepatitis B serologic testing

d. HIV-1 and HIV-2 antibody test, syphilis serology, and hepatitis B vaccination

e. HIV-1 and HIV-2 antibody test, syphilis serology, and hepatitis A and B vaccination

Answers

1.   Answer d.
The first and third patients should be screened at age 50, and if the screening is negative, screening should continue at intervals according to the screening strategy selected. Thus, if colonoscopy is used for screening, the next colonoscopy would be advised in 10 years. The second and fourth patients should undergo colonoscopy in their 40s, ideally 10 years before the index family case. If the colonoscopy is negative, the next screening colonoscopy is advised in 5 years.

2.   Answer b.
This patient has a clean, minor wound, which is not a tetanus-prone injury. Nonetheless, he requires a Td booster injection because it has been more than 10 years since he last received tetanus toxoid, which presumably would have been given during military service.

He does not require TIG because he has had 1 and possibly 2 primary series of tetanus toxoid.

3.   Answer d.
A PPD skin test reaction of 10 mm or more at 48 to 72 hours is considered positive for recent arrivals from countries with high TB prevalence. Therefore, this patient's initial skin test was positive. She had appropriate further screening for active tuberculosis, including questions about symptoms suggesting active TB as part of the medical history, a physical examination, and chest radiography. She has no symptoms or physical findings to suggest active tuberculosis. However, chest radiographic findings are abnormal, showing fibrotic changes in both upper lobes, suggesting old TB. In addition, she has a small nodule in the right upper lobe. She would be a candidate

for INH therapy, 300 mg daily for 9 months, as treatment for latent TB infection. However, before starting this treatment, further evaluation is necessary to rule out active pulmonary tuberculosis as a cause for the indeterminate nodule in her right upper lobe. Further evaluation should include induced sputum specimens for mycobacterial smear and culture daily for 3 days. If induced sputum tests are negative, further evaluation should be considered with CT of the chest, bronchoscopy, or chest radiography repeated in 3 to 6 months. Waiting 12 months to repeat chest radiography would not be an appropriate initial evaluation, because the patient could spread tuberculosis in the community while awaiting follow-up chest radiography if she has active pulmonary tuberculosis. It is important to consider active tuberculosis in individuals who have resided in countries of high TB prevalence. Further evaluation for active pulmonary or extrapulmonary tuberculosis is always appropriate in the presence of suspicious symptoms, physical findings, or radiographic findings, regardless of PPD status.

4. Answer e.

Insectivorous bats in the upper Midwest of the United States are known to be a reservoir of rabies virus. This patient has had a potential exposure. He is uncertain about skin cuts or breaks on his hands when he handled the bat 3 months ago. The bat is not available for rabies testing. The incubation period for rabies is usually 3 to 8 weeks, but it can be as short as 9 days or as long as 7 years. The incubation period for rabies depends on many factors, including wound severity, location of wound site in relation to nerve supply and distance from the brain, viral inoculum, protection provided by clothing, and possible other factors. In this situation, the safest course would be to provide immediate protection with rabies immune globulin and a full 5-dose series of rabies vaccine. Administration of rabies immune globulin alone would not provide adequate long-term protection against rabies. The 3-dose series of rabies vaccine is recommended only for preexposure vaccination before prolonged travel or residence in countries with hyperendemic rabies and for veterinarians, animal control officials, and others with potential occupational exposure to rabid animals. The 5-dose series of rabies vaccine administered without rabies immune globulin would not provide adequate short-term immunity while awaiting development of an active immune response in the patient.

5. Answer c.

Primary varicella zoster infection often causes more severe symptoms in nonimmune adults, including high fever and constitutional symptoms. In addition, primary infection in adults is associated with an increased risk of complications, including pneumonia, encephalitis, and death. Secondary bacterial infection of vesicles may result in necrotizing fasciitis or septicemia. In addition, infection early in pregnancy may result in congenital varicella syndrome (low birth weight, atrophy of extremities with skin scarring, and neurologic abnormalities). Administration of varicella zoster immune globulin within 96 hours of exposure may prevent or modify disease in a susceptible close contact of a patient with known chickenpox or herpes zoster. Waiting for the results of varicella serology would delay administration of VZIG and possibly decrease its effectiveness. Postexposure varicella vaccination would not be appropriate in this setting because a live virus vaccine is contraindicated during pregnancy. Treatment with acyclovir would be appropriate if the patient had symptoms of chickenpox, which typically occurs after an incubation period of 2 to 3 weeks.

6. Answer c.

The risk of a large abdominal aortic aneurysm is increased in men, in persons who have a family history of abdominal aortic aneurysms, and in current or former smokers. Screening and repair of an aneurysm 5.5 cm or greater is estimated to reduce cause-specific mortality by 43%. The other screening tests might be considered from this man's cardiovascular risk profile. However, no significant decrease in cardiovascular mortality has been attributed to use of these screening tests to guide risk reduction therapy.

7. Answer d.

The patient admits to having multiple sexual partners during the past 5 years. He has had 2 recent sexually transmitted infections. Therefore, it would be appropriate to recommend testing for other sexually transmitted diseases, including HIV-1, HIV-2, and syphilis. The Centers for Disease Control and Prevention (CDC) national immunization strategy to eliminate transmission of hepatitis B virus (HBV) infection includes vaccination of adolescents and adults at increased risk of infection. This includes persons with a history of a sexually transmitted disease and persons who have had multiple sexual partners. Prevaccination serologic testing may be cost-effective in adult populations with a high prevalence of hepatitis B virus infection, which includes injectable drug users, men who have sex with men, sexual contacts of persons with chronic HBV infection, and persons from countries with endemic HBV infection. The CDC currently recommends hepatitis A vaccination for men who have sex with men (including those who report having minimal or no current sexual activity) but not for heterosexual men.

22

Psychiatry

Bruce Sutor, MD

An understanding of psychiatric illness is critical to the practice of internal medicine. Since 30% to 40% of ambulatory primary care visits have a psychiatric component to the chief complaint, successful disease management often hinges on successful treatment of comorbid psychiatric illness. A comprehensive psychiatric evaluation is essential because many psychiatric symptoms are nonspecific. This situation is analogous to a patient presenting in general internal medicine with fever or nausea. The presence of a single symptom (eg, depressed mood) is never pathognomonic of a specific disorder. All psychiatric disorders are based on a set of inclusion and exclusion criteria outlined in the *Diagnostic and Statistical Manual of Mental Disorders (DSM)*, which is periodically updated by the American Psychiatric Association. For patients with psychiatric symptoms, the biopsychosocial model is widely used. With this approach, the biologic, psychologic, and social factors contributing to the patient's clinical presentation are evaluated. Some psychiatric symptoms indicate severe problems, whereas others are much less important to the extent that they may not be clinically relevant. A key concept is whether the symptom interferes with a patient's functioning or causes distress. For example, a patient may have a fear of heights. If this acrophobia never causes an alteration in activity, then intervention likely is not necessary. However, if a patient hesitates to visit offices on higher floors of an office building, the distress during the visits or avoidance of these situations warrants intervention.

The common psychiatric disorders confronting general physicians in outpatient settings are anxiety disorders, mood disorders, substance abuse, somatoform disorders, adjustment disorders, and dementia. In the general hospital setting, the common psychiatric conditions are mood disorders, adjustment disorders, substance abuse, delirium, and dementia. (Suicide, a leading cause of death in the United States, has been reported to occur in all psychiatric conditions.)

The Suicidal Patient

Emergency medicine physicians are often the first to deal with patients who have suicidal ideation or who have attempted or completed suicide. The recognition of risk factors for suicide, a thorough assessment of the psychiatric and medical factors, and urgent intervention are critically important. Although the patient who overdoses with a benzodiazepine may be very serious about the intent to die, the person who overdoses with acetaminophen is more at risk of serious medical complications.

Recognition of a suicidal gesture is essential in evaluating a patient in an emergency department. Although drug overdoses are the commonest form, alcohol intoxication, single-vehicle accidents, and falls from heights may merit further investigation. Many suicidal patients see a physician the week before the attempt. Some of the risk factors to be aware of include recent psychiatric hospitalization, an older divorced or widowed man, unemployment, poor physical health, past suicide attempts, family history of suicide (especially a parent), psychosis, alcoholism, drug abuse, chronic pain syndrome, sudden life changes, loneliness, and anniversary of significant loss. Almost without exception, patients come to an emergency department with intense suicidal ideation or gestures. These patients should not be sent home alone.

- In evaluating patients in an emergency department, it is important to recognize a suicidal gesture.
- Many patients see a physician the week before they attempt suicide.
- Patients who come to an emergency department with intense suicidal ideation or gestures should not be sent home alone.
- Typical clinical scenario: A 68-year-old, lonely, divorced man has a sudden life change.

Mood Disorders

Mood disorders are common, with a prevalence of 8% in the general US population, and are divided into the following subtypes:
1. Depressive disorders
   a) Major depression
   b) Dysthymia
2. Bipolar disorders (manic depression)
   a) Bipolar I
   b) Bipolar II
   c) Cyclothymia
3. Substance-induced mood disorders due to a medical condition

a) Depression
b) Hypomania, mania

The essential feature of mood disorders is a disturbance of mood in the context of symptoms related to cognitive, psychomotor, vegetative, and interpersonal difficulties. Mood disorders may also be related to a general medical condition or be substance induced.

* Mood disorders: the essential feature is disturbance of mood in a constellation of other symptoms.
* Mood disorders are accompanied by related cognitive, psychomotor, vegetative, and interpersonal difficulties.
* Mood disorders may also be related to a general medical condition or be substance induced.

Depressive Disorders

Major Depression

Major depression is a serious psychiatric disorder that must be distinguished from an adjustment disorder and dysthymia by the severity of the mood and cognitive disturbances and potentially by the presence of major physical somatic complaints. The primary symptoms of major depression include depressed mood, diminished interest or pleasure in many activities, notable weight loss or weight gain (>5% of body weight in a month), decrease or increase in appetite, insomnia or hypersomnia, psychomotor agitation or retardation, fatigue or loss of energy, feelings of worthlessness or of excessive or inappropriate guilt, diminished ability to concentrate, recurrent thoughts of death or suicidal ideation, or a suicide attempt. These must be present for at least 2 weeks. This time frame helps in differentiating major depression from acute changes in mood seen in delirium or medical processes (eg, acute blood loss).

If delusions or hallucinations are also present, they are less prominent than in a primary psychotic disorder, and the disorder is referred to as *major depression with psychotic features*. The presence of psychotic symptoms increases the likelihood of treatment resistance. Another severe type of major depression is the melancholic type. In addition to the symptoms listed above, this form is characterized by the lack of reactivity to pleasurable stimuli (does not feel better even temporarily if involved in what is usually a pleasurable activity), diurnal mood variation (depression regularly worse in the morning), and early morning awakening (≥2 hours before the usual time of awakening).

* Major depression: symptoms include depressed mood, diminished interest or pleasure in all or almost all activities, and notable weight loss or weight gain.
* Major depression with psychotic features: presence of hallucinations or delusions, which are often subtle.
* Major depression, melancholic type: characterized by lack of reactivity to pleasurable stimuli, diurnal mood variation, and early morning awakening.
* Typical clinical scenario: A 43-year-old woman who has lost weight and has fatigue and feelings of worthlessness and excessive guilt is much less interested in many things that used to attract her. Her ability to concentrate has decreased.

The lifetime prevalence of depression is 20% for women and 12% for men. The peak age at onset of depression in women is 33 to 45 years and in men, more than 55 years. Among those who seek treatment from a physician, the diagnosis is not made in as many as one-third or sometimes it is a misdiagnosis because patients often present primarily with physical or somatic complaints. As the population ages and more elderly patients seek medical care, diagnosing and treating their mood disorders become more complicated because many of these patients often have overlapping medical and neurologic problems. Patients occasionally present with the combination of a dementing process and depression. When the depressive symptoms are treated effectively in these patients, cognitive performance may also improve.

* Among persons seeking treatment for major depression, the diagnosis is not made in as many as one-third or it is a misdiagnosis.
* In elderly patients, diagnosing and treating mood disorders become more complicated because of possible comorbid psychiatric and medical conditions.
* The prevalence of depression among women is twice as high as among men.

Seasonal affective disorder is a subtype of major depression usually characterized by the onset of depression in autumn or winter. It is twice as common in women as in men and is associated with psychomotor retardation, hypersomnia, overeating (carbohydrate craving), and weight gain. To establish the diagnosis, winter episodes of depression must recur for 3 or more consecutive years. These episodes must resolve during spring or summer. Treatment has relied primarily on phototherapy, using a full-spectrum light source of 10,000 lux, which must be used for a minimum of 30 minutes a day. Antidepressant agents are also of benefit in treating this disorder.

* Seasonal affective disorder: onset of depression in autumn or winter; it resolves in the spring.
* It is twice as common among women as among men.
* It is associated with psychomotor retardation, hypersomnia, and overeating.
* Treatment: phototherapy and antidepressant agents.
* Typical clinical scenario: A 45-year-old woman has had recurrent depression in the winter for three consecutive winters.

Postpartum depression affects 10% of mothers. Although it occurs in all socioeconomic groups, single or poor mothers are at greater risk. Left untreated, postpartum depression can adversely affect parent-child bonding and positive interaction between mother and child. Treatment with antidepressants, although effective, must be balanced with the possible effect on a developing fetus or breast-fed infant, but it is generally accepted that in moderate to severe depression, the risks of not treating depression outweigh the risk of treatment with most antidepressants. Prescribing clinicians should be cognizant of the pregnancy category of the agent they prescribe in this patient group.

* Postpartum depression affects 10% of mothers.

- Postpartum depression can be prevented in some women by taking antidepressants.
- Risks to the developing fetus or breast-fed infant must be taken into account when prescribing antidepressants to women in their reproductive years.

Because depressive disorders are heterogeneous in clinical presentation, the cause is expected to be multifactorial. There is probably no single etiologic agent. According to current theories, depression appears to be related to alterations of several neurotransmitter systems and neuropeptides, effects on presynaptic and postsynaptic receptors, neurohormonal alterations, and, in general, an alteration in the overall balance of these systems, which are interdependent on one another. Adverse life events (eg, marital discord, bankruptcy, professional setbacks, and failure) can initiate or perpetuate a depressive episode by overwhelming a person's coping mechanisms.

Dysthymia

Dysthymia is chronic depression that is milder in severity than major depression. It may have either an early onset or a late onset, as defined by onset before or after age 21 years. It can be disabling for the person because the depressed mood is present most of the time during at least a 2-year period. Many patients have 1 or 2 associated vegetative signs, such as disturbance of sleep and appetite. Also, patients often feel inadequate, have low self-esteem, and struggle with interpersonal relationships. If onset is in late adolescence, the dysthymia may become intertwined with the person's personality, behavior, and general attitude toward life. Treatment is usually a combination of psychotherapy (cognitive or interpersonal) and pharmacotherapy. Psychopharmacotherapy may be particularly useful for patients with a family history of mood disorders or for those who have the early-onset form of dysthymia. In patients with dysthymia, superimposed major depressive episodes may develop. Also, some are prone to turn to alcohol or other substance abuse to "treat" their dysphoria.

- Dysthymia: a form of chronic depression.
- Depressed mood is present most of the time during at least a 2-year period.
- Treatment is usually a combination of psychotherapy and pharmacotherapy.
- Major depressive episodes may develop in patients with dysthymia.
- Typical clinical scenario: A 25-year-old woman has had disturbed sleep, appetite changes, low self-esteem, and issues with interpersonal relationships for 3 years.

Adjustment Disorder With Depressed Mood

Adjustment disorder with depressed mood is a reaction that develops in response to an identifiable psychosocial stressor (eg, divorce, job loss, or family or marital problems). The severity of the adjustment disorder (degree of impairment) does not always parallel the intensity of the precipitating event. The critical factor appears to be the relevance of the event or stressor to the patient and his or her ability to cope with the stress. In general, these reactions are relatively transient. Although patients generally can be managed by an empathic primary care physician, the development of extreme withdrawal, suicidal ideation, or failure to improve as the circumstances improve may prompt psychiatric referral. Treatment includes supportive psychotherapy, psychosocial interventions, and, sometimes, use of antidepressant agents.

Treatment of Depression

There are 3 common major groups of treatment modalities for depression: psychotherapy, pharmacotherapy, and electroconvulsive therapy (ECT). Generally, these therapeutic modalities are used in some combination.

Psychotherapy

There are multiple forms of psychotherapy, many of which can be used in the treatment of depression. However, the 2 forms that have been used extensively for treating depression are cognitive therapy and interpersonal therapy. *Cognitive therapy* strives to help patients have a better integration of cognition (thoughts), emotion, and behavior. This therapy is based on the premise that thoughts have a profound effect on emotions, which have an effect on behavior. For example, if a patient repeatedly thinks that he or she is failing professionally because of striving for unrealistic, perfectionist goals, then over time that person's emotions and behavior will be affected. If patients can perceive themselves in more realistic or adaptive ways, their general outlook will be expected to improve. Ultimately, they may experience an increase in a sense of worth and self-esteem. *Interpersonal therapy* focuses on current interpersonal functioning. It is based on the concept that depression is associated with impaired social relationships that either precipitate or perpetuate the disorder.

- Cognitive therapy: helps patients achieve a better integration of cognition (thoughts), emotion, and behavior.
- Interpersonal therapy: focuses on current interpersonal functioning.

Pharmacotherapy

The selection of medication is based on the side-effect profile of the medication and the clinical profile of the patient (Table 22-1).

Initially, use a relatively low dose, and then titrate to a therapeutic dose based on clinical assessment. Blood level determinations of a drug are meaningful only for tricyclic antidepressants. The duration of treatment is usually a minimum of 6 to 12 months, counting from the time the patient attained noticeable improvement. Patients with a severe depressive episode or who have experienced 2 or more depressive episodes are at high risk of symptom recurrence if they are not receiving prophylactic medication. In such cases, continuing the use of antidepressants is advisable, but if use is discontinued, the patient should be monitored regularly for symptom recurrence. Antidepressant use should be tapered rather than stopped abruptly when treatment is discontinued. If the response to the first antidepressant agent is minimal, reevaluate the diagnosis, change to a different class of drug, or treat with ECT, which is still probably the most consistently effective treatment for severe depression. ECT is especially valuable if psychotic symptoms complicate the major depression. ECT is described in detail in the last section of this chapter.

Table 22-1 Commonly Used Antidepressants

Drug	Daily Dose Range, mg	Receptor Affinity	Comments
Tricyclic antidepressants			Obtain electrocardiogram
Imipramine	75-300	S, 5, H, α, M	Establish treatment dose through blood levels
Amitriptyline	75-300	S, 5, H, α, M	Helpful in neuropathic pain
Nortriptyline	75-300	N, H, α, M	
Doxepin	50-300	N, 5, H, α, M	
SSRIs			Dose of SSRIs should be titrated gradually when starting
Fluoxetine[a]	20-60	S	Taper gradually when stopping
Sertraline	75-200	S, D	Manage sexual side effects by avoiding use of SSRI
Paroxetine[a]	20-60	S, M[b]	with long half-life on weekends (use short half-life
Citalopram	20-60	S	agents only), addition of sustained-release form of
Escitalopram	10-20	S	bupropion 150 mg daily, & dose reduction
Venlafaxine[a]	75-375	S, N[b]	See the 3 items listed immediately above
			Can increase blood pressure
Bupropion[a]	300-450	D	Avoid in patients with seizure disorder or active eating disorders
			No sexual side effects
Mirtazapine	15-45	5, H	Few sexual side effects
			Low doses are more sedating than high doses
			Weight gain is common
Duloxetine	40-60	S, N	Also indicated for certain neuropathic pain problems

Abbreviations: α, $α_1$-adrenergic receptor; D, dopamine transporter; 5, 5-hydroxytryptamine$_{2A}$; M, muscarinic; N, norepinephrine transporter; S, serotonin transporter; SSRI, selective serotonin reuptake inhibitor.

[a] Available in extended-release forms.

[b] At high therapeutic doses.

Data from Richelson E. Pharmacology of antidepressants. Mayo Clin Proc. 2001;76:511-27.

Mania and Bipolar Disorder

The essential features of a manic episode are the presence of an abnormally euphoric, expansive, or irritable mood associated with some of the following features: inflated self-esteem or grandiosity, decreased need for sleep, pressured speech, flight of ideas, distractibility, increase in goal-directed activity or psychomotor agitation, and excessive involvement in pleasurable activities that have a high potential for painful consequences (eg, unrestrained buying sprees, sexual indiscretions, or inappropriate financial investments). These episodes must last a minimum of 1 week (unless the course is altered by treatment). To establish the diagnosis of bipolar disorder, the patient must have had at least 1 episode of mania. Most bipolar patients have had recurrent depressive episodes in addition to manic episodes, although rarely patients have mania exclusively. The prevalence of bipolar disorder is estimated to be about 1%. Bipolar disorder occurs about as frequently in women as in men, and the usual age at onset is from the teens to 30 years. A family history of bipolar or other mood disorder is more common for patients with bipolar disorder than for other mood disorders. Some patients do not experience a fully developed manic episode but have fewer symptoms. The term *hypomania*

has been introduced to describe this form of bipolar disorder (type II), which generally is challenging to clinicians because its more subtle features make it more difficult to recognize, and it may be confused with other psychiatric disorders.

- Mania: the essential feature is an abnormally euphoric, expansive, or irritable mood.
- The prevalence of bipolar disorder is estimated to be about 1%.
- Bipolar disorder occurs about as frequently in women as in men.
- The usual age at onset is from the teens to 30 years.
- A family history of bipolar or other mood disorder is more common for patients with bipolar disorder than for other mood disorders.
- Typical clinical scenario: For more than 1 week, a 25-year-old man has had a euphoric mood, flight of ideas, decreased need for sleep, and unrestrained buying sprees.

Treatment is aimed at mood stabilization with medication and improved social and occupational functioning. Pharmacotherapy of mania includes lithium carbonate, valproic acid, carbamazepine, and next-generation neuroleptics. Lithium has the added benefit of being useful in prevention or treatment of bipolar depression. Lamotrigine is also effective in treating bipolar depression. Patients with bipolar disorder and depression may be treated with ECT, lithium carbonate, lamotrigine, or an antidepressant (used simultaneously with a mood-stabilizing agent to prevent mania).

* Treatment of mania and bipolar disorder is aimed at stabilizing mood and improving social and occupational functioning.
* Primary pharmacologic treatment: lithium carbonate, valproic acid, carbamazepine, and next-generation neuroleptics.

Mood Disorders Caused by a General Medical Condition

The essential feature of mood disorders caused by a general medical condition is depression or mania—including potential depressive symptoms such as energy, sleep, and appetite changes—that is attributable to the physiologic effects of the specific medical condition. The full criteria for 1 of these episodes regarding the number of symptoms and time course need not be met. Many medical conditions may induce mood changes, so the clinical interview needs to identify coexisting symptoms such as excessive guilt, social withdrawal, or suicidal ideation, which are more specific for a depressive disorder. Medical conditions that may cause mood symptoms include endocrinopathies (Cushing syndrome, Addison disease, hyperthyroidism, hypothyroidism, hyperparathyroidism, and hypoparathyroidism), certain malignancies (lymphomas, pancreatic carcinoma, and astrocytomas), neurologic conditions (Parkinson disease and Huntington disease), autoimmune conditions (systemic lupus erythematosus), and infections (chronic hepatitis C, encephalitis, mononucleosis, and human immunodeficiency virus [HIV] infection).

* In mood disorders due to a general medical condition, the essential feature is a disturbance of mood attributable to the physiologic effects of a specific medical condition.
* Many medical conditions may induce mood changes, so the clinical interview needs to identify coexisting symptoms such as excessive guilt, social withdrawal, or suicidal ideation, which are more specific for a depressive disorder.
* Some potential depressive symptoms such as energy, sleep, and appetite changes may be due to a medical condition in the absence of a depressive disorder.

Substance-Induced Mood Disorders

The essential feature of a substance-induced mood disorder is a disturbance of mood, either depressed or manic, that is judged to be due to the direct physiologic effects of a substance. Many substances can induce mood changes, including medications, toxins, and drugs of abuse. The mood symptoms may occur during the use of or exposure to the substance or during withdrawal from the substance. Medications that have been implicated in inducing mood disturbances include corticosteroids, interferon, reserpine, methyldopa, carbonic anhydrase inhibitors, stimulants, sedative-hypnotics, benzodiazepines, and narcotics as well as the long-term use or abuse of alcohol or hallucinogens. Recent studies have demonstrated that β-adrenergic agents are less likely to cause depressive disorders than previously thought.

* In substance-induced mood disorders, the essential feature is a disturbance of mood due to the physiologic effects of a substance.
* Many medications and drugs of abuse may induce mood changes.

Anxiety Disorders

Anxiety disorders are encountered most frequently in the outpatient setting. Anxiety symptoms may be misinterpreted as those of medical illness because many of the symptoms overlap, (eg, tachycardia, diaphoresis, tremor, shortness of breath, nausea, abdominal pain, and chest pain). Autonomic arousal and anxious agitation in a medically ill patient can also be attributed quickly to stress or anxiety when the symptoms may represent pulmonary embolus or cardiac arrhythmia. Common sources of anxiety in the medical setting are related to fears of death, abandonment, loss of function, pain, dependency, and loss of control. When to treat or to seek psychiatric consultation depends on the assessment of the degree of anxiety. Is the patient able to function in his or her role without distress or avoidance?

* Anxiety symptoms may be misinterpreted as those of medical illness.
* Common sources of anxiety in the medical setting are related to fears of death, abandonment, loss of function, and pain.

Panic Disorder With or Without Agoraphobia

Panic disorder refers to recurrent, discrete episodes of extreme anxiety accompanied by various somatic symptoms such as dyspnea, unsteady feelings, palpitations, paresthesias, hyperventilation, trembling, diaphoresis, chest pain or discomfort, or abdominal distress. *Agoraphobia* refers to extreme fear of being in places or situations from which escape may be difficult or embarrassing. This may lead to avoidance of such situations as driving, travel in general, being in a crowded place, and many other situations, ultimately causing severe limitations in daily functioning for the patient. Panic disorder is more common in women (prevalence, 2%-3%) than in men (prevalence, 0.5%-1.5%). The usual age at onset is from the late teens to the early 30s. A history of childhood separation anxiety is reported in 20% to 50% of patients. The incidence is higher in first- and second-degree relatives. Most patients describe their first panic attack as spontaneous. They generally go to an emergency department after the first attack, believing they are having a heart attack or a severe medical problem.

* Panic disorder: recurrent, discrete episodes of extreme anxiety accompanied by various somatic symptoms.
* Agoraphobia: extreme fear of being in places or situations from which escape may be difficult.
* Panic disorder is more common in women than in men.
* Patients generally go to an emergency department after their first panic attack, believing they are having a heart attack or a severe medical problem.

Patients with panic attacks may be prone to episodes of major depression. The differential diagnosis of panic disorder includes several medical disorders, such as endocrine disturbances (eg, hyperthyroidism, pheochromocytoma, and hypoglycemia), gastrointestinal tract disturbances (eg, colitis and irritable bowel syndrome), cardiopulmonary disturbances (eg, pulmonary embolism, exacerbation of chronic obstructive pulmonary disease, and acute allergic reactions), and neurologic conditions (especially conditions like seizures that are episodic or are associated with paresthesias, faintness, or dizziness).

Several substances of abuse may cause or exacerbate anxiety symptoms. Stimulants (eg, cocaine, amphetamines, and caffeine) can fuel anxiety, as can withdrawal from sedating agents (eg, alcohol, benzodiazepines, and narcotics). Patients may use alcohol or benzodiazepines to prevent or treat panic symptoms, but regular or high-dose use may result in a cycle of tolerance and withdrawal, paradoxically causing an increase in anxiety symptoms.

Treatment with antidepressants, cognitive behavioral therapy, benzodiazepines, or a combination of these modalities is effective for most patients.

* Patients with panic attacks may be prone to episodes of major depression.
* Alcohol and benzodiazepines may reduce the distress of panic attacks, but symptoms may rebound, potentially leading to the abuse of these substances.

Posttraumatic Stress Disorder

Posttraumatic stress disorder can be a brief reaction that follows an extremely traumatic, overwhelming, or catastrophic experience, or it may be a chronic condition that produces severe disability. The syndrome is characterized by intrusive memories, flashbacks, nightmares, avoidance of reminders of the event, and often a restricted range of affect. It may occur in adults or children. There is increased comorbidity with substance abuse, depression, and other anxiety disorders. Patients may be more prone to impulsivity, including suicide. As for other anxiety disorders, treatment is usually a combination of behavioral, psychotherapeutic, and, if necessary, pharmacologic interventions.

* Posttraumatic stress disorder may be a brief reaction or a chronic condition that produces severe disability.
* Patients may be prone to impulsivity, including suicide.
* Typical clinical scenario: A 30-year-old man who is a military veteran has flashbacks, nightmares, and depression.

Generalized Anxiety Disorder

Generalized anxiety disorder is characterized by chronic excessive anxiety and apprehension about life circumstances accompanied by somatic symptoms of anxiety, such as trembling, restlessness, autonomic hyperactivity, and hypervigilance. Treatment is usually a mixture of behavioral, progressive muscle relaxation, psychotherapeutic, and adjunctive psychopharmacologic modalities.

Obsessive-Compulsive Disorder

Obsessive-compulsive disorder is characterized by recurrent obsessions or compulsions that are severe enough to disrupt daily life. The obsessions are distressing thoughts, ideas, or impulses experienced as unwanted. Compulsions are repetitive, intentional behaviors usually performed in response to an obsession. The obsessions cause

marked anxiety or distress, and the compulsions serve to neutralize the anxiety. Prevalence rates are about 2% to 3% and are about equal in men and women. The onset of this disorder is usually in adolescence or early adulthood. Obsessive traits are often present before onset of the disorder. The predominant neurobiologic theory for the cause of obsessive-compulsive disorder involves dysfunction of brain serotonin systems. Pharmacologic treatment of this disorder is with antidepressants that are more selective for effects on the serotonin transmission system. These include clomipramine and selective serotonin reuptake inhibitors (SSRIs) (fluvoxamine, fluoxetine, paroxetine, and sertraline); occasionally, lithium or neuroleptic augmentation is used with any of these agents. In extremely severe, debilitating cases for which other treatments have failed, neurosurgical procedures such as cingulotomy, stereotactic limbic leukotomy, or anterior capsulotomy may be of some benefit. The effectiveness of these procedures is thought to be related to disruption of the efferent pathways from the frontal cortex to the basal ganglia. Behavioral therapies and some forms of psychotherapy can also be helpful as primary or adjunctive therapy. As with the treatment of many psychiatric disorders, a combination of treatments is most often used. For obsessive-compulsive disorder, the pharmacologic treatments are generally less effective than for major depressive episodes. Also, higher doses of antidepressants may be needed for longer trial periods to see effectiveness in reducing symptoms of obsessive-compulsive disorder.

* Obsessive-compulsive disorder is characterized by recurrent obsessions (distressing thoughts) and compulsions (repetitive behaviors) that are recognized as unreasonable but irresistible.
* Treatment consists primarily of antidepressants with serotonergic activity and behavioral therapy.

Adjustment Disorder With Anxious Mood

Adjustment disorder with anxious mood is a maladaptive reaction to an identifiable environmental or psychosocial stress accompanied primarily by symptoms of anxiety that interfere with the patient's usual functioning. Treatment may include supportive counseling and help with identifying the stressor. However, in some cases, the anxiety may be so severe as to require short-term use of anxiolytic agents. However, these should be used with caution to avoid problems of long-term use and possible dependence.

* Adjustment disorder with anxious mood is characterized by a maladaptive reaction to an identifiable environmental or psychosocial stress accompanied by symptoms of anxiety.
* This disorder may require short-term use of anxiolytic agents.

Psychotic Disorders

Psychosis is a generic term used to describe altered thought and behavior in which the patient is incapable of interpreting his or her situation rationally and accurately. Psychotic symptoms can occur in various medical, neurologic, and psychiatric disorders. Many psychotic reactions seen in medical settings are associated with the use of recreational or prescription drugs (Table 22-2). Some of these drug-induced psychotic reactions are nearly indistinguishable from schizophrenia in terms of hallucinations and paranoid delusions (eg, amphetamine and phencyclidine [PCP] psychoses). When evaluating psychotic patients, exploring temporal relationships between illness, medication, and the onset of symptoms is often helpful in determining the cause. As an example, it would be unusual for schizophrenia to initially present in a 70-year-old patient; thus, psychotic symptoms that develop at this age likely have a metabolic, medical, or substance-induced cause. Many brain regions may be involved with the production of psychotic symptoms, but abnormalities in the frontal, temporal, and limbic regions are more likely than others to produce psychotic features.

- Psychosis: a generic term describing altered thought and behavior in which the patient is incapable of interpreting his or her situation rationally and accurately.
- Many psychotic reactions may be associated with the use of recreational or prescription drugs.
- Some drug-induced psychotic reactions have symptoms similar to those found in schizophrenia.

Various disorders throughout a person's life may be associated with schizophrenia-like psychoses. These include genetic abnormalities (eg, a microdeletion of chromosome 22, the velocardiofacial syndrome), childhood neurologic disorders (eg, autism and epilepsy), adult neurologic disorders (eg, narcolepsy), medical and metabolic diseases (eg, infections, inflammatory disorders, endocrinopathies, nutritional deficiencies, uremia, and hepatic encephalopathy), drug abuse, and psychologic stressors.

Schizophrenia may have multifactorial causes, but a large body of functional neuroimaging studies have shown a wide array of anatomical and functional alterations in the central nervous systems of schizophrenic patients. Both genetic and environmental factors are thought to have a role in these changes. Psychotic symptoms and altered interpersonal skills typically become evident initially in the teenage years. Symptoms have been subdivided into positive (delusions and hallucinations) and negative (apathy and amotivation) symptoms. Current diagnostic criteria are divided into inclusion and exclusion criteria. Inclusion criteria include the presence of delusions and hallucinations; marked decrement in functional level in areas

Table 22-2 Classes of Drugs That Can Produce Psychotic Symptoms

Stimulants
Hallucinogens
Phencyclidine (PCP)
Catecholaminergic drugs
Anticholinergic drugs
Central nervous system depressants
Glucocorticoids
Heavy metals (eg, lead, mercury, manganese, arsenic, thallium)
Others (eg, digitalis, disulfiram, cimetidine, bromide, tacrolimus)

such as work, school, social relations, and self-care; and continuous signs of the disturbance for at least 6 months. Exclusion criteria include consistent mood disorder component and evidence of an organic factor that produces the symptoms. The 5 subtypes of schizophrenia are catatonic, disorganized, paranoid, undifferentiated, and residual. These subtypes are not used extensively in clinical practice because of diagnostic overlap during the course of a patient's illness.

- Schizophrenia may be a neurodevelopmental disorder resulting from possible environmental or genetic factors occurring before birth.
- The psychotic symptoms and altered interpersonal skills typically become evident initially in the teenage years.

Somatoform Disorders, Factitious Disorders, and Malingering

Somatoform disorders, factitious disorders, and malingering represent medical symptoms that are excessive for the degree of objective disease. These conditions differ with regard to whether the symptoms and motivations for their persistence are conscious or unconscious.

Somatoform Disorders

Somatoform disorders include somatization disorder, conversion disorder, hypochondriasis, chronic pain disorder, and body dysmorphic disorder. In all these conditions, the patient experiences physical complaints because of an effort to satisfy unconscious needs. These patients are not deliberately seeking to appear ill.

Somatization Disorder

Somatization disorder is a heterogeneous disorder that begins in early life, is characterized by recurrent multiple somatic complaints, and is seen more commonly in women. It is often best managed by collaborative work with an empathic primary care physician and mental health professional. Regularly scheduled appointments with the primary care physician are a cost-effective strategy that lessens "doctor shopping" and frequent visits to an emergency department.

- Somatization disorder begins in early life and is characterized by recurrent multiple physical complaints.
- It mostly affects women.
- It is associated with high use of health care.

Conversion Disorder

Conversion disorder is a loss or alteration of physical functioning suggestive of a medical or neurologic disorder that cannot be explained on the basis of known physiologic mechanisms. The disorder is not limited to pain or sexual dysfunction. It is seen most often in the outpatient setting. Patients frequently respond to any of several therapeutic modalities that suggest hope of a cure. When conversion disorder becomes chronic, it carries a poorer prognosis and is difficult to treat. Treatment focuses on management of the symptoms rather than cure, much as in somatization or chronic pain disorder.

- Conversion disorder is characterized by a loss or alteration of physical functioning.

- It cannot be explained by known physiologic mechanisms.
- It is usually seen in the outpatient setting.
- Treatment focuses on managing the symptoms and encouraging the patient to resume normal functioning.

Chronic Pain Disorder

Chronic pain somatoform disorder (ie, somatoform, chronic pain syndromes) may occur at any age but most often develops in the 30s or 40s. It is diagnosed twice as often in women as in men and is characterized by preoccupation with pain for at least 6 months. No organic lesion is found to account for the pain, or if there is a related organic lesion, the complaint of pain or resulting interference with usual life activities is in excess of what would be expected from the physical findings. A thorough assessment is essential before this diagnosis can be established. Treatment is usually multidisciplinary (eg, primary care, psychiatry, psychology, and physiatry) and focused on helping the patient manage or live with the pain rather than continuing with the expectation of "cure." Avoidance of long-term dependence on addictive substances is an important goal.

- Chronic pain disorder: occurs at any age but usually develops in the 30s or 40s.
- It is diagnosed twice as often in women as in men.
- It is characterized by preoccupation with pain for at least 6 months.
- Treatment: usually multidisciplinary, ideally with involvement of primary care, psychiatry, psychology, and physiatry.
- Typical clinical scenario: A 33-year-old woman has been preoccupied with pain for 8 months, and this has interfered with normal function. An extensive medical evaluation has not found any organic lesion.

Hypochondriasis

Hypochondriasis is an intense preoccupation with the fear of having or the belief that one has a serious disease despite the lack of physical evidence to support the concern. It tends to be a chronic problem for the patient. The differential diagnosis includes obsessive-compulsive disorder (somatic presentation) and delusional disorder (somatic type). Patients with hypochondriasis and obsessive-compulsive disorder tend to have fleeting insight into their excessive concern for their health, unlike patients with delusional thinking. The treatment of hypochondriasis, similar to that of obsessive-compulsive disorder, depends on a combination of serotonergic antidepressants and cognitive-behavioral psychotherapy.

Factitious Disorders

Factitious disorders are characterized by the deliberate production of signs or symptoms of disease. The diagnosis of these disorders requires that the physician maintain a high degree of suspicion and look for objective data at variance with the patient's history (eg, surgical scars that are inconsistent with past surgical history). The more common form of factitious disorder generally occurs among socially conforming young women of a higher socioeconomic class who are intelligent, educated, and frequently work in a medically related field. The possibility of a coexisting medical disorder or intercurrent illness needs to be appreciated in the diagnostic and therapeutic man-

agement of these difficult cases. Factitious disorders are often found in patients with a history of childhood emotional traumas. These patients, through their illness, may be seeking to compensate for childhood traumas and secondarily to escape from and make up for stressful life situations. The most extreme form of the disorder is Munchausen syndrome, which is characterized by the triad of simulating disease, pathologic lying, and wandering. This syndrome has been recognized primarily in men of lower socioeconomic class who have a lifelong pattern of poor social adjustment.

- Factitious disorder: the voluntary production of signs or symptoms of disease to assume the sick role.
- Common form: occurs among socially conforming young women of a higher socioeconomic class.
- Munchausen syndrome is the most extreme form of factitious disorder, with the characteristic triad of simulating disease, pathologic lying, and wandering.
- Factitious disorders often occur in patients with a history of childhood emotional traumas.
- Typical clinical scenario: A 32-year-old woman who is a registered nurse has recurrent fevers but no other presenting signs or symptoms, with a documented double-organism bacteremia due to self-injection.

Malingering

The essential feature of malingering is the intentional production of false or exaggerated physical or psychologic symptoms. It is motivated by external incentives such as avoiding military service or work, obtaining financial compensation or drugs, evading criminal prosecution, or securing better living conditions. Malingering should be suspected in cases in which a medicolegal context overshadows the clinical presentation, a marked discrepancy exists between the person's claimed stress or disability and the objective findings, a lack of cooperation exists during the diagnostic evaluation and in complying with prescribed treatments, and an antisocial personality disorder is present. The person who is malingering is much less likely to present his or her symptoms in the context of emotional conflict, and the presenting symptoms are less likely to be related symbolically to an underlying emotional conflict.

- Malingering is the intentional production of false or exaggerated physical or psychologic symptoms.
- It is motivated by external incentives such as disability payments, housing, release from jail, or avoiding court appearances.

Delirium and Dementia

The primary distinguishing feature between delirium and dementia is the retention and stability of alertness in dementia.

Delirium: An Acute Confusional State

Delirium is characterized by a fluctuating course of an altered state of awareness and consciousness. Although the onset typically is abrupt, the symptoms of this disorder may occasionally be insidious. It may be accompanied by hallucinations (tactile, auditory, visual, or olfactory), illusions (misperceptions of sensory stimuli), delusions, emotional lability, paranoia, alterations in the sleep-wake cycle, and psychomotor slowing or hyperactivity. The symptoms can be dramatic and mimic primary psychotic disorders. Delirium is usually reversible with correction of the underlying cause. It often is related to an external toxic agent, medication side effect, metabolic abnormality, central nervous system abnormality, or withdrawal of a medication or drug. Delirium is relatively common (range, 10%-30%) in medical or surgical inpatients older than 65 years. The diagnosis is made primarily by clinical assessment and changes in the results of a patient's mental status examination. Patients may present with either agitation or withdrawal, the latter being more difficult to recognize. High-risk groups include elderly patients with medical illness (especially congestive heart failure, urinary tract infection, renal insufficiency, hyponatremia, dehydration, or stroke), postcardiotomy patients, patients with dementia, patients in drug withdrawal, patients with severe burns, and patients with AIDS.

- Delirium is characterized by a fluctuating course of inattention and altered level of consciousness.
- Delirium usually is reversible with correction of the underlying cause.
- It often is related to an external toxic agent, medication side effect, metabolic abnormality, central nervous system abnormality, or withdrawal of a medication or drug.
- Delirium is relatively common in medical or surgical patients older than 65 years.

Common causes of delirium in the elderly are infection and intoxication with psychotropic drugs, especially drugs with sedative and anticholinergic side effects. The first step in management is determining whether a specific cause can be identified. Comprehensive medical investigations are frequently warranted. After the cause of the delirium has been recognized, a treatment is selected that can reverse the disease process. If the cause is unknown and the patient's behavior interferes with safety and medical care, several categories of intervention can be considered. Management aspects include monitoring vital signs, electrolytes, and fluid balance and giving neuroleptic agents such as haloperidol. Environmental supports aid orientation; these include calendars, clocks, windows, and family and other persons. Also, psychosocial support, including family or other care providers, is helpful. Severely agitated patients may require physical restraints to prevent injury to themselves or others if medications are not yet effective. Restraints should be avoided whenever possible.

- Common causes of delirium in the elderly are infection and intoxication with psychotropic drugs.
- Typical clinical scenario: A 70-year-old man hospitalized for renal insufficiency and hyponatremia has abrupt onset of visual hallucinations and paranoia accompanied by alternation of his sleep-wake cycle.

Dementia

Dementia is a syndrome of acquired persistent impairment of mental function involving at least 3 of the following 5 domains: memory, language, visuospatial skills, personality or mood, and cognition (including abstraction, judgment, calculations, and executive function). The most common form of cortical dementia is Alzheimer disease. The lifetime prevalence for patients reaching age 65 is estimated at 5% to 10% and for those over age 85, 15% to 20%. Dementia with Lewy bodies is a progressive neurodegenerative disorder that typically has a faster rate of decline than Alzheimer disease. Patients have parkinsonism, visual hallucinations, cognitive impairment, dream enactment, and waxing and waning of symptoms similar to delirium. Treatment of the hallucinations with traditional neuroleptics may worsen the hallucinations and the parkinsonism. There is some evidence that donepezil is rapidly effective in treating some symptoms of dementia with Lewy bodies. Another common type of dementia is multi-infarct dementia, which represents 15% of the cases of dementia in a pure form and an additional 10% in a mixed form.

Dementia may be associated with HIV infection, multiple sclerosis, amyotrophic lateral sclerosis, vitamin B_{12} deficiency, hypothyroidism, and Wilson disease. Other rare types of dementia include Pick disease, Creutzfeldt-Jakob disease, and Huntington disease.

- Alzheimer disease is the most common form of dementia.
- Dementia with Lewy bodies is characterized by parkinsonism, visual hallucinations, cognitive impairment, dream enactment, and waxing and waning of symptoms.

Dementia is differentiated from delirium by appropriate levels of arousal, more preserved attention, and persistence of the cognitive changes. Some forms may be reversible, as in dementia related to hypothyroidism, and some may be "treatable" without reversing the intellectual deficits, for example, preventing further ischemic injury in patients with vascular dementia. Dementia may be a chronic progressive form in which treatment is generally related to improved control of the behavioral disturbances.

Psychologic Aspects of AIDS

From the early to the terminal phases of AIDS and its sequelae, many psychiatric symptoms and complications are possible. The organic mental disorders associated with this process can be primary (ie, directly induced by HIV infection), secondary (ie, related to the effects of the HIV infection leading to immunodeficiency and opportunistic infections or tumors systemically or within the central nervous system), or iatrogenic (ie, resulting from the treatment of HIV or its sequelae). The delirium of AIDS often has a multifactorial cause, similar to delirium in general, namely, electrolyte imbalance, encephalopathy from intracranial or systemic infections, hypoxemia, or medication side effects. HIV itself can cause encephalopathy. The dementia of AIDS can result from the chronic sequelae of most of the causes of delirium. However, direct cerebral infection with HIV probably causes much of the dementia. Other psychiatric symptoms are more nonspecific, such as anger, depression, mania, psychosis, and the general problems of dealing with a terminal illness. Also, all these might be complicated by undiagnosed and, thus, untreated alcohol or drug dependence, especially in the early phases of the disease. A patient who contracted HIV infection through intravenous drug abuse may need chemical dependency treatment as well as thoughtful management of pain complaints.

- AIDS has many possible psychiatric symptoms and complications.
- Organic mental disorders can be primary (due to HIV infection), secondary (due to immunodeficiency and opportunistic infections), or iatrogenic.
- Delirium in AIDS is multifactorial.
- Dementia in AIDS can result from the chronic sequelae of most of the causes of delirium.

Eating Disorders

The 2 common eating disorders are anorexia nervosa and bulimia. Both are markedly more prevalent among women than men. Onset is usually in the teenage or young adult years; rarely, it starts prepubertally. Eating disorders are increasingly found across all income, racial, and ethnic groups. Both disorders have a primary symptom of preoccupation with weight and distortion of body image. For example, the patient perceives herself to look less attractive than an observer would. The disorders are not mutually exclusive, and about 50% of patients with anorexia nervosa also have bulimia. Many patients with bulimia previously had at least a subclinical case of anorexia nervosa.

- The 2 common eating disorders are anorexia nervosa and bulimia.
- They are markedly more prevalent among women than men.
- Primary symptom: preoccupation with weight and a desire to be thinner.

Anorexia Nervosa

To meet the diagnostic criteria of anorexia nervosa, weight must be 15% below that expected for age and height. However, weight of 30% to 40% below normal is not uncommon and leads to the medical complications of starvation, such as depletion of fat, muscle wasting, bradycardia, arrhythmias, ventricular tachycardia and sudden death, constipation, abdominal pain, leukopenia, hypercortisolemia, and osteoporosis. In extreme cases, patients develop lanugo (fine hair on the body) and metabolic alterations to conserve energy. Thyroid effects include low levels of triiodothyronine (T_3), cold intolerance, and difficulty maintaining core body temperature. Reproductive effects include a pronounced decrease or cessation of the secretion of luteinizing hormone and follicle-stimulating hormone, resulting in secondary amenorrhea.

Bulimia

Patients with bulimia frequently lose control and consume large quantities of food. Many patients may have a concurrent depressive or anxiety disorder. Physical complications of the binge-purge cycle may include fluid and electrolyte abnormalities, hypochloremic-hypokalemic metabolic alkalosis, esophageal and gastric irritation and bleeding, colonic abnormalities from laxative abuse, marked erosion of dental enamel with associated decay, parotid and salivary gland hypertrophy, and amylase levels 25% to 40% higher than normal. If bulimia is untreated, it often becomes chronic. Some patients have a gradual spontaneous remission of some symptoms.

- Patients with bulimia may have a concurrent depressive or anxiety disorder.
- The binge-purge cycle causes physical complications.

Alcoholism and Substance Abuse Disorders

Alcoholism and substance abuse disorders are a major concern in all age groups and across all ethnic, socioeconomic, and racial groups. Despite national and international efforts to curb the problem and to make treatment more readily available, the condition is not diagnosed in many persons and less than 10% of persons with addiction are involved in some form of treatment, either self-help groups or professional supervision. The lifetime incidence of alcohol and drug abuse approaches 20% of the population. These disorders have devastating effects on families and other persons and contribute to social problems such as motor vehicle accidents and fatalities, domestic violence, suicide, and increased health care costs. Untreated alcoholics have been estimated to generate twice the general health care costs of nonalcoholics. Persons with addictive disorders are a heterogeneous group and may present in many different ways. Recognizing addictive disorders is critically important. The current definition of *alcoholism* approved by the National Council on Alcoholism and Drug Dependence may also be applicable to other drugs of abuse: alcohol abuse and dependence are primary, chronic diseases with genetic, psychosocial, and environmental factors influencing their development and manifestations. The disease is often progressive and fatal. It is characterized by continuous or periodic impaired control over drinking, preoccupation with the drug alcohol, the use of alcohol despite adverse consequences, and distortions in thinking, most notably denial.

- Less than 10% of persons with addiction receive some form of treatment.
- Persons with addictive disorders are a heterogeneous group.
- The lifetime incidence of alcohol and drug abuse approaches 20% of the population.
- Untreated alcoholics generate twice the general health care costs of nonalcoholics.

The adverse consequences of alcohol and substance abuse disorders cross over into several domains. Physical health issues include alcohol withdrawal syndromes, liver disease, gastritis, anemia, and neurologic disorders. Psychologic functioning issues include impaired cognition and changes in mood and behavior. Interpersonal functioning issues include marital problems, child abuse, and impaired social relationships. Occupational functioning issues include academic, scholastic, or job problems. Legal, financial, and spiritual problems also occur.

Several different pharmacologic agents are now available to help diminish the craving for alcohol and other drugs or to serve as a deterrent to relapse. Although medications such as disulfiram, acamprosate, and naltrexone, among others, may be helpful in preventing relapse, they should be viewed as adjunctive therapy to chemical dependency treatment and should never be used instead of formal chemical dependency treatment.

- Chemical dependency can be viewed as continued problematic chemical use despite life consequences.
- Pharmacologic agents can be useful adjuncts to chemical dependency treatment, but they should never replace chemical dependency treatment.

Alcoholism
Medical data from physical examination and laboratory tests can be helpful. However, most of the pertinent findings are not apparent until after several years (often up to 5 years) of notable alcohol use and, thus, do not reflect the earliest stages of the disease. Two of the earlier detectable signs are increases in serum γ-glutamyltransferase level and mean corpuscular volume. In both men and women, the combination of increased γ-glutamyltransferase level and mean corpuscular volume can identify up to 90% of alcoholics. Carbohydrate-deficient transferrin is the most sensitive screening test. Other abnormal laboratory findings include increased levels of alkaline phosphatase, bilirubin, uric acid, and triglycerides. However, because of the number of false-negative results, it is not practical to rely on laboratory data alone to establish the diagnosis of alcoholism. The CAGE questions (related to attempts to cut down on alcohol use, other persons expressing annoyance, experiencing guilt, and early-morning drinking) have excellent sensitivity and specificity. Alcohol withdrawal can range from mild to quite severe, with the occurrence of withdrawal seizures or delirium tremens (or both). The medical complications of alcoholism can affect nearly every organ system, but the liver, gastrointestinal tract, pancreas, and central nervous system are particularly susceptible to the effects of alcohol.

- Increased γ-glutamyltransferase level and mean corpuscular volume can identify up to 90% of alcoholics.
- It is not practical to rely on laboratory data alone to diagnose alcoholism.
- Medical complications of alcoholism can affect nearly every organ system.

Benzodiazepines, Sedative-Hypnotics, and Anxiolytics
Benzodiazepines, sedative-hypnotics, and anxiolytics are widely prescribed in many areas of medicine, so abuse and dependence are often iatrogenic. However, 5 characteristics may help distinguish medical use from nonmedical use:
1. Intent—What is the purpose of the use?
2. Effect—What is the effect on the user's life?
3. Control—Is the use controlled by the user only or does a physician share in the control?
4. Legality—Is the use of the drug legal or illegal? Medical drug use is legal.
5. Pattern—In what settings is the drug used?

These same characteristics may also be used to distinguish between the medical and nonmedical use of opioids. Withdrawal from use of benzodiazepines and barbiturates, in particular, may be serious because of the increased risk of withdrawal seizures.

- Withdrawal of the use of benzodiazepines and barbiturates, in particular, can be serious because of the increased risk of withdrawal seizures.

Psychopharmacology
The use of a pharmacologic treatment of a psychiatric disorder or the use of psychoactive medications in other disorders is a decision that generally is made after considering multiple factors in the case. Medication alone is rarely the sole treatment of a psychiatric disorder but rather a component of a comprehensive treatment plan. Because psychoactive medications are used in various circumstances for many different indications, the major groups of these medications—antidepressants, antipsychotics, antimanic agents, anxiolytics, and sedative drugs—are discussed below in general terms rather than for treatment of specific disorders. The choice of a medication usually is based on its side-effect profile and the clinical profile of the patient. There are many effective drugs in each of the major groups, but they differ in terms of pharmacokinetics, side effects, and available routes of administration.

- Medication alone is rarely the sole treatment for a psychiatric disorder.
- The choice of a medication generally is based on its side-effect profile and the clinical profile of the patient.

Antidepressants
In the United States, more than 30 antidepressants are available to treat depression, and several others have been approved by the US Food and Drug Administration. First-generation antidepressants include tricyclic agents and monoamine oxidase inhibitors. Newer-generation antidepressants are not easily grouped by their chemical structure or function; they are instead a diverse group of compounds. Currently, the most widely used of this group of agents are SSRIs.

Although older-generation antidepressants were effective in treating depression, they were associated with important side effects that limited their use in certain groups of patients, especially those with other medical problems. In particular, tricyclic agents are associated with orthostatic hypotension, anticholinergic side effects, and altered cardiac conduction. Monoamine oxidase inhibitors are effective antidepressants but require special dietary restrictions and attention to interactions with other medications. Because the newer-generation antidepressants have fewer potential side effects and drug interactions than older agents, they are prescribed more widely, but they are not optimal for all patients.

Types of antidepressants with examples include the following:
1. Tricyclics—tertiary amines (including amitriptyline, doxepin, imipramine, and trimipramine) and secondary amines (including desipramine, nortriptyline, and protriptyline)
2. Monoamine oxidase inhibitors—pargyline, phenelzine, and tranylcypromine
3. SSRIs—citalopram, fluoxetine, fluvoxamine, paroxetine, sertraline, and escitalopram
4. Newer-generation antidepressants—bupropion, nefazodone, trazodone, venlafaxine, and duloxetine

The mechanism of action of antidepressants is related to their neurochemical activity at central nervous system receptors for serotonin, norepinephrine, and dopamine, among others. Side effect profiles are related to half-life and receptor affinity in the central nervous system and other organ systems (Tables 22-3 and 22-4). While it is not practical for clinicians to know the pharmacologic properties of all antidepressants, knowing several agents of each class well will be sufficient to treat the majority of depressed patients in a busy practice.

Antidepressants have been approved primarily for use in the treatment of depression. However, they are useful in several other disorders, including panic disorder, obsessive-compulsive disorder, generalized anxiety disorder, social anxiety disorder, posttraumatic stress disorder, enuresis, bulimia, and attention-deficit/hyperactivity disorder. Tricyclic agents and duloxetine can be beneficial for the treatment of certain pain syndromes.

A complete trial of antidepressant medication consists of 4 to 6 weeks of therapeutic doses before considering refractoriness. If improvement has occurred with the initial trial of the medication but the patient's condition has not returned to baseline, it may be worthwhile to increase the dose of the medication or augment it with low-dose lithium or a low dose of another antidepressant that has a different mechanism of action. After clinical improvement has been noted, the medication may need to be maintained for an extended period. Another option is to switch to an antidepressant with a different mechanism of action that interacts with different neurochemical pathways.

- Antidepressants work at various receptors, primarily serotonergic and noradrenergic.
- Side effects can typically be predicted from receptor affinity.
- A trial of at least 4 weeks is necessary before one can judge the efficacy of an antidepressant.

Glucose intolerance, weight changes, and electrophysiologic cardiac changes have been associated with next-generation antipsychotics (Table 22-5). Additionally, these medications are frequently used off-label for treatment of agitation in dementia patients. Several studies have shown a lack of efficacy in this population, and safety concerns have arisen concerning an increased risk of death among dementia patients treated with antipsychotic agents.

Monoamine Oxidase Inhibitors

Monoamine oxidase inhibitors are now seldom used because of concerns about drug-drug and drug-food interactions. The mechanism of action is to inhibit irreversibly the enzyme monoamine oxidase A or B, which degrades catecholamines, serotonin, and the neurotransmitter amino acid precursor tyramine. Most clinical concerns about the use of monoamine oxidase inhibitors are related to reactions from the ingestion of tyramine, which is not metabolized because of the inhibition of intestinal monoamine oxidase. Tyramine may act as a false transmitter and displace norepinephrine from synaptic vesicles. Patients should be instructed in a tyramine-restricted diet, especially to avoid aged cheeses, smoked meats, pickled herring, beer, red wine, yeast extracts, fava beans, and overripe bananas and avocados. Certain general anesthetics and drugs with sympathomimetic activity should be avoided; patients should beware especially of over-the-counter cough and cold preparations, decongestants, and appetite suppressants. Meperidine (Demerol) is absolutely contraindicated because of its potentially lethal interaction with monoamine oxidase inhibitors.

- Clinical concerns about monoamine oxidase inhibitors: reactions due to ingestion of tyramine, which is not metabolized.
- Tyramine is a false neurotransmitter that displaces norepinephrine from synaptic vesicles.
- Meperidine (Demerol) is absolutely contraindicated because of its potentially lethal interaction with monoamine oxidase inhibitors.

Treatment of hypertensive reactions relies on administering drugs with α-adrenergic blocking properties, such as intravenous administration of phentolamine.

Antipsychotic Agents

Next-generation "atypical" antipsychotic agents are now widely used and are replacing "standard" antipsychotics such as chlorpromazine and haloperidol. The currently available newer-generation antipsychotics include aripiprazole, clozapine, olanzapine, quetiapine, risperidone, and ziprasidone.

The choice of medication is based on the patient's clinical situation, side-effect profile of the chosen agent, history of previous response, and issues related to compliance. The prevailing theory about the mechanism of action of these agents is that they cause blockade of postsynaptic dopamine receptors. This is related to both the antipsychotic activity and the other side effects, depending on which dopamine pathways in the brain are affected and which type of dopamine receptor is preferentially affected. If the nigrostriatal dopaminergic system (involved with motor activity) is affected, extrapyramidal symptoms may result. Blockade of the dopamine pathways in the pituitary and hypothalamus causes increased release of prolactin and changes in appetite and temperature regulation. The effects of these drugs on the limbic system, midbrain tegmentum, septal nuclei, and mesocortical dopaminergic projections are thought to be responsible for their antipsychotic action. Atypical antipsychotic medications combine dopaminergic and serotonergic antagonism, which appears to minimize extrapyramidal side effects.

- The theory about the mechanism of action of antipsychotic agents is that they cause blockade of postsynaptic dopamine receptors.
- The antipsychotic effects of these agents are due to their actions on the limbic system, midbrain tegmentum, septal nuclei, and mesocortical dopaminergic projections.

Side Effects: Extrapyramidal Reactions

Atypical antipsychotic agents have a lower rate of extrapyramidal side effects. Yet, because these events are still reported occasionally, it is important to recognize these possible complications of therapy. Acute dystonic reactions occur within hours or days after treatment is initiated with antipsychotic drugs. These reactions are characterized by uncontrollable tightening of the face and neck muscles with spasms. The effect on the eyes may cause an oculogyric crisis, and the effect on the laryngeal muscles may cause respiratory or ventilatory difficulties. Treatment is usually with intravenous or intramuscular administration of an anticholinergic agent, followed by the use of an oral anticholinergic agent for a few days.

Table 22-3 Receptor Activity and Possible Side Effects

Drug	Therapeutic Effect	Adverse Effect
Norepinephrine transporter	Antidepressant	Tremors Tachycardia Blockade of antihypertensive effects of guanethidine & guanadrel Augmentation of pressor effects of sympathomimetic amines
Serotonin transporter	Antidepressant	Gastrointestinal tract disturbances (including weight loss early in treatment & weight gain late in treatment) Increase or decrease in anxiety (dose dependent) Sexual dysfunction (including decreased libido) Extrapyramidal adverse effects Interactions with tryptophan, monoamine oxidase inhibitors, & fenfluramine
Dopamine transporter	Antidepressant Antiparkinsonian	Psychomotor activation Precipitation or aggravation of psychosis
α_1-Adrenergic receptors	Unknown	Potentiation of antihypertensive effect of prazosin, terazosin, doxazosin, & labetalol Postural hypotension & dizziness Reflex tachycardia
Dopamine D_2 receptor	Amelioration of signs & symptoms of psychosis	Extrapyramidal movement disorders: dystonia, parkinsonism, akathisia, tardive dyskinesia, rabbit syndrome Endocrine effects: prolactin elevation (galactorrhea, gynecomastia, menstrual changes, sexual dysfunction in men)
Histamine H_1 receptor	Sedation	Sedation Drowsiness Weight gain Potentiation of central depressant drugs
Muscarinic receptor	Antidepressant	Blurred vision Attack or exacerbation of narrow-angle glaucoma Dry mouth Sinus tachycarida Constipation Urinary retention Memory dysfunction
5-Hydroxytryptamine$_{2A}$ receptor	Antidepressant Reduction of anxiety Promotion of deep sleep Prophylaxis of migraine headaches Antipsychotic	Unknown

Modified from Richelson E. Pharmacology of antidepressants. Mayo Clin Proc. 2001;76:511-27. Used with permission of Mayo Foundation for Medical Education and Research.

- Acute dystonic reactions occur within hours or days after treatment is initiated with antipsychotic drugs.
- Reactions include uncontrollable tightening of the face and neck muscles with spasms.
- Treatment: intravenous or intramuscular administration of an anticholinergic agent.

Parkinsonian syndrome has a more gradual onset and can be treated with oral anticholinergic agents or decreased doses of the antipsychotic agent (or both). *Akathisia* is an unpleasant feeling of restlessness and the inability to sit still. It often occurs within days after treatment is initiated with an antipsychotic agent. Akathisia is sometimes mistaken for exacerbation of the psychosis. Treatment, if possible, is to

Table 22-4 Side Effects of the Major Groups of Antidepressants

Orthostatic hypotension—The cardiovascular side effect that most
  commonly results in serious morbidity, especially in the elderly
Anticholinergic effects—Dry mouth, blurred vision, urinary
  retention; beware of these side effects in patients with prostatic
  hypertrophy & narrow-angle glaucoma
  Drugs with more anticholinergic side effects also seem to be more
  sedating (eg, tertiary amine tricyclics)
Cardiac conduction effects—Most of the tricyclics prolong PR &
  QRS intervals; thus, these drugs need to be used with caution in
  patients with preexisting heart block, such as second degree heart
  block or markedly prolonged QRS & QT intervals
  The tricyclics are potent antiarrhythmic agents because of their
  quinidine-like effect
  Newer-generation antidepressants have considerably fewer cardiac
  interactions
Sedation—Tertiary amine tricyclics & trazodone
Potential stimulation—Secondary amine tricyclics, bupropion,
  fluoxetine, sertraline, & paroxetine

Table 22-5 Potentially Serious Side Effects of Next-Generation
            Antipsychotic Agents

Hyperglycemia & diabetes mellitus
Weight gain
Neuroleptic malignant syndrome
Tardive dyskinesia
Extrapyramidal symptoms
Prolonged QT interval (ziprasidone only)
Increased mortality in dementia-related psychosis

Clozapine-specific side effects
Agranulocytosis
Seizures
Myocarditis
Orthostatic hypotension

decrease the dose of the antipsychotic agent or to try using a β-adrenergic blocking agent such as propranolol, if not contraindicated.

Tardive dyskinesia has an incidence of 3% to 5% annually and
consists of involuntary movements of the face, trunk, or extremities.
The most consistent risk factors for its development are long-term
use (>6 months) of typical antipsychotics and older age. Prevention
is the most important aspect of management because no reliable
treatment is available. It is best if treatment with the antipsychotic agent
can be discontinued because the dyskinesia is sometimes reversible,
although the involuntary movements may increase temporarily.

* Tardive dyskinesia is involuntary movements of the face, trunk,
  or extremities.
* Prevention is the most important aspect of management.

Neuroleptic malignant syndrome is a potentially life-threatening disorder that may occur after the use of any antipsychotic agent, although
it is more common with rapid increases in the dosage of high-potency
antipsychotic agents. Its clinical presentation is characterized by severe
rigidity, fever, leukocytosis, tachycardia, tachypnea, diaphoresis, blood
pressure fluctuations, and marked increase in creatine kinase levels
because of muscle breakdown. Treatment consists of discontinuing the
use of the antipsychotic agent and providing life-support measures
(ventilation and cooling). Pharmacologic interventions may include
the use of 1 or both of the following: dantrolene sodium, which is a
direct-acting muscle relaxant, or bromocriptine, which is a centrally
acting dopamine agonist. Often, one of the most effective treatments
is ECT, which likely increases presynaptic dopamine release markedly;
this reverses the extreme degree of dopamine receptor blockade present in neuroleptic malignant syndrome.

* Neuroleptic malignant syndrome is potentially life-threatening.

* It may occur after the use of any antipsychotic agent.
* Characteristics include severe rigidity, fever, leukocytosis, tachycardia, tachypnea, diaphoresis, blood pressure fluctuations, and
  marked increase in creatine kinase levels (from muscle breakdown).

Side effects other than extrapyramidal effects of antipsychotic agents
are listed in Table 22-6.

Next-Generation ("Atypical") Antipsychotic Agents

The atypical antipsychotic agents are different from their predeces-
sors in terms of potential mechanisms of action and side-effect profiles. They are less likely to cause bothersome extrapyramidal side
effects, and their potential for causing tardive dyskinesia may be less.
The evidence for the latter will take time to establish because the
onset of the symptoms is delayed and the drugs have not been widely used long enough to determine the risk of tardive dyskinesia.
Neuroleptic malignant syndrome has been reported to occur with
clozapine and risperidone. Clozapine has a 1% to 2% risk of producing agranulocytosis, which is reversible if use of the medication
is withdrawn immediately. Because of this serious potential side
effect, a specific requirement is that blood cell counts be made regularly (weekly for the first 6-18 months).

Antianxiety Medications

Antianxiety medications are used most appropriately to treat time-
limited anxiety or insomnia related to an identifiable stress or change
in sleep cycle. After long-term use (>2-3 months), the use of benzodiazepines and related substances should be tapered rather than
discontinued abruptly to avoid any of the 3 "discontinuation syndromes," which include relapse, rebound, and withdrawal.

Relapse is the return of the original anxiety symptoms, often after
weeks to months. *Rebound* is the intensification of the original symptoms, which usually last several days and appear within hours to days
after abrupt cessation of drug use. *Withdrawal* may be mild to severe
and includes autonomic and central nervous system symptoms that
are different from the original presenting symptoms of the disorder.

Table 22-6 Side Effects Other Than Extrapyramidal Effects of Antipsychotic Agents

Anticholinergic
Orthostatic hypotension—related to α-adrenergic receptor blockade
Hyperprolactinemia—gynecomastia possible in men & women, galactorrhea (rare), amenorrhea, weight gain, breast tenderness, decreased libido
Sexual dysfunction
Dermatologic—pigmentary changes in the skin, photosensitivity
Decreased seizure threshold

Benzodiazepines are well absorbed orally but have unpredictable availability with intramuscular use, except for lorazepam. There is great variability in the pharmacokinetics of benzodiazepines. Several of these drugs have metabolites with a long half-life. Therefore, much smaller doses need to be used in the elderly, in patients with cognitive dysfunction, and in children. All these patient groups are prone to paradoxical reactions (anxiety, irritability, aggression, agitation, and insomnia), especially patients with known brain damage.

- Benzodiazepines have great variability in their half-life, which directly determines the duration of action and side effects.

Buspirone is a non-benzodiazepine anxiolytic drug whose mechanism of action is well understood. However, the drug has effects on many neurotransmitter systems, especially the serotonergic and dopaminergic systems. Cross-tolerance does not exist between benzodiazepines and buspirone. It generally takes 2 to 3 weeks for the drug to become effective. Patient compliance can be an issue because of the long latency to effectiveness and the need for divided doses daily.

- Buspirone is a non-benzodiazepine anxiolytic drug.
- It takes 2 to 3 weeks for the drug to become effective.

Lithium

For many years, lithium carbonate was the drug of choice for treating bipolar disorders. It may also be effective in patients with recurrent unipolar depression and as an adjunct for maintenance of remission of depression after ECT. Acute manic symptoms usually respond to treatment with lithium within 7 to 10 days; during this time, the adjunctive use of antipsychotic agents and benzodiazepines may be helpful. Lithium is well absorbed from the gastrointestinal tract, with peak levels in 1 to 2 hours. Its half-life is about 24 hours. Levels are generally checked 10 to 12 hours after the latest dose. Relatively common side effects include resting tremor, diarrhea, polyuria, polydipsia, thirst, and nausea, which is often improved by taking the medication on a full stomach. Lithium is contraindicated in the first trimester of pregnancy because of its potential for causing defects in the developing cardiac system. Renal effects generally can be reversed with discontinuation of lithium therapy. The most noticeable renal

effect is the vasopressin-resistant effect leading to impaired concentrating ability and nephrogenic diabetes insipidus with polyuria and polydipsia. Most patients who take lithium develop some degree of polyuria, but not all develop the more severe manifestations of nephrogenic diabetes insipidus. Renal function should be followed in all patients receiving maintenance lithium therapy. However, whether lithium has severe nephrotoxic effects is a matter of controversy. A hematologic side effect is benign leukocytosis. Hypothyroidism may occur in as many as 20% of patients taking lithium because of the direct inhibitory effects on thyroid hormone production or increased antithyroid antibodies.

- Lithium carbonate: the common side effects are hand tremor, diarrhea, polyuria, polydipsia, thirst, and nausea.
- Renal effects generally can be reversed with discontinuation of lithium therapy.
- The most noticeable renal effect is impaired concentrating ability.
- Hypothyroidism occurs in as many as 20% of patients taking lithium.

Because the range between the therapeutic and toxic levels of lithium in the plasma is narrow, patients and physicians should be familiar with conditions that may increase or decrease lithium levels and with the signs and symptoms of lithium toxicity so it can be recognized and treated promptly (Tables 22-7 and 22-8).

Other Mood Stabilizers

Valproic acid, carbamazepine, and several next-generation antipsychotics are effective in the treatment of acute manic episodes and in prophylactic maintenance therapy for bipolar disorder. Valproic acid is now the most commonly prescribed mood stabilizer. The mechanism of action for valproic acid is not clear. The side effect of most concern with valproic acid is hepatotoxicity, which has occurred mostly in children receiving treatment with multiple anticonvulsants. Carbamazepine has also been used in this context, and because its chemical structure is similar to that of tricyclic antidepressants, it has a quinidine-like effect.

- Lamotrigine is helpful in treating bipolar depression without risk of inducing hypomania or mania.
- Valproic acid, carbamazepine, and next-generation antipsychotics are effective in treating mania in bipolar disorder.

Electroconvulsive Therapy

ECT is the most effective treatment for severely depressed patients, especially those with psychotic features. It is also helpful in treating catatonia and mania and may be used in children and adults. Also, ECT can be administered safely to pregnant women, provided fetal monitoring is available. It may be effective in patients with overlapping depression and Parkinson disease or dementia. ECT induces rapid changes in several transmitter-receptor systems simultaneously, particularly acetylcholine, norepinephrine, dopamine, and serotonin. ECT is administered with the patient under barbiturate anesthesia, with succinylcholine or a similar muscle relaxant to minimize peripheral

Table 22-7 Conditions That Increase or Decrease Lithium Levels in the Plasma

Increase Levels	Decrease Levels
Dehydration	Increased caffeine consumption
Overheating & increased perspiration with exercise or hot weather	Theophylline
Nonsteroidal anti-inflammatory drugs	
Thiazide diuretics	
Angiotensin-converting enzyme inhibitors	
Certain antibiotics—tetracycline, spectinomycin, & metronidazole	

manifestations of the seizure. An anticholinergic agent such as atropine is generally given to decrease secretions and to prevent bradycardia caused by central stimulation of the vagus nerve. A usual course of treatment is 6 to 12 sessions given over 2 to 4 weeks.

- ECT is the most effective treatment for severely depressed patients, especially those with psychotic features.
- It is also helpful in treating catatonia and mania.
- ECT can be administered to pregnant women.
- It may be helpful in cases of overlapping depression and Parkinson disease or dementia.
- Mechanism of action—ECT induces rapid changes in several transmitter-receptor systems simultaneously, particularly acetylcholine, norepinephrine, dopamine, and serotonin.

ECT no longer has any absolute contraindications, although it has several relative contraindications. Previously, the only absolute contraindication was the presence of an intracranial space-occupying lesion and increased intracranial pressure. Serious complications or mortality is generally reported as less than 1 per 10,000, which makes this therapy one of the safest interventions that uses general anesthesia. Morbidity and mortality usually are due to cardiovascular complications, such as arrhythmia, myocardial infarction, or hypotension. The major risks are those associated with the brief general anesthesia. Medical evaluations performed before ECT is administered should pay particular attention to cardiovascular function, pulmonary function, electrolyte balance, neurologic disorder (epilepsy), and the patient's previous experiences with anesthesia.

- ECT no longer has any absolute contraindications.
- It has several relative contraindications.
- Morbidity and mortality are usually due to cardiovascular complications.

Table 22-8 Signs and Symptoms of Lithium Toxicity

Mild to Moderate Toxicity (Plasma Level, 1.5-2.0 mEq/L)	Moderate to Severe Toxicity (Plasma Level, 2.0-2.5 mEq/L)	Severe Toxicity (Plasma Level >2.5 mEq/L)
Vomiting	Persistent nausea & vomiting	Generalized seizures
Abdominal pain	Anorexia	Oliguria & renal failure
Dry mouth	Blurred vision	Death
Ataxia	Muscle fasciculations	
Slurred speech	Hyperactive deep tendon reflexes	
Nystagmus	Delirium	
Muscle weakness	Convulsions	
	Electroencephalographic changes	
	Stupor & coma	
	Circulatory system failure	
	Decreased blood pressure	
	Cardiac arrhythmias	
	Conduction abnormalities	

Modified from Silver JM, Hales RE, Yudofsky SC. Biological therapies for mental disorders. In: Stoudemire A, editor. Clinical psychiatry for medical students. Philadelphia: JB Lippincott Company; 1990. p. 459-96. Used with permission.

Psychiatry Pharmacy Review
Julie L. Cunningham, PharmD, BCPP

Review of Antipsychotic Agents

Drug	Toxic/Adverse Effects	Drug Interactions/Comments

Typical agents
Chlorpromazine
Fluphenazine
Mesoridazine
Perphenazine
Thioridazine
Trifluoperazine
Haloperidol
Loxapine
Molindone
Thiothixene
	EPS—dystonia, pseudoparkinsonism, akathisia; TD, NMS
	Anticholinergic effects, sedation, orthostatic hypotension, galactorrhea, amenorrhea, gynecomastia, weight gain, sexual dysfunction, photosensitivity, risk of seizures
	Pigmentary retinopathy—thioridazine
		Thioridazine—contraindicated in patients with QTc interval >450 msec & coadministration of other drugs that cause QTc prolongation
		Drug interactions:
		  Additive sedative effects with CNS depressants
		  Decreased concentrations in the presence of carbamazepine, barbiturates, cigarette smoking
		  Increased concentrations in the presence of quinidine, fluoxetine, & paroxetine
		  Antihypertensive agents may produce additive hypotensive effects
		  Haloperidol & fluphenazine—available as depot, long-acting injections

Atypical agents Aripiprazole (Abilify) Clozapine (Clozaril) Olanzapine (Zyprexa) Quetiapine (Seroquel) Paliperidone (Invega) Risperidone (Risperdal) Ziprasidone (Geodon)	Increased risk of DM & hyperglycemia Increased incidence of mortality in dementia patients treated for behavioral disorders EPS & prolactin elevation risk highest with risperidone (dose-related) Anticholinergic effects greatest with clozapine & olanzapine Orthostatic hypotension risks greatest with clozapine, risperidone, & quetiapine Sedative risks greatest with clozapine, olanzapine, & quetiapine Weight gain greatest with clozapine & olanzapine Hypertriglyceridemia with clozapine & olanzapine Increased risk of seizures with clozapine (dose-related) Mandatory WBC monitoring with clozapine (risk of agranulocytosis)	Decreased risk of EPS, TD, & prolactin effects than with typical agents Drug interactions—all have lower levels when used concurrently with carbamazepine; additive orthostatic hypotension with trazodone Aripiprazole, risperidone—increased levels with use of paroxetine, fluoxetine, duloxetine Clozapine—increased risk of agranulocytosis with captopril, carbamazepine, sulfonamides Clozapine/olanzapine—increased levels with cimetidine, erythromycin, fluoroquinolones, fluoxetine, fluvoxamine; decreased levels with cigarette smoking Quetiapine—increased levels with ketoconazole & nefazodone; decreased levels with phenytoin Paliperidone—cytochrome P450 interactions unlikely Ziprasidone—contraindicated for patients with QTc prolongation or with other agents that prolong the QTc interval Risperidone—available as a depot, long-acting injectable Aripiprazole—unique mechanism with both dopamine antagonist & agonist activity

Abbreviations: CNS, central nervous system; DM, diabetes mellitus; EPS, extrapyramidal symptoms; NMS, neuroleptic malignant syndrome; TD, tardive dyskinesia; WBC, white blood cell count.

Psychiatry Pharmacy Review (continued)

Review of Antidepressants[a][b]

Drug	Toxic/Adverse Effects	Drug Interactions/Comments
NDRI Bupropion (Wellbutrin)	Can cause agitation, insomnia, psychosis, confusion, weight loss	Contraindicated in patients with seizure or history of anorexia, bulimia, or MAOIs Low incidence of sexual dysfunction & minimal drug interactions Also available as SR & XL formulations

MAOI
  Phenelzine (Nardil)
  Tranylcypromine (Parnate)
  Selegiline (Emsam) transdermal patch
	Associated with weight gain, orthostatic hypotension, sexual dysfunction
	Hypertensive crisis may occur with tyramine-containing foods
		Limited use because of drug/food interactions
		Contraindicated with use of other antidepressants, alcohol, meperidine, or general anesthesia
		Selegiline patch applied once daily; doses ≤6 mg do not require dietary restrictions

Mirtazapine (Remeron)	Low risk of sexual dysfunction May cause weight gain & increase serum cholesterol & triglycerides Rare incidence of agranulocytosis Can lower seizure threshold	Avoid use with MAOIs, clozapine, or carbamazepine Unique mechanism of action Lower doses more sedating than higher doses
Nefazodone	Low risk of sexual dysfunction Some sedative, orthostatic hypotensive, & anticholinergic effects Liver failure	May improve symptoms of anxiety & insomnia Contraindicated with triazolam, alprazolam, MAOIs, & cisapride because nefazodone inhibits their metabolism

SSRIs
  Citalopram (Celexa)
  Escitalopram (Lexapro)
  Fluoxetine (Prozac)
  Paroxetine (Paxil)
  Sertraline (Zoloft)
	Common: insomnia, GI upset, HA, sexual dysfunction, & tremors
	Rare: extrapyramidal symptoms & hyponatremia/SIAD
	May impair platelet aggregation & increase risk of bleeding
		No significant anticholinergic effects, minimal weight gain, & relatively safe in overdose
		Avoid with use of MAOIs, tramadol, & migraine agents (may precipitate serotonin syndrome)
		Fluoxetine—long half-life & active metabolites; available in a weekly formulation
		Paroxetine—also available in a CR formulation

Tricyclic antidepressants
  Tertiary amines
    Amitriptyline (Elavil)
    Imipramine (Tofranil)
    Doxepin (Sinequan)
  Secondary amines
    Nortriptyline (Pamelor)
    Desipramine (Norpramin)
	Potentially fatal in overdose
	Increased risk of seizures & conduction abnormalities
	Common anticholinergic effects, weight gain, sedation, sexual dysfunction, & orthostatic hypotension
		Secondary amine agents generally have milder side effects
		Blood levels are useful for monitoring
		Contraindicated with use of MAOIs & in patients with recent myocardial infarction
		SSRIs may inhibit metabolism & cause toxicity

SNRIs
  Duloxetine (Cymbalta)
  Venlafaxine (Effexor)
	Can cause insomnia, GI upset, HA, sexual dysfunction, sustained increase in blood pressure
	Minimal weight gain
		No significant anticholinergic effects
		Avoid with use of MAOIs
		May be beneficial for resistant cases because of dual mechanism of action (venlafaxine at doses >200 mg daily)
		Duloxetine also approved for DPN

Mood stabilizer Lithium (Lithobid, Eskalith)	Hand tremor, nausea, polyuria, polydipsia, diarrhea, weight gain, & hypothyroidism	Adjust for renal function Monitor trough levels Contraindicated in severe CV or renal disease, dehydration, sodium depletion Use cautiously with drugs that affect sodium—diuretics, NSAIDs, ACEIs (lithium toxicity) Caffeine use may decrease lithium levels

Abbreviations: ACEI, angiotensin-converting enzyme inhibitor; CR, continuous release; CV, cardiovascular; DPN, diabetic peripheral neuropathy; GI, gastrointestinal tract; HA, headache; MAOI, monoamine oxidase inhibitor; NDRI, norepinephrine-dopamine reuptake inhibitor; NSAID, nonsteroidal anti-inflammatory drug; SIAD, syndrome of inappropriate antidiuresis; SNRI, serotonin-norepinephrine reuptake inhibitor; SR, sustained release; SSRI, selective serotonin reuptake inhibitor; XL, extended release.

[a] Avoid abrupt discontinuation of use, which may cause withdrawal effects.

[b] All antidepressants have the potential to cause switch to mania in bipolar patients.

Psychiatry Pharmacy Review (continued)

Review of Anxiolytics

Drug	Toxic/Adverse Effects	Drug Interactions	Comments

Benzodiazepines
    Alprazolam (Xanax)
    Chlordiazepoxide (Librium)
    Clonazepam (Klonopin)
    Clorazepate (Tranxene)
    Diazepam (Valium)
    Estazolam (ProSom)
    Flurazepam (Dalmane)
    Lorazepam (Ativan)
    Midazolam (Versed)
    Oxazepam (Serax)
    Quazepam (Doral)
    Temazepam (Restoril)
    Triazolam (Halcion)
	CNS effects—drowsiness, fatigue, light-headedness, confusion, impairments in memory & attention, headaches
	Tachycardia, palpitations
	Nausea, diarrhea
	Blurred vision
		Additive CNS effects with other CNS agents, including alcohol
		CYP3A4 inhibitors may increase concentration of many BZDs (erythromycin, clarithromycin, ketoconazole, itraconazole, diltiazem, verapamil, grapefruit)
		CYP3A4 inducers may decrease concentration of many BZDs (carbamazepine, rifampin)
			DEA schedule IV substances
			Elderly may be more susceptible to adverse effects
			Doses should be adjusted in hepatic & renal failure
			Adolescents & patients with MR may have a paradoxical disinhibition effect
			Avoid abrupt discontinuation (withdrawal effects)

Buspirone (BuSpar)	Dizziness, nervousness, headaches, excitement, anger/hostility, confusion, nausea, diarrhea	Risk of serotonin syndrome with SSRIs & serotonin agents Contraindicated with MAOIs CYP3A4 inhibitors may increase concentration of buspirone (see above) CYP3A4 inducers may decrease concentration of buspirone (see above)	Not controlled by DEA Give with food for increased tolerability Adjust dose in hepatic & renal failure

Abbreviations: BZD, benzodiazepine; CNS, central nervous system; DEA, Drug Enforcement Administration; MAOI, monoamine oxidase inhibitor; MR, mental retardation; SSRI, selective serotonin reuptake inhibitor.

Questions

Multiple Choice (choose the best answer)

1. A 50-year-old man reports drinking 2 to 3 drinks a night. Which of the following questions would *not* be helpful in diagnosing alcoholism?

    a. Have you felt the need to cut down on your drinking?
    b. Have you lost your job because of your drinking?
    c. Has your family expressed anger about your use of alcohol?
    d. Do you feel guilty about your use of alcohol?
    e. Have you had a drink in the morning?

2. An obese, 20-year-old patient is evaluated in the psychiatric unit for possible schizophrenia. What would be the appropriate treatment?

    a. Olanzapine
    b. Haloperidol
    c. Chlorpromazine
    d. Risperidone
    e. Fluphenazine

3. You are seeing a 76-year-old man with a history of paranoid schizophrenia, who was recently admitted to a nursing home. He has a history of type 2 diabetes mellitus, mild congestive heart failure, and osteoarthritis. He has no history of dementia. His psychotic symptoms have been largely controlled with risperidone, 6 mg orally daily. Which of the following is *false* regarding the use of risperidone in this patient?

    a. He is at increased risk of sudden death from cardiovascular disease or stroke.
    b. He is at increased risk of parkinsonism.
    c. He is at increased risk of tardive dyskinesia.
    d. He is at increased risk of poorly controlled diabetes mellitus.
    e. He is at increased risk of neuroleptic malignant syndrome.

4. A 33-year-old woman has recently received a diagnosis of bipolar disorder and is now taking lithium carbonate, 600 mg orally twice daily. She wants to know some of the long-term risks of taking this medication. Which of the following is *not* true about long-term management of bipolar disorder with lithium?

    a. Nonsteroidal anti-inflammatory drugs (NSAIDs) should be avoided because of nephrotoxicity associated with taking the combination of an NSAID and lithium.
    b. There is an increased risk of birth defects in children of women taking lithium during pregnancy.
    c. Thyroid function needs to be monitored because of the potential for thyrotoxicity.
    d. Acetaminophen should be avoided because of hepatotoxicity associated with taking the combination of acetaminophen and lithium.

    e. Lithium doses may need to be decreased temporarily if an acute illness develops and leads to dehydration.

5. A 42-year-old woman presents to your office again after 16 years of intermittent severe left lower quadrant abdominal pain. She denies any weight loss, fever, or chills. No distinct cause for her symptoms was apparent from previous workups, including a complete blood cell count, electrolyte evaluations, urinalysis, CT scan of the abdomen and pelvis, colonoscopy, and gynecologic examination. She has been thoroughly evaluated for episodic dizziness, headaches, flulike syndromes, and back pain; all findings were negative. What is the most likely diagnosis?

    a. Conversion disorder
    b. Somatization disorder
    c. Hypochondriasis
    d. Body dysmorphic disorder
    e. Factitial disorder

6. A 24-year-old first-year medical student presents with 2 months of progressive heightened anxiety punctuated by discrete episodes during which he experiences light-headedness, shortness of breath, dry mouth, tachycardia, chest pain, and tingling in the hands. These usually occur when he is trying to study. He says, "It feels like I am going to die!" He has read about angina and Sjögren syndrome, and he asks you if he has these disorders. What is the most likely diagnosis?

    a. Angina pectoris
    b. Somatization disorder
    c. Conversion disorder
    d. Panic disorder
    e. Posttraumatic stress disorder

7. Diagnostic evaluation of the patient in question 6 includes electrocardiography, electrolytes, liver function tests, urine drug-abuse screen, complete blood cell count, and thyroid tests. All results were negative. He asks you about the advisability of cardiac catheterization (which you wisely opt not to order). Which of the following would *not* be considered a reasonable treatment option?

    a. A trial of sertraline, titrating up to 100 mg daily
    b. A trial of low-dose scheduled lorazepam, 0.5 mg twice a day, with additional dosing available as needed for anxiety episodes
    c. A trial of valproic acid, titrating up to 1,000 mg daily in divided doses
    d. Cognitive behavioral psychotherapy
    e. A combination of fluoxetine, 20 mg daily and cognitive behavioral psychotherapy

Answers

1.   Answer b.
The CAGE questions (Have you ever felt the need to *cut* down on drinking, had family express *a*nger about your drinking, felt *g*uilty about drinking, or had an *eye*-opener?) are used to identify individuals with an increased risk of alcoholism. Patients rarely report job loss due to alcohol use because their work provides the funds to continue drinking.

2.   Answer d.
The patient is obese and likely will experience further weight gain with olanzapine. Research suggests an association between weight gain and hyperglycemia in patients treated with olanzapine. Another atypical antipsychotic such as risperidone would be optimal because of decreased extrapyramidal symptoms and decreased risk of tardive dyskinesia.

3.   Answer a.
Dementia patients treated with antipsychotics are at increased risk of sudden death from cardiac disease or stroke, but this association has not been found for elderly patients with schizophrenia. Next-generation antipsychotics are associated with hyperglycemia and an increased risk of diabetes mellitus. Similar to traditional neuroleptics, next-generation antipsychotics may cause extrapyramidal symptoms, tardive dyskinesia, and neuroleptic malignant syndrome.

4.   Answer d.
Lithium is not hepatotoxic and may be used safely with acetaminophen. Lithium can cause nephrotoxicity, an effect that can be increased when taken concomitantly with NSAIDs. Lithium is a pregnancy category D medication (associated with cardiac and facial structural abnormalities) and should be avoided if possible during pregnancy, especially in the first trimester. Lithium can cause thyrotoxicity. Because it is a positive ion with a valence similar to that of sodium, lithium will be retained by the kidney during periods of dehydration, rapidly reaching toxic levels in some patients. Renal function, thyroid function, and electrolytes should be checked periodically (at least annually) for all patients taking lithium.

5.   Answer b.
Somatization disorder is characterized by physical symptoms without an identifiable organic cause. The patients believe that they have a physical problem and are not consciously generating the symptoms or pretending to have them. Somatization disorder entails a history of multiple somatic complaints over many years, including 4 pain symptoms, 2 gastrointestinal symptoms, 1 sexual symptom, and 1 neurologic symptom. Conversion disorder is marked by a neurologic symptom such as a motor or sensory deficit and is unconscious in origin (unlike factitial disorder, in which the symptoms are consciously produced). Body dysmorphic disorder is characterized by a perception that a normally appearing body part is in some way misshapen or otherwise appears abnormal. Hypochondriasis is characterized by an irrational fear that one has an illness or serious disease.

6.   Answer d.
Panic disorder typically occurs in the third decade of life, with patients usually engaged in ordinary activities. Patients experience light-headedness, shortness of breath, dry mouth, tachycardia, chest pain, and tingling in the hands. Attacks typically last 5 to 25 minutes. Illnesses in the somatization disorder spectrum (see the answer to question 5) would not be pertinent at this juncture, but if the patient continues to believe he has a primary medical illness that is driving his symptoms, despite negative diagnostic findings, a somatization disorder type illness would become more likely in the differential diagnosis.

7.   Answer c.
Selective serotonin reuptake inhibitors, benzodiazepines, and cognitive behavioral therapy have been shown to be effective in treating panic disorder and would all be considered first-line therapies. Valproic acid is not a common therapy for panic disorder. The combination of behavioral therapy and pharmacotherapy is effective in treating panic disorder. Although not all antidepressants are approved by the Food and Drug Administration for treating panic disorder, most are effective, with the exception of bupropion.

23

Pulmonary Diseases

John G. Park, MD
Timothy R. Aksamit, MD
Karen L. Swanson, DO
Charles F. Thomas, Jr., MD
Sean M. Caples, DO

Part I

John G. Park, MD

Symptoms and Signs

Cough

Cough is an explosive expiration that clears and protects the airways. It is 1 of the most common presenting complaints encountered in an outpatient practice. A cough is under both voluntary and involuntary control. The latter is the cough reflex, which has 5 components: cough receptors, afferent nerves, cough center (medulla), efferent nerves, and effector organs. The afferent limb of the cough reflex includes the sensory branches of the trigeminal, glossopharyngeal, and vagus nerves. Inflammatory, mechanical, chemical, or thermal stimulation of the receptors and sensory pathways can trigger cough. The efferent limb includes the recurrent laryngeal and spinal nerves that innervate the expiratory and laryngotracheobronchial musculature. Lesions in the nose, pharynx, larynx, bronchi, lungs, pleura, or abdominal viscera can cause cough. Common causes of cough include postnasal drip (due to infectious and noninfectious causes) and chronic obstructive pulmonary disease (COPD) exacerbations.

- Cough is 1 of the most common symptoms in an outpatient practice.
- Lesions in the nose, pharynx, larynx, bronchi, lungs, pleura, or abdominal viscera can cause cough.
- Common causes of cough include postnasal drip and COPD exacerbations.

Chronic cough is cough that lasts 3 weeks or more. The most common causes of chronic cough are postinfectious (viral, *Mycoplasma*, *Chlamydia pneumoniae* TWAR, or *Bordetella pertussis*), postnasal drip, asthma, gastroesophageal reflux, and COPD. Patients with

connective tissue diseases such as giant cell arteritis, rheumatoid bronchiolitis, and Sjögren syndrome may also present with cough. Cough can be the presenting manifestation or the only manifestation of asthma in up to 57% of asthmatic patients. Cough is a complication in up to 10% of patients who take angiotensin-converting enzyme inhibitors (ACEIs). There is a decrease of up to 10-fold in the incidence of cough associated with angiotensin II receptor blockers (ARBs). Up to 90% of the patients with persistent cough may have more than 1 cause for the cough. Initial treatment is often empirical based on history, physical examination, and the more common causes of chronic cough. Initial diagnostic testing may include computed tomography (CT) of the sinuses and ear-nose-throat consultation, sputum analysis, methacholine inhalation challenge, 24-hour esophageal pH monitoring, or esophagography. If no chest radiographic (CXR) abnormalities are detected, bronchoscopy has a low (4%) diagnostic yield. In cough syncope, a hard cough produces increased intrathoracic pressure, which decreases cardiac output and cerebral perfusion. Other complications include rib fracture, seizures, and pneumothorax.

- Postnasal drip, asthma, gastroesophageal reflux, COPD, and ACEI use account for 80%-90% of cases of chronic cough.
- Cough can be the presenting manifestation or the only manifestation of asthma.
- ACEIs cause cough in 10% of patients.
- Up to 90% of patients may have more than 1 cause of chronic cough.
- Initial treatment is often empirical.
- Bronchoscopy: low diagnostic yield if CXR is normal.
- Complications of cough: cough syncope, rib fracture, pneumothorax.

Sputum

Purulent sputum is found in bronchiectasis and lung abscess. The sputum is frothy pink in pulmonary edema. Expectoration of bronchial casts, mucous plugs, or thin strings occurs in asthma, bronchopulmonary aspergillosis, and mucoid impaction syndrome. Plastic bronchitis is the formation of thick bronchial casts in asthma, bronchopulmonary aspergillosis, and other conditions. Bronchorrhea (expectoration of thin serous fluid >100 mL daily) occurs in 20% of patients with diffuse alveolar cell carcinoma. Sputum analysis may identify eosinophils, Charcot-Leyden crystals, and Curschmann spirals, which are seen with asthma. The most important cause of broncholithiasis is histoplasmosis.

- Bronchorrhea is uncommon in diffuse alveolar cell carcinoma.
- The most common cause of broncholithiasis: histoplasmosis.
- Sputum analysis may identify eosinophils, Charcot-Leyden crystals, and Curschmann spirals in patients with asthma.

Hemoptysis

Hemoptysis is the expectoration of blood or blood-streaked sputum that originates below the level of the larynx. *Pseudohemoptysis* is expectoration of blood previously aspirated into the airways from the gastrointestinal tract, nose, or supraglottic areas. History, examination, and CXR findings are important in the diagnosis of hemoptysis. Bronchial arterial bleeding occurs in chronic bronchitis, bronchiectasis, malignancies, and broncholithiasis and with the presence of foreign bodies. Pulmonary arterial bleeding occurs in pulmonary arteriovenous malformations, fungus ball, tumors, vasculitis, pulmonary hypertension, and lung abscess. Pulmonary capillary bleeding occurs in mitral stenosis, left ventricular failure, pulmonary infarction, vasculitis, Goodpasture syndrome, and idiopathic pulmonary hemosiderosis. A common cause of streaky hemoptysis is acute exacerbation of chronic bronchitis. Airway-vessel fistula (eg, tracheoinnominate) can cause massive hemoptysis (>200 mL in 24 hours). The cause of death in massive hemoptysis is asphyxiation, not exsanguination.

- History, examination, and CXR findings are important in the diagnosis of hemoptysis.
- Common cause of streaky hemoptysis: acute exacerbation of chronic bronchitis.
- The cause of death in massive hemoptysis is asphyxiation, not exsanguination.

Dyspnea

Dyspnea is the subjective awareness of breathlessness. It usually is the result of increased work of breathing. Other mechanisms include abnormal activation of respiratory centers, voluntary hyperventilation, and Cheyne-Stokes respiration. Dyspnea may be due to cardiopulmonary disease or to disorders of the skeletal (eg, kyphoscoliosis), endocrine, metabolic, neurologic, or hematologic systems. Other causes are physiologic dyspnea of pregnancy, drugs, psychogenic, deconditioning, and obesity. Recent studies have suggested that an increased serum level of B-type natriuretic peptide (BNP) (>100 pg/mL) differentiates dyspnea due to congestive heart failure from that due to pulmonary dysfunction.

- Disease in any organ can cause dyspnea, but the most common cause is cardiopulmonary dysfunction.
- Increased levels of BNP may help differentiate the cause of dyspnea.

A medical history, physical examination, CXR, electrocardiography (ECG), complete blood count, and pulmonary function tests (PFTs) are required for most patients. Arterial blood gases and cardiopulmonary physiologic testing may also be required. *Tachypnea* is breathing more than 20 breaths/min, and *bradypnea* is fewer than 10 breaths/min. *Orthopnea* is dyspnea in the supine posture, as in congestive heart failure, bilateral diaphragmatic paralysis, severe COPD, asthma, sleep apnea, or severe gastroesophageal reflux disease. *Trepopnea* is dyspnea in the lateral decubitus position, as occurs with tumors of the main bronchi, unilateral pleural effusion, or after pneumonectomy. *Platypnea* is dyspnea in the upright posture and is due to an increased right-to-left shunt in lung bases; it is seen in liver disease, severe lung fibrosis, or after pneumonectomy. *Paroxysmal nocturnal dyspnea* is nocturnal episodes of dyspnea, resulting in frequent waking up (associated with pulmonary edema and asthma).

Treatment is based on suspected cause, but supplemental oxygen or surgical intervention should be considered. For some patients in whom organic cause cannot be identified, patient education and cognitive behavior therapy may need to be considered.

Chest Pain

Pulmonary causes of chest pain are often difficult to distinguish from cardiac and other causes. Tightness of the chest and dyspnea are also described as "chest pain" by some patients. Pleuritic pain is encountered in pleuritis, pleuropericarditis, pericarditis, pneumothorax, pleural effusion, mediastinitis, pulmonary embolism, pulmonary infarction, esophageal disease, aortic dissection, and chest wall trauma. Subdiaphragmatic diseases that produce chest pain include pancreatitis, cholecystitis, and colonic distention.

Cyanosis

Cyanosis, the bluish discoloration of the skin and mucous membranes that appears when the capillary content of deoxygenated hemoglobin is greater than 5 g/dL, may be difficult to detect clinically. The causes of central cyanosis are severe hypoxia (arterial oxygen tension [PaO_2] is usually <55 mm Hg), anatomical right-to-left shunt, mild hypoxia with polycythemia ("red cyanosis"), shock, and abnormal hemoglobin. Methemoglobinemia and sulfhemoglobinemia cause cyanosis in the setting of normal PaO_2. Certain systemic diseases, such as argyria (silver deposition) can cause blue-gray discoloration of the nails which is not cyanosis. Cherry-red flush (not cyanosis) is caused by carboxyhemoglobinemia. Anemia does not cause cyanosis. Peripheral cyanosis (ie, cyanosis detected in the extremities only) results from decreased peripheral perfusion with increased oxygen extraction. Any cause of central cyanosis, however, will cause peripheral cyanosis.

- Cyanosis occurs when deoxygenated hemoglobin is >5 g/dL.
- Central cyanosis should be distinguished from peripheral cyanosis.
- Polycythemia vera causes "red cyanosis."

- Methemoglobinemia and sulfhemoglobinemia: cyanosis in the setting of normal PaO2.
- Cherry-red flush (not cyanosis) is caused by carboxyhemoglobinemia.

Clubbing

Clubbing is the bulbous enlargement of the distal segment of a digit (fingers or toes) caused by increased soft tissue mass. Its mechanisms are neurogenic, humoral/hormonal, hereditary, and idiopathic. The mnemonic *CLUBBING* is a reminder of common causes for clubbing including the following: *c*yanotic heart diseases and cystic fibrosis; *l*ung cancer and lung abscess; *u*lcerative colitis; *b*ronchicctasis; *b*enign mesothelioma; *i*nfective endocarditis, idiopathic pulmonary fibrosis, idiopathic, and inherited; *n*eurogenic tumors; and *g*astrointestinal tract diseases (eg, cirrhosis and regional enteritis). Clubbing can be the presenting manifestation of any of the above entities, and it may precede other clinical features of lung cancer. Clubbing is present in 30% of patients with non–small cell lung cancer; it is more common in women than in men (40% vs 19%).

- Clubbing may precede other clinical features of lung cancer.
- Common causes: pulmonary fibrosis, congenital heart disease with right-to-left shunt, cystic fibrosis, and idiopathic.

Hypertrophic Pulmonary Osteoarthropathy

Hypertrophic pulmonary osteoarthropathy (HPO) is characterized by clubbing, painful periosteal hypertrophy of long bones, and symmetrical arthralgias of large joints (usually knees, elbows, and wrists). Other features include gynecomastia, fever, and an increased erythrocyte sedimentation rate (ESR). The mechanisms of HPO are neurogenic (vagal afferents), hormonal, and idiopathic. The most common cause is bronchogenic carcinoma, usually adenocarcinoma or large cell carcinoma. HPO is an early sign of pulmonary metastasis from nasopharyngeal carcinoma. Radiographs of long bones show thickened and raised periosteum. Bone scans show increased uptake of radionuclide by the affected periosteum. If HPO does not resolve after tumor resection, treatment options include the administration of a somatostatin analogue or ipsilateral vagotomy.

- Common causes of HPO: idiopathic and adenocarcinoma or large cell carcinoma of the lung.
- Radionuclide bone scans show characteristic changes.
- Therapy: resection of the tumor, somatostatin analogue, or ipsilateral vagotomy.
- Typical clinical scenario: An adult with clubbing, pain in the long bones, symmetrical arthralgias of large joints, increased ESR, and fever.

Horner Syndrome

Horner syndrome consists of ipsilateral miosis, anhidrosis, and ptosis on the side of the lesion. It is a complication of a superior sulcus tumor (Pancoast tumor) of the lung.

- Horner syndrome: ipsilateral miosis, anhidrosis, and ptosis.
- Superior sulcus tumor (Pancoast tumor).

Other Signs and Symptoms of Pulmonary Disease

Conjunctival suffusion is seen in severe hypercarbia, superior vena cava syndrome, and conjunctival sarcoidosis. Mental obtundation is seen with hypercarbia. Asterixis is seen in severe acute or subacute hypercarbia. Telangiectasia of the skin and mucous membranes occurs in patients with pulmonary arteriovenous malformation. Skin lesions of various types occur in patients with pulmonary involvement of Langerhans cell granulomatosis (eosinophilic granuloma or histiocytosis X), tuberous sclerosis, sarcoidosis, or lung cancer.

- Asterixis is seen in severe acute or subacute hypercarbia.
- Mental obtundation is seen with hypercarbia.

History and Examination

An approach to the history and physical examination of patients with pulmonary disease is outlined in Table 23-1. Percussion and auscultation findings associated with various pulmonary conditions are also listed in Table 23-1.

Diagnostic Tests

Radiology

The radiologic tests performed in the diagnosis of chest diseases include plain CXR, CT, magnetic resonance imaging (MRI), pulmonary angiography, and bronchial angiography.

Plain Chest Radiography

Many of the radiographic diagnoses such as pneumothorax, pleural effusion, and lung nodule can be established by CXR. It is essential to correlate clinical and other laboratory data with CXR findings. It is also important to compare the present film with previous films, particularly in assessing the seriousness of a newly identified abnormality. A lateral CXR is of most help in identifying retrocardiac and retrodiaphragmatic abnormalities.

- Obtain earlier CXRs for comparison.
- Lateral CXRs are important in identifying retrocardiac and retrodiaphragmatic abnormalities.

The ability to identify normal radiographic anatomy is essential. A routine step-by-step method of interpretation should be developed so that subtle abnormalities are not missed (Table 23-2). Initially, the CXR should be globally assessed, without focusing on any 1 area or abnormality. This is to ensure that the technical aspects are adequate and the patient identification markers and the orientation of the CXR (identification of the left and right sides) are correct. Next, the extrapulmonary structures are viewed. For instance, destructive arthritis of a shoulder joint seen on a CXR may be the result of rheumatoid arthritis and may prompt the CXR reader to look for pulmonary manifestations of this disease. The absence of a breast shadow on the CXR of a female patient suggests the need to look for signs of pulmonary metastases. The visualization of a tracheostomy stoma or cannula on the CXR may indicate previous laryngeal cancer, suggesting the possibility of complications such as aspiration pneumonia

Table 23-1 History and Physical Examination of Patients With Pulmonary Disease

History
    Smoking
    Occupational exposure
    Exposure to infected persons or animals
    Hobbies & pets
    Family history of diseases of lung & other organs
    Past malignancy
    Systemic (nonpulmonary) diseases
    Immune status (corticosteroid therapy, chemotherapy,
      cancer)
    History of trauma
    Previous chest radiography
Examination
    Inspection
        Respiratory rate, hoarseness of voice
        Respiratory rhythm (abnormal breathing pattern)
        Accessory muscles in action (FEV_1 <30%)
        Postural dyspnea (orthopnea, platypnea, trepopnea)
        Intercostal retraction
        Paradoxical motions of abdomen/diaphragm
        Cough (type, sputum, blood)
        Wheeze (audible with or without stethoscope)
        Pursed lip breathing/glottic wheeze (patients with
          chronic obstructive pulmonary disease)
        Cyanosis (central vs peripheral)
        Conjunctival suffusion (CO_2 retention)
        Clubbing
        Thoracic cage (eg, anteroposterior diameter,
          kyphoscoliosis, pectus carinatum)
        Trachea, deviation
        Superior vena cava syndrome
        Asterixis, central nervous system status
        Cardiac impulse, jugular venous pressure, pedal edema
          (signs of cor pulmonale)
    Palpation
        Clubbing
        Lymphadenopathy
        Tibial tenderness (hypertrophic pulmonary osteoarthropathy)
        Motion of thoracic cage (hand or tape measure)
        Chest wall tenderness (costochondritis, rib fracture,
          pulmonary embolism)
        Tracheal deviation, tenderness
        Tactile (vocal) fremitus
        Subcutaneous emphysema
        Succussion splash (effusion, air-fluid level in thorax)
    Percussion
        Thoracic cage (dullness, resonance)
        Diaphragmatic motion (normal, 5-7 cm)
        Upper abdomen (liver)
    Auscultation
        Tracheal auscultation
        Normal breath sounds
        Bronchial breath sounds
        Expiratory slowing
        Crackles
        Wheezes
        Pleural rub
        Mediastinal noises (mediastinal crunch)
        Heart sounds
        Miscellaneous (muscle tremor, etc; see text—"Other
          Signs and Symptoms of Pulmonary Disease" subsection)

Percussion/Auscultation Finding	Chest Expansion	Fremitus	Resonance	Breath Sounds	Egophony	Bronchophony
Pleural effusion	Decreased	Decreased	Decreased	Decreased	Absent>>present	Absent>>present
Consolidation	Decreased	Increased	Decreased	Bronchial	Present	Present
Atelectasis	Decreased	Decreased	Decreased	Decreased	Absent>present	Absent>present
Pneumothorax	Variable	Decreased	Increased	Decreased	Absent	Absent

Note: The trachea is shifted ipsilaterally in atelectasis and contralaterally in effusion. Whispered pectoriloquy is present in consolidation.
Abbreviation: FEV_1, forced expiratory volume in 1 second.

and lung metastases. Infradiaphragmatic abnormalities such as calcifications in the spleen, displacement of the gastric bubble and colon, and signs of upper abdominal surgery (eg, metal staples or feeding tubes) may indicate the cause of a pleuropulmonary process.

- Initially look at the entire CXR.
- Look for extrapulmonary abnormalities before focusing on any obvious parenchymal findings.

The skeletal thorax should be viewed to exclude rib fracture, osteolytic and other lesions of the ribs, rib notching, missing ribs, and vertebral abnormalities. Changes due to a previous thoracic surgical procedure such as coronary artery bypass, thoracotomy, lung resection, or esophageal surgery may provide clues to the pulmonary disease. Next, the intrathoracic but extrapulmonary structures such as the mediastinum (including the great vessels, esophagus, heart, lymph nodes, and thymus) should be assessed. The superior

Table 23-2 Systematic Approach to Evaluation of a Chest Radiograph

1. Check for patient identifier
2. Evaluate extrapulmonary structures
   Destructive arthritis
   Absence of breast shadow
   Evidence of previous surgery: sternal wires, valvular prosthesis, surgical staples demarking previous lobectomy, etc.
   Tracheostomy
3. Infradiaphragmatic abnormalities
4. Skeletal changes: rib fractures, notching, osteolytic lesions, etc.
5. Intrathoracic, extrapulmonary structures: mediastinum, thyroid calcification, achalasia, aortopulmonary window, hilum, calcified adenopathy
6. Pleural region: blunting, calcification
7. Lung parenchyma: infiltrates, air bronchogram, nodules, cysts, abscess, pneumothorax
8. Lateral views to evaluate retrocardiac & retrodiaphragmatic spaces

mediastinum should be viewed to see whether the thyroid gland extends into the thoracic cage. A calcified mass in the region of the thyroid almost always indicates a goiter. The esophagus can produce important abnormalities in the CXR. A large esophagus, as in achalasia, may mimic a mass, and a large hiatal hernia with an air-fluid level may mimic a lung abscess. The aortopulmonary window (a notch below the aortic knob on the left, just above the pulmonary artery), if obliterated, may indicate a tumor or lymphadenopathy. Right paratracheal and paramediastinal lymphadenopathy can be subtle. Hilar regions are difficult to interpret because lymphadenopathy, vascular prominence, or tumor may make the hila appear larger. The retrocardiac region may show hiatal hernia with an air-fluid level; this may be helpful in the diagnosis of reflux or aspiration.

- Rib lesions: osteolytic, expansile, notching, or absence of a rib.
- Note changes due to previous surgical procedures.
- Assess the mediastinum: the esophagus, thyroid, thymus, and great vessels.

The pleural regions should be examined for pleural effusion, pleural thickening (particularly in the apices), blunting of costophrenic angles, pleural-based lesions such as pleural plaques or masses, and pneumothorax. A lateral decubitus film may be necessary to confirm the presence of free fluid in the pleural space. An air bronchogram depicting the major airways may indicate a large tumor (cut-off of air bronchogram), deviation of airways, signs of compression or stenosis, and the relation of major airways to the esophagus. Finally, the lung parenchyma should be evaluated. Nearly 15% of the pulmonary parenchyma is located behind the heart and diaphragm; a lateral CXR is helpful in examining this region. It is important not to overinterpret increased interstitial lung markings.

Oligemia of the lung fields is difficult to assess because the clarity of the film depends on the duration of the exposure of the film. Generally, bronchovascular markings should be visible throughout the lung parenchyma. The complete absence of any markings within the lung parenchyma should suggest a bulla or an air-containing cyst. Apical areas should be evaluated carefully for the presence of pleural thickening, pneumothorax, small nodules, and subtle infiltrates. If the apices cannot be visualized properly with a standard CXR, a lordotic view should be obtained.

- Look for small pneumothorax, nodules, and large airway lesions.
- Examine the apices for thickening, pneumothorax, nodules, and subtle infiltrates.
- Examine the lung parenchyma behind the heart and diaphragm.

Some of the common CXR abnormalities are depicted in Figures 23-1 through 23-26.

Fluoroscopy
Fluoroscopy is useful in localizing lesions during biopsy and aspiration procedures. It also is valuable in assessing diaphragmatic motion and in diagnosing diaphragmatic paralysis by the sniff test. Paradoxic motion of the diaphragm suggests diaphragmatic paralysis (but it is present in up to 6% of healthy subjects).

- Up to 6% of healthy subjects exhibit paradoxic diaphragmatic motion.

Computed Tomography
Standard CT is useful in the staging of lung cancer and in assessing mediastinal and hilar lesions, solitary nodules, calcification in nodules, diffuse lung disease, and pleural processes. High-resolution CT (HRCT) demonstrates characteristic findings in pulmonary bronchiectasis (HRCT has replaced bronchography for diagnosing bronchiectasis), Langerhans cell granulomatosis (nodular-cystic spaces in the upper lung fields), lymphangitic carcinomatosis (nodular interlobular septal thickening), lymphangioleiomyomatosis (well-defined cystic spaces in lung parenchyma), and idiopathic pulmonary fibrosis (subpleural honeycombing). HRCT findings in pulmonary fibrotic diseases are more than 90% accurate; honeycombing may be seen in up to 90% of patients, as compared with 30% with traditional CXR. HRCT is also helpful in diagnosing certain granulomatous lung diseases (sarcoidosis and mycobacterial infections), asbestosis, pulmonary alveolar phospholipoproteinosis, chronic eosinophilic pneumonia, and bronchiolitis obliterans. Ultrafast CT with contrast media is better than a ventilation-perfusion ($\dot{V}/\dot{Q}$) scan in detecting pulmonary emboli in the main and lobar arteries.

- HRCT demonstrates characteristic features in pulmonary Langerhans cell granulomatosis, lymphangioleiomyomatosis, idiopathic pulmonary fibrosis, and lymphangitic pulmonary metastasis.
- HRCT has replaced bronchography for diagnosing bronchiectasis.
- CT is helpful in the staging of lung cancer.

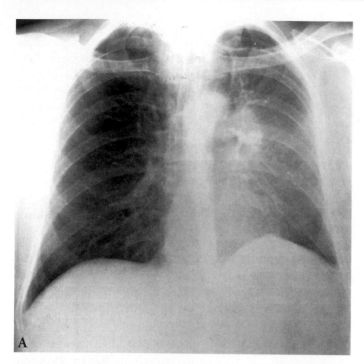
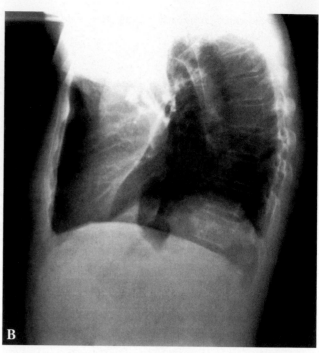

Figure 23-1. Collapsed Left Upper Lobe. A, Posteroanterior chest radiograph (CXR) and, B, lateral CXR. The ground-glass haze over the left hemithorax is typical of a partially collapsed left upper lobe. In more than 50% of patients with collapsed lobes, loss of volume is evidenced by left hemidiaphragmatic elevation; the mediastinum is shifted to the left and the left hilus is pulled cranially. Also, the left main bronchus deviates cranially. Calcification in the left hilar mass represents an unrelated, old granulomatous infection. In panel B, the density from the left hilus down toward the anterior portion of the chest represents the partially collapsed left upper lobe. The radiolucency substernally is the right lung.

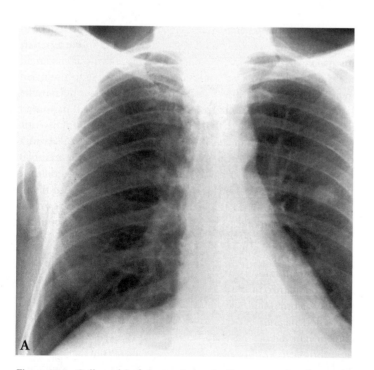
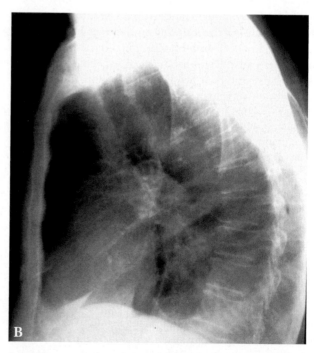

Figure 23-2. Collapsed Left Lower Lobe. A, Posteroanterior chest radiograph (CXR) and, B, lateral CXR. Note nodule in left mid lung field plus collapsed left lower lobe, seen as a density behind the heart. This entity represents 2 separate primary lung cancers: synchronous bronchogenic carcinomas. Do not stop with the first evident abnormality, such as the nodule in the mid lung field, without looking carefully at all other areas. Panel B demonstrates an increased density over the lower thoracic vertebrae without any obvious wedge-shaped infiltrate. Over the anterior portion of the hemidiaphragm, the small wedge-shaped infiltrate is not fluid in the left major fissure because the left major fissure is pulled away posteriorly. Instead, it is an incidental normal variant of fat pushed up into the right major fissure.

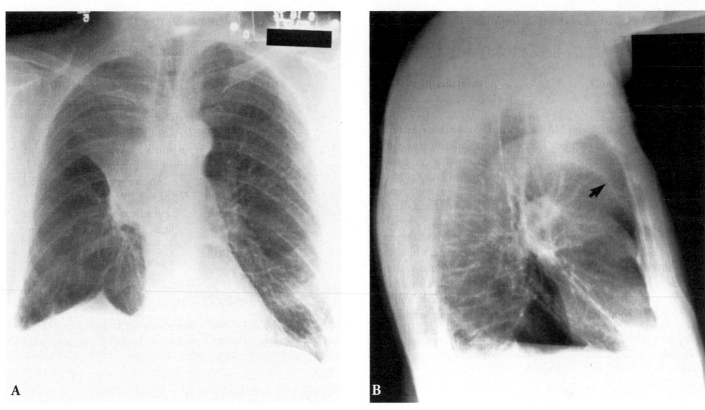

Figure 23-3. Collapsed Right Upper Lobe. A, Posteroanterior chest radiograph (CXR) and, B, lateral CXR. A, This is a classic "reversed S" mass in the right hilus with partial collapse of the right upper lobe. Loss of volume is evident with the elevation of the right hemidiaphragm. In panel B, the partially collapsed right upper lobe is faintly seen in the upper anterior portion of the hemithorax (arrow).

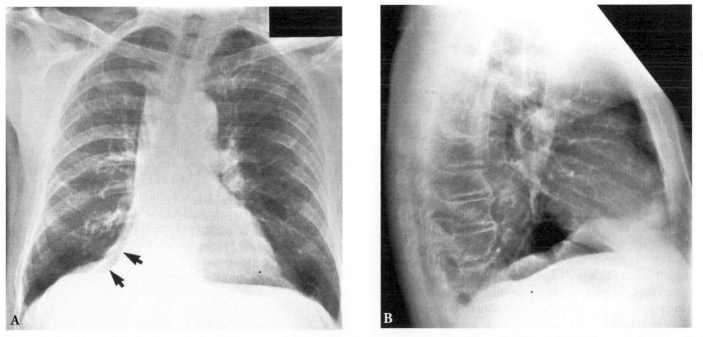

Figure 23-4. Collapsed Right Lower Lobe. A, Posteroanterior chest radiograph (CXR) and, B, lateral CXR. A, This 75-year-old smoker had hemoptysis for 1.5 years; his CXR had been read as "normal" on several occasions. Note the linear density (arrows) projecting downward and laterally along the right border of the heart. It projects below the diaphragm and is not a normal line. Also, the right hilus is not evident; it has been pulled centrally and downward because of carcinoma obstructing the bronchus of the right lower lobe. Note the very slight shift in the mediastinum to the right, indicative of some loss of volume. B, In the lateral view, in spite of notable collapse of the right lower lobe, only a subtle increased density over lower thoracic vertebrae represents this collapse.

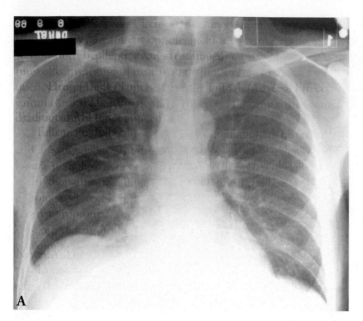
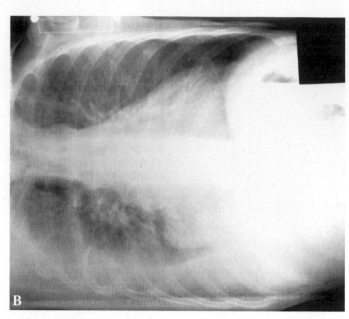

Figure 23-5. Effusion. A, Posteroanterior chest radiograph (CXR) and, B, decubitus CXR. A, "Elevated right hemidiaphragm" that is really an infrapulmonic effusion, or subpulmonic, as seen on the decubitus film. B, For unknown reasons, a meniscus is not formed in some people with infrapulmonic pleural effusion. Thus, any seemingly elevated hemidiaphragm should be examined with the suspicion that it could be an infrapulmonic effusion. Subpulmonic effusions occur more frequently in patients with nephrotic syndrome. Decubitus CXR or ultrasonography would disclose the free fluid.

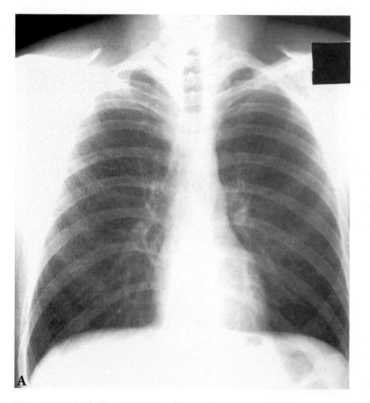
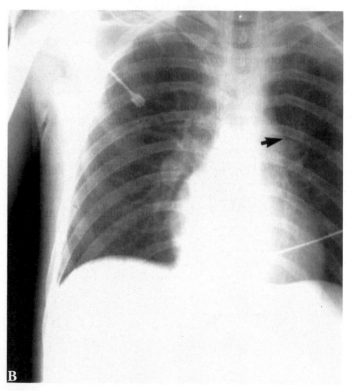

Figure 23-6. Embolism. A, Normal, prepulmonary embolism on posteroanterior chest radiograph (CXR); B, pulmonary embolism. The CXR is read as "normal" in up to 30% of patients with angiographically proven pulmonary embolism. In comparison with panel A, panel B shows a subtle elevation of the right hemidiaphragm. In panel A, the right and left hemidiaphragms are equal. In some series, an elevated hemidiaphragm is the most common finding with acute pulmonary embolism. Also, note the plumpness of the right pulmonary artery, prominent pulmonary outflow tract on the left (arrow), and subtle change in cardiac diameter. At the time of CXR, this 28-year-old man was in shock from massive pulmonary emboli as a result of major soft tissue trauma produced by a motorcycle accident 7 days earlier.

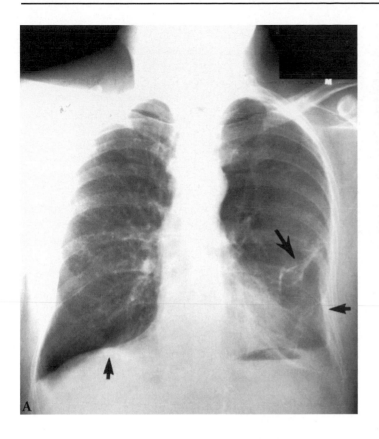

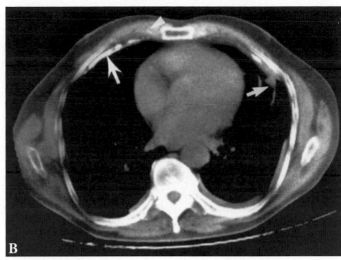

Figure 23-7. Asbestos Exposure. Abnormal chest radiograph, A, in a 68-year-old asymp-tomatic man. Small arrows indicate areas of pleural calcification, particularly on the right hemidiaphragm. This is a tip-off to previous asbestos exposure. The process in the left mid lung was worrisome (large arrow), perhaps indicating a new process such as bronchogenic carcinoma in this smoker. However, computed tomography, B, disclosed rounded atelectasis (small arrow). The "comma" extending from this mass is characteristic of rounded atelectasis, which is the result of subacute-to-chronic pleural effusion resolving and trapping some lung as it heals. Also note pleural calcification in panel B (large arrow).

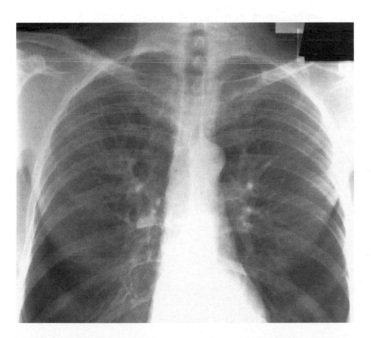

Figure 23-8. Panlobular Emphysema at the Bases Consistent With the Diagnosis of α_1-Antitrypsin Deficiency. Emphysema should not be read into a chest radiograph because all it usually represents is hyperinflation that can occur with severe asthma as well. However, in this setting, there are markedly diminished interstitial markings at the bases, with radiolucency. Also, blood flow is increased to the upper lobes because that is where most of the viable lung tissue is.

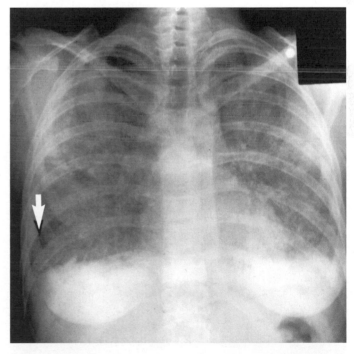

Figure 23-9. Lymphangitic Carcinoma in a 27-Year-old Woman. She had a 6-week history of progressive dyspnea and weight loss. Because of her young age, neoplasm may not be considered initially. However, the chest raddiographic features suggest it: bilateral pleural effusions, Kerley B lines as evident in the right base (arrow), and mediastinal and hilar lymphadenopathy in addition to diffuse parenchymal infiltrate.

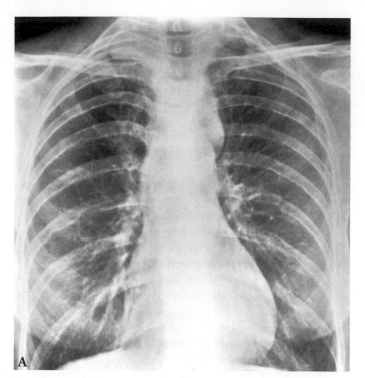

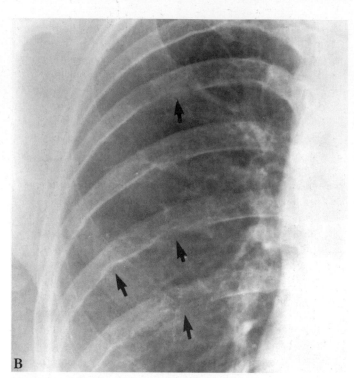

Figure 23-10. Coarctation. A and B, Posteroanterior chest radiographs showing coarctation with a tortuous aorta mimicking a mediastinal mass. This occurs in about one-third of patients with coarctation. Rib notching is indicated by the arrows in panel B.

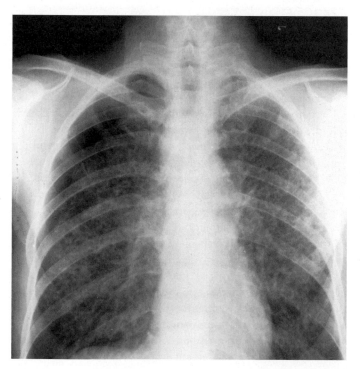

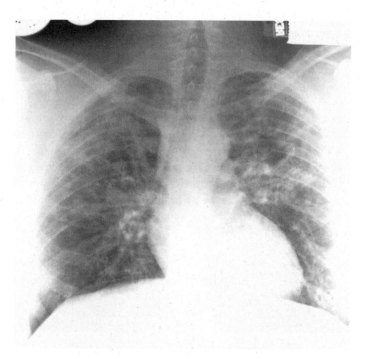

Figure 23-11. Histiocytosis X (or Eosinophilic Granuloma). Extensive change is predominantly in the upper two-thirds of the lung fields. Eventually 25% of these patients have pneumothorax, as seen on this chest radiograph (right side). The honeycombing, also described as microcysts, is characteristic of advanced histiocytosis X.

Figure 23-12. Sarcoidosis in a 35-Year-Old Patient. This chest radiograph shows the predominant upper two-thirds parenchymal pattern seen in many patients with stage II or III sarcoidosis. The pattern can be interstitial, alveolar (which this one is predominantly), or a combination. There probably is some residual adenopathy in the hila and right paratracheal area.

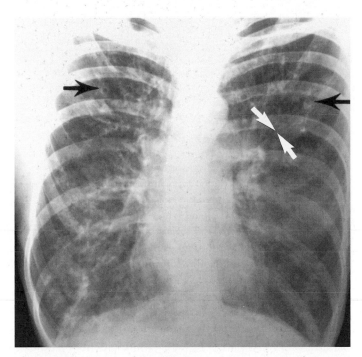

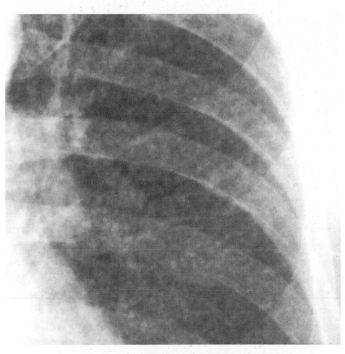

Figure 23-13. Advanced Cystic Fibrosis. Chest radiograph shows hyperinflation with low-lying hemidiaphragms, bronchiectasis (white arrows pointing to parallel lines), and microabscesses (black arrows) representing small areas of pneumonitis distal to the mucous plug that has been coughed out. Cystic fibrosis almost always begins in the upper lobes.

Figure 23-14. Miliary Tuberculosis. Chest radiograph shows a miliary pattern of relatively discrete micronodules, with little interstitial (linear or reticular) markings. Disseminated fungal disease has a similar appearance, as does bronchoalveolar cell carcinoma; however, the patients do not usually have the systemic manifestations of miliary tuberculosis. Other, less common differential diagnoses include lymphoma, lymphocytic interstitial pneumonitis, and pulmonary edema. *Pneumocystis carinii* pneumonia usually has a more interstitial reaction.

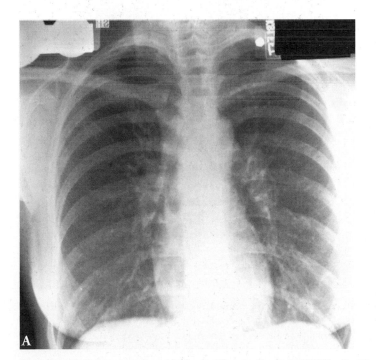

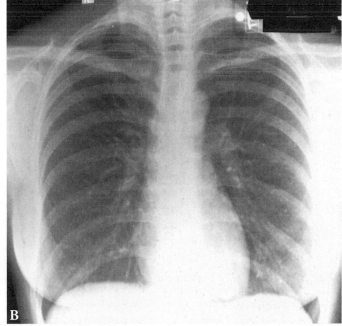

Figure 23-15. Pulmonary Sarcoidosis. A, Chest radiograph (CXR) of a 30-year-old woman with stage I pulmonary sarcoidosis with subtle bilateral hilar and mediastinal adenopathy, particularly right paratracheal and left infra-aortic adenopathy. B, CXR 1 year later, after spontaneous regression of sarcoidosis.

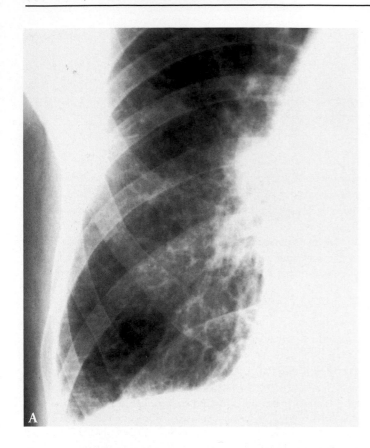

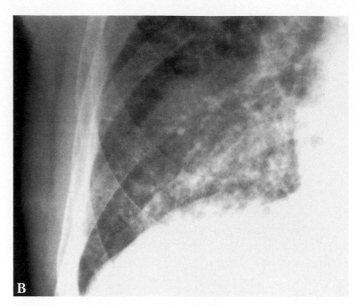

Figure 23-16. Kerley B Lines. A and B, Two examples that can be helpful in interpreting chest radiographs. A, Kerley B lines in a 75-year-old man with colon cancer. B, Kerley B lines are from metastatic adenocarcinoma of the colon and were a tip-off that the parenchymal process in this patient was due to metastatic carcinoma and not to a primary pulmonary process such as pulmonary fibrosis, which was the working diagnosis.

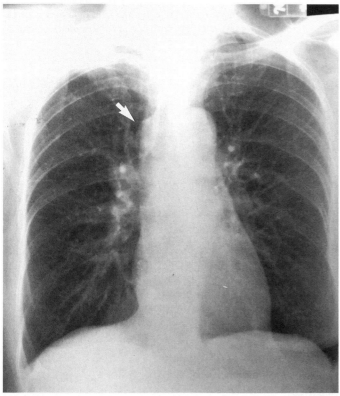

Figure 23-17. Metastatic Carcinoma of the Breast. Chest radiograph from a 55-year-old woman who had had a right mastectomy for breast carcinoma now shows subtle but definite right paratracheal (arrow) and right hilar adenopathy from metastatic carcinoma of the breast.

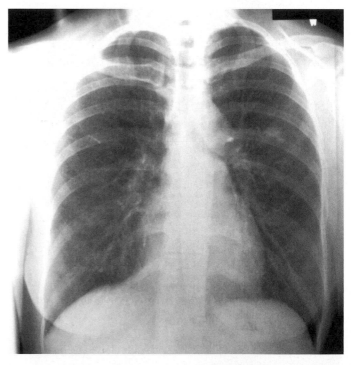

Figure 23-18. "Solitary Pulmonary Nodule." The nodule in the left mid lung field is technically not a solitary pulmonary nodule because of another abnormality in the thorax that might be related to it, left infra-aortic adenopathy. The differential diagnosis would be bronchogenic carcinoma with hilar nodal metastasis or, as in this case, acute primary pulmonary histoplasmosis. Had this patient been in an area with coccidioidomycosis, it would also be included in the differential diagnosis.

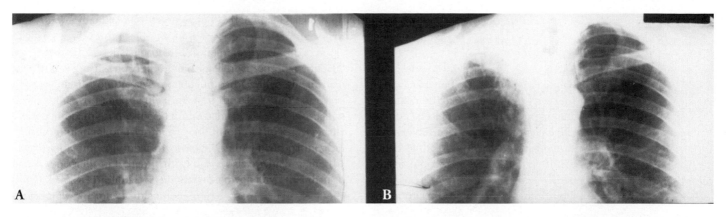

Figure 23-19. Pancoast Tumor. A, Subtle asymmetry at the apex of the right lung was more obvious 3.5 years later, B, at the time the Pancoast lesion (primary bronchogenic carcinoma) was diagnosed. The patient was symptomatic at the time of the initial chest radiograph, with the symptoms attributed to a cervical disk.

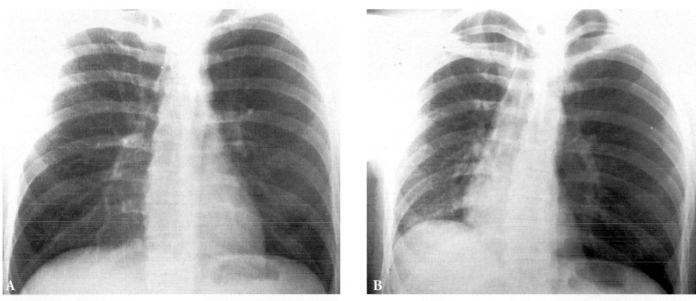

Figure 23-20. Bronchial Carcinoid. The adage that "not all that wheezes is asthma" should be remembered every time a patient with asthma is encountered and the condition does not seem to improve. In the case shown here, A, wheezes were predominant over the left hemithorax. The forced expiration film, B, showed air trapping in the left lung. Bronchial carcinoid of the left main bronchus was diagnosed at bronchoscopy.

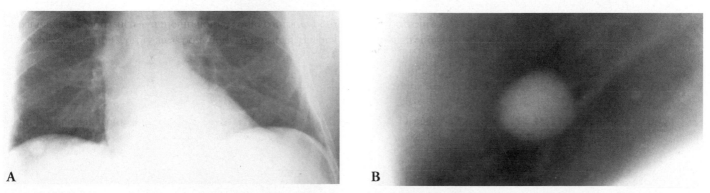

Figure 23-21. Adenocarcinoma. A, A solitary pulmonary nodule is evident below the right hemidiaphragm, where at least 15% of the lung is obscured. B, Tomography shows that the nodule has a discrete border but is noncalcified. It was not present 18 months earlier.

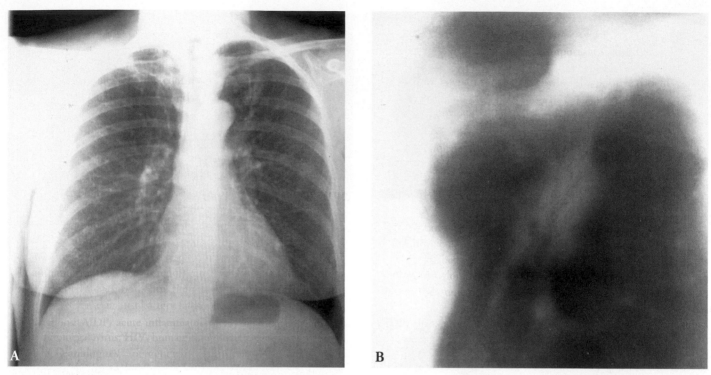

Figure 23-22. Infiltrate. A, Solitary infiltrate in the left upper lobe with air bronchogram, as evident on tomography or computed tomography. B, Air bronchogram should be considered a sign of bronchoalveolar cell carcinoma or lymphoma until proved otherwise.

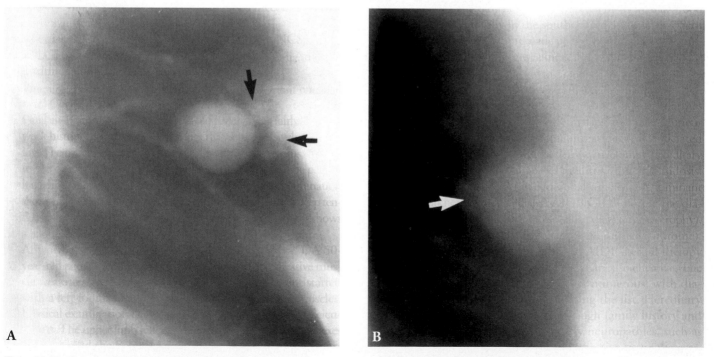

Figure 23-23. Granuloma. A and B, Tomography of solitary pulmonary nodules shows characteristic satellite nodules (arrows).

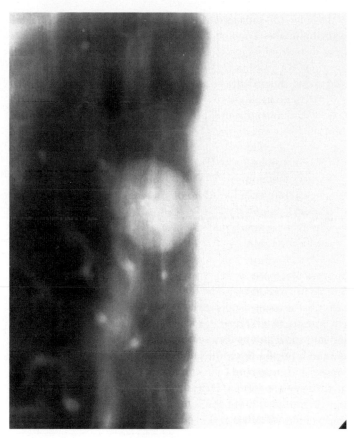

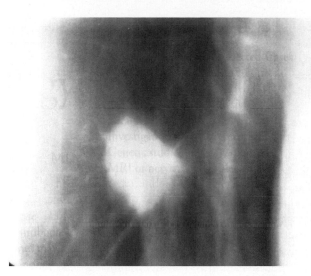

Figure 23-25. Primary Bronchogenic Carcinoma. Tomography of a solitary nodule shows characteristic spiculation or sunburst effect. Spicules represent extension of the tumor into septa. Computed tomography showed a similar appearance.

Figure 23-24. Popcorn Calcification of Hamartoma. This can be seen also in granuloma and represents a benign process.

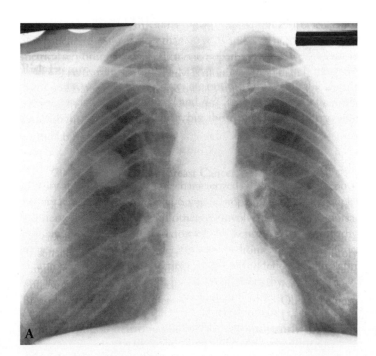

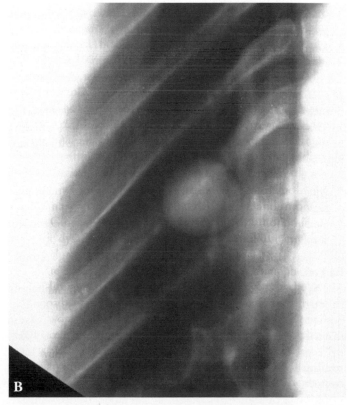

Figure 23-26. Bull's-eye Calcification Characteristic of Granuloma in a Solitary Pulmonary Nodule (A and B). These nodules occasionally enlarge but even then almost never warrant removal.

- CT is useful in evaluating the presence of solitary pulmonary nodules, multiple lung nodules (metastatic), and calcification in nodules.
- Ultrafast CT with contrast media is better than a $\dot{V}/\dot{Q}$ scan for diagnosing pulmonary emboli.

Magnetic Resonance Imaging

MRI is recommended for the initial evaluation of superior sulcus tumors (Pancoast tumor), lesions of the brachial plexus, and paraspinal masses that on CXR appear most consistent with neurogenic tumors. MRI is superior to CT in the evaluation of chest wall masses and in the search for small occult mediastinal neoplasms (eg, ectopic parathyroid adenoma). Magnetic resonance angiography is useful when CT with contrast media is contraindicated for patients with renal failure or contrast allergy. MRI may be superior to CT in evaluating pulmonary sequestration, arteriovenous malformation, vascular structures, and tumor recurrence in patients with total pneumonectomy.

- MRI: useful for the evaluation of superior sulcus tumors and neurogenic tumors.

Pulmonary Angiography

The main indication for pulmonary angiography is to detect pulmonary emboli. However, small peripheral emboli may not be seen. Pulmonary angiography is also useful in the diagnosis of pulmonary arteriovenous fistulas and malformations, and it is usually a prerequisite if embolotherapy is planned.

- Common indications: pulmonary embolism and pulmonary arteriovenous malformations and fistulas.
- Pulmonary angiography may not detect a peripheral or tiny pulmonary embolism.

Bronchial Angiography

Bronchial angiography is used to determine whether the bronchial arteries are the cause of massive pulmonary hemorrhage or massive hemoptysis. It is a prerequisite if bronchial arterial embolotherapy is planned.

- Main indication: suspected bronchial arterial bleeding in massive hemoptysis.
- Both pulmonary and bronchial angiography may be needed for some patients who have massive hemoptysis.

Radionuclide Lung Scans

The $\dot{V}/\dot{Q}$ scan is still used in the diagnosis of pulmonary embolism, although CT angiography is assuming an increasingly larger diagnostic role. The likelihood of pulmonary embolism in a $\dot{V}/\dot{Q}$ scan that shows "high probability" and a scan that shows "low probability" is greater than 90% and less than 5%, respectively. An "intermediate probability" scan usually is an indication for a CT scan with contrast medium or for pulmonary angiography. However, clinical suspicion of pulmonary embolism should guide the decision. The quantitative $\dot{V}/\dot{Q}$ scan is used to assess unilateral and regional pulmonary function by measuring $\dot{V}/\dot{Q}$ relationships in different regions of the lungs. It is indicated for patients who are poor surgical candidates for lung resection because of underlying pulmonary dysfunction. If the lung region to be resected shows minimal or no lung function on a quantitative $\dot{V}/\dot{Q}$ scan, the resection is unlikely to further impair the patient's pulmonary reserve. The gallium scan is of minimal or no use in the diagnosis of diffuse lung diseases. The technetium 99m scan is useful in detecting diffuse pulmonary calcification associated with chronic hemodialysis.

- Quantitative $\dot{V}/\dot{Q}$ scan is used to assess unilateral or regional pulmonary function.
- The gallium scan has no role in the diagnosis of diffuse lung disease.
- The technetium 99m lung scan detects diffuse pulmonary calcification.

Sputum Microscopy

Simple microscopy with a "wet" slide preparation of sputum is helpful in assessing the degree of sputum eosinophilia and detecting the presence of Charcot-Leyden crystals. Gram staining of sputum should be used to evaluate suspected bacterial infections. Induced sputum is helpful in identifying mycobacteria, fungi, *Pneumocystis jiroveci*, and malignant cells. Gastric washings are used to identify mycobacteria and fungi. Hemosiderin-laden macrophages in sputum do not always indicate alveolar hemorrhage; smokers can have a large number of hemosiderin-laden macrophages in their sputum.

- A sputum "wet prep" detects eosinophilia and Charcot-Leyden crystals.
- Induced sputum is helpful for identifying *P jiroveci*.

Pulmonary Function Tests

The major indication for PFTs is dyspnea. PFT results do not diagnose lung disease, but they are used to assess the mechanical function of the respiratory system and to quantify the loss of lung function. They can be used to separate obstructive dysfunction, which indicates airflow limitation (as in asthma, bronchitis, and emphysema) from restrictive phenomena. In restrictive phenomena, the lungs cannot fully expand because of a large pleural effusion or disease in the lung parenchyma, chest wall, or diaphragm, and the volumes are diminished. A combination of obstructive and restrictive patterns is also possible (eg, COPD with pulmonary fibrosis). Bronchoprovocation testing with agents such as methacholine is useful in detecting airway hyperresponsiveness. An increase in flow rates (>12% and 200 mL) after bronchodilator therapy suggests reversible component airway disease, although the absence of response does not preclude a clinical trial with inhaled bronchodilator medications. Results of previous PFTs are helpful in following the course of lung disease.

- Obstructive dysfunction: indicates airflow limitation, as in asthma, bronchitis, and emphysema.
- An increase in flow rates (>12% and 200 mL) after bronchodilator therapy suggests reversible component airway disease, although the absence of response does not preclude a clinical trial with inhaled bronchodilator medications.

- Restrictive dysfunction: limitation to full expansion of the lungs because of a large pleural effusion or disease in the lung parenchyma, chest wall, or diaphragm; volumes are diminished.
- A combination of obstructive and restrictive patterns is also possible (eg, COPD with pulmonary fibrosis).

Provocation Inhalational Challenge

Provocation inhalational challenge is useful when the diagnosis of asthma or hyperreactive airway disease is uncertain. The test uses agents that elicit a bronchospastic response, for example, methacholine, carbachol, histamine, industrial irritants, exercise, isocapneic hyperventilation, and cold air. A 20% decrease in forced expiratory volume in 1 second (FEV_1) from baseline is considered a positive test result. Up to 10% of healthy subjects may exhibit a positive response to provocation challenge without symptoms of asthma. Thus, the strength of the test is in its high negative predictive value. A positive test is not diagnostic for asthma since airways may become hyperreactive owing to recent infection or inflammation.

- A 20% decrease in FEV_1 from baseline is considered a positive test result.
- Up to 10% of healthy subjects exhibit a positive response to an inhalational challenge.
- A negative test is helpful in ruling out hyperreactive airway disease.

Interpretation of Pulmonary Function Tests

A simplified step-by-step approach to interpretation of PFT results is as follows:

1. Evaluate volumes and flows separately.
2. Look at the flow volume curve to see whether it suggests an obstructive ("scooped out" appearance) or a restrictive (high peak with narrow curve) pattern.
3. Look at the FEV_1/forced vital capacity (FVC) ratio. An FEV_1/FVC ratio <70% suggests airflow obstruction. Look at FEV_1, which is used to classify the severity of airflow obstruction (Table 23-3).
4. If FEV_1/FVC is >70% but FEV_1 is reduced, look at total lung capacity (TLC). Reduced TLC suggests a restrictive defect (Table 23-3).
5. TLC, functional residual capacity (FRC), and residual volume (RV) indicate volumes. TLC = VC (vital capacity) + RV. Increases in TLC and RV suggest hyperinflation (asthma or COPD). If TLC and VC are decreased, consider restrictive lung disease (fibrosis) or loss of lung volume (surgery, diaphragmatic paralysis, or skeletal problems).
6. VC measured during a slow (not forced) expiration is not affected by airway collapse in COPD. FVC may be low with forced expiration because of airway collapse. In healthy subjects, VC = FVC.
7. FEV_1 and forced expiratory flow (FEF) between 25% and 75% of VC ($FEF_{25\%-75\%}$) indicate flow rates. Flow rates are diminished in COPD, but smaller decreases can occur if lung volumes are low. Decreased FEV_1/FVC (<70%) indicates obstruction to airflow.

8. The maximal voluntary ventilation (MVV) test requires rapid inspiratory and expiratory maneuvers and, thus, tests airflow through major airways and muscle strength. Disproportionately reduced MVV ($MVV = FEV_1 \times 35$) may be from poor effort, variable extrathoracic obstruction, and respiratory muscle weakness. Respiratory muscle weakness can be assessed by maximal inspiratory pressure (PImax) and maximal expiratory pressure (PEmax). Clinical features should be correlated with the results of PFTs.
9. Diffusing capacity for carbon monoxide (DLCO) is dependent on the thickness of the alveolocapillary membrane (T); the area of the alveolocapillary membrane (A), which is also influenced by number of capillaries and blood volume/flow; and the driving pressure (ie, the difference in carbon monoxide tension between the alveolar gas and venous blood (ΔP_{CO})). Thus, DLCO is represented by the following:

$$DLCO \sim \frac{A \times \Delta P_{CO}}{T}$$

DLCO is low in anatomical emphysema ($\downarrow A$), anemia (effectively $\downarrow A$), restrictive lung diseases ($\downarrow A$ or $\downarrow T$ in pulmonary fibrosis or other interstitial lung diseases), pneumonectomy ($\downarrow A$), pulmonary hypertension (effectively $\downarrow T$), and recurrent pulmonary emboli (effectively $\downarrow A$). DLCO is increased in the supine posture ($\uparrow A$ due to

Table 23-3 Interpretation of Pulmonary Function Testing

Obstruction is indicated by FEV_1/FVC <70% of predicted value

FEV_1, % of predicted value	Severity of airflow obstruction
>80	Borderline
<80 & >60	Mild
<60 & >40	Moderate
<40	Severe

Restriction is indicated by TLC <80% of predicted value (restrictive defect is only suggested by reduced vital capacity; TLC is needed for confirmation)

TLC, % of predicted value	Severity of restrictive defect
<80 & >60	Mild
<60 & >50	Moderate
<50	Severe

Bronchodilator response

Requires both 12% & 200-mL improvement in FEV_1 after bronchodilator therapy

Methacholine challenge

Requires 20% decrease in FEV_1 after challenge to be considered positive

Abbreviations: FEV_1, forced expiratory volume in 1 second; FVC, forced vital capacity; TLC, total lung capacity.

increased blood volume in upper lobes), after exercise (↑A due to increased blood volume), in polycythemia (↑A), in obesity (↑A due to increased blood volume), in left-to-right shunt (↑A), and in some patients with asthma. Isolated low DLCO (with normal results on PFT) is seen in pulmonary hypertension, multiple pulmonary emboli, combined diseases such as pulmonary fibrosis with COPD, and anemia. A decrease in hemoglobin by 1 g diminishes DLCO by 7%.

10. Flow-volume curves are helpful to distinguish between intrathoracic and extrathoracic major airway obstructions. Flattening of the expiratory flow curve with a normal inspiratory flow curve suggests intrathoracic airway obstruction. Flattening of the inspiratory flow curve alone suggests extrathoracic airway obstruction. Flattening of both flow curves suggests fixed airway obstruction, and the location cannot be determined.

* Respiratory muscle weakness can be assessed by PImax and PEmax.
* Clinical features should be correlated with the results of PFTs.
* DLCO is decreased in anatomical emphysema.
* An isolated decrease in DLCO (normal volumes and flows) may occur in pulmonary hypertension, multiple pulmonary emboli, combined restrictive and obstructive lung diseases, and severe anemia.
* A decrease in hemoglobin by 1 g diminishes DLCO by 7%.
* Flow-volume curves are helpful to distinguish between intrathoracic and extrathoracic major airway obstructions.

Explanations for Table 23-4

Patient 1. The patient has typical features of emphysema. The FEV_1/FVC ratio indicates obstruction. The FEV_1 indicates that the obstruction is severe. The TLC indicates hyperinflation. The reduced DLCO suggests emphysema. The clinical diagnosis is severe obstructive disease with anatomical emphysema.

Patient 2. As in the first case, the PFTs suggest emphysema. In a young nonsmoker, other causes of emphysema must be considered. The clinical diagnosis is severe emphysema caused by familial deficiency of α_1-antitrypsin.

Patient 3. Flow rates and lung volumes are decreased only slightly but are within normal limits. MVV is severely decreased. In this patient, PImax and PEmax were severely decreased, suggesting muscle weakness. The clinical diagnosis is severe thyrotoxicosis with proximal muscle weakness (ie, thyrotoxic myopathy). This pattern of PFT results can also occur in neuromuscular diseases such as amyotrophic lateral sclerosis and myasthenia gravis.

Patient 4. As indicated by the FEV_1/FVC ratio and FEV_1, there is a moderately severe airflow obstruction. The normal TLC and residual volume suggest an absence of air trapping. The normal DLCO excludes anatomical emphysema or other parenchymal problems. Bronchodilator testing that was performed elicited improvement in lung volumes and flow rates. The clinical diagnosis is typical asthma.

Patient 5. This patient has normal lung volumes and flow rates (80%-120% of predicted normal). A former "superathlete," he recently noted cough and chest tightness after exertion. Previous PFT results were unavailable. The following are important points: 1) In a young, otherwise healthy patient, the lung volumes and flow rates are usually above normal, more so in an athlete. 2) This patient may have had very high volumes and flow rates in the past, but without previous PFT results, no comparison can be made (if earlier PFT results were available, the new results might represent a severe decrease in pulmonary function). 3) The history suggests the possibility of exercise-induced asthma; spirometry after an exercise test showed a 28% reduction in flow rates 5 to 10 minutes after termination of exercise. 4) Note the relatively high DLCO in this

Table 23-4 Try to Interpret These Results of Pulmonary Function Tests Before Reading the Explanations[a]

Patient	1	2	3	4	5	6	7	8	9
Age, y; sex	73 M	43 M	53 F	43 M	20 M	58 F	40 M	28 F	44 M
Weight, kg	52	53	50	63	80	59	75	52	148
Tobacco	63PY	NS	NS	NS	NS	NS	NS	NS	NS
Total lung capacity, %	140	128	84	118	100	56	68	108	90
Vital capacity, %	52	75	86	78	95	62	58	106	86
Residual volume, %	160	140	90	110	90	65	80	98	90
FEV_1, %	35	38	82	48	90	85	42	112	96
FEV_1/FVC, %	40	34	80	40	85	88	50	85	78
$FEF_{25\%-75\%}$	18	14	80	35	88	82	24	102	88
Maximal voluntary ventilation, %	62	48	40	60	120	108	62	88	90
Diffusing capacity	9	10	20	28	32	8	8	6	40
(normal)	(22)	(28)	(20)	(28)	(34)	(26)	(28)	(32)	(28)

Abbreviations: $FEF_{25\%-75\%}$, forced expiratory flow between 25% and 75% of vital capacity; FEV_1, forced expiratory volume in 1 second; FVC, forced vital capacity; NS, nonsmoker; PY, pack-years of smoking.
[a] Values of 80%-120% of predicted are considered normal.

patient, a phenomenon seen in patients with asthma. The clinical diagnosis is exercise-induced asthma.

Patient 6. This patient has a moderately severe decrease in lung volumes and normal flow rates. MVV is normal, but DLCO is severely diminished. These suggest severe restrictive lung disease. The slightly diminished flow rates are the result of decreased lung volumes. The clinical diagnosis is biopsy-proven idiopathic pulmonary fibrosis. Patients who have had lung resection also have low lung volumes and decreased DLCO.

Patient 7. The reduction in the FEV_1/FVC ratio suggests the presence of obstructive dysfunction. TLC is also decreased, which suggests additional restrictive lung disease. MVV is also reduced, and DLCO is severely decreased. Compared with patient 6, this patient has obstructive disease plus severe restrictive lung disease. A very low DLCO suggests parenchymal disease. CXR showed bilaterally diffuse nodular interstitial changes, especially in the upper two-thirds of the lungs. Biopsy specimens of the bronchial mucosa and lung showed extensive endobronchial sarcoidosis. The clinical diagnosis is severe restrictive lung disease from parenchymal sarcoidosis and obstructive dysfunction caused by endobronchial sarcoidosis.

Patient 8. This patient has normal lung volumes and flow rates. MVV is slightly reduced but within normal limits. DLCO is very low. PaO_2 is 56 mm Hg. The clinical diagnosis is primary pulmonary hypertension.

Patient 9. This patient has normal lung volumes and flow rates. DLCO is abnormally high. This patient was extremely obese. Abnormally high DLCO is reported to be a result of increased VC. The clinical diagnosis is obesity-related pulmonary dysfunction.

Preoperative Evaluation of Lung Function

If patients scheduled to undergo lung resection have suspected or documented lung disease, PFT results should be obtained preoperatively. A patient can tolerate pneumonectomy if the values are more than 50% of predicted for FEV_1, MVV, RV/TLC, and DLCO. If the values are less than 50% of predicted, a quantitative $\dot{V}/\dot{Q}$ scan will help assess regional lung functions. Preoperative bronchodilators, chest physiotherapy, incentive spirometry, and physical conditioning decrease the risk of postoperative pulmonary complications. Increased morbidity and mortality are associated with severe COPD and arterial carbon dioxide tension ($PaCO_2$) greater than 45 mm Hg (hypoxemia is not a reliable indicator). Upper abdominal operations (gallbladder and abdominal aortic aneurysm repair) have higher rates of pulmonary complications than lower abdominal procedures.

It would also be advisable to obtain smoking history and recommend smoking cessation ideally several weeks before elective surgery. Also, screening for and treatment of sleep-related breathing disorder (especially for the postoperative period) would be beneficial.

Exercise Testing

Exercise testing can assess cardiopulmonary function. Indications for cardiopulmonary exercise testing include unexplained dyspnea or effort intolerance, ability-disability evaluation, quantification of severity of pulmonary dysfunction, differentiation of cardiac from pulmonary causes of disability, evaluation of progression of a disease process, estimation of operative risks before cardiopulmonary surgery

(lung resection or heart-lung or lung transplant), rehabilitation, and evaluation of need for supplemental oxygen. Special equipment and expertise are required to perform an optimal cardiopulmonary exercise study.

Blood Gases and Oximetry

The interpretation of blood gas abnormalities is discussed in Chapter 18 ("Nephrology").

Overnight oximetry may be helpful in screening for sleep-related breathing disorders. Owing to a decrease in oxygen reserve during sleep, a brief episode of insufficient respiration can result in desaturation. Frequent oscillatory desaturations suggest sleep-related breathing disorder.

Bronchoscopy

Common diagnostic indications for bronchoscopy include persistent cough, hemoptysis, suspected cancer, lung nodule, atelectasis, diffuse lung disease, and lung infections. Diagnostic yield is low in pleural effusion. Therapeutic indications include atelectasis, retained secretions, tracheobronchial foreign bodies, airway stenosis (dilatation), and obstructive lesions (laser therapy or stent placement). Bronchoscopy may be helpful in the staging of lung cancer. Complications from bronchoscopy are minimal and include bleeding from mucosal or lung biopsy, pneumothorax (from lung biopsy), and hypoxemia.

* Bronchoscopy: low diagnostic yield in pleural effusion.
* Useful in the diagnosis and staging of lung cancer.

Bronchoalveolar Lavage

Bronchoalveolar lavage (BAL) is performed by instilling 100 to 150 mL of sterile normal saline into diseased segments of the lung. The instilled saline is aspirated through the bronchoscope. The aspirated effluent can be analyzed for cells, chemical constituents, and cultures for infectious agents. BAL in healthy subjects shows alveolar macrophages (93%±3%) and lymphocytes (7%±1%). Other types of leukocytes (neutrophils <1%) are rarely found in healthy subjects.

* BAL can quantify and identify cell morphology at the alveolar level.
* Healthy subjects: macrophages (93%), lymphocytes (7%), and neutrophils (<1%).

BAL may be helpful in diagnosing alveolar hemorrhage, alveolar proteinosis, pulmonary Langerhans cell granulomatosis, and lymphangitic pulmonary metastasis. The CD4/CD8 ratio in BAL effluent is reversed in patients with acquired immunodeficiency syndrome (AIDS) complicated by lymphocytic interstitial pneumonitis and in many patients with hypersensitivity pneumonitis. BAL is helpful in the diagnosis of infections in immunocompromised hosts, *P jiroveci* infection, tuberculosis, mycoses, and other infections. BAL has a limited role in the diagnosis of sarcoidosis and idiopathic pulmonary fibrosis. It is diagnostic in more than 60% of patients with pulmonary lymphangitic carcinomatosis.

- BAL is helpful in diagnosing opportunistic lung infections.
- BAL has a limited role in the diagnosis of sarcoidosis and idiopathic pulmonary fibrosis.
- BAL is diagnostic in >60% of patients with pulmonary lymphangitic carcinomatosis.

Lung Biopsy

Lung biopsy can be performed by means of bronchoscopy, thoracoscopy, or thoracotomy. The indications for lung biopsy in diffuse lung disease should be based on the clinical features, treatment planned, and risks from biopsy and from treatment without a pathologic diagnosis. Bronchoscopic lung biopsy can provide a diagnostic yield of up to 80% to 90% in sarcoidosis, pulmonary Langerhans cell granulomatosis, eosinophilic pneumonitis, lymphangioleiomyomatosis, infections, pulmonary alveolar proteinosis, lymphangitic carcinomatosis, and hypersensitivity pneumonitis, especially when performed in combination with special stains. The major complications after bronchoscopic lung biopsy are pneumothorax (<2%) and hemorrhage (<3%).

Obstructive Lung Diseases

A common pathophysiologic feature of obstructive lung diseases is the obstruction to flow of air. Obstructive lung diseases include emphysema, bronchitis, asthma, bronchiectasis, cystic fibrosis, bronchiolitis, bullous lung disease, and airway stenosis. The 3 most prevalent obstructive lung diseases are emphysema, chronic bronchitis, and asthma; they affect at least 25 to 30 million people in the United States. The salient features of these diseases are compared in Table 23-5. COPD represents the fourth leading cause of chronic morbidity and mortality in the United States. The current working definition of *COPD* is a disease state characterized by airflow limitation that is not fully reversible. This implies that asthma, which is considered fully reversible (at least in its early stages), is separate from COPD. Although there is airway inflammation in both diseases, the inflammation characteristics of COPD appear to be different from those of asthma. In some instances, however, the 2 diseases can coexist. A classification of the severity of COPD has been proposed and should guide management at various stages of the disease (Table 23-6). Note the difference in clinical staging of COPD from the classification of severity of airflow obstruction on the PFT.

Etiology

Tobacco smoking is the major cause of COPD. Nearly 10% to 20% of smokers exhibit an accelerated rate of decrease in FEV_1. This decrease is proportional to the number of pack-years of smoking. Smokers have 10 times the risk of nonsmokers of dying of COPD. Pipe and cigar smokers have between 1.5 and 3 times the risk of nonsmokers. Smoking increases the risk of developing COPD in persons who have α_1-antitrypsin deficiency. Smokers have an increased incidence of COPD, atherosclerosis, abdominal aortic aneurysm, and carcinoma of the lung, larynx, esophagus, and bladder. Diseases associated with or aggravated by smoking include asthma, some forms of interstitial lung diseases, calcification of pleural plaques in asbestosis, pulmonary alveolar phospholipoproteinosis, pulmonary

Table 23-5 Salient Differential Features of Bronchial Asthma, Chronic Bronchitis, and Emphysema[a]

Differential Feature	Bronchial Asthma	Chronic Bronchitis	Emphysema
Onset	70% <30 y old	≥50 y old	≥60 y old
Cigarette smoking	0	++++	++++
Pattern	Paroxysmal	Chronic, progressive	Chronic, progressive
Dyspnea	0 to ++++	+ to ++++	+++ to ++++
Cough	0 to +++	++ to ++++	+ to +++
Sputum	0 to ++	+++	+ to ++
Atopy	50% (adult)	15%	15%
Infections	↑ Symptoms	↑↑↑ Symptoms	↑ Symptoms
Chest radiograph	Usually normal	↑ Marking	Hyperinflation
$PaCO_2$	Normal or ↓ in attack	↑	Normal or ↑
PaO_2	Normal or ↓ in attack	Low	Low
DLCO	Normal	Normal or slight ↓	↓
FEV_1, %	↓↓ in attack or normal	↓↓	↓↓
Total lung capacity	Normal or ↑ in attack	Normal or slight ↑	↑↑↑
Residual volume	Normal or ↑ in attack	Normal or slight ↑	↑↑↑
Cor pulmonale	Rare	Common	Rare
Hematocrit	Normal	Normal or ↑	Normal or ↑

Abbreviations: DLCO, diffusion capacity to total lung capacity ratio; FEV_1, %, percentage of vital capacity expired in 1 second.

[a] ↑ indicates increase; ↓, decrease; ↑↑, increased more; ↓↓, decreased more; ↑↑↑, increased greatly; ↓↓↓, decreased greatly; +, present; ++, bothersome; +++, major problem; ++++, significant problem.

From Kaliner M, Lemanske R. Rhinitis and asthma. JAMA. 1992;268:2807-29. Used with permission.

Table 23-6 Practical Aspects of Managing Chronic Obstructive Pulmonary Disease (COPD)

Steps in management
   Identify the type of COPD
   Identify pathophysiology
   Assess lung dysfunction
   Eliminate causative/exacerbating factors
   Aim drug therapy at underlying pathophysiology
   Anticipate & treat complications
   Enroll in a rehabilitation program
   Educate patient & family
Stepped care approach
   Mild COPD (FEV$_1$/FVC <70%, FEV$_1$ ≥80% of predicted)
      Short activity bronchodilators as needed
   Moderate COPD (FEV$_1$/FVC <70%, 50% ≤FEV$_1$ <80% of predicted)
      Scheduled use of long-acting bronchodilators, short-acting bronchodilator as needed, rehabilitation
   Severe COPD (FEV$_1$/FVC <70%, 30% ≤FEV$_1$ <50% of predicted)
      Scheduled use of bronchodilators with or without inhaled steroids if repeated exacerbations or lung function response, short-acting bronchodilator as needed, rehabilitation
   Very severe COPD (FEV$_1$/FVC <70%, FEV$_1$ <30% of predicted or presence of respiratory failure or right heart failure)
      Regular use of bronchodilators with or without inhaled steroids, rehabilitation, long-term oxygen if respiratory failure; consider surgical treatments

Abbreviations: FEV$_1$, forced expiratory volume in 1 second; FVC, forced vital capacity.

Langerhans cell granulomatosis, and lung hemorrhage in Goodpasture syndrome. Sidestream tobacco exposure (secondhand smoke) is also carcinogenic. Other increased risks (particularly in children) include infections of the lower respiratory tract, fluid collection in the middle ear, decreased lung function, increased severity of preexistent asthma, and increased risk of asthma.

* Nearly 10%-20% of smokers exhibit an accelerated rate of decrease in FEV$_1$.
* Pulmonary Langerhans cell granulomatosis and pulmonary alveolar proteinosis are more common in smokers.
* Sidestream smoke is also carcinogenic.

Air pollution caused by oxidants, oxides of nitrogen, hydrocarbons, and sulfur dioxide has an important role in exacerbating COPD. Occupational exposures, heredity (α_1-antitrypsin deficiency), infections, allergy (in asthma), and other factors are also involved in the etiology of COPD.

Pathology
Obstruction to airflow in COPD can result from damage of lung tissue by mucus hypersecretion and hypertrophy, airway narrowing

(bronchospasm) and fibrosis, destruction of lung parenchyma, and pulmonary vascular changes. The premature collapse of airways leads to air-trapping and hyperinflation of the lungs (barrel chest). Bronchospasm in susceptible persons occurs from increased bronchomotor tone in the smooth muscles of the airways. Bronchospasm can occur as a result of many underlying complex mechanisms mediated by the vagus nerve, extrinsic allergens, release of intrinsic chemicals, external physical and chemical injury, hypothermia of airways, and other factors. Mucous gland hypertrophy occurs in chronic bronchitis, asthma, and other airway diseases as a result of direct or indirect stimulation of mucous glands. Increased bronchomotor tone can be elicited by the provocation inhalational challenge (see above). Histologically, centrilobular emphysema is the most common type of COPD and usually starts in the upper lobes. The panlobular type usually starts in the lower lobes and is often seen in COPD associated with α_1-antitrypsin deficiency.

* Causes of airway obstruction: expiratory collapse of airways, bronchospasm, mucosal inflammation, pulmonary vascular changes, and mucous gland hypertrophy.
* Upper lobe centrilobular emphysema is the most common type of emphysema in susceptible smokers.
* Lower lobe panlobular emphysema is the usual pattern in patients with α_1-antitrypsin deficiency.

Physiology
Decreased flow rates are characteristic of COPD. Lung compliance is increased in emphysema, and elastic recoil of the lung is decreased (the opposite occurs in restrictive lung disease). DLCO is diminished in emphysema (as well as in most restrictive lung diseases). Hyperexpansion is manifested by increased total lung capacity and residual volume. As COPD progresses, continued parenchymal destruction and pulmonary vascular abnormalities result in hypoxemia, which eventually may progress to hypercapnia.

* Lung compliance is increased in emphysema (decreased in restrictive lung disease).

Emphysema
Emphysema, a pathology term, is characterized by enlargement of the airspaces distal to the terminal bronchioles and destruction of the alveolar walls. This entity describes only 1 of several structural abnormalities present in patients with COPD. CT of the lungs can identify emphysema and bullous lung disease. Severe weight loss is a relatively common finding in severe emphysema. Carbon dioxide retention does not occur until late in the disease.

Bullous Lung Disease
Small apical bullae are present in many healthy persons. Bullous lung disease can be congenital or acquired. Bullous changes may be seen in Marfan and Ehlers-Danlos syndromes, burned-out sarcoidosis, and cadmium exposure. Panlobular emphysema may look like a bulla. Lack of communication with bronchi may cause air-trapping. Complications include pneumothorax, COPD, infection and formation of lung abscess, bleeding into a bulla, and compression of

adjacent normal lung. Surgical therapy may improve lung function by 5% to 10% in 10% to 15% of patients. The incidence of lung cancer is increased in patients with bullous emphysema.

- Panlobular emphysema may look like a bulla.
- Bullous changes may be seen in Marfan and Ehlers-Danlos syndromes, burned-out sarcoidosis, and cadmium exposure.
- Bullous lung disease is associated with an increased risk of lung cancer.

α_1-Antitrypsin Deficiency

The synthesis of α_1-antitrypsin, a secretory glycoprotein, by hepatocytes is determined by the α_1-antitrypsin gene on chromosome 14. α_1-Antitrypsin inhibits many proteolytic enzymes and, thus, protects the lungs from destructive emphysema. α_1-Antitrypsin deficiency is an autosomal recessive disease; the phenotypes are normal (P_1MM), heterozygote (P_1MZ), homozygote (P_1ZZ), and null (P_1Null). Other phenotypes with either no increased risk or a slightly increased risk of disease are P_1SS and P_1SZ, respectively. The threshold for disease is set at a plasma α_1-antitrypsin level of less than 11 mcmol/L (normal, 20-53 mcmol/L). The prevalence of P_1ZZ in the United States is 1:1,670 to 1:5,097. Up to 10% of patients with P_1ZZ α_1-antitrypsin deficiency do not develop lung disease. Up to 95% of those with the P_1ZZ phenotype may have an unrecognized deficiency because they are asymptomatic or the disease is unrecognized. In nonsmoking P_1ZZ persons, lung function decreases with increasing age, especially after age 50. Men are at greater risk of deterioration of lung function than women. Smoking hastens the onset of emphysema. Signs and symptoms may appear during the third or fourth decade of life. Features include basal emphysema on CXR, absence of α_1-globulin on protein electrophoresis, patient with COPD, and family history of COPD. Hepatic cirrhosis develops in up to 3% of patients. In young patients with clinical features of COPD, consider asthma, α_1-antitrypsin deficiency, cystic fibrosis, ciliary dyskinesia, and bronchiectasis. A lack of α_1-antitrypsin seems to increase the propensity to develop asthma. Replacement therapy for symptomatic persons with the P_1ZZ phenotype should be considered when the serum level of α_1-antitryptsin is less than 11 mcmol/L. α_1-Antitrypsin derived from human plasma has been used as replacement therapy; minimal decreases in the rate of decrease of FEV_1 (~27 mL per year) have been observed in patients with severe emphysema.

- In α_1-antitrypsin deficiency, smoking hastens the onset of emphysema.
- Features of the disease: basal emphysema on CXR, absence of α_1-globulin on protein electrophoresis, patient with COPD, and family history of COPD.
- Hepatic cirrhosis develops in up to 3% of patients.
- In young patients with clinical features of COPD, consider asthma, α_1-antitrypsin deficiency, cystic fibrosis, ciliary dyskinesia, and bronchiectasis.
- Replacement therapy for symptomatic persons with the P_1ZZ phenotype should be considered when the serum level of α_1-antitrypsin is <11 mcmol/L.

Asthma

Asthma is discussed in Chapter 2 ("Allergy").

Treatment of COPD

The therapeutic approach to COPD consists of reducing risk factors (eg, smoking cessation), identifying the severity of COPD, quantification of pulmonary dysfunction and response to bronchodilator therapy, selection of appropriate bronchodilators, anticipation and appropriate treatment of complications, and initial as well as continued education of the patient and family about long-term therapy. Proper inhalation technique is essential in optimal treatment. Pulmonary rehabilitation decreases disability and improves the handicap, but PFT results show minimal improvement.

Reducing Risk Factors

Because cigarette smoking represents a major risk factor in the development and progression of COPD, smoking cessation should be discussed and programs offered to those who continue to smoke. Smoking cessation can prevent or delay the onset of symptoms in persons without disease and slow the progression in those with disease. Brief physician intervention can be effective in 5% to 10% of smokers. A formal multidisciplinary program with the use of skills training, problem solving, social support, and medications (nicotine replacement therapy, bupropion, or varenicline) can increase smoking cessation in up to 35% of smokers. Reduction in occupational dusts, gases, and fumes and other pollutants is also important in the management of COPD.

- Smoking cessation is vital in the treatment of COPD.
- Minimize exposure to other occupational and environmental pollutants.
- Formal smoking cessation programs can be effective in up to 35% of smokers.

Bronchodilators

Bronchodilator drugs are administered to reverse bronchoconstriction (bronchospasm). They can be divided into β-adrenergic agonists (β_2-selective agonists), anticholinergics (ipratropium), adrenergic agonists (sympathomimetics), phosphodiesterase inhibitors (theophylline), mast cell inhibitors (cromolyn), leukotriene modifiers, antihistamines, anti-inflammatory agents (corticosteroids and methotrexate), and other agents (troleandomycin, gamma globulin, and mucolytics).

Short-Acting β-Adrenergic (β_2-Selective) Agonists

Short-acting β-adrenergic agonists are the most commonly used bronchodilators. They include albuterol, bitolterol, metaproterenol, pirbuterol, and terbutaline. In most patients, single doses of these agents produce clinically important bronchodilatation within 5 minutes, a peak effect 30 to 60 minutes after inhalation, and a beneficial effect that lasts for 3 to 4 hours. The standard dosage for inhalation therapy is 2 inhalations 4 times daily. It is essential to tailor the dosage on the basis of the clinical features and the potential side effects. Adverse effects include tremor, anxiety, restlessness, tachycardia, palpitations, increased blood pressure, and cardiac arrhythmias. Prostatism may become exacerbated. Side effects are more likely in the elderly and in the presence of cardiovascular, liver, or neurologic disorders and in patients taking other medications for nonpulmonary diseases (eg, β-blockers for cardiac disease). Rarely, paradoxic bronchospasm may result from tachyphylaxis (a rapidly decreasing response to a drug after a few doses) or from exposure to preservatives and propellants. A newer single-isomer β-agonist, levalbuterol, binds to β-adrenergic receptors with 100-fold greater affinity than albuterol. Because of the narrow therapeutic window for methylxanthines (ie, theophylline) and the wide range of toxic effects (eg, cardiac arrhythmias and grand mal convulsions) and drug interactions, the use of theophylline has decreased. The use of inhaled bronchodilators is preferred.

* Standard dosage: 2 inhalations 4 times daily.
* Side effects: tremor, anxiety, tachycardia, palpitations, increased blood pressure, cardiac arrhythmias, exacerbated prostatism.

Long-Acting β-Adrenergic (β2-Selective) Agonists

Long-acting β-adrenergic agonists include salmeterol and formoterol. Salmeterol is more β_2-selective than isoproterenol, a short-acting bronchodilator that has approximately equal agonist activity on β_1- and β_2-adrenergic receptors. Albuterol has a β_2- to β_1-adrenergic receptor selectivity ratio of 1:1,400. Salmeterol is at least 50 times more selective for β_2-adrenergic receptors than albuterol. Salmeterol is highly lipophilic (albuterol is hydrophilic), hence the depot effect in tissues. Salmeterol has a prolonged duration of action (10-12 hours) and inhibits the release of proinflammatory and spasmogenic mediators from respiratory cells. It has a persistent effect in inhibiting histamine release for up to 20 hours, as compared with the short duration of action of isoproterenol and albuterol. Salmeterol and formoterol are also effective in preventing exercise-induced asthma, methacholine-induced bronchospasm, and allergen challenge. The dosage of salmeterol is 2 inhalations (100 mcg) twice daily. The dosage of formoterol is 1 inhalation (12 mcg capsule) twice daily. The longer duration of action may aid in the management of nocturnal asthma. The side effects are similar to those of other β-adrenergic agents. However, tachyphylaxis is distinctly uncommon. Salmeterol and other β-adrenergic bronchodilators may potentiate the actions of monoamine oxidase inhibitors and tricyclic antidepressants. There is controversy in the use of these agents, but a recent Cochrane review has confirmed benefit of these agents in patients with COPD.

* Salmeterol is lipophilic (albuterol is hydrophilic).
* Salmeterol and formoterol: long-acting bronchodilator (>12 hours).
* Salmeterol dosage: 2 inhalations (100 mcg) twice daily.
* Formoterol dosage: 1 inhalation (12 mcg) twice daily.

Anticholinergic Agents

Anticholinergic agents (eg, ipratropium, tiotropium, and atropine) are useful in treating chronic bronchitis or asthmatic bronchitis. As a single agent, ipratropium is only modestly effective in the management of acute or chronic airway disease. Ipratropium prevents bronchoconstriction caused by cholinergic agents such as methacholine and carbachol. It does not protect against bronchoconstriction produced by tobacco smoke, citric acid, sulfur dioxide, or carbon dust.

Allergen-induced bronchospasm also responds poorly to ipratropium therapy. Ipratropium has no effect on mucus production, mucus transport, or ciliary activities. The usual dosage is 2 inhalations 4 times daily. The duration of action is 3 to 5 hours. No more than 12 inhalations should be permitted in 24 hours. Side effects include nervousness, headache, gastrointestinal tract upset, dry mouth, and cough. The drug may aggravate narrow-angle glaucoma, prostatic hypertrophy, and bladder neck obstruction.

Tiotropium has been shown to improve bronchodilation in patients with asthma or COPD. It appears to be more effective than ipratropium in asthma and in reducing the number of COPD exacerbations. The usual dosage is 1 inhalation (18-mcg capsule) once daily.

* Ipratropium inhibits vagally mediated reflexes by blocking the effects of acetylcholine.
* It has minimal or no benefit in pure emphysema.
* It is only modestly effective if used alone.
* Tiotropium appears to be more effective than ipratropium in asthma and COPD.

Phosphodiesterase Inhibitors

Theophylline (methylxanthine) is the main phosphodiesterase inhibitor. Overall, the use of theophylline has diminished, with β-agonists being given more often in its place. Theophylline is effective in combination with β_2-agonists in the management of moderate and severe asthma. It increases the contractility of respiratory muscles in a dose-related fashion. The effects of various substances and circumstances on the clearance of theophylline are shown in Table 23-7.

* The exact mechanism of action of theophylline is unclear.
* Theophylline is effective in combination with β_2-agonists.

The recommended blood level of theophylline is 10 to 15 mcg/mL. The loading dose is 6 mg/kg (range, 5-7 mg/kg); the maintenance dosage is 0.5 mg/kg per hour or 1.15 g in 24 hours. The normal

Table 23-7 Theophylline Clearance

Increased By	Decreased By
β-Agonists	Allopurinol
Carbamazepine	Antibiotics—macrolides,
Dilantin	ciprofloxacin, norfloxacin,
Furosemide	isoniazid
Hyperthyroidism	β-Blocker—propranolol
Ketoconazole	Caffeine
Marijuana	Cirrhosis
Phenobarbital	Congestive heart failure
Rifampin	H_2-blocker—cimetidine
Tobacco smoke	Mexiletine
	Oral contraceptives
	Viral infection

adult dosage is usually less than 1,000 mg daily. Longer-acting preparations may be given in a single dose of 300 to 600 mg. The dose should be decreased by 50% if the patient has received theophylline in the preceding 24 hours or has heart failure, severe hypoxemia, hepatic insufficiency, or seizures. Each dose should be increased by 50 to 100 mg if the therapeutic effect is suboptimal and in smokers who can tolerate the increased dose. Each dose should be decreased by 50 to 100 mg if toxic effects develop or if progressive heart or liver failure develops. Tobacco smoking decreases the efficacy (half-life) of theophylline. In clinical practice, it is not necessary to measure frequently the serum levels of theophylline. The main side effects are tremor, aggravation of prostatism, tachycardia, and arrhythmias. Owing to its narrow therapeutic window, theophylline should be used with caution.

- Tobacco smoking decreases the half-life of theophylline.
- The recommended blood level is 10-15 mcg/mL.
- In clinical practice, it is not necessary to measure frequently the serum levels of theophylline.

Antileukotrienes

The efficacy of antileukotrienes in the treatment of COPD is not known.

Corticosteroids

Corticosteroids have no bronchodilating effect in patients with emphysema. Patients with bronchitis, however, may benefit from the anti-inflammatory action. Systemic corticosteroid therapy in nonasthmatic COPD has a limited role; only about 15% of patients have improvement. Inhaled corticosteroids can be given in conjunction with systemic (oral) corticosteroids, especially during the weaning period of long-term or high-dose systemic (oral) corticosteroids. All inhaled corticosteroids, when given at higher doses, are associated with greater side effects and fewer benefits. The most common side effect with aerosolized corticosteroids is oral candidiasis. Inhaled corticosteroids in dosages greater than 1.5 mg per day (0.75 mg daily for fluticasone propionate) may lead to slowing of linear growth velocity in children, decrease in bone density (particularly in perimenopausal women), posterior subcapsular cataracts, or glaucoma. The use of corticosteroids, inhaled or oral, in the treatment of stable COPD is limited. A short course of oral corticosteroids may be tried for stable COPD, but studies have suggested that, unlike in patients with asthma, the response to a short course of treatment is a poor predictor of a long-term response in patients with COPD. Steroid myopathy in those receiving long-term treatment with oral corticosteroids may lead to worsening respiratory muscle function and eventually to hastened respiratory failure. Several large studies on the use of inhaled corticosteroids have suggested that their regular use may be appropriate for patients who have a documented FEV_1 response to inhaled corticosteroids or for those with moderate to severe COPD who have repeated exacerbations requiring oral corticosteroid therapy. A short course of systemic corticosteroid is essential in the treatment of acute COPD exacerbation since it has been shown to reduce duration and severity of the illness.

- Oropharyngeal candidiasis is a complication of aerosolized corticosteroids.
- The use of corticosteroids in the treatment of stable COPD is limited, whereas systemic corticosteroids are very effective in the treatment of acute exacerbation of COPD.

Adjuvant Therapy

Antibiotic therapy is helpful for patients with symptoms suggestive of bacterial infection, especially during COPD exacerbations. Maintenance of good oral hydration, avoidance of tobacco smoking and other respiratory irritants, annual influenza vaccination, and prompt treatment of respiratory infections are equally important.

Oxygen

Low-flow oxygen (<2 L/min) therapy is recommended when the PaO_2 is 55 mm Hg or less, arterial oxygen saturation (SaO_2) is 88% or less, or PaO_2 is 59 mm Hg or less if there is polycythemia or clinical evidence of cor pulmonale. The lack of carbon dioxide retention should be assured before recommending oxygen. Continuous oxygen therapy is more useful than nocturnal-only treatment. The need for chronic or indefinite oxygen therapy should be reassessed after 3 months of treatment. For each liter of oxygen administered, the fraction of inhaled oxygen (FIO_2) is increased by approximately 3%. This amount, however, is variable and depends on the amount of entrained room air during respiration. Exercise therapy (ie, pulmonary rehabilitation) improves exercise tolerance and maximal oxygen uptake but does not improve PFT results.

- Oxygen therapy is recommended if PaO_2 is ≤55 mm Hg or SaO_2 is ≤88%.
- FIO_2 increases by approximately 3% for each liter of supplemental oxygen.
- An exercise program does not improve PFT results.

Practical aspects of managing COPD are outlined in Table 23-6.

Complications and Causes of Exacerbation of COPD

The complications and causes of exacerbation of COPD include viral and bacterial respiratory infections (commonly *Haemophilus influenzae*, *Moraxella catarrhalis*, and *Streptococcus pneumoniae*), cor pulmonale, myocardial infarction, cardiac arrhythmias, pneumothorax, pulmonary emboli, bronchogenic carcinoma, environmental exposure, oversedation, neglect of therapy, excessive oxygen use (suppression of hypoxemic drive and worsening $\dot{V}/\dot{Q}$ mismatch), and excessive use of β_2-agonist (tachyphylaxis). Nocturnal oxygen desaturation is common in those with emphysema as are premature ventricular contractions and episodic pulmonary hypertension. A decrease in SaO_2 correlates with an increase in pulmonary artery pressure. Severe weight loss, sometimes more than 50 kg, is noted in 30% of patients with severe COPD.

- Bacterial infections in COPD are caused by *H influenzae*, *M catarrhalis*, and *S pneumoniae*.
- Nocturnal oxygen desaturation is more common in those with emphysema.

- A decrease in SaO_2 correlates with an increase in pulmonary artery pressure.
- Severe weight loss is seen in 30% of patients with severe COPD (emphysema).

Other Topics in COPD

Nicotine gum and patch help maintain nicotine blood levels while a smoker tries to cope with the psychologic and other aspects of nicotine addiction. Nearly 25% of smokers require treatment for more than 12 months to remain tobacco-free. Nicotine from gum is absorbed more slowly from the buccal mucosa and stomach than from the airways with inhaled smoke. Side effects include mucosal burning, light-headedness, nausea, stomachache, and hiccups. The patch causes a rash in a large number of patients. Use of the nicotine patch with continued smoking aggravates heart problems. Bupropion has been shown to be effective either as a single agent or in combination with nicotine replacement therapy in achieving smoking cessation. This medication is contraindicated for persons who have a seizure disorder, anorexia nervosa, or bulimia. The most common side effects of bupropion include insomnia, headache, and dry mouth. Varenicline is a partial nicotine agonist that was recently approved for use in smoking cessation. The most common side effects are nausea, insomnia, and headache.

- Nicotine gum and patch are important aspects of a tobacco cessation program.
- The simultaneous use of cigarette and nicotine products aggravates heart problems.
- Bupropion is effective in achieving smoking cessation, but its use is contraindicated for those who have a seizure or eating disorder.

Lung volume reduction surgery (resection of 20%-30% of peripheral lung parenchyma) in patients with emphysema appears to improve pulmonary function in selected individuals with COPD. The benefit is thought to be the result of regaining normal or near-normal mechanical function of the thoracic cage that was compromised by the severe hyperinflation of the lungs. However, lung volume reduction surgery is associated with increased mortality for patients whose FEV_1 is less than 20% of predicted and who have either DLCO less than 20% of predicted or homogeneous changes on chest CT. Lung transplant is used to treat various end-stage pulmonary diseases. It does not confer a survival advantage for patients with advanced emphysema, but it may confer a survival advantage for patients with cystic fibrosis or idiopathic pulmonary fibrosis. Regardless of the underlying disease for which a transplant is performed, the procedure improves the quality of life.

- Lung volume reduction surgery is beneficial in selected individuals with COPD.
- It is associated with increased mortality for those with severe disease.

Cystic Fibrosis

Cystic fibrosis is the most common lethal autosomal recessive disease among whites in the United States. The locus of the responsible gene is on the long arm of chromosome 7. This gene codes for cystic fibrosis transmembrane conductance regulator (CFTR), a protein that regulates the function of epithelial cell chloride channels. The most common genetic mutation is the DeltaF(508) mutation, which results in the omission of a phenylalanine residue at the regulatory site. Cystic fibrosis develops in 1 in 2,000 to 3,500 live births among whites; about 1 in 20 (2%-5%) whites is a heterozygous carrier. There is no sex predominance. Occurrence in African Americans is 1 in 15,300 and in Asian Americans, 1 in 32,100. Siblings of such a child have a 50% to 65% chance of being heterozygotes. The diagnosis is made in 80% of patients before the age of 10 years. Obstruction of exocrine glands, with the exception of sweat glands, by viscous secretions causes almost all the clinical manifestations. Mucociliary clearance is normal in patients with minimal pulmonary dysfunction and is decreased in those with obstructive phenomena.

- Cystic fibrosis: the most common lethal autosomal recessive disease among whites.
- In 20% of patients, the diagnosis is not made until the adolescent years.
- Siblings of children with cystic fibrosis have a 50%-65% chance of being heterozygotes.
- All exocrine glands, except sweat glands, are affected; this accounts for the majority of symptoms.

Up to 10% of patients with cystic fibrosis and heterozygous carriers demonstrate nonspecific airway hyperreactivity and an increased susceptibility to asthma and atopy. Because of chronic airway obstruction from viscous secretions, bacteria such as *H influenzae*, *Staphylococcus aureus*, and *Pseudomonas aeruginosa* often colonize the airways. Also, defective CFTR protein may be responsible for the ineffective clearance of *P aeruginosa*. Positive serologic reactions to *Aspergillus* species and *Candida albicans* occur with higher frequency in patients with cystic fibrosis than in those with asthma. Allergic bronchopulmonary aspergillosis occurs in up to 10% of patients with cystic fibrosis, and up to 57% of patients with cystic fibrosis become colonized with *Aspergillus fumigatus*.

- Up to 10% of patients with cystic fibrosis and carriers exhibit increased airway response.
- Up to 10% of patients show increased susceptibility to asthma and atopy.
- Allergic bronchopulmonary aspergillosis occurs in up to 10% of patients.
- Organisms such as *H influenzae*, *S aureus*, *P aeruginosa*, and *A fumigatus* often colonize the airways.

There is no evidence for a primary defect in sodium transport. However, the epithelial cells in cystic fibrosis are poorly permeable to chloride ions because of the defect in CFTR protein in most cases. There is a marked increase in the electrical potential difference across the nasal and tracheobronchial epithelium compared with that of healthy subjects and heterozygote relatives. The normally negative potential difference across the cell membrane becomes more negative (because of chloride impermeability) in cystic fibrosis.

This leads to defects in intracellular chloride and, secondarily, to sodium homeostasis.

* No evidence for a primary defect in sodium transport.
* Because of a defect in CFTR protein, chloride ion transport is defective.
* There is a marked increase in the electrical potential difference across the nasal and tracheobronchial epithelium compared with that of healthy subjects and heterozygote relatives.

Diagnosis in adults requires at least 3 of the following: clinical features of cystic fibrosis, positive family history, sweat chloride >80 mEq/L, and pancreatic insufficiency. Quantitative pilocarpine iontophoresis is helpful in making the diagnosis; abnormal results on at least 2 tests are necessary for the diagnosis (abnormal sweat chloride: adult, >80 mEq/L; child, >60 mEq/L). Note that normal sweat chloride values do not exclude cystic fibrosis. This test must be performed with extreme care because inaccurate collection is a common source of misdiagnosis. Conditions associated with high levels of sodium and sweat chloride include smoking, chronic bronchitis, malnutrition, hereditary nephrogenic diabetes insipidus, adrenal insufficiency, hypothyroidism, hypoparathyroidism, pancreatitis, hypogammaglobulinemia, and ectodermal dysplasia. The concentrations of sodium and sweat chloride increase with age. Heterozygotes may have normal sodium and sweat chloride values. False-negative test results are common in edematous states or in persons receiving corticosteroids. When sweat chloride levels are normal in a patient in whom cystic fibrosis is highly suspected, alternative diagnostic tests (eg, nasal transepithelial voltage measurements and genotyping) should be considered. Respiratory manifestations include sinusitis, nasal polyps, progressive cystic bronchiectasis, purulent sputum, atelectasis, hemoptysis, and pneumothorax.

* Diagnosis in adults requires at least 3 of the following: clinical features of cystic fibrosis, positive family history, sweat chloride >80 mEq/L, and pancreatic insufficiency.
* Respiratory manifestations: sinusitis, nasal polyps, progressive cystic bronchiectasis, purulent sputum, atelectasis, hemoptysis, and pneumothorax.

Cystic fibrosis is the most common cause of COPD and pancreatic deficiency in the first 3 decades of life in the United States. COPD is present in 97% of adults with cystic fibrosis, and COPD is the major cause of morbidity and mortality in adults. Men constitute 55% of the adult patients. Adults with cystic fibrosis have a higher incidence of minor hemoptysis (60% of patients), major hemoptysis (5%), pneumothorax (16%), and sinusitis and nasal polyposis (48%). Pancreatic insufficiency is present in 95% of patients, but it is seldom symptomatic. Acute or chronic pancreatitis can develop, however. Intussusception and fecal impaction (similar to meconium ileus) are more frequent (21%) in adults than in children. Both hyperinflation of lungs on CXR and lobar atelectasis are less frequent in adults than in children. The mean age at onset of massive hemoptysis is 19 years, and median survival from the initial episode of hemoptysis is about 3.5 years. The mean age at occurrence of

pneumothorax in adults is 22 years. Azoospermia occurs in 95% of male patients.

* COPD is present in 97% of adults with cystic fibrosis; COPD is the major cause of morbidity and mortality.
* Adults with cystic fibrosis: minor hemoptysis (60% of patients), major hemoptysis (5%), pneumothorax (16%), and sinusitis and nasal polyposis (48%).
* Pancreatic insufficiency occurs in 95% of patients; it is seldom symptomatic, but acute or chronic pancreatitis can develop.

Nearly 50% of patients with cystic fibrosis survive to age 25, and the overall survival rate for patients older than 17 years is approximately 50%. Survival and quality of life are improved with aggressive chest physical therapy, prompt treatment of upper and lower respiratory tract infections, intensive nutritional support, and conditioning. Poor prognostic factors include female sex, residence in a non-northern climate, pneumothorax, hemoptysis, recurrent bacterial infections, presence of B cepacia, and systemic complications.

Respiratory therapy for cystic fibrosis includes management of obstructive lung disease, chest physiotherapy, postural drainage, immunization against influenza, and hydration. P aeruginosa is the dominant organism and is difficult to eradicate. The presence of Burkholderia cepacia is associated with rapid deterioration in lung function. Inhaled antipseudomonal antibiotic therapy, such as inhaled tobramycin, is an option; it has been associated with an increase in FEV_1 and a decrease in the likelihood of hospitalization. Its role in management of acute exacerbation is not well defined. The sputum of patients with cystic fibrosis contains high concentrations of extracellular DNA, a viscous material released by leukocytes. Aerosolized recombinant human DNase I (dornase alfa) reduces sputum viscosity by degrading the DNA. Results of DNase I therapy have shown decreased risk of lung infections, improvement in FEV_1, and reduced antibiotic requirement. The usual dosage is 2.5 mg once daily with a nebulizer; patients older than 21 years may benefit from 2.5 mg twice daily. However, recent studies have suggested that alternate-day dosing may have equivalent clinical outcomes. Serum antibodies to dornase alfa develop in about 2% to 4% of patients, but anaphylaxis has not been noted. Side effects of dornase alfa have included voice alteration, hoarseness, rash, chest pain, pharyngitis, and conjunctivitis. Although systemic glucocorticoids are administered during acute exacerbations or to those with allergic bronchopulmonary aspergillosis, routine use has been associated with notable side effects and is not recommended. Small studies have shown some benefit with inhaled glucocorticoids, which may be beneficial for patients with airway hyperreactivity. If examination of the sputum does not show nontuberculous mycobacteria, treatment with azithromycin (500 mg 3 times weekly) appears to sustain the improvement in FEV_1 and to decrease the frequency of pulmonary exacerbations. The risk of death from cystic fibrosis is 38% to 56% within 2 years when FEV_1 has reached 20% to 30% of predicted. Patients younger than 18 years have worse survival rates after FEV_1 deteriorates. Bilateral lung transplant is an option for patients with declining lung function. Survival rates are comparable to those of patients who undergo lung transplant for other reasons. Presence of

B cepacia, however, is a contraindication for transplant. The 5-year survival rate is between 40% and 60%.

- Nearly 50% of patients with cystic fibrosis survive to age 25.
- The overall survival rate for patients older than 17 years is approximately 50%.
- Aggressive chest physical therapy, prompt treatment of upper and lower respiratory tract infections, intensive nutritional support, and conditioning improve survival and quality of life.
- Poor prognostic factors: female sex, residence in a non-northern climate, pneumothorax, hemoptysis, recurrent bacterial infections, presence of *B cepacia*, and systemic complications.
- Bilateral lung transplant is an option for patients with declining lung function.

Bronchiectasis

Bronchiectasis is ectasia, or dilatation, of the bronchi due to irreversible destruction of bronchial walls. Its clinical features are similar to those of COPD. Airway inflammation in bronchiectasis is characterized by tissue neutrophilia, a mononuclear cell infiltrate composed mainly of CD4+ T cells and CD68+ macrophages, and increased interleukin-8 expression. Bronchiectasis is reversible when it results from severe bronchitis, acute pneumonia, or allergic bronchopulmonary aspergillosis. Bronchiectasis most commonly occurs in the lower lung fields. Mild cylindrical bronchiectasis seen in many heavy smokers with chronic bronchitis may be diffuse. Distal bronchial segments (second- to fourth-order bronchi) are involved in most cases of bronchiectasis. An exception is proximal bronchial involvement in allergic bronchopulmonary aspergillosis. Disease is bilateral in 30% of patients. Upper lobes are involved in cystic fibrosis and chronic mycotic and mycobacterial infections, and lower lobe involvement predominates in idiopathic bronchiectasis. Perihilar involvement is suggestive of allergic bronchopulmonary aspergillosis.

- Bronchiectasis is reversible in chronic bronchitis, acute pneumonia, and allergic bronchopulmonary aspergillosis.
- Upper lobes are involved in cystic fibrosis and chronic mycotic and mycobacterial infections.
- Central (perihilar) involvement is suggestive of allergic bronchopulmonary aspergillosis.
- Lower lobe predominance is suggestive of idiopathic bronchiectasis.

Most cases are diagnosed on clinical grounds (chronic cough with purulent sputum expectoration). Some patients with *dry bronchiectasis* caused by tuberculosis do not have productive cough, but episodes of severe hemoptysis may develop (this presentation is uncommon). Many mildly symptomatic or asymptomatic patients with atelectatic segments of the right middle lobe (*right middle lobe syndrome*) and lingular segments of the left upper lobe have minor degrees of bronchiectasis. Other signs suggestive of bronchiectasis include fetor oris, anorexia, weight loss, clubbing, and HPO. CXR shows segmental atelectasis, loss of lung volume, dilated and thickened airways (manifested as "tram tracks" or parallel lines), and air-fluid levels (if cystic bronchiectasis is present). HRCT can have a diagnostic sensitivity as high as 97%; it is the preferred test to confirm the presence of bronchiectasis. Findings include signet-ring shadows (ie, a dilated bronchus, with bronchial artery forming the "stone"), bronchial wall thickening, dilated bronchi extending to the periphery (lack of tapering), bronchial obstruction due to inspissated purulent secretions, loss of volume, and air-fluid levels if cystic or saccular changes are present. The HRCT diagnosis of *nodular bronchiectasis* usually indicates peribronchial granulomatous infiltration caused by secondary infection by *Mycobacterium avium* complex. High seroprevalence of *Helicobacter pylori* has been reported in active bronchiectasis, but the clinical implications are unclear.

- Nonpulmonary symptoms: fetor oris, anorexia, weight loss, arthralgia, clubbing, and HPO.
- HRCT of the chest has replaced bronchography in making the diagnosis.
- PFT results usually indicate obstructive phenomena.
- Typical clinical scenario: A patient has asymptomatic or chronic cough, and HRCT shows signet-ring shadows and bronchial wall thickening.
- Dry bronchiectasis with episodes of marked hemoptysis without sputum is usually due to bronchiectasis in an area of old tuberculous damage.

Causes and Associations of Bronchiectasis

Infections

In adults, many cases of bronchiectasis are related to adenoviral or bacterial infections (measles, influenza, adenovirus, or pertussis) in childhood. Various infections, including *Mycoplasma pneumoniae*, nontuberculous mycobacteria, and anaerobic organisms, have also been associated with bronchiectasis. Tuberculosis is a common cause of bronchiectasis, particularly in the upper lobes. Occasionally, chronic histoplasmosis and coccidioidomycosis cause bronchiectasis. However, in patients with chronic stable bronchiectasis, *P aeruginosa* is the predominant organism in respiratory secretions.

- Bronchiectasis may result from a chronic infection or be a complication of a previous viral infection.

Ciliary Dyskinesia (Immotile Cilia) Syndrome

Cilia are normally present in many organs, and their absence or abnormality may cause clinical problems (which are listed in parentheses): nasal mucosa (nasal polyps), paranasal sinuses (chronic sinusitis), eustachian tube (inner ear infection or deafness), and tracheobronchial tree (chronic bronchitis or bronchiectasis). Many types of ciliary abnormalities (loss of radial spokes, eccentric tubules, absence of tubules, and adhesion of multiple cilia) occur. Although the term *immotile cilia* is commonly used, the cilia do move, but their motion is abnormal; thus, the preferred term is *primary ciliary dyskinesia* (PCD).

- Many forms of ciliary abnormalities can occur.
- Ciliary dyskinesia—not ciliary immotility—is the main abnormality.

Kartagener syndrome, a classic example of PCD, is an autosomal recessive disorder that involves the triad of situs inversus, sinusitis, and bronchiectasis or at least bronchitis. Loss of the dynein arm—the fundamental defect—is an inherited abnormality involving a single protein. The prevalence of Kartagener syndrome is 1 in 40,000 to 60,000 persons, whereas the prevalence of PCD is approximately 1 in 20,000 to 40,000 persons. The loss of the dynein arm results in sinusitis and otitis (less common in adults), nasal polyposis, bronchiectasis (in 75% of adults), situs inversus, and infertility in males. Infertility is not a universal phenomenon, and, in fact, approximately 50% of women with PCD are often fertile. Kartagener syndrome accounts for 0.5% of the cases of bronchiectasis and 15% of the cases of dextrocardia.

* Kartagener syndrome is an autosomal recessive disorder.
* Loss of the dynein arm is the fundamental defect.
* Typical clinical scenario: A patient presents with situs inversus, sinusitis, and bronchiectasis.

Diagnosis of PCD depends on the clinical features and documentation of ciliary abnormalities by electron microscopic examination of the nasal mucosa, bronchial mucosa, or semen. At least 20 types of axonemal defects have been described. Ciliary defects are not always inherited; acquired forms occur in smokers and patients with bronchitis, viral infections, or other pulmonary diseases. However, these acquired defects are different from those of PCD.

* Ciliary defects are not always inherited but are separate from PCD.
* Acquired ciliary defects occur in smokers, in patients with bronchitis, and after viral infections.

Hypogammaglobulinemia

Bruton agammaglobulinemia (X-linked agammaglobulinemia) predisposes to recurrent bacterial infections and bronchiectasis. The bacteria that are isolated include *H influenzae*, *S aureus*, and *S pneumoniae*. Acquired (common variable) agammaglobulinemia may be manifested as sinopulmonary infections in the second or third decade. Selective IgA deficiency is the most common immunoglobulin deficiency; most of these patients are asymptomatic. IgA deficiency is frequently associated with IgG subclass (IgG2 and IgG4) deficiency. Despite the inability to form antibody, most patients have a normal number of circulating B cells, which fail to dedifferentiate into plasma cells that make immunoglobulins. Pulmonary disease occurs more commonly and is more severe than in patients with X-linked agammaglobulinemia. Infections caused by encapsulated bacteria are more common. Bronchiectasis and obstructive airway disease occur in up to 73% of patients.

* The overall incidence of bronchiectasis in hypogammaglobulinemia and agammaglobulinemia can be as high as 73%.
* Typical clinical scenario: Selective IgA deficiency is the most common immunoglobulin deficiency; most of these patients are asymptomatic or minimally symptomatic.

Right Middle Lobe Syndrome

Right middle lobe syndrome is recurrent atelectasis associated with localized bronchiectasis of the right middle lobe. Mechanisms include compression of the middle lobe bronchus by lymph nodes, acute angulation of the origin of the bronchus, narrow opening of the bronchus, lengthy bronchus, and lack of collateral ventilation. CXR usually points to the diagnosis, although many patients are asymptomatic.

* Typical clinical scenario for right middle lobe syndrome: An asymptomatic patient has chronic atelectasis and volume loss in the right middle lobe.
* The diagnosis is frequently made as an incidental CXR finding.

Allergic Bronchopulmonary Aspergillosis

Central bronchiectasis is present in 85% of patients with allergic bronchopulmonary aspergillosis at the time of the initial diagnosis and has been used as a diagnostic criterion of the disease.

Allergic bronchopulmonary aspergillosis also occurs in about 10% of patients with cystic fibrosis. The disease is caused by both IgG- and IgE-mediated immune responses directed at *Aspergillus* species. Type I (bronchospasm), type III (pulmonary-destructive changes), and type IV (parenchymal granuloma and mononuclear cell infiltrates) reactions are involved. The major criteria are asthma, blood eosinophilia ($>1 \times 10^9$/L), immediate skin reactivity (type I reaction—IgE dependent) to *Aspergillus* antigen, IgG antibodies (type III reaction) to *Aspergillus* antigen, high IgE titer (>1,000 ng/mL), transient or fixed pulmonary infiltrates, and central bronchiectasis (noted in 85% of patients). A normal IgE level in a symptomatic patient virtually excludes allergic bronchopulmonary aspergillosis.

Minor criteria include the presence of *Aspergillus* in sputum, expectoration of brownish mucous plugs, and late-phase (Arthus) skin test reactivity to *Aspergillus* antigen. CXR shows fleeting infiltrates ("gloved finger" sign, "tram-track" line lesions, and "toothpaste shadows") in 85% of patients, mucoid impaction in 15% to 40%, atelectasis, and central bronchiectasis. Although generally associated with *A fumigatus*, allergic bronchopulmonary mycosis can be caused by *C albicans*, *Aspergillus terreus*, *Curvularia lunata*, *Helminthosporium* species, and *Stemphylium lanuginosum*. Systemic corticosteroid therapy for more than 6 months is required for most patients.

* Allergic bronchopulmonary aspergillosis may develop in 10% of patients with cystic fibrosis.
* Types I, III, and IV immune reactions may be involved.
* An increased IgE level is the most useful laboratory finding.
* Presence of *A fumigatus* is only a minor criterion for the diagnosis.
* Therapy consists of long-term systemic corticosteroids.
* Typical clinical scenario: A patient has refractory asthma, expectoration of brownish mucous plugs, segmental atelectasis, and eosinophilia.

Miscellaneous Causes and Associations

Bronchiectasis develops in approximately 20% of patients with yellow nail syndrome. This syndrome is thought to arise from lymphatic hypoplasia or atresia. It consists of yellow-green discoloration of the nails (with a thickened and curved appearance) of all extremities, lymphedema of the lower extremities, and lymphocyte-predominant pleural effusion.

Nearly 10% of patients with bronchiectasis may have an abnormal α_1-antitrypsin phenotype, with serum levels less than 66% of normal. Other causes and associations include rheumatoid arthritis (Felty syndrome), toxic chemicals, recurrent aspiration, heroin, inflammatory bowel disease, foreign body, sequestrated lung, relapsing polychondritis, chronic tracheoesophageal fistula, heart-lung transplant, chronic granulomatous disease of childhood, obstructive azoospermia (Young syndrome), unilateral hyperlucent lung syndrome (Swyer-James or Macleod syndrome), and postobstructive status (tumors, long-standing foreign body, or stenosis).

* Uncommon causes of bronchiectasis include α_1-antitrypsin deficiency, Felty syndrome, inflammatory bowel disease, toxic inhalation, and chronic tracheobronchial stenosis.

Complications of Bronchiectasis

Complications of bronchiectasis include hemoptysis from bronchial vessels (in 50% of patients), progressive respiratory failure with hypoxemia and cor pulmonale, and secondary infections by fungi and noninfectious mycobacterioses. The presence of these organisms usually represents a saprophytic state, but active infection has to be excluded. The most commonly isolated bacterium in bronchiectasis is *P aeruginosa*. As in cystic fibrosis, it is impossible to eradicate this bacterium. Patients with bronchiectasis infected by *P aeruginosa* have more extensive bronchiectasis than those without this infection. Routine culture of respiratory secretions is not warranted for all patients.

* The source of bleeding in bronchiectasis is the bronchial (systemic) circulation; hence, it can be brisk.
* The presence of mycobacteria and fungi may represent saprophytic growth.

Treatment

Treatment of bronchiectasis is aimed at controlling the symptoms and preventing complications. Predisposing conditions should be sought and treated aggressively (gamma globulin injections, removal of foreign body or tumor, control of aspiration, and treatment of infections of paranasal sinuses, gums, and teeth). Postural drainage, chest physiotherapy, humidification, bronchodilators, and cyclic antibiotic therapy are effective in many patients. Surgical treatment is reserved for patients with troublesome symptoms, localized disease, and severe hemoptysis. High-dose inhaled corticosteroid therapy (fluticasone) is reportedly effective in reducing the sputum inflammatory indices in bronchiectasis.

Occupational Lung Disease

The points to remember about occupational lung diseases are summarized in Table 23-8.

Pleural Effusion

The normal volume of pleural fluid is 0.2 to 0.3 mL/kg of body weight. Excess pleural fluid collects in the pleural space when fluid

Table 23-8 Pulmonary Diseases: Causes and Associations

Pulmonary Disease	Causes and Associations
Progressive massive fibrosis	Silicosis, coal, hematite, kaolin, graphite, asbestosis
Autoimmune mechanism	Silicosis, asbestosis, berylliosis
Monday morning sickness	Byssinosis, bagassosis, metal fume fever
Metals & fumes producing asthma	Bakers' asthma, meat wrappers' asthma, printers' asthma, nickel, platinum, toluene diisocyanate, cigarette cutters' asthma
Increased incidence of tuberculosis	Silicosis, hematite lung
Increased incidence of carcinoma	Asbestos, hematite, arsenic, nickel, uranium, chromate
Welder's lung	Siderosis, pulmonary edema, bronchitis, emphysema
Centrilobular emphysema	Coal, hematite
Generalized emphysema	Cadmium
Silo filler's lung	Nitrogen dioxide
Farmer's lung	*Thermoactinomyces, Micropolyspora*
Asbestos exposure	Mesothelioma, bronchogenic cancer, gastrointestinal tract cancer
Eggshell calcification	Silicosis, sarcoid
Sarcoid-like disease	Berylliosis
Diaphragmatic calcification	Asbestosis (also ankylosing spondylitis)
Nonfibrogenic pneumoconioses	Tin, emery, antimony, titanium, barium
Minimal abnormality in lungs	Siderosis, baritosis, stannosis
Bullous emphysema	Bauxite lung
Occupational asthma	Toluene diisocyanate, laboratory animals, grain dust, biologic enzymes, gum acacia, tragacanth, silkworm, anhydrides, wood dust, platinum, nickel, formaldehyde, Freon, drugs

collection exceeds normal removal mechanisms. Hydrostatic, oncotic, and intrapleural pressures regulate fluid movement in the pleural space. Any of the following mechanisms can produce pleural effusion: changes in capillary permeability (inflammation), increased hydrostatic pressure, decreased plasma oncotic pressure, impaired lymphatic drainage, increased negative intrapleural pressure, and movement of fluid (through diaphragmatic pores and lymphatic vessels) from the peritoneum. The principal causes of pleural effusion are listed in Table 23-9. The diagnosis may be suggested by certain characteristics of the effusion. For example, obvious pus suggests empyema; lupus erythematosus cells and a ratio of pleural fluid to serum antinuclear antibody greater than 1 suggests lupus pleuritis; a high level of salivary amylase level with pleural fluid acidosis suggests esophageal rupture; and a ratio of pleural fluid hematocrit to blood hematocrit greater than 0.5 suggests hemothorax. On the basis of clinical suspicion, testing of the effusion should be selective. Despite thorough testing of pleural fluid, the cause of up to one-third of pleural effusions is unknown.

Transudate Versus Exudate

Traditionally, an effusion with any *one* of the following is considered an exudate:

1. Ratio of pleural fluid protein to serum protein >0.5
2. Ratio of pleural fluid lactate dehydrogenase (LDH) to serum LDH >0.6
3. Pleural fluid LDH greater than two-thirds of the upper limit of the reference range for serum LDH

A recent meta-analysis found that any *one* of the following findings can also be used to identify the fluid as an exudate:

1. Pleural fluid protein >2.9 g/dL
2. Pleural fluid cholesterol >45 mg/dL
3. Pleural fluid LDH >60% of the upper limit of the reference range for serum LDH

An increased level of LDH in the fluid is nonspecific, but it is increased in pulmonary embolism, rheumatoid effusion, lymphoma, and most exudative effusions. The classification of pleural fluid into transudates and exudates does not permit the consideration of all causes. The most common cause of a transudate is congestive heart failure (pulmonary artery wedge pressure >25 mm Hg). The most common cause of an exudate is pneumonia (parapneumonic effusion).

- It is not necessary to perform all the above tests to differentiate a transudate from an exudate.
- Clinically, it is more useful to classify the cause by considering the source (organ system) of the fluid (Table 23-9).
- The classification of pleural fluid into transudates and exudates does not permit the consideration of all causes.
- The most common cause of a transudate is congestive heart failure (pulmonary artery wedge pressure >25 mm Hg).
- The most common cause of an exudate is pneumonia (parapneumonic effusion).

Table 23-9 Principal Causes of Pleural Effusion

Osmotic-hydraulic[a]
   Congestive heart failure
   Superior vena caval obstruction
   Constrictive pericarditis
   Cirrhosis with ascites
   Hypoalbuminemia
   Salt-retaining syndromes
   Peritoneal dialysis
   Hydronephrosis
   Nephrotic syndrome
Infections[b]
   Parapneumonic (bacterial) effusions
   Bacterial empyema
   Tuberculosis
   Fungi
   Parasites
   Viruses & mycoplasma
Neoplasms[b]
   Primary & metastatic lung tumors
   Lymphoma & leukemia
   Benign & malignant tumors of pleura
   Intra-abdominal tumors with ascites
Vascular disease[b]
   Pulmonary embolism
   Wegener granulomatosis
Intra-abdominal diseases[b]
   Pancreatitis & pancreatic pseudocyst
   Subdiaphragmatic abscess
   Malignancy with ascites
   Meigs syndrome[a]
   Hepatic cirrhosis with ascites[a]
Trauma[b]
   Hemothorax
   Chylothorax
   Esophageal rupture
   Intra-abdominal surgery
Miscellaneous
   Drug-induced effusions[b]
   Uremic pleuritis[b]
   Myxedema[a]
   Yellow nail syndrome[b]
   Dressler syndrome[b]
   Familial Mediterranean fever[b]

[a] Usually a transudate.
[b] Usually an exudate.

Glucose and pH

When the pleural fluid glucose concentration is high, the pH is usually high, and when the glucose concentration is low, the pH is usually low. Pleural fluid hypoglycemia (<60 mg/dL or ratio of fluid glucose to plasma glucose <0.5) is found in rheumatoid effusion, malignant mesothelioma, empyema, systemic lupus erythematosus, esophageal rupture, and tuberculous pleurisy. In some cases of rheumatoid pleurisy and empyema, pleural fluid glucose may not be detectable. The pH of normal pleural fluid, which should be determined with a blood gas machine instead of a pH meter, is approximately 7.60. A pleural fluid pH less than 7.30 is found in empyema, esophageal rupture, rheumatoid effusion, tuberculosis, malignancy, and trauma. If the pH is low (<7.20) and clinical suspicion is high for infection, drainage with a chest tube should be considered. Empyema caused by *Proteus* species produces a pH greater than 7.8 (because of the production of ammonia).

* The pleural fluid glucose concentration and pH usually go together (ie, if glucose is low, so is pH).
* Glucose levels are low in rheumatoid effusion, malignant mesothelioma, and empyema.

Amylase

The concentration of amylase in the pleural fluid is increased (ratio of pleural fluid amylase to serum amylase >1.0) in pancreatitis, pseudocyst of the pancreas, malignancy (typically a primary tumor in the lung), and rupture of the esophagus (with leakage of salivary amylase) or abdominal viscera. The amylase level in the fluid remains higher for longer periods than in the serum. Rare causes include ruptured ectopic pregnancy, hydronephrosis, cirrhosis, and pneumonia. In any unexplained left-sided effusion, consider pancreatitis and measure the amylase level in the pleural fluid.

* The concentration of amylase in the pleural fluid is increased in esophageal rupture because of leakage of salivary amylase.
* In any unexplained left-sided effusion, consider pancreatitis and measure the amylase level in the pleural fluid.

Chylous Effusion

Chylous effusion is suggested by a turbid or milky white appearance of the fluid. However, chylothorax is confirmed by the presence of chylomicrons. Supportive evidence includes a pleural fluid triglyceride concentration greater than 110 mg/dL. A concentration less than 50 mg/dL excludes chylothorax. Chylous effusions occur in numerous conditions: Kaposi sarcoma with mediastinal adenopathy, after Valsalva maneuver, during childbirth, amyloidosis, esophagectomy, esophageal sclerotherapy, tuberous sclerosis (lymphangiomyomatosis), and thrombosis of the superior vena cava or the innominate or subclavian vein. Lymphoma is the most common nontraumatic cause of chylothorax. Cholesterol effusions (fluid cholesterol >250 mg/dL, triglyceride <110 mg/dL, and absence of chylomicrons) are not true chylous effusions but are known as *pseudochylothorax*. They are seen with chronic pleural effusions and in some cases of nephrotic syndrome; the more common causes are old tuberculous effusions and rheumatoid effusions.

* A mnemonic for the occurrence of chylous effusions is *5 T's*: thoracic duct, *t*rauma, *t*umor (lymphoma), *t*uberculosis, and *t*uberous sclerosis (lymphangiomyomatosis).
* True chylous effusions contain chylomicrons.
* Cholesterol effusions are not true chylous effusions.

Complement

Total complement and C3 and C4 components in the pleural fluid are decreased in systemic lupus erythematosus (80% of patients), including the drug-induced form, and in rheumatoid arthritis (40%-60% of patients), carcinoma, pneumonia, and tuberculosis. Increased pleural fluid antinuclear antibody (>1:160) is strongly suggestive of lupus erythematosus. The presence of lupus erythematosus cells in the pleural fluid is diagnostic of systemic lupus erythematosus. Rheumatoid factor is greater than 1:320 in rheumatoid pleural effusion.

* Low pleural fluid complement: systemic lupus erythematosus (also in the drug-induced form).

Cell Counts

A hemorrhagic effusion (pleural fluid hematocrit >50% of serum hematocrit) is seen in trauma, tumor, asbestos effusion, pancreatitis, pulmonary embolism with infarctions, and other conditions. A bloody effusion in lung cancer usually denotes pleural metastasis, even if the cytologic results are negative. Pleural fluid eosinophilia (>10%) is nonspecific and occurs in trauma (air or blood in the pleural space), pulmonary infarction, psittacosis, drug-induced effusion, pulmonary infiltrate with eosinophilia-associated effusions, benign asbestos pleural effusion, and malignancy. Pleural fluid lymphocytosis occurs in tuberculosis, chronic effusions, lymphoma, sarcoidosis, chylothorax, and some collagenoses such as yellow nail syndrome and chronic rheumatoid pleurisy.

* A bloody effusion in lung cancer usually denotes pleural metastasis, even if the cytologic results are negative.

Cytology

Most effusions in adults should be examined cytologically if the clinical features do not suggest an obvious benign cause. Cytologic findings are positive in 60% of all malignant effusions, and pleural biopsy results are positive in less than 50%. Cytologic examination and biopsy give a slightly higher yield than either one alone, and repeated cytologic examination from sequential thoracentesis increases the diagnostic yield. Cytologic examination is less helpful in malignant mesothelioma and lymphoma, and an open biopsy is often necessary. Positive fluid cytologic findings in primary lung carcinoma imply unresectability (stage IIIB disease).

* Cytologic examination is an important test in most adults with an "unknown" effusion.
* The overall yield from a cytologic examination is 60%, less in cases of mesothelioma and lymphoma.

Cultures

Tuberculous effusions (fluid alone) yield positive cultures in less than 15% of cases. Pleural biopsy (histology and culture) has a higher (>75%) diagnostic yield in tuberculosis. Culture is of value if the effusion is due to actinomycosis or *Nocardia* infection. Culture is less helpful in mycoses, but if fungal infection of the pleural space is suspected, the pleural fluid should be cultured.

Cultures for viruses and certain bacteria (influenza A, chlamydia, coxsackievirus B, and mycoplasma) are often negative. Paragonimiasis causes pleural effusion. The diagnosis of tuberculous pleuritis is strongly suggested by a high adenosine deaminase level in the pleural fluid. Another relatively sensitive test for the diagnosis of tuberculous pleuritis is the level of interferon-γ in the pleural fluid.

* In tuberculosis, it is important to culture pleural biopsy specimens.
* The adenosine deaminase level is increased in tuberculous pleural effusion.
* Poor yield in viral infections.

Pleural Biopsy

Pleural biopsy, now most commonly performed through a thoracoscope, is indicated if tuberculous involvement of the pleural space is suspected. The diagnostic rate from pleural biopsy in tuberculosis is greater than 75%, whereas pleural fluid alone has a much lower yield (<15%). With thoracoscopy, the overall diagnostic yield is higher in pleural effusion of unknown cause, mesothelioma, and lung cancers than with pleural fluid analysis alone. Use of the thoracoscope also offers the advantage of being able to proceed to pleurodesis depending on the findings during the procedure.

* Pleural biopsy is indicated if tuberculous pleural disease is suspected.
* Pleural biopsy through a thoracoscope improves the diagnostic yield of pleural effusions.

Miscellaneous

Nearly 30% of all effusions are undiagnosed despite extensive studies, including open pleural biopsy. At least 350 to 400 mL of fluid must be present to be seen on CXR. It is important to look for subpulmonic effusions, elevated hemidiaphragms, and blunting of the costophrenic angle. When in doubt, obtain a lateral decubitus CXR. Ultrasonography is helpful in tapping small amounts of fluid and loculated fluid collections. Small effusions are common after abdominal operations and the normal labor of pregnancy; almost all resolve spontaneously. Assess for signs of trauma (eg, rib fracture), abdominal surgery, acute abdomen, pancreatitis, and cirrhosis. Asbestos-induced effusions frequently mimic malignant pleural mesothelioma, with pain, bloody fluid, and recurrence. Mesothelioma should be excluded by repeated thoracentesis, pleural biopsy, or thoracotomy. Consider drug-induced pleural effusion (nitrofurantoin, methysergide, drug-induced systemic lupus erythematosus, and busulfan) on the basis of an accurate history of all medications used, suggestive correlation of symptom onset with initiation of the suspected drug, and pleural fluid eosinophilia (>10%) with or without peripheral eosinophilia.

* Small effusions are common after abdominal operations and the normal labor of pregnancy; almost all resolve spontaneously.
* Drug-induced pleural effusion: nitrofurantoin, methysergide, drug-induced systemic lupus erythematosus, and busulfan.
* Nearly 30% of all effusions are undiagnosed despite extensive studies, including open pleural biopsy.

Complications

Complications of thoracentesis include pneumothorax (in 3%-20% of patients), hemothorax, pulmonary edema, intrapulmonary hemorrhage, hemoptysis, vagal inhibition, air embolism, subcutaneous emphysema, bronchopleural fistula, empyema, seeding of a needle tract with malignant cells, and puncture of the liver or spleen.

Sleep-Related Breathing Disorders

Sleep-related breathing disorders (SRBD) encompass various abnormal breathing patterns that occur during sleep. These patterns can be in the form of reduced tidal volumes with or without resultant hypoventilation or complete cessation of airflow resulting in apnea. Complications from SRBD can include sleepiness, an increase in cardiovascular morbidity, an influence on various endocrine factors, and increase in overall mortality (Table 23-10). Diagnosis is confirmed through an overnight polysomnogram (PSG), which defines the presence and severity of SRBD and, in many cases, helps with treatment by titration of noninvasive positive pressure devices.

Obstructive Sleep Apnea Hypopnea Syndrome

Obstructive sleep apnea (OSA) is defined as periodic cessation of airflow (≥10 seconds in duration) during sleep due to obstruction of the upper airway in the setting of continued respiratory effort. This event is typically terminated with a temporary arousal from sleep and return of normal upper airway patency. *Hypopnea* is defined as reduction in airflow for at least 10 seconds, usually with resultant desaturation of at least 4%, which is also typically terminated by an arousal. Such periodic episodes of apnea and hypopnea usually result in fragmented sleep and periodic desaturations. This entity should be suspected in those who are obese (although not always), known to snore, and complain of daytime sleepiness. An overnight PSG is required to make the diagnosis of OSA, which is defined as having more than 5 episodes of apnea and hypopnea per hour of sleep. *Obstructive sleep apnea hypopnea syndrome* implies the presence of OSA accompanied by other symptoms such as excessive daytime sleepiness. Although overnight oximetry may suggest the presence of OSA, it alone is neither sensitive enough nor specific enough for confirmation of the diagnosis.

OSA has been associated with multisystemic dysfunction as noted in Table 23-10. Several studies suggest there is an increase in postoperative complications and overall mortality for those with OSA who remain untreated.

Central Sleep Apnea

Central sleep apnea (CSA) is defined as periodic cessation of airflow (≥10 seconds) during sleep in the absence of upper airway obstruction, presumably due to lack of respiratory muscle stimulation. Airflow is gradually resumed and is not always associated with an arousal from sleep. This entity may be seen in those with neurologic abnormalities (eg, cerebrovascular accident, amyotrophic lateral sclerosis, and postpolio syndrome) or endocrine dysfunctions (eg, acromegaly and hypothyroidism), or it may be idiopathic. Within CSA, a specific respiratory pattern cycles between crescendo-decrescendo respirations followed by a pause. This pattern is known as *Cheyne-Stokes respiration* or *periodic respiration* and is often seen in those with

Table 23-10 Systemic Disorders That Have Been Associated With Sleep-Related Breathing Disorders

Central nervous system
  Cerebrovascular accidents
  Cognitive impairments
  Excessive sleepiness
  Lower seizure threshold
  Recurrent headaches
Cardiovascular
  Myocardial infarcts
  Hypertension
  Cardiac arrhythmia
  Acceleration of atherosclerosis
  Pulmonary hypertension
Endocrine
  Insulin insensitivity
  Suppression of growth hormone release
  Alteration of progesterone & testosterone release
  Obesity
Gastrointestinal
  Gastroesophageal reflux disease
Respiratory
  Hypercapnia
  Dyspnea
  Reduced exercise tolerance
Psychiatric
  Depression
  Insomnia
  Nocturnal panic disorders

congestive heart failure (especially during acute exacerbation), at high altitude, and after a cerebrovascular event.

Sleep Hypoventilation Syndrome

Sleep hypoventilation syndrome is characterized by a reduction in respiration, resulting in hypercapnia and usually hypoxemia during sleep, but is most pronounced during rapid eye movement (REM) sleep. Most affected persons have daytime hypercapnia and pulmonary hypertension or even cor pulmonale. Sleep hypoventilation syndrome may be seen in those who are significantly obese (known as *obesity-hypoventilation syndrome*) or who have severe respiratory (including chest wall defects) or neurologic diseases.

Treatment

Treatment typically involves use of noninvasive positive pressure devices such as continuous positive airway pressure (CPAP) and bilevel positive airway pressure (BiPAP) devices. Adequate titration can be achieved during a polysomnogram, but, in certain circumstances, an autotitrating CPAP device may be used. In severe cases, tracheostomy may be required, but, in most cases, these disorders can be managed noninvasively with or without addition of supplemental oxygen. Treatment of CSA, however, can be difficult, and positive airway pressure devices may not always be effective.

Part II

Timothy R. Aksamit, MD

Diffuse Lung Disease

Diffuse lung disease includes a wide range of parenchymal lung diseases that have infectious, inflammatory, malignant, drug, occupational/environmental, and other causes. Although many identifiable causes are recognized, the cause of most cases of diffuse lung disease in many published series is idiopathic. The clinical course may be acute or prolonged and may progress rapidly to life-threatening respiratory failure with death, or it may be indolent over many years. In most instances, a differential diagnosis can readily be formulated by obtaining the medical history, with emphasis on the nature of the symptoms, duration, and pertinent environmental, occupational, drug, and travel exposures. The physical examination, laboratory tests, pulmonary function tests (PFTs), chest radiography (CXR), and computed tomography (CT) often provide clues to the diagnosis. The diagnosis may be confirmed on clinical grounds but may also require bronchoscopy with bronchoalveolar lavage (BAL) and transbronchial biopsy or open lung biopsy via video-assisted thoracoscopy (VATS).

This overview of diffuse lung disease emphasizes the differential diagnosis, classification schemes, clinical clues to diagnosis, and available diagnostic tools and summarizes a diagnostic strategy for approaching diffuse lung disease in clinical practice.

Some of the causes of diffuse lung disease and the diseases associated with them are listed in Figure 23-27. The numerous idiopathic causes are listed in Table 23-11. The relative proportions of the causes of diffuse lung disease are given in Table 23-12. In a typical internal medicine practice, approximately three-fourths of the cases of diffuse lung disease represent 1 of 3 diagnoses: idiopathic pulmonary fibrosis (IPF) (also called *usual interstitial pneumonia* [UIP]), sarcoidosis,

or collagen vascular disease–associated interstitial lung disease (especially nonspecific interstitial pneumonia [NSIP]). Many of the causes of diffuse lung disease usually described in textbooks are uncommon in clinical practice.

The abbreviations and clinicopathologic correlates of diffuse lung disease are listed in Tables 23-13 and 23-14, respectively. In most instances, the histopathologic findings alone are not sufficient to establish a specific clinical diagnosis of diffuse lung disease. The pathology findings are common to several diagnostic possibilities and need to be correlated with the clinical history and laboratory test and radiographic results to establish the diagnosis. Similarly, different disease entities have overlapping histopathologic features. The histopathologic features of IPF-UIP or NSIP may be found separately or together, as in collagen vascular disease–associated interstitial diffuse lung disease. In other instances, the histopathologic features are specific for a particular diagnosis (eg, lymphangioleiomyomatosis). The histopathologic features may also have prognostic and therapeutic implications. For example, the histopathologic findings of IPF-UIP, compared with those of NSIP, are consistently correlated with less responsiveness to corticosteroid therapy and poorer prognosis. In contrast, NSIP–interstitial diffuse lung disease is more common in younger persons, is often associated with drug-induced or collagen vascular disease–associated diffuse lung disease, and has a more cellular inflammatory process.

Thus, the physician needs to formulate a systematic approach to diffuse lung disease that involves a complete medical history, physical examination, PFTs, blood tests, and radiographic studies before considering bronchoscopy with BAL and transbronchial biopsy or open lung biopsy via VATS. Occasionally, specific patterns of diagnostic test results provide additional clues to assist the physician. In this way,

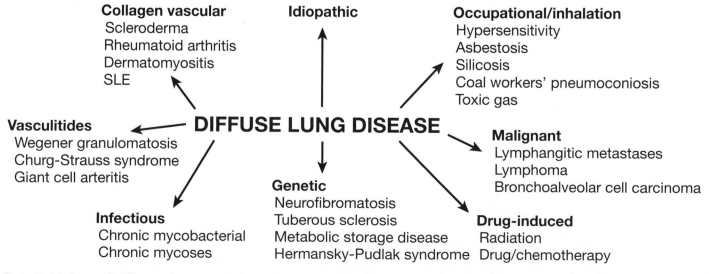

Figure 23-27. Causes of Diffuse Lung Disease. SLE indicates systemic lupus erythematosus.

Table 23-11 Idiopathic Diffuse Lung Disease

Idiopathic pulmonary fibrosis–usual interstitial pneumonia (IPF-UIP)

Nonspecific interstitial pneumonia (NSIP)

Sarcoidosis

Bronchiolitis obliterans with organizing pneumonia/cryptogenic organizing pneumonia (BOOP/COP)

Eosinophilic lung diseases

Lymphocytic interstitial pneumonia (LIP)

Alveolar microlithiasis

Lymphangioleiomyomatosis (LAM)

Langerhans cell histiocytosis/eosinophilic granulomatosis

Pulmonary alveolar proteinosis

Acute respiratory distress syndrome/acute lung injury

Others

Table 23-12 Epidemiology of Diffuse Lung Disease[a,b]

Diagnosis	%
IPF	12-42
Sarcoidosis	8-41
ILD-CVD	10-17
Hypersensitivity	2-8
Vasculitides	2-8
Histiocytosis	1-11
Drug/radiation	1-10
Pneumoconioses	5-10
BOOP	1-3
LAM	1-2
Lymphangitic cancer	1-2
LIP	1-2

Abbreviations: BOOP, bronchiolitis obliterans with organizing pneumonia; CVD, collagen vascular disease; ILD, interstitial lung disease; IPF, idiopathic pulmonary fibrosis; LAM, lymphangioleiomyomatosis; LIP, lymphocytic interstitial pneumonia.

[a] Prevalence is 2 to 200 per 100,000 persons.

[b] Prevalence of IPF is higher among males and the elderly.

Data from American Thoracic Society (ATS), European Respiratory Society (ERS). Idiopathic pulmonary fibrosis: diagnosis and treatment. International consensus statement. Am J Respir Crit Care Med. 2000;161:646-64; Coultas DB, Zumwalt RE, Black WC, Sobonya RE. The epidemiology of interstitial lung diseases. Am J Respir Crit Care Med. 1994;150:967-72; Grenier P, Chevret S, Beigelman C, Brauner MW, Chastang C, Valeyre D. Chronic diffuse infiltrative lung disease: determination of the diagnostic value of clinical data, chest radiography, and CT and Bayesian analysis. Radiology. 1994;191:383-90.

close working interactions between clinicians, radiologists, and pathologists have been demonstrated to be the most efficient and accurate approach to patients with diffuse lung disease.

In diffuse lung disease, PFTs generally demonstrate restrictive change, with various degrees of gas exchange abnormalities and hypoxemia. A component of obstructive change may be found in some cases. Specifically, the causes of diffuse lung disease that demonstrate various degrees of airflow obstruction on PFTs with or without restrictive change and gas exchange abnormalities include rheumatoid arthritis, Langerhans cell histiocytosis, lymphangioleiomyomatosis, tuberous sclerosis, sarcoidosis, bronchiectasis, cystic fibrosis, eosinophilic pneumonia, and hypersensitivity pneumonitis.

The CXR is the initial radiographic study for virtually all patients who present with respiratory symptoms attributed to diffuse lung disease. The findings may include interstitial or alveolar patterns or both. However, the differences between alveolar and interstitial infiltrates can be subtle; also, they are sufficiently nonspecific to be of limited usefulness. Nonetheless, alveolar infiltrates generally predominate in processes of diffuse lung disease that include diffuse alveolar damage (which is the histopathologic diagnosis that corresponds to acute respiratory distress syndrome [ARDS], the clinical diagnosis), pulmonary edema (cardiogenic and noncardiogenic), aspiration pneumonia, alveolar hemorrhage syndromes, pulmonary alveolar proteinosis, bronchoalveolar cell carcinoma, toxic gas exposure, desquamative interstitial pneumonia, infectious pneumonia, and hematogenous metastases. Infiltrates may be nodular, cavitary, or mixed. An upper versus lower predominance may be suggestive of specific diagnoses. Upper predominance often occurs in diffuse lung disease related to ankylosing spondylitis, silicosis/coal workers' pneumoconiosis, sarcoidosis, Langerhans cell histiocytosis, tuberculosis and mycotic lung disease, cystic fibrosis, and allergic bronchopulmonary aspergillosis. Basilar predominance is common in IPF-UIP, asbestosis, desquamative interstitial pneumonia, lymphocytic interstitial pneumonitis, and hematogenous metastatic disease.

Chest CT, including high-resolution chest CT (HRCT, thin-section CT), is commonly used to evaluate patients who present with diffuse lung disease. In conjunction with a "characteristic" clinical history, physical examination, blood tests, and PFTs, HRCT findings may obviate the need for bronchoscopy or VATS open lung biopsy (or both) to establish the clinical diagnosis, to outline a therapeutic strategy, and to provide prognostic information. Similarly, specific chest CT findings alone may suggest the diagnosis of Langerhans cell histiocytosis, lymphangioleiomyomatosis, IPF-UIP, and lymphangitic metastases and, occasionally, sarcoidosis, bronchiolitis obliterans with organizing pneumonia (BOOP), eosinophilic pneumonia, asbestosis, and mycobacterial disease. Ground-glass opacities seen with HRCT are patchy, hazy areas of increased attenuation with preserved bronchial and vascular margins. They may represent air-space or interstitial abnormalities, although rarely they are seen in nondisease states because of technical limitations. In the case of air-space opacification and interstitial lung disease, ground-glass opacities have been correlated with increased cellularity, as in NSIP. In contrast, interlobular septal thickening and subpleural "reticular" honeycombing with traction bronchiectasis reflect a less cellular lesion that is more fibrotic and has scattered fibroblastic foci, which are characteristic of IPF-UIP. Both ground-glass opacities and peripheral reticular honeycombing occur in many cases of interstitial diffuse lung disease.

Table 23-13 Abbreviations for Diffuse Lung Disease

AIP	Acute interstitial pneumonia (Hamman-Rich syndrome)
BOOP/COP	Bronchiolitis obliterans with organizing pneumonia/cryptogenic organizing pneumonia
DAD	Diffuse alveolar damage (acute respiratory distress syndrome)
DIP	Desquamative interstitial pneumonia
GIP	Giant cell pneumonitis
ILD	Interstitial lung disease
IPF	Idiopathic pulmonary fibrosis
NSIP	Nonspecific interstitial pneumonia
RB-ILD	Respiratory bronchiolitis–associated interstitial lung disease
UIP	Usual interstitial pneumonia

Flexible fiberoptic bronchoscopy has dramatically improved the ability to sample the airway and lung in stabilized outpatients as well as in inpatients with hypoxemic respiratory failure due to diffuse lung disease. BAL generally can be performed safely in most settings, and the findings may be used to quickly identify the cause of diffuse lung disease, especially atypical or typical infectious causes or lymphangitic metastases. BAL is safe for patients who have thrombocytopenia or hypoxemia. Nonetheless, BAL has a limited role in establishing many other specific diagnoses of diffuse lung disease, including IPF, NSIP, sarcoidosis, hypersensitivity pneumonitis, and asbestosis. In many cases, transbronchial biopsy can be performed in combination with BAL, resulting in a diagnostic yield greater than 70% for sarcoidosis, hypersensitivity pneumonitis, Langerhans cell histiocytosis, pulmonary alveolar proteinosis, lymphangitic metastases, diffuse pulmonary lymphoma, bronchoalveolar cell carcinoma, mycobacterial and mycotic lung disease, pneumoconioses, and lung rejection after transplant. The complication rates with transbronchial biopsy are 1% to 5% for pneumothorax, 1% to 2% for hemorrhage,

and less than 0.2% for death. In comparison, the mortality rate with BAL is 0.04%.

In most cases, the results of blood tests provide supportive but not definitive diagnostic information for diffuse lung disease. Results that are often abnormal but nonspecific, and thus not helpful diagnostically, include the leukocyte count, antinuclear antibody (ANA) titer, rheumatoid factor (RF), and gamma globulins. Moreover, an increase in the angiotensin-converting enzyme (ACE) level is neither specific nor sensitive enough to establish the diagnosis of sarcoidosis. The level may be increased in many other causes of granulomatous lung disease. When the ACE level is increased in sarcoidosis, it may be a marker of disease activity and thus be helpful in follow-up evaluations. In other cases, blood test abnormalities are specific but lack sensitivity; these include fungal serologic tests (for histoplasmosis, blastomycosis, coccidioidomycosis, and cryptococcal disease), serum precipitins (for hypersensitivity pneumonitis), and specific autoantibody titers in connective tissue diseases or vasculitis. An exception is the test for cytoplasmic antinuclear cytoplasmic antibody (cANCA), which has an estimated overall sensitivity of 81% and a specificity of 98% for Wegener granulomatosis when performed in an experienced laboratory. This antibody is directed specifically against proteinase 3 (PR3). The perinuclear antinuclear cytoplasmic antibody (pANCA) is directed against myeloperoxidase and may also be positive in Wegener granulomatosis as well as in microscopic polyangiitis, Churg-Strauss syndrome, and other vasculitides. Higher sensitivity and specificity rates may be expected during disease activity.

The pretest probability, including medical history and laboratory data, and radiographic findings need to be combined to optimize the diagnostic yield. The diagnostic yield increases from 27% to 53% and 61% when clinical information is added to CXR and HRCT findings, respectively. An algorithm for diagnosing diffuse lung disease is given in Figure 23-28. With this strategy, including HRCT, the diagnostic yield may approach 90% if the diffuse lung disease is rapidly progressive. The likelihood of establishing a specific diagnosis using this algorithm is greatest for sarcoidosis, Langerhans cell histiocytosis, hypersensitivity pneumonitis, asbestosis, lymphangitic metastases, silicosis, and possibly IPF-UIP.

Table 23-14 Clinicopathologic Classification of Diffuse Lung Disease

Idiopathic pulmonary fibrosis–usual interstitial pneumonia (IPF-UIP) > collagen-vascular disease, others
Nonspecific interstitial pneumonia (NSIP): collagen-vascular disease, drugs
DIP/RB-ILD: smokers
Lymphocytic interstitial pneumonitis: Sjögren syndrome, AIDS, lymphoma, dysproteinemia, inflammatory bowel disease/Crohn disease, primary biliary cirrhosis, lymphomatoid granulomatosis
Acute interstitial pneumonia: Hamman-Rich syndrome, diffuse alveolar damage-ARDS
BOOP (idiopathic): also drugs, collagen-vascular disease
Hypersensitivity pneumonitis: drugs, avian, mold

Abbreviations: ARDS, acute respiratory distress syndrome; BOOP, bronchiolitis obliterans with organizing pneumonia; DIP, desquamative interstitial pneumonia; RB-ILD, respiratory bronchiolitis–associated interstitial lung disease.

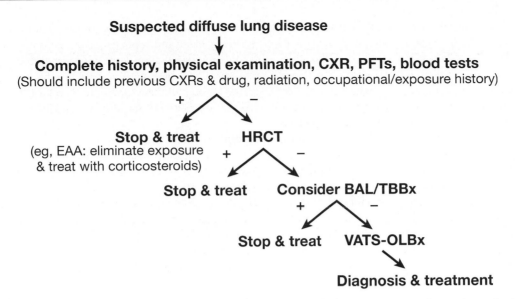

Figure 23-28. Strategy for Diagnosing Diffuse Lung Disease. BAL indicates bronchoalveolar lavage; CXR, chest radiography; EAA, extrinsic allergic alveolitis; HRCT, high-resolution computed tomography; OLBx, open lung biopsy; PFT, pulmonary function test; TBBx, transbronchial biopsy; VATS, video-assisted thoracoscopy.

VATS open lung biopsy may still be required in up to one-third of patients.

Specific Diagnoses

Idiopathic Pulmonary Fibrosis–Usual Interstitial Pneumonia

The onset of IPF-UIP is insidious and involves a dry progressive cough. It generally affects persons 50 to 70 years old. Serologic tests are too nonspecific to be helpful diagnostically. Antinuclear antibody, erythrocyte sedimentation rate, rheumatoid factor, and gamma globulins are often mildly abnormal. HRCT findings vary but typically include lower lobe predominance of interlobular septal thickening with subpleural fibrosis and honeycombing with few, if any, ground-glass opacities. In many cases of IPF-UIP, peripheral honeycombing and ground-glass opacities are seen together. Classic HRCT findings in combination with a compatible clinical presentation suggest IPF-UIP and may obviate the need for bronchoscopy or biopsy. PFTs are expected to demonstrate restrictive abnormalities, with reduced diffusing capacity and abnormal gas exchange with various degrees of hypoxemia. By the time the diffusing capacity is about 50% of predicted or less, hypoxemia with exercise is usually present. As a rule, the response to treatment is poor. Corticosteroids, other immunosuppressive agents (eg, azathioprine and cyclophosphamide), and antifibrotic drugs (eg, colchicine and penicillamine) have not been shown clearly to be of benefit. Some data suggest that corticosteroids worsen the outcome of IPF-UIP if more than a low dose (prednisone equivalent of ≥10 mg per day) is administered. Recent multicenter trial results suggest that interferon-γ does not improve outcome in IPF-UIP. Ongoing multicenter trials are expected to confirm preliminary results that *N*-acetylcysteine (NAC) improves the rate of decline in lung function. The overall prognosis is poor, with 5-year survival from the time of diagnosis estimated to be 20%.

Nonspecific Interstitial Pneumonia

Nonspecific interstitial pneumonia (NSIP) represents a distinct histopathologic type of interstitial lung disease. Its pathologic features often are found in drug-induced or collagen vascular disease–associated interstitial diffuse lung disease. However, in many cases, it appears to be idiopathic. NSIP generally occurs in younger patients (≤50 years) and has a female to male ratio of 2:1. HRCT often shows ground-glass opacities, in contrast to the basilar subpleural honeycombing, fibrosis, and traction bronchiectasis typical of IPF-UIP. The course usually includes various degrees of cough, dyspnea, and fever over weeks or months. The cellularity detected with BAL and the inflammatory components seen in biopsy specimens tend to be greater than those of IPF-UIP. Thus, NSIP tends to be more responsive to corticosteroid therapy and to have a better prognosis overall, with a 5-year survival rate of approximately 65% to 80%.

Sarcoidosis

Sarcoidosis is a granulomatous disease of patients who generally are younger than 50 years. They may present with lung disease, either acute inflammatory disease or chronic end-stage diffuse fibrotic lung disease. The development of sarcoidosis has not been linked to tobacco use. Although the lungs and lymph nodes are the most commonly involved organs, the disease can affect virtually any organ, including the heart, liver, spleen, eye, bone, skin, bone marrow, parotid glands, pituitary, reproductive organs, and the nervous system. If the disease is systemic, hypercalcemia, anemia, and increased liver enzyme levels may be noted. Familial clusters of sarcoidosis have been reported. The incidence, clinical course, and prognosis are influenced by ethnic and genetic factors. Stages 0 through IV correlate with the severity of pulmonary disease and the prognosis. Radiographic stage 0 indicates a normal CXR; stage I, hilar adenopathy; stage II, hilar adenopathy with pulmonary infiltrates; stage III, infiltrates without adenopathy; and stage IV, fibrotic lung disease. CXRs may also demonstrate characteristic right paratracheal, bilateral hilar, or mediastinal lymphadenopathy (or a combination of these) with or without eggshell calcification. Chest CT may show small nodules with a bronchovascular and subpleural distribution, thickened intralobular septa, architectural distortion, or conglomerate masses.

A diagnosis of acute sarcoidosis (ie, Löfgren syndrome) can be made on the basis of clinical findings in a young patient who presents with fever, erythema nodosum, polyarthritis, and hilar adenopathy. For the diagnosis in most other cases, granulomatous histopathologic features need to be demonstrated and other causes of granulomatous inflammation need to be excluded, primarily infectious (mycotic and mycobacterial) causes. If hilar adenopathy and parenchymal infiltrates are present, bronchoscopy with biopsy confirms granulomatous changes in more than 90% of cases. Thus, sarcoidosis must be considered a diagnosis of exclusion after other causes of granulomatous disease have been ruled out.

Although rales may be present when acute parenchymal interstitial changes occur, the lung fields typically are clear on auscultation even if parenchymal infiltrates are substantial. The serum levels of ACE are not sufficiently sensitive or specific to be of diagnostic value, but they may be helpful as a marker of disease activity.

Corticosteroids are first-line therapy. However, whether any immunosuppressive therapy, including corticosteroids, alters the natural course of the disease is debated. Other immunosuppressive regimens used as second-line therapy for pulmonary sarcoidosis have included methotrexate, azathioprine, pentoxifylline, and cyclosporine. Treatment is reserved for progressive disease or advanced-stage disease with active granulomatous inflammation. In up to 90% of patients with stage I pulmonary sarcoidosis, the disease is expected to remain stable or to resolve spontaneously with no treatment. Stage III pulmonary sarcoidosis is expected to spontaneously remit in only 10% of patients. Pregnancy does not alter disease activity, although a flare in disease activity may occur post partum. Pulmonary sarcoidosis is expected to progress within 2 to 5 years after diagnosis, although increased disease activity can occur at any time. Indefinite long-term follow-up is recommended for patients with stage II or higher pulmonary or extrapulmonary sarcoidosis.

Desquamative Interstitial Pneumonia and Respiratory Bronchiolitis–Associated Interstitial Lung Disease

Desquamative interstitial pneumonia (DIP) and respiratory bronchiolitis–associated interstitial lung disease (RB-ILD) likely represent similar entities along a spectrum of disease. Both are diagnosed universally in current or former smokers who present with worsening cough and dyspnea over weeks or months. Crackles may be present. In DIP, chest CT demonstrates diffuse ground-glass opacities, but in RB-ILD, it shows a mix of diffuse, fine reticular, or nodular interstitial abnormalities. PFTs may show restrictive, obstructive, or mixed abnormalities, with various degrees of reduced diffusing capacity and hypoxemia. Macrophages are thought to be an integral part of the disease process. Abnormal accumulations of macrophages are seen in the alveoli in DIP and in the peribronchiolar airway–respiratory bronchioles in RB-ILD. Mild fibrosis of the peribronchiolar area is more prominent in RB-ILD than in DIP, in which little fibrosis is noted. Cellularity, including lymphocytic infiltration, is also more prominent in the airway-oriented lesions of RB-ILD than the relatively bland macrophage accumulations seen in the alveoli in DIP. Smoking cessation is the mainstay of therapy, although corticosteroids have been used in some instances. Overall, prognosis is better for both of these conditions than for IPF-UIP. The expected 10-year mortality rate for DIP is approximately 30%.

Lymphangioleiomyomatosis

Lymphangioleiomyomatosis (LAM) is a disease of women of childbearing age. It is characterized clinically by a history of recurrent pneumothoraces, chylous pleural effusions, diffuse infiltrates with hypoxemia, and airflow obstruction. HRCT typically demonstrates well-defined cysts scattered throughout the lungs, without nodules or interstitial fibrosis. Hemoptysis is common. Pregnancy or exogenous estrogens may worsen the course of the disease. The histopathologic features, similar to those of tuberous sclerosis, include a distinctive proliferation of atypical interstitial smooth muscle and thin-walled cysts within the lung. Extrapulmonary involvement may include uterine leiomyomas and renal angiomyolipomas. The response to treatment with hormonal manipulation has been limited. Currently, lung transplantation is the definitive treatment.

Langerhans Cell Histiocytosis

Langerhans cell histiocytosis is a rare diffuse lung disease mostly affecting young white smokers. Spontaneous pneumothoraces are common. CXR demonstrates diffuse interstitial infiltrates with classic cystic and nodular changes, predominantly in the upper lobe. The distinctive nodular component with cystic change seen on HRCT differentiates Langerhans cell histiocytosis from lymphangioleiomyomatosis. Airflow obstruction with decreased diffusing capacity and hypoxemia is expected. In the systemic variant of the disease, bone may be involved, especially in children. Pituitary insufficiency with central diabetes insipidus has been described, as it has been for other granulomatous processes, including sarcoidosis. Peripheral blood eosinophilia is not expected, although eosinophilia may be detected on BAL. PFTs often demonstrate restrictive, obstructive, or mixed changes, with reduced diffusing capacity and various degrees of gas exchange abnormality and hypoxemia. Aggregates of Langerhans cells interspersed with normal lung parenchyma are the characteristic histopathologic finding. An increase in the number of Langerhans cells can be detected by staining BAL specimens for OKT6, which is overexpressed in these cells. Absolute cessation from smoking is mandatory. The response to abstinence from all tobacco products varies, with stabilization or improvement noted in as many as two-thirds of patients. Langerhans cell histiocytosis increases the risk of bronchogenic cancer. The success of corticosteroid treatment and chemotherapy has been limited. Transplant is reserved for advanced, progressive disease.

Hypersensitivity Pneumonitis (Extrinsic Allergic Alveolitis): Farmer's Lung Disease, Hot-Tub Lung, and Bird Fancier's Lung Disease

Hypersensitivity pneumonitis is an uncommon but often discussed form of diffuse lung disease. It respresents an allergic sensitization to various organic antigens, including molds, grain dusts (farmer's lung), pets and birds (bird fancier's lung), and mycobacterial antigens (hot-tub lung). Serum precipitins for specific antigens are inconsistently specific and have poor sensitivity for diagnostic purposes. In many cases, serum precipitins are tested but the results are not helpful diagnostically except for patients who have a clear history of exposure to birds and positive serologic results to testing with an avian panel of antigens. Other blood tests are expected to demonstrate nonspecific and various degrees of leukocytosis, eosinophilia, an increase in the erythrocyte sedimentation rate and rheumatoid factor, and a mild increase in antinuclear antibodies. Patients may present with acute inflammatory disease, subacute mixed inflammatory–fibrotic disease, or chronic fibrotic lung disease. The symptoms and clinical course are related temporally to antigen exposure. Acutely, patients may experience dyspnea, cough, fever, chest pain, headache, malaise, fatigue, and flulike illness. Clinically, radiographically, histopathologically, or bronchoscopically, chronic diffuse fibrotic lung disease may be indistinguishable from IPF-UIP.

The histopathologic features of hypersensitivity pneumonitis show a range of bronchiolar-oriented, loosely organized, noncaseating granulomas with lymphocytic-predominant centrilobular infiltrates and various degrees of fibrosis, depending on how long the disease has been present. PFTs show restrictive abnormalities, although an airway component may also be present and result in an obstructive component. Gas exchange abnormalities and hypoxemia may be profound in more severe cases of acute or chronic disease. Bronchodilators may be needed to treat airflow obstruction. CXR generally demonstrates reticulonodular changes, with various amounts of alveolar infiltrates. HRCT findings often include nonspecific nodules and ground-glass opacities, predominantly in the upper lobe. Diffuse fibrotic changes indistinguishable from those of IPF-UIP may be seen in chronic disease. Acute symptoms generally improve after the patient is removed from antigen exposure. Severe cases require treatment with corticosteroids.

Asbestos-Related Lung Disease

Asbestos-related lung disease manifests as diffuse interstitial lung disease (asbestosis), but it may also present as benign pleural plaques and effusions, malignant mesothelioma, pulmonary nodules, or rounded atelectasis. The asbestos fibers usually associated with the disease are the amphibole type, of which the crocidolite subtype is the most fibrogenic and carcinogenic. A dose-response relation has been reported consistently between the intensity and duration of exposure to asbestos fibers and the development of asbestosis. A long dormant period between exposure and symptomatic disease is common. The dormant period for interstitial disease, pleural plaques, and malignant mesothelioma is generally longer (20-40 years) than for the development of benign pleural effusions (<15 years). Progressive isolated pleural disease may lead to restrictive pulmonary function without parenchymal change. Asbestos-related interstitial lung disease is characterized by a progressive course of dry cough, dyspnea, and basilar rales in association with restrictive abnormalities detected with PFTs, decreased diffusing capacity, and hypoxemia. Smoking greatly increases the risk of bronchogenic cancer for patients with asbestos-related interstitial disease and may accelerate the rate of progression of parenchymal lung disease. A basilar predominance of interstitial infiltrates seen on CXR resembles that of IPF-UIP. Pleural plaques, when present, may differentiate asbestosis from IPF-UIP. Although HRCT is not needed as often to establish the diagnosis of asbestosis as it is for IPF-UIP, it is able to detect parenchymal changes earlier than CXR and it demonstrates the characteristic subpleural lines, parenchymal bands, thickened interlobular septal lines, and honeycombing. Treatment, including corticosteroids, is not effective.

Silicosis

Silicosis-related diffuse lung disease may result from acute or chronic exposure to silica dust. Generally, the disease affects predominantly the upper lobe, with typical 1- to 3-mm nodular infiltrates. Coalescence may lead to conglomerate masses and fibrosis. Dry cough and dyspnea are typical symptoms. Eggshell calcifications of mediastinal and hilar lymph nodes may be seen, as in sarcoidosis. The antinuclear antibodies are often high titer, but their role in disease progression is unclear. PFTs are usually normal, unless the disease is advanced. Restrictive changes and a decrease in diffusing capacity without obstructive change are expected. Patients with silicosis are at increased risk of *Mycobacterium tuberculosis* infection and should have screening tests for latent tuberculosis infection and active disease. The risk of bronchogenic cancer is less for silicosis than for asbestosis.

Bronchiolitis Obliterans With Organizing Pneumonia/Cryptogenic Organizing Pneumonia

BOOP is a specific histopathologic entity that can occur with collagen vascular- and drug-induced diffuse lung disease, various infections, radiation injury, and other conditions. Idiopathic BOOP appears to represent a distinct clinical diagnosis, assuming that other secondary causes have been excluded. It generally affects men and women between 50 and 70 years old. The presentation is more acute, occurring over days or weeks, than that of IPF-UIP, which occurs over months or years. Approximately 75% of cases of idiopathic BOOP present within 8 weeks after symptoms appear. Most often, the symptoms are cough, dyspnea, fever, fatigue, and flulike illness not responsive to antibiotics. CXR findings include consolidation, interstitial infiltrates, alveolar infiltrates, or mixed infiltrates. Often, the infiltrates are predominantly peripheral, resembling chronic eosinophilic pneumonia. Diagnosis is usually confirmed by transbronchial or VATS open lung biopsy. The response to corticosteroid therapy is generally dramatic. Overall, the prognosis is favorable. Long-term outcome studies do not usually indicate progression.

Diffuse Alveolar Damage, ARDS, and Acute Interstitial Pneumonitis

Diffuse alveolar damage is a specific pathologic diagnosis made on the basis of lung biopsy findings. When diffuse alveolar damage is found in combination with causes of the systemic inflammatory response syndrome, including sepsis, pneumonia, pancreatitis, and trauma, the clinical diagnosis is ARDS or, if it is less severe, acute lung injury. If a patient presents with acute or subacute hypoxemic respiratory failure and diffuse lung disease without any identifiable cause and the histopathologic features of diffuse alveolar damage, the diagnosis is acute interstitial pneumonitis. The mortality rate is high (>50%-80%), and the disease is not very responsive to treatment, including high-dose corticosteroids or other aggressive immuno-suppressive regimens. Treatment is largely supportive.

Eosinophilic Pneumonia

Acute and chronic eosinophilic pneumonias are 2 of several forms of eosinophilic lung disease. Acute eosinophilic pneumonia has an acute onset (days) of severe dyspnea and cough associated with fulminant hypoxemic respiratory failure and diffuse alveolar and interstitial infiltrates and, usually, pleural effusions. Peripheral blood eosinophilia is not necessarily present, but marked eosinophilia is expected in BAL and pleural fluid specimens. Typically, the response to corticosteroid therapy is complete and without relapse. The long-term prognosis for acute eosinophilic pneumonia is excellent. In comparison, patients with chronic eosinophilic pneumonia present with cough, dyspnea, and fever over months or years and, clinically and radiographically, may be essentially indistinguishable from patients with IPF-UIP or chronic BOOP. In the subacute form of the disease, CXR typically shows pulmonary edema, which may also be seen in some cases of BOOP and occasionally in sarcoidosis and drug reactions. BAL fluid eosinophilia with peripheral blood eosinophilia (88% of patients) is expected. Usually, long-term corticosteroid therapy is required to prevent disease relapse.

Lymphocytic Interstitial Pneumonia

Lymphocytic interstitial pneumonia (LIP) is an unusual form of interstitial diffuse lung disease that is related to several hematologic diseases (eg, lymphoma), autoimmune disorders (eg, Sjögren syndrome), dysproteinemia, human immunodeficiency virus infection, and transplant rejection (graft-versus-host disease). The response to treatment is highly variable and depends primarily on the underlying disease process.

Giant Cell Pneumonitis

Another rare form of interstitial diffuse lung disease, giant cell pneumonitis (GIP) is most often associated with hard-metal (eg, cobalt) pneumoconioses.

Pulmonary Alveolar Proteinosis

Pulmonary alveolar proteinosis is a rare and idiopathic form of diffuse lung disease characterized by the filling of alveoli with proteinaceous material consisting mostly of phospholipoprotein (dipalmitoyl lecithin). A defect in the signaling of granulocyte-macrophage colony-stimulating factor is thought to contribute to the clinical manifestations. Most patients are smokers younger than 50 years, with a male predominance (male to female ratio of 3:1). Symptoms of dyspnea, cough, and low-grade fever are common. Many infectious, occupational, inflammatory, and environmental secondary causes of pulmonary alveolar proteinosis-like presentations have been recognized. Increased predisposition to *Nocardia* infections has been reported. CXR may demonstrate an alveolar filling pattern infiltrate that resembles "bat wings," mimicking pulmonary edema. A nonspecific but characteristic alveolar filling pattern seen with HRCT, described as a "crazy paving" pattern with airspace consolidation and thickened interlobular septa, is suggestive of pulmonary alveolar proteinosis. A milky white return of BAL fluid or lung biopsy findings usually indicate the diagnosis. In addition to smoking cessation, therapy has involved whole lung lavage and, more recently, trials of granulocyte-macrophage colony-stimulating factor.

Alveolar Microlithiasis

Alveolar microlithiasis, a rare form of idiopathic familial (autosomal recessive) diffuse lung disease, is characterized by interstitial infiltrates. Fine miliary nodular changes due to the deposition of microliths occur throughout all lung fields. Most patients are asymptomatic through the third to fourth decades of life. Symptoms of dyspnea may progress to cor pulmonale as the disease advances. No therapy has been shown to be effective.

Summary

Diffuse lung disease represents a wide range of idiopathic and secondary lung disease processes that have various presentations and prognoses. A focused, complete medical history and physical examination in combination with judicious use of laboratory data, PFTs, chest imaging, bronchoscopy, and open lung biopsy when needed can considerably narrow the differential diagnosis and provide important therapeutic and prognostic information.

Part III

Karen L. Swanson, DO

Pulmonary Neoplasms

Solitary Pulmonary Nodule

A *solitary pulmonary nodule* is defined as a solitary lesion seen on plain chest radiography (CXR). It is less than 4 cm in diameter and is round, ovoid, or slightly lobulated. The lesion is located in lung parenchyma, is at least moderately circumscribed, and is uncalcified on plain CXRs. It is not associated with satellite lesions or other abnormalities on plain CXRs. Common causes include carcinoma of the lung (15%-50% of patients), mycoses (5%-50%), tuberculosis, uncalcified granulomas, resolving pneumonia, hamartoma, and metastatic lesions. Granulomas and hamartomas make up 40% to 60% of all solitary pulmonary nodules and 90% of nonmalignant solitary pulmonary nodules. Hamartomas alone comprise less than 10% of nonmalignant nodules. Uncommon causes include carcinoid tumors, bronchogenic cysts, resolving infarction, rheumatoid and vasculitic nodules, and arteriovenous malformations.

- Granulomas and hamartomas make up 40%-60% of all solitary pulmonary nodules and 90% of nonmalignant solitary pulmonary nodules.
- Hamartomas alone comprise <10% of nonmalignant nodules.

Clinical Evaluation

The following are important in the evaluation of solitary pulmonary nodules: age of patient, availability of previous CXRs, smoking history, previous malignancy, exposure to tuberculosis, travel to areas endemic for mycoses, recent respiratory infection, recent pulmonary embolism (suggestive of infarction), recent trauma to the chest, asthma, mucoid impaction, systemic diseases (congestive heart failure or rheumatoid arthritis), ear-nose-throat symptoms (Wegener granulomatosis), exposure to mineral oil or oily nose drops, immune defense mechanisms, and family history (arteriovenous malformation seen in hereditary hemorrhagic telangiectasia).

- History: old CXRs for comparison, age, smoking history, previous malignancy, and exposure history are important.

Diagnosis

Physical examination, routine blood tests, chemistry group, and the exclusion of obvious causes (eg, congestive heart failure, vasculitis, and rheumatoid arthritis) are important for making the diagnosis. Obtain an earlier CXR for comparison if possible. Generally, sputum cytology, skin tests, serologic studies, and cultures are unrewarding in evaluating asymptomatic patients. Bronchoscopy has a 60% diagnostic yield in cancer. Transthoracic needle aspiration with computed tomographic (CT) or fluoroscopic guidance has an 85% diagnostic yield in cancer but a 20% risk of pneumothorax. CT detects 30% more nodules than CXR and is helpful in assessing the location of a solitary pulmonary nodule, calcification, cavitation,

satellite lesions, margins, density, and multiple nodules (particularly in evaluating metastatic malignancy) and in the staging of lung cancer. A nodule is more likely to show contrast enhancement on CT if it is malignant. For nodules larger than 1 cm, dynamic positron emission tomography (PET) with fludeoxyglucose F 18 imaging reportedly differentiates malignant from benign pulmonary lesions more accurately than CT and may be helpful in evaluation and staging. It is important to remember that enhancement on PET scanning can be seen with malignancy as well as with inflammatory or infectious processes, so it is not diagnostic. Similarly, carcinoid tumors and bronchoalveolar cell carcinoma may not enhance on PET scanning, leading to a false-negative result. For asymptomatic patients who have a single lung nodule, extensive studies (gastrointestinal tract series, intravenous pyelography, and scans of bone, brain, liver, and bone marrow) are not indicated because of the low diagnostic yield (<3%).

- CT detects 30% more nodules than CXR.
- A nodule is more likely to show contrast enhancement on CT if it is malignant.
- Bronchoscopy has a 60% diagnostic yield in cancer.
- Transthoracic needle aspiration (CT- or fluoroscopy-guided) has an 85% diagnostic yield in cancer but a 20% risk of pneumothorax.

Decision Making

General guidelines for decision making are given in Table 23-15. If a benign cause cannot be firmly established after complete clinical, imaging, culture, and biopsy evaluations, the following clinical decisions advocate surgical resection: 1) the solitary pulmonary nodule is probably malignant because little or no other clinical information is available to indicate a benign diagnosis or 2) the nodule may be benign but must be resected now because the benign nature cannot be established. If the clinical information firmly indicates a benign cause, follow-up CXR is recommended. If the nodule is followed clinically, serial CXR or CT (or both) should be performed for at least 2 years to ensure no change. If the patient is a poor surgical risk, repeat CXR or CT (or both) every 3 to 6 months (enlargement of the lesion may alter the decision).

- If the nodule is followed clinically, serial CXR or CT (or both) should be performed for at least 2 years to ensure no change.
- If the patient is a poor surgical risk, repeat CXR or CT (or both) every 3-6 months (enlargement of the lesion may alter the decision).

Primary Lung Cancer

Lung cancer is the most common malignant disease and the most common cause of cancer death in the United States. The estimated incidence of new lung cancer cases in 2004 was 13% (of all cancers) for both men and women. It was estimated that more than 170,000

Table 23-15 Likelihood of Benign or Malignant Single
Pulmonary Nodule According to Clinical and
Radiographic Variables

Clinical Factor or Radiographic Result	More Likely Benign	More Likely Malignant
Patient age, y	<35	≥35
Sex	Female	Male
Smoking	No	Yes
Symptoms	No	Yes
Exposure to tuberculosis, cocci, etc	Yes	No
Previous malignancy	No	Yes
Nodule size, cm	<2.0	≥2.0
Nodule age, y	≥2	<2
Doubling time, d	<30	≥30
Nodule margins	Smooth	Irregular
Calcification	Yes	No
Satellite lesions	Yes	No

new cases would be diagnosed and more than 160,000 deaths would be attributable to lung cancer. The risk factors include cigarette smoking (25% of cancers may result from passive smoking), other carcinogens, cocarcinogens, radon exposure (uranium mining), arsenic (glass workers, smelters, and pesticides), asbestos (insulation, textile, and asbestos mining), coal dust (coke oven, road work, and roofing work), chromium (leather, ceramic, and metal), vinyl chloride (plastic), chloromethyl ether (chemical), and chronic lung injury (idiopathic pulmonary fibrosis and chronic obstructive pulmonary disease [COPD]). Genetic and nutritional factors (perhaps deficiency of vitamin A) have been implicated.

The World Health Organization (WHO) classification of pathologic types of pulmonary neoplasms is given in Table 23-16 and the TNM classification for staging of non–small cell lung carcinoma, in Table 23-17.

Small cell carcinoma is staged as follows:
1. Limited: single hemithorax, mediastinum, ipsilateral supraclavicular nodes
2. Extensive: anything beyond limited stage

Overall Survival

The overall 5-year survival for all stages of lung cancer is 14%. The overall survival rate for patients with occult and in situ cancers is greater than 70%. The overall survival for other stages is as follows: stage I, 50%; stage II, less than 20%; and stage III, less than 10%. One-year survival for stage I cancer is greater than 80%. In small cell cancer, the median survival is less than 12 months; the 5-year survival for limited cancer is 15% to 20%; and for extensive disease, 1% to 5%.

- The overall 5-year survival for all lung cancers is 14%.

Cell Types

Primary lung cancer is broadly divided into non–small cell lung carcinoma (adenocarcinoma, 35%; squamous cell carcinoma, 30%; and large cell carcinoma, 1%-15%), small cell carcinoma (20%-25%), mixed (small and large cell), and others (metastatic lesions).

Clinical Features

Most patients are older than 50 years. Only 5% of patients with lung cancer are asymptomatic. The presentation is highly variable and depends on the cell type, location, rate of growth, paraneoplastic syndromes, systemic symptoms, and other factors. Cough is the most frequent symptom and is more likely in squamous cell carcinoma and small cell lung carcinoma than in other types of lung cancer. Hemoptysis occurs in 35% to 50% of patients and is more common with squamous cell, small cell, carcinoid, and endobronchial metastases than with other types of tumors. Wheezing is due to intraluminal tumor or extrinsic compression. Dyspnea depends on the extensiveness of the tumor, COPD, degree of bronchial obstruction, and other factors. Persistent chest pain may suggest rib metastasis, local extension, or pleural involvement. Superior vena cava syndrome may suggest small cell carcinoma, lymphoma, squamous cell carcinoma, or Pancoast tumor. Horner syndrome is indicative of Pancoast tumor. Fever, postobstructive pneumonitis, nonthoracic skeletal pain, central nervous system symptoms, abdominal pain or discomfort, and hepatomegaly are indicative of possible distant metastases. During the course of the disease, central nervous system metastasis is found in 15% of patients with squamous cell carcinoma, in 25% with

Table 23-16 World Health Organization Classification of
Pulmonary Neoplasms

Type	Histologic Type
I	Squamous cell carcinoma
II	Small cell carcinoma
	Oat cell carcinoma
	Intermediate cell carcinoma
	Combined oat cell carcinoma
III	Adenocarcinoma
	Acinar adenocarcinoma
	Papillary adenocarcinoma
	Bronchoalveolar carcinoma
	Solid carcinoma with mucus formation
IV	Large cell carcinoma
	Giant cell carcinoma
	Clear cell carcinoma
V	Combined cell types
VI	Carcinoid
VII	Bronchial gland tumors
	Cylindroma
	Mucoepidermoid
VIII	Papillary tumors

Table 23-17 Staging of Lung Cancer: TNM Classification

T, primary tumor

T0	No evidence of primary tumor
TX	Cancer cells in respiratory secretions; no tumor on chest radiographs or at bronchoscopy
Tis	Carcinoma in situ
T1	Tumor ≤3 cm in greatest dimension, surrounded by lung tissue; no bronchoscopic evidence of tumor proximal to lobar bronchus
T2	Tumor >3 cm in diameter, or tumor of any size that involves visceral pleura, or associated with atelectasis extending to hilum (but not involving entire lung); must be ≥2 cm from main carina
T3	Tumor involves chest wall, diaphragm, mediastinal pleura, or pericardium, or is <2 cm from main carina (but does not involve it)
T4	Tumor involves main carina or trachea, or invades mediastinum, heart, great vessels, esophagus, or vertebrae, or malignant pleural effusion

N, nodal involvement

NX	Regional lymph nodes cannot be assessed
N0	No demonstrable lymph node involvement
N1	Ipsilateral peribronchial or hilar lymph nodes involved
N2	Metastasis to ipsilateral mediastinal lymph nodes or to subcarinal lymph nodes
N3	Metastasis to contralateral mediastinal &/or hilar lymph nodes or to scalene &/or supraclavicular lymph nodes

M, metastasis

MX	Presence of distant metastasis cannot be assessed
M0	No known distant metastasis
M1	Distant metastasis present (specify site or sites)

Stage Grouping—TNM Subsets[a]

Stage	TNM	Stage	TNM
Stage 0	Carcinoma in situ	Stage IIIB	T4 N0 M0
			T4 N1 M0
Stage IA	T1 N0 M0		T4 N2 M0
Stage IB	T2 N0 M0		T1 N3 M0
			T2 N3 M0
Stage IIA	T1 N1 M0		T3 N3 M0
Stage IIB	T2 N1 M0		T4 N3 M0
	T3 N0 M0		
		Stage IV	Any T, any N, M1
Stage IIIA	T3 N1 M0		
	T1 N2 M0		
	T2 N2 M0		
	T3 N2 M0		

[a] Staging is not relevant for occult carcinoma, designated TX N0 M0.

adenocarcinoma, in 28% with large cell carcinoma, and in 30% with small cell carcinoma.

- Cough and hemoptysis are more common in squamous cell carcinoma and carcinoid.
- Chest pain may indicate pleural effusion, pleural metastasis, or rib lesion.
- Nonpulmonary symptoms may indicate distant metastases or paraneoplastic syndromes.
- Central nervous system metastasis is more common with small cell carcinoma.

Squamous Cell Carcinoma

Two-thirds of squamous cell carcinomas arise in the proximal tracheobronchial tree (first 4 subdivisions). They also may arise in the upper airway and esophagus. Symptoms appear early in the course of the disease because of proximal bronchial involvement and consist of cough, hemoptysis, and lobar or segmental (or both) collapse with postobstructive pneumonia. CXR findings include atelectasis (23% of patients), obstructive pneumonitis (13%), hilar adenopathy (38%), and cavitation (35%). One-third of patients present with peripheral masses. Bronchoscopy is indicated in almost all patients. One-third of squamous cell carcinomas have thick-walled irregular cavities. Treatment is resection in combination with either irradiation or chemotherapy (or both). Laser bronchoscopy and endobronchial brachytherapy are palliative measures.

- Squamous cell carcinoma: proximal airway disease in 66% of cases, peripheral mass in 33%, and cavitation in 35%.
- Bronchoscopy is an important test.

Adenocarcinoma

Most adenocarcinomas arise in the periphery and, thus, remain asymptomatic and undetected until they have spread locally or distally. This means that the chance of dissemination to extrapulmonary sites is higher for these tumors. However, incidentally detected peripheral carcinomas tend to be in an early stage. Adenocarcinoma is the most common type of peripheral primary lung cancer. Sputum cytology has a low diagnostic yield. The most common presentation is as a solitary peripheral nodule. A small number cavitate. Clubbing and hypertrophic pulmonary osteoarthropathy are more common than in other kinds of primary lung cancer. The response to radiotherapy and chemotherapy is generally poor.

- Adenocarcinoma: a solitary pulmonary nodule in the periphery of the lung.
- The symptomatic stage usually denotes advanced disease.
- Sputum cytology has a low diagnostic yield.
- Clubbing and hypertrophic pulmonary osteoarthropathy are more common than in squamous cell carcinoma.

Bronchoalveolar Cell Carcinoma

Bronchoalveolar cell carcinoma is thought to arise from alveolar type II pneumocytes or Clara cells (or both) and is unrelated to tobacco smoking. The tumor presents in 2 forms: as a localized solitary nodular lesion and as a diffuse alveolar process. More than 60% of patients are asymptomatic. The cancer presents as a solitary nodule in the majority of patients and as lobar pneumonitis or a diffuse infiltrate in a minority. The solitary form carries the best prognosis of all types of lung cancer, with a 1-year survival rate greater than 80% after resection. Patients with the diffuse form have a mean survival of less than 6 months. Bronchorrhea (>100 mL of a thin, serous mucous secretion in 24 hours) is seen in 20% of patients (usually with the diffuse form). CXR shows a solitary nodule, localized infiltrate with vacuoles (on tomography), or pneumonic lesions. Both forms of bronchoalveolar cell carcinoma can mimic ordinary pneumonia. Because of the slow growth, the chronic course of the disease may suggest a benign process; thus, close surveillance is imperative. The treatment of a solitary lesion is resection. The response to radiotherapy and chemotherapy is poor, although bronchorrhea seems to respond to radiotherapy in some patients.

- Bronchoalveolar cell carcinoma: unrelated to tobacco smoking.
- The solitary form grows slowly and may mimic a benign lung nodule.
- Patients with the solitary (localized) form have a 1-year survival rate >80% after resection.
- Patients with the diffuse form have a mean survival of <6 months.

- Bronchorrhea occurs in 20% of patients (usually with the diffuse form).

Large Cell Carcinoma

Large cells are seen on histologic examination, and CXR shows large masses. Large cell carcinoma grows more rapidly than adenocarcinoma. Cavitation occurs in 20% to 25% of patients. Clubbing and hypertrophic pulmonary osteoarthropathy are more common than in other tumors except for adenocarcinoma. The treatment is surgical. The response to irradiation and chemotherapy is poor.

- Large cell carcinoma: a large, rapidly growing lung mass, with cavitation in 25% of patients; clubbing and hypertrophic pulmonary osteoarthropathy are common.

Small Cell Carcinoma

Small cell carcinoma (oat cell carcinoma) accounts for 25% of all bronchogenic carcinomas. Smokers and uranium miners are at high risk. It is associated with many paraneoplastic syndromes, including the syndrome of inappropriate antidiuretic hormone (SIADH), corticotropin (ACTH) production, and myasthenic syndrome (Eaton-Lambert syndrome). The tumor originates from neuroendocrine cells, invades the tracheobronchial tree, and spreads submucosally. Later, it breaks through the mucosa and produces changes similar to those seen in squamous cell carcinoma. CXR shows a unilateral, rapidly enlarging hilar or perihilar mass or widening of the mediastinum. Less than 20% of these tumors are peripheral. Bronchoscopy may show heaped-up or thickened mucosa. This tumor responds better to radiotherapy and chemotherapy than do other lung tumors. Brain metastasis is common. Prophylactic brain irradiation is standard at many medical centers; this decreases the frequency of brain metastasis but does not prolong survival. Peripheral nodules that are found after resection to be small cell carcinoma should be treated as any small cell carcinoma.

- Small cell carcinoma: smokers and uranium miners are at high risk; it is associated with many paraneoplastic syndromes, including SIADH, ACTH production, and myasthenic syndrome (Eaton-Lambert syndrome).
- Surgical treatment is not a standard therapeutic option; radiotherapy and chemotherapy are.

Carcinoid

Carcinoid arises from the same cells as small cell carcinoma, but its clinical behavior is different. Typically, carcinoid presents with cough, with or without hemoptysis, in young adults. CXR may show a solitary nodule or segmental atelectasis. Paraneoplastic syndromes in pulmonary carcinoid are rare (occurring in <1% of patients with bronchial carcinoid) but can develop from hormonal secretion (ACTH and parathyroid hormone [PTH]). Treatment is surgical resection of the tumor without lung resection. The diagnosis of malignant carcinoid is based on the extent of spread noted at resection or on clinical behavior.

- Typical clinical scenario for carcinoid: A young adult presents with cough and hemoptysis; symptoms may be related to the

production of ACTH (Cushing syndrome and hypertension) and PTH (hypercalcemia).
* Carcinoid "syndrome" is rare, occurring in <1% of patients with bronchial carcinoid.

Bronchial Gland Tumors
Cylindroma (adenoid cystic carcinoma) and mucoepidermoid tumors usually are located centrally and cause cough, hemoptysis, and obstructive pneumonia. Distant metastasis is unusual. Cylindromas arising in salivary glands can metastasize to the lungs after many years. Surgical treatment is used for lesions causing major airway obstruction. The response to radiotherapy and chemotherapy is poor.

* Cylindromas arising in salivary glands can metastasize to the lungs after many years.

Mesenchymal Tumors
This group of tumors includes lymphoma, lymphosarcoma, carcinosarcoma, fibrosarcoma, mesothelioma, and soft tissue sarcomas. Many of these present as large peripheral masses, homogeneous densities, and cavitated lesions.

Lymphoma
Patients with Hodgkin or non-Hodgkin lymphoma may have pulmonary involvement. CXR findings include bilateral hilar adenopathy, chylous pleural effusion, segmental atelectasis from endobronchial lesions, a diffuse nodular process, fluffy infiltrates, and diffuse interstitial or alveolar infiltrates (or both). Almost all cases of lymphocytic interstitial pneumonitis represent low-grade lymphomas that originate from the mucosa-associated lymphoid tissue (MALToma). They are very responsive to chemotherapy.

* Intrathoracic involvement is common in Hodgkin lymphoma.
* Bilateral hilar lymphadenopathy and chylous pleural effusion may occur.
* Hodgkin lymphoma can produce any type of CXR abnormality.

Diagnostic Tests
Sputum cytology findings are positive in up to 60% of patients with squamous cell carcinoma, in 21% with small cell carcinoma, in 16% with adenocarcinoma, and in 13% with large cell carcinoma. More tumors are diagnosed with CXR than with sputum cytology, but CXR is not recommended as a surveillance tool for all patients. Lung cancer screening using chest CT scanning continues to be studied but is currently not endorsed by the American Cancer Society. Bronchoscopy is helpful in diagnosing the cell type, in assessing staging and resectability, in using laser treatment for large airway tumors, and in brachytherapy. Transthoracic needle aspiration has an 85% to 90% yield, but the incidence of pneumothorax is 25%. CT is helpful in assessing the number of nodules in patients with pulmonary metastasis and in examining the hila and mediastinum. Positive results on pleural fluid cytology establish stage IIIB disease. Mediastinoscopy and mediastinotomy (Chamberlain procedure) are staging procedures that are often used before thoracotomy is performed.

* More lung tumors are diagnosed with CXR than with sputum cytology.
* Sputum cytology findings are positive in up to 60% of patients with squamous cell cancer.
* Routine surveillance of all susceptible persons (heavy smokers) with CXR and sputum cytology or with chest CT is not recommended.

Paraneoplastic Syndromes
As a group, primary lung tumors are the most common cause of paraneoplastic syndromes. The presence of a paraneoplastic syndrome does not indicate metastatic spread of lung cancer. It is more helpful to consider paraneoplastic manifestations based on each organ system (see below).

* Primary lung tumors cause most of the paraneoplastic manifestations.
* A paraneoplastic syndrome does not indicate metastatic spread of lung cancer.

Endocrine
Small cell carcinoma is associated with SIADH and ACTH production. Hypokalemia, muscle weakness, and CXR abnormality should suggest ACTH production. These patients do not survive long enough for the typical Cushing syndrome to develop. The ACTH levels are high and not suppressed by dexamethasone. ACTH is also produced by bronchial carcinoid. Hypercalcemia is not associated with small cell carcinoma. The overall frequency of hypercalcemia is 13%, with squamous cell cancer as the cause in 25% of patients, large cell carcinoma in 13%, and adenocarcinoma in 3%. Bony metastasis may also cause hypercalcemia. Hyperpigmentation from melanocyte-stimulating hormone occurs in small cell carcinoma. Calcitonin is secreted in 70% of patients with small cell carcinoma and in adenocarcinoma. SIADH is also seen in some patients with alveolar cell carcinoma and adenocarcinoma. Hypoglycemia with insulin-like polypeptide is found in patients with squamous cell carcinoma and mesothelioma. The human chorionic gonadotropin, luteinizing hormone, and follicle-stimulating hormone secreted by adenocarcinoma and large cell carcinoma may be responsible for gynecomastia.

* Abnormal CXR, hypokalemia, and muscle weakness: small cell carcinoma (ACTH).
* ACTH is also produced by bronchial carcinoid.
* Hypercalcemia: squamous cell carcinoma and carcinoid.

Nervous System
The mechanisms for encephalopathy, myelopathy, sensorimotor neuropathies, and polymyositis are unknown but may include toxic, nutritional, autoimmune, and infectious causes. Cerebellar ataxia is similar to alcohol-induced ataxia and is more common with squamous cell carcinoma. Myasthenic syndrome (Eaton-Lambert syndrome) is closely associated with small cell carcinoma; the proximal muscles are initially weak, but strength returns to normal with repeated stimulation on electromyography. This differentiates Eaton-Lambert syndrome from myasthenia gravis. Focal neurologic signs should

suggest central nervous system metastasis. Acute and rapidly progressive lower extremity signs should indicate spinal cord compression by tumor. Antineuronal nuclear antibody (ANNA)-1 is positive in many patients with small cell carcinoma.

- Myasthenic syndrome may precede the clinical detection of small cell carcinoma.
- Cerebellar ataxia (similar to alcohol-induced ataxia) is more common in squamous cell carcinoma.

Skeletal

Hypertrophic pulmonary osteoarthropathy (HPO) indicates periosteal bone formation and is associated with clubbing and symmetrical arthralgias. Other features include fever, gynecomastia, and an increased erythrocyte sedimentation rate (ESR). The proposed mechanisms include neural (vagal afferents), hormonal, and others. HPO is more common in adenocarcinoma and large cell carcinoma than in squamous cell and small cell lung carcinoma, and it may precede detection of the tumor by months. Clubbing may be the only feature. Removal of the tumor relieves the HPO, but ipsilateral vagotomy may be indicated if the HPO persists after resection of the tumor. Octreotide appears to be effective in treating HPO.

- HPO is more common in adenocarcinoma and large cell carcinoma.
- Tumor resection relieves HPO.
- Treatment: octreotide (somatostatin analogue) or ipsilateral vagotomy if the HPO persists after resection of the tumor.

Others

Other paraneoplastic manifestations include malignant cachexia, marantic endocarditis, increased incidence of thrombophlebitis, fever, erythrocytosis, leukocytosis, lymphocytopenia, eosinophilia, thrombocytosis, leukemoid reaction, disseminated intravascular coagulation, dysproteinemia, fever, acanthosis nigricans (adenocarcinoma), epidermolysis bullosa (squamous cell carcinoma), and nephrotic syndrome.

Pulmonary Metastases

Nearly 30% of all cases of malignant disease from extrapulmonary sites metastasize to the lung. More than 75% present with multiple lesions, and the rest may present as a solitary pulmonary nodule, a diffuse process, lymphangitic spread (breast, stomach, thyroid, pancreas, and the lung itself), or endobronchial metastases (kidney, colon, Hodgkin lymphoma, and breast). Solitary metastases are more common with carcinoma of the colon, kidneys, testes, and breast and with sarcoma and melanoma. The estimated occurrence of pulmonary metastasis by primary tumor is as follows: choriocarcinoma, 80%; osteosarcoma, 75%; kidney, 70%; thyroid, 65%; melanoma, 60%; breast, 55%; prostate, 45%; nasopharyngeal, 20%; gastrointestinal tract, 20%; and gynecologic malignancies, 20%.

Vascular Diseases

Pulmonary Embolism

Pulmonary embolism (PE) is the cause of death of 5% to 15% of patients who die in hospitals in the United States. In a multicenter study of PE, the mortality rate at 3 months was 15% and important prognostic factors included age older than 70 years, cancer, congestive heart failure, COPD, systolic arterial hypotension, tachypnea, and right ventricular hypokinesis. PE is detected in 25% to 30% of routine autopsies. Antemortem diagnosis is made in less than 30% of cases. Among hospitalized patients, the prevalence of PE is 1%. The risk of death from untreated PE is 8%. In about 90% of patients who die of PE, death occurs within 1 to 2 hours. The risk of fatal PE is greater among patients with severe deep venous thrombosis (DVT).

- PE is a common problem; consider PE in all patients who have lung problems.
- Antemortem diagnosis is made in <30% of cases.
- The risk of death from untreated PE is 8%.

Etiology

The factor responsible for most PEs is DVT of the lower extremities. Among patients with fatal PE, DVT has been identified clinically in only 40%. In those with a large angiographically diagnosed PE, DVT is detected in about 35%. About 60% of patients with PE have asymptomatic lower extremity DVT. Approximately 45% of femoral and iliac DVTs embolize to the lungs. Other sources of emboli include thrombi in the upper extremities, right ventricle, and indwelling catheters. In up to 20% of patients, DVTs from the calves propagate to the thigh and iliac veins, and up to 10% of cases of superficial thrombophlebitis are complicated by DVT. The risk of recurrent DVT is similar among carriers of factor V Leiden and patients without this mutation. The primary and secondary coagulation abnormalities that predispose to the development of DVT and PE are listed in Table 23-18.

- DVT is detected in only 40% of cases of PE.
- Consider factor V Leiden mutation and deficiencies of antithrombin III, protein S, and protein C and the presence of lupus anticoagulant among predisposing factors for DVT and PE.

The incidence of DVT in various clinical circumstances is listed in Table 23-19. Idiopathic DVT, particularly when recurrent, may indicate the presence of neoplasm in 10% to 20% of patients. The presence of varicose veins does not increase the risk of DVT.

- In idiopathic, recurrent DVT, look for an occult neoplasm.
- Risk of DVT: thoracic surgery, 25%-60%; hip surgery, 50%-75%; myocardial infarction, 20%-40%; congestive heart failure, 70%; and stroke with paralysis, 50%-70%.

DVT is diagnosed in only 50% of clinical cases. A diagnosis based on physical examination findings is unreliable. The Homan sign (pain and tenderness on dorsiflexion of the ankle) is elicited in less than 40% of cases of DVT, and a false-positive Homan sign occurs in 30% of high-risk patients. Impedance plethysmography (IPG) and duplex ultrasonography together are the most commonly used noninvasive tests and have a diagnostic accuracy of 90% to 95% in detecting iliac and femoral DVTs. They are clinically unreliable in the diagnosis of calf vein thrombosis. Serial (daily) IPG or duplex

Table 23-18 Coagulation Disorders Predisposing to the Development of Deep Venous Thrombosis and Pulmonary Embolism

Primary hypercoagulable states	Secondary hypercoagulable states
Activated protein C resistance[a] (factor V Leiden carriers)	Cancer
Antithrombin III deficiency[b]	Postoperative states (stasis)
Protein C deficiency[b]	Lupus anticoagulant syndrome
Protein S deficiency[b]	Increased factor VII & fibrinogen
Fibrinolytic abnormalities	Pregnancy
Hypoplasminogenemia	Nephrotic syndrome
Dysplasminogenemia	Myeloproliferative disorders
TPA release deficiency	Disseminated intravascular coagulation
Increased TPA inhibitor	Acute stroke
Dysfibrinogenemia	Hyperlipidemias
Homocystinuria	Diabetes mellitus
Heparin cofactor deficiency	Paroxysmal nocturnal hemoglobinuria
Increased histidine-rich glycoprotein	Behçet disease & vasculitides
	Anticancer drugs (chemotherapy)
	Heparin-induced thrombocytopenia
	Oral contraceptives
	Obesity

Abbreviation: TPA, tissue plasminogen activator.
[a] Prevalence of factor V Leiden in patients with deep venous thrombosis is 16%; presence of factor V Leiden is associated with a 40% risk of recurrent deep venous thrombosis (N Engl J Med. 1997;336:399-403).
[b] Prevalence of these protein deficiencies in patients with deep venous thrombosis is 5% to 10%.
From Prakash UBS. Pulmonary embolism. In Murphy JG, editor. Mayo Clinic Cardiology Review. 2nd ed. Philadelphia: Lippincott Williams & Wilkins; 2000. p. 379-406. Used with permission of Mayo Foundation for Medical Education and Research.

ultrasonography (or both) is recommended for high-risk patients because of a 15% detection rate of DVT after an initial negative study. Currently, IPG is performed less often than ultrasonography. Duplex ultrasonography is less accurate for the diagnosis of chronic DVT and less useful in pelvic DVT than in the diagnosis of acute femoral DVT. Venography is considered nearly 100% sensitive and specific. Venography should be performed when other tests are nondiagnostic or cannot be performed. Magnetic resonance imaging (MRI) has a high sensitivity and specificity for the diagnosis of pelvic DVT.

* DVT is diagnosed in only 50% of clinical cases.
* IPG plus duplex ultrasonography is up to 95% accurate for detecting iliac and femoral DVTs.

Clinical Features

PE has no pathognomonic clinical symptoms and signs. Tachypnea and tachycardia are observed in nearly all patients. Other symptoms include dyspnea in 80% of patients, pleuritic pain in up to 75%, hemoptysis in less than 25%, pleural friction rub in 20%, and wheezing in 15%. The differential diagnosis of PE includes myocardial infarction, pneumonia, congestive heart failure, pericarditis, esophageal spasm, asthma, exacerbation of COPD, intrathoracic malignancy, rib fracture, pneumothorax, pleurisy from any cause, pleurodynia, and nonspecific skeletal pains. Acute cor pulmonale occurs if more than 65% of the pulmonary circulation is obstructed

by emboli. PE should be suspected in the setting of syncope or acute hypotension.

* PE has no pathognomonic signs or symptoms.
* Acute cor pulmonale occurs when >65% of the pulmonary circulation is obstructed by PE.

Diagnostic Tests

Clinical examination, electrocardiography, CXR, blood gas abnormalities, and increased plasma D-dimer level have low specificity and sensitivity for the diagnosis of PE. Clinical suspicion is the most important factor in steering a clinician toward the appropriate tests to diagnose PE. CXR may show diaphragmatic elevation in 60% of patients, infiltrates in 30%, focal oligemia in 10% to 50%, effusion in 20%, an enlarged pulmonary artery in 20%, and normal findings in 30%. Nonspecific electrocardiographic changes are noted in 80%, ST and T changes in 65%, T inversion in 40%, S_1Q_3 pattern in 15%, right bundle branch block in 12%, and left axis deviation in 12%. In patients in critical condition, echocardiography should be performed early to assess right ventricular hypokinesia or dysfunction.

* Normal CXR in 30% of patients with PE.
* The classic S_1Q_3 pattern is seen in only 15% of patients.

Both the partial pressure of arterial oxygen (PaO_2) and the alveolar-arterial difference in partial pressure of oxygen, $P(A-a)O_2$ gradient,

Table 23-19 Incidence of Deep Venous Thrombosis (DVT) in
Various Clinical Circumstances

Clinical Circumstance	Incidence of DVT, %
Major abdominal surgery[a]	14-33
Thoracic surgery	25-60
Gynecologic surgery	
Patient age ≤40 y	<3
Patient age >40 y	10-40
Patient age >40 y + other risks	40-70
Urologic surgery	10-40
Hip surgery	50-75
Myocardial infarction	20-40
Congestive heart failure	70
Stroke with paralysis	50-70
Postpartum	3
Trauma	20-40

[a] Odds are 1:20 without prophylaxis and 1:50 with prophylaxis.

may be normal in 15% to 20% of patients. The $P(A-a)O_2$ gradient shows a linear correlation with the severity of PE. A normal $P(A-a)O_2$ gradient does not exclude PE. Indeed, in the Prospective Investigation of Pulmonary Embolism Diagnosis (PIOPED) study, about 20% of patients with angiographically documented PE had a normal $P(A-a)O_2$ gradient (≤20 mm Hg). Most patients with acute PE demonstrate hypocapnia.

* The $P(A-a)O_2$ gradient correlates linearly with the severity of PE.
* Of patients with PE, 20% have a normal $P(A-a)O_2$ gradient (≤20 mm Hg).

The plasma levels of D dimer (a specific fibrin degradation product) are increased in DVT and in PE. However, high levels themselves have no positive predictive value for PE. A normal level of D dimer does not exclude PE but makes it unlikely in patients with a low pretest probability of PE. Age and pregnancy are associated with increased levels. Levels less than 300 mcg/L (by enzyme-linked immunosorbent assay [ELISA]) or less than 500 mcg/L (by latex agglutination) are considered to reliably exclude PE in patients with an abnormal but not high-probability ventilation-perfusion ($\dot{V}/\dot{Q}$) lung scan. A plasma concentration of D dimer of less than 500 mcg/L allows the exclusion of PE in less than 30% of patients with suspected PE. Currently, the D-dimer test cannot be recommended as a standard part of the PE or DVT diagnostic algorithm.

* Increased D-dimer levels have no positive predictive value for PE.
* Normal D-dimer levels (<500 mcg/L) exclude PE in <30% of cases.

Echocardiography can identify thrombi in the right side of the heart in up to 15% of patients with PE. Dysfunction of the right ventricle, frequently seen in massive as well as recurrent PE, can be detected with echocardiography. Although the echocardiographic findings are

abnormal in more than 80% of patients with documented PE, the findings are nonspecific. The presence of associated abnormalities (intracardiac tumors or myxoma) poses a difficulty in distinguishing among the lesions. A highly mobile intracavitary thrombus-in-transit has a 98% risk of acute PE and a 1-week mortality of 50%. Transesophageal echocardiography is reportedly 97% sensitive and 86% specific for the diagnosis of centrally located pulmonary arterial thrombi. Currently, the role of echocardiography in the diagnosis of acute PE is undefined.

The $\dot{V}/\dot{Q}$ scan is commonly used in the diagnosis of PE. A "high-probability" lung scan has a sensitivity of 41% and a specificity of 97%. A "low-probability" lung scan excludes the diagnosis of PE in more than 85% of patients. A normal lung scan excludes PE in 100% of cases. An "intermediate-probability" or "indeterminate-probability" scan is associated with PE in 21% to 30% of patients. Therefore, patients with an intermediate-probability lung scan usually require pulmonary angiography. A negative or normal perfusion-only scan (excluding ventilation scan) rules out PE with a very high probability.

* High-probability scan: 90% probability of PE.
* Intermediate-probability scan: 30% probability of PE.
* Low-probability scan: 15% probability of PE.
* Normal scan excludes PE in 100% of cases.

CT permits ultrafast scanning of pulmonary arteries during contrast injection. In some institutions, spiral (helical) CT with intravenous contrast (CT angiography) is being used more frequently than $\dot{V}/\dot{Q}$ scans to detect PE. Sensitivity and specificity rates greater than 95% have been reported. Spiral CT has the greatest sensitivity in the diagnosis of PE in the main, lobar, or segmental arteries. Lymph node enlargement may result in false-positive studies. MRI may have the advantage of detecting both DVT and PE.

* Spiral CT has the greatest sensitivity in the diagnosis of PE in the main, lobar, or segmental arteries.

Pulmonary angiography is the best diagnostic test. It should be performed within 24 to 48 hours after the diagnosis has been considered. However, it is nondiagnostic in 3% of cases. Major and minor complications following pulmonary angiography occur in 1% and 2% of patients, respectively, and mortality from the procedure is 0.5%. Pulmonary angiography followed by therapy with tissue plasminogen activator (tPA) is associated with a 14% risk of major hemorrhage.

* Major and minor complications from pulmonary angiography are 1% and 2%, respectively.

Treatment
The therapy for uncomplicated DVT is identical to that for PE. For acute disease, treatment can begin simultaneously with both heparin (low-molecular-weight heparin [LMWH] or unfractionated heparin [UFH]) and warfarin unless warfarin is contraindicated. When treatment with both drugs is begun simultaneously, an overlap for 4 to 5 days is recommended. For patients with acute disease, UFH (80

IU/kg) is administered as a bolus, followed by a maintenance dose of 18 IU/kg per hour intravenously. The dose should be adjusted to maintain an activated partial thromboplastin time (aPTT) of 1.5 to 2 times the control value. With LMWH regimens, indications for outpatient therapy include stable proximal DVT or PE, normal vital signs, low risk of bleeding, and availability of appropriate monitoring.

* In acute DVT or PE, heparin (LMWH or UFH) and warfarin treatment can begin simultaneously.
* UFH dose: bolus, 80 IU/kg; maintenance, 18 IU/kg per hour.
* aPTT in uncomplicated cases: 1.5-2 times normal.

Long-term anticoagulant therapy can be maintained with either heparin or warfarin. LMWH has been prescribed for patients who have difficulty monitoring the aPTT. Warfarin at a dose to achieve an international normalized ratio (INR) of 2.0 to 3.0 is recommended. The loading dose of warfarin is usually 10 mg daily for 1 or 2 days, followed by adjustment of the dose to maintain an INR of 2.0 to 3.0. Recurrent and complicated cases (eg, coagulopathies) may require lifelong anticoagulation, maintenance of higher aPTT or prothrombin time (PT), and other measures such as the inferior vena cava filter. The recommended duration of treatment of venous thromboembolic disease is given in Table 23-20.

* PT in uncomplicated cases: INR of 2.0-3.0.
* Duration of treatment for first episode of idiopathic DVT or PE: 3-6 months.

Thrombolytic agents are administered in cases of massive PE and massive iliofemoral thrombosis. The indications are debated, although these drugs generally are indicated for patients with massive DVT or PE (or both). The 1-year mortality among those treated with heparin alone is 19% and among those treated with thrombolytic agents, 9%. The rate of recurrent PE in heparin-alone therapy is 11% and in thrombolytic therapy, 5.5%. Ideally, thrombolytic agents should be administered within 24 hours after PE. The doses for different agents are as follows: streptokinase, loading dose of 250,000 international units infused over 30 minutes, followed by a maintenance dose of 100,000 international units per hour for up to 24 hours; urokinase, loading dose of 4,400 IU/kg infused over 10 minutes, followed by continuous infusion of 4,400 IU/kg per hour for 12 hours; and TPA, a total dose of 100 mg given intravenously over a 2-hour period. The adequacy of thrombolytic therapy is monitored with the thrombin time. Heparin infusion is begun or resumed if the aPTT is less than 80 seconds after thrombolytic therapy.

* Thrombolytic agents should be administered within 24 hours after PE.
* Heparin therapy is necessary after thrombolytic therapy.

Among patients receiving chronic warfarin therapy, the cumulative incidence of fatal bleeding is 1% at 1 year and 2% at 3 years. A greater risk of major hemorrhage exists when anticoagulation is continued indefinitely. The presence of malignant disease at the initiation of warfarin therapy is significantly associated with major hemorrhage.

Patients with PE treated with thrombolytic drugs have about a 1% risk of intracranial bleeding.

* Thrombolytic therapy: 1% risk of intracranial bleeding.

Drugs that prolong the effect of warfarin include, among others, salicylates, heparin, estrogen, antibiotics, clofibrate, quinidine, and cimetidine. Drugs that decrease the effect of warfarin include glutethimide, rifampin, barbiturates, and etchlorvynol. This is only a partial list of drugs that interfere with warfarin metabolism. Therefore, the physician recommending warfarin therapy should ascertain the drug-drug interaction or consult a pharmacist.

* Knowledge of the interaction of warfarin with other drugs is important.

Inferior Vena Cava Interruption

Inferior vena cava interruption is aimed at preventing PE while maintaining blood flow through the inferior vena cava. It is indicated if anticoagulant therapy is contraindicated, complications result from anticoagulant therapy, anticoagulant therapy fails, a predisposition to bleeding is present, chronic recurrent PE and secondary pulmonary hypertension occur, or surgical pulmonary thromboendarterectomy has been performed or is intended to be performed. Inferior vena cava plication does not replace anticoagulant therapy; many patients require both. After the filter has been inserted, anticoagulant therapy is aimed at preventing DVT at the insertion site, inferior vena cava thrombosis, cephalad propagation of a clot from an occluded filter, and propagation or recurrence of lower extremity DVT. PE occurs in 2.5% of patients despite inferior vena cava interruption.

* Inferior vena cava plication does not replace chronic anticoagulant therapy.
* PE occurs in 2.5% of patients despite inferior vena cava interruption.

Table 23-20 Recommended Duration of Treatment of Venous Thromboembolic Disease

Patient Characteristic	Duration of Treatment, mo
First event, with a reversible or time-limited risk factor[a]	≥3
First episode of idiopathic DVT or PE	3-6
Recurrent idiopathic DVT or PE or a continuing risk factor[b]	≥12

Abbreviations: DVT, deep venous thrombosis; PE, pulmonary embolism.
[a] Surgery, trauma, immobilization, or estrogen use.
[b] Cancer, antithrombin deficiency, anticardiolipin antibody syndrome.
Modified from Hyers TM, Agnelli G, Hull RD, Morris TA, Samama M, Tapson V, et al. Antithrombotic therapy for venous thromboembolic disease. Chest. 2001;119:176S-93S. Used with permission.

Prophylaxis

Prophylaxis against DVT and PE includes early ambulation after surgery or immobilization, intermittent pneumatic compression of the lower extremities, active and passive leg exercises, and a low dose of heparin given subcutaneously. A low dose of heparin decreases the incidence of DVT from 25% to 8%. Prophylactic enoxaparin, 40 mg daily subcutaneously, safely reduces the risk of DVT in patients with acute medical illnesses. LMWH has been approved in the United States for prophylaxis against DVT and PE after total hip arthroplasty and total knee arthroplasty. A postoperative, fixed-dose LMWH (enoxaparin, 30 mg subcutaneously every 12 hours) is more effective than adjusted-dose warfarin (INR, 2.0-3.0) in preventing DVT after total hip or knee arthroplasty. LMWH has a rapid onset of action, is safe, and is approximately 50% more effective than standard heparin. Also, heparin-induced thrombocytopenia is reduced with LMWH. Because of a more predictable dose response to LMWH, it is not necessary to monitor the aPTT.

* LMWH has been approved in the United States for DVT and PE prophylaxis after total hip arthroplasty.
* LMWH therapy does not require measuring aPTT.
* Heparin-induced thrombocytopenia is reduced with LMWH.

Complications of PE

Pulmonary infarction occurs in less than 10% of patients with PE. Pulmonary infarction and hemorrhage occur more frequently in patients with disseminated intravascular coagulation. Complications of pulmonary infarction include secondary infection, cavitation, pneumothorax, and hemothorax. Recurrent PE (in 8% of patients) is a common cause of secondary pulmonary hypertension (in 0.5% of patients). Mechanical obstruction of one-half to two-thirds of the pulmonary vascular bed by emboli is necessary for this complication to develop.

* Pulmonary infarction occurs in <10% of patients.
* Recurrent PE occurs in 8%.
* Secondary pulmonary hypertension occurs in 0.5%.

Pulmonary Vasculitides

The vasculitides are a heterogeneous group of disorders of unknown cause characterized by various degrees of inflammation and necrosis of the arteries and, sometimes, veins. Immunologic factors, the absence or deficiency of certain chemical mediators in the body, and mycotic infectious processes, particularly those caused by *Aspergillus* and *Mucor*, are associated with vasculitis. The common vasculitides and their frequency in North America are as follows: giant cell (temporal) arteritis, 26.5%; polyarteritis nodosa, 14.6%; Wegener granulomatosis, 10.5%; Schönlein-Henoch purpura, 10.5%; Takayasu arteritis, 7.8%; and Churg-Strauss syndrome, 2.5%.

Wegener Granulomatosis

Wegener granulomatosis is a systemic vasculitis of arteries and veins characterized by necrotizing granulomatous vasculitis of the upper and lower respiratory tract, glomerulonephritis, and variable degrees of small-vessel vasculitis. The Wegener triad consists of necrotizing granulomas of the upper or lower respiratory tract (or both), generalized focal necrotizing vasculitis of arteries and veins in the lungs, and glomerulonephritis. Bronchiolitis obliterans with organizing pneumonia (BOOP), bronchocentric inflammation, a marked eosinophilic infiltrate, and alveolar hemorrhage are atypical features. Pulmonary capillaritis occurs in up to 40% of patients. Eosinophilic infiltrates are seen in tissue samples, but peripheral blood eosinophilia is not a feature of Wegener granulomatosis. The term *limited Wegener granulomatosis* is used to describe the disease involving the lungs only.

* Typical clinical scenario for Wegener granulomatosis: systemic disease with major respiratory manifestations and renal involvement with focal segmental glomerulonephritis.

The cause of Wegener granulomatosis is unknown. Occupational exposure has been suggested as an etiologic factor; a 7-fold risk for development of Wegener granulomatosis was observed in persons with a history of inhalation of silica-containing compounds and grain dust. Heterozygotes for the P_I*Z variant of the α_1-antitrypsin gene are reported to have a 6-fold greater risk of developing the disease than the general population. The prevalence of Wegener granulomatosis in the United States is approximately 3 per 100,000 persons. Some have noted associations between disease exacerbations during the winter months and during pregnancy.

The mean age at the onset of symptoms is 45.2 years (the male to female ratio is 2:1); 91% of the patients are white. The initial symptoms are nonspecific: fever, malaise, weight loss, arthralgias, and myalgias. The organs affected are the ear, nose, and throat (initial complaints in 90% of patients are rhinorrhea, purulent or bloody nasal discharge, sinus pain, nasal mucosal drying and crust formation, epistaxis, and otitis media); skin (40%-50% of patients); and eyes (43%) and the central nervous system (25%). Arthralgias occur in 58% of patients and frank arthritis in 28%. Patients older than 60 have a relatively low incidence of upper respiratory tract complaints but a high incidence (4.5-fold) of neurologic involvement. Two important signs of Wegener granulomatosis are nasal septal perforation and ulceration of the vomer bone. The differential diagnosis of the saddle-nose deformity includes Wegener granulomatosis, relapsing polychondritis, and leprosy.

* Major organs affected are represented by the mnemonic *ELKS* (*e*ar, nose, and throat; *l*ungs; *k*idney; and *s*kin).
* Ear, nose, and throat symptoms are the initial complaints in 90% of patients.
* Nasal septal perforation and ulceration of the vomer bone are 2 important signs.
* Differential diagnosis of saddle-nose deformity: Wegener granulomatosis, relapsing polychondritis, and leprosy.

Ulcerated lesions of the larynx and trachea occur in 30% of untreated patients, and subglottic stenosis occurs in 8% to 18% of treated patients. The pulmonary parenchyma is affected in more than 60% of patients. Symptoms include cough, hemoptysis, and dyspnea. The clinical manifestations can range from subacute to rapidly progressive respiratory failure. Most patients with pulmonary symptoms have associated nodular infiltrates on CXR. Hemoptysis is seen in 98% of patients and CXR abnormalities are seen in 65% (unilateral in 55% and bilateral in 45%), including infiltrates (63%), nodules (31%), infiltrates with cavitation (8%), and nodules with cavitation (10%). CXR shows rounded opacities (from a few millimeters to several centimeters large). The nodules are usually bilateral and one-third cavitate. Solitary nodules occur in 30% to 40% of patients. Pneumonic infiltrates, lobar consolidation, and pleural effusions are also seen. Diffuse alveolar infiltrates indicate alveolar hemorrhage. Massive pulmonary alveolar hemorrhage is occasionally a life-threatening emergency. Benign stenoses of the tracheobronchial tree (15% of patients) are more likely in chronic cases and in patients whose disease is stable. The shape of the inspiratory and expiratory flow volume loop should be assessed.

* Hemoptysis occurs in almost all patients.
* CXR: multiple nodules in 31% of patients or masses with cavitation in 10% of patients who have CXR abnormalities.
* Diffuse alveolar infiltrates indicate alveolar hemorrhage.
* Tracheobronchial stenosis occurs in 15% of patients. Assess the shape of the inspiratory and expiratory flow volume loop.

Laboratory tests demonstrate mild or moderate normochromic normocytic anemia, mild leukocytosis, mild thrombocytosis, positive rheumatoid factor, and elevations of immunoglobulins IgG and IgA and circulating immune complexes. A highly increased ESR (often >100 mm in 1 hour) is a consistent finding. Peripheral blood eosinophilia is not a feature. All these abnormalities are nonspecific. Urinalysis is an important test because hematuria, proteinuria, and red cell casts are found in 80% of patients.

* Increased ESR.
* Hematuria, proteinuria, and red cell casts occur in 80% of patients.

The antineutrophil cytoplasmic autoantibodies (ANCAs) are used to corroborate the diagnosis of Wegener granulomatosis. The 2 main patterns of ANCA are cytoplasmic (c-ANCA) and perinuclear (p-ANCA). Almost all c-ANCAs are directed to proteinase 3 (PR3), whereas myeloperoxidase (MPO) is the major target antigen of p-ANCA. Also, c-ANCA is highly specific and sensitive for Wegener granulomatosis and is present in more than 90% of patients with systemic Wegener granulomatosis. In active disease, the sensitivity and specificity are 91% and 98%, respectively, whereas in inactive disease, the values are 63% and 99.5%. The following points are important:

1. A positive c-ANCA without clinical evidence of disease does not establish the diagnosis.
2. Some patients with active disease have negative results for c-ANCA.
3. Some patients have persistently positive c-ANCA results despite inactive disease or disease in remission.
4. c-ANCA titers may increase without evidence of an increase in disease activity.
5. c-ANCA is present in other diseases, such as hepatitis C virus infection, some cases of microscopic polyangiitis,

and ulcerative colitis and as a manifestation of sulfasalazine toxicity.

* c-ANCA is generally considered specific for Wegener granulomatosis.
* Positive c-ANCA without clinical evidence of disease does not establish the diagnosis.
* c-ANCA can be positive in other diseases.

p-ANCA is positive in various diseases, including inflammatory bowel disease, autoimmune liver disease, rheumatoid arthritis, and many other vasculitides. Reportedly, p-ANCA with specificity against MPO is closely associated with microscopic polyangiitis, mononeuritis multiplex, leukocytoclastic vasculitis of the skin, pauci-immune necrotizing-crescentic glomerulonephritis, and other vasculitides affecting small vessels. Some cases of Churg-Strauss syndrome may demonstrate p-ANCA with specificity for MPO.

* p-ANCA has been noted in other vasculitides and collagen diseases.
* p-ANCA with specificity for MPO should suggest small-vessel vasculitis (microscopic polyangiitis).

The combination of corticosteroids and cyclophosphamide produces complete remission in more than 90% of patients. The usual dosage of each drug is up to 2 mg/kg daily orally. In milder cases, corticosteroids alone may be sufficient. Because of immunosuppression, the overall incidence of *Pneumocystis jiroveci* (formerly *Pneumocystis carinii*) pneumonia in these patients is approximately 6%. Respiratory infection, particularly from *Staphylococcus aureus*, is more common. The nasal carriage rate for this bacteria is higher in patients with Wegener granulomatosis. Disease relapse usually is associated with viral or bacterial infections. A combination of trimethoprim, 160 mg daily, and sulfamethoxazole, 800 mg daily, is an effective prophylactic regimen to prevent disease relapse; 82% of treated patients remain in remission for 24 months compared with 60% who do not receive prophylaxis. Stenosis of large airways may require bronchoscopic interventions, including dilation by rigid bronchoscope, YAG-laser treatment, and placement of silicone airway stents.

* Cyclophosphamide and corticosteroids are effective.
* Trimethoprim-sulfamethoxazole is effective in preventing relapse.

Giant Cell (Temporal) Arteritis

Giant cell arteritis, also known as *temporal arteritis, cranial arteritis,* and *granulomatous arteritis,* is a vasculitis of unknown cause. It usually affects middle-aged or older persons. Pulmonary complications include cough, sore throat, and hoarseness. Nearly 10% of the patients have prominent respiratory symptoms, and respiratory symptoms are the initial manifestation in 4%. Giant cell arteritis should be considered in older patients who have a new cough or throat pain without obvious cause. Pulmonary nodules, interstitial infiltrations, pulmonary artery occlusion, and aneurysms have been described. Virtually all patients have a favorable response to systemic corticosteroid therapy.

- Giant cell arteritis: nearly 10% of patients have prominent respiratory symptoms.
- Cough, sore throat, and hoarseness may be the presenting features.

Churg-Strauss Syndrome

Churg-Strauss syndrome, also called *allergic granulomatosis* and *angiitis*, is among the least common of the vasculitides. It is characterized by pulmonary and systemic vasculitis, extravascular granulomas, increased levels of IgE, and eosinophilia, which occur exclusively in patients with asthma or a history of allergy. Patients have progressive respiratory distress. Allergic rhinitis, nasal polyps, nasal mucosal crusting, and septal perforation occur in more than 70% of patients. Nasal polyposis is a major clinical finding. The chief pulmonary manifestation is refractory asthma, which is noted in almost all patients. CXR abnormalities are noted in more than 60% of patients: patchy and occasionally diffuse alveolar-interstitial infiltrates in the perihilar area, with a predilection for the upper two-thirds of the lung fields. Up to one-third of patients with Churg-Strauss vasculitis develop pleural effusions. A dramatic response can be expected with high doses of systemic corticosteroids.

- Churg-Strauss syndrome: refractory asthma, progressive respiratory distress, allergic rhinitis, nasal polyps, nasal mucosal crusting, septal perforation in >70% of patients, tissue and blood hypereosinophilia, and increased IgE.

Behçet Disease

Behçet disease is a chronic, relapsing, multisystemic inflammatory disorder characterized by aphthous stomatitis along with 2 or more of the following: aphthous orogenital ulcerations (in >65% of patients), uveitis, cutaneous nodules or pustules, synovitis, and meningoencephalitis. Superficial venous thrombosis and DVT of the upper and lower extremities and thrombosis of the inferior and superior venae cavae occur in 7% to 37% of patients. Pulmonary vascular involvement produces severe hemoptysis. Severe hemoptysis, initially responsive to therapy with corticosteroids, tends to recur; death is due to hemoptysis in 39% of patients. CXR may show lung infiltrates, pleural effusions, prominent pulmonary arteries, and pulmonary artery aneurysms. Aneurysms of the pulmonary artery communicating with the bronchial tree (bronchovascular anastomosis) should be considered in patients with Behçet disease and massive hemoptysis. Because of the high incidence of DVT of the extremities and the venae cavae, PE commonly occurs in these patients. Corticosteroids and chemotherapeutic agents have been used to treat Behçet disease. The prognosis is poor if marked hemoptysis develops.

- Behçet disease: aphthous stomatitis, uveitis, cutaneous nodules, and meningoencephalitis.
- Severe hemoptysis is the cause of death in 39% of patients.
- A fistula between the airway and vascular structures is common.
- High incidence of DVT and PE.

Takayasu Arteritis

Takayasu arteritis, also known as *pulseless disease*, *aortic arch syndrome*, and *reversed coarctation*, is a chronic inflammatory disease of unknown cause that affects primarily the aorta and its major branches, including the proximal coronary arteries and renal arteries and the elastic pulmonary arteries. The pulmonary arteries are involved in more than 50% of patients, with lesions in medium-size and large arteries. Early abnormalities occur in the upper lobes, whereas the middle and lower lobes are involved in later stages of the disease. Perfusion lung scans have shown abnormalities in more than 75% of patients; pulmonary angiography has demonstrated arterial occlusions in 86%. Corticosteroid therapy has produced symptomatic remission within days to weeks. Pulmonary involvement signifies a poor prognosis.

- Takayasu arteritis: pulmonary artery involvement in >50% of patients.

Mixed Cryoglobulinemia

Mixed cryoglobulinemia is characterized by recurrent episodes of purpura, arthralgias, weakness, and multiorgan involvement. Frequently, levels of cryoglobulin and rheumatoid factor are increased. Biopsy findings in vascular structures are similar to those in leukocytoclastic vasculitis. The most serious complication is glomerulonephritis caused by deposition of immune complexes. Pulmonary insufficiency, Sjögren syndrome-like illness with lung involvement, subclinical T-lymphocytic alveolitis, diffuse pulmonary vasculitis with alveolar hemorrhage, BOOP, and bronchiectasis have been described in isolated cases.

- Mixed cryoglobulinemia: lymphocytic alveolitis, BOOP, alveolar hemorrhage.

Polyarteritis Nodosa

Polyarteritis nodosa is characterized by a necrotizing arteritis of small and medium-size muscular arteries involving multiple organ systems. This disease seldom affects the lungs. Arteritis affecting bronchial arteries and producing diffuse alveolar damage has been reported. Lung involvement is rare also in Schönlein-Henoch purpura.

- Polyarteritis nodosa and Schönlein-Henoch purpura rarely affect the lungs.

Secondary Vasculitis

Many of the rheumatologic diseases (eg, systemic lupus erythematosus, rheumatoid arthritis, and scleroderma) demonstrate secondary vasculitic processes in the tissues involved. Certain infectious processes, particularly mycoses, may cause secondary vasculitis. For treatment of vasculitic lesions, the well-known etiologic agents such as drugs and chemicals should be considered.

- Collagen diseases are common causes of secondary vasculitis.

Alveolar Hemorrhage Syndromes

Diffuse hemorrhage into the alveolar spaces is called *alveolar hemorrhage syndrome*. Disruption of the pulmonary capillary lining may result from damage caused by different immunologic mechanisms (eg, Goodpasture syndrome, renal-pulmonary syndromes, glomerulonephritis, and systemic lupus erythematosus), direct chemical or toxic injury (eg, toxic or chemical inhalation, penicillamine, mitomycin, abciximab, all-*trans*-retinoic acid, trimellitic anhydride, and smoked crack cocaine), physical trauma (pulmonary contusion), and increased vascular pressure within the capillaries (mitral stenosis and severe left ventricular failure). The severity of hemoptysis, anemia, and respiratory distress depends on the extent and rapidity with which bleeding occurs in the alveoli. Alveolar hemorrhage is indicated, reportedly, if hemosiderin-laden macrophages constitute more than 20% of the total alveolar macrophages recovered with bronchoalveolar lavage. Pulmonary alveolar hemorrhage is strongly associated with thrombocytopenia ($\leq 50 \times 10^9$/L), other abnormal coagulation variables, renal failure (creatinine ≥ 2.5 mg/dL), and a history of heavy smoking.

* Alveolar hemorrhage syndrome is caused by different mechanisms.
* Hemoptysis is not a consistent feature.
* Increased risk with platelets $\leq 50 \times 10^9$/L, other coagulopathy, creatinine ≥ 2.5 mg/dL, and heavy smoking.
* Drugs that cause alveolar hemorrhage: penicillamine, abciximab, all-*trans*-retinoic acid, and mitomycin.

Goodpasture Syndrome

Goodpasture syndrome is a classic example of a cytotoxic (type II) disease. The Goodpasture antigen (located in type IV collagen) is the primary target for the autoantibodies. The highest concentration of Goodpasture antigen is in the glomerular basement membrane (GBM). The alveolar basement membrane is affected by cross-reactivity with the GBM. Lung biopsy specimens show diffuse alveolar hemorrhage. Immunofluorescent microscopy shows linear deposition of IgG and complement along basement membranes. Anti-GBM antibody is positive in more than 90% of patients, but it is also present in persons exposed to influenza virus, hydrocarbons, or penicillamine and in some patients with systemic lupus erythematosus, polyarteritis nodosa, or Schönlein-Henoch purpura. The cause of Goodpasture syndrome is unknown, but influenza virus, hydrocarbon exposure, penicillamine, and unknown genetic factors are known to stimulate anti-GBM antibody production. Inadvertent exposure to hydrocarbons has resulted in the exacerbation of Goodpasture syndrome. The treatment of rheumatoid arthritis and other diseases with penicillamine and carbimazole has been associated with Goodpasture syndrome, circulating anti-GBM antibodies, and focal necrotizing glomerulonephritis with crescents. Azathioprine hypersensitivity may mimic pulmonary Goodpasture syndrome.

* Goodpasture syndrome: a classic example of a cytotoxic (type II) disease.
* Anti-GBM antibody is positive in >90% of patients.
* Anti-GBM antibody is also present in persons exposed to influenza virus, hydrocarbons, or penicillamine and in some patients with collagen diseases.
* Exposure to hydrocarbons may exacerbate the disease.

Patients with anti-GBM antibody–mediated nephritis demonstrate 2 principal patterns of disease: 1) young men presenting in their 20s with Goodpasture syndrome (glomerulonephritis and lung hemorrhage) and 2) elderly patients, especially women, presenting in their 60s with glomerulonephritis alone. In the classic form (in younger

patients) of Goodpasture syndrome, men are affected more often than women (male to female ratio, 7:1) and the average age at onset is approximately 27 years. Recurrent hemoptysis, pulmonary insufficiency, renal involvement with hematuria and renal failure, and anemia are the classic features. Pulmonary hemorrhage almost always precedes renal manifestations. Active cigarette smoking increases the risk of alveolar hemorrhage. Frequent initial clinical features include hemoptysis, hematuria, proteinuria, and an increased serum level of creatinine.

* Typical clinical scenario for the classic form: A young man with glomerulonephritis and lung hemorrhage.
* Typical clinical scenario for the atypical form: An elderly patient, especially a woman, with glomerulonephritis alone.
* Pulmonary hemorrhage almost always precedes renal manifestations.
* Active cigarette smoking increases the risk of alveolar hemorrhage.

CXR demonstrates a diffuse alveolar filling process, with sparing of the costophrenic angles. One-third of the patients with anti-GBM disease (Goodpasture syndrome) test positive for p-ANCA–MPO. These patients are more prone to develop fulminant pulmonary hemorrhage than those who are p-ANCA–negative. Plasmapheresis is the treatment of choice for Goodpasture syndrome. Although complete recovery can be expected in most patients treated with systemic corticosteroids, immunosuppressive agents, or plasmapheresis, relapse occurs in up to 7% of them. A previous history of pulmonary hemorrhage markedly decreases the diffusing capacity of the lung for carbon monoxide without affecting other variables of pulmonary function.

* One-third of the patients with anti-GBM disease test positive for p-ANCA–MPO.
* Patients with positive p-ANCA–MPO are more likely to have fulminant pulmonary hemorrhage.
* Plasmapheresis is the treatment of choice.

Glomerulonephritis

Rapidly progressive glomerulonephritis, in the absence of anti-GBM antibody, is a major cause of pulmonary alveolar hemorrhage. Nearly 50% of the patients with alveolar hemorrhage syndromes caused by a renal mechanism do not have anti-GBM antibody. Alveolar hemorrhage is mediated by immune-complex disease. Several vasculitic syndromes, including Wegener granulomatosis and microscopic polyangiitis, belong to this group. ANCAs have been detected in patients with idiopathic crescentic glomerulonephritis and alveolar hemorrhage syndrome. The alveolar hemorrhage syndrome in systemic lupus erythematosus and other vasculitides is discussed elsewhere.

* Glomerulonephritis: a major cause of pulmonary alveolar hemorrhage.
* Alveolar hemorrhage is mediated by immune-complex disease.

Vasculitides

Diffuse alveolar hemorrhage is present sometimes in patients with vasculitis. Alveolar hemorrhage is rare as an initial symptom of Wegener granulomatosis and is more common in Churg-Strauss syndrome and Schönlein-Henoch purpura. Alveolar hemorrhage is more common in Behçet disease than in other vasculitides. Pulmonary capillaritis is a distinct histologic lesion characterized by extensive neutrophilic infiltration of the alveolar interstitium, and subclinical alveolar hemorrhage may occur in patients with this disease. This lesion can be seen in various vasculitides such as Wegener granulomatosis, microscopic polyarteritis, systemic lupus erythematosus, and other collagen diseases.

Microscopic Polyangiitis

Microscopic polyangiitis is distinct from classic polyarteritis nodosa, which typically affects medium-size arteries. Pulmonary capillaritis is the most common lesion in microscopic polyangiitis but does not occur in classic polyarteritis nodosa. Microscopic polyangiitis is a systemic vasculitis associated with renal involvement in 80% of patients, characterized by rapidly progressive glomerulonephritis. Other features include weight loss (70% of patients), skin involvement (60%), fever (55%), mononeuritis multiplex (58%), arthralgias (50%), myalgias (48%), and hypertension (34%). Males are affected more frequently than females; the median age at onset is 50 years. Pulmonary alveolar hemorrhage is observed in 12% to 29% of patients and is an important contributory factor to morbidity and mortality. ANCA is detected in 75% of patients with microscopic polyangiitis, and the majority are the p-ANCA–MPO type.

* Microscopic polyangiitis: progressive glomerulonephritis is a major feature.
* Pulmonary alveolar hemorrhage is observed in 12%-29% of patients.
* p-ANCA–MPO is positive in 75% of patients.

Mitral Valve Disease

Diffuse alveolar hemorrhage is a well-known feature of mitral stenosis, even though the possibility is rarely considered in clinical practice. Severe mitral insufficiency can also produce alveolar hemorrhage. Hemoptysis can be the presenting feature. It is caused by the rupture of dilated and varicose bronchial veins early in the course of mitral stenosis, or it is the result of stress failure of pulmonary capillaries. In patients not treated surgically, recurrent episodes of alveolar hemorrhage may lead to chronic hemosiderosis of the lungs, fibrosis, and punctate calcification or ossification of the lung parenchyma.

* Mitral stenosis is an important cause of alveolar hemorrhage syndrome.

Idiopathic Pulmonary Hemosiderosis

Idiopathic pulmonary hemosiderosis is a rare disorder of unknown cause. The term *idiopathic pulmonary hemorrhage* has been suggested instead of the traditional name. Idiopathic pulmonary hemosiderosis is a diagnosis of exclusion. It manifests as recurrent intra-alveolar hemorrhage, hemoptysis, transient infiltrates on CXR, and secondary iron deficiency anemia. The cause is unknown, but many factors have been implicated: heritable defect, an immunologic mechanism based on the presence of antibodies to cow's milk (Heiner syndrome),

cold agglutinins, increased serum IgA, viral infections, a primary disorder of airway epithelial cells, and a structural defect of pulmonary capillaries. Idiopathic pulmonary hemosiderosis has been described in association with idiopathic thrombocytopenic purpura, autoimmune hemolytic anemia, and nontropical sprue (celiac disease). A pediatric form of pulmonary hemosiderosis, presumed to be caused by the toxins of a spore growing in humid basements, has been described.

* Idiopathic pulmonary hemosiderosis: a diagnosis of exclusion.

Most cases begin in childhood. Although this disease is often fatal, a prolonged course is common. In children, the male to female ratio is 1:1 and in adults, 3:1. Pathologic features include hemosiderin-laden macrophages. No autoimmune phenomena are noted. Some patients have cold agglutinins. The iron content in the lung depends on the duration of the disease. Clinical features are chronic cough with intermittent hemoptysis, iron deficiency anemia, fever, weight loss, generalized lymphadenopathy (25% of patients), hepatosplenomegaly (20%), clubbing (15%), and eosinophilia (10%). The kidneys are not involved. CXR shows transient, blotchy, perihilar alveolar infiltrates in the mid and lower lung fields. Small nodules, fibrosis, and cor pulmonale may also be found. Intrathoracic lymphadenopathy occurs in up to 25% of patients. Treatment is repeated blood transfusions, iron therapy, corticosteroids, and, possibly, cytotoxic agents. A 30% mortality rate within 5 years after disease onset has been reported.

* Generalized lymphadenopathy in 25% of patients, hepatosplenomegaly in 20%, and clubbing in 15%.
* The kidneys are not involved.
* Eosinophilia in 10% of patients.

Toxic Alveolar Hemorrhage

Dust or fumes of trimellitic anhydride (a component of certain plastics, paints, and epoxy resins) cause acute rhinitis and asthma symptoms if exposure is minor. With greater exposure, alveolar hemorrhage occurs. The trimellitic anhydride–hemoptysis anemia syndrome (pulmonary hemorrhage–anemia syndrome) occurs after "high-dose exposure" to fumes. Antibodies to trimellitic anhydride, human proteins, and erythrocytes have been found in these patients. Isocyanates have caused lung hemorrhage. Other toxins known to cause alveolar hemorrhage syndromes are penicillamine and mitomycin C. Lymphangiography has been complicated by pulmonary alveolar hemorrhage. Pulmonary lymphangioleiomyomatosis is an uncommon cause of alveolar hemorrhage syndrome. Alveolar hemorrhage occurs in many patients who have pulmonary veno-occlusive disease. Anticardiolipin antibody syndrome, tumor emboli, and bone marrow transplant are other causes of alveolar hemorrhage.

* Alveolar hemorrhage occurs with penicillamine and mitomycin C.
* Trimellitic anhydride can cause pulmonary hemorrhage–anemia syndrome.
* Alveolar hemorrhage occurs with tumor emboli and after bone marrow transplant.

Pulmonary Arterial Hypertension

Pulmonary arterial hypertension (PAH) is present when the mean pulmonary arterial pressure (MPAP) is greater than 25 mm Hg at rest (or >35 mm Hg with exercise). Pathologically, PAH is characterized by vasoconstriction, pulmonary vascular remodeling, and thrombosis in situ that leads to progressive increases in pulmonary vascular resistance, right-heart failure, and death. There are many causes of pulmonary hypertension, and Table 23-21 illustrates the revised clinical classification of pulmonary hypertension.

Typically a diagnosis of PAH is made initially with the finding of increased right ventricular systolic pressure on transthoracic echocardiography and is confirmed with right-heart catheterization. Hemodynamic measurements at right-heart catheterization are important to exclude pulmonary hypertension due to fluid overload (increased pulmonary capillary wedge pressure) or contributions from a high cardiac output (such as seen in liver disease). Nonspecific symptoms include progressive dyspnea, lower extremity edema, and fatigue. Patients who exhibit vasoreactivity at right-heart catheterization (a decrease in MPAP or pulmonary vascular resistance by 20% with vasodilator challenge) may benefit from a trial of calcium channel blockers.

To date, no cure exists; however, several treatment options are available that have been shown to improve quality of life and survival. Oxygen, diuretics, digoxin, and anticoagulation may be useful in the treatment of PAH. Other treatment options approved by the Food and Drug Administration include intravenous, subcutaneous, and inhaled prostanoids (epoprostenol, treprostinil, iloprost), and oral endothelin receptor antagonists (bosentan). Phosphodiesterase type 5 inhibitors (sildenafil) are currently being studied and may be efficacious in the treatment of PAH.

- Consider the diagnosis of pulmonary hypertension in patients with a new onset of dyspnea.
- Transthoracic echocardiography can suggest the presence of PAH; however, right-heart catheterization is the diagnostic procedure of choice.
- Several treatment options for PAH may improve quality of life and survival.

Table 23-21 Revised Clinical Classification of Pulmonary Hypertension (Venice 2003)[a]

1. Pulmonary arterial hypertension (PAH)
    1.1. **Idiopathic** (IPAH)
    1.2. Familial (FPAH)
    1.3. Associated with (APAH):
        1.3.1. Collagen vascular disease
        1.3.2. Congenital systemic-to-pulmonary shunts[b]
        1.3.3. Portal hypertension
        1.3.4. Human immunodeficiency virus infection
        1.3.5. Drugs & toxins
        1.3.6. **Other** (thyroid disorders, glycogen storage disease, Gaucher disease, hereditary hemorrhagic telangiectasia, hemoglobinopathies, myeloproliferative disorders, splenectomy)
    1.4. **Associated with significant venous or capillary involvement**
        1.4.1. Pulmonary veno-occlusive disease (PVOD)
        1.4.2. Pulmonary capillary hemangiomatosis (PCH)
    1.5. Persistent pulmonary hypertension of the newborn
2. Pulmonary hypertension with left heart disease
    2.1. Left-sided atrial or ventricular heart disease
    2.2. Left-sided valvular heart disease
3. Pulmonary hypertension associated with lung disease &/or hypoxemia
    3.1. Chronic obstructive pulmonary disease
    3.2. Interstitial lung disease
    3.3. Sleep-disordered breathing
    3.4. Alveolar hypoventilation disorders
    3.5. Chronic exposure to high altitude
    3.6. Developmental abnormalities
4. Pulmonary hypertension due to chronic thrombotic &/or embolic disease
    4.1. Thromboembolic obstruction of proximal pulmonary arteries
    4.2. Thromboembolic obstruction of distal pulmonary arteries
    4.3. Nonthrombotic pulmonary embolism (tumor, parasites, foreign material)
5. **Miscellaneous**
    Sarcoidosis, histiocytosis X, lymphangiomatosis, compression of pulmonary vessels (adenopathy, tumor, fibrosing mediastinitis)

Table 23-21 (continued)

[a] Main modifications to the previous Evian clinical classification are set in **bold** in the table body. These include idiopathic pulmonary hypertension instead of primary hypertension; some newly identified possible risk factors and associated conditions have been added in the APAH subgroup (glycogen storage disease, Gaucher disease, hereditary hemorrhagic telangiectasia, hemoglobinopathies, myeloproliferative disorders, splenectomy); another subgroup has been added in the PAH category: PAH associated with significant venous or capillary involvement (PVOD and PCH); the last group, now termed "miscellaneous," includes some conditions associated with pulmonary hypertension of various and multiple etiologies (histiocytosis X, lymphangiomatosis, compression of pulmonary vessels by adenopathy, tumor, fibrosing mediastinitis).

[b] Guidelines for classification of congenital systemic-to-pulmonary shunts:

1. Type
    Simple
        Atrial septal defect (ASD)
        Ventricular septal defect (VSD)
        Patent ductus arteriosus
        Total or partial unobstructed anomalous pulmonary
            venous return
    Combined
        Describe combination and define prevalent defect if any
    Complex
        Truncus arteriosus
        Single ventricle with unobstructed pulmonary blood flow
        Atrioventricular septal defects
2. Dimensions
    Small (ASD ≤2.0 cm and VSD ≤1.0 cm)
    Large (ASD >2.0 cm and VSD >1.0 cm)
3. Associated extracardiac abnormalities
4. Correction status
    Noncorrected
    Partially corrected (age)
    Corrected: spontaneously or surgically (age)

From Simonneau G, Galiè N, Rubin LJ, Langleben D, Seeger W, Domenighetti G, et al. Clinical classification of pulmonary hypertension. J Am Coll Cardiol. 2004;43:5S-12S. Used with permission.

Part IV

Charles F. Thomas, Jr., MD
Sean M. Caples, DO

Pulmonary Infections

Viral Infections

The common cold is caused by rhinovirus, parainfluenza virus, adenovirus, respiratory syncytial virus, and coxsackievirus. The temporary interference with mucociliary clearance caused by acute viral infection may increase the risk of other infections. Viral respiratory tract infections constitute 80% of all acute infections. Nearly one-half of the general population has a viral respiratory tract infection in December through February and only 20% in June through August. Respiratory syncytial virus is an important cause of acute lower respiratory tract disease among children and the elderly. Coxsackieviruses are a more frequent cause of viral respiratory tract infections in the summer and autumn.

- Coxsackieviral infections are more frequent in the summer and autumn.
- Typical clinical scenario: Coxsackievirus B causes pleurodynia (Bornholm disease or "devil's grip")—fever, headache, malaise, and severe pleuritic pain lasting from several days to weeks.

Viral Pneumonia

Common causes of viral pneumonia are parainfluenza virus, adenovirus, and influenza viruses A and B. In adults, varicella (chickenpox) pneumonia is a severe illness, the resolution of which may be followed by nodular pulmonary calcification. In adults with chickenpox, cough (25% of patients), profuse rash, fever for more than 1 week, and age older than 34 years are the most important predictors of varicella pneumonia. Early aggressive therapy with intravenous acyclovir is recommended for patients at risk of pneumonia. Corticosteroids reportedly are of value in the treatment of previously well patients with life-threatening varicella pneumonia; however, this has not been tested in a large controlled trial since this condition is uncommon. Herpes simplex virus may cause pneumonia in an immunocompromised host or in patients with extensive burns. Cytomegalovirus (CMV) is seen more commonly in immunocompromised patients such as those with CD4 counts less than 50/mcL from acquired immunodeficiency syndrome (AIDS) (also associated with *Pneumocystis jiroveci* [formerly *Pneumocystis carinii*] infection) or transplant recipients, in hematologic malignancy, and after multiple blood transfusions and cardiopulmonary bypass. Diffuse, small nodular, or hazy infiltrates are seen on chest radiography (CXR) in 15% of patients with pneumonia caused by CMV, but interstitial pneumonia due to CMV is seen in 50% of bone marrow graft recipients. Diagnosis of CMV is made by finding inclusion bodies in affected cells, isolating the virus, or detecting CMV antigens or nucleic acids.

- Typical clinical scenario for varicella pneumonia: An adult with a characteristic chickenpox rash has cough and fever lasting more than 1 week; acyclovir is recommended for patients at risk.

- CMV infection is associated with immunocompromised patients, such as those with AIDS (CD4 count <50/mcL).
- Isolation of CMV from respiratory tract secretions does not always establish that infection is present.

Influenza

Influenza epidemics occur during winter in the United States and cause approximately 40,000 deaths per year. Worldwide pandemics can lead to increased morbidity and mortality from influenza. Although the rates of influenza infection are highest among children, the rates of serious morbidity and death are highest among adults older than 65 years and persons of any age with serious underlying medical conditions. These conditions include chronic cardiovascular disease such as rheumatic valvular disease, chronic pulmonary disease (asthma, chronic bronchitis, or emphysema), diabetes mellitus, kidney disease, chronic anemia, or immunosuppression due to medications or human immunodeficiency virus (HIV) infection. Women who are pregnant during the influenza season are at risk of infection. Influenza A and B cause human disease, but only influenza A is categorized into subtypes on the basis of the expression of the surface antigens hemagglutinin (H) and neuraminidase (N). Influenza is spread from person to person through respiratory secretions, and the average incubation period is 2 days. Adults are usually infectious until 5 days after symptom onset; however, virus shedding can be prolonged for weeks in immunocompromised patients. In the majority of adults, the symptoms of influenza (fever, myalgias and malaise, headaches, nonproductive cough, pharyngitis, and rhinitis) resolve after several days without specific treatment. In some patients, however, secondary bacterial pneumonia, primary influenza viral pneumonia, or coinfections may develop. Deaths due to influenza can result from pneumonia or from exacerbations of underlying cardiopulmonary diseases or other chronic conditions. Antiviral agents can decrease the duration of influenza A illness by several days if therapy is started within 2 days of infection. Because of increasing rates of resistance, amantadine and rimantadine are not recommended for treatment or prophylaxis unless susceptibility is confirmed. Zanamivir and oseltamivir are effective against both influenza A and influenza B. It is uncertain whether antiviral agents have a role in preventing the development of serious complications from influenza. The use of the influenza vaccine is efficacious for preventing the disease and its complications. Vaccination is recommended for adults who have any of the following risk factors for influenza:

1. Age 50 years or older
2. Chronic cardiopulmonary diseases
3. Chronic diseases such as diabetes mellitus, kidney disease, chronic anemia, or immunosuppression due to medications or human immunodeficiency virus infection
4. Resident of nursing home or long-term care facility
5. Pregnant during the influenza season
6. Health care worker

Both the inactivated influenza vaccine and the live attenuated influenza intranasal vaccine are available for use in the United States. Persons with a history of hypersensitivity to eggs or the components of the vaccines should not receive either vaccine. Persons older than 50 years, pregnant women, immunocompromised patients, persons with a history of Guillain-Barré syndrome, persons with chronic cardiopulmonary diseases, and persons with chronic diseases should not receive the live attenuated influenza vaccine.

* Typical clinical scenario for influenza A pneumonia: A 73-year-old woman with underlying valvular heart disease presents with fever, dyspnea, cyanosis, and mid-lung infiltrates.

Avian Influenza A (H5N1)
With birds serving as the original reservoir for avian influenza A, the first reported human infection was reported in 1997 in Hong Kong. Since then, the highly pathogenic avian influenza A (H5N1), posessing genetic similarities to the virus linked to the 1918 influenza pandemic, has spread westward to infect poultry and rodents in central Europe. Bird-to-human transmission is the usual route of infection, but at least 1 case of person-to-person spread has been confirmed. By mid-2007, more than 300 cases of human infection had been documented, most in southern and eastern Asia, with a mortality rate of more than 50%. Infections characteristically occur in young, previously healthy individuals who present initially with pulmonary infiltrates and hypoxic respiratory failure consistent with acute respiratory distress syndrome (ARDS) followed by progression to multiorgan failure. Since avian influenza A (H5N1) is generally resistant to amantadine and rimantadine, the recommended first-line treatment is oseltamivir. Corticosteroids have been used adjunctively, but high-level studies have not been performed to confirm their efficacy. Vaccines are not yet available.

Hantavirus Pulmonary Syndrome
Hantavirus pulmonary syndrome, first recognized in the southwestern United States in 1993, is caused by an RNA virus (family, Bunyaviridae; genus, *Hantavirus*). The rodent reservoir for this virus is the deer mouse (*Peromyscus maniculatus*). Infection occurs by inhalation of rodent excreta. No human-to-human transmission has been documented. The syndrome is more common in the southwestern United States. The demographic features are the following: median age of patients, 32 years (range, 12-69 years); males (52%); and Native Americans (55%). The illness is characterized by a short prodrome of fever, myalgia, headache, abdominal pain, nausea or vomiting (or both), and cough, followed by the abrupt onset of respiratory distress. Bilateral pulmonary infiltrates (noncardiogenic pulmonary edema) that occur within 48 hours after the onset of illness have been reported in all patients. Pleural effusions are common and can be transudates or exudates. Hemoconcentration, thrombocytopenia, and prolonged activated partial thromboplastin time (aPTT) are common; however, disseminated intravascular coagulation is rare. Early thrombocytopenia may provide a clue to the diagnosis of the infection. Myocardial suppression is an important component of the infection. Autopsy has routinely documented serous pleural effusions and heavy edematous lungs, with interstitial mononuclear cells in the alveolar septa, alveolar edema, focal hyaline

membranes, and occasional alveolar hemorrhage. *Hantavirus* antigens are detected with immunohistochemistry. Serologic (*Hantavirus*-specific IgM or increasing titers of IgG), polymerase chain reaction, and other studies are available. Treatment is entirely supportive. The mortality rate is as high as 50%.

* The reservoir for *Hantavirus* is the deer mouse.
* Typical clinical scenario for hantavirus pulmonary syndrome: After a prodrome, a Native American male has abrupt onset of respiratory distress, shock, and hypoxemia. CXR demonstrates bilateral pulmonary infiltrates and pleural effusion. Laboratory studies demonstrate a left-shift neutrophilia, hemoconcentration, thrombocytopenia, and circulating immunoblasts.

Severe Acute Respiratory Syndrome
Severe acute respiratory syndrome (SARS) is a viral respiratory infection caused by a novel coronavirus that previously had infected only animals. SARS transmission is through aerosol and possibly fecal-oral routes. The majority of patients with SARS have been adults 25 to 70 years old who were previously healthy. Many of the cases have been reported in Asia, particularly Hong Kong, Taiwan, and the People's Republic of China; however, cases have been reported in other countries in Asia as well as in North America and Europe. Notably, no new cases have been documented since 2004. SARS has an incubation period of 2 to 7 days and as long as 10 days in some patients. The illness begins with fever (>38.0°C) and associated chills and rigors. Other frequent symptoms are headache, malaise, and myalgia. Within the first 7 days, a dry nonproductive cough and dyspnea develop, with hypoxemia. This worsens in 20% of patients, who require mechanical ventilation and treatment in an intensive care unit. Currently, the fatality rate is approximately 15%. Leukocyte counts generally have been normal or decreased, with more than 50% of patients having lymphopenia and thrombocytopenia. Increased levels of liver aminotransferases and creatine kinase have been noted. Treatment is primarily supportive, with no role for antivirals.

* SARS is caused by a coronavirus.
* No new cases have been documented since 2004.
* Typical clinical scenario for SARS: After a febrile prodrome with associated myalgias, a dry nonproductive cough with dyspnea and hypoxemia develop in a 39-year-old traveler from Asia. CXR demonstrates bilateral interstitial pulmonary infiltrates. Laboratory studies demonstrate leukopenia, thrombocytopenia, and elevated levels of creatine kinase and liver aminotransferases.

Bacterial Infections

Sinusitis
Most bacterial sinus infections occur after an acute viral infection of the nasal mucosa. Bacteria in acute and chronic sinusitis are listed in Table 23-22. Most cases of acute sinusitis are due to viral infections and do not need treatment with antibiotics. However, distinguishing viral sinusitis from bacterial sinusitis is often difficult. Although multiple sinuses are commonly affected, the maxillary sinus is most commonly involved. Approximately 10% of the cases of maxillary

sinusitis are related to odontogenic infections. Sinus involvement is also seen in asthma, chronic bronchitis, bronchiectasis, cystic fibrosis, Kartagener syndrome, and Wegener granulomatosis. Cultures of the nasal secretions from more than 90% of patients with chronic rhinosinusitis are positive for fungi. Computed tomography (CT) of the sinuses is better than traditional radiography for detecting sinusitis but is not routinely indicated in these patients unless persistent or recurrent symptoms develop. Iatrogenic nasal obstruction with nasogastric tubes or nasotracheal tubes can result in nosocomial sinusitis and serious infection. In these instances, a high degree of awareness is needed and CT of the sinus may be indicated for prompt diagnosis.

- Sinus involvement is also seen in asthma, chronic bronchitis, bronchiectasis, cystic fibrosis, Kartagener syndrome, and Wegener granulomatosis.
- Fungal sinusitis is common in chronic rhinosinusitis.

Otitis Media

The relation between otitis media and common viral infections is strong, especially in children. Nearly 10% of children with measles have otitis media. Bacteria are isolated from 70% to 80% of patients with otitis media and include pneumococci (25%-75% of patients), *Haemophilus influenzae* (15%-30%), anaerobes, peptococci and propionibacteria (20%-30%), group A streptococci (2%-10%), and *Staphylococcus aureus* (1%-5%). Ampicillin-resistant *H influenzae* is found in 15% to 40% of patients. Otitis media in adults occurs in the setting of diabetes mellitus and cystic fibrosis.

- Otitis media in adults occurs with diabetes mellitus and cystic fibrosis.

Pharyngitis

Pharyngitis is caused by group A *Streptococcus pyogenes* (>30% of patients), *Neisseria gonorrhoeae*, *Corynebacterium diphtheriae*, and *Mycoplasma pneumoniae* (5%). Sore throat is also caused by adenovirus, Epstein-Barr virus, and other viruses.

Pneumonia

Streptococcus pneumoniae

Streptococcus pneumoniae is the most commonly isolated pathogen

Table 23-22 Bacteria in Acute and Chronic Sinusitis

Bacteria	Sinusitis, % of Patients	
	Acute	Chronic
Pneumococci	20-35	5-15
Haemophilus influenzae	15-30	3-10
Streptococcus, anaerobes & aerobes	5-35	10-25
Staphylococcus aureus	3-6	5-15
No growth	2-25	25-60

(identified in 20%-60% of cases) in adults with community-acquired pneumonia. In community-acquired pneumonia, a specific pathogen is not identified in as many as 50% of patients, even when extensive testing is performed. The incidence peaks in the winter and spring, when carrier rates in the general population may be as high as 70%. It is most common in infants and the elderly and in alcoholic or immunocompromised patients. At high risk are persons with cardiopulmonary disease (especially pulmonary edema), viral respiratory tract infections, or hemoglobinopathy and immunosuppression, including patients with hyposplenism. The incidence of bacteremic pneumonia among hospitalized patients is 25%, and the mortality rate is 20%. Of the elderly with bacteremic pneumonia, 30% do not have fever and 50% have minimal respiratory symptoms. Leukocytosis is common. Sputum may be blood-streaked or rusty. Early in the disease, CXR findings may be normal, but later, they may show classic lobar pneumonia. Pleurisy or effusion is common, and cavitation is rare. *Streptococcus pneumoniae* urinary antigen has a sensitivity of 80% and a specificity of 97% in patients with bacteremic pneumococcal pneumonia. The emergence of drug-resistant *S pneumoniae* (DRSP) is an increasing problem in the United States. By in vitro measures of resistance, more than 40% of pneumococci are resistant to penicillin; however, in the absence of meningitis, treatment failure with high-dose β-lactam antibiotics is thought to be unlikely.

- *Streptococcus pneumoniae*: the mortality rate is about 20% among hospitalized patients with bacteremic pneumonia.
- Of the elderly with bacteremic pneumonia, 30% do not have fever and 50% have minimal respiratory symptoms, 50% have altered mental state, and 50% have volume depletion.
- Typical clinical scenario for streptococcal pneumonia: A patient with cardiopulmonary disease has a recent viral respiratory tract infection, leukocytosis, and rusty sputum.

The pneumococcal vaccine consists of purified capsular polysaccharide from the 23 pneumococcal types accounting for at least 90% of pneumococcal pneumonias. It offers as much protection against drug-resistant pneumococci as against drug-sensitive ones. Vaccination decreases serious complications of pneumococcal infection by about one-half and reduces the carrier state among the general population. The overall efficacy of the pneumococcal vaccine is 60% for preventing invasive infections. Vaccine efficacy rates vary for certain diseases (diabetes mellitus, 84%; coronary artery disease, 73%; congestive heart failure, 69%; chronic obstructive pulmonary disease [COPD], 65%; and anatomical asplenia, 77%). The pneumococcal vaccine decreases the incidence of pneumonia by 79% to 92%. Pneumococcal vaccination is recommended for elderly persons (older than 65) and for those with diabetes mellitus, heart and lung diseases, renal insufficiency, hepatic insufficiency, sickle cell anemia, asplenia or hyposplenia, hematologic and other malignancies, alcoholism, cerebrospinal fluid leakage, immunodeficiency states, organ transplants, or AIDS. Some recommend pneumococcal vaccination for all adults, especially health care workers. Guidelines for subsequent vaccinations are controversial. Patients with nephrotic syndrome and other protein-losing nephropathies rapidly lose pneumococcal antibody and, thus, should receive the vaccine every 5 or 6 years. For persons older than 65, a single revaccination is suggested if the primary immunization was more than 5 years ago. The pneumococcal vaccine should be given to pregnant women only if clearly needed.

- The overall efficacy of the pneumococcal vaccine is 60% for preventing invasive infections.
- Vaccine efficacy rates vary for certain diseases (diabetes mellitus, 84%; coronary artery disease, 73%; congestive heart failure, 69%; COPD, 65%; and anatomical asplenia, 77%).
- The pneumococcal vaccine decreases the incidence of pneumonia by 79%-92%.

Staphylococcus aureus

Staphylococcus aureus may be isolated from the nasal passages of 20% to 40% of healthy adults, but pneumonia is uncommon. *Staphylococcus aureus* pneumonia is more likely to occur in patients with severe diabetes mellitus or an immunocompromised state, in patients receiving dialysis, in drug abusers, and in those with influenza or measles. In drug addicts, it may begin as septic emboli from right-sided endocarditis. It is a nosocomial type of pneumonia. Consolidation, bronchopneumonia, abscess with air-fluid level, pneumatocele, pneumothorax, empyema, and a high mortality rate characterize staphylococcal pneumonia.

- Lung abscess and pneumatoceles are more common complications of *S aureus* pneumonia.
- Associations with *Staphylococcus* pneumonia: diabetes mellitus, immunocompromised host, dialysis patients, influenza or measles infection, or drug abuse.

Pseudomonas aeruginosa

Pseudomonas aeruginosa is a ubiquitous organism commonly isolated from patients with cystic fibrosis and bronchiectasis. Colonization may be difficult to distinguish from true infection. Pneumonia may occur in patients with COPD, congestive heart failure, diabetes mellitus, kidney disease, alcoholism, malignant otitis media, tracheostomy, or prolonged ventilation. It also may develop postoperatively and in immunocompromised hosts. *Pseudomonas* pneumonia results in microabscess, alveolar hemorrhage, and necrotic areas.

- *Pseudomonas aeruginosa*: colonization may be difficult to distinguish from true infection.
- It is an important pathogenic organism in cystic fibrosis, bronchiectasis, malignant otitis media, immunocompromised state, and ventilator-associated pneumonia.

Klebsiella pneumoniae

Pneumonia due to *K pneumoniae* is more likely in persons who are alcoholic, diabetic, or hospitalized and receiving mechanical ventilation. It is more common in males. Dependent lung lobes are affected most frequently and CXR may show a "bulging fissure." Complications include abscess and empyema.

- Typical clinical scenario for *K pneumoniae* pneumonia: A patient is alcoholic, diabetic, or hospitalized and has a "bulging fissure" sign on CXR.

Haemophilus influenzae

Unencapsulated strains of *H influenzae* are present in the sputum of 30% to 60% of normal adults and 58% to 80% of patients with COPD. In contrast, bacteremia is almost always associated with encapsulated strains. Both strains cause pulmonary infections and otitis, sinusitis, epiglottitis, and pneumonia. Many patients with pneumonia have underlying COPD or alcoholism, even though *H influenzae* pneumonia develops in healthy military recruits. Pneumonia is detected in the lower lobes more often than in the upper lobes. CXR findings are typical for bronchopneumonia or lobar pneumonia. Pleural effusions occur in 30% of patients, and cavitation is rare.

- Typical clinical scenario for *H influenzae* pneumonia: A patient has COPD or is alcoholic; 30% of patients have pleural effusions, and cavitation is rare.

Moraxella catarrhalis

Moraxella catarrhalis, a gram-negative diplococcus, is part of the normal flora. Colonization is more common in the winter. It causes sinusitis, otitis, and pneumonia. The latter is more likely in patients who have alcoholim, COPD, diabetes mellitus, or immunocompromised status. Bacteremia is rare. Infection produces segmental patchy bronchopneumonia in the lower lobes. Cavitation and pleural effusion are rare. These bacteria produce β-lactamase, and most are resistant to penicillin and ampicillin.

- Typical clinical scenario for *M catarrhalis* pneumonia: A patient has COPD, immunocompromised status, or alcoholism and has gram-negative diplococci that are β-lactamase–positive.

Legionella pneumophila

Legionella is a gram-negative bacillus whose natural habitat is water. Infection results from the inhalation of aerosolized organisms, aspiration, and contaminated respiratory equipment; human-to-human transmission has not been described. Epidemics have occurred from contaminated air-conditioning cooling towers, construction or excavation in contaminated soil, and contaminated hospital showers. Most cases occur in the summer and early autumn. Risk factors include COPD, smoking, cancer, diabetes mellitus, immunosuppression, and chronic heart and kidney diseases. Almost all cases of pneumonia are caused by *L pneumophila* (85% of patients) and *Legionella micdadei* (10%). *Legionella* is the most common atypical organism resulting in severe pneumonia. Bacteria can be demonstrated in tissue with the Dieterle and fluorescent antibody stains. The incubation period is 2 to 10 days. Symptoms, in decreasing order of frequency, are abrupt onset of cough (hemoptysis in 30% of patients), chills, dyspnea, headache, myalgia, arthralgia, diarrhea, and relative bradycardia. Common signs include high fever, diarrhea, and change in mental status. Measurement of the *Legionella* urinary antigen is diagnostically valuable, since it is positive in the majority of patients with acute *Legionella* pneumonia. The fluorescent antibody stain is positive in the sputum in 20% of infected patients. Bacteria can be cultured from tissue or other samples. Serologic testing takes from 1 to 3 weeks before a titer of 1:64 is seen; the peak titer is reached in 5 to 6 weeks. A titer of 1:128 is suspicious, and a 4-fold increase in titer is diagnostic. A false-positive serologic titer can be seen in plague, tularemia, leptospirosis, and adenovirus infections.

- Typical clinical scenario for *L pneumophila* pneumonia: A 67-year-old with COPD, diabetes mellitus, and chronic heart failure presents with hyponatremia and hypophosphatemia, lobar consolidations on CXR, leukocytosis ($>10\times10^9$/L), proteinuria, and increased serum level of aspartate aminotransferase (AST).
- The *Legionella* urinary antigen is detected in the majority of patients with acute *Legionella* pneumonia.
- A false-positive serologic titer can be seen in plague, tularemia, leptospirosis, and adenovirus infections.

Anaerobic Bacteria

Bacteroides melaninogenicus, *Fusobacterium nucleatum*, anaerobic cocci, and anaerobic streptococci are responsible for most cases of anaerobic pneumonia. *Bacteroides fragilis* is recovered from 15% to 20% of patients with anaerobic pneumonia. Most of these anaerobes reside in the oropharynx as saprophytes. Common factors responsible for aspiration of anaerobes include altered consciousness, tooth extraction, poor dental hygiene, oropharyngeal infections, and drug overdose. Anaerobic bacterial infections may complicate underlying pulmonary problems (eg, cancer, bronchiectasis, or foreign body). More than 50% of patients have foul-smelling sputum. Patchy pneumonitis in dependent segments may progress to lung abscess and empyema.

- Typical clinical scenario for anaerobic bacterial pneumonia: Aspiration of anaerobes is facilitated by altered consciousness, tooth extraction, poor dental hygiene, oropharyngeal infections, and drug overdose; the patient has cavitated lung abscesses in dependent lobes.

Community-Acquired "Atypical" Pneumonia

The classification of pneumonia into "atypical" and "typical" arose from the clinical observation that in some patients pneumonia had a different course from that of pneumococcal pneumonia. The appreciation that numerous organisms, each with varied manifestations, can cause atypical pneumonia limits the clinical usefulness of such a classification. Organisms causing atypical community-acquired pneumonia include *L pneumophila*, *M pneumoniae*, *Chlamydia psittaci*, *Chlamydia pneumoniae*, *Coxiella burnetii*, and *Francisella tularensis*. In atypical pneumonia, the CXR abnormalities are often disproportionate to the pulmonary symptoms, and sputum analysis may reveal numerous leukocytes and no organisms. Community-acquired typical pneumonias are caused by *S pneumoniae* (45% of patients), gram-negative bacilli (15%), and *H influenzae* (15%). For patients not admitted to the hospital, the mortality from community-acquired pneumonia is less than 1%. However, the overall mortality for patients admitted to the hospital is 14%; for elderly patients, 18%; and for those with bacteremia, 20%. The mortality of patients with community-acquired pneumonia who are admitted to an intensive care unit is 37%.

- Community-acquired atypical pneumonia is caused by *M pneumoniae*, *C psittaci*, *C pneumoniae*, *C burnetii*, and *Legionella* species.

Mycoplasma

Mycoplasma species is spread from person to person by droplet nuclei. Infections occur in epidemic and endemic forms, and outbreaks occur in closed populations (eg, military camps and colleges). Epidemics are more common in the summer and autumn. Illness is more common in school-aged children and young adults. The incubation period is 2 to 3 weeks. Clinical features include cough (>95% of patients), fever (85%), pharyngitis (50%), coryza, and tracheobronchitis. Bullous myringitis (20%) is a rare but unique feature of this disease. Other rare complications include pleural effusion, hemolytic anemia, erythema multiforme, hepatitis, thrombocytopenia, and Guillain-Barré syndrome. Nearly 20% of all community-acquired pneumonias and 50% of all pneumonias in healthy young adults in close living quarters (eg, military recruits and dormitory students) may be caused by *M pneumoniae*. Pneumonia occurs in only 3% to 10% of infected persons and is more likely in younger adults (military recruits or children in summer camps); it causes interstitial pneumonia and acute bronchiolitis. CXR shows unilateral bronchopneumonia, lower lobe involvement (65% of patients), and pleural effusion (5%). Cold agglutinins (>1:64 in 50% of patients) appear during the second or third week after the onset of symptoms, and the titer decreases to insignificant levels by 4 to 6 weeks. With complement fixation serologic testing, a 4-fold increase in titer is noted in 50% to 80% of patients.

- Typical clinical scenario for *Mycoplasma* pneumonia: Cough, fever, pharyngitis, coryza, and tracheobronchitis, with bullous myringitis, hemolytic anemia, erythema multiforme, or Guillain-Barré syndrome; it causes interstitial pneumonia and acute bronchiolitis.
- Cold agglutinins (>1:64 in 50% of patients) appear during the second or third week.

Chlamydia pneumoniae *(TWAR Strain)*

Chlamydia pneumoniae is confined to the human respiratory tract; no reservoirs are known. Person-to-person spread occurs among schoolchildren, family members, and military recruits. The incubation period is 10 to 65 days (mean, 31 days). Reinfection is common, with cycles of disease every few years. *Chlamydia pneumoniae* is the cause of at least 10% of all cases of community-acquired pneumonia. About 15% of patients are symptomatic and have clinical features that include pharyngitis (90% of patients), pneumonia (10%), bronchitis (5%), and sinusitis (5%). Pharyngeal erythema and wheezing are common. CXR shows unilateral segmental patchy opacity. The complement fixation test is insensitive and nonspecific. *Chlamydia pneumoniae* is considered an etiologic agent in coronary artery disease.

- *Chlamydia pneumoniae*: person-to-person spread among schoolchildren, family members, and military recruits.
- Pneumonia in 10% of patients, and bronchitis in 5% of symptomatic patients.
- *Chlamydia pneumoniae* is considered an etiologic agent in coronary artery disease.

Chlamydia psittaci

Chlamydia psittaci causes psittacosis (ornithosis) in humans. The organism is found in psittacine birds (parrots and lories), turkeys, pigeons, and other birds. Asymptomatic infection of these birds with continued shedding of the organism is common. Infected birds have anorexia, weight loss, diarrhea, ruffled feathers, conjunctivitis, and rhinitis, and they are not able to fly. In humans, the incubation period is 1 to 6 weeks. Clinical features include myalgias, fever, headache, pharyngitis, lethargy, confusion, delirium, neutropenia (in 25% of patients), and splenomegaly (in 1%-10%). Pulmonary symptoms are late and mild. CXR shows patchy unilateral or bilateral lower lobe pneumonia and an occasional small pleural effusion. Laboratory findings include a normal leukocyte count, increased creatine kinase level, and a 4-fold increase in complement fixation over more than 2 weeks. Whereas psittacosis is transmitted from birds to humans, *C pneumoniae* pneumonia is transmitted between people. Pigeon-breeder's lung (bird fancier's lung) is hypersensitivity pneumonitis caused by an immune reaction to avian proteins.

* Typical clinical scenario for psittacosis: Exposure to sick birds that harbor *C psittaci*; patients have myalgias, fever, headache, lethargy, confusion, delirium, and splenomegaly.
* Note the differences: *C pneumoniae* pneumonia (human-to-human transmission), psittacosis (bird-to-human transmission), and pigeon-breeder's or bird fancier's lung (hypersensitivity pneumonitis caused by immune reaction to avian proteins).

Coxiella burnetii

Coxiella burnetii, a rickettsia shed in the urine, feces, milk, and birth products of sheep, cattle, goats, and cats, is responsible for Q fever (named for the *query* associated with an outbreak in an Australian slaughterhouse in 1935). However, epidemiologic factors such as contact with cats or farm animals are identified for only 40% of patients. Humans are infected by inhalation of dried aerosolized material. The incubation period is 10 to 30 days. Clinical features include fever, myalgias, chills, chest pain, and cough (late). The leukocyte count is normal, and the erythrocyte sedimentation rate is increased. CXR findings may be normal or show unilateral bronchopneumonia and small pleural effusions. Lobar consolidation is seen in 25% of patients. Hepatitis and endocarditis can occur. Hyponatremia occurs in more than 25% of patients. Liver enzyme levels may increase. Indirect immunofluorescence is the immunologic test of choice.

* *C burnetii*: rickettsial illness (Q fever).
* Inhalation of dried inoculum from urine, feces, milk, or birth products of sheep, cattle, goats, or cats.
* Bronchopneumonia and pleural effusion.

Francisella tularensis

Francisella tularensis is a gram-negative bacillus transmitted to humans from wild animals and by bites of ticks or deer flies. An analysis of an outbreak in Martha's Vineyard showed that the highest identifiable risk was associated with lawn mowing and brush cutting. Aerosol inhalation can occur (eg, laboratory workers), and it is a potential bioterrorism agent. The incubation period for tularemia is 2 to 5 days. Cutaneous ulcer and lymphadenopathy are common features. Cough, fever, and chest pain are frequent, but many patients are asymptomatic. CXR shows unilateral lower lobe patchy infiltrates (bilateral in 30% of patients) and pleural effusion (30% of patients). The leukocyte count is normal; the organism is not seen with Gram staining of the sputum. Serologic testing (agglutinins) is considered diagnostic if it shows a 4-fold increase in titer in paired samples 2 to 3 weeks apart or a single titer greater than 1:160.

* Tularemia: transmitted from wild rabbits, squirrels, and other wild animals. Mowing grass and cutting brush have also been identified as risk factors in outbreaks of tularemia.
* Typical clinical scenario for tularemia: Patients may be asymptomatic or have cough and fever, with cutaneous ulcer, lymphadenopathy, bronchopneumonia, and pleural effusion.

Yersinia pestis

Yersinia pestis is a gram-negative bacillus that causes plague. It is more prevalent in New Mexico, Arizona, Colorado, and California than in other states. It is spread from wild rodents (occasionally cats), either directly or by fleas, usually in May to September. Because it is endemic to largely rural and uninhabited areas, the incidence of disease is low. The incubation period is 2 to 7 days. Clinical features include fever, headache, bubo (groin or axilla), cough, and tachypnea. Pneumonia occurs in 10% to 20% of patients. Pneumonic plague is the most serious and fulminant form of this disease. CXR shows bilateral lower lobe alveolar infiltrates. Pleural effusion is common, and nodules and cavities can occur. The leukocyte count is higher than 15×10^9/L. The organism is seen with Giemsa or direct fluorescent antibody staining and in cultures of blood, lymph node, or sputum. Serologic testing gives positive results.

* Typical clinical scenario for *Y pestis* pneumonia: A patient from the southwestern United States has alveolar infiltrates and pleural effusion; the leukocyte count is >15×10^9/L.

Burkholderia pseudomallei

Burkholderia pseudomallei is a gram-negative rod responsible for melioidosis. The disease is most prevalent in parts of Southeast Asia; sporadic cases have been reported in the United States. The organism is widely distributed in water and soil, and infection occurs after direct inoculation through the skin or, less commonly, by inhalation. Although the incubation period can be as short as 3 days, the disease remains latent and may become evident months to years later. Up to 2% of US Army personnel stationed in Vietnam were seropositive for *B pseudomallei*, even though the majority of them were free of clinical disease. Clinical features include acute community-acquired pneumonia, pleurisy, subacute presentation with upper lobe lesions (sometimes with cavitation), or chronic cavitary lung disease that resembles tuberculosis. Diagnosis is by positive findings on culture.

* Melioidosis may resemble chronic cavitary tuberculosis.

Nocardia *Pneumonia*

Nocardia asteroides, *Nocardia brasiliensis*, and *Nocardia otitidis-caviarum* can cause pneumonia in susceptible persons. *N asteroides* is a weakly acid-fast saprophytic bacteria present in the soil, dust, plants, and water. Infection is more common in immunosuppressed patients and in those with pulmonary alveolar proteinosis. Primary infection leads to necrotizing pneumonia with abscess formation. No inflammatory response or granuloma formation occurs. Pulmonary nodules suggestive of cancer metastases and dense alveolar infiltrates are common CXR findings. Infection may produce pleural effusion. Lymphohematogenous spread occurs in 20% of patients; nearly all such patients develop a brain abscess. The diagnosis is made at autopsy in 40% of cases. Isolation of the organism from the sputum of immunocompetent patients might represent colonization since the saprophytic state is well recognized; however, in an immunocompromised patient, this should be considered a true infection.

- Typical clinical scenario for *Nocardia* pneumonia: An immunocompromised patient or a patient with pulmonary alveolar proteinosis, necrotizing pneumonia, and lung abscess.
- Brain abscess is common in those with disseminated infection.

Actinomycosis

Actinomycosis is caused by *Actinomyces israelii* or *Actinomyces bovis*. The organism is easily isolated from scrapings around the teeth, gums, and tonsils in subjects with poor dental or oral hygiene. It is an opportunistic organism and becomes invasive with severe caries, tissue necrosis, and aspiration. In tissue, the organism grows into a sulfur granule caused by mycelial clumps in a matrix of calcium phosphate. The disease is more common in rural areas and has a male to female ratio of 2:1. Infection is always mixed with anaerobes. Skin abscesses, ulcers, sinus tracts, and cervicofacial node involvement are found in up to 40% of patients. Pulmonary involvement is seen in 20% of patients, along with cough, fever, pulmonary consolidation, pleurisy with effusion, and, eventually, draining sinuses.

- Typical clinical scenario for actinomycosis: A patient has severe dental caries, tissue necrosis, and aspiration, with cough, fever, pulmonary lesions, pleural effusion, and fistula and sinus tracts.

Hospital-Acquired (Nosocomial) Pneumonia

About 60% of the cases of nosocomial pneumonia are caused by aerobic gram-negative bacilli, 20% by *S aureus*, 10% by *S pneumoniae*, and the rest by anaerobes, *Legionella* species, and others. Risk factors include coma, hypotension, shock, acidosis, azotemia, prolonged treatment with antibiotics, major surgical operations, lengthy procedures, mechanical ventilation, and immunosuppressive therapy. Methicillin-resistant *Staphylococcus aureus* (MRSA) has become a prevalent nosocomial pathogen in the United States. By definition, MRSA is resistant to methicillin, oxacillin, penicillin, and amoxicillin. This infection occurs most frequently among patients with weakened immunity in hospitals, nursing homes, dialysis centers, or other long-term care facilities. Colonized patients are the most important reservoirs of MRSA in hospitals, and the main transmission of MRSA is by hands (particularly those of health care workers).

Standard precautions (eg, hand washing and use of gloves, masks, and gowns) should be implemented to control the spread of MRSA. Recently, community-associated MRSA (CA-MRSA) has been identified in persons who have not been hospitalized or had a medical procedure within the past year. Clusters of CA-MRSA skin infections have occurred among athletes, military recruits, children, prisoners, and others. Close contact seems to be a major risk factor. The identified CA-MRSA strains seem to have properties that differ from those of hospital-acquired MRSA.

- About 60% of cases of nosocomial pneumonia are caused by gram-negative bacilli, 20% by *S aureus*, and 10% by *S pneumoniae*.
- In hospital outbreaks involving a single type of organism, consider contaminated respiratory equipment.

Aspiration Pneumonia

Aspiration pneumonia can be either acute or chronic. The acute type usually results from aspiration of a volume larger than 50 mL, with a pH less than 2.4. It produces classic aspiration pneumonia that is usually sterile and does not require the use of antibiotics. Predisposing factors include nasogastric tube, anesthesia, coma, seizures, central nervous system problems, diaphragmatic hernia with reflux, and tracheoesophageal fistula. Nosocomial aspiration pneumonia is caused by *Escherichia coli*, *S aureus*, *K pneumoniae*, and *P aeruginosa*. Community-acquired aspiration pneumonias are caused by infections due to anaerobes (*B melaninogenicus*, *F nucleatum*, and gram-positive cocci). Preventive measures are important. Chronic aspiration pneumonia results from recurrent aspiration of small volumes. Examples include patients with reflux aspiration who develop mineral oil granuloma. Symptoms include chronic cough, patchy lung infiltrates, and nocturnal wheeze.

- Acute aspiration pneumonia: from the aspiration of a volume >50 mL, with a pH <2.4. Usually sterile and antibiotics are not needed.
- Chronic aspiration pneumonia: from recurrent aspiration of small volumes.

Lung Abscess

Lung abscess is a circumscribed collection of pus in the lung that leads to cavity formation; the cavity has an air-fluid level on CXR. Lung abscess usually is caused by bacteria, particularly anaerobic bacilli (30%-50% of cases), aerobic gram-positive cocci (25%), and aerobic gram-negative bacilli (5%-12%). Polymicrobial infections are most common. Suppuration leading to lung abscess can result from primary, opportunistic, and hematogenous lung infection. Primary lung abscess is caused by oral infection; aspiration accounts for up to 90% of all abscesses. Alcohol abuse and dental caries also contribute. Lung abscesses caused by opportunistic infections are seen in elderly patients with a blood dyscrasia and in patients with cancer of the lung or oropharynx. In patients with advanced HIV infection, lung abscess can develop in association with a broad spectrum of pathogens, including opportunistic organisms. These patients have a poor prognosis. Hematogenous lung abscesses occur with septicemia, septic embolism, and sterile infarcts (3% of patients). A history of any of these conditions in association with fever, cough with purulent or bloody sputum, weight loss, and leukocytosis suggests the diagnosis. CXR may show cavitated lesions. The abscess may rupture into the pleural space and cause empyema. Bronchoscopy may be necessary to obtain cultures, to drain the abscess, and to exclude obstructing lesions. High rates of morbidity and mortality (20%) are associated with lung abscess despite antibiotic therapy. The prognosis is worse for patients with a large abscess and for those infected with *S aureus*, *K pneumoniae*, and *P aeruginosa*. Treatment includes drainage (physiotherapy, postural, and bronchoscopic), antibiotics for 4 to 6 weeks, and surgical treatment if medical therapy fails.

- Typical clinical scenario for primary lung abscess: A 54-year-old alcoholic male presents with fever. CXR demonstrates a cavity with an air-fluid level.
- Hematogenous lung abscess is seen in septicemia and septic embolism.
- Cause is often polymicrobial and prolonged antibiotic therapy is often needed.

Mycobacterial Diseases

Mycobacterium tuberculosis
Mycobacterium tuberculosis causes the most common type of human-to-human chronic infection by mycobacteria worldwide. The most common mode of transmission is by inhalation of droplet nuclei from expectorated respiratory secretions. Of those exposed to *M tuberculosis*, 30% become infected, and among the latter group, less than 5% develop active primary disease and less than 5% develop active disease from reactivation. Active infection is diagnosed by documenting the presence of *M tuberculosis* in respiratory secretions or other body fluids or tissues. Sputum and gastric washings have approximately a 30% diagnostic yield. Bronchoscopy with bronchoalveolar lavage has an approximately 40% diagnostic yield, which increases to almost 95% if biopsy is performed. Culture of pleural fluid alone provides the diagnosis in less than 20% of cases, but culture of pleural biopsy specimens has a 70% diagnostic yield. Faster culture results are available with the use of broth culture systems (1.5-2 weeks) and nucleic acid amplification (8 hours). Culture-positive pulmonary tuberculosis with normal CXR findings is not uncommon, and the incidence of this presentation is increasing. *Latent tuberculosis infection* (LTBI) is the current term for a person who does not have active tuberculosis but has a positive purified protein derivative (PPD) skin test. Such a person is infected with mycobacteria but does not have active disease.

- The PPD skin test indicates infection with mycobacteria and not active disease.
- Active infection should be confirmed by the growth of *M tuberculosis* in respiratory secretions or other body fluids or tissues.
- Bronchoscopically obtained specimens have a higher diagnostic yield.
- CXR findings can be normal in active tuberculosis.

A positive PPD tuberculin skin test is an example of a delayed (T-cell–mediated) hypersensitivity reaction. The test can be positive within 4 weeks after exposure to *M tuberculosis*. The PPD test is negative in 25% of patients with active tuberculosis. A false-negative PPD result is also seen in infections with viruses or bacteria, live virus vaccinations, chronic renal failure, nutritional deficiency, lymphoid malignancies, leukemias, corticosteroid and immunosuppressive drug therapy, newborn or elderly patients, recent or overwhelming infection with mycobacteria, and acute stress. The specificity of a positive PPD reaction is variable and is dependent on the prevalence of infection with nontuberculous mycobacteria. The annual risk of active tuberculosis for those who are PPD-positive depends on the underlying medical condition (annual risk in parentheses): HIV-positive (8%-10%), recent converters (2%-5%), abnormal CXR (2%-4%), intravenous drug abuse (1%), end-stage renal disease (1%), and diabetes mellitus (0.3%). PPD skin testing should use a 5-tuberculin unit (TU) preparation; the widest induration is read at 48 and 72 hours. Prior vaccination with BCG is not a contraindication for the PPD skin test. There is no reliable method to distinguish positive PPD results caused by BCG vaccination from those caused by mycobacterial infections, although large reactions (≥20 mm) are not likely caused by BCG. The role of the serum assay, QuantiFERON-TB Gold, continues to evolve and has the promise of increasing the specificity of testing to identify latent tuberculosis. QuantiFERON-TB Gold may help in distinguishing tuberculous infection from nontuberculous mycobacterial infection and BCG vaccination since it measures interferon-γ production from a patient's blood sample incubated with the *M tuberculosis*–specific antigens ESAT-6 and CFP-10. Initiatives are under way to incorporate the test into established guidelines. However, the principles of targeted testing (ie, identifying groups at highest risk of progressing to active tuberculosis) will not change.

- The PPD reaction is a delayed type of hypersensitivity reaction.
- The PPD skin test can become positive within 4 weeks after exposure to *M tuberculosis*.
- The PPD skin test is negative in 25% of patients with active tuberculosis.

Targeted tuberculin testing for LTBI identifies persons at high risk of tuberculosis who would benefit from treatment of LTBI. Indications for the PPD skin test include persons with signs and symptoms suggestive of current tuberculous infection, recent contacts with known or suspected cases of tuberculosis, abnormal CXR findings compatible with past tuberculosis, patients with diseases that increase the risk of tuberculosis (silicosis, gastrectomy, diabetes mellitus, immune suppression, and HIV infection), and groups at high risk of recent infection with *M tuberculosis* (immigrants and long-time residents and workers in hospitals, nursing homes, or prisons). The following criteria are used to diagnose LTBI (ie, a positive PPD skin test):

1. Reaction ≥5 mm—persons with HIV infection, close contact with infectious cases, patients with organ transplants and other immunosuppressed patients (receiving the equivalent of 15 mg daily of prednisone for ≥1 month), and those with fibrotic lesions on CXR consistent with prior tuberculosis

2. Reaction ≥10 mm—immigrants within the past 5 years from high-prevalence countries; injection drug users;

mycobacteriology laboratory workers; children younger than 4 years, or infants, children, and adolescents exposed to adults at high risk of tuberculosis; and employees and residents of high-risk congregate facilities including prisons, nursing homes, hospitals and other health care facilities, residential facilities for patients with AIDS, and homeless shelters; and patients with high-risk clinical conditions (eg, diabetes mellitus, silicosis, chronic renal failure, leukemias and lymphomas, carcinoma of the head or neck and lung, weight loss ≥10% of ideal body weight, gastrectomy, and jejunoileal bypass)

3. Reaction ≥15 mm—any person without a defined risk factor for tuberculosis

Pleural tuberculosis used to be more common in younger (<40 years) patients; now, it is more common among the elderly. In the United States, 4% of all tuberculous patients have pleural involvement, and pleural tuberculosis constitutes 23% of the cases with extrapulmonary tuberculosis. Effusions usually occur 3 to 6 months after the primary infection. Acute presentation (cough, fever, and pleuritic chest pain) is more common in younger patients. Bilateral exudative effusions occur in up to 8% of patients, and the PPD skin test is positive in more than 66%. The effusions typically have high protein levels (>5g/dL), lymphocytosis (>50%), and low levels of glucose (<50 mg/dL). A low pleural fluid pH occurs in 20% of patients. Measurement of levels of the enzyme adenosine deaminase (ADA) in the pleural fluid has a sensitivity of 70% to 90% for pleural tuberculosis, with a specificity that varies from less than 50% to 90%. The test is not diagnostic for pleural tuberculosis, and its main utility is to suggest tuberculosis infection if the ADA level is very high or to rule out the diagnosis of pleural tuberculosis if the ADA level is very low. Pleural biopsy specimens show caseous granulomas in up to 80% of patients, and cultures of biopsy specimens are positive in more than 75%. Cultures of pleural fluid are positive in only 20% to 40% of patients and the sputum is positive in 40%. Bronchopleural fistula is a complication.

- Pleural tuberculosis is more common among the elderly.
- Effusion occurs 3 to 6 months after primary infection.

Miliary tuberculosis constitutes 10% of cases of extrapulmonary tuberculosis. It is characterized by the diffuse presence of small (<2 mm) nodules throughout the body. The spleen, liver, and lung are frequently involved. The disease can be acute and fatal or insidious in onset and slowly progressive. CXR shows typical miliary lesions in more than 65% of patients. Sputum findings are negative in up to 80% of patients and the PPD skin test is negative in approximately 50% of patients with miliary tuberculosis. Mortality is high (30%) even with therapy. *Tuberculous lymphadenitis* (ie, scrofula) is the most common form of extrapulmonary tuberculosis. It is more common in children and young adults than in older persons. Cervical lymph nodes are affected most commonly; 1 or more nodes (painless, nontender, and rubbery) may be palpable. Abscess and sinus formation may occur. *Skeletal tuberculosis* is becoming less common; when seen, it is more common in the young than in older adults. Any bone can be involved, but the vertebrae are involved in 50% of cases. Pott disease is *tuberculous spondylitis* and may produce severe kyphosis.

Tuberculous meningitis is the most common form of central nervous system involvement and is localized mainly to the base of the brain. It occurs more commonly in intravenous drug users who are HIV-positive and in immunocompromised patients. Tuberculous meningitis is often insidious in onset. *Abdominal tuberculosis* frequently affects the peritoneum. *Ileocecal tuberculosis* can lead to ulcerative enteritis, strictures, and fistulas. *Genitourinary tuberculosis* is responsible for up to 13% of extrapulmonary disease. It is usually a late manifestation of the infection and is more common in older patients. The renal cortex is affected initially, and the infection can then spread to the renal pelvis, ureter, bladder, and genitalia. Sterile pyuria is an important feature. *Laryngeal tuberculosis* is usually a complication of pulmonary tuberculosis. *Pericardial tuberculosis* is usually due to hematogenous spread. Pericardial constriction may begin subacutely and become a chronic problem.

- Miliary tuberculosis is responsible for 10% of cases of extrapulmonary tuberculosis.
- Tuberculous lymphadenitis is the most common form of extrapulmonary tuberculosis.
- Tuberculous meningitis is often insidious in onset.

Tuberculosis is particularly prone to develop in HIV-positive persons. In this group of patients, a CD4 count less than 200/mcL and a PPD-positive status increase the risk. Furthermore, there is an increased rate of reactivation, increased rate of progressive primary infection, increased incidence of multidrug resistance, atypical clinical features, and increased progression of HIV disease. Among those who are HIV-positive and are exposed to *M tuberculosis*, nearly 40% develop primary tuberculosis, and the rate of reactivation is 8% to 10% per year. Tuberculous pleurisy and hilar and mediastinal lymphadenopathy are more common in AIDS than in non-AIDS patients with tuberculosis. The diagnosis of tuberculosis in a patient with AIDS can be difficult owing to the varied manifestations. These patients may lack cavitation and granuloma formation and have negative sputum findings and negative PPD skin tests. Treatment of tuberculosis in HIV-negative and HIV-positive patients is essentially identical with a few notable exceptions. Certain treatment schemes are contraindicated in HIV-infected patients because of a high rate of relapse due to resistant organisms or an increased risk of toxicity. Management of these patients is complex and requires expertise with both HIV and tuberculosis. Rifampin-containing regimens are effective in curing tuberculosis in HIV-positive patients. Initiation of HIV protease inhibitor therapy in patients who are HIV-positive or who have AIDS increases the symptoms and signs of the underlying mycobacterial infection. Rifampin accelerates the metabolism of protease inhibitors (decreased plasma levels) and leads to HIV resistance. Isoniazid prophylaxis for 12 months decreases the incidence of tuberculosis and increases the life expectancy for HIV-infected patients.

- Tuberculosis is particularly prone to develop in HIV-positive persons.
- The simultaneous presence of HIV and tuberculosis leads to increased severity of both infections.
- HIV protease inhibitor therapy may lead to worsening of the signs and symptoms of tuberculosis.

Definitive therapy is indicated for all patients with culture-positive tuberculosis. Treatment usually should include multidrug therapy (>2 drugs) for all patients who have active tuberculosis (Tables 23-23 to 23-25; Figures 23-29 and 23-30). With rigidly administered 6-month regimens, more than 90% of patients are smear-negative after 2 months of therapy, more than 95% are cured, and less than 5% have relapse. A 9-month regimen provides a cure rate higher than 97% and a relapse rate less than 2%. All treatment programs should be recommended and preferably undertaken by physicians and health care workers experienced in the management of mycobacterial diseases. The most important impediment to lack of adequate therapy worldwide is the lack of adherence to the treatment.

Extrapulmonary tuberculosis can be treated effectively with either a 6- or 9-month regimen. However, miliary tuberculosis, bone and joint tuberculosis, and tuberculous meningitis in infants and children may require treatment for 12 or more months. Cavitary tuberculosis is often treated for 9 months. Systemic corticosteroid therapy may be useful in the prevention of pleural fibrosis, pericardial constriction, neurologic complications from tuberculous meningitis, tuberculous bronchial stenosis, and adrenal insufficiency caused by tuberculosis. Extrapulmonary tuberculosis confined to lymph nodes has no effect on obstetrical outcomes, but tuberculosis at other sites adversely affects the outcome of pregnancy.

- Miliary, skeletal, and meningeal tuberculosis may require >12 months of therapy.
- Corticosteroids are helpful in treating extrapulmonary tuberculosis.

Drug-resistant tuberculosis is a problem in many large cities; for example, a rate of 30% has been reported in New York City. Drug resistance can develop against a single drug or multiple drugs. Multidrug resistance is usually defined as *M tuberculosis* resistance to at least isoniazid and rifampin. Multidrug resistance is more likely in the following settings: nonadherence to treatment guidelines and treatment errors by physicians and health care workers, lack of compliance by patients, homelessness, drug addiction, and exposure to multidrug-resistant tuberculosis (MDR-TB) in high-prevalence countries with inadequate tuberculosis control programs. Multidrug resistance occurs rapidly in HIV-infected persons. The American Thoracic Society (ATS) and the Centers for Disease Control and Prevention (CDC) recommend an intensive phase of therapy with 4 drugs if the local rate of resistance to isoniazid is more than 4%. Even though the mortality from MDR-TB is high in HIV-positive and HIV-negative patients, appropriate treatment produces a favorable outcome (>80%). MDR-TB is often treated for 18 to 24 months.

- Drug-resistant tuberculosis may require multidrug (≥4 drugs) therapy.

To prevent drug resistance and to effectively decrease the number of cases of tuberculosis, many health care organizations recommend administration of antituberculous drugs by directly observed therapy (DOT) in which a health care provider monitors each patient as every dose of a 6-month regimen is taken. This approach makes a cure almost certain with drug-sensitive tuberculosis. The DOT regimen is particularly important for the homeless, chronic alcoholics, intravenous drug abusers, AIDS patients, and prison inmates. A fixed-dose combination should be considered in cases of newly diagnosed disease. Even though fixed-dose combinations of antituberculous drugs (Rifamate and Rifater) are available and have been strongly recommended by the World Health Organization, CDC, ATS, and the International Union Against Tuberculosis and Lung Disease, less than 25% of rifampin-containing therapies use the fixed-dose regimen. Treatment completion rates for pulmonary tuberculosis are most likely to exceed 90% with DOT. However, DOT may not increase the cure rate in areas where the rate of cure is high (without DOT).

- DOT for 6 months is effective in preventing relapses and emergence of drug-resistant tuberculosis.
- DOT is also useful in the treatment of drug-resistant tuberculosis and tuberculosis in immunocompromised patients.
- A fixed-dose combination should be considered in cases of newly diagnosed disease.

Treatment of LTBI is indicated for persons with a positive PPD skin test who do not have active infection (Table 23-25). If an isoniazid-sensitive organism is suspected to have caused LTBI, the treatment options include isoniazid 300 mg daily or 900 mg biweekly. Rifampin (600 mg daily) is an alternative option. If isoniazid resistance is suspected or known, the options include rifampin (600 mg daily) or rifabutin (300 mg daily). A short course of therapy (4 months) with rifampin and pyrazinamide was an alternative regimen for LTBI, but this is no longer routinely recommended because of the increased frequency of cases of fatal hepatitis. Therapy with this combination should be supervised by a specialist. The recommended duration for LTBI therapy is outlined below:

1. Isoniazid for HIV-positive adults and children: 12 months
2. Isoniazid for HIV-negative adults: at least 6 months
3. Isoniazid for HIV-negative children: 9 months
4. Rifampin or rifabutin: 12 months
5. Silicosis or old fibrotic lesion on CXR without active tuberculosis: 4-month therapy with isoniazid and rifampin, although 12 months of isoniazid alone is an acceptable alternative

In the United States, BCG vaccine is recommended for PPD-negative persons in the following categories:

1. Infants and children who are at high risk of intimate and prolonged exposure to persistently untreated or ineffectively treated patients with infectious pulmonary tuberculosis, who cannot be removed from the source of exposure, and who cannot be given long-term prophylactic therapy
2. Health care workers in settings in which the likelihood of transmission and subsequent infection with *M tuberculosis* strains resistant to isoniazid and rifampin is high, provided comprehensive tuberculosis infection-control precautions have been implemented in the workplace and have not been successful.

BCG is not recommended for HIV-positive children and adults.

Table 23-23 Drug Regimens for Culture-Positive Pulmonary Tuberculosis Caused by Drug-Susceptible Organisms

	Initial Phase			Continuation Phase				Rating[a] (Evidence[b])	
Regimen	Drugs	Interval and Doses[c] (Minimal Duration)	Regimen	Drugs	Interval and Doses[c,d] (Minimal Duration)	Range of Total Doses (Minimal Duration)		HIV−	HIV+
1	INH RIF PZA EMB	7 d/wk for 56 doses (8 wk) *or* 5 d/wk for 40 doses (8 wk)[e]	1a	INH/RIF	7 d/wk for 126 doses (18 wk) *or* 5 d/wk for 90 doses (18 wk)[e]	182-130 (26 wk)		A (I)	A (II)
			1b	INH/RIF	Twice weekly for 36 doses (18 wk)	92-76 (26 wk)		A (I)	A (II)[f]
			1c[g]	INH/RPT	Once weekly for 18 doses (18 wk)	74-58 (26 wk)		B (I)	E (I)
2	INH RIF PZA EMB	7 d/wk for 14 doses (2 wk), *then* twice weekly for 12 doses (6 wk) *or* 5 d/wk for 10 doses (2 wk)[e], *then* twice weekly for 12 doses (6 wk)	2a	INH/RIF	Twice weekly for 36 doses (18 wk)	62-58 (26 wk)		A (II)	B (II)[f]
			2b[g]	INH/RPT	Once weekly for 18 doses (18 wk)	44-40 (26 wk)		B (I)	E (I)
3	INH RIF PZA EMB	3 times weekly for 24 doses (8 wk)	3a	INH/RIF	3 times weekly for 54 doses (18 wk)	78 (26 wk)		B (I)	B (II)
4	INH RIF EMB	7 d/wk for 56 doses (8 wk) *or* 5 d/wk for 40 doses (8 wk)[e]	4a	INH/RIF	7 d/wk for 217 doses (31 wk) *or* 5 d/wk for 155 doses (31 wk)[e]	273-195 (39 wk)		C (I)	C (II)
			4b	INH/RIF	Twice weekly for 62 doses (31 wk)	118-102 (39 wk)		C (I)	C (II)

Abbreviations: EMB, ethambutol; INH, isoniazid; PZA, pyrazinamide; RIF, rifampin; RPT, rifapentine.

[a] Definitions of evidence ratings: A, preferred; B, acceptable alternative; C, offer when A and B cannot be given; E, should never be given.

[b] Definitions of evidence ratings: I, randomized clinical trial; II, data from clinical trials that were not randomized or were conducted in other populations; III, expert opinion.

[c] When directly observed therapy is used, drugs may be given 5 d/wk and the necessary number of doses adjusted accordingly. Although there are no studies that compare 5 with 7 daily doses, extensive experience indicates this would be an effective practice.

[d] Patients with cavitation on initial chest radiograph and positive cultures at completion of 2 months of therapy should receive a 7-month (31 weeks; either 217 doses [daily] or 62 doses [twice weekly]) continuation phase.

[e] Five-day-a-week administration is always given by directly observed therapy. Rating for 5 d/wk regimens is A (III).

[f] Not recommended for human immunodeficiency virus (HIV)-infected patients with CD4+ cell counts <100 cells/mL.

[g] Options 1c and 2b should be used only in HIV-negative patients who have negative sputum smears at the time of completion of 2 months of therapy and who do not have cavitation on the initial chest radiograph. For patients receiving this regimen and found to have a positive culture from the 2-month specimen, treatment should be extended an extra 3 months.

From Blumberg HM, Burman WJ, Chaisson RE, Daley CL, Etkind SC, Friedman LN, et al. American Thoracic Society/Centers for Disease Control and Prevention/Infectious Diseases Society of America: treatment of tuberculosis. Am J Respir Crit Care Med. 2003;167:603-62. Used with permission.

- BCG is indicated for children who are at high risk of intimate and prolonged exposure to *M tuberculosis*.
- BCG is not recommended for HIV-positive adults or children.

Nontuberculous Mycobacteria

Mycobacteria other than *M tuberculosis* and *Mycobacterium leprae* are commonly classified as *nontuberculous mycobacteria* (NTM) even though tubercle formation occurs. Most NTM have been isolated from natural water and soil. Human-to-human spread has not been documented. Natural waters are the source for most human infections caused by *Mycobacterium avium* complex; some cases are likely acquired from hospital tap water. Colonization or a saprophytic state of NTM is uncommon. NTM disease is not reportable in the United States.

Table 23-24 First-Line Drugs for Tuberculosis[a,b]

Drug	Daily Children[d]	Daily Adults	2 Times Weekly[c] Children[d]	2 Times Weekly[c] Adults	3 Times Weekly[c] Children[d]	3 Times Weekly[c] Adults	Adverse Reactions	Monitoring
INH[e] (maximal dose, mg)	10-20 (300)	5 (300)	20-40 (900)	15 (900)	20-40 (900)	15 (900)	Liver enzyme elevation, hepatitis, peripheral neuropathy, mild effects on central nervous system, drug interactions	Baseline measurements of liver enzymes for adults. Repeat measurements if baseline results are abnormal, if patient is at high risk of adverse reactions, if patient has symptoms of adverse reactions
RIF[f] (maximal dose, mg)	10-20 (600)	10 (600)	10-20 (600)	10 (600)	10-20 (600)	10 (600)	GI upset, drug interactions, hepatitis, bleeding problems, flulike symptoms, rash	Baseline measurements for adults: complete blood cell count, platelets, liver enzymes. Repeat measurements if baseline results are abnormal, if patient has symptoms of adverse reactions
PZA[g] (maximal dose, g)	15-30 (2)	15-30 (2)	50-70 (4)	50-70 (4)	50-70 (3)	50-70 (3)	Hepatitis, rash, GI upset, joint aches, hyperuricemia, gout (rare)	Baseline measurements for adults: uric acid, liver enzymes. Repeat measurements if baseline results are abnormal, if patient has symptoms of adverse reactions
EMB[h]	15-25	15-25	50	50	25-30	25-30	Optic neuritis	Baseline & monthly tests: visual acuity, color vision
SM[i] (maximal dose, g)	20-40 (1)	15 (1)	25-30 (1.5)	25-30 (1.5)	25-30 (1.5)	25-30 (1.5)	Ototoxicity (hearing loss or vestibular dysfunction), renal toxicity	Baseline & repeat as needed: hearing, kidney function

Abbreviations: EMB, ethambutol; GI, gastrointestinal tract; INH, isoniazid; PZA, pyrazinamide; RIF, rifampin; SM, streptomycin.
[a] Adjust weight-based dosages as weight changes.
[b] INH, RIF, PZA, and EMB are administered orally; SM is administered intramuscularly.
[c] Directly observed therapy should be used with all regimens administered 2 or 3 times weekly.
[d] Younger than 12 years.
[e] Hepatitis risk increases with age and alcohol consumption. Pyridoxine can prevent peripheral neuropathy.
[f] Severe interactions with methadone, oral contraceptives, and many other drugs. Drug colors body fluids orange and may permanently discolor soft contact lenses.
[g] Treat hyperuricemia only if patient has symptoms.
[h] Not recommended for children too young to be monitored for changes in vision unless tuberculosis is drug resistant.
[i] Avoid or decrease dose in adults older than 60 years.
From Centers for Disease Control and Prevention, Division of Tuberculosis Elimination: core curriculum on tuberculosis. 3rd ed. 1994.

Table 23-25 Targeted Tuberculin Testing for Latent Tuberculosis Infection

Prophylactic Group Description	PPD, mm
Persons with known or suspected HIV infection	≥5
Close contacts of person with infectious TB	≥5
Persons with chest radiographic findings suggestive of previous TB & inadequate or no treatment[a]	≥5
Persons who inject drugs & are known to be HIV-negative	≥10
Persons with certain medical conditions or factors	≥10
Diabetes mellitus, silicosis, prolonged corticosteroid or other immunosuppressive therapy, cancer of the head & neck, hematologic & reticuloendothelial diseases (eg, leukemia & Hodgkin disease), end-stage renal disease, intestinal bypass or gastrectomy, chronic malabsorption syndromes, low body weight (≥10% below ideal)	
Persons in whom PPD converted from negative to positive within the past 2 y	[b]
Age <35 y in the following high-prevalence groups:	≥10
Foreign-born persons from areas of the world where TB is common (eg, Asia, Africa, Caribbean, & Latin America)	
Medically underserved, low-income populations including high-risk racial & ethnic groups (eg, Asians & Pacific Islanders, African Americans, Hispanics, & American Indians)	
Residents of long-term care facilities (eg, correctional facilities & nursing homes)	
Children <4 y	
Other groups identified locally as having an increased prevalence of TB (eg, migrant farm workers or homeless persons)	
Persons <35 y with no known risk factors for TB	≥15
Occupational exposure to TB (eg, health care workers & staff of nursing homes, drug treatment centers, or correctional facilities)	[c]
Close contacts with an initial PPD <5 mm & normal findings on chest radiography	<5
Circumstances suggest a high probability of infection	
Evaluation of other contacts with a similar degree of exposure demonstrates a high prevalence of infection	
Child or adolescent	
Immunosuppressed (eg, HIV infection)	

Abbreviations: HIV, human immunodeficiency virus; PPD, purified protein derivative of tubercle bacillus; TB, tuberculosis.

[a] Isolated calcified granulomas are excluded.

[b] Increase of ≥10 mm if person is younger than 35 years or is a health care worker; increase of ≥15 mm if person is 35 years or older.

[c] Appropriate cutoff for defining a positive reaction depends on the employee's individual risk factors for TB and on the prevalence of TB in the facility.

From Van Scoy RE, Wilkowske CJ. Antimicrobial therapy. Mayo Clin Proc. 1999;74:1038-48. Used with permission of Mayo Foundation for Medical Education and Research.

- Human-to-human spread has not been documented.
- NTM disease is not reportable in the United States.

Chronic pulmonary disease is caused most frequently by *M avium* complex and *Mycobacterium kansasii*. Pulmonary disease is more common in older adults, those with underlying COPD, smokers, alcohol abusers, and some children with cystic fibrosis. Another group of patients who develop pulmonary infection from *M avium* complex are white women in their 60s who are HIV-negative without preexisting lung disease. Most of these patients (>90%) demonstrate bronchiectasis or small nodules without predilection for any lobe. High-resolution CT may show associated multifocal bronchiectasis with small (<5 mm) nodular infiltrates. Bilateral nodular or interstitial lung disease (or both) or isolated disease in the right middle lobe or lingular disease is more predominant in elderly nonsmoking women. Hypersensitivity pneumonitis caused by exposure to *M avium* complex growing in a hot tub has been reported. *M*

avium complex is responsible for 5% of the cases of mycobacterial lymphadenitis in adults and more than 90% of the cases in children. Lymphadenopathy is usually unilateral and nontender. Disseminated disease caused by NTM presents as a fever of unknown origin in immunocompromised patients without AIDS.

- *M avium* complex infection occurs in bronchiectasis.

HIV-infected persons are at high risk of NTM infections. More than 95% of NTM disease in HIV-infected persons is caused by *M avium* complex. In those with AIDS, disseminated infection occurs in up to 40% and localized infection in 5%; dissemination is more likely in those with a CD4 cell count less than 50/mcL. The risk of disseminated infection is 20% per year when the CD4 cell count is less than 100/mcL. High fever and sweats are common, as are anemia and increased alkaline phosphatase levels. Dissemination is usually documented with positive blood cultures (sensitivity, 90%).

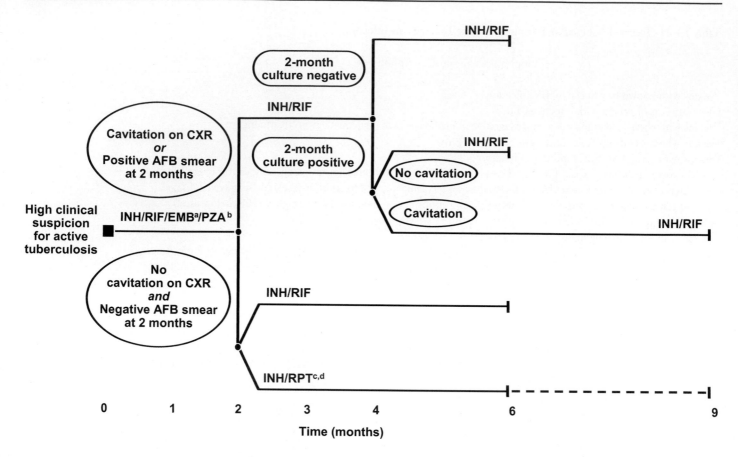

Figure 23-29. Treatment Algorithm for Tuberculosis. Patients in whom tuberculosis is proved or strongly suspected should have treatment initiated with isoniazid (INH), rifampin (RIF), pyrazinamide (PZA), and ethambutol (EMB) for the initial 2 months. Another smear and culture should be performed when 2 months of treatment has been completed. If cavities were seen on the initial chest radiograph (CXR) or if the acid-fast smear is positive at completion of 2 months of treatment, the continuation phase of treatment should consist of INH and RIF daily or twice weekly for 4 months (total of 6 months of treatment). If cavitation was present on the initial CXR and if the culture at the completion of 2 months of therapy is positive, the continuation phase should be lengthened to 7 months (total of 9 months of treatment). If the patient has HIV infection and the CD4+ cell count is <100/mcL, the continuation phase should consist of daily or 3-times-weekly doses of INH and RIF. In HIV-uninfected patients having no cavitation on CXR and negative acid-fast smears at completion of 2 months of treatment, the continuation phase may consist of either once-weekly doses of INH and rifapentine (RPT), or daily or twice-weekly doses of INH and RIF (total of 6 months) (bottom of figure). Patients receiving INH and RPT and whose 2-month cultures are positive should have treatment extended by an additional 3 months (total of 9 months). [a]EMB may be discontinued when results of drug susceptibility testing indicate no drug resistance. [b]PZA may be discontinued after it has been taken for 2 months (56 doses). [c]RPT should not be used in HIV-infected patients with tuberculosis or in patients with extrapulmonary tuberculosis. [d]Therapy should be extended to 9 months if the 2-month culture is positive. (From Blumberg HM, Burman WJ, Chaisson RE, Daley CL, Etkind SC, Friedman LN, et al. American Thoracic Society/Centers for Disease Control and Prevention/Infectious Diseases Society of America: treatment of tuberculosis. Am J Respir Crit Care Med. 2003;167:603-62. Used with permission.)

- Disseminated *M avium* complex in AIDS is more likely when the CD4 count is <50/mcL.
- A single blood culture in disseminated *M avium* complex infection has a sensitivity of 90%.

Mycobacterium kansasii is the second most common cause of non-tuberculous mycobacterial pulmonary disease in the United States. It primarily affects adult white men. Approximately 90% of patients with *M kansasii* disease have cavitary infiltrates. *Mycobacterium kansasii* infection can be clinically indistinguishable from tuberculosis;

however, symptoms may be less severe and more chronic than with tuberculosis. In HIV-negative patients, common symptoms are cough (90%), purulent sputum (85%), weight loss (55%), and dyspnea (50%). In immunocompromised patients, including those with AIDS, the lung is most commonly involved and symptoms include fever, chills, night sweats, cough, weight loss, dyspnea, and chest pain. Disseminated *M kansasii* infection occurs in 20% of HIV-positive patients who have *M kansasii* pulmonary disease.

- Cavitation occurs in 90% of patients with *M kansasii* infection.

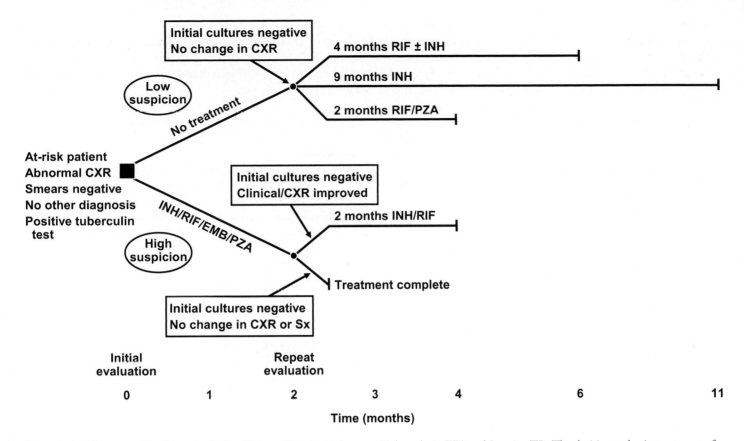

Figure 23-30. Treatment Algorithm for Active, Culture-Negative Pulmonary Tuberculosis (TB) and Inactive TB. The decision to begin treatment of a patient with sputum smears that are negative depends on the degree of suspicion that the patient has TB. If the clinical suspicion is high (bottom of figure), multidrug therapy should be initiated before acid-fast smear and culture results are known. If the diagnosis is confirmed by a positive culture, treatment can be continued to complete a standard course of therapy (see Figure 23-29). If initial cultures remain negative and treatment has consisted of multiple drugs for 2 months, there are 2 options depending on reevaluation at 2 months (bottom of figure): 1) If the patient demonstrates symptomatic or radiographic improvement without another apparent diagnosis, a diagnosis of culture negative tuberculosis can be inferred. Treatment should be continued with isoniazid (INH) and rifampin (RIF) alone for an additional 2 months. 2) If the patient demonstrates neither symptomatic nor radiographic improvement, prior TB is unlikely and treatment is complete after treatment including at least 2 months of RIF and pyrazinamide (PZA) has been administered. In low-suspicion patients not initially receiving treatment (top of figure), if cultures remain negative, the patient has no symptoms, and the chest radiograph is unchanged at 2-3 months, the 3 treatment options are 1) INH for 9 months, 2) RIF with or without INH for 4 months, or 3) RIF and PZA for 2 months. The RIF/PZA 2-month regimen should be used only for patients who are not likely to complete a longer course of treatment and can be monitored closely. CXR indicates chest radiograph; EMB, ethambutol; Sx, signs and symptoms. (From Blumberg HM, Burman WJ, Chaisson RE, Daley CL, Etkind SC, Friedman LN, et al. American Thoracic Society/Centers for Disease Control and Prevention/Infectious Diseases Society of America: treatment of tuberculosis. Am J Respir Crit Care Med. 2003;167:603-62. Used with permission.)

Specific skin tests are not available for the diagnosis of NTM. Routine cultures of sputum, blood, or stool are not recommended for asymptomatic patients. All specimens positive for acid-fast bacilli must be considered to indicate *M tuberculosis* until final culture results are available. Bronchoscopy or open lung biopsy is required for diagnosis in nearly half the cases. Therapy fails in half the patients. More than 80% of patients remain symptomatic, and 60% do not tolerate the initial multidrug regimen. Treatment of infections caused by NTM should be undertaken by a physician who specializes in infections caused by mycobacteria. The macrolides azithromycin and clarithromycin are important in the treatment of infections with *M avium* complex. Isoniazid is not used to treat infection with *M avium* complex. The current recommendation for treatment of pulmonary

disease caused by *M kansasii* in adults is to use isoniazid, rifampin, and ethambutol. In patients who are unable to tolerate 1 of these 3 drugs, clarithromycin can be substituted. Pyrazinamide is avoided because all isolates are resistant.

- Isoniazid is not used to treat infection with *M avium* complex.
- Macrolides are important in the therapy for infections with *M avium* complex, and rifampin is clinically useful for *M kansasii*.

Toxicity From Antituberculous Drugs
Isoniazid, rifampin, ethambutol, and pyrazinamide are considered first-line antituberculous medications. These 4 medications are the foundation of numerous treatment regimens for tuberculosis. Each

has its own potential toxicity, and each can potentiate toxicity when used in combination. Hepatitis (AST usually >5 times normal value) is the most common important adverse effect from antituberculous medications and is distinct from the mild elevation in transaminases which occur in up to 20% of patients receiving these medications (AST usually <3 times normal value). In adults receiving these medications, it is important to assess baseline liver function, creatinine level, complete blood cell count, and uric acid (if pyrazinamide is used) and to perform an ophthalmic examination (if ethambutol is used) before antituberculous therapy is begun. All patients should be evaluated periodically for adverse reactions to the drugs (Table 23-24).

Isoniazid

Clinically significant hepatitis is seen in less than 1% of patients receiving isoniazid, with the incidence increasing with age. Middle-aged and black females are at higher risk. Hepatitis is more likely in patients who are "rapid acetylators," and neuritis is more likely in those who are "slow acetylators." Isoniazid also causes skin rash, purpura, drug-induced systemic lupus erythematosus, seizures, optic neuritis, and arthritis. The addition of pyridoxine is recommended for patients with neuropathy (eg, patients with diabetes mellitus, uremia, alcoholism, or malnutrition), pregnancy, or seizure disorder. Before initiating treatment of LTBI, baseline laboratory testing is indicated in patients with known liver disease or HIV infection, in pregnant women, in women in the immediate postpartum period (within 3 months after delivery), and in persons who drink alcohol regularly. Routine monitoring of liver function during treatment is recommended for patients with abnormal baseline liver function tests or those at risk of liver disease. Therapy should be stopped if the AST value is more than 5 times normal or 3 times more than the baseline value. Alcohol consumption should be avoided.

- The incidence of isoniazid-induced hepatitis increases with age.
- Isoniazid causes hepatitis and peripheral neuropathy.
- Stop therapy if AST is >5 times normal or 3 times above baseline.

Rifampin

The overall incidence of serious side effects with rifampin is 1%. Gastrointestinal tract upset is the most common reaction. Larger or intermittent doses (>10 mg/kg) (or both) are associated with thrombocytopenia, flulike syndrome, hemolytic anemia, and cholestatic jaundice. Skin rash can occur, and use of the drug needs to be stopped for persistent rash. Hepatitis can also occur. Harmless orange discoloration of body secretions occurs. Rifampin induces liver microsomal enzymes, and it increases the metabolism of contraceptive pills, corticosteroids, warfarin, oral hypoglycemic agents, theophylline, anticonvulsant agents, ketoconazole, cyclosporine, methadone, and antiarrhythmic drugs (digitalis, quinidine, verapamil, and mexiletine); therefore, dosages of these drugs may have to be increased.

- Rifampin: gastrointestinal tract upset is the most common side effect.
- Rifampin induces liver microsomal enzymes.

Pyrazinamide

The most serious adverse reaction of pyrazinamide is liver damage. Hyperuricemia is common but gout is not, although arthralgias are reported occasionally. Skin rash and gastrointestinal tract upset are sometimes encountered.

- Pyrazinamide: liver damage is the most serious adverse reaction.

Ethambutol

Ethambutol in doses greater than 25 mg/kg causes retrobulbar neuritis in less than 3% of patients; symptoms usually are observed 2 months after therapy has been initiated. Because ophthalmoscopic findings are normal in these patients, symptoms are important (blurred vision, central scotoma, and red-green color blindness). These symptoms precede changes in visual acuity. Optic neuritis is best prevented by giving a lower dose (15 mg/kg) during the maintenance phase of treatment. Renal failure prolongs the half-life of the drug and increases the frequency of ocular toxicity.

- Ethambutol: Retrobulbar neuritis (dose-related) is the most frequent and serious side effect.
- Renal failure prolongs the half-life of the drug and increases the frequency of ocular toxicity.

Streptomycin

Because streptomycin is excreted by the kidneys, the dosage should be decreased in renal insufficiency. The most common adverse side effect is vestibular toxicity, which causes vertigo. Hearing loss may also occur. These side effects are more likely in the elderly (>60 years). Ototoxicity and nephrotoxicity are related to both the cumulative dose and the peak serum concentration. Streptomycin should be avoided in pregnancy.

- Streptomycin: nephrotoxicity and vestibular toxicity are more common in persons >60 years.
- Streptomycin should be avoided in pregnancy.

Fungal Diseases of the Lung

Serious fungal infections are found at autopsy in 2% of patients overall, in up to 10% of those with solid tumors, and in up to 40% of those dying of leukemia. Among renal transplant patients, 15% have a fungal infection at some time during the posttransplant course. Almost all fungi produce granulomas. The saprophytic state of fungi is a common problem, particularly with *Aspergillus* species. Pulmonary manifestations are described here. Treatment of the mycoses is discussed in Chapter 15 ("Infectious Diseases").

Histoplasmosis

Histoplasma capsulatum infections are more common in the Mississippi, Ohio, and St. Lawrence river valleys than elsewhere. Infection is by inhalation of fungal spores, which are especially numerous in chicken coops, dusty areas, starling roosts, bat-infested caves, and decayed wood. Clinically, patients may present with asymptomatic infection, acute pneumonia or acute respiratory distress syndrome (ARDS), disseminated infection (AIDS or other immunocompromised hosts), chronic cavitary disease (underlying lung structural defects), or late complications of mediastinal granuloma, mediastinal fibrosis, broncholithiasis, or residual pulmonary nodules seen on CXR. The nodules may be calcified, and hilar adenopathy may be seen.

- Typical clinical scenario for *Histoplasma* pneumonitis: Exposure to chicken coops, dusty areas, starling roosts, bat-infested caves, and decayed wood in the Mississippi River Valley, with late complications that include chronic cavitary disease, mediastinal granulomas, calcified hilar adenopathy, and hilar adenopathy.

Coccidioidomycosis

The endemic zone for *Coccidioides immitis* extends from northern California to Argentina. Infections are more common when dry windy conditions exist, with epidemics occurring in the dry hot months after the rainy season, often after the soil has been disturbed. Clinically, patients may be asymptomatic, with CXR showing nodules or thin-walled cavities, or they may have a range of symptomatic disease: valley fever (erythema nodosum, erythema multiforme, arthralgia, arthritis, and eosinophilia), acute pneumonia (mildly symptomatic flulike illness in 40% of patients), disseminated disease (more common in Filipinos, African Americans, Mexicans, and immunocompromised patients), and chronic cavitary disease. Infection acquired late during pregnancy is associated with higher maternal and fetal mortality. Chronic thin-walled cavities are associated with increased risk of hemoptysis.

- Typical clinical scenario for coccidioidomycosis pneumonitis: A patient from the southwestern United States presents with erythema nodosum, arthalgias and arthritis, acute pneumonia, and chronic cavitary disease.

Blastomycosis

Blastomyces dermatitidis infections occur most commonly in the southern, south-central, and Great Lakes states. Persons and animals (canines) in contact with soil are more likely to be infected. The male to female ratio is 10:1. Patients with pulmonary infections can be asymptomatic or have acute pneumonia (mimicking an acute bacterial pneumonia), chronic progressive pneumonia, or extrapulmonary dissemination (typically to skin, bone, prostate, or central nervous system). The most characteristic CXR finding is a perihilar mass that mimics carcinoma. Sputum analysis with 10% potassium hydroxide is helpful in diagnosis. Laryngeal blastomycosis can resemble cancer.

- Typical clinical scenario for blastomycosis pneumonitis: A person has contact with the soil, lives in 1 of the Great Lakes states, and has the CXR finding of a perihilar mass mimicking carcinoma.

Cryptococcosis

Cryptococcus neoformans is a unimorphic fungus that is widely distributed in the soil and excreta of pigeons and other animals. In humans, it may exist as a saprophyte in preexisting lung disease, but one-third to one-half of patients with cryptococcosis are immunosuppressed. The lung is the portal of entry, but the most common clinical presentation is subacute or chronic meningitis (the common cause of death). Diseases that predispose to cryptococcosis include an immunocompromised state, Hodgkin and non-Hodgkin lymphomas, leukemia, sarcoidosis, and diabetes mellitus. The onset of neurologic symptoms, fever, nausea, and anorexia is insidious. Pulmonary features include chest pain (45%), dyspnea (25%), night sweats (25%), cough with scant sputum (15%), and hemoptysis (7%). Nodular infiltrates with cavitation, especially in the lower lobes, occasional hilar adenopathy, and a solitary mass may be found. In non-AIDS patients with pulmonary cryptococcosis, masses and air space consolidation are common and atelectasis, lymphadenopathy, and pleural effusion or empyema are relatively rare. The cerebrospinal fluid should be examined in almost all patients who have organisms in respiratory secretions.

- Typical clinical scenario for *C neoformans* pneumonitis: An immunocompromised patient or a patient with diabetes who has nodular, cavitary, and patchy infiltrates on CXR, fever, and pulmonary and neurologic symptoms.
- The cerebrospinal fluid should be examined in almost all patients who have organisms in respiratory secretions.

Aspergillosis

Aspergillus fumigatus, A flavus, and *A niger* are responsible for several pulmonary manifestations. The clinical forms include 1) allergic bronchopulmonary aspergillosis, 2) hypersensitivity pneumonitis in red cedarwood workers, 3) mycetoma or fungus ball in preexisting lung disease, 4) locally invasive (chronic necrotizing) aspergillosis of lung tissue, 5) tracheobronchial form in immunocompromised or HIV-infected persons and lung transplant recipients (at anastomotic site), 6) disseminated, 7) bronchocentric granulomatosis, and 8) saprophytic. The organism frequently colonizes the respiratory tract in patients with lung disease. Invasive aspergillosis in immunosuppressed hosts is the most serious form of infection and occurs mainly in granulocytopenic patients with a hematologic malignancy. The occurrence of life-threatening complications in patients with invasive fungal pneumonia is closely related to rapid granulocyte recovery. The presence of *Aspergillus* in respiratory secretions is not diagnostic; tissue invasion should be documented. Generally, diagnosis of invasive infection is based on microscopic examination of tissue. However, for patients in whom tissue confirmation is risky (eg, patients with thrombocytopenia following bone marrow transplant), clinical grounds may be sufficient to institute antifungal therapy. Recently, a serum assay to detect a product of hyphae growth (galactomannan) has become available. Its role in the diagnostic algorithm of invasive aspergillosis is evolving: The test appears to have value in ruling out the diagnosis, but it has limited sensitivity in confirming active disease.

Aspergilloma is a mass of fungal hyphae in preexisting lung cavities, almost always in the upper lobes. The major symptoms include hemoptysis, cough, low fever, and weight loss. CXR and CT show a meniscus of air around the fungus ball. Because surgical therapy of aspergilloma has a high morbidity and mortality, another therapeutic option is the intracavitary instillation of amphotericin.

- Typical clinical scenario for pulmonary invasive aspergillosis: Fever and pulmonary infiltrates with prolonged neutropenia in acute leukemias and Hodgkin disease.

- Aspergillosis: tissue invasion should be documented.
- Aspergilloma (fungus ball) occurs in previously damaged lung; hemoptysis is a serious complication.

Zygomycosis (Mucormycosis)

Zygomycosis is caused by fungi in the order Mucorales (class Phycomycetes). Serious infections of the upper respiratory tract, lungs, central nervous system, and skin occur in patients with severe diabetes mellitus, hematologic malignancy, skin or mucosal injury, or immunocompromised status. The organism invades blood vessels in the lungs and causes hemoptysis. CXR may show patchy infiltrates, consolidation, cavitation, and effusions. Bronchial stenosis is a peculiar complication of zygomycosis.

- Zygomycosis: immunocompromised and diabetic patients.
- Propensity to invade blood vessels; hemoptysis is common.

Candidiasis

Candida species are present in the oropharynx of 30% of normal persons, in the gastrointestinal tract of 65%, and in the vagina of up to 70% of women. Systemic candidiasis is found at autopsy in as many as 25% of patients with leukemia. Risk factors for developing candidiasis include diabetes mellitus, cancer, cirrhosis, renal failure, blood dyscrasia, cytotoxic therapy, intravenous or urinary catheters, intravenously administered antibiotics, prostheses, cachexia, burns, and HIV infection. Lung involvement is relatively rare, and CXR shows patchy or diffuse infiltrates. *Candida* bronchitis, an occupational disease of tea tasters, is manifested by low-grade fever, cough, and patchy infiltrates.

- Typical clinical scenario for candidiasis: A patient with hematologic malignancy and prolonged granulocytopenia.
- Lung involvement is uncommon; patchy or diffuse lung infiltrates.

Sporotrichosis

Sporothrix schenckii is a dimorphic fungus that exists as a saprophyte in soil, plants, wood, straw, sphagnum moss, decaying vegetation, cats, dogs, and rodents. Sporotrichosis is an occupational hazard of farmers, florists, gardeners, horticulturists, and forestry workers. Infection is by cutaneous inoculation and inhalation. Cutaneous nodules along lymphatic vessels may appear in 75% of patients. Hematogenous dissemination to the lungs is rare, but inhalation-induced pulmonary disease mimics cavitary tuberculosis.

- Sporotrichosis: occupational hazard of florists, horticulturists, and gardeners.
- Lymphangitis of the skin and subcutaneous nodules.
- Pulmonary infection mimics chronic tuberculosis.

Pneumocystis jiroveci *Infection*

Pneumocystis jiroveci (formerly *Pneumocystis carinii*) is a fungus with trophic and cyst forms. *Pneumocystis jiroveci* infections occur in immunosuppressed patients, especially those with AIDS (CD4 <200/mcL) or malignancy, and after organ transplant. Infection causes alveolar and interstitial inflammation and edema with plasma cell infiltrates. Clinical features in patients with AIDS include the gradual onset of dyspnea, fever, tachypnea, and hypoxia. In patients without AIDS, the onset is more abrupt and progression to respiratory failure occurs quickly. Patients typically have relatively normal findings on lung examination and a patchy or diffuse interstitial or alveolar process on CXR. An upper lobe process is seen on CXR of patients receiving pentamidine aerosolized prophylaxis. The typical CT finding is ground-glass attenuation. However, this classic radiographic presentation is less frequent now and is being replaced by cystic lung disease, spontaneous pneumothorax, and an upper lobe distribution of parenchymal opacities. Routine laboratory data are unhelpful. The diagnosis can be made with induced sputum, bronchoalveolar lavage, or lung biopsy. Induced sputum or bronchoalveolar lavage is an excellent method for diagnosis, and the cyst stains best with methenamine silver nitrate. The number of organisms present in immunocompromised patients without AIDS is smaller and overall mortality is greater.

- Typical clinical scenario: AIDS patient with CD4 <200/mcL and gradual onset of dyspnea, fever, tachypnea, hypoxia, cyanosis, cough; relatively normal findings on lung examination; and a patchy or diffuse interstitial or alveolar process on CXR.
- An upper lobe process is seen on CXR of patients receiving pentamidine aerosolized prophylaxis.

Parasitic Diseases

Parasitic infections of the lung are less common in the United States than in other parts of the world. Travelers to regions where parasitic infestations are endemic may become infected and, when they return to the United States, present with difficult diagnostic problems. However, dirofilariasis is indigenous to the eastern and southeastern United States. Other parasitic infections, including helminthic infestations, also occur in the United States. The parasites most likely to cause pulmonary infections include *Paragonimus westermani* (paragonimiasis), *Echinococcus granulosus* (echinococcosis or hydatid disease), *Dirofilaria immitis* (dirofilariasis), *Schistosoma japonicum* and *Schistosoma mansoni* (schistosomiasis), and *Entamoeba histolytica* (amebiasis). Protozoal infections are more likely in patients whose cellular immunity is suppressed.

Dirofilariasis, caused by the heartworm that infects dogs, is transmitted to humans by mosquitoes. The disease is endemic to the Mississippi River Valley, the southeastern United States, and the Gulf Coast. Characteristically, the infection manifests as a well-defined solitary lung nodule or multiple lung nodules 1.5 to 2.5 cm in diameter. Eosinophilia occurs in less than 15% of patients. Serologic tests may aid in the diagnosis.

Echinococcosis has occurred in Alaska and the southwestern United States. Lung disease presents with the CXR findings of well-defined round or oval cystic or solid lesions up to 15 cm in diameter. Rupture of the cysts can cause anaphylactic shock, hypersensitivity reactions, and seeding of adjacent anatomical areas. Liver involvement (in 40% with lung disease) and positive serologic findings are common.

Paragonimiasis is more likely in immigrants from Southeast Asia, but sporadic cases occur in the United States. It is transmitted typically through consumption of raw or undercooked crabs or crayfish. Respiratory features resemble those of chronic bronchitis, bronchiectasis, or tuberculosis. Profuse brown-colored sputum and hemoptysis can be seen. Pleural effusion is relatively common, and peripheral eosinophilia is common. Ova can be found in pleural fluid, bronchial wash, or sputum.

Schistosomiasis is not acquired in the United States. The infection leads to gradual development of secondary pulmonary hypertension caused by occlusion of the pulmonary arterial tree by the parasite. Cor pulmonale develops in 5% of patients.

Amebiasis may present as lobar pneumonia or lung abscess (pleuropulmonary complications are almost always right-sided). Rupture into the bronchial tree (hepatobronchial fistula) may be followed by expectoration of sputum that resembles anchovy paste or chocolate. Rupture of the liver abscess into the pleural space causes empyema along with respiratory distress in many patients. Pericardial involvement can also occur.

Strongyloidiasis involving the lungs can mimic asthma with eosinophilia. Risk factors include corticosteroid use, age older than 65, chronic lung disease, and chronic debilitating illness. Pulmonary signs and symptoms include cough, shortness of breath, wheezing, and hemoptysis in more than 90% of patients and pulmonary infiltrates in 90%. In a series of 20 patients with pulmonary strongyloidiasis, ARDS developed in 9 patients (45%). Preexisting chronic lung disease and the development of ARDS are important predictors of a poor prognosis.

- Typical clinical scenario for dirofilariasis: A patient from the Mississippi River Valley, southeastern United States, or Gulf Coast has a solitary lung nodule or multiple nodules. Dirofilariasis is transmitted by mosquitoes.
- Schistosomiasis: pulmonary hypertension.
- Amebiasis: pleuropulmonary complications are almost always right-sided; rupture into the bronchial tree, with sputum that resembles anchovy paste or chocolate.
- Strongyloidosis: mimics asthma with eosinophilia.

Noninfectious Pulmonary Complications in AIDS

Infectious pulmonary complications are discussed in Chapter 15 ("Infectious Diseases"). The noninfectious pulmonary complications in AIDS are discussed below (also see Chapter 12, "HIV Infection").

Nonspecific interstitial pneumonitis represents 30% to 40% of all episodes of lung infiltrates in patients with AIDS. Its incidence has decreased with the institution of highly active antiretroviral therapy (HAART). More than 25% of patients with this problem have concurrent Kaposi sarcoma, previous experimental treatments, or a history of *P jiroveci* pneumonia or drug abuse. The clinical features are similar to those of patients with *P jiroveci* pneumonia. Histologic examination of the lung may show various degrees of edema, fibrin deposition, and interstitial inflammation with lymphocytes and plasma cells. This condition is self-limited and often needs no therapy.

- Nonspecific interstitial pneumonitis occurs in up to 40% of patients with AIDS, and *P jiroveci* pneumonia should be excluded.

Lymphocytic interstitial pneumonitis is caused by pulmonary infiltration with mature polyclonal B lymphocytes and plasma cells. It occurs most commonly in children and is diagnostic of AIDS when it occurs in a child younger than 13 years who is seropositive for HIV. Corticosteroid therapy may produce marked improvement. Pulmonary lymphoid hyperplasia has been reported in 40% of children with AIDS.

- Lymphocytic interstitial pneumonitis is diagnostic of AIDS when it occurs in a child younger than 13 years who is seropositive for HIV.

Cystic lung disease is more common in patients with *P jiroveci* infections and in those receiving aerosolized pentamidine therapy. Cystic lesions are more common in the upper and mid lung zones. Chest CT identifies these small or medium-size cystic lesions.

- Cystic lung disease is more common in patients with *P jiroveci* pneumonia receiving aerosolized pentamidine therapy.

Bilateral synchronous pneumothorax occurs with increasing frequency in patients with *P jiroveci* pneumonia and in those receiving aerosolized pentamidine therapy. Other causes of pneumothorax include Kaposi sarcoma, tuberculosis, and other infections. Pneumothorax in patients with AIDS has a poor prognosis.

- High incidence of bilateral synchronous pneumothoraces.

Pleural effusion is found in 25% of hospitalized patients with AIDS. Nearly one-third of the pleural effusions are due to noninfectious causes. Hypoalbuminemia is the leading cause of these effusions. Other important noninfectious causes include Kaposi sarcoma and atelectasis. Among the infectious causes, bacterial pneumonias, *P jiroveci* pneumonia, and *M tuberculosis* are important. Fungal infections can also produce pleural effusion. Large effusions are caused by tuberculosis and Kaposi sarcoma.

- Pleural effusion is caused by infections in two-thirds of hospitalized patients with AIDS.
- Kaposi sarcoma and tuberculosis cause large effusions.

Pulmonary hypertension has been found in patients with AIDS. It is more common in those with HLA-DR6 alleles. The mechanism is not clear, but HIV is thought to affect the endothelium directly and to cause vascular changes. The clinical, physiologic, and pathologic features are identical to those of primary pulmonary hypertension.

- Pulmonary hypertension is clinically identical to idiopathic pulmonary hypertension.

Kaposi sarcoma occurs with greater frequency among homosexuals with AIDS than among other patients with AIDS. It is believed to be caused by human herpesvirus 8. The incidence of its occurrence has diminished. Cutaneous lesions usually precede pulmonary Kaposi sarcoma. Previous or concurrent pulmonary opportunistic infections have been noted in more than 70% of patients with Kaposi sarcoma. Kaposi sarcoma occurs in the lungs of up to 35% of patients who have this tumor. The lung may be the only site in about 15% of patients. In most patients, the diagnosis of pulmonary Kaposi sarcoma is established only at autopsy. The diagnostic yield from bronchoscopy is 24% and from lung biopsy, 56%. Hemoptysis is an uncommon complication of Kaposi sarcoma, although endobronchial metastasis develops in 30% of patients. Multiple, discrete, raised, violaceous, or bright red tracheobronchial lesions can be seen on bronchoscopy. Bronchoscopic biopsy is associated with a high incidence of significant bleeding. CXR may show typical nodular infiltrates in less than 10% of patients. Pleural effusion is present in more than two-thirds of patients with lung involvement with Kaposi sarcoma. Clinically, pulmonary Kaposi sarcoma is indistinguishable from *P jiroveci* pneumonia or opportunistic pneumonia.

- Pulmonary Kaposi sarcoma is usually preceded by cutaneous lesions.
- Lung involvement due to Kaposi sarcoma occurs in up to 35% of patients with this neoplasm.
- Clinically, pulmonary Kaposi sarcoma is indistinguishable from *P jiroveci* pneumonia or opportunistic pneumonia.
- Multiple, discrete, raised, violaceous, or bright red tracheobronchial lesions can be seen on bronchoscopy.

Non-Hodgkin lymphoma involving the lungs is seen in less than 10% of patients with AIDS who develop lymphoma. The lymphoma in these patients is usually extranodal non-Hodgkin B-cell lymphoma. Lung involvement is a late occurrence. Nodules, masses, and infiltrates can be seen on CXR. A 6.5-fold increased incidence of primary lung cancer has been noted among HIV-infected and AIDS patients.

Pulmonary Diseases Pharmacy Review
Todd M. Johnson, PharmD

Drugs for Pulmonary Disease

Drug	Toxic/Adverse Effects	Drug Interactions	Comment
Bronchodilators 　Albuterol (Proventil HFA, 　　Ventolin HFA, Vospire ER) 　Epinephrine (Primatene) 　Formoterol (Foradil) 　Isoetharine (Bronkosol) 　Isoproterenol (Isuprel) 　Levalbuterol (Xopenex) 　Metaproterenol (Alupent) 　Pirbuterol (Maxair) 　Salmeterol (Serevent) 　Terbutaline (Brethine)	Palpitations, tachycardia, hyper-tension, arrhythmia, tremor, nervousness, headache, insomnia, gastroesophageal reflux disease, or pharyngitis	β-Blockers may inhibit effect of bronchodilators in asthmatic patients Tricyclic antidepressants & sympathomimetics may cause hypertension Isoproterenol or epinephrine may sensitize the myocardium to the effects of general anesthetic	Bronchodilators must be used with caution in patients with diabetes mellitus, cardiovas-cular disorders, hyperthyroid-ism, or seizure Use of β-blockers in asthmatics may precipitate asthma
Ipratropium 　　(Atrovent) 　Ipratropium with albuterol 　　(Combivent, Duoneb) 　Tiotropium (Spiriva)	Ipatropium may cause blurred vision & dry mouth		
Leukotriene receptor 　antagonists 　Montelukast 　　(Singulair) 　Zafirlukast 　　(Accolate) 　Zileuton (Zyflo)	Rarely may cause systemic eosinophilia with vasculitis, consistent with Churg-Strauss syndrome	Zafirlukast & zileuton can increase warfarin effects Zileuton can double theophylline concentrations	
Anti-inflammatory 　inhalant products 　Beclomethasone (QVAR) 　Budesonide (Pulmicort) 　Budesonide with formoterol 　　(Symbicort) 　Flunisolide (Aerobid) 　Fluticasone (Flovent HFA) 　Fluticasone with salmeterol 　　(Advair Diskus) 　Triamcinolone (Azmacort) 　Cromolyn (Intal) 　Nedocromil (Tilade)			Corticosteroids, cromolyn, & nedocromil are not effective for the relief of acute bronchospasm When systemic corticosteroids are withdrawn, inhaled corticosteroids do not provide systemic effects necessary to prevent symptoms of adrenal insufficiency

Pulmonary Diseases Pharmacy Review (continued)

Drugs for Pulmonary Tuberculosis

Drug	Toxic/Adverse Effects	Drug Interactions
Isoniazid	Hepatitis, hypersensitivity reactions, lupus-like reactions, peripheral neuropathy	Carbamazepine, cycloserine, phenytoin, levodopa, prednisone, rifampin, theophylline, warfarin
Rifampin	Orange discoloration of body fluids, leukopenia, thrombocytopenia, proteinuria, hypersensitivity	Aminosalicylic acid, anticoagulants, azole antifungals, barbiturates, benzodiazepines, contraceptives (oral), corticosteroids, cyclosporine, delavirdine, digoxin, estrogens, haloperidol, hydantoins, isoniazid, macrolides, progestins, protease inhibitors, quinine, sulfones, tacrolimus, theophylline, thyroid replacement
Rifabutin (Mycobutin)	Neutropenia, body fluid discoloration, GI intolerance, rash, uveitis, increased liver enzymes	Anticoagulants, azole antifungals, cyclosporine, delavirdine, hydantoins, macrolides, methadone, nelfinavir, quinine, theophylline
Pyrazinamide	Hepatitis, hyperuricemia, nausea, anorexia, polyarthralgia	Ethionamide, probenecid, zidovudine
Ethambutol (Myambutol)	Optic neuritis, hyperuricemia	Aluminum salts
Cycloserine (Seromycin)	CNS (somnolence, headache, tremor, psychosis, seizures)	Isoniazid
Para-aminosalicylic acid	Skin rash, GI intolerance, hypersensitivity	
Acyclovir (Zovirax)	Malaise, nausea, vomiting, diarrhea, phlebitis (IV)	
Famciclovir (Famvir)	Headache, dizziness, nausea, diarrhea, fatigue	Probenecid
Valacyclovir (Valtrex)	Nausea, headache, diarrhea, dizziness	
Amantadine	Nausea, dizziness, light-headedness, insomnia	
Rimantadine (Flumadine)	Insomnia, dizziness, nervousness, nausea, vomiting	
Foscarnet (Foscavir)	Renal impairment, leukopenia, electrolyte disturbances, seizures, fever, anemia, headache, nausea, vomiting	Nephrotoxic drugs
Cidofovir (Vistide)	Renal impairment, neutropenia, ocular hypotony, headache, asthenia, alopecia, rash, GI distress, anemia, infection, fever	Nephrotoxic drugs
Oseltamivir (Tamiflu)	Nausea, vomiting, diarrhea, bronchitis, abdominal pain, dizziness	
Zanamivir (Relenza)	Nausea, diarrhea, nasal signs & symptoms, bronchitis	

Abbreviations: CNS, central nervous system; GI, gastrointestinal tract; IV, intravenous.

Questions

Multiple Choice (choose the best answer)

1. A 56-year-old man who smokes 1 pack of cigarettes per day presents to your clinic with chronic cough and dyspnea. He has been smoking for 30 years. You suspect chronic obstructive pulmonary disease (COPD), and pulmonary function testing confirms this. Which of the following is true about the management of COPD?

   a. Inhaled glucocorticoid should be given to all patients to reduce airway inflammation.
   b. Bronchodilators must be given on a regular basis to prevent or reduce symptoms.
   c. Long-acting bronchodilators are just as effective as short-acting bronchodilators.
   d. The combinination of an inhaled β_2-agonist and an inhaled anticholinergic has been shown to result in greater and more sustained improvement in forced expiratory volume in 1 second (FEV_1) than either alone.
   e. Regular use of a β_2-agonist can modify the long-term decline in lung function.

2. A 45-year-old obese woman who smokes 1 pack of cigarettes per day presents to your emergency department with a sudden onset of dyspnea. She has a history of inflammatory bowel disease. She is febrile (temperature 38.0°C) and tachycardic (heart rate, 110 beats per minute). Her lung fields sound clear. A chest radiograph appears normal. Her only current medication is hormone replacement therapy, which she began after undergoing hysterectomy several days ago. You suspect pulmonary embolism (PE). Which of the following is *not* considered a definite risk factor for venous thromboembolism?

   a. Age
   b. Obesity
   c. Smoking history
   d. Inflammatory bowel disease
   e. Hormone replacement therapy

3. For the patient in question 2, you proceeded with a CT scan of the chest with contrast medium and followed a PE protocol. The CT angiogram, however, was negative for PE. What should you do next?

   a. PE has been ruled out and no further testing is needed.
   b. Repeat CT angiography in 2 days.
   c. Proceed with pulmonary angiography.
   d. Perform duplex ultrasonography of the lower extremities.
   e. Perfom magnetic resonance angiography of the chest.

4. A 54-year-old man is being evaluated for dyspnea. Results of pulmonary function testing are as follows:

Component	Value	Percentage of Predicted Value
Total lung capacity (TLC), %	7.28	98
Residual volume (RV), %	2.57	102
Forced vital capacity (FVC), %	4.69	93
FEV_1, %	3.59	90
FEV_1/FVC, %	76.5	
Diffusing capacity for carbon monoxide (DLCO), %	8.8	34

These findings are most consistent with which of the following?

   a. Normal findings
   b. Pulmonary vascular abnormality
   c. Asthma
   d. Emphysema
   e. Late-stage interstitial lung disease (ILD) or usual interstitial pneumonitis (UIP)

5. A 47-year-old obese man presents with fatigue. His wife describes very loud and disruptive snoring, witnessed episodes of apnea, and frequent naps during permissive situations. His current medical conditions include hypertension, insulin resistance, hypogonadism, gastroesophageal reflux disease, and peripheral vascular disease. You suspect he has significant obstructive sleep apnea (OSA). Which of his medical conditions has *not* been independently associated with OSA?

   a. Hypertension
   b. Insulin resistance
   c. Hypogonadism
   d. Gastroesophageal reflux disease
   e. Peripheral vascular disease

6. A 20-year-old woman who has never smoked presents to your clinic for recurrent respiratory infections and recurrent sinusitis. She is presenting after her second bout of pancreatitis. On examination, she appears chronically malnourished. Pulmonary function testing suggests mild airflow obstruction that has progressed since last year. Which factor is *not* associated with accelerated decline in lung function?

   a. Female sex
   b. Respiratory tract colonization with methicillin-resistant *Staphylococcus aureus*
   c. Secondhand smoke exposure
   d. Poor nutritional status
   e. Pancreatic insufficiency

7. A 64-year-old man with emphysema presents to your clinic asking about possible surgical intervention for his significant

dyspnea at rest and exercise. You initially recommend a pulmonary rehabilitation program, in which he participated for 6 months. You then perform pulmonary function testing. The results are as follows (expressed as percentages of the predicted values): TLC 140%, FVC 40%, FEV_1 18%, and DLCO 19%. A CT scan of the chest shows a homogeneous distribution of emphysema. What would you now recommend?

a. Proceed with lung volume reduction surgery.
b. Proceed with lung volume reduction surgery, but use video-assisted thoracoscopy.
c. Repeat 6 months of pulmonary rehabilitation and reassess.
d. Try a 3-month trial of oral corticosteroids and then reassess.
e. Continue medical management without surgery.

8. A 54-year-old presents with progressive dyspnea. A chest radiograph shows a right-sided effusion. Results of thoracentesis and laboratory tests include the following:

Component	Value
Fluid glucose, mg/dL	45
Fluid protein, g/dL	3
Fluid lactate dehydrogenase (LDH), U/L	85
Serum LDH, U/L	200
Serum protein, g/dL	5.5

What is the most likely diagnosis?

a. Congestive heart failure
b. Uncomplicated parapneumonic effusion
c. Rheumatoid effusion
d. Benign asbestos-related pleural effusion
e. Pancreatitis

9. A 72-year-old woman who is a current smoker presents to the emergency department with worsening dyspnea and orthopnea over the past week. She has a previous history of congestive heart failure, but she has not been taking any β-blockers, angiotensin-converting enzyme inhibitors, or diuretics. Her room air oxygen saturation is 86%. A chest radiograph shows bilateral effusion that is worse on the right. You immediately begin administration of supplemental oxygen and intravenous furosemide. You later proceed with a right-sided thoracentesis because of persistent dyspnea. Results of thoracentesis and laboratory tests include the following:

Component	Value
Fluid glucose, mg/dL	85
Fluid protein, g/dL	2.5
Fluid LDH, U/L	75
Fluid triglyceride, mg/dL	20
Serum protein, g/dL	4.7

What is the next appropriate step in management?

a. Continue with diuresis.
b. Obtain a CT scan of the chest.
c. Insert a chest tube on the right.
d. Initiate therapy with a nonsteroidal anti-inflammatory drug.
e. Obtain a positron emission tomographic scan.

10. A 25-year-old woman who is a nonsmoker presents with a 1-week history of mild cough and dyspnea following a flulike illness with fever, arthralgias, and tender erythematous lesions on the anterior aspects of the legs. She has no history of asthma or notable past medical history. No environmental or occupational high-risk exposures are noted. Physical examination reveals clear lung fields without other abnormality. Chest radiography (CXR) demonstrates bilateral interstitial infiltrates with prominent bihilar adenopathy. On pulmonary function tests (PFTs), vital capacity (VC) is 88% of predicted and FEV_1 is 76% of predicted, with an FEV_1/VC ratio of 68%. Diffusing capacity for carbon monoxide (DLCO) is 83% of predicted. What would be the most appropriate therapy?

a. Systemic corticosteroids
b. Methotrexate
c. Cyclosporine
d. Azathioprine
e. Nonsteroidal anti-inflammatory medication

11. One year later, a right-sided Bell palsy and left arm weakness developed in the patient in question 10. On the basis of physical examination, cerebrospinal fluid findings, and MRI, the Bell palsy and arm weakness were most consistent with neurosarcoidosis. What would be the most appropriate first therapy?

a. Systemic corticosteroids
b. Methotrexate
c. Cyclosporine
d. Azathioprine
e. Nonsteroidal anti-inflammatory medication

12. A 62-year-old man, a former smoker, presents with a 2-year history of progressive dry cough and dyspnea. No occupational or environmental exposures are noted. Findings on physical examination include bibasilar Velcro rales and clubbing. CXR reveals prominent interstitial infiltrates in the middle and lower lung fields. The antinuclear antibody (ANA) titer is minimally elevated at 1:40. Serum protein electrophoresis demonstrates a polyclonal increase. Rheumatoid factor is also minimally elevated at 1:40. High-resolution chest CT demonstrates subpleural honeycombing with thickened alveolar septa in the lower lobes with bilateral mediastinal lymph nodes of 1.5 cm and no ground-glass opacities. On PFTs, VC is 62% of predicted, FEV_1 is 69% of predicted, the FEV_1/VC ratio is 78%, and DLCO is 52% of predicted. Which of the following treatments is likely to result in clinical improvement?

a. Interferon-γ
b. Systemic corticosteroids
c. Cyclophosphamide
d. Colchicine
e. No treatment has been found effective.

13. A 36-year-old man, a nonsmoker without prior known pulmonary disease or respiratory symptoms, presents with a several-hour history of dyspnea, dry cough, fever, chills, malaise, headache, and wheezing. The symptoms began while he was on the job at a plastic manufacturing company. His vital signs are stable. Scattered wheezes and bilateral crackles are detected on physical examination. CXR demonstrates bilateral mixed interstitial and alveolar reticular nodular infiltrates with apical sparing. Oxygen saturation is 94% on room air at rest. DLCO is 78% of predicted. On spirometry, VC is 65% of predicted, FEV_1 is 58% of predicted, and forced expiratory flow ($FEF_{25\%-75\%}$) is 25% of predicted. After the patient has been removed from the workplace and bronchodilator therapy started, which of the following treatments is likely to be needed for a period of months?

a. Levofloxacin
b. Azithromycin
c. Interferon-γ
d. N-acetylcysteine (NAC)
e. None of the above

14. A 52-year-old man, a current 75-pack-year smoker, is evaluated for acute dyspnea and right-sided chest pain. He denies having fever, chills, sweats, cough, sputum production, or hemoptysis. On physical examination, diminished breath sounds are noted throughout, on the right more than the left. On previous PFTs, FVC was 4.0 L (72% of predicted) and FEV_1 was 2.5 L (53% of predicted). CXR and chest CT demonstrated scattered interstitial changes with cystic and nodular abnormalities in addition to a right-sided pneumothorax. What is the best initial therapy?

a. Interferon-γ
b. Smoking cessation
c. Cyclophosphamide
d. Systemic corticosteroids
e. Azithromycin

15. A 68-year-old man, an ex-smoker, presents with a 6- to 12-month history of dry cough and dyspnea. He denies having fever, chest pain, or hemoptysis. No reflux or dysphagia are reported. His past medical history is notable for diabetes, hyperlipidemia, and benign prostatic hypertrophy. No important hobby, travel, or environmental exposures are noted. His past occupational history includes ship refurbishing while in the armed services. Medications include pravastatin, glyburide, and prazosin. His vital signs are stable. He is afebrile. No adenopathy is noted. Bibasilar crackles are present. Heart rhythm is regular.

The abdomen is normal, and no edema is noted. Clubbing is present. Blood test results are normal. PFTs demonstrate mild restriction and a low DLCO. CXR and high-resolution chest CT demonstrate bilateral lower lobe infiltrates, with some honeycombing, pleural thickening, diaphragmatic calcification, and an area of consolidation in the right lower lobe consistent with rounded atelectasis. What would you do next?

a. Begin therapy with systemic corticosteroids.
b. Begin therapy with interferon-γ.
c. Begin therapy with methotrexate.
d. Perform open lung biopsy via video-assisted thoracoscopy.
e. Observe only.

16. A 43-year-old woman, a nonsmoker, has had a several-month history of progressive dyspnea, cough, and chest tightness. No important occupational, travel, environmental, or hobby exposures are noted. Arthralgias are present. She denies having any reflux or dysphagia and is not taking any medication. The past medical history is notable for a left lower extremity deep venous thrombosis and pulmonary embolism following pregnancy at age 25. Her vital signs are stable. Examination reveals bibasilar crackles. Heart rhythm is regular. No murmurs are present. Joint examination is normal. No rashes, clubbing, cyanosis, or edema is present. CXR demonstrates bibasilar peripheral interstitial infiltrates. High-resolution chest CT confirms prominent ground-glass opacities without peripheral honeycombing or subpleural fibrosis. Results of the following are normal: complete blood cell count, manual differential, liver-associated enzymes, and renal function. Urinalysis demonstrates a rare leukocyte and hyaline cast. The ANA titer is elevated at 1:640. Serum protein electrophoresis demonstrates a polyclonal increase. Rheumatoid factor is also minimally elevated at 1:40. On PFTs, VC is 60% of predicted, FEV_1 is 56% of predicted, total lung capacity is 72% of predicted, residual volume is 75% of predicted, and DLCO is 62% of predicted. After proceeding with diagnostic bronchoscopy or video-assisted thoracoscopy (or both), which of the following medications should this patient begin using?

a. Systemic corticosteroids
b. Azathioprine
c. Azithromycin
d. Cyclophosphamide
e. Interferon

17. A 55-year-old man, a current cigarette smoker who has a 30-pack-year history, presents for evaluation of chronic cough. CXR shows a 1.3-cm nodule in the left upper lobe that was not present 3 years previously. Results of the physical examination and routine laboratory testing are unremarkable. Spirometry demonstrates moderate airflow obstruction with notable response to bronchodilator administration. The nodule enhances markedly on positron emission tomography (PET) scanning. Which of the following is the most appropriate next step in the evaluation of this pulmonary nodule?

a. Bronchoscopy with transbronchial biopsy
b. CXR and PET scan repeated in 1 year
c. Surgical resection
d. Transthoracic needle aspiration
e. Tuberculin skin test and fungal serology

18. A 62-year-old man with a 40-pack-year history of smoking presents with hemoptysis. On physical examination, temperature is 38.4°C, pulse rate is 100 beats per minute, respirations are 24 per minute, and blood pressure is 168/92 mm Hg. Signs of consolidation in the right upper lobe are detected on physical examination. No clubbing is noted. Laboratory findings include the following: hematocrit 35%, leukocyte count 14 × 10^9/L, serum creatinine 1.2 mg/dL, and serum calcium 11.4 mg/dL. CXR shows a 3-cm cavitated right upper lobe mass. What is the most likely diagnosis?

a. Small cell carcinoma
b. Adenocarcinoma
c. Non-Hodgkin lymphoma
d. Squamous cell carcinoma
e. Bronchoalveolar carcinoma

19. A 69-year-old man is brought to the emergency department because of increasing confusion, nausea, and vomiting for 1 week. On physical examination, the pulse rate is 110 beats per minute, blood pressure is 103/62 mm Hg, and temperature is 37.4°C. The patient is lethargic but responds to questions. Auscultation of the lungs is normal. Laboratory findings include the following: hemoglobin 11.0 g/dL, leukocyte count 8.6 × 10^9/L, serum sodium 115 mEq/L, serum potassium 4 mEq/L, serum creatinine 1.1 mg/dL, and serum osmolality 265 mOsm/kg. On urinalysis, sediment is normal, urinary sodium is 40 mEq/L, and urine osmolality is 600 mOsm/kg. CXR shows a large left hilar mass. What is the most likely diagnosis?

a. Small cell carcinoma
b. Adenocarcinoma
c. Lymphoma
d. Squamous cell carcinoma
e. Bronchoalveolar carcinoma

20. A 67-year-old woman is brought to the emergency department with chest pain and shortness of breath. Her husband states that she received a diagnosis of metastatic breast cancer 2 months ago. On physical examination, the pulse rate is 130 beats per minute, blood pressure is 84/40 mm Hg, and respirations are 30 per minute. Helical (spiral) CT angiography demonstrates an occlusive thrombus in the main pulmonary artery trunk extending into the right lower lobe and left upper lobe pulmonary arteries. Echocardiographic assessment reveals right-heart dilatation with an estimated right ventricular systolic pressure of 50 mm Hg. Which of the following is the most appropriate next step in the management of this patient?

a. Placement of a vena cava filter
b. Surgical pulmonary thromboendarterectomy
c. Thrombin inhibitor therapy
d. Thrombolytic therapy
e. Treatment with warfarin

21. A 35-year-old man complains of progressive dyspnea on exertion, nonproductive cough, and sinus congestion. His dyspnea is so severe that he is unable to play basketball. He denies hemoptysis. On physical examination, blood pressure is 130/70 mm Hg, pulse rate is 76 beats per minute, and respirations are 20 per minute. On examination, there is expiratory wheezing on forced expiration, nasal crusting, and saddle-nose deformity. His cytoplasmic–antineutrophil cytoplasmic autoantibody (c-ANCA) serology is 1:240 with a positive proteinase 3 (PR3) antibody. CXR shows several cavitary pulmonary nodules. The inspiratory flow-volume loop is normal, and the expiratory flow-volume loop is shown in the accompanying figure. What test is indicated next?

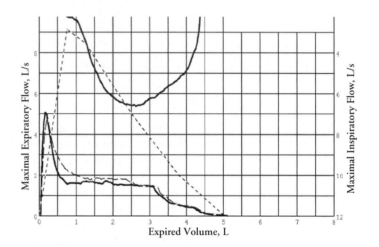

Question 21

a. PFTs repeated with methacholine challenge
b. Bronchoscopy
c. Rhinoscopy
d. Chest CT
e. Surgical biopsy of the pulmonary nodules

22. A 45-year-old woman is evaluated because of hemoptysis, photophobia, and loss of vision in the left eye. Seronegative rheumatoid arthritis was diagnosed 4 years ago. On physical examination, blood pressure is 138/84 mm Hg, pulse rate is 92 beats per minute, and respirations are 20 per minute. Physical examination reveals aphthous ulceration of the oral mucosa. Auscultation of the chest is normal. Laboratory findings include the following: leukocyte count, 11 × 10^9/L (with 85% neutrophils, 10% lymphocytes, 0% eosinophils, and 5% monocytes) and serum creatinine 1.1 mg/dL. CXR demonstrates bilateral upper lobe infiltrates. Which of the following diagnoses is most likely?

a. Behçet disease
b. Wegener granulomatosis
c. Churg-Strauss syndrome
d. Giant cell arteritis
e. Allergic bronchopulmonary aspergillosis

23. A 43-year-old man with acute promyelocytic anemia (M3) treated with all-*trans*-retinoic acid in addition to initial chemotherapy 2 weeks ago is admitted for hemoptysis. On physical examination, respirations are 24 per minute, pulse rate is 100 beats per minute, blood pressure is 112/64 mm Hg, and oxygen saturation is 85% on 2 L/min of oxygen. Bilateral crackles are noted on chest examination. CXR demonstrates extensive bilateral alveolar infiltrates. Laboratory findings include the following: hemoglobin 5.8 g/dL, leukocyte count 1.1×10^9/L, platelet count 9,000, serum creatinine 1.3 mg/dL, and c-ANCA and perinuclear-ANCA (p-ANCA) negative. The antistreptococcal O titer and anti–glomerular basement membrane antibody are normal. Urinalysis results are normal. Which of the following diagnoses is most likely?

a. Acute poststreptococcal glomerulonephritis
b. Microscopic polyarteritis
c. Wegener granulomatosis
d. Goodpasture syndrome
e. Diffuse alveolar hemorrhage

24. A 75-year-old woman is transferred to the intensive care unit for respiratory failure. She was admitted to the hospital 2 days earlier for dyspnea, cough, and fever of 2 weeks' duration. She is a current smoker; she has smoked for 30 years. She has underlying diabetes mellitus treated with an oral hypoglycemic agent. Her admission CXR shows consolidation of the left lower lobe, and she has been receiving intravenous levofloxacin. Blood cultures have been negative; however, a urine antigen test for *Legionella* species is positive. Despite several days of antimicrobial therapy, the patient continues to have fever and requires oxygen therapy. Which antibiotic could be added?

a. Trimethoprim-sulfamethoxazole
b. Penicillin G
c. Isoniazid
d. Rifampin
e. Gentamicin

25. A 32-year-old man with AIDS is receiving mechanical ventilation for severe hypoxemic respiratory failure due to *Pneumocystis jiroveci* pneumonia (PCP). Use of trimethoprim-sulfamethoxazole is stopped after 4 days because of a severe skin rash. Which of the following would you administer at this time?

a. Atovaquone
b. Primaquine plus clindamycin
c. Pentamidine

d. Dapsone
e. Trimethoprim

26. A 56-year-old woman who currently smokes one-half pack of cigarettes per day presents with worsening dyspnea on exertion, fever, and a cough that is productive with purulent sputum. Her symptoms started 5 days ago. COPD was diagnosed last year and her only medication is an albuterol inhaler, which she is using 2 to 3 times daily. Her vital signs are as follows: temperature of 38.3°C, blood pressure 135/70 mm Hg, pulse 102 beats per minute, and respiratory rate 18 per minute. She has crackles over the right lower lobe with increased egophony and faint wheezes anteriorly. Her room air oxygen saturation is 97% and her CXR shows a patchy right lower lobe infiltrate. You decide to treat her pneumonia on an outpatient basis with antibiotics, bronchodilators, smoking cessation, and a short course of oral corticosteroids. Which of the following antibiotics would *not* be appropriate?

a. Azithromycin
b. Cefuroxime
c. Ciprofloxacin
d. Levofloxacin
e. Amoxicillin/clavulanate

27. Which of the following persons has latent tuberculosis infection (LTBI) and should receive isoniazid therapy?

a. A diabetic patient 6 months after bariatric surgery who has 7 mm of induration on a tuberculin test and normal CXR findings
b. A third-year medical student with 8 mm of induration on a tuberculin test and normal CXR findings
c. A store clerk with 12 mm of induration on a tuberculin test and normal CXR findings
d. An elementary school teacher with 10 mm of induration on a tuberculin test and a left mid-lung calcified granuloma on CXR
e. A hemodialysis patient who has 12 mm of induration on a tuberculin test and pleural effusions on CXR

28. Influenza B is diagnosed in a 67-year-old man who has underlying asthma. Which is the most appropriate treatment for this patient?

a. Oseltamivir
b. Amantadine
c. Zanamivir
d. Rimantadine
e. Ribavirin

29. A 19-year-old woman received a bone marrow transplant for acute lymphocytic leukemia 2 weeks ago. She has had increasing dyspnea, dry cough, and intermittent fevers for the past 3 days. Her CXR shows diffuse interstitial infiltrates without

pleural effusions or nodules. She undergoes bronchoscopy with bronchoalveolar lavage, which demonstrates enlarged atypical cells with prominent intranuclear inclusions. What is the most likely cause of this patient's illness?

a. *Candida albicans*
b. *Pneumocystis jiroveci*
c. Cytomegalovirus
d. *Mycobacterium avium* complex
e. *Rhodococcus equi*

30. A 66-year-old woman with COPD has had progressive dyspnea on exertion, cough, mild weight loss, and low-grade fevers for the past 3 months. Symptoms began after she explored caves on her summer vacation. Recently she saw streaks of bright red blood mixed in her sputum. A CXR shows a new infiltrate in the right upper lobe with associated pleural thickening. A bronchoscopic biopsy sample of the infiltrate shows necrotizing granulomatous inflammation with small ovoid yeast forms visualized with methenamine silver stain. Culture results are not yet available. Which would be the most appropriate treatment for this patient?

a. Amphotericin B
b. Ketoconazole

c. Itraconazole
d. Fluconazole
e. Voriconazole

31. A 44-year-old diabetic woman is seen for fever and productive cough that have been present for 1 week along with severe headache and fluctuating mental status. She received a kidney-pancreas transplant 6 weeks ago. Her medications include prednisone, cyclosporine, and azathioprine. Results of laboratory studies include the following: white blood cell count 22×10^9/L with an increased number of neutrophils, hemoglobin 10.6 g/dL, and platelet count 317×10^9/L. A CT scan of the chest shows consolidation involving the right lower lobe and MRI of the head shows multiple enhancing lesions. A Gram-stained sputum specimen shows an increased number of neutrophils and normal bacterial flora. What organism is most likely to cause this constellation of findings?

a. *Mycobacterium kansasii*
b. *Staphylococcus aureus*
c. *Aspergillus fumigatus*
d. *Legionella pneumophila*
e. *Nocardia asteroides*

Answers

1. Answer d.

These are statements modified from the GOLD (Global Initiative for Chronic Obstructive Lung Disease) document. Inhaled glucocorticoid therapy is appropriate only for patients with symptomatic severe COPD with repeated exacerbations. Bronchodilators can be given either as needed or as scheduled to prevent or reduce symptoms. Regular use of long-acting bronchodilators has been shown to be more effective than treatment with short-acting bronchodilators. As of 2005, inhaled bronchodilators had not been shown to affect the long-term decline in lung function.

2. Answer c.

All the listed risk factors except smoking have clearly been shown to be a risk factor for development of venous thromboembolism. Smoking, however, remains controversial. Although the Nurses' Health Study suggested a correlation, several other studies, including the Framingham Study, failed to show a clear association. Several studies have highlighted the increased risk of thromboembolism in persons with inflammatory bowel disease (see NEJM 2003;349:1247-56).

3. Answer d.

This patient has a high clinical probability of PE. Since the CT angiogram was negative for PE, you should proceed with lower extremity duplex ultrasonography. If that is negative for PE, the recommendation is to proceed with pulmonary angiography. If the pulmonary angiogram is negative for PE, the diagnosis of PE is ruled out. The algorithm for patients with a low clinical probability of PE is slightly different: For these patients, if CT angiography is negative, the diagnosis of PE is considered to be ruled out and no further testing is necessary. (See the article cited in the answer to question 2.)

4. Answer b.

The results of pulmonary function testing show an isolated reduction in DLCO with normal lung volumes and spirometry results. Thus, the results are not normal and cannot suggest COPD, asthma, or late-stage ILD. Patients with ILD can present with isolated reduction in DLCO and normal spirometry results, but in the late stages of ILD/UIP, one would expect the total lung volumes to be reduced because of extensive fibrosis. Although asthmatics may have normal lung volumes and spirometry results, the DLCO should be normal to increased.

5. Answer e.

Although OSA has been independently associated with an increased risk of cardiovascular morbidity and numerous studies have shown the presence of endothelial dysfunction, it has not been associated with peripheral vascular disease. OSA, however, has been clearly associated with hypertension, insulin resistance, gastroesophageal reflux disease, and hypogonadism. Other independently associated conditions include atrial fibrillation and mood disorders.

6. Answer b.

This patient most likely has cystic fibrosis on the basis of the recurrent sinopulmonary infections and pancreatic insufficiency (as evidenced by recurrent pancreatitis and signs of chronic malnutrition). Ideally, any of the following should be performed to establish the diagnosis: sweat chloride test, transmembrane conductance regulator (CFTR) gene mutation analysis, or ion transport anaylsis. In addition to the factors listed in the question, the following factors have been identified as contributing to accelerated decline in lung function: poor physical fitness and respiratory tract colonization with *Pseudomonas aeruginosa* or *Burkholderia cepacia*.

7. Answer e.

This patient has severe emphysema and is considered a high-risk patient for lung volume reduction surgery. The National Emphysema Treatment Trial identified factors that increase the risk of death when surgery is compared with medical management: FEV_1 ≤20% of the predicted value and either DLCO ≤20% of the predicted value or a homogeneous distribution of emphysema. Thus, medical management is recommended for patients who meet those criteria.

8. Answer c.

The ratio of pleural fluid protein to serum protein indicates that the effusion is an exudate. This essentially eliminates choices *a* and *b*. Although the others would result in exudative effusion, the low glucose level limits the choices. The differential diagnosis for low pleural fluid glucose includes rheumatoid effusion, systemic lupus erythematosus empyema, esophageal rupture, malignant mesothelioma, and tuberculous pleurisy.

9. Answer a.

Although by the Light criteria the fluid is considered an exudate (ie, the ratio of fluid protein to serum protein is >0.5), the patient has received diuretics for the first time. The protein ratio can be affected by short-term use of diuretics, resulting in false elevation of the fluid protein level. In such cases, the fluid cholesterol level may be helpful: if it is less than 45 mg/dL, the fluid should be considered a transudate. Other findings that support the fluid being a transudate are the low LDH and the history consistent with short-term exacerbation of congestive heart failure.

10. Answer e.

Sarcoidosis is a granulomatous disease that most often affects the lung and lymph nodes. It can occur following a flulike illness, and it may be diagnosed on the basis of a specific constellation of symptoms and signs of Löfgren syndrome (erythema nodosum, bihilar adenopathy, fever, and polyarthritis) when present. In most other cases, the diagnosis of sarcoidosis requires a compatible history, findings of noncaseating granulomas in a biopsy specimen, and the exclusion of other possible causes of disease. Blood tests may show abnormalities, including hypercalcemia, anemia, and elevated liver enzymes if systemic involvement is present. ACE levels are neither specific nor sensitive as a diagnostic tool, but they may be helpful in following disease activity when they are elevated. Bronchoscopy can confirm granulomatous disease in more than 90% of patients with hilar adenopathy and parenchymal lung involvement. Although rales may be present when acute parenchymal interstitial changes occur, the typical examination finding is clear lung fields. The incidence, clinical course, and prognosis of sarcoidosis are also influenced by ethnic and genetic factors. CT findings may demonstrate small nodules with a bronchovascular and subpleural distribution, thickened intralobular septa, architectural distortion, or conglomerate masses. Viruses, mycobacteria, mycoplasma, and other environmental factors are possible etiologic risk factors for developing sarcoidosis. Tobacco use has not been associated with the development of sarcoidosis. Extrapulmonary involvement may include the heart, liver, spleen, eye, bone, skin, bone marrow, parotid glands, pituitary gland, and reproductive organs. This patient's presentation is most consistent with Löfgren syndrome, which should be treated symptomatically with a nonsteroidal anti-inflammatory agent. For progressive pulmonary and extrapulmonary disease, corticosteroids or immunosuppressive therapy should be considered.

11. Answer a.
Bell palsy is the most common manifestation of neurosarcoidosis. It occurs in 49% to 67% of patients with neurologic involvement. Treatment of Bell palsy as an isolated manifestation of neurosarcoidosis is controversial, but when treatment is required, the initial treatment of choice is systemic corticosteroids. Neurosarcoidosis, other than Bell palsy, clearly warrants immunosuppressive therapy, including cyclosporine, methotrexate, azathioprine, chlorambucil, or cyclophosphamide for patients who do not have a response to systemic corticosteroid therapy or who cannot tolerate the treatment because of adverse side effects.

12. Answer e.
The combination of lower lung field interstitial lung disease, lack of occupational exposure, duration of symptoms, and peripheral honeycombing make the diagnosis of idiopathic pulmonary fibrosis (IPF)–usual interstitial pneumonia (UIP) most likely. Favorable prognostic factors in IPF-UIP include age younger than 50, female sex, shorter duration of symptoms before presentation, presence of ground-glass opacities on chest CT, and lymphocytic bronchoalveolar lavage. PFTs in IPF-UIP show restrictive abnormalities. No more than 20% to 30% of patients with IPF-UIP are expected to have a response to corticosteroids or other immunosuppressive therapy. Oxygen has been shown to extend survival in COPD but not in IPF-UIP. Familial clusters of IPF-UIP suggest a potential genetic predisposition in some cases. Although subjective improvement in patients with IPF-UIP may be expected to be as high as 70%, objective improvement in PFTs occurs in no more than 20% to 30% of patients. Most studies require single-parameter improvements of at least 15% to 20% in VC, total lung capacity, or DLCO to be considered a response. Radiographic improvement generally does not occur. Currently, no treatment is available. Recent studies have not demonstrated benefit with the use of interferon-γ in the treatment of IPF-UIP. Ongoing studies are evaluating the role of NAC in the treatment of IPF-UIP. In a recently published preliminary study,

there was a suggestion of preserved lung function in IPF-UIP patients given NAC instead of placebo. All participants had also received prednisone and azathioprine.

13. Answer e.
Symptoms of acute hypersensitivity pneumonitis usually resolve 8 to 12 hours after exposure ceases but are likely to recur if exposure is repeated. Airflow obstruction may occur if occupational asthma and airway disease develop. Corticosteroid therapy is seldom required but may accelerate improvement in symptoms and gas exchange in severe cases. The use of bronchodilators is indicated when airflow obstruction occurs. Other immunomodulatory therapies, including interferon-γ, azithromycin (and other macrolides), and NAC, have not been shown to be effective for hypersensitivity pneumonitis. Isocyanates used in plastic manufacturing and automobile body repair can cause both occupational asthma and hypersensitivity pneumonitis. Skin testing, an IgE-mediated reaction, is not usually helpful for the diagnosis of hypersensitivity pneumonitis. In contrast, serum precipitins, with precipitating IgG antibodies, indicate a host response to specific antigens and may be correlated with disease activity in some patients. After removal from the offending antigen, physiologic abnormalities are expected to resolve within a few days for acute hypersensitivity pneumonitis and within a month for chronic hypersensitivity pneumonitis. The prognosis is generally excellent if permanent radiographic or physiologic abnormalities are not present at the onset of acute hypersensitivity pneumonitis.

14. Answer b.
This patient's presentation is most consistent with Langerhans cell histiocytosis. Absolute smoking cessation is the primary form of treatment. Stabilization or improvement with smoking cessation alone is expected to occur in up to two-thirds of patients. Other therapies, including systemic corticosteroids and immunosuppressive agents, have been used with limited success. No role has been described for plasmapheresis.

15. Answer e.
Asbestosis, in contrast to all other likely diagnoses, typically has a basilar predominance. Rounded atelectasis is suggestive of asbestos exposure. It should be noted that known or remembered histories of occupational asbestos exposure may not always be elicited, although when they are, they can be helpful. Common findings would include pleural plaques or diaphragmatic calcification (or both). Malignant mesothelioma is strongly associated with asbestos exposure but not with smoking. Pleural surfaces are generally abnormal and involved with asbestos-related parenchymal lung disease. However, in some instances, pleural and parenchymal abnormalities may occur independently of each other. Asbestos fibers typically are dormant for decades before pulmonary fibrosis develops. No clinical response is expected to corticosteroids or other medication for treatment of asbestos-related pulmonary fibrosis. Smoking in the setting of asbestos-related pulmonary fibrosis increases the rate of progression of fibrosis and the risk of developing bronchogenic carcinoma. Tuberculosis is not a common complication of asbestosis. No therapy has been shown to be effective in preventing progressive pulmonary fibrosis due to asbestos exposure.

16. Answer a.

This patient's presentation, medical history, physical examination findings, laboratory data, and radiographic findings are most consistent with nonspecific interstitial pneumonia (NSIP)-IPF, most likely related to a connective tissue disease. Therefore, therapy with systemic corticosteroids would be appropriate. PFTs are expected to demonstrate decreased VC with a preserved FEV_1/VC ratio, decreased lung volumes (including total lung capacity and residual volume), and decreased DLCO. Hypoxemia at rest or with exercise may also be present. Blood tests may demonstrate an elevated ANA, polyclonal gammopathy, slightly elevated rheumatoid factor, and elevated ESR. Serum precipitants for farmer's lung battery, including thermophilic actinomycetes, are not expected to be positive. The important differentiation is whether this patient has IPF-UIP, a steroid-unresponsive process, or NSIP-IPF, generally a steroid-responsive process. If there had been historical elements, examination findings, or laboratory data that did not suggest collagen vascular disease–associated or drug-induced lung disease, one would consider a diagnosis of idiopathic NSIP. The gound-glass opacities seen on high-resolution chest CT and the short duration of symptoms are more consistent with a steroid-responsive process such as NSIP-IPF in this relatively young female patient. Proceeding with additional diagnostic tests, including bronchoscopy or video-assisted thoracoscopy, would be the next appropriate step to confirm a diagnosis before treatment.

17. Answer c.

This patient presents with a new pulmonary nodule that was not present 3 years earlier as assessed by previous CXR. This is a new nodule that enhances on PET scanning in a patient with a notable smoking history. Thus, this nodule should be surgically resected.

18. Answer d.

Squamous cell carcinoma is the type of lung cancer most likely to be cavitated and to be associated with hypercalcemia caused by production of parathyroid hormone–related protein secreted by tumor cells. Proximal tracheobronchial involvement occurs in 65% of these malignancies, resulting in the earlier onset of symptoms such as cough, hemoptysis, and obstructive pneumonitis.

19. Answer a.

The patient has the syndrome of inappropriate antidiuretic hormone (SIADH), which is associated most commonly with small cell carcinoma. It is characterized by hyponatremia in association with euvolemia, low serum osmolality, and high urine osmolality. Other paraneoplastic syndromes associated with small cell carcinoma include Cushing syndrome, Lambert-Eaton myasthenic syndrome, and cerebellar degeneration.

20. Answer d.

Thrombolytic therapy is the initial treatment of choice for a hemodynamically unstable patient with a large occlusive pulmonary embolism. Anticoagulation with heparin would also be indicated; however, warfarin therapy would not be the next step. The patient is too unstable hemodynamically to consider surgical pulmonary thromboendarterectomy, which is usually reserved for patients with chronic thromboembolic pulmonary hypertension.

21. Answer b.

The combination of sinus congestion, saddle-nose deformity, and cavitated lung nodules with positive c-ANCA serology and PR3 antibody all confirm the diagnosis of Wegener granulomatosis. Surgical biopsy is not necessary. The flow-volume loop shows a normal inspiratory curve and flattening, with plateau of the expiratory curve that is consistent with a variable intrathoracic obstruction. Bronchoscopy is indicated because tracheobronchial stenosis occurs in 15% of patients who have Wegener granulomatosis. Bronchoscopic intervention, including dilation by rigid bronchoscopy, YAG laser treatment, or placement of silicone airway stents (or a combination of these) may be necessary to relieve the obstruction and the patient's dyspnea. Chest CT does not replace bronchoscopy, and there is no indication for methacholine challenge, which may be dangerous given the tracheal stenosis. Rhinoscopy would not be helpful in explaining the abnormal flow-volume loop.

22. Answer a.

The patient has features of Behçet disease. Her presenting symptoms consist of hemoptysis, seronegative arthritis, uveitis, and aphthous stomatitis. Arthritis occurs in about two-thirds of patients, and death due to severe hemoptysis occurs in 39%. Although the disease is typically characterized by remissions and exacerbations, a dramatic response can be expected with high doses of systemically administered corticosteroids and immunosuppressive therapy. This presentation would not be consistent with Wegener granulomatosis, giant cell arteritis, or allergic bronchopulmonary aspergillosis. Patients with Churg-Strauss syndrome usually have peripheral eosinophilia.

23. Answer e.

The most likely diagnosis is diffuse alveolar hemorrhage. The patient has received all-*trans*-retinoic acid as part of his chemotherapy induction, which increases the risk of diffuse alveolar hemorrhage. He is also thrombocytopenic. The diagnosis is established by bronchoscopy with bronchoalveolar lavage exhibiting progressively bloody return and showing more than 20% hemosiderin-laden macrophages. The normal results for antistreptococcal O titer and anti–glomerular basement membrane antibody essentially exclude poststreptococcal glomerulonephritis and Goodpasture syndrome.

24. Answer d.

The 3 most common organisms in patients with community-acquired pneumonia who require care in an intensive care unit are *Streptococcus pneumoniae*, *Legionella*, and *Haemophilus influenzae*. Macrolides and quinolones are the mainstays of therapy for legionellosis. Rifampin is highly active in this infection and is recommended as part of combination therapy (with a macrolide or a quinolone) for severely ill patients, especially those who are immunosuppressed.

25. Answer b.

Trimethoprim-sulfamethoxazole is the most effective treatment for severe PCP. Unfortunately, patients with allergies to sulfa cannot tolerate it and the incidence of side effects is high. Primaquine plus clindamycin is recommended instead of pentamidine in patients with severe PCP who cannot take trimethoprim-sulfamethoxazole. Atovaquone can be used in mild cases of PCP, and dapsone is recommended only for prophylaxis. The addition of corticosteroids benefits HIV-infected patients with PCP who have room air PaO_2 <70 mm Hg or an alveolar-arterial (A-a) oxygen gradient >35 mm Hg.

26. Answer c.

This current smoker with community-acquired pneumonia has underlying COPD. The most common pathogens to cause pneumonia in this setting include *Streptococcus pneumoniae*, followed by *Mycoplasma pneumoniae* and *Chlamydia pneumoniae*, *Haemophilus influenzae*, enteric gram-negatives, *Legionella* species, *Moraxella* species, and viruses. Of the antibiotics listed, ciprofloxacin has poor activity against *S pneumoniae* and would not be a good option.

27. Answer e.

Targeted tuberculin testing is designed to identify persons at high risk of active tuberculosis who would benefit from treatment of LTBI. Three cut-off levels define a positive tuberculin skin reaction based on the size of the skin induration. A patient with chronic renal failure would have a positive skin test with at least 10 mm of induration.

28. Answer a.

Amantadine and rimantadine can be used to treat and prevent influenza A infections but are not active against influenza type B viruses. Zanamivir and oseltamivir can be used to treat both influenza A and B infections, and oseltamivir can also be used for prevention of influenza A and B. Inhaled zanamivir is not recommended for use in persons with underlying lung disease such as COPD and asthma, since bronchospasm and decreased respiratory function have been reported with its use. Treatment with any of these drugs can shorten the duration of illness by approximately 1 day if treatment is started within the first 2 days of illness.

29. Answer c.

Diffuse lung infiltrates in an immunocompromised host are most likely of an infectious cause. In these patients, performing bronchoscopy with bronchoalveolar lavage can direct therapy if a specific infectious agent is found. Additionally, noninfectious causes (such as alveolar hemorrhage) can be diagnosed by bronchoalveolar lavage in these patients. The finding of large atypical cells with prominent intracellular inclusion bodies is consistent with cytomegalovirus infection.

30. Answer c.

The exposure history, clinical presentation, and biopsy are characteristic of a granulomatous lung infection with the dimorphic fungus *Histoplasma capsulatum*. Patients with non–life-threatening symptoms that persist beyond 1 month are candidates for treatment, and itraconazole is the medication of choice. Severely ill patients should be treated initially with Amphotericin B.

31. Answer e.

The cell-mediated immunity of this immunocompromised patient has been altered by the immunosuppressive medications she takes to prevent organ rejection. Lung and brain lesions have developed. Of the organisms listed, *Nocardia asteroides* would cause these findings. *Nocardia* are rod-shaped, opportunistic bacteria that are usually not identified with Gram stain. Instead, they are weakly acid-fast, and morphologically they can appear as beaded, branching filaments. The central nervous system will be involved in approximately 30% of the patients. Trimethoprim-sulfamethoxazole is the treatment of choice.

24

Rheumatology

Clement J. Michet, Jr., MD
Kevin G. Moder, MD
William W. Ginsburg, MD

Part I

Clement J. Michet, Jr., MD
Kevin G. Moder, MD

Rheumatoid Arthritis

Rheumatoid arthritis is a chronic systemic inflammatory disease characterized by joint destruction. It affects 0.03% to 1.5% of the population worldwide. Its incidence peaks between the ages of 35 and 45 years; however, the age-related prevalence continues to increase even after age 65. It occurs 3 times more frequently in women than men. The cause remains unknown. The presentation of an unknown antigen to genetically susceptible persons is believed to trigger rheumatoid arthritis.

There is an immunogenetic predisposition to the development of rheumatoid arthritis. Class II major histocompatibility complex molecules on the surface of antigen-presenting cells are responsible for initiating cellular immune responses and for stimulating the differentiation of B lymphocytes into plasma cells that produce antibody. Most white patients with rheumatoid arthritis have class II major histocompatibility complex type HLA-DR4 or HLA-DR1 or both. HLA-DR4 can be divided into 5 subtypes, 2 of which independently promote susceptibility to rheumatoid arthritis ("shared epitope"). The risk of rheumatoid arthritis is increased 3 to 5 times in white Americans with HLA-DR4. The concordance of rheumatoid factor–positive rheumatoid arthritis is increased 6 times among dizygotic twins. The risk of rheumatoid arthritis in a monozygotic twin is increased 30 times when a sibling has the disease.

- Rheumatoid arthritis affects 0.03%-1.5% of the population.
- Most white patients with rheumatoid arthritis have class II major histocompatibility complex type HLA-DR4 or HLA-DR1 or both.
- The concordance of rheumatoid factor–positive rheumatoid arthritis is increased 6 times among dizygotic twins.

- The risk of rheumatoid arthritis in a monozygotic twin is increased 30 times when a sibling has the disease.

Pathogenesis of Rheumatoid Arthritis

The immune reaction begins in the synovial lining of the joint. The earliest pathologic changes in the disease are microvascular injury that increases vascular permeability and the accumulation of inflammatory cells (CD4+ lymphocytes, polymorphonuclear leukocytes, and plasma cells) in the perivascular space. Pro-inflammatory cytokines are released. Mediators of inflammation promote synovial angiogenesis and synovial cell proliferation, the accumulation of neutrophils in synovial fluid, and the maturation of B cells into plasma cells. Plasma cells in the joint locally synthesize rheumatoid factor and other antibodies that promote inflammation. Immune complexes activate the complement system, releasing chemotactic factors and promoting vascular permeability and opsonization. Phagocytosis releases lysosomal enzymes and fosters the digestion of collagen, cartilage matrix, and elastic tissues. The release of oxygen-free radicals injures cells. Damaged cell membranes set free phospholipids that fuel the arachidonic acid cascade.

The local inflammatory response becomes self-perpetuating. Cytokines continue to play an important role, including tumor necrosis factor-α, interleukin-1, and interleukin-6. Proliferating synovium of activated macrophages and fibroblasts polarizes into a centripetally invasive pannus, destroying the weakened cartilage and subchondral bone. Chondrocytes, stimulated in the inflammatory milieu, release their own proteases and collagenases.

Patients have swelling, pain, and joint stiffness with the onset of vascular injury of the synovial lining, angiogenesis, and cellular proliferation. Joint warmth, swelling, pain, and limitation of motion worsen as the synovial membrane proliferates and the inflammatory reaction builds. Histologic and radiographic evidence of rheumatoid synovitis is found in clinically unaffected joints, suggesting that the disease may be present for a period of time before clinical manifestations appear.

Rheumatoid factor is an immunoglobulin not specific for rheumatoid arthritis. Rheumatoid factor may be detected in other inflammatory diseases such as primary Sjögren syndrome, systemic lupus erythematosus, hepatitis C, and systemic vasculitis. It also occurs with aging.

Anti-citrullinated protein antibodies (anti-CCP) are detected in the majority of patients with rheumatoid arthritis. These target antigens are found in peptides containing citrulline, an amino acid resulting from posttranslational enzyme modification of arginine. Unlike rheumatoid factor, these antibodies seem to be highly specific for rheumatoid arthritis. They are present at the onset of disease, and in a high titer they are associated with progressive erosive disease.

- Swelling, pain, and joint stiffness occur with the onset of immune-mediated vascular injury of the synovial lining, angiogenesis, and cellular proliferation.
- Anti-CCP antibodies are equally sensitive and more specific than rheumatoid factor for the diagnosis of early, erosive rheumatoid arthritis.
- Cytokines, in particular tumor necrosis factor-α, and immune complexes, including rheumatoid factor, are important components of the joint inflammatory reaction.

Clinical Features of Rheumatoid Arthritis

The joints most commonly involved (more than 85% of patients) in rheumatoid arthritis are the metacarpophalangeal, proximal interphalangeal, wrist, and metatarsophalangeal joints (Figure 24-1). The distal interphalangeal joints are typically spared. The distribution of involvement is symmetric and polyarticular (5 or more joints); predominantly, small joints are involved. Ultimately, the

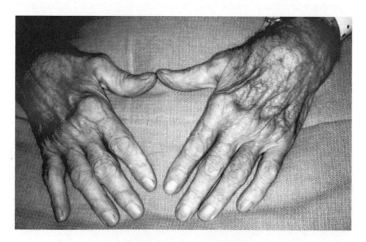

Figure 24-1. Moderately Active Seropositive Rheumatoid Arthritis. The patient has soft tissue swelling across the entire row of metatarsophalangeal joints and proximal interphalangeal joints bilaterally and soft tissue swelling mounding up over the wrists. Note the nearly complete lack of change at the distal interphalangeal joints.

knees (80% of patients), ankles (80%), shoulders (60%), elbows (50%), hips (50%), acromioclavicular joints (50%), atlantoaxial joint (50%), and temporomandibular joints (30%) can be involved. The sternoclavicular joints, cricoarytenoid joints, and the ear ossicles are affected infrequently. Joints affected with rheumatoid arthritis are warm and swollen. The joint enlargement feels spongy and occurs with the thickening of the synovium. An associated joint effusion may make the joint feel fluctuant. Patients describe deep aching and soreness in the involved joints, which are aggravated by use and can be present at rest. Prolonged morning joint stiffness and "gelling" throughout the body and recurrence of this stiffness after resting are some of the many constitutional features that complicate rheumatoid arthritis.

- The joints most commonly involved in rheumatoid arthritis are the metacarpophalangeal, proximal interphalangeal, wrist, and metatarsophalangeal joints.
- The distribution of involvement is symmetric and polyarticular; predominantly, small joints are involved.
- Hallmarks of joint inflammation: stiffness, heat, redness, soft tissue swelling, pain, and dysfunction.

Constitutional Features of Rheumatoid Arthritis

Fatigue, weight loss, muscle pain, excessive sweating, or low-grade fever may be reported by patients presenting with rheumatoid arthritis. Adult seropositive rheumatoid arthritis is not a cause of fever of unknown origin because temperatures greater than 38.3°C cannot be attributed to the disease. A high temperature should raise concern about another problem, such as infection or malignancy. Most patients with *active* arthritis have more than 1 hour of morning stiffness. The musculoskeletal complications of rheumatoid arthritis are listed in Table 24-1.

Musculoskeletal Complications of Rheumatoid Arthritis

Cervical Spine

Half of all patients with chronic rheumatoid arthritis have radiographic involvement of the atlantoaxial joint. It is diagnosed with cervical flexion and extension radiographs showing subluxation. Alternatively, some patients have subaxial subluxations, typically at 2 or more levels. The cervical instability is usually asymptomatic; however, patients may have pain and stiffness in the neck and occipital region. Patients may present dramatically with drop attacks or tetraplegia, but more commonly progression can be slow and subtle with symptoms of hand weakness or paresthesias or signs of cervical myelopathy. Interference with blood flow by ischemic compression of the anterior spinal artery or vertebral arteries (vertebrobasilar insufficiency) causes the neurologic symptoms. All patients with destructive rheumatoid arthritis should be managed with intubation precautions and the assumption that cervical instability is present. New neurologic symptoms mandate urgent neurologic evaluation, including magnetic resonance imaging of the cervical spine and consideration of surgical intervention. Indications for surgical treatment include neurologic or vascular compromise and intractable pain. In active patients, prophylactic cervical spine stabilization is recommended

Table 24-1 Musculoskeletal Complications of Rheumatoid Arthritis

Characteristic deformities include
>   Boutonnière deformity of the finger, with hyperextension of the distal interphalangeal joint & flexion of the proximal interphalangeal joint
>   Swan-neck deformity of the finger, with hyperextension at the proximal interphalangeal joint & flexion of the distal interphalangeal joint
>   Ulnar deviation of the metacarpophalangeal joints; it can progress to complete volar subluxation of the proximal phalanx from the metacarpophalangeal head
>   Compression of the carpal bones & radial deviation at the carpus
>   Subluxation at the wrist
>   Valgus of the ankle & hindfoot
>   Pes planus
>   Forefoot varus & hallux valgus
>   Cock-up toes from subluxation at the metatarsophalangeal joints

when there is evidence of extreme (>8 mm) subluxation of C1 over C2. The probability of cervical involvement is predicted by the severity of peripheral arthritis.

- Half of all patients with chronic rheumatoid arthritis have radiographic involvement of the atlantoaxial joint.
- Patients with cervical spine involvement may present with occipital pain, signs of myelopathy, weakness and paresthesias of the hands, or drop attacks.
- Indications for surgical treatment: neurologic or vascular compromise or intractable pain.
- The probability of cervical involvement is predicted by the severity of peripheral arthritis.

Popliteal Cyst

Flexion of the knee markedly increases the intra-articular pressure of a swollen joint. This pressure produces an out-pouching of the posterior components of the joint space, termed a *popliteal* or a *Baker* cyst. Ultrasonographic examination of the popliteal space can be diagnostic. A popliteal cyst should be distinguished from a popliteal artery aneurysm, lymphadenopathy, phlebitis, and (more rarely) a benign or malignant tumor. The cyst can rupture down into the calf or, rarely, superiorly into the posterior thigh. Rupture of the popliteal cyst with dissection into the calf may resemble acute thrombophlebitis and is called *pseudophlebitis*. Fever, leukocytosis, and ecchymosis around the ankle (crescent sign) can occur with the rupture. Treatment of an acute cyst rupture includes bed rest, elevation of the leg, ice massage or cryocompression, and an intra-articular injection of corticosteroid. Treatment of the popliteal cyst requires improvement in the knee arthritis.

- Popliteal cyst is also called Baker cyst.

- Rupture of a popliteal cyst may resemble acute thrombophlebitis (pseudophlebitis).
- Ultrasonography can distinguish a cyst from a popliteal artery aneurysm, lymphadenopathy, phlebitis, and tumor.

Tenosynovitis

Tenosynovitis of the finger flexor and extensor tendon sheaths is common. It presents with diffuse swelling between the joints and a palpable grating within the flexor tendon sheaths in the palm with passive movement of the digit. Other tenosynovial syndromes in rheumatoid arthritis include de Quervain and wrist tenosynovitis. Persistent inflammation can produce stenosing tenosynovitis, loss of function, and, ultimately, rupture of tendons. Treatment of acute tenosynovitis includes immobilization, warm soaks, nonsteroidal anti-inflammatory drugs, and local injections of corticosteroid in the tendon sheath.

- Tenosynovitis of the finger flexor and extensor tendon sheaths is common and can lead to tendon rupture.

Carpal Tunnel Syndrome

Rheumatoid arthritis is a common cause of carpal tunnel syndrome (pregnancy is the commonest cause). The sudden appearance of bilateral carpal tunnel syndrome should raise the question of an early inflammatory arthritis. This syndrome is associated with paresthesias of the hand in a typical median nerve distribution. Discomfort may radiate up the forearm or into the upper arm. The symptoms worsen with prolonged flexion of the wrist and at night. Late complications include thenar muscle weakness and atrophy and permanent sensory loss. Treatment includes resting splints, control of inflammation, and local injection of glucocorticosteroid. Surgical release is recommended for persistent symptoms.

- Rheumatoid arthritis is a common cause of carpal tunnel syndrome.
- Carpal tunnel syndrome: paresthesias of the hand in a typical median nerve distribution.

Extra-articular Complications of Rheumatoid Arthritis

Extra-articular complications of rheumatoid arthritis occur almost exclusively in patients who have high titers of rheumatoid factor. In general, the number and severity of the extra-articular features vary with the duration and severity of disease.

Rheumatoid Nodules

Rheumatoid nodules are the most common extra-articular manifestation of seropositive rheumatoid arthritis. More than 20% of patients have rheumatoid nodules, which occur over extensor surfaces and at pressure points. They are rare in the lungs, heart, sclera, and dura mater. The nodules have characteristic histopathologic features. A collagenous capsule and a perivascular collection of chronic inflammatory cells surround a central area of necrosis encircled by palisading fibroblasts. Breakdown of the skin over rheumatoid nodules, with ulcers and infection, can be a major source of morbidity. The infection can spread to local bursae, infect bone, or spread hematogenously to joints.

- Extra-articular complications in rheumatoid arthritis occur almost exclusively in seropositive rheumatoid arthritis.
- Rheumatoid nodules are the most common extra-articular complication.
- Rheumatoid nodules occur over extensor surfaces and at pressure points and are prone to ulceration and infection.

Rheumatoid Vasculitis

Rheumatoid vasculitis usually occurs in persons with severe, deforming arthritis and a high titer of rheumatoid factor. The vasculitis is mediated by the deposition of circulating immune complexes on the blood vessel wall. At its most benign, it occurs as rheumatoid nodules, with small infarcts over the nodules and at the cuticles. Proliferation of the vascular intima and media causes this obliterative endarteropathy, which has little associated inflammation. It is best managed by controlling the underlying arthritis. Leukocytoclastic or small vessel vasculitis produces palpable purpura or cutaneous ulceration, particularly over the malleoli of the lower extremities. This vasculitis can cause pyoderma gangrenosum or peripheral sensory neuropathy. Secondary polyarteritis, which is clinically and histopathologically identical to polyarteritis nodosa, results in mononeuritis multiplex. Occasionally, the vasculitis occurs after the joint disease appears "burned out."

- Rheumatoid vasculitis usually occurs in the setting of severe, deforming arthritis and a high titer of rheumatoid factor.
- Rheumatoid vasculitis is mediated by the deposition of circulating immune complexes on the blood vessel wall.
- Rheumatoid vasculitis comprises a spectrum of vascular disease, including rheumatoid nodules and obliterative endarteropathy, leukocytoclastic or small vessel vasculitis, and secondary polyarteritis (systemic necrotizing vasculitis).

Neurologic Manifestations

Neurologic manifestations of rheumatoid arthritis include mild peripheral sensory neuropathy. Painful sensory-motor neuropathy (mononeuropathy) suggests vasculitis or nerve entrapment (eg, carpal tunnel syndrome). Cervical vertebral subluxation can cause myelopathy. Erosive changes may promote basilar invagination of the odontoid process of C2 into the underside of the brain, causing spinal cord compression and death.

Pulmonary Manifestations

Pleural disease has been noted in more than 40% of autopsies in cases of rheumatoid arthritis, but clinically significant pleural disease is less frequent. Characteristically, rheumatoid pleural effusions are asymptomatic until they become large enough to interfere mechanically with respiration. The pleural fluid is an exudate with a concentration of glucose that is low (10-50 mg/dL) because of impaired transport of glucose into the pleural space. Pulmonary nodules appear singly or in clusters. Single nodules have the appearance of a coin lesion. Nodules typically are pleural-based and may cavitate and create a bronchopleural fistula. Pneumoconiosis complicating rheumatoid lung disease, or Caplan syndrome, results in a violent fibroblastic reaction and large nodules.

Acute interstitial pneumonitis is a rare complication that may begin as alveolitis and progress to respiratory insufficiency and death. Interstitial fibrosis is a chronic, slowly progressive process. It has physical findings of diffuse dry crackles on lung auscultation and a reticular nodular radiographic pattern affecting both lung fields, initially in the lung bases. A decrease in the diffusing capacity for carbon dioxide and a restrictive pattern are characteristic pulmonary function test findings. Interstitial disease is highly associated with smoking. Bronchiolitis obliterans with or without organizing pneumonia may occur with rheumatoid arthritis or its treatment. It produces an obstructive picture on pulmonary function testing and typically responds to corticosteroid treatment. High-resolution computed tomography is useful for distinguishing these different interstitial rheumatoid lung syndromes and predicting treatment response. Methotrexate treatment causes a hypersensitivity lung reaction in 1% to 3% of patients. It can present insidiously with a dry cough or with life-threatening pneumonitis.

- Rheumatoid pleural disease is common but asymptomatic until pleural effusions interfere with respiration.
- The exudative pleural fluid is remarkable for low levels of glucose.
- High-resolution computed tomography helps to distinguish among rheumatoid-associated interstitial lung diseases, including interstitial pneumonitis, interstitial fibrosis, and bronchiolitis obliterans with or without organizing pneumonia.
- Methotrexate hypersensitivity pneumonitis may be a life-threatening complication of therapy.

Cardiac Complications

Pericarditis has been noted in 50% of autopsies in cases of rheumatoid arthritis. However, patients rarely present with acute pericardial symptoms or cardiac tamponade. Recurrent effusive pericarditis without symptoms may evolve to chronic constrictive pericarditis. Signs of unexplained edema or ascites may be the presenting manifestations. Untreated constrictive pericarditis has a very high 1-year mortality of 70%. It will not respond to medical therapies. Surgical pericardiectomy is necessary.

- Patients rarely present with acute pericardial symptoms despite frequent serous pericarditis.
- Rheumatoid pericardial disease frequently presents with edema or ascites due to occult constrictive disease.
- Chronic constrictive pericarditis necessitates surgical treatment.

Liver Abnormalities

Patients with rheumatoid arthritis can have increased levels of liver enzymes, particularly alkaline phosphatase. Increased levels of aspartate aminotransferase, γ-glutamyltransferase, and acute-phase proteins and hypoalbuminemia also occur in active rheumatoid arthritis. Liver biopsy shows nonspecific changes of inflammation. Nodular regenerative hyperplasia is rare and causes portal hypertension and hypersplenism. Many medications used to treat rheumatoid arthritis may cause increased levels of the transaminases.

- Increased levels of liver enzymes, particularly alkaline phosphatase, may occur in rheumatoid arthritis.

- Nodular hyperplasia of the liver can complicate rheumatoid arthritis and lead to portal hypertension and hypersplenism.
- Many medications used to treat rheumatoid arthritis increase the levels of transaminases.

Ophthalmic Abnormalities

Keratoconjunctivitis sicca, or secondary Sjögren syndrome, is the most common ophthalmic complication in rheumatoid arthritis. Episcleritis and scleritis also occur independently of the joint inflammation and are usually treated topically. Severe scleritis progressing to scleromalacia perforans causes blindness. Infrequent ocular complications of rheumatoid arthritis include episcleral nodules, palsy of the superior oblique muscle caused by tenosynovitis of its tendon sheath (Brown syndrome), and uveitis. Retinopathy is an infrequent complication of antimalarial drug treatment.

- Keratoconjunctivitis sicca, or secondary Sjögren syndrome, is the most common ophthalmic complication in rheumatoid arthritis.
- Severe scleritis progressing to scleromalacia perforans causes blindness.

Laboratory Findings of Rheumatoid Arthritis

Nonspecific alterations in many laboratory values are common. In very active disease, normocytic anemia (hemoglobin value about 10 g/dL), leukocytosis, thrombocytosis, hypoalbuminemia, and hypergammaglobulinemia are common. Rheumatoid factor (IgM) occurs in 90% of patients, but its presence may not be detected for months after the initial joint symptoms occur. A positive rheumatoid factor is not specific for rheumatoid arthritis. Diseases in boldface type in Table 24-2 are most likely to have high titers of rheumatoid factor. Five percent of the general population has a low titer of rheumatoid factor. Anti-CCP antibodies are more specific for rheumatoid arthritis and may be present when rheumatoid factor is absent. Antinuclear antibodies are common in seropositive rheumatoid disease. C-reactive protein correlates with disease activity, but it is not more helpful than the erythrocyte sedimentation rate. Active rheumatoid arthritis is associated with low iron-binding capacity, low plasma levels of iron, and an increased ferritin value, unless they are iron-deficient.

- Normocytic anemia, leukocytosis, thrombocytosis, and hypoalbuminemia are common in active rheumatoid arthritis.
- Rheumatoid factor is not specific for the diagnosis of rheumatoid arthritis.
- Anti-CCP antibodies may be present when rheumatoid factor is absent. They are not present in the other diseases associated with a factor.

Synovial fluid is cloudy and light yellow, has poor viscosity, and typically contains 10,000 to 75,000 leukocytes/mcL, predominantly neutrophils.

Radiographic Findings of Rheumatoid Arthritis

The radiographic findings in early rheumatoid arthritis are normal or show soft tissue swelling and periarticular osteopenia. Later, the characteristic changes of periarticular osteoporosis, symmetric narrowing of the joint space, and marginal bony erosions become obvious. These signs are most common in radiographs of the hands and forefeet. Radiographic changes at end-stage rheumatoid arthritis include subluxation and other deformities, joint destruction, fibrous ankylosis, and, rarely, bony ankylosis.

- The characteristic radiologic changes in rheumatoid arthritis include periarticular osteoporosis, symmetric narrowing of the joint space, and bony erosions of the joint margin. These occur earliest in the hands and metatarsal phalangeal joints.

Diagnosis of Rheumatoid Arthritis

Adult rheumatoid arthritis should be considered in a person older than 16 years with inflammatory joint symptoms lasting for more than 6 weeks. The time criterion is important because there are viral arthropathies, such as parvovirus B19 infection, that mimic acute rheumatoid arthritis. Morning stiffness lasting for more than 30 minutes, small joint involvement in the metatarsophalangeal joints (morning metatarsalgia), metacarpophalangeal joints with tenderness and swelling, and more than 3 joints affected are clues to an early rheumatoid arthritis presentation. Of the 7 criteria of the American

Table 24-2 Diseases That May Have Positive Rheumatoid Factor[a]

Rheumatoid arthritis
Sjögren syndrome
Systemic lupus erythematosus
Scleroderma
Sarcoidosis
Idiopathic pulmonary fibrosis
Mixed cryoglobulinemia
Hypergammaglobulinemic purpura
Asbestosis
Malignancies
Infectious mononucleosis
Influenza
Chronic active hepatitis
Vaccinations
Tuberculosis
Syphilis
Subacute bacterial endocarditis
Brucellosis
Leprosy
Salmonellosis
Malaria
Kala-azar
Schistosomiasis
Filariasis
Trypanosomiasis

[a] Diseases in boldface type are the most likely to have high-titer rheumatoid factor.

Rheumatism Association, listed in Table 24-3, 4 are used to classify cases as definite rheumatoid arthritis for research studies, but the vast majority of patients with rheumatoid arthritis do not meet these criteria at early presentation.

Natural History of Rheumatoid Arthritis

The majority of patients have insidious onset of the joint disease, occurring over weeks to months. However, in a third of patients, the onset is rapid, occurring in days or weeks. Early in the course of the disease, most patients have oligoarthritis. Their disease becomes polyarticular with time. From 10% to 20% of patients have relentlessly progressive arthritis, and 70% to 90% have persistent, chronic, progressive arthritis. The course may be slow, fluctuating, or rapid, but the end point is the same: disabling, destructive arthritis. Seventy percent of patients experience polycyclic disease, with repeated flares interrupted by partial or complete remissions. Spontaneous remissions in the polycyclic or progressive group almost never occur after 2 years of disease. Patients who experience a persisting polyarthritis with increased acute-phase reactants and a positive rheumatoid factor or anti-CCP antibody are at high risk for early erosive disease within 1 to 2 years of symptom onset and early disability. The relationship between disease duration and inability to work is nearly linear. After 15 years of rheumatoid arthritis, 15% of patients are completely disabled. Life expectancy in seropositive rheumatoid arthritis is shortened, but it may be improving with more aggressive early intervention in the illness. Age, disease severity, comorbid cardiovascular disease, and functional status predict mortality. Educational level and socioeconomic factors also influence mortality.

- In a third of patients, the onset of rheumatoid arthritis is rapid (days or weeks).
- Among patients with rheumatoid arthritis, 70%-90% have persistent, chronic, progressive arthritis.
- The relationship between disease duration and inability to work is nearly linear.

Table 24-3 American Rheumatism Association Criteria for the Diagnosis of Rheumatoid Arthritis[a]

One or more hours of morning stiffness in & around the joints
Arthritis of 3 or more joint areas involved simultaneously
Arthritis of at least 1 area in the wrist, metacarpophalangeal or proximal interphalangeal joints
Symmetric arthritis involving the same joint areas on both sides of the body
Rheumatoid nodules
Serum rheumatoid factor
Radiographic changes typical of rheumatoid arthritis, including periarticular osteoporosis, joint-space narrowing, & marginal erosions

[a] 1987 revision.

Treatment of Rheumatoid Arthritis

The management of patients with rheumatoid arthritis requires making the correct diagnosis, determining the functional status of the patient, and selecting the goals of management with the patient. Goals of management include relieving inflammation and pain and maintaining function.

The principles emphasized by physical medicine include bed rest or rest periods, improving nonrestorative sleep, and joint protection (including modification of activities of daily life, range-of-motion exercises, orthotics, and splints, if they help the pain). Exercise should begin with range of motion and stretching to overcome contracture. Strengthening and conditioning exercises should be prescribed carefully, depending on the activity of the patient's disease.

Initial treatment includes but is not limited to a nonsteroidal anti-inflammatory drug given at anti-inflammatory doses. If the response is inadequate after 3 or 4 weeks, a trial of a second, chemically unrelated nonsteroidal anti-inflammatory drug is used. Low-dose prednisone (≤7.5 mg daily) may be necessary to reduce symptoms while disease-modifying therapies are initiated. Intra-articular cortico-steroids are effective for symptomatic joints not responding to oral anti-inflammatory drugs. A disease-modifying agent of rheumatic disease (DMARD) is also known as a second-line agent, slow-acting antirheumatic drug, or remittive agent. The goal of DMARD therapy is to slow disease progression (erosive damage) and maintain joint function. A goal of disease remission will be possible as new therapies are introduced. Disease-modifying agents include the following:

- Methotrexate
- Hydroxychloroquine
- Sulfasalazine
- Minocycline
- Leflunomide
- Cyclosporine
- Azathioprine
- Anticytokine therapies, including anti-tumor necrosis factor and interleukin-1 inhibitors
- Rituximab
- Abatacept

DMARD therapy should be started early, once rheumatoid arthritis is diagnosed. The choice of first DMARD is empiric, but usually consists of methotrexate, sulfasalazine, hydroxychloroquine, or minocycline. Uninterrupted treatment with a disease-modifying agent for 3 to 6 months is usually necessary to assess its effect. Traditionally, DMARDs have been used sequentially, although recent studies have shown an enhanced benefit with combination DMARD treatments that include methotrexate. A second disease-modifying drug is substituted or added to the first one when a therapeutic or toxic roadblock is reached. Evidence supporting the pivotal pro-inflammatory role of tumor necrosis factor-α in rheumatoid arthritis has been exploited clinically with the development of several effective tumor necrosis factor-α antagonists. These generally are reserved for patients not responding to trials of more traditional and less expensive DMARDs. Abatacept, a T-cell co-stimulatory inhibitor, and rituximab, an anti-CD20 B-cell–depleting agent, are used in treatment failures.

- Goals of management include relieving inflammation and pain and maintaining function.
- A disease-modifying regimen is started when rheumatoid arthritis is diagnosed.
- Low-dose prednisone may be necessary to preserve function during initiation of DMARD therapy.
- With disease-modifying agents, uninterrupted treatment for 3 to 6 months is needed to assess efficacy. Combination DMARD therapy has become more common.

Surgery in the Treatment of Rheumatoid Arthritis

An orthopedic surgical procedure for resistant rheumatoid arthritis remains the most important therapeutic option for preserving or enhancing function. Synovectomy of the wrist and nearby tendon sheaths is beneficial when medication alone fails to control the synovitis. The operation preserves joint function and prevents the lysis of extensor tendons that can result in a loss of function. Synovectomy of the knee, either open or through an arthroscope, can delay the progression of rheumatoid arthritis from 6 months to 3 years. Removal of nodules and treatment for local nerve entrapment syndromes are also important surgical treatments for rheumatoid arthritis. Arthroplasty is reserved for patients in whom medical management has failed and in whom intractable pain or compromise in function developed because of a destroyed joint. Arthroplasty, arthrodesis (wrist), and synovectomy are important components of well-balanced rheumatology treatment programs. Total joint arthroplasty has a slightly poorer long-term outcome in rheumatoid arthritis than in osteoarthritis. Nevertheless, joint replacement has had a major impact on reducing patient disability.

- Orthopedic surgery is the most important advance in the treatment of medically resistant rheumatoid arthritis.
- Total joint arthroplasty has a slightly poorer long-term outcome in rheumatoid arthritis than in osteoarthritis.
- Typical clinical scenarios:
  Rheumatoid arthritis—A patient presents with bilateral inflammation of metacarpophalangeal and proximal interphalangeal joints and considerable morning stiffness. The joint involvement is symmetric. Laboratory tests are positive for rheumatoid factor.
  Baker cyst—A patient with a known history of rheumatoid arthritis who is receiving therapy presents with acute pain and swelling in the posterior aspect of the right knee. Mild fever and leukocytosis are present.

Conditions Related to Rheumatoid Arthritis

Seronegative Rheumatoid Arthritis

Rheumatoid factor-negative (seronegative) rheumatoid arthritis is not associated with extra-articular manifestations. However, the arthritis usually is destructive, deforming, and otherwise indistinguishable from seropositive rheumatoid arthritis.

- Seronegative rheumatoid arthritis is not associated with extra-articular manifestations.

Seronegative Rheumatoid Arthritis of the Elderly

A subgroup of patients older than 60 years with seronegative rheumatoid arthritis may have milder arthritis. In this subgroup, polyarticular inflammation suddenly develops and is controlled best with low doses of prednisone. The presence of anti-CCP antibodies may help to distinguish this condition from polymyalgia rheumatica. Minimal destructive changes and deformity occur. Some elderly patients with seronegative arthritis (men in their 70s) present with acute polyarthritis and pitting edema of the hands and feet, so-called RS3PE (remitting symmetric seronegative synovitis with pitting edema). They have a prompt and gratifying response to low doses of prednisone.

- Typical clinical scenario: In a patient older than 60 years, rheumatoid factor-negative polyarticular arthritis suddenly develops. It is best controlled initially with low doses of prednisone.

Adult-Onset Still Disease

Systemic *juvenile* rheumatoid arthritis is known as Still disease. It has quotidian (fever spike with return to normal all in 1 day) high-spiking fevers, arthralgia, arthritis, seronegativity (negative rheumatoid factor and antinuclear antibody), leukocytosis, macular evanescent rash, serositis, lymphadenopathy, splenomegaly, and hepatomegaly. Fever, rash, and arthritis are the classic triad of Still disease.

Adult-onset Still disease has a slight female predominance. Its onset commonly occurs between ages 16 and 35 years. Temperature more than 39°C occurs in a quotidian or double quotidian pattern in 96% of patients. The rash has a typical appearance: a macular salmon-colored eruption on the trunk and extremities. The transient rash is usually noticed at the time of increased temperature. Arthritis occurs in 95% of these patients, and in about a third the joint disease is progressive and destructive. Adult-onset Still disease has a predilection for the wrists, shoulders, hips, and knees. Sixty percent of patients complain of sore throat, which can confuse the diagnosis with rheumatic fever; however, the course is much more prolonged than that of acute rheumatic fever. Weight loss is common. Lymphadenopathy occurs in two-thirds of patients and hepatosplenomegaly in about half. Pleurisy, pneumonitis, and abdominal pain occur in less than a third of patients. The serum ferritin level is markedly increased.

Treatment of adult-onset Still disease includes high doses of aspirin or indomethacin. Corticosteroids may be needed to control the systemic symptoms. Half of patients require methotrexate to control the systemic and articular features.

- Typical clinical scenario: A patient presents with the classic triad of fever, rash, and arthritis.
- Rheumatoid factor and antinuclear antibodies are absent in Still disease.
- There is a predilection for the wrists, shoulders, hips, and knees.
- Sore throat occurs in 60% of patients.

Felty Syndrome

Felty syndrome has the classic triad of rheumatoid arthritis, leukopenia, and splenomegaly. (Classic Felty syndrome usually occurs after 12 years or more of rheumatoid arthritis.) It occurs in less than 1% of patients with seropositive rheumatoid arthritis. Splenomegaly either may not be clinically apparent or may manifest only after the arthritis and leukopenia have been present for some time. Other features of Felty syndrome are listed in Table 24-4. Patients with this syndrome frequently have bacterial infections, particularly of the skin and lungs. Infection related to the cytopenia is the major cause of mortality. High titers of rheumatoid factor are the rule, and a positive antinuclear antibody occurs in two-thirds of patients. Hypocomplementemia often occurs with active vasculitis. Patients often die of sepsis despite vigorous antibacterial treatment. Treatment can include corticosteroids, methotrexate, granulocyte colony-stimulating factor, and splenectomy.

- Felty syndrome occurs in <1% of patients with seropositive rheumatoid arthritis.
- Felty syndrome has the classic triad of rheumatoid arthritis, leukopenia, and splenomegaly.
- High titers of rheumatoid factor are the rule.
- Patients with Felty syndrome frequently die of infection.

Sjögren Syndrome

Sjögren syndrome has a triad of clinical features: keratoconjunctivitis sicca (with or without lacrimal gland enlargement), xerostomia (with or without salivary gland enlargement), and connective tissue disease (usually rheumatoid arthritis). Histologically, CD4 lymphocytic infiltration and destruction of lacrimal salivary glands characterize it. Clinically, it manifests with dry eyes and dry mouth. Primary Sjögren syndrome is diagnosed predominantly in middle-aged women. Additional features of primary Sjögren syndrome are listed in Table 24-5. Most patients have a polyclonal hypergammaglobulinemia. Autoantibodies typically are present, including

Table 24-4 Features of Felty Syndrome

Classic triad
    Rheumatoid arthritis
    Leukopenia
    Splenomegaly
Other features
    Recurrent fevers with & without infection
    Weight loss
    Lymphadenopathy
    Skin hyperpigmentation
    Lower extremity ulcers
    Vasculitis
    Neuropathy
    Keratoconjunctivitis sicca
    Xerostomia
    Other cytopenias

Table 24-5 Features of Sjögren Syndrome

Classic triad
    Arthritis: typically episodic polyarthritis
    Dry eyes
    Dry mouth (& other dry mucous membranes)
Other features
    Constitutional features: fatigue, malaise, myalgia
    Raynaud phenomenon
    Cutaneous vasculitis
    CNS abnormalities
        Cerebritis, CNS vasculitis
        Stroke
        Multiple sclerosis-like illness
    Peripheral neuropathy
    Sensory
    Autonomic
    Interstitial lung disease
    Pleurisy

Abbreviation: CNS, central nervous system.

rheumatoid factor, antinuclear antibodies, and antibodies to extractable nuclear antigens (SS-A and SS-B).

Patients can present with primary Sjögren syndrome without any additional connective tissue disease. The primary syndrome typically has episodic and nondeforming arthritis. More commonly, rheumatoid arthritis, systemic lupus erythematosus, scleroderma, polyarteritis nodosa, or polymyositis accompanies Sjögren syndrome. There is no perfect definition for Sjögren syndrome, and no test is completely diagnostic. Simple dry eyes of the elderly, benign sicca syndrome, is distinguished from Sjögren syndrome by the absence of SSA antibodies. Patients with Sjögren syndrome, but not the seronegative sicca syndrome, have an increased risk for development of non-Hodgkin lymphoma.

Treatment of primary Sjögren syndrome is mainly symptomatic. Pilocarpine, 5 mg orally 4 times daily, improves salivary and lacrimal gland function in the majority of the patients. Side effects, including flushing and sweating, limit its usefulness. In addition to hydration, systemic therapy is indicated if there is evidence of systemic inflammation. A Sjögren-like syndrome has been described in patients with human immunodeficiency virus (HIV) infection.

- Typical clinical scenario: A patient presents with dry eyes, dry mouth, and a connective tissue disorder (usually rheumatoid arthritis).
- Sjögren syndrome can exist by itself or with another formal connective tissue disease such as rheumatoid arthritis, systemic lupus erythematosus, scleroderma, or myositis.
- Treatment focuses on control of inflammation and symptoms of dryness.
- A Sjögren-like syndrome has been described in patients with HIV infection.

Osteoarthritis

Osteoarthritis is the failure of articular cartilage and subsequent degenerative changes in subchondral bone, bony joint margins, synovium, and para-articular fibrous and muscular structures. Osteoarthritis is the most common rheumatic disease; 80% of patients have some limitation of their activities, and 25% are unable to perform major activities of daily living. More than 10% of the population older than 60 years has osteoarthritis. Annually, symptomatic hip or knee osteoarthritis develops in half a million new patients.

- Osteoarthritis is the most common rheumatic disease.
- More than 10% of the population older than 60 years has osteoarthritis.

Pathogenesis of Osteoarthritis

Two principal changes associated with osteoarthritis are the progressive focal degeneration of articular cartilage and the formation of new bone in the floor of the cartilage lesion at the joint margins (osteophytes). Not all the mechanisms causing osteoarthritis have been identified. Current theories include 1) mechanical process: cartilage injury, particularly after impact loading, and 2) biochemical process: failure of cartilage repair processes to adequately compensate for injury. A combination of mechanical and biochemical processes likely contributes in most cases of osteoarthritis. It must be emphasized that osteoarthritis is not just the consequence of "wear and tear."

- Osteoarthritis: progressive focal degeneration of articular cartilage, with subsequent degeneration of surrounding soft tissues and proliferation (osteophytosis) of bone.
- Osteoarthritis is not the consequence of normal use ("wear and tear").

Clinical Features of Osteoarthritis

The pain of an osteoarthritic joint is usually described as a deep ache. Subchondral bone edema may contribute to the pain. The pain occurs with use of the joint and is relieved with rest and cessation of weight bearing. As the disease progresses, the involved joint may be symptomatic with minimal activity or even at rest. The pain originates in the structures around the disintegrating cartilage (there are no nerves in cartilage). There may be stiffness in the joint with initial use, but this initial stiffness is not prolonged as it is in inflammatory arthritis, such as rheumatoid arthritis. Although the symptoms are related predominantly to mechanical failure and motion limits, joint debris and the associated repair process promote mild inflammation, accumulation of synovial fluid, and mild hypertrophy of the synovial membrane. Acute inflammation can transiently occur at Heberden nodes (distal interphalangeal joints with prominent osteophytes as a consequence of osteoarthritis) or at the knee with tearing of a degenerative meniscal cartilage.

- Osteoarthritic pain is usually described as a deep ache with joint use and is improved with rest.
- The stiffness with initial use of the joint is not prolonged in osteoarthritis as it is in inflammatory arthritis (rheumatoid arthritis).

Physical examination documents joint margin tenderness, fine crepitance, limits to motion, and enlargement of the joint. The enlargement is usually bony (proliferation of cartilage and bone to form osteophytes), but it can include effusions and mild synovial thickening. Deformity is a late consequence of the osteoarthritis and is associated with atrophy or derangement of the local soft tissues, ligaments, and muscles. Radiographic or physical examination evidence of the severity of osteoarthritis does not reliably predict a patient's symptoms.

Clinical Subsets of Osteoarthritis

Primary Osteoarthritis

Primary osteoarthritis is cartilage failure without a known cause that would predispose to osteoarthritis. It almost never affects the shoulders, elbows, ankles, metacarpophalangeal joints, or ulnar side of the wrist. It is divided into several clinical patterns, as described below.

Generalized osteoarthritis involves the distal interphalangeal joints, proximal interphalangeal joints, first carpometacarpal joints, hips, knees, and spine (Figure 24-2). It occurs most frequently in middle-aged postmenopausal women.

Isolated nodal osteoarthritis is primary osteoarthritis that affects only the distal interphalangeal joints. It occurs predominantly in women and has a familial predisposition.

Isolated hip osteoarthritis is more common in men than in women. It has no clear association with obesity or activity.

Erosive osteoarthritis affects only the distal and proximal interphalangeal joints. Patients with erosive osteoarthritis have episodes of local inflammation. Mucous cyst formation at the distal interphalangeal joint is common. Painful flare-up of the disease recurs for years. Symptoms usually begin about the time of menopause. Bony erosions and collapse of the subchondral plate—features not

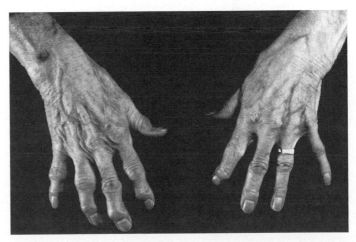

Figure 24-2. Generalized Osteoarthritis. Note prominent bony swelling at the proximal (Bouchard nodes) and distal (Heberden nodes) interphalangeal joints. The metacarpophalangeal joints are spared. Early hypertrophic changes are seen on profile at the first carpometacarpal joint, giving a slight squaring of the hand deformity, appreciated best on the left.

usually seen in primary osteoarthritis—with osteophytes are markers of erosive osteoarthritis. Joint deformity can be severe. In many cases, bony ankylosis develops. Ankylosis is usually associated with relief of pain. The synovium is intensely infiltrated with mononuclear cells. This condition may be confused with rheumatoid arthritis.

Diffuse idiopathic skeletal hyperostosis is a variant of primary osteoarthritis. It occurs chiefly in men older than 50 years. It is also known as Forestier disease. The diagnosis requires finding characteristic exuberant, flowing osteophytosis that connects 4 or more vertebrae with preservation of the disk space. Diffuse idiopathic skeletal hyperostosis must be distinguished from typical osteoarthritis of the spine with degenerative disk disease and from ankylosing spondylitis. Extraspinal sites of disease involvement include calcification of the pelvic ligaments, exuberant osteophytosis at the site of peripheral osteoarthritis, well-calcified bony spurs at the calcaneus, and heterotopic bone formation after total joint arthroplasty. Patients with diffuse idiopathic skeletal hyperostosis are often obese, and 60% have diabetes mellitus or glucose intolerance. Symptoms include mild back stiffness and, occasionally, back pain. Pathologically and radiologically, diffuse idiopathic skeletal hyperostosis is distinct from other forms of primary osteoarthritis.

* Primary osteoarthritis almost never affects the shoulders, elbows, ankles, metacarpophalangeal joints, or the ulnar side of the wrist.
* Generalized osteoarthritis involves the distal interphalangeal joints, proximal interphalangeal joints, first carpometacarpal joints, hips, knees, and spine.
* Isolated nodal osteoarthritis is primary osteoarthritis affecting only the distal interphalangeal joints.
* Isolated hip osteoarthritis is more common in men than in women.
* Erosive osteoarthritis affects only the distal and proximal interphalangeal joints.
* Diffuse idiopathic skeletal hyperostosis is a variant of primary osteoarthritis and should be distinguished from ankylosing spondylitis.

Secondary Osteoarthritis

Secondary osteoarthritis is cartilage failure caused by some known disorder, trauma, or abnormality. Any patient with an unusual distribution of osteoarthritis or widespread chondrocalcinosis should be considered to have secondary osteoarthritis. Secondary osteoarthritis frequently complicates trauma and the damage caused by inflammatory arthritis. Inherited disorders of connective tissue and several metabolic abnormalities, including ochronosis, hemochromatosis, Wilson disease, and acromegaly, are complicated by secondary osteoarthritis. Paget disease of bone, involving the femur or pelvis about the hip joint, can predispose to osteoarthritis.

* Osteoarthritis involving the shoulder, metacarpophalangeal joints, or isolated large joints or with chondrocalcinosis should prompt physicians to consider secondary causes of osteoarthritis.

Trauma or injury to a joint and supporting periarticular tissues predisposes persons to the most common type of secondary osteoarthritis. Stress from repeated impact loading could weaken subchondral bone.

Internal joint derangement with ligamentous laxity or meniscal damage alters the normal mechanical alignment of the joint. Isolated large joint involvement is a clue to posttraumatic osteoarthritis. Chronic rotator cuff tear with subsequent loss of shoulder joint cartilage (cuff arthropathy) and knee osteoarthritis that develops years after meniscal cartilage damage are examples of secondary osteoarthritis.

Congenital malformations of joints, such as congenital hip dysplasia and epiphyseal dysplasia, lead to premature osteoarthritis. Other developmental abnormalities, including slipped capital femoral epiphysis and Legg-Calvé-Perthes disease (idiopathic avascular necrosis of the femoral head), may first present as premature osteoarthritis years after they occur. Inherited disorders of connective tissue frequently predispose the afflicted person to premature osteoarthritis. Table 24-6 describes several inherited disorders, including their gene defects and characteristics.

* Injury to a joint or supporting periarticular tissues can predispose to osteoarthritis.
* Posttraumatic osteoarthritis is the most common form of secondary osteoarthritis.
* Isolated large joint involvement is a clue to posttraumatic osteoarthritis.

Alkaptonuria/ochronosis is a rare autosomal recessive disorder of tyrosine metabolism. Deficiency of the enzyme homogentisic acid oxidase leads to excretion of large amounts of homogentisic acid in the urine. Black, oxidized, polymerized homogentisic acid pigment collects in connective tissues (ochronosis). The diagnosis may go unrecognized until middle life. The first manifestation can be secondary osteoarthritis. The patient's urine darkens when allowed to stand or with the addition of sodium hydroxide. Ochronotic arthritis affects the large joints (eg, the hips, knees, and shoulders) and is associated with calcium pyrophosphate crystals in the synovial fluid. The radiographic finding of calcified intervertebral disks at multiple levels is characteristic of ochronosis. Other manifestations include grayish brown scleral pigment and generalized darkening of the ear pinnae.

* Alkaptonuria/ochronosis is a rare autosomal recessive disorder of tyrosine metabolism.
* Ochronosis: black, oxidized, polymerized homogentisic acid pigment collects in connective tissues.
* Ochronotic arthritis affects the large joints: the hips, knees, and shoulders.

Hemochromatosis was formerly considered an unusual autosomal recessive disorder of white males. It is now considered the commonest inherited disease. The full clinical spectrum of hemochromatosis includes hepatomegaly, bronze skin pigmentation, diabetes mellitus, the consequences of pituitary insufficiency, and degenerative arthritis. The arthropathy affects up to 50% of patients with hemochromatosis and generally resembles osteoarthritis; however, it involves the metacarpophalangeal joints and shoulders, joints not typically affected by generalized primary osteoarthritis. Attacks of acute pseudogout arthritis may occur in relation to deposition of calcium pyrophosphate dihydrate crystals. Chondrocalcinosis is commonly superimposed

Table 24-6 Inherited Disorders of Connective Tissue

Condition	Gene Defect	Characteristics
Marfan syndrome (autosomal dominant)	Fibrillin gene	Hypermobile joints: osteoarthritis, arachnodactyly, kyphoscoliosis Lax skin, striae, ectopic ocular lens Aortic root dilatation (aortic insufficiency), mitral valve prolapse, aneurysms, & aortic dissection
Ehlers-Danlos syndrome (10 subtypes)	Type I & type III collagen gene defects	Joint hypermobility, friable skin, osteoarthritis Type III collagen defects associated with vascular aneurysms
Osteogenesis imperfecta (autosomal dominant & recessive variations; the most common heritable disorder of connective tissue: 1:20,000; 4 subtypes)	Type I collagen gene defects	Brittle bones, blue sclerae, otosclerosis & deafness, joint hypermobility, & tooth malformation
Type II collagenopathies: Achondrogenesis type II Hypochondrogenesis Spondyloepiphyseal dysplasia Spondyloepimetaphyseal dysplasia Kniest dysplasia Stickler syndrome Familial precocious osteoarthropathy	Type II collagen gene defects	Spectrum from lethal (achondrogenesis) to premature osteoarthritis (Stickler syndrome)
Achondroplasia (autosomal dominant)	Fibroblast growth factor III receptor gene defect	Dwarfism, premature osteoarthritis
Pseudoachondroplasia	Cartilage oligomeric matrix protein (COMP) gene defect	Short stature, premature osteoarthritis
Multiple epiphyseal dysplasia (autosomal dominant)		

on chronic osteoarthritic change in hemochromatosis. The pathogenesis of joint degeneration in hemochromatosis is not clear.

- Arthropathy affects up to 50% of patients with hemochromatosis.
- It involves the metacarpophalangeal joints and shoulders.

Wilson disease is a rare autosomal recessive disorder. Arthropathy occurs in 50% of adults with Wilson disease. This disease is suspected in anyone younger than 40 years with unexplained hepatitis, cirrhosis, or movement disorder. The diagnosis is suggested when the serum level of ceruloplasmin is less than 200 mg/L. Arthropathy is unusual in children with the disease. The radiologic appearance varies somewhat from that of primary osteoarthritis; there are more subchondral cysts, sclerosis, cortical irregularities, and radiodense lesions, which occur centrally and at the joint margins. Focal areas of bone fragmentation occur, but they are not related to neuropathy. Although chondrocalcinosis occurs, calcium pyrophosphate dihydrate crystals have not been observed in the synovial fluid.

- Arthropathy occurs in 50% of adults with Wilson disease.
- Arthropathy is unusual in children with Wilson disease.

Apatite microcrystals are associated with degenerative arthritis and are found in patients with hypothyroidism, hyperparathyroidism, and acromegaly. They occur without an associated endocrinopathy. The role of microcrystalline disease in the progression of osteoarthritis is unclear, especially in the absence of acute recurrent flares of pseudogout.

Neuroarthropathy (Charcot joint) commonly affects patients with diabetes mellitus. Men and women are equally affected. Patients with diabetic neuroarthropathy have had diabetes an average of 16 years. Frequently, the diabetes is poorly controlled. Diabetic peripheral neuropathy causes blunted pain perception and poor proprioception. Repeated microtrauma, overt trauma, small vessel occlusive disease (diabetes), and neuropathic dystrophic effects on bone contribute to neuroarthropathy.

Patients can present with an acute arthritic condition that includes swelling, erythema, and warmth. The foot, particularly the tarsometatarsal joint, is involved most commonly in patients with diabetes. Patients usually describe milder pain than suggested by the clinical condition and radiographic appearances. They walk with an antalgic limp. Callus formation occurs over the weight-bearing site of bony damage, and the callus subsequently blisters and ulcerates. Infection can spread from skin ulcers to the bone. Osteomyelitis frequently complicates diabetic neuroarthropathy. Radiography shows disorganized normal joint architecture. Bone and cartilage fragments later coalesce to form characteristic sclerotic loose bodies. There is an attempt at reconstruction with new bone formation. This periosteal new bone is inhibited by small vessel ischemic change in some patients with diabetes. Diabetic osteopathy is a second form of neuroarthropathy. Osteopenia of para-articular areas, particularly the distal metacarpals and proximal phalanges, results in rapidly progressive osteolysis and juxta-articular cortical defects. This can be associated with osteomyelitis.

Initial treatment in patients with diabetes includes good local foot care, treatment of infection, and protected weight bearing. Involvement of the knee, lumbar spine, and upper extremity is uncommon. Classically, hip and spinal neuroarthropathy is caused by tertiary syphilis, and shoulder neuroarthropathy is associated with cervical syringomyelia.

* Neuroarthropathy (Charcot joint) most commonly affects the feet and ankles of patients with diabetes mellitus.
* Neuroarthropathy is a consequence of peripheral neuropathy and local injury.
* Osteomyelitis is caused by skin ulcers extending to the bone and should be suspected when an affected diabetic has sudden worsening of his or her glucose control.

Aseptic necrosis of the bone, also known as avascular necrosis of bone, may lead to collapse of the articular surface and subsequent osteoarthritis. It usually occurs in the hip after femoral neck fracture. Systemic corticosteroid therapy increases the risk of aseptic necrosis. Aseptic necrosis of the bone has other causes, including alcoholism, sickle cell disease, and systemic lupus erythematosus (Table 24-7). No underlying cause can be identified in 10% to 25% of patients.

Table 24-7 Mnemonic Device for Causes of Aseptic Necrosis of Bone

A	Alcohol, atherosclerotic vascular disease
S	Steroids, sickle cell anemia, storage disease (Gaucher disease)
E	Emboli (fat, cholesterol)
P	Postradiation necrosis
T	Trauma
I	Idiopathic
C	Connective tissue disease (especially SLE), caisson disease

Abbreviation: SLE, systemic lupus erythematosus.

Aseptic necrosis of bone usually affects the hips, shoulders, knees, or ankles. Treatment is conservative, including reduced weight bearing and analgesics. Some investigators have treated patients successfully with vascularized bone grafts in the bed of necrotic trabecular bone, although controlled studies are not available. Core decompression may help with pain but does not influence progression to gonarthritis. When there is evidence of cortical bone collapse, progression to advanced osteoarthritis is inevitable. The most sensitive test for aseptic necrosis is magnetic resonance imaging. Plain radiography is insensitive to early aseptic necrosis.

* Aseptic necrosis usually occurs in the hip after femoral neck fracture and may lead to osteoarthritis.
* Alcoholism and corticosteroid use are other common causes of avascular necrosis.

Hypertrophic osteoarthropathy is characterized by clubbing of the fingernails and painful distal long bone periostitis. The patient may have a noninflammatory arthritis at the ankles, knees, or wrists. This condition complicates primary and metastatic pulmonary malignancies, chronic pulmonary infections, cystic fibrosis, and hypoxic congenital heart disease. Treatment is usually symptomatic.

Hemophilic arthropathy, a type of progressive degenerative arthropathy, is more destructive than primary osteoarthritis. Patients with hemophilia and recurrent hemarthroses are at risk for hemophilic arthropathy. Widening of the intercondylar notch of the knees is an early radiographic feature suggesting the diagnosis of this condition.

Radiographic Features of Osteoarthritis

The radiographic features of osteoarthritis do not always predict the extent of symptoms. With aging, radiographic osteoarthritis is far more prevalent than the clinical illness. Common radiographic features include osteophyte formation, asymmetric joint-space narrowing, subchondral bony sclerosis, and subchondral cysts. Later bony changes include malalignment and deformity (Figure 24-3). In the spine, the radiographic finding called spondylosis includes anterolateral spinous osteophytes, degenerative disk disease with disk-space narrowing, and facet sclerosis. A defect in the bony structure of the posterior neural arch produces spondylolysis. With bilateral spondylolysis, subluxation of 1 vertebra on another may occur, a condition called spondylolisthesis. The causes of spondylolisthesis are trauma, osteoarthritis, and congenital. No laboratory studies of blood are useful in the diagnosis of osteoarthritis.

* Common radiographic features of osteoarthritis include osteophyte formation, asymmetric joint-space narrowing, subchondral bony sclerosis, subchondral cysts, and buttressing of angle joints.
* No laboratory studies of blood are useful in the diagnosis of osteoarthritis.

Therapy for Osteoarthritis

Therapeutic goals include relieving pain, preserving joint motion and function, and preventing further injury and wear of cartilage. Weight loss (especially in knee osteoarthritis), use of canes or crutches, correction of postural abnormalities, and proper shoe support are helpful

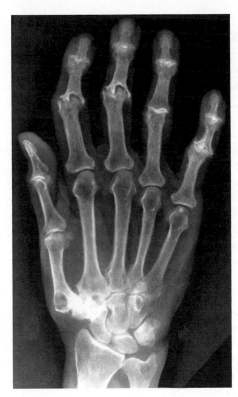

Figure 24-3. Severe Osteoarthritis. Hypertrophic changes, asymmetric joint-space narrowing, and subchondral sclerosis are prominent at the interphalangeal joints and at the first carpometacarpal joint. Note that the metacarpophalangeal joints are completely spared, distinguishing this arthritis from rheumatoid arthritis. Also, there is joint-space narrowing and sclerosis at the base of the thumb at the first carpometacarpal joint and between the trapezium and the scaphoid. Osteoarthritis does not affect the entire wrist compartment equally. The involvement seen here is the most common. An additional interesting feature seen here is central erosions at the second and third proximal interphalangeal joints. This variant occasionally has been called erosive osteoarthritis.

measures. Isometric or isotonic range-of-motion exercises and muscle strengthening provide para-articular structures with extra support and help reduce symptoms. Relief of muscle spasm with local application of heat or cold to decrease pain can help. Addressing the patient's ability to cope with the illness may be more helpful than medication therapy alone.

Initial drug therapy should be analgesics, such as acetaminophen (1 g 4 times daily as needed). Nonsteroidal anti-inflammatory drugs are beneficial for inflammatory flares of osteoarthritis and usually do not need to be taken in anti-inflammatory doses every day. Selective use of opioid analgesics can be considered for disabling pain, especially in persons who are not surgical candidates. Intra-articular corticosteroids offer some temporary relief but should be used only if there is a symptomatic effusion or synovitis. Injections of hyaluronic acid into the knee joint may provide short-term improvement in symptomatic osteoarthritis in selected patients.

Joint arthroplasty may relieve pain, stabilize joints, and improve function. Total joint arthroplasty is very successful at the knee or hip. Table 24-8 describes the indications for total joint arthroplasty in radiographically advanced osteoarthritis. Surgical treatment for osteoarthritis of the shoulder is usually reserved for patients with intractable pain. Tibial osteotomy redistributes knee-joint forces. Arthroscopy removes loose bodies and trims torn menisci to correct lockup or giving way of the joint. Herniated disks or spinal stenosis with radicular symptoms may require decompression.

- Simple analgesics such as acetaminophen are the first choice for treating osteoarthritis.

Arthritis in Chronic Renal Failure

Up to 75% of patients undergoing chronic renal dialysis have musculoskeletal complaints after 4 years of dialysis. Renal failure arthritis affects the interphalangeal joints, metacarpophalangeal joints, wrists, shoulders, and knees. Symmetric joint-space narrowing and para-articular osteoporosis, subchondral cysts, and erosions have been described. There is no osteophytosis to confuse this condition with osteoarthritis. The synovial fluid is noninflammatory, and the synovitis on biopsy is nonspecific. Possible causes of this arthritis include apatite microcrystal deposition, hyperparathyroidism, and renal failure amyloidosis. Aseptic necrosis occasionally affects large joints.

After 10 years of hemodialysis, 65% of patients have pathologic or radiologic evidence of amyloid deposition (renal failure amyloid arthropathy). The amyloid is composed of β_2-microglobulin, is arthrotropic, and results in complete joint-space loss that occurs over a 3- to 12-month period. Shoulder pain and stiffness syndrome and carpal tunnel syndrome are strongly related to this amyloid deposition. Currently, treatment is aimed at relieving the symptoms.

- Up to 75% of patients undergoing chronic renal dialysis have musculoskeletal complaints after 4 years of dialysis.
- Destructive arthritis, shoulder pain and stiffness syndrome, and carpal tunnel syndrome are strongly related to amyloid deposition.

Nonarticular Rheumatism

Fibromyalgia
Fibromyalgia is a condition characterized by chronic widespread musculoskeletal pain. Older terms used to describe this condition include fibrositis, tension myalgias, generalized nonarticular rheumatism, and psychogenic rheumatism. For the diagnosis, the pain should be present for at least 3 months and should involve areas on both sides of the body above and below the waist and some part of the

Table 24-8 Indications for Total Joint Arthroplasty

Radiographically advanced osteoarthritis
Night pain that cannot be modified by changing position
Lockup or giving way of the weight-bearing joint associated with falls or near falls
Joint symptoms compromise activities of daily living

axial skeleton. Symptoms should not be explainable on the basis of other coexisting diseases or conditions. To meet classification criteria for fibromyalgia, 11 of 18 tender points must be present. Fibromyalgia affects 2% to 10% of populations studied. This condition accounts for 15% of all visits to general internists in the United States; 75% to 95% of all patients are women. It is unusual for the diagnosis to be made in a person younger than 12 years or after age 65. Of the patients (or their parents), 60% recall childhood growing pains (leg pains). Fibromyalgia is associated with psychosocial stress.

* Fibromyalgia is characterized by chronic widespread musculoskeletal pain.
* Fibromyalgia affects 2%-10% of populations studied; 75%-95% of patients are women.

Symptoms

Patients typically describe pain all over the body and use qualitatively different descriptions of the pain and discomfort than used by patients with rheumatoid arthritis. Patients localize the pain poorly, referring it to muscle attachment sites or muscles. The discomfort may be worse late in the day after activity. Some patients report morning stiffness, but it is usually not as long or as severe as in patients with inflammatory arthritis. Physical activity or changes in the weather typically aggravate the symptoms. Most patients describe nonrestorative, nonrestful sleep. Psychosocial stress, anxiety, and depression frequently are present. Other patient complaints can include subjective joint swelling (without objective synovitis on examination), arthralgias, headaches, and paresthesias. About a third of patients have multiple somatic visceral symptoms, including urinary irritability, pelvic pain, temporomandibular joint symptoms, and irritable bowel syndrome.

* Patients with fibromyalgia typically describe pain all over the body.
* Physical activity or weather changes typically aggravate the symptoms.
* Multiple somatic symptoms, including headaches, paresthesias, numbness, and irritable bowel symptoms, are common.
* Widespread chronic musculoskeletal pain is associated with psychosocial stress.

Diagnosis

A detailed history and physical examination exclude most rheumatologic and neurologic diseases (Table 24-9). The finding of painful points at muscle attachment sites supports the diagnosis of fibromyalgia. Laboratory evaluation should include a complete blood count, erythrocyte sedimentation rate, thyroid function studies, and baseline chemistry studies of electrolytes, creatinine, calcium, and liver function. Vitamin D levels have been reported to be low in some patients with chronic pain syndromes, including fibromyalgia. It is reasonable to check for vitamin D deficiency, although the response of symptoms to replacement is variable. In select cases, if liver transaminase values are increased, then creatine kinase and hepatitis serologic tests may be indicated. Radiographs are sometimes helpful for excluding other diseases. There is no diagnostic test for fibromyalgia. If sleep disturbance is prominent, sometimes sleep studies are helpful in that some patients with sleep apnea have fibromyalgia symptoms.

* Chronic widespread musculoskeletal pain not explained by physical findings of a rheumatic disease supports the diagnosis of fibromyalgia.
* No laboratory test confirms the diagnosis of fibromyalgia.

Natural History

Fibromyalgia is a chronic waxing and waning condition. Patients have periods of pain and dysfunction alternating with variable periods of feeling reasonably well. Over a period of years, a patient's symptoms and concerns can shift considerably from musculoskeletal concerns to fatigue or other associated symptoms. There is no increased physical disability in patients who have had fibromyalgia for longer periods in comparison with those for whom the diagnosis is recent. Treatment includes reassurance and education, addressing sleep problems, and establishing an exercise program. Nonsteroidal anti-inflammatory drugs, simple analgesics, and medications to help with sleep (such as tricyclic antidepressants) have a role in some patients. Chronic pain management techniques may be helpful for patients with impaired life skills.

Several recent controlled trials have shown that the new antidepressant agent duloxetine is efficacious for patients with fibromyalgia

Table 24-9 Differential Diagnosis of Fibromyalgia

Characteristic	Fibromyalgia	PMR	RA	Polymyositis
Age	Usually young	>50 years	Any	Any
Chief complaint	Pain all over	Pain around shoulders, hips	Joint pain	Weakness
Morning stiffness	<15 minutes	>1 hour	>1 hour	Variable
Physical examination findings	Tender points	Hip, shoulder girdle tenderness & limited ROM	Synovitis	Muscle weakness
ESR	Normal	Increased	Increased or normal	Normal or increased
CPK	Normal	Normal	Normal	Normal
Response to prednisone	No response	Prompt and dramatic	Gradual response	Gradual response

Abbreviations: CPK, creatine phosphokinase; ESR, erythrocyte sedimentation rate; PMR, polymyalgia rheumatica; RA, rheumatoid arthritis; ROM, range of motion.

with or without depression. This agent seems to be efficacious in female patients but less so in males with fibromyalgia. Another new agent, pregabalin, which is used for treatment of peripheral neuropathy, has also been shown to be beneficial in some patients with fibromyalgia. Pramipexole has also been shown to be beneficial in a subset of patients with fibromyalgia.

- In fibromyalgia, symptoms wax and wane.
- There is no progressive physical disability; however, patients may feel that they are unable to function normally.

Low Back Pain

One-third of all people older than 50 years have episodes of acute low back pain. Chronic low back pain is the number 1 compensable work-related injury. The many causes of low back pain include mechanical, neurologic, inflammatory, infectious, neoplastic, and metabolic and referred pain from the viscera. The vast majority of episodes of acute low back pain cannot be explained on a structural basis. Only 3% of patients presenting with acute low back pain have a cause that is not apparent after the initial interview and physical examination. Clinical suspicion of acute spinal cord compromise, spinal infection, or neoplasm requires immediate evaluation and prompt therapy. More than 90% find relief on their own or with the help of a medical practitioner within the first 6 weeks after symptoms occur.

- Only 3% of patients presenting with acute low back pain have a cause that is not apparent after the initial interview and physical examination.

Diagnosis

The most important consideration during the initial evaluation of acute low back pain is the possibility of severe compromise of the spinal cord or cauda equina. In the absence of evidence for acute spinal cord compromise, spinal infection, or neoplastic involvement, immediate pursuit of a cause for the acute back pain is often not helpful. Objective leg weakness or bladder or bowel dysfunction is an indication for more extensive examination and possible surgical decompression. Substantial weight loss or pain that increases with recumbency suggests a neoplastic or infectious process. Pain that worsens with coughing, straining, or sneezing suggests irritation of the dura mater. Radiating pain, weakness, or numbness in an extremity implicates irritation of a spinal nerve root. Exertional calf or thigh cramping but normal peripheral pulses suggest pseudoclaudication (spinal stenosis). Pseudoclaudication symptoms improve with leaning forward on a shopping cart while walking or with sitting (not standing still). Typically, pseudoclaudication also begins in the back or buttock and gradually radiates down the thigh into the leg. This is in contrast to claudication, which usually begins distally and then gradually spreads proximally. Referred pain from an abdominal, pelvic, or hip area suggests an extra-axial cause. An insidious onset with prominent morning stiffness suggests an inflammatory axial arthropathy.

- Objective leg weakness or bladder or bowel dysfunction is an indication for more extensive examination.

- Substantial weight loss or pain that interferes with sleep suggests a neoplastic or infectious process.
- Exertional calf or thigh cramping but normal peripheral pulses suggest pseudoclaudication.
- An insidious onset with prominent morning stiffness suggests an inflammatory axial arthropathy.

Clinical suspicion of acute spinal cord compromise, spinal infection, or neoplasm requires immediate evaluation and prompt therapy. In the absence of specific historical or physical examination findings, laboratory or plain radiographic findings often are unrevealing. The radiographic findings of spondylosis, disk degeneration, facet osteoarthritis, transitional lumbosacral segments, Schmorl nodes, spina bifida occulta, or mild scoliosis are often incidental findings not relevant to a patient's complaints of acute back pain. The routine use of bone scanning, electromyography, computed tomography, or magnetic resonance imaging is usually not necessary to evaluate acute low back pain. More than 20% of asymptomatic adults older than 65 years may have evidence of spinal stenosis on magnetic resonance imaging. The indications for spinal radiography in patients with acute low back pain are listed in Table 24-10.

Treatment

The treatment of acute nonspecific low back pain begins with reassuring the patient, because 90% of all patients with acute low back pain have considerable improvement in 6 weeks. Temporary modification of activities by empowering the patient to adjust lifestyle and demands works best. Bed rest should never be prescribed for more than 3 days to treat acute nonspecific low back pain, because longer bed rest has not been shown to be more beneficial. Short-term use of narcotic analgesics or tramadol can supplement the use of acetaminophen, nonsteroidal anti-inflammatory drugs, and muscle relaxants such as cyclobenzaprine. Physical therapy measures include local heat and ice massage. Pelvic traction and transcutaneous electrical nerve stimulation add little to the management of acute nonspecific low back pain. Epidural glucocorticosteroid injections are best suited to acute disk herniation, although their role is controversial. Injections into the facets are helpful occasionally, particularly if the patient describes a locking or catching as part of the pain syndrome.

Table 24-10 Indications for Spinal Radiography in Patients With Acute Low Back Pain

First episode of acute back pain is after age 50 years
History of back disease
History of back surgery
History of neoplasm
Acute history of direct trauma to the back
Fever
Weight loss
Severe pain unrelieved in any position
Neurologic symptoms or signs

- Clinical suspicion of acute spinal cord compromise, spinal infection, or neoplasm requires immediate evaluation and prompt therapy.
- In 90% of patients, acute low back pain (local or sciatic presentations) remits within 6 weeks.
- Pelvic traction and transcutaneous electrical nerve stimulation add little to the management of acute nonspecific low back pain.

Bursitis

A bursa is a fluid-filled sac lined with a membrane. Bursae are present in the areas where tendons and muscles move over bony prominences. Additional bursae form in response to irritative stimuli. Trauma or overuse, microcrystalline disease, chronic inflammatory arthritis, and infection cause bursitis. Treatment of aseptic bursitis involves strict immobilization, ice compresses, nonsteroidal anti-inflammatory drugs, bursal aspiration, corticosteroid injections, and, occasionally, physical therapy. Glucocorticosteroids should not be given if there is a clinical suggestion of sepsis.

- Always consider infection or microcrystalline disease in the differential diagnosis of acute bursitis.

Septic bursitis may result from puncture wounds or cellulitis or occur after a local injection. In half of the cases, there is no portal of entry for infection in septic superficial bursitis (olecranon and prepatellar bursae). The organisms frequently responsible for infection are staphylococci and streptococci. Patients with septic superficial bursitis present with localized pain and swelling. Warmth about the area of the superficial bursa should raise the possibility of a septic bursa. If there is doubt, the bursa should be aspirated with strict aseptic technique. The needle should enter from the side through uninvolved skin—not at the point of maximal fluctuance—to avoid creating a chronic draining fistula.

When infection is suspected, patients should be treated empirically with antistaphylococcal and antistreptococcal oral antibiotics, pending the microbiologic results. Gram stains are positive in only 40% to 60% of patients. The number of leukocytes in infected bursal fluid can be low compared with that in infected joint fluid. This may be due to the modest blood supply of the bursae compared with that of joints. Patients with more severe infections or with associated cellulitis frequently do not respond to outpatient management. They should be hospitalized and given antibiotics intravenously, and the affected part should be immobilized for 3 or 4 days. Repeated aspirations or even surgical débridement is necessary in some cases.

- Septic bursitis frequently occurs without evidence of a portal of entry.
- Bursal warmth is the best predictor of infection.
- Gram stains are positive in only 40%-60% of patients.
- The number of leukocytes in infected bursal fluid can be low.
- Patients with more severe infections should be hospitalized.

Polymyalgia Rheumatica

Polymyalgia rheumatica is a clinical syndrome usually characterized by the onset of aching and morning stiffness in the proximal musculature (hip and shoulder girdles). It is more common in females than males and usually occurs in patients older than 60 years. Patients usually have an increased erythrocyte sedimentation rate; autoantibody results, including rheumatoid factor, CCP antibodies, and antinuclear antibody, are usually negative or normal. Many patients have a mild normochromic anemia. A small number of patients may have a normal sedimentation rate at presentation. The C-reactive protein value is usually increased in these cases. In patients in whom the acute-phase reactants are normal and there is not certainty about the diagnosis, radionucleotide joint scanning can be done. In patients with active polymyalgia rheumatica, radionuclide joint scanning confirms hip and shoulder synovitis, a finding supporting synovitis as the cause of the symptoms. The presence of other specific diseases such as rheumatoid arthritis, chronic infection, inflammatory myositis, or malignancy should be excluded. Patients with polymyalgia rheumatica have prompt (within 24-72 hours) response to small doses of prednisone (10-20 mg daily).

- Typical clinical scenario: An elderly patient presents with aching and morning stiffness in the proximal musculature and increased erythrocyte sedimentation rate.

Features and Differential Diagnosis

Patients with polymyalgia rheumatica complain of stiffness and pain. This stiffness is most prominent in the mornings and after prolonged sitting. They also have problems getting comfortable at night to sleep. They occasionally have mild constitutional symptoms, including sweats, fevers, anorexia, and weight loss. Very prominent constitutional features and markedly increased erythrocyte sedimentation rate could suggest associated giant cell arteritis. Extremity edema or oligoarticular synovitis can occur, particularly at the knees, wrists, and shoulders. Polyarticular small joint arthritis is not a feature. Table 24-11 summarizes the rheumatic syndromes and other diseases that occasionally present with a polymyalgia rheumatica-like syndrome. Clinical evaluation and screening laboratory tests usually distinguish polymyalgia rheumatica from these other conditions. A variant known as the RS3PE syndrome (remitting symmetric seronegative synovitis with pitting edema) can occur, primarily in older men. Patients with this present with symptoms of polymyalgia rheumatica but also synovitis and marked edema in the hands or feet.

- In polymyalgia rheumatica, stiffness is more prolonged in the mornings, and patients describe gelling (ie, stiffening again after prolonged inactivity).
- Prominent constitutional features and markedly increased erythrocyte sedimentation rate could suggest associated giant cell arteritis.
- Extremity edema or oligoarticular synovitis can occur.

Pathogenesis and Relationship to Giant Cell Arteritis

Polymyalgia rheumatica can begin before, appear simultaneously with, or develop after the symptoms of giant cell arteritis. The pathogenesis of polymyalgia rheumatica is unknown. Clinicians appreciate the close relationship between giant cell arteritis and polymyalgia rheumatica. Up to 15% of patients with polymyalgia rheumatica also have giant cell arteritis. Familial aggregation and increased

Table 24-11 Systemic Illnesses Presenting With a Polymyalgia-like Syndrome

Rheumatic Syndromes	Other Systemic Illnesses
Systemic vasculitis	Paraneoplastic syndromes
Myositis	Systemic amyloidosis
Systemic lupus erythematosus	Infectious endocarditis
Seronegative rheumatoid arthritis	Hyperthyroidism
	Hypothyroidism
Polyarticular osteoarthritis	Hyperparathyroidism
Fibromyalgia	Osteomalacia
Remitting seronegative, symmetric synovitis & peripheral edema	Depression

incidence in patients of northern European background suggest a genetic predisposition. HLA-DR4 is associated with these conditions more commonly than would be expected by chance. Among patients with giant cell arteritis, 40% have symptoms of polymyalgia rheumatica during the course of their disease.

- Up to 15% of patients with polymyalgia rheumatica also have giant cell arteritis.
- Among patients with active giant cell arteritis, 40% have symptoms of polymyalgia rheumatica.
- Polymyalgia rheumatica can begin before, appear simultaneously with, or develop after the symptoms of giant cell arteritis.

Treatment

All patients with polymyalgia rheumatica should respond completely after 3 to 5 days of treatment with prednisone, 10 to 20 mg/day. Sometimes, split-dose (5 mg 3 times daily) prednisone is more effective than a single daily dose of 15 mg. Patients should be followed clinically, and usually the erythrocyte sedimentation rate should be measured monthly to confirm the disease flare. Polymyalgia rheumatica is thought to be a self-limited disease, although relapses occur. Prednisone treatment is discontinued in more than half of patients within 2 years. A minority of patients may be at risk of later appearance of giant cell arteritis.

- All patients with polymyalgia rheumatica should respond completely after 3-5 days of treatment with prednisone.
- Polymyalgia rheumatica is thought to be a self-limited disease, although relapses occur and a small risk of late appearance of giant cell arteritis exists.

Vasculitic Syndromes

Vasculitis, or angiitis, is an inflammatory disease of blood vessels. Damage to the vessel wall and stenosis or occlusion of the vessel lumen by thrombosis and progressive intimal proliferation of the vessel result in the clinical manifestations of the illness. The distribution of the vascular lesions and the size of the blood vessels involved vary considerably in different vasculitic syndromes and in different patients with the same syndrome. Vasculitis can be transient, chronic, self-limited, or progressive. It can be the primary abnormality or due to another systemic process. Histopathologic classification does not distinguish local from systemic illness or secondary from primary insult. The key clinical features suggestive of vasculitis are listed in Table 24-12. Vasculitis "look-alikes," or simulators, are listed in Table 24-13. These diseases and conditions should be considered whenever a patient's condition suggests vasculitis. Clinical features of vasculitis are outlined in Table 24-14. The ability to recognize characteristic clinical patterns of involvement is very helpful in making the diagnosis of systemic necrotizing vasculitis (Figure 24-4).

- Vasculitic symptoms reflect the nonspecific systemic features of inflammation (constitutional features) and the ischemic consequences of vascular occlusion.

Specific Vasculitic Syndromes

Giant Cell Arteritis

Giant cell arteritis, also known as temporal arteritis, predominantly affects persons older than 50 years. The prevalence exceeds 223 cases per 100,000 persons older than 50. It is most common in persons of northern European ancestry. Females outnumber males by 3:1. Polymyalgia rheumatica symptoms may develop in 40% to 50% of all patients with giant cell arteritis. Up to 15% of patients with polymyalgia rheumatica have temporal artery biopsy findings positive

Table 24-12 **Clinical Features That Suggest Vasculitis**

Constitutional features
  Fatigue, fever, weight loss, & anorexia
Skin lesions
  Palpable purpura, necrotic ulcers, livedo reticularis, urticaria, nodules, & digital infarcts
Arthralgia or arthritis
Myalgia or prominent fibrositis
  Polymyalgia rheumatica symptoms
Claudication or phlebitis
Headache
Cerebrovascular accident
Neuropathy
  Mononeuritis multiplex
Hypertension
Abnormal renal sediment
Pulmonary abnormalities
  Pulmonary hemorrhage, pulmonary nodules with cavities
Abdominal pain or intestinal hemorrhage
Nonspecific indicators of inflammation
  Anemia, thrombocytosis, low levels of albumin, elevated erythrocyte sedimentation rate, increased levels of liver enzymes, or eosinophilia

Table 24-13 Syndromes That Mimic Vasculitis

Cardiac myxoma with embolization
Infective endocarditis
Thrombotic thrombocytopenic purpura
Atheroembolism: cholesterol or calcium emboli
Ergotism
Pseudoxanthoma elasticum
Ehlers-Danlos type 4
Neurovasculopathy secondary to antiphospholipid syndrome
Arterial coarctation or dysplasia
Infectious angiitis
    Lyme disease
    Rickettsial infection
    HIV infection

Abbreviation: HIV, human immunodeficiency virus.

Table 24-14 Clinical Features of Systemic Vasculitis

Common Features	Uncommon Features
Fever, fatigue, weight loss	Coronary arteritis
Arthralgia, arthritis	Myocardial infarction
Myalgia	Congestive heart failure
Mononeuritis multiplex	Central nervous system
Focal necrotizing glomerulo-	abnormalities
nephritis	Seizures
Abnormal renal sediment	Cerebrovascular accident
Hypertension	Lung (interstitial pneumonitis)
Skin abnormalities	Eye (retinal hemorrhage)
Palpable purpura	Testicular pain
Livedo reticularis	
Cutaneous infarctions	
Abdominal pain/ischemic	
bowel	
Liver enzyme abnormalities	

for giant cell arteritis. There is considerable morbidity with this disease; however, the rate of blindness is declining. Affected patients are at higher subsequent risk of aortic aneurysms. The mortality rate for patients with giant cell arteritis is similar to that for the general population.

- Giant cell arteritis is most common in persons of northern European ancestry.
- Polymyalgia rheumatica develops in 40%-50% of patients with giant cell arteritis.
- Up to 15% of patients with polymyalgia rheumatica have temporal artery biopsy findings positive for giant cell arteritis.

Pathology
Giant cell arteritis involves the primary and secondary branches of the aorta in a segmental or patchy fashion. However, any artery, and occasionally veins, can be affected. It is unusual for intracranial arteries to be involved. Histopathologically, all layers of the vessel wall are extensively disrupted, with intimal thickening and a prominent mononuclear and histiocytic infiltrate. Multinucleated giant cells infiltrate the vessel wall in 50% of cases. Fragmentation and disintegration of the internal elastic membrane, the other characteristic features, are closely associated with the accumulation of giant cells and vascular occlusive symptoms.

- Giant cell arteritis affects primary and secondary branches of the aorta in a segmental or patchy fashion.

Clinical Features
Early clinical features of giant cell arteritis include temporal headache, polymyalgia rheumatica symptoms, fatigue, and fever. The classic features of this disease are included in Table 24-15. Arteritis of the branches of the ophthalmic or posterior ciliary arteries causes ischemia of the optic nerve (ischemic optic neuritis) and blindness. Less often, retinal arterioles are occluded. Blindness occurs in fewer than 15% of untreated patients. Large peripheral artery involvement in giant

cell arteritis occurs in about 10% of patients. Extremity claudication, Raynaud phenomenon, aortic dissection, decreased pulses, and vascular bruits suggest large peripheral artery involvement. Patients with large peripheral artery involvement do not differ from those with more classic giant cell arteritis, either histologically or with regard to laboratory findings. Patients who have had giant cell arteritis are at increased risk for the development of aneurysms. Because of this risk, guidelines exist for periodic screening of patients with a history of giant cell arteritis.

- Typical clinical scenario: A 60-year-old patient presents with temporal headache, polymyalgia rheumatica-like symptoms, fatigue, and fever. The sedimentation rate is markedly increased. Physical examination shows scalp tenderness.
- Blindness occurs in <15% of untreated patients.

Diagnosis
The necessary length of an adequate temporal artery biopsy specimen is controversial. However, because of patchy involvement and skip lesions, a length of at least 1 cm is recommended. In 15% of

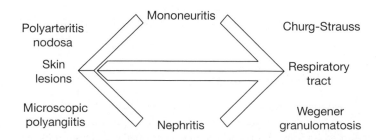

Figure 24-4. Common Organ Involvement in Systemic Vasculitis.

Table 24-15 Classic Clinical Features of Giant Cell Arteritis

Fever, weight loss, fatigue
Polymyalgia rheumatica symptoms
Temporal headache
Jaw or tongue claudication
Ocular symptoms
    Blindness
    Diplopia
    Ptosis
Scalp tenderness
Dry cough
Peripheral large vessel vasculitis (10%)

patients, the biopsy is positive on the opposite side if that on the initial side is negative. Typical laboratory abnormalities in acute active giant cell arteritis include a markedly increased erythrocyte sedimentation rate, moderate normochromic anemia, and thrombocytosis. A mild increase in liver enzyme values, most typically alkaline phosphatase, occurs in one-third of patients because of granulomatous hepatitis. The erythrocyte sedimentation rate is rarely normal in patients with active giant cell arteritis. The classification criteria for giant cell arteritis are given in Table 24-16.

- The temporal artery biopsy specimen should be at least 1 cm long to compensate for patchy involvement.
- In 15% of patients, the biopsy is positive on the opposite side if that on the initial side is negative.
- Typical laboratory abnormalities in giant cell arteritis are markedly increased erythrocyte sedimentation rate, moderate normochromic anemia, and thrombocytosis.

Treatment

Treatment is initiated with corticosteroids when the diagnosis of giant cell arteritis is considered and the biopsy is requested. A temporal artery biopsy specimen remains positive for disease even after several weeks of corticosteroid treatment. Initial treatment includes prednisone, typically 40 to 60 mg/day. A higher dose of corticosteroids can be given parenterally in cases of visual or life-threatening symptoms. A recent study suggested parenteral corticosteroids initially may lessen the total duration and cumulative dose needed. Most symptoms of giant cell arteritis begin to respond within 24 hours after corticosteroid therapy is initiated. Visual changes that are present for more than a few hours are often irreversible. Alternate-day administration of corticosteroids does not control symptoms in at least half of patients.

- Treatment is initiated with corticosteroids when the diagnosis of giant cell arteritis is considered and the biopsy is requested.
- Initial treatment of giant cell arteritis includes prednisone, typically 40-60 mg/day.
- Alternate-day administration of corticosteroids does not initially control symptoms in at least half of patients.

Outcome

Giant cell arteritis typically has a self-limited course. In 24 months, half of patients are able to discontinue treatment with corticosteroids. An effective steroid-sparing agent has not been identified, but methotrexate or azathioprine has been used in some patients. The diagnosis of giant cell arteritis does not influence mortality rates. Relapse may occur in a third of patients, and a thoracic or abdominal aneurysm develops in a third.

- Giant cell arteritis typically has a self-limited course over about 2 years, although relapses and late consequences, including aortic aneurysms, occur.

Takayasu Arteritis

Takayasu arteritis is also known as aortic arch syndrome or pulseless disease. Each year, about 2.6 new cases per 1,000,000 population occur. Most patients are between the ages of 15 and 40 years. At least 80% of them are female. This disease is more common in Asia, Latin America, and Eastern Europe. Its pathologic features cannot be distinguished from those of giant cell arteritis. Takayasu arteritis affects the aorta and its primary branches. The arterial wall is irregularly thickened, with luminal narrowing, dilatations, aneurysms, and distortions. The aortic valve and coronary ostia can be involved.

- Among patients with Takayasu arteritis, most are female and between the ages of 15 and 40 years.
- The aorta and its primary branches are most commonly affected.

Clinical and Laboratory Features

The constitutional features of fever, weight loss, fatigue, and arthralgia can precede symptoms of ischemia to the brain or claudication of the extremities. Renovascular hypertension, pulmonary hypertension, and coronary artery insufficiency can complicate Takayasu arteritis. Cutaneous vasculitis, erythema nodosum, and synovitis occasionally occur in cases of active Takayasu arteritis. Compromise of the cerebral vasculature can lead to dizziness, blurry or fading vision, syncope, and, occasionally, stroke. Physical examination findings confirm vascular bruits, absence of peripheral pulses, and, occasionally, fever. When the disease is active, results of laboratory studies usually show increased erythrocyte sedimentation rate, normochromic anemia, and thrombocytosis. However, in some cases

Table 24-16 Classification Criteria for Giant Cell Arteritis

Temporal artery biopsy findings positive for classic giant cell arteritis

or

Four of the 5 following criteria:
    Tender, swollen temporal artery
    Jaw claudication
    Blindness
    Polymyalgia rheumatica symptoms
    Rapid response to corticosteroids

of active disease, the erythrocyte sedimentation rate is normal. The diagnosis can be confirmed with conventional angiography, although magnetic resonance angiography may become the imaging method of choice.

- Renovascular hypertension, pulmonary hypertension, and coronary artery insufficiency can complicate Takayasu arteritis.
- Typical clinical scenario: A young patient presents with fever, weight loss, fatigue, and arthralgia. Physical examination shows carotid bruits and absence of peripheral pulses. On laboratory testing, the erythrocyte sedimentation rate is increased.

Treatment and Outcome

Corticosteroid therapy alone is usually adequate for controlling the inflammation. Methotrexate or cyclophosphamide treatment is indicated in resistant cases. On average, patients receive corticosteroids for about 2 years. Late stenotic complications are amenable to vascular operation and bypass grafting. Survival is more than 90% at 10 years. Congestive heart failure from previous coronary artery involvement and cerebrovascular accidents are major causes of mortality.

- Survival in patients with Takayasu arteritis is >90% at 10 years.

Classic Polyarteritis Nodosum and Microscopic Polyangiitis

Systemic necrotizing vasculitis occurs alone or in association with several diseases (secondary). When it occurs as a primary vasculitis, it is most commonly a small vessel antineutrophil cytoplasmic antibody (ANCA)-associated disease of Wegener granulomatosis or microscopic polyangiitis. Medium-vessel polyarteritis nodosa, frequently associated with hepatitis B, is far less common. A secondary necrotizing vasculitis can occur in association with rheumatoid arthritis, systemic lupus erythematosus, other connective tissue diseases, cryoglobulinemia, hepatitis C infection, hairy cell leukemia, and other malignant conditions.

- Systemic necrotizing vasculitis occurs alone or in association with several diseases.

Pathology

These diseases are characterized by transmural inflammation and necrosis of blood vessels. Classic polyarteritis nodosa affects medium-sized muscular arteries. ANCA-associated vasculitis affects arterioles, venules, and capillaries. The size of the affected vessels plays a large part in determining the clinical manifestations of the syndromes.

- Systemic vasculitis may affect a spectrum of vessel sizes.

Clinical Features

Systemic vasculitis usually is associated with prominent constitutional features, including fever, fatigue, weight loss, and, occasionally, myalgia or arthralgia, along with manifestations of multisystem organ involvement. Virtually any organ can be affected eventually. Occasionally, vasculitis is limited to a single organ or found incidentally associated with

cancer at the time of operation and cured by surgical removal. Other cases are limited to isolated involvement of the skin or peripheral nerves.

Classic polyarteritis nodosa is a necrotizing vasculitis of small and medium-sized arteries and is associated with vascular nephropathy (usually without glomerulonephritis), causing multiple renal infarctions, hypertension, and renal failure. Hypertension develops as a result of angiographically demonstrable renal artery compromise or, less commonly, glomerular involvement. Lung involvement is very uncommon.

Microscopic polyangiitis is distinguished from polyarteritis nodosa as a necrotizing vasculitis that affects capillaries, venules, and arterioles and most frequently presents with pauci-immune and sometimes rapidly progressive necrotizing glomerulonephritis. Proteinuria is common, and, rarely, a nephritic syndrome may develop. There is an active urinary sediment, with red blood cells and red cell casts characteristic of glomerular involvement. Renal insufficiency is frequently noted at presentation, and glomerulonephritis causes oliguric renal failure in one-third of all patients. Renal angiography in microscopic polyangiitis is usually normal. Hypertension is uncommon. Lung involvement, including pulmonary capillaritis and hemorrhage, eventually may affect up to a third of patients with microscopic polyangiitis.

Systemic vasculitis may be a manifestation or complication of other diseases. This secondary vasculitis complicates hepatitis C infection, rheumatoid arthritis, Sjögren syndrome, mixed cryoglobulinemia, hairy cell leukemia, myelodysplastic syndrome, and other hematologic malignancies. Some forms of secondary vasculitis have more favorable clinical presentations. For example, systemic rheumatoid vasculitis most commonly manifests with constitutional symptoms, skin lesions, and neuropathy. It rarely causes a necrotizing glomerulonephritis or pulmonary hemorrhage.

- Systemic vasculitis is associated with prominent constitutional features, including fever, fatigue, weight loss, and, occasionally, myalgia or arthralgia, along with manifestations of multisystem organ involvement.
- ANCA-associated vasculitis disorders of Wegener granulomatosis and microscopic polyangiitis are more common than classic polyarteritis nodosa.
- Secondary vasculitis may be a complication of other diseases.

Diagnosis

Abnormal laboratory findings include normocytic anemia, increased erythrocyte sedimentation rate, and thrombocytosis. Microscopic polyangiitis presents with a myeloperoxidase-specific perinuclear (p-) ANCA in 90% of cases. Complement consumption is not part of primary systemic vasculitis. Low complement may be evident if immune complexes such as cryoglobulins are part of the pathogenesis of secondary vasculitis. Hepatitis B infection occurs in a small proportion of patients with ANCA-negative (classic) polyarteritis nodosa and should always be sought, because treatment is directed against the infection. Hepatitis C is associated with the secondary vasculitis that is the cause of some cases of mixed cryoglobulinemia.

Evaluation should document the extent and severity of the condition. The confirmatory test typically is angiography or biopsy of involved tissue showing vasculitis. The biopsy should be of accessible symptomatic tissue. If medium-sized vessel polyarteritis nodosa is suspected, visceral angiography, including views of the renal and mesenteric arteries, shows saccular or fusiform aneurysm formation coupled with smooth, tapered stenosis alternating with normal or dilated blood vessels (Figure 24-5).

- Microscopic polyangiitis often presents with positive myeloperoxidase-specific p-ANCA.
- Hepatitis B infection occurs in a small proportion of patients with ANCA-negative (classic) polyarteritis nodosa and should always be sought, because treatment is directed against the infection.
- Hepatitis C is associated with some cases of mixed cryoglobulinemia.
- Confirmatory diagnostic tests include angiography or biopsy of involved tissue showing vasculitis.
- Visceral angiography shows saccular or fusiform aneurysm formation coupled with smooth, tapered stenosis.
- Consider visceral angiography for diagnosis when the patient has significant gastrointestinal symptoms or markedly increased liver enzyme values and no tissue or organ system (nerve, skin) is affected or easily sampled by biopsy.

Treatment

The cornerstone of treatment is early diagnosis and corticosteroid therapy. Cytotoxic or antimetabolite drugs such as cyclophosphamide,

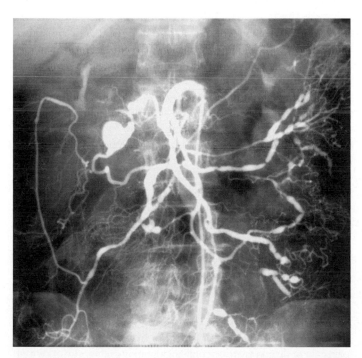

Figure 24-5. Visceral Polyarteritis Nodosa. Angiography shows the classic features of smooth tapers followed by normal or dilated vessels. Note the large saccular aneurysm in the hepatic artery. (From Audiovisual Aids Subcommittee of the Education Committee of the American College of Rheumatology. Syllabus: revised clinical slide collection on the rheumatic diseases and 1985, 1988, and 1989 slide supplements. Atlanta [GA]: American College of Rheumatology. Used with permission.)

methotrexate, and azathioprine are used in combination with corticosteroids. The choice of the second agent is usually determined according to the severity of organ involvement. A new treatment that has shown promise in some patients with systemic vasculitis, especially those with Wegener granulomatosis, is rituximab. More information on this agent is included in the section of this chapter dealing with medications. When a patient's condition deteriorates in the face of potent treatment, consider possible progression of disease, superimposed infection, or noninflammatory, proliferative, occlusive vasculopathy. Hepatitis-associated vasculitis is treated best with antiviral drugs after a short course of systemic corticosteroids.

- Cyclophosphamide, methotrexate, and azathioprine are often used in conjuction with corticosteroids.

Outcome

In the first year after diagnosis of systemic vasculitis, deaths are related to the extent of disease activity, particularly gastrointestinal tract ischemia and renal insufficiency. Distinguishing classic polyarteritis nodosa from microscopic polyangiitis and type of organ involvement may influence treatment, complications, relapse rate, and mortality (Table 24-17).

After 1 year, complications of treatment, including infections in the immunocompromised patient, contribute most to mortality rates. With treatment, survival at 5 years is between 55% and 60% for microscopic polyangiitis and between 75% and 90% for classic polyarteritis nodosa.

- In the first year after diagnosis, deaths are related to the extent of disease activity, particularly gastrointestinal tract ischemia and renal insufficiency.
- Complications from treatment affect long-term mortality.
- Typical clinical scenario: A patient presents with fever, fatigue, weight loss, arthralgia, mononeuritis multiplex, and renal failure. Renal angiography shows saccular and fusiform aneurysm formation with smooth, tapered stenosis of the vessels. Laboratory testing shows increased sedimentation rate and negative antimyeloperoxidase antibodies. Chest radiography is normal.

Churg-Strauss Vasculitis

Churg-Strauss vasculitis, or Churg-Strauss syndrome, is similar to microscopic angiitis and Wegener granulomatosis in that it involves small vessels and may be associated with ANCA antibodies. The median age at onset is about 38 years (range, 15-69 years). Churg-Strauss vasculitis is defined by 1) a history of, or current symptoms of, asthma, 2) peripheral eosinophilia ($>1.5 \times 10^9$ eosinophils/L), and 3) systemic vasculitis of at least 2 extrapulmonary organs. There is a slight male predominance. The histopathologic features of the disease include eosinophilic extravascular granulomas and granulomatous or nongranulomatous small vessel necrotizing vasculitis. It typically involves the small arteries, veins, arterioles, and venules.

- Churg-Strauss vasculitis: asthma, eosinophilia, systemic vasculitis involving at least 2 extrapulmonary systems.
- It involves small arteries, veins, arterioles, and venules.

Table 24-17 Features of Polyarteritis Nodosa and Microscopic
Polyangiitis

Characteristic	Polyarteritis Nodosa	Microscopic Polyangiitis
Vessels involved	Small & medium-sized	Capillaries, venules, arterioles
ANCA	Often negative	Usually p-ANCA (MPO)-positive
Renal involvement	Ischemic nephropathy	Often glomerulonephritis
Pulmonary involvement	Seldom	Alveolar hemorrhage in 1/3

Abbreviations: ANCA, antineutrophil cytoplasmic antibody; MPO, myeloperoxide; p-ANCA, perinuclear ANCA.

Clinical Features

Churg-Strauss syndrome is thought to evolve in 3 stages. Patients need not progress in an orderly manner from 1 stage to another. There usually is a prodrome of allergic rhinitis, nasal polyposis, or asthma. In the second stage, peripheral blood and tissue eosinophilia develops, suggesting Löffler syndrome. Chronic eosinophilic pneumonia and gastroenteritis may remit or recur over years. The third stage is life-threatening vasculitis. Transient, patchy pulmonary infiltrates or nodules, pleural effusions, pulmonary angiitis and cardiomegaly, eosinophilic gastroenteritis, extravascular necrotizing granulomata of the skin, mononeuritis multiplex, and polyarthritis can complicate Churg-Strauss syndrome. A Churg-Strauss–like syndrome has been reported in some patients treated with the asthma medication zafirlukast.

- Churg-Strauss syndrome: prodrome of allergic rhinitis, nasal polyposis, or asthma.
- Peripheral blood and tissue eosinophilia develops.
- Transient, patchy pulmonary infiltrates, extravascular necrotizing granulomata of the skin, and mononeuritis multiplex can complicate Churg-Strauss syndrome.

Treatment and Outcome

The 1-year survival with treated Churg-Strauss syndrome is similar to that with microscopic polyangiitis. There is more cardiac involvement but fewer renal deaths than in polyarteritis nodosa. Treatment includes corticosteroids with or without the addition of cytotoxic agents. The eosinophilia resolves with treatment.

- In Churg-Strauss syndrome, there is more cardiac involvement but fewer renal deaths than in polyarteritis nodosa.
- Typical clinical scenario: A patient presents with a history of bronchial asthma with recent worsening of pulmonary symptoms and development of mononeuritis multiplex. There is a history of nasal polyposis. Physical evaluation reveals palpable

purpura. On laboratory testing, the eosinophil count is markedly increased.

Buerger Disease

Buerger disease, or thromboangiitis obliterans, occurs almost exclusively in young adult smokers. There is a male predominance. Patients usually present with ischemic injury to fingers or, less commonly, toes. Buerger disease affects the small and medium-sized arteries and veins of the extremities. Acute vasculitis in Buerger disease is accompanied by characteristic intraluminal thrombus that contains microabscesses. Usually, the disease is arrested when smoking is stopped. In contrast to other forms of vasculitis, Buerger disease is best thought of as a vasculopathy in that it does not require immunosuppressive therapy.

- Buerger disease occurs almost exclusively in young adult smokers.
- Patients present with ischemic injury to fingers or toes.
- The disease is arrested when smoking is stopped.

Isolated (Primary) Angiitis of the Central Nervous System

Clinical Features

Isolated, or primary, angiitis of the central nervous system, once thought to be rare, has a chronic fluctuating and progressive course. The average age of patients presenting with this disease is 45 years. Forty percent of patients have had symptoms for less than 4 weeks at presentation, and another 40% present with symptoms that have been noted for more than 3 months. The most common symptom is headache (mild or severe), often associated with nausea or vomiting. Nonfocal neurologic abnormalities (including confusion, dementia, drowsiness, or coma) may interrupt prolonged periods of apparent remission. Acute stroke-like focal neurologic presentations are increasingly described. Cerebral hemorrhage occurs in fewer than 4% of patients. Focal and nonfocal neurologic abnormalities coexist in half of patients. Systemic features—fever, weight loss, arthralgia, and myalgia—are uncommon and occur in fewer than 20% of patients; seizures occur in about 25%.

- Isolated angiitis of the central nervous system has a chronic fluctuating and progressive course, most commonly without evidence of systemic inflammation.
- Most common symptom is headache.
- Complications include acute strokes, with or without nonfocal neurologic abnormalities (decreased consciousness or cognition).
- Cerebral hemorrhage occurs in <4% of patients.

Diagnosis

There are no reliable noninvasive tests for making the diagnosis. The mainstays of diagnosis are cerebral angiography and biopsy of central nervous system tissues, including the leptomeninges. The cerebrospinal fluid is abnormal in most patients with pathologically documented primary angiitis of the central nervous system. Computed tomography of the head is not specific or sensitive for the condition. Magnetic resonance imaging may be sensitive but does not distinguish this primary angiitis from other vasculopathic or demyelinating lesions of the brain, and it is not useful for following the condition. Patients with a chronic progressive course are more likely to have the diagnosis made pathologically and have abnormal results on examination of the cerebrospinal fluid.

* The mainstays of diagnosis of isolated angiitis are cerebral angiography and biopsy of central nervous system tissues, including the leptomeninges.

Rheumatologic syndromes that may produce a clinical picture similar to that of primary angiitis of the central nervous system include Cogan syndrome (nonsyphilitic keratitis and vestibular dysfunction), Behçet syndrome (uveitis, oral and genital ulcers, meningitis, and vasculitis), systemic lupus erythematosus, and polyarteritis. Drug-induced vasculopathy (particularly cocaine), demyelinating disease, human immunodeficiency virus (HIV) infection, Lyme disease, syphilis, carcinomatous meningitis, angiocentric immunoproliferative lesions, and antiphospholipid antibody syndrome are also part of the differential diagnosis in patients presenting with a syndrome suggesting primary angiitis of the central nervous system.

Treatment

The treatment for primary angiitis of the central nervous system may be influenced by the clinical subset. Younger patients with acute disease in whom the diagnosis was made with angiography may have a benign course and typically respond well to a short course of treatment with corticosteroids and calcium channel blockers to prevent vasospasm. Patients with a protracted course, abnormal cerebrospinal fluid, and diagnosis made with brain and leptomeningeal biopsy are best treated with combination therapy, including corticosteroids and cytotoxic agents. If untreated, this clinical subset has a high mortality rate.

* The mortality rate is high among patients with histopathologically confirmed or recurrent symptoms treated without cytotoxic agents.

Wegener Granulomatosis

Clinical Features

Wegener granulomatosis is a well-recognized pathologic triad of upper and lower respiratory tract necrotizing granulomatous inflammation and focal segmental necrotizing glomerulonephritis. Wegener granulomatosis occurs in less than 1 person annually per 100,000 population. The peak incidence of the disease occurs in the fourth and fifth decades of life. There is a slight male predominance. Eighty-five percent of the patients have generalized disease, including glomerulonephritis; 15% can present with local inflammation involving only the upper respiratory tract or kidneys. The clinical features of this disease are summarized by the mnemonic ELKS: involvement of *e*ar/nose/throat, *l*ung, *k*idney, and *s*kin. Lung involvement most commonly includes thick-walled, centrally cavitating pulmonary nodules. Alveolitis and pulmonary hemorrhage occur in up to 20% of patients. Biopsy in patients with renal involvement shows focal segmental necrotizing glomerulonephritis and, occasionally, granulomatous vasculitis. Skin involvement may

include urticaria, petechiae, papules, vesicles, ulcers, pyoderma, and livedo reticularis. Inflammatory arthritis is usually oligoarticular and transient, occurring early in the clinical presentation. Central nervous system involvement includes distal sensory neuropathy, mononeuritis multiplex, and cranial nerve palsies. Conjunctivitis, uveitis, and proptosis are not unusual. Neurosensory hearing loss has been described together with serous otitis and inner ear vasculitis. Wegener granulomatosis-associated subglottic tracheal stenosis due to chondritis should be distinguished from primary polychondritis. Laboratory testing shows a positive cytoplasmic (c-) ANCA test.

* Typical clinical scenario: A 50-year-old patient presents with the triad of upper and lower respiratory tract necrotizing granulomatous inflammation and focal segmental necrotizing glomerulonephritis. Laboratory testing shows a positive c-ANCA test.
* ELKS: involvement of *e*ar/nose/throat, *l*ung, *k*idney, and *s*kin.
* Alveolitis and pulmonary hemorrhage occur in up to 20% of patients.
* Central nervous system involvement includes distal sensory neuropathy, mononeuritis multiplex, and cranial nerve palsies.

Pathologic Diagnosis

The diagnosis of Wegener granulomatosis may require finding characteristic pathologic features in biopsy specimens. Biopsy of the upper respiratory tract suggests the diagnosis in 55% of patients, but only 20% have granulomata or vasculitis associated with necrosis. An open lung biopsy has a higher diagnostic yield than transbronchial biopsy. Renal biopsies usually show only a focal segmental necrotizing glomerulonephritis. The renal biopsy thus is not specific for Wegener granulomatosis. Infrequently, renal biopsy shows vasculitis. Relevant laboratory findings in active Wegener granulomatosis include non-specific increases in the erythrocyte sedimentation rate and platelet count, normocytic anemia, and low levels of albumin. A positive c-ANCA directed against proteinase 3 test in a patient with the clinical features of Wegener granulomatosis may be sufficient for diagnosis, especially if tissue is not easily obtained.

* Laboratory findings in Wegener granulomatosis include non-specific increases in erythrocyte sedimentation rate and platelet count and normocytic anemia.
* Diagnosis: positive proteinase 3, c-ANCA test and granulomatous inflammation on biopsy.

ANCA

c-ANCA is directed against proteinase 3, a serine protease from azurophilic granules. c-ANCA occurs in more than 90% of active cases of generalized Wegener granulomatosis. Occasionally, it is found in idiopathic crescentic glomerulonephritis, microscopic polyarteritis nodosa, and Churg-Strauss syndrome. The antibody titer tends to correlate with disease activity in an individual patient.

p-ANCA is directed against myeloperoxidase and other neutrophil cytoplasmic constituents. p-ANCA (anti-myeloperoxidase-specific) is found in idiopathic crescentic glomerulonephritis, microscopic polyarteritis nodosa, Churg-Strauss syndrome, Wegener granulomatosis, and other connective tissue diseases. p-ANCA directed against other antigens can occur in patients with inflammatory bowel disease, autoimmune liver disease, other connective tissue diseases, malignancies, and even drug-induced syndromes.

* Proteinase 3, c-ANCA occurs in >90% of active cases of Wegener granulomatosis.
* Non-myeloperoxidase p-ANCA is found in many different conditions.

Treatment and Outcome

If untreated, generalized Wegener granulomatosis is associated with a mean survival of 5 months and 95% mortality in 1 year. More than 95% of patients eventually have clinical remission with oral cyclophosphamide treatment. Corticosteroids are useful initially, and the dose can be tapered quickly after the disease is controlled. Mortality in the first year of disease is related primarily to the inflammatory process, with pulmonary hemorrhage or renal failure. In subsequent years, drug toxicity may dominate, with opportunistic infection and increasing risk of neoplasm and hemorrhagic cystitis related to the use of cyclophosphamide. Relapses even years after treatment are not uncommon.

Recent studies have suggested that rituximab may be efficacious in the treatment of patients with Wegener granulomatosis. Studies are currently under way to better define the optimal patients and regimens for use of this agent in ANCA-associated vasculitis, including Wegener granulomatosis.

There is also a role for use of trimethoprim-sulfamethoxazole, in addition to its antimicrobial action and use for PCP prophylaxis.

* If untreated, generalized Wegener granulomatosis is associated with a mean survival of 5 months.
* Cyclophosphamide has revolutionized the treatment of Wegener granulomatosis and dramatically altered the natural history.
* Corticosteroids are useful initially, and the dose can be tapered quickly after the disease is controlled.

Small Vessel Vasculitis and Cutaneous Vasculitis

Clinical Features

Small vessel vasculitis occurs by itself or complicates many infectious, neoplastic, and connective tissue diseases. The most common cause of isolated cutaneous vasculitis is drugs. It manifests with urticaria, palpable purpura, livedo reticularis, or skin ulceration. Small vessel vasculitis occurs with many illnesses; a partial listing is given in Table 24-18.

* The most common cause of isolated cutaneous vasculitis is drugs.
* Isolated cutaneous vasculitis manifests with urticaria, palpable purpura, livedo reticularis, or skin ulceration.
* It can complicate most types of primary and secondary systemic vasculitis.

Histopathology

A neutrophilic- or (uncommonly) lymphocytic-predominant infiltrate surrounds small arteries, veins, arterioles, or venules. The histopathologic picture called "leukocytoclastic vasculitis" includes immune complexes deposited in vessel walls, along with fibrin deposition, endothelial cell swelling and necrosis, and a polymorphonuclear leukocytoclasis with scattering of nuclear fragment or nuclear dust. A classic clinical correlate of leukocytoclastic vasculitis is palpable purpura. This is a pathologic diagnosis and not a specific clinical condition.

* A classic clinical correlate of leukocytoclastic vasculitis is palpable purpura.

Diagnosis

The clinician must interpret small vessel or cutaneous vasculitis as a clinical finding and not a diagnosis. These various conditions are distinguished clinically and pathologically. For instance, Schönlein-Henoch vasculitis is suggested by the clinical features of abdominal pain or gastrointestinal hemorrhage in addition to the classic picture of lower extremity purpura, arthritis, and hematuria. Schönlein-Henoch vasculitis has IgA deposition in vessel walls and normal complement levels. Mixed cryoglobulinemia has circulating cryoglobulins and evidence of complement consumption. Complement levels, especially C4, may be low transiently in hypersensitivity vasculitis. Hypersensitivity vasculitis is almost always a nonsystemic small vessel vasculitis temporally related to infection, ingestion of drugs, or, less commonly, malignancy. The results of other laboratory studies are nonspecific. The leukocyte count and platelet count may be increased. Eosinophilia may be present. The erythrocyte sedimentation rate usually is increased.

Table 24-18 Conditions With Small Vessel Vasculitis

Systemic small vessel vasculitis
    Systemic vasculitis
        Wegener granulomatosis
        Polyarteritis (primary and secondary)
        Churg-Strauss vasculitis
        Takayasu arteritis
        Schönlein-Henoch purpura/vasculitis
    Serum sickness
    Goodpasture syndrome
Nonsystemic small vessel vasculitis
    Hypocomplementemic urticarial vasculitis
    Leukocytoclastic vasculitis related to:
        Rheumatoid arthritis
        Sjögren syndrome
        Systemic lupus erythematosus
        Other connective tissue diseases
    Drug-induced & postinfectious angiitis
    Mixed cryoglobulinemia
    Malignancy-associated vasculitis
    Inflammatory bowel disease
    Organ transplant-associated vasculitis
    Hypergammaglobulinemic purpura of Waldenström

- Complement levels may be low in mixed cryoglobulinemia and hypersensitivity vasculitis.
- Schönlein-Henoch vasculitis has 4 classic clinical features: lower extremity purpura, arthritis, gastrointestinal hemorrhage, and nephritis. IgA is noted on biopsy.

Treatment and Outcome

The outcome of nonsystemic small vessel vasculitis depends on the underlying condition. Control of the infection or discontinuation of the offending drug may be all that is required. In other cases, corticosteroids or nonsteroidal anti-inflammatory drugs are beneficial. Hypersensitivity vasculitis is usually self-limited, but it may recur with repeated exposure to the antigen or drug.

- Nonsystemic small vessel vasculitis: the outcome is good.
- Hypersensitivity vasculitis may recur with repeated exposure to the antigen or drug.

Cryoglobulinemia

Cryoglobulins are immunoglobulins that reversibly precipitate at reduced temperatures. They are grouped into 2 major categories. *Type I cryoglobulins* are aggregates of a single monoclonal immunoglobulin and generally are associated with multiple myeloma, Waldenström macroglobulinemia, and lymphomas. They usually are found in high concentrations (1-5 g/dL). Patients with type I cryoglobulins are often asymptomatic. Symptoms of type I cryoglobulinemia are usually related to increased viscosity and include headaches, visual disturbances, nosebleeds, Raynaud phenomenon, and ischemic ulceration from occlusion of arterioles and venules by precipitated immune complexes. Vasculitis is rare.

- Type I cryoglobulins are aggregates of a single monoclonal immunoglobulin.
- Patients with type I cryoglobulins are often asymptomatic.
- Symptoms are usually related to increased viscosity.
- Vasculitis is rare.

Type II and *type III cryoglobulins* consist of more than 1 class of immunoglobulin (mixed cryoglobulinemia) and can occur alone (essential, primary) or be due to another disease. Type II cryoglobulinemia involves a monoclonal immunoglobulin (usually IgM) with anti-immunoglobulin specificity (rheumatoid factor). Type III cryoglobulinemia involves polyclonal immunoglobulins (usually IgM) directed against other polyclonal immunoglobulins (usually IgG). Not all rheumatoid factors are cryoglobulins. Other components of the immune complexes formed in mixed cryoglobulinemia include hepatitis C antigen, other infectious agents, cellular/nuclear antigens, and complement. These immune complexes precipitate slowly and are present in smaller quantities (50-500 mg/dL) than type I cryoglobulins.

Type II cryoglobulins frequently are associated with chronic infections (most commonly hepatitis C), autoimmune disorders, and, occasionally, lymphoma. The immune complexes that form precipitate on endothelial cells in peripheral blood vessels and fix complement, promoting vasculitic inflammation. The size of immune complexes, ability to fix complement, persistent IgM production,

and many other factors may influence the clinical presentation of mixed cryoglobulinemia. The typical presentation is that of nonsystemic small vessel vasculitis with palpable purpura, urticaria, and cutaneous ulceration. Peripheral neuropathy, arthralgia, and arthritis are common. Less commonly, mixed cryoglobulinemia is complicated by hepatosplenomegaly, pneumonitis or pulmonary hemorrhage, focal segmental necrotizing glomerulonephritis, serositis (pleurisy, pericarditis), and thyroiditis.

- Type II cryoglobulins frequently are associated with chronic infections (most often hepatitis C) and immune disorders.
- Typical presentation: nonsystemic small vessel vasculitis with palpable purpura, urticaria, and cutaneous ulceration.
- Peripheral neuropathy, arthralgia, and arthritis are common.

Laboratory Studies

Patients with type II cryoglobulinemia and small vessel vasculitis usually have an increased erythrocyte sedimentation rate, increased immunoglobulin levels, positive rheumatoid factor, and low levels of complement. Evidence of chronic hepatitis infection (particularly hepatitis C) frequently is identified. For cryoglobulin testing, it is important to draw blood into a warmed syringe and to keep it warm until transferred to a cryocrit tube. Cooled specimens must be kept for up to 3 days to identify type II cryoglobulins. Serum protein electrophoresis, immunoelectrophoresis, and quantitative immunoglobulin determinations can be helpful in some cases.

- Immunoglobulin levels and the erythrocyte sedimentation rate are increased, rheumatoid factor is positive, and complement levels are low.
- Evidence of chronic hepatitis infection (particularly hepatitis C) frequently is identified.

Outcome

The clinical course depends on the underlying associated conditions and on the organs involved. Progressive renal disease is the most common systemic complication. Pulmonary hemorrhage can be life-threatening.

- Outcome depends on associated conditions and organs involved.
- Progressive renal disease is the most common systemic complication.

Vasculitis Associated With Connective Tissue Diseases

Obliterative Endarteropathy

Vascular involvement in rheumatoid arthritis can have various presentations. Vasculitis in patients with rheumatoid arthritis usually occurs only in seropositive (rheumatoid factor-positive) patients. Digital nail fold and nodule infarcts occur in some patients with active rheumatoid arthritis. Histopathologically, this is a bland, obliterative endarteropathy with intimal proliferation. Managing the rheumatoid arthritis itself is all that is needed, because these vasculopathic changes require no other therapy. A process similar to that of obliterative endarteropathy occurs in scleroderma and systemic lupus erythematosus. A renal arcuate artery vasculopathy is responsible for scleroderma renal crisis.

* Rheumatoid factor is invariably present in patients with rheumatoid arthritis who have vasculitis.

Small and Medium-Sized Vessel Vasculitis
Small vessel vasculitis or leukocytoclastic vasculitis with palpable purpura and systemic vasculitis (polyarteritis) can occur with seropositive nodular rheumatoid arthritis. A systemic necrotizing vasculitis, histopathologically indistinguishable from polyarteritis nodosa, complicates some cases of seropositive rheumatoid arthritis. Systemic lupus erythematosus can present with leukocytoclastic vasculitis or a polyarteritis-like picture. Sjögren syndrome uncommonly includes small vessel vasculitis, with either a polymorphonuclear leukocyte or a lymphocyte predominance. Type II cryoglobulins and vasculitis may complicate many different connective tissue diseases. Cryoglobulins should be assayed in any patient with an autoimmune disease in whom vasculitis develops.

* Rheumatoid arthritis, Sjögren syndrome, and systemic lupus erythematosus can present with skin-limited vasculitis or a polyarteritis-like picture.
* Cryoglobulins should be assayed in any patient with an autoimmune disease in whom vasculitis develops.

Large Vessel Vasculitis
Aortitis, an inflammation of the aortic root with dilatation and aortic insufficiency, occurs in a minority of patients with HLA-B27–associated spondyloarthropathies. Patients present with aortic valve insufficiency.

Atypical Vasculitic Syndromes: Differential Diagnosis
Patients may present with the classic features of one of the vasculitic syndromes described above. When they do not, a diagnostic approach to determine what type of vasculitis is present may prove difficult. Some patterns suggesting vasculitic disease and their differential diagnoses are listed in Tables 24-19 and 24-20 and Figure 24-6.

Skin Lesions Associated With Vasculitis
Palpable purpura suggests leukocytoclastic vasculitis, but this pathologic diagnosis does not define the clinical syndrome. Table 24-20 outlines the differential diagnosis of palpable purpura. Nodules or papules diagnosed as necrotizing granuloma on biopsy occur in Churg-Strauss syndrome, Wegener granulomatosis, rheumatoid arthritis, and, occasionally, systemic lupus erythematosus. Other nodules or papules without necrotizing granulomata can be the sign of angiocentric lymphoproliferative disorders or sarcoidosis or they may be related to inflammatory bowel disease. Urticarial or pustular lesions complicate hypocomplementemic vasculitis, inflammatory bowel arthritis syndrome, and Behçet syndrome. Livedo reticularis, which is associated with proliferative endarteropathy, occurs in connective tissue diseases and antiphospholipid antibody syndrome and in association with cholesterol emboli and many systemic necrotizing vasculitides.

* Urticarial or pustular lesions complicate hypocomplementemic vasculitis, inflammatory bowel arthritis syndrome, and Behçet syndrome.
* Livedo reticularis occurs in connective tissue diseases and antiphospholipid antibody syndrome.

Sinusitis and Vasculitis
Included in the differential diagnosis of sinusitis and presumed vasculitis are Wegener granulomatosis, Churg-Strauss syndrome, relapsing polychondritis, angiocentric lymphoproliferative disorders, sarcoidosis, nasopharyngeal carcinoma, and, occasionally, systemic bacterial or fungal infection.

Antirheumatic Drug Therapies

Colchicine and allopurinol treatments are considered in the section on gout.

Nonsteroidal Anti-Inflammatory Drugs (NSAIDs)
NSAIDs are among the most commonly prescribed medications in the world. There are no clear guidelines for selecting a particular NSAID on the basis of toxicity or efficacy. Patients vary in their responsiveness to different drugs. The various NSAIDs available permit individualization of therapy. All of them are equivalent to aspirin with regard to efficacy. They are all potent cyclooxygenase (COX) inhibitors or prodrugs of COX inhibitors. Clinical studies have not consistently found greater efficacy or tolerance for any 1 of these medications. NSAIDs are used to treat all types of arthritis and many types of soft tissue rheumatism.

Table 24-19 Acute Pulmonary-Renal Syndrome: Differential Diagnosis

Common
    Wegener granulomatosis
    Churg-Strauss syndrome
    Goodpasture syndrome
    Systemic small vessel vasculitis
        Systemic lupus erythematosus (SLE)
        Cryoglobulinemic vasculitis
Uncommon
    Schönlein-Henoch purpura/vasculitis
    Connective tissue disease (other than SLE)-associated vasculitis
        Rheumatoid arthritis
        Mixed connective tissue disease
        Polychondritis
        Behçet syndrome
    Thrombotic thrombocytopenic purpura
    Thromboembolic disease
    Infectious pneumonia-associated hypersensitivity vasculitis
        Streptococcus
        Mycoplasma
        Legionella

Table 24-20 Palpable Purpura: Differential Diagnosis

Polyarteritis
Churg-Strauss syndrome
Wegener granulomatosis
Schönlein-Henoch purpura/vasculitis
Cryoglobulinemic vasculitis
Connective tissue disease-associated vasculitis (rheumatoid arthritis,
  Sjögren syndrome, systemic lupus erythematosus)
Hypersensitivity vasculitis
    Drugs, infection, malignancy

- Patients vary in their responsiveness to different drugs.
- NSAIDs are all potent COX inhibitors or prodrugs of COX inhibitors.

Mechanisms of Action of NSAIDs

The mechanism of action of NSAIDs is incompletely understood. They decrease prostaglandin synthesis by inhibiting COX conversion of arachidonic acid to prostaglandin precursors. Prostaglandins cause vasodilatation, mediate pain, and potentiate the inflammatory effects of histamines and bradykinin. Furthermore, prostaglandins act as immunomodulators, influencing cellular and humoral immune responses. NSAIDs have potent analgesic effects that are related to their suppression of prostaglandin synthesis. Decreased levels of prostaglandin decrease the sensitivity of peripheral nerve receptors

and may affect pain transmission. Acetaminophen is not a potent prostaglandin inhibitor in peripheral tissue. However, it does affect prostaglandin concentrations in neural tissue. This may explain the analgesic effect of acetaminophen. Acetaminophen, salicylates, and other NSAIDs are potent antipyretic medications.

- NSAIDs decrease prostaglandin synthesis by inhibiting COX conversion of arachidonic acid to prostaglandin precursors, explaining most of their therapeutic effects.
- Prostaglandins cause vasodilatation, mediate extravasation and pain sensation, potentiate inflammatory mediators, and influence cellular and humoral immunity.
- Acetaminophen is not a potent prostaglandin inhibitor in peripheral tissue.

Mechanisms of Toxicity of NSAIDs

Toxic reactions are due primarily to inhibition of COX-1 and prostaglandin production. Recent investigation has uncovered 2 forms of COX: COX-1 and COX-2. COX-1 is constitutively expressed in most tissues and produces the prostaglandin precursors needed for "housekeeping function." Prostaglandins protect the gastric mucosal barrier from autodigestion. Patients with renal insufficiency or liver or cardiac disease may have prostaglandin-dependent renal blood flow. NSAIDs interfere with the synthesis of thromboxane via COX-1, which influences vascular tone, platelet aggregation, and hemostasis. COX-2 is not found in resting cells but is rapidly induced in activated fibroblasts, endothelial cells, and smooth muscle cells by cytokines, growth factors, and lipopolysaccharide. Simply viewed, the acute anti-inflammatory effects of NSAIDs relate

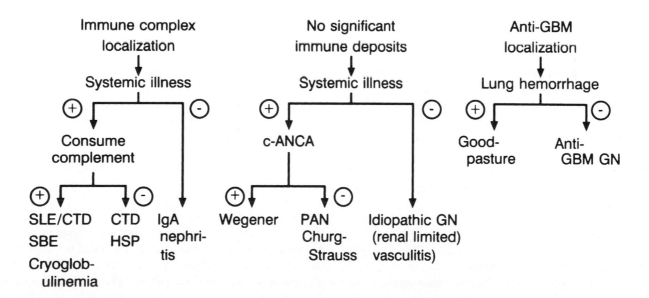

Figure 24-6. Diagnostic Approach to Vasculitis. Disease pattern recognition. Focal segmental necrotizing glomerulonephritis (kidney biopsy). c-ANCA indicates antineutrophil cytoplasmic antibody with cytoplasmic staining; CTD, connective tissue disease; GBM, glomerular basement membrane; GN, glomerulonephritis; HSP, Henoch-Schönlein purpura; PAN, polyarteritis nodosa; SBE, subacute bacterial endocarditis; SLE, systemic lupus erythematosus. (Modified from Rosen S, Falk RJ, Jennette JC. Polyarteritis nodosa, including microscopic form and renal vasculitis. In: Churg A, Churg J, editors. Systemic vasculitides. New York: Igaku-Shoin Medical Publishers; 1991, p. 57-77. Used with permission.)

to their ability to inhibit COX-2. The side effects of NSAIDs reside mostly with their ability to inhibit COX-1 and the "housekeeping function" associated with the prostaglandins synthesized by COX-1. Selective COX-2 inhibitors were developed to reduce the risk of gastrointestinal toxicity.

Blocking COX with currently available NSAIDs augments conversion of arachidonic acid to leukotrienes. Leukotrienes (previously known as "slow-reacting substance of anaphylaxis") aggravate asthma, rhinitis, hives, and nasal polyps.

- The acute anti-inflammatory action of NSAIDs is mediated by COX-2 inhibition.
- Toxic reactions are due primarily to inhibition of COX-1.
- Selective COX-2 inhibitors are available to reduce the risk of gastrointestinal toxicity.
- NSAIDs interfere with the synthesis of thromboxane and influence platelet function.
- Leukotrienes aggravate asthma, rhinitis, hives, and nasal polyps. NSAIDs may increase the production of leukotrienes.

NSAIDs are bound extensively to plasma proteins. Protein binding has obvious implications for other medications that are also protein-bound. Indomethacin, diclofenac, and piroxicam decrease lithium excretion. NSAIDs also can influence methotrexate toxicity at high doses (>50 mg/week) by interfering with the renal clearance of methotrexate. At the dose range of methotrexate used in rheumatic diseases, this is not a concern.

Most NSAIDs attenuate the effects of antihypertensive medications. Diuretics, β-adrenergic blockers, and angiotensin-converting enzyme inhibitors are the drugs affected most by the influence of NSAIDs on renal prostaglandins. Aspirin irreversibly inhibits COX-1. The effect of all the other NSAIDs on COX-1 is reversible. These drugs prolong bleeding time. Aspirin therapy needs to be discontinued for up to 10 days before the bleeding time returns to normal. NSAID therapy should be discontinued at least 4 drug half-lives before invasive procedures in which bleeding is a concern. NSAIDs with a short half-life are best when an acute effect (eg, treatment of acute gout) is required. The half-life is proportional to the onset of maximal clinical benefit. The common side effects of NSAIDs are listed in Table 24-21.

- Diuretics, β-blockers, and angiotensin-converting enzyme inhibitors are the drugs affected most by the influence of NSAIDs on renal prostaglandins.
- Aspirin irreversibly inhibits COX-1.
- NSAIDs usually prolong the bleeding time.

Gastrointestinal Side Effects of NSAIDs
Twenty percent of chronic users of NSAIDs have gastric ulcer noted on endoscopy, and 15% to 35% report dyspepsia, but this complaint does not appear to be related to abnormal findings on endoscopy. Nausea and abdominal pain are described in up to 40% of users of NSAIDs. Stomach upset or pain forces discontinuation of therapy with these drugs in more than 10% of patients. Gastrointestinal blood loss related to these drugs is most often

occult and can result in iron deficiency anemia. The true incidence of significant gastrointestinal bleeding requiring hospitalization or operation or resulting in death is unknown. However, the elderly, persons with considerable cardiovascular morbidity, and persons with a previous history of NSAID-associated ulcer are at greatest risk for significant gastrointestinal toxicity related to NSAIDs. These patients are the most likely candidates to benefit from the risk reduction of selective COX-2 inhibitors. Alcohol, corticosteroid, or tobacco use also predisposes to the development of gastrointestinal toxicity.

- Of chronic users of NSAIDs, 20% have gastric ulcer and 15%-35% have dyspepsia.
- Stomach upset or pain forces discontinuation of therapy with these drugs in >10% of patients.
- Gastrointestinal blood loss related to these drugs is most often occult.
- A small number of NSAID users are at risk of increased gastrointestinal toxicity and may be candidates for a selective COX-2 inhibitor.

Other Toxic Effects of NSAIDs
Central nervous system symptoms such as headaches, dizziness, mood alterations, blurred vision, and confusion are reported most frequently with the use of indomethacin. Ibuprofen, tolmetin, and sulindac have been associated with aseptic meningitis in patients with systemic lupus erythematosus. All the central nervous system effects resolve when the use of NSAIDs is discontinued. Rashes, urticaria, exfoliative dermatitis, erythema multiforme, and scalded skin syndrome or toxic epidermal necrolysis all occur, albeit rarely, with the use of NSAIDs. Easy bruisability is a common complaint of chronic users of these drugs. Dependent petechiae may develop if platelet function is already compromised. Pulmonary infiltrates, bronchospasm, and anaphylaxis may occur with all NSAIDs, including aspirin. Although it is not IgE-mediated, anaphylaxis occurs most commonly in patients who have the classic triad of asthma, nasal polyps, and aspirin sensitivity. Combination therapy with NSAIDs should be avoided. Whereas toxicity is additive, there is no evidence that the therapeutic effect is additive. Recently, selective COX-2 inhibitors have been associated with increased cardiovascular complications. As a result, some agents have been removed from the market.

- Combination therapy with 2 different NSAIDs should be avoided.

Nonacetylated Salicylates
Careful studies have not identified significant differences in efficacy of nonacetylated salicylates compared with NSAIDs. Nonacetylated salicylates (eg, salsalate) minimally inhibit COX-1 and are about half as potent as aspirin for inhibiting COX-2. Although their use decreases the incidence of gastrointestinal bleeding, they can cause many of the gastrointestinal symptoms that influence patient compliance. Tinnitus remains a potential problem. Nonacetylated salicylates do not interfere with renal blood flow, and they do not inhibit platelet function. They usually can be safely prescribed for patients with aspirin allergy.

Table 24-21 Common Side Effects of Nonsteroidal Anti-inflammatory Drugs

Gastrointestinal
  Nausea
  Abdominal pain
  Constipation or diarrhea
  Occult blood loss & iron deficiency anemia
  Peptic ulcer disease
  Colitis and colonic hemorrhage
Renal
  Reduced renal blood flow
  Reduced glomerular filtration rate
  Increased creatinine clearance
  Pyuria
  Interstitial nephritis
  Papillary necrosis
  Nephrotic syndrome
  Hyperkalemia & type IV renal tubular acidosis
  Fluid retention
Hematologic
  Bone marrow suppression
      Agranulocytosis
      Aplastic anemia
  Iron deficiency anemia
  Platelet-aggregating defect
Neurologic
  Delirium/confusion
  Headache
  Dizziness
  Blurred vision
  Mood swings
  Aseptic meningitis
Dermatologic
  Urticaria
  Erythema multiforme
  Exfoliative syndromes (toxic epidermal necrolysis)
  Oral ulcers
  Dermatitis
Pulmonary
  Pulmonary infiltrates
  Noncardiac pulmonary edema (aspirin toxicity)
  Anaphylaxis & bronchospasm
  Nasal polyps
Drug interactions
  Augment hemostatic effect of warfarin
  Attenuate antihypertensive effect of diuretics, β-blockers, angiotensin-converting enzyme inhibitors
  Influence drug metabolism
      Methotrexate (high doses only)
      Lithium
      Oral hypoglycemic agents

- Nonacetylated salicylates minimally inhibit COX-1.
- Nonacetylated salicylates do not interfere with renal blood flow, and they do not inhibit platelet function.
- Nonacetylated salicylates can cause stomach upset or tinnitus.

Disease-Modifying Antirheumatic Drugs

Antimalarial Compounds (Hydroxychloroquine)

Open and randomized placebo-controlled studies have confirmed the benefit of hydroxychloroquine in the management of rheumatoid arthritis and systemic lupus erythematosus. The dose typically does not exceed 4.5 mg/kg daily. Retinopathy is the major toxic effect associated with the use of hydroxychloroquine. The risk of irreversible retinopathy is small (<3%) in patients taking less than 4.5 mg/kg daily. The elderly may be at somewhat increased risk. Regular eye examinations can identify the premaculopathy stage of the toxic reaction, which is reversible. Permanent symptomatic retinopathy is preventable when patients have eye examinations every 6 to 12 months.

- Retinopathy is the major toxic effect associated with the use of hydroxychloroquine.
- The risk of irreversible retinopathy is small (<3%) in patients taking <4.5 mg/kg daily.

The clinical response to hydroxychloroquine does not appear before 8 weeks. Improvement may not occur until 6 months of continuous therapy. Approximately 40% to 60% of patients with rheumatoid arthritis may respond (based on established criteria for response). It is used most commonly in combination with NSAIDs or low doses of corticosteroids in patients with early or mild polyarthritis.

- The clinical response to hydroxychloroquine does not appear before 8 weeks and may not occur until 6 months of continuous therapy.

Sulfasalazine

Enteric-coated tablets of sulfasalazine have reduced some of the immediate gastrointestinal upset associated with this drug. The metabolites of sulfasalazine include 5-aminosalicylic acid and sulfapyridine. The results of short-term randomized trials indicate significant efficacy in mild-to-moderate rheumatoid arthritis. Rheumatologists also recommend treatment with sulfasalazine for seronegative spondyloarthropathies and psoriatic arthritis; however, peripheral arthritis responds more effectively than axial or spinal inflammation. The benefit of this drug in rheumatoid arthritis is equal to that of intramuscular injections of gold but with fewer toxic effects. Sulfasalazine treatment is usually reserved for early or milder cases of inflammatory polyarthritis. Although the onset of efficacy occurs as early as 8 weeks, the effect may not be documented for as long as 6 months. The toxic effects include nausea, vomiting, gastric ulcers, and, more rarely, hepatitis or cholestasis. Ten percent of patients complain of headache or sense of fatigue. Recently, a combination of sulfasalazine, hydroxychloroquine, and methotrexate was found to be superior to single-drug therapy for patients with rheumatoid arthritis in whom treatment with at least 1 DMARD had failed.

- Sulfasalazine treatment is usually reserved for early or milder cases of inflammatory polyarthritis.
- Sulfasalazine is used in combination with methotrexate and hydroxychloroquine for refractory rheumatoid arthritis.

Methotrexate

Methotrexate is a structural analogue of folic acid and is considered an antimetabolite rather than a cytotoxic agent. It is used extensively in rheumatoid arthritis and also has a place in the treatment of psoriatic arthritis and peripheral arthritis of seronegative spondyloarthropathies. Methotrexate may have a role in the treatment of arthritis in systemic lupus erythematosus and scleroderma. Its mechanism of action includes inhibition of folate metabolism (critical in nucleotide production), inhibition of leukotriene B_4, and increasing intracellular adenosine. It has both immunomodulatory and anti-inflammatory effects. Its strongest effect is on rapidly dividing cells, particularly those in the S phase of the cell cycle. Methotrexate is unique among the first-line disease-modifying antirheumatic drugs because its antirheumatic effect occurs within 4 to 6 weeks. Oral, subcutaneous, intramuscular, and intravenous routes are equally effective for low dosages.

- Methotrexate is used extensively in rheumatoid arthritis and has a place in the treatment of psoriatic arthritis, peripheral arthritis of seronegative spondyloarthropathies, and the arthritis in systemic lupus erythematosus and scleroderma.
- The antirheumatic effect occurs within 4-6 weeks.

In patients with rheumatoid arthritis receiving methotrexate, 80% have substantial improvement within the first year of therapy. At 5 years, it is estimated that at least 35% of patients treated with methotrexate still take it. No other DMARD has this combination of efficacy and tolerability. Most patients with rheumatoid arthritis have a severe flare of their disease within 3 weeks after discontinuation of methotrexate therapy. This drug should not be used in patients with significant renal dysfunction (creatinine >2.0 mg/dL). Coadministration of trimethoprim-sulfamethoxazole and methotrexate increases the risk of hematologic toxicity.

- 80% of rheumatoid arthritis patients taking methotrexate have substantial improvement within the first year of treatment.
- Most patients with rheumatoid arthritis have a severe flare of their disease within 3 weeks after discontinuation of methotrexate therapy.

Gastrointestinal toxic reactions are common side effects of methotrexate. Nausea and vomiting may persist for 24 to 48 hours after ingestion. Stomatitis and diarrhea are insurmountable problems for some patients. Methotrexate treatment should be withheld from patients with significant gastric ulceration until their ulcers have healed. Methotrexate should not be used in patients with significant liver disease. Increased liver enzyme levels suggest a subclinical hepatic toxic effect due to methotrexate. Persistent increase in aspartate aminotransferase levels or decreasing albumin levels are markers for developing hepatic fibrosis and, potentially, cirrhosis. Cryptic cirrhosis may develop without liver enzyme abnormalities being detected. Stomatitis and the less common hematologic abnormalities such as leukopenia, thrombocytopenia, and pancytopenia may respond to folic acid supplementation. Pulmonary toxic side effects include chemical pneumonitis and insidious pulmonary fibrosis, beginning with a dry cough. Acute pneumonitis due to methotrexate may be associated with eosinophilia. Neurologic features such as headache and seizure are uncommon. Methotrexate is teratogenic and should be withheld for 3 months before the patient attempts to conceive.

Supplemental folic acid, 1 mg daily, is provided to patients taking methotrexate. This strategy often reduces mild side effects and may help to prevent cytopenia and liver toxicity.

- Gastrointestinal toxic reactions are common side effects of methotrexate.
- Methotrexate should not be used in patients with significant liver disease.
- Stomatitis and diarrhea are insurmountable problems for some patients.

Leflunomide

Leflunomide is an immunoregulatory agent that interferes with pyrimidine synthesis and is approved for the treatment of rheumatoid arthritis. Its efficacy may be comparable to that of methotrexate and is noted within 12 weeks after initiation of therapy. Toxic effects are also comparable to those of methotrexate, although no pulmonary complications have been reported. The most common side effects include gastrointestinal distress, rashes, and alopecia. The monitoring of side effects, including cytopenias and liver toxicity, that is recommended currently is the same as that recommended for methotrexate. This drug is a teratogen and must be avoided in pregnancy. A protocol with cholestyramine is used to accelerate the clearance of leflunomide.

Azathioprine

Azathioprine and its metabolites are purine analogues. It is considered a cytotoxic agent. Azathioprine is metabolized by xanthine oxidase and thiopurine methyltransferase. Allopurinol, an inhibitor of xanthine oxidase, delays the metabolism of azathioprine and can lead to toxic reactions if the dose of azathioprine is not decreased by 50% to 66%. Thiopurine methyltransferase can be assayed; low levels of this enzyme predict the 1 in 300 patients in whom a severe hematologic reaction to azathioprine will develop. Controlled studies have documented the efficacy of azathioprine in the treatment of rheumatoid arthritis and systemic lupus erythematosus.

The most common toxic effects of azathioprine are gastrointestinal effects and cytopenias. An idiosyncratic, acute pancreatitis-like attack is an absolute contraindication to further treatment with this drug. Cholestatic hepatitis is rare, but if it occurs, it generally does so within the first several weeks after drug administration. If tolerated initially, hematologic toxic effects become the most significant concern. In patients who have undergone organ transplant, azathioprine treatment increases the risk of neoplasia, particularly lymphomas, leukemias, and skin and cervical malignancies. Azathioprine does not alter fertility, but it may have some teratogenic potential. For pregnant women, azathioprine should be reserved for those with severe or life-threatening rheumatic diseases.

- Azathioprine is a cytotoxic agent.
- The most common toxic effects of azathioprine are gastrointestinal effects and cytopenias.
- Allopurinol should be avoided in patients taking azathioprine.

Cyclophosphamide

Cyclophosphamide is a potent alkylating agent. It acts on dividing and nondividing cells, interfering with cellular DNA function. It depletes T cells and B cells, causing considerable immunosuppression. Oral cyclophosphamide is well absorbed and completely metabolized within 24 hours, and most of its metabolites are excreted in the urine. Allopurinol increases the risk of leukopenia in patients taking cyclophosphamide. Short-term studies document significant efficacy of this drug in the treatment of rheumatoid arthritis at doses of 1 to 2 mg/kg daily. Unequivocal healing and arrest of erosive change occur. The considerable toxicity associated with chronic administration of cyclophosphamide limits its use in rheumatoid arthritis to very severe cases, often with complicating vasculitis. It is the drug of choice in the treatment of generalized Wegener granulomatosis. Intravenous administration of cyclophosphamide is efficacious in managing systemic necrotizing vasculitis and severe systemic lupus erythematosus, including proliferative glomerulonephritis. Short-term advantages of intravenous pulse of cyclophosphamide may include fewer toxic effects on the bladder and perhaps a lower risk of infection.

- Cyclophosphamide depletes T cells and B cells, causing considerable immunosuppression.
- Cyclophosphamide is efficacious in managing systemic necrotizing vasculitis and severe systemic lupus erythematosus.

Dose-related bone marrow suppression is common in patients receiving cyclophosphamide and requires close laboratory monitoring. Immunosuppression from treatment with cyclophosphamide increases the risk of infection. Herpes zoster infection occurs in most patients receiving the drug orally. Cyclophosphamide directly affects ovarian and testicular function. Premature ovarian failure frequently occurs in premenopausal lupus patients taking the drug. Spermatogenesis also can be affected by this drug, which causes atrophy of seminiferous tubules. Cyclophosphamide has teratogenic potential. Alopecia, stomatitis, cardiomyopathy (with drug doses used to treat cancer), and pulmonary fibrosis may complicate cyclophosphamide therapy. The metabolites of this drug, including acrolein, accumulate in the bladder. Acrolein has direct mucosal toxic effects and causes hemorrhagic cystitis. This complication is potentially life-threatening. The chronic use of cyclophosphamide taken orally is associated with an increased risk of neoplasia, including hematologic and bladder malignancies. The risk of malignancy with intravenous pulse therapy has not been established. All patients who have had cyclophosphamide therapy should have urinalysis and urine cytology performed at regular intervals for life.

- Dose-related bone marrow suppression is common in patients receiving cyclophosphamide.

- Cyclophosphamide directly affects ovarian and testicular function.
- The chronic use of cyclophosphamide is associated with an increased risk of neoplasia.

Glucocorticosteroids

Glucocorticosteroids modify the inflammatory response dramatically. They are potent inhibitors of neutrophil function. Glucocorticosteroids suppress cellular immune activity and, to a lesser extent, inhibit the humoral response. Low doses of glucocorticosteroids (<10 mg of prednisone per day) are frequently used in the day-to-day management of the articular manifestations of rheumatoid arthritis. At least one-third of all patients with rheumatoid arthritis take glucocorticosteroids chronically. High doses of glucocorticosteroids (1-2 mg of prednisone per kilogram of body weight) may be required for life-threatening or serious inflammatory disorders, including systemic vasculitis and complications of systemic lupus erythematosus. Prednisone doses of more than 30 mg/day are associated with a higher risk of infection, including *Pneumocystis carinii*. This is particularly the case if prednisone is given in addition to cyclophosphamide, azathioprine, or methotrexate. Many clinicians add 1 double-strength trimethoprim-sulfamethoxazole tablet twice weekly to these immunosuppressive regimens as prophylaxis against *Pneumocystis* infection.

- Glucocorticosteroids are potent inhibitors of neutrophil function.
- They suppress cellular immune activity and, to a lesser extent, inhibit the humoral response.
- One-third of all patients with rheumatoid arthritis take glucocorticosteroids chronically.

These drugs have many side effects; these are not idiosyncratic but actually unwanted effects of the medication. The duration of treatment and the dose used determine how fast an unwanted effect appears. Many patients with rheumatoid arthritis tolerate prednisone doses of 1 to 5 mg/day for years without having serious side effects. Patient concerns about glucocorticosteroids include weight gain from increased appetite, water retention, and hirsutism. Longer-term concerns include thinning of the skin, easy bruising, progressive osteoporosis (unclear if this happens with physiologic doses of prednisone) and compression fractures, high blood pressure, glucose intolerance, cataract formation, and aggravation of glaucoma. Glucocorticosteroids interfere with wound healing and increase the risk of opportunistic infection. Steroid-induced osteoporosis should be anticipated, and patients should be treated with calcium, vitamin D supplementation, and oral bisphosphonates. The psychoactive potential of high doses of glucocorticosteroids is an additional factor in treating older patients. Glucocorticosteroid psychosis can complicate the diagnosis of neuropsychiatric lupus.

- Many patients with rheumatoid arthritis tolerate prednisone doses in the 1-5 mg/day range for years without having serious side effects.
- Long-term concerns: thinning of the skin, progressive osteoporosis and compression fractures, high blood pressure, glucose intolerance, cataract formation, and aggravation of glaucoma.
- Glucocorticosteroid psychosis can complicate the diagnosis of neuropsychiatric lupus.

- Glucocorticosteroids interfere with wound healing and increase the risk of opportunistic infection.
- Bisphosphonates, calcium, and vitamin D are used to reduce the risk of glucocorticoid osteoporosis.

Biological Agents

Appreciation of the role of tumor necrosis factor-α and interleukin-1 in the inflammatory process in rheumatoid arthritis has led to the development of specific inhibitors of these cytokines. Tumor necrosis factor antagonists include neutralizing antibodies (infliximab and adalimunab) and soluble receptor recombinant fusion protein (etanercept). Anakinra is a recombinant interleukin-1 receptor antagonist. Anti-cytokine therapies are very expensive. Their roles in the management of rheumatoid arthritis are still being defined. Because of evidence that they delay radiographic progression, they are usually added to other therapies such as methotrexate when the disease has not been adequately controlled. The primary risk of these agents, especially the tumor necrosis factor inhibitors, is infection. Reactivation of latent tuberculosis is a major concern, and potential candidates for tumor necrosis factor inhibitors must be evaluated with tuberculin testing before treatment. Infection is also a concern with abatacept.

Part II

William W. Ginsburg, MD

Crystalline Arthropathies

Hyperuricemia and Gout

Hyperuricemia has been described in 2% to 18% of normal populations. Hyperuricemia is associated with hypertension, renal insufficiency, obesity, and arteriosclerotic heart disease. The prevalence of clinical gouty arthritis ranges from 0.1% to 0.4%. There is a family history of gout in 20% of patients with gouty arthritis. Genetic studies suggest a multifactorial inheritance pattern. Of patients with hyperuricemia whose uric acid level is more than 9 mg/dL, gout develops in 5 years in approximately 20%.

* Hyperuricemia is associated with hypertension, renal insufficiency, obesity, and arteriosclerotic heart disease.
* The prevalence of gouty arthritis is 0.1%-0.4%.
* 20% of patients with gouty arthritis have a family history of gout.
* In patients with a uric acid level >9 mg/dL, gout develops in 20% in 5 years.

Ninety percent of patients with gout have underexcretion of uric acid. They have reduced filtration of uric acid, enhanced tubular reabsorption, or decreased tubular secretion. Overproduction of uric acid is the cause of hyperuricemia in approximately 10% of patients with primary gout. Of these 10%, about 15% have 1 of the 2 X-linked inborn errors of purine metabolism: 1) hypoxanthine-guanine phosphoribosyltransferase deficiency (Lesch-Nyhan syndrome) and 2) 5-phosphoribosyl-1-pyrophosphate synthetase overactivity. Of the remaining 85% of patients who have overproduction, most are

obese, but the cause of overproduction and the relationship between obesity and overproduction of uric acid remain unknown.

* ≤10% of patients with gout have overproduction of uric acid.

Events leading to initial crystallization of monosodium urate in a joint after many years of asymptomatic hyperuricemia are unknown. Trauma with disruption of microtophi in cartilage may lead to release of urate crystals into synovial fluid. The urate crystals become coated with immunoglobulin and then complement. They are then phagocytosed by leukocytes with subsequent release of chemotactic protein, activation of the kallikrein system, and disruption of the leukocytes, which release lysosomal enzymes into synovial fluid.

Important Enzyme Abnormalities in the Uric Acid Pathway (Figure 24-7)

Lesch-Nyhan syndrome is a complete deficiency of hypoxanthine-guanine phosphoribosyltransferase. It is characterized by an X-linked disorder in young boys, hyperuricemia, self-mutilation, choreoathetosis, spasticity, growth retardation, and severe gouty arthritis.

Overactivity of 5-phosphoribosyl-1-pyrophosphate synthetase is associated with hyperuricemia, X-linked genetic inheritance, and gouty arthritis.

Adenosine deaminase deficiency is inherited in an autosomal recessive pattern. It causes a combined immunodeficiency state with severe T-cell and mild B-cell dysfunction. There is a buildup of deoxyadenosine triphosphate in lymphocytes, which is toxic to immature lymphocytes. Features of the disorder are hypouricemia,

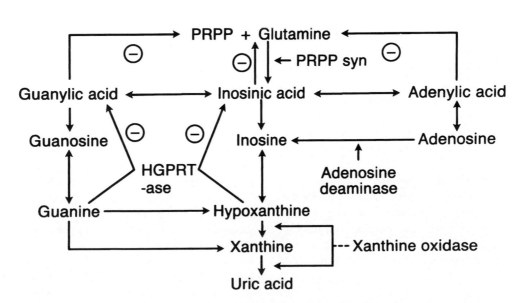

Figure 24-7. Purine Metabolism. HGPRTase indicates hypoxanthine-guanine phosphoribosyltransferase; PRPP, phosphoribosylpyrophosphate; PRPP syn, phosphoribosylpyrophosphate synthetase; ⊖, feedback inhibition.

recurrent infection, chondro-osseous dysplasia, and an increased deoxyadenosine level in plasma and urine. Treatment for the disorder is with irradiated frozen red blood cells or marrow transplant.

Xanthine oxidase deficiency is also inherited in an autosomal recessive pattern. It is characterized by hypouricemia, xanthinuria with xanthine stones, and myopathy associated with deposits of xanthine and hypoxanthine.

Causes of Secondary Hyperuricemia

Secondary hyperuricemia can be attributed to overproduction or underexcretion of uric acid (Table 24-22).

- Important causes of overproduction of uric acid include cancer, psoriasis, and sickle cell anemia.
- Important causes of underexcretion of uric acid include chronic renal insufficiency, lead nephropathy, alcohol, diabetic ketoacidosis, and drugs, notably thiazide diuretics, nicotinic acid, and cyclosporine.

Causes of Hypouricemia

Increased urinary excretion of uric acid contributes to hypouricemia. It can develop in healthy persons with an isolated defect in tubular reabsorption of uric acid. It also can be related to diminished reabsorption of urate, such as in Fanconi syndrome, Fanconi syndrome associated with Wilson disease, carcinoma of the lung, acute myelogenous leukemia, light-chain diseases, and use of outdated tetracycline. Malignant neoplasms, such as carcinoma, Hodgkin disease, and sarcoma, also are associated with increased excretion of uric acid. Hypervolemia caused by inappropriate secretion of antidiuretic hormone also can be a factor. Drugs involved in increased excretion of uric acid are high-dose aspirin, probenecid and other uricosuric agents, and glyceryl guaiacolate. Radiographic contrast agents that can cause hypouricemia are iopanoic acid (Telopaque), iodipamide meglumine (Cholografin), and diatrizoate sodium (Hypaque). It also can occur in severe liver disease.

Decreased synthesis of uric acid also can cause hypouricemia. The drug allopurinol inhibits the enzyme xanthine oxidase, causing hypouricemia. The decrease also can be caused by congenital deficiencies in enzymes involved in purine biosynthesis: 5-phosphoribosyl-1-pyrophosphate synthetase deficiency, adenosine deaminase deficiency, purine nucleoside phosphorylase deficiency, and xanthine oxidase deficiency (xanthinuria). Acquired deficiency in xanthine oxidase activity (metastatic adenocarcinoma of lung) also can cause decreased synthesis of uric acid, as can acute intermittent porphyria.

Factors Predisposing to Gout and Pseudogout

The following can predispose to an attack of gout or pseudogout: trauma, operation (3 days after), major medical illness (eg, myocardial infarction, cerebrovascular accident, pulmonary embolus), fasting, alcohol use, infection, and acidosis. The attacks are precipitated by changes in the urate equilibrium between the blood and joints.

- Factors that precipitate gout and pseudogout include trauma, operation, alcohol use, and acidosis.

Table 24-22 Causes of Secondary Hyperuricemia

Overproduction of uric acid
   Myeloproliferative disorders
      Polycythemia, primary or secondary
      Myeloid metaplasia
      Chronic myelocytic leukemia
   Lymphoproliferative disorders
      Chronic lymphocytic leukemia
   Plasma cell proliferative disorders
      Multiple myeloma
   Disseminated carcinoma & sarcoma
   Sickle cell anemia, thalassemia, & other forms of chronic
    hemolytic anemia
   Psoriasis
   Cytotoxic drugs
   Infectious mononucleosis
   Obesity
   Increased purine ingestion
Underexcretion of uric acid
   Intrinsic renal disease
      Chronic renal insufficiency of diverse cause
      Saturine gout (lead nephropathy)
   Drug-induced
      Thiazide diuretics, furosemide, ethacrynic acid,
       ethambutol, pyrazinamide, low-dose aspirin, cyclosporine,
       nicotinic acid, laxative abuse, levodopa, rasburicase
   Endocrine conditions
      Adrenal insufficiency, nephrogenic diabetes insipidus,
       hyperparathyroidism, hypoparathyroidism,
       pseudohypoparathyroidism, hypothyroidism
   Metabolic conditions
      Diabetic ketoacidosis, lactic acidosis, starvation,
       ethanolism, glycogen storage disease type I, Bartter
       syndrome
   Other
      Sarcoidosis
      Down syndrome
      Beryllium disease

Clinical Manifestations of Acute Gout

In 50% of patients with gout, the metatarsophalangeal joint of the great toe is involved initially (podagra), and this joint is eventually involved in more than 75% of patients. Rapid joint swelling is associated with extreme tenderness. Uric acid crystals, which are needle-shaped and strongly negatively birefringent under polarized light, are always found in the joint during an acute attack. The diagnosis of gout is established by the demonstration of uric acid crystals in the joint aspirate. The joint fluid is usually inflammatory, and the polymorphonuclear neutrophil count is between 5 and 75×10^9/L.

Gout occurs most commonly in middle-aged men, but, after menopause, the incidence of gout in women increases. Although gout is usually monarticular and usually involves the joints in the lower extremity, attacks may become polyarticular over time in some patients.

- Podagra is the initial presentation of gout in 50% of cases.
- Uric acid crystals are negatively birefringent under polarized light microscopy.
- Gout is usually monarticular and most often involves the joints in the lower extremities.
- Typical clinical scenario: Pain, swelling, redness, and tenderness develop over the right metatarsophalangeal joint of the great toe 3 days after myocardial infarction in an elderly patient. Aspiration of the joint shows needle-like crystals, which are strongly negatively birefringent under polarized light. Joint fluid has a polymorphonuclear neutrophil value of $50 \times 10^9/L$.

Treatment of Acute Gouty Arthritis

Indomethacin or other nonsteroidal anti-inflammatory drugs (NSAIDs) are the drugs of choice for the treatment of acute gouty arthritis and should be used for a 7- to 10-day course. These drugs are relatively contraindicated in patients with congestive heart failure, active peptic ulcer disease, or renal insufficiency. NSAIDs should not be used in patients with nasal polyps and aspirin sensitivity because they may cause bronchospasm.

- NSAIDs are the initial drugs of choice for an acute attack of gouty arthritis.
- NSAIDs should be avoided in patients with congestive heart failure, peptic ulcer disease, and renal insufficiency.

Intra-articular or oral corticosteroids and subcutaneous adrenocorticotropic hormone are other treatments, especially in patients who have contraindications to colchicine and NSAIDs. Oral corticosteroids may need to be given for 10 days to avoid relapses. Allopurinol or probenecid therapy should not be initiated until the acute attack completely subsides. If patients are already receiving these medications, their use should be continued. Because of severe gastrointestinal side effects, high-dose oral colchicine is rarely used for an acute attack. Intravenously administered colchicine in a single dose (1-2 mg) has no gastrointestinal side effects. It has increased toxicity in patients with renal insufficiency, bone marrow depression, sepsis, and immediate prior use of oral colchicine. Repeat dosages should be avoided. It can cause severe skin necrosis if it infiltrates into subcutaneous tissues.

- Colchicine has the potential for gastrointestinal side effects with the oral form, but there are no gastrointestinal side effects with single-dose intravenous administration.
- Avoid intravenous colchicine in patients with renal insufficiency, bone marrow depression, sepsis, or immediate prior use of oral colchicine.

Treatment During Intercritical Period

Oral colchicine, 0.6 mg twice daily, should be given prophylactically with probenecid or allopurinol for 6 to 12 months to prevent exacerbation of acute gout. Long-term use of low-dose colchicine can

be associated with a myopathy and neuropathy, especially in patients with renal insufficiency. A myoneuropathy may rapidly appear in patients taking medications that affect colchicine metabolism via the cytochrome P450 system. These include simvastatin, lovastatin, atorvastatin, diltiazem, cimetidine, verapamil, and amiodarone. If a statin is needed in conjunction with colchicine in a patient with renal insufficiency, fluvastatin and pravastatin are not handled by the cytochrome P450 system.

Probenecid inhibits tubular reabsorption of filtered and secreted urate, thereby increasing urinary excretion of uric acid. It should not be used if the patient has a creatinine clearance less than 50 mL/minute or a history of kidney stones or if the 24-hour uric acid value is more than 1,000 mg (normal, <600 mg/day). Probenecid delays the renal excretion of indomethacin and thereby increases its blood level. Probenecid delays the renal excretion of acetylsalicylic acid (ASA), and ASA completely blocks the uricosuric effect of probenecid. ASA also blocks tubular secretion of urates. Probenecid should not be used with methotrexate because probenecid increases methotrexate blood levels, increasing toxicity.

- Probenecid inhibits tubular reabsorption of filtered and secreted urate.
- Probenecid should not be used if the patient has a creatinine clearance <50 mL/minute or a history of kidney stones or if 24-hour uric acid value is >1,000 mg.
- Probenecid delays renal excretion of indomethacin and ASA.

Allopurinol is a xanthine oxidase inhibitor. It is the drug of choice to prevent gouty attacks if the patient has a history of renal stones, tophi, or renal insufficiency. Allopurinol also can precipitate gout. Allopurinol and probenecid usually are not used simultaneously unless the patient has extensive tophaceous gout with good renal function. Allopurinol can cause a rash and a severe toxicity syndrome consisting of eosinophilia, fever, hepatitis, decreased renal function, and an erythematous desquamative rash. This syndrome usually occurs in patients with decreased renal function. Allopurinol should be given in the lowest dose possible to keep the uric acid value less than 6 mg/dL. In patients with chronic renal disease, the starting dose should always be low (50-100 mg) and increased slowly. If allopurinol is used in conjunction with 6-mercaptopurine or azathioprine, the dose of 6-mercaptopurine or azathioprine needs to be reduced at least 25% or bone marrow toxicity can occur. Both of these drugs are metabolized by xanthine oxidase, which allopurinol inhibits. Patients who have had transplant frequently receive both medications.

- Allopurinol is a xanthine oxidase inhibitor.
- Allopurinol can precipitate gout.
- It is the drug of choice if patient has a history of renal stones, tophi, or renal insufficiency.
- Allopurinol can cause a severe toxicity syndrome: eosinophilia, fever, hepatitis, decreased renal function, and erythematous desquamative rash.

The indications for use of allopurinol rather than probenecid for lowering the uric acid level are tophaceous gout, gout complicated by renal insufficiency, uric acid excretion more than 1,000 mg/day, history of uric acid calculi, use of cytotoxic drugs, and allergy to uricosuric agents. Allopurinol should be used before treatment of rapidly proliferating tumors. The nucleic acid liberated with cytolysis is converted to uric acid and can cause renal failure due to precipitation of uric acid in collecting ducts and ureters (acute tumor lysis syndrome). Patients also should have adequate hydration and alkalinization of the urine before chemotherapy.

* Indications for allopurinol include tophaceous gout, gout complicated by renal insufficiency, history of uric acid calculi, and use of cytotoxic drugs.

Renal Disease and Uric Acid

Renal function is not necessarily adversely affected by an increased serum urate concentration. The incidence of interstitial renal disease and renal insufficiency is no greater than that in patients of comparable age with similar degrees of hypertension, arteriosclerotic heart disease, diabetes, and primary renal disease. Correction of hyperuricemia (to ≤10 mg/dL) has no apparent effect on renal function.

Most rheumatologists do not treat asymptomatic hyperuricemia if the uric acid level is less than 10.0 mg/dL (normal, to 8.0). When hyperuricemia is associated with a urinary uric acid of more than 1,000 mg/24 hours, which increases the risk of uric acid stones, renal function should be monitored closely. Excessive exposure to lead may contribute to the renal disease found in some patients with gout.

* Renal function is not necessarily adversely affected by an increased serum urate concentration.
* Correction of hyperuricemia (to ≤10 mg/dL) has no apparent effect on renal function.

Miscellaneous Points of Importance

* Positive diagnosis of a crystalline arthritis requires identification of crystal by polarization microscopy.
* Allopurinol therapy should not be started during an acute attack of gout.
* 30% of patients with chronic tophaceous gout are positive for rheumatoid factor (usually weakly positive).
* 10% of patients with acute gout are positive for rheumatoid factor (usually weakly positive).
* 5%-10% of patients will have a gout and a pseudogout attack simultaneously.
* 50% of synovial fluids aspirated from first metatarsophalangeal joints of asymptomatic patients with gout have crystals of monosodium urate.
* Up to 20% of patients with acute gout have a normal level of serum uric acid at the time of the acute attack.
* Gout in a premenopausal female is very unusual.
* Sulfinpyrazone is also uricosuric and potentially therapeutic.
* There have been many recent reports of superimposed gout occurring in Heberden and Bouchard nodes in older women taking thiazide diuretics.
* A septic joint can trigger a gout or pseudogout attack in a pre-

disposed person. Synovial fluid should always be analyzed for crystals, Gram stain, and culture.
* The frequency of gout in patients who have had cardiac transplant is high (25%). (Both cyclosporine and diuretics cause hyperuricemia.)

Calcium Pyrophosphate Deposition Disease

Etiologic Classification

Calcium pyrophosphate deposition (CPPD) is classified as idiopathic, hereditary, or associated with metabolic disease. The associated diseases include hyperparathyroidism, hemochromatosis-hemosiderosis, hypothyroidism, gout, hypomagnesemia, hypophosphatasia, Wilson disease, and ochronosis.

* CPPD associations include hyperparathyroidism, hemochromatosis-hemosiderosis, hypothyroidism, and hypomagnesemia.

Pseudogout

When CPPD causes an acute inflammatory arthritis, the term *pseudogout* is applied. CPPD crystals are weakly positively birefringent and are rhomboid. Pseudogout rarely involves the first metatarsophalangeal joint. It most commonly affects the knees, but the wrists, elbows, ankles, and intervertebral disks may be involved. It usually occurs in older individuals. Most patients with pseudogout have chondrocalcinosis on radiography. The presence of chondrocalcinosis does not necessarily mean that a patient will have pseudogout or even CPPD.

* Pseudogout is an acute inflammatory arthritis caused by CPPD.
* CPPD crystals are weakly positively birefringent under polarized light microscopy.
* Pseudogout most commonly affects the knees, but the wrists, elbows, ankles, and intervertebral disks can be affected.
* Chondrocalcinosis is found on radiographs in most patients with pseudogout.
* Chondrocalcinosis does not mean that patients will have pseudogout or even CPPD.

Treatment of Pseudogout

For treatment of acute attacks, NSAIDs or injection of a steroid preparation can be used. Intravenously administered colchicine is effective for acute attacks, but oral administration is not consistently effective. Prophylactic oral colchicine (0.6 mg 2-3 times daily) can lead to a decrease in the frequency and severity of pseudogout attacks. In patients with underlying metabolic disease, the frequency of acute attacks of pseudogout does not necessarily decrease with treatment of the underlying disease (eg, hypothyroidism, hemochromatosis, or hyperparathyroidism).

* Treatment of acute attacks of pseudogout: NSAIDs, injection of steroid preparation, or colchicine given intravenously.
* Prophylactic oral colchicine can lead to a decrease in the frequency and severity of attacks.
* Typical clinical scenario: An elderly patient presents with acute pain,

swelling, and redness over the right knee joint. Radiographic examination shows chondrocalcinosis. Aspiration of joint fluid shows rhomboid crystals that are weakly positively birefringent on polarized light examination.

Basic Calcium Phosphate Disease (Hydroxyapatite Deposition Disease)

Presentation
Clinical presentations of hydroxyapatite deposition disease include 1) acute inflammation, including calcific tendinitis, osteoarthritis with inflammatory episodes, periarthritis or arthritis dialysis syndrome, and calcinotic deposits in scleroderma and 2) chronic inflammation, including severe osteoarthritis and Milwaukee shoulder or knee: advanced glenohumeral and knee osteoarthritis, rotator cuff tear, noninflammatory paste-like joint fluid containing hydroxyapatite.

* Hydroxyapatite deposition disease can present as acute or chronic inflammation.

Diagnosis and Treatment
Individual crystals cannot be seen on routine polarization microscopy (Table 24-23). Small, round (shiny coin) bodies 0.5 to 100 mcm are seen. On electron microscopy, these represent lumps of needle-shaped crystals. Positive identification requires transmission electron microscopy or elemental analysis. Alizarin red stain showing calcium staining provides a presumptive diagnosis (if CPPD is excluded). Treatment involves NSAIDs and intra-articular steroids.

* In hydroxyapatite deposition disease, individual crystals are not seen on polarization microscopy.
* Positive identification requires transmission electron microscopy.

Calcium Oxalate Arthropathy
Calcium oxalate arthropathy occurs in patients with primary oxalosis and in patients undergoing chronic hemodialysis. It can cause acute inflammatory arthritis. Crystals are large, bipyramidal, and birefringent. Calcium oxalate can cause chondrocalcinosis or large soft tissue calcifications.

* Calcium oxalate arthropathy occurs in patients with primary oxalosis and patients undergoing chronic hemodialysis.

Other Crystals Implicated in Joint Disease
Cholesterol crystals are a nonspecific finding and have been found in the synovial fluid of patients with various types of chronic inflammatory arthritis. Cryoglobulin crystals are found in essential cryoglobulinemia and paraproteinemia. Corticosteroid crystals are found in an arthritis flare after a corticosteroid injection, and Charcot-Leyden crystals have been found in hypereosinophilic syndromes. In patients undergoing hemodialysis, aluminum phosphate crystals can develop.

Spondyloarthropathies

Conditions that form the spondyloarthropathies include ankylosing spondylitis, reactive arthritis, enteropathic spondylitis, and psoriatic arthritis.

Spondyloarthropathies are characterized by involvement of the sacroiliac joints (uncommon in rheumatoid arthritis), peripheral arthritis that is usually asymmetric and oligoarticular, absence of rheumatoid factor, and an association with HLA-B27 in more than 90% of cases. They are enthesopathic disorders.

The HLA region of chromosome 6 contains genes of the human histocompatibility complex. Every person has 2 of chromosome 6, 1 inherited from each parent. On each of these there is an HLA-A and HLA-B allele. Therefore, everyone has 2 HLA-A types and 2 HLA-B types. With regard to inheritance, an offspring has a 50% chance of acquiring a specific HLA-A or HLA-B antigen from a parent (Figure 24-8). Siblings have a 25% chance of being identical for all 4 HLA-A and HLA-B alleles.

The frequency of HLA-B27 in control populations is as follows: whites (United States), 8%; African blacks, 0%; Asians, 1%; Haida (North American Indian), 50%.

The rheumatic diseases associated with HLA-B27 are ankylosing spondylitis (HLA-B27 in more than 90%), reactive arthritis (more than 80%), enteropathic spondylitis (approximately 75%), and psoriatic spondylitis (approximately 50%).

* Ankylosing spondylitis is associated with HLA-B27 in more than 90% of cases.

Table 24-23 Differential Diagnosis According to Results of Synovial Fluid Analysis

Diagnosis	Leukocyte Count, ×10⁹/L	Differential	Polarization Microscopy
Degenerative joint disease	<1	Mononuclear cells	Negative
Rheumatoid arthritis	5-50	PMNs	Negative
Gout	5-100	PMNs	Monosodium urate
Pseudogout	5-100	PMNs	CPPD
Hydroxyapatite	5-100	PMNs	Negative
Septic arthritis	≥100	PMNs	Negative

Abbreviations: CPPD, calcium pyrophosphate deposition disease; PMN, polymorphonuclear leukocytes.

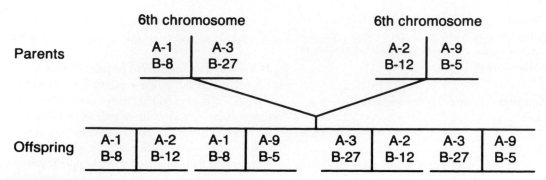

Figure 24-8. Inheritance of HLA Antigens.

Many theories have been proposed to explain the association between HLA-B27 and the spondyloarthropathies: B27 may act as a receptor site for an infective agent, may be a marker for an immune response gene that determines susceptibility to an environmental trigger, and may induce tolerance to foreign antigens with which it cross-reacts.

An offspring of a person with HLA-B27 has a 50% chance of carrying the antigen. In randomly selected persons with HLA-B27, the chance of the disease developing is 2%. In B27-positive relatives of B27-positive patients with ankylosing spondylitis, the risk of the disease developing is 20%.

Ankylosing Spondylitis

Ankylosing spondylitis is a chronic systemic inflammatory disease that affects the sacroiliac joints, the spine, and the peripheral joints. Sacroiliac joint involvement and low back pain define this disease, and decreased spinal motion and reduced chest expansion also are often found.

* Sacroiliac joint involvement and low back pain define ankylosing spondylitis, and decreased spinal motion and reduced chest expansion also are often found.

Features

Characteristic features of low back pain in ankylosing spondylitis are age at onset usually between 15 and 40 years, insidious onset, duration of more than 3 months, morning stiffness, improvement with exercise, family history, involvement of other systems, and diffuse radiation of back pain.

* Typical clinical scenario: A 20-year-old man has a history of low back pain of insidious onset that improves with exercise. He has diminished chest expansion, iritis, and tenderness over the sacroiliac joints. Laboratory testing shows an increased sedimentation rate. Rheumatoid factor is negative. Radiographic examination shows sclerosis and erosions of the sacroiliac joints and squaring of the vertebral bodies with the presence of syndesmophytes.

Findings of ankylosing spondylitis on physical examination are listed in Table 24-24. Other physical findings in ankylosing spondylitis are listed in Table 24-25.

The radiographic findings in ankylosing spondylitis are 1) sacroiliac involvement with erosions, "pseudo widening" of joint space, sclerosis (both sides of sacroiliac joint; this finding is needed for diagnosis), and fusion and 2) spine involvement with squaring of superior and inferior margins of vertebral body, syndesmophytes, and bamboo spine.

In patients with early disease, magnetic resonance imaging can detect inflammation in the sacroiliac joints even when radiographs of the sacroiliac joints are normal.

* Radiographic findings in ankylosing spondylitis include sacroiliac sclerosis and possible erosions, spine involvement with squaring of the vertebral bodies, syndesmophytes, and bamboo spine.

Laboratory Findings

The erythrocyte sedimentation rate may be increased, there may be an anemia of chronic disease, rheumatoid factor is absent, and 95% of white patients are positive for HLA-B27.

Extraspinal Involvement

Enthesopathic involvement distinguishes spondyloarthropathies from rheumatoid arthritis and consists of plantar fasciitis, Achilles tendinitis, and costochondritis. Hip and shoulder involvement are common (up to 50%), but peripheral joints can be affected, usually with asymmetric involvement of the lower extremities. Some patients in whom juvenile rheumatoid arthritis is diagnosed, especially male

Table 24-24 Findings in Ankylosing Spondylitis

Characteristic	Finding
Scoliosis	Absent
Decreased range of movement	Symmetric
Tenderness	Diffuse
Hip flexion with straight-leg raising	Normal
Pain with sciatic nerve stretch	Absent
Hip involvement	Frequently present
Neurodeficit	Absent

Table 24-25 Results of Testing in Ankylosing Spondylitis

Test	Method	Results
Schober	Make a mark on the spine at level of L5 & 1 at 10 cm directly above with the patient standing erect. Patient then bends forward maximally & the distance between the 2 marks is measured	An increase of <5 cm indicates early lumbar involvement
Chest expansion	Measure maximal chest expansion at nipple line	Chest expansion of <5 cm is clue to early costovertebral involvement
Sacroiliac compression	Exert direct compression over sacroiliac joints	Tenderness or pain suggests sacroiliac involvement

adolescents, may have juvenile ankylosing spondylitis in which peripheral arthritis preceded the axial involvement.

* Enthesopathic involvement is characteristic of ankylosing spondylitis and the other spondyloarthropathies and consists of plantar fasciitis, Achilles tendinitis, and costochondritis.
* Hip and shoulder involvement are common (up to 50%).

Extraskeletal Involvement
Other findings in active disease include 1) fatigue, 2) weight loss, 3) low-grade fever, and 4) iritis (25% of patients). Iritis is an important clinical clue in the diagnosis of spondyloarthropathies. It is not found in adults with rheumatoid arthritis.

* Iritis is an important clue to the diagnosis of spondyloarthropathies and is not found in adults with rheumatoid arthritis.
* Osteoporosis is a common complication of ankylosing spondylitis and can occur in early stages of the disease. It is largely confined to the axial skeleton to involve the spine and hips.

Late complications can include 1) traumatic spinal fracture leading to cord compression, 2) cauda equina syndrome (symptoms include neurogenic bladder, fecal incontinence, radicular leg pain), 3) fibrotic changes in upper lung fields, 4) aortic insufficiency in 3% to 5% of patients, 5) complete heart block, and 6) secondary amyloidosis.

* Late complications of ankylosing spondylitis include traumatic spinal fractures leading to cord compression, cauda equina syndrome, fibrotic changes in upper lung fields, and aortic insufficiency.

Ankylosing Spondylitis in Men and Women
Ankylosing spondylitis has been thought to be a disease primarily of men, but it is now recognized that the incidence in women is higher than originally thought, although women have less tendency for spinal ankylosis. The ratio of men to women is approximately 3:1. Women more frequently have osteitis pubis and peripheral joint involvement.

Differential Diagnosis
The differential diagnosis includes diffuse hypertrophic skeletal hyperostosis, osteitis condensans ilii, fusion of sacroiliac joint seen in paraplegia, osteitis pubis, infection, and degenerative joint disease. The clinical symptoms of diffuse hypertrophic skeletal hyperostosis are "stiffness" of spine and relatively good preservation of spine motion. It generally affects middle-aged and elderly men. Patients with diffuse hypertrophic skeletal hyperostosis can have dysphagia related to cervical osteophytes. Criteria for the condition are "flowing" ossification along the anterolateral aspect of at least 4 contiguous vertebral bodies, preservation of disk height, absence of apophyseal joint involvement, absence of sacroiliac joint involvement, and extraspinal ossifications, including ligamentous calcifications.

Osteitis condensans ilii usually affects young to middle-aged females with normal sacroiliac joints. Radiography shows sclerosis on the iliac side of the sacroiliac joint only.

The sacroiliac joint also can be involved with 1) tuberculosis, 2) metastatic disease, 3) gout, 4) Paget disease, or 5) other infections (eg, *Brucella, Serratia, Staphylococcus*).

* Osteitis condensans ilii usually affects young to middle-aged females; radiography shows sclerosis on the iliac side of the sacroiliac joint only.
* The sacroiliac joint can be involved with metastatic disease, gout, Paget disease, or infection (eg, *Brucella, Serratia, Staphylococcus*).

Treatment
Treatment involves physical therapy (upright posture is very important), exercise (swimming), cessation of smoking, genetic counseling, and drug therapy with NSAIDs such as indomethacin. Tumor necrosis factor inhibitors etanercept, infliximab, and adalimumab recently were approved, and they can provide benefit for spinal and peripheral joint symptoms.

Reactive Arthritis
This is an aseptic arthritis induced by a host response to an infectious agent rather than direct infection. HLA-B27 is associated in 80% of cases. The condition develops after infections with *Salmonella*

organisms, *Shigella flexneri*, *Yersinia enterocolitica*, and *Campylobacter jejuni*, which cause diarrhea, and *Chlamydia* and *Ureaplasma urealyticum*, which cause nonspecific urethritis. Inflammatory eye disease (conjunctivitis or iritis) and mucocutaneous disease (balanitis, oral ulcerations, or keratoderma) also can occur. Keratoderma blennorrhagicum is a characteristic skin disease on the palms and soles which is indistinguishable histologically from psoriasis. Joint predilection is for the toes and asymmetric large joints in the lower extremities. It can cause "sausage" toe, as can psoriatic arthritis. The distal interphalangeal joints in the hands can be affected also. Cardiac conduction disturbances and aortitis can develop. Sacroiliitis (sometimes unilateral) can occur. Long-term studies indicate that the disease remains episodically active in 75% of patients and that disability is a frequent outcome.

- Reactive arthritis is an aseptic arthritis induced by a host response to an infectious agent rather than direct infection.
- HLA-B27 is associated in 80% of cases.
- Reactive arthritis develops after infections with *Salmonella*, *Shigella flexneri*, *Yersinia enterocolitica*, *Campylobacter jejuni*, *Chlamydia*, *Ureaplasma urealyticum*.

Treatment is with NSAIDs (indomethacin). Sulfasalazine and methotrexate are used in patients with chronic disease. Treatment with tetracycline or erythromycin-type antibiotics may decrease the duration and severity of illness in some cases of *Chlamydia*-triggered reactive arthritis.

Arthritis Associated With Inflammatory Bowel Disease

Two distinct types of arthritis are associated with chronic inflammatory bowel disease: 1) a nondestructive oligoarthritis of the peripheral joints tending to correlate with the activity of the bowel disease and 2) ankylosing spondylitis (enteropathic spondylitis). The spondylitis is not a complication of the bowel disease. It may be diagnosed many years before the onset of bowel symptoms, and its subsequent progress bears little relationship to the bowel disease. Approximately 75% of patients with enteropathic spondylitis and inflammatory bowel disease are HLA-B27–positive. Patients with inflammatory bowel disease alone do not have an increased frequency of HLA-B27 and are not at increased risk for development of spondylitis.

- Patients with inflammatory bowel disease may have a nondestructive oligoarthritis of the peripheral joints which tends to correlate with the activity of the bowel disease.

Psoriatic Arthritis

Psoriatic arthritis develops in 7% or less of patients with psoriasis. Pitting of nails is strongly associated with joint disease. Patients with more severe skin disease are at higher risk for the development of arthritis. A "sausage" finger or toe is characteristic of psoriatic arthritis and is very uncommon in rheumatoid arthritis. Radiographic evidence of involvement of the distal interphalangeal joint with erosions is common in psoriasis and uncommon in rheumatoid arthritis. Psoriatic arthritis also can, in severe cases, cause a characteristic "pencil-in-cup" deformity of the distal interphalangeal and proximal interphalangeal joints on radiography.

- Psoriatic arthritis develops in 7% or less of patients with psoriasis.
- Pitting of nails is strongly associated with joint disease.
- "Sausage" finger or toe is characteristic.
- "Pencil-in-cup" deformity of the distal and proximal interphalangeal joints is found on radiography.

There are 5 clinical groups of psoriatic arthritis: 1) predominantly distal interphalangeal joint involvement, 2) asymmetric oligoarthritis, 3) symmetric polyarthritis-like rheumatoid arthritis but negative for rheumatoid factor, 4) arthritis mutilans, and 5) psoriatic spondylitis (HLA-B27–positive in 50%-75% of cases). Treatment is with NSAIDs, methotrexate, and tumor necrosis factor inhibitors.

Iritis and Rheumatologic Diseases

Various rheumatologic diseases are associated with iritis, particularly the seronegative spondyloarthropathies. Iritis is uncommon in rheumatoid arthritis and systemic lupus erythematosus. Nongranulomatous iritis without any other associated symptoms may be associated with HLA-B27 in almost 50% of patients.

Behçet Syndrome

Behçet syndrome is most common in Middle Eastern countries and Japan. HLA-B51 is associated with the syndrome. In addition to oral and genital ulcerations, uveitis, synovitis, cutaneous vasculitis, and meningoencephalitis may be present. The pathergy reaction (hyperreactivity of the skin in response to superficial trauma) also occurs. Migratory, superficial thrombophlebitis and erythema nodosum also have been associated with this syndrome. The combination of recurrent aphthous dermatitis, similar ulcerations in the genital area, and uveitis is most common. Treatment is with corticosteroids, although more aggressive immunosuppression often is required.

- Common manifestations of Behçet syndrome include oral and genital ulcers and uveitis.

Osteoid Osteoma

Osteoid osteoma is a benign bone tumor. It usually occurs in males and females between the ages of 5 and 30 years. The classic symptom is bone pain at night, which is relieved completely with aspirin or another NSAID. The diagnosis may be made with routine radiography, but often this is negative and bone scanning may be helpful for localizing the tumor. Tomography or computed tomography then can be done for better visualization. Radiography shows a small nidus, usually less than 1 cm, varying from radiolucent to radiopaque, depending on the age of the lesion. There is usually a lucent ring around the nidus and adjacent bone sclerosis. Definitive treatment includes excision, which is curative.

- Osteoid osteoma is a benign bone tumor.
- Bone pain at night is relieved by aspirin or another NSAID.
- Treatment includes excision, which is curative.

Bypass Arthritis

Bypass arthritis occurs in patients who have undergone intestinal bypass operations, including jejunocolic or jejunoileal. The arthritis may be acute or subacute, is usually intermittent, and can last occasionally for short periods, only to recur. The most commonly affected joints are the metacarpophalangeal, proximal interphalangeal, wrists, knees, and ankles. It commonly is associated with a dermatitis, which can be pustular. Circulating immune complexes composed of bacterial antigens have been found in both the circulation and the synovial fluid and are thought to be the cause of this disorder. Treatment consists of NSAIDs and antibiotics such as tetracycline, but reanastomosis may be necessary for complete resolution of symptoms.

- Bypass arthritis occurs in patients who have had intestinal bypass operations.
- Most commonly affected joints are metacarpophalangeal, proximal interphalangeal, wrists, knees, and ankles.
- Bypass arthritis is commonly associated with a dermatitis.

Systemic Lupus Erythematosus

Systemic lupus erythematosus (SLE) is a chronic inflammatory disease of unknown cause with a wide spectrum of clinical manifestations and variable course characterized by exacerbations and remissions. Antibodies that react with nuclear antigens commonly are found in patients with the disease. Genetic, hormonal, and environmental factors seem to be important in the cause.

- SLE is characterized by exacerbations and remissions.

Diagnosis
Findings in patients with SLE are listed in Table 24-26. At least 4 of the findings are needed for the diagnosis of SLE.

Epidemiology
The female to male ratio is 8:1 during the reproductive years. The first symptoms usually occur between the second and fourth decades of life. The disease seems to be less severe in the elderly. In SLE with onset at an older age, the female to male ratio is equal. The frequency of SLE is increased in American blacks, Native Americans, and Asians.

- Female to male ratio in SLE is 8:1 during the reproductive years.
- The frequency of SLE is increased in American blacks, Native Americans, and Asians.

Etiology
In human disease, viral-like particles in glomeruli of patients with SLE have been reported; however, attempts to isolate viruses have been unsuccessful. A direct causal relationship between virus and SLE has not yet been established. Patients with SLE have increased viral antibody titers to a wide range of antigens without much sign of specificity for a particular viral agent.

Table 24-26 Criteria for the Classification of Systemic Lupus Erythematosus

Malar rash
Discoid lupus
Photosensitivity
Oral ulcers
Nonerosive arthritis
Proteinuria (protein >0.5 g/day) or cellular casts
Seizures or psychosis
Pleuritis or pericarditis
Hemolytic anemia, leukopenia, lymphopenia, or thrombocytopenia
Antibody to native DNA, antibody to Sm (Smith), immunoglobulin G or M antiphospholipid antibodies, positive test for lupus anticoagulant, or false-positive result of VDRL test
Positive results of fluorescent antinuclear antibody test

- In SLE, there are increased viral antibody titers to a wide range of antigens without much sign of specificity for a particular viral agent.

Genetics
Among relatives of patients with SLE, 20% have a different immunologic disease. Another 25% have antinuclear antibodies, circulating immune complexes, antilymphocyte antibodies, or a false-positive result on VDRL test without clinical disease. Concordance for SLE among monozygotic twins is much greater than among dizygotic twins. Multiple genetic and environmental factors are important in the development of SLE. Immune complex levels are much higher in persons with close contact to SLE patients than in unexposed consanguineous relatives. The frequency of HLA-B8, HLA-DR2, and HLA-DR3 is increased.

- 20% of relatives of patients with SLE have a different immunologic disease.
- In SLE, the frequency of HLA-B8, HLA-DR2, and HLA-DR3 is increased.

Pathogenesis
There is a change in the activity of the cellular immune system with an absolute decrease in T-suppressor cells. There is an increase in the activity of the humoral immune system with B-cell hyperactivity resulting in polyclonal activation and antibody production.

Circulating immune complexes (anti-native DNA) may contribute to glomerulonephritis and skin disease, among other manifestations. Immune complexes bind complement, which initiates the inflammatory process. Organ-specific autoantibodies also contribute to the pathophysiology of the disease and include antibodies that are 1) antierythrocyte, 2) antiplatelet, 3) antileukocyte, 4) antineuronal, and 5) antithyroid.

- Circulating immune complexes (anti-native DNA) are responsible for glomerulonephritis and certain skin manifestations.

- Organ-specific autoantibodies also may contribute to the pathophysiology.

Late complications of SLE are related to vascular damage, sometimes in the relative absence of active immunologic disease. Damage to the intima during active disease ultimately may result in various thrombotic, ischemic, and hypertensive manifestations.

Clinical Manifestations

Fever in SLE usually is caused by the disease, but infection must be ruled out. Shaking chills and leukocytosis strongly suggest infection.

Articular

The arthritis is characteristically inflammatory but nondeforming and nonerosive. Avascular necrosis of bone occurs, and not only in patients taking steroids. The femoral head, navicular bone, and tibial plateau are most commonly affected.

Dermatologic

Discoid lupus involves the face, scalp, and extremities. There is follicular plugging with atrophy leading to scarring. Subacute cutaneous LE is a subset of SLE that primarily has skin involvement with psoriasiform or annular erythematous lesions. Patients may be negative for antinuclear antibodies but frequently are positive for antibodies to the extractable nuclear antigen SS-A (Ro) (Sjögren syndrome A).

Cardiopulmonary

Cardiac involvement in SLE is manifested by pericarditis, myocarditis, valvular involvement, accelerated coronary atherosclerosis, and coronary vasculitis. An association between SLE and premature coronary artery disease has also been established. The prevalence of subclinical coronary artery disease is approximately 35%. Therefore, in a young woman with chest pain, coronary artery disease must be strongly considered. Besides known cardiovascular risk factors such as hypertension and hyperlipidemia, SLE itself is an independent risk factor, possibly through immune-mediated chronic vascular inflammation common to the pathogenesis of SLE and atherosclerosis.

Pulmonary involvement in SLE is manifested by any of the following: pleurisy, pleural effusions, pneumonitis, pulmonary hypertension, hemorrhage, and diaphragmatic dysfunction.

Neuropsychiatric

Central nervous system lupus is a most variable and unpredictable phenomenon. Manifestations such as impaired cognitive function, seizures, long tract signs, cranial neuropathies, psychosis, and migraine-like attacks occur with little apparent relationship to each other or to other systemic manifestations. Immune complexes in the choroid plexus are *not* specific for central nervous system disease because they also occur in patients without central nervous system disease. Patients may have increased cerebrospinal fluid protein immunoglobulin (Ig) G, pleocytosis, and antineuronal antibodies.

Results of electroencephalography can be abnormal. Magnetic resonance imaging usually shows areas of increased signal in the periventricular white matter, similar to those found in multiple sclerosis.

Magnetic resonance imaging findings are often nonspecific and sometimes can be seen in patients who have SLE without central nervous system manifestations. Pathologic examinations of autopsy specimens usually reveal microinfarcts, nerve cell loss, rarely vasculitis, or no detectable abnormalities.

Proposed pathogenetic mechanisms causing neuropsychiatric manifestations include autoneuronal antibodies, vasculitis, leukoagglutination, antiphospholipid-associated hypercoagulability, and cytokine effect.

Psychosis caused by steroid therapy is probably rarer than previously thought. When there is doubt about the cause of the psychosis in patients with SLE, the steroid dose can be increased and the patient observed. Patients rarely can have isolated central nervous system involvement and normal results of cerebrospinal fluid examination and no other organ involvement.

Particularly with neuropsychiatric symptoms or respiratory symptoms, secondary causes must be considered, especially infection, hypertension, anemia, and hypoxia. Fever should be considered due to infection until proved otherwise.

- Central nervous system lupus is a most variable and unpredictable phenomenon.
- Immune complexes in the choroid plexus are not specific for central nervous system disease.
- Magnetic resonance imaging findings are nonspecific.
- Particularly with neuropsychiatric symptoms or respiratory symptoms, secondary causes must be considered, especially infection, hypertension, anemia, and hypoxia.
- Fever should be considered due to infection until proved otherwise.

Pregnancy and SLE

Women with SLE who become pregnant have a high prevalence of spontaneous abortion. Because abortion itself may lead to a flare of the disease, therapeutic abortion ordinarily is not recommended after the first trimester. Flares of disease should be treated with steroids, particularly during the postpartum period.

In infants of mothers with SLE, thrombocytopenia and leukopenia can develop from passive transfer of antibodies. They also can have transient cutaneous lesions and complete heart block. Mothers usually have anti-SS-A (Ro), which crosses the placenta and is transiently present in the infant. Mothers usually are HLA-B8/DR3-positive, but there is no HLA association in the child.

Renal Involvement

The types of renal disease in SLE are 1) mesangial, 2) focal glomerulonephritis, 3) membranous glomerulonephritis, 4) diffuse proliferative glomerulonephritis, 5) interstitial nephritis with defects in the renal tubular handling of K+, and 6) renal vein thrombosis with nephrotic syndrome.

Treatment of renal disease depends in part on the results of renal biopsy. Patients with high activity indices on biopsy such as active inflammation, proliferation, necrosis, and crescent formation are considered for aggressive therapy. Patients with high chronicity indices such as tubular atrophy, scarring, and glomerulosclerosis are less likely to respond to aggressive therapy. Patients with mesangial changes alone do not require aggressive therapy. Active diffuse proliferative glomerulonephritis is treated with high-dose steroids and cyclophosphamide. Recently, mycophenolate mofetil has shown efficacy equivalent to cyclophosphamide with fewer side effects and can be considered an alternative to induction and maintenance therapy in lupus nephritis. Immunosuppressive agents lower the incidence of renal failure in patients with diffuse proliferative glomerulonephritis and may improve overall survival. Appropriate treatment for focal proliferative glomerulonephritis and membranous glomerulonephritis is controversial because the prognosis is more favorable.

In patients with chronic proteinuria even without evidence of active renal disease, angiotensin-I converting enzyme inhibitors should be used. They have been shown to lower proteinuria and have renoprotective effects.

* Renal biopsies are helpful for directing therapy in renal disease associated with SLE.
* Patients with mesangial changes alone do not require aggressive therapy.
* Active diffuse proliferative glomerulonephritis is treated with high-dose steroids and immunosuppressive agents.

Laboratory Findings

Anemia of chronic disease and hemolytic anemia (Coombs positive) can occur. Leukopenia usually does not predispose to infection. Anti-lymphocyte antibodies cause lymphopenia in SLE. Idiopathic thrombocytopenic purpura with the presence of platelet antibodies can be the initial manifestation of SLE. Polyclonal gammopathy due to hyperactivity of the humoral immune system is common. The erythrocyte sedimentation rate usually correlates with disease activity.

Hypocomplementemia (CH$_{50}$, C3, C4) usually correlates with active disease. Hypocomplementemia with increased anti-nDNA antibodies usually implies renal disease (or skin disease). Complement split products (such as C3a, C5a, Ba/BB) are increased in active disease. A total complement value too low to measure with normal C3 and C4 values suggests a hereditary complement deficiency. Familial C2 deficiency is the most common complement deficiency in SLE, but C1r, C1s, C1q, C4, C5, C7, and C8 deficiencies also have been reported.

Patients with SLE may have false-positive results of the VDRL test as a result of antibody to phospholipid, which cross-reacts with VDRL. Patients with SLE also can have false-positive results of the fluorescent treponemal antibody test, but they usually have the "beaded pattern" of fluorescence. LE cells are present in approximately 70% of patients with SLE and are caused by antibody to deoxyribonucleoprotein (DNP). This test is not specific and is no longer performed in many centers. Anti-DNP also is detected by the fluorescent antinuclear antibody test in a homogeneous pattern.

Anti-native DNA levels fluctuate with disease activity, whereas levels of other autoantibodies (ribonucleoprotein, Sm, antinuclear antibody) show *no* consistent relationship to levels of anti-native DNA or disease activity. Methods used to measure anti-native DNA are 1) an immunofluorescent method using *Crithidia lucilia*, an organism with a kinetoplast that contains helical native DNA free of other nuclear antigens—therefore, there is no single-stranded DNA

contamination, and 2) radioimmunoassay and enzyme-linked immunosorbent assay, which suffer from the difficulty of maintaining DNA in its native double-stranded state and so are contaminated with single-stranded DNA.

Although all patients with lupus should have positive results of antinuclear antibody tests, a positive result is by no means specific for lupus. Antinuclear antibody patterns are outlined in Table 24-27. Other autoantibodies and disease associations are outlined in Table 24-28.

* Hemolytic anemia (Coombs positive) can occur in SLE.
* Idiopathic thrombocytopenic purpura can be the initial manifestation of SLE.
* Hypocomplementemia (CH50, C3, C4) usually correlates with active disease.
* Hypocomplementemia with increased anti-native DNA antibodies usually implies renal disease (or skin disease).
* Anti-native DNA levels fluctuate with disease activity, but other associated antibodies do not.
* A positive result of an antinuclear antibody test is by no means specific for lupus.

Treatment

Treatment should match the activity of SLE in the individual patient. Serial monitoring of organ function and appropriate laboratory evaluation (anti-native DNA, C3, erythrocyte sedimentation rate) allow rapid recognition and treatment of flares and appropriate tapering of steroid dose during periods of disease quiescence. Table 24-29 provides guidelines for treatment, and Table 24-30 outlines the complications of treatment.

Outcome

The 10-year survival rate is 90% in newly diagnosed SLE. Prognosis is worse in blacks and Hispanics than in whites. Prognosis is worse in patients with creatinine values more than 3.0 mg/dL. The major causes of death are 1) renal disease, 2) infection, 3) central nervous system involvement, and 4) vascular disease (such as myocardial infarction).

* The 10-year survival rate is 90% in newly diagnosed SLE.
* The prognosis is worse in blacks and Hispanics.

Table 24-27 Antinuclear Antibody Patterns

Fluorescent Pattern	Antigen	Disease Association
Rim, peripheral, shaggy	nDNA	SLE
Homogeneous	DNP	SLE, others
Speckled	ENA	MCTD, SLE, others
Nucleolar	RNA	Scleroderma

Abbreviations: DNP, deoxyribonucleoprotein; ENA, extractable nuclear antigen; MCTD, mixed connective tissue disease; nDNA, native DNA; SLE, systemic lupus erythematosus.

Table 24-28 Autoantibodies in Rheumatic Diseases

Antibody	Disease Association
Anti-nDNA	SLE, 50%-60%
Anti-Sm (Smith)	SLE, 30%
Anti-RNP (ribonucleoprotein)	MCTD, 100% high titer
	SLE, 30% titer
	Scleroderma, low frequency, low titer
Anti-SS-A (Sjögren syndrome A)	Sjögren, 70%
	SLE, 35%
	Scleroderma + MCTD, low frequency, low titer
Anti-SS-B (Sjögren syndrome B)	Sjögren, 60%
	SLE, 15%
Antihistone	Drug-induced SLE, 95%
	SLE, 60%
	RA, 20%
Anti-Scl-70 (antitopoisomerase I)	Scleroderma, 25%
Anticentromere	CREST, 70%-90%
	Scleroderma, 10%-15%
Anti-PM1	PM, 50%
Anti-Jo1 (histidyl-tRNA synthetase)	PM/interstitial lung disease, 30%

Abbreviations: CREST, syndrome of calcinosis cutis, Raynaud phenomenon, esophageal dysmotility, sclerodactyly, telangiectasia; MCTD, mixed connective tissue disease; nDNA, native DNA; PM, polymyositis; RA, rheumatoid arthritis; SLE, systemic lupus erythematosus.

Table 24-29 Treatment of Manifestations of Systemic Lupus Erythematosus

Manifestation	Treatment
Arthritis, fever, mild systemic symptoms	ASA, NSAID
Photosensitivity, rash	Avoidance of sun, use of sunscreens
Rash, arthritis	Hydroxychloroquine (Plaquenil)
Significant thrombocytopenia, hemolytic anemia	Steroids
Renal disease, CNS disease, pericarditis, other significant organ involvement	Steroids
Rapidly deteriorating renal function	Cyclophosphamide, mycophenolate mofetil

Abbreviations: ASA, acetylsalicylic acid; CNS, central nervous system; NSAID, nonsteroidal anti-inflammatory drug.

Table 24-30 Complications of Treatment for Systemic Lupus Erythematosus

Treatment	Complication
Ibuprofen	Aseptic meningitis (headache, fever, stiff neck, CSF pleocytosis)
NSAID	Decreased renal blood flow
ASA	Salicylate hepatitis (common), benign
Cyclophosphamide	Hemorrhagic cystitis, alopecia, opportunistic lymphomas, infection, increased incidence of lymphomas (CNS)
Hydroxychloroquine (Plaquenil)	Retinal toxicity

Abbreviations: ASA, acetylsalicylic acid; CNS, central nervous system; CSF, cerebrospinal fluid; NSAID, nonsteroidal anti-inflammatory drug.

- Typical clinical scenario: A young woman presents with malar rash and photosensitivity. She has a history of oral ulcers and arthralgias. Laboratory results are significant proteinuria and red blood cell casts in the urine. There is a normochromic normocytic anemia with a positive Coombs test. Antibody to native DNA is present. Results of the VDRL test are positive.

Drug-Induced Lupus

Many drugs have been implicated in drug-induced lupus. The most common drugs are listed in Table 24-31. One must differentiate between the clinical syndrome of drug-induced lupus and only a positive antinuclear antibody result without clinical symptoms. Many drugs can cause a positive antinuclear antibody result without ever causing the clinical syndrome of drug-induced lupus. Only hydralazine and procainamide have been strongly implicated in drug-induced lupus. A drug-induced lupus syndrome develops in approximately 5% of persons taking hydralazine and in 15% to 25% of those who take procainamide. Virtually all patients taking procainamide for 1 year will have a positive result of the antinuclear antibody test.

- Only hydralazine and procainamide are strongly implicated in drug-induced lupus.
- Virtually all patients taking procainamide for 1 year have a positive result of the antinuclear antibody test.

Clinical Features

The clinical manifestations of drug-induced lupus include arthralgias and polyarthritis, which occur in approximately 80% of cases. Malaise is common, and fever has been reported in up to 40% of cases. Cardiopulmonary involvement is also common, and approximately 30% of patients have pleural-pulmonary manifestations as their presenting symptoms. Pericarditis has been reported in approximately 20% of cases. Diffuse interstitial pneumonitis has been noted. Asymptomatic pleural effusions may be found on routine chest radiography. A few cases of pericardial tamponade have been reported. In contrast to SLE, the incidence of renal and central nervous system involvement is low in drug-induced lupus. Therefore, it is regarded as more benign than SLE. Other clinical differences include a lower

Table 24-31 Implicated Agents in Drug-Induced Lupus

Definite	Probable
Common	Phenytoin
Procainamide	Carbamazepine
Hydralazine	Ethosuximide
Uncommon	Propylthiouracil
Isoniazid	Penicillamine
Methyldopa	Sulfasalazine
Chlorpromazine	Lithium carbonate
Quinidine	Acebutolol
Minocycline	Lovastatin

incidence of skin manifestations, lymphadenopathy, and myalgias in drug-induced disease.

- In drug-induced lupus, arthralgias and polyarthritis occur in about 80% of cases.
- Malaise is common, and fever occurs in up to 40% of cases.
- About 30% of patients have pleural-pulmonary manifestations on presentation.
- Pericarditis is reported in about 20% of cases.
- The incidence of renal and central nervous system involvement is low.

SLE is predominantly a disease of premenopausal females, whereas drug-induced disease has an almost equal sex distribution and occurs in an older population. This disparity in age reflects the use of hydralazine and procainamide primarily in an older population.

Laboratory Abnormalities

Virtually all patients with SLE and drug-induced lupus have antinuclear antibodies. Although patients with SLE and drug-induced lupus are serologically similar in many respects, there are notable differences. Antibodies to native DNA are found in only a small percentage of cases of drug-induced lupus but in approximately 60% of cases of SLE. Serum total hemolytic complement, C3, and C4 are usually normal in drug-induced disease, in contrast to SLE. Antibodies such as anti-Sm (Smith), SS-A, SS-B, and RNP (ribonucleoprotein) are also unusual in drug-induced lupus. The frequency of antihistone antibodies in drug-induced lupus is high (>95% of cases), but these also occur in approximately 60% of cases of SLE. Other, less frequent laboratory abnormalities in drug-induced lupus can include a positive LE preparation, positive Coombs test, positive rheumatoid factor, false-positive result of serologic test for syphilis, circulating anticoagulants, and cryoglobulins.

Metabolism

Drugs involved in drug-induced lupus have different chemical structures, but 3 of them—isoniazid, procainamide, and hydralazine—contain a primary amine that is acetylated by the hepatic N-acetyltransferase system. Persons who are taking 1 of these drugs and who are *slow* acetylators have a much higher incidence of serologic abnormalities and clinical disease than rapid acetylators. These manifestations also occur over a shorter period in slow acetylators than in rapid acetylators.

- Slow acetylators have a much higher incidence of serologic abnormalities and clinical disease.

Treatment

When possible, patients with drug-induced lupus should stop using the offending drug. Symptoms usually subside within several weeks, although the duration for complete resolution varies depending on the drug. Serologic abnormalities can remain for years after resolution of clinical symptoms. Patients taking procainamide are most likely to have a rapid remission once use of the drug is stopped, but patients taking hydralazine might have prolonged clinical manifestations.

Treatment depends on the clinical manifestations and could include NSAIDs or possibly low-dose prednisone if needed.

- Typical clinical scenario: A patient presents with a history of fever, arthralgias, fatigue, and a rash. The patient is taking procainamide for suppression of a ventricular arrhythmia. Laboratory results are a positive antinuclear antibody test and negative anti-native DNA antibody.

Overlap Syndromes

An overlap syndrome is a disease characterized by features of more than 1 connective tissue disease. Secondary Sjögren syndrome accompanying another connective tissue disease is not classified as an overlap syndrome.

Mixed Connective Tissue Disease

This is a distinct disease with variable features of SLE, polymyositis, systemic sclerosis, and rheumatoid arthritis. The incidence of renal disease is low. It is serologically characterized by a positive antinuclear antibody and by a high titer of the autoantibody anti-RNP. Anti-native DNA antibodies usually are not present. Raynaud phenomenon is common.

Undifferentiated Connective Tissue Disease

This category includes patients with symptoms that do not fulfill the diagnostic criteria for a definite or specific connective tissue disease. Common symptoms include Raynaud phenomenon, arthralgias, fatigue, and variable joint or soft tissue swelling. The antinuclear antibody may be positive, but other autoantibodies are not present. Patients need to be observed to determine whether progression to a distinct connective tissue disease occurs.

Antiphospholipid Antibody Syndrome

The diagnosis of the antiphospholipid antibody syndrome is made on the basis of 1) a history of venous or arterial thrombosis, fetal loss after 10 weeks' gestation, or recurrent fetal loss before 10 weeks' gestation and 2) the presence of medium to high levels of IgG or IgM antiphospholipid antibodies or the lupus anticoagulant on 2 occasions at least 12 weeks apart. Antiphospholipid antibodies may be either the IgG or the IgM class. The hallmark of the antiphospholipid antibody syndrome is prolongation on all phospholipid-dependent coagulation tests. The antibodies prolong the partial thromboplastin time at the level of the prothrombin activator complex of the clotting cascade. The antiphospholipid antibodies are thought to interact with the β_2-glycoprotein-1 that binds to phospholipid, interfering with the calcium-dependent binding of prothrombin factor Xa to the phospholipid. The failure of normal plasma to correct the prolonged clotting time distinguishes the lupus anticoagulant and antiphospholipid antibody clotting factors from clotting factor deficiencies. In the usual coagulation screening tests, the lupus anticoagulant results in prolongation of the activated partial thromboplastin time without prolongation of the prothrombin time (Table 24-32).

- Antiphospholipid antibodies are of either the IgG or the IgM class.
- Prolongation on all phospholipid-dependent coagulation tests is the laboratory hallmark of the antiphospholipid antibody syndrome.
- Activated partial thromboplastin time is prolonged and not corrected by adding normal plasma, but it is corrected with the addition of platelet-rich plasma, and this is the laboratory hallmark of a lupus anticoagulant.

Various other tests are reported to be sensitive for detection of lupus anticoagulants, including the plasma clotting time, kaolin clotting time, a platelet neutralization procedure, and modified Russell viper venom time.

Many, but not all, patients with the lupus anticoagulant also have increased IgG or IgM antiphospholipid antibody levels.

The lupus anticoagulant and antiphospholipid antibodies are associated with SLE, but they also have been reported in various other autoimmune, malignant, infectious, and drug-induced diseases. Other associated diseases include Sjögren syndrome, rheumatoid arthritis, idiopathic thrombocytopenic purpura, Behçet syndrome, myasthenia gravis, and mixed connective tissue disease. The antibodies are also found in persons with no apparent disease but in whom recurrent thrombosis develops. This is the primary antiphospholipid antibody syndrome, which represents approximately 50% of cases.

- Lupus anticoagulant and antiphospholipid antibodies also have been reported in various other autoimmune, malignant, infectious, and drug-induced diseases.
- The primary antiphospholipid antibody syndrome represents 50% of cases.

Clinical Features

There is an association between the presence of the lupus anticoagulant and antiphospholipid antibodies and recurrent venous or arterial thrombosis. Thrombotic events described have included stroke, transient ischemic attacks, myocardial infarctions, brachial artery thrombosis, deep venous thrombophlebitis, retinal vein thrombosis, hepatic vein thrombosis resulting in Budd-Chiari syndrome, and pulmonary hypertension. Other manifestations include recurrent fetal loss, thrombocytopenia, positive results of Coombs test, migraines, chorea, epilepsy, chronic leg ulcers, livedo reticularis, and progressive dementia resulting from cerebrovascular accidents. Recently, acquired valvular heart disease, especially aortic and mitral

Table 24-32 Coagulation Tests Characterizing the Lupus Anticoagulant

Screening tests
Prothrombin time normal
PTT prolonged
Plasma clot time prolonged
Tests identifying the lupus anticoagulant
Prolonged PTT not corrected by adding normal plasma

Abbreviation: PTT, partial thromboplastin time.

insufficiency, has been described. The mechanism or mechanisms by which antiphospholipid antibodies are associated with thromboembolic manifestations remain unclear. Blocking the production of prostacyclin from vascular endothelial cells, inhibition of the prekallikrein activity protein C pathway and fibrinolysis, and decreased plasminogen activator release have all been described.

Although many patients with lupus and other diseases can have a lupus anticoagulant or antiphospholipid antibodies, of either the IgG or the IgM class, thrombosis will not necessarily develop. In general, patients with the highest levels of antiphospholipid antibodies are more prone to thrombosis than those with lower levels. Also, the IgG antiphospholipid antibody is more strongly associated with recurrent thrombosis than is the IgM antiphospholipid antibody. In patients with a lupus anticoagulant or increased antiphospholipid antibodies without a history of thrombosis, most physicians are reluctant to provide treatment other than aspirin. In patients with either antiphospholipid antibodies or the lupus anticoagulant, even if they have not had a thrombotic event, the use of estrogen-containing oral contraceptive pills should be avoided because they may put the patient at higher risk for thrombosis.

* There is an association between the presence of the lupus anticoagulant and antiphospholipid antibodies and recurrent venous or arterial thrombosis.
* Other manifestations: recurrent fetal loss, thrombocytopenia, positive Coombs test, migraines, chorea, epilepsy, chronic leg ulcers, livedo reticularis, and progressive dementia from cerebrovascular accidents.
* Acquired valvular heart disease, especially aortic insufficiency, has been described.
* Patients with the highest levels of antiphospholipid antibodies are more prone to thrombosis.
* IgG antiphospholipid antibody is more strongly associated with recurrent thrombosis.

Treatment

For most patients who have recurrent thrombosis and high-titer anticardiolipin antibody, warfarin is prescribed in doses sufficient to yield international normalized ratio values close to 3 and will need to be taken for life. Low-dose aspirin and subcutaneous heparin have been used in pregnant women to prevent fetal loss. Corticosteroids have not been clearly shown to be efficacious for preventing thrombosis.

* Typical clinical scenario: A young patient presents with recurrent deep venous thrombosis. In the absence of anticoagulant therapy, the activated partial thromboplastin time is prolonged. Laboratory tests show that this prolongation is not corrected by the addition of normal plasma.

Raynaud Phenomenon

This is biphasic or triphasic color changes (pallor, cyanosis, erythema) accompanied by pain and numbness in the hands or feet. Cold is a common precipitating agent. Associated factors are listed in Table 24-33.

* Cold is a common precipitating agent for Raynaud phenomenon.

Raynaud phenomenon is related to an abnormality of the microvasculature associated with intimal fibrosis. In male patients with Raynaud phenomenon, a rare occurrence, a connective tissue disease may develop. Although Raynaud phenomenon is common in females, it usually is not associated with a connective tissue disease unless the patient has positive results for antinuclear antibody, which suggest that a connective tissue disease may develop in the future.

Skin capillary microscopy reveals tortuous, dilated capillary loops in systemic sclerosis, mixed connective tissue disease, and polymyositis. They also may be present in patients with Raynaud phenomenon who will go on to have systemic sclerosis, polymyositis, or mixed connective tissue disease.

Treatment involves smoking cessation, wearing gloves, biofeedback, 2% nitrol paste, and antihypertensive agents (prazosin or the calcium channel blockers amlodipine besylate or nifedipine). A stellate ganglion block, digital nerve block, or surgical digital sympathectomy is used if ischemia is severe. β-Adrenergic blockers and serotonin agonists such as sumatriptan can increase spasm and should be avoided.

To differentiate primary Raynaud phenomenon from the secondary form (resulting from a connective tissue disease), clinical features are considered. In primary Raynaud phenomenon, females are usually affected, the onset is at menarche, usually all digits are involved, and attacks are very frequent. The severity of symptoms is mild to moderate, and they can be precipitated by emotional stress. Digital ulceration and finger edema are rare, as is periungual erythema. Livedo reticularis is frequent.

`Table 24-33 Causes of Secondary Raynaud Phenomenon

Chemotherapeutic agents
Bleomycin
Vinblastine
Toxins
Vinyl chloride
Vibration-induced injuries
Jackhammer use
Vascular occlusive disorders
Thoracic outlet obstruction
Atherosclerosis
Vasculitis
Connective tissue diseases
Scleroderma, 90%-100%
Mixed connective tissue disease, 90%-100%
Systemic lupus erythematosus, 15%
Rheumatoid arthritis, <10%
Polymyositis
Miscellaneous
Cryoglobulinemia
Cold agglutinins
Increased blood viscosity

In persons with Raynaud phenomenon due to a connective tissue disease, both males and females are affected. The onset of Raynaud phenomenon is in the mid-20s or later. It often begins in a single digit, and attacks are usually infrequent (0-5 a day). It is moderate to severe, and the disorder is not precipitated by emotional stress. Digital ulceration, finger edema, and periungual erythema are frequent. Livedo reticularis is uncommon.

Systemic Sclerosis (Scleroderma)

Systemic sclerosis (scleroderma) can be subdivided into several categories: 1) diffuse systemic sclerosis (diffuse scleroderma); 2) limited cutaneous scleroderma, which includes the CREST (calcinosis cutis, Raynaud phenomenon, esophageal dysmotility, sclerodactyly, telangiectasias) syndrome; 3) localized scleroderma, which includes morphea and linear scleroderma; and 4) overlap and undifferentiated connective tissue diseases, which include some component of scleroderma in conjunction with a manifestation of another connective tissue disease. For the diagnosis of systemic sclerosis, 1 major criterion or 2 or more minor criteria need to be present. The major criterion is symmetric induration of the skin of the fingers and the skin proximal to metacarpophalangeal or metatarsophalangeal joints. The minor criteria are sclerodactyly, digital pitting scars or loss of substance from the finger pad, and bibasilar pulmonary fibrosis.

* Systemic sclerosis is characterized by symmetric induration of the skin of the fingers and the skin proximal to metacarpophalangeal or metatarsophalangeal joints, sclerodactyly, fingertip pitting or scarring, and bibasilar pulmonary fibrosis.

Clinical Manifestations

Skin
Patients are at risk for the development of rapidly progressive acral and trunk skin thickening and early visceral abnormalities. Skin and visceral changes tend to parallel each other in severity, but not always. Some patients have rapid progression for 2 to 3 years and then arrest of the disorder, allowing for some improvement of the disorder.

Raynaud Phenomenon
Raynaud phenomenon occurs in almost all patients. It usually occurs more than 2 years before skin changes. The vasospasm in the hands can be associated with reduced perfusion to the heart, lungs, kidneys, and gastrointestinal tract. If Raynaud phenomenon is not present but skin findings are suggestive of scleroderma, another disease such as eosinophilic fasciitis should be considered.

Articular
Nondeforming symmetric polyarthritis similar to rheumatoid arthritis may precede cutaneous manifestations by 12 months. Patients can have both articular erosions and nonarticular bony resorptive changes of ribs, mandible, radius, ulna, and distal phalangeal tufts which are unique to systemic sclerosis. Up to 60% of patients have "leathery" crepitation of the tendons of the wrist.

Pulmonary
A considerable decrease in diffusing capacity can be present with a normal chest radiograph. Diffuse interstitial fibrosis occurs in approximately 70% of patients and is the most common pulmonary abnormality. Patients who have active alveolitis demonstrated by 1) bronchopulmonary lavage, 2) high-resolution computed tomography showing ground-glass appearance without honeycombing, or 3) lung biopsy are most likely to respond to prednisone and cyclophosphamide therapy with improvement of pulmonary function. Pleuritis (with effusion) is very rare. Pulmonary hypertension is more common in patients with CREST variant.

* A considerable decrease in diffusing capacity can be present with a normal chest radiograph.
* Diffuse interstitial fibrosis occurs in approximately 70% of patients and is the most common pulmonary abnormality.
* Pleuritis is very rare.
* Pulmonary hypertension is more common in patients with CREST variant.

Cardiac
Cardiac abnormalities occur in up to 70% of patients. Conduction defects and supraventricular arrhythmias are most common. Pulmonary hypertension with cor pulmonale is the most serious problem.

* Cardiac abnormalities occur in up to 70% of patients. Pulmonary hypertension with cor pulmonale is a serious potential problem.

Gastrointestinal
Esophageal dysfunction is the most frequent gastrointestinal abnormality. It occurs in 90% of patients and often is asymptomatic. Lower esophageal sphincter incompetence with acid reflux may produce esophageal strictures or ulcers. Medications to reduce acid production are important. Reduced esophageal motility may respond to therapy with metoclopramide, cisapride, or erythromycin. Small bowel hypomotility may be associated with pseudo-obstruction, bowel dilatation, bacterial overgrowth, and malabsorption. Treatment with tetracycline may be helpful, but promotility agents are less effective. Colonic dysmotility also occurs, and wide-mouthed diverticuli may be found.

Renal
Renal involvement may result in fulminant hypertension, renal failure, and death if not treated aggressively. Proteinuria, newly diagnosed *mild* hypertension, microangiopathic hemolytic anemia, vascular changes on renal biopsy, and rapid progression of skin thickening may precede overt clinical findings of renal crisis. Renal involvement with hyperreninemia necessitates the use of angiotensin-converting enzyme inhibitors. Aggressive early antihypertensive therapy can extend life expectancy.

Laboratory Findings
Antinuclear antibodies are found in 95% or more of patients. Antitopoisomerase I antibody (anti-Scl-70) is found in approximately

25% of patients with scleroderma, and anticentromere antibody occurs in 10% to 20%.

Treatment

No remissive or curative therapy is available. Retrospective studies suggest that D-penicillamine (62.5 mg daily) may decrease skin thickness, prevent or delay internal organ involvement, and perhaps prolong life expectancy, but enthusiasm for this treatment has faded. Aggressive nutritional support, including hyperalimentation, may be required for extensive gastrointestinal disease.

* No remissive or curative therapy is available for systemic sclerosis.

CREST Syndrome

This is characterized by *c*alcinosis cutis, *R*aynaud phenomenon, *e*sophageal dysmotility, *s*clerodactyly, and *t*elangiectasias. Skin involvement progresses slowly and is limited to the extremities. Development of internal organ involvement occurs but is delayed. Lung involvement occurs in 70% of patients. Diffusing capacity may be low, and pulmonary hypertension can develop. The latter is more common in CREST than in diffuse scleroderma. Bosentan and sildenafil were recently approved for pulmonary hypertension in scleroderma and CREST syndrome. Onset of Raynaud phenomenon occurs less than 2 years before skin changes. Anticentromere antibody is found in 70% to 90% of patients and antiscleroderma-70 antibody in 10%. The incidence of primary biliary cirrhosis is increased.

* In CREST syndrome, 70% of patients have lung involvement.
* The diffusing capacity may be low, and pulmonary hypertension can develop.
* Anticentromere antibody is present in 70%-90% of patients.
* There is an increased incidence of primary biliary cirrhosis.

The clinical manifestations of limited and systemic scleroderma are listed in Table 24-34.

Scleroderma-like Syndromes

Disorders Associated With Occupation or Environment

This group includes polyvinyl chloride disease, organic solvents, jackhammer disease, silicosis, and toxic oil syndrome.

Eosinophilic Fasciitis

Clinical features of this disorder include tight bound-down skin of the extremities, characteristically sparing the hands and feet. Peau d'orange skin changes can develop. Onset after vigorous exercise is common. Raynaud phenomenon does not occur, and there is no visceral involvement. Flexion contractures and carpal tunnel syndrome can develop.

Laboratory findings are peripheral eosinophilia, increased sedimentation rate, and hypergammaglobulinemia. The diagnosis is based on the findings of inflammation and thickening of the fascia on deep fascial biopsy. Treatment is with prednisone (40 mg daily). The response is usually good. Associated conditions are aplastic anemia and thrombocytopenia (both antibody-mediated) as well as leukemia and myeloproliferative diseases.

* Eosinophilic fasciitis is characterized by tight bound-down skin of the extremities, usually sparing the hands and feet.
* Raynaud phenomenon does not occur.
* There is no visceral involvement.
* Laboratory findings include peripheral eosinophilia.
* Treatment with prednisone provides good response.

Metabolic Causes of Scleroderma-like Syndrome

This group includes porphyria, amyloidosis, carcinoid, and diabetes mellitus (flexion contractures of the tendons in the hands, cheiropathy, can develop).

Table 24-34 Clinical Findings in Limited and Diffuse Scleroderma

Clinical Finding	Cutaneous Disease	
	Limited	Diffuse
Raynaud phenomenon	Precedes other symptoms by years	Onset associated with other symptoms within 1 year
Nailfold capillaries	Dilated	Dilated with dropout
Skin changes	Distal to elbow	Proximal to elbow with involvement of trunk
Telangiectasia, digital ulcers, calcinosis	Frequent	Rare early, but frequent later in the course
Joint & tendon involvement	Uncommon	Frequent (tendon rubs)
Visceral disease	Pulmonary hypertension	Renal, intestinal, & cardiac disease; pulmonary interstitial fibrosis
Autoantibodies	Anticentromere (70%-90%)	Antitopoisomerase 1 (anti-Scl-70) (25%)
10-year survival	>70%	<70%

Other Causes

As a manifestation of *graft-versus-host disease*, skin induration develops in up to 30% of patients who receive a bone marrow transplant. *Drug-induced disorders* are caused by carbidopa, bleomycin, and bromocriptine. *Eosinophilic myalgia syndrome* is associated with ingestion of contaminated L-tryptophan. Eosinophilia, myositis, skin induration, fasciitis, and peripheral neuropathy develop. Skin changes are similar to those of eosinophilic fasciitis. There is a poor response to steroids. *Scleredema* frequently occurs after streptococcal upper respiratory tract infection in children. It is usually self-limiting. Swelling of the head and neck is common. In adults, diabetes mellitus often is associated. *Scleromyxedema* is associated with IgG monoclonal protein. Cocaine use and appetite suppressants also cause scleroderma-like illness. Nephrogenic fibrosing dermopathy, a recently described cutaneous fibrosing disorder, is caused by exposure to gadolinium-containing contrast agents during magnetic resonance imaging, especially in patients with renal insufficiency.

The Inflammatory Myopathies

Inflammatory myopathies can be classified into several categories, including polymyositis, dermatomyositis, myositis associated with malignancy, childhood-type, and overlap connective tissue disease. Polymyositis is an inflammatory myopathy characterized by proximal muscle weakness. Patients with dermatomyositis have an associated rash that includes a heliotrope hue of the eyelids, a rash on the metacarpophalangeal and proximal interphalangeal joints (Gottron papules), and photosensitivity dermatitis of the face. Most patients have an increased creatine kinase level, a characteristic electromyogram, and a characteristic muscle biopsy.

Electromyography is characteristic but not diagnostic of inflammatory myopathies. It shows decreased amplitude and increased spike frequency, it is polyphasic, and conduction speed is normal. Fibrillation potentials are not specific for inflammatory myopathies, but when present they indicate active disease. Loss of fibrillation potentials usually means the inflammatory myopathy is under control, but if the electromyographic result is still myopathic, it suggests an associated steroid myopathy caused by treatment. The muscle biopsy, which is mandatory in all patients with inflammatory myopathy, shows degeneration, necrosis, and regeneration of myofibrils with lymphocytic and monocytic infiltrate in a perivascular or interstitial distribution.

In patients older than 40 years, perhaps 10% to 20% of those with dermatomyositis and polymyositis have an associated malignancy. The antibody anti-Jo1 is associated with polymyositis and dermatomyositis in approximately 25% of cases. This antibody is associated with inflammatory arthritis, progressive interstitial lung disease, Raynaud phenomenon, and increased mortality primarily due to respiratory failure. The autoantibody anti-Mi-2 is associated with dermatomyositis in 2% to 20% of patients.

* Polymyositis is an inflammatory myopathy characterized by proximal muscle weakness.
* Dermatomyositis is an inflammatory myopathy plus a rash that includes heliotrope hue of eyelids.
* Electromyography is characteristic but not diagnostic of polymyositis.

* Perhaps 10%-20% of patients older than 40 years with dermatomyositis and polymyositis have associated malignancy.
* Anti-Jo1 is associated with polymyositis and dermatomyositis, pulmonary disease, and increased mortality.
* Typical clinical scenario: A 50-year-old patient presents with bilateral progressive proximal muscle weakness. There is a history of arthralgias. On physical examination there is a rash on the eyelids bilaterally. Laboratory testing shows positive anti-Jo1 antibody and increased creatine kinase level.

Treatment of polymyositis includes prednisone (60 mg daily), usually for 1 to 2 months, until the muscle enzyme values normalize. The dosage is slowly reduced thereafter, and the clinical course and creatine kinase values are monitored. In severe or steroid-resistant cases, either azathioprine (1-2 mg/kg daily) or methotrexate can be used.

Aspiration pneumonia can occur as a result of pharyngeal weakness. If so, a liquid diet, feeding tube, or feeding gastrostomy is needed until there is clinical improvement.

Inclusion Body Myositis

Inclusion body myositis needs to be considered in the differential diagnosis of inflammatory myopathies. This usually occurs in the older age group. The onset of weakness is more insidious, occurring over many years. The creatine kinase value often is only minimally to several times increased, and distal and proximal weakness occur. The electromyogram, besides showing a myopathic picture, also has an associated neuropathic picture. The diagnosis of inclusion body myositis is made from biopsy. Histopathologic findings are indistinguishable from those of polymyositis except for the presence of eosinophilic inclusions and rimmed vacuoles with basophilic enhancement. Inclusion body myositis responds poorly to prednisone and immunosuppressive therapy, and the course is one of slow, progressive weakness.

* Inclusion body myositis usually occurs in the older age group.
* Diagnosis is made from biopsy.
* It responds poorly to prednisone.

Drug-Induced Myopathies

Muscle Disease

Drugs may cause an inflammatory myopathy. The myopathy associated with colchicine mimics polymyositis, and patients have muscle weakness and an increased creatine kinase level. This often occurs in the setting of a patient with gout and renal insufficiency receiving long-term therapy with colchicine. Lipid-lowering drugs such as the statins, other drugs including zidovudine, D-penicillamine, and hydroxychloroquine, and addictive drugs such as heroin or cocaine have all been associated with myopathy. Corticosteroids cause a steroid myopathy with proximal muscle weakness and a normal creatine kinase value.

Infectious Arthritis

An infectious cause should be ruled out immediately in a patient with acute monarticular arthritis. Approximately 5% to 10% of patients with septic arthritis present with multiple joint involvement.

Bacterial Arthritis

Nongonococcal bacterial arthritis is caused by hematogenous spread of bacteria, direct inoculation (which is usually traumatic), or extension of soft tissue infection with osteomyelitis into the joint space. Large joints are more commonly affected. Patients who are elderly or immunosuppressed are predisposed to septic arthropathy, including patients with cancer, diabetes mellitus, chronic renal failure, liver disease, or sickle cell anemia. Patients with chronic inflammatory and degenerative arthritis are also at increased risk for septic arthritis, and the possibility of septic arthritis should be considered in patients with a preexisting polyarthritis who have a single joint flare that is out of proportion to the rest of their joint symptoms. In any patient with a septic joint, the possibility of infectious endocarditis, other septic joints, or a disk space infection should be considered.

Septic arthritis is a medical emergency. A thorough search for a source of infection is important. Joint aspiration is required. Gram staining of centrifuged synovial fluid and appropriate cultures should be performed. Typically, patients with nongonococcal septic arthritis have a leukocyte value of more than 50,000/mcL in the synovial fluid. Low glucose levels in synovial fluid and high levels of lactic acid are common but not specific for septic arthritis. Blood cultures should be performed when septic arthritis is considered. Radiographs of an involved joint may show an associated osteomyelitis or previous local trauma, but radiographic findings of infection usually lag considerably behind clinical symptoms.

Staphylococcus aureus is the most common pathogen in adult patients with nongonococcal bacterial arthritis. In sickle cell anemia, *Salmonella* is the organism commonly causing septic arthritis. *Pseudomonas* should be considered in the context of cat or dog bites, and an anaerobic infection should be considered in cases of human bites. Intravenous drug users may have bacteremia with unusual organisms, such as *Pseudomonas* or *Serratia*, and this may present with septic arthritis in unusual locations, such as the sternoclavicular or sacroiliac joints. The portal of entry may help predict the infecting organism; for example, gram-negative bacilli, such as *Escherichia coli* and *Klebsiella*, may cause septic arthritis in older patients with gastrointestinal or genitourinary infections or instrumentation.

Broad-spectrum antibiotics should be used until culture results are available. Daily aspiration and lavage of the affected joint should be performed until clinical improvement is obvious. Synovial fluid leukocytes and volume should decrease, or orthopedic arthroscopic or even open drainage should be considered. Such drainage usually is indicated in joints such as the hip, which are not readily accessible. The duration of treatment depends on the virulence of the organisms, but antibiotics usually are given intravenously for at least 2 weeks.

* Nongonococcal bacterial arthritis usually is caused by hematogenous spread of bacteria, direct inoculation (which is usually traumatic), or extension of soft tissue infection or osteomyelitis.
* Synovial fluid Gram stain and culture are essential.
* The portal of entry may predict the organism causing septic arthritis.
* Antibiotic therapy should be initiated even before culture results are available.
* If repeated aspiration and antibiotics do not lead to clinical

improvement as well as a decrease in synovial fluid volume and leukocytosis, then arthroscopic or open drainage and débridement may be necessary.

* Typical clinical scenario: A patient presents with acute swelling of the right knee, fever, and constitutional symptoms. The joint is tender and painful.

Gonococcal Arthritis

Disseminated gonococcal infection develops in approximately 0.2% of patients with gonorrhea. The male to female ratio is 3:1. This is the most common form of septic arthritis in younger, sexually active persons who may be asymptomatic carriers of gonococci. When gonococcal infection is suspected, specimens from the pharynx, joints, rectum, blood, and genitourinary tract should be cultured. Females present with gonococcal arthritis commonly during pregnancy or within 1 week after onset of menses, possibly related to the pH of vaginal secretions. The most common form of gonococcal arthritis is the disseminated gonococcal arthritis syndrome with fever, dermatitis, and an inflammatory tenosynovitis. Approximately 50% of these patients present with an inflammatory arthritis, commonly of the knee, wrist, or ankle. Tenosynovitis is more common than large joint effusions. Rash, sometimes with pustules or hemorrhagic vesicles, is common. The second form of gonococcal arthritis commonly begins as a migratory polyarthralgia, which subsequently localizes to 1 or more joints.

Synovial fluid cultures are positive in only 30% of patients with known disseminated gonococcal infection. Culture of the skin lesion is positive for gonococcus in 40% to 60% of patients with disseminated gonococcal infection. The leukocyte count in the joint fluid may be lower than in the other types of septic arthritis. Joint effusions in patients with disseminated gonococcal infection may be related to a *reactive* postinfectious response rather than to bacterial invasion. Rare patients who have recurrent disseminated gonococcal infection may have an associated terminal complement component deficiency (C5-C9).

Most patients with disseminated gonococcal arthritis are treated as outpatients. Current treatment recommendations suggest a later third-generation cephalosporin, such as ceftriaxone, 1.0 g daily. Treatment involves a minimal 7-day course. Treatment should include an antichlamydial antibiotic.

* Gonococcal arthritis develops in 0.2% of patients with gonorrhea.
* In the disseminated gonococcal arthritis syndrome, fever, dermatitis, and tenosynovitis are common.
* In the nonbacteremic form of gonococcal arthritis, migratory polyarthralgias are followed by inflammation localizing to 1 or more joints.
* Synovial fluid cultures are positive in 30% of patients with known disseminated gonococcal infection.
* Joint fluid leukocyte counts may be lower than in other types of septic arthritis.
* Joint effusions may be related to a reactive or postinfectious arthritis.
* Treatment recommendations are the use of a later third-generation cephalosporin (eg, ceftriaxone).
* Treatment should include an antichlamydial antibiotic.

Mycobacterial and Fungal Joint Infections

These types of organisms usually cause chronic bone and joint infections. Months are required for radiographic changes to be obvious. A synovial biopsy and culture may be required to document these infections. Tuberculous arthritis is often otherwise asymptomatic and usually is caused by direct extension from adjacent bony infection. Atypical mycobacterial infection may cause an inflammatory arthritis and tenosynovitis frequently involving the hand and wrist. Surgical excision and prolonged treatment with multiple drug regimens are often required. Sporotrichosis and blastomycosis are the fungi most likely to have osteoarticular manifestations.

- Tuberculous arthritis is often otherwise asymptomatic and is caused by direct extension from adjacent bony infection.
- Atypical mycobacterial infection may cause an inflammatory arthritis and tenosynovitis most commonly affecting the hand and wrist.
- Sporotrichosis and blastomycosis are the fungi most likely to have osteoarticular manifestations.

Spinal Septic Arthritis

This condition should be suspected in patients with acute or chronic, unrelenting back pain associated with fever and marked local tenderness. The thoracolumbar region is most commonly affected. An antecedent infection or procedure predisposing to bacteremia may help suggest this diagnosis. Imaging studies usually have evidence for infection crossing the disk space. In tuberculous spinal septic arthritis (Pott disease), the site of involvement is most commonly T10-L2, and there is usually an associated paraspinal abscess.

Intravertebral disk infection is often a difficult diagnosis to establish because pain patterns may be unusual and localizing signs may be absent. Bone scanning may be helpful, but magnetic resonance imaging may be very helpful, particularly because of the ability to show extension of infection into surrounding tissues.

Infected Joint Prostheses

Infection in joint prostheses occurs in 1% to 5% of all joint replacements. Symptoms and signs of infection may be difficult to detect during the postoperative period. Fever may not be present, and laboratory findings are often unhelpful, although the erythrocyte sedimentation rate may be increased. There may or may not be evidence of loosening of the cement holding the new joint in place, and radiographs may reveal lytic changes around the prosthesis. A negative bone scan is reassuring. Aspiration of fluid from the prosthetic joint is necessary to confirm infection. Prosthetic joint infection usually is caused by gram-positive organisms, particularly *Staphylococcus aureus* and *Staphylococcus epidermidis*, in the first 6 months after the replacement operation and by gram-negative and fungal organisms after 6 months. In long-standing prosthetic joints, return of pain and evidence of prosthetic loosening may be the only signs and symptoms. Patients with prosthetic joints do not require antibiotic prophylaxis before invasive dental, gastrointestinal, or genitourinary procedures according to the recent guidelines, unless obvious immunosuppression is present.

- Prosthetic joint infection usually is caused by a gram-positive organism within the first 6 months after joint replacement.

- Prosthetic joint infections usually are caused by gram-negative or fungal organisms beyond the initial 6 months after joint replacement.

Lyme Disease

Lyme disease is a tick-borne spirochetal illness with acute and chronic manifestations primarily affecting the skin, heart, joints, and nervous system. Diagnosis is important because treatment with appropriate antibiotics at an early stage of disease can prevent chronic sequelae. Even some chronic symptoms are treatable. Endemic areas in the United States include Connecticut, Delaware, Maryland, Massachusetts, New Jersey, New York, Pennsylvania, Rhode Island, Minnesota, Wisconsin, California, Nevada, Oregon, and Utah.

- Lyme disease is a tick-borne spirochetal illness.
- Acute and chronic manifestations affect skin, heart, joints, and nervous system.

The Tick

Ticks that transmit Lyme disease include *Ixodes dammini* in the northeastern and midwestern United States and *Ixodes pacificus* in the western United States. *Amblyomma americanum* ("lone star" tick) is a possible vector in the eastern, southern, and western United States. *Ixodes scapularis* is the common deer tick. It has a wide distribution. Humans are accidental hosts.

The Spirochete

Borrelia burgdorferi was an unknown organism until isolated initially from ticks by Burgdorfer in 1983. It is similar to an organism causing relapsing fever. It apparently exists only in the digestive tract of tick vectors.

Clinical Stages

Signs and symptoms occur in stages that may overlap. Later stages may occur without evidence of previous disease.

Stage I

About 50% to 67% of patients experience erythema chronicum migrans. Flu-like symptoms, including fever, headache, malaise, and adenopathy, can occur. They usually occur several days to a month after the tick bite.

- In stage I Lyme disease, 50%-67% of patients experience erythema chronicum migrans.

Stage II

Symptoms begin weeks to months after the initial symptoms in stage I. Disseminated infection develops and can include symptoms of the skin, musculoskeletal system, heart, and nervous system. In approximately 15% of untreated patients, neurologic symptoms develop, including Bell palsy, meningoencephalitis, and sensory and motor radiculoneuritis. Approximately 5% of untreated patients have cardiac abnormalities, including heart block. About 30% to

50% of untreated patients have arthritis. This usually affects large joints, primarily the knees, and joint fluid analysis shows a leukocytosis similar to that in rheumatoid arthritis. Baker cysts may form early and are prone to rupture in patients who have arthritis of the knees.

- In stage II Lyme disease, symptoms begin weeks to months after initial symptoms of stage I.
- Disseminated infection develops.
- 15% of untreated patients have neurologic symptoms.
- 5% of untreated patients have cardiac abnormalities.
- 0%-50% of untreated patients have arthritis.

Stage III

This usually occurs several years after the initial onset of illness. Episodes of arthritis can develop and become chronic. Histologically, the synovium resembles that in rheumatoid arthritis, although a unique feature of Lyme arthritis is the finding of an obliterative endarteritis. Spirochetes occasionally are seen in and around the blood vessels. Patients in whom chronic joint disease develops have increased frequency of HLA-DR4, often in combination with HLA-DR2. Patients with chronic arthritis have a poor response to antibiotics.

- Stage III Lyme disease occurs several years after initial onset of illness.
- Episodes of arthritis can be chronic.
- Synovium resembles that in rheumatoid arthritis.
- A unique feature of Lyme arthritis is obliterative endarteritis in the synovium.
- Patients with chronic joint disease have increased frequency of HLA-DR4, often in combination with HLA-DR2.

Diagnosis

Culturing the organism is difficult and of low yield. Antibody to spirochete can be measured by several techniques. The enzyme-linked immunosorbent assay (ELISA) is most commonly performed, but there is a substantial frequency of false-positive results. Patients with other autoimmune disease can have false-positive results. Also, such results may occur in syphilis, relapsing fever, and Rocky Mountain spotted fever. Up to 25% of patients with lupus and rheumatoid arthritis have false-positive results of Lyme test by ELISA. It is important to remember that test results remain negative for up to 4 to 6 weeks after infection. Also, if patients are treated early with tetracycline or another antibiotic, the results might never be positive, although symptoms of chronic Lyme disease can result. The Western blot assay for Lyme disease is now being used as a confirmatory test if the ELISA test result is positive.

- In Lyme disease, culturing the organism is difficult and of low yield.
- The ELISA assay is commonly performed but there is a substantial frequency of false-positive results.
- False-positive ELISA results may occur in syphilis, relapsing fever, and Rocky Mountain spotted fever.
- Up to 25% of patients with lupus and rheumatoid arthritis have false-positive results of Lyme test by ELISA.

- Patients treated early with tetracycline or other antibiotics may never have positive results.

Treatment

For early treatment of Lyme disease, either oral tetracycline or doxycycline, or amoxicillin in children, for 14 to 21 days can prevent later complications. The optimal treatment for patients with neurologic, cardiac, and arthritic symptoms of Lyme disease includes ceftriaxone, 2 g intravenously daily for 28 days. Patients with Lyme disease can experience worsening of symptoms analogous to the Jarisch-Herxheimer reaction and can be treated with acetaminophen.

- Early treatment of Lyme disease is either oral tetracycline or doxycycline (amoxicillin in children) for 14-21 days.
- Treatment for neurologic, cardiac, and arthritic symptoms of Lyme disease includes ceftriaxone for 28 days.

Rheumatic Fever and Poststreptococcal Reactive Arthritis

Arthritis affects two-thirds of all patients with rheumatic fever. One-third of patients with acute rheumatic fever have no obvious antecedent pharyngitis. In adults, arthritis may be the only clinical feature of acute rheumatic fever and often occurs early. The arthritis usually involves the large joints, particularly the knees, ankles, elbows, and wrists. The arthritis may be migratory, with each joint remaining inflamed for approximately 1 week. The arthritis of rheumatic fever is nonerosive; however, repeated attacks may result in a Jaccoud deformity, in which the metacarpophalangeal joints are in ulnar deviation as a result of tendon laxity rather than bony damage.

Patients with joint symptoms without carditis may be treated with high-dose salicylates (3-6 g daily). Corticosteroids may be required if patients do not respond to salicylates. Joint symptoms may rebound when anti-inflammatory therapy is discontinued.

- The arthritis in rheumatic fever may be migratory and usually involves the large joints, particularly the knees, ankles, elbows, and wrists.
- Repeated attacks of rheumatic fever may result in Jaccoud deformity.
- The mainstay treatment for the arthritis of rheumatic fever is high-dose salicylates (3-6 g daily).

Viral Arthritis

Viruses associated with arthralgia and arthritis include human immunodeficiency virus (HIV), hepatitis B, rubella, parvovirus, and, less commonly, mumps, adenovirus, herpesvirus, and enterovirus. Most viral-related arthritides have joint symptoms with a semiacute onset, but fortunately they are usually of brief duration. The arthritis is nondestructive.

Although *parvovirus* infection in children is usually mild, in adults associated arthralgias and arthritis are common, and the distribution of involved joints is symmetric and may mimic rheumatoid arthritis. Joint symptoms in adults are usually self-limited, but chronic disease develops in some patients. The diagnosis of parvovirus infection is made by demonstrating the presence of anti-B19 IgM antibodies, but these may be increased in patients for only 2 months after acute infection. Because the joint symptoms usually occur approximately 1 to 3 weeks after the initial infection, the antibodies are usually present at the time of onset of rash or joint symptoms. Treatment is usually conservative and includes anti-inflammatory medications, but in more chronic infections more aggressive treatment such as low-dose corticosteroids may be warranted. Parvovirus infection also has been associated rarely with significant hematologic abnormalities.

Hepatitis B virus infection has been associated with an immune complex-mediated arthritis, which can be dramatic. The arthritis is usually limited to the pre-icteric prodrome, although patients with chronic types of hepatitis may have recurrent arthralgias or arthritis. Polyarteritis nodosa has been associated with chronic hepatitis. *Hepatitis B* and more commonly *hepatitis C* are associated with mixed cryoglobulinemia. Hepatitis C virus infections can mimic autoimmune diseases, including rheumatoid arthritis, Sjögren syndrome, and SLE, both clinically and serologically. Numerous autoantibodies may be detected in hepatitis C virus infection, including a positive rheumatoid factor, antinuclear antibody, anti-SSA and -SSB, and antiphospholipid antibodies. *Rubella* virus infection is frequently associated with joint complaints in young adults. In a few patients, the symptoms have persisted for months to years. Joint symptoms may occur just before or after the appearance of the characteristic rash.

* Parvovirus infection in adults may cause a symmetric polyarthritis mimicking rheumatoid arthritis.
* Parvovirus infection can be documented by demonstrating the presence of anti-B19 IgM antibodies.
* Hepatitis B virus infection has been associated with an arthritis limited to the pre-icteric prodrome.
* Hepatitis B and C viremia have been associated with cryoglobulinemia and vasculitis.
* Rubella virus infection frequently is associated with joint complaints in young adults.

Rheumatologic Manifestations of HIV Infection (Table 24-35)

Musculoskeletal complaints can be among the first manifestations of HIV infection. Articular manifestations can be extremely debilitating. Epidemiologic studies have not concluded whether HIV infection predisposes to arthritis or whether other viral or new mechanisms associated with HIV infection have a role in the pathogenesis of arthritis.

Reactive Arthritis and Undifferentiated Spondyloarthropathy
Signs and symptoms of reactive arthritis, psoriatic arthritis, or a nonspecific enthesopathy and related destructive arthritis may occur before or simultaneously with the onset of HIV infection. The prevalence of these conditions in HIV-infected patients varies from 0.5% to 10% in reports. These HIV-associated spondyloarthropathies have a predisposition for patients who are HLA-B27–positive and frequently are associated with severe enthesopathy and dactylitis. Progressive axial involvement is less common in HIV-associated

arthritides. The foot and ankle are common sites of enthesopathy in reactive arthritis, which may be severe. Symptoms may be episodic. Most HIV-infected patients with reactive arthritis have skin and mucocutaneous manifestations, including urethritis, keratoderma blennorrhagicum, circinate balanitis, or painless oral ulcers, but conjunctivitis is unusual. In approximately one-third of patients, the onset of HIV-associated reactive arthritis has been linked to a documented infection with specific enteric organisms known to precipitate reactive arthritis. Genitourinary tract infection with *Ureaplasma* or *Chlamydia* is less common.

* Enthesopathy and dactylitis may be severe in HIV-infected patients.
* Mucocutaneous features are common, but conjunctivitis is unusual.

Lupus-Like Illnesses in HIV Infection
Some of the features of systemic lupus erythematosus are similar to those in HIV infection. Fever, lymphadenopathy, mucous membrane lesions, rashes, arthritis, and hematologic abnormalities are common to both lupus and HIV infection. HIV infection also may be associated with polyclonal B-cell activation resulting in autoantibody production, including antinuclear and antiphospholipid antibodies. HIV infection should be considered in the differential diagnosis of systemic lupus erythematosus in any patient who is at risk for HIV. Antinuclear antibodies in high titer have not been found in HIV infection, and antibodies to double-stranded DNA are absent.

* Although some features of HIV infection may resemble lupus, antinuclear antibodies are present in low titer only, and antibodies to double-stranded DNA are absent.

HIV-Associated Vasculitis
Different types of vasculitic syndromes have been described in association with HIV infection. Primary angiitis of the central nervous system, angiocentric lymphoproliferative lesions related to lymphomatoid granulomatosis, and polyarteritis nodosa have been

Table 24-35 Rheumatologic Manifestations of Human Immunodeficiency Virus (HIV)

Arthralgia
Painful articular syndrome
HIV arthropathy
Reactive arthritis
Psoriatic arthritis
Undifferentiated spondyloarthropathy
Myositis
Vasculitis
Raynaud phenomenon
Sjögren-like syndrome (diffuse infiltrative lymphocytosis syndrome)
Septic arthritis
Fibromyalgia
Serologic abnormalities

reported. It has not been established whether the association of vasculitis and HIV infection is coincidental, related to comorbidities such as drugs or other infections, or represents a direct pathogenetic role for HIV. All patients with primary angiitis of the central nervous system and lymphoproliferative angiocentric vasculopathies should be tested for HIV. Any person with known HIV infection who presents with new mononeuritis should be evaluated for vasculitis.

Other HIV-Associated Rheumatic Syndromes

The diffuse, infiltrative lymphocytosis syndrome is manifested by xerostomia, xerophthalmia, and salivary gland swelling mimicking Sjögren syndrome. The glands are infiltrated with CD8 lymphocytes. In contrast to Sjögren syndrome, HIV-positive patients usually do not have antibodies to SS-A or SS-B and are usually rheumatoid factor-negative.

There is an inflammatory articular syndrome associated with HIV infection which is distinct from any resemblance to spondyloarthropathy.

Usually this is an oligoarthritis affecting joints of the lower extremities and is short-lived.

There is an acquired immunodeficiency syndrome-associated myopathy that may be viral. There is also a myopathy due to zidovudine therapy. Fibromyalgia also has been reported in up to 25% of HIV-infected patients.

Other Types of Infectious Arthritis

Whipple disease is a rare cause of arthropathy and usually is associated with constitutional symptoms, fever, neurologic symptoms, malabsorption, lymphadenopathy, and hyperpigmentation. There may be a slow, progressive dementia. The arthritic symptoms may precede the gastrointestinal manifestations. The infectious agent is *Tropheryma whippelii*. Polymerase chain reaction on small bowel or synovial biopsy or synovial fluid may be necessary to establish the diagnosis. Treatment is usually with doxycycline or trimethoprim-sulfamethoxazole, often required for a year.

Rheumatology Pharmacy Review
Christopher M. Wittich, PharmD, MD, Jennifer D. Lynch, PharmD

Drug	Toxic/Adverse Effects	Drug Interactions	Comments
Nonsteroidal anti-inflammatory drugs (NSAIDs), by chemical group			

Acetic acids
  Diclofenac potassium
  Diclofenac sodium
  Etodolac
  Indomethacin
  Ketorolac
  Sulindac
Propionic acids
  Flurbiprofen
  Ibuprofen
  Ketoprofen
  Naproxen
  Naproxen sodium
Salicylates
  Aspirin
  Diflunisal
  Salicylate
Fenamates
  Mefanamic acid
Enolic acids
  Meloxicam
  Piroxicam
	Central nervous system: dizziness, headache, drowsiness
	Gastrointestinal: constipation, dyspepsia, nausea, abdominal pain, gastrointestinal bleeding
	Hematologic: irreversible platelet inhibition (salicylates)
	Renal: decreased renal perfusion & glomerular filtration
		ACE inhibitors: antihypertensive effects may be reduced
		Antacids: antacids may decrease effectiveness of enteric coating
		Anticoagulants: coadministration may increase bleeding risk
		Cyclosporine: coadministration may increase nephrotoxicity
		Digoxin: serum digoxin levels may increase
		Diuretics: decreased effects
		Lithium: serum lithium levels may increase
		Methotrexate: methotrexate clearance may be reduced
		Phenytoin: serum phenytoin levels may increase
			If an NSAID from 1 chemical group is not effective, 1 from another chemical group may be more effective
			Use with caution in patients with asthma

COX-2 inhibitor Celecoxib			Use with caution in patients with known cardiovascular disease
Glucocorticosteroids			
Betamethasone Dexamethasone Methylprednisolone Prednisone	Cardiovascular: fluid retention, hypertension Central nervous system: euphoria, depression, insomnia, mania, hallucinations, anxiety, pseudotumor cerebri Dermatologic: acneiform eruptions, bruising, atrophy, hirsutism, impaired wound healing, striae, telangiectasia Endocrine: hypothalamic-pituitary-adrenal axis suppression, central obesity, moon facies, buffalo hump, growth suppression, hyperglycemia	Cyclosporine: plasma clearance may be decreased by certain glucocorticoids NSAIDs: concomitant use may cause gastrointestinal ulcerations or perforation Diuretics: concomitant use may cause increased potassium loss Anticholinesterase agents: concomitant use may cause weakness in patients with myasthenia gravis Vaccines: glucocorticoids may decrease response to vaccines Anticoagulants: concomitant use can increase or decrease anticoagulant effects	

Rheumatology Pharmacy Review (continued)

Drug	Toxic/Adverse Effects	Drug Interactions	Comments
Glucocorticosteroids (continued)			
	Gastrointestinal: candidiasis, perforations, ulcers Hematologic: increased absolute granulocyte count, decreased lymphocyte & monocyte counts Musculoskeletal: myopathy, osteoporosis Ocular: posterior subcapsular cataracts, increased intraocular pressure		
Disease-modifying antirheumatic drugs (DMARDs)			
Hydroxychloroquine	Ocular: macular damage Dermatologic: accumulation in melanin-rich tissues, pruritus	Decreased digoxin levels Gold compounds lead to an increase in dermatologic adverse effects	Initial ophthalmologic exam, then every 6 to 12 mo Periodic CBC Hemolysis possible in G-6-PD–deficient patients
Gold salts	Dermatologic: rash, stomatitis, alopecia Hematologic: blood dyscrasias Gastrointestinal: diarrhea, worse with oral gold Renal: hematuria, proteinuria Special senses: metallic taste, may be a precursor to other reactions	Increased phenytoin levels Use with immunosuppressants, penicillamine, or antimalarials increases risk of blood dyscrasias	Before initiation of therapy: CBC, UA, renal & liver function Before each injection: CBC & UA
D-Penicillamine	Dermatologic: stomatitis, rashes Hematologic: possible induction of autoimmune diseases, myelosuppression Renal: glomerulonephritis, proteinuria Special senses: hypogeusia	Antacids & iron decrease penicillamine absorption Decreased digoxin concentrations Increased gold concentrations	UA and CBC every wk for 1 mo, then monthly LFT every 6 mo
Sulfasalazine	Genitourinary: crystalluria, urine discoloration Gastrointestinal: nausea, vomiting, diarrhea, anorexia Dermatologic: hypersensitivity	Increased effect of warfarin Antibiotics & iron decrease absorption Decreased folic acid absorption Decreased digoxin absorption	CBC w/diff at initiation CBC w/diff & LFT should be done every 2 wk for 3 mo, then every mo for 3 mo, then every 3 mo Can lead to folic acid deficiencies
Methotrexate	Hepatotoxicity: hepatic fibrosis & cirrhosis Hematologic: myelosuppression Gastrointestinal: mucositis, stomatitis Pulmonary: pneumonitis	NSAIDs, salicylates, cisplatin, cyclosporine, & penicillamine delay methotrexate excretion, leading to toxicities	Initial CBC, LFT, & renal function tests CBC monthly LFT & renal function tests every 1 to 2 mo

Rheumatology Pharmacy Review (continued)

Drug	Toxic/Adverse Effects	Drug Interactions	Comments
Disease-modifying antirheumatic drugs (DMARDs) (continued)			
Leflunomide	Liver: hepatotoxicity Cardiovascular: hypertension Dermatologic: alopecia, rash Pregnancy: teratogen with a long half-life & dangerous blood levels for up to 2 years after therapy	Cytochrome P450 inhibitor Increased methotrexate concentrations Rifampin increases leflunomide Cholestyramine decreases leflunomide	Baseline LFTs followed by monthly LFTs until the enzyme levels are stable
Azathioprine	Hematologic: myelosuppression Liver: hepatotoxicity Gastrointestinal: nausea, vomiting, diarrhea	Allopurinol increases concentration of azathioprine; reduce the dose of azathioprine by 70% ACE inhibitors & methotrexate increase azathioprine Decreased anticoagulant concentrations	CBC every wk for 1 mo, then every 2 wk for 2 mo, then monthly Periodic LFTs
Cyclophosphamide	Genitourinary: cystitis Hematologic: leukopenia (nadir at 8-15 days) Dermatologic: alopecia Gastrointestinal: nausea, vomiting Cardiovascular: cardiotoxicity	Phenytoin & barbiturates induce liver enzymes, which increase conversion to the active metabolite, leading to cyclophosphamide toxicities Allopurinol & thiazide diuretics can increase cyclophosphamide concentrations Doxorubicin can increase cardiotoxic potential Increased anticoagulant effects Decreased digoxin effects	Initial UA & CBC, then every wk for 1 mo, then every 2-4 wk The risk for hemorrhagic cystitis from high-dose cyclophosphamide may be reduced by the coadministration of mesna
Cyclosporine	Renal: nephrotoxicity Liver: hepatotoxicity Cardiovascular: hypertension	Carbamazepine, phenytoin, phenobarbital, rifamycin decrease effect Increased toxicities are azoles, macrolides, grapefruit juice, protease inhibitors, immunosuppressants, calcium channel blockers, & oral contraceptives NSAIDs & aminoglycosides increase nephrotoxic potential	Initial monitoring of blood pressure & serum creatinine; then monitor every 2 wk for 3 mo, then monthly

Rheumatology Pharmacy Review (continued)

Drug	Toxic/Adverse Effects	Drug Interactions	Comments
Immunologic agents			
Etanercept Infliximab Adalimumab	Cardiovascular: hypertension, exacerbation of congestive heart failure Dermatologic: injection site reaction, rash Immunologic: antibody development, antinuclear antibody development Neurologic: headache Hematologic: aplastic anemia, erythrocytosis, leukopenia, pancytopenia ID: tuberculosis, invasive fungal infections, opportunistic infections	Coadministration with abatacept or anakinra increases risk for infection Do not give with live vaccines	Mechanism of action: TNF-α inhibitor Monitor: signs of worsening heart failure, CBC periodically during long-term therapy Prior to initiation: tuberculin skin test, latent tuberculosis should be treated before initiating therapy
Anakinra	Dermatologic: injection site reactions ID: serious infection Hematologic: blood dyscrasias, formation of antibodies	Do not give with live virus vaccines Coadministration with adalimumab, etanercept, infliximab increases risk for serious infections	Mechanism of action: interleukin-1 receptor antagonist Monitor: neutrophil count before initiation of therapy, monthly for the first 3 mo, & then at 6, 9, & 12 mo
Abatacept	Gastrointestinal: nausea Neurologic: headache Respiratory: acute exacerbation of COPD, nasopharyngitis, upper respiratory infection ID: Urinary tract infection, other infections Other: malignancy	Adalimumab, anakinra, etanercept, infliximab: increased risk for infection Live virus vaccines: concurrent use within 3 mo may result in reduced efficacy of vaccine	Mechanism of action: cytotoxic T-lymphocyte antigen immunoglobulin that downregulates T-cell activation Monitor: C-reactive protein, ESR, infections, respiratory status, signs & symptoms of malignancy Before initiation: tuberculin skin test, latent tuberculosis should be treated before initiating therapy

Rheumatology Pharmacy Review (continued)

Drug	Toxic/Adverse Effects	Drug Interactions	Comments
Rituximab	Dermatologic: severe mucocutaneous reactions, pruritus Cardiovascular: arrhythmias, infusion hypotension ID: Serious infection Neurologic: dizziness, headache Hematologic: cytopenias Gastrointestinal: nausea, vomiting	Do not administer with live vaccines Coadministration with DMARDs other than methotrexate can increase risk of serious infection	Mechanism of action: monoclonal antibody that binds to CD20 on B lymphocytes Warning: fatal infusion reactions are reported Used in combination with methotrexate after TNF-α agent failure Monitor: CBC w/diff, platelets, vital signs during infusion

Abbreviations: ACE, angiotensin-converting enzyme; CBC, complete blood count; COPD, chronic obstructive pulmonary disease; COX, cyclooxygenase; DMARD, disease-modifying agent of rheumatic disease; ESR, erythrocyte sedimentation rate; exam, examination; G-6-PD, glucose-6-phosphate dehydrogenase; ID, infectious disease; LFT, liver function tests; PVC, polyvinyl chloride; TNF-α, tumor necrosis factor-α; UA, urinalysis; w/diff, with differential.

Questions

Multiple Choice (choose the best answer)

1. A 76-year-old white woman presents to you because of complaints of new-onset headache. She thinks it has been present for about 2 months. It occurs daily. She also has had some fatigue and has lost about 5 pounds during the past month. On further questioning, she complains of morning stiffness lasting about 1 hour. Physical examination is essentially within normal limits for her age. Results of initial laboratory studies show a mild normochromic anemia and an increased erythrocyte sedimentation rate (55 mm in 1 hour). Which of the following would be the next most appropriate step?

   a. Temporal artery biopsy
   b. Bone marrow biopsy
   c. Initiation of prednisone therapy 15 mg/day orally
   d. Electromyography
   e. Upper aortic arch angiography

2. A 29-year-old white woman presents to your office because she aches all over. She tells you that this condition has been present for several years but has gotten worse during the past 6 months. She has problems getting to sleep and does not feel rested when she wakes up. She denies depression. On examination, her muscle strength is normal and there is no synovitis. She has multiple tender points. Her laboratory studies include normal complete blood count, chemistry panel, and erythrocyte sedimentation rate, and a positive antinuclear antibody titer of 1.1. Of the following, which would be the most appropriate next step?

   a. Sensitive thyroid-stimulating hormone test
   b. Extractable nuclear antigen panel
   c. A trial of prednisone 5 mg orally 3 times daily
   d. A trial of pregabalin initially at 50 mg orally 3 times daily
   e. A trial of duloxetine initially at 20 mg orally daily

3. A 22-year-old woman presents to your office with a 2-week history of abdominal pain, rash on the legs, and joint pain. She had an upper respiratory tract infection several weeks earlier. On examination, she has palpable purpura on her legs and synovitis of the ankles and knees. She has normal posterior tibial and dorsalis pedis pulses. Her laboratory study results show a mild normochromic anemia (hemoglobin, 11.5 mg/dL), an increased erythrocyte sedimentation rate of 33 mm in 1 hour, normal chemistry values including creatinine, and trace proteinuria and 4 to 10 red blood cells per high-power field on urinalysis. The antinuclear antibody titer is positive at 1.1, but double-stranded DNA is negative. Which of the following tests would help confirm the diagnosis?

   a. Biopsy of the kidney
   b. Biopsy of the skin
   c. Temporal artery biopsy
   d. Aspiration of the knee effusion
   e. Arteriography of the lower extremities

4. A 69-year-old woman presents to your office with complaints of shoulder and hip pain that has come on during the past 8 weeks. She reports stiffness lasting 1.5 hours in the morning. She denies headache, jaw claudication, or visual loss. She is having trouble falling asleep, which she thinks is from the pain. She has also noted increased fatigue. On examination, she is normotensive and afebrile and weighs 62 kg (body mass index of 23 kg/m^2). There is some tenderness over both glenohumeral joints bilaterally but she has normal strength, allowing for pain. Laboratory study results show a mild normochronic anemia (hemoglobin, 10.6 mg/dL) and an increased erythrocyte sedimentation rate of 59 mm in 1 hour. What is the next most appropriate step in her care?

   a. Initiate therapy with prednisone 60 mg/day.
   b. Obtain a temporal artery biopsy.
   c. Determine the creatine phosphokinase level.
   d. Initiate therapy with prednisone 5 mg 3 times daily.
   e. Perform overnight oximetry.

5. A 51-year-old man comes to the emergency department for evaluation of abdominal pain. He describes the pain as worse after he eats and better when his stomach is empty. He has lost about 30 pounds during the past 3 months since the pain started. He has also noted some joint pains in the hands and feet. On examination his abdomen is diffusely tender to deep palpation. Bowel sounds are present. He has a purpuric rash on the lower extremities bilaterally and mild synovitis of several of the metacarpophalangeal and proximal interphalangeal joints of both hands. He is hypertensive (blood pressure, 180/100 mm Hg). Laboratory study results include a normochromic anemia (hemoglobin, 10.9 g/dL), an increased erythrocyte sedimentation rate (94 mm in 1 hour), and increased C-reactive protein level (1.7 mg/ dL). Urinalysis shows only trace protein. Which of the following tests would be most helpful in establishing a diagnosis?

   a. Temporal artery biopsy
   b. Renal biopsy
   c. Antineutrophil cytoplasmic antibody (ANCA) tests
   d. Otolaryngologic examination
   e. Abdominal angiography

6. A 39-year-old woman presents to your office with arthralgias and myalgias. She has had Raynaud symptoms in the hands bilaterally. She denies use of alcohol or intravenous drugs. She has a 20 pack-year history of smoking but stopped smoking last year. She denies a history of asthma or respiratory complaints. On examination she has good peripheral pulses in all 4 extremities. You do not detect fibromyalgia tender points or active synovitis. Several tattoos are noted on the trunk. Her lower extremities have a livedo-type rash. Laboratory study

results include a normal complete blood count including leukocyte differential. The erythrocyte sedimentation rate is increased at 39 mm in 1 hour. Chemistry values are normal except for an increased aspartate aminotransferase value of 44 U/L (normal, 12-30). ANCA tests are negative. Of the following, which is the most likely diagnosis?

a. Churg-Strauss vasculitis
b. Buerger disease
c. Wegener granulomatosis
d. Cryoglobulinemia
e. Fibromyalgia

7. A 47-year-old man comes to your office because he has been short of breath for the past several weeks and has had several episodes of hemoptysis. He has also had a 30-pound weight loss during the past 3 months and has felt fatigued. He is a nonsmoker and does not have a history of asthma. On examination he is afebrile. There are diffuse crackles on auscultation of the lungs but no wheezing. Laboratory study results include a normochromic anemia, normal leukocyte count with normal differential, increased erythrocyte sedimentation rate of 67 mm in 1 hour, and normal chemistry values except for an increased creatine value of 1.7 mg/dL. Chest radiography shows diffuse pulmonary infiltrates consistent with alveolar hemorrhage. On urinalysis, trace proteinuria and red blood cell casts are found. He has a positive perinuclear-ANCA and positive myeloperoxidase antibodies. What is the most likely diagnosis?

a. Wegener granulomatosis
b. Giant cell arteritis
c. Churg-Strauss vasculitis
d. Classic polyarteritis
e. Microscopic polyarteritis

8. A 45-year-old white man has a 5-year history of gout being treated with allopurinol 300 mg daily. Three days after laparoscopic cholecystectomy, he noticed the onset of pain and swelling in his right ankle, and now the entire foot is infected. He was taking ibuprofen 2 to 4 tablets daily and had minimal relief. The uric acid level is 6.1 mg/dL (normal, <8 mg/dL). He has no fever and is otherwise well. On radiography, soft tissue swelling is seen but findings are otherwise normal. He has no other joint involvement. Which of the following is the most likely diagnosis?

a. Gouty arthritis
b. Pseudogout
c. Rheumatoid arthritis
d. Stress fracture
e. Septic arthritis

9. Which of the following types of arthritis is associated with hemochromatosis?

a. Gout
b. Pseudogout
c. Oxalate arthritis
d. Basic calcium phosphate disease (calcium hydroxyapatite)
e. Avascular necrosis

10. A 32-year-old man has had ankylosing spondylitis for 3 years. He has been taking naproxen 500 mg twice daily with some benefit, but he continues to have low back pain with morning stiffness, and radiographs have shown progression of disease. Which of the following is the best therapeutic option at this time?

a. Change therapy from naproxen to indomethacin.
b. Change therapy from naproxen to celecoxib.
c. Begin methotrexate therapy.
d. Begin low-dose prednisone therapy, 10 mg daily.
e. Begin therapy with an antitumor necrosis factor drug.

11. A 33-year-old woman with a 12-year history of ulcerative colitis presents with a 2-month history of pain and swelling of the right ankle and left knee. Analysis of synovial fluid from the knee shows 15,000 leukocytes with negative culture. She has no history of low back pain and is negative for HLA-B27. Her ulcerative colitis has been more symptomatic during the past several months. Which of the following is the most likely diagnosis?

a. Spondyloarthropathy with peripheral joint involvement
b. Reactive arthritis
c. Enteropathic arthritis due to ulcerative colitis
d. Gout
e. Rheumatoid arthritis

12. A 32-year-old man presents for evaluation of recurrent Achilles tendinitis. There is no history of injury or overuse. He considers himself in otherwise good health. At age 25 years, he had an episode of iritis, which has not recurred. He has no history of rash. He does have some low back pain with morning accentuation. He is an avid hunter. Which of the following is most likely to account for his Achilles tendinitis?

a. Rheumatoid arthritis
b. Spondyloarthropathy
c. Idiopathic Achilles tendinitis
d. Sarcoidosis
e. Lyme disease

13. A 35-year-old man has a history of progressive ankylosing spondylitis nonresponsive to nonsteroidal anti-inflammatory drugs. He considers himself otherwise healthy. You recommend treatment with an antitumor necrosis factor drug. Before starting the therapy, which of the following should be done?

a. Baseline echocardiography
b. Positron emission tomography

c. Skin test for tuberculosis
d. Serum protein electrophoresis
e. Testing for human immunodeficiency virus (HIV)

14. Which of the following drugs can cause acute gouty arthritis by decreasing urinary excretion of uric acid?

a. Pravastatin
b. Cyclosporine
c. Etanercept
d. Enalapril
e. Cyclosphosphamide

15. A 68-year-old woman has been found to have severe pulmonary hypertension. She has a long history of Raynaud phenomenon. She has a 10-year history of non–insulin-dependent diabetes treated with metformin. She used omeperazole 20 mg for dyspepsia. She considers herself otherwise healthy. She was recently found to have a positive antinuclear antibody titer (1:640). She denies photosensitivity and pleurisy, and there is no history of renal disease. On physical examination, she has several small telangiectasias on her fingers. Sclerodactyly is present. Which of the following is the most likely diagnosis to account for her pulmonary hypertension?

a. Lupus
b. Primary pulmonary hypertension
c. Scleroderma
d. Antiphospholipid antibody syndrome
e. CREST syndrome (calcinosis cutis, Raynaud phenomenon, esophageal dysmotility, sclerodactyly, and telangiectasias)

16. A 32-year-old woman with known lupus has a flare of her disease to include diffuse proliferative glomerulonephritis. Her creatinine level is 1.5 mg/dL. She has no children and does not want to consider cyclophosphamide therapy. Which of the following is the best treatment to use in conjunction with high-dose prednisone?

a. Mycophenolate mofetil
b. Hydroxychloroquine
c. Azathioprine
d. Etanercept
e. Methotrexate

17. A patient with systemic lupus erythematosus has sudden onset of nephrotic syndrome, dyspnea, and pleuritic chest pain. Urinalysis shows +4 protein without red blood cells. Oxygen saturation is 84%. Which of the following tests will help identify an underlying cause of the acute symptoms?

a. Antiphospholipid antibody test
b. Antinuclear antibody test
c. Anti–double-stranded DNA test
d. Anti-ribonucleoprotein test
e. C3 complement test

18. A 25-year-old woman has been referred because of positive results of the VDRL test when she applied for a marriage license. Her primary care physician had performed a fluorescent treponemal antibody (FTA) test, results of which were negative. She denies a history to suggest syphilis. She is otherwise healthy. Antinuclear antibody test was negative. Which of the following tests is likely to be positive?

a. Antiphospholipid antibodies
b. Anti-ribonucleoprotein
c. Anti-Smith (Sm) antigen test
d. Anti-native DNA
e. HIV

19. A 65-year-old woman with scleroderma presents with progressive shortness of breath. Chest radiography shows interstitial changes. Dry bibasilar rales are heard on examination. Diffusing capacity is reduced. High-resolution CT shows diffuse bibasilar ground-glass appearance. In addition to prednisone, which of the following is the best treatment for her lung involvement?

a. Azathioprine
b. Cyclophosphamide
c. Methotrexate
d. Mycophenolate mofetil
e. Plasmapharesis

20. A 42-year-old woman presents with a 3-month history of violaceous rash of her face and difficulty getting up from a seated position. She has significant proximal muscle weakness. Laboratory study results are as follows:

Component	Value
Hemoglobin	11.1 g/dL
Leukocytes	6.4 × 10⁹/L
Sedimentation rate	62 mm in 1 hour
Antinuclear antibody titer	1:160
Creatine kinase	4,210 U/L (normal <200)
Electromyography	Inflammatory myopathy

Which of the following studies would be most likely to aid diagnosis of an underlying condition to account for her disease?

a. Sensitive thyroid-stimulating hormone
b. Skin biopsy
c. CT of chest, abdomen, and pelvis
d. MRI of proximal muscles in legs
e. Muscle biopsy

21. A 36-year-old man has a several-month history of dry eyes and mouth and parotid gland swelling. He has no joint symptoms

or rash. He did have thrush 1 month ago. Laboratory studies included negative results of antinuclear antibody, anti-Sjögren syndrome A (SSA), and rheumatoid factor tests. Which of the following is the most likely cause of his parotid swelling and sicca syndromes?

a. Sjögren syndrome
b. Sarcoidosis
c. Amyloidosis
d. HIV
e. Lymphoma

Answers

1. Answer a.

In women of this age with a new onset of headache, anemia, and increased sedimentation rate, one would be concerned about the possibility of giant cell arteritis, and the appropriate next step would be a temporal artery biopsy. A bone marrow biopsy would be inappropriate as the next step because the anemia is likely one of chronic disease rather than a primary hematologic process. If giant cell arteritis is highly suspected, prednisone therapy could be considered, but the dose for giant cell arteritis typically would be 1 mg/kg daily as opposed to lower doses that could be used for polymyalgia rheumatica. Electromyography would be done if myopathy was suspected; this patient does not describe weakness, and on examination there is no mention of muscle weakness. Upper aortic arch angiography could be done if there was a marked blood pressure difference in the arms or the patient described symptoms of arm claudication.

2. Answer a.

This patient has fibromyalgia. Before treatment is initiated, it would be appropriate to determine the sensitive thyroid-stimulating hormone level because her symptoms have worsened recently. An extractable nuclear antigen test is unlikely to be helpful given the paucity of evidence suggesting a connective tissue disease. A trial of prednisone would also be inappropriate for a patient with fibromyalgia. Both pregabalin and duloxetine have been shown in clinical trial to be helpful for patients with fibromyalgia.

3. Answer b.

The patient has Henoch-Schönlein purpura. It presents usually at a young age and features include purpuric rash, arthralgias or arthritis, abdominal pain, and often nephritis. It often follows an upper respiratory tract infection. Skin biopsy shows vasculitis with immunoglobulin A deposition. Given the mild renal involvement, which often resolves, a renal biopsy would not be necessary at this time in this patient. This patient is the wrong age for giant cell arteritis and has no symptoms to warrant a temporal artery biopsy. Aspiration of the knee effusion would likely show inflammation

but would not be specific. Arteriography would not be helpful because she has normal pulses, and this is a small vessel vasculitis.

4. Answer d.

This patient has classic polymyalgia rheumatica. Treatment with moderate to low doses of prednisone (about 15 mg daily) is appropriate, but higher doses are usually not necessary. Because she has no symptoms to suggest giant cell arteritis, a temporal artery biopsy would not be necessary. Larger doses of prednisone such as 1 mg/kg daily, which would be used for giant cell arteritis, are not necessary for patients with polymyalgia rheumatica. Determining the creatine phosphokinase level would be appropriate for evaluation of polymyositis but not for polymyalgia rheumatica. Patients with polymyositis usually present with complaints of muscle weakness rather than pain. She has no complaint of this or any weakness on examination. The patient is not overweight, and her sleep disturbance is likely related to pain, and thus the yield from overnight oximetry would be low. Also, although patients with sleep apnea can have fibromyalgia-like symptoms, they would not typically have an increased erythrocyte sedimentation rate.

5. Answer e.

The patient has polyarteritis nodosa. He does not have features of temporal arteritis and is younger than most patients with this form of vasculitis. Also, temporal arteritis seldom affects the abdominal vessels. He does not have an active renal sediment, and polyarteritis nodosa typically does not cause a glomerulonephritis but may cause renal failure on a vasculopathic basis. With hypertension, the renal biopsy would also be relatively contraindicated. Often, the ANCA is negative in a patient with polyarteritis nodosa. Wegener granulomatosis can cause upper airway symptoms, but this patient has none, and thus an otolaryngologic examination would likely be of low yield. He is describing intestinal angina, and thus an abdominal angiogram may be diagnostic with radiographic changes including narrowing of vessels with poststenotic dilatation and even aneurysm formation.

6.   Answer d.

Cryoglobulinemia can occur in association with hepatitis C infection. It can cause a livedo-type rash, arthralgias, and Raynaud symptoms. Churg-Strauss vasculitis occurs in patients with a history of asthma and who have eosinophilia. Buerger disease is more common in men and occurs in current smokers. Wegener granulomatosis classically involves the upper and lower respiratory system and kidneys, and usually patients have a positive cytoplasmic ANCA. Although the patient described some athralgias and myalgias, she does not have fibromyalgia tender points. Furthermore, patients with hepatitis C virus and with cryoglobulinemia can have diffuse musculoskeletal symptoms.

7.   Answer e.

Patients with Wegener granulomatosis usually have a positive cytoplasmic ANCA with positive proteinase 3 on enzyme-linked immunosorbent assay. Classically, they have upper and lower respiratory tract and renal disease. Giant cell arteritis would not occur in this age group and typically would not cause alveolar hemorrhage or glomerulonephritis. Churg-Strauss vasculitis occurs in patients with asthma and typically patients have eosinophilia. Classic polyarteritis nodosa does not affect the lungs. It can affect the kidney, but usually as a vasculopathic nephropathy and not a glomerulonephritis. Most patients with classic polyarteritis nodosa are also ANCA-negative. The findings in this patient fit best with microscopic polyarteritis nodosa. Patients with this condition frequently have alveolar hemorrhage, glomerulonephritis, and a positive perinuclear-ANCA with myeloperoxidase.

8.   Answer a.

Although the uric acid level is normal, gout occurs with a normal uric acid level in 20% of cases. Even patients taking allopurinol can be prone to gouty attacks, although these are much less frequent the longer the allopurinol therapy. Gout and pseudogout can be precipitated by surgery and characteristically occur 3 days postoperatively. Radiography was done after 1 month of symptoms. If septic arthritis had been present, joint space narrowing and destructive changes would have been noted. Also, a stress fracture would have been seen in 1 month's time. There was no mention of chondrocalcinosis, thus pseudogout is unlikely. Rheumatoid arthritis rarely causes monoarticular disease.

9.   Answer b.

Hemochromatosis is associated with chondrocalcinosis, which can lead to pseudogout. It is also associated with a secondary degenerative arthritis, usually involving the second and third metacarpophalangeal joints with hooklike osteophytes.

10.   Answer e.

This patient has active ankylosing spondylitis with continued low back pain and morning stiffness. Changing therapy to another anti-inflammatory drug would be unlikely to provide significant benefit. Methotrexate has not been shown to be beneficial for ankylosing spondylitis. The anti-tumor necrosis factor drugs such as etanercept and infliximab have been shown to provide good symptomatic relief both for spinal symptoms and for the peripheral arthritis of ankylosing spondylitis.

11.   Answer c.

An inflammatory arthritis, usually involving the lower extremities and usually asymmetric, develops in 15% to 20% of persons with ulcerative colitis. Absence of low back pain and negative HLA-B27 status would make spondyloarthropathy or reactive arthritis unlikely. Similarly the absence of birefringent uric acid crystals on joint fluid analysis would make the diagnosis of gout unlikely in this case. Crystals were not found on synovial fluid analysis, and thus gout could not be diagnosed. Rheumatoid arthritis usually is symmetric and polyarticular.

12.   Answer b.

The spondyloarthropathies are associated with iritis and enthesopathic symptoms characteristically involving the Achilles tendon. This patient also has low back pain with morning stiffness, characteristic of sacroiliitis. Rheumatoid arthritis, sacroidosis, and Lyme disease do not typically cause Achilles tendinitis. Sarcoidosis can cause iritis.

13.   Answer c.

Skin tests for tuberculosis should be done in all patients in whom treatment with 1 of the anti-tumor necrosis factor drugs is being considered. These drugs can reactivate latent tuberculosis; if a patient has positive results of the skin test, therapy with isoniazid 300 mg daily for 9 months would be needed. Severe congestive heart failure is also a relative contraindication for anti-tumor necrosis factor drugs, but because the history does not suggest congestive heart failure, baseline echocardiography is not required. Patients who have chronic infections also should not be given anti-tumor necrosis factor drugs; because there is no mention of an infection in the history, HIV testing would not be necessary unless there was a clinical indication.

14.   Answer b.

Cyclosporine decreases urinary excretion of uric acid and can lead to gouty arthritis. Approximately 25% of patients who have had a cardiac transplant and are receiving cyclosporine will have gouty arthritis.

15.   Answer e.

This patient has telangiectasias, Raynaud phenomenon, and sclerodactyly. She also gave a history of dyspepsia. CREST syndrome is associated with pulmonary hypertension. Patients with antiphospholipid antibody syndrome can also have pulmonary hypertension as a result of recurrent pulmonary emboli, but there was no mention of positive tests for antiphospholipid antibodies. This patient did not meet criteria for scleroderma, which would include tightening of the skin of the fingers and the skin proximal to the metacarpophalangeal joints. Patients with scleroderma are more prone to interstitial lung disease than pulmonary hypertension, which is more common in CREST syndrome.

16.   Answer a.

Mycophenolate mofetil is efficacious for the treatment of active diffuse proliferative glomerulonephritis. Although methotrexate and hydroxychloroquine are used in lupus, they have not been found to be beneficial for renal disease and are usually used for joint and skin manifestations. Azathioprine is usually used for maintenance therapy in renal disease and not as an initial agent to induce a remission.

17. Answer a.

Antiphospholipid antibodies can predispose to clotting. The history of sudden onset nephrotic syndrome suggests acute renal vein thrombosis due to clotting of the renal vein. Pulmonary emboli can also develop from the renal vein thrombosis and cause shortness of breath and chest pain.

18. Answer a.

One of the antigenic components in the VDRL test is a phospholipid, so there is cross-activity with antiphospholipid antibodies, causing a false-positive result on the VDRL test. The FTA test, which is much more specific for syphilis, is usually negative, but on occasion there will be a false-positive result with a so-called beaded pattern. Patients with antiphospholipid antibodies might or might not have an underlying connective tissue disease such as lupus.

19. Answer b.

Ground-glass appearance on chest CT correlates with active alveolitis. This finding can be responsive to cyclophosphamide treatment. A honeycomb appearance on CT is more indicative of fibrosis, which is not responsive to medication.

20. Answer c.

This patient has dermatomyositis. Approximately 20% to 30% of patients will have an underlying malignancy and require a workup to include CT. Although any malignancy can be associated with dermatomyositis, there is an increased frequency of ovarian cancer relative to other malignancies. Hypothyroidism is associated with an increased creatine kinase level but not rash. A skin biopsy would show inflammatory changes consistent with dermatomyositis. MRI of muscles will show inflammation but would not lead to an underlying diagnosis. A muscle biopsy would confirm the diagnosis of dermatomyositis but would not aid diagnosis of an underlying malignancy.

21. Answer d.

Although this patient had symptoms suggestive of Sjögren syndrome with dry eyes and dry mouth, results of laboratory studies included negative antinuclear antibody, rheumatoid factor, and SSA, all of which would have been expected to be positive in patients with Sjögren syndrome. HIV can mimic Sjögren syndrome with parotid swelling and dry eyes and dry mouth, but laboratory results are negative for antinuclear antibody, rheumatoid factor, and SSA. The clinical clue that HIV might be causing the symptoms was the history of thrush in a 36-year-old man. Sarcoidosis and lymphoma can also cause parotid swelling but would not be associated with the history of thrush.

25

Vascular Diseases

Peter C. Spittell, MD

Peripheral vascular diseases are prevalent in current medical practice. Characteristic clinical features, accurate diagnostic techniques, and improved treatment of peripheral vascular disease further emphasize the need for increased awareness of this group of disorders.

Disease of the Aorta

Aneurysmal Disease

Thoracic Aortic Aneurysm

Thoracic aortic aneurysms are caused most commonly by atherosclerosis, but they also occur in patients with systemic hypertension, inherited disorders of connective tissue (eg, Marfan syndrome), giant cell arteritis (cranial and Takayasu disease), and infection and as a result of trauma. There is also a familial tendency. Most thoracic aortic aneurysms are asymptomatic and are discovered incidentally on chest radiography (Figure 25-1). Symptoms, when present, may include chest or back pain, vocal hoarseness, cough, dyspnea, stridor,

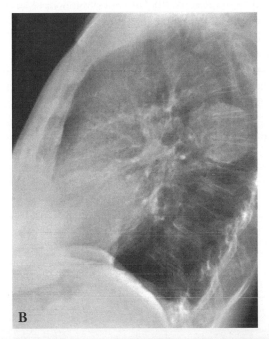

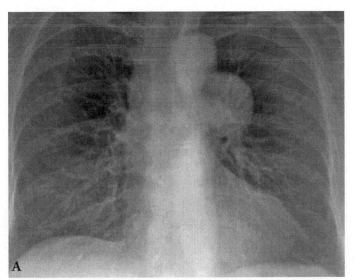

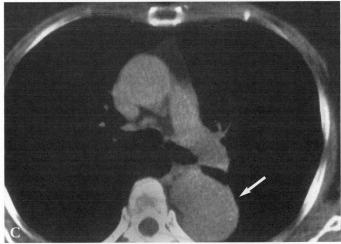

Figure 25-1. A and B, Chest radiographs (A, anteroposterior; B, lateral) show a large mass in the left posterior chest. C, Computed tomogram shows a saccular aneurysm in the mid-descending thoracic aorta.

and dysphagia. Findings on physical examination may include systemic hypertension, fixed distention of a neck vein(s), aortic regurgitation, a fixed vocal cord, signs of cerebral or systemic embolism, and other aneurysmal disease (ie, abdominal aortic aneurysm). Complications of thoracic aortic aneurysm include rupture, dissection, embolism, pressure on surrounding structures, infection, and, rarely, thrombosis. Factors that seem to worsen the prognosis include diastolic hypertension, aneurysm size (critical hinge point for rupture >6 cm ascending aorta and >7 cm descending thoracic aorta), traumatic aneurysm, and associated coronary and carotid artery disease. The overall cumulative risk of rupture after 5 years is 20%, but rupture risk is a function of aneurysm size at recognition (0% for aneurysms <4 cm in diameter, 16% for aneurysms 4.0-5.9 cm, and 31% for aneurysms ≥6.0 cm). Computed tomography (CT), magnetic resonance imaging (MRI) (Figure 25-2), and transesophageal echocardiography (TEE) are all accurate in the diagnosis of thoracic aortic aneurysm. Medical management of thoracic aortic aneurysm includes control of systemic hypertension (preferably with a β-adrenergic blocking agent), discontinuation of tobacco use, diagnosis and treatment of associated coronary and carotid artery disease, and follow-up combining clinical assessment and noninvasive imaging tests. Indications for surgical resection include the presence of symptoms attributable to the aneurysm, an aneurysm rapidly enlarging under observation (particularly if the patient has poorly controlled hypertension), traumatic aneurysm, pseudoaneurysm, mycotic aneurysm, and an aneurysm 6 cm or more in diameter (5.5-6 cm in low-risk patients). In patients with Marfan syndrome, operation is indicated when the ascending aortic diameter exceeds 4.5 to 5 cm.

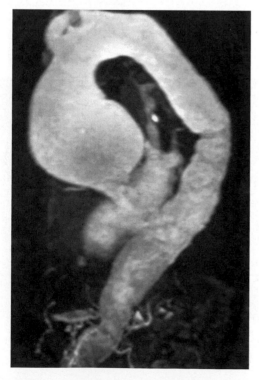

Figure 25-2. Magnetic resonance angiogram (longitudinal view) shows a large ascending aortic aneurysm and moderate aortic regurgitation.

Abdominal Aortic Aneurysm

Approximately three-fourths of all atherosclerotic aneurysms involve the abdominal aorta. Most abdominal aortic aneurysms (AAAs) are infrarenal, and 2% to 5% are suprarenal, usually the result of distal extension of a thoracic aneurysm (thoracoabdominal aneurysm). Men are affected more frequently than women (9:1), and the majority of patients are older than 50 years. There is a familial tendency for development of AAA, and both sex-linked and autosomal patterns of inheritance are involved. There is a strong association with current or prior chronic tobacco exposure. Infection and trauma are additional causes of AAA.

The majority of patients with AAA are asymptomatic. The most common physical examination finding is the presence of a pulsatile abdominal mass. The sensitivity of abdominal palpation for the detection of AAA is 43% overall (57% for aneurysms ≥4.0 cm in diameter, 29% for aneurysms <4.0 cm in diameter). A tortuous abdominal aorta, transmitted pulsation from an abdominal mass, or a horseshoe kidney anteriorly displacing the abdominal aorta are conditions that can mimic AAA on physical examination. Because physical examination for the detection of AAA lacks sensitivity, screening tests are indicated in high-risk subsets of patients. Early detection of AAA can reduce mortality. Furthermore, single screening ultrasonography for men older than 65 years can identify the majority of AAAs. The United States Preventive Services Task Force recommends a 1-time screening ultrasonography in men ages 65 to 75 years who have ever smoked. Screening of siblings and first-degree relatives of patients with aneurysm generally begins at age 50 years.

When AAAs are symptomatic without rupture, the most common complaint is abdominal pain. New low back pain can occur and may be due to dissection within the aneurysm or retroperitoneal hematoma. Abdominal pain radiating to the flank, groin, or testes also may occur. Livedo reticularis, blue toes with palpable pulses, hypertension, renal insufficiency, increased erythrocyte sedimentation rate, and transient eosinophilia characterize atheroembolism in association with AAA (Figure 25-3). Atheroembolism can occur spontaneously or as a result of anticoagulants (warfarin or thrombolytic therapy) or angiographic or surgical procedures. Treatment of choice is surgical resection of the symptomatic AAA if feasible.

The most frequent complication of AAA is rupture, which is related to aneurysm size: 1-year incidence of rupture for AAA diameter 5.5 to 5.9 cm is 9.4%; diameter 6.0 to 6.9 cm, 10.2%; diameter 7.0 cm or more, 32.5%. The triad of severe abdominal pain, hypotension, and a tender abdominal mass characterizes rupture of an AAA. The pain is acute in onset, constant, and severe, most commonly located in the lumbar area or diffusely throughout the abdomen, with radiation into the flanks, genitals, or legs. The abdominal aorta is usually tender, and there may be peritoneal signs if free rupture into the peritoneal cavity has occurred. Less common presentations of AAA include obstructive uropathy due to ureteral compression, gastrointestinal hemorrhage when the aneurysm ruptures into the intestinal tract, high-output congestive heart failure due to an aortocaval fistula, and disseminated intravascular coagulation.

AAA can be diagnosed reliably with ultrasonography, CT and CT angiography, or MRI and MR angiography (Figure 25-4).

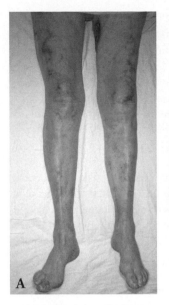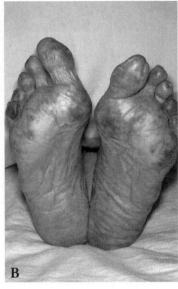

Figure 25-3. A and B, Patient with atheroembolism, characterized by livedo reticularis (upper thighs, plantar surface of feet) and multiple blue toes.

Angiography is not required unless the renal or peripheral arterial circulation needs to be visualized to plan treatment.

Medical management of AAA includes control of systemic hypertension (preferably with a β-adrenergic blocking agent), discontinuation of tobacco use, treatment of associated coronary and carotid artery disease, and serial noninvasive imaging tests. Noninvasive imaging should be used to assess both absolute aneurysm size and growth rate. The frequency of surveillance is based on aneurysm size at initial detection (Table 25-1).

In a good-risk patient, selective surgical treatment of AAA should be considered for aneurysms 5.0 to 5.5 cm in diameter. When the patient has considerable comorbid conditions (pulmonary, cardiac, renal, or liver disease), surgical therapy is individualized. Endovascular repair of AAA with stent grafts that are delivered intraluminally by

catheters is an alternative to open surgical repair, particularly in patients at increased risk of perioperative complications, and early results are comparable to those of open repair. At tertiary care centers, more than 30% of AAA repairs are accomplished with an endovascular approach. With extended follow-up, however, postoperative complications and graft failures have been reported in some patients, resulting in reintervention, conversion to open repair, or death. The high incidence of secondary interventions brings into question the relative durability of endograft repair and emphasizes the need for detailed long-term follow-up care.

Inflammatory AAA accounts for approximately 2% to 4% of all AAAs. An inflammatory AAA is suggested by the triad of abdominal or back pain, weight loss, and increased erythrocyte sedimentation rate. Obstructive uropathy may occur with ureteral involvement. The findings on CT are diagnostic. The treatment is surgical resection regardless of aneurysm size. The role of corticosteroids is not well defined.

Operation is also indicated for AAAs that are symptomatic, traumatic, infectious in origin, or rapidly expanding (>0.5 cm a year).

- Elective surgical repair is definitely indicated when the AAA diameter is >5.0 cm in good-risk patients.
- Surgical treatment is also indicated for AAAs that are symptomatic, traumatic, infectious in origin, or are rapidly expanding (>0.5 cm a year).
- The triad of back pain, weight loss, and increased erythrocyte sedimentation rate suggests an inflammatory AAA. The findings on CT are diagnostic. Treatment is surgical resection regardless of aneurysm size.

Aortic Dissection

Etiology

The most common predisposing factors for aortic dissection are advanced age, male sex, hypertension, Marfan syndrome, and congenital abnormalities of the aortic valve (bicuspid or unicuspid valve). When aortic dissection complicates pregnancy, it usually occurs in

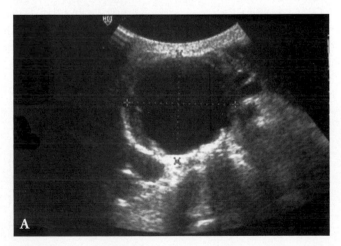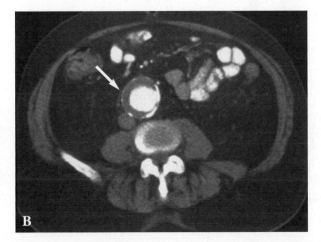

Figure 25-4. A, Ultrasonogram (transverse view) shows a 4.7-cm abdominal aortic aneurysm. B, Computed tomogram (contrast-enhanced) shows an abdominal aortic aneurysm with moderate mural thrombus.

Table 25-1 Surveillance of Abdominal Aortic Aneurysm

Size at Initial Detection, cm	Surveillance Interval
3.0-3.4	3 y
3.5-3.9	1 y
4.0-4.9	6 mo
≥5.0	3 mo[a]

[a]If surveillance is ongoing (vs surgery).
Data from McCarthy RJ, Shaw E, Whyman MR, Earnshaw JJ, Poskitt KR, Heather BP. Recommendations for screening intervals for small aortic aneurysms. Br J Surg. 2003;90:821-6.

the third trimester. Iatrogenic aortic dissection, as a result of cardiac operation or invasive angiographic procedures, also can occur.

Classification

Aortic dissection involving the ascending aorta is designated as type I or II (proximal, type A), and dissection confined to the descending thoracic aorta is designated as type III (distal, type B) (Figure 25-5).

Clinical Features

The sudden onset of severe pain (often migratory) in the anterior aspect of the chest, back, or abdomen occurs in 70% to 80% of patients and has a sensitivity of 90% and specificity of 84%. Hypertension is present in 60% to 80%. Additional findings include aortic diastolic murmur (15%-20%), pulse deficits (10%-40%), and neurologic changes (10%-30%). Syncope in association with aortic dissection occurs when there is rupture into the pericardial space, producing cardiac tamponade. Congestive heart failure is most commonly due to severe aortic regurgitation. Acute myocardial infarction (most commonly inferior infarction due to right coronary artery ostial involvement), pericarditis, and complete heart block are additional cardiac presentations.

Clues to type I aortic dissection include substernal pain, aortic valve incompetence, decreased pulse or blood pressure in the right arm, decreased right carotid pulse, pericardial friction rub, syncope, ischemic electrocardiographic changes, and Marfan syndrome.

Clues to type III aortic dissection include interscapular pain, hypertension, and left pleural effusion.

- In a patient with a catastrophic presentation, systemic hypertension, and unexplained physical findings of vascular origin, especially in the presence of chest pain and an aortic murmur, aortic dissection should always be included in the differential diagnosis and an appropriate screening test performed on an emergency basis.

Laboratory Tests

Chest radiography may show widening of the superior mediastinum and supracardiac aortic shadow, deviation of the trachea from the midline, a discrepancy in diameter between the ascending and descending aorta, and pleural effusion (Figure 25-6). Normal findings on chest radiography do not exclude aortic dissection.

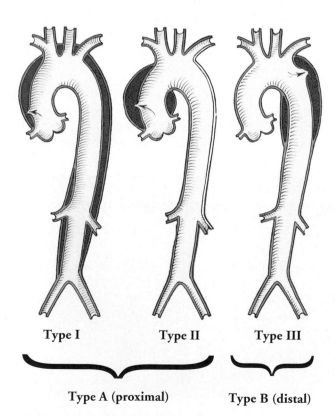

Type I   Type II   Type III

Type A (proximal)   Type B (distal)

Figure 25-5. Classification System for Aortic Dissection.

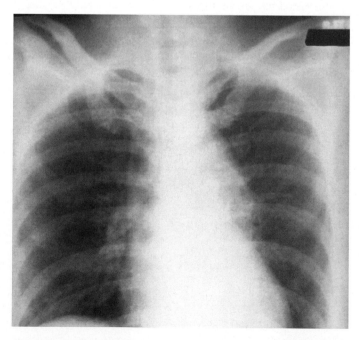

Figure 25-6. Chest radiograph in a patient with aortic dissection shows widening of the superior mediastinum.

Electrocardiography most commonly shows left ventricular hypertrophy, but ST-segment depression, ST-segment elevation, T-wave changes, and the changes of acute pericarditis and complete heart block occur in up to 55% of patients.

Diagnosis

Aortic dissection can be definitively diagnosed with any of the following imaging methods: echocardiography, CT, MRI, and aortography (Figure 25-7).

Combined transthoracic and transesophageal echocardiography (TTE/TEE) can identify an intimal flap, entry and reentry sites, aortic root dilatation (>4 cm), thrombosis of the false lumen, aortic regurgitation, pericardial effusion or cardiac tamponade, pleural effusion, involvement of the left common carotid or left subclavian arteries, and proximal abdominal aortic involvement. Multiplane transducers have markedly improved the accuracy of TEE. Advantages of TEE include portability, safety, accuracy, rapid diagnosis, ability to provide a comprehensive cardiac assessment, ability to use in patients with hemodynamic instability, and intraoperative applications.

CT can accurately detect the intimal flap, identify 2 lumina, and show displaced intimal calcification, a disparate size between the ascending and descending aortic lumina, hemopericardium, pleural effusion, and abdominal aortic involvement. Disadvantages of CT include nonportability (limiting use in patients with hemodynamic instability) and the need for intravenous contrast agents.

MRI is highly accurate for the diagnosis of aortic dissection. Demonstration of the intimal flap, entry or exit sites, thrombus formation, aortic regurgitation, pericardial effusion, pleural effusion, and abdominal aortic involvement is possible. MRI is also able to delineate involvement of aortic arch vessels. Disadvantages of MRI include cost, nonportability, and other standard MRI contraindications.

Aortography can accurately diagnose aortic dissection by showing the intimal flap, opacification of the false lumen, and deformity of the true lumen. Also, associated aortic regurgitation and coronary artery anatomy can be visualized, in addition to branch vessel involvement. The disadvantages include invasive risks, exposure to intravenous contrast agents, and nonportability.

The choice of test (TTE/TEE, CT, MRI, or aortography) in a patient with suspected acute aortic dissection depends on which is most readily available and the hemodynamic stability of the patient.

The initial management of suspected acute aortic dissection is shown in Figure 25-8.

The most common cause of death is rupture into the pericardial space, with subsequent cardiac tamponade. Cardiac tamponade due to aortic dissection is a surgical emergency, and pericardial fluid should be removed only in the operating room after cardiopulmonary bypass has been instituted. Echocardiographically guided pericardiocentesis in a patient with cardiac tamponade complicating aortic dissection is associated with an increased risk of aortic rupture and death. Other causes of death in aortic dissection include acute congestive heart failure due to severe aortic regurgitation, rupture through the aortic adventitia, rupture into the left pleural space, and occlusion of vital arteries.

- Aortic dissection can be diagnosed with TTE/TEE, CT, MRI, or aortography.

Treatment

Pharmacologic therapy should be instituted as soon as the diagnosis of aortic dissection is suspected (Table 25-2). Emergency operation is indicated in types I and II (proximal, type A) aortic dissection. Continued pharmacologic therapy in the coronary care unit is the preferred initial management in type III (distal, type B) aortic dissection, and surgical therapy is delayed (2-3 weeks) for select patients whose general medical condition permits operation, especially patients with partial thrombosis of the false lumen. When long-term pharmacologic therapy for type III aortic dissection is used, indications for operation include development of saccular aneurysm, increasing aortic diameter, or symptoms related to chronic dissection.

- Emergency operation is indicated in types I and II aortic dissection.

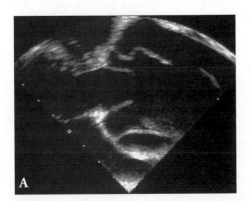
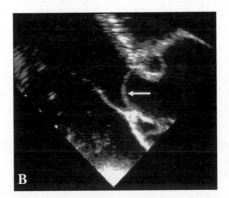
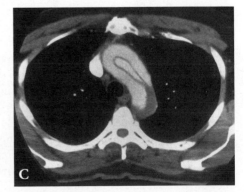

Figure 25-7. A, Multiplane transesophageal echocardiogram (longitudinal view) shows an intimal flap in the ascending aorta. B, In diastole, the intimal flap prolapses through the aortic valve (*arrow*). C, Computed tomogram (contrast-enhanced) shows a spiraling intimal flap in the transverse aortic arch.

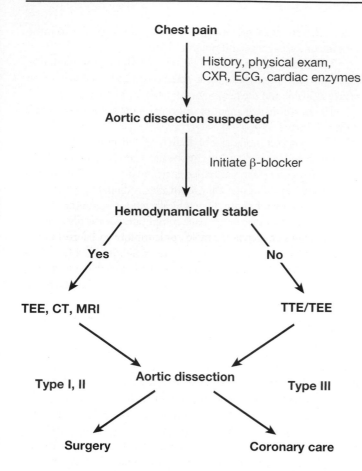

Chest pain

History, physical exam,
CXR, ECG, cardiac enzymes

Aortic dissection suspected

Initiate β-blocker

Hemodynamically stable

Yes   No

TEE, CT, MRI   **TTE/TEE**

Type I, II   **Aortic dissection**   **Type III**

Surgery   **Coronary care**

Figure 25-8. Algorithm for Initial Management of Suspected Acute Aortic Dissection. CT indicates computed tomography; CXR, chest radiography; ECG, electrocardiography; MRI, magnetic resonance imaging; TEE, transesophageal echocardiography; TTE, transthoracic echocardiography.

- Pharmacologic treatment is the preferred initial management in type III aortic dissection.

Penetrating Aortic Ulcer

Penetrating aortic ulcer occurs when an atherosclerotic plaque undergoes ulceration and penetrates the internal elastic lamina. It results in 1 of 4 possible consequences: 1) formation of an intramural hematoma, 2) formation of a saccular aneurysm, 3) formation of a pseudoaneurysm, or 4) transmural aortic rupture. Penetrating aortic ulcer most commonly involves the mid or distal descending thoracic aorta, less often the ascending or abdominal aorta. The clinical features of penetrating aortic ulcer are similar to those of aortic dissection and include acute onset of pain in the anterior or posterior chest (or both) and hypertension. Pulse deficits, neurologic signs, and acute cardiac disease (aortic regurgitation, myocardial infarction, pericardial effusion) do not occur in penetrating aortic ulcer, as they do in classic aortic dissection.

The treatment of penetrating aortic ulcer is usually nonoperative if only an intramural hematoma is present. With control of hypertension, the intramural hematoma tends to resolve spontaneously over

time. Surgical therapy is indicated for patients who have ascending aortic involvement, patients in whom a saccular aneurysm or pseudoaneurysm develops, or patients with intramural hematoma who have persistent symptoms, increasing aortic diameter, or poorly controlled hypertension. The most common serious complication of surgical therapy for penetrating aortic ulcer is paraplegia.

Aortic Intramural Hematoma

Aortic intramural hematoma is characterized by the absence of an intimal tear and also is associated with cystic medial necrosis. Aortic intramural hematoma is increasingly recognized, largely due to advances in noninvasive imaging techniques. The exact cause of aortic intramural hematoma is not well defined. Aortic intramural hematoma is diagnosed in the same manner as aortic dissection. The classification schemes are also identical, and traditionally the management has been similar—operation for type A intramural hematoma and medical treatment for type B lesions.

Incomplete Aortic Rupture

Incomplete rupture of the thoracic aorta (in the region of the aortic isthmus) results from a sudden deceleration injury. It occurs most often in victims of motor vehicle accidents and should be suspected when there is evidence of chest wall trauma, decreased or absent leg pulses, left-sided hemothorax, or widening of the superior mediastinum on chest radiography. Affected patients are usually hypertensive at initial presentation. TEE, CT, MRI, or angiography can confirm the diagnosis (Figure 25-9). Treatment is emergency surgical repair in patients who are suitable surgical candidates. At initial presentation, the condition of 40% to 50% of patients is unstable. No clinical or imaging criteria accurately predict future complete rupture, so even if a patient presents with a chronic incomplete rupture, operation is still indicated. Most patients are young, and the risk of elective surgical repair is low, with an otherwise good prognosis for long-term survival if aortic repair is successful.

- Incomplete rupture of the thoracic aorta (in the region of the aortic isthmus) results from a sudden deceleration injury, frequently a motor vehicle accident.

Thoracic Aortic Atherosclerosis

Atherosclerosis of the thoracic aorta usually involves the origin of the brachiocephalic arteries, principally the left subclavian and occasionally the innominate artery. Although atherosclerotic disease of the aortic arch branches is usually asymptomatic, stenosis of the origin of the left or right subclavian artery may cause intermittent claudication of the arm of sufficient degree to warrant surgical treatment. With complete occlusion of the origin of either subclavian artery, collateral blood flow to the arm may be derived principally from the cerebral circulation via reversed flow through the ipsilateral vertebral artery, so-called subclavian steal. This may result in episodes of transient cerebral ischemia, especially when the ipsilateral arm is exercised. A similar situation may occur on the right side if the obstruction occurs at the origin of the innominate artery, in which case flow in the right vertebral artery can "reverse" to enter the right subclavian artery. In addition to the symptoms

Table 25-2 Initial Pharmacologic Therapy for Acute Aortic Dissection

Hypertensive patients

    Sodium nitroprusside intravenously (2.5-5.0 mcg/kg per minute)

      with

    Propranolol intravenously (1 mg every 4-6 h)

      • Goal: Systolic blood pressure in the range of 110 mm Hg (or the lowest level maintaining a urine output of 25-30 mL/h) until oral medication is started

    Or Esmolol, metoprolol, or atenolol intravenously (in place of propranolol)

    Or Labetolol intravenously (in place of sodium nitroprusside & a β-blocker)

Normotensive patients

    Propranolol 1 mg intravenously every 4-6 h or 20-40 mg orally every 6 h (metoprolol, atenolol, esmolol, or labetolol may be used in place of propranolol)

---

of transient cerebral ischemia, physical signs of this condition include reduced arm and wrist pulses and reduced blood pressure on the affected side. The astute examiner, when palpating both radial pulses simultaneously, also may detect a delay in pulsation on the affected side.

Furthermore, a coronary-subclavian steal phenomenon may occur in patients who have undergone prior coronary artery bypass grafting in which the internal mammary artery is used. When a hemodynamically significant subclavian artery stenosis is present ipsilateral to the internal mammary artery graft, flow through the internal mammary artery may reverse or "steal" during upper extremity exercise.

Acquired coarctation of the thoracic aorta due to focally obstructive calcific atherosclerotic disease is rare. Symptomatic patients present with upper extremity hypertension and reduced blood pressure in the lower extremities, with or without intermittent claudication.

Microemboli or macroemboli from atherosclerotic plaque and thrombus in the thoracic aorta are important causes of cerebral and systemic embolism. Aortic atheroma occurs in approximately 27% of patients with previous embolic events and is also a strong predictor of coronary artery disease. Thoracic aortic atherosclerotic plaque is most accurately assessed with TEE. Plaque thickness more than 4 mm or mobile thrombus (of any size) is associated with an increased risk of embolism. Embolism can occur spontaneously, in relation to invasive angiographic procedures, as a result of warfarin or thrombolytic therapy, and from cardiac surgical procedures requiring cardiopulmonary bypass. Treatment is surgical resection if a focal source of embolism is present and the patient's general medical condition permits. Antiplatelet agents and a statin medication should be used for the management of all patients unless an absolute contraindication is present. Warfarin therapy may be beneficial for reducing subsequent embolic events, but further randomized trials are required.

• Emboli from atherosclerotic plaque and thrombus in the thoracic aorta are important causes of cerebral and systemic embolism.

Peripheral Arterial Occlusive Disease

Intermittent Claudication

Clinical Features

Lower extremity arterial occlusive disease affects 8 to 12 million Americans, but 75% have no significant symptoms. Despite an overall incidence of 30% in high-risk groups (age >70 years, diabetes, tobacco use), the condition is frequently not diagnosed (>30%). Furthermore, peripheral arterial disease can provide an

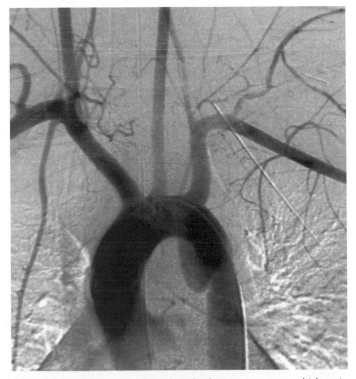

Figure 25-9. Aortogram in a patient involved in a severe motor vehicle accident shows a contained rupture of the proximal descending thoracic aorta just distal to the origin of the left subclavian artery.

important clue to systemic atherosclerosis and identify persons at increased risk for left ventricular systolic dysfunction, myocardial infarction, and cerebrovascular accident. Variable presentations occur with lower extremity arterial occlusive disease, including no symptoms (or atypical symptoms), intermittent claudication, and critical limb ischemia (rest pain, ulceration, gangrene). The degree of functional limitation varies depending on the degree of arterial stenosis, collateral circulation, exercise capacity, and comorbid conditions. Intermittent claudication (aching, cramping, or tightness) is always exercise-induced and may involve 1 or both legs, and symptoms occur at a fairly constant walking distance. Relief is obtained by standing still. Supine ankle to brachial systolic pressure indices before and after exercise testing (treadmill walking or active pedal plantar flexion) can confirm the diagnosis (Table 25-3). Furthermore, a low ankle to brachial systolic pressure index (<0.9) is associated with an increased risk of stroke, cardiovascular death, and all-cause mortality.

* The discomfort of intermittent claudication is always exercise-induced; standing still provides relief.

Pseudoclaudication

Pseudoclaudication, due to lumbar spinal stenosis, is the condition most commonly confused with intermittent claudication. Pseudoclaudication is usually described as a "paresthetic" discomfort that occurs with standing or walking (variable distances). Symptoms are almost always bilateral and are relieved by sitting or leaning forward. The patient often has a prior history of chronic back pain or lumbosacral spinal operation. The diagnosis of lumbar spinal stenosis can be confirmed with normal or minimally abnormal ankle to brachial systolic pressure indices before and after exercise, in combination with characteristic findings on electromyography and CT or MRI of the lumbar spine (Table 25-4).

* Pseudoclaudication occurs with standing or walking.

Natural History

Peripheral arterial occlusive disease is associated with considerable mortality because of its association with coronary and carotid atherosclerosis. The 5-year mortality rate in patients with intermittent claudication is 29%, and the overall amputation rate over 5 years is 4%. More than half of patients have stable or improved symptoms over this same period. Continued use of tobacco results in a 10-fold increase in the risk for major amputation and a more than 2-fold increase in mortality. The effect of diabetes mellitus on patients with intermittent claudication deserves special mention; it accounts for the majority of amputations in a community (12-fold increased risk of below-knee amputation and a cumulative risk of major amputation exceeding 11% over 25 years). Independent predictors of a decline in the ankle to brachial systolic pressure index include advanced age, current tobacco use, hypertension, diabetes mellitus, and increased level of low-density lipoprotein cholesterol. Other clinical features that predict an increased risk of limb loss in lower extremity arterial occlusive disease include ischemic rest pain, ischemic ulceration, and gangrene.

* The 5-year mortality rate in patients with intermittent claudication is 29%, predominantly due to associated coronary atherosclerosis.
* Tobacco use, diabetes mellitus, ischemic rest pain, ulceration, and gangrene are associated with an increased risk of limb loss in patients with intermittent claudication.
* Independent predictors of a decline in the ankle to brachial systolic pressure index include advanced age, current tobacco use, hypertension, diabetes mellitus, and increased level of low-density lipoprotein cholesterol.

Diagnosis

Peripheral angiography is rarely needed to diagnose intermittent claudication. Semi-quantification of the severity of peripheral arterial disease can readily be obtained with noninvasive testing (determination of ankle:brachial systolic pressure indices before and after exercise or duplex ultrasonography). Angiography is indicated to define arterial anatomy before operation or endovascular therapy. Angiography also is indicated when an "uncommon" type of arterial disease is suspected. Magnetic resonance angiography is an accurate alternative to standard angiography and is especially useful for preoperative planning in patients with contraindications to invasive angiography (ie, renal insufficiency or severe allergy to contrast media).

Table 25-3 Grading System for Lower Extremity Arterial Occlusive Disease[a]

Grade	ABI	
	Supine Resting	Postexercise
Normal	1.0-1.4	No change or increase
Mild disease	0.8-0.9	>0.5
Moderate disease	0.5-0.8	>0.2
Severe disease	<0.5	<0.2

Abbreviation: ABI, ankle to brachial systolic pressure index.
[a] After treadmill exercise, 1-2 mph, 10% grade, 5 minutes or symptom-limited or active pedal plantar flexion, 50 repetitions or symptom-limited.

Table 25-4 Differential Diagnosis of Intermittent Claudication and Pseudoclaudication

	Claudication	Pseudoclaudication
Onset	Walking	Standing & walking
Character	Cramp, ache	"Paresthetic"
Bilateral	+/-	+
Walking distance	Fairly constant	More variable
Cause	Atherosclerosis	Spinal stenosis
Relief	Standing still	Sitting down, leaning forward

- Peripheral angiography is rarely needed to diagnose intermittent claudication.

Treatment

Medical management of lower extremity arterial occlusive disease involves 3 areas: risk factor reduction, exercise training, and pharmacologic therapy. In addition, weight reduction (if obese), foot care and protection, and avoidance of vasoconstrictive drugs are of benefit. Foot care and protection are of paramount importance in patients with diabetes who have peripheral arterial disease. The combination of peripheral neuropathy, small vessel disease, or peripheral arterial disease in patients with diabetes makes foot trauma more likely to be associated with a nonhealing wound or ulcer.

All patients with peripheral arterial disease should be prescribed an antiplatelet agent. Aspirin (81-325 mg daily) is effective, resulting in a decreased risk of limb loss, reduced need for vascular surgery, and a decreased incidence of major coronary and cerebrovascular events. Clopidogrel (75 mg daily) has been shown to be more effective than aspirin for preventing major atherosclerotic vascular events. The Clopidogrel for High Atherothrombotic Risk and Ischemic Stabilization, Management, and Avoidance (CHARISMA) trial found that dual-antiplatelet use (aspirin and clopidogrel) is more effective than either agent alone for preventing ischemic events in patients with peripheral vascular disease.

Exercise training is of significant benefit in intermittent claudication. A regular walking program (level ground, walking the distance to claudication, stopping to rest for relief, repeatedly for 45-60 minutes per session, 4 or more days a week, continued for 6 months) can result in a significant (often more than 180%) improvement in initial distance to claudication in many patients. For patients who do not adequately respond to a walking program, cilostazol may be useful. Cilostazol, a phosphodiesterase III inhibitor, results in a significant improvement in walking ability (an approximate doubling of initial and absolute distance to claudication) compared with placebo and pentoxifylline. Cilostazol seems to be more effective than pentoxifylline, but it is contraindicated in patients with congestive heart failure of any severity. The dose is 100 mg orally daily (50 mg orally twice daily in patients taking diltiazem, ketoconazole, or other inhibitors of cytochrome P450 3A4). Propionyl-L-carnitine seems to improve alterations in carnitine metabolism in patients with a severe functional impairment from intermittent claudication, resulting in improvement in maximal walking distance and quality of life. The dose is 1 g orally twice daily.

Statins should be considered in patients with peripheral arterial disease and have been shown to improve the symptoms of intermittent claudication and to reduce the incidence of adverse cardiovascular and cerebrovascular events. In hypercholesterolemic patients with symptomatic peripheral arterial occlusive disease, simvastatin in high doses (40 mg daily) may improve walking performance and the symptoms of intermittent claudication. Angiotensin-converting enzyme inhibitors also reduce the risk of ischemic cardiovascular events in patients with peripheral arterial disease and have nephroprotective effects in patients with diabetes.

Indications for endovascular or surgical revascularization in a patient with peripheral arterial occlusive disease are "disabling" (lifestyle-limiting) symptoms despite optimal medical therapy, diabetes mellitus with symptoms, or critical limb ischemia (ischemic rest pain, ischemic ulceration, or gangrene).

Revascularization is *elective* in nondiabetic patients with intermittent claudication because 1) it does not improve coronary or cerebrovascular disease, the major cause of mortality, and consequently does not affect overall long-term survival; 2) the incidence of severe limb-threatening ischemia is relatively low because runoff is usually adequate; 3) perioperative complications of peripheral vascular operation, although infrequent, do occur; and 4) reocclusion may occur.

Revascularization in patients with ischemic rest pain or ischemic ulceration or in those with diabetes mellitus and progressive symptoms of intermittent claudication is *indicated* because 1) the incidence of limb loss is increased without revascularization, 2) operation may permit a lower anatomical level of amputation, and 3) the risks of the procedure are generally less than the risk of amputation.

Percutaneous intervention (balloon angioplasty and stents) is an effective alternative to surgical therapy in patients with proximal disease, short, partial occlusions, and good distal runoff. The ideal lesion for angioplasty is an iliac stenosis less than 5 cm. Advantages of angioplasty over operation include less morbidity, shorter convalescence, lower cost, and preservation of the saphenous vein for future use. Percutaneous transluminal angioplasty in aortic or iliac disease also may allow for an infrainguinal surgical procedure to be performed at reduced perioperative risk (compared with intra-abdominal aortic operation).

- For intermittent claudication, medical management is important as initial therapy, including antiplatelet agents, cessation of tobacco use, lipid reduction, foot care and protection, a walking program, and, in selected cases, cilostazol.
- Diabetes mellitus with progressive claudication symptoms and critical limb ischemia (ischemic rest pain, ischemic ulceration, and gangrene) are associated with an increased risk of limb loss in patients with lower extremity arterial occlusive disease. The presence of these features warrants an invasive approach (angiography followed by endovascular or surgical revascularization).

Cardiac Risk and Vascular Surgery

Patients with peripheral arterial disease (AAA, lower extremity arterial occlusive disease, and cerebrovascular disease) have an approximate 60% incidence of significant coronary artery disease (>70% stenosis of 1 or more epicardial coronary arteries). Up to 30% of patients have severe correctable 3-vessel coronary artery disease with reduced left ventricular function, the group most likely to benefit from coronary artery bypass grafting. Clinical markers that identify patients who are at increased risk for a perioperative cardiac event when undergoing vascular operation include age older than 70 years, angina, diabetes mellitus, ventricular ectopy, Q waves on electrocardiography, and a carotid bruit. If the preoperative clinical evaluation indicates that further noninvasive cardiac testing is indicated, pharmacologic stress (ie, dobutamine, dipyridamole, or adenosine) is usually performed because patients with intermittent claudication often cannot achieve an adequate double product during standard treadmill exercise. The presence of reversible defects (thallium-201 or sestamibi scintigraphy) or new regional wall motion abnormalities on stress echocardiography predicts an increased perioperative cardiac risk (30% and 53%, respectively). In contrast, the absence of perfusion abnormalities or stress-induced regional wall motion abnormalities predicts a perioperative cardiac risk of 3% and less than 1%, respectively. An assessment of resting left ventricular function alone, by either radionuclide angiography or echocardiography, is not predictive of perioperative cardiac risk during vascular operation.

• Clinical markers that identify patients who are at increased risk for a perioperative cardiac event when undergoing vascular operation include age older than 70 years, angina, diabetes mellitus, ventricular ectopy, pathologic Q waves on electrocardiography, and carotid bruit.
• An assessment of resting left ventricular function alone is not predictive of perioperative cardiac risk during vascular operation.

Acute Arterial Occlusion

The symptoms of acute arterial occlusion are sudden in onset (<5 hours) and include the "5 Ps": pain, pallor, paresthesia (numbness), poikilothermy (coldness), and absent pulse(s).

Features that suggest a *thrombotic* cause of acute arterial occlusion include previous occlusive disease in the involved limb, occlusive disease involving other extremities, acute aortic dissection, hematologic disease, arteritis, inflammatory bowel disease, neoplasm, and ergotism.

An *embolic* cause of acute arterial occlusion is suggested by the presence of cardiac disease (valvular, ischemic), atrial fibrillation, proximal aneurysm, or proximal atherosclerotic disease.

After confirmation by angiography, the initial therapeutic options for acute arterial occlusion include intra-arterial thrombolysis and surgical therapy (thromboembolectomy). If thrombolysis is the initial treatment, percutaneous treatment or surgical therapy is usually indicated to treat the underlying stenosis (if present) to improve long-term patency rates.

• The "5 Ps" suggestive of acute arterial occlusion include pain, pallor, paresthesia, poikilothermy (coldness), and absent pulse(s).

Peripheral Arterial Aneurysms

Because aneurysms are most commonly caused by atherosclerosis, they are more common in men 60 years or older. Coronary and carotid occlusive disease are frequent comorbid conditions. Other predisposing factors for aneurysmal disease include hypertension, familial tendency, connective tissue disease, trauma, infection, and inflammatory disease.

Most aneurysms are asymptomatic. Complications of aneurysms include embolization, pressure on surrounding structures, infection, and rupture. Aneurysms of certain arteries develop specific complications more often than other complications. For example, the most common complication of aortic aneurysms is rupture, whereas embolism is a more common complication of femoral and popliteal artery aneurysms.

An iliac artery aneurysm usually occurs in association with an AAA, but it may occur as an isolated finding. Iliac artery aneurysms

may cause atheroembolism, obstructive urologic symptoms, unexplained groin or perineal pain, or iliac vein obstruction. CT with intravenous contrast agent and MRI are the preferred diagnostic procedures. Surgical resection is indicated when the aneurysm is symptomatic or larger than 3 cm in diameter.

Thrombosis, venous obstruction, embolization, popliteal neuropathy, popliteal thrombophlebitis, rupture, and infection can complicate popliteal artery aneurysm. Popliteal artery aneurysms are bilateral in 50% of patients, and 40% of patients have 1 or more aneurysms at other sites, usually the abdominal aorta. The diagnosis is readily made with ultrasonography, but angiography is necessary before surgical treatment to evaluate the proximal and distal arterial circulation. When a popliteal aneurysm is diagnosed, operation is the treatment of choice to prevent serious thromboembolic complications.

• An iliac artery aneurysm usually occurs in association with an AAA, but it may occur as an isolated finding.
• Popliteal artery aneurysms are bilateral in 50% of patients, and 40% of patients have 1 or more aneurysms at other sites.

Uncommon Types of Arterial Occlusive Disease

The clinical features that suggest an uncommon type of peripheral arterial occlusive disease include young age, acute ischemia without a history of arterial occlusive disease, and involvement of the upper extremity or digits (Figure 25-10). Uncommon types of arterial occlusive disease include thromboangiitis obliterans, arteritis associated with connective tissue disease, giant cell arteritis (cranial and Takayasu disease), and arterial occlusive disease due to blunt trauma or arterial entrapment.

Thromboangiitis Obliterans (Buerger Disease)

The diagnostic clinical criteria for thromboangiitis obliterans (Buerger disease) are listed in Table 25-5. More definitive diagnosis of thromboangiitis obliterans requires angiography, which usually shows multiple, bilateral focal segments of stenosis or occlusion with normal

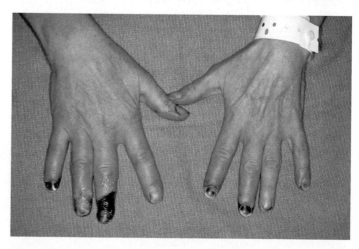

Figure 25-10. Patient with thromboangiitis obliterans has gangrene of the tips of multiple upper extremity digits.

proximal vessels. Treatment of thromboangiitis obliterans is the same as for other types of occlusive peripheral arterial disease, but particular emphasis is placed on the need for permanent abstinence from all forms of tobacco. Smoking cessation ameliorates the course of the disease but does not invariably stop further exacerbations. Abstinence from tobacco also substantially reduces the risk of ulcer formation and amputation, thus improving quality of life in patients with thromboangiitis obliterans. Because the arteries involved are small, arterial reconstruction for ischemia in patients with Buerger disease is technically challenging. Distal arterial reconstruction, if necessary, is indicated to prevent ischemic limb loss. Collateral artery bypass is an option when the main arteries are affected by the disease. A patent but diseased artery should be avoided as a target for reconstruction. Sympathectomy may be useful in severe digital ischemia with ulceration to control pain and to improve cutaneous blood flow. Therapeutic angiogenesis with phVEGF$_{165}$ gene transfer may be beneficial in patients with advanced Buerger disease that is unresponsive to standard medical or surgical treatment methods.

- Treatment of thromboangiitis obliterans is the same as for other types of occlusive peripheral arterial disease, but particular emphasis is placed on the need for permanent abstinence from all forms of tobacco.

Popliteal Artery Entrapment

Popliteal artery entrapment (PAE) is an uncommon congenital abnormality that is often overlooked clinically. PAE is important because repeated compression of the popliteal artery can lead to localized atherosclerosis, poststenotic dilatation, or thrombosis resulting in serious ischemia in the distal leg or foot. PAE occurs most often in young men, who may present with a complaint of intermittent claudication in the arch of the foot or calf. If the popliteal artery is not already occluded, the finding of reduced pedal pulses with sustained active plantar flexion should increase suspicion of the disorder.

PAE can occur by several mechanisms. The artery can be compressed because of its anomalous relationship to the medial head of the gastrocnemius muscle (looping around and under or through the muscle), by its displacement by an anomalous insertion of the plantaris muscle, or by passing beneath rather than behind the popliteal muscle.

The diagnosis of PAE can be made noninvasively with duplex ultrasonography, CT, and MRI. MRI is superior to ultrasonography and CT for defining the exact abnormality in PAE, with results similar to those with digital subtraction angiography. The combined morphologic and functional evaluation of the popliteal fossa makes MRI the investigation of choice in the management of young adults with intermittent claudication. MRI is particularly useful when the popliteal artery is occluded, in which situation ultrasonography and angiography are of limited value.

Angiographic findings in PAE include irregularity of the wall of the popliteal artery in an otherwise normal arterial tree, often associated with prestenotic or poststenotic dilatation. If the artery is still patent, medial displacement of the popliteal artery from its normal position in the popliteal space and popliteal artery compression with

Table 25-5 Clinical Criteria for Thromboangiitis Obliterans

Age	<40 years (often <30 years)
Sex	Males most often
Habits	Tobacco, cannabis use
History	Superficial phlebitis
	Claudication, arch or calf
	Raynaud phenomenon
	Absence of atherosclerotic risk factors other than smoking
Examination	Small arteries involved
	Upper extremity involved (positive Allen test)
	Infrapopliteal artery disease
Laboratory	Normal glucose, blood counts, sedimentation rate, lipids, & screening tests for connective tissue disease & hypercoagulable disorders
Radiography	No arterial calcification

extension of the knee and dorsiflexion of the foot are diagnostic angiographic findings. If the mechanism of compression is by the plantaris or popliteal muscle, the position of the artery may appear normal on angiography. If PAE has been diagnosed in 1 limb, the contralateral limb should be screened because bilateral disease occurs in more than 25% of patients.

The management of PAE depends on the clinical presentation and anatomical findings. Although the natural history of PAE is not well defined, surgery has been advocated to prevent progression of the disease from repetitive arterial trauma. Detection and treatment of PAE at an early stage appear to permit better long term results.

Thoracic Outlet Compression Syndrome

Compression of the subclavian artery in the thoracic outlet (thoracic outlet compression syndrome) can occur at several points, but the most common site of compression is in the costoclavicular space between the uppermost rib (cervical rib, or first rib) and the clavicle. If the patient is symptomatic, the presentation may be any 1 of the following: Raynaud phenomenon in 1 or more fingers of the ipsilateral hand, digital cyanosis or ulceration, and "claudication" of the arm or forearm. Occlusive arterial disease in the affected arm or hand is readily detected on examination of the arterial pulses and with the Allen test. Compression of the subclavian artery in the thoracic outlet can be determined by noting a decreased or absent pulse in the ipsilateral radial artery during performance of thoracic outlet maneuvers. Venous compression resulting in edema and deep venous thrombosis, and neurologic compression resulting in paresthesias or pain, also can occur. The diagnosis is confirmed with duplex ultrasonography, magnetic resonance angiography, or angiography, with the involved arm in the neutral and hyperabducted position.

The optimal therapy for thoracic outlet compression is controversial. In general, treatment depends on the severity of symptoms. In minimally symptomatic patients, physical therapy and education regarding the relationship of arm and body position to arterial compression may be sufficient treatment. In patients who have more severe symptoms, aneurysm formation, distal embolization, or digital ischemia, surgical treatment is indicated. Surgical resection of the first thoracic or cervical rib is the most effective way to relieve the arterial compression. In some cases, thrombectomy and reconstruction of the subclavian artery in patients with subclavian artery stenosis, thrombosis, or occlusion are also indicated. Sympathectomy may be used as an adjunctive surgical procedure when there is extensive digital or hand ischemia. Stent placement in residual subclavian artery stenoses has been successful but needs to be performed after surgical decompression of the costoclavicular space to decrease the likelihood of recurrent symptoms or damage to the stent.

It is important to remember that all of the connective tissue disorders and giant cell arteritides can involve peripheral arteries and that symptoms of peripheral arterial involvement may dominate the clinical picture. Other than the medical measures already discussed for ischemic limbs, therapy is directed mainly at the underlying disease. Only after the inflammatory process is controlled should surgical revascularization or endovascular therapy of chronically ischemic extremities be performed.

Heparin-Induced Thrombocytopenia

Heparin-induced thrombocytopenia (HIT) affects between 5% and 10% of patients who receive heparin therapy, but the incidence of arterial or venous thrombosis is less than 1% to 2%. HIT (type II) typically occurs 5 to 14 days after heparin exposure and is associated with arterial thrombosis (arterial occlusion, ischemic strokes, myocardial infarction) and venous thrombosis (pulmonary embolism, phlegmasia cerulea dolens [venous gangrene], and sagittal sinus thrombosis) (Figure 25-11). The diagnosis of HIT is primarily clinical (occurrence of thrombocytopenia during heparin therapy, resolution of thrombocytopenia when heparin therapy is discontinued, and exclusion of other causes of thrombocytopenia) and can be confirmed by demonstration in vitro of a heparin-dependent platelet antibody. Treatment of HIT includes discontinuation of all forms of heparin exposure (subcutaneous, intravenous, or heparin flushes and heparin-coated catheters), including low-molecular-weight

heparins. The current anticoagulant of choice for HIT is a direct thrombin inhibitor, that is, lepirudin or argatroban.

Vasospastic Disorders

Vasospastic disorders are characterized by episodic color changes of the skin resulting from intermittent spasm of the small arteries and arterioles of the skin and digits. Vasospastic disorders are important because they frequently are a clue to another underlying disorder such as arterial occlusive disease, connective tissue disorders, neurologic disorders, or endocrine disease. Vasospastic disorders also can appear as side effects of drug therapy, specifically of ergot preparations, estrogen replacement therapy, and certain β-blockers.

Raynaud Phenomenon

When Raynaud phenomenon is present, several clinical features can help to differentiate primary Raynaud disease from secondary Raynaud phenomenon (Table 25-6).

Primary Raynaud disease is more common in women than men and usually has its onset before age 40 years. Episodes are characterized by triphasic color changes (white, blue, then red). Symptoms are usually bilateral and often symmetric and precipitated by cold exposure or emotion. Ischemic or gangrenous changes are not present. The absence of any causal condition and the presence of symptoms for at least 2 years are required for diagnosis. Raynaud disease is generally a benign condition; treatment emphasizes protection from cold exposure and other vasoconstrictive influences. Patients with severe symptoms not controlled by local measures may benefit from a trial of a calcium-channel blocker or an α_1-adrenergic receptor antagonist.

Secondary Raynaud phenomenon affects men more often than women, and in most patients the onset is after age 40 years. It is usually unilateral or asymmetric at onset. Associated pulse deficits, ischemic changes, and systemic signs and symptoms are often present. Identification of the underlying cause is basic to appropriate treatment for secondary Raynaud phenomenon.

The initial laboratory evaluation in a patient with Raynaud phenomenon includes a complete blood count, determination of the erythrocyte sedimentation rate, urinalysis, serum protein electrophoresis, antinuclear antibody test, tests for cryoglobulin, cryofibrinogen, and cold agglutinins, and chest radiography to detect disorders not identified by the medical history and physical examination.

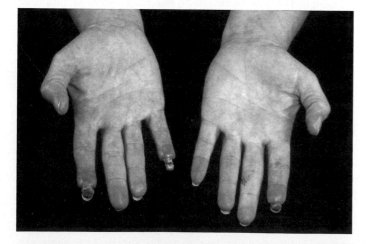

Figure 25-11. Multiple gangrenous upper extremity digits in a patient with heparin-induced thrombocytopenia.

Table 25-6 Characteristic Clinical Features of Primary and Secondary Raynaud Phenomenon

	Primary	Secondary
Age at onset, y	<40	>40
Sex	Women	Men
Bilateral	+	+/-
Symmetric	+	+/-
Toes involved	+	-
Ischemic changes	-	+
Systemic manifestations	-	+

- Primary Raynaud disease is a benign condition more common in women than men, and its onset is usually before age 40 years.
- Secondary Raynaud phenomenon affects men more often than women, and in most patients the onset is after age 40 years.

Livedo Reticularis

Spasm or occlusion of dermal arterioles causes livedo reticularis, the bluish mottling of the skin in a lacy, reticular pattern. Primary livedo reticularis is idiopathic and not associated with an identifiable underlying disorder. Secondary livedo reticularis is suggested by an abrupt, severe onset of symptoms, ischemic changes, and systemic symptoms. Most commonly, it is the result of embolism of atheromatous debris from thrombus within a proximal aneurysm or from proximal atheromatous plaques. The appearance of livedo reticularis in a patient older than 50 years should suggest the possibility of atheroembolism. Other causes of secondary livedo reticularis include connective tissue disease, vasculitis, myeloproliferative disorders, dysproteinemias, reflex sympathetic dystrophy, cold injury, and as a side effect of amantadine hydrochloride therapy.

- The appearance of livedo reticularis in a patient older than 50 years should suggest the possibility of atheroembolism.

Chronic Pernio

Chronic pernio is a vasospastic disorder characterized by sensitivity to cold in patients (usually women) with a past history of cold injury. Chronic pernio presents with symmetric blueness of the toes in the autumn and resolution of the discoloration in the spring (Figure 25-12). Without treatment, the cyanosis may be accompanied by blistering of the skin of the affected toes. The cyanosis can often be relieved in a few days after instituting treatment with an α_1-adrenergic receptor antagonist, which can then be used to prevent recurrence.

Erythromelalgia

Erythromelalgia is the occurrence of red, hot, painful, burning extremity digits on exposure to warm temperatures or after exercise. It is not a vasospastic disorder but is associated with color change of the skin. It may be primary (idiopathic) or be due to an underlying disorder, most commonly myeloproliferative disorders (eg, polycythemia rubra vera), diabetes mellitus, or small fiber neuropathy. Treatment of the primary form includes avoidance of exposure to warm temperatures, aspirin, and a nonselective β-blocker, which is helpful in some patients. In persons with secondary erythromelalgia, treatment of the underlying disorder usually relieves the symptoms.

Edema

Lower extremity edema is commonly encountered in clinical practice. Aside from edema due to underlying cardiac disease, other causes of regional edema usually can be identified from characteristic clinical features (Table 25-7).

Lymphedema

Lymphedema can be primary (idiopathic) or due to an underlying disorder. Primary lymphedema (lymphedema praecox) usually affects young women (9 times more frequently than men) and begins before the age of 40 years (often before age 20 years). In women, the symptoms often first appear at the time of menarche or with the first pregnancy. Edema is bilateral in about half the cases. The initial evaluation in a young woman with lymphedema should include a complete history and physical examination (including pelvic examination and Papanicolaou smear) and CT of the abdomen and pelvis to exclude a neoplastic cause of lymphatic obstruction.

- In a healthy young woman with painless progressive swelling of 1 or both lower extremities in a pattern consistent with lymph edema, lymphedema praecox is the most likely diagnosis.

Secondary lymphedema is broadly classified into obstructive (postsurgical, postradiation, neoplastic) and inflammatory (infectious) types. Obstructive lymphedema due to neoplasm typically begins after the age of 40 years and is due to pelvic neoplasm or non-Hodgkin lymphoma. The most frequent cause in men is prostate cancer.

- In a man older than 60 years with painless progressive swelling of 1 leg, the diagnosis is prostate cancer until proved otherwise.

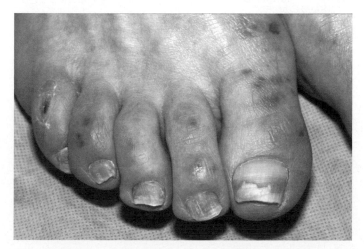

Figure 25-12. Characteristic Lesions of Chronic Pernio.

Table 25-7 Differential Diagnosis of Regional Types of Edema

Feature	Venous	Lymphedema	Lipedema
Bilateral	Occasional	+/-	Always
Foot involved	+	+	0
Toes involved	0	+	0
Thickened skin	0	+	0
Stasis changes	+	0	0

Inflammatory (infectious) lymphedema occurs as a result of chronic or recurring lymphangitis or cellulitis (or both). The portal of entry for infection is usually dermatophytosis (tinea pedis), which is often overlooked. The diagnosis of lymphedema can be confirmed noninvasively with lymphoscintigraphy.

Medical management of lymphedema includes edema reduction therapy, followed by daily use of custom-fitted graduated compression (usually 40-50 mm Hg compression) elastic support. Manual lymphatic drainage is a type of massage used in combination with skin care, support and compression therapy, and exercise in the management of lymphedema. A combined multimethod approach may substantially reduce excess limb volume and improve quality of life. Antifungal treatment is essential if dermatophytosis is present. Weight reduction in obese patients is also beneficial. Surgical treatment of lymphedema (lymphaticovenous anastomosis, lymphedema reduction) is indicated in highly selected patients.

Venous Disease

Deep vein thrombosis (DVT) is the third most common cardiovascular disease, after acute coronary syndromes and stroke. Approximately 1 in 1,000 individuals is affected by venous thromboembolism each year, and more than 200,000 new cases occur in the United States annually. Of these, 30% of patients die within 30 days; one-fifth suffer sudden death due to pulmonary embolism. The Virchow triad of stasis, hypercoagulability, and vascular endothelial damage contributes in varying degrees to the development of DVT. Independent risk factors for venous thromboembolism include increasing age, male sex, surgery, trauma, hospital or nursing home confinement, malignancy, neurologic disease with extremity paresis, central venous catheter or transvenous pacemaker, prior superficial vein thrombosis, varicose veins, and liver disease; among women, additional risk factors include pregnancy, oral contraceptive use, and hormone replacement therapy. A major clinical risk factor (immobility, trauma, or recent operation) is present in approximately half of patients with confirmed DVT. A family history of thrombophilia is important, because there are several identifiable and treatable inherited disorders of coagulation.

Causes of recurrent DVT are listed in Table 25-8.

Protein C Deficiency

Protein C deficiency is characterized by recurrent venous thrombosis and is inherited as an autosomal dominant trait. Episodes of thrombosis are generally spontaneous and usually begin before the age of 30 years. Protein C levels are about 50% of normal. Treatment is lifelong oral anticoagulation, and there is a potential risk of warfarin necrosis. Acquired protein C deficiency can develop in patients with liver disease or disseminated intravascular coagulation, or it can occur postoperatively. Purpura fulminans occurs in persons homozygous for this condition.

Protein S Deficiency

Protein S deficiency also causes recurrent venous thrombosis and is inherited as an autosomal dominant trait. Onset of episodes usually begins before the age of 35 years, and the episodes are generally spon-

taneous. Protein S levels are about 50% of normal. Treatment is lifelong oral anticoagulation, and there is no risk of warfarin necrosis. Acquired protein S deficiency can occur in association with the nephrotic syndrome, warfarin therapy, pregnancy, antiphospholipid antibody syndrome, and disseminated intravascular coagulation.

Antithrombin III Deficiency

Antithrombin III deficiency, characterized by recurrent venous and arterial thrombosis, is also inherited as an autosomal dominant trait. The first thrombotic episode is usually after age 20 years and is usually provoked by infection, trauma, operation, or pregnancy. Antithrombin III levels are usually 40% to 60% of normal. Treatment is lifelong oral anticoagulation. An acquired form of antithrombin III deficiency can occur in patients with nephrotic syndrome or severe liver disease and in those receiving estrogen therapy.

Factor V (Leiden) Mutation

Factor V Leiden mutation, the genetic defect underlying resistance to activated protein C, is the most common risk factor for venous thrombosis. Heterozygous carriers of a mutation in factor V (factor V Leiden) are at increased risk for venous thrombosis (ie, activated protein C resistance). This mutation may occur in 5% to 10% of the general population and may account for as many as 50% of patients with recurrent venous thromboembolism. Heterozygous carriers of factor V mutation have an 8-fold increased risk of venous thromboembolism, whereas homozygous carriers have an 80-fold increased risk. Of interest, in patients who have had myocardial infarction without significant coronary artery stenosis, the prevalence of factor V Leiden is considerably higher than in controls, suggesting that factor V Leiden mutation is an independent risk factor for myocardial infarction. Factor V Leiden mutation also increases the risk of cerebrovascular accident and paradoxic embolism (in patients with a patent foramen ovale).

Table 25-8 Causes of Recurrent Deep Vein Thrombosis

Primary
    Idiopathic
Secondary
    Neoplasm
    Connective tissue disease
    Inflammatory bowel disease
    Myeloproliferative disorder
    Thromboangiitis obliterans
    Oral contraceptives
Coagulation disorders
    Antithrombin III deficiency
    Protein C deficiency
    Protein S deficiency
    Activated protein C resistance
    Prothrombin 20210 G-A mutation
    Antiphospholipid antibody syndrome
    Hyperhomocystinemia

Prothrombin 20210 G-A Mutation

A mutation in the prothrombin gene has been identified in some patients with venous thromboembolism. The mechanism whereby this abnormality might cause thrombosis has been assumed to be an increase in prothrombin levels. Available data indicate that this mutation may be associated with an increased risk of venous thrombosis but not arterial thrombosis (with a possible exception for myocardial infarction).

Hyperhomocysteinemia

Hyperhomocysteinemia, a disorder of methionine metabolism, is a risk factor for premature atherosclerosis and recurrent DVT. Inherited forms (disorders of transsulfuration and remethylation) and acquired forms (chronic renal failure, organ transplantation, acute lymphoblastic leukemia, psoriasis, vitamin deficiencies [vitamins B_6 and B_{12} and folate], and medications [phenytoin, carbamazepine, theophylline]) occur. Hyperhomocysteinemia is an independent risk factor for stroke, coronary artery disease, peripheral arterial disease, and DVT. A normal plasma homocysteine level is 5 to 15 mcmol/L. Folic acid at a dosage of 0.4 mg daily reduces homocysteine levels, but higher doses of folate are required in patients with chronic renal failure. Prospective treatment trials are lacking. Screening for hyperhomocysteinemia should be considered in patients with premature atherosclerotic disease, a strong family history of premature atherosclerosis, idiopathic DVT, chronic renal failure, systemic lupus erythematosus, or severe psoriasis and in organ transplant recipients.

Clinical Evaluation of DVT

Symptoms of DVT include extremity pain, redness, and swelling, although many patients may be asymptomatic. Signs of DVT include pitting edema, warmth, erythema, tenderness, and a dilated superficial venous pattern in the involved extremity. Although leg veins are the most common location of DVT, upper extremity DVT may occur, especially in patients with a central venous line or transvenous permanent pacemaker. Extensive DVT involving an entire extremity may lead to venous gangrene (phlegmasia cerulea dolens), most commonly in association with an underlying malignancy. The clinical diagnosis of DVT is neither sensitive (60%-80%) nor specific (30%-72%), and three-fourths of patients who present with suspected acute DVT have other causes of leg pain such as cellulitis, leg trauma, muscular tear or rupture, postphlebitic syndrome, or Baker cysts. Therefore, objective noninvasive tests are required to establish a diagnosis of DVT.

Important historical features in a patient with DVT which should increase suspicion of a hypercoagulable disorder include spontaneous event, unusual site (mesenteric or cerebral), young age, positive family history, and recurrent events.

Although venography is the reference standard for the diagnosis of DVT and is highly accurate for both proximal and calf DVT, it is invasive, expensive, and technically inadequate in about 10% of patients, and it may precipitate a DVT in approximately 3% of patients. Noninvasive tests (duplex ultrasonography, magnetic resonance venography) for diagnosing DVT are accurate for proximal DVT but not calf vein thrombosis. If the results of noninvasive testing

are nondiagnostic or are discordant with the clinical assessment, venography is indicated.

- Noninvasive tests for diagnosing DVT are accurate for proximal DVT but not calf vein thrombosis.
- If the results of noninvasive testing are nondiagnostic or are discordant with the clinical assessment, venography is indicated.

Continuous-Wave Doppler

Doppler assessment at the bedside, which evaluates each limb systematically for spontaneous venous flow, phasic flow with respiration, augmentation with distal compression, and venous competence with the Valsalva maneuver and proximal compression, is useful in the diagnosis of proximal DVT. Continuous-wave Doppler is relatively insensitive to calf vein thrombosis.

Impedance Plethysmography and Strain-Gauge Outflow Plethysmography

Impedance plethysmography and strain-gauge outflow plethysmography both reliably detect occlusive thrombi in the proximal veins (popliteal, femoral, and iliac veins) but are less reliable for detecting nonocclusive thrombi and are insensitive for calf DVT. False-positive results do occur (extrinsic venous obstruction, increased central venous pressure). The reported sensitivity of impedance plethysmography for proximal DVT ranges from 70% to 90%.

Compression Ultrasonography

Compression ultrasonography (venous noncompressibility is diagnostic of DVT; venous compressibility excludes DVT) is highly sensitive and specific for detecting proximal DVT. It is currently the most accurate noninvasive test for the diagnosis of a first symptomatic proximal DVT. Compression ultrasonography is less accurate for symptomatic patients with isolated calf vein thrombosis. It should be noted that both impedance plethysmography and compression ultrasonography have decreased sensitivity when used to evaluate asymptomatic patients (22% and 58%, respectively). Withholding anticoagulant therapy in symptomatic patients with suspected DVT who have normal results on serial compression ultrasonography or impedance plethysmography is safe.

D Dimer

Plasma levels of D dimer, a product of fibrin degradation, are increased in patients with acute DVT. D Dimer functions as an exclusionary test in patients with suspected DVT. For example, in a patient with both a negative objective test (compression ultrasonography or impedance plethysmography) and normal results of D dimer test, a diagnosis of DVT becomes highly unlikely. D Dimer is also useful to exclude DVT in patients with a low clinical suspicion of DVT. D Dimer may also be useful at the end of therapy to ascertain which patients might benefit from a more prolonged course of anticoagulation.

Evaluation of Idiopathic DVT

In a patient with idiopathic DVT, a clinical evaluation that includes a complete history and physical examination, routine laboratory testing (hematology group with differential count, chemistry profile, urinalysis, fecal hemoglobin test), and chest radiography seems to be appropriate for detecting cancer. Mammography, pelvic examination, and Papanicolaou smear should be included in a woman with idiopathic DVT. Additional testing should be guided by any abnormalities detected by the initial clinical evaluation.

Treatment of DVT

Treatment options for acute DVT include anticoagulant therapy (heparin, warfarin), thrombolytic therapy, vena cava filter, and surgical thrombectomy.

Initial inpatient treatment of DVT is with low-molecular-weight heparin (LMWH) rather than unfractionated heparin whenever possible. Either unfractionated heparin or LMWH is appropriate for the initial treatment of pulmonary embolism. Outpatient treatment of DVT, and possibly pulmonary embolism, with LMWH is safe and cost-effective for carefully selected patients and should be considered if the required support services are in place.

Use of heparin is discontinued when the internal normalized ratio is more than 2.0. The optimal duration of warfarin anticoagulation for a first episode of DVT is controversial. Available data suggest that it is necessary to tailor the duration of anticoagulation individually according to the topography of DVT and the presence of continuing risk factors. For proximal DVT, a short course seems sufficient in patients with temporary risk factors (6 months), and a longer course (more than 6 months) is recommended for patients with continuing risk factors or idiopathic DVT. Compression stockings should be used routinely to prevent postthrombotic syndrome, beginning within 1 month of diagnosis of proximal DVT and continuing for a minimum of 1 year after diagnosis.

The inherited or acquired hypercoagulable states can be divided into those that are common and associated with a modest risk of recurrent DVT (ie, isolated factor V Leiden or 20210 G-A prothrombin gene mutation) and those that are uncommon but associated with a high risk of recurrence (ie, antithrombin III, protein C or S deficiencies, and antiphospholipid antibodies). The presence of 1 of the latter abnormalities favors more prolonged anticoagulant therapy. For patients with a high risk of recurrent DVT, there is a paucity of evidence, particularly for patients with thrombophilia, and randomized controlled trials in this population are required. An assessment of low- or fixed-dose oral anticoagulation is also needed to reduce hemorrhagic complications.

When problems with anticoagulation (ie, contraindications, complications, failed effect, or unacceptable risk) are present, insertion of a vena cava filter may be indicated. Vena cava filters are also indicated for prophylactic use in patients at high risk of pulmonary embolism and as an adjunct to an urgent surgical procedure in the patient with acute DVT. Complications of vena cava filters include pulmonary embolism (1%-4%), caval thrombus (19%-24%), penetration of the cava (9%), filter migration (6%), fracture (2%), and lower extremity edema (25%).

Thrombolytic therapy may be indicated when DVT is extensive, with thrombosis extending into the iliac veins or inferior vena cava, or in upper extremity DVT. Thrombolytic therapy has the best results when initiated less than 7 days after the onset of DVT, and it may decrease the incidence of the postphlebitic syndrome by salvaging venous valve function. Catheter-directed delivery of the thrombolytic agent directly into the thrombus is used. Surgical thrombectomy is reserved for patients with limb-threatening DVT (ie, phlegmasia cerulea dolens).

Reduction of limb edema, initially by leg elevation and woven elastic (Ace) wrapping, is an integral part of the initial therapy of acute DVT. When edema has been reduced, a graduated compression elastic support stocking is required to both control edema and prevent development of the postphlebitic (postthrombotic) syndrome. A 30- to 40-mm Hg graduated elastic support garment is usually sufficient. Customized, graduated compression stockings significantly reduce the occurrence of the postphlebitic syndrome in patients with a first episode of proximal DVT.

Postphlebitic Syndrome

Chronic venous insufficiency (postphlebitic syndrome) is a common disorder that results in significant morbidity. In approximately 30% of patients with DVT, postphlebitic syndrome develops within 20 years after the initial DVT. Chronic venous insufficiency most commonly results in swelling, pain, fatigue, and heaviness in the involved extremity. Secondary varicose vein formation, venous stasis changes, and cutaneous ulceration can occur in untreated cases (Figure 25-13). Venous claudication in the setting of prior iliofemoral or vena cava thrombosis causes discomfort, fullness, tiredness, and aching of the extremity during exercise. In contrast to patients with intermittent claudication, patients with venous claudication must sit down and elevate the extremity for relief. Postphlebitic syndrome due to chronic deep venous incompetence is frequently misdiagnosed as recurrent DVT. The correct diagnosis is suggested by the clinical

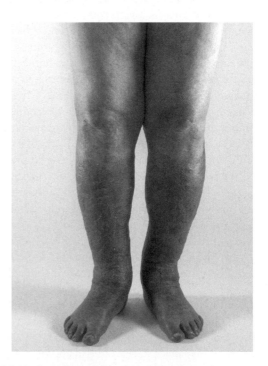

Figure 25-13. A patient with severe deep venous incompetence and perforator vein incompetence with severe venous stasis changes and indurated cellulitis.

findings of chronic venous insufficiency (edema, venous stasis changes, secondary varicose vein formation) and confirmed by exclusion of new thrombus formation by objective testing (eg, compression ultrasonography). "Side-by-side" comparison of current ultrasonographic studies with previous ultrasonographic or venographic studies is invaluable for documenting new venous thrombosis.

Treatment of postphlebitic syndrome includes initial aggressive efforts at edema reduction with woven elastic (Ace) wrapping and pumping devices until edema is reduced, followed by fitting with a graduated compression elastic support stocking (30-40 mm Hg). Periodic leg elevation during the day and weight reduction in obese patients are also beneficial.

- The treatment of postphlebitic syndrome includes initial aggressive efforts at edema reduction with woven elastic (Ace) wrapping and pumping devices until edema is reduced, followed by fitting with a graduated compression elastic support stocking (30-40 mm Hg).
- Periodic leg elevation during the day and weight reduction in obese patients are also beneficial.

Leg Ulcer

The cause of lower extremity ulceration usually can be determined with clinical examination. Clinical features of the four most common types of leg ulcer are summarized in Table 25-9.

Table 25-9 Clinical Features of the 4 Most Common Types of Leg Ulcer

	Type of Ulcer			
Feature	Venous	Arterial	Arteriolar	Neurotrophic
Onset	Trauma +/-	Trauma	Spontaneous	Trauma
Course	Chronic	Progressive	Progressive	Progressive
Pain	No (unless infected)	Yes	Yes	No
Location	Medial aspect of leg	Toe, heel, foot	Lateral, posterior aspect of leg	Plantar
Surrounding skin	Stasis changes	Atrophic	Normal	Callous
Ulcer edges	Shaggy	Discrete	Serpiginous	Discrete
Ulcer base	Healthy	Eschar, pale	Eschar, pale	Healthy or pale

Vascular Diseases Pharmacy Review
Kevin W. Odell, PharmD

Drug	Dosage	Toxic/Adverse Effects	Comments
Warfarin	Patient-specific	Bleeding, skin necrosis in patients who have protein C deficiency, purple toe syndrome, osteoporosis, alopecia, rash	Anticoagulant effect reversible with vitamin K 2.5-5 mg orally or fresh frozen plasma Lab monitor: PT, INR Pregnancy category X
Aspirin	81-325 mg once daily	Bleeding, hypoglycemia (high doses), dyspepsia, gastric ulcers, dysgeusia, hepatotoxicity (rare), urticaria, rash	Lab monitor: bleeding time Use with caution in children & teens with viral infections (risk of Reye syndrome) Use with caution in patients with asthma (risk of bronchospasm)
Clopidogrel	75 mg once daily	Bleeding, rash, urticaria, edema, hypertension, gastrointestinal upset, increased liver function values, rare decrease in platelets, leukocytes, & hemoglobin	Lab monitor: platelet aggregation if suspected adverse effects Rare cases of thrombotic thrombocytopenic purpura have been reported with use
Pentoxifylline	400 mg 3 times daily with meals	Bleeding, dizziness, headache, dyspepsia, GI bleed, nausea & vomiting, rash, brittle fingernails, leukopenia (rare)	Decrease dose to twice daily if GI or CNS side effects Consider discontinuing if GI or CNS side effects persist
Cilostazol	100 mg twice daily	Palpitations, tachycardia, dizziness, vertigo, headache, diarrhea, rash	No effect on PT, INR, or bleeding time
Heparin	Dose usually based on weight	Bleeding, thrombocytopenia, skin necrosis, disseminated intravascular coagulation, erythematous plaques, alopecia, osteoporosis	Lab monitor: aPTT, platelet counts Anticoagulant effect reversible with protamine

Low-molecular-weight heparins
  Dalteparin
  Enoxaparin
  Tinzaparin
	Once or twice daily subcutaneously based on weight or condition	Bleeding, pain or bruising at injection site, osteoporosis, rash	Lab monitor: antifactor Xa activity
			Anticoagulant effect partially reversible with protamine
			Use with caution in patients with history of heparin-induced thrombocytopenia

Fondaparinux	Once daily subcutaneously based on weight or condition	Bleeding, pain or bruising, rash, pruritus at injection site, fever, anemia	Lab monitor: antifactor Xa activity Recombinant factor VIIa reverses anticoagulant effect

Abbreviations: aPTT, activated partial thromboplastin time; CNS, central nervous system; GI, gastrointestinal; INR, international normalized ratio; Lab, laboratory; PT, prothrombin time.

Questions

Multiple Choice (choose the best answer)

1. A 61-year-old man complains of right leg tiredness that has been present for the past 3 months. It occurs when he walks rapidly for approximately 3 blocks. He has no other complaints. He has modified hyperlipidemia and modified systemic hypertension. Medications include aspirin 81 mg daily, simvastatin 40 mg at bedtime, and lisinopril 10 mg daily. He quit smoking 5 years ago (45 pack-year history). On physical examination the blood pressure is 143/84 mm Hg, and other results are unremarkable. Resting ankle to brachial systolic pressure index is (right/left) 0.7/0.9. What is the next most appropriate step in the management of this patient?

    a. Increase aspirin dose to 325 mg daily.
    b. Obtain an MR angiogram of the lower extremities.
    c. Begin therapy with cilostazol 100 mg twice daily.
    d. Initiate a walking program for intermittent claudication.
    e. Obtain a CT scan of the lumbosacral spine.

2. A 68-year-old woman is brought to the emergency department after the sudden development of severe chest pain followed by a syncopal spell. On initial examination, blood pressure is 82/35 mm Hg and pulse rate is 130 beats per minute and regular. Heart sounds are distant, jugular venous distention is present, and there are bilateral moist rales at the lung bases. Portable chest radiography shows moderate cardiomegaly and interstitial edema. Emergency transthoracic echocardiography shows a moderate pericardial effusion and findings of cardiac tamponade. There is moderate to severe aortic regurgitation, and the ascending aorta is 4.9 cm in diameter. What is the next most appropriate step in the management of this patient?

    a. CT of the chest
    b. Coronary angiography
    c. Echocardiography-guided pericardiocentesis
    d. Emergency cardiac surgery
    e. Bedside transesophageal echocardiography

3. A 70-year-old woman with acute ST-segment elevation myocardial infarction (anterior location, ejection fraction by transthoracic echocardiography is 52%) underwent emergency percutaneous coronary intervention. The next morning she has worsening hypertension and discoloration of multiple toes on each foot; the results of the rest of the examination are unchanged. On hematologic testing, leukocytosis and increased serum creatinine level (2.3 mg/dL) are found. Troponin-T level is increased, but the creatine kinase-MB level is trending downward. All of the following are indicated in the management of this patient *except*:

    a. Provide foot protection and keep legs level or dependent.
    b. Perform noninvasive imaging of the thoracic and abdominal aorta.

    c. Initiate anticoagulation therapy with warfarin for a minimum of 3 months.
    d. Determine ankle to brachial systolic pressure indices.
    e. Discontinue the use of the angiotensin-converting enzyme inhibitor.

4. A 48-year-old woman complains of episodic color changes of the long finger on the right hand and first and fifth fingers of the left hand, present for the past 2 months. The episodes have been worse since winter began. She also complains of progressive dyspnea on exertion and early satiety. The patient could be expected to have any of the following conditions *except*:

    a. Primary pulmonary hypertension
    b. Scleroderma
    c. Hypothyroidism
    d. Ehlers-Danlos syndrome
    e. Dermatomyositis

5. A 72-year-old man presents for an annual examination. He complains of new right groin pain that is intermittent, but he otherwise feels well. He has a history of chronic systemic hypertension and chronic obstructive pulmonary disease (he discontinued tobacco use 10 years earlier —55 pack-years). He is relatively inactive because of severe arthritis of the left hip and right knee. On physical examination, blood pressure is 135/85 mm Hg and there is a prominent pulsation in the mid abdomen; results of the examination are otherwise normal. Ultrasonography of the abdomen and pelvis shows a 4.9-cm abdominal aortic aneurysm and bilateral iliac artery aneurysms (4.2 cm diameter on the right, 3.8 cm on the left). What is the next most appropriate step in the management of this patient?

    a. Initiate therapy with a β-adrenergic blocker.
    b. Repeat ultrasonography in 3 months.
    c. Obtain a vascular surgical consultation.
    d. Obtain a CT angiogram of the abdomen.
    e. Perform pharmacologic stress testing (ie, dobutamine echocardiography).

6. A 61-year-old woman presents to a large tertiary-care facility complaining of a swollen and painful left calf. This developed after she had flown from California to Minnesota on a nonstop flight. On examination, the left calf is warm and slightly erythematous and there is prominence of the superficial veins below the knee. Results of the examination are otherwise normal. Ultrasonography shows an acute-appearing thrombus within the left superficial femoral vein. What is the most appropriate next step in the initial management of this patient?

    a. Bed rest, leg elevation, heat, and nonsteroidal anti-inflammatory drug

b. Outpatient therapy with low-molecular-weight heparin concurrent with warfarin

c. Inpatient intravenous unfractionated heparin

d. Inpatient low-molecular-weight heparin

e. Warfarin 5 mg daily until the international normalized ratio is 2.0 to 3.0

7. An 83-year-old man comes to your office complaining of a swollen left leg. This has been getting progressively worse during the prior 4 months. The swelling improves slightly overnight. There is no pain and no prior history of trauma or infection. On physical examination, grade 2 edema involving the left thigh, calf, foot, and toes is found. Ultrasonography of the left lower extremity veins is negative for deep vein thrombosis. What is the next most appropriate step in the management of this patient?

a. MRI of the left lower extremity

b. Ultrasonography of the pelvis

c. Lymphoscintigraphy and determination of the serum prostate-specific antigen level

d. A knee-high compression stocking (20-30 mm Hg)

e. CT of the abdomen and pelvis

Answers

1.   Answer d.

The diagnosis of intermittent claudication is often apparent from the clinical history and physical examination and can be verified with noninvasive testing (ankle to brachial systolic pressure index before and after exercise). This patient's history is compatible with intermittent claudication, and resting ankle to brachial indices are mildly to moderately abnormal on the right. The patient is already receiving aspirin, and a dose increase is not likely to be beneficial. MR angiography is not warranted to establish the diagnosis, and surgery is not currently indicated. CT of the lumbosacral spine is useful to evaluate for spinal stenosis (pseudoclaudication), but this patient's history is not suggestive of spinal stenosis. A walking program for intermittent claudication is very effective if performed regularly (≥4 days weekly) over a 3- to 4-month period. Cilostazol may be indicated after an initial trial of a walking program if exercise training is of insufficient benefit.

2.   Answer d.

The clinical presentation of sudden and severe chest pain suggests an acute aortic event (eg, aortic dissection, aortic intramural hematoma, penetrating aortic ulcer). When syncope occurs in association with acute aortic dissection, it is usually due to hemopericardium and cardiac tamponade. The transthoracic echocardiogram is highly suggestive of an acute aortic event involving the ascending aorta, which warrants emergency cardiac surgery. Intraoperative transesophageal echocardiography can be performed during preparation for surgery to verify the diagnosis and provide additional surgical information. CT of the chest is not indicated in this highly unstable patient with an acute aortic event because the delay in diagnosis would increase mortality. Echocardiography-guided pericardiocentesis should be avoided in cardiac tamponade complicating aortic dissection. Relief of tamponade may lead to a rapid increase in systemic pressure and extension of the dissecting process. Coronary angiography, with its inherent risks and delays, is associated with increased mortality and is not indicated.

3.   Answer c.

Clinical features of atheroembolism include livedo reticularis, multiple blue toes, systemic hypertension, renal insufficiency, leukocytosis, transient eosinophilia, and an increased erythrocyte sedimentation rate. Proximal atherosclerosis and aneurysmal disease are the source of embolic material, and episodes can occur spontaneously or be provoked with medication (eg, warfarin, thrombolytic therapy), invasive angiographic procedures, cardiac surgery, or trauma. Initial management includes foot care and protection of the ischemic extremity(s), keeping the legs level or dependent, and initiation of therapy with an antiplatelet agent, a statin, and intravenous heparin. Subsequent tests usually include ankle to brachial indices and noninvasive evaluation of the thoracic and abdominal aorta for the source of embolism. Discontinuing therapy with an angiotensin-converting enzyme inhibitor is warranted given progressive acute renal failure. Currently, there is no indication for warfarin anticoagulation; in fact, it may precipitate atheroembolism.

4.   Answer d.

Features suggestive of secondary Raynaud phenomenon include male sex, onset after 40 years of age, asymmetric symptoms, pulse deficits, ischemic changes, and systemic symptoms. The differential diagnosis of secondary Raynaud phenomenon is extensive and includes occupation-related injury (eg, pneumatic hammer disease, occupational arterial occlusive disease of the hand, occupational acro-osteolysis, vasospasm of typists and pianists), neurologic conditions (eg, Buerger disease, postembolic or thrombotic arterial occlusion), and miscellaneous conditions (eg, scleroderma, systemic lupus erythematosus, rheumatoid arthritis, dermatomyositis, Fabry disease, paroxysmal nocturnal hemoglobinuria, cold agglutinins or cryoglobulinemia, primary pulmonary hypertension, myxedema, certain neoplasms, having had combination chemotherapy for testicular cancer, hepatitis B antigenemia, pheochromocytoma, and ergotism). Ehlers-Danlos syndrome is not known to be a cause of secondary Raynaud phenomenon.

5.   Answer e.

This patient has large iliac artery aneurysms, likely symptomatic on the right (groin pain). Indications for surgical repair of iliac artery aneurysm include diameter more than 3 cm or symptoms attributable to the aneurysm. In addition, the patient's abdominal aortic aneurysm is 4.9 cm and would likely be repaired concurrently with the iliac aneurysms (ie, aorto-iliac artery graft). The next most appropriate step in the management of this patient would be a functional cardiac study to ascertain perioperative cardiac risk (the presence of aneurysmal disease increases the likelihood of significant coronary artery disease). β-Adrenergic blockers may attenuate aneurysm growth rate and reduce perioperative cardiac events, but until ischemic heart disease burden is known the best course of action is not defined. Vascular surgical consultation would be indicated after the preoperative cardiac assessment is completed. Repeat ultrasonography in 3 months is not warranted because the aneurysmal disease in the iliac territory has already achieved surgical size. CT angiography of the abdomen may be warranted to identify the options for endovascular repair if preoperative stress test and other comorbidities deem a patient to be at an unacceptable risk for open surgical repair.

6.   Answer b.

This patient has an uncomplicated deep vein thrombosis involving the left superficial femoral vein (this is a deep vein, not a superficial vein). Current guidelines recommend low-molecular-weight heparin for initial outpatient management of uncomplicated deep venous thrombosis, as long as required support services are in place, such as would be the case in this large tertiary-care facility. If necessary support services were not available, inpatient treatment with either low-molecular-weight heparin or intravenous unfractionated heparin would be used. Warfarin therapy is started concurrently with low-molecular-weight heparin until the international normalized ratio is more than 2.0. Unopposed warfarin anticoagulation is contraindicated as initial treatment of deep vein thrombosis because of the transient hypercoagulable state that occurs early in treatment (without concurrent heparin use). Additional measures for this patient would include leg elevation and fitting with graduated elastic support (knee-high length, 30-40 mm Hg compression) to prevent the postphlebitic syndrome.

7.   Answer c.

This patient likely has secondary lymphedema and, given the absence of trauma, infection, or prior surgery involving the pelvis or left lower extremity, the diagnosis is most likely prostate cancer, until proved otherwise. MRI of the extremity may show dermal edema characteristic of lymphedema, but lymphoscintigraphy would more precisely establish the diagnosis and level of lymphatic obstruction. CT of the pelvis or ultrasonography of the pelvis may be indicated if the prostate-specific antigen level is increased, but they would not be the initial tests of choice. Lymphedema responds well to elastic compression and requires a minimum compression strength of 30 to 40 mm Hg. Graduated elastic support of 20 to 30 mm Hg is inadequate to control lymphedema and is generally prescribed for patients with superficial venous incompetence.

26

Women's Health

Lynne T. Shuster, MD
Deborah J. Rhodes, MD

The science and practice of women's health have evolved considerably during the past 10 years. Increasingly, internal medicine physicians will be expected to manage diseases or conditions unique to women, more prevalent or more serious in women, or for which risk factors or interventions are different in women than in men.

Menstruation and Menopause

Menstruation

The normal menstrual cycle is comprised of 3 phases: follicular (proliferative), periovulatory, and luteal (secretory). Menses start at the onset of the follicular cycle, when circulating levels of estrogen and progesterone are low and signal the hypothalamus and pituitary to release follicle-stimulating hormone (FSH). FSH initiates maturation of the follicle, which then increases estrogen production and new endometrial growth. At periovulation, the mature follicle triggers a surge in luteinizing hormone, causing release of an ovum. Luteinizing hormone then stimulates the residual ovarian follicle to transform into a corpus luteum. During the luteal phase, progesterone secretion from the corpus luteum leads to a thickened, enriched endometrium. The corpus luteum then regresses if fertilization does not occur, estrogen and progesterone levels decline, and menses occurs. Menstrual cycle length is determined by the rate and quality of follicular growth and development. It is most variable in the early teenage years and the years preceding menopause. Most women have cycles lasting from 24 to 35 days, but about 20% of women have irregular cycles on an ongoing basis. Women at the extremes of body mass index tend to have longer mean cycle lengths. Women within 5 to 7 years after menarche and 10 years before menopause have greater cycle variability.

Premenstrual Syndrome

Premenstrual syndrome (PMS) is defined as the cyclic occurrence of symptoms that are of sufficient severity to interfere with some aspects of life and that appear with consistent and predictable relationship to the luteal phase. Typical symptoms include mood irritability, abdominal bloating, breast tenderness, appetite changes, fatigue, or decreased concentration. Up to 85% of menstruating women report 1 or more premenstrual symptoms, but only 5% to 10% have symptoms of sufficient severity to interfere with life, meeting the diagnostic criteria for PMS.

Premenstrual dysphoric disorder differs from PMS in the severity of the emotional symptoms. Typically, emotional symptoms predominate over physical symptoms in premenstrual dysphoric disorder and may include markedly depressed mood, anxiety, persistent anger or emotional lability, lethargy, difficulty concentrating, insomnia or hypersomnia, and feeling out of control. These symptoms occur during the last week of the luteal phase and remit within a few days of the onset of menses. They must markedly interfere with work, school, or usual social activities and relationships with others to be considered for the diagnosis of premenstrual dysphoric disorder. Other disorders that could cause the symptoms must be considered before making the diagnosis, and prospective daily rating during at least 2 consecutive cycles should be completed to confirm the diagnosis.

Reducing the intake of caffeine, salt, and alcohol and increasing complex carbohydrates during the luteal phase may be helpful for some women with mild to moderate PMS symptoms. Calcium carbonate (1,200-1,600 mg daily in divided doses) has been found to reduce the severity of PMS symptoms. Some studies have found vitamin B_6 (50-100 mg daily) or magnesium (200-400 mg daily) to be helpful for PMS symptoms, but the evidence is less strong than for calcium.

For women with more severe premenstrual symptoms or premenstrual dysphoric disorder, selective serotonin reuptake inhibitors are the treatment of choice. They may be prescribed continuously or cyclically during the luteal phase when symptoms occur. Oral contraceptives, used to suppress ovulation, may improve physical symptoms of PMS but have not been proved to help with mood.

- 5% to 10% of women have symptoms severe enough to meet diagnostic criteria for PMS.
- Selective serotonin reuptake inhibitors are the treatment of choice for severe premenstrual dysphoric disorder.
- Oral contraceptives may improve physical symptoms but do not help mood.

Abnormal Vaginal Bleeding

Bleeding that is excessive in amount or outside the normal cyclic bleeding pattern is considered abnormal uterine bleeding (Table 26-1). Following are some commonly used terms: *amenorrhea*, absence of bleeding for 3 usual cycles; *oligomenorrhea*, decreased frequency of menstrual periods; *menorrhagia*, excessive or prolonged bleeding at regular intervals of menstruation; *metrorrhagia*, bleeding that occurs between periods; and *menometrorrhagia*, frequent bleeding that is excessive and irregular in amount and duration. Heavy menstrual bleeding is the most common concern in women with abnormal uterine bleeding.

Evaluation of abnormal vaginal bleeding includes taking a meticulous history with regard to date of last menstrual period; timing, duration, and amount of bleeding; pattern of bleeding; associated pain; evidence of ovulatory cycling (regular menses; cyclic symptoms such as breast tenderness, fluid retention, menstrual cramps, mood changes; midcycle cervical mucus); contraceptive history; medical conditions such as thyroid disease or blood dyscrasias; current medications; and the impact of bleeding on quality of life, which may determine treatment options.

Physical examination, in addition to breast and pelvic examination, includes assessing the body habitus and hair distribution and thyroid and skin examination. Obese women can have irregular, anovulatory bleeding because of increased circulating levels of estrogen from androgen conversion in adipose tissue. Patients under the 10th percentile in body weight may have oligomenorrhea due to hypothalamic dysfunction. Hirsutism can suggest polycystic ovary syndrome, a cause of infrequent and sometimes very heavy menstrual periods associated with anovulation. Petechiae can suggest abnormal clotting disorders. Vaginal atrophy and cervical lesions can cause postcoital spotting or bleeding. Rectal examination can identify hemorrhoids that may have bled and been mistaken by the patient as vaginal bleeding.

In women of reproductive age, pregnancy always needs to be considered first when abnormal bleeding is evaluated. In reproductive women with vaginal bleeding along with unilateral pelvic pain, particularly after an episode of amenorrhea, ectopic pregnancy needs to be considered. In postmenopausal women with vaginal bleeding, endometrial cancer needs to be ruled out.

Table 26-1 Possible Causes of Abnormal Uterine Bleeding

Pregnancy	Endometrial carcinoma
Anovulation or oligo-ovulation	Coagulation disorders
Fibroids	Hyperprolactinemia
Polyps, endometrial or endocervical	Liver disease
Adenomyosis	Thyroid dysfunction
Endometriosis	Obesity
Infection, including pelvic inflammatory disease	Anorexia
	Rapid fluctuations in weight
	Corticosteroids
Endometrial hyperplasia	Hormonal contraceptives
	Tamoxifen

When history, physical examination, and pregnancy testing do not reveal the cause of abnormal uterine bleeding, further evaluation may be indicated, including the following:

1. Blood tests, including complete blood count and thyroid function
2. Endometrial biopsy, to exclude endometrial cancer or atypical hyperplasia, particularly if there is intermenstrual bleeding and in women 45 years or older.
3. Ultrasonography, the first-line diagnostic tool for identifying structural abnormalities
4. Hysteroscopy, to obtain direct visualization of the endometrial cavity, particularly if ultrasonography results are inconclusive or to determine the exact nature of an endometrial abnormality

Dysfunctional Uterine Bleeding

Abnormal, excessive uterine bleeding not due to a specific identifiable cause is considered dysfunctional uterine bleeding. It is a term frequently used to refer to noncyclic, anovulatory bleeding. Dysfunctional uterine bleeding is most commonly observed at the extremes of reproductive age (ie, at menarche and perimenopause). Useful therapies include hormonal contraception (most commonly with combination oral contraceptive pills), cyclic oral progestins (mostly commonly medroxyprogesterone acetate 10 mg daily for 10-13 days), and nonsteroidal anti-inflammatory drugs (which may reduce menorrhagia blood loss up to 50%).

Menopause

Menopause is a natural biologic process that occurs when the supply of ovarian follicles is depleted, resulting in permanent cessation of menses. Menopause is a clinical diagnosis, confirmed when a woman has had no menstrual periods for 12 months. It occurs naturally between the ages of 42 and 58 (average age, 51), or it may be induced by surgery, chemotherapy, or pelvic radiation. It tends to occur earlier in women who smoke and women who are nulliparous.

Hot flashes, characterized by the abrupt onset of warmth and red skin blotching typically involving the chest, face, and neck, often associated with transient anxiety, palpitations, and profuse sweating, are considered the hallmark of menopause. Most menopausal women experience hot flashes, but only 10% to 15% report that they are frequent or severe. Hot flashes usually begin 2 or more years before menopause, tend to peak within 2 to 3 years after menopause, but may continue in some women for many years. The frequency, duration, and intensity of hot flashes vary for each woman. Hot flashes coincide with declining estrogen levels, but they are not specifically due to hypoestrogenism. Their mechanism is attributed to dysfunction of the thermoregulatory center in the hypothalamus, likely due to complex neuroendocrine pathways involving norepinephrine, serotonin, estrogen, and testosterone.

Other postmenopausal symptoms may include vaginal dryness and irritation, urinary urgency and frequency, discomfort with sex and other changes in sexual function, mood swings, and cognitive changes. Menopausal symptoms tend to be more intense after surgically induced menopause than natural menopause. Differential diagnosis of hot flashes includes thyroid dysfunction, infection, carcinoid syndrome, pheochromocytoma, autoimmune disorders, mast cell disorders, malignancies, and, rarely, seizure disorders. When hot flashes occur in a healthy woman of typical menopausal age, no diagnostic testing is necessary. If the clinical scenario is atypical, an increased FSH level may sometimes be helpful and thyroid function is commonly assessed.

- Menopause is a clinical diagnosis confirmed when a woman has had no menstrual periods for 12 months.
- Hot flashes are considered the hallmark of menopause.

After menopause, any vaginal bleeding (with the exception of predictable bleeding associated with hormone therapy) is abnormal and needs diagnostic evaluation.

Perimenopause
Perimenopause is characterized by erratic hormone levels and irregular menstrual periods. Symptoms such as hot flashes, vaginal dryness, and sleep disturbances may begin even while menses still occur. Anovulation is common during this interval and contributes to the irregular menstrual bleeding patterns typical of perimenopause. Despite a decline in fertility, pregnancy is still possible until menopause is reached, confirmed either by 12 months of no menstrual periods or consistently increased FSH levels (>30 mIU/mL).

Menstrual changes during perimenopause may include lighter or heavier bleeding, bleeding that is shorter (less than 2 days) or longer (more than 4 days) in duration, or skipped menstrual periods. Certain patterns of bleeding warrant further evaluation: very heavy flow, especially with clots; menstrual bleeding lasting more than 7 days; intervals less than 21 days from the onset of 1 period to the next; spotting or bleeding between periods; or uterine bleeding after sexual intercourse.

Hormonal contraceptives may be useful for menstrual regulation, dysmenorrhea, menorrhagia, and hot flashes in perimenopausal women. For treatment of hot flashes during perimenopause, oral contraceptives are preferred over menopausal regimens of estrogen-progestogen therapy, because postmenopausal hormone therapy does not suppress endogenous ovarian function and irregular bleeding can result.

The decision about when to stop use of oral contraceptives or switch to postmenopausal hormone therapy is not straightforward. Clinical signs of menopause are masked by taking hormonal contraceptives. FSH levels are labile in perimenopause, and unless they are consistently increased to more than 30 mIU/mL, menopause is not confirmed. Additionally, hormonal contraceptives may lower FSH levels, confounding interpretation in women taking oral contraceptives. Even measuring the FSH level on the seventh pill-free day is not sensitive for confirming menopause. If certainty in establishing menopause is needed for a woman taking oral contraceptives, FSH testing after a pill-free interval of 1 to 2 months, while using alternative contraception, is appropriate.

Hormone Therapy
Estrogen is the most effective treatment for hot flashes and other troublesome menopausal symptoms, but it carries potential risks. The Women's Health Initiative found an increased risk of cardiovascular

events, venous thromboembolism, stroke, and breast cancer in women treated with a combination of estrogen and progesterone hormone. The US Food and Drug Administration advises that postmenopausal hormone therapy is appropriate only for women with moderate to severe symptoms of menopause, including vasomotor symptoms (hot flashes) and urogenital symptoms (eg, vaginal dryness and discomfort, urinary frequency and burning). It should be prescribed at the lowest dose needed for symptom relief and for the shortest duration needed for treatment goals.

There is great controversy about the applicability of these recommendations for women early in menopause or women receiving long-term estrogen therapy after surgical menopause. Accumulating evidence suggests that the timing of initiation of estrogen therapy is an important determinant of the balance of benefits and risks. When the therapy is started early in menopause, there may be notable cardiovascular benefits. Clotting risks can be reduced by the use of transdermal instead of oral estrogen.

Prescribing Menopausal Hormone Therapy
If clinical indications are appropriate for estrogen therapy and if contraindications do not exist (Table 26-2), the following general guidelines are used when prescribing hormone therapy: 1) the risk of venous thromboembolism is increased by oral estrogens; 2) combination estrogen plus progestogen is needed if the woman has not had a hysterectomy, to provide adequate protection against endometrial hyperplasia or cancer; 3) unopposed estrogen therapy is prescribed if the woman's uterus has been removed; 4) transdermal estrogen is preferred over oral in the setting of hypertriglyceridemia, headaches, liver or gallbladder disease, or history of phlebitis; and 5) vaginal estrogen therapy is preferred for treatment of urogenital atrophy.

Table 26-2 Contraindications to Use of Estrogen-Containing Oral Contraceptives

Absolute contraindications
- History of deep vein thrombosis or pulmonary embolism
- History of arterial vein thrombosis
- Active liver disease
- Cardiovascular disease such as congestive heart failure, myocardial infarction or coronary artery disease, atrial fibrillation, mitral stenosis, mechanical heart valve
- Systemic diseases that affect the vascular system (such as systemic lupus erythematosus, diabetes with retinopathy or nephropathy)
- Cigarette smoking by women older than 35 years
- Uncontrolled hypertension
- History of breast cancer
- Undiagnosed amenorrhea

Relative contraindications
- Classic migraine
- Hypertriglyceridemia
- Depression

Contraception, Infertility, and Pregnancy

Contraception

A woman's life expectancy is inversely proportional to the number of pregnancies she has. At least 50% of pregnancies in the United States are unintended. Contraceptive methods include hormonal, intrauterine, barrier, chemical, or physiologic approaches. None are 100% effective, and all are associated with some degree of risk. However, nearly all contraceptive methods are safer than carrying a pregnancy to term.

Factors that should be considered in counseling women regarding choice of contraceptive methods include efficacy, convenience, duration of action, reversibility and time to return of fertility, effect on uterine bleeding, risk of adverse events, affordability, and protection against sexually transmitted diseases. Balancing the advantages and disadvantages of each method will guide each woman's individual decision (Table 26-3). Methods consistent with her values and lifestyle are most likely to be successful.

Effective contraceptive management requires education and counseling regarding appropriate use. It is particularly important for internists to be familiar with the medical aspects of oral contraceptives.

Oral Contraceptives

The main types of oral contraceptives are fixed-dose estrogen-progestin pills, phasic estrogen-progestin pills, and daily progestin-only pills. Combination estrogen-progestin pills are most effective for preventing ovulation and are highly effective (97%-99%) for preventing pregnancy. Oral contraceptives prohibit ovulation by inhibing the midcycle surge of gonadotropin secretion. They also act on cervical mucus and tubal motility to interfere with sperm transport. Progestins also alter the endometrium, thereby interfering with implantation of fertilized ovum.

Noncontraceptive benefits of oral contraceptives include a reduction in dysmenorrhea, menstrual flow, and development of functional ovarian cysts; an increase in bone mineral density; a reduced risk of ovarian cancer (by 40%-80% depending on duration of use) and endometrial cancer (by 50%); and reduced risk for pelvic inflammatory disease and ectopic pregnancy. Other uses of oral contraceptives include the treatment of acne, hirsutism, and perimenopausal symptoms (Table 26-4).

The synthetic estrogens used in oral conceptives cause an increase in the hepatic production of proteins that affect thrombosis, including factors V, VIII, X, and fibrinogen, and an increase in angiotensinogen, which may affect blood pressure. Blood pressure should be monitored in all women taking oral contraceptives, particularly estrogen-containing oral contraceptives. Although there is an increased risk of venous thromboembolism with all estrogen-containing oral contraceptives, the absolute risk is low. The risk is reduced with lower-dose estrogen-containing oral contraceptives, and the excess risk is lower after the first year of use. Women with inherited coagulopathies are at further increased risk for venous thromboembolism from use of combination oral contraceptives, but screening for thrombophilias currently is not recommended unless the woman has a personal or strong family history of thrombotic events. Use of low-dose oral contraceptives by nonsmoking women without hypertension is not associated with a significantly increased risk for myocardial infarction or stroke. Women older than 35 years who smoke cigarettes have a relative contraindication to combination oral contraceptives, because of an increased risk for myocardial infarction and stroke (Table 26-2).

Progestins have adverse lipid effects, including a decrease in high-density lipoprotein and an increase in low-density lipoprotein, related to the amount and potency of the progestin. Estrogens increase high-density lipoprotein and decrease low-density lipoprotein. Newer combination oral contraceptives with lower-androgenic progestins have a less adverse effect on lipids. The net effect of newer combination oral contraceptives is little or no change in total cholesterol, high-density lipoprotein, or low-density lipoprotein levels, although there is a substantial increase in triglyceride levels from the synthetic estrogen component.

The relationship between use of oral contraceptives and breast cancer risk remains controversial. There may be a slight increase in breast cancer risk that decreases after discontinuation of use. There has been concern that the large increase in the rate of breast cancer

Table 26-3 Currently Available Contraceptive Methods

Reversible methods
  Intrauterine devices, contraceptive implants, & injectable
    contraceptives
      Very low pregnancy rate
      Minimally influenced by compliance
  Oral contraceptives
    Very low pregnancy rate if taken consistently & correctly
    Actual pregnancy rates are increased because of incorrect use
  Other methods, including diaphragms, cervical caps, condoms,
    spermicides, withdrawal, & periodic abstinence
      Actual pregnancy rates are much higher than perfect-use
      rates
Permanent methods
  Tubal ligation
  Vasectomy

Table 26-4 Noncontraceptive Benefits of Oral Contraceptives

Reductions in:
  Dysmenorrhea
  Menorrhagia
  Iron deficiency anemia
  Acne
  Ectopic pregnancy
  Ovarian cysts
  Ovarian cancer
  Uterine cancer
  Hirsutism
  Bone loss
  Perimenopausal symptoms

in the developed parts of the world may be due to hormonal contraception, but most studies have not confirmed a significant association.

Progestin-only pills are an option for women who request a contraceptive pill but need to avoid estrogen. They are associated with a slightly higher failure rate than combined oral contraceptives and there is a higher frequency of breakthrough bleeding. Conditions for which they are commonly considered include migraine headaches, age older than 35 years, smoking, hypertension, diabetes, history of thromboembolism, cardiac disease such as coronary artery disease or congestive heart failure, cerebrovascular disease, and hypertriglyceridemia.

* Combination estrogen-progestin pills prevent pregnancies at a rate of 97%-99%.
* Other benefits of oral contraceptives include an increase in bone mineral density, a 40%-80% reduced risk of ovarian carcinoma, and a 50% reduction in the risk of endometrial carcinoma.
* Women older than 35 years who take oral combination contraceptives and smoke cigarettes are at an increased risk for myocardial infarction and stroke.

Infertility

Infertility is defined as the inability to conceive after 1 year of intercourse without contraception. It may be due to male or female factors, or a combination of the 2, but the cause is often difficult to elucidate. The most commonly identified causes of female infertility include ovulatory disorders (such as from polycystic ovary syndrome, hypothyroidism, hyperprolactinemia, eating disorders, extreme stress), endometriosis, pelvic adhesions, and tubal blockage or other tubal abnormalities. Decreasing oocyte quality with advanced age has become a major cause of infertility as an increasing portion of women delay childbearing.

Initial evaluation of the woman commonly includes assessment of ovulation by basal body temperature charting for 1 month and mid-luteal progesterone level testing, assessment of ovarian reserve by measuring day 3 FSH level, assessment of fallopian tube patency with hysterosalpingography, and exclusion of endocrinologic causes by measurement of prolactin and thyroid-stimulating hormone levels.

Medical Issues of Pregnancy

Preconception Counseling

Good prenatal care is associated with improved pregnancy outcomes. In addition to recommending a healthful diet, exercise, and avoidance of smoking and illicit drugs, preconception counseling should address the following:

Supplementation with folic acid before conception decreases the risk of neural tube defects. For women with no history of neural tube defects in prior pregnancies, 0.4 mg is adequate and can be obtained in most over-the-counter multivitamins or in prenatal vitamins.

Alcohol abuse during pregnancy is the third leading cause of mental retardation and also is associated with early spontaneous abortion, placental abruption, and possibly attention deficit disorder in children of moderate drinkers. The greatest negative impact is at the time of conception through the first month of pregnancy.

Avoiding alcohol prevents fetal alcohol syndrome. There is no agreement about the lowest safe level of alcohol consumption for pregnant women or women planning pregnancy.

Smoking is associated with low birth weight, perinatal mortality, infertility, spontaneous abortion, ectopic pregnancy, placenta previa and placental abruption, and subsequent sudden infant death syndrome.

Caffeine intake limited to 1 to 2 cups of coffee or caffeinated beverage daily is not associated with miscarriage or birth defects.

* Alcohol abuse during pregnancy is the third leading cause of mental retardation and is associated with early spontaneous abortion and placental abruption.
* Smoking is associated with low birth weight, perinatal mortality, infertility, spontaneous abortion, ectopic pregnancy, placenta previa and placental abruption, and sudden infant death syndrome.

Immunizations and Pregnancy
* Tetanus-diphtheria: Tetanus immunization is indicated routinely for pregnant women. All patients should be given a tetanus booster if they have not had one in 10 years.
* Measles, mumps, and rubella vaccine should not be given to pregnant women because of a theoretical risk to the fetus from live virus vaccine. For persons born before 1957 in the United States, immunity is usually established. Nonpregnant women of childbearing age should be given the combined measles, mumps, and rubella vaccine if there is uncertainty about immunity. There is little risk to receiving the vaccine even if immunity already exists.
* Rubella: Measles, mumps, and rubella vaccine should not be given to pregnant women. All nonpregnant women of childbearing age should be vaccinated if no documentation exists of prior immunization or if rubella antibody testing is negative.
* Influenza: Women who will be pregnant during the influenza season should be vaccinated, regardless of trimester of pregnancy.
* Hepatitis B: Neither pregnancy nor lactation is a contraindication to vaccination of women at risk.
* Pneumococcal: Women at increased risk, such as those who are asplenic and those with cardiopulmonary, chronic kidney, or liver disease, should be vaccinated. It is preferable to wait until after the first trimester.
* Varicella: Pregnant women should not be vaccinated, because the effects on the fetus from this vaccine are unknown. For nonpregnant persons, having a pregnant household contact is not a contraindication to vaccination.

Hypertension and Pregnancy
Hypertension, complicating up to 15% of pregnancies, is the most common medical problem in pregnancy and an important cause of maternal and fetal morbidity and mortality worldwide. Hypertension may precede pregnancy or develop during pregnancy. Chronic hypertension predating pregnancy is associated with an increased risk for preeclampsia, placental abruption, fetal growth retardation, and prematurity, but 85% of women with chronic hypertension have an uncomplicated pregnancy. Preeclampsia is associated with an increased risk for cardiovascular disease later in a woman's life.

Hypertension originating during pregnancy is diagnosed when the blood pressure after 20 weeks of gestation increases more than 30 mm Hg systolic or 15 mm Hg diastolic, or when the blood pressure is persistently 140/90 mm Hg or more in a woman who was previously normotensive. Although treatment for mild gestational hypertension is not of proven benefit, monitoring for the development of preeclampsia and intervening before complications develop is very important for reducing serious maternal and perinatal complications.

During normal pregnancy, intravascular volume increases by 40% and cardiac output increases by 20%, but peripheral vascular resistance decreases. There is a net decrease in blood pressure in the second trimester, but in the third trimester blood pressure tends to increase to pre-pregnancy or first-trimester levels. With preeclampsia, which occurs after 20 weeks of gestation, both cardiac output and plasma volume are reduced, but systemic vascular resistance is increased, resulting in worsening hypertension, proteinuria, hyperuricemia, and sometimes coagulation abnormalities. Perfusion to the placenta, kidneys, liver, and brain is reduced. Risks include seizures, stroke, placental abruption with disseminated intravascular coagulation, pulmonary edema, renal failure, liver hemorrhage, and death.

Methyldopa, β-adrenergic blockers, and vasodilators are preferred medications when treatment is needed for hypertension during pregnancy. Diuretics should be used with caution because of their potential risk of volume depletion. Angiotensin-converting enzyme inhibitors and angiotensin-receptor blockers should be avoided for pregnant women or women likely to become pregnant because of associated risks for miscarriage, fetal death, fetal malformations, and neonatal renal failure. Risks from these agents primarily are associated with use in the second and third trimesters.

Thromboembolic Disease and Pregnancy

Pregnancy is associated with multiple changes that increase clot formation, yet thromboembolism is uncommon during pregnancy. However, women with hereditary thrombophilias are at high risk for thrombosis during pregnancy, with potentially serious complications. Women with antiphospholipid antibodies are prone to arterial or venous thromboemboli, placental infarction, recurrent pregnancy loss, preeclampsia, fetal growth retardation, or fetal death.

Low-molecular-weight heparin is usually the preferred treatment for thromboembolism during pregnancy or for prevention in high-risk women. Warfarin should be avoided during pregnancy because of its teratogenicity. Aspirin is recommended before conception for women with antiphospholipid antibodies. Once pregnancy is established, additional treatment with heparin, glucocorticoids, or other medications may be indicated.

* Low-molecular-weight heparin is the preferred treatment for thromboembolism during pregnancy or for prophylaxis.

Thyroid Disorders and Pregnancy

Maternal hypothyroidism is associated with infertility, miscarriage, stillbirth, placental abruption, preeclampsia, and motor and mental retardation in the infant. Thyroid-stimulating hormone should be measured early in pregnancy. Women taking thyroid hormone should be monitored each trimester; approximately 20% will require a dose increase during pregnancy. Thyroid-stimulating hormone levels are altered only slightly by pregnancy and remain useful for the detection of hypothyroidism or for monitoring thyroid hormone replacement.

Hyperthyroidism is the second most common endocrine disorder (after diabetes) during pregnancy and occurs in about 0.2% of pregnancies. Signs of hyperthyroidism such as tachycardia, a sensation of warmth, and fatigue can be a part of normal pregnancy, and an inappropriately low weight gain may be the only clue. Mild hyperthyroidism is generally well tolerated, but poorly controlled hyperthyroidism can be associated with spontaneous abortion, premature delivery, low birth weight, preeclampsia, and congestive heart failure. Propylthiouracil is the treatment of choice, given in the smallest doses necessary, in order to prevent fetal goiter and hypothyroidism. Radioiodine is absolutely contraindicated, and surgery is relatively contraindicated for gestational hyperthyroidism. In many women, the dose of propylthiouracil can be tapered or use can be discontinued in the last trimester.

Postpartum thyroid dysfunction occurs in up to 10% of women during the year after delivery, and it mostly occurs in women with goiters. Transient hyperthyroidism followed by hypothyroidism is typical. Hypothyroidism is often temporary, warranting thyroid hormone replacement for just several months.

Diseases of the Uterus and Adnexa

Endometriosis

Endometriosis is a common condition in which endometrial glands and stroma occur outside the endometrial cavity and uterine wall, commonly in the ovary or on the pelvic peritoneal surfaces such as the cul-de-sac and rectovaginal septum. Commonly associated symptoms include dysmenorrhea, dyspareunia, and premenstrual spotting. It is found in 20% to 40% of women with infertility and up to 65% of women with chronic pelvic pain. The amount of endometriosis does not correlate with the severity of symptoms.

Treatment depends primarily on the severity of symptoms and the desire for future fertility. Nonsteroidal anti-inflammatory drugs, by inhibiting prostaglandins, help reduce menstrual bleeding and pain. Oral contraceptive pills reduce menstrual bleeding and pain and also may slow disease progression. Oral progestogens such as medroxyprogesterone acetate, given cyclically, likewise can slow progression of endometriosis. When symptoms are more severe, treatment with gonadotropin-releasing hormone agonists (eg, leuprolide) can provide relief from pain and involution of endometriosis implants by causing temporary castration. If fertility is desired and other treatments have failed, resection of endometriomas and lysis of tubal adhesions may be recommended. Even with minimal endometriosis, laparoscopic resection can improve fertility. For severe endometriosis, when fertility is desired, preoperative or postoperative treatment with danazol or a gonadotropin-releasing hormone agonist may be given to further improve the likelihood of subsequent fertility.

* 20% to 40% of women with infertility and up to 65% of women with chronic pelvic pain have endometriosis.

Uterine Fibroids

Leiomyomata uteri, also known as fibroids, are the most common pelvic tumors in women, occurring in 50% to 80% of women. Fibroids are benign tumors that arise from smooth muscle cells and can be intramural, benign, monoclonal tumors of the smooth muscle cells of the myometrium. They are most prevalent during reproductive years and regress after menopause. Most fibroids cause no symptoms; approximately 25% are symptomatic. Symptoms may include dysmenorrhea, menorrhagia, recurrent miscarriage, pelvic pain and pressure, and obstetric complications. Submucous fibroids are associated with decreased fertility, and their removal increases fertility to baseline. Large fibroids may increase the risk of premature labor, and a fibroid under the placenta increases the risk of placental abruption.

Late menarche and increased parity are associated with a reduced risk of fibroids. Obesity is associated with an increased risk. The relative risk of fibroids is 2- to 3-fold greater in black women than white women.

Clinically significant fibroids can usually be diagnosed by the finding of an enlarged, irregularly shaped, firm, nontender uterus on pelvic examination. If the diagnosis is uncertain, ultrasonography, saline-infusion sonography, hysteroscopy, or magnetic resonance imaging is sometimes used. On ultrasonography, fibroids frequently appear as symmetric, well-defined, hypoechoic, and heterogeneous masses.

Treatment of fibroids is necessary only if they are symptomatic. Abnormal uterine bleeding is the most common symptom. Fibroids typically cause prolonged or excessively heavy menstruation but not intermenstrual bleeding. The bleeding pattern is influenced more by location of the fibroids than by size: submucosal fibroids are more likely to cause heavy bleeding. If treatment is needed (because of bleeding, anemia, or pain), a trial of medical therapy before surgical therapy is reasonable to determine whether symptoms can be controlled. Gonadotropin-releasing hormone agonists lead to amenorrhea and a reduction in uterine size in most cases. They usually are used only as a temporizing measure to reduce blood loss before definitive surgery or in women approaching menopause who are expected to require no more than 6 months of treatment. Adverse effects (including a reduction in bone density) often preclude long-term use. Pretreatment patterns of bleeding and uterine size usually return rapidly after cessation of treatment. Danazol, an androgenic steroid, can be used to control anemia and decrease bleeding but does not reduce uterine volume. Low-dose oral contraceptives do not cause fibroids to grow and thus are not contraindicated in premenopausal women with fibroids. However, oral contraceptives and progestational agents have little efficacy in treating uterine fibroids.

Surgical treatment is indicated when significant symptoms persist despite medical treatment, when there is a suspicion of malignancy, or when infertility or recurrent pregnancy loss is thought to be related to fibroids. Surgical options include hysterectomy or myomectomy (removal of the myomas with uterine conservation). Myomectomy is a good option for women who want to preserve childbearing potential. One disadvantage is the high risk of new fibroid formation after myomectomy (approximately 50% at 5 years). Other, less invasive options in women who have completed childbearing include endometrial ablation, myolysis (laparoscopic thermal coagulation or cryoablation of fibroids), uterine artery embolization, and magnetic resonance-guided focused ultrasound ablation.

Endometrial Cancer

Endometrial cancer is the most common gynecologic malignancy in the United States and accounts for 6% of all cancers in women. The incidence of endometrial cancer increases with age. The average age at diagnosis is 60 years, and 75% of cases occur in postmenopausal women. Fewer than 5% of cases occur in women before the age of 40 years. Table 26-5 lists factors that affect the risk of endometrial cancer. Most cases of endometrial cancer are related to estrogen stimulation; thus, many of the risk factors reflect both endogenous and exogenous sources of estrogen. There are some familial associations with endometrial cancer, but the risk incurred by family history is not as strong as in some other cancers, such as breast cancer. An increased risk of uterine cancer has been found in families with hereditary nonpolyposis colorectal cancer (Lynch syndrome II) and *BRCA1* mutations. Screening for uterine cancer in asymptomatic women is not warranted, except in women with known or suspected mutations associated with hereditary nonpolyposis colorectal cancer.

The most common type of endometrial cancer is endometrioid adenocarcinoma. Clear cell and serous carcinomas are rarer and more aggressive. The classic symptom of endometrial carcinoma is abnormal uterine bleeding, which occurs in 90% of cases. The possibility of endometrial cancer needs to be excluded in any postmenopausal woman with any amount of vaginal bleeding (with the exception of predictable bleeding related to hormone therapy). Atypical endometrial cells found on Papanicolaou smear may also

Table 26-5 Factors That Affect the Risk of Endometrial Cancer

Risk factors
- Increasing age
- Obesity
- High-fat diet
- Unopposed estrogen therapy
- Infertility
- Nulliparity
- Chronic anovulation (including polycystic ovary syndrome)
- Early menarche
- Late menopause (age >52 years)
- Obesity
- Diabetes mellitus
- Hypertension
- Tamoxifen
- First-degree relative with endometrial cancer
- Hereditary nonpolyposis colorectal cancer (Lynch syndrome II)
- *BRCA1* mutation

Protective factors
- Combination oral contraceptive therapy
- Smoking
- Physical activity

herald endometrial carcinoma: atypical endometrial cells are twice as likely to be associated with cancer as benign-appearing endometrial cells. An endometrial biopsy is recommended for women 40 years or older with any endometrial cells noted on Papanicolaou smear unless the test was done during an episode of bleeding.

The initial diagnostic test of choice to exclude endometrial cancer is endometrial biopsy. Hysteroscopy with dilation and curettage is an acceptable alternative. Transvaginal ultrasonography is often used in postmenopausal women with vaginal bleeding to differentiate atrophy (the most common cause of bleeding in this age group) from other causes that require further evaluation. In postmenopausal women, an endometrial thickness of less than 4 to 5 mm is associated with a low risk of endometrial disease; a thicker lining should prompt further evaluation, such as endometrial biopsy or hysteroscopy with dilation and curettage. Endometrial biopsy also may be used as the initial diagnostic test to evaluate abnormal uterine bleeding. Transvaginal ultrasonography is never sufficient to exclude endometrial cancer in premenopausal women with abnormal vaginal bleeding, given the cyclic variability in the thickness of the endometrium.

Uterine sarcoma accounts for only 5% of uterine cancers, and the prognosis is poorer than for other types of uterine cancer. It can arise from the endometrium or myometrium. Risk factors include race (risk higher in blacks), pelvic irradiation, and tamoxifen.

* Endometrial cancer is the most common gynecologic malignancy in the United States and accounts for 6% of all cancers in women.
* Average age at diagnosis is 60 years.
* Risk factors include increasing age, unopposed estrogen therapy, infertility, nulliparity, chronic anovulation, late menopause, obesity, diabetes mellitus, and tamoxifen therapy.

Adnexal Masses

Adnexal masses occur in females of all ages, and 90% are benign. The differential diagnosis and management of an adnexal mass depend on the patient's age and menstrual status.

The differential diagnosis of an adnexal mass includes both ovarian and extraovarian masses. Examples of adnexal masses are listed in Table 26-6.

The most probable cause of an adnexal mass differs depending on the patient's age. The most common adnexal mass in a premenopausal woman is a physiologic ovarian cyst. Pregnancy should always be excluded in a premenopausal woman with an adnexal mass, because an ectopic pregnancy necessitates urgent treatment. In women of reproductive age, only 5% to 18% of adnexal masses are malignant. In women older than 50 years, 30% to 60% of adnexal masses are malignant. The median age at diagnosis of ovarian cancer is 63. In postmenopausal women, any solid enlargement of an ovary must be considered to be cancer until proved otherwise.

Many of the risk factors for epithelial ovarian cancer relate to the total number of ovulatory cycles. Thus, gravida 0, early age at menarche, and late age at menopause increase the risk of ovarian cancer. Other risk factors include Caucasian race, age older than 34 years at first birth, use of postmenopausal hormone therapy for more than 10 years, and family history of ovarian or endometrial cancer. Protective factors associated with a reduced risk of ovarian cancer include oral contraceptive therapy, multiparity, tubal ligation, and breastfeeding.

Several features of the history may assist in the diagnosis. Patients with ovarian cancer often present with vague complaints such as back pain, fatigue, bloating, constipation, abdominal pain, and urinary symptoms. The combination of bloating, increased abdominal size, and urinary symptoms was found in almost half of women with ovarian cancer. The onset of mid-cycle pain in premenopausal women suggests a follicular or corpus luteum cyst. Pain during or after intercourse may be related to a ruptured cyst. Chronic dysmenorrhea and dyspareunia often occur with endometriosis. The sudden onset of severe pain, often with fever, nausea, and vomiting, suggests ovarian torsion. Pelvic pain with fever suggests pelvic inflammatory disease, appendicitis, diverticulitis, or torsion. Renal colic also should be considered in the differential diagnosis of pelvic pain.

Pelvic ultrasonography is the best radiologic test to evaluate adnexal masses and can distinguish whether they are cystic or solid. Both transvaginal and transabdominal ultrasonography may be necessary. Transvaginal ultrasonography provides better resolution of pelvic structures, whereas transabdominal ultrasonography is better for visualizing abdominal structures. The normal ovary is typically 3.5 cm in greatest dimension in the premenopausal patient and 1.5 cm in greatest dimension after menopause. A palpable ovary in a postmenopausal woman should be considered suspicious, as should an ovary that on ultrasonography is twice the size of the contralateral ovary in a postmenopausal woman. Ultrasonographic features that increase the likelihood of malignancy include septations, mural or septal nodules, thickened or irregular walls, and partially solid or solid masses.

Table 26-6 Differential Diagnosis of Adnexal Mass

Ovarian mass
    Physiologic cyst, simple or hemorrhagic
        Follicular
        Corpus luteum
    Polycystic ovary syndrome
    Benign ovarian neoplasm
        Leiomyoma (fibroid)
        Endometrioma
        Dermoid cyst (cystic teratoma); most common ovarian tumor in women in their second & third decades
        Cystadenoma
    Metastatic carcinoma (ie, colon, endometrium, breast); non-Hodgkin lymphoma
    Ovarian carcinoma
Extraovarian mass
    Ectopic pregnancy
    Tubo-ovarian abscess
    Paraovarian cyst
    Peritoneal inclusion cyst
    Diverticular abscess
    Cancer of the fallopian tube

Follicular and corpus luteum cysts are typically solitary, thin-walled, unilocular, and less than 10 cm in diameter. Corpus luteum cysts may be associated with hemorrhage. In the premenopausal woman, a cyst with no solid component that is less than 10 cm in size can be managed with follow-up ultrasonography after several cycles. Approximately 70% resolve spontaneously. If the cyst is unchanged or larger after an interval of observation, surgery is required. Prescribing oral contraceptives during the observation period helps to prevent formation of new cysts. Masses more than 10 cm require surgical exploration, as do masses that are solid, fixed, or bilateral. Surgical exploration also is needed in women who present with ascites, suspicion of metastatic disease, or a family history of breast or ovarian cancer in a first-degree relative.

Benign ovarian cysts also can occur in postmenopausal women, but the management differs because of the higher risk of ovarian cancer. A postmenopausal woman with a simple unilocular cyst on ultrasonography which is less than 5 cm can be followed with serial ultrasonography examinations and determination of CA 125 levels at 3-month intervals. Most cysts resolve spontaneously within 1 year. Postmenopausal women with complex cysts or cysts more than 5 cm should be referred for surgical consultation, as should women with a symptomatic adnexal mass. Other factors that should prompt surgical consultation in a postmenopausal woman with an adnexal mass are an increased CA 125 level, suspicion of metastatic disease, ascites, or a family history of breast or ovarian cancer in a first-degree relative. Surgical management of suspicious adnexal masses should be guided by the potential risk of tumor spill by rupture of the ovarian capsule during laparoscopic removal of the tumor. Thus, open laparotomy may be more prudent when neoplasm is suspected.

The CA 125 level may contribute to the diagnostic evaluation of an adnexal mass but is not sufficient to establish or exclude a diagnosis of ovarian cancer. Many conditions unrelated to ovarian cancer can increase the CA 125 level, including endometriomas, uterine fibroids, pelvic inflammatory disease, pancreatic and other malignancies, and cirrhosis. The specificity of CA 125 is low in premenopausal women, thus its usefulness as a diagnostic tool is limited. In contrast, the combination of a suspicious finding on pelvic ultrasonography and an increased CA 125 level is highly specific and sensitive for ovarian cancer in postmenopausal women. The CA 125 test should not be used as screening for ovarian cancer in the general population. However, screening with transvaginal ultrasonography and tests for CA 125 levels is appropriate in women with a family history of ovarian cancer or a known *BRCA1* or *BRCA2* mutation. Determining the CA 125 level is most useful as a surveillance test in women with an established diagnosis of ovarian cancer. When the CA 125 level is increased at the time of diagnosis, it can be followed to gauge response to chemotherapy and to monitor for recurrence.

- 30% to 60% of adnexal masses are malignant.
- In postmenopausal women, any enlargement of an ovary must be considered malignant until proved otherwise.
- Risk factors for ovarian carcinoma include gravida 0, early age at menarche, and late age at menopause.
- A suspicious result on pelvic ultrasonography and an increased CA 125 level are highly specific and sensitive for ovarian carcinoma.

- Typical clinical scenario of ovarian carcinoma: A 63-year-old woman has an adnexal mass and an increased CA 125 level.

Breast Conditions

Evaluation of the Palpable Breast Mass

Breast lumps are common and most are benign: in 1 study, 11% of women presenting with a palpable breast mass were found to have cancer. The challenge of distinguishing benign from malignant lumps should be guided by 2 principles: benign characteristics by history or on physical examination are not sufficient to exclude a cancer, and negative findings on mammography and ultrasonography do not definitively exclude a cancer if the clinical suspicion is high.

Elements of the history that are important in evaluating the palpable breast lump are precise location of the lump, when the patient first noted the lump, the association of any pain or skin or nipple changes (such as discharge), whether the lump has changed in size, and whether the size of the lump fluctuates with the menstrual cycle. The patient's risk factors for breast cancer also should be assessed, particularly in regard to prior history of breast cancer, prior history of atypia or lobular carcinoma in situ of the breast, or family history of breast cancer.

The physical examination should be done in both the sitting and the supine position and should begin with a visual inspection of the breasts for asymmetry, puckering, dimpling, nipple lesions or retraction, erythema, and peau d'orange. Palpation of the breast should include all tissue from the clavicle to the inframammary area and from the sternum to the mid-axillary line. Palpation of the axillary and supraclavicular areas also should be part of the clinical breast examination.

Diagnostic mammography is recommended as part of the evaluation in all women 30 to 35 years or older who have a palpable breast mass. Initial mammography in younger women is often difficult to interpret because the density of the breast tissue reduces the sensitivity of mammography. Although mammography may be useful in younger women when the suspicion of cancer is high on clinical examination, the negative predictive value of mammography is limited in this setting.

Ultrasonography is most useful as the initial imaging method in the evaluation of women younger than 30 years who have a palpable breast mass, as an adjunct to mammography in women 30 to 35 years or older with a palpable breast mass and normal mammography, and as an adjunct to mammography to clarify whether a nodule found on mammography is solid or cystic. A palpable mass or mammographic nodule that corresponds to a simple cyst on ultrasonography does not require further diagnostic evaluation. A complex cyst should be aspirated under ultrasonographic guidance to confirm complete resolution of the cyst.

There are 3 primary diagnostic methods for tissue evaluation of breast masses: fine-needle aspiration (FNA), core needle biopsy, and excisional biopsy. FNA is inexpensive to perform and can be done in an office setting, but the sensitivity and specificity vary according to the skill of the operator and cytopathologist. FNA should be distinguished from cyst aspiration, which has as its goal removal of cystic fluid that does not need to be sent for cytologic analysis provided that it is nonbloody. Bloody fluid or cells aspirated from a solid mass should be sent for cytologic analysis. A negative FNA result is not sufficient to exclude cancer if suspicion is high on the basis of clinical examination or imaging.

In a core needle biopsy, a larger needle is used, thereby providing adequate tissue for histologic diagnosis. This technique is often done in conjunction with imaging guidance and has a higher sensitivity and better specimen quality than FNA. Concordance between core needle biopsy and excisional biopsy exceeds 90%. Core needle biopsy is also used to confirm the diagnosis in women with locally advanced breast cancer before administration of neoadjuvant chemotherapy.

Excisional biopsy is reserved for cases in which FNA and core biopsy are technically unfeasible or when the findings on FNA or core biopsy are discordant with the findings on physical examination or imaging. Excisional biopsy also should be done when FNA shows atypical cells or a core biopsy shows atypical ductal or lobular hyperplasia or lobular carcinoma in situ to exclude the presence of ductal carcinoma in situ or invasive carcinoma in the surrounding tissues.

Evaluation of Nonpalpable Mammographic Abnormalities

Calcifications found on mammography generally are classified into 3 categories: benign, intermediate concern, or high suspicion for malignancy. Round and oval calcifications that are also uniform in size and shape are more likely to be benign, whereas pleomorphic calcifications are more likely to be malignant. Biopsy must be done for suspicious calcification, whereas intermediate calcification may be reassessed with mammography in 6 months or biopsy done. For nodules found on mammography which are not palpable, biopsy can be done under stereotactic guidance, under ultrasonographic guidance (if visible on ultrasonography), or by wire localization excisional biopsy.

- Benign characteristics on history or physical examination do not exclude breast cancer.
- Negative findings on mammography and ultrasonography do not definitively exclude breast cancer.
- Pleomorphic calcifications are most likely malignant.

Breast Pain

Breast pain can be classified into 3 categories: cyclic, noncyclic, and extramammary. Cyclic mastalgia occurs in premenopausal women: pain generally begins in the luteal phase of the menstrual cycle (2 weeks before the onset of menstruation) and resolves with menstruation. This type of mastalgia is usually diffuse and bilateral, but it may be more severe in 1 breast and most concentrated in the upper outer aspect of the breast.

Noncyclic mastalgia is defined as constant or intermittent breast pain that is not associated with the menstrual cycle. It typically presents in women in their fourth or fifth decade of life. The cause of most cases of noncyclic breast pain is elusive, but some cases may be attributed to pregnancy, duct dilatation, cysts, fibroadenomas, injury, prior breast surgery, breast infections, and exogenous estrogen exposure. Fewer than 10% of women who present with breast pain have cancer. The risk of subsequent breast cancer after normal findings

on clinical examination and mammography for breast pain is estimated to be only 0.5%; thus, patients can be reassured in this setting.

Extramammary pain has numerous possible causes; the most common are costochondritis and other chest wall syndromes. Therapy should be directed at the underlying cause of pain.

The evaluation of focal breast pain should include mammography; if the result is negative, ultrasonography is done in the area of the pain. Ultrasonography often is used alone to evaluate focal breast pain in younger women.

Reassurance that the pain is not due to cancer is often the only necessary treatment. For persistent breast pain, there is overlap in the initial treatment strategies for cyclic and noncyclic breast pain: a properly fitted brassiere, the application of heat or cold, gentle massage, dietary restrictions (eg, caffeine, sodium, dietary fat), relaxation techniques, and exercise. Over-the-counter analgesics also may be effective. Eliminating or adjusting doses of exogenous estrogen may alleviate breast pain. Other hormonal agents may be effective in patients with severe cyclic breast pain. Danazol is the only medication approved by the US Food and Drug Administration for treatment of mastalgia, but the incidence of adverse androgenic effects limits its use. Several studies have shown a reduction in mastalgia with tamoxifen and bromocriptine, but adverse effects also limit their use.

- Fewer than 10% of women who present with breast pain are found to have cancer.

Nipple Discharge

Nipple discharge is a common complaint in women of reproductive age. Nipple discharge most often is due to benign causes, but it must be evaluated to exclude 2 rare but serious causes: a pituitary tumor and breast cancer. Approximately 5% of all cases of nipple discharge are due to breast cancer. It is helpful to classify nipple discharge into 2 categories: nipple discharge due to galactorrhea and nipple discharge due to ductal lesions.

Galactorrhea is defined as milk production more than 1 year after weaning or in any nulligravid or menopausal woman. Galactorrhea usually appears as a spontaneous, milky discharge from multiple ducts of both breasts. It results from a relative or absolute increase in serum prolactin. The evaluation and treatment of galactorrhea are discussed in the endocrinology chapter.

Nipple discharge not due to galactorrhea is caused by ductal lesions, either benign or malignant. Benign nipple discharge is typically bilateral, guaiac-negative, and multiductal and is yellow, green, gray, blue, brown, or clear. Thyroid-stimulating hormone and prolactin should be checked to exclude galactorrhea. Discharge due to cancer is typically bloody, serosanguineous, or, rarely, watery. The most common cause of bloody nipple discharge is papilloma (35%-48%) followed by ductal ectasia (defined as ductal dilatation with or without inflammation; 17%-36%) and then carcinoma (5%-21%). Ductal carcinoma in situ and papillary carcinoma are the most common types of breast cancer associated with bloody nipple discharge. Factors associated with an increased likelihood that nipple discharge is due to cancer are detailed in Table 26-7.

If the discharge can be reproduced on examination, it should be characterized as unilateral or bilateral, spontaneous or expressible, and emanating from a single or multiple ducts. The discharge should be assessed for gross or occult blood (using Hemoccult testing). Discharge that is grossly bloody or Hemoccult-positive may be sent for cytologic analysis; this has a high positive predictive value but a low negative predictive value.

Mammography should be done in all nonlactating women with nipple discharge, with the exception of women younger than 30 years in whom ultrasonography may be a reasonable substitute. If mammography shows a suspicious mass, then surgical consultation should be obtained. If mammography is negative, ultrasonography should be considered in the subareolar area to determine whether an intraductal lesion is visible. Galactography and ductoscopy are not routinely used in the evaluation of bloody nipple discharge.

Patients who have nipple discharge that is neither bloody nor galactorrhea and who have normal mammographic and ultrasonographic results can be reassured and followed. Patients with bloody or watery (clear) discharge that can be localized to 1 duct require surgical duct excision even if the mammographic and ultrasonographic results are negative. Patients with normal results on imaging studies who report bloody or watery nipple discharge that cannot be reproduced on clinical examination require close interval follow-up. Surgical duct excision should be performed if the involved duct subsequently can be identified. Figure 26-1 contains a suggested algorithm for the evaluation of spontaneous nipple discharge.

* Approximately 5% of all cases of nipple discharge are due to cancer.
* Typical clinical scenario for nipple discharge associated with cancer: A 56-year-old woman with recurrent, spontaneous, guaiac positive discharge from a single duct.

Benign Breast Disease

Simple cysts are the most common cause of discrete benign breast lumps. They occur most often in women between the ages of 35 and 50 years. Fibroadenomas are the most common cause of solid benign masses. The median age at diagnosis is 30 years, but fibroadenomas also can be found in postmenopausal women. There are many other histologic classifications of benign breast disease. The main significance of these distinctions lies in whether they confer an increased risk for the subsequent development of breast cancer. Patients with findings that confer a significantly increased risk should be counseled about options to reduce the risk of breast cancer. In a

Table 26-7   Factors That Increase the Likelihood of Cancer Associated With Nipple Discharge

Associated palpable mass
Age >40 y
Grossly bloody, guaiac-positive, serosanguineous, or watery discharge
Unilateral
Spontaneous
Persistent
Single duct

recent study of women with a diagnosis of benign breast disease on prior biopsy, the relative risk of breast cancer was 1.56 overall. The relative risk associated with a diagnosis of atypia was 4.24, proliferative breast disease without atypia 1.88, and nonproliferative lesions 1.27. Table 26-8 lists histologic diagnoses associated with these 3 categories of benign breast disease. This study also found that the degree of risk associated with some of these histologic diagnoses was modified by the age at diagnosis and the degree of family history of breast cancer. For instance, no increased risk of breast cancer was found among women who had a nonproliferative breast lesion unless a strong family history of breast cancer was present.

Breast Cancer: Risk Assessment and Prevention

Women at increased risk for breast cancer should be identified and counseled about options for risk reduction. The most widely used method of risk assessment is the National Cancer Institute Risk Assessment Tool, a computerized version of the Gail model that incorporates some but not all risk factors for breast cancer: current age, age at menarche, age at first live birth, number of previous breast biopsies, presence of atypical hyperplasia, and number of first-degree relatives affected by breast cancer. The relative risks associated with these risk factors are listed in the oncology chapter. The tool cannot be applied to women younger than 35 years old or to women with a history of breast cancer, ductal carcinoma in situ, or lobular carcinoma in situ. The tool overestimates the risk of breast cancer in women with numerous previous biopsies for nonproliferative breast disease and underestimates the risk of breast cancer in women with a family history of breast cancer that includes early-onset breast cancer or numerous second-degree relatives affected by breast cancer. Alternative risk assessment models, such as the Claus model, are more appropriate in women whose predominant risk factor is a family history of breast cancer. Neither the Gail nor the Claus model takes into account breast density, which has been found in numerous studies to be independently associated with an increased risk of breast cancer.

Only 5% to 10% of all breast cancers are due to an inherited gene mutation. Approximately one-third of hereditary breast cancers are due to a mutation in the *BRCA1* gene and approximately one-third are due to a mutation in the *BRCA2* gene. Both genes follow an autosomal dominant inheritance pattern. Women with a mutation in either of these genes have a lifetime risk of breast cancer ranging from 55% to 80% and a lifetime risk of ovarian cancer of 15% to 40%. Risk factors for *BRCA* involvement include onset of breast cancer at age younger than 50 years, breast and ovarian cancer within the same individual or family, multiple cases of breast cancer in a family, bilateral breast cancer, male breast cancer, and breast cancer in a family of Ashkenazi Jewish heritage. Multiple statistical models exist to estimate the probability of carrying a *BRCA1* or *BRCA2* mutation, the most common of which is the BRCAPRO tool. Women with family histories suggestive of an inherited gene mutation should be referred for genetic counseling and consideration of gene testing.

Management Options for Women at Increased Risk of Breast Cancer

Once an increased risk of breast cancer has been confirmed, options for surveillance and risk reduction should be reviewed, depending on

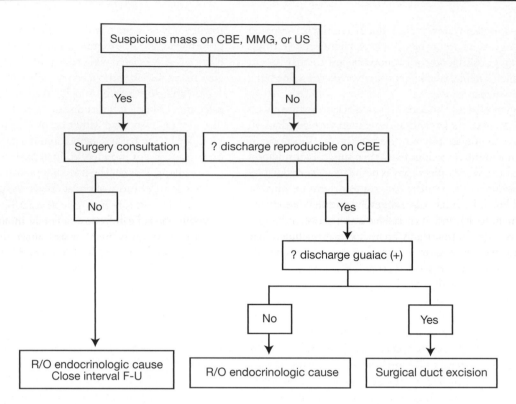

Figure 26-1. Algorithm for Evaluation of Spontaneous Nipple Discharge. CBE indicates clinical breast examination; F-U, follow-up; MMG, mammography; R/O, rule out; US, ultrasonography.

the woman's preferences and level of risk. Women at increased risk may adopt 1 or more of the options for risk reduction discussed below.

Table 26-8 Categories of Benign Breast Disease

Nonproliferative breast lesions
    Duct ectasia
    Fibroadenoma without proliferative epithelial changes
    Fibrosis
    Mastitis
    Mild hyperplasia without atypia
    Cysts
    Simple apocrine metaplasia
    Squamous metaplasia
Proliferative breast lesions without atypia
    Fibroadenoma with proliferative epithelial changes
    Moderate or florid hyperplasia without atypia
    Sclerosing adenosis
    Papilloma
    Radial scar
Atypia
    Atypical ductal hyperplasia
    Atypical lobular hyperplasia

Lifestyle Modification

Factors found to be associated with an increased risk of breast cancer include postmenopausal weight gain, alcohol intake more than 2 drinks per day, and physical inactivity. Corresponding lifestyle modifications may have a beneficial effect on the risk of breast cancer. Although an association between the risk of breast cancer and use of oral contraceptives is controversial, postmenopausal combination hormone therapy (estrogen and progestogen) has been shown in numerous studies to increase slightly the risk of breast cancer. In general, it is prudent to avoid the use of combination hormone therapy in women at significantly increased risk of breast cancer. Although the Women's Health Initiative study did not find an increased risk of breast cancer associated with use of estrogen alone in women with prior hysterectomy, this result may not be generalizable to women with a significantly increased risk of breast cancer.

Close Surveillance

According to guidelines from the US Preventive Services Task Force, women with a known or suspected *BRCA1* or *BRCA2* mutation should begin monthly breast self-examination by age 18 to 21 years, annual or semiannual clinical breast examinations by age 25 to 35 years, and annual mammography beginning at age 25 to 35 years. *BRCA1* mutation carriers should begin annual or semiannual screening with transvaginal ultrasonography and tests of CA 125 serum levels at age 25 to 35 years. This ovarian cancer screening is considered optional for *BRCA2* mutation carriers. Women with 2 or more first-degree relatives with ovarian cancer should be offered prophylactic oophorectomy after completion of childbearing or at age 35 years.

Women with a family history of breast cancer that is not consistent with a *BRCA* mutation should begin annual screening mammography 10 years before the age at which their youngest relative was diagnosed with breast cancer, but no later than age 40 years.

The American Cancer Society recommends annual breast magnetic resonance imaging in addition to annual mammography for women with any of the following characteristics: 1) known *BRCA* mutation, 2) unknown *BRCA* status with a first-degree relative with a proven *BRCA* mutation, 3) lifetime risk of breast cancer of 20% to 25% or more (as calculated from 1 of several accepted breast cancer risk-assessment tools), and 4) chest irradiation between the ages of 10 and 30 years. The American Cancer Society concluded that there was insufficient evidence to recommend magnetic resonance imaging screening for women with 1) a prior history of breast cancer, 2) dense breast parenchyma, or 3) a history of atypia or lobular carcinoma in situ.

Chemoprevention

Tamoxifen is currently the only drug approved by the US Food and Drug Administration for reducing the incidence of breast cancer in high-risk women. Tamoxifen reduces the risk of breast cancer by 50% among women at increased risk. Women must weigh this potential benefit against the risks of tamoxifen, which include an increased risk of endometrial cancer, deep vein thrombosis, pulmonary embolus, stroke, and cataracts. Because most cases of tamoxifen-associated endometrial cancer present with vaginal bleeding, women taking tamoxifen should be asked about vaginal bleeding but do not need routine surveillance with pelvic ultrasonography or endometrial biopsy.

Like tamoxifen, raloxifene is a selective estrogen-receptor modifier. In the Study of Tamoxifen and Raloxifene (STAR), raloxifene was found to work as well as tamoxifen for reducing the risk of invasive breast cancer in postmenopausal women at increased risk for development of breast cancer. Whereas tamoxifen has been shown to reduce by half the risk of both invasive and noninvasive breast cancer (including ductal carcinoma in situ and lobular carcinoma in situ), raloxifene did not have an effect on the incidence of noninvasive breast cancer. Both groups had similar incidences of ischemic heart and cerebrovascular events, osteoporotic fractures, and mortality. The incidence of cataracts, thromboembolism (including pulmonary embolism), and endometrial hyperplasia was significantly lower in the raloxifene group. Uterine cancer was also less common in the raloxifene group, although this difference was not statistically significant. The raloxifene group experienced more musculoskeletal problems, dyspareunia, and weight gain, whereas the tamoxifen group experienced more vasomotor symptoms, leg cramps, and bladder and gynecologic problems. Quality of life was the same for both drugs. Because selective estrogen-receptor modulators reduce the incidence of estrogen-receptor–positive breast cancer but not estrogen-receptor–negative breast cancer, they are not as effective in the subset of women with *BRCA1* mutations whose tumors are more likely to be estrogen-receptor–negative.

Studies are now in progress to assess the role of aromatase inhibitors in the chemoprevention of breast cancer.

Prophylactic Surgery

Prophylactic surgery is an option usually reserved for women with a significantly increased risk of breast cancer. Prophylactic mastectomy is associated with a 90% reduction in the risk of breast cancer. Bilateral oophorectomy in women younger than 40 years is associated with a decrease in the risk of breast cancer of approximately 50% and perhaps even more among women with *BRCA* mutations.

* 5% to 10% of all breast cancers are due to an inherited gene mutation.
* Factors that increase the likelihood of a *BRCA* mutation include onset of breast cancer at age <50 years, breast and ovarian cancer within the same individual or family, multiple cases of breast cancer in a family, bilateral breast cancer, male breast cancer, and breast cancer in a family of Ashkenazi Jewish heritage.
* One-third of hereditary breast cancers are due to mutations in the *BRCA1* gene and one-third are due to mutations in the *BRCA2* gene.
* In women who are *BRCA*-positive, the lifetime risk of breast cancer is 55%-80% and of ovarian carcinoma 15%-40%.

Cardiovascular Disease in Women

Although cardiovascular disease (CVD) is the leading cause of death among women in the United States, it is underrecognized and undertreated in women. Critical differences exist between men and women in the epidemiology, prevention, clinical presentation, diagnosis, and treatment of CVD. A thorough understanding of the differences may assist in early diagnosis of CVD in women.

One in 2.5 women dies of CVD, whereas 1 in 30 women die of breast cancer. Coronary heart disease, which includes coronary atherosclerotic disease (CAD), myocardial infarction, acute coronary syndromes, and angina, accounts for the largest proportion of CVD deaths. The prevalence of CAD in premenopausal women is much lower than the prevalence among similarly aged men. The incidence of CAD in women lags 10 to 15 years behind the incidence in men until the seventh decade of life. The overall number of coronary deaths in men in the United States has declined, but the number of coronary deaths in women has stabilized or increased, depending on the study referenced.

Risk factors for men and women are similar. However, the magnitude of the effect of certain risk factors differs by sex. Low high-density lipoprotein cholesterol level, rather than high low-density lipoprotein cholesterol level, is more predictive of coronary risk in women than in men. In the Women's Health Initiative, the total cholesterol to high-density lipoprotein cholesterol level was the lipid factor most predictive of cardiovascular events. The Women's Health Initiative study also found that serum C-reactive protein was a strong independent risk factor for CVD in women that added to the predictive value of traditional risk factors. The relative risk of death from coronary heart disease is greater in female patients with diabetes than male patients with diabetes. Smoking seems to confer a higher risk of coronary heart disease in women than men. Among patients presenting with a first myocardial infarction, women are more likely than men to be older and more likely to have a history of diabetes, hypertension, hyperlipidemia, and heart failure. Women also are more likely to underestimate the impact of CVD risk factors on their health.

The mortality rate from CVD is higher in women than in men: 38% of women and 25% of men will die within 1 year after a heart attack. The mortality rate from CVD is higher in African-American women than in white women. Underrecognition of CAD risk in women contributes to this higher mortality rate. Physicians tend to rate women as being at lower risk than men, even in patients with equivalent risks. Physicians are also less likely to recommend established preventive therapies (such as statin medications) to women, which may be due to the false perception of lower risk. Furthermore, sex-specific data on effective primary and secondary CVD prevention are limited. In 1 recent study of primary prevention of CVD in women, low-dose aspirin lowered the risk of stroke without affecting the risk of myocardial infarction or death from CVD.

Underdiagnosis of CAD also contributes to the higher post-myocardial infarction mortality rate among women. Women having a heart attack are less likely to have a correct diagnosis than men. This difference is due, in part, to the higher likelihood of atypical symptoms in women. Up to 50% of women present with atypical symptoms of heart disease and heart attack, which may include any of the following: pain in the neck, shoulder, upper back or abdomen; indigestion; belching; "gas" pains; nausea or vomiting; weakness; unexplained fatigue; shortness of breath; or a sense of doom. Women are more likely than men to avoid or delay seeking medical care for cardiac symptoms. In addition, because women tend to be older when symptoms of CAD develop, comorbid conditions (ie, arthritis) may cause symptoms that mask cardiac symptoms.

Women are less likely than age-matched men to have obstructive CAD, particularly triple-vessel or left main coronary artery CAD. The higher prevalence of nonobstructive CAD and single-vessel disease in women results in a decreased accuracy of treadmill electrocardiography. Additional factors also may contribute to the decreased accuracy of treadmill electrocardiographic findings in women, including more frequent resting ST-T changes, lower electrocardiographic voltage, and hormonal factors. The false-positive rate of treadmill electrocardiographic testing is higher in women than in men (particularly in young women with a low likelihood of CVD) and the false-negative rate is also higher. Exercise electrocardiography does have a high negative predictive value in women with a low pretest probability of CAD and a low-risk Duke treadmill score.

Despite these limitations, guidelines still support the use of exercise testing in women at intermediate pretest risk of CAD on the basis of symptoms and risk factors who have normal results of resting electrocardiography and are capable of maximal exercise. Exercise stress echocardiography is recommended for symptomatic women with an intermediate to high pretest probability of CAD, and dobutamine stress echocardiography is recommended for women with normal or abnormal electrocardiographic results who are incapable of exercise. Imaging stress tests (echocardiography, nuclear perfusion) have similar sensitivity and specificity in women and men.

The Women's Ischemia Syndrome Evaluation (WISE) study identified an important subset of women with stress test results suggestive of ischemia but no significant obstruction at coronary angiography.

These patients were typically labeled as having false-positive stress test results. However, the WISE study suggested that these women have true ischemia, likely due to mechanisms that are more common in women than in men, such as diffuse atherosclerosis that is not detected by angiography, coronary microvascular dysfunction, or reduced myocardial perfusion due to high left ventricular filling pressures related to hypertension or diastolic dysfunction. Another finding from this study is that women with persistent nonspecific chest pain and normal coronary arteries have a higher risk of future adverse coronary events than women with nonspecific chest pain that resolves. This study suggested that negative results on coronary angiography cannot definitively exclude ischemia in women with persistent symptoms suggestive of ischemia or positive results on stress imaging test. Because these women are at increased risk for adverse events, interventions to modify risk factors, relieve symptoms, and improve microvascular and macrovascular function should be considered.

In regard to invasive testing, women are less likely than men to be referred for coronary angiography. Women also are more likely to require urgent or emergency coronary artery bypass grafting. In-hospital mortality after coronary artery bypass grafting is higher in women than men, which is largely explained by their higher risk profile: compared with men, women undergoing coronary artery bypass grafting are older and have more comorbidities, such as diabetes, hypertension, and obesity. Long-term outcomes after coronary artery bypass grafting are similar for women and men. Women with multivessel disease treated with coronary artery bypass grafting have better long-term survival than women treated medically.

For secondary prevention, the Cholesterol and Recurrent Events (CARE) study found that cholesterol lowering with a statin drug was more effective in women than in men. Prospective studies have shown that hormone therapy should not be used for the purpose of secondary prevention. The HERS (Heart and Estrogen/Progestin Replacement Study) trial found no overall effect of 4.1 years of hormone therapy on risk of myocardial infarction or fatal coronary artery events in women with known CAD; coronary events increased in the first year after randomization. The Estrogen Replacement and Atherosclerosis trial showed no benefit of hormone therapy on angiographic progression in postmenopausal women with documented coronary stenosis.

The Women's Health Initiative study was the first randomized trial to investigate the effects of hormone therapy as primary prevention for CVD in healthy postmenopausal women. For women receiving combination therapy (conjugated equine estrogen and medroxyprogesterone acetate), the rate of coronary events increased (an additional 7 events per 10,000 person-years of use) and the rate of stroke increased (an additional 8 strokes per 10,000 person-years of use). For women receiving unopposed conjugated equine estrogen, there was no effect on the incidence of coronary events but an increased risk of stroke (12 additional strokes per 10,000 person-years of use). As a result of these prospective, randomized, controlled trials that contradicted the results of numerous prior observational studies, hormone therapy is not currently recommended for primary or secondary prevention of CVD. Hormone therapy should be discontinued if a CVD event occurs. Studies are ongoing to assess whether hormone therapy has a differential effect on atherogenesis depending on when it is initiated, because some studies suggest that initiation of hormone therapy at the time of menopause reduces the risk of subsequent atherogenesis.

The lipid alterations associated with hormone therapy are complex and include both favorable and unfavorable changes. Hormone therapy leads to reductions in low-density lipoprotein cholesterol and lipoprotein (a) levels and increases in high-density lipoprotein cholesterol levels. Oral estrogen (but not transdermal estrogen) leads to increases in triglyceride and C-reactive protein levels.

- Cardiovascular disease is the leading cause of death in women in the United States.
- The magnitude of diabetes mellitus and tobacco use as risk factors is higher in women than in men.
- 38% of women compared with 25% of men will die within 1 year after a myocardial infarction.
- Up to 50% of women present with atypical symptoms of heart disease.
- Hormone therapy should not be used for the purpose of primary or secondary prevention.

Heart Failure in Women

Heart failure (HF) affects approximately 2.5 million women in the United States. Women account for nearly 50% of all hospital admissions for HF. HF tends to develop at an older age in women than men. During the past 50 years, the incidence of HF has declined among women but not among men. Sex-related differences in the pathophysiologic mechanisms of heart failure likely exist. Women with HF are more likely to have hypertension, diabetes, obesity, tobacco use, and atrial fibrillation; men with HF are more likely to have CAD and left ventricular systolic dysfunction. Relative to men, women tend to have diastolic HF with a preserved ejection fraction. In general, women survive longer than men with HF, but they have more dyspnea on exertion and functional impairment. Depression frequently is associated with HF and is more common in women than men.

Atrial Fibrillation

Atrial fibrillation is less common in women than men, but women with atrial fibrillation are at higher risk for stroke. This difference may be due to women being less likely to receive treatment with anticoagulation.

Depression and Anxiety in Women

The lifetime prevalence of depression is 21% in women and 12% in men. The peak age at onset of depression is 33 to 45 years in women and more than 55 years in men. Women are less likely to commit suicide but twice as likely to make a suicide attempt. Caucasian women are twice as likely to commit suicide as African-American women. The lifetime prevalence rate for dysthymia is 8% in women and 4.8% in men. There is no sex difference for bipolar disorder.

Recent studies have found that the risk of depressive symptoms and clinical depression increases in the perimenopausal years. Studies have not found an association between natural or surgical menopause and rate of depression in women. Hormone therapy has been associated with improved scores on the Beck Depression Inventory for nondepressed women but not for clinically depressed women. Estrogen may improve symptoms in women with mild depressive symptoms, but hormone therapy alone is not sufficient therapy for clinical depression in postmenopausal women.

Postpartum depression affects approximately 10% to 15% of women. It develops during the first 4 weeks after childbirth, although it often is not recognized by the woman or health-care provider. Risk factors for postpartum depression include prior history of major depression, prior postpartum depression, depression during the pregnancy, unmarried status, or unplanned pregnancy. Because of overlap in the symptoms of postpartum depression and thyroid disease, it is essential to measure thyroid-stimulating hormone in all women who present with symptoms of postpartum depression. In a small fraction of women with postpartum depression, psychosis develops, and this usually requires acute hospitalization.

Anxiety disorders that are more prevalent in women than in men include panic disorder, agoraphobia, social phobia, generalized anxiety disorder, and posttraumatic stress disorder. Women with a panic disorder frequently present with a comorbid psychiatric condition, such as major depression, generalized anxiety disorder, or substance abuse. An anxiety disorder may underlie persistent somatic complaints. If nonpharmacologic measures do not provide sufficient relief, combined medication and cognitive behavioral therapy should be offered. The risks and benefits of pharmacologic therapy need to be measured carefully in the woman who is breastfeeding: tricyclic antidepressants and some selective serotonin reuptake inhibitors seem to be relatively safe, although there are isolated adverse reports in infants exposed through breast milk.

- The lifetime risk of depression in women is 21% and 12% in men.

Intimate Partner Violence

Intimate partner violence (IPV) is defined as intentional controlling or violent behavior by a person who is or was in an intimate relationship with the victim. The controlling behavior may include physical or emotional abuse, sexual assault, economic control, or social isolation of the victim. Of reported IPV cases, 95% involve a male perpetrator and a female victim. Over a lifetime, at least 1 of 3 American women is physically assaulted by a partner. Female victims of this abuse most often present for care that is not directly related to abuse injuries. Battered women use health services 6 to 8 times more than nonbattered women and have a higher incidence of headaches, sexually transmitted diseases, irritable bowel syndrome, depression, and anxiety. Aspects of the history that may suggest IPV include chronic pain syndromes, gastrointestinal complaints, an overprotective partner, injuries during pregnancy, frequent visits for injuries, a history of depression, or a history of childhood abuse. All women should be asked about IPV. Routine prenatal screening for IPV is particularly important, because abuse occurs in 1 of 6 pregnancies and often begins or escalates in early pregnancy.

Physical examination findings that are suggestive of IPV include injuries incompatible with a given history, multiple injuries in various stages of healing, injuries suggestive of a defensive posture (such as ulnar fractures), and pattern injuries (such as burns, choking marks, bite marks, or wrist or ankle abrasions).

Documentation of IPV in the medical record is essential and may provide evidence to help the victim separate from the perpetrator. If the victim consents, photographs of injuries should be obtained, which may be helpful in court proceedings. Physical evidence, such as torn or bloody clothes or sexual assault evidence, should be preserved.

Victims need treatment of their injuries, support and reassurance that the abuse is not their fault, safety assessment, and referral to appropriate resources to prevent further abuse. A safety assessment is a critical part of the evaluation. When possible, it should be done by a victim's advocate, social worker, or law enforcement personnel. When these services are not available, it should be done by the clinician or nurse. An immediate psychiatric referral should be arranged for any patient expressing suicidal or homicidal intentions. The assessment also must include inquiries regarding children in the home: any child abuse must be reported to child abuse authorities. Some jurisdictions require reporting to the child abuse authorities of any IPV in a home where children reside. Because IPV homicides are more likely to occur immediately after separation, ensuring the safety of the victim during separation is critical. Strategies include relocation of the victim or arrest of the perpetrator.

Referral to a victim's advocate group, women's shelter, or social worker should be arranged. Immediate contact with the referral source is best, because this is the time when the victim is more likely to make a change.

Questions

Multiple Choice (choose the best answer)

1. A 50-year-old woman comes in with concerns of vaginal dryness and painful intercourse. She had breast cancer at age 48 years and underwent a mastectomy for a 0.5-cm infiltrating ductal adenocarcinoma, grade 2, with sentinel lymph nodes negative for metastases. She completed a course of chemotherapy and now is taking anastrazole (Arimidex, an aromatase inhibitor). Results of examination are as follows: breasts, right mastectomy; left breast, negative; axillae, negative; pelvis, pale, mottled vaginal mucosa, friable to examination. Which of the following is true, in considering treatment options for her symptoms?

   a. Treatment with usual doses of vaginal estrogen cream results in increased estradiol levels for at least 2 months after treatment.
   b. Even small doses of vaginal estrogen cream can reach the systemic circulation.
   c. If the patient elects to use vaginal estrogen cream, she will need to take a progestogen to adequately protect the endometrium from hyperplasia or endometrial cancer.
   d. Vaginal moisturizers (such as Replens) are nearly as effective as vaginal estrogen therapy for atrophic vaginitis.
   e. Switching therapy from anastrazole to tamoxifen would be helpful.

2. A 42-year-old woman with very heavy, painful periods comes in to discuss treatment options. Treatment with oral contraceptives and endometrial ablation have not provided lasting benefit. A gynecologist recommends the option of hysterectomy, which your patient welcomes for relief from her symptoms. She has been advised to have her ovaries removed at the same time and asks for your opinion. With regard to advising her about the long-term effects of elective oophorectomy with hysterectomy, all of the following risks or benefits apply *except*:

   a. Increased risk for breast cancer
   b. Decreased risk for ovarian cancer
   c. Increased risk for cardiovascular disease
   d. Increased risk for osteoporosis
   e. Increased overall mortality

3. A 40-year-old woman comes in for recheck of hyperlipidemia and an annual preventive health check. She has heard that she might no longer need to have annual Papanicolaou smear. Her mother had cervical cancer at age 45 years. Her last Papanicolaou smear was 1 year ago, and results were normal. Results of routine Papanicolaou smears since age 21 years have been normal. The patient is gravida 2, para 2, has hyperlipidemia, has been married for 20 years (monogamous), has had 4 sexual partners in her lifetime, and is a past smoker (10 pack-year × 10 years). Multiple paternal relatives have hyperlipidemia.

   Current medications are levonorgestrel and ethinyl estradiol (Alesse, for birth control) and atorvastatin 40 mg daily (Lipitor, for lipid lowering). On examination, her heart and lungs are normal. Genitalia are normal, cervix is normal-appearing, and bimanual examination is negative. What should you recommend for the patient with regard to frequency of cervical cytologic screening?

   a. She may decrease screening frequency to every 3 years because her Papanicolaou smears have been consistently normal and she is in a stable, monogamous relationship.
   b. She should continue annual cervical cytologic testing because smoking puts her at increased risk for cervical cancer.
   c. She needs cervical cytologic testing yearly because she takes an oral contraceptive.
   d. She should continue annual screening because of her mother's history of cervical cancer.
   e. Human papillomavirus (HPV) testing should be completed annually in place of the Papanicolaou smear.

4. A 48-year-old woman presents for evaluation of nipple discharge. On several occasions during the past 3 months, she has noticed a drop of straw-colored fluid spontaneously emerging from 1 area on her right nipple. Current medication is norgestimate/ethinyl estradiol (Ortho Tri-Cyclen, for birth control). On examination, her breasts appear symmetric. There is no erythema, ulceration, or crusting of nipples and skin dimpling or palpable breast lump. With minimal pressure on the right areola, a drop of straw-colored fluid is expressed from 1 duct in the 9:00 position of the right breast. The fluid is guaiac-positive. Mammography and right breast ultrasonography are negative. What is the appropriate next step in evaluating this patient?

   a. Reassure the patient that the discharge is consistent with benign physiologic nipple discharge.
   b. Repeat right breast mammograpphy and ultrasonography in 6 months.
   c. Measure serum thyroid-stimulating hormone level.
   d. Discontinue use of oral contraceptive and assess for recurrence of nipple discharge.
   e. Obtain surgical consultation for anticipated duct excision.

5. A 49-year-old woman comes in for her annual pelvic and breast examination and screening mammography. She denies breast concerns. She had menarche at age 14 years. She is gravida 2, para 2. A right breast biopsy at age 32 years showed mild hyperplasia without atypia. Current medication is ethinyl estradiol and drospirenone (Yasmin, for menstrual regulation). A paternal aunt had breast cancer at age 60 years. Bilateral screening mammography shows an extremely dense pattern. There are a few scattered benign calcifications in the right breast and a metal clip identified at the site of prior core needle biopsy. There are no mammographic features of malignancy. What

aspect of this patient's presentation poses the greatest risk for sub-sequent development of breast cancer?

a. Prior breast biopsy
b. Breast density
c. Family history of breast cancer
d. Age at menarche
e. Oral contraceptive use

6. Which of the following factors in a patient's family history is the most important for determining risk for a clinically significant *BRCA1* or *BRCA2* gene mutation?

a. Young age at breast cancer diagnosis in a first-degree relative
b. Multiple cases of breast cancer in a family
c. Family history of breast and ovarian cancer
d. Family history of breast, endometrial, and colon cancer
e. Ashkenazi Jewish heritage

7. A 49-year-old woman presents with questions about menopause. She has not had a menstrual period for 9 months. Menstrual periods were irregular for about a year before that time. She describes some hot flashes during the day, sweats at night, and troublesome vaginal dryness. She wonders whether she is menopausal, whether she can stop use of birth control (diaphragm with spermicidal gel), and what treatment she can take for her symptoms. Results of examination are normal. On laboratory testing, the sensitive thyroid-stimulating hormone level is normal, and the follicle-stimulating hormone (FSH) level is 30 IU/mL (postmenopausal, >10 mIU/mL). What do you advise for this patient?

a. She and her husband may discontinue contraception because she can no longer become pregnant.
b. There is no single test of ovarian function that will predict or confirm menopause.
c. She should switch to an oral contraceptive for better efficacy at preventing pregnancy.
d. She should wait until she has gone 12 months without a menstrual period before starting use of vaginal estrogen.
e. She can start menopausal hormone replacement therapy with estrogen and progesterone, which will help vasomotor symptoms and prevent pregnancy.

Answers

1.   Answer b.

For women with a history of breast cancer who experience troublesome symptoms from urogenital atrophy, over-the-counter moisturizers are the safest option but not as effective as vaginal estrogen therapy. Even small doses of vaginal estrogen cream can reach the systemic circulation, but the increase in serum estradiol is transient and the risk for recurrence of her breast cancer is exceedingly low. There is not enough systemic absorption from currently used regimens of vaginal estrogen to require a progestogen for endometrial protection.

2.   Answer a.

Prophylactic oophorectomy is associated with a reduced incidence of ovarian cancer by more than 95%. The risk of breast cancer is also reduced by about half when oophorectomy is performed before the age of 50 years. Women who undergo removal of the ovaries before natural menopause have been found, however, to be at increased risk for cardiovascular disease (some studies have reported a doubling of the risk of myocardial infarction), osteoporosis, and osteoporotic fracture (50% increased risk of hip fracture) and have an excess overall mortality (9% excess mortality in women undergoing oophorectomy before age 55 years). Ovarian cancer is rare; the lifetime risk is 1.48%. Benefits of reducing cancer risk need to be balanced against long-term effects of loss of ovarian function.

3.   Answer a.

Cervical cancer is a sexually transmitted disease; virtually all cases of squamous cell cervical cancer arise from prior infection with a high-risk type of HPV. Her mother's history of cervical cancer does not increase her personal risk. Behavioral risk factors for cervical cancer include early age at onset of sexual intercourse and greater number of lifetime partners. Smoking increases the risk approximately 2-fold but does not alter recommended screening intervals. Screening should be performed at least every 3 years. Testing for high-risk types of HPV is most useful in evaluating abnormal Papanicolau test results such as atypical squamous cells of undetermined significance. HPV testing may also be used for screening women aged 30 years or older, but no more frequently than every 3 years.

4.   Answer e.

Serous, serosanguineous, and grossly bloody nipple discharge have the same significance. Most cases are due to a benign papilloma or duct ectasia, but a malignant cause should be excluded by surgical duct excision if the involved duct can be identified. The risk of cancer is greater when nipple discharge is bloody or guaiac-positive or unilateral or occurring in a woman older than 40 years. Repeat mammography and ultrasonography do not exclude the possibility of cancer. They would be a reasonable option only if the nipple discharge resolved and could not be reproduced, precluding localization of the involved duct. Galactorrhea is usually milky and bilateral but occasionally can present as unilateral yellow or clear discharge. Both hypothyroidism and oral contraceptive therapy can cause galactorrhea; however, the milky secretion is not guaiac-positive.

5.   Answer b.

Breast density has been called the most undervalued and underutilized risk factor in studies investigating the causes of breast cancer. The sensitivity of mammography in women with extremely dense breast tissue is as low as 30%, and specificity is also reduced. Also, breast density is an independent risk factor for the development of breast cancer, increasing risk by approximately 4-fold. The relative risk for women with a family history of breast cancer in a first-degree relative is 2.1 and for current users of oral contraceptives, 1.24. In the absence of proliferative changes or atypia, the prior biopsy does not confer an increased risk.

6.   Answer c.

In 2005, the US Preventive Services Task Force published recommendations for genetic risk assessment and *BRCA* mutation testing for breast and ovarian cancer susceptibility. Clinically significant mutations of the *BRCA1* or *BRCA2* gene increase a woman's lifetime risk for breast cancer to 60% to 85% and ovarian cancer to 26% (*BRCA1*) or 10% (*BRCA2*). Of the characteristics associated with an increased likelihood of *BRCA1* or *BRCA2* mutations, family history of breast and ovarian cancer on 1 side (maternal or paternal) is the most important factor. Other important factors include young age at breast cancer diagnosis, bilateral breast cancer, multiple cases of breast cancer in a family, and Ashkenazi Jewish heritage. In addition to female breast and ovarian cancer risk, *BRCA1* and *BRCA2* mutations are associated with an increased risk for pancreatic cancer, and *BRCA2* mutations are associated with increased risk for pancreatic cancer, stomach cancer, male breast cancer, and melanoma.

7.   Answer b.

Women should be advised that pregnancy is possible until menopause occurs, which is confirmed either by 12 consecutive months of amenorrhea or by consistently increased levels of FSH ($\geq$30 mIU/mL). FSH and estradiol levels can be labile during perimenopause, and a single increased FSH level does not confirm menopause. In fact, there is no single test of ovarian function that will predict or confirm menopause. Although postmenopausal hormone replacement therapy relieves vasomotor and urogenital symptoms, it does not suppress ovulation and so does not prevent pregnancy. If women during perimenopause need hormone treatment for relief from symptoms, typically a low-dose oral contraceptive is used.

Index

D

Daily refractory headaches, 761

Dalfopristin/quinupristin, 643

Daptomycin, 643

de Quervain tenosynovitis, 973

de Quervain thyroiditis, 212

Death

definition, 676

leading causes in United States, 840t

Debulking, ovarian tumors, 811

Decongestants, rhinitis, 21

Deep venous thrombosis (DVT), 1050-1053, 1052i

causes, 1050t

clinical evaluation, 1051

incidence in various clinical circumstances, 930t

and pulmonary embolism, 928-929

treatment, 1052

Degenerative aortic valve disease, 42

Dehydroepiandrosterone (DHEA), 229, 230

Delayed hemolytic transfusion reactions, 427-428

Delirium, 390, 390t, 868-869

Delirium, postoperative, 514, 514t

Delta gap formula, metabolic acidosis, 724-725

Dementia, 752-754, 869

differential diagnosis, 753t

in elderly, 388-390

neurologic diagnostic testing, 749-750

Dementia with Lewy bodies, 389, 869

Dementia with Parkinson disease, 389

Demyelinating diseases, 779-780

Depression

adjustment disorder with depressed mood, 863

major, 862-863

treatment, 863

in women, 1073

Dermatitis herpetiformis, 177-178, 178i

Dermatology

autoimmune bullous diseases, 176-179, 182

cutaneous T-cell lymphoma, 174

drug reactions, 179-180

erythema multiforme, 179

erythema nodosum, 179, 182

general cutaneous conditions, 173-182

HIV manifestations, 189-190

malignancy manifestation, 180-182

malignant melanoma, 173-174

nail clues in systemic disease, 189

psoriasis, 174-175

systemic disease manifestations, 182-189

skin cancer, 173

Dermatomyositis, 181-182, 182i, 814-815

Desquamative interstitial pneumonia, 920

Diabetes insipidus, 209, 718-719

Diabetes mellitus, 234-239

cardiac effects, 58

coronary artery disease, 58, 92, 92t, 855

cutaneous manifestation, 187-188, 188i

hypoglycemia, 237

neuroarthropathy, 981

neuropathies, 766, 767t, 770

in pregnancy, 238-239

Diabetic ketoacidosis, 237-238

Diabetic nephropathy (DN), 698-699

stages, 699t

Diagnostic tests

2×2 table, 329t, 330-331, 331t

interpretation, 329-333

likelihood ratio (LR), 331-332, 332t

outcomes, 329t

relative risk reduction, 332-333

Dialysis

ARF, 711-712

drug overdoses, 715t

ESRD, 714

Diarrhea, 267-268

acute, 268-269

bacterial, 272-274, 273t, 618t, 618-620

bacterial overgrowth, 272

carcinoid tumors, 271-272

chronic, 269-270

hospital-acquired, 513

infectious, 272-280

laxative abuse, 272

malabsorption, 269-270, 272, 274-275

organic vs functional, 269t

osmotic, 270t, 270-271

secretory, 270t, 271

small bowel/colonic contrast, 269t

systemic illnesses causing, 271t

tuberculosis, 282

viral, 279-280

Dietary Approaches to Stop Hypertension (DASH), 529, 531t

Diffuse alveolar damage, 921-922

Diffuse cerebral symptoms, 747-748

Diffuse esophageal spasm, 259

Diffuse lung disease

abbreviations, 918t

causes, 916i

classification, 918t

epidemiology, 917t

overview, 916-919

specific diagnoses, 919-922

Diffusing capacity for carbon monoxide (DLCO), 899-900

Digoxin

atrial fibrillation, 83

heart failure, 119

Dilated cardiomyopathy, 113-121, 114i, 116t, 308

device therapy, 120

drug effects, 118i

heart replacement therapy, 120-121

pharmacologic therapy, 117-120

Diphtheria, 573-574

vaccination, 849

Diphtheria-tetanus-pertussis (DTP) vaccination, 853

Direct thrombin inhibitors, 459-460

Directly observed therapy (DOT), TB, 948

Dirofilariasis, 956

Discoid lupus erythematosus, 186, 187i

Disease-modifying agent of rheumatic disease (DMARD) therapy, 976-977, 999-1001

Disease severity scoring, 164

Disk disease, neurologic diagnostic testing, 749

Diskitis, 623-624

Disseminated intravascular coagulopathy and fibrinolysis (DIC/ICF), 450-451

causes, 450t

Distributive shock, 161, 161t

Diuretics

dilated cardiomyopathy, 119

hypertension, 532-533

Diverticular disease, colon, 284

Dizziness, 763

multisensory, 763t, 764

psychophysiologic, 763t, 764

types, 763t

"Do Not Resuscitate" orders, 676

Dopamine agonists, pituitary tumors, 207

Doppler-color Doppler echocardiography, 63-64